P9-CBK-451

Abrams' Angiography

Vascular and Interventional Radiology

Abrams' Angiography

Vascular and Interventional Radiology

FOURTH EDITION

Stanley Baum, MD

EDITOR

Eugene P. Pendergrass Professor of Radiology
and Chairman, Department of Radiology
University of Pennsylvania School of Medicine
Chairman, Department of Radiology
Hospital of the University of Pennsylvania
Philadelphia

VOLUME I

With Introductory Comments by

Herbert L. Abrams, M.D.
Professor of Radiology
Stanford University School of Medicine
Stanford, California
Philip H. Cook Professor of Radiology, Emeritus
Harvard Medical School
Boston

Little, Brown and Company

BOSTON NEW YORK TORONTO LONDON

Fourth Edition

Library of Congress Cataloging-in-Publication Data

Abrams' angiography : vascular and interventional radiology. — 4th ed. / Stanley Baum, editor.
p. cm.
"With introductory comments by Herbert L. Abrams."
Includes bibliographical references and index.
ISBN 0-316-08408-5 (v. 1). — ISBN 0-316-08409-3 (v. 2). — ISBN 0-316-08467-0 (set)
1. Angiography. 2. Interventional radiology. I. Abrams, Herbert L. II. Baum, Stanley, 1929– .
[DNLM: 1. Angiography. WG 500 A157a 1997]
RC691.6.A53A27 1997
616.1′307572—dc20
DNLM/DLC
for Library of Congress 96-24525
CIP

Vol. I ISBN 0-316-08408-5
Set ISBN 0-316-08467-0

Printed in the United States of America

EB-M

Editorial: Nancy E. Chorpenning, Deeth K. Ellis
Production Services: Julie Sullivan
Indexer: AlphaByte, Inc.
Production Supervisor: Michael A. Granger
Designer: Marty Tenney
Cover Designer: Louis C. Bruno, Jr.

To **Jeanne**

Contents

Volume I

I. General Considerations

II. The Central Nervous System

III. The Thorax

Section A: Thoracic Aortography

Section B: Coronary Arteriography

Section C: Pulmonary Arteriography

Section B: Renal Angiography

Section C: Adrenal Angiography

Section D: Pancreatic, Hepatic, and Splenic Arteriography

Section E: Mesenteric Arteriography

Section F: Bladder and Pelvic Arteriography

Section G: Retroperitoneal Angiography

V. The Extremities and Lymphangiography

Section A: Angiography of the Extremities

Section B: Lymphangiography

Contributing Authors

HERBERT L. ABRAMS, M.D.
Professor of Radiology, Stanford University School of Medicine, Stanford, California; Formerly, Philip H. Cook Professor and Chairman of Radiology, Harvard Medical School, and formerly, Chairman of Radiology, Brigham and Women's Hospital, Boston

MARJORIE A. AMBOS, M.D.
Private practice, Atmore, Alabama

KURT AMPLATZ, M.D.
Director and Professor of Radiology, Department of Cardiovascular/Interventional Radiology, University of Minnesota Hospital and Clinic, Minneapolis

JOHN E. ARUNY, M.D.
Assistant Professor of Radiology, Eastern Virginia Medical School; Director of Vascular and Interventional Radiology, DePaul Medical Center, Norfolk, Virginia

ROBERT J. ASHENBURG, M.D.
Clinical Assistant Professor of Radiology, SUNY Health Science Center at Syracuse; Director of Interventional Radiology, Crouse Irving Memorial Hospital, Syracuse, New York

ROBERT E. BARTON, M.D.
Assistant Professor, Dotter Interventional Institute, Oregon Health Sciences University; Department of Interventional Therapy, Oregon Health Sciences University, Portland

RICHARD A. BAUM, M.D.
Assistant Professor, Department of Radiology, and Assistant Professor of Radiology in Surgery, University of Pennsylvania; Staff Interventional Radiologist, Department of Radiology, Hospital of the University of Pennsylvania, Philadelphia

STANLEY BAUM, M.D.
Eugene P. Pendergrass Professor of Radiology and Chairman, Department of Radiology, University of Pennsylvania; Chairman, Department of Radiology, Hospital of the University of Pennsylvania, Philadelphia

YORAM BEN-MENACHEM, M.D.
Professor of Radiology, UMDNJ-New Jersey Medical School; Chief, Trauma Radiology, Department of Radiology, UMDNJ-University Hospital, Newark, New Jersey

MICHAEL A. BETTMANN, M.D.
Professor of Radiology, Dartmouth Medical School, Hanover, New Hampshire; Chief, CVIR, Director of Clinical Research, Department of Radiology, Dartmouth-Hitchcock Medical Center/Dartmouth Medical School, Lebanon, New Hampshire

ERIK BOIJSEN, M.D.
Professor Emeritus and Former Director, Department of Radiology, University Hospital, Lund, Sweden

INGEMAR BERGSTRAND, M.D.
Associate Professor of Diagnostic Radiology (retired), Department of Radiology, University of Lund, Lund, Sweden

SCOTT J. BOLEY, M.D.
Professor, Department of Surgery/Pediatrics, Albert Einstein College of Medicine; Chief of Pediatric Surgical Services, Department of Surgery, Montefiore Medical Center, Bronx, New York

JOSEPH J. BOOKSTEIN, M.D.
Professor Emeritus, Department of Radiology, University of California, San Diego; Research Professor, Department of Radiology, University of California Medical Center, San Diego

MORTON A. BOSNIAK, M.D.
Professor of Radiology, New York University School of Medicine; Chief of Uroradiology, New York University Medical Center, New York

LAWRENCE J. BRANDT, M.D.
Professor of Medicine, Albert Einstein College of Medicine; Director of Gastroenterology, Moses Division of Montefiore Medical Center, Bronx, New York

KLAUS M. BRON, M.D.
Professor of Radiology, University of Pittsburgh School of Medicine; Senior Staff, Department of Medicine, University of Pittsburgh Medical Center-Presbyterian-University Hospital, Pittsburgh

DANA R. BURKE, M.D.
Interventional Radiology, Easton Hospital, Easton, Pennsylvania

JEFFREY P. CARPENTER, M.D.
Assistant Professor, Department of Surgery, University of Pennsylvania; Assistant Professor of Surgery in Radiology, Hospital of the University of Pennsylvania, Philadelphia

RONALD A. CASTELLINO, M.D.
Chairman, Department of Radiology, Memorial Sloan Kettering Cancer Center; Professor of Radiology, Cornell University Medical College, New York

ARNOLD CHAIT, M.D.
Clinical Professor of Radiology, University of Pennsylvania School of Medicine; Director, Section of Vascular and Interventional Radiology, Graduate Hospital, Philadelphia

CONSTANTIN COPE, M.D.
Professor of Radiology and Staff, Angiography and Interventional Radiology, University of Pennsylvania School of Medicine, Philadelphia

MARTIN R. CRAIN, M.D.
Assistant Professor, Section of Vascular/Interventional Radiology, Medical College of Wisconsin and Affiliated Hospitals, Milwaukee

DEWITTE T. CROSS III, M.D.
Assistant Professor of Radiology, Washington University School of Medicine, St. Louis; Director of Interventional Neuroradiology, Mallinckrodt Institute of Radiology, St. Louis

ANDREW B. CRUMMY, M.D.
Professor of Radiology, Angio/Interventional Section, University of Wisconsin Hospital & Clinics, Madison, Wisconsin

J. A. GORDON CULHAM, M.D.
Professor of Radiology, University of British Columbia; Head, Cardiovascular and Interventional Radiology, British Columbia's Children's Hospital, Vancouver, British Columbia, Canada

JOHN L. DOPPMAN, M.D.
Chief of Radiology, National Institutes of Health, Bethesda, Maryland

BENJAMIN B. FAITELSON, M.D.
Radiologist, Christian Hospital, St. Louis, Missouri

KENNETH E. FELLOWS, M.D.
Professor of Radiology, Department of Radiology, University of Pennsylvania; Radiologist-in-Chief, Children's Hospital of Philadelphia, Philadelphia

ERNEST J. FERRIS, M.D.
Professor and Chairman, University of Arkansas for Medical Sciences; Chief, Department of Radiology, University Hospital of Arkansas, Little Rock, Arkansas

RICHARD G. FISHER, M.D.
Associate Professor, Department of Radiology, Baylor College of Medicine; Director, Vascular/Interventional Radiology, Ben Taub General Hospital, Houston

WALTER A. FUCHS, M.D.
Professor, Department of Medical Radiology, University Hospital of Zurich; Director, Institute of Diagnostic Radiology, University Hospital of Zurich, Zurich, Switzerland
Deceased

GEOFFREY A. GARDINER, JR., M.D.
Associate Professor, Department of Radiology, Jefferson Medical College; Director, Cardiovascular/Interventional Radiology, Thomas Jefferson University Hospital, Philadelphia

MARYELLYN GILFEATHER, M.D.
Instructor in Radiology, University of Pennsylvania School of Medicine, Philadelphia

CLEMENT J. GRASSI, M.D.
Assistant Professor of Radiology, Harvard Medical School; Attending Interventional and Cardiovascular Radiologist, Department of Radiology, Brigham and Women's Hospital, Boston

RICHARD H. GREENSPAN, M.D.
Professor Emeritus, Diagnostic Radiology, Yale University Medical School; Attending, Diagnostic Radiology, Yale New Haven Hospital, New Haven, Connecticut

DIANA F. GUTHANER, M.D.
Clinical Associate Professor and Clinical Faculty, Department of Diagnostic Radiology, Stanford University Medical Center, Stanford, California

MICHAEL J. HALLISEY, M.D.
Assistant Clinical Professor, Vascular and Interventional Radiology, University of Connecticut School of Medicine, Farmington, Connecticut; Hartford Hospital, Hartford, Connecticut

SAMUEL J. HESSEL, M.D.
Senior Clinical Lecturer, Department of Radiology, University of Arizona College of Medicine, Tucson, Arizona; Radiologist, Scottsdale Memorial Hospital, Scottsdale, Arizona

GEORGE A. HOLLAND, M.D.
Assistant Professor, Department of Radiology, University of Pennsylvania, Philadelphia

ROBERT W. HURST, M.D.
Associate Professor of Radiology, and Associate Professor of Radiology in Surgery, University of Pennsylvania; Director of Interventional Radiology, Hospital of the University of Pennsylvania, Philadelphia

KRASSI IVANCEV, M.D.
Assistant Professor, Department of Radiology, University of Lund, Malmö, Sweden

GUNNAR JÖNSSON, M.D.
Director Emeritus, Roentgendiagnostic Department, Sodersjukhuset, Stockholm, Sweden
Deceased

MELVIN P. JUDKINS, M.D.
Professor of Radiology, Loma Linda University School of Medicine, Loma Linda, California
Deceased

PAUL R. JULSRUD, M.D.
Associate Professor of Diagnostic Radiology, Mayo Medical School; Co-Director, Cardiac Catheterization Laboratory, St. Mary's Hospital, Rochester, Minnesota

KRISHNA KANDARPA, M.D., Ph.D.
Associate Professor of Radiology, Harvard Medical School; Co-Director, Cardiovascular and Interventional Radiology, Department of Radiology, Brigham and Women's Hospital, Boston

BARRY T. KATZEN, M.D.
Clinical Professor of Radiology, Department of Radiology, University of Miami School of Medicine; Medical Director, Miami Vascular Institute, Baptist Hospital, Miami

DANIEL K. KIDO, M.D.
Professor and Chief, Neuroradiology Section, Washington University Medical School; Chief, Neuroradiology Section, Mallinckrodt Institute of Radiology, Washington University Medical Center, St. Louis

PAUL C. LAKIN, M.D.
Assistant Professor, Dotter Interventional Institute, Oregon Health Sciences University; Attending Physician, Vascular/Interventional Radiology, University Hospital and Clinics, Portland, Oregon

ERICH K. LANG, M.D.
Professor of Radiology, UMDNJ, Newark, New Jersey and Louisiana State University Medical School, New Orleans; Professor of Urology, Louisiana State University Medical School, New Orleans

RICHARD S. LEFLEUR, M.D.
Associate Professor of Clinical Radiology, New York University School of Medicine; Director, Vascular and Interventional Radiology, Bellevue Hospital Medical Center, New York

JANIS GISSEL LETOURNEAU, M.D.
Professor, Departments of Surgery and Radiology, Louisiana State University Medical School; Director, Diagnostic Ultrasound, Medical Center of Louisiana, New Orleans

DAVID C. LEVIN, M.D.
Professor of Radiology, Jefferson Medical College; Chairman, Department of Radiology, Thomas Jefferson University Hospital, Philadelphia

JONATHAN M. LEVY, M.D.
Senior Clinical Lecturer, Department of Radiology, University of Arizona, Tucson, Arizona; Radiologist, Scottsdale Memorial Hospital, Scottsdale, Arizona

DEBORAH G. LONGLEY, M.D.
St. Paul Radiology; Staff Radiologist, United Hospital, St. Paul, Minnesota

ANDERS LUNDERQUIST, M.D.
Professor Emeritus, Department of Radiology, University of Lund, Lund, Sweden

ALAN H. MATSUMOTO, M.D.
Associate Professor of Radiology, University of Virginia Health Sciences Center, Charlottesville, Virginia

JOHN B. MAWSON, M.B., Ch.B.
Lecturer, Department of Medical Imaging, University of Toronto; Staff Radiologist, Department of Diagnostic Imaging, The Hospital for Sick Children, Toronto

JOHN C. MCDERMOTT, M.D.
Professor of Radiology, Angio/Interventional Section, University of Wisconsin Hospital & Clinics, Madison, Wisconsin

STEVEN G. MERANZE, M.D.
Associate Professor, Department of Radiology, Vanderbilt University; Section Chief, Cardiovascular and Interventional Radiology, Vanderbilt University, Nashville, Tennessee

MARK W. MEWISSEN, M.D.
Associate Professor and Director, Section of Vascular/Interventional Radiology, Medical College of Wisconsin, Milwaukee, Wisconsin

MICHAEL F. MEYEROVITZ, M.D.
Associate Professor, Department of Radiology, Harvard Medical School; Co-Director, Cardiovascular and Interventional Radiology, Brigham and Women's Hospital, Boston

CHRISTOPHER J. MORAN, M.D.
Associate Professor, Mallinckrodt Institute of Radiology, Washington University School of Medicine, St. Louis, Missouri

STEVEN B. OGLEVIE, M.D.
Assistant Professor, Department of Radiology, University of California, San Diego School of Medicine; Director of Interventional Radiology, Department of Radiology, San Diego Department of Veterans Affairs Medical Center, San Diego

SVEN PAULIN, M.D., Ph.D.
Miriam H. Stoneman Distinguished Professor of Radiology, Department of Radiology, Harvard Medical School; Radiologist-in-Chief, Emeritus, Department of Radiology, Beth Israel Hospital, Boston

RACHEL R. PHILLIPS, MRCP, FRCR
Honorary Senior Lecturer, The Department of Medicine, University College London, London; Senior Fellow in Pediatric Radiology, British Columbia's Children's Hospital, Vancouver, British Columbia, Canada

JOSEPH F. POLAK, M.D., M.P.H.
Associate Professor of Radiology, Harvard Medical School, Boston; Director, Noninvasive Vascular Imaging, and Codirector, Vascular Diagnostic Laboratory, Brigham and Women's Hospital, Boston

PATRICIA ANN RANDALL, M.D.
Professor of Radiology and Chief of Cardiac Radiology, SUNY-Health Science Center, Syracuse, New York

DOUGLAS C.B. REDD, M.D.
Assistant Professor of Radiology, University of Pennsylvania School of Medicine, Philadelphia

MICHAEL R. REES, M.D.
Professor and Head of Department of Clinical Radiology, Bristol University; Honorary Consultant, Department of Radiology, University of Bristol, Bristol, England

JOSEF RÖSCH, M.D.
Director and Professor, Research Laboratory, Dotter Interventional Institute, Oregon Health Sciences University, Portland, Oregon

ALEXANDER ROSENBERGER, M.D.
Professor of Diagnostic Radiology, Technion-Israel Institute of Technology; Former Chairman of Diagnostic Radiology, Rambam Medical Center, Haifa, Israel

HEMENDRA R. SHAH, M.D.
Associate Professor, Departments of Radiology and Urology, University of Arkansas for Medical Sciences; Director of Body CT/MRI, Department of Radiology, University Hospital, Little Rock, Arkansas

MARCELLE J. SHAPIRO, M.D.
Assistant Professor of Radiology, Jefferson Medical College; Assistant Professor, Cardiovascular-Interventional Radiology, Thomas Jefferson University Hospital, Philadelphia

RICHARD D. SHLANSKY-GOLDBERG, M.D.
Assistant Professor of Radiology and Surgery, University of Pennsylvania Medical School; Staff Interventional Radiologist, University of Pennsylvania Medical School, Philadelphia

MORRIS SIMON, M.D.
Professor of Radiology, Harvard Medical School; Director of Clinical Radiology, Department of Radiology, Beth Israel Hospital, Boston

DAVID J. SPINOSA, M.D.
Interventional Radiologist, Peninsula Radiology Associates, Peninsula Regional Medical Center, Salisbury, Maryland

CHARLES J. TEGTMEYER, M.D.
Director and Professor, Division of Angiography and Interventional Radiology, University of Virginia Health Sciences Center, Charlottesville, Virginia
Deceased

MICHAEL S. VAN LYSEL, Ph.D.
Associate Professor, Departments of Medicine and Medical Physics, University of Wisconsin Medical School; Technical Director, Cardiac Catheterization Laboratories, Cardiology Section, Department of Medicine, University of Wisconsin Hospital and Clinics, Madison, Wisconsin

FELIX W. WEHRLI, Ph.D.
Professor of Radiology, University of Pennsylvania, Philadelphia

LEWIS WEXLER, M.D.
Professor of Radiology and Member, Section of Cardiovascular Radiology, Stanford University School of Medicine, Stanford, California

Introductory Comments

Abrams' Angiography was published in 1961 as the first multivolume work in the field, responding both to rapid technological developments and to the perceived need for a comprehensive reference work. The second edition appeared in 1972 and the third in 1983, each reflecting the extraordinary advances that had taken place in the intervening years.

To my great pleasure and the readers' great profit, Dr. Stanley Baum, a former fellow of mine in cardiovascular radiology and now the chairman of one of the most renowned university departments in the world, agreed to serve as editor of the fourth edition. This was a project of daunting magnitude, since the field has widened to include a new set of remarkable achievements in interventional radiology. Dr. Baum has organized and edited this edition with a keen eye for noteworthy progress and for the finest contributors worldwide, and it is certain to receive the wide circulation accorded the first three editions.

I am pleased to note my own modest contribution in the revisions of some of the chapters of my authorship, always a learning experience in the light of clinical and research progress and the recent literature.

There is, then, the pleasure of continuity both in the renewed efforts of prior contributors and in the editorship of Dr. Baum. The reader will find these volumes a treasure chest of information, fully encompassing the present state of the art and encouraging another generation to go forward, learning and leading the way in cardiovascular and interventional radiology.

Herbert L. Abrams, M.D.

Preface

The publication of this fourth edition of *Abrams' Angiography* coincides with the centennial of Roentgen's discovery of the x-ray. Roentgen would indeed be surprised if he had the opportunity to read the three volumes of this fourth edition. He could not have imagined the advances and innovations that have been made with the "mysterious rays" described in 1896.

In just 13 years since the previous edition of *Abrams' Angiography,* there has been remarkable growth in the entire field of radiology. As major advances in imaging were made, interventional radiology grew from a field of "useful medical photography" to a clinical specialty that is indispensable to the practice of modern medicine. It began in areas that had traditionally been the domain of the vascular radiologist. Once the angiographer demonstrated the bleeding lesion by injecting a catheter that had been positioned in the appropriate artery, it was a logical extension to attempt to stop the bleeding by either infusing a vasoconstrictor or injecting an embolus. Then, as angiographic skills improved and catheters were manipulated in diseased vessels, attempts were made to mechanically increase lumen diameter, thereby increasing blood flow. This attempt was first described by Dotter and Judkins, who used stiff, straight catheters, and later by Gruentzig, who used specially designed balloon catheters with unique expansion characteristics. This later technique allowed for dilation in diseased vessels that were not readily accessible to stiff, compressing catheters.

As interest in angiography and interventional radiology soared in the past 20 years, these approaches became widely used in both major medical centers and community hospitals. Since many radiologists in the United States, Europe, and Asia were devoting most of their professional effort to the study of cardiovascular disease and interventional radiology, a need for a forum arose in which different investigators could examine, evaluate, and share their experiences. Around the world, cardiovascular and interventional radiology societies grew from small, informal "clubs" to major societies. In the United States, the specialty received further recognition in 1993 when the American Board of Radiology began to issue Certificates of Added Qualification in Cardiovascular and Interventional Radiology. Diplomats of the American Board of Radiology can apply for the special examination leading to these certificates after demonstrating satisfactory completion of an approved fellowship program following radiology residency training. In offering these certificates, the American Board of Radiology has acknowledged cardiovascular and interventional radiology as a legitimate subspecialty of radiology.

The new fourth edition has been completely updated to reflect the dynamic change and growth of the specialty since 1983. The first two volumes are dedicated to diagnostic angiography and the expanding role of ultrasonography, computed tomography, and, more recently, magnetic resonance imaging in the visualization of the vascular system. Seventy-five chapters in the first two volumes are either new or have been completely rewritten to reflect the changes of conventional and noninvasive modalities in vascular diagnosis.

The third volume of the fourth edition, with Dr. Michael Pentecost serving as coeditor, is dedicated solely to interventional radiology. This volume consists of 63 new chapters describing the most recent advances made in this field.

One approaches the task of updating and reediting a classic text with a great deal of humility and caution. I hope that the result captures some of the excitement and scope that has been the hallmark of the previous editions. The first edition of this text was published in 1961 when the specialty of angiography was coalescing and there was a need for such a work. We are in a similar position today with interventional radiology, and it is hoped that these volumes will provide the same authoritative voice in the emergence of this new specialty. Attempts have been made to avoid redundancy and to present a coherent and easily readable text. As a result, I have at times altered the format, organization, and language of some of the contributors. Hopefully, the fourth edition will not squander its inheritance and will live up to its predecessors.

I am indebted to Herb Abrams for the role that he has played in my career as advisor, mentor, and friend. His impact on the field of angiography and interventional radiology has been enormous and through his trainees at Stanford and later at Harvard, he has dominated the specialty for three decades. Herb was tireless in his efforts to preserve angiography as a part of radiology during the era of the 1960s and 1970s, when radiologists were viewed by their medical and surgical colleagues as shadow gazers who were incapable of assuming major clinical responsibilities. Indeed, in most hospitals, orders for premedication could be written on patients' charts by diagnostic radiologists only if they were countersigned by "a real doctor." Herb also understood the importance of basic and clinical research very early in the development of the specialty. At a time when most radiology research was in radiologic physics and radiobiology, he insisted on having in his department research laboratories that attempted to answer basic physiologic questions. His was the first laboratory to describe and study the lack of response of tumor vessel to vasoconstrictors. The observation that tumor vessels do not constrict after the intraarterial administration of epinephrine became clinically important because it allowed the angiographer to differentiate small renal cell carcinomas from normal parenchyma during diagnostic arteriography. As the field of cell biology began to expand, Herb's laboratory at Harvard embarked on studies to better understand the process of angiogenesis as it relates to cancer as well as to chronic ischemia. The environment that he created in his department influenced many of his trainees at Stanford and Harvard to pursue academic- and research-oriented careers in diagnostic radiology.

I was honored that Herb Abrams suggested that I edit this edition, and I am grateful for his continuing encouragement from the time of planning to the final days of completion.

My wife Jeanne deserves special credit for her willingness to put up with my working vacations and the hours of preparation that this edition required. Without her encouragement, this work would not have happened.

I am also indebted to my vice-chairman, Michael Pentecost, who has served as coeditor of the volume on interventional radiology.

An authoritative text of this magnitude required the willingness of over 100 authors to meet deadlines, conform to the editorial changes required, and, throughout the process, tolerate my sometimes weekend calls. I do not believe that I have lost many friends in the process, and I am appreciative and thankful to all of them.

I am also thankful to my assistant, Flora Cauley, who somehow managed to keep track of the 143 individual chapters, and to Mary Frawley, who is an outstanding editorial assistant. Additional thanks go to the editorial staff of Little, Brown and Company for their help and encouragement. Nancy Chorpenning, Executive Editor, was wonderful to work with, as were Deeth Ellis, Development Editor, and Julie Sullivan, Project Manager.

Last, but not least, I would like to thank the contributors from the faculty of the Radiology Department at the University of Pennsylvania. Drs. Richard Baum, Constantin Cope, Kenneth Fellows, Ziv Haskal, George Holland, Robert Hurst, Parvati Ramchandani, Douglas Redd, Richard Shlansky-Goldberg, Michael Soulen, and Felix Wehrli willingly took up the slack and added this responsibility to their already demanding clinical and academic schedules. I have also asked favors of many of my longtime friends and colleagues. I am grateful to all of you.

Stanley Baum, M.D.

Abrams' Angiography

Vascular and Interventional Radiology

Notice

The indications and dosages of all drugs in this book have been recommended in the medical literature and conform to the practices of the general medical community. The medications described do not necessarily have specific approval by the Food and Drug Administration for use in the diseases and dosages for which they are recommended. The package insert for each drug should be consulted for use and dosage as approved by the FDA. Because standards for usage change, it is advisable to keep abreast of revised recommendations, particularly those concerning new drugs.

I

General Considerations

1

Historical Notes

HERBERT L. ABRAMS

Angiography is the study of blood vessels in living subjects by roentgen contrast methods. To trace its development, we must go back to the discovery of x-rays.

On November 8, 1895, Roentgen, while experimenting with the Hittorf-Crookes tube, observed a bright fluorescence of barium platinocyanide crystals. He assumed initially that the fluorescence might be caused by cathode (beta) rays. Using a fluorescent screen, he removed it beyond the range of cathode rays; when the fluorescence persisted, he became aware that the effect was produced by a new kind of ray. Not long afterward, he replaced the screen by a recording photographic plate. One of the dramatic results of this experiment was a picture of his wife's hand. On December 28, 1895, after 8 weeks of intensive investigation, he delivered the manuscript reporting his discovery of x-rays to the Physical Medical Society of Würzburg. Printed as a preliminary communication in the annals of the society, it was a remarkably succinct and careful description of the behavior of x-rays.[1] His two classic papers of March 1896 and May 1897 completed the recording of many fundamental observations to which little was added for many years.

By early January 1896, word of Roentgen's discovery and its import had spread around the world.[2] Almost immediately the possibilities of applying the new "photography" to traumatic lesions of bone fired the imaginative, and within a month x-rays of fractures had been obtained and published. Early in the year, Edison and many others began intensive work on the fluoroscope. By the end of March 1896, Becher had outlined the stomach and intestines of a sacrificed guinea pig with lead subacetate and had mentioned the idea of delineating fistulas in this way.[3] In the fall of 1896, Walter B. Cannon, a physiologist who was interested in the motor activities of the stomach, undertook a study in cats suggested to him by H. P. Bowditch of Boston. Mixing bismuth subnitrate with the food, he observed the movements of the opaque mass in the stomach and subsequently described in detail the nature and site of peristaltic activity as he saw it on the fluoroscopic screen.[4] He noted in particular the "extreme sensitiveness" of the cat stomach to anxiety or rage and the marked inhibition of peristalsis that resulted. The usefulness of contrast agents was already becoming apparent. Before the year ended, the first textbook on the subject of x-rays had been published.

Visualization of the blood vessels in humans was achieved early in the year. In January 1896, the month after the announcement of Roentgen's discovery, Haschek and Lindenthal injected Teichman's mixture into the blood vessels of an amputated hand.[5] A photograph of their original roentgenogram was published in the January issue of the *Wiener klinische Wochenschrift* (Fig. 1-1) and showed clearly the potential of the method for visualizing the vascular bed. A volume by Morton written in 1896 is of interest in this regard. Morton, a "Professor of Diseases of the Mind and Nervous System" at the New York Post-Graduate Medical School, was fascinated by the new field of roentgenology. In collaboration with an electrical engineer named Hammer, he wrote a text entitled *The X-ray, or, Photography of the Invisible and Its Value in Surgery*.[6] In it were not only chapters on normal anatomy, fractures and dislocations, stiff joints, and foreign objects in the body, but also a section on medicolegal applications of x-rays. His remarks concerning contrast studies are intriguing:

> In teaching the anatomy of the blood vessels, the x-ray opens out a new and feasible method. The arteries and veins of dead bodies may be injected with a substance opaque to the x-ray and thus, their distribution may be more accurately followed than by any possible dissection. The feasibility of this method applies equally well to the study of the structures and organs of the dead body. To a certain extent, therefore, x-ray photography may replace both dissection and vivisection, and in the living body, the location and size of a hollow organ, as for instance the stomach, may be ascertained by causing the subject to drink a harmless fluid more or less opaque to the x-ray, or an effervescing mixture which will cause distention, and then taking the picture.

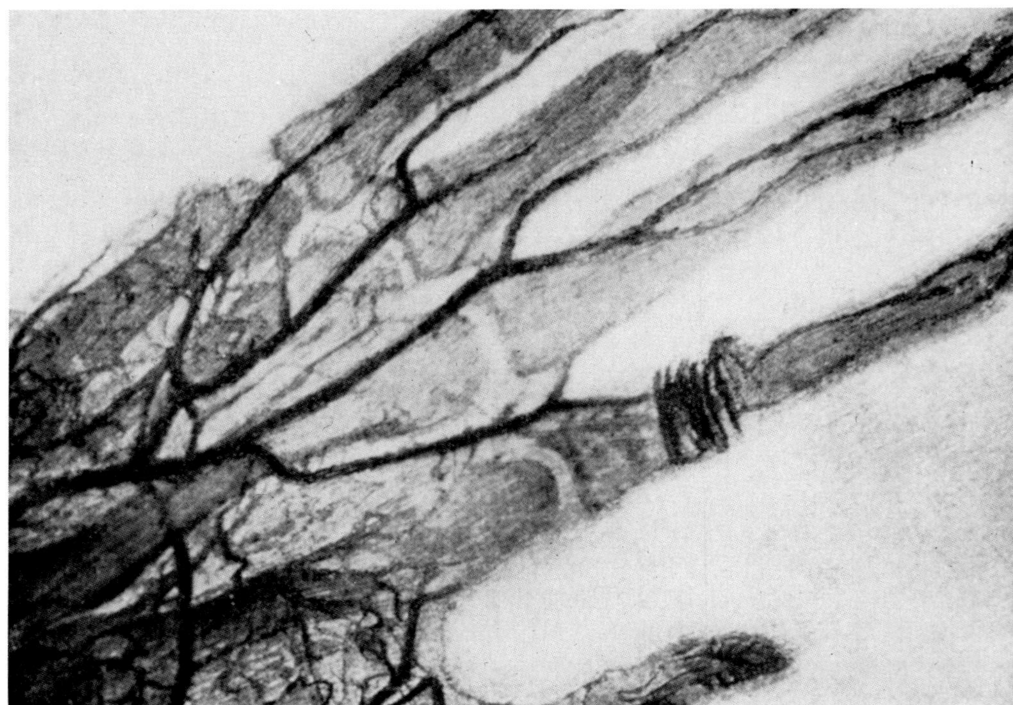

Figure 1-1. A roentgenogram made by Haschek and Lindenthal after the injection of Teichman's mixture into the blood vessels of an amputated hand. (From Haschek E, Lindenthal OT. A contribution to the practical use of the photography according to Röntgen. Wien Klin Wochenschr 1896;9:63.)

By 1900 an entire volume entitled *The Use of the Roentgen Ray by the Medical Department of the U.S. Army in the War with Spain*[7] had been published. Gunshot fragments in the soft tissues and traumatic lesions of bone were illustrated in large plates in this volume.

At the time that Voelcker and von Lichtenberg introduced retrograde pyelography to the field of urographic diagnosis in 1906,[8] a number of medical schools had organized departments of roentgenology. In Kassabian's voluminous textbook of 1907, *Röntgen Rays and Electrotherapeutics,* the chapters on diseases of the thorax and diseases of the abdominal organs warranted 60 pages for adequate description.[9] His comments regarding the blood vessels deserve consideration:

> I have studied the blood vessels of infants and adults by injecting into them a substance opaque to the x-rays. The substance used is a concentrated emulsion of bismuth subnitrate, a strong solution of litharge (red oxide of lead) or metallic mercury. In order to demonstrate sharply the arterial tree, the injection must be done carefully and slowly. By some it is deemed advisable first to empty the arterial system of all its blood, and then to inject a solution of zinc chloride so as to get rid of any existing clots. This solution should be removed by washing, or by forcing water into the arterial system, followed by an injection of metallic mercury by a force pump connected to the external carotid artery.

Kassabian also studied the blood vessels of the kidney, heart, brain, spleen, liver, and stomach in cadavers.

In 1920 an x-ray atlas devoted only to the systemic arteries of the body was published in England.[10,11] In it were roentgenographic reproductions that showed the blood vessels in cadavers with great clarity (Fig. 1-2).

Meanwhile Franck and Alwens, in 1910, introduced a suspension of bismuth and oil into the hearts of dogs and rabbits directly through the large veins.[12] They were able to observe the passage of the oily droplets from the heart into the lungs. The work of Sicard and Forestier, 12 years later, represented the next major advance. They had employed Lipiodol to study first the bronchial tree and then the spinal subarachnoid space in 1922. A year later, they decided to try the oil in the cardiovascular system.[13] Working with dogs, they slowly injected 5 ml of Lipiodol into the femoral vein and, with the aid of fluoroscopy, watched the droplets move with increasing speed from the iliac vein

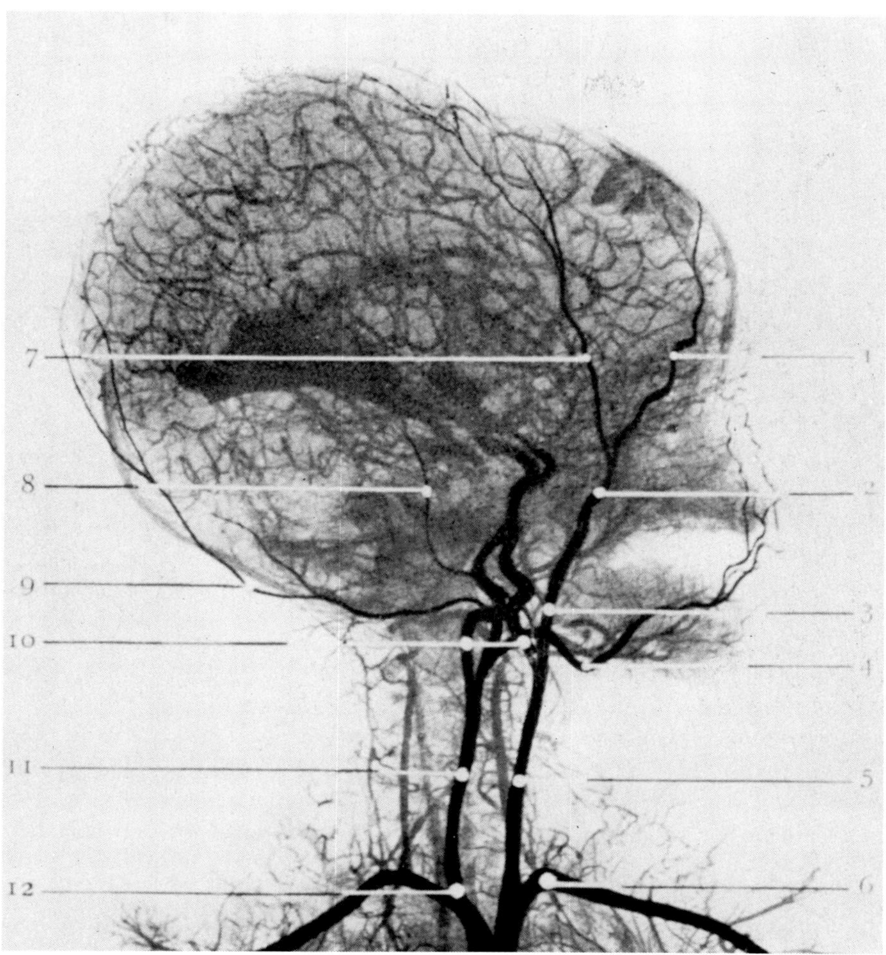

Figure 1-2. Reproduction of a 1920 roentgenogram of a cadaver after the injection of opaque medium into the cerebral vessels. *1,* anterior temporal artery; *2,* temporal artery; *3,* external carotid; *4,* facial artery; *5,* left common carotid; *6,* subclavian artery; *7,* posterior temporal artery; *8,* posterior auricular artery; *9,* occipital artery; *10,* right and left internal carotid arteries; *11,* right common carotid artery; *12,* innominate artery. (From Orrin HC. The x-ray atlas of the systemic arteries of the body. London: Ballière, Tindall, and Cox, 1920.)

into the heart. The Lipiodol was then "pulverized" by ventricular contraction, thrown with great speed into the pulmonary artery, and finally spread as multiple emboli into the small vessels of the lung, disappearing in 10 to 12 minutes. Emboldened by their success in dogs, they repeated the experiment with human subjects, in whom they carefully observed the course of the opaque oil from the antecubital vein to the pulmonary capillaries. Their patients coughed as the oil reached the lungs but suffered no other ill effects. They also injected Lipiodol into the femoral artery and the carotid artery of dogs; the latter studies produced respiratory distress and death.

In the same year, 1923, Berberich and Hirsch reported the first arteriograms and venograms obtained in humans with 20 percent strontium bromide.[14] The quality of the films, showing arteries and veins of the upper extremity, was respectable, and vessel detail was good (Fig. 1-3). One year later, in 1924, Brooks reported the intraarterial injection of sodium iodide as a means of demonstrating the vessels of the lower extremity in humans.[15] His studies were comparable in quality to good modern arteriograms (Fig. 1-4). He considered his technique useful for delineating the precise anatomy of the arteries, for showing atheromatous change, and for indicating when amputation had to be done in the presence of a compromised blood supply. Subsequently Carnett and Greenbaum used Lipiodol for arteriography, but its viscosity and globulation rendered it an unsatisfactory agent.[16] Saito et al., to eliminate the globule formation, emulsified Lipiodol and used as much as 20 ml for arteriography in

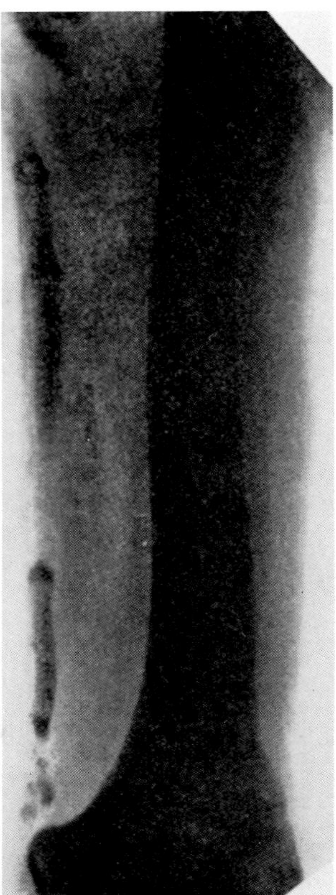

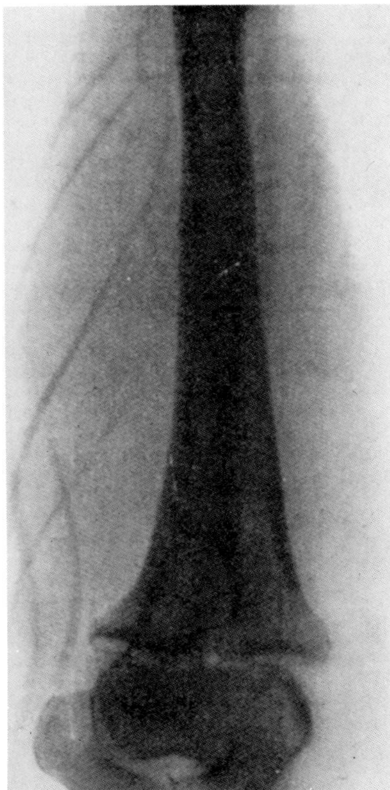

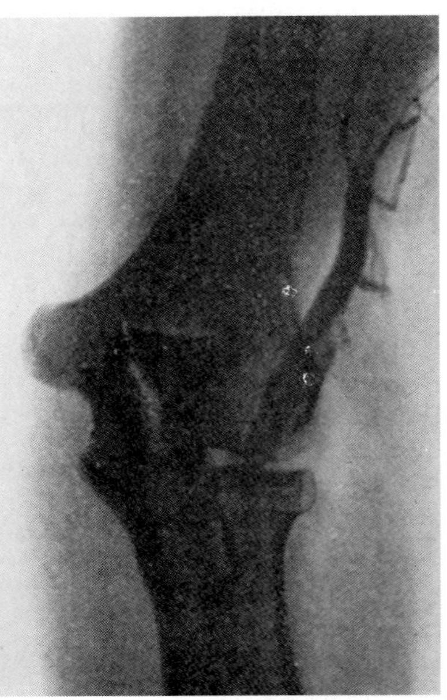

Figure 1-3. Venographic studies obtained by Berberich and Hirsch in 1923. They injected 20 percent strontium bromide into the veins of the upper extremity. (From Berberich J, Hirsch S. Die roentgenographische Darstellung der Arterien und Venen am Lebenden. Munchen Klin Wochenschr 1923;49:2226.)

patients.[17] Their studies were clear, and the detail was satisfactory. No severe reactions were reported. Charbonnel and Massé reported their experience with sodium iodide in arteriography in 1929 but emphasized the irritating qualities of the agent.[18] Dos Santos et al., however, considered sodium iodide an effective arteriographic agent.[19,20] During this period McPheeters and Rice investigated varicose veins with Lipiodol and followed its course under fluoroscopy.[21] Their diagrams are intriguing, even today, but they were confronted with the same problem of fragmentation of the opaque column noted by other workers.

The decade of the 1920s was an exciting developmental period for the entire field of angiography. In 1928 Moniz et al. described the technique of carotid angiography and its application to the study of cerebral lesions (Fig. 1-5).[22] During the same year, Forssmann, having practiced on a cadaver, inserted a catheter into his own antecubital vein until he felt that it had reached the right atrium. A roentgenogram confirmed his supposition. Originally he conceived of this as a method of infusing therapeutic substances into the heart, but in 1931 he undertook to visualize the right heart and the pulmonary vessels with Uroselectan.[23] He succeeded in dogs but not in human subjects. Dos Santos et al. in 1929 showed that satisfactory opacification of the abdominal aorta and its branches could be obtained using translumbar needle puncture and injection (Fig. 1-6).[19]

The Portuguese, pioneers in the field of angiography, also addressed themselves to the problem of showing the pulmonary vessels in disease. In 1931, using sodium iodide, Moniz and his colleagues devised the technique of "angiopneumography," as they called it, and described the appearance of the pulmonary vessels in a variety of conditions.[24] Initially they injected sodium iodide directly into the right ventricle of a rabbit to opacify the pulmonary vessels. Subsequently they injected the medium into the jugular vein of the rabbit, the dog, and the monkey and obtained excellent visualization of the pulmonary arteries. In humans, using Forssmann's technique of cardiac catheterization, they were able to increase the opacity of the pulmonary vessels as recorded roentgenographi-

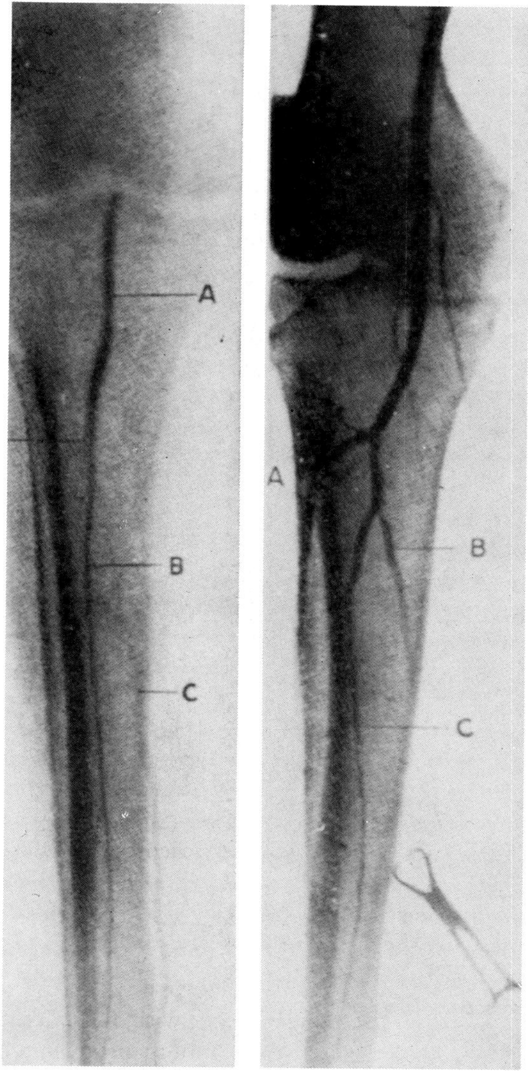

Figure 1-4. The first femoral arteriogram obtained in a human subject. Brooks used sodium iodide as a means of demonstrating the vessels of the lower extremities in 1924. (From Brooks B. Intraarterial injection of sodium iodide. JAMA 1924;82:1016.)

cally. They could not distinguish the arteries from the veins, and they were unable to visualize the cardiac chambers.

It is of great interest that during this period intravenous urography was not employed to a significant degree for the study of renal disease. In 1923 Osborne et al. described the visualization of the collecting system of the kidney by the intravenous and oral administration of large amounts of sodium iodide.[25] Within the next few years a number of observers repeated the observations with sodium iodide; but delineation was not satisfactory, and there were reactions to the large amounts of inorganic iodide employed. Roseno, using an agent that combined urea with sodium iodide,[26] obtained satisfactory studies in 1927, but the medium was too toxic.

In 1929 Swick reported the use of an organic iodide, synthesized by Binz and Rath,[27,28] known as Selectan.[29] This drug had been applied to the treatment of mastitis in cows and was known to be excreted in the urine and in the bile. Because of its iodine content, Swick thought it might opacify the collecting structures of the kidney during its excretion after intravenous injection. This supposition proved to be correct.[29,30]

The discovery of an opaque organic iodide that was moderately well tolerated when administered intravenously was of immense importance to the field of angiography. When set against the background of rising interest in delineating specific segments of the vascular bed in humans, it proved to be a catalyst of significant proportions. Selectan was supplemented by Neoselectan (Iopax) and then by Uroselectan B (Neo-Iopax). Soon thereafter, Abrodil (Skiodan) was synthesized, to be replaced by Per-Abrodil (Diodrast).

By 1931 Skiodan had been employed in arteriography[31,32] and venography[33,34] with gratifying results, and within the next few years a number of studies of varicose veins were reported.[35,36] The organic iodides, then, were introduced at a time when femoral, brachial, and carotid arteriography, venography, and translumbar aortography had all been accomplished but depended in large measure on a relatively noxious agent, sodium iodide. Satisfactory opacification of the heart and great thoracic arteries had not yet been attained.

In 1933 Rousthöi, working with the experimental animal, described the opacification of the cardiac chambers and the aorta in an important paper called "Über Angiokardiographie."[37] During succeeding years a number of investigators[38-40] attempted to opacify the heart in humans before Ameuille et al. in 1936 finally succeeded in doing so using the catheter method.[41] A year later the first practical method of angiocardiography was described.[42]

As far back as 1931 Castellanos had been intrigued by the possibility of studying congenital cardiac anomalies with the opaque media. He found sodium iodide too toxic for satisfactory intravenous use in humans and discontinued his studies until a more satisfactory substance was available. Satisfied at length that Per-Abrodil (iodopyracet or Diodrast) combined adequate contrast with relatively slight toxicity, he tried it in human subjects.

Late in 1937 Castellanos, Pereiras, and García re-

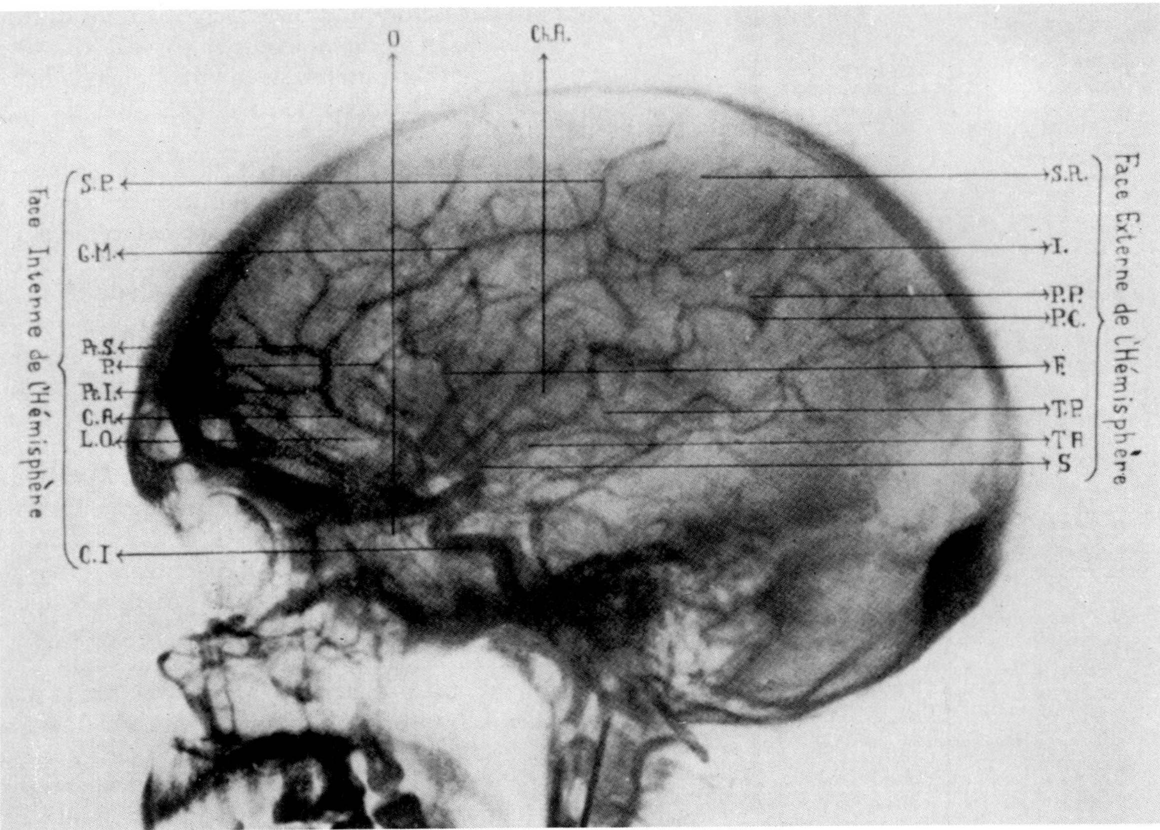

Figure 1-5. Reproduction of a cerebral arteriogram. (From Moniz E, de Carvalho L, Lima A. La radioartériographie et la topographie cranioencephalique. J Radiol Electrol Med Nucl 1928;12:72.)

ported the first successful roentgen contrast diagnosis of a number of congenital cardiac anomalies during life. Between September 1937 and July 1938, they issued many reports; published illustrations of atrial and ventricular septal defects, pulmonic stenosis, the tetralogy of Fallot, and transposition of the great vessels; suggested and performed biplane studies; and devised an automatic injection device which they described in detail.[43–45] One gap in their method of investigating the heart in the living subject was that they were able to opacify adequately only the right heart chambers.

Robb and Steinberg in 1938 introduced the use of ether and cyanide circulation times as a guide to the timing of successive exposures to obtain sequential opacification of the right and left heart.[46] Their technique was applicable to adults, and they further suggested the possibility of using cineroentgenography and rapid serial roentgenography, as well as coordinating the exposure with the heartbeat.[47]

Not until 10 years after Castellanos et al. and Robb and Steinberg had published their initial papers was there a significant change in angiocardiographic technique. Chávez and his coworkers described intracardiac injection in clinical subjects in 1947,[48] and Jönsson and his associates used this method of "selective" angiocardiography extensively during subsequent years.[49]

The development of thoracic aortography paralleled that of angiocardiography. Using the direct puncture technique that had been applied to animals, Nuvoli in 1936 studied the aorta in humans, showing aneurysm, tortuosity, and other conditions (Fig. 1-7).[50] Countercurrent or retrograde brachial aortography was described in 1939 by Castellanos and Pereiras (Fig. 1-8),[51] and catheter aortography by Radner in 1948.[52]

The study of the abdominal aorta depended on the translumbar approach advocated by dos Santos until 1941, when Fariñas reported the retrograde passage of a catheter from the femoral artery for aortography.[53]

With the introduction of the percutaneous trans-

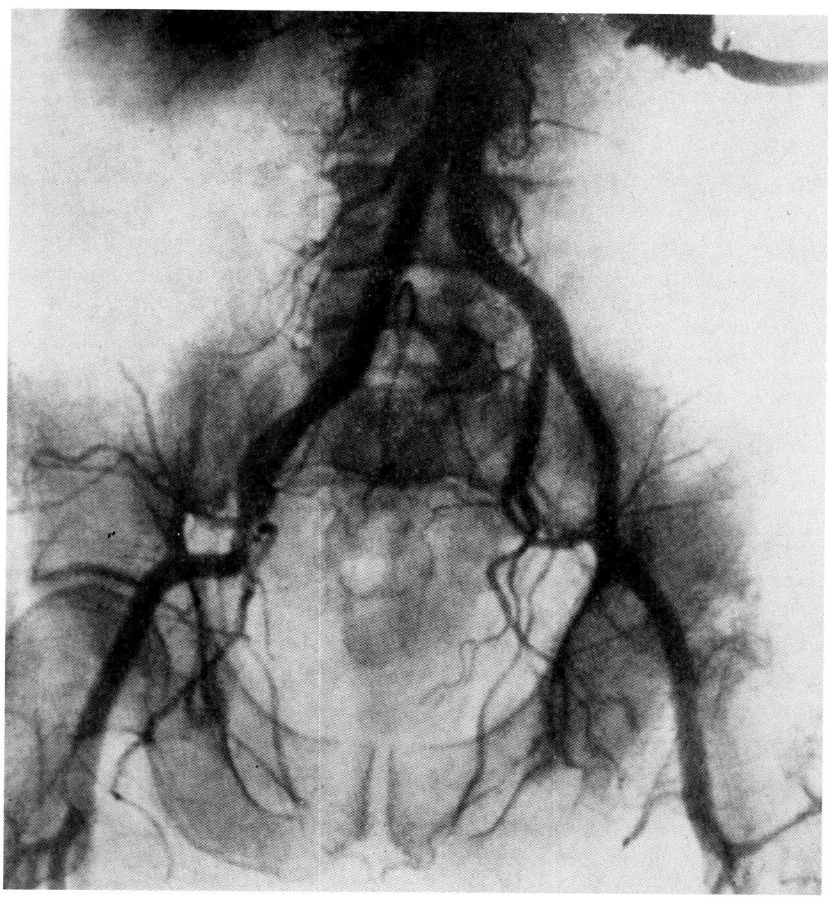

Figure 1-6. Translumbar aortogram, one of the early studies of the abdominal aorta. (From dos Santos R, Lamas AC, Pereira-Caldas J. Arteriografia da aorta e dos vasos abdominais. Bull Mem Soc Natl Chir 1929;47:93.)

femoral catheterization method in 1953 by Seldinger, the groundwork of the modern method of angiography was well established.[54]

Technical advances during this period included the development of a rapid film changer by Gidlund[55] and of biplane film changers by Axen and Lind,[56] the application of cineangiocardiography,[57,58] and the movement toward practical image amplification suggested by Chamberlain in 1942[59] and subsequently developed by Coltman in 1948[60] and Sturm and Morgan in 1949.[61] Chapman and his coworkers described the use of biplane cinefluorography to evaluate ventricular volume in 1958,[62] and in the same year Abrams introduced biplane *image-amplified* cineangiography,[63] which has become the most widely applied method of studying children with congenital heart disease.

During the past four decades, angiography has developed into a series of polished and versatile techniques applicable to virtually all of the viscera. This progress has paralleled the advances in vascular surgery and surgical techniques in general and has derived much of its stimulus from them. The vertebral and azygos venous systems have been subjected to detailed study in vivo. The circulation of the myocardium has been repeatedly explored in a revealing manner by roentgen contrast study. The approach to the renal vessels, formerly requiring large amounts of heavily concentrated medium injected directly into the aorta, can now be accomplished by direct catheterization of the renal artery with relatively small volumes of opaque medium. The study of the pancreas, liver, and spleen by angiography yielded definitive diagnoses never before available before surgery. A major episode in the history of angiography was the development of coronary arteriography in humans, first described by Gunnar Jönsson in 1948,[64] amplified by Dotter and Frische with aortic occlusion in 1958,[65] and finally applied to humans as a selective technique in 1959 by F. Mason

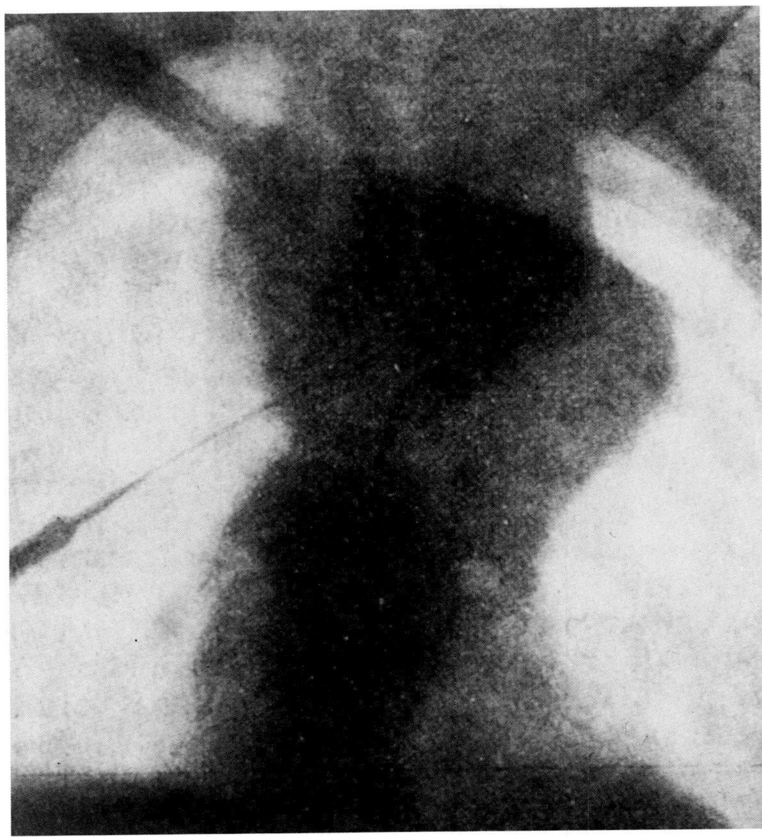

Figure 1-7. Thoracic aortography. Nuvoli used the direct puncture technique in 1936 to study the thoracic aorta. This poor reproduction of one of his original studies demonstrates an aortogram in the presence of a thoracic aortic aneurysm. (From Nuvoli I. Arteriografia dell'aorta toracica mediante punctura dell'aorta ascendente o del ventricolos. Policlinico (Prat) 1936;43:227.)

Sones.[66] In 1961, Ricketts and Abrams first performed percutaneous transfemoral selective coronary arteriography with preformed catheters,[67] and 5 years later Judkins modified transfemoral preformed catheters with thermoplastic material to provide what has become the most widely applied method of coronary arteriography throughout the world.[68]

The past few decades have witnessed major changes in the field of pharmacoangiography, used not only for diagnostic purposes but also to manage gastrointestinal bleeding or to increase blood flow in the presence of vasospasm. Interventional radiology, which figures so largely in these volumes, was just beginning to emerge at the time of the second edition of *Angiography* in 1971.

No sophisticated surgery has ever been able to develop in the history of modern medicine without a preceding sophisticated radiology to provide a road map. This is as true of surgery of the brain, lungs, gastrointestinal tract, kidneys, and bone as it is of the cardiovascular system. By the time open heart surgery became feasible in the mid-1950s, angiography had graduated from the status of an experimental investigative procedure with little clinical applicability to a highly refined diagnostic method. It was thus able immediately to be put to use to provide for the surgeon the kind of morphologic information that was essential not only to successful surgery at the time but also to the development of new methods of handling more and more complicated lesions. Angiography was the forerunner of interventional radiology.

Improvements in angiography have been designed to decrease the dangers and improve the quality of the studies. As a consequence, new media have been synthesized, and meticulous preangiographic and postangiographic care has become a central and important focus. These complex and immensely revealing diagnostic procedures can now be performed with a minimum of hazard to the patient and with a maximum of critical information on which to base the clinical management of the patient.

Angiography occupies a unique place in medicine.

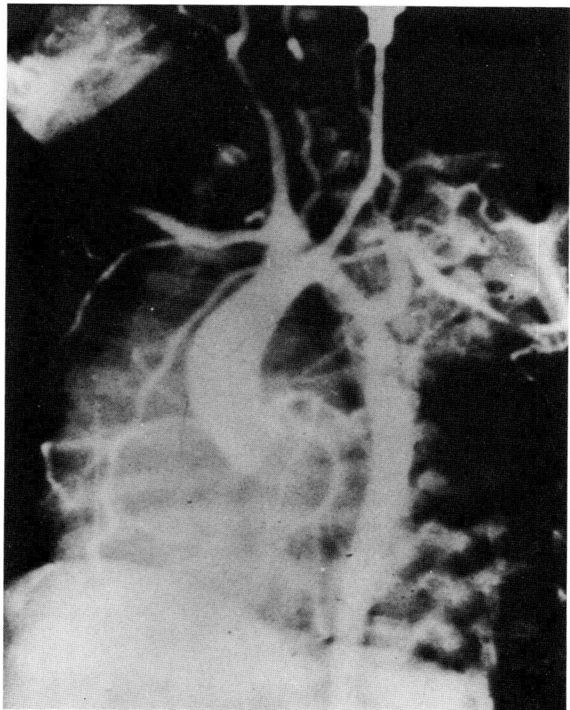

Figure 1-8. Retrograde brachial aortography in coarctation of the aorta. This examination was performed in 1938 by Augustus Castellanos, M.D., who has graciously provided a copy of the original examination.

It is an invaluable aid in the diagnosis of diseases of the viscera, such as tumors. It is a definitive method of showing congenital vascular malformations in all parts of the human body. The wear and tear on arteries caused by atheromatous change is reflected in the arteriogram as in no other study, and when this results in thrombosis, the site of block can usually be delineated.

The development of new imaging methods, such as ultrasound, computed tomography, and magnetic resonance imaging, has clearly affected the utilization of angiography in specific areas. Nevertheless, there is no substitute for angiography in many of its applications.

In the pages to follow, an attempt has been made to define the present status of angiographic procedures, to assess their value and their limitations, and to assess the possible hazards that may attend them.

References

1. Roentgen WC. On a new kind of ray. Sitz Ber Phys-Med Ges (Wurzburg) 1895;137.
2. Glasser O. Wilhelm Conrad Roentgen and the early history of the x-rays. Springfield, IL: Thomas, 1934.
3. Becher W. Zur Anwendung des roentgenischen Verfahrens in der Medizin. Deutsch Med Wochenschr 1896;22:202.
4. Cannon WB. The movements of the stomach studied by means of the roentgen ray. Am J Physiol 1898;1:359.
5. Haschek E, Lindenthal OT. A contribution to the practical use of the photography according to Röntgen. Wien Klin Wochenschr 1896;9:63.
6. Morton WG, Hammer WE. The x-ray, or, photography of the invisible and its value in surgery. New York: American Technical Book Co., 1896.
7. Borden WC. The use of the roentgen ray by the Medical Department of the U.S. Army in the war with Spain. Washington: GPO, 1924.
8. Voelcker F, von Lichtenberg A. Pyelographie (Roentgenographie des nierenbeckens nach kollargolfullung). Munchen Med Wochenschr 1906;53:105.
9. Kassabian MK. Röntgen rays and electrotherapeutics with chapters on radium and phototherapy. Philadelphia: Lippincott, 1907.
10. Orrin HC. The x-ray atlas of the systemic arteries of the body. London: Baillière, Tindall, and Cox, 1920.
11. Orrin HC. First aid x-ray atlas of the arteries. New York: Hoeber, 1923.
12. Franck O, Alwens W. Kreislaufstudien am Röntgenschirm. Munchen Med Wochenschr 1910;51:950.
13. Sicard JA, Forestier G. Injections intravasculaires d'huile iodée sous controle radiologique. C R Soc Seances Soc Biol Fil (Paris) 1923;88:1200.
14. Berberich J, Hirsch S. Die roentgenographische Darstellung der Arterien und Venen am Lebenden. Munchen Klin Wochenschr 1923;49:2226.
15. Brooks B. Intraarterial injection of sodium iodide. JAMA 1924; 82:1016.
16. Carnett JB, Greenbaum SS. Blood vessel visualization. JAMA 1927;89:2039.
17. Saito M, Kamikawa K, Yanagizawa K. Blood vessel visualization in vivo. Am J Surg 1930;10:225.
18. Charbonnel, Massé. Artériographie des membres avec l'iodure de sodium, spécialment dans les artérites. Bull Mem Soc Natl Chir 1929;55:735.
19. dos Santos R, Lamas AC, Pereira-Caldas J. Arteriografia da aorta e dos vasos abdominais. Bull Mem Soc Natl Chir 1929; 47:93.
20. dos Santos R, Lamas AC, Pereira-Caldas J. L'artériographie des membres de l'aorte et de ses branches abdominales. Bull Mem Soc Natl Chir 1929;55:587.
21. McPheeters HO, Rice CO. Varicose veins—the circulation and direction of venous flow. Surg Gynecol Obstet 1929;49:29.
22. Moniz E, de Carvalho L, Lima A. La radioartériographie et la topographie cranioencephalique. J Radiol Electrol Med Nucl 1928;12:72.
23. Forssmann W. Ueber Kontrastdarstellung der Höhlen des levenden rechten Herzens und der Lungenschlagader. Munchen Med Wochenschr 1931;78:489.
24. Moniz E, de Carvalho L, Lima A. Angiopneumographie. Presse Med 1921;53:996.
25. Osborne ED, Southerland CG, Scholl AJ, et al. Roentgenography of the urinary tract during excretion of sodium iodide. JAMA 1923;80:368.
26. Roseno A. Die intravenose Pyelographie: II. Mitteilung Klinische Ergebnisse. Klin Wochenschr 1929;8:1165.
27. Binz A. Geschichte des Uroselectans. Z Urol Nephrol 1937; 31:73.
28. Binz A, Rath C. Über biochemische Eigenschaften von Derivaten des Pyridins und Chinolins. Biochem Z 1928;203: 218.
29. Swick N. Darstellung der Niere und Harnwege in Röntgenbild durch intravenöse Einbringung eines neuen Kontraststoffes, des Uroselectans. Klin Wochenschr 1929;8:2087.
30. Swick N. Intravenous urography by means of Uroselectan. Am J Surg 1930;8:405.
31. Pearse HE, Warrne SL. The röntgenographic visualization of the arteries of the extremities in peripheral vascular disease. Ann Surg 1931;94:1094.

32. Schüller J. Zweijährige Erfahrung mit der Arteriographie. Arch Orthop Unfallchir 1931;30:233.
33. Frey S, Zwerg HG. Die röntgenologische Darstellung der Gefässe am lebenden Eiere und Menschen. (Vasographie.) Deutsch Z Chir 1931;232:173.
34. Wohleben T. Venographie. Klin Wochenschr 1932;112: 1786.
35. Barber THT, Orley A. Some x-ray observations in varicose disease of the leg. Lancet 1932;2:175.
36. Edwards EA. The status of vasography. N Engl J Med 1933; 209:1337.
37. Rousthöi P. Über Angiokardiographie. Acta Radiol (Stockh) 1933;14:419.
38. Conte E, Costa A. Angiopneumography. Radiology 1933;21: 461.
39. Ravina A. L'exploration radiologique des vaisseaux pulmonaires par l'injection de substances de contraste. Prog Med (Paris) 1934;3:1701.
40. Reboul H, Racine M. La ventriculographie cardiaque expérimentale. Presse Med 1933;41:763.
41. Ameuille P, Ronneaux G, Hinault V, et al. Remarques sur quelques cas d'artériographie pulmonaire chez l'homme vivant. Bull Mem Soc Med Hop Paris 1936;52:729.
42. Castellanos A, Pereiras R, Garcia A. La angiocardiografia radio-opaca. Arch Soc Estud Clin (Habana) 1937;31:523.
43. Castellanos A, Pereiras R, Garcia A. Angio-cardiographies in newborn. Bol Soc Cuba Pediatr 1938;10:225.
44. Castellanos A, Pereiras R, Garcia A, et al. On the factors intervening in the obtention of perfect angiocardiograms. Bol Soc Cuba Pediatr 1938;10:217.
45. Castellanos A, Pereiras R, Vasquez-Paussa A. On a special automatic device for angiocardiography. Bol Soc Cuba Pediatr 1938;10:209.
46. Robb GP, Steinberg I. A practical method of visualization of chambers of the heart, the pulmonary circulation, and the great blood vessels in man. J Clin Invest 1938;17:507.
47. Robb GP, Steinberg I. Visualization of the chambers of the heart, the pulmonary circulation and the great blood vessels in man. AJR 1939;41:1.
48. Chávez I, Dorbecker N, Celis A. Direct intracardiac angiocardiography: its diagnostic value. Am Heart J 1947;33:560.
49. Jönsson G, Brodén B, Karnell J. Selective angiocardiography. Acta Radiol (Stockh) 1948;29:536.
50. Nuvoli I. Arteriografia dell'aorta toracica mediante punctura dell'aorta ascendente o del ventricolos. Policlinico (Prat) 1936; 43:227.
51. Castellanos A, Pereiras R. Countercurrent aortography. Rev Cuba Cardiol 1939;2:187.
52. Radner S. Thoracic aortography by catheterization from the radial artery. Acta Radiol (Stockh) 1948;29:178.
53. Fariñas PL. A new technique for the arteriographic examination of the abdominal aorta and its branches. AJR 1941;46:641.
54. Seldinger SI. Catheter replacement of needle in percutaneous arteriography: new technique. Acta Radiol (Stockh) 1953;39: 368.
55. Gidlund AS. New apparatus for direct cineroentgenography. Acta Radiol (Stockh) 1949;32:81.
56. Axen O, Lind J. Electrocardiographic recording in angiocardiography with synchronous serial photography at right angled planes. Cardiologia (Basel) 1950;16:60.
57. Janker R, Hallerbach H. Die angiocardiokinematographie als Mittel zur Bestimmung der Lungenkreislaufzeit. ROEFO 1951;75:290.
58. Ramsey GHS, Watson JS Jr, Steinhausen TB, et al. Cinefluorography: a progress report on technical problems, dosage factors, and clinical impressions. Radiology 1919;52:684.
59. Chamberlain WE. Fluoroscopes and fluoroscopy; Carman lecture. Radiology 1942;38:383.
60. Coltman JW. Fluoroscopic image brightening by electronic means. Radiology 1948;51:359.
61. Sturm RE, Morgan RH. Screen intensification systems and their limitations. AJR 1949;62:617.
62. Chapman CB, Baker O, Reynolds J, et al. Use of biplane cinefluorography for measurement of ventricular volume. Circulation 1958;18:1105.
63. Abrams HL. An approach to biplane cineangiocardiography. Radiology 1958;73:531.
64. Jönsson G. Visualization of the coronary arteries: preliminary report. Acta Radiol (Stockh) 1948;29:536.
65. Dotter CT, Frische LH. Visualization of the coronary circulation by occlusion aortography: a practical method. Radiology 1958;71:502.
66. Sones FM Jr, Shirey EK. Cine coronary arteriography. Mod Concepts Cardiovasc Dis 1962;31:735.
67. Ricketts HJ, Abrams HL. Percutaneous selective coronary cine-arteriography. JAMA 1962;181:620.
68. Judkins MP. Selective coronary arteriography, a percutaneous transfemoral technique. Radiology 1967;89:815.

2

Radiographic Contrast Agents: History, Chemistry, and Variety

MICHAEL A. BETTMANN

Many compounds are available for use as angiographic contrast agents, and the field of contrast agent development is far from static. This chapter reviews the history of contrast agents, the chemistry of the various classes of agents, and the variety of currently available contrast media, as well as those likely to be clinically available over the next decade.

The development of contrast agents has been reviewed extensively by Grainger[1] and by Sovak.[2] The advantages of having contrast agents for visualization of arteries and veins were first recognized shortly after the description of x-rays. Haschek and Lindenthal published angiography of an amputated hand in 1896, using bismuth, lead, and barium salts. Subsequently, many investigators attempted to find compounds with sufficiently low toxicity to be injected for visualizing arteries, veins, and, by excretion, the hepatobiliary and urinary tracts. It is curious that over time success has been achieved in the vascular and urinary systems but is still somewhat elusive in the hepatobiliary tract.

Many elements were investigated. The first glimmering of success, perhaps, was seen in the work of von Lichtenberg, who in 1905 used a colloidal silver preparation for retrograde cystography and pyelography.[3] Von Lichtenberg's passion, for at least the next 25 years, was to develop an agent that could be administered intravenously for visualizing the urinary tract, a passion he shared with others. The first clinical success occurred in 1923.[4] Osborne and coworkers from the Mayo Clinic, in search of a cure for syphilis, noted that the urine of patients treated with large oral and intravenous doses of sodium iodide was radiopaque. It was evident, however, that intravenous sodium iodide was too toxic to be used clinically. Other avenues were being explored simultaneously. In 1921 in France, Sicard and Forestier introduced iodinated poppy seed oil, Lipiodol, as a contrast agent for myelography.[5] An interesting sidelight is that this material is still in limited clinical use for lymphangiography. Almost simultaneously, Berberich and Hirsch performed experimental femoral angiography with strontium bromide,[6] and Brooks performed the first clinical femoral arteriogram using sodium iodide.[7] Both primitive contrast agents were too toxic for real clinical utility. These investigators also were the first to perform successful pulmonary angiography in a living patient, who survived.[6,7]

At this juncture, Egas Moniz began to make contributions to the area of research. Moniz was a Portuguese neurologist, psychiatrist, scholar, and diplomat who in 1949 received the Nobel Prize for medicine and biology for developing the therapeutic prefrontal lobotomy, a technique now discredited. His interest in contrast agents centered on the visualization of the cerebral circulation. He succeeded by developing what still remains in many ways (but, unfortunately and even tragically, not in all ways) the ideal contrast agent, thorium dioxide.[8] Moniz settled on this compound after extensive animal experiments using bromine and iodine salts of various elements, including sodium, potassium, lithium, strontium, and rubidium, all of which proved highly toxic. Thorium dioxide was radiopaque, was essentially painless on intravascular injection, and had little acute toxicity. Unfortunately, it had two major drawbacks: it was largely sequestered by the reticuloendothelial system, and it is a long-lived alpha emitter. Despite its advantages and initial clinical success, thorium led to the late development of sarcomas, and was recognized as unsuitable as a contrast agent by the late 1930s.

In the mid-1920s, the chemists Binz and Raeth, at the Berlin Agricultural College, developed many organic iodine–containing compounds, with the aim of developing improved antisyphilitic and antibacterial agents. They discovered that placing atoms such as arsenic or iodine on a heterocyclic pyridine ring markedly lowered toxicity. Such a ring consists of six atoms distributed as five carbons and one nitrogen, and becomes pyridone with the addition of an oxygen as a side element. Many of the pyridines and pyridones developed by Binz and Raeth were distributed to collab-

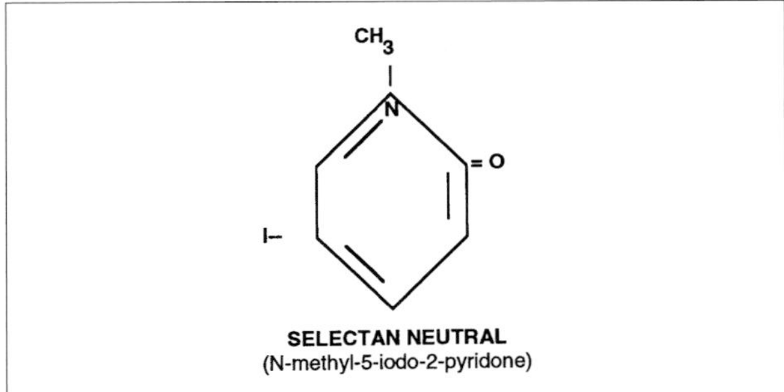

Figure 2-1. Selectan Neutral, a monoiodopyridone, precursor of the first viable intravascular contrast agents.

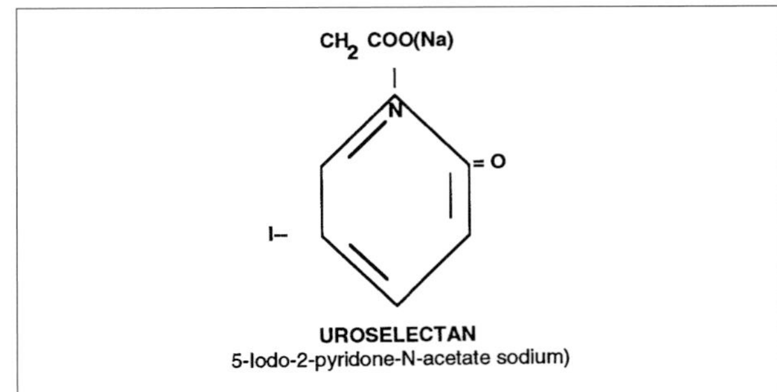

Figure 2-2. Uroselectan, the di-iodinated pyridone that was the first successful intravascular contrast agent for visualization of the urinary tract. A result of work by Binz and Raeth, it was first used in animals by Swick.

orators for evaluation of their clinical utility. One pyridone, which was called "Selectan Neutral" and had a methyl group at the 1 position, oxygen at 2, and a single iodine at 5, was used by Lichtwitz in Hamburg for the treatment of gallbladder infections (Fig. 2-1). Moses Swick, a young New Yorker, was working with Lichtwitz and, as a budding urologist, became interested in the urographic possibilities of this compound. He began animal studies on Selectan Neutral and related compounds in the laboratory of Professor von Lichtenberg in Berlin. Simultaneously the Viennese urologist Hryntschalk was investigating numerous compounds for urography and had some success with a particular unidentified compound,[9] which may have been the formulation subsequently used by Swick as the first successful clinical urographic agent.

In 1929, Swick, after discussions with von Lichtenberg and Binz, suggested that Selectan Neutral would be less toxic if the methyl group were removed. As an alternative, Binz provided a pyridone with CH_2COOH at the 1 position. The carboxyl group, —COOH, led to a marked improvement in solubility. Sodium was subsequently substituted for the hydrogen, and this became Uroselectan (Fig. 2-2), a compound actually patented by Binz's assistant Raeth in 1927,[10] but investigated first in animals by Swick in 1929 and 1930.[11] As detailed by Grainger,[1] it is perhaps not surprising that extensive and not entirely positive discussions occurred regarding who would present the initial stunning success with Uroselectan. This dispute involved primarily von Lichtenberg, the established professor who had long attempted to find an agent for clinical urography and in whose laboratory and with whose contacts success was achieved, and Swick, the young investigator who actually came up with the idea for the chemical alterations and accomplished the goal. Swick was allowed to make the initial presentation, but his contribution and achievement were then essentially forgotten, with credit accruing to von Lichtenberg until 1965. Swick was finally recognized with the award of a medal for outstanding contributions to urology by the New York Academy of Medicine. It is interesting that, at the same time in the same center (Berlin, 1929), Forsmann was the first to perform right heart catheterization, a procedure he performed on himself using a urologic catheter passed via the left arm.[12] Forsmann was ridiculed and essentially banished from Berlin for his work, but was recognized in 1956 with the award of the Nobel Prize in medicine and biology.

Evolution from Uroselectan, which had good clinical utility but relatively high toxicity, was rapid. Variants of the monoiodo pyridone, such as Uroselectan B, and Diodrast, with two iodine atoms rather than one and altered side chains, were developed and widely used clinically (Fig. 2-3). A nonaromatic (i.e., not a carbon ring) series of compounds was developed, including Abrodil, an iodinated methanesulfonate extensively used for myelography through the 1930s (Fig. 2-4). The next major advance toward reaching a combination of good radio-opacity and low toxicity came in 1933 with the development by Moses Swick and Vernon Wallingford, at Mallinckrodt Chemical Works in St. Louis, of a monoiodinated, partially substituted, six-carbon molecule, instead of the five-carbon and one-nitrogen heterocyclic pyridone ring. This molecule was sodium monoiodohippurate (Fig. 2-5).[13,14] Although this was too toxic for clinical use, use of the six-carbon benzene ring as the basic vehicle for iodine has become the avenue of all subsequent major developments to date. It was recognized that adding additional iodine atoms to the molecule would increase clinical utility for both angiography and urography by increasing radio-opacity. Wallingford accomplished this by adding an amine (—NH_2) group. Based on the work of Binz and Raeth, the conversion of a

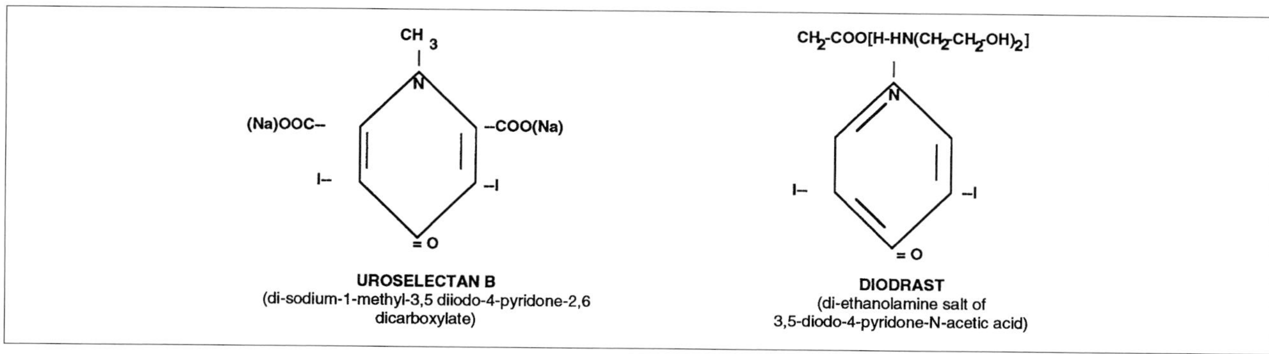

Figure 2-3. Uroselectan B and Diodrast. These pyridone derivatives were less toxic than Uroselectan and equally effective. They were developed in the early 1930s and were widely used clinically.

six-atom ring into a salt, using a dissociating carboxyl group (COO^-) and sodium, increased solubility, but with relatively high toxicity as manifest in a low LD_{50}. Substituting an amine lowered the toxicity, but adding an iodine atom raised it. By placing the amine at C2 or C4, Wallingford noted that a second iodine atom could be added. If the amine was placed at C3, three iodine atoms could be added, but the toxicity of the molecule was increased more than tenfold (Fig. 2-6).[14]

Subsequent developments came quickly during the early 1950s. Hoppe from Sterling-Winthrop noted that the amine group could be acetylated, creating sodium acetrizoate, which had a tenfold decrease in toxicity, as measured by LD_{50} (Fig. 2-6).[15] It was then noted by Hoppe and Larsen, as well as by Langenecker of Schering, that a second amino group could be added to the benzene ring and acetylated.[2,16] This compound, called sodium diatrizoate, had still lower toxicity (Fig. 2-6). This tri-iodinated, fully substituted benzene ring was introduced as Hypaque and as Urografin; also sold as Renografin, it has been the basis of all ionic monomers in clinical use since that time. It is an acid that is combined with a sodium or, subsequently, with a methylglucamine ion as a cation, but that dissociates in solution to leave two charged particles.

The developments over the next decade and a half were relatively minor. They centered on altering one or both of the acetrizoate (or acetylated amine) side chains. The intent of these alterations was to improve tolerance, in large part by improving solubility, or hydrophilicity: that is, the more water-soluble and less lipid-soluble a compound is, the less likely it is that it will interact with lipid cell membranes. Similarly, full substitution of the benzene ring decreases the likelihood of chemical interaction of the contrast molecule. All developments, then, were and continue to be directed at making the iodine-containing moiety as inert as possible.[17,18] These ionic monomers were widely recognized as generally safe and effective, but it was also realized that substantial side effects occurred, ranging from pain to, rarely, sudden death.

In the 1960s, a young Swedish radiologist, Torsten Almen, became interested in attempting to decrease the pain caused by contrast agents in arteriography. Almen reasoned that ionic monomeric contrast agents were markedly hypertonic to blood, and this "osmotoxicity" caused the pain. He supported this hypothesis with the following mental picture: "When you swim in the ocean with eyes open, the hypertonic salt

Figure 2-4. Abrodil. Representative of a series of nonaromatic compounds, this agent was widely used for myelography.

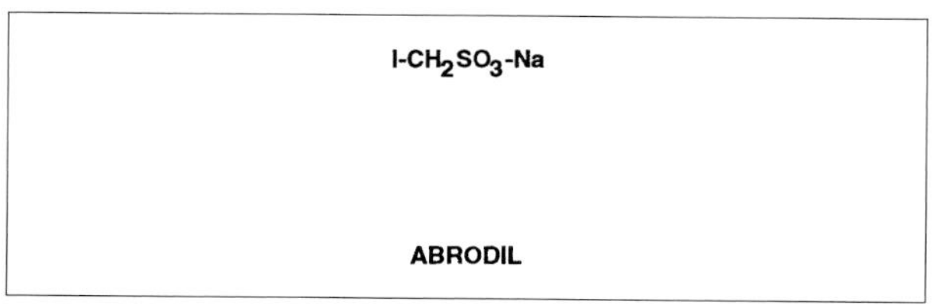

Figure 2-5. Sodium monoiodohippurate, the first six-carbon-based contrast agent. This compound was too toxic for clinical use but served as a model for subsequent development.

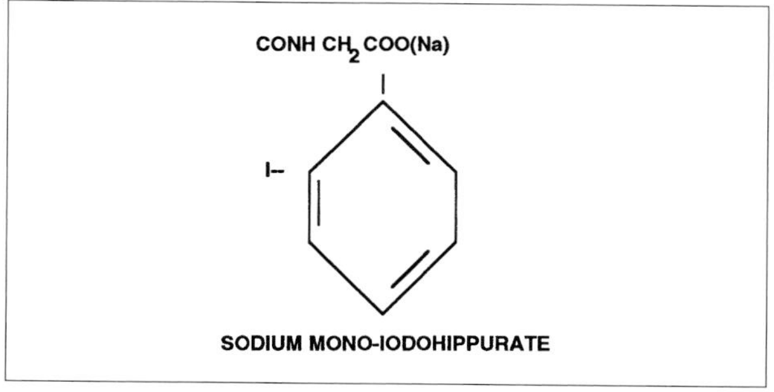

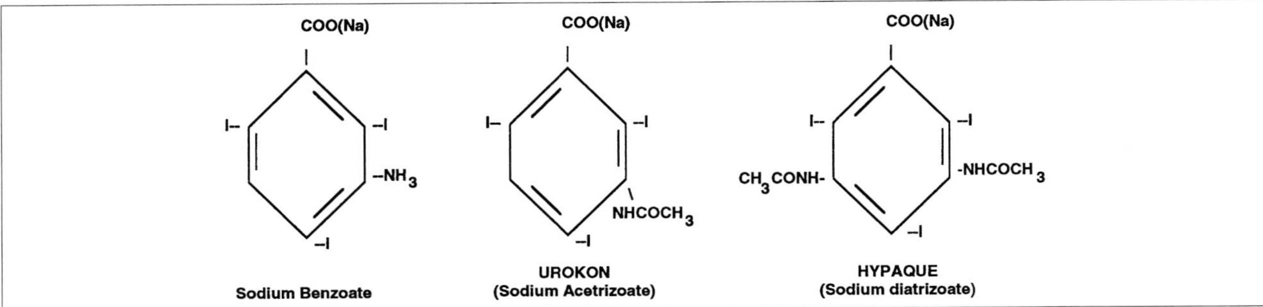

Figure 2-6. Three compounds derived primarily from the work of Wallingford. They evolved from the initial aromatic (six-carbon-ring) compound; the additions of side chains led to progressively (from *left* to *right*) decreased toxicity.

water of the ocean flowing over your eyes draws water out of your conjunctivae and you feel pain to your eyes. Analogously, in arteriography a hypertonic CM [contrast medium] flowing over endothelial cells of the vessels draws water out of the vessel wall and causes pain."[18] He provided evidence for this hypothesis with the observation that thorium dioxide (Thorotrast) did not cause pain when injected intraarterially, and it had an osmolality of 500 mOsm. This contrasted to the marked pain experienced with Hypaque and similar agents, which were injected at osmolalities of 1500 to 2100 mOsm. Similarly, an oily emulsion used for angiography in Japan in the 1930s was isotonic to plasma (with an osmolality of 300 mOsm) and caused no pain.[19] Almen's aim, then, was to markedly lower the osmolality of the ionic monomers. While working as a research fellow in the United States, he recognized that this could be accomplished either by converting the monomer to a dimer or by making the ionic formulation into a nonionic one; in theory, both approaches would halve the osmolality. This had to be accomplished, however, without markedly increasing viscosity or, through altering the carboxyl (—COOH) group, decreasing water solubility. The approach that Almen took was to eliminate the dissociating carboxyl group, which eliminated the ionicity of the molecule, and then to add hydroxyl groups (—OH) at various points on the benzene ring to preserve full substitution (thereby lowering toxicity) and increase water solubility (thereby hopefully improving tolerance). The first nonionic contrast agent, metrizamide, was made by substituting an amide bonded to glucosamine for the carboxyl group. The molecule was otherwise identical (in the iodine content and the other side chains) to metrizoate, an ionic monomer that is closely related to diatrizoate (Fig. 2-7). After several years of trying to arouse interest among chemical companies, Almen finally found an interested partner in Nyegaard (now Nycomed), at that time a small Norwegian company and now a much larger multinational one. In 1965, Nycomed began the synthesis of water-soluble non-ionic contrast media.[20] Metrizamide had significant limitations for use in clinical studies because it was very expensive to produce, and also because it was not stable in solution. It was, therefore, supplied as a lyophilized powder and was reconstituted before use. Initial studies in the subarachnoid space showed that metrizamide, sold as Amipaque, was far less toxic than ionic contrast agents, and had the significant advantage over oily iodinated emulsions that it was water-soluble and did not have to be removed.[21] It was not until several years later that metrizamide was used for angiography and, as Almen had predicted, proved far less painful than ionic monomers.[22]

A parallel approach to improving the tolerance of contrast agents was the development of dimeric formulations, which would similarly decrease osmolality by half at an equal iodine concentration. The first dimers were developed in the early 1950s. They were low in osmolality but consisted of incompletely substituted benzene rings, much like early contrast agents but with three iodine molecules, a carboxyl group, and one additional side chain (instead of two) on each of the rings. Such compounds were characterized by marked protein binding, biliary rather than renal excretion, and high toxicity. One representative, iodipamide, is still available. About the time that metrizamide began to be used in clinical trials, another ionic dimer, sodium meglumine ioxaglate, was developed (Fig. 2-8).[23] This compound consists of two slightly altered ionic monomers linked together. In one, the carboxyl group is replaced by a substituted amine. This is linked to the second, which has the carboxyl group preserved by a glycyl bridge. This compound, available as Hexabrix, is now extensively used worldwide. Unlike iodipamide, which carries two negative charges in

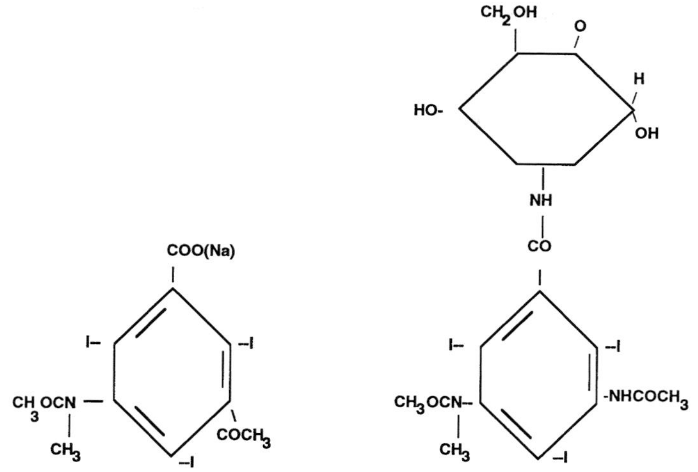

METRIZOATE

METRIZAMIDE
(Amipaque)

Figure 2-7. Metrizoate and metrizamide. An ionic contrast agent, metrizoate is very similar to diatrizoate. It was widely used in Europe and formed the basis for Almen's development of nonionic contrast media. Metrizamide, which was the first clinically used nonionic agent, consists of metrizoate with an eliminated ionic carboxyl group and two altered side chains.

solution, Hexabrix has only one. As with other low-osmolality agents, the measured osmolality is substantially less than predicted—that is, less than half that of ionic monomers. This lowered osmolality is thought to be related to the formation of aggregates or to stearic reorganization.

Subsequently, many other nonionic formulations have been developed. The first to follow metrizamide were iopamidol, developed by Bracco of Italy, and iohexol, also developed by Nycomed. Sovak independently and in collaboration with Schering developed several nonionic monomers. Much as the ionic monomers such as diatrizoate, metrizoate, and iothalamate differed little from each other chemically, and as metrizamide was a derivative of the ionic monomer metrizoate, most of the nonionic formulations differ in relatively minor ways. As elucidated by Almen,[18] one principle in the improvement of tolerance of contrast agents is to increase hydrophilicity. This is done by adding hydroxyl groups (—OH) to the substituent side chains. It appears, in part because of the experience with metrizamide, that the mere presence of hydroxyl groups is not sufficient. A distribution of these groups around the molecule in such a way as to shield

Figure 2-8. Sodium ioxaglate. This molecule represents an alternative approach to toxicity. It is an ionic dimer, with an osmolality equal to that of nonionic monomers.

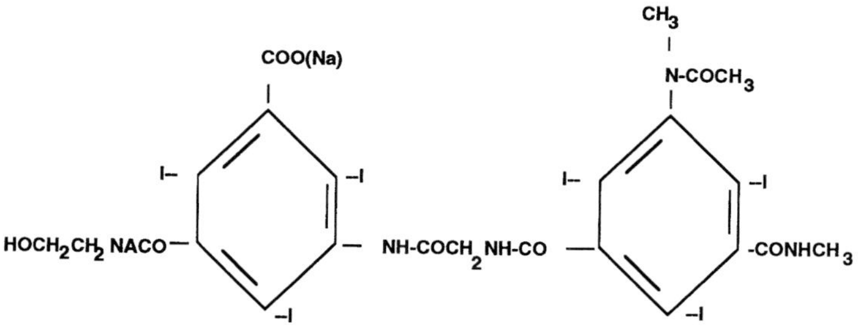

SODIUM IOXAGLATE
(Hexabrix)

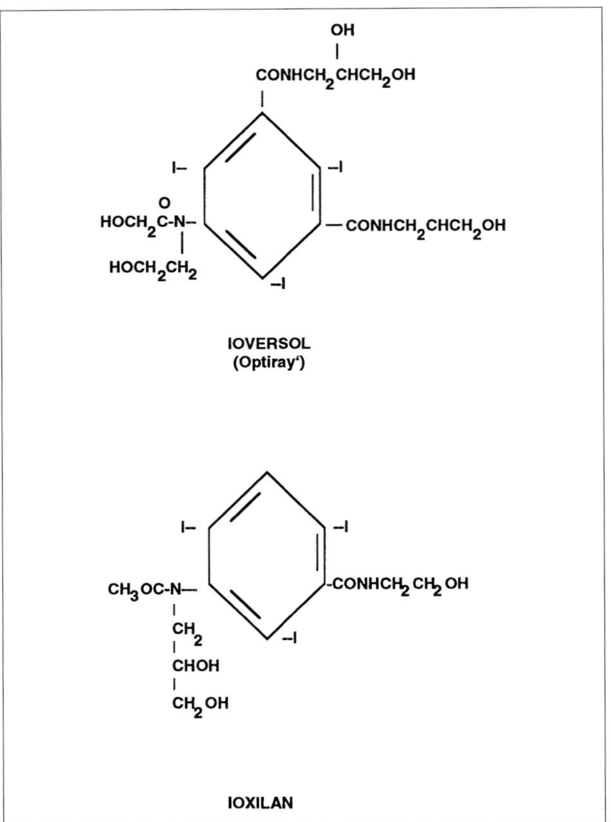

Figure 2-9. Ioversol and ioxilan, examples of the second generation of nonionic monomeric agents. They are stable in solution and have improved stoichiometry.

the iodine atoms appears to improve hydrophilicity, a readily measured parameter, as well as clinical tolerance, which is harder to quantitate. Using ioxithalamate, another diatrizoate variant, Sovak in 1983 developed ioxilan. This compound has a hydrophobic region that is masked hydrophilically, leading to a theoretical increase in water solubility and subarachnoid tolerance.[24] Similarly, ioversol was developed by Mallinckrodt with the aim of improving water solubility, and thus clinical tolerance (Fig. 2-9). Various side chains were produced in an attempt to increase hydrophilicity, most of which were not viable clinically (e.g., because of very high viscosity)[25] or were little different from previously produced nonionic monomers. The basic principle of development of nonionic monomers, as elucidated by Hoey[23] and by Almen,[18] are that low toxicity and high hydrophilicity go hand in hand. This combination is achieved through combining the six-carbon benzene ring with a coupler, such as an amide (—CONR), which links to a moiety with multiple hydroxyl groups. With a huge variety of couplers and polyhydroxyl groups, and three possible sites for side chains, the potential number of compounds based on this single concept is huge. It is not surprising, then, that many nonionic monomers are clinically available and that others are in various stages of development and testing.

Other avenues were explored to improve the toxicity profile of contrast agents still further. Gries and Speck of Schering synthesized a series of compounds with, in essence, three sugars as side chains on the benzene ring. These tri-carboxyl-triiodobenzenes were highly hydrophilic and had very low toxicity, but their viscosity was so high that intravascular delivery was problematic.[26] Another approach was to develop radiopaque cations, rather than anions, but the toxicity of such compounds was relatively high.[2,24]

Perhaps the final branch on this road of development of contrast agents is the concept of nonionic polymers. A series of nonionic dimers was initially developed by Pfeiffer and Speck[27] in 1978, but water sol-

Figure 2-10. Iotrolan, one of several nonionic dimers in clinical use. This class of agents is essentially isotonic to plasma but has increased viscosity compared to nonionic monomers.

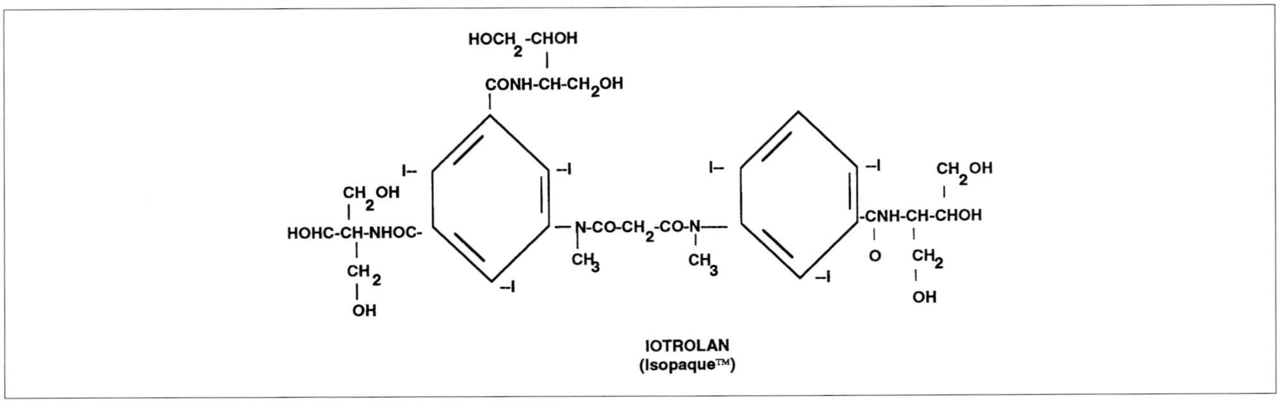

IOTROLAN
(Isopaque™)

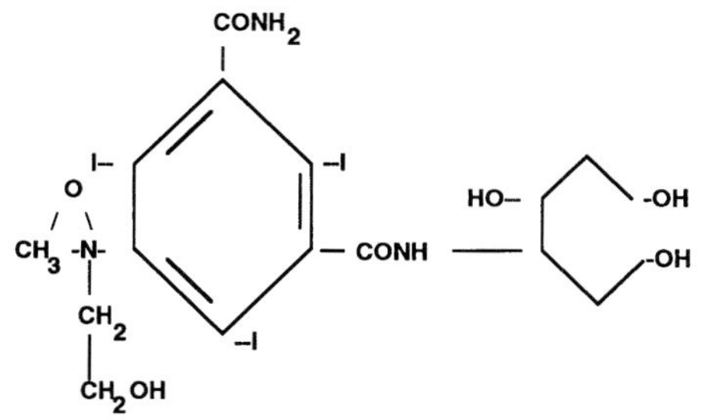

5-[N-(2-Hydroxyethyl)] acetylamino-2-4-6-triodo-3-[N-threo-1,3,4-trihydroxy-but-2-yl] carbamoyl beazamide.
PRIMARY CARBOXAMIDE (29).

Figure 2-11. A primary carboxamide as developed by Sovak and associates.[29] It has theoretically decreased toxicity because of its decreased lipid solubility and protein binding. Such compounds are promising because of their low viscosity and low osmolality.

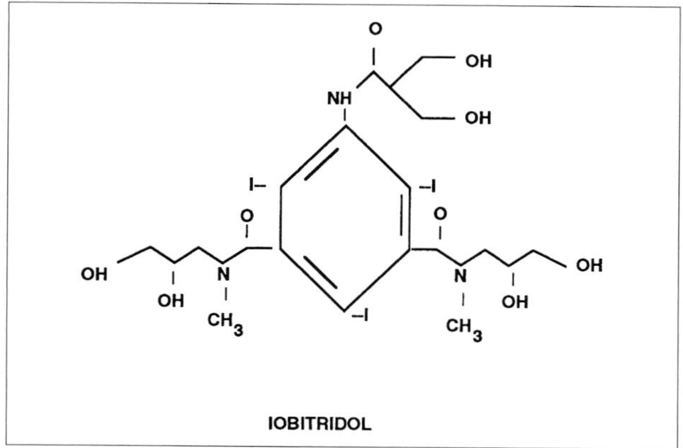

Figure 2-12. Iobitridol, a third-generation nonionic monomer. It was designed with symmetrically placed hydroxyl groups to decrease protein binding and increase hydrophilicity.

ubility was too low for clinical use. The first example of this group that had low toxicity, high solubility, and sufficiently low viscosity to allow injection was iotrolan, which has been widely used in the subarachnoid space and has been investigated in various intravascular studies, with promising results (Fig. 2-10). This compound was developed by Sovak and Ranganathan in 1979,[28] but full clinical work did not begin until nearly a decade later. Another successful variant in this category is iodixanol, developed by Nycomed. Both have been used extensively in clinical studies. They are both safe and effective, although the extent to which they are truly an improvement over nonionic monomers, particularly in light of their high viscosity and high production costs, is not yet clear.

A further development in nonionic monomers extending from these developments is based on the observations of Almen and Sovak. Almen noted that eliminating the carboxyl (—COOH) group and adding stable hydroxyl groups had three effects: reduced osmolality, increased hydrophilicity, and decreased toxicity, most notably in the subarachnoid space.[18] In addition, Sovak[29] observed that with ionic carboxyl-containing contrast agents, osmolality increases in a linear fashion with increasing concentration. With nonionic agents, however, the increase is less than linear, suggesting that aggregations occur. Sovak suggested that one could improve biologic tolerance by producing agents that were more hydrophilic but also more transiently aggregated in solution. Achieving this would decrease osmolality and also decrease interaction with cell membranes and macromolecules, thus decreasing toxicity. Some of these suggestions have been adopted in various compounds. To increase aggregation, Sovak posited that the inherent hydrophobicity of the iodine-containing benzene ring could be used: hydrophobic regions must be exposed to increase aggregation and decrease osmolality, but must be masked with hydrophilic regions to limit protein binding and interaction with lipid cell membranes. To this end, Sovak and colleagues developed a series of nonionic agents based on carboxamides as side chains (—$CONH_2$). Such compounds, which are not currently undergoing clinical evaluation, are nonetheless promising because of their relatively low viscosity, isotonicity to plasma at 300 mgmI/ml, and general intravenous toxicity equivalent to earlier nonionic monomers (Fig. 2-11).[29,30] The carboxamide side chain, which is small, is thought to expose the benzene ring to allow aggregation in solution; multiple hydroxyl groups attached to carboxamide increase water solubility and decrease interactions on injection. Another new nonionic, iobitridol (Fig. 2-12), is constructed with hydroxyl groups placed in a stable symmetric distribution around the benzene ring, to achieve the same aim of increasing hydrophilicity and decreasing toxicity. This compound has shown promise in clinical studies.

Both the development of contrast agents and the understanding of their advantages and disadvantages have gone through evolution and revolution. Many distinguished investigators have made major contributions. In concert with the development of radiology in general, earlier developments in contrast agents were achieved by nonradiologists such as Swick and Moniz. It was not until the 1960s that radiologists, notably

Table 2-1. Contrast Agents

Class	Molecule	Cations	Additives	Vendor/ Manufacturer	Proprietary Name
Ionic monomer	Diatrizoate	Sodium and methylglucamine	$CaNa_2EDTA$	Nycomed	Hypaque
			NaEDTA	Mallinckrodt	MD
			NaCitrate	Mallinckrodt	MD
			$CaNa_2EDTA$	Bracco	Renografin
			$CaNa_2EDTA$	Berlex	Angiovist
	Iothalamate	Sodium and methylglucamine	$CaNa_2EDTA$	Mallinckrodt	Conray
	Ioxithalamate	Sodium and methylglucamine	$CaNa_2EDTA$	Guerbet	Telebrix
	Metrizoate	Sodium and methylglucamine	$CaNa_2EDTA$	Nycomed	
Ionic dimer	Ioxaglate	Sodium and methylglucamine	$CaNa_2EDTA$	Mallinckrodt/ Guerbet	Hexabrix
Nonionic monomer	Metrizamide		$CaNa_2EDTA$	Nycomed	Amipaque
	Iohexol		$CaNa_2EDTA$	Nycomed	Omnipaque
	Iopamidol		$CaNa_2EDTA$	Bracco	Isovue Iopamiro
	Ioversol		$CaNa_2EDTA$	Mallinckrodt	Optiray
	Ioxilan		NaEDTA NaCitrate	Cook	
	Iopromide		$CaNa_2EDTA$	Berlex/Schering	Ultravist
	Iobitridol		$CaNa_2EDTA$	E-Z Em/Guerbet	Xenetix
Nonionic dimer	Iotrol		$CaNa_2EDTA$	Berlex/Schering	Isovist
	Iodixanol		$CaNa_2EDTA$	Nycomed	Visipaque

Almen and later Sovak, made major contributions. The revolutionary achievements of the earlier investigators have been succeeded in the last decade by more evolutionary achievements. Progress in improving contrast agents is occurring in the development and evaluation of nonionic monomers, or perhaps of dimers. A better understanding of the mechanisms of contrast agent–caused adverse events will lead to improvements in design.

Another important direction being actively investigated is the development of more specific agents. There is a clear role for intravascular contrast media that remain in the blood pool, or that can be targeted to specific tissues, such as hepatocytes or the reticuloendothelial system. Although they are unlikely to play a major role in angiography directly, such agents are likely to be important in computed tomography, perhaps hastening the demise of diagnostic angiography.

Many contrast agents (Table 2-1) are available, and the advantages and disadvantages of broad categories of these agents are discussed in Chapter 3. Many features of their clinical performance, however, are obvious from a consideration of their chemistry and their developmental history.

References

1. Grainger RG. Intravascular contrast media—the past, the present and the future. Br J Radiol 1982;55:1–18.
2. Sovak M. From iodide to iotrolan: history and argument, an introductory address. European Radiol 1995; in press.
3. Voelker F, von Lichtenberg A. Pyelographie (Roentgenographie des Nierenbeckeas nach Kollargolfuelluag). Munchen Med Wochenschr 1906;53:105–106.
4. Osborne ED, Sutherland CG, Scholl AJ Jr, Rowntree LG. Roentgenography of the urinary tract during excretion of sodium iodide. JAMA 1923;80:368–373.
5. Sicard JA, Forestier G. Injections intravasculaire d'huite iodée sous controle radiologique. C R Soc Biol 1923;88:1200.
6. Berberich J, Hirsch S. Die Roentgenographische Darstellung cler Arterien aund Venen au Lebenden. Munchen Klin Wochenschr 1923;49:2226.
7. Brooks B. Intraarterial injection of sodium iodide. JAMA 1924; 82:1016.
8. Veiga-Pires JA, Grainger RG. The Portuguese pioneers in angiography. Lancaster, UK: MTP Press, 1982.
9. Hryntschalk T. Studiem zur Roentgenologischen Darstellung von Niaerenparenchym und Nierenbec ken auf intravenoesem Wege. Z Urol 1929;23:893–906.
10. Binz A. The chemistry of Uroselectan. J Urol 1931;25:297–301.
11. Swick M. Darstellung der Niere und Harnwege in Roentgenbild direkt intravenose Einbringung eines neuen Kontraststoffes: des Uroselectans. Klin Wochenschr 1929;8:2087–2089.
12. Forsmann W. Die Sondierung des rechten Herzens. Klin Wochenschr 1929;8:2085–2087.

13. Swick M. Excretion urography by means of the intravenous and oral administration of sodium ortho-iodo-hippurate with some physiologic considerations. Surg Gynecol Obstet 1933;56:62–65.
14. Wallingford VH. The development of organic iodide compounds as x-ray contrast media. J Am Pharmacol Assoc (Scientific Edition) 1953;42:721–728.
15. Hoppe JO, Larsen HA, Coulston FJ. Observations on the toxicity of a new urographic contrast medium, sodium 3,5-diacetamido-2,4,6 tri-iodobenzoate (Hypaque sodium) and related compounds. J Pharmacol Exp Ther 1956;116:394–403.
16. Hoey GB, et al. Organic iodine compounds as x-ray contrast media. In: International encyclopedia of pharmacology and therapeutics. Oxford: Pergamon Press, 1971;1:23–132.
17. Eloy R, Corot C, Belleville J. Contrast media for angiography: physicochemical properties, pharmacokinetics and biocompatibility. Clin Materials 1991;7:89–197.
18. Almen T. Relations between chemical structure, animal toxicity and clinical adverse effects of contrast media. In: Enge I, Edgren F, eds. Patient safety and adverse events in contrast medium examinations. Amsterdam: Elsevier, 1989:25–45.
19. Saito M, Kawikawa K, Yanagizaua H. A new method for blood vessel visualization (arteriography, veinography, angiography) in vivo. Am J Surg 1930;10:225.
20. Almen T. Contrast agent design, some aspects on the synthesis of water-soluble contrast agents of low osmolality. J Theor Biol 1969;24:216–226.
21. Salvesen S. Acute toxicity tests of metrizamide. Acta Radiol 1973;335(Suppl):5–13.
22. Almen T, Boijsen E, Lindell SE. Metrizamide in angiography: 1. Femoral angiography. Acta Radiol Diagn 1977;18:33–38.
23. Hoey GB, Smith KR, El-Antably S, Murphy GP. Chemistry of x-ray contrast media. In: Sovak M, ed. Radiocontrast agents. Berlin: Springer Verlag, 1984:23–125.
24. Sovak M, Ranganathan R, Lang JH, Lasser EC. Concepts in design of improved intravascular contrast agents. Ann Radiol 1978;21:283–289.
25. Speck U, Gries H, Klieger E, Muetzel W, Press WR, Heinmann HJ. New contrast media developed at Schering AG: first experience. Invest Radiol 1984;19:S144.
26. Sovak M, Nahlorsky B, Lang J, Lasser EC. Preliminary evaluation of Di-iodo-triglucosyl benzene: an approach to the design of nonionic water-soluble radiographic contrast media. Radiology 1975;117:717–719.
27. Speck U, Mutzel W, Mannesman G, Pfeiffer H, Siefer HM. Pharmacology of nonionic dimers. Invest Radiol 1980;15:5317.
28. Sovak M, Ranganathan R, Speck U. Nonionic dimer: development and partial testing of an intrathecal contrast agent. Radiology 1982;142:115–118.
29. Sovak M. Contrast media: a journey almost sentimental. Invest Radiol 1994;29:54–514.
30. Sovak M, Terry RC, Douglass JG, Schwertzer L. Primary carboxamides: nonionic isotonic monomers. Invest Radiol 1991; 16(Suppl 1):5159–5161.

3

Physiologic Effects and Systemic Reactions

MICHAEL A. BETTMANN

In a very real sense angiography began shortly after the discovery of x-rays by Roentgen, when various substances were injected into cadaver specimens to visualize vascularity.[1] As reviewed in the prior chapter, contrast agents evolved from the time of Roentgen to the late 1920s, with the adoption of iodine as the standard atom to block penetration of the roentgen ray through the structure to be defined. By the 1930s, iodine was linked to the benzene ring to lower toxicity.[2] Over the next few years, it was realized that complete substitution of the benzene ring lowered toxicity still further.[3] With this evolution, there was then relatively little change until the 1970s, when it was recognized that hypertonicity and the presence of ions might both contribute to adverse events, with the resultant development of dimeric compounds and nonionic compounds.[4] With the development of nonionic dimers, brought to clinical utility in the 1990s, there is a general feeling that iodinated contrast agents for general intravascular use have progressed as far as they can.[5]

Iodinated contrast agents are widely used, primarily in peripheral, visceral, and cardiac angiography and for enhancement of vascular structures and perfused areas during computed tomography (CT). In terms of volume, they are among the most widely used, as well as among the safest, of all medications. Because of the noninvasive nature of CT, contrast agents are responsible for most of the adverse events that occur with this procedure. Conversely, because of the invasive nature of angiography, adverse events related to contrast agents are at least relatively less important than procedural considerations themselves. Further, it is often difficult to determine clearly whether an adverse event is related to the contrast agent specifically, to the procedure itself, or to general considerations such as the underlying health of the patient and related risk factors.[6] These difficulties of attribution notwithstanding, adverse events related to contrast agents are important to angiography and require both definition and understanding.

The use of contrast agents depends on two factors: the type of imaging used (cut film versus digital subtraction angiography, DSA) and the specific vascular bed to be imaged. Because of its inherent improvement in contrast resolution as compared to cut film, DSA offers the opportunity for using either lower volumes of contrast or a lower iodine concentration. Initially, this was recognized as one of its advantages. Perhaps as a function of the improved resolution capability of newer DSA units (i.e., finer matrix size), the trend recently has been toward using higher volumes and higher iodine concentrations for DSA. In many ways, this obviates the advantages inherent to this imaging approach.

The iodine content necessary to achieve satisfactory opacification is, to a large extent, subjective. In angiography, the aim of employing contrast is generally to achieve good definition of the luminal surface of the vessel. In some situations, such as in peripheral venography, it is preferable to use an iodine content that is high enough to visualize the vessel wall, but low enough to facilitate seeing through the vessel to define clots.[7] The same consideration is true to a lesser extent in angiography, in which definition of luminal detail is important, but less so than definition of luminal size. In general, the smaller the vessel to be imaged, the higher the iodine content must be to allow satisfactory imaging. This also is a function of the site of injection of contrast: that is, the closer the vessel to be imaged is to the injection site, the tighter the bolus of contrast injected and therefore the higher the functional iodine content of the contrast agent. For example, to visualize the abdominal aorta with digital subtraction angiography, an iodine content of 100 to 150 mg/ml is generally satisfactory. This same iodine concentration may be satisfactory for visualizing pedal vessels if there is no obstruction, and particularly if contrast is injected into the common femoral or external iliac arteries rather than into the aorta. Conversely, if a distal aortic injection is made to visualize pedal arteries in a patient with long segment occlusion of the superficial femoral artery, an iodine content of 200 to 320 mg/ml may be necessary. Similarly, if cut film angiography is being performed for definition of the abdominal aorta, an iodine content of 280 to 320 mg/ml is generally satisfactory. For good visualization of distal pedal vessels with cut film angiography, an iodine content of 350 to 370 mg/ml is generally necessary. As with any medications, it is advantageous to use as low a dose and as low a volume of contrast material as is consistent with obtaining the necessary clinical results.

Complications of Contrast Agents

There are several important general principles related to complications. First, the margin of safety with all currently available contrast agents is very high. Second, certain risk factors exist that predispose to adverse reactions, as will be discussed subsequently. Third, the most important single etiologic factor in most contrast agent reactions is the degree of hypertonicity.

With this as background, adverse events can be considered in four distinct but overlapping categories: (1) renal, (2) vascular and hematologic, (3) cardiac, and (4) systemic.

Renal Effects

Experimental studies have demonstrated that contrast agents have substantial nephrotoxicity. Although these effects are not as great as with certain other drugs, such as gentamicin, they are nonetheless considerable and of significant clinical concern. One major difficulty in understanding the nephrotoxicity of contrast agents is that no good animal model exists. In large part, this is due to the involvement of multiple factors whenever contrast-related renal failure occurs.[8,9] Studies in both animal models and in humans have demonstrated that iodinated contrast agents are excreted by glomerular infiltration alone, without tubular secretion or resorption. Studies have also demonstrated that contrast agents cause significant alterations in renal hemodynamics, in general with a transit increase in renal blood flow, followed by a prolonged decrease.[10] This decrease is both larger in magnitude and more prolonged with high-osmolality agents than with low-osmolality agents. It has also been shown that morphologic changes occur in the tubules after contrast injection.[11] Whether these are relevant to clinical adverse events, however, is still not clear.

Many studies have examined the clinical effects of contrast agents, but substantive questions remain. The lack of clarity is probably related to the relative infrequency of contrast-related renal failure, as well as to the many variables that exist in attempting to define this complication. Unlike many other complications, transient renal failure generally is evident only when looked for; patients are rarely symptomatic with this complication. Further, the definitions of contrast-related renal failure vary widely from study to study. Some studies rely on a fixed rise of serum creatinine, such as 0.5 or 1.0 mg/dl, whereas others assess the percentage change in serum creatinine, such as a 25 or 50 percent increase from baseline.[12] Studies also vary widely in regard to when the serum creatinine level is measured. Since the course of contrast-related renal failure is not well defined, measurements ranging from 12 hours to 5 days may lead to markedly different results.[13]

Equally important are patient-related factors, such as route of administration, the coexistence of diabetes, the degree of hydration of the patient, and, most importantly, the coexistence of underlying renal dysfunction. It is likely that the same volume of contrast injected intravenously has less effect on the kidneys than if the injection is intraarterial, because in the latter case the kidneys will be faced with a higher concentration of the contrast. The degree of hydration may also play a major role, because it will affect the rate of washout of the contrast from the kidneys. It is important to consider approaches to hydration when comparing various studies, and hydration is also an important consideration clinically. Because it is common practice to keep patients NPO before angiography, it is likely that many patients are somewhat dehydrated, and this may play a major role in contrast-related renal failure.

Other comorbid factors, such as the presence of diabetes, congestive heart failure, or hepatic failure, have been thought to play a role. In general, the data suggest that only diabetes is an independent risk factor.[14] The major comorbid consideration is underlying renal failure,[13–17] which is clearly the major and perhaps the only significant determinant of contrast-related renal failure. That is, the presence of totally normal renal function all but rules out the occurrence of renal failure with the administration of contrast. It is possible that preexistent renal failure has not been clinically noted (e.g., in patients with long-standing hypertension) or that acute renal failure may occur secondary to a severe systemic reaction such as cardiovascular collapse. It is important to recognize that in such situations, renal failure is not primarily due to the effect of the contrast agent on the kidneys.

The largest, most comprehensive study of contrast-related renal failure was performed in about 1200 patients undergoing cardiac catheterization.[18] Hydration was uniform and adequate in all patients, and levels of serum creatinine as well as creatinine clearance and urine enzymes were obtained at baseline over at least 24 hours after contrast administration and, in many patients, over 72 hours. Several different definitions of contrast-related renal failure were examined. The results showed that clinically significant renal failure did not occur in patients who had entirely normal serum creatinine levels and creatinine clearance before contrast injection. Further, it was evident that there was a risk of a rise in serum creatinine level among patients with an initially elevated creatinine level, and the risk increased if patients also had insulin-dependent diabetes mellitus. In comparing high-osmolality (HOCA) and low-osmolality (LOCA) nonionic contrast agents, there was a statistically significant difference between the two classes, both overall and among patients with preexistent renal failure, in favor of LOCAs. Interestingly, only nine patients in each of the HOCA and LOCA groups experienced what were considered clinically significant adverse renal events; all of these occurred in patients with significantly elevated baseline serum creatinine levels. This suggests that there is a disparity between a rise in serum creatinine after the administration of contrast, which occurred (as a function of the definition used) in up to 30 percent of the patients, and clinically significant adverse renal effects. Such events occurred only among patients who had a significant creatinine elevation before contrast administration, and in less than 3 percent of these patients. This raises an interesting, as yet still unanswered, question regarding the significance of a rise in serum creatinine secondary to contrast administration, or the administration of other nephrotoxic drugs. An increase in creatinine reflects an adverse effect on the kidneys, but if this rise is self-limited and, as is almost invariably true, there is a return to baseline levels, is this effect clinically important or even relevant?

In terms of clinical practice, several points can be made. First, it is good practice to ensure that all patients are well hydrated, rather than dehydrated, before contrast administration.[19,20] Second, given adequate hydration and the absence of a process that would predispose to acute tubular necrosis, such as cardiogenic shock, there is cause for concern only among patients with underlying renal dysfunction, either with or without diabetes. The worse the underlying renal failure, the greater the level of concern should be. Third, experience suggests that the risk of the underlying renal failure worsening increases with age, particularly over age 60. Finally, the volume of contrast employed plays a significant role.[18,21] Somewhat surprisingly, as already noted, although the differences between HOCAs and LOCAs in terms of serum creatinine and in terms of experimental results are clear, clinically relevant differences remain unclear.[14,18,22] What is clearly important is to ensure that patients are well hydrated and that the volume of contrast is limited as much as possible. Whether nonionic dimers will play a role among patients with underlying renal failure is not yet known, although experimental results suggest that they should.[23] Similarly, carbon dioxide as a contrast agent may have a substantial role among patients with underlying renal failure.[24]

Vascular and Hematologic Effects

Over the past decade, there has been increasing awareness that the blood vessel wall is not a passive system responding merely to alterations in blood pressure, but is instead a complex metabolic organ. The endothelium and the media play a very large role in both vascular homeostasis and in thrombosis. In the normal healthy state, the single-cell-layer endothelium contains substances that exert major control on vessel tone, alter the response of the vessel to injury, play a large role in preventing thrombosis, and actively participate in clot lysis.[25,26] Many of these functions alter over time. Similarly, the smooth muscle cell layers of the media are not merely controlled by distant neural impulses or gross changes in flow and pressure. Contrast agents, like all other substances injected in large quantities, have a significant effect on endothelial and other vessel wall functions. At this time, these effects are difficult to quantitate because many of them are transient and minor, in terms of systemic manifestations. Nonetheless, it is important to be aware of the possible interactions among blood vessel wall, flowing blood, and contrast agents.

In early studies of the effects of contrast agents, it was noted that it is possible to cause gross endothelial damage.[27,28] This occurred, however, in models in which high doses of contrast agents were employed in the absence of flowing blood. More recently, it has been difficult to demonstrate any gross effect of contrast agents on endothelium if the doses used are in a range that is clinically relevant and if blood flow is maintained.[29] It has been possible to examine the effect of contrast agents on endothelial function by using in vitro experimental approaches. In a series of studies on cultured porcine endothelial cells, for example, the author was able to demonstrate changes in cellular function with relatively brief perfusion by contrast agents. These effects were primarily related to the osmolality of the perfusate. At equal osmolality, increased effect was noted with longer perfusion (Fig. 3-1). Such alterations in function, manifest by release of prostaglandins or adenine nucleotides and nucleosides, may be clinically relevant both in terms of local effects and in terms of the induction of systemic effects. Because of the relatively low concentrations at which such substances are released, however, docu-

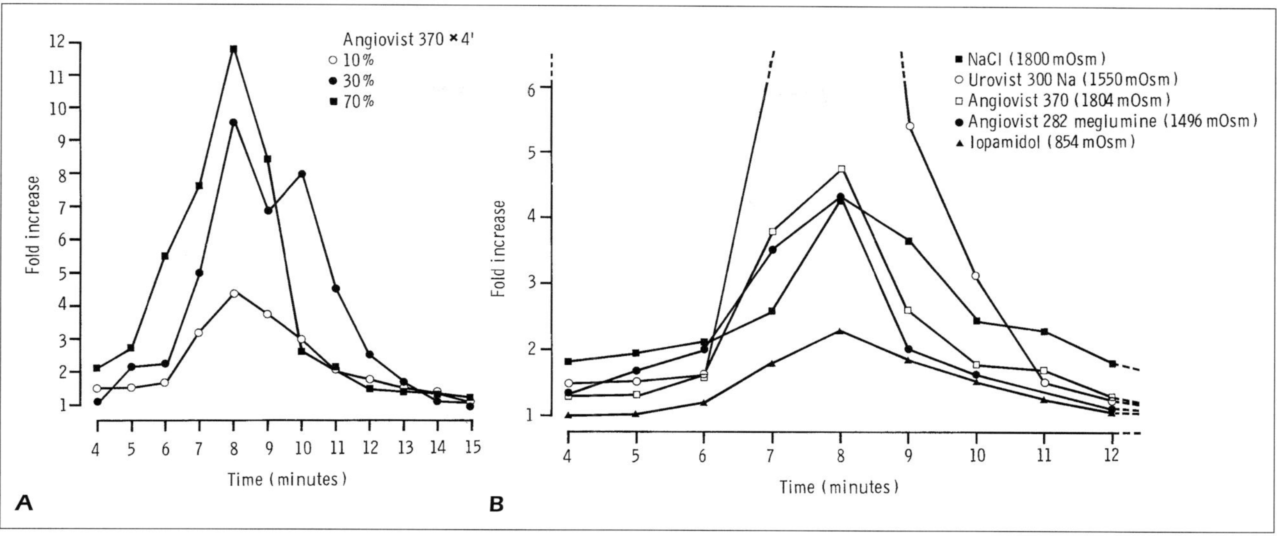

Figure 3-1. Effect of perfusion of human umbilical vein endothelial cells with various contrast agents. *Y* axis: increased release of the stable metabolite of prostacyclin. (A) Perfusion with increasing concentrations of a high-osmolality contrast agent. (B) Perfusion with various contrast agents (iopamidol is nonionic; other contrast agents are ionic; NaCl was used as a control) at various osmolalities. Note that the major, but not sole, determinant of prostacyclin release by endothelial cells is osmolality.

mentation of anything other than local effects is difficult.

Additional studies have examined the endothelial effects of contrast agents.[29,30] In one study, the effect of relatively long exposures of very low concentrations of contrast on cultured endothelial cells was assessed.[29] Alterations in DNA, RNA, and protein production were used as end points. It was found that at clinically relevant levels there was little alteration in these functional parameters, with the exception of depression of protein synthetic capability. The observed effects were not altered by concurrent exposure to ionizing radiation. There were minor differences between HOCAs and LOCAs that were almost exclusively related to osmolality per se, with little obvious effect of different formulations.

The hematologic effects of contrast agents are similarly difficult to evaluate because of the multiplicity of variables that must be taken into consideration. All contrast agents appear to interact with the coagulation system, although such interactions are, in general, minor. Studies to date have examined various aspects of the coagulation cascade. In most, there appears to be more perturbation with higher-osmolality agents.[31] Perhaps more importantly, there is a retardation of coagulation with ionic agents, which is not seen with nonionic contrast media.[32] This effect appears to be minor and largely reversible. It is thus possibly beneficial. Conversely, one study suggested that the fibrin polymer that is the end point of the coagulation cascade is altered more by nonionic agents, making a less stable molecule and thus a less effective clot.[33]

The effects on platelets are difficult to define. The effects on red blood cells have been somewhat easier to examine. Aspelin and coworkers showed that contrast agents lead to an alteration in the deformability of red cells, making them less able to move through capillaries.[34] This work suggests that this limitation of deformability is greater with HOCAs than with LOCAs. This effect does not appear to be related to ionic strength.[35]

In clinical terms, the effects of contrast agents on the vessel wall and on thrombosis must be considered together. Although this is largely true in regard to thrombosis, it is also true in regard to hemostasis and to generalized systemic effects. For example, it has been widely postulated that adverse reactions that occur with contrast administration are more frequent with venous than with arterial administration. The explanation offered for this unproven observation is that, because of the high degree of vascularity and thus the large number of endothelial cells in the lung, there is greater exposure of the endothelium to contrast agents with intravenous as compared to intraarterial administration. Such an explanation clearly requires further proof, but it rests on an understanding that contrast agents affect both the vessel wall and flowing blood.

In terms of clinical implications, the effects of contrast agents on venous administration are readily recognized with the pain that occurs during large-volume venous injections of HOCAs, for example, during contrast-enhanced CT examinations or upper or lower extremity venography. It has been shown in clinical studies that slow, high-volume intravenous infusion may lead to not only pain but also to venous thrombosis, and the frequency of such effects has been quantitated.[36–39] With the use of HOCAs, in the range of 1200 to 1500 mOsm/kg, the incidence of venous thrombosis after venography was as high as 30 percent. If the osmolality of the contrast agent was reduced to 500 to 1000 mOsm/kg, a marked reduction in the incidence of postvenographic thrombosis occurred, to 5 to 7 percent.[38] By objective criteria, no difference in the incidence of venous thrombosis was observable with the use of the nonionic contrast agent at near isotonicity as compared to a dilute conventional contrast agent with an osmolality of approximately 1000 mOsm.[39]

These findings are relevant in terms of venous injection because of the relatively slow flow and long exposure time; arterial effects are presumably somewhat different. Although endothelial function is largely the same, other wall functions are different because of the presence of a thicker media in arteries as compared to veins. Additionally, flow is clearly much more rapid on the arterial side, leading to an inherently shorter exposure time of the contrast to the vessel wall. Arterial thrombosis does not appear to occur as a function of damage to the underlying endothelium. It has been observed, however, in low-flow situations when contrast is exposed to static blood for relatively long periods of time, such as in selective coronary angiography in the presence of much underlying disease.[40] The clinical importance of such observations is unclear: that is, even in the presence of anticoagulation, if there is prolonged stasis of blood, thrombosis will occur. It is possible that such thrombosis is made more likely if a nonionic contrast agent remains in contact with blood for prolonged periods of time, as compared to an ionic contrast agent. Ionic contrast agents, in an experimental setting, clearly retard thrombosis to a greater extent.[41] The differences experimentally, however, are not great. It is likely, then, that in the clinical setting differences between ionic and nonionic agents are less important than appropriate technique. In other words, contrast agents should not be considered inherently anticoagulants and should not be used for flushing catheters. Also, it must be recognized that catheters are inherently somewhat thrombogenic, as are guidewires, and the possibility of a thrombus forming increases in the presence of underlying vessel wall disease.

The vascular and hematologic effects of contrast agents are clearly complex and incompletely understood. It must be kept in mind that thrombosis, hemostasis, and vessel wall function are interactive, and that contrast agents have effects on all three. These effects are, in general, minor and probably inconsequential. In certain situations, such as long exposure of static blood to contrast, or prolonged exposure of vessels to high concentrations of contrast, the potentially relevant clinical effects may be vessel wall damage, formation of thrombi, or even release of substances (e.g., prostaglandins) that cause systemic manifestations such as severe hypotension.

Cardiac Effects

As with the effects on blood and the endothelium, the heart is exposed to contrast whenever and wherever it is injected and physiologic effects are essentially ubiquitous. That is, if a careful evaluation is undertaken, changes in heart rate and blood pressure invariably accompany contrast injection. In general, such changes have relatively little importance. In two situations, however, the physiologic effects on the heart are of clear importance. First, when contrast agents are injected into or near the heart, as for pulmonary angiography or inferior vena cavography, the alterations may be substantial. Second, in patients with compromised or borderline cardiac function, any physiologic changes may become clinically important.

Extensive experimental investigations have been undertaken to evaluate the effects of contrast agents on the heart. Such studies have focused on several primary factors: osmolality, viscosity, free ions, chemical formulation, and additives. Each of these factors has been shown to play some role in the effects that contrast agents have on the heart. Any attempt to assess the importance of any isolated factor and what can broadly be considered contrast toxicity is heavily influenced by the model that is used. It is important to recognize that no single factor explains toxicity, but rather that multiple factors interact with each other. Further, the effect of any single factor is strongly influenced by the model in which it is examined. Extensive experimental work, although limited in direct applicability, has shed substantial light on the effects of contrast agents on the heart, and on the relationships between these effects and clinical events.

Osmolality is clearly the most important single factor in terms of cardiac toxicity, as has been noted in regard to renal and vascular and hematologic effects. Numerous investigations have been undertaken to quantitate the effect of osmolality, with somewhat confusing results.[42,43] Perhaps the clearest results can be gleaned from a study using an isolated perfused heart preparation,[44] which allows separation of effects on the myocardium from effects on the coronary arteries. In general, in this model, solutions that are moderately to markedly hypertonic, in the absence of ions, appear to have a positive ionotropic effect. Conversely, ionic solutions, such as sodium chloride, at the same osmolality have a negative ionotropic effect. The effect on coronary arteries is somewhat different. All hypertonic solutions, with essentially no difference between ionic and nonionic ones, lead to a dilatation of the coronary arteries. This suggests that osmolality alone, in the absence of ions, stimulates myocardial contractility in a dose-dependent effect and depresses vascular contractility in a similarly dose-related effect. The addition of ions alters the direct myocardial effect, to induce depression of contractility, but does not alter the depression of contractility of the vascular smooth muscle cells. Contrast agents, both ionic and nonionic, somewhat surprisingly behave very much as do ionic hypertonic solutions such as sodium chloride. That is, all contrast agents suppress both myocardial contractility and coronary artery contractility in an osmolality-related fashion. The only exception is the nonionic dimer iotrolan, which at an osmolality equivalent to that of plasma has a positive effect on myocardial contractility and a minor negative effect on coronary artery contractility.[44]

Other studies have examined the effect of osmolality in different models, with somewhat conflicting results. In open chest models, nonionic contrast agents appear to have a positive ionotropic effect, and ionic hypertonic contrast agents produce a negative ionotropic effect.[42,43,45] In a close chest model, however, the results are similar to those seen in the isolated perfused heart experiments, with a depression of myocardial contractility in an osmotically dependent fashion.[46] Even nonionic contrast agents that are hypertonic cause a moderate decrease in myocardial contractility.

The effect of viscosity as an isolated variable is also difficult to define. In essence, the major effect of viscosity should be to alter the period of exposure of the contrast agent to the heart. Again using the isolated perfused heart model, viscosity per se appears to have no effect on myocardial contractility.[44] Viscosity may have an effect in terms of the ability to inject the contrast agent, but this is likely to be minor, particularly if a power injector is used.[47]

As already indicated, it is difficult to separate the different components of contrast toxicity. Ions in contrast agents have long been recognized to have an effect on the heart. This was perhaps most dramatically demonstrated in the 1970s, with the observation that eliminating sodium from a hypertonic, ionic contrast agent precipitated an increased incidence of ventricular fibrillation.[48] That is, in the presence of other ions, the absence of sodium increases contrast toxicity. More recently, experiments have suggested that the same may be true for nonionic agents. In one particular model, high-dose, prolonged infusions of nonionic agents with ions added led to a lower incidence of ventricular arrhythmias than infusion of a solution identical but for the absence of ions.[49] These observations led to further studies, which again had somewhat conflicting results. Overall, they appear to suggest that in a situation that mimics human use, and particularly concerning the conduction system and induction of arrhythmias, the presence or absence of ions per se has relatively little impact.[50] The degree of hypertonicity, again, seems to be more important, so limiting osmolality is the major consideration.

The single important exception to this, however, regards calcium binding. It has long been recognized that a sudden drop in serum ionized calcium can lead to electromechanical dissociation.[51] This clinical picture is identical to an anaphylactoid response, with a sudden cessation of effective cardiac function. Experimentally, contrast agents lower serum ionized calcium, with both cardiac and noncardiac injection.[52–54] This may lead to minor effects, such as relatively minor alterations in contractility and conduction. On the one hand, it is reasonable to consider the addition of ions, particularly calcium and sodium, to contrast agents to prevent such effects.[53] On the other hand, it is clearly better to attempt to understand why such alterations in ion concentration have discernible effects, and then to prevent such effects from occurring. In the case of sodium ions, it is difficult to determine exactly why alterations in sodium levels might occur, and how they might be prevented. With regard to calcium ions, however, it is clear that alterations in concentration are primarily due to the additives to contrast agents, many of which are avid calcium binders.[54] For example, several of the currently available formulations of standard ionic HOCAs contain sodium citrate and sodium EDTA to sequester ions and to stabilize the solution. Both of these chelate calcium, as has long been recognized, and they are used clinically to inhibit coagulation of blood samples. The calcium-binding effects of such contrast agents are primarily related to these additives. The elimination of these additives, as has occurred in most contrast agents, both high and low osmolality, clearly lessens the amount of calcium chelation that occurs, and thus the possible fall in ionized calcium. It does not, however, totally eliminate such changes from occurring. Newer formulations, then, may still cause electromechanical dissociation, but with a much lower incidence.

The formulation per se may also play a significant

role in regard to cardiac and other effects of contrast agents. Although most contrast agents are similar, differing primarily in osmolality and in additives, minor differences do exist, which lead to differences in lipid solubility and in protein binding. Both of these factors are likely to play a relatively small but significant role in contrast toxicity.[55] Because of the marked similarity between contrast agents, it has been difficult to isolate the effects of the formulation alone, either experimentally or clinically. At this time, it is reasonable to assume that the effect of different formulations within a specific category, such as high-osmolality ionic or low-osmolality nonionic, are far outweighed by other considerations, such as osmolality and specific additives.

The clinically relevant effects of contrast agents on the heart follow from the experimental studies. With injection of any contrast agent into a coronary artery, there is a fall in blood pressure and a fall in heart rate, which begins approximately 3 seconds after the injection, with return to baseline levels within 20 to 60 seconds.[56] More subtle changes in electrical pattern have been extensively investigated, but their relationship to clinical events remains unclear.[57,58] With injection into the left ventricle, there is a more delayed fall in heart rate, a rise in diastolic pressure (suggesting decreased compliance of the myocardial cells), and a fall in blood pressure, which is probably compensatory and mediated by peripheral receptors. These changes return to baseline within 30 to 180 seconds. All of these changes are related to osmolality, in that they are less severe with lower-osmolality agents, but qualitatively similar changes are invariably observed. By extension, similar hemodynamic and conduction alterations are also observed with other injections of contrast agents, such as for peripheral angiography, but are less marked. In various clinical studies, clear differences between HOCAs and LOCAs have been observed in terms of the hemodynamic and electrical effects.[56,59–62] These differences in large patient series are often fairly striking. What is also striking, however, is that the large hemodynamic differences do not generally translate into differences in major complication rates.[56,62] It is somewhat speculative as to why this disparity between hemodynamic changes and adverse clinical effects occurs. One possible explanation lies in an examination of the patient and physician expectations. As shown in Table 3-1, if HOCAs and LOCAs are compared in double-blind prospective randomized studies, in this report[63] as in others, the incidence of both hemodynamic alterations and of contrast-related adverse events is significantly higher with the HOCAs. If two LOCAs are compared in similar prospective randomized trials, there is little difference between the two. There is, however, a significantly lower incidence of adverse events when the two LOCAs are compared than when an LOCA is compared to an HOCA. The incidence of both hemodynamic changes and contrast-related adverse events, in this and in other studies, is higher when an HOCA is compared to an LOCA than when an LOCA is compared to another LOCA.

Table 3-1. Adverse Events as a Function of Type of Study

Contrast Comparison	Percentage of Patients with: Change in Blood Pressure	Change in Cardiac Function	Contrast Reaction
Open (nonionic)	3.3	0	6.7
Nonionic a	2.5	3.7	0
vs.			
Nonionic b	2.6	1.3	0
Nonionic a	37.5	26.2	6.2
vs.			
HOCA	65.8	49.4	18.9

From Bettmann MA. Clinical experience with ioversol for angiography. Invest Radiol 1989;S24:S61–S66. Used with permission.

An alternative explanation for the major hemodynamic but relatively small clinical differences relates to the patient population studied. Most such studies have involved relatively stable, healthy patients, patients who ordinarily would not be expected to have adverse events. In general, in stable patients, without significant risk factors, cardiac events that are serious are relatively rare and differences between HOCAs and LOCAs are primarily in the hemodynamic changes and in relatively minor adverse events, such as heat and pain. In the few studies that have examined unstable patients, differences between HOCAs and LOCAs do emerge.[61,64] It is, perhaps, not surprising that this less stable population has not been extensively examined in prospective randomized trials, since the expectation that LOCA will cause a lower incidence of adverse effects is very strong. As suggested, however, by studies of HOCA versus LOCA and LOCA versus LOCA (see Table 3-1), the physician expectation may play a substantial role in this outcome.

Hemodynamic and conduction abnormalities occur whenever contrast agents are injected. Such changes are generally of little importance but may lead to significant adverse events in patients with underlying cardiac abnormalities. This even, and perhaps especially, includes asymptomatic patients with lesions such as tight aortic stenosis, who may be unable to compensate sufficiently for a sudden drop in blood pressure.

It also includes patients with significant arrhythmias, those with marked limitation of cardiac function, those with severe coronary artery disease, and those with severe pulmonary hypertension.

Patients undergoing pulmonary angiography fall into a special category. In large series, pulmonary angiography has been shown to be generally safe.[65] Patients appear to tolerate pulmonary angiography even when there is marked elevation in pulmonary artery and right ventricular peak systolic pressure. Again, there is relatively little clinical difference between HOCAs and LOCAs, although hemodynamic changes are clearly greater with HOCAs. Further, because of discomfort on injection, patients often cough during injection of high concentrations of HOCAs (i.e., cut-film angiography using a high iodine–content HOCA). This potentially makes the examination less than diagnostic. Such a response can be avoided either by using an LOCA with cut-film angiography,[66] or by using a dilute HOCA (e.g., Conray 43 or any sodium meglumine diatrizoate preparation diluted to an iodine content of 125–200 mg iodine/ml) with digital subtraction angiography. Patients who appear to be at greatest risk of significant adverse events during pulmonary angiography are those with an acute rise in pulmonary artery pressure to a range of 60 to 80 mmHg peak systolic. In such patients, a sudden rise in pulmonary pressure related to contrast injection, mediated by the volume load, by myocardial depression, and by increased pulmonary vascular resistance, may lead to sudden cardiac decompensation. In such patients, selective injections of a low volume of contrast and low-osmolality contrast material are of paramount importance.

Systemic Effects

The systemic effects of contrast agents have been extensively discussed in the literature, with the general view that most contrast agent adverse events must be considered systemic.[67] As evident from the preceding discussion, many if not most contrast reactions that are of significance are not truly systemic in etiology, but are rather related to endothelial, hematologic, or cardiac interactions. Immune-mediated systemic reactions clearly occur, but they are rarely, if ever, allergic in a classic sense, because antibodies to contrast agents or their components have been documented only once or twice.[68] Further, in patients with typical immune-mediated adverse events, repeat injection of a contrast agent leads to recurrent reaction in only 20 to 50 percent of cases. If a classic allergic mechanism were involved, such reexposure would be expected to cause an equivalent or more severe reaction. Systemic reactions, then, must be considered both in terms of focal etiologies, such as cardiac effects, and in terms of unpredictable but immune-mediated responses.

The overall incidence of systemic reactions has been thought to be lower with arterial than with venous injections.[69,70] Examination of the relatively sparse data that relate to this, however, shows that this is probably not true. The overall incidence of adverse events with arteriography is clearly higher than with venous injection, in large part because of catheter- and other procedure-related aspects of angiography.[63] Although the data are surprisingly sparse, it appears that the incidence of contrast-related adverse events is essentially equivalent with arterial and venous injections.

Systemic reactions of concern range from pain and a feeling of heat to cardiorespiratory arrest. Because of the subjective nature of most of the minor reactions, such as pain, and the infrequency of the major reactions, systemic reactions have been difficult to evaluate, both experimentally and clinically. It has become evident that pain and heat are related primarily, but not solely, to osmolality. Below a certain osmolality, pain is markedly decreased. At isotonicity, there is essentially no pain. Interestingly, a feeling of heat may occur with isotonic contrast agents, such as iotrolan. Further, in the midrange of osmolality, approximately 600 to 900 mOsm/kg, the amount of discomfort experienced by patients appears to vary not only with osmolality, but also with the specific formulation.[71,72] This may in part be related to the lipophilicity versus hydrophilicity of contrast media, but the exact mechanism of these feelings of discomfort is not understood.

Other minor reactions such as nausea and vomiting and urticaria also appear to be related in large part to osmolality; in general they occur less frequently with LOCAs than with HOCAs. One interesting exception is that histaminelike reactions, such as urticaria, appear to be more frequent with the low-osmolality ionic agent ioxaglate than with nonionic formulations of the same osmolality.[73] Again, experimental studies as to the etiology of these reactions are relatively sparse and inconclusive. Although fairly extensive investigations of the immune effects of contrast agents have been undertaken, direct connection with the clinical experience is still lacking.[74,75]

The rare, more severe adverse reactions, such as bronchospasm, laryngotracheal edema, and a full-blown anaphylactoid response, are of major concern to physicians who use contrast agents. It is important to recognize that, to a large extent, such reactions cannot be predicted, but they can be successfully treated. In regard to mortality from contrast agents, although it is clear that patients do experience reactions that cause death, such reactions appear to occur in less than 1 in 165,000 cases.[76] Most deaths that occur during angiography are probably in part related to the contrast agent, but are generally more related to underlying risk factors, ranging from preexistent severe trauma to severe cardiac disease, combined with other procedural factors such as catheter-induced ischemia. It is also apparent that a prior reaction to a contrast agent increases the likelihood of a reaction, but does not appear to be helpful in predicting reactions that will be severe or fatal.[69,77,78] Other risk factors for contrast reactions are severe allergies, active asthma, and underlying cardiac disease. Although a connection has long been thought to exist between shellfish allergies and contrast reactions, available data suggest that this is no stronger a risk factor than any other severe allergy.[69]

In contradistinction to defining the frequency and etiology of severe systemic reactions, the treatment is fairly straightforward. These reactions fall into three different general categories: vasovagal, respiratory, and cardiorespiratory. Vasovagal reactions, which may be related to causes as diverse as generalized anxiety, catheter placement, or contrast injection, are characterized by hypotension accompanied by bradycardia or a lack of tachycardia. Such reactions are generally mild and require no treatment other than leg elevation and infusion of fluids. Should such reactions become more severe, with substantial fall in blood pressure and heart rate, the treatment consists of intravenous administration of atropine at a dose of 0.4 to 1 mg intravenously. The major importance of such reactions is that they cannot be ignored. If untreated, some vagal reactions may persist and worsen.[79] If effectively treated, however, such reactions almost invariably resolve quickly, without a tendency to recur during the procedure or during subsequent arteriograms.

Respiratory reactions, such as laryngeal edema or bronchospasm, are generally self-limited, but may progress to significant or complete respiratory compromise and at least cause moderate anxiety for both the patient and the physician. Such reactions can be treated with adrenergic inhalers such as albuterol as a first step. If this therapy cannot be employed or is ineffective, epinephrine can be administered at a dose of 0.5 to 1.0 ml intramuscularly at a dilution of 1:1000 or at 0.5 to 1.0 ml of 1:10,000 dilution intravenously.[80] Epinephrine must be administered with care because of its potent vasoconstrictive and positive adrenergic effects. Severe cardiovascular reactions, with hypertension and tachycardia or with complete cardiorespiratory collapse, must be treated with appropriate cardiopulmonary resuscitation. The occurrence, albeit infrequent, of such reactions, regardless of precise etiology, makes it imperative that contrast injections be performed only in facilities where personnel fully trained in resuscitation practices are readily available.

Other adverse systemic reactions, such as generalized edema or focal skin rashes, are similarly of concern but are rare. They require symptomatic treatment and generally resolve without sequelae. Recent reports of delayed reactions to nonionic agents are of interest,[81] but such reactions may well be related to other concomitant medications.

The role of corticosteroid pretreatment in preventing reactions is controversial. If corticosteroids are to be used, a dose regimen similar to that suggested by Lasser et al[69,82] of 32 mg of methyl prednisolone given in two doses 12 and 2 hours before the procedure should be used. Even with severe reactions, it is clear that corticosteroid treatment alone is ineffective immediately. Similarly, the use of antihistamines to treat acute reactions is effective in achieving symptomatic relief of histamine-mediated manifestations, such as urticaria, but ineffective in terms of more severe reactions. Studies suggest that corticosteroid or other immune-suppressant therapy may help decrease the incidence of certain milder reactions.[69,82,83] There is no evidence to suggest that it prevents severe reactions. The most effective way to prevent severe reactions is simply to screen patients at high risk, to reassure such patients, and to be prepared to treat any reactions that occur.

High- Versus Low-Osmolality Contrast Agents

The use of these two categories of agents is controversial, with some advocating universal use of low-osmolality agents and others advocating very limited use. The major resistance to the use of low-osmolality agents, both ionic and nonionic, is that they are significantly more expensive, and the data to date suggest that they do not change the incidence of severe reactions.[84–88] On careful review, however, it is reasonable to conclude that LOCAs decrease the incidence of certain reactions among certain high-risk patients. Selective use of LOCAs, therefore, is both rational and helpful in patient care. Although it is difficult to define the specific patients who are most likely to benefit from LOCAs, in general terms, certain guidelines can be followed. These are shown in Table 3-2.

Several new contrast agents as well as other developments are likely to alter the pattern of use of contrast

Table 3-2. Indications for Use of Low-Osmolality Contrast Agents

1. Prior significant contrast reaction
2. Severe allergies
3. Active asthma
4. Significant cardiac disease (coronary artery disease or severe angina, severe congestive heart failure, active significant arrhythmia, tight aortic stenosis, pulmonary hypertension)
5. Significant renal failure (serum creatinine ≥2.5 mg/dcL)
6. Otherwise painful examination
7. Patients who would possibly be harmed by minor reactions (e.g., suspected spinal cord injury) or who would otherwise be unable to deal with such reactions (e.g., excessively anxious or anxious and psychotic patients).

media for angiography. Magnetic resonance angiography and other noninvasive modalities are likely to further decrease contrast use as they replace angiography for many purely diagnostic procedures. Conversely, the number of interventional angiographic procedures is likely to increase, with a concomitant increase in the use of contrast agents for these procedures. Over the next few years, patents expire on several of the nonionic contrast agents approved by the FDA for use in the United States in 1985. This may lead to the availability of generic versions, which are likely to be available at lower cost. Several new LOCAs are being investigated, and their availability may also decrease contrast cost. Nonionic dimeric contrast agents, which are potentially isotonic to blood, may also play a role because of their potentially increased safety and comfort. Whether there is a true or significant safety advantage over currently available low-osmolality agents remains to be seen. Finally, alternatives are also worthy of consideration, such as carbon dioxide or iodinated contrast agents targeted to specific organs.

Contrast agents provide a huge amount of useful information to all physicians, but carry certain drawbacks. Further investigations are warranted to continue to understand and improve the role that these agents play in angiography and in all imaging. However, contrast agents remain central to medical practice, and continue to be remarkable for their overall safety.

References

1. Grainger RG. Intravascular contrast media—the past, the present and the future. Br J Radiol 1982;55:1–18.
2. Wallingford VH. The development of organic iodide compounds as x-ray contrast media. J Am Pharmacol Assoc (Scientific Edition) 1953;42:721–728.
3. Hoppe JO, Larsen HA, Coulston FJ. Observations on the toxicity of a new urographic contrast medium, sodium 3,5-diacetamido-2,4,6-tri-iodobenzoate (Hypaque sodium) and related compounds. J Pharmacol Exp Ther 1956;116:394–403.
4. Almen T. Contrast agent design: some aspects on the synthesis of water-soluble contrast agents of low osmolality. J Theor Biol 1969;24:216–226.
5. Sovak M. Contrast media: a journey almost sentimental. Invest Radiol 1994;29:54–514.
6. Hildner FJ, Javier RP, Ramaswamy K, Samet P. Pseudo-complications of cardiac catheterization. Chest 1973;63:15–17.
7. Bettmann MA, Paulin S. Lower limb phlebography: the incidence, nature and modification of undesirable side effects. Radiology 1977;122:101–104.
8. Shasterman N, Strom BL, Murray TG, Morrison G, West SL, Maislin G. Risk factors and outcome of hospital-acquired acute renal failure: clinical epidemiologic study. Am J Med 1987;83: 65–71.
9. Dorph S. The effect of contrast media on renal function. European Radiol 1995;in press.
10. Katzberg RW, Morris TW, Casser EC, Merguerian PA, Ventura JA, Babico RC, McKeana BA, Dimarco PL. Acute systemic and renal hemodynamic effects of meglumine/sodium diatrizoate 76% and iopamidol in euvolemic and dehydrated dogs. Invest Radiol 1986;21:793–797.
11. Messana JM, Cielnisky DA, Nguyen VD, Humes HD. Comparison of the toxicity of the radiocontrast agents iopamidol and diatrizoate, to rabbit renal proximal tubule cells in vitro. J Pharmacol Exp Ther 1988;244:1139–1144.
12. Bettmann MA. The evaluation of contrast-related renal failure. AJR 1991;157:66–68.
13. Idee JM, Beanfils H, Bonnemain B. Iodinated contrast media–induced nephropathy: pathophysiology, clinical aspects and prevention. Fundam Clin Pharmacol 1994;8:193–206.
14. Moore RD, Steinberg EP, Powe NR, Briaher JA, Fishman EK, Grazrano S, Gopaleu R. Nephrotoxicity of high-osmolality versus low-osmolality contrast media: randomized clinical trial. Radiology 1992;182:649–655.
15. Brezis M, Epstein FH. A closer look at radiocontrast-induced nephropathy. NEJM 1989;320:179–181.
16. Cronin RE. Renal failure following radiologic procedures. Am J Med Sci 1989;298:342–356.
17. Katholy RE, Taylor GJ, Woods WT, et al. Nephrotoxicity of nonionic low-osmolality versus high-osmolality contrast media: a prospective double-blind randomized comparison in human beings. Radiology 1993;186:183–187.
18. Rudnick MR, Goldfarb S, Wexler L, et al. Nephrotoxicity of ionic and nonionic contrast media in 1196 patients: a randomized trial. Kidney Int 1995;47:254–261.
19. Eisenberg RL, Bank WO, Hedgcock MW. Renal failure after major arteriography can be avoided with hydration. AJR 1981; 136:859–861.
20. Becker JA. Evaluation of renal function. Radiology 1991;179: 337–338.
21. Ciqarroa RC, Lange RA, Williams RH, Hillis LD. Dosing of contrast material to prevent contrast nephropathy in patients with renal disease. Am J Med 1989;86:649–652.
22. Barreff BJ, Carlisle EJ. Metanalysis of the relative nephrotoxicity of high and low osmolality iodinated contrast media. Radiology 1993;188:171–178.
23. Claus W. Iotrolan in patients with renal failure. European Radiol 1995;in press.
24. Bettmann MA, D'Agnostino R, Juravsky LI, Jeffrey RF, Tottle AJ, Goudey CP. Carbon dioxide as an angiographic contrast agent: a prospective randomized trial. Invest Radiol 1994;29: 434–546.
25. Vanhoutte PM. The endothelium-modulator of vascular smooth-muscle tone. NEJM 1988;319:512–513.
26. Loscalzo J, Braunwald E. Tissue plasminogen activator. NEJM 1988;319:925–931.
27. Merseredu WA, Robertson HR. Observations on venous endothelial injury following the injection of various radiographic contrast media in the rat. J Neurosurg 1961;18:289–294.

28. Laerum F. Cytotoxic effects of six angiographic contrast media on human endothelium in culture. Acta Radiol 1987;28:99–105.
29. Morgan DML, Bettmann MA. Effects of x-ray contrast media and radiation on human vascular endothelial cells in vitro. Cardiovasc Intervent Radiol 1989;12:154–160.
30. Thiesea B, Muetzer W. Effects of angiographic contrast media on venous endothelium of rabbits. Invest Radiol 1990;25:121–126.
31. Stormorken H, Skalpe IO, Testart MC. Effects of various contrast media on coagulation, fibrinolysis and platelet function: an in vitro study. Invest Radiol 1986;21:348–354.
32. Mamoa JF, Hoppensteadt MS, Fareed J, Moncada R. Biochemical evidence for a relative lack of inhibition of thrombin formation by nonionic contrast media. Radiology 1991;179:399–402.
33. Kopko PM, Smith DC, Bull BS. Thrombin generation in nonclottable mixtures of blood and nonionic contrast agents. Radiology 1990;174;459–461.
34. Aspelin P. Effect of ionic and non-ionic contrast media on morphology of human erythrocytes. Acta Radiol Diagn 1978;19:675–687.
35. Aspelin P, Schmid-Schoenberg H, Malotta H. Do non-ionic contrast media increase red cell aggregation and clot formation? Invest Radiol 1988;23:5326–5333.
36. Albrechtsson U, Olsson C-G. Thrombotic side effects of lower limb phlebography. Lancet 1976;1:723–724.
37. Laeram F, Holm HA. Postphlebographic thrombosis: a double blind study with methylglucamine metrizoate and metrizamide. Radiology 1981;140:651–654.
38. Bettmann MA, Salzman EW, Rosenthal D, et al. Reduction of venous thrombosis complicating phlebography. AJR 1980;134:1169–1172.
39. Bettmann MA, Robbins A, Braun SD, Wetzner S, Dunnick NR, Finkelstein J. Comparison of the diagnostic efficacy, tolerance and complication rates of a nonionic and an ionic contrast agent for leg phlebography. Radiology 1987;165:113–116.
40. Grollman JF, Liu CK, Astone RA, Lurie MD. Thromboembolic complication in coronary angiography associated with the use of nonionic contrast medium. Cathet Cardiovasc Diagn 1988;14:159–164.
41. Ing JJ, Smith DC, Ball BS. Differing mechanisms of clotting inhibition by ionic and nonionic contrast agents. Radiology 1989;172:345–348.
42. Higgins CB, Sovak M, Schmidt WS, Kelley MJ, Newell JD. Direct myocardial effects of intracoronary administration of new contrast materials with low osmolality. Invest Radiol 1980;15:39–46.
43. Kozeny GA, Murdock DK, Euler DE, Hano JE, et al. In vivo effects of acute changes in osmolality and sodium concentration on myocardial contractility. Am Heart J 1984;109:290–296.
44. Fleetwood G, Bettmann MA, Gordon JL. The effects of radiographic contrast media on myocardial contractility and coronary resistance: osmolality, ionic concentration, and viscosity. Invest Radiol 1990;25:254–260.
45. Newell JD, Higgins CB, Kelley MJ, Green CE, et al. The influence of hyperosmolality on left ventricular contractile state: disparate effects of nonionic and ionic solutions. Invest Radiol 1980;15:363–370.
46. Bourdillon PD, Bettmann MA, McCracken S, et al. Effects of a new nonionic and a conventional ionic contrast agent on coronary sinus ionized calcium and left ventricular hemodynamics in dogs. J Am Coll Cardiol 1985;6:845–853.
47. Halsell RD. Heating contrast media: role in contemporary angiography. Radiology 1987;164:276–278.
48. Paulin S, Adams DF. Increased ventricular fibrillation during coronary arteriography with a new contrast medium preparation. Radiology 1971;101:45–50.
49. Morris TW. Ventricular fibrillation during right coronary arteriography with ioxaglate, iohexol and iopamidol in dogs. Radiology 1988;23:205–208.
50. Booth L, Besjahov J, Oksendal A. Sodium-calcium balance in nonionic contrast media. Invest Radiol 1993;28:223–227.
51. Caulfield JB, Zir L, Harthorn JW. Blood calcium levels in the presence of arteriographic contrast material. Circulation 1975;52:119–123.
52. Morris TW, Lawrence GS, Fischer HW. Calcium binding by radiopaque media. Invest Radiol 1982;17:501–505.
53. Mallette LE, Gomez LS. Systemic hypocalcemia after clinical injections of radiographic contrast media: amelioration by omission of calcium chelating agents. Radiology 1983;147:677–679.
54. Bourdillon PD, Bettmann MA, McCracken S, Poole-Wilson PA, Grossman W. Effects of a new ionic and a conventional ionic contrast agent on coronary sinus ionized calcium and left ventricular hemodynamics in dogs. J Am Coll Cardiol 1985;6:845–853.
55. Almen T. Relations between chemical structure, animal toxicity and clinical adverse effects of contrast media: patient safety and adverse events in contrast medium examinations. In Enge I, Edgren J (eds). Excerpta medica. Amsterdam: Elsevier, 1989, pp. 25–45.
56. Bettmann MA, Bourdillon PD, Barry WH, Brush KA, Levin DC. Contrast agents for cardiac angiography: effects of a nonionic agent vs. a standard ionic agent. Radiology 1984;153:583–587.
57. Morris TW, Dukovic D, Pagani E. The effects of coronary injections of iodixanol, iopamidol and ioxaglate on contractility and electrophysiology. Invest Radiol 1994;29:S99–S101.
58. Besjakov J, Chai CM, Baath L, Almen T. Comparison between oxygenated iohexol solution enriched with electrolytes and other low osmotic contrast media. Invest Radiol 1994;29:S238–S241.
59. Bettmann MA, Higgins CB. Comparison of an ionic with a nonionic contrast agent for cardiac angiography: results of a multicenter trial. Invest Radiol 1985;20:S70–S74.
60. Hirshfield JW, Wieland J, Davis CA, Giles BD, et al. Hemodynamic and electrocardiographic effects of ioversol during cardiac angiography, comparison with iopamidol and diatrizoate. Invest Radiol 1989;24:138–144.
61. Hill JA, Winniford M, Cohen MB, Van Fossen DB, Murphy MJ, Halpern EF, Ludbrook PA, Wexler L, Rudnick MR, Goldfarb S. Multicenter trial of ionic versus nonionic contrast media for cardiac angiography. Am J Cardiol 1993;72:770–775.
62. Steinberg EP, Moore RD, Gopalau R, et al. Safety and cost effectiveness of high osmolality as compared with low osmolality contrast material in patients undergoing cardiac angiography. NEJM 1992;326:425–540.
63. Bettmann MA. Clinical experience with ioversol for angiography. Invest Radiol 1989;S24:S61–S66.
64. Feldman RL, Jalowiec DA, Hill JA, Lambert CR. Contrast media-related complications during cardiac catheterization using Hexabrix or Renografin in high-risk patients. Am J Cardiol 1988;61:1334–1337.
65. Stein PD, Athanasoulis C, Alavi A, Greenspan RH, Hales CA, Saltzman HA, Vreim CE, Terrin ML, Weg JG. Complications and validity of pulmonary angiography in acute pulmonary embolism. Circulation 1992;85:462–468.
66. Smith DC, Lois JF, Gomes AS, Maloney MD, Yahiku PY. Pulmonary arteriography: comparison of cough stimulation effects of diatrizoate and ioxaglate. Radiology 1987;162:617–618.
67. Lasser EC, Berry CC, Mishkin MM, Williamson B, Zheutlin N, Silverman JM. Pretreatment with corticosteroids to prevent adverse reactions to nonionic contrast media. AJR 1994;162:523–526.
68. Brasch RC. Allergic reactions to contrast media: accumulated evidence. AJR 1980;134:797–801.
69. Lasser EC, Berry CC, Talner LB, et al. Pre-treatment with corticosteroids to alleviate reactions to intravenous contrast material. NEJM 1987;317:845–849.
70. Shehadi WH, Tonlolo G. Adverse reactions to contrast media. Radiology 1980;137:229–302.
71. Smith DC, Yakiku PY, Maloney MD, et al. Three new low os-

molality agents: a comparative study of patient discomfort. AJNR 1988;9:137–139.
72. Sovak M, Deutsch JA, Ranganathan R. Evaluation of intrathecal contrast media by aversion conditioning in rats. Invest Radiol 1982;17:5101–5106.
73. Eloy R, Corot C, Belleville J. Contrast media for angiography: physicochemical properties, pharmacokinetics and biocompatibility. Clin Materials 1991;7:89–197.
74. Lasser EC. A coherent biochemical basis for increased reactivity to contrast material in allergic patients: a novel concept. AJR 1987;149:1281–1285.
75. Herd CM, Robertson AR, Frewin DB, Taylor WB. Adverse reactions during intravenous urography: are these due to histamine release? Br J Radiol 1988;61(721):5–11.
76. Katayama H, Yamaguchi K, Kozuka T, Takashima T, Seez P, Matsuura K. Adverse reactions to ionic and nonionic contrast media. Radiology 1990;175:621–628.
77. Bettmann MA. Radiographic contrast agents—a perspective. NEJM 1987;317:891–893.
78. Bettmann MA. Ionic versus nonionic contrast agents for intravenous use: are all the answers in? Radiology 1990;175:616–618.
79. van Sonnenberg E, Neff CC, Pfister RC. Life-threatening hypotensive reactions to contrast media administration: comparison of pharmacologic and fluid therapy. Radiology 1987;162:15–19.
80. Manual on iodinated contrast media. Reston, VA: American College of Radiology, 1991.
81. Gavant ML, Siegle RL. Iodixanol in excretory urography: initial clinical experience with a nonionic, dimeric (ratio 6:1) contrast medium. Radiology 1992;183:515–518.
82. Lasser EC, Berry CC, Mishkin MM, Williamson B, Zheutlin N, Silverman JM. Pretreatment with corticosteroids to prevent adverse reactions to nonionic contrast media. AJR 1994;162:523–526.
83. Greenberger PA, Patterson R, Tapio CM. Prophylaxis against repeated radiocontrast media reactions in 857 cases: adverse experience with cimetidine and safety of β-adrenergic antagonists. Arch Intern Med 1985;145:2197–2200.
84. Jacobson PD, Rosenquist J. The introduction of low-osmolar contrast agents in radiology. JAMA 1988;260:1586–1592.
85. Powe NR. Low- versus high-osmolality contrast media for intravenous use: a health care luxury or necessity? Radiology 1992;183:21–22.
86. Steinberg EP, Moore RD, Powe NR, Gopalan R, Davidoff AJ, Litt M, Graziano, Brinker JA. Safety and cost effectiveness of high-osmolality as compared with low-osmolality contrast material in patients undergoing cardiac angiography. NEJM 1992;326(7):425–430.
87. Barrett BJ, Parfrey PS, Vavasour HM, O'Dea F, Kent G, Stone E. A comparison on nonionic low-osmolality radiocontrast agents with ionic, high-osmolality agents during cardiac catheterization. NEJM 1992;326:431–436.
88. Hirshfeld JW Jr. Low-osmolality contrast agents—who needs them? NEJM 1992;326(7):482–484.

4

The Emergency Treatment of Reactions to Contrast Media

STANLEY BAUM

For Quick Reference

As a radiologist, you must (1) be prepared to deal with both the common and uncommon reactions to iodinated contrast material, (2) be able to take a rational and effective therapeutic approach toward minor and major reactions, and (3) set up lines of communication with consulting physicians who could be called on to treat your patients with advanced diagnostic and resuscitative measures. Certainly you would do well to acquaint yourself with the information presented in this chapter *before* an untoward event occurs.

The availability of the National Standards for Cardiopulmonary Resuscitation[1] and the training programs in Basic and Advanced Life Support offered by the American Heart Association have enabled every practicing physician to become proficient in resuscitation. This chapter, while following the basic format of its predecessor,[2] relies heavily on, and is derived primarily from, the National Standards for Cardiopulmonary Resuscitation.[1] These uniform standards for resuscitation being taught nationwide have, no doubt, improved the chances for survival of all patients suffering cardiopulmonary arrest of whatever cause.[3–8]

Question all patients regarding previous drug reactions, with particular emphasis on the specific drug or test substance to be administered.[9] Even the most insignificant prior reaction must be given careful consideration before that drug or any medication chemically related to it is administered. Attempt to elicit a personal or family history of atopy (hay fever, asthma, or eczema). Persons so afflicted experience serious drug reactions more frequently than do those with no history of atopy.

The incidence of adverse reactions to iodinated contrast media varies considerably, depending on the series studied as well as on the type of examination.[10] Thus, deaths from intravenous pyelography have been

General Precautions

Before injecting contrast media
- Review patient's chart and take history:
  - Allergy? Reactions? Previous injections? Pulmonary edema?
- Read label (drug, strength).
- Reduce dose for children.
- Have epinephrine and syringe ready.

After injecting
- Be readily available for 5 minutes.
- Be generally available for 30 to 60 minutes.

reported to occur in the range of 1 in 100,000[11] to 1 in 40,000 examinations.[12] Although serious reactions to contrast media are rare, occurring in 1 in 1000 to 5000 examinations, depending on the series, minor adverse reactions occur in 6 to 9 percent of patients receiving these agents. Among people who have had a previous reaction, the recurrence rate is about 20 percent.[13]

Unnecessary tests must be avoided. Careful selection of patients for x-ray studies will help reduce reactions. Slower infusion of the media, adequate hydration before the procedure, premedication with antihistamines, and the use of a test dose have all been advocated as measures to reduce or prevent reactions to contrast media.[14-16] For immediate treatment of reactions, have 1 mg of epinephrine (1 ml, 1:1000 solution, or 10 ml, 1:10,000 solution) available in a syringe with a needle attached.[17,18]

Although most reactions occur during the first five minutes, some may take place as long as an hour after the injection. Be on guard (and be available) for these delayed reactions.

Treatment of reactions to contrast media must begin without delay. This is of greatest importance when resuscitation is required. The goal of cardiopulmonary resuscitation is to prevent irreversible brain damage. If nothing is done, such damage will begin after 3 minutes of cerebral anoxia, possibly sooner in some cases.[19] Therefore go to the patient immediately, and along the way collect others to help. Even the unskilled can lift the patient, bring emergency drugs and equipment, and serve as messengers.

Evaluate the patient as you enter the room. Is the patient awake or unconscious? Gather information from the conscious patient. If the patient is unconscious, question personnel. The radiology request form or the patient's chart may offer clues regarding medications taken and whether the patient suffers from diabetes, epilepsy, a cardiac condition, or the like. *Has the patient had a minor reaction or a major reaction?*

When Called in an Emergency

Go to patient at once.
Recruit others to help.
Start evaluation as you enter room.
Gather information from patient and chart.
Determine if reaction is minor (usually allergic and requiring drugs) or major (usually requiring cardiopulmonary resuscitation).

Minor (Allergic) Reaction: Symptoms and Treatment

Conjunctivitis
Erythema
Pruritus
Rhinitis
Urticaria
Immediate treatment
- Epinephrine, 0.3 ml of 1:1000 solution IM
- Diphenhydramine, 50 mg IV

Supportive measures
- Diphenhydramine, 50 mg q6h
- Observe for response to therapy

The common manifestations and treatment of minor reactions have been summarized briefly here. For a detailed presentation of the management of minor reactions, see Chapter 3.

If on first inspection the patient's condition indicates an immediate or a likely need for cardiopulmonary resuscitation, call for the necessary personnel, drugs, and equipment. The well-established trend toward using cardiac arrest teams has resulted in a better survival rate,[20] especially as such teams have gained experience in basic and advanced life support. Note well, however, that using a team approach in no way reduces your initial responsibility as the first physician on the scene.

Basic life support is an emergency first-aid procedure that consists of recognizing respiratory and car-

Major Reaction: Apparent Need for Cardiopulmonary Resuscitation

Have emergency drugs and equipment brought.
Call for additional help (cardiac arrest team, anesthesiologist, internist, surgeon).
Begin basic life support (see subsequent discussion).
- Airway opened and cleared.
- Breathing restored.
- Circulation restored.
- Definitive therapy.
  - Drugs.
  - Intravenous line.
  - Defibrillation.
  - Electrocardiogram.

Establish Vital Functions

Airway
- Look for and correct upper airway obstruction.
- Establish head-tilt position.
- Clear airway of vomitus and foreign bodies.

Breathing
- Start artificial ventilation if patient is apneic or if there is inadequate air exchange.

Circulation
- Palpate carotid pulse; absence or questionable presence of pulse requires external cardiac compression.

diac arrest and starting the proper application of cardiopulmonary resuscitation to maintain life until the patient recovers sufficiently to be transported elsewhere or until advanced life support is available.[1] Do not fail to act because the patient has dilated pupils. The size of the pupils is noted as an indication of the duration of cerebral anoxia and as an aid in the assessment of the effectiveness of the resuscitation efforts. Thus, fully dilated pupils indicate at least 2 minutes of cerebral anoxia; the prognosis for recovery of cerebral function when the pupils are fully dilated is not as favorable as it is when the pupils are constricted. Pupils that constrict during cardiopulmonary resuscitation are evidence that the brain is being oxygenated.[21]

Determine immediately the adequacy or absence of breathing and circulation. If only breathing is inadequate or absent, artificial ventilation may be all that is necessary.[22] If circulation is also absent, start artificial circulation in combination with artificial ventilation.

In the unconscious patient, the jaw muscles that normally support the tongue are relaxed. If the patient is supine, the base of the tongue falls back against the posterior wall of the pharynx, obstructing the flow of air into the trachea. You can relieve this upper airway obstruction easily and quickly by tilting the patient's head backward as far as possible. Sometimes this simple maneuver is all that is required for breathing to resume spontaneously.[22] To perform the head-tilt maneuver, place one hand beneath the patient's neck and the other hand on the forehead. Then lift the neck with one hand and tilt the head backward by pressure with your other hand on the forehead. You must keep the head in this position at all times.

Another cause of upper airway obstruction is the presence of vomitus or a foreign body, which must be removed. Use suction or forceps, or turn the patient on his or her side and forcibly strike the patient on the back between the shoulder blades.

If the patient does not promptly resume adequate spontaneous breathing after the airway is opened, you must start artificial ventilation with a ventilation bag and mask.

Open your mouth widely, take a deep breath, make a tight seal with your mouth around the patient's mouth, and blow air into the patient's mouth. Watch the chest rise. Then remove your mouth and allow the patient to exhale passively. Watch the chest fall. Adequate artificial ventilation on each breath is shown by feeling in your own airway the resistance and compliance of the patient's lungs as they expand and by hearing and feeling the air escape from the patient's lungs during exhalation. The initial maneuver should be four quick, full breaths with no time allowed for full lung deflation between breaths. Repeat the cycle every 5 seconds as long as respiratory inadequacy persists.

For an infant or a small child, cover both the mouth and nose of the infant or child with your mouth and use small breaths to inflate the lungs every 3 seconds. A newborn infant requires only a puff of air from the rescuer's cheeks. Do not exaggerate the head-tilt position, because the infant's neck is so pliable that forceful backward tilting of the head may cause upper airway obstruction.

Quickly determine whether the heart is beating. Cardiac arrest is evidenced by pulselessness in large arteries in an unconscious patient who has a deathlike appearance and absent breathing. Check the carotid pulse as quickly as possible when cardiac arrest is suspected. Palpation of the carotid pulse rather than other pulses is recommended because (1) you are already at the patient's head to perform artificial ventilation, (2) you have immediate access to the neck area and do not need to remove any clothing, and (3) the carotid pulse will persist when the more peripheral pulses are no longer palpable. The pulse area is located lateral to the larynx, in the groove between the trachea and the muscles at the side of the neck. Palpate the area gently; do not compress!

Rate of Artificial Ventilation

Adults: Once every 5 seconds
Infants: Once every 3 seconds

Rate of External Cardiac Compression

Adults: 80 and 60 per minute for one-rescuer and two-rescuer resuscitation, respectively
Infants: 100 per minute.

Absence of the pulse is the indication for starting artificial circulation by external cardiac compression. Apply pressure rhythmically over the lower half of the sternum but not over the xiphoid process. Intermittent pressure applied to the sternum compresses the heart and produces a pulsatile artificial circulation.

External cardiac compression must always be accompanied by artificial ventilation. Compression of the sternum produces some ventilation, but the volumes are insufficient for adequate oxygenation of the blood. Therefore, artificial ventilation is always required when external cardiac compression is used.

If you are the only person available for cardiopulmonary resuscitation (Fig. 4-1), you must perform both artificial ventilation and artificial circulation using a 15:2 ratio.[1] Deliver two very quick lung inflations after each 15 chest compressions. Because of the interruptions for lung inflations, you must perform each series of 15 chest compressions at the faster rate of 80 compressions per minute to achieve an actual compression rate of 60 per minute. Deliver the two full lung inflations in rapid succession, within 5 seconds, without allowing full exhalation between breaths.

Figure 4-1. One-rescuer cardiopulmonary resuscitation—15 chest compressions (rate of 80 per minute), two quick lung inflations. (From American Heart Association and National Academy of Sciences–National Research Council. Standards for cardiopulmonary resuscitation (CPR) and emergency cardiac care (ECC). JAMA 1974;227 (Suppl): 833. Used with permission.)

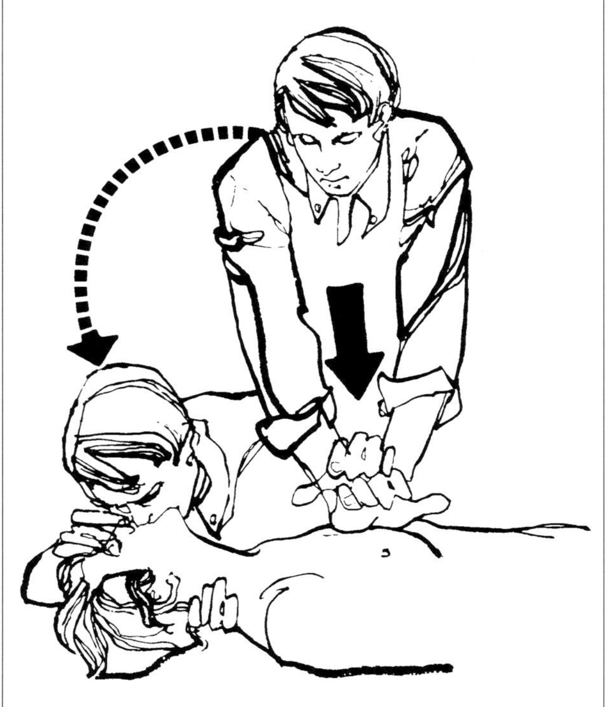

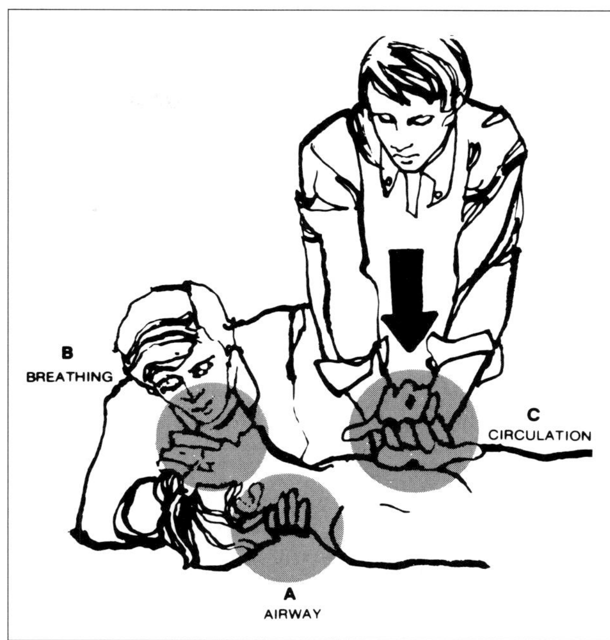

Figure 4-2. Two-rescuer cardiopulmonary resuscitation—five chest compressions at a rate of 60 per minute with no pause for ventilation; one lung inflation after each five compressions, interposed between compressions. (From American Heart Association and National Academy of Sciences–National Research Council. Standards for cardiopulmonary resuscitation (CPR) and emergency cardiac care (ECC). JAMA 1974;227 (Suppl):833. Used with permission.)

Because artificial circulation must always be combined with artificial ventilation, two-person cardiopulmonary resuscitation (Fig. 4-2) is preferable.[1] One person is positioned at the patient's side and performs external cardiac compression while the other person is positioned at the patient's head and maintains the head-tilt position and performs artificial ventilation. The compression rate is 60 per minute. This rate is practical because it avoids fatigue, simplifies timing (one compression per second), and allows optimum artificial ventilation and circulation to be achieved by quickly interposing one inflation after each five chest compressions without any pause in compressions (5:1 ratio).

The various mechanical resuscitation units that are available may be useful during prolonged resuscitation, which may involve transporting the patient from one hospital to another. However, valuable time may be spent applying the equipment, and direct contact with the patient is lost.

The most common error in resuscitation is failure to establish adequate artificial ventilation. There is little point in pumping desaturated blood through the body. Further, a heart that has developed a bradycardia

Artificial Ventilation Methods

Exhaled-air technique
Bag-valve-mask unit
Tracheal intubation
Cricothyreotomy

or some other life-threatening dysrhythmia will frequently resume normal rhythm when its oxygen supply has improved. Various devices and techniques are available to assist in providing artificial ventilation.

Airway adjuncts (Fig. 4-3) include various tubes that are inserted into the pharynx, a mask that covers the mouth and nose, and an esophageal airway.[23] The esophageal airway is a tube that is inserted into the esophagus without the aid of a laryngoscope. An inflated balloon in the esophagus prevents vomitus from entering the pharynx and air from entering the esophagus. The upper end of the tube passes through a face mask. When one blows into the tube, air travels out the holes in the tube, into the upper airway, and then into the trachea. Self-inflating bag-valve-mask units are desirable not only because they overcome the esthetic deficiency of the mouth-to-mouth or mouth-to-nose method and the concern about HIV transmission, but also because they can be combined with

Figure 4-3. Pulmonary resuscitation. (A) If there is no airway, the chin must be pulled forward and the neck extended to free the tongue from obstructing the airway. Note that the rescuer's cheek occludes the victim's nostrils. (B) Convenient resuscitation with double-ended airway that keeps two sizes available in a single device. The patient's lips should be sealed against the airway. Rise and fall of the chest wall indicates effective air movement. (C) One type of hand-operated respirator. The mask must be pressed firmly against the face. If an airway is not inserted, the position of the head and neck must be the same as that in mouth-to-mouth resuscitation. (D) The asterisk (*) marks the location of the cricothyroid membrane just below the thyroid cartilage where a large-bore needle can be inserted (see text). The plus sign (+) marks the location below the cricoid cartilage where a quick tracheotomy can be performed. (E) Final position of esophageal airway and mask. (Parts A to D modified from Barnhard HJ, Barnhard FM. The emergency treatment of reactions to contrast media. In: Abrams HL, ed. Angiography. 2nd ed. Boston: Little, Brown, 1971. Part E from Goldberg AH. Adjuncts for airway and breathing [ventilation]. In: Sladen A, ed. Advanced cardiac life support manual. Dallas: American Heart Association. Used with permission.)

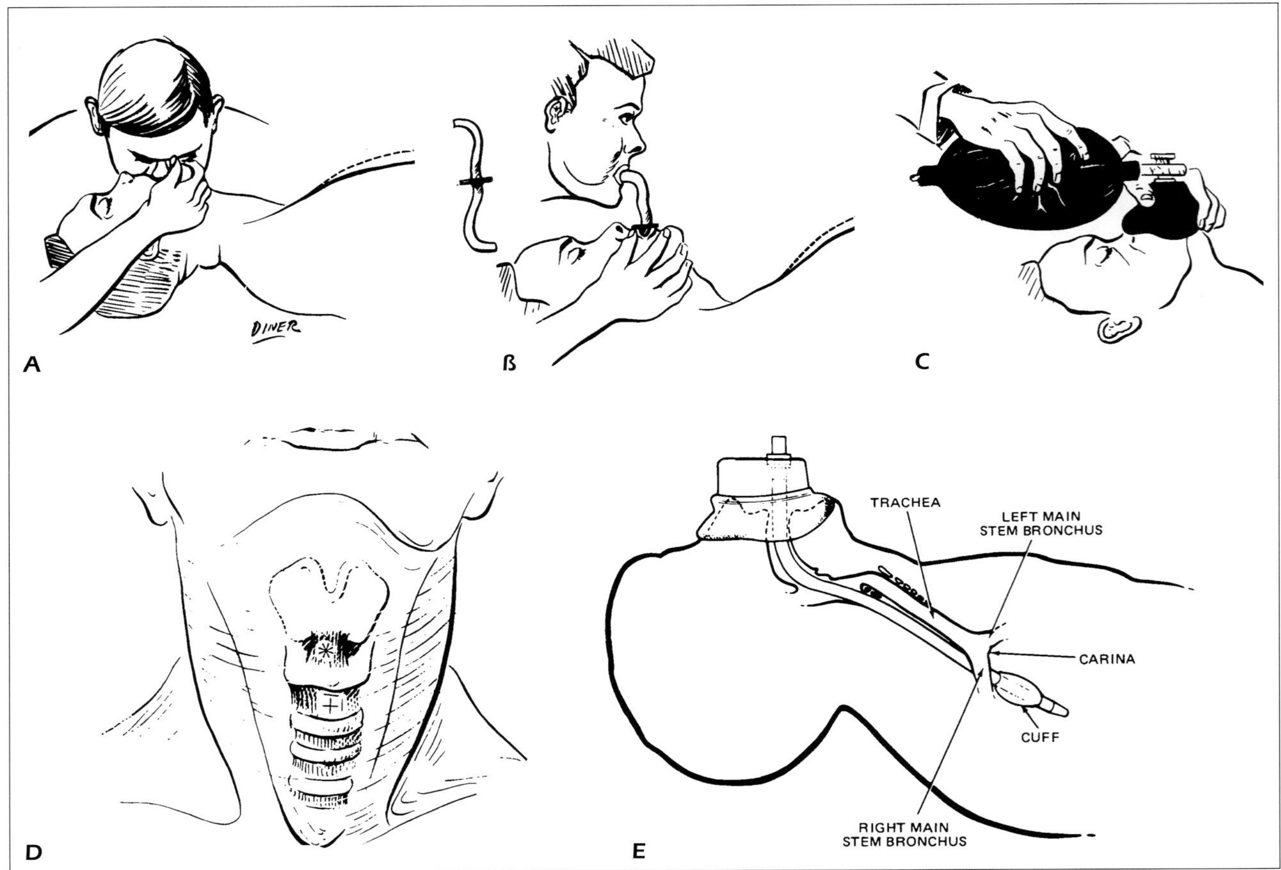

supplementary oxygen to increase the fraction of inspired oxygen delivered to the patient.

If there is difficulty in maintaining patency of the airway, you can use either tracheal intubation or cricothyreotomy (see Fig. 4-3). You should not attempt tracheal intubation unless you are familiar with the technique. Radiologists may feel more comfortable performing cricothyreotomy. Locate the cricothyroid membrane just below the thyroid cartilage in the midline, and either thrust a large-bore (12-gauge) needle through the membrane or make a stab wound with a pointed scalpel blade. Insert a plastic cannula and attach it to a bag-valve unit with appropriately sized connectors. Cricothyreotomy is not without potential complications. Hemorrhage, false passage, perforation of the esophagus, subcutaneous or mediastinal emphysema, or tracheal stenosis may follow.

A patient requiring prolonged cardiopulmonary resuscitation or postresuscitation artificial ventilation certainly should be intubated, but only after the patient has been well ventilated by other means and only by persons skilled in the technique. Tracheal intubation will help prevent aspiration of foreign material, facilitate positive pressure ventilation, and allow a high oxygen concentration to be administered.

Provide oxygen in as high a concentration as possible. Establish and maintain an intravenous infusion to administer drugs and fluids; a percutaneous puncture of the subclavian or internal jugular vein is preferable, but standard peripheral venipuncture may suffice if no one trained in the former technique is present. Give sodium bicarbonate, 1 mEq/kg initially (may be repeated once) and 0.5 mEq/kg at 10-minute intervals, to combat metabolic acidosis, which invariably develops during cardiac arrest.[24] Administer epinephrine early in cardiac arrest to convert "fine" ventricular fibrillation to "coarse" ventricular fibrillation, to restore myocardial contractility in the presence of electromechanical dissociation or asystole, and to facilitate direct current (D.C.) countershock. The usual adult dose is 0.5 to 1.0 mg (0.5–1.0 ml of a 1:1000 solution or 5–10 ml of a 1:10,000 solution) given intravenously. Because of its rapid biodegradation, epinephrine can be given every 5 minutes.

To be effective, external cardiac compression must be done correctly (Fig. 4-4). Place the patient in the horizontal position during external cardiac compression. During cardiac arrest, even with properly performed cardiopulmonary resuscitation there is reduced or absent blood flow to the brain when the body is in the vertical or the head-elevated position. Elevate the lower extremities to promote venous return and to augment artificial circulation during external cardiac compression. Effective cardiac compression must be performed with the patient on a firm surface.

Position yourself close to the patient's side and place the heel of one hand over the lower half of the sternum. You must exercise great care not to place your hand over the lower tip of the sternum (the xiphoid process), which extends downward over the upper abdomen. The other hand is then placed on top of the first hand (the fingers are interlocked). Bring your shoulders directly over the patient's sternum, keep your arms straight, and exert pressure vertically downward to depress the lower sternum a minimum of 1½ to 2 inches. Do not remove your hand from the chest during relaxation but release pressure on the sternum to allow it to return to the normal resting position.

For small children, use only the heel of one hand. For infants, use only the tips of the index and middle fingers (see Fig. 4-4). Because the ventricles of infants and small children lie higher in the chest, you should exert external pressure over the midsternum. Infants require ½- to ¾-inch compressions of the sternum; young children require ¾- to 1½-inch compressions. The compression rate should be 80 to 100 per minute, with breaths delivered as quickly as possible after each five compressions.

Because backward tilt of the head lifts the back of an infant or small child, provide firm support beneath

External Cardiac Compression in Adults

Patient in horizontal position on firm surface
Rescuer close to patient's side, with shoulders at arm's length directly over patient's sternum
Heel of one hand over lower third of sternum, other hand over that hand
Fingers off chest wall
Thrust 1½ to 2 inches vertically downward

Cardiac Resuscitation in Infants and Children

Infants
- Tips of index and middle fingers over midsternum or
- Fingers interlaced behind back with thumbs superimposed over midsternum
- ½- to ¾-inch compressions of sternum

Children
- Heel of one hand over midsternum
- ¾- to 1½-inch compressions of sternum

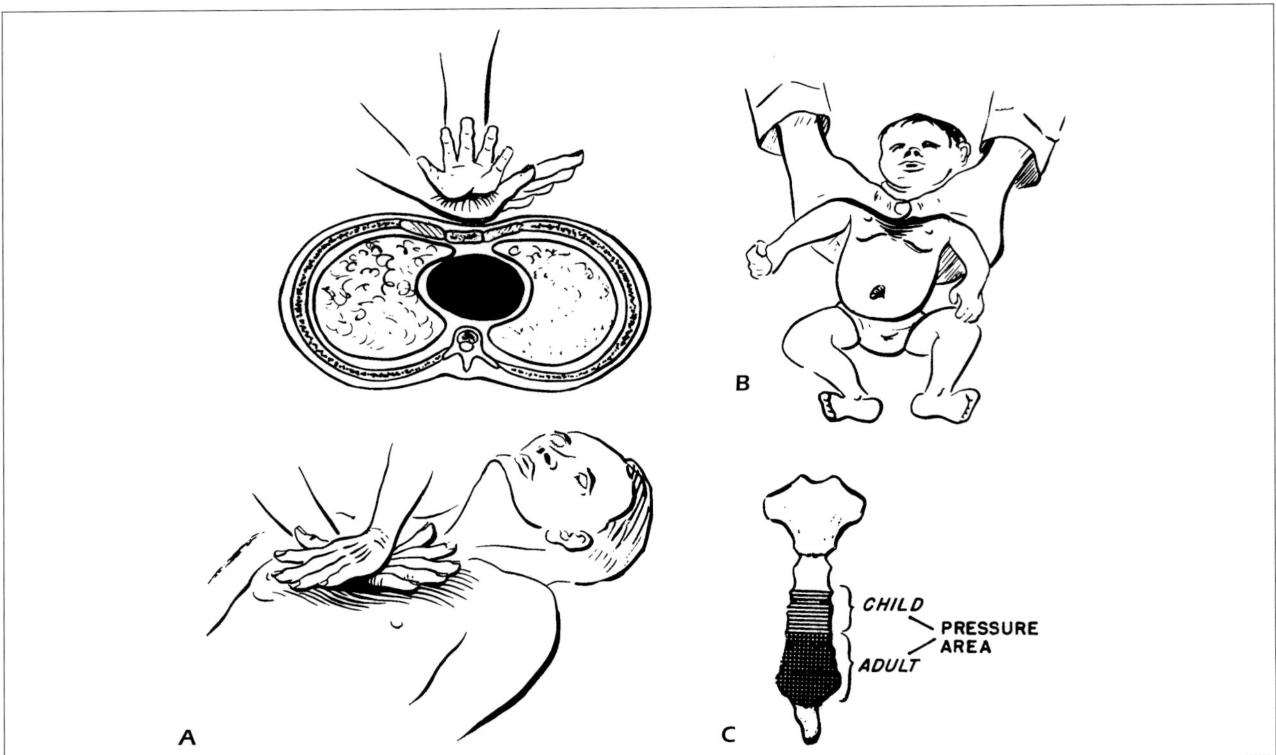

Figure 4-4. External cardiac compression. (A) In an adult, the hands are placed on the chest so that the sternum is pressed against the heart without compression of the ribs. (B) In a child, the fingers are interlaced behind the back while superimposed thumbs transmit pressure to the sternum. (C) The pressure area in the adult is just above the xiphisternum, while the pressure area in a child is at the midsternum. (From Barnhard HJ, Barnhard FM. The emergency treatment of reactions to contrast media. In: Abrams HL, ed. Angiography. 2nd ed. Boston: Little, Brown, 1971. Used with permission.)

the back for external cardiac compression by slipping one hand beneath the child's back while using the other hand to compress the chest. For a small infant, an alternative method is to encircle the chest with the hands and compress the midsternum with both thumbs.

Although many complications of closed-chest cardiac compressions have been described,[25,26] fractured ribs and liver damage due to incorrect hand placement and the use of too much force remain the most common ones.

If external cardiac compression does not appear to be effective, open chest cardiac massage may be required.[19] It should be performed only by skilled personnel who use the required equipment. Indications for open chest cardiac massage include (1) situations in which the chest must be opened (penetrating chest wounds, severe crush injuries, hemothorax, and cardiac tamponade) and (2) chest deformities that make external cardiac compression impossible (flail chest and severe emphysema). Open chest cardiac massage has the definite advantage of providing increased cardiac output.

Check the reaction of the pupils periodically during cardiopulmonary resuscitation. Pupil reaction is the best indication of the delivery of oxygenated blood to the brain. Pupils that constrict when exposed to light indicate adequate oxygenation and blood flow to the brain.[21] If the pupils remain widely dilated and do not react to light, serious brain damage is imminent. Note

Criteria of Effective Cardiopulmonary Resuscitation

Constricted pupils
Carotid pulse palpable
Spontaneous gasping
Swallowing
Movement of extremities
Improved color

that normal pupillary reactions may, however, be altered in the aged and frequently are altered in any patient by the use of drugs.

Palpate the carotid pulse periodically during cardiopulmonary resuscitation to check the effectiveness of external cardiac compression and to search for the return of a spontaneous heartbeat. Palpate the pulse after the first minute of cardiopulmonary resuscitation and every few minutes thereafter.

If resuscitation efforts are going well, improvement should be seen. If they are not, you must reevaluate the airway, breathing, and circulation, step by step, to look for areas that can be improved. Continue the administration of oxygen in maximum concentrations, sodium bicarbonate, 1.0 mEq/kg initially (repeat once), followed by 0.5 mEq/kg every 10 minutes, and epinephrine, 0.5 to 1.0 mg, 1:1000 solution, every 5 minutes.

In the clinically apparent cardiac arrest, you may perform electrical defibrillation with a maximal shock of 200 to 400 watt-seconds before the dysrhythmia is diagnosed.[27,28] "Blind" (unmonitored) defibrillation carries little risk and is justified because 75 percent[29] of the patients in whom cardiac arrest occurs are in ventricular fibrillation rather than cardiac standstill (asystole).

After you have begun immediate lifesaving treatment, the consulting physicians decided on previously should be summoned to aid in ongoing efforts to resuscitate the patient. In-hospital radiologists will call on the cardiac arrest team or will "code blue" for help. Radiologists outside the hospital will call on nearby internists or surgeons for help. Additional drugs and diagnostic and therapeutic equipment should be readily available[30] (see Appendix to this chapter).

Information about recognizing and treating dysrythmias,[31] as well as a complete list and discussion of the American Heart Association's "essential" and "useful" drugs,[1] is given later in the Appendix.

When the patient has been resuscitated (i.e., has a spontaneous, effective heartbeat and spontaneous or assisted ventilations) and when his or her condition has been stabilized, the radiologist and the consulting physicians should have him transported to an intensive care unit. Measures that may be required during transportation to an intensive medical unit include supplemental oxygen therapy, monitoring for cardiac dysrhythmias, repeated defibrillation, and the administration of drugs to (1) stabilize rhythm, (2) maintain adequate perfusion, and (3) relieve pain.

In clinical practice, care after resuscitation has not been adequately emphasized.[21,32] Approximately two-thirds of patients successfully resuscitated die in the hospital. Recurrent cardiac arrest is frequent in the immediate survival period; it indicates not only the severity of the underlying pathology in such patients but also the need for further improvement in therapy.

When to Stop Trying

Cardiac death

Persistent asystole or ventricular fibrillation, or a slow sinusoidal "agonal" rhythm unresponsive to electrical or drug therapy

The period after resuscitation should be one of anticipating complications, which unfortunately are frequent, particularly recurrent cardiac arrest. Factors of importance during the first 24 hours after cardiac arrest include (1) admission to an intensive care unit for proper monitoring and attention, (2) determination and treatment of the primary cause of the arrest, (3) provision of adequate ventilation and circulatory support, (4) continuous ECG monitoring with rapid correction of dysrythmias, (5) utilization of the central venous pressure or the pulmonary artery catheter to monitor cardiac and circulatory status, (6) serial determinations of arterial pH, PO_2, and PCO_2, (7) correction of electrolyte abnormalities, (8) hourly checks of urine output, (9) treatment of hypertension, (10) treatment of hypotension with a view toward improving flow to tissues, (11) chest x-rays to detect fractured ribs, pneumothorax, and other complications of cardiopulmonary resuscitation, and (12) prevention or attenuation of cerebral edema by use of corticosteroids, potent diuretic agents, hypothermia, or controlled hyperventilation.[21]

Unfortunately, many patients do not respond to proper resuscitation and the decision to terminate efforts must be made. You may discontinue cardiopulmonary resuscitation if evidence of brain or cardiac death persists throughout 1 hour of adequate basic and advanced cardiac life support.[19,21,24] The criterion for cardiac death is persistent asystole or ventricular fibrillation or a slow sinusoidal "agonal" rhythm that is unresponsive to electrical or drug therapy. The criteria for brain death are dilated, unresponsive pupils; absence of any spontaneous activity (spontaneous movements or gasping respirations); and complete lack of responsiveness (to such stimuli as pain, touch, sound, or light) in the absence of hypothermia or drug intoxication. When these criteria for brain death are present, further resuscitative efforts either are futile or may produce a patient with only a vegetative existence.

Acknowledgments

This chapter appeared in the third edition coauthored by Drs. Howard Barnhard and F. Allen White. It was updated for this edition by Dr. Stanley Baum.

References

1. American Heart Association and National Academy of Sciences–National Research Council. Standards for cardiopulmonary resuscitation (CPR) and emergency cardiac care (ECC). JAMA (special issue); October 1992.
2. Barnhard HJ, Barnhard FM. The emergency treatment of reactions to contrast media. In: Abrams HL, ed. Angiography. 2nd ed. Boston: Little, Brown, 1971.
3. Manual on Iodinated Contrast Media. Reston, VA: American College of Radiology, 1993.
4. Bush WH. Risk factors and clinical considerations in the management of contrast-induced adverse reactions. In: Parvez Z, Moncada R, Sovak M, eds. Contrast media: biologic effects and clinical application. 3 vols. Boca Raton: CRC Press, 1987: 137–149.
5. Cohan RH, Dunnick NR. Intravascular contrast media: adverse reactions. AJR 1987;149:665–670.
6. Cohan RH, Dunnick NR, Bashore TM. Treatment of reactions to radiographic contrast material. AJR 1988;151:263–270.
7. Greenberger PA, Halwig JM, Patterson R, Wallemark CB. Emergency administration of radiocontrast media in high-risk patients. J Allergy Clin Immunol 1986;77:630–634.
8. Lasser EC, Berry CC, Talner LB, et al. Pretreatment with corticosteroids to alleviate reactions to intravenous contrast material. N Engl J Med 1987;317:845–849.
9. Sheffer AL. Therapy of anaphylaxis. N Engl J Med 1966;275: 1059.
10. Lockey RF, Bukantz SC. Allergic emergencies. Med Clin North Am 1974;58:147.
11. Shehadi WH. Clinical problems and toxicity of contrast agents. AJR 1966;97:762.
12. Ansell G. Adverse reactions to contrast agents, scope of problem. Invest Radiol 1970;5:374.
13. Goldfrank L, Mayer A. Anaphylaxis—the IVP emergency. Hosp Physician 1978;14(8):28.
14. Millbern SM, Bell SD. Prevention of anaphylaxis to contrast medium. Anesthesiology 1979;50:56.
15. Patterson R, Schatz M. Administration of radiographic contrast medium after a prior adverse reaction. Ann Intern Med 1975; 83:277.
16. Zweiman B, Mishkin MM, Hildreth EA. An approach to the performance of contrast studies in contrast material—reactive persons. Ann Intern Med 1975;83:159.
17. Kelly JF, Patterson R. Anaphylaxis, course, mechanisms and treatment. JAMA 1974;227:1431.
18. Morrow DH, Luther RR. Anaphylaxis: etiology and guidelines for management. Anesth Analg 1976;55:493.
19. Goldberg AH. Cardiopulmonary arrest. N Engl J Med 1974; 290:381.
20. Lemire JG, Johnson AL. Is cardiac resuscitation worthwhile? A decade of experience. N Engl J Med 1972;286:970.
21. Grossman JI, Rubin IL. Cardiopulmonary resuscitation: II. Am Heart J 1969;78:709.
22. Grossman JI, Rubin IL. Cardiopulmonary resuscitation: I. Am Heart J 1969;78:569.
23. White RD. Cardiopulmonary resuscitation: a technical and pharmacological update. Wkly Anesthesiol Update 1978;3:1.
24. Hodgkin JE, Foster GL, Nicolay LI. Cardiopulmonary resuscitation: development of an organized protocol. Crit Care Med 1977;5:93.
25. Baldwin JJ, Edwards JE. Rupture of right ventricle complicating closed chest cardiac massage. Circulation 1976;53:562.
26. Patterson RH, Burns WA, Jannotta FS. Complications of external cardiac resuscitation: a retrospective review and survey of the literature. Med Ann DC 1974;43:389.
27. Loeb HS. Cardiac arrest. JAMA 1975;232:845.
28. Shoemaker WC. A patient care algorithm for cardiac arrest. Crit Care Med 1976;4:157.
29. Rosenberg MB, Goldberg MJ, Bourke DL. Cardiac arrest. Orthop Clin North Am 1978;9:733.
30. Safar P, ed. Advances in cardiopulmonary resuscitation. New York: Springer, 1977.
31. Sladen A, ed. Advanced cardiac life support manual. Dallas: The American Heart Association, 1975.
32. Zoll PM. Rational use of drugs for cardiac arrest and after cardiac resuscitation. Am J Cardiol 1971;27:645.
33. White RD. Drugs in cardiac supportive care. Anesth Analg 1976;55:633.

Appendix

Dysrythmia Recognition and Treatment

1. Analyze each ECG rhythm strip in a systematic fashion.
   Is the rate too fast or slow? Are the atrial and ventricular rates equal?
   Are the P-to-P and R-to-R wave intervals regular or irregular? If the rhythm is irregular, is it consistent or is it irregularly irregular?
   Is there a P wave before each QRS complex? Are the P waves and the QRS complexes identical and normal in configuration?
   Are the P-R and the QRS intervals within normal limits?
   What is the significance of the dysrhythmia when it is correlated with clinical observation of the patient?
2. Identify the ECG patterns (Fig. 4-5). Rhythms may include the following:
   Normal sinus rhythm.
   Sinus tachycardia.
   Sinus bradycardia.
   Premature atrial contractions.
   Atrial flutter.
   Atrial fibrillation.
   Atrioventricular block: first, second, third degree.
   Premature ventricular contractions.
   Ventricular tachycardia.
   Ventricular fibrillation, fine.
   Ventricular fibrillation, coarse.
   Cardiac standstill.
3. Recognize the significance of the rhythms and begin treatment.[31,33]
   Normal sinus rhythm
      Significance: Normal. No therapy.
   Sinus tachycardia.
      Significance: The rapid rate may increase cardiac output and precipitate congestive heart failure in the damaged heart.
      Therapy: Treat underlying cause.
   Sinus bradycardia.
      Significance: A common finding in the early period of acute myocardial infarction (MI), which may predispose to premature beats.
      Therapy: Atropine sulfate, to decrease vagal tone, 0.5 mg as a bolus; the dose may be repeated if needed at 5-minute intervals up to a maximum dose of 2 mg. If this fails, try isoproterenol, 1 mg in 500 ml dextrose in water, 1 to 10 ml per minute, titrated. Consider temporary transvenous pacemaker if isoproterenol fails to restore adequate circulation.
   Premature atrial contractions (PACs).
      Significance: Isolated PACs may occur in normal persons. Frequent PACs may indicate organic heart disease and possibly initiate atrial tachydysrhythmias.
      Therapy: Sedation; omission of "stimulants" (alcohol, caffeine, tobacco); occasionally digitalis, quinidine, propranolol, and procainamide may be employed.
   Atrial flutter.
      Significance: Atrial flutter is most common in the presence of organic heart disease.
      Therapy: Directed at slowing ventricular rate. D.C. countershock is effective, especially if clinical status suggests urgency. Digitalis may slow ventricular rate; propranolol is useful.
   Atrial fibrillation.
      Significance: Atrial fibrillation is usually the result of underlying heart disease.
      Therapy: Digitalis, the traditional initial treatment, effectively slows ventricular rate. D.C. shock is usually effective if conversion to normal sinus rhythm (NSR) is essential. Quinidine or propranolol may also be used to convert to NSR.
   Atrioventricular block, first degree.
      Significance: May be the warning of more advanced forms of atrioventricular block in acute MI. It may also be due to digitalis excess.
      Therapy: Usually none. Atropine, isoproterenol, occasionally temporary pacemaker for acute MI.
   Atrioventricular block, second degree, Mobitz type I.
      Significance: It is the less serious type of second-degree atrioventricular block, but it is still quite common in patients with acute inferior MI. Generally transient, the type I block does not necessarily require a pacemaker.
      Therapy: Observation; if ventricular rate very slow, atropine, isoproterenol; rarely, a pacemaker.
   Atrioventricular block, second degree, Mobitz type II.
      Significance: Type II block occurs in large anterior MIs and is commonly a forerunner of sudden complete atrioventricular block.
      Therapy: Standby pacemaker insertion; atropine, etc., only until definitive therapy can be employed.
   Atrioventricular block, third degree.
      Significance: The ventricular rate may be so slow

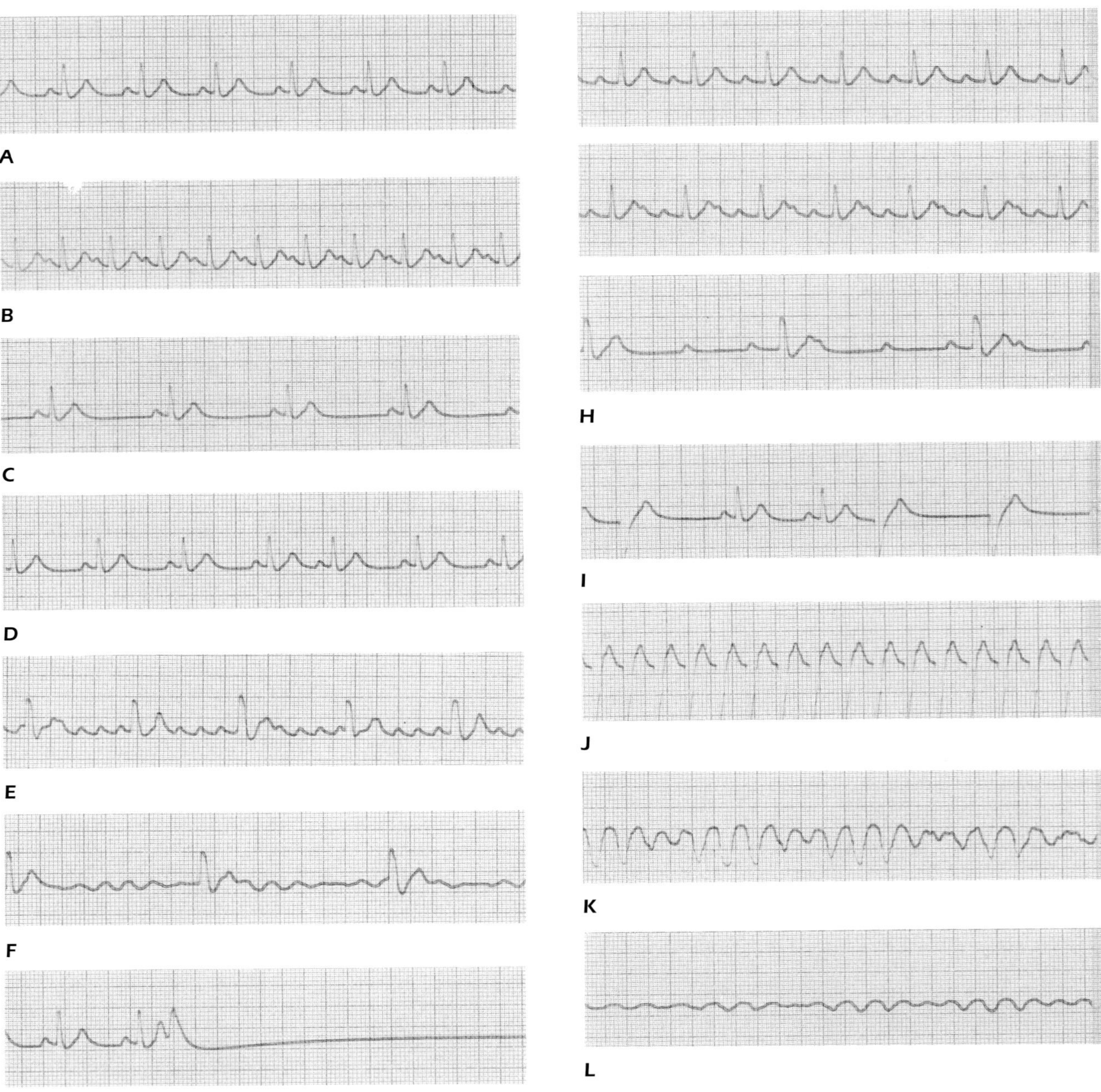

Figure 4-5. ECG rhythms that are commonly seen during cardiopulmonary resuscitation. (A) Normal sinus rhythm; (B) sinus tachycardia; (C) sinus bradycardia; (D) premature atrial contractions; (E) atrial flutter; (F) atrial fibrillation; (G) cardiac standstill; (H) atrioventricular block: first, second, third degree; (I) premature ventricular contractions; (J) ventricular tachycardia; (K) ventricular fibrillation, coarse; (L) ventricular fibrillation, fine.

that circulation cannot be maintained, and syncope, congestive heart failure, or angina may occur.

Therapy: Pacemaker as soon as possible; atropine and/or isoproterenol to try to maintain ventricular rate of 60.

Premature ventricular contractions (PVCs).

Significance: Dangerous signs are frequent PVCs, runs of PVCs, multifocal PVCs, and the R-on-T phenomenon.

Therapy: Lidocaine, 50- to 100-mg bolus, may be repeated once if necessary. Lidocaine infusion, 500 mg in 500 ml dextrose in water, titrated to control the PVCs but not more rapidly than 3 to 4 mg per minute. Other medications—procainamide, phenytoin, propranolol, quinidine, digitalis—may be required.

Ventricular tachycardia.

Significance: A most serious and dangerous dysrhythmia. Ventricular tachycardia may be the precursor of ventricular fibrillation.

Therapy: Lidocaine intravenous bolus, 1 mg/kg, followed by infusion of 500 mg in 500-ml dextrose in water. D.C. countershock, beginning with 50 joules.

Ventricular fibrillation.

Significance: The patient is clinically dead without effective cardiac output.

Therapy: *Immediate* D.C. defibrillation at maximum setting, 400 joules; otherwise, cardiopulmonary resuscitation until defibrillation is available. Sodium bicarbonate IV 50 to 100 mEq (1 mEq/kg), followed by a second dose 5 to 10 minutes later if needed and then by one-half dose every 10 minutes if needed. Epinephrine, 5 ml of 1:10,000 solution, repeated every 5 minutes if needed. Lidocaine, 50- to 100-mg bolus, followed by second identical dose if needed.

Cardiac standstill.

Significance: No cardiac output; the patient is clinically dead.

Therapy: Cardiopulmonary resuscitation, epinephrine, sodium bicarbonate, isoproterenol, calcium chloride intravenously; finally, a pacemaker.

Essential Drugs and Useful Drugs

The national standards for cardiopulmonary resuscitation[13] classify seven drugs as "essential" and nine drugs as "useful." In practice, this distinction does not necessarily apply because useful drugs may suddenly become essential ones. The intent of the distinction is to recognize the drugs most frequently required in emergency cardiac care that are likely to be essential to survival.

1. The objectives of drug treatment during cardiopulmonary resuscitation include the following:
   Correcting hypoxia.
   Correcting metabolic acidosis.
   Increasing perfusion pressure during cardiac compression.
   Stimulating spontaneous or more forceful myocardial contraction.
   Accelerating cardiac rate.
   Suppressing ventricular ectopic activity.
2. The following medications (Table 4-1) must be readily available:

Essential drugs	Useful drugs
Oxygen	Vasoactive drugs
Sodium bicarbonate	Norepinephrine
Epinephrine	Metaraminol
Atropine	Dopamine
Lidocaine	Isoproterenol
Calcium chloride	Propranolol
Morphine sulfate	Procainamide
	Corticosteroids
	Diuretic agents
	Furosemide
	Ethacrynic acid

3. Discussion
   Oxygen heads the list of essential drugs since it protects the brain and other vital organs from irreversible damage. Hypoxia is likely to occur during cardiac arrest because of reduced cardiac output, increased intrapulmonary shunting, and ventilation-perfusion abnormalities. Because oxygen intoxication does not occur for many hours, the concentration of oxygen should be as high as possible until resuscitation is complete or until arterial blood gases and pH indicate that the inspired oxygen concentration can be safely reduced.
   Sodium bicarbonate is used to correct the metabolic acidosis that invariably develops during oxygen deprivation. The usual initial adult dose is 1 mEq/kg IV. The dose can be repeated once; thereafter, one-half the initial dose can be given at 10-minute intervals until resuscitation is complete or until arterial blood gases and pH are satisfactory. Avoid mixing sodium bicarbonate with either epinephrine or calcium because inotropic agent inactivation will result.

Epinephrine should always be administered early in cardiac arrest to convert fine ventricular fibrillation to coarse ventricular fibrillation, to restore myocardial contractility in the presence of electromechanical dissociation or asystole, and to increase the efficacy of D.C. countershock. The usual adult dose is 0.5 to 1.0 mg (0.5–1.0 ml of a 1:1000 solution or 5–10 ml of a 1:10,000 solution) IV. Because of its rapid biodegradation, it can be given every 5 minutes. Epinephrine can be injected directly into the ventricles of the heart (a dangerous procedure), and it is also rapidly ab-

Table 4-1. Recommended Intravenous Dosage

Drug	Adults	Infants/Children	Comments
Essential			
Sodium bicarbonate	1 mEq/kg initially (repeat once); 0.5 mEq/kg at 10-min intervals or as indicated by blood gases	1 ml (0.9 mEq)/kg diluted 1:1 with sterile water (repeat after pH obtained and base deficit calculated)	Do not mix with epinephrine, calcium
Epinephrine	0.5–1.0 ml of 1:1000 solution (repeat at 5-min intervals as needed)	0.1–0.5 ml of 1:1000 solution (repeat at 5-min intervals as needed)	
Atropine	0.5-mg bolus to be given slowly (repeat at 5-min intervals to total dose of 2 mg)	0.01 mg/kg	Total dose in adults can equal 3 mg when third-degree atrioventricular block present
Lidocaine	1 mg/kg bolus (repeat once); dose then continued as IV drip (1–4 ml/min of 0.1% solution)	Infants: 0.5 mg/kg; children: 5 mg (repeat as needed); dose then continued as IV drip	In adults, infusion rate maximum 4 mg/min; infants and children, rate maximum 100 mg/hr
Calcium chloride 10%	2.5–5.0 ml (3.4–6.8 mEq Ca^{++}); dose may be repeated at 10-min intervals	1 ml/5 kg maximum dose	Calcium salts should never be mixed with sodium bicarbonate
Morphine sulfate	1.0–1.5 ml (3.0–4.5 mg) of 3 mg/ml distilled water solution		
Useful			
Norepinephrine	Mix 4 mg in 250 ml D5W; start 4 μg/min (¼ ml) and increase to desired effect	Infants: 0.5 mg 1:250 ml D5W; children: 1 mg in 250 ml D5W; titrate to desired effect	First correct blood volume when hypovolemia has led to cardiac arrest
Metaraminol	2–5-mg bolus given slowly; dose may be continued as drip	25 mg/100 ml D5W	Titrate to desired effect
Dopamine	2–20 μg/kg/min in D5W		Titrate to desired effect
Isoproterenol	Mix 1 mg in 500 ml D5W; start 4 μg/min (2 ml) and titrate to desired effect		
Propranolol	0.5–1.0 mg slowly (repeat as needed to maximum of 3 mg)		Lidocaine should be given first; propranolol is given only if lidocaine fails to establish stable cardiac rhythm
Procainamide	25–50 mg/min; total dose range 0.2–1.0 mg		Lidocaine should be given first

Data from Cohen MR, Turco SJ. Parenteral drugs used in cardiopulmonary resuscitation. Bull Parenter Drug Assoc 1975;29:39; and from Hodgkin JE, Foster GL, Nicolay LI. Cardiopulmonary resuscitation: development of an organized protocol. Crit Care Med 1977;5:93. Used with permission.

sorbed by the tracheobronchial tree. The dose when the drug is given by the latter route is 1 to 2 mg in 10 ml of sterile distilled water.

Atropine sulfate is indicated mainly in hemodynamically significant bradycardia, especially that associated with MI or that complicated by hypotension and PVCs. The initial dose is 0.5 mg given as a bolus, with repeated doses given at 5-minute intervals until the ventricular rate reaches 60 per minute or a maximum dose of 2 mg is reached.

Lidocaine is indispensable in most attempts at cardiac resuscitation although it is of no use to the patient in cardiac standstill. Lidocaine may prevent ventricular fibrillation in the presence of frequent or multifocal PVCs. Control of ventricular tachycardia may be effected with lidocaine, but electrical cardioversion is preferred if the patient also has hypotension. The initial dose of lidocaine is 1 mg/kg IV. Because of the drug's short therapeutic effect, a second bolus may be given, to be followed by a continuous infusion of 1 to 4 ml/min. Rates faster than 4 ml/min may cause convulsions.

Calcium chloride is effective in reversing electromechanical dissociation because it increases myocardial contractility. It is also useful in asystole and in converting fine fibrillation to coarse fibrillation. The adult dose is 2.5 to 5.0 ml of a 10 percent calcium chloride solution (3.4–6.8 mEq Ca^{++}). As mentioned previously, calcium precipitates with sodium bicarbonate and produces an insoluble salt.

Morphine sulfate is the narcotic of choice for relief of pain in patients with suspected MI. The drug may be prepared by diluting 1 ml (15 mg) morphine sulfate with distilled water to a total volume of 5 ml (3 mg morphine sulfate per ml water). Then 1.0 to 1.5 ml (3.0–4.5 mg) of the solution should be given as an initial dose and repeated as necessary.

The drugs classified as useful are most often administered in the postresuscitation period, but they may be indicated in impending arrest situations or as part of the immediate therapy of cardiac resuscitation.

Vasoactive drugs, such as norepinephrine and metaraminol, are useful when systemic peripheral resistance is low, as in the hypotension that often accompanies or follows resuscitation.

Norepinephrine in low doses stimulates beta cardiac receptors, which increases the cardiac output and improves the coronary blood flow. In higher doses, the alpha (vasoconstrictive) effect increases peripheral resistance, causing the heart to work harder. Norepinephrine is administered as an IV drip by preparing a solution of 4 mg in 250 ml of 5 percent dextrose in water (D5W). Administration should begin at a rate of 4 μg/min (¼ ml) and the rate increased until a systolic blood pressure of 90 to 100 mmHg is achieved.

Metaraminol will, in a similar fashion, improve inadequate coronary and cerebral blood flow. It may be given as a bolus of 2 to 5 mg and then continued as a drip.

Dopamine increases beta receptor activity, which increases the cardiac output. In low doses (2–10 μg/kg/min) dopamine may increase the heart rate. In high doses (10–20 μg/kg/min), dopamine stimulates alpha receptors, causing peripheral vasoconstriction and an increase in blood pressure. Splanchnic perfusion is increased by specific dopamine receptors, especially in the kidney. The 5 percent dextrose drip should be titrated to obtain the desired effect.

Isoproterenol is a very useful drug when atropine fails to increase the heart rate in patients with profound sinus bradycardia. Isoproterenol increases cardiac output through its chronotropic and inotropic effects, but because of its tendency to produce dysrhythmias, especially PVCs, it is a difficult drug to use. It is given IV and is prepared as a solution, 1 mg in 500 ml D5W. It should be begun at a rate of 0.4 μg/min and increased to achieve a heart rate of 60 beats per minute.

Propranolol is used to treat specific dysrhythmias, such as ventricular tachycardia and ventricular fibrillation, that after initially responding to standard (lidocaine) therapy repeatedly revert to their original life-threatening character. Propranolol is administered IV at a rate not to exceed 1 mg/min. The usual adult dose is 0.5 to 1.0 mg to a maximum of 3 mg.

Procainamide depresses excitation and conduction in the myocardium. It is useful in treating PVCs and ventricular tachycardia that fail to respond to lidocaine and after countershock when NSR reverts to ventricular fibrillation. Procainamide is infused IV at a maximal rate of 25 to 50 mg/min during ECG monitoring.

Corticosteroids and diuretics may be useful in specific conditions, such as adult respiratory distress syndrome, aspiration, or pulmonary edema, and during the postresuscitation period.

Emergency Cart Equipment and Drugs

We cannot overemphasize the desirability of having emergency equipment and drugs available in your department. Although every hospital certainly possesses such equipment and medications, the nonhospital-based radiologist needs to assemble these materials beforehand, just as the radiologist needs to choose the consulting physicians he or she wishes to call on in the event of cardiac arrest. Emergency carts range in complexity from the most simple, locally designed and stocked carts to the commercially available prefilled cardiopulmonary resuscitation kits (Banyan Emergency Kits). We strongly recommend that the following "essential" equipment be kept close at hand to be used in the event of an emergency; the drugs that are "useful" in providing advanced life support are listed in Table 4-2.

Respiratory Equipment

For airway management and artificial ventilation, the following equipment is essential:

- Oxygen cylinders (two E cylinders) with reducing valves capable of delivering 15 liters per minute
- Mask for mask-to-mouth ventilation
- Oropharyngeal airways
- Laryngoscope with blades (curved and straight, for adult, child, and infant) and extra batteries and bulbs
- Assorted adult-size (cuffed) and child-size (uncuffed) endotracheal tubes with stylet and 15-mm/22 adapters
- Syringe with clamp or plastic valve for endotracheal tube cuff
- Bag-valve-mask with provisions for 100 percent oxygen ventilation

Table 4-2. Strengths and Volumes of Drugs Commonly Used for Emergency Treatment

Drug	Strength	Volume
Essential		
Atropine	0.4 mg	1-ml ampule
Calcium chloride	10%	10-ml ampule
Epinephrine	1:1000	1-ml ampule
Lidocaine HCl	2%	5-ml syringe
Sodium bicarbonate	50 mEq	50-ml bottle
Useful		
Aminophylline	500 mg	20-ml ampule
Calcium gluconate	10%	10-ml ampule
Dexamethasone sodium phosphate (Decadron)	4 mg/ml	5-ml vial
Dextrose solution	50%	50-ml ampule
Digoxin	0.25 mg/ml	2-ml ampule
Diphenhydramine HCl (Benadryl)	10 mg/ml	10-ml vial
Dopamine HCl (Intropin)	40 mg/ml	5-ml ampule
Ephedrine sulfate	50 mg/ml	1-ml ampule
Furosemide (Lasix)	10 mg/ml	2-ml ampule
Hydrocortisone sodium succinate (Solu-Cortef)	250 mg	2-ml Mix-O-Vial
Isoproterenol	1:5000 (0.2 mg/ml)	1- or 5-ml ampule
Levarterenol bitartrate (Levophed)	1 mg/ml	5-ml ampule
Meperidine HCl (Demerol)	50 mg/ml	1-ml ampule
Metaraminol bitartrate (Aramine)	1%	1-ml vial
Methylprednisolone sodium succinate (Solu-Medrol)	125 mg	2-ml Mix-O-Vial
Morphine sulfate	15 mg/ml	20-ml vial
Naloxone HCl (Narcan)	0.4 mg/ml	1-ml ampule
Pancuronium bromide (Pavulon)	1 mg/ml	10-ml vial
Phenylephrine (Neo-Synephrine)	1%	1-ml ampule
Potassium chloride	40 mEq	20-ml ampule
Procainamide HCl (Pronestyl)	100 mg/ml	10-ml vial
Propranolol HCl (Inderal)	1 mg/ml	1-ml ampule
Succinylcholine chloride (Anectine)	20 mg/ml	10-ml vial

Suction device with catheters
Padded tongue depressors
Needle (12-gauge) for cricothyreotomy

The following equipment is optional:

Oxygen reserve equipment (two E cylinders)
Nasogastric tube
Esophageal obturator airway
Tracheotomy tray

Circulatory Equipment

For management of the circulatory system, the following equipment is essential:

Intravenous infusion sets
Indwelling venous catheters
Intravenous solutions (D5W, lactated Ringer)
Cutdown set
Sterile gloves
Assorted syringes and needles, stopcocks, venous extension tubes
Intracardiac needles
Tourniquets, adhesive tape, disposable razor
Sphygmomanometer, stethoscope
Sterile towels, 4 × 4 gauze pads

The following equipment is optional:

Portable defibrillator—monitor with ECG electrode—defibrillator paddles or portable D.C. defibrillator and portable ECG monitor
Portable ECG machine, direct writing, with connection to monitor
Central venous pressure catheters
Urinary catheters
Thoracotomy tray

5

Diagnostic Pharmacoangiography

DOUGLAS C. B. REDD

Pharmacoangiography involves the use of drugs, typically vasoconstrictive or vasodilatory, to modulate blood flow through an organ or vascular bed. This action may enhance the diagnostic value of an angiographic study or modify the outcome of a therapeutic or interventional procedure. This chapter defines the principles that underlie the use of selected pharmacologic agents; examines their toxicities, limitations, and clinical indications; and reviews their diagnostic potential. This discussion also briefly reviews the cell biology and vascular physiology of blood vessels and the pharmacology of readily available agents most germane to angiography, and introduces some topics under investigation in the basic science laboratory that may find future clinical utility. Other chapters present more detailed accounts of the use of selected agents in specific diagnostic or therapeutic angiographic applications.

General Characteristics of Pharmacologic Agents

The general characteristics important for any agent used for pharmacoangiography are efficacy, safety, availability, and reasonable cost. It is essential that the response to an agent be extremely predictable, because diagnostic information may be erroneous if a system fails to respond. Each agent has its own dose-response curve and should be of sufficient potency and safety to be effective in virtually all patients.

The toxicity of any agent can be classified as hypersensitivity (allergic), dose-related, or idiosyncratic.[1] *Hypersensitivity* reactions represent the most common form of toxicity and result from previous sensitization to a particular agent or related compound. Foreign macromolecules may function effectively in the induction of an immune response; however, in order for drugs of lower molecular weight to induce a similar antigenic response, the drug or a metabolite acting as a hapten must bind to an endogenous protein to form an antigenic complex, which then induces antibody formation. Upon subsequent exposure to the antigen, reaction with a cell-fixed IgE antibody results in an immunologic response typical of allergy.[2] Hypersensitivity reactions may be further categorized as anaphylactic (immediate), accelerated, or delayed. Anaphylactic reactions typically occur within 30 minutes after the administration of an agent; accelerated reactions occur within the first few hours. Both of these reactions involve the release of biologically active substances (e.g., histamine, heparin, leukotrienes, eosinophil chemotactic factor of anaphylaxis, neutrophil chemotactic factor, and neutral proteases) from the secretory granules of blood basophils, or their tissue equivalent (mast cells), resulting in a physiologic response of variable magnitude.[3]

To circumvent *dose-related* toxicity, an agent should be highly specific for the system under study and have minimal effects on other organ systems at dosages required for pharmacoangiography. Some agents (e.g., acetylcholine, bradykinin, and the prostaglandins) are rapidly degraded by local or systemic mechanisms. Other agents, like papaverine, are metabolized more slowly; thus accumulation may result, which increases the likelihood of a systemic response.[4] Additional safety is conferred when a specific, competitive antagonist may be administered for the treatment of systemic or cardiovascular side effects. For example, phentolamine binds reversibly to the alpha-adrenergic receptor, blocking the systemic actions of sympathomimetic amines.[5]

Idiosyncrasy is the genetically determined abnormal reactivity to certain chemicals or agents; the observed physiologic response is qualitatively similar among persons of like genetic predisposition.[2,6] For example, in approximately 10 percent of black males who receive primaquine, an antimalarial drug, a serious hemolytic anemia follows as a result of erythrocytic deficiency of glucose-6-phosphate dehydrogenase.

Cell Biology and Physiology of Blood Vessels

Endothelial cells (ECs) line the vascular tree, forming a monolayer whose long axis is oriented in the direction of blood flow.[7] These cells may be identified by specific morphologic characteristics and by staining for factor VIII–related antigen (von Willebrand factor).[8] ECs contribute to the formation and maintenance of subendothelial components of the vessel wall by synthesizing components of both the basement membrane (e.g., types IV and V collagen, laminin, and proteoglycans) and extracellular matrix (e.g., fibronectin).[9] They modify the processes of thrombolysis and hemostasis actively by releasing substances locally (e.g., heparin, prostacyclin, and plasminogen activator), and passively by preventing contact between blood elements and subendothelial components of the vessel wall. ECs participate in the vasomotor response of the vessel wall through the local production and release of both vasodilators (e.g., endothelium-derived relaxing factor [EDRF] and prostacyclin) and vasoconstrictors (e.g., the endothelins and a local renin–angiotensin II system).[10,11]

The pharmacologic response of an agent upon the vasculature may be through an endothelium-independent mechanism (e.g., nitrodilators) that acts directly upon the vascular smooth muscle cells (SMCs) or indirectly through processes that depend on an intact, functional endothelium. Such endothelium-dependent substances include acetylcholine, adenosine phosphate, arachidonic acid, arginine vasopressin, bradykinin, epinephrine, histamine, norepinephrine, serotonin, and thrombin (Fig. 5-1). Agents acting through an endothelium-dependent mechanism may involve an agent-specific receptor and result in the ultimate release of one or more mediators (e.g., EDRF or endothelium-derived hyperpolarizing factor) that induce relaxation of the subjacent vascular smooth muscle.[12–14]

EDRF shares pharmacologic similarity with nitrodilator drugs and may be identical to nitric oxide (NO), which is synthesized by the endothelial cell from L-arginine.[15–17] Following diffusion of EDRF (NO) into the vascular smooth muscle cell, enzymatic activation

Figure 5-1. Proposed sites of action of various vasoactive agents acting through endothelium-dependent mechanisms. By the activation of specific receptors on or within endothelial cells, endothelial-derived relaxing factor(s) (EDRF) and nitric oxide (NO) are released, which in turn promote relaxation of the subjacent vascular smooth muscle cells. *ACh*, acetylcholine; *M*, muscarinic receptors; H_2, histaminergic receptors; *AVP*, arginine vasopressin; VP_1, vasopressinergic receptors; *A*, adrenaline (epinephrine); *NA*, noradrenaline (norepinephrine); α_2, alpha$_2$-adrenergic receptor; *AA*, arachidonic acid; *ADP*, adenosine diphosphate; P_1, purinergic receptors; 5-HT, 5-hydroxytryptamine (serotonin); S_1, serotonergic receptors; *T*, thrombin receptors. (Adapted from Vanhoutte PM. Endothelium and control of vascular function: state of the art lecture. Hypertension 1989;13(6):658–667. Copyright 1989 American Heart Association.)

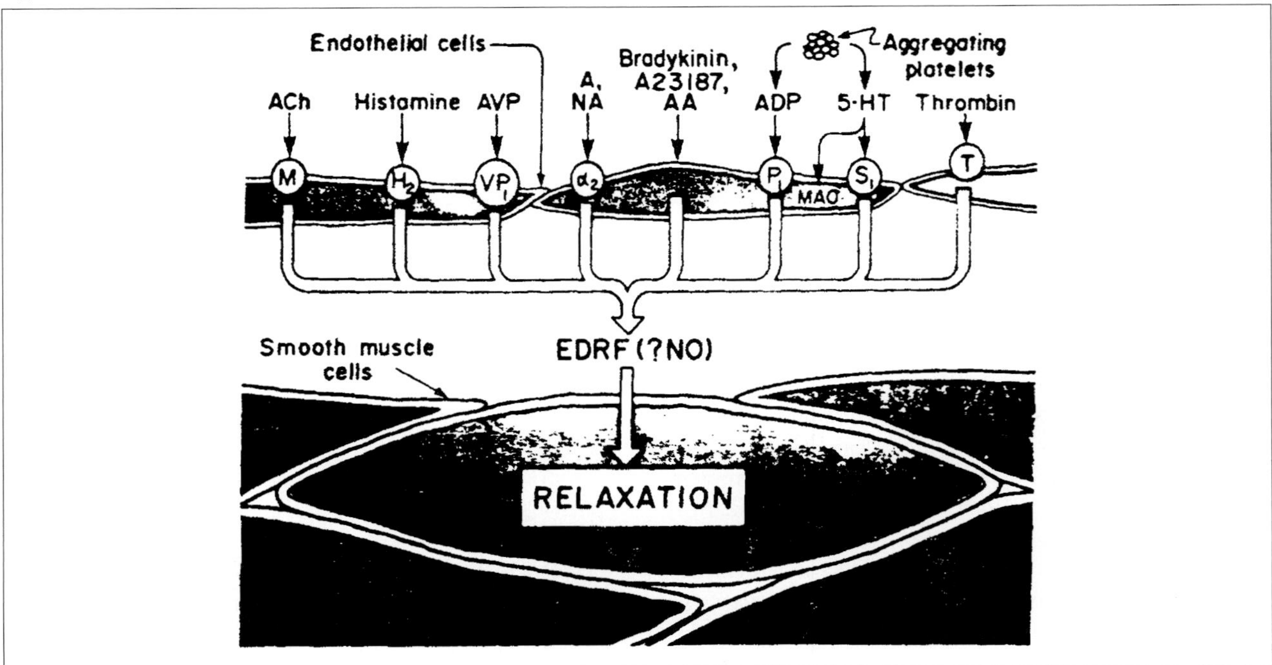

promotes conversion of cyclic guanosine triphosphate (cGTP) into cyclic guanosine monophosphate (cGMP), resulting in sequestration of intracellular calcium ion (Ca^{++}). As the concentration of free cytoplasmic Ca^{++} decreases, vascular smooth muscle relaxation ensues. As with nitrate therapy, vasodilatation results as long as there is diffusion of EDRF into the underlying vascular SMCs.

The endothelins represent an important class of vasoconstrictor agents that are synthesized and released by ECs. Endothelin-1, a subtype, has a pressor potency ten times greater than that of angiotensin II.[18] Circulating levels of endothelin, although not altered after diagnostic angiography, are significantly increased after angioplasty and thus may represent an important mediator of vasospasm after interventions like percutaneous transluminal angioplasty (PTA).[19]

Vascular smooth muscle is capable of responding to a wide variety of agents that induce alterations in either blood flow or vessel capacitance. SMCs constitute a variable percentage of the composition of the vessel wall and are in highest concentration in the arterioles,[20] where they are maintained in a contractile phenotype under a myriad influences, including the local release of heparin from the overlying ECs.[21] This functional state is characterized by a diminished ability to divide, sparse endoplasmic reticulum and synthetic organelles, and decreased production of extracellular matrix.[10,22] Following vascular injury, vascular SMCs are converted into a synthetic phenotype with diminished contractile capability and a markedly increased intracellular apparatus for synthetic function.[23] In addition to their vasoconstrictor action in vivo, agents like angiotensin II also promote hypertrophy of cultured vascular smooth muscle cells.[24] For this reason, angiotensin-converting enzyme (ACE) inhibitors are being evaluated for the prevention of restenosis following percutaneous transluminal coronary angioplasty (PTCA).

The sympathetic nervous system provides major control over peripheral vascular resistance through action at the postganglionic $alpha_1$-adrenergic receptors. Upon stimulation, norepinephrine is released at the neuromuscular junction and mediates an influx of Ca^{++} into the vascular SMC that is followed by contraction, an effect that is independent of both adenylate cyclase activity and intracellular cyclic adenosine monophosphate (cAMP) concentration. This vasoconstrictive action is of greatest functional importance in the arterioles, smaller veins, and microcirculation, where tonic activity maintains most vessels at one-half of their maximal diameter.[25] Capacitance vessels show greater response to sympathetic stimulation than do resistance vessels, and require a lower threshold of stimulation for maximal constriction. Smooth muscle relaxation and passive vasodilatation are observed as cytoplasmic Ca^{++} is sequestered after uptake by the sarcoplasmic reticulum.[26] Many other humoral factors (e.g., local and circulating hormones) are capable of modulating the local release of neurotransmitters from the nerve terminal, thereby eliciting a variable response in different vascular beds.[27] Table 5-1 details the vascular response to the stimulation of adrenergic and cholinergic receptors at various sites within the vascular system.

The beta-adrenergic receptor mediates a vasodilator response in peripheral vascular beds, especially within skeletal muscle. Activation results in increased cytoplasmic concentration of cAMP with resultant smooth muscle relaxation.[28] Additional vasodilatory effects result from sympathetic cholinergic innervation of resistance vessels of both skeletal muscle and skin. Excitement or apprehension activates this system, inducing vasodilatation, especially in skeletal muscle, in anticipation of their use. Most vascular SMCs have uninnervated muscarinic (cholinergic) receptors that also effect vasodilatation; the mesenteric and renal vascular

Table 5-1. Vascular Response to Adrenergic and Cholinergic Receptors

Vascular Site	Receptor Type	Response
Coronary arteriole	Alpha-adrenergic	Constriction +
	$Beta_2$-adrenergic	Dilatation[a] ++
	Cholinergic	Dilatation ±
Skin and mucosa arteriole	Alpha-adrenergic	Constriction +++
	Cholinergic	Dilatation[b]
Skeletal muscle arteriole	Alpha-adrenergic	Constriction ++
	$Beta_2$-adrenergic	Dilatation[a,c] ++
	Cholinergic	Dilatation[d] +
Pulmonary arteriole	Alpha-adrenergic	Constriction +
	$Beta_2$-adrenergic	Dilatation[a]
	Cholinergic	Dilatation[b]
Renal arteriole	$Alpha_1$-adrenergic	Constriction +++
	$Beta_1$, $beta_2$-adrenergic	Dilatation[c] +
Abdominal viscera arteriole	Alpha-adrenergic	Constriction +++
	$Beta_2$-adrenergic	Dilatation[c] +
Systemic vein	$Alpha_1$-adrenergic	Constriction ++
	$Beta_2$-adrenergic	Dilatation ++

[a]Dilatation predominates in situ because of metabolic regulatory phenomena.
[b]Cholinergic vasodilatation at these cites is of questionable physiologic significance.
[c]Over the usual concentration range of physiologically released, circulating epinephrine, beta-adrenergic receptor response (vasodilatation) predominates in blood vessels of skeletal muscle and liver, whereas alpha-adrenergic receptor response (vasoconstriction) predominates in blood vessels of other abdominal viscera. The renal and mesenteric vessels also contain specific dopaminergic receptors, activation of which causes vasodilatation.
[d]Sympathetic cholinergic system causes vasodilatation in skeletal muscle, but this is not involved in most physiologic responses.
Adapted from Weiner N, Taylor P. Neurohumoral transmission: the autonomic and somatic motor nervous systems. In: Gilman AG, et al, eds. The pharmacological basis of therapeutics. 7th ed. New York: Macmillan, 1985: 66–99. Used with permission.

beds also contain dopaminergic receptors, which also result in vasodilatation.[29]

Pharmacoangiographic Agents

Since the first use of epinephrine as a vasoconstrictor some 30 years ago to enhance the visualization of renal tumors,[30,31] many vasoconstrictor agents have been evaluated in other vascular beds for both diagnostic imaging and therapeutic intervention. For example, vasopressin has been shown to be useful in controlling gastrointestinal hemorrhage[32] and portal hypertension,[33] and ergonovine has found application during coronary arteriography in the evaluation of Prinzmetal angina.[34] Vasodilators (e.g., tolazoline [Priscoline] and papaverine) have been employed to reverse vasoconstriction associated with nonocclusive intestinal ischemia.[35,36] Tables 5-2 through 5-4 summarize the preparation and administration of a variety of pharmacologic agents, including vasoconstrictor and vasodilator agents, useful in the practice of diagnostic and therapeutic angiography.

Vasoconstrictors

Pharmacologic maneuvers directed at manipulating a visceral vascular bed during angiography have been explored in great detail in the kidney. Both microscopic and microangiographic studies have shown that malignant tumors are supplied by both normal, preformed vessels and by primitive vessels that lack elastic tissue and muscle elements.[37] Thus early pharmacoangiographic application was in the use of vasoconstrictor agents (e.g., the catecholamines, epinephrine and norepinephrine, and angiotensin) to separate normal vessels from the abnormal neovasculature of tumors. However, this pharmacologic maneuver lacks sensitivity and specificity because the vascular anatomy in more highly differentiated tumors may be relatively preserved and thereby retain the ability to respond to these pharmacologic agents;[38] in contrast, less well differentiated tumors with a highly primitive neovascular structure may be more readily detectable because of their lack of response to a pharmacologic or neurohumoral challenge.

Diagnostic and therapeutic considerations that may dictate the use of a vasoconstrictor agent or combination of agents include the attempt to further define a questionable area of neovascularity shown on a control angiogram; to better delineate the margins of a highly vascular tumor; to ascertain the vasoreactivity of suspected tumor vessels; to enhance filling of pancreaticoduodenal branches when superselective injection is not feasible;[39] and to control acute gastrointestinal bleeding.

Table 5-2. Vasoconstrictor Agents Used During Pharmacoangiography

Agent	Dosage and Preparation
Epinephrine	Preparation: mix 1 ml epinephrine (1:1000) in 500 ml 5% dextrose in water or normal saline (2 μg/ml). Celiac and mesenteric arteriography: 8–12 μg/min infused intraarterially over 2 min followed by 5–10 ml saline flush immediately prior to contrast injection. Renal arteriography: 3–6 μg diluted in 10 ml normal saline infused intraarterially followed by 5–10 ml saline flush 30 sec prior to contrast injection; for demonstrating neoplastic vessels, contrast injection rate should be decreased by 30%.
Epinephrine	Renal venography: 10–12 μg infused into the renal artery followed by 5–10 ml saline flush; contrast then injected retrograde into the renal vein. Duration of action: diagnostic effects of epinephrine last approximately 2 min.
Norepinephrine	Preparation: dilute a 4-ml ampule (4 mg norepinephrine) into 1000 ml 5% dextrose and water or saline (4 μg/ml). Therapy for blood pressure support: intravenous infusion should be initiated into a large vein centrally at a rate of 2–3 ml/min (8–12 μg norepinephrine/min); titrate to the desired blood pressure response (e.g., 80–100 mmHg) sufficient to maintain perfusion of vital organs.
Vasopressin	Preparation: mix 100–200 units of vasopressin in 500 ml normal saline or 5% dextrose in water (0.2–0.4 units/ml). Dosage and method: infuse intraarterially by constant infusion pump; initial rate of 60 ml/hr (0.2–0.4 units/min) for superior mesenteric arterial infusion; dosage lowered for inferior mesenteric arterial infusion.

Catecholamines

Two synaptic neurotransmitter substances, norepinephrine or acetylcholine, are released by the sympathetic and parasympathetic nervous system; fibers that secrete norepinephrine are termed *adrenergic*, and those secreting acetylcholine are termed *cholinergic*. Adrenergic receptors regulate vascular, cardiac, bronchiolar, and gastrointestinal smooth muscle tone and were first described by Ahlquist in 1948.[40] Three types of adrenergic receptors have been described: alpha-adrenergic ($alpha_1$ and $alpha_2$), beta-adrenergic ($beta_1$ and $beta_2$), and dopaminergic.[41–43] Stimulation of the dopaminergic receptor by low-dose dopamine results in increased mesenteric and renal blood flow, and higher doses of dopamine induce alpha-adrenergic ef-

Table 5-3. Vasodilator Agents Used During Pharmacoangiography

Agent	Dosage and Preparation
Papaverine	Treatment of mesenteric ischemia: supplied in ampules or vials containing 30 mg/ml, papaverine is administered intraarterially by injection (30-mg single dose) or continuous infusion (30–60 mg/hr) over several hours.
Tolazoline (Priscoline)	Diagnostic arteriography: intraarterial infusion (25–50 mg diluted in 5% dextrose in water or normal saline) delivered slowly intraarterially over 2–3 min immediately before contrast injection.
Phentolamine (Regitine)	Prevention and control of hypertensive episodes: intravenous injection, 5 mg intraarterially, 100 μg/min.
Nitroglycerine	Preparation: dilute 15 mg in 150 ml 5% dextrose in water for concentration of 100 μg/ml; protect from light until use. Angina pectoris and cardiac ischemia: 0.3 mg orally or sublingually, 10–100 μg/min intravenous infusion. Percutaneous angioplasty: intraarterial bolus (100–200 μg) is beneficial to prevent or treat vasospasm caused by catheter or guidewire manipulation.
Reserpine	Antihypertensive: oral dose (0.1–1.0 mg/d) usually in two divided doses.
Nifedipine	Percutaneous angioplasty: sublingual administration (10 mg) before angioplasty.
Iodinated contrast media	Iodinated contrast agent: a bolus priming dose of 10–15 ml of iodinated contrast medium (e.g., 76%) injected over 1–2 sec, 30–40 sec before selective arteriography.

fects resulting in mesenteric and renal vasoconstriction.

Alpha$_1$ receptors are present in the postsynaptic region of neurons and vascular SMCs, where stimulation leads to vasoconstriction. Presynaptic alpha$_2$ receptors modulate alpha-receptor tone in large blood vessels and provide a counterregulatory mechanism for alpha$_1$ receptor activity through the inhibition of release and accumulation of neurotransmitter (norepinephrine). Postsynaptic alpha$_2$ receptors are also capable of mediating venous and arteriolar vasoconstriction, an action blunted by calcium channel blockers.[44] Different tissues may possess both beta$_1$ and beta$_2$ receptors in varying proportions, with beta$_1$ receptors predominating in cardiac tissues and beta$_2$ receptors predominating in smooth muscle and gland cells.[45] The relative composition of alpha- and beta-adrenergic receptors within a vascular bed determines the overall response to catecholamines. Over the range of physiologically released, circulating epinephrine, beta-receptor response (vasodilatation) predominates in blood vessels of skeletal muscle and liver. In the mesenteric and renal arteries, catecholamines function as vasoconstrictors through preferential alpha-adrenergic activity.[46]

Table 5-4. Use of Glucagon During Pharmacoangiography

Agent	Dosage and Preparation
Glucagon	Preparation: dissolve lyophilized glucagon in diluent solution provided. Adjunct for visceral arteriography: intravenous infusion of 0.5–1.0 mg a few minutes before visceral angiography; onset of action is 1 min and duration 9–17 min.

Epinephrine is an endogenous catecholamine with both alpha- and beta-adrenergic activity. Epinephrine elicits a complex pharmacologic response in the cardiovascular system that includes an increase in systemic vascular resistance, arterial blood pressure, heart rate, myocardial contractility, and coronary and cerebral blood flow. Norepinephrine differs chemically from epinephrine in that it lacks a methyl group on the terminal amine. These neurohormones are equipotent at the beta$_1$-adrenergic receptor; epinephrine is equal to or more potent than norepinephrine at the alpha$_1$-adrenergic receptor. At the beta$_2$-adrenergic receptor, epinephrine is much more potent than norepinephrine. At the alpha$_2$-receptor, epinephrine is either more or less potent than norepinephrine, depending on the tissue.[45] Epinephrine exerts a profound effect on the peripheral blood vessels, where it induces arterial and venous vasoconstriction. In skeletal muscle, low concentrations of epinephrine increase blood flow by dilating resistance vessels (beta-adrenergic effect), whereas in skin only vasoconstriction is elicited. The primary effect of norepinephrine in most vascular beds is vasoconstriction (alpha-adrenergic effect).

Epinephrine and norepinephrine have a rapid onset of action (minutes) and short duration when administered intravascularly; when administered subcutaneously, onset is rapid but action may be prolonged (hours). Since they are naturally occurring neurohormones, these substances never evoke an allergic response. Two principal mechanisms are responsible for inaction of catecholamines: first, they are reaccumulated by the nerve terminal where the catecholamines are stored; second, they are degraded primarily by monoamine oxidase (MAO) and catechol-O-methyltransferase (COMT) upon circulation through the liver. In large doses, systemic effects may be encountered; these include a hypertensive response due to increased systemic vascular resistance, tachycardia, increased myocardial oxygen consumption, and increased ventricular contractility. Because of the rapid peripheral inactivation of catecholamines, treatment of acute toxicity is mainly supportive. Rarely, a rapidly acting alpha-adrenergic blocking agent (e.g., phentolamine) may be required to counteract the pressor effect.

The clinical indications for epinephrine administration during diagnostic pharmacoangiography include differentiation of normally vasoconstricting vessels from abnormal vasculature, where the vasoactive response may be variable. The failure of vessels within a neoplastic or inflammatory lesion to constrict following epinephrine administration helps in the detection of renal neoplasms, since normal renal vessels maximally constrict after intraarterial epinephrine infusion into the renal vascular bed.[30,31] By reducing renal blood flow, retrograde injection into the corresponding renal vein gives excellent visualization of the renal venous system. This may be of value in evaluating patients with suspected renal inflammatory disease, renal neoplasm, or renal vein thrombosis.[47–49] The literature on the use of epinephrine to enhance tumor diagnosis is extensive; for example, epinephrine is used to distinguish inflammatory from neoplastic gastrointestinal lesions and to improve visualization of tumor vessels, including ovarian carcinomas, bone and soft tissue sarcomas, and pancreatic neoplasms.[31,50–55] In an experimental animal model, epinephrine has been shown to increase hepatic arterial and portal venous resistance, which is followed by a concomitant diminution of oxygen consumption, liver weight, and bile flow. With the exception of decrease in bile flow, these effects are inhibited by alpha-adrenergic antagonists, the most potent of which is phenoxybenzamine.[56]

Catecholamines may also be useful in visualizing adjacent structures that are otherwise hypoperfused relative to a more vascular structure. For example, if blood flow is diverted away from a vasoconstricted kidney, there is enhanced visualization of the adrenal gland following intrarenal epinephrine administration.[57] Because the results with commonly used vasoconstrictors are inconsistent, in particular within the mesenteric circulation, some authors have investigated the combined action of a beta-adrenergic blocking agent (propranolol) together with epinephrine.[39,58,59]

Norepinephrine (Levophed) is useful for the treatment of hemodynamically significant hypotension that is refractory to other sympathomimetic amines. It is also useful when systemic vascular resistance is low, as may be encountered in sepsis.

In general, catecholamines are contraindicated in patients with organic brain damage and narrow-angle glaucoma. When catecholamines are used, adverse reactions must always be anticipated and appropriate medical therapy must be implemented as dictated by the clinical situation. Known reactions following catecholamine administration include dizziness, headache, anxiety, palpitations, respiratory difficulty, hypertension, tachycardia, and ventricular arrhythmias.

Angiotensin

Potent, naturally occurring vasoconstrictive peptide hormones have been identified. These include the endothelins and angiotensin, a product of the renin-angiotensin system.[60–62] After the intravenous administration of angiotensin I, a decapeptide, peptidase activity rapidly converts it into angiotensin II, an octapeptide, resulting in both agents having an indistinguishable pharmacologic response. Angiotensin II is rapidly degraded by amino peptidases in both tissues and plasma and has a half-life of approximately 20 seconds. After intraarterial administration for visceral arteriography, most of the angiotensin effect is dissipated within 1 to 2 minutes.[63] After injection of angiotensin II into the renal artery, Jekell et al. observed the onset of vasoconstrictive effects within 4 to 8 seconds, which reached a maximum at 90 seconds and dissipated by 3 minutes. They noted a 5 percent reduction in renal length 90 seconds after the injection with a return to baseline length by 8 minutes.[63] Alterations in renal length appear to be due to vasoconstriction, as well as to changes in the glomerular filtration rate (GFR) and tubular reabsorption. When infused in a dose of 10 ng/kg of body weight, significant decreases in renal blood flow and GFR are observed, suggesting an effect on both pre- and postglomerular renal vessels.[63]

Local infusion of angiotensin can be used in evaluating renal tumors because this agent provokes a vasoconstrictive effect in normal renal vessels, an action that usually does not occur in tumor vessels; thus renal tumors may be rendered more visible by selective intraarterial infusion during renal arteriography.[63–67] This agent has also been employed in attempts to enhance visualization of other tumors (e.g., bone and soft tissue neoplasms[51,68]), as well as to improve visualization of pancreatic,[62] celiac, mesenteric, and peripheral vessels.[69] Sasaki et al. report that an intraarterial infusion of angiotensin II (10 μg/min) is effective in transiently increasing tumor blood flow in human hepatic cancers relative to nontumor regions (tumor-nontumor blood flow ratio 3:3); a peak effect occurs approximately 100 seconds after infusion.[70]

The drug angiotensin amide (Hypertensin, Ciba Pharmaceutical) is available in Europe but not in the United States, and may be administered by slow IV infusion (0.01–0.20 μg/kg/min) for the treatment of hypotensive crises, when cardiac dysrhythmias induced by sympathomimetic amines are potentially hazardous.[60] Because it occurs naturally in humans, allergic reaction is unlikely following intravascular administration. Desensitization to angiotensin may occur in clinical situations in which the renin–angiotensin system is activated (e.g., cirrhosis and congestive heart failure); however, little information is available to determine whether this effect is of clinical significance.

Antidiuretic Hormone

Antidiuretic hormone (ADH), or 8-arginine vasopressin, is a nonapeptide that is a product of the posterior pituitary and is found in all mammals except swine.[71] This hormone alters the permeability of the renal tubules to water and urea. Pitressin (Parke-Davis) is an aqueous solution of synthetic 8-arginine vasopressin standardized to contain 20 pressor units/ml. In the splanchnic bed, this agent results in contraction of smooth muscles of the GI tract with accompanying vasoconstriction of the splanchnic circulation. Its action at the small arteriolar and capillary level results in diminished mesenteric, gastric, and splenic arterial blood flow.[72] Such action is desirable in the treatment of acute gastrointestinal hemorrhage, when constriction of bleeding vessels promotes hemostasis.[32]

In an experimental portal hypertension model in dogs, Nusbaum et al. demonstrated that the infusion of fractionated doses of vasopressin directly into the superior mesenteric artery resulted in a significant decrease in both the superior mesenteric arterial flow and in portal venous pressure with no evidence of decrease in cardiac output. Additionally, continuous or repeated fractionated doses of vasopressin maintained these actions without causing tachyphylaxis, as is observed with catecholamines.[33] After initial animal experiments suggested that intravenous infusions of vasopressin were as effective as intraarterial infusion in reducing gastrointestinal blood flow,[73,74] intravenous therapy of gastrointestinal hemorrhage in humans was evaluated in anticipation of permitting greater ease of administration with fewer complications than are associated with intraarterial infusion.[75,76] The effect of selective mesenteric arterial infusion of vasopressin is usually evaluated by comparing a mesenteric arteriogram performed 15 to 20 minutes after beginning the infusion with a preliminary control arteriogram. In humans, the postinfusion arteriogram demonstrates a reduction in caliber of major mesenteric arterial branches; the degree of constriction is thought to correlate with a reduction in arterial blood flow. Proximal arterial vasoconstriction is not a constant response to intraarterial vasopressin infusion, and both site-[77] and species-specific effects have been described.[78]

Like other peptide hormones, vasopressin has a fairly rapid onset of action (15–30 minutes) when used to control gastrointestinal bleeding. Because of its short half-life (minutes), continuous infusion is required to control gastrointestinal hemorrhage. Vasopressin must be used with caution because adverse hemodynamic effects upon the heart and systemic circulation may be observed (e.g., myocardial ischemia and infarction, cardiac dysfunction and ventricular arrhythmias) as a result of decreased coronary artery blood flow and increased systemic blood pressure. Simultaneous nitroglycerin (NTG) administration may minimize the cardiotoxic effects of vasopressin and benefit selected patients.[79] Additional contraindications to the use of vasopressin for control of gastrointestinal hemorrhage include chronic nephritis with renal dysfunction (elevated BUN), hyponatremia resulting from the ADH effect of vasopressin, and hypersensitivity to the drug. Other transient side effects of vasopressin therapy include blanching of skin, abdominal cramps, and nausea, which spontaneously resolve minutes after the infusion is discontinued.

Desmopressin (dDAVP), a synthetic analogue of ADH, has been useful in the control of bleeding in patients with uremia.[80] This unexpected action may relate to an increase in the levels of factor VIII.[81] Desmopressin acetate may be administered by slow infusion over 15 to 30 minutes (0.3 μg/kg diluted in sterile saline) and aids in achieving hemostasis after diagnostic or therapeutic interventions in patients with hemophilia, von Willebrand disease, or uremia.

Ergot Alkaloids

Ergot alkaloids and their dihydrogenated derivatives have a wide range of biologic activity reflecting mixed agonist and antagonist properties at different receptor sites. In vascular smooth muscle, their actions are mediated through agonist activity at the alpha-adrenergic receptor, and by antagonist and partial agonist effect upon the serotonin receptor.[82,83] Their effects in the central nervous system (CNS) produce a complex combination of both stimulation and depression, with toxic doses inducing sedation and respiratory depression. The natural amino acid alkaloids, particularly ergotamine, produce vasoconstriction in both arteries and veins via stimulation of vascular smooth muscle. Vasospasm induced by ergot alkaloid overdose may be prolonged and severe and is not reversible by alpha-antagonists or serotonin antagonists. These agents may also induce capillary endothelial damage with resultant vascular stasis, thrombosis, and gangrene.[82] The action of dihydroergotamine is far more effective upon capacitance than upon resistance vessels, a property of value in the treatment of postural hypotension and of risk in the patient with congestive heart failure (CHF). Ergotamine tartrate preparations, administered orally or sublingually, are useful in the treatment of migraine headache, an action mediated by alpha-adrenergic blockade.

Intravenous administration of ergonovine maleate has been used in the evaluation of variant angina pectoris during coronary angiography in an effort to provoke coronary artery spasm,[34] a use that is controversial because of the documented risks of this agent (e.g., exacerbation of CHF due to decreased pulmonary venous capacitance). Ergonovine maleate may be delivered by serial administration of bolus intravenous injection of 0.1, 0.2, and 0.3 mg separated by 3- to 10-minute observation intervals with cineangiography performed in multiple projections 5 minutes after the bolus is given, or earlier if angina or ECG changes develop. The administration of ergonovine may either require a higher dose or be delayed if given following the administration of nitroglycerin. Safety precautions for the use of ergonovine maleate include the immediate availability of intravenous nitroglycerin and nitroprusside, continuous ECG and arterial pressure monitoring, and prophylactic temporary pacing catheter when the history includes syncope or bradycardia with chest pain.[84]

Side effects from ergotamine therapy include nausea and vomiting in approximately 10 to 20 percent of patients following oral or parenteral administration. Numbness, tingling, weakness, and muscle pain may be present in the extremities. Precordial discomfort and transient tachycardia or bradycardia may also occur. Contraindications to the use of ergotamine include sepsis, thrombophlebitis, Raynaud or Buerger disease, and advanced vascular disease.[82]

Digitalis

Digitalis is useful in increasing myocardial contractility and in controlling the ventricular response to atrial fibrillation and flutter. For these reasons it is used to treat congestive heart failure and to slow ventricular response with atrial arrhythmia. The positive inotropic action of digitalis is mediated by inhibition of the membrane-bound Na^+K^+ATPase pump and by an increase in the slow inward current during the action potential, which increases cytosolic Ca^{++} ion concentration with resultant increased contractility.[85] Because mean systemic arterial pressure is elevated without increase in cardiac output, digitalis causes an increase in systemic vascular resistance, which results from contraction of vascular smooth muscle in arterial resistance vessels as well as vasoconstriction in the mesenteric and coronary vascular beds. Digitalis also acts directly on vascular smooth muscles in veins, causing constriction. In dogs, a prominent effect is noted in the hepatic veins with pooling of mesenteric venous blood in the portal system.[85]

The drug may be delivered either orally or parenterally as digoxin or digitoxin. Digitoxin is metabolized by hepatic microsomal enzymes to digoxin, which is excreted by the kidneys with a 1.6-day half-life.[85]

Somatostatin

Somatostatin and its long-acting analogue, octreotide acetate, suppress the secretion of serotonin, growth hormone, and a variety of other gastroenteropancreatic peptides (e.g., glucagon, gastrin, motilin, pancreatic polypeptide, secretin, and vasoactive intestinal peptide). The agents are administered by intravenous infusion and cause a decrease in hepatosplanchnic blood flow and a lowering of portal venous pressure. In a number of clinical trials, somatostatin and octreotide have been as effective as vasopressin in the treatment of acute variceal hemorrhage, but with fewer side effects because of their route of delivery. At a dose of 250 μg/hr IV, somatostatin reduces total hepatic blood flow by approximately 25 percent in conscious humans.[86] A similar dose is effective in controlling bleeding from peptic ulcer hemorrhage. Somatostatin (250 μg/hr IV) has been noted to be as effective in controlling acute variceal bleeding as injection sclerotherapy and a safe alternative;[87] a similar dose is also noted to be effective in controlling bleeding following injection sclerotherapy of esophageal varices, esophageal ulcers, and esophagitis.[88]

In an animal model of hepatic metastases, Hemingway et al. have shown that after intravenous administration of octreotide acetate (4.7 μg/kg) total hepatic arterial blood flow is reduced by over 40 percent. They note a significant increase in the tumor-liver blood flow ratio due predominantly to a reduction in hepatic arterial flow to normal liver with no significant change in tumor blood flow.[89]

Vasodilators

A variety of pharmacologic agents function as vasodilators, either through local action or systemic effect, and may be used when vasospasm detracts from the examination, or to augment blood flow when increased arterial flow or enhanced venous opacification is desired. These agents are useful in differentiating fixed vascular pathology from functional vasospastic disorders and in improving the diagnostic accuracy of arteriographic studies by verifying the hemodynamic significance of a vascular lesion before treatment. Vasodilator agents also find application in treating nonocclusive mesenteric ischemia and in alleviating vasospasm, thereby initiating a return to normal function.

Papaverine

Papaverine, an alkaloid derived from opium, is a nonspecific smooth muscle relaxant of relatively low potency that has been effective in reversing vasoconstriction in experimental models[90] and in reversing nonocclusive intestinal ischemia.[4,36,90–93] Nonocclusive mesenteric ischemia occurs frequently in elderly individuals with heart disease and with associated low cardiac output syndromes (e.g., congestive heart failure, cardiac arrhythmia, or digitalis administration) and diminished splanchnic blood flow.

Papaverine relaxes all smooth muscle, especially that which has been spasmodically contracted (e.g., bronchial musculature; biliary, urinary, and gastrointestinal tracts). It is effective in dilating larger arteries of the vascular system, including the splanchnic, cerebral, coronary, peripheral, and pulmonary arteries. The antispasmodic effect is due to a direct action upon smooth muscle, unrelated to muscular innervation. It has been suggested that this vasodilator action is caused by inhibition of cyclic nucleotide phosphodiesterase.[94] Unlike tolazoline, papaverine is not a coronary vasoconstrictor and may be administered by constant infusion through an arterial catheter. The usual dosage is 30 mg infused intraarterially in a single dose, or 30 to 60 mg/hr infused intraarterially for several hours.

Although detailed knowledge of its metabolism is not available, it is known that papaverine is not degraded on a single passage through an organ, and thus drug levels may accumulate and cause hypotension. Other side effects related to papaverine use include depression of atrioventricular and intraventricular conduction, and induction of transient ectopic rhythms of ventricular origin;[4] thus papaverine is contraindicated in the presence of complete heart block.

Normal erection in the male involves both an increase in blood flow to the corpora cavernosum and a relative decrease in venous drainage from the corpora, an action mediated by the release of vasoactive substances from the nerves that feed the corpora. Intracorporal injection of a vasodilator (e.g., papaverine or prostaglandin E_1) is useful in evaluating vasculogenic erectile dysfunction. This diagnosis is suspected if the patient fails to achieve erection within 30 minutes following intracorporal injection of papaverine.[95]

Imidazoline Derivatives

An enormous number of substituted imidazoline derivatives have been synthesized and studied pharmacologically.[96,97] These agents offer high potency, with slight changes in molecular structure producing striking differences in pharmacologic effect. Agents of this chemical group are marketed for their antihistaminic, sympathomimetic, vasodilator, and alpha-adrenergic blocking effects. Most agents lack specificity, producing several of these effects at comparable doses. Tolazoline (Priscoline, Ciba Pharmaceutical), phentolamine (Regitine, Ciba Pharmaceutical), and phenoxybenzamine (Dibenzyline, SmithKline Beecham Pharmaceuticals) are synthetic alpha-adrenergic antagonists that are useful as vasodilators. These agents produce vasodilatation through alpha-adrenergic blockade and by direct action on vascular smooth muscle, an effect produced at a lower dose than is required for alpha-adrenergic blockade. Phentolamine is at least six times more potent than tolazoline as an alpha-adrenergic antagonist; it is relatively short-acting, having a 19-minute half-life following IV administration. Phenoxybenzamine is a long-acting agent that can induce a "chemical sympathectomy"; it can have a duration of action lasting days.

Tolazoline is rapidly cleared by the kidney and has been employed for mesenteric vasodilatation to improve visualization of the portal vein[98] and for imaging the pancreas.[99] In the extremities its vasodilator properties are valuable in investigating peripheral vascular disease,[100] as well as bone and soft tissue tumors.[51] For use in diagnostic angiography, tolazoline hydrochloride, 25 to 50 mg, may be diluted and delivered slowly intraarterially over a period of 2 to 3 minutes immediately before the injection of contrast agent. Selective injection of tolazoline into vascular beds may be therapeutically useful in the treatment of vasospasm or mesenteric ischemia, as suggested by Aakhus.[35] In the newborn, tolazoline is useful in treating persistent fetal circulation when systemic arterial oxygenation cannot be maintained through routine supportive measures. In each of these cases, the pharmacoangiographic value of this agent is as a vasodilator rather than an alpha-adrenergic antagonist.

Tolazoline increases venous capacitance, decreases peripheral and pulmonary vascular resistance, and functions as a coronary vasoconstrictor; thus it must be used cautiously in patients with ischemic heart disease and mitral stenosis. Adverse reactions following tolazoline administration include systemic hypotension, tachycardia, oliguria, nausea, vomiting, and skin flushing. Side effects may be reversed by the Trendelenburg position and intravenous fluids. Alpha-adrenergic agonists (epinephrine or norepinephrine) should not be used for treatment of hypotension due to tolazoline overdosage.

Phentolamine has been employed largely as an alpha-adrenergic receptor antagonist to control hypertensive episodes that may occur in patients with pheochromocytoma. It has been investigated as an agent to reverse the hepatorenal syndrome by direct renal arterial infusion,[101] to improve renal perfusion in essential hypertension,[102] and to improve visualization of the splanchnic vasculature during diagnostic angiography.[39,103] Phenoxybenzamine may be administered by both oral and intravenous routes and is useful in producing and maintaining a "chemical sympathectomy," which may be beneficial in the management of pheochromocytoma. Locally injected into the mesenteric vascular system, it may provide prolonged vasodilation in the setting of nonocclusive mesenteric ischemia without inducing systemic side effects.[104]

The side effects encountered with the use of this and other substituted imidazoline derivatives reflect their nonspecificity of action: cardiac effects include tachycardia, arrhythmias, and angina; gastrointestinal stimulation by these agents may result in abdominal pain, nausea, vomiting, and diarrhea; and cholinergiclike side effects include myosis, stimulation of salivary, pancreatic, and respiratory tract secretions, and profuse sweating.

Sodium Nitroprusside

Sodium nitroprusside is a potent vasodilator that has been used over the past four decades to induce an acute reduction in arterial blood pressure.[105] Nitroprusside is metabolized by red blood cells into hydrocyanic acid, which is then converted to thiocyanate by the liver and excreted by the kidneys. It acts to reduce blood pressure by reducing arterial resistance and increasing venous capacitance; thus cardiac preload is decreased. Reduction in arterial pressure is dose-dependent and transient because of the rapid peripheral conversion of nitroprusside into thiocyanate. If employed for several days, toxicity may develop from accumulation of the cyanide moiety. Acute toxicity manifests as hypotension secondary to excessive vasodilatation. This is rapidly reversible following the discontinuation of the drug. The vasodilator properties of this agent are somewhat more prominent in the mesenteric and somatic vascular beds and have less action on the renal vasculature.[105]

Sodium nitroprusside has been employed with dramatic effect in the treatment of ergotism, reversing diffuse vascular spasm. This action is due to its diffuse activity in a number of vascular beds. Its ease in use allows the dose to be titrated to achieve a desired blood pressure response.[105–107] Treatment usually begins with an infusion rate of 0.5 μg/kg/min and the drip is titrated to the desired end point; average therapeutic doses range between 0.5 and 8.0 μg/kg/min.

Nitrates

The nitrates were among the first vasodilators identified and continue to have an important role in diagnosis and therapy in coronary artery and peripheral vascular disease.[4] Nitrites, organic nitrates, nitroso-compounds, and other nitrogen- and oxygen-containing compounds (e.g., nitroprusside) activate guanylate cyclase and increase the synthesis of cGMP in smooth muscle and other tissues.[94] This action is mediated by nitric oxide; hence the term *nitrodilators*. It occurs directly at the vascular smooth muscle level and is independent of vascular endothelium (see Fig. 6-1). Nitric oxide is rapidly inactivated by hemoglobin, conferring safety in the use of systemic nitrodilator agents.[18]

Within the venous system, nitrates induce vasodilatation (increased capacitance), which decreases venous return and leads to diminished ventricular volume, pressure, and wall tension. Nitrates dilate smaller arterioles, thereby increasing blood flow; they also produce sustained dilatation of the larger epicardial coronary arteries and increased collateral blood flow within the heart. Intravenous delivery of nitroglycerin may be useful when prompt initiation of therapy is indicated for treatment of angina pectoris. High drug concentrations in the systemic circulation may be rapidly attained and titrated for a desired clinical effect.[94] Nitroglycerin has been employed during coronary and peripheral angiography to differentiate arterial spasm from a fixed vascular lesion and to reverse ergonovine-induced coronary artery spasm.[4,34] It has been used to discriminate between functional and organic abnormalities of the renal blood supply.[37] During percutaneous transluminal angioplasty, a 100- to 200-μg intraarterial bolus is beneficial to prevent or treat vasospasm caused by catheter or guidewire manipulation.

In humans, peak plasma concentrations of nitroglycerin are found within 4 minutes of sublingual administration; the plasma half-life is approximately 1 to 3 minutes, and an undetectable clinical effect occurs within 1 hour. Oral delivery of organic nitrates (e.g., isosorbide dinitrate) may provide prolonged antiangina prophylaxis in a more convenient drug form than sublingual nitroglycerin. This preparation has a peak effect 60 to 90 minutes following administration and a duration of action of 3 to 6 hours. The topical administration of nitroglycerin ointment is useful for prolonged prophylactic purposes. Onset of action is within 60 minutes, and the effect persists for 4 to 8 hours.

Acetylcholine

Acetylcholine (ACh) is a neurotransmitter that is active in the autonomic and parasympathetic nervous systems and motor endplate of skeletal muscle.[108] This neurohormone is rapidly degraded into its inactive precursors, acetate and choline, by acetylcholinesterase and butyryl cholinesterase within tissues and plasma. ACh also acts as a potent vasodilator agent following intravenous infusions. In humans, intravenous injection of 20 to 50 μg/min causes peripheral vasodilatation with a reduction in systemic blood pressure and a reflex increase in heart rate.[109] Higher systemic doses decrease arteriovenous nodal conduction velocity, resulting in bradycardia (negative chronotropy) and hypotension.[110] When ACh is injected into the coronary artery, immediate cardiac arrest is produced, an effect exploited by Dotter for visualization of the coronary circulation during occlusion aortography.[111]

The dose-response curve to ACh in most organ systems is characterized by vasodilatation at low to moderate doses; at high doses, ACh results in the release of epinephrine, with resultant vasoconstriction.[37] ACh has been shown useful for renal pharmacoangiography,[102,112–114] during which intraarterial infusion (e.g., 1–100 μg/min) induces vasodilatation and increased renal blood flow. These changes result angiographically in an increase in the size of the kidney, a decrease in the arterial washout time, and an early appearance of contrast in the renal vein, along with an increase in the maximal contrast density in this vein. Because of an ACh-induced diuretic effect, the maximal density of the nephrogram is often decreased. In patients with severe small-vessel renal disease (e.g., nephrosclerosis or chronic pyelonephritis), the vasodilator response to ACh may be blunted; a potentiated ACh response occurs in patients with uncomplicated essential hypertension. This suggests a fixed, organic lesion in the former and a functional abnormality in the latter.[102] Although safe and effective as a vasodilator for investigating the renal vasculature, ACh appears to have little other practical utility because of its rapid hydrolysis and its diffuse action at remote sites.[114,115]

Reserpine

Reserpine acts by depleting stores of catecholamines and serotonin in many organs, including the brain, the adrenal medulla, and the peripheral sympathetic nerves.[5] In the central nervous system, this tends to produce sedation, whereas in the cardiovascular system it promotes an antihypertensive effect. The antihypertensive action of reserpine is largely due to depletion of peripheral nerve stores of catecholamines; as an antihypertensive agent, it has a prolonged duration of action measured in days. A superimposed direct vasodilator effect may also be contributory in the peripheral circulation. The oral antihypertensive dose of reserpine ranges from 0.1 to 1.0 mg/d, usually in two divided doses.[5] Intraarterially administered reserpine has been shown to produce vasodilatation in both normal and sympathectomized human limbs and to induce a sustained reversal of vasoconstriction, especially in Raynaud disease and in scleroderma.[116]

Major side effects associated with prolonged use of reserpine include severe postural hypotension, central nervous system depression, exacerbation of peptic ulcer disease, extrapyramidal disturbances, and increased gastrointestinal tone and motility with consequent cramps and diarrhea.

Isoproterenol

Isoproterenol, a beta-adrenergic agonist, has been shown to be an effective vasodilator and also causes pronounced relaxation of smooth muscle of the bronchi and alimentary tract. In the heart, isoproterenol induces positive inotropic and chronotropic effects. It results in decreased pulmonary and systemic vascular resistance and increases in coronary and renal arterial blood flow. Isoproterenol is metabolized primarily in the liver; its action is slightly longer than that of epinephrine but is still brief. Use of isoproterenol is contraindicated in patients with angina pectoris, tachyarrhythmias, heart block caused by digitalis intoxication, and ventricular arrhythmias that require inotropic therapy.[117]

After a 2-minute intraarterial infusion into the celiac or superior mesenteric artery (3.8 μg/min), a consistent vasodilator effect is observed during visceral arteriography, resulting in more rapid transit of contrast material through the vascular bed, diminished aortic reflux, improved opacification of the bowel wall, and better visualization of the portal venous circulation.[39]

Calcium Channel Blockers

Calcium channel blockers promote vasodilatation of vascular smooth muscle through the inhibition of Ca^{++} ion influx into cells or its mobilization from intracellular stores. This action results in a decrease in arterial tone, which lowers both blood pressure and peripheral vascular resistance (afterload). In the cardiac myocyte, these agents result in a negative inotropic effect and antiarrhythmic effects. They may be indicated during angioplasty to prevent or treat vasospasm caused by catheter or guidewire manipulation.

Nifedipine, an antianginal drug, is useful in preventing coronary and peripheral artery vasospasm. The drug is supplied as a 10-mg capsule and may be administered sublingually after a hole is punctured in the capsule and its contents are expressed sublingually, after which the patient swallows the capsule. After oral administration, about 50 percent of the drug is rapidly absorbed. Generally, the drug is well tolerated as a one-time 10-mg dose, although hypotension may be observed. Plasma half-life is approximately 2 to 4 hours, with 80 percent of the drug and its metabolites excreted by the kidney. Clearance may be delayed with impaired renal function.[94] Significant hypotension following nifedipine administration may require cardiovascular support, including monitoring of cardiac and respiratory function or elevation of extremities. Attention to circulating fluid volume and urine output is essential because the additional use of a vasoconstrictor (e.g., norepinephrine) may be required. The drug is contraindicated if there is known hypersensitivity.

Verapamil is efficiently absorbed after oral administration but is extensively metabolized in the liver, resulting in a low bioavailability (about 20 percent). Effects of verapamil are evident 1 to 2 hours after oral administration; plasma half-life averages 5 hours.[94] The drug is given intravenously as a single 5- to 10-mg dose over 2 minutes to interrupt supraventricular arrhythmias. This can be repeated 30 minutes later if necessary.

Iodinated Contrast Media

Iodinated contrast media have reproducible vasodilator effects following intraarterial injection. In an animal model, following a 3-second priming injection of 12 ml of Renografin, 76 percent into the superior mesenteric artery, Steckel et al. describe an initial flow reduction (about 6–8 seconds) followed by a prolonged increase in arterial flow 1.5 to 2.5 times above baseline lasting 20 to 30 seconds. Mesenteric blood flow returns to baseline approximately 4 to 5 minutes after the injection.[39] Arteriographically, the changes are manifest by diminished aortic reflux, dilatation of mesenteric artery branches, decreased contrast transit time, improved contrast density in the bowel wall, and improved opacification of the mesenteric and portal venous branches.

Other Pharmacologic Agents

Prostaglandins

The prostaglandins are endogenous, 20-carbon unsaturated fatty acids derived from arachidonic acid that serve as attractive pharmacoangiographic agents. Several classes of prostaglandins (e.g., A, B, C, D, E, I, and F) have been identified with astonishingly diverse ranges of biologic activity. Synthesis involves a series of microsomal enzymes known collectively as prostaglandin synthetase, or cyclooxygenase.[118] Prostaglandins are released following synthesis and then rapidly degraded by tissue-bound enzymes. Most prostaglandins are almost completely (about 90 percent) metabolized during a single passage through the liver or lung; thus accumulation following local infusion is unlikely. These agents are found in nearly every tissue and body fluid and, given their natural occurrence, are unlikely to evoke an allergic response following parenteral administration.

Prostaglandin E functions as a potent vasodilator in most vascular beds, exceeding the effects of both acetylcholine and histamine. Systemic blood pressure usually drops and blood flow to most organs increases after parenteral prostaglandin E administration. Prostaglandin E_1 (PGE_1), available from Upjohn as alprostadil, is supplied as 500 μg in 1 ml of dehydrated alcohol and causes vasodilatation and inhibition of platelet aggregation, and also stimulates intestinal and uterine smooth muscle.[117] Intravenous doses of 1 to 10 μg/kg lower blood pressure by decreasing peripheral vascular resistance. The drug is rapidly metabolized, with 80 percent being inactivated in a single pass through the lung. It has been used to enhance angiographic visualization in the extremities, to intensify the pressure gradient across a stenosis, to improve visualization of hepatic and pancreatic tumors,[119,120] and to enhance renal blood flow.[112] Bolus injection of PGE_1 (0.5 μg/kg) into the superior mesenteric artery in dogs produces a 92 percent increase in superior mesenteric arterial blood flow along with enhanced opacification of the mesenteric and portal veins; this action is achieved with only a small decrease (about 5 mmHg) in systolic blood pressure.[121] By optimizing the venous phase during mesenteric angiography, PGE_1 may also be useful in evaluating the degree of venous invasion in the setting of colon carcinoma.[122]

Prostaglandin $F_{2\alpha}$ has also been employed to enhance visualization during visceral angiography. Injection of $PGF_{2\alpha}$ into the superior mesenteric artery of humans (80 μg diluted in 10 ml saline) results in a doubling of superior mesenteric arterial blood flow, diminished aortic reflux on arteriography, and improved mesenteric venous contrast density, which is as good or better than obtained by a similar intraarterial injection of 10 μg of bradykinin.[123] $PGF_{2\alpha}$ injected intraarterially (60 μg over 15–20 seconds) during selective hepatic arterial catheterization in humans has been employed to enhance the visualization of the liver and to improve detection of hepatic metastases and gallbladder carcinomas.[124]

The pulmonary vasculature, especially the ductus arteriosus in neonates, is especially sensitive to the vasodilatory effects of PGI_2 (prostacyclin) and PGE_1. PGI_2 (available in Europe as epoprostenol), unlike PGE_1, is not inactivated on passage through the pulmonary circulation and is equally effective when given intravenously or intraarterially. When used for maintaining patency of the ductus arteriosus, PGE_1 is administered by intravenous infusion at an initial rate of 0.1 μg/kg/min with subsequent reduction in dose to the lowest level that achieves the desired effect. Intravenous administration of PGI_2 causes prominent hypotension by inducing vasodilatation in the coronary, mesenteric, renal, skeletal, and pulmonary circulation. This response is mediated at the level of the arteriolar precapillary sphincters and postcapillary venules. Both agents have been used to increase pulmonary blood flow and oxygenation in infants with congenital heart disease and to decrease pulmonary vascular resistance, thereby improving exercise tolerance in the setting of primary pulmonary arterial hypertension.[125,126] When given to patients with severe peripheral vascular disease, PGE_1 and PGI_2 infused intravenously or intraarterially have been shown to provide dramatic and long-lasting benefit in relieving symptoms in patients in whom total occlusion is absent.[125–128]

PGI_2 is also useful in preventing platelet aggregation by counterbalancing the effects of thromboxane A_2. By stimulating adenyl cyclase, it causes a decrease in intracellular Ca^{++} with inhibition of platelet secretion and aggregation.[129] In extracorporeal circulation systems (e.g., cardiopulmonary bypass and hemodialysis), prostacyclin may be used in place of heparin in selected patients when heparin is contraindicated.[128]

Dopamine

Dopamine, the biosynthetic precursor of norepinephrine, stimulates dopaminergic, $beta_2$- and alpha-adrenergic receptors. It is unique in that it can produce renal and splanchnic vasodilatation at low doses (e.g., 2–10 μg/kg/min) while maintaining a primary vasoconstrictor influence on other vascular beds, an action mediated by the alpha-adrenergic receptor.[130] The alpha-adrenergic effect predominates at higher doses (e.g., above 10 μg/kg/min), with resultant renal, mesenteric, peripheral arterial, and venous vasoconstriction.

A major advantage of dopamine when used during renal arteriography is its excellent response following intravenous infusion. A dose that may be infused without effecting a hypertensive response in normal patients is 3 μg/kg/min. The renal arteries dilate and renal blood flow increases approximately 50 percent by 2 to 3 minutes, with a maximum response (about 70–100 percent increase in renal blood flow) by 10 to 15 minutes.[37] There is an associated increase in renal size, a decrease in the arterial washout time, and an early appearance of contrast in the renal vein, although these actions are somewhat less than the maximal response observed with ACh.[112,131] As with ACh, this response may be useful for further evaluating functional abnormalities of the renal vasculature in both humans[102] and animals.[132] Dopamine stimulates the heart directly, resulting in increased cardiac output, an action that is useful in the treatment of low cardiac output and low blood pressure syndromes.

As is true of other endogenous substances employed in pharmacoangiography, allergy is very unlikely. Toxicity is dose-related and is primarily cardiovascular in nature because of the agent's pressor effect. At large dosages, cardiac arrhythmias may occur.

Glucagon

Glucagon, a hormone secreted by pancreatic alpha cells, has a hyperglycemic effect: it promotes the breakdown of hepatic glycogen and inhibits the breakdown of glucose to lactate; as such, it opposes the actions of insulin.[133,134] It is a single-chain polypeptide of 29 amino acid residues (molecular weight of 3485 Daltons) with an identical amino acid sequence in all mammals.[135] As with other polypeptide hormones, glucagon is rapidly degraded by a number of proteolytic enzymes and is extensively degraded in the liver, kidney, and plasma, and at tissue receptor sites. Plasma half-life is approximately 3 to 6 minutes, similar to that of insulin. When administered intravenously, the onset of action of a 0.5-mg dose is 1 minute with a duration of 9 to 17 minutes.

The vasodilator properties of glucagon are useful for visceral and renal angiography. Glucagon is as effective as ACh in dilating the intrarenal vasculature.[112,136,137] Danford et al. describe the effect of glucagon on the renal circulation in dogs.[138] Following an intraarterial infusion of 0.5 mg, increase in renal blood flow and vasodilatation of the entire renal arterial tree are observed in a fashion similar to ACh. However, glucagon differs from ACh in that the vasodilatory response is prolonged (about 120 minutes), which is a surprising response in view of its short biologic half-life.

In large doses, glucagon induces profound relaxation in intestinal smooth muscle, an action that is useful for hypotonic duodenography and during digital subtraction arteriography.[135,139] Glucagon has a variety of clinical uses, including the treatment of severe hypoglycemia in insulin-dependent diabetics when dextrose solutions are not available[139] and in the evaluation of selected endocrine disorders (e.g., pheochromocytoma). It is as effective as other anticholinergic drugs but has fewer side effects. The agent is relatively free of severe adverse reactions but should be used with caution in patients with diabetes, insulinomas, or pheochromocytoma. Glucagon also induces nausea and vomiting at dosages not much greater than required to achieve a maximal renal vascular response.

Bradykinin

Bradykinin is an endogenous peptide formed from high-molecular-weight kininogen by a group of enzymes in plasma, body fluids, cells, and tissues collectively known as kininogenases. Bradykinin has a plasma half-life of about 15 seconds, and, in a single passage through the pulmonary vascular bed, approximately 80 to 90 percent is deactivated by angiotensin-converting enzyme.[118] Therefore, patients treated with ACE inhibitor antihypertensive agents may show a potentiated response.[140] The kinins, including bradykinin, are about ten times more potent as vasodilators than is histamine, an action that is endothelial-dependent.[60] At very low concentration, increased capillary permeability is produced, resulting in edema. Intravenous injection in humans causes flushing with vasodilatation of kidney, muscle, other viscera, and various glands. Dilatation of resistance arterioles results in a decrease in total peripheral resistance, which may produce a sharp drop in systolic and diastolic blood pressure. By contrast, large arteries and most veins vasoconstrict in response to the kinins.

Bradykinin has been employed for a wide variety of pharmacoangiographic maneuvers, including attempts to enhance visualization of the pancreatic,[141] peripheral,[69] celiac and mesenteric,[69,142,143] and renal vascular beds.[69,112,144,145] In dogs, Freed et al. reported the optimum dose of bradykinin to be 0.1 μg/kg intraarterially injected into the renal artery (diluted in 2 ml saline). This dose resulted in marked arterial dilatation, increased density of the early cortical nephrogram, early intense opacification of the renal vein, and marked decrease in aortic reflux following renal arterial contrast injection.[144]

References

1. Melmon KL, Morelli HF. Drug reactions. In: Melmon KL, Morelli HF, eds. Clinical pharmacology: basic principles in therapeutics. New York: Macmillan, 1972:585–604.
2. Klaassen CD. Principles of toxicology. In: Gilman AG, et al, eds. The pharmacological basis of therapeutics. New York: Macmillan, 1985:1592–1604.
3. Douglas WW. Histamine and 5-hydroxytryptamine (serotonin) and their antagonists. In: Gilman AG, et al, eds. The pharmacological basis of therapeutics. New York: Macmillan, 1985:605–638.
4. Nickerson M. Vasodilator drugs. In: Goodman LS, Gilman A, eds. The pharmacological basis of therapeutics. New York: Macmillan, 1975:727–743.
5. Weiner N. Drugs that inhibit adrenergic nerves and block adrenergic receptors. In: Gilman AG, et al, eds. The pharmacological basis of therapeutics. New York: Macmillan, 1985: 181–214.
6. Goldstein A, Aronow L, Kalman SM. Principles of drug action: the basis of pharmacology. 2nd ed. New York: Wiley, 1974.
7. Levesque MJ, Nerum RM. The elongation and organization of cultured endothelial cells in response to shear. J Biomech Eng 1985;107:341.
8. Jaffe EA. Endothelial cells and the biology of factor VIII. N Engl J Med 1977;296:377–383.
9. Cox DA, Liu MW, Roubin GS. Mechanical intervention: endothelial and smooth muscle cell biology. In: Roubin GS, et al, eds. Interventional cardiovascular medicine: principles and practice. New York: Churchill-Livingstone, 1994:17–32.
10. Stary H, Blankenhorn DH, Chandler AB, Glagov S, et al. A definition of the intima of human arteries and of its atherosclerosis-prone regions. Circulation 1992;85:391–405.
11. Webb DJ, Cockroft JR. Circulating and tissue renin-angiotensin systems: the role of endothelium. In: Warren JB, ed. The endothelium: an introduction to current research. New York: Wiley-Liss, 1990:65.
12. Furchgott RF, Zawadzki JV. The obligatory role of endothelial cells in the relaxation of arterial smooth muscle by acetylcholine. Nature 1980;288:373–376.
13. Vanhoutte PM. Endothelium and control of vascular function. Hypertension 1989;13:658–667.
14. Feletou M, Vanhoutte PM. Endothelium-dependent hyperpolarization of canine coronary smooth muscle. Br J Pharmacol 1988;93:515–524.
15. Palmer RMJ, Ferrige AG, Moncada AS. Nitric oxide accounts for the biological activity of endothelium-derived relaxing factor. Nature 1987;327:524–526.
16. Palmer RMJ, Ashton DS, Moncada S. Vascular endothelial cells synthesize nitric oxide from L-arginine. Nature 1988; 333:664–666.
17. Wennmalm A. Endothelial nitric oxide and cardiovascular disease. J Int Med 1994;235:317–327.
18. Vane JR, Anggard EE, Botting RM. Regulatory functions of the vascular endothelium. N Engl J Med 1990;323:27–36.
19. Ameli S, Kaul S, Castro L, Arora C, et al. Effect of percutaneous transluminal coronary angioplasty on circulating endothelin levels. Am J Cardiol 1993;72(18):1352–1356.
20. Burton AC. Relation of structure to function of the tissues of the wall of blood vessels. Physiol Rev 1954;34(4):619–642.
21. Clowse AW, Schwartz SM. Significance of quiescent smooth

muscle migration in the injured rat carotid artery. Circ Res 1985;56:139–145.
22. Liu MW, Roubin GS, King SB. Restenosis after coronary angioplasty: potential biologic determinants and role of intimal hyperplasia. Circulation 1989;79:1374–1387.
23. Schwartz SM, Campbell GR, Campbell JH. Replication of smooth muscle cells in vascular disease. Circ Res 1986;58:427–444.
24. Berk BC, Vekshtein V, Gordon HM, Tsuda T. Angiotensin II-stimulated protein synthesis in cultured vascular smooth muscle cells. Hypertension 1989;13:305–314.
25. Guyton AC. Local control of blood flow by the tissues, and nervous and humoral regulation. In: Guyton AC, ed. Textbook of medical physiology. Philadelphia: Saunders, 1986: 230–243.
26. Bolton TB. Mechanisms of action of transmitters and other substances on smooth muscle. Physiol Rev 1979;59:606–718.
27. Mellander S, Johansson B. Control of resistance, exchange, and capacitance functions in the peripheral circulation. Pharmacol Rev 1968;20:117–196.
28. Hoffman BB. Adrenergic receptor activating drugs. In: Katzung BG, ed. Basic and clinical pharmacology. Los Altos: Lange, 1984:86–96.
29. Katzung BG. Introduction to autonomic pharmacology. In: Katzung BG, ed. Basic and clinical pharmacology. Los Altos: Lange, 1984:53–63.
30. Abrams HL, Boijsen E, Borgstrom KE. Effect of epinephrine on renal circulation, angiographic observations. Radiology 1962;79:911–922.
31. Abrams HL. The response of neoplastic renal vessels to epinephrine in man. Radiology 1964;82:217–224.
32. Baum S, Nusbaum M. The control of gastrointestinal hemorrhage by selective mesenteric arterial infusion of vasopressin. Radiology 1971;98:497–505.
33. Nusbaum M, Baum S, Sakiyalak P, Blakemore WS. Pharmacologic control of portal hypertension. Surgery 1967;62:299–310.
34. Fester A. Ergonovine maleate—a provocative test. Cathet Cardiovasc Diagn 1980;6:217.
35. Aakhus T, Brabrand G. Angiography in acute superior mesenteric arterial insufficiency. Acta Radiol (Stockh) 1967;6:1–12.
36. Boley SJ, Siegelman SS. Experimental and clinical nonocclusive mesenteric ischemia: pathophysiology, diagnosis and management. In: Hilal SK, ed. Small vessel angiography. St. Louis: Mosby, 1973:438–453.
37. Abrams HL, Obrez I, Hollenberg NK, Adams DF. Pharmacoangiography of the renal vascular bed. Curr Probl Diagn Radiol 1971;1:1–50.
38. Day ED. Vascular relationships of tumor and host. Prog Exp Tumor Res 1964;4:57.
39. Steckel RJ, Rosch J, Ross G, Grollman JH Jr. New developments in pharmacoangiography (and arterial pharmacotherapy) of the gastrointestinal tract. Invest Radiol 1971;6:199–211.
40. Ahlquist RP. A study of adrenotropic receptors. Am J Physiol 1948;153:586–600.
41. Lands AM, Arnold A, McAuliff JP. Differentiation of receptor systems activated by sympathomimetic amines. Nature 1967; 214:597–598.
42. Langer SZ. Presynaptic receptors and their role in the regulation of transmitter release. Sixth Gaddum memorial lecture, National Institute for Medical Research. Br J Pharmacol 1977;60:481–497.
43. Lefkowitz RJ. Beta-adrenergic receptors: recognition and regulation. N Engl J Med 1976;295:323–328.
44. Mehta J, Lopez LM. Calcium-blocker withdrawal phenomenon: increase in affinity of $alpha_2$ adrenoreceptors for agonist as a potential mechanism. Am J Cardiol 1986;58:242–246.
45. Weiner N. Norepinephrine, epinephrine, and the sympathomimetic amines. In: Gilman AG, et al, eds. The pharmacological basis of therapeutics. New York: Macmillan, 1985:145–180.
46. Ekelund L, Gerlock J Jr, Goncharenko V. The epinephrine effect in renal angiography revisited. Clin Radiol 1978;29: 387–392.
47. Olin T, Reuter SR. A pharmacological method for improving nephrophlebography. Radiology 1964;85:1036–1042.
48. Smith JC, Rosch J, Athanasoulis CA, Baum S, et al. Renal venography in the evaluation of poorly vascularized neoplasms of the kidney. AJR 1975;123(3):552–556.
49. Goldman ML, Gorelkin L, Rude JC III, Sybers RG, et al. Epinephrine renal venography in severe inflammatory disease of the kidney. Radiology 1978;127:93–101.
50. Boijsen E, Reuter SR. Mesenteric angiography in evaluation of intestinal disease. Radiology 1966;87:1028.
51. Ekelund L, Laurin S, Lunderquist A. Comparison of a vasoconstrictor and a vasodilator in pharmacoangiography of bone and soft-tissue tumors. Radiology 1977;122:95–99.
52. Clouse ME, Costello P, Legg MA, Soeldner SJ, et al. Subselective angiography in localizing insulinomas of the pancreas. AJR 1977;128:741–746.
53. Rockoff SD, Doppman J, Block JB, Ketcham A. Variable response of tumor vessels to intra-arterial epinephrine: an angiographic study in man. Invest Radiol 1966;1:205–213.
54. Boijsen E, Redman H. Effect of epinephrine on celiac and superior mesenteric angiography. Invest Radiol 1967;2:184.
55. Kahn PC, Frates WJ, Paul RE. Epinephrine effect in angiography of gastrointestinal tract tumors. Radiology 1967;88:686.
56. Martinkova J, Bulas J, Krejci V, Hartman M, et al. A study of the inhibition of adrenaline-induced vasoconstriction in the isolated perfused liver of rabbit. Hepatology 1990;12(5): 1157–1165.
57. Winkler SS, Kahn PC. Pharmacologic aids in adrenal angiography. Invest Radiol 1967;2:48–52.
58. Ross G. Effects of epinephrine and norepinephrine on the mesenteric circulation of the cat. Am J Physiol 1967;212: 1037–1042.
59. Steckel RJ, Ross G, Grollman JH Jr. A potent drug combination for producing constriction of the superior mesenteric artery and its branches. Radiology 1968;91:579.
60. Douglas WW. Polypeptides—angiotensin, plasma kinins and others. In: Gilman AG, et al, eds. The pharmacological basis of therapeutics. New York: Macmillan, 1985:639–659.
61. Ohno K, Yamashita M, Yamakawa N, Akinoto S, et al. Effectiveness of pharmacoangiography using nitroglycerin and angiotensin II. Nippon Igaku Hoshasen Gakkai Zasshi 1989; 49(11):1436–1438.
62. Kaplan JH, Bookstein JJ. Abdominal visceral pharmacoangiography with angiotensin. Radiology 1972;103:79–83.
63. Jekell K, Sandqvist S, Castenfors J. Angiotensin effect in the human kidney. Acta Radiol (Stockh) 1978;19:329–336.
64. Ekelund L, Gothlin J, Lunderquist A. Diagnostic improvement with angiotensin in renal angiography. Radiology 1972; 105:33.
65. Elkin M, Meng CH. The effects of angiotensin on renal vascularity in dogs. AJR 1966;98:927–934.
66. Hollenberg NK, Adams DF. Vascular factors in the pathogenesis of acute renal failure in man. In: Friedman EA, Eliahou HE, eds. Proceedings: acute renal failure conference. Washington, DC: GPO, 1973:209–230.
67. Ekelund L, Karp W. Evaluation of solitary renal cystic lesions. Acta Radiol (Stockh) 1978;19:321–328.
68. Gaussin G, Garnier JP, Gruchy D, D'Aboville M. Faits cliniques. Artériographie des métastases rénales d'origine bronchique. Intérêt de l'angiotensine. J Radiol Electrol Med Nucl 1978;59:505.
69. Weber J, Novak D. Abdominale und periphere Pharmakoangiographie mit Angiotensin und Bradykinin. Radiologe 1976; 6:524.
70. Sasaki Y, Imaoka S, Hasegawa Y, Nakano S, et al. Changes in distribution of hepatic blood flow induced by intra-arterial

infusion of angiotensin II in human hepatic cancer. Cancer 1985;55:311–316.
71. Hays RM. Agents affecting the renal conservation of water. In: Gilman AG, et al, eds. The pharmacological basis of therapeutics. New York: Macmillan, 1985:908–919.
72. Nusbaum M, Baum S, Kuroda K, Blakemore WS. Control of portal hypertension by selective mesenteric arterial drug infusion. Arch Surg 1968;97:1005–1013.
73. Davis GB, Bookstein J, Hagan PL. The relative effects of selective intra-arterial and intravenous vasopressin infusion. Radiology 1976;120:537–538.
74. Barr JW, Larkin RC, Rosch J. Similarity of arterial and intravenous vasopressin on portal and systemic hemodynamics. Gastroenterology 1975;69:13–19.
75. Johnson WC, Widrich WC, Ansell JE, Robbins AH, et al. Control of bleeding varices by vasopressin: a prospective randomized study. Ann Surg 1977;186:369–374.
76. Fogel MR, Kinauer CM, Andres LL, Mahal AS, et al. Continuous intravenous vasopressin in active upper gastrointestinal bleeding. Ann Intern Med 1982;96:565–569.
77. Baum S, Athanasoulis CA, Waltman AC. Angiographic diagnosis and control of gastrointestinal bleeding. In: Welch C, ed. Advances in Surgery. Chicago: Year Book, 1973.
78. Ring EJ, Oleaga JA, Freiman DB, Dann RW, et al. Comparison of the effect of vasopressin infusions on the mesenteric arteries of different species. Invest Radiol 1978;13:138–142.
79. Groszmann RJ, Kravetz D, Bosdch J, Glickman M, et al. Nitroglycerin improves the hemodynamic response to vasopressin in portal hypertension. Hepatology 1982;2:757–762.
80. Mannucci PM, Remuzzi G, Pusineri F, Lombardi R, et al. Deamino-8-D-arginine vasopressin shortens the bleeding time in uremia. N Engl J Med 1983;308:8–12.
81. Mannucci PM, Pareti FI, Ruggeri ZM, Capitano A. 1-deamino-8-D-arginine vasopressin: a new pharmacological approach to the management of haemophilia and von Willebrand's disease. Lancet 1977;1:869–872.
82. Rall TW, Schleifer LS. Drugs affecting uterine motility. In: Gilman AG, et al, eds. The pharmacological basis of therapeutics. New York: Macmillan, 1985:926–945.
83. Burkhalter A, Frick OL. Histamine, serotonin, and the ergot alkaloids. In: Katzung BC, ed. Basic and clinical pharmacology. Los Altos: Lange, 1984:189–206.
84. Conti RC, Levin DC, Grossman W. Coronary angiography. In: Grossman W, ed. Cardiac catheterization and angiography. Philadelphia: Lea & Febiger, 1980:147–169.
85. Hoffman BF, Bigger JT Jr. Digitalis and allied cardiac glycosides. In: Gilman AG, et al, eds. The pharmacological basis of therapeutics. New York: Macmillan, 1985:716–747.
86. Keller U, AP, Kayasseh L, Gyr N. Effect of therapeutic doses of somatostatin (SST) on splanchnic blood flow in man. Eur J Clin Invest 1978;8:335.
87. Sheilds R, Jenkins SA, Baxter JN, Kingsnorth AN. A prospective randomized controlled trial comparing the efficacy of somatostatin with injection sclerotherapy in the control of bleeding oesophageal varices. J Hepatol 1992;16:128–137.
88. Jenkins SA. Somatostatin in acute bleeding oesophageal varices. Clinical evidence. Drugs 1992;2:36–55.
89. Hemingway DM, Jenkins SA, Cooke TG. The effects of sandostatin (Octreotide, SMS 201-995) infusion on splanchnic and hepatic blood flow in an experimental model of hepatic metastases. Br J Cancer 1992;65:396–398.
90. Siegelman SS, Sprayregen S, Boley SJ. Angiographic diagnosis of mesenteric arterial vasoconstriction. Radiology 1974;112: 533–542.
91. Widrich WC, Nordahl DL, Robbins AH. Contrast enhancement of the mesenteric and portal veins using intra-arterial papaverine. AJR 1974;121:374–379.
92. Bookstein JJ, Goldberger L, Niwayama G, Naderi MJ, et al. Angiographic aspects of experimental nonocclusive intestinal ischemic injury. AJR 1977;128:923–930.
93. Athanasoulis CA. Bowel ischemia, management with intra-arterial papaverine infusion and transluminal angioplasty. In: Interventional radiology. Philadelphia: Saunders, 1982, chap. 24.
94. Needleman P, Corr PB, Johnson EM Jr. Drugs used for the treatment of angina: organic nitrates, calcium channel blockers, and β-adrenergic antagonists. In: Gilman AG, et al, eds. The pharmacological basis of therapeutics. New York: Macmillan, 1985:806–826.
95. Bookstein JJ, Fellmeth B, Moreland S, Lurie AL. Pharmacoangiographic assessment of the corpora cavernosa. Cardiovasc Intervent Radiol 1988;11(4):218–224.
96. Nickerson M, Hollenberg NK. Blockade of alpha-adrenergic receptors. In: Root W, ed. Physiological pharmacology. New York: Academic, 1967:243–305.
97. Nickerson M, Collier B. Drugs inhibiting adrenergic nerves and structures innervated by them. In: Goodman LS, Gilman AG, eds. The pharmacological basis of therapeutics. New York: Macmillan, 1975:533–564.
98. Redman HC, Reuter SR, Miller WJ. Improvement of superior mesenteric and portal vein visualization with tolazoline. Invest Radiol 1969;4:24.
99. Schmarsow VR, Keifer H. Der pankreatographische Effekt bei der Pankreasangiographie nach Verabreichung von Dopamin und Tolazolin. ROFO: Fortschr Geb Rontgenstr Nuklearmedizin Verfahr 1978;129(4):429–435.
100. Neubauer B. Intraarterial tolazoline in angiography of the foot. Acta Radiol (Stockh) 1978;19:793–798.
101. Epstein M, Berk DP, Hollenberg NK, Adams DF, et al. Renal failure in the patient with cirrhosis: the role of active vasoconstriction. Am J Med 1970;49:175–185.
102. Hollenberg NK, Adams DF, Solomon H, Chenitz WR, et al. Renal vascular tone in essential and secondary hypertension: hemodynamic and angiographic responses to vasodilators. Medicine 1975;54:29–44.
103. Cioffi CM, Ruzicka FF Jr, Carillo FJ, Gould HR. Enhanced visualization of the portal system using phentolamine and isoproterenol in combination. Radiology 1973;108:43–49.
104. Habboushe F, Wallace HW, Nusbaum M, Baum S, et al. Nonocclusive mesenteric vascular insufficiency. Ann Surg 1974;6:819–822.
105. Rudd P, Blaschke TF. Antihypertensive agents and the drug therapy of hypertension. In: Gilman AG, et al, eds. The pharmacological basis of therapeutics. New York: Macmillan, 1985:784–805.
106. Carliner NH, Denune DP, Finch CS Jr, Goldberg LI. Sodium nitroprusside treatment of fergotamine-induced peripheral ischemia. JAMA 1974;227:308–309.
107. O'Dell CW Jr, Davis GB, Johnson AD, Safdi MA, et al. Sodium nitroprusside in the treatment of ergotism. Radiology 1977;124:73–74.
108. Koelle GB. Parasympathomimetic agents. In: Goodman LS, Gilman A, eds. The pharmacological basis of therapeutics. New York: Macmillan, 1975:467–476.
109. Watanabe AM. Cholinergic receptor stimulants. In: Katzung BG, ed. Basic and clinical pharmacology. Los Altos: Lange, 1984:64–76.
110. Furchgott RF. The requirement for endothelial cells in the relaxation of arteries by acetylcholine and some other vasodilators. Trends Pharmacol Sci 1981;2:173–176.
111. Dotter CT, Frische LH. Visualization of the coronary circulation by occlusion aortography: a practical method. Radiology 1958;71:502–523.
112. Ozer H, Hollenberg NK. Renal angiographic and hemodynamic responses to vasodilators: a comparison of five agents in the dog. Invest Radiol 1974;9:473–478.
113. Freed TA, Hager H, Vinik M. Effects of intra-arterial acetylcholine on renal arteriography in normal humans. AJR 1968; 104:312–318.
114. Chuang VP, Fried AM. High-dose pharmacoangiography in the assessment of hypovascular renal neoplasms. AJR 1978; 131:807–811.

115. Taylor P. Cholinergic agonists. In: Gilman AG, et al, eds. The pharmacological basis of therapeutics. New York: Macmillan, 1985:100–109.
116. Arneklo-Nobin B, Albrechtsson U, Eklof B, Tylen U. Indications for angiography and its optimal performance in patients with Raynaud's phenomenon. Cardiovasc Intervent Radiol 1985;8(4):174–179.
117. Physician's desk reference. Montvale, NJ: Medical Economics Data Production Company, 1995:2575–2576.
118. Douglas WW. Polypeptides—angiotensin, plasma kinins, and other vasoactive agents: prostaglandins. In: Goodman LS, Gilman A, eds. The pharmacological basis of therapeutics. New York: Macmillan, 1975:630–652.
119. Jonsson K, Wallace S, Jacobson ED, Anderson JH, et al. The use of prostaglandin E_1 for enhanced visualization of the splanchnic circulation. Radiology 1977;125:373–378.
120. Jonsson K, de Santos, LA, Wallace S, Anderson JH. Prostaglandin E_1 (PGE_1) in angiography of tumors of the extremities. AJR 1978;130:7–11.
121. Davis LJ, Anderson JH, Wallace S, Gianturco C, et al. The use of prostaglandin PGE_1 to enhance the angiographic visualization of the splanchnic circulation. Radiology 1975;114: 281–286.
122. Iijima T. Pharmacoangiographic diagnosis of venous invasion of carcinoma of the colon with reference to liver metastases. Dis Colon Rectum 1988;31(9):718–722.
123. Dencker H, Gothlin J, Hedner P, Lunderquist A, et al. Superior mesenteric angiography and blood flow following intraarterial injection of prostaglandin F_2-alpha. Am J Roentgenol 1975;125:111–118.
124. Legge D. The use of prostaglandin F_2 alpha in selective hepatic angiography. Radiology 1977;124:331–335.
125. Higgenbottam T, Wheeldon D, Wells F, Wallwork J. Long-term treatment of primary pulmonary hypertension with continuous intravenous epoprostenol (prostacyclin). Lancet 1984;1:1046–1047.
126. Moncada S, Flower RJ, Vane JR. Prostaglandins, prostacyclin, thromboxane A_2, and leukotrienes. In: Gilman AG, et al, eds. The pharmacological basis of therapeutics. New York: Macmillan, 1985:660–673.
127. Olsson AG, Carlsson AL. Clinical, hemodynamic and metabolic effects of intraarterial infusions of prostaglandin E_1 in patients with peripheral vascular disease. Adv Prostaglandin Thromboxane Res 1976;1:429–432.
128. Zusman RM, Rubin RH, Cato AE, Cocchetto DM, et al. Hemodialysis using prostacyclin instead of heparin as the sole antithrombotic agent. N Engl J Med 1981;304:934–939.
129. Weiss HJ, Turitto VT, Baumgartner HR. Effect of shear rate on platelet interaction with subendothelium in citrated and native blood. J Lab Clin Med 1978;92:750–764.
130. Innes IR, Nickerson M. Norepinephrine, epinephrine, and the sympathomimetic amines. In: Goodman LS, Gilman A, eds. The pharmacological basis of therapeutics. New York: Macmillan, 1975:477–513.
131. Hollenberg NK, Adams DF, Mendell P, Abrams HL, et al. Renal vascular responses to dopamine: hemodynamic and angiographic observations in normal man. Clin Sci 1973;45: 733–742.
132. Borgersen A, Ayers CR. Effect of dopamine on renal vasculature of dogs with experimental renovascular hypertension. Invest Radiol 1968;3:1–5.
133. Lehninger A. Hormones. In: Principles of biochemistry. New York: Worth, 1982:721–752.
134. Larner J, Haynes RC Jr. Insulin and oral hypoglycemic drugs; glucagon. In: Goodman LS, Gilman A, eds. The pharmacological basis of therapeutics. New York: Macmillan, 1975: 1507–1533.
135. Karam JH. Pancreatic hormones and antidiabetic drugs. In: Katzung BG, ed. Basic and clinical pharmacology. Los Altos: Lange, 1984:491–502.
136. Danford RO. The effect of glucagon on renal hemodynamics and renal arteriography. AJR 1970;108:665–673.
137. Danford RO, Davidson AJ. The use of glucagon as a vasodilator in visceral angiography. Radiology 1969;93:173–175.
138. Danford RO. The effect of glucagon on renal hemodynamics and renal arteriography. Am J Roentgenol 1970;108:665–673.
139. Larner J. Insulin and oral hypoglycemic drugs; glucagon. In: Gilman AG, et al, eds. The pharmacological basis of therapeutics. New York: Macmillan, 1985:1490–1516.
140. Williams GH, Hollenberg NK. Accentuated vascular and endocrine response to SQ 20881 in hypertension. N Engl J Med 1977;297:184–188.
141. Pokieser H. Pharmacoangiography. In: Anacker H, ed. Efficiency and limit of radiologic examination of the pancreas. Stuttgart: Thieme, 1975.
142. Aspelin P, Nylander G, Petterson H. Bradykinin-induced changes in caliber of portal vein during splanchnic angiography. Invest Radiol 1976;11:10–19.
143. Boijsen E, Redman HC. Effect of bradykinin on celiac and superior mesenteric angiography. Invest Radiol 1966;1:422–430.
144. Freed TA, Neal MP Jr, Vinik M. The effect of bradykinin on renal arteriography: experimental observations. AJR 1968; 102:776–782.
145. Dollery CT, Goldberg LI, Pentecost BL. Effects of intrarenal infusions of bradykinin and acetylcholine on renal blood flow in man. Clin Sci 1965;29:433.

6

Rapid Film Changers

KURT AMPLATZ

Historical Considerations

Progress in angiography is intimately linked to the development of better contrast media and improved radiographic equipment. The development of rapid film changers, which permitted a filming rate of two or more radiographs per second, represented a major advance in the angiographic diagnosis of congenital and acquired heart disease.

Numerous homemade machines were constructed by pioneers in this field because the x-ray companies showed little interest in the development of rapid film changers. The first roll-film changer was described by Howard Ruggles[1] and was demonstrated before the 11th Annual Meeting of the Radiological Society of North America in Cleveland, Ohio, December 7–11, 1925. This amazing machine was used by Edward Chamberlain[2] a year later for the study of the heart action. The apparatus was, for all practical purposes, identical to modern angiographic equipment and surpassed it with its high filming rate of 15 exposures per second. Eight-inch-wide and 30-foot-long x-ray roll film was transported intermittently by rubber-covered rollers between intensifying screens. The film was compressed between the intensifying screens, and x-ray exposures were accomplished by a high-tension, oil-immersed switch operated from the shaft of the machine.

H. Jarre, M.D.,[3] designed a similar roll-film device in 1929 (Fig. 6-1). His cinex camera was used for the study of physiologic phenomena such as spasm of the tracheobronchial tree, motor function of the urinary tract, and functional alterations as in hysterosalpingography. This ingenious pioneer also predicted the modern trend in radiology in general and concluded:[3]

> Physiology has been a step-child in our roentgenographic laboratories. Very much in contrast to our advanced knowledge on roentgen anatomy, efforts to collect information on physiology roentgenologically have been badly neglected.

He finished his address by saying:

> When you resume work remember this thought: Apparent anatomic normalcy is not of necessity associated with normal function. Pathologic function does not necessitate demonstrable anatomical alteration; therefore, we must bend our efforts to the investigation of anatomy and physiology, whenever the occasion arises and information of incalculable value is to be obtained.

Jarre's paper also reflected the frustrations of many x-ray pioneers at the lack of support from either their colleagues or equipment manufacturers.

> I tried in vain to interest one of the manufacturing companies building radiologic equipment in the task of designing and building a camera. Those approached considered the idea impractical or too extravagant, but now appear willing to utilize our designs without the intention of meeting any of its developmental expenses.

Jarre's advanced apparatus used 10-inch roll film, which was intermittently transported between intensifying screens at a rate of four frames per second.[3,4] Dr. Jarre presented his paper to the American Radiological Society of North America in December 1929 and had prepared an extensive exhibit showing radiographic demonstration of physiologic phenomena such as bronchial spasm, peristalsis of the ureter, and others. Unfortunately, he was not allowed to show his audience the results obtained with his amazing machine because the fire marshal forbade the showing of nitrocellulose films.

Neither Dr. Ruggles's nor Dr. Jarre's machine came to commercial production, although each could have influenced greatly the progress of angiography in this country.

A cassette changer described for the first time by J. Pereira Caldas[5] in 1934 represented in some respects a step backward because it had a much lower filming rate, but it probably afforded better radiographic definition because of better film-to-screen contact. The radio-carousel invented by Caldas was a manual

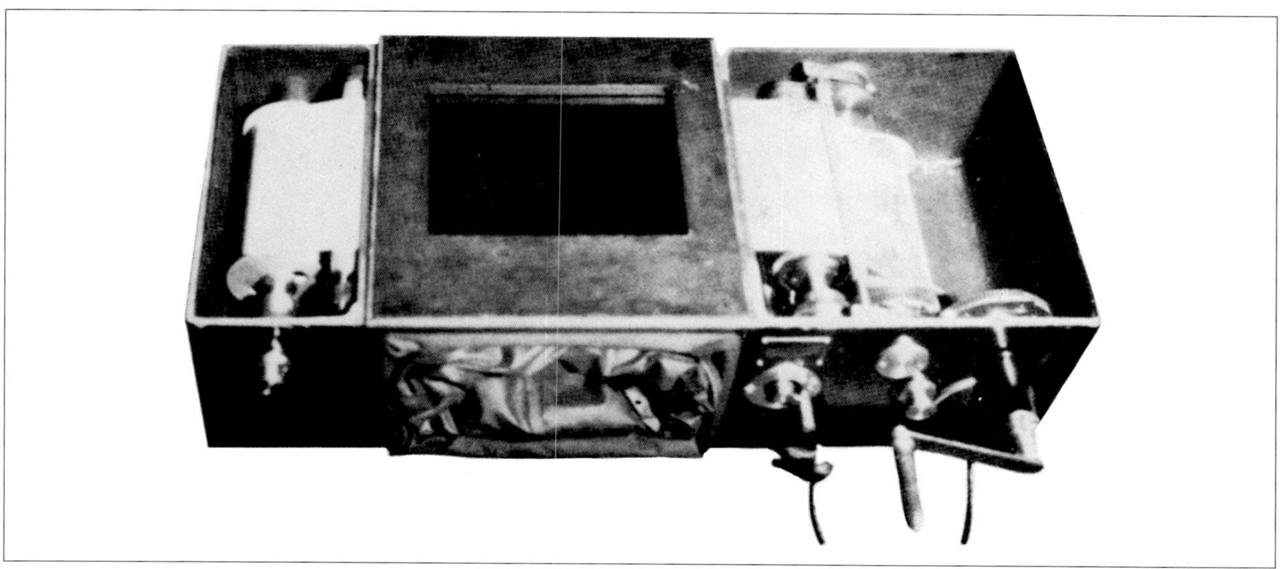

Figure 6-1. Roll-film camera of H. A. Jarre, M.D., constructed in 1929. (From Jarre HA. Roentgenologic studies of physiologic motor phenomena [with the aid of the cinex-camera]. Radiology 1930;15:377.)

device consisting of a heavy turntable with 24 × 30 cm cassettes mounted about its periphery (Fig. 6-2). An exposure rate of one per second could be achieved. In 1938 Van de Maele[6] described a rapid film changer using perforated roll film that was transported by a Maltese cross mechanism. The unit was capable of producing six exposures per second and had an off-center rotating grid to absorb secondary radiation. The rotating-wheel idea of Caldas was revived in 1942 by Sussman et al.,[7] who described a device with 10 × 12 inch cassettes mounted on the periphery of a large wheel with a maximum exposure rate of one per second.

The idea of placing cassettes on the periphery of a rotating wheel was a poor mechanical solution because the cassettes and the turntable had to be intermittently accelerated, limiting the exposure rate to one or two per second. Therefore Fredzell et al.[8] in 1950 abandoned the turntable and two-stage cassette changer and constructed a single-stage rotating-wheel mechanism that is of particular interest because it was used in biplane fashion (Fig. 6-3). The apparatus could take up to 12.5 roentgenograms per second on 18 × 24 cm cassettes in two planes at right angles. Up to 60 cassettes could be placed into two magazines, which were held by a strong spring against a rotating disk with a radial slit. After exposure, the cassette was ejected into a collecting receptacle.

Egas Moniz[9] deviated from the turntable idea and in 1934 built a manually operated cassette changer for cerebral angiography which he termed *Escamoteur.* Two cassettes were held together by coil springs, and the lower one was protected from exposure by a sheath of lead. After the exposure of the top cassette, it was pulled out manually into a lead-protected receiving bin. Sanchez-Perez, who had spent a year studying with Moniz, returned to this country and was forced to build his own seriograph, a similar manually operated unit using four cassettes. In 1943 Sanchez-Perez

Figure 6-2. The radio-carousel of Caldas, a heavy turntable with cassettes arranged in radial fashion. It was manually rotated with a maximum exposure rate of one per second. (From Caldas JP. Artériographies en série avec l'appareil radio-carrousel. J Radiol Electrol Med Nucl 1934;18:34.)

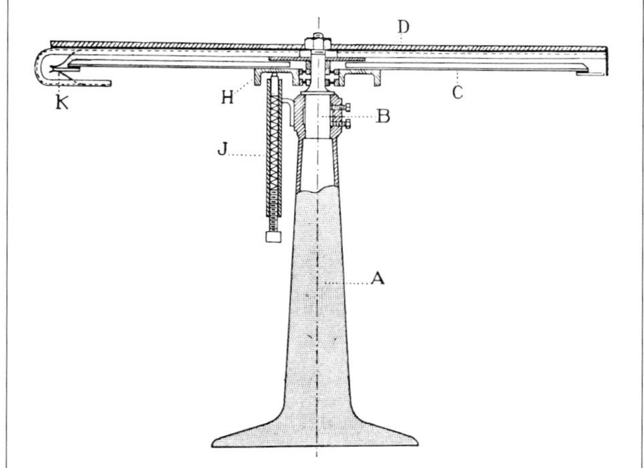

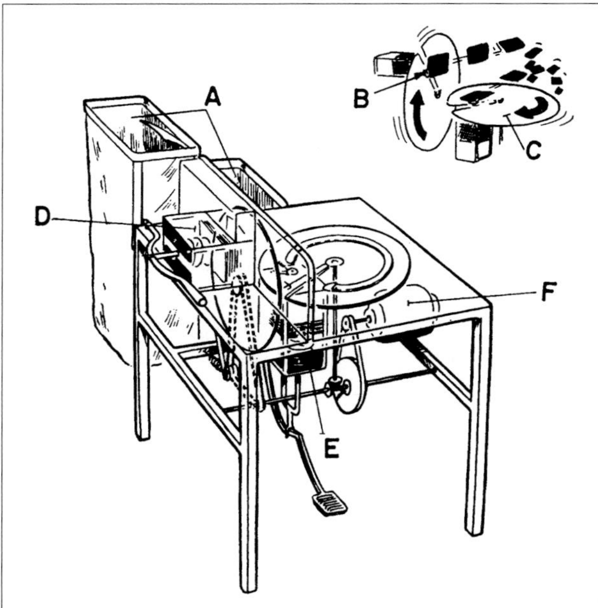

Figure 6-3. Single-stage rapid cassette changer of Fredzell et al. described in 1950.[8] *A,* collecting receptacles for exposed cassettes; *B,* spring wheel to eject exposed cassettes into collecting receptacles; *C,* rotating metal disk with radial slit to catch one cassette every revolution; *D,* magazine of cassettes in the vertical plane; *E,* magazine of cassettes in the horizontal plane; *F,* motor driving both rotating disks synchronously.

and Carter[10] described an improved model that eventually developed into the motor-driven cassette changer, the most widely used in this country.

The roll-film changer described by Gidlund[11] in 1949 is interesting because it was apparently a forerunner of the well-known Elema-Schönander apparatus and was very similar in construction to the cinex camera of Jarre. The prototype of the widely used American-made roll-film changer was developed by Rigler and Watson[12] at the University of Minnesota in 1953. The film was transported in intermittent fashion by a Geneva drive piercing the film edge by sharpened phonograph needles. After the exposure, an automatic cutting knife transformed the roll film into cut film, which was stored in the receiver bin. This changer represented distinct progress because at that time the available manual or semiautomatic film development limited the usefulness of roll film. The apparatus was used for several years at the University of Minnesota Heart Hospital and later was produced commercially by Franklin X-Ray Corporation.

In addition to the described major developments in the field of film changers, numerous homemade devices were developed that used the described mechanical principles in addition to gravity and spring-driven devices.[4,6,8,13–19] For a more complete review of the subject, the reader is referred to the excellent paper of Wendell G. Scott.[20]

General Remarks

Cineradiography and digital radiography have dramatically improved in quality, largely replacing film changers. The resolution capability of these newer techniques approaches that of radiographs made with high-speed screens. The minor resolution difference in cineradiography is offset by a much faster sampling rate (60 frames per second as compared to a maximum of 8 to 12 frames). Cine recordings, therefore, are superior in the demonstration of dynamic events and allow simultaneous viewing and recording on tape or disk. With the increasingly high cost of silver, it is likely that fewer and fewer angiograms will be recorded on cut film rather than digital radiography. However, for certain applications—cerebral angiography, renal angiography, pulmonary angiography, etc.—the use of film changers remains superior. The spatial resolution limit of digital angiography is less than half that for film (2 line pair/mm versus 5 line pair/mm).[21]

Because many readers do not have cineradiography or digital radiography equipment, this chapter presents a comprehensive review of the basic principles of all film changers that were or are commercially available.

Roll-Film Versus Cut-Film Changers

Rapid film changers can best be classified into roll-film and cut-film changers, depending on the type of film used. Before deciding which film changer may be useful for a specific angiographic laboratory, one must decide whether roll film or cut film is more practical; each film has certain advantages.

From the engineering standpoint, roll film is more attractive because it can be transported more easily; consequently, the apparatus tends to be more reliable mechanically. The main advantage of cut film, however, is that it can be stored easily in a regular film jacket. Roll film, on the other hand, cannot be stored with plain films. The film rolls are more bulky and require a larger space and a special filing system.

Viewing of roll film is less time-consuming, and the angiograms are always in sequential order. There is also less possibility that films will disappear. With the advent of automatic developing, roll film can be processed simply (previously one of the major obstacles to its use).

Considering the large volume of angiography performed at the University of Minnesota School of Medicine, roll-film changers are preferred because of their higher mechanical reliability. To eliminate the storage problem, the film is cut and the individual angiograms are taped together. This procedure preserves the sequential order and allows rapid viewing of an entire set of films.

Basic Principles of Film Changers

Two main systems are in use: (1) the rapid transport and mechanical changing of radiographic cassettes, and (2) rapid film transport with intermittent closure of intensifying screens. Both systems have merits. Cassette changers ensure perfect film-to-screen contact, but because of the weight and inertia of the radiographic cassettes, these changers have a limited exposure rate. Furthermore, the rapid acceleration and deceleration of cassettes may cause vibration of the angiographic apparatus. The vibration of these machines tends to occur at a right angle to the x-ray beam, and thus the vibration is more noticeable than it is in machines using intermittent closure of intensifying screens.

The main technical problems in equipment using intermittent closure of intensifying screens are inadequate film-to-screen contact and static electricity. The main obstacle to perfect film-to-screen contact is the trapping of air: Two perfectly flat metallic plates cannot be brought in good apposition because invariably a small air layer is trapped between the plates. Three different approaches have been used to solve this problem:

1. The lower plate on which the intensifying screen is mounted is slightly curved so it makes contact with the upper plate in the center first (Fig. 6-4A), allowing the air to escape toward the periphery.
2. Closure of the intensifying screens is like that of a book, so the air escapes toward one side (Fig. 6-4B).
3. The intensifying screens are mounted on Mylar membranes that are forced against each other; they meet in the center first and force the air uniformly toward the periphery (Fig. 6-4C). This system has the further advantage of operating without vibration.

Technical Considerations on the Use of Film Changers

To obtain optimal results, it is of paramount importance that the angiographer be entirely familiar with the technical aspects of angiography and the use of modern angiographic equipment. The radiologist should accept the responsibility for proper patient positioning, determination of exposure factors, selection of a proper program, and delivery of contrast medium.

Common mistakes causing poor studies include the following:

1. Improper exposure factors, particularly overexposures. A scout film invariably should be obtained and studied carefully with the x-ray technician. Generally speaking, the kilovoltage should be held at the range of 70 to 85, and the exposure time should be as short as possible, particularly in angiocardiography. For coronary arteriography, extremely short exposures, 1/60 or, better, 1/120 of a second, are mandatory. For abdominal and renal arteriography, in which

Figure 6-4. Methods of avoiding air entrapment. (A) Closure of intensifying screens with one of the plates slightly curved. (B) Closure of intensifying screens at one edge first. (C) Closure of intensifying screens by air pressure from both sides.

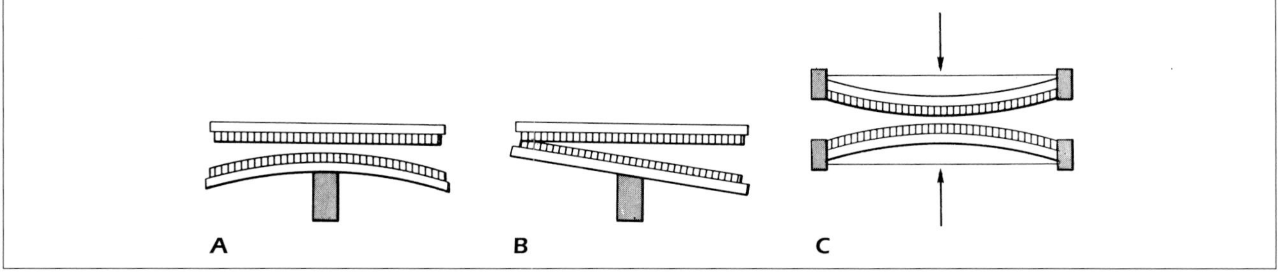

there is little or no motion, a longer exposure time is acceptable.

2. Improper coning. Maximal coning is an absolute necessity to reduce secondary radiation. Commonly, the full field of a 14 × 14 inch cut film, for example, is exposed, causing deterioration of the radiographic image. On a selective renal arteriogram or angiocardiogram, the exposed area should not extend more than 1 inch beyond the organ of interest. In coronary arteriography, maximal coning can be achieved by taping a lead mask on the chest wall over the heart. A nongrid technique can be used to reduce further the exposure times and consequently to eliminate unsharpness due to heart motion. The improvement of the radiographic image by maximal coning is striking.

3. Biplane technique. The use of biplane angiographic technique is almost indispensable to evaluate congenital heart disease in children, but it gives poor results in the adult patient. Despite the use of cross-hatched grids, there is considerable cross-fogging, particularly in heavier patients. In heavy adult patients, it is advantageous to perform two injections rather than simultaneous biplane exposures. The use of biplane angiography should be limited to children and slim adults. If it is used at all, maximal coning is the best means of obtaining acceptable biplane angiograms.

4. Inadequate delivery rate of the contrast medium.

Almost invariably a poor angiogram is caused by one of the errors just listed rather than by the film changer. Modern angiographic equipment yields excellent results provided the operator is entirely familiar with the technical aspects of angiography.

Cassette Changers

Cassette changers can be divided into single-stage and two-stage design (Fig. 6-5). In the single-stage changer, radiographic cassettes are held together in a stack by a strong coil spring and the underlying cassettes are protected from exposure by lead (Fig. 6-5A). After the cassette has been exposed, it is pulled or pushed into the receiver bin and the next cassette is pushed into exposure position by the coil spring. A typical example of this design is the well-known Sanchez-Perez cassette changer.

In the two-stage changer, radiographic cassettes are also held together by spring pressure, but the cassette is moved into the exposure area, exposed, and transported rapidly into the exposure bin (Fig. 6-5B). This design eliminates the need for lead protection of the underlying cassettes. Consequently, the radiographic cassettes can be much lighter. The disadvantage of this system, of course, is the additional motion of the cassettes into the exposure area. Classic examples of this basic construction are drum mechanisms for femoral arteriography and the radio-carousel of Caldas.[5]

Modern Cassette Changers

The classic single-stage cassette changer originally described by Moniz and later perfected by Sanchez-Perez and Carter developed into a widely used commercial apparatus (Fig. 6-6). Up to twelve 10 × 12 inch radiographic cassettes can be loaded and automatically changed at a maximal rate of two per second. The unit can be raised and lowered by motor drive and is easily tilted manually into the vertical position; thus it is par-

Figure 6-5. Cassette changer principles. (A) Single-stage changer with lead protection of each individual cassette. (B) Two-stage changer, which eliminates lead backing of cassette but requires additional transport motion of cassettes into exposure area.

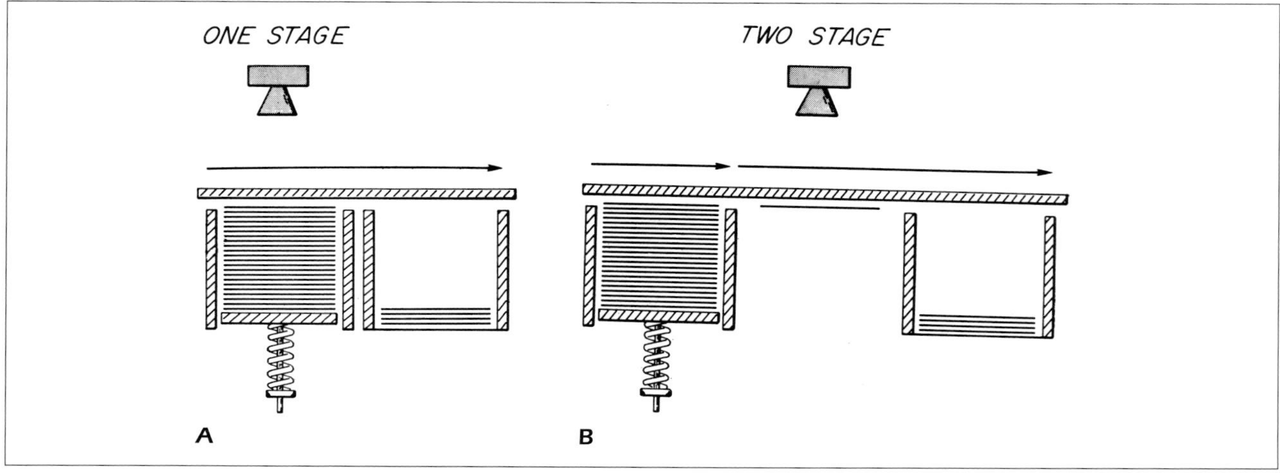

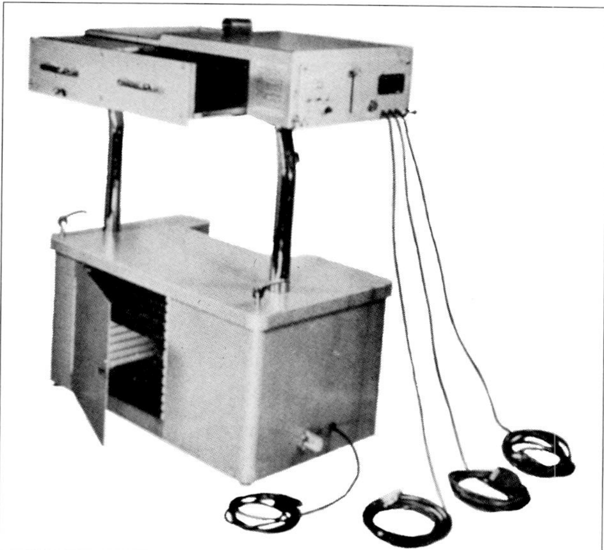

Figure 6-6. The Sanchez-Perez cassette changer. This unit can be raised and lowered and easily tilted into the vertical position.

ticularly useful for cerebral angiography. An automatic change in exposure rate can be accomplished by a program selector. The unit is the oldest commercial American-made cassette changer and is still used, especially for cerebral angiography. In 1963[22] a similar but spring-driven cassette changer that employed a newly designed ultrathin and ultralight vacuum cassette was developed for cerebral angiography at the University of Minnesota. With vacuum cassettes, atmospheric pressure holds the film-and-screen combination in uniform ultimate contact and thus eliminates the rigid, heavy frame of the standard cassette. This is a great advantage in transport and allowed Picker Corporation to construct a cassette changer with a maximal speed of four per second. This unit is no longer produced.

In the Picker-Amplatz vacuum contact system, the film-and-screen combination was placed in a black polyethylene bag and heat-sealed in a special vacuumatic sealing unit (Fig. 6-7). The loaded envelope, which could be 8 × 10, 14 × 14, or 14 × 17 inches, was placed in receiving tray *A* of the vacuumatic unit. By closing its lid, *B*, one automatically applied a vacuum, and the air was wiped out from the film-and-screen sandwich by a neoprene diaphragm. At the same time, the metal jaws of the lid were automatically heated and permanently sealed the polyethylene bag in 4.5 seconds. Because of the rather low leakage rate of the polyethylene envelope, the cassettes could be presealed and stored for as long as 1 week.

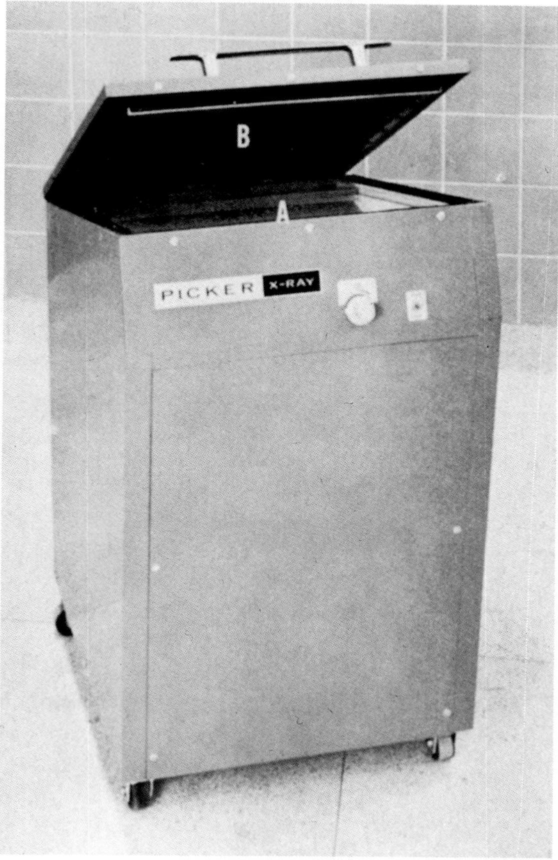

Figure 6-7. The Picker-Amplatz system. Vacuumatic sealing unit in this contact system allows evacuation and heat sealing of vacuum cassettes in 4.5 seconds.

The Picker Cassette Changer with Computer Programmer

This unit is designed according to the single-stage cassette changer principle (Fig. 6-8; see Fig. 6-5). In the feed chamber, up to 21 vacuum cassettes are stacked on a spring-loaded platform. The cassettes are pressed firmly by springs against the exposure plate. At the end of each exposure, the compression spring releases, and the exposed film is removed by a push-bar arrangement. Programming of the unit, the table, and the injection syringe is accomplished by inserting IBM cards into a simple computer. The apparatus may be used for any type of angiography and is available in biplane arrangements. The thin vacuum cassette allows a changing rate of four per second, a distinct advantage over the Sanchez-Perez cassette changer.

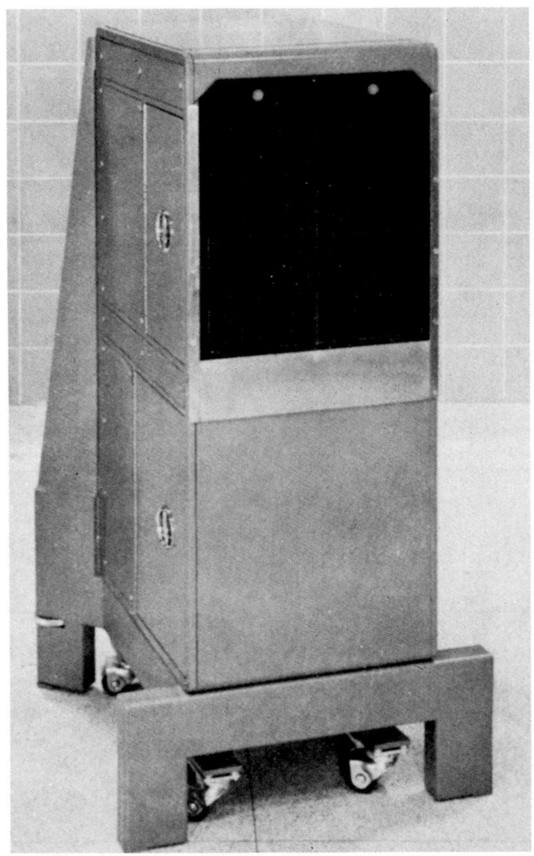

Figure 6-8. Picker cassette changer in vertical position. The maximum changing rate is four per second with vacuum cassettes.

Rapid Film Changers

The lower weight of radiographic roll and cut film as compared to cassettes makes it possible to achieve a much higher exposure rate (up to 12 per second in one of the commercially available units). As the changing rate increases, the longest permissible exposure time must become shorter and shorter, so that high-powered generators are required. The manufacturer recommends a maximal permissible exposure time for the various film-changing rates. This has important practical implications because it determines the top possible changing rate at a certain exposure time.

In all rapid film changers, a certain part of the cycle is allowed for film transport, whereas during another part of the cycle the film is clamped in a stationary position between the intensifying screens. In all film changers, the film is in motion slightly longer than 50 percent of the cycle. For the Schönander cut-film changer and the Elema roll-film changer, for example, the film's stationary time coincides with the closure of the intensifying screens and is approximately 40 percent of the cycle. For the Franklin film changer, the closure time is only 37 percent of the total cycle. Theoretically, this stationary time, during which the film is firmly compressed between the intensifying screens, would be available for exposure. This, however, is not the case because certain delays have to be taken into consideration.

Zero Time

The film changer signals the generator as to when the exposure should occur by closing a switch. Once the changer has given the signal, the exposure occurs after a small delay. One portion of this delay is constant within each machine and is due to the time it takes to close relays, build up voltages to proper height, and so forth, in the x-ray control. This constant and predictable delay has been termed the *zero time of the x-ray apparatus.* Because the zero time of the x-ray apparatus is constant, it is possible to compensate for the delay by presetting the exposure on the film changer. If the zero time of the x-ray apparatus is 60 milliseconds, the exposure switch on the film changer can give the signal 60 milliseconds before the film is actually in full compression. In other words, the actual exposure can be anticipated by the exposure switch; therefore, this time has also been termed *anticipation time.* Switches in the film changer must be adjusted so that the zero time is constant regardless of changing rate. For the newer three-phase generators with electronic contractors, the zero time may be so short that it can be disregarded.

Phasing-in Time

There is another delay in the x-ray apparatus, which is not constant. This variable delay has been termed *phasing-in* or *interrogation time* and depends on the moment when the film changer signals the generator to expose in relation to the phase of the alternating current.

The x-ray generators are constructed in such a fashion that the exposure can start only when the cycle of the line voltage passes through zero. If the film changer closes its exposure switch at this very moment, the exposure can start immediately and the phasing-in time is zero. On the other hand, if the exposure switch closes just after the cycle has passed through zero, there may be a full cycle of delay before the exposure can start. The maximum duration of the phasing-in time is 1/60 of a second or 16.7 milliseconds. For

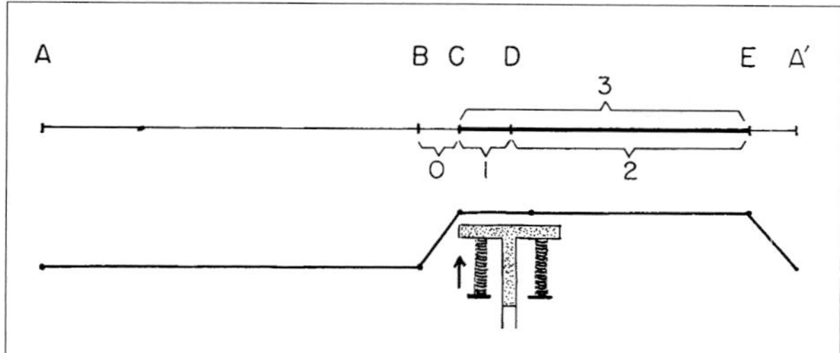

Figure 6-9. Diagram showing timing cycle of film changers. Film stationary time, *C–E;* zero time, *B–C;* phasing-in time, *C–D;* film cycle, *A–A′*.

all film changers, therefore, at least 16.7 milliseconds must be subtracted from the stationary time of the film to allow calculation of the maximal permissible exposure time.

The sequence of events is summarized in Figure 6-9. The time between *A* and *A′* represents the film cycle, which repeats itself at a preset frequency. At point *C,* the film is in full compression and stationary, and theoretically exposure could be started. During the other time of the cycle, from *E* to *C* (usually 60 percent or more of the entire film cycle), the film is in motion. Because of the fixed delay in the x-ray apparatus, the exposure release can be initiated slightly before *C* at point *B* (*B–C* zero time). Because of the phase-in time, *C–D* exposure can be started only at point *D,* which gives the longest permissible exposure time, *D–E.* From the film stationary time *C–E,* the phase-in time *C–D* of 16.7 milliseconds has therefore been subtracted.

From these theoretical considerations the longest permissible exposure time can be calculated for a certain type of film changer. If the film changer transport time is 60 percent and the stationary time is 40 percent of the film cycle, the maximal permissible exposure time for a rate of 12 per second is calculated in the following way: For an exposure rate of 1 per second, the stationary time would be 400 milliseconds; for a rate of 12 per second, divide 400 by 12 (33.3 milliseconds). From the stationary time, the maximum phase-in time or interrogation time of the generator (one full cycle or 16.7 milliseconds) must be subtracted: 33.3 milliseconds minus 16.7 is 16.6 milliseconds. The maximal available exposure time is therefore 16.6 milliseconds when the fixed zero time of the x-ray apparatus is compensated for by anticipating the exposure.

Because the calculated maximal permissible exposure time of 16.6 milliseconds may not be available as a step on the x-ray control and a slight safety margin must be allowed, the manufacturer invariably suggests a shorter than calculated exposure time. To improve radiographic quality, some manufacturers suggest a much shorter exposure time to allow the air to escape after screen closure. For the Franklin roll-film changer, the short exposure time of 1/60 second is recommended at a filming rate of six per second.

The Schönander Cut-Film Changer

The Schönander cut-film changer in film sizes 14 × 14 and 10 × 12 inches is also referred to as *AOT,* an abbreviation for "*a*ngi*o*-*t*able," because the apparatus was once part of an examination table. The radiologist does not need to be familiar with the technical details of construction but should have an understanding of the basic function of this apparatus, which is shown in the simplified drawing of Figure 6-10.

Basically, film is transported from the feeding magazine *A* through the exposure area *C* into the receiving magazine *B.* The transport is accomplished by rubberized rollers that touch the films only at both edges. The most important and most delicate part of the film changer is the lower compression plate, *D,* on which one of the intensifying screens is mounted. The compression plate is lowered by cam *E* and suddenly released. Actual compression of the film between the screens is achieved by forcing the precision-machined plate *D* upward by coil springs *F.*

After inserting the feeding magazine *A,* which may contain up to 30 films, the technician pushes the "advance" button on the program selector, causing the motor to turn. The magazine *A* moves into the position *A′* because the lead screw *G* is turned by the motor. The lid of the magazine and two small ports on the bottom of the magazine are opened, allowing levers *H* to enter the magazine. The advancement of the magazine is controlled by a set of microswitches until the tips of the ejection levers *H* come to rest immediately beneath the first film, which is now in line with the rubber-covered transport wheel *J* and pinch-roller *K.* The film is ejected from the magazine by levers *H* and transported into the exposure area by rollers *K* and *J* (*arrows*). Breaking of the film is accomplished by a leaf spring (not shown in this drawing) and a cam-operated lever *L.* Pressure plate *D,* which had been pulled down by cam *E,* now releases and compresses the film between the two intensifying screens by springs *F.* The exposure is initiated. After the film has been exposed, plate *D* is pulled down by cam *E,* the stop lever *L* lowers, and the pinch-roller *M* engages the film against the rotating rubberized transport wheel *J′*. The film is transported at high velocity into the receiving magazine *B,* where it is braked by a leaf spring and foam-rubber cushion at the floor of the magazine. At the same time the lead screw *G* has further advanced maga-

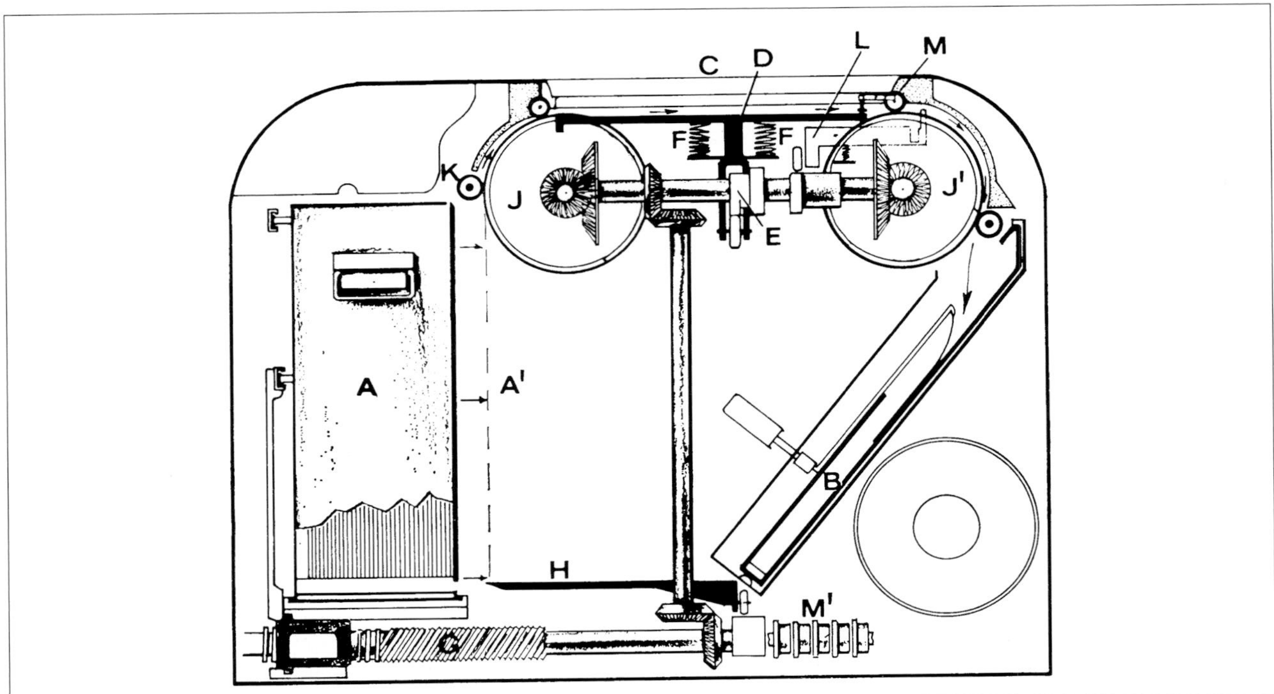

Figure 6-10. Simplified schematic drawing of Schönander cut-film changer. *A,* feeding magazine; *B,* receiving magazine; *C,* exposure area; *D,* compression plate; *E,* compression plate cam; *F,* compression coil springs; *G,* feeding magazine lead screw; *H,* ejection lever; *J* and *J′,* rubberized transport wheels; *K,* pinch-roller; *L,* film stop lever; *M,* pinch-roller; *M′,* exposure switches.

zine *A* to such a degree that the ejection levers *H* come to rest beneath the second film in order to be ejected, and the cycle is repeated. After the program has been completed, the direction of the motor reverses and transports feeding magazine *A* to its original position. The spring-loaded cover of receiving magazine *B* closes to allow removal of the magazine from the apparatus in daylight.

The apparatus is amazingly trouble-free, but there is a tendency toward jamming, particularly in the spring and fall, because changing humidity may cause curling of sheet film. Under ideal conditions, the film should be perfectly straight. Production of static electricity in the exposure area has been lessened by various antistatic sprays and a protective antistatic coating of the intensifying screens. This protective coating wears off with time and requires periodic replacement of the intensifying screens. Excessive friction of film in the receiver magazine *B* can be alleviated by leaving one film in the receiving magazine.

The apparatus can be used in biplane fashion (Fig. 6-11), or it can be tilted into the vertical position by a hand crank or a modified power drill. The unit is sturdy and will operate for many years without major adjustments.

The Puck Film Changer

The Puck film changer is a lightweight versatile unit (Fig. 6-12) that can be mounted on a hydraulic stand for horizontal or vertical operation (Figs. 6-12, 6-13) and lowered for magnification radiography. For exact positioning it can be moved over the image intensifier by using the Amplatz see-through principle. Because of the light weight and low profile, it is usually mounted on C arms and parallelograms, allowing for angle angiography without turning the patient (Fig. 6-14).

The cut-film changer uses either 24 × 30 cm or 35 × 35 cm (14 × 14 inch) film. Maximal loading capacity is 20 films, with a changing rate of up to 3 films per second. A simple magazine allows daylight loading and unloading. As with the Picker film changer, the program is controlled by punch cards; the filming sequence, start of exposure, and injector can be integrated.

The apparatus works according to the two-stage changer principle, basically transporting cut film from a feeding magazine into the exposure area and from there into the receiving magazine (Fig. 6-15). The magazine *A* is preloaded in the darkroom with at most

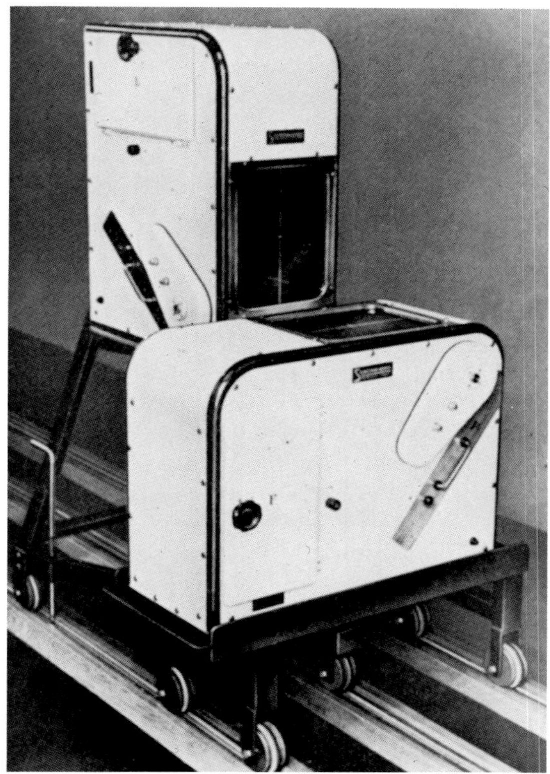

Figure 6-11. Schönander cut-film changer in biplane arrangement.

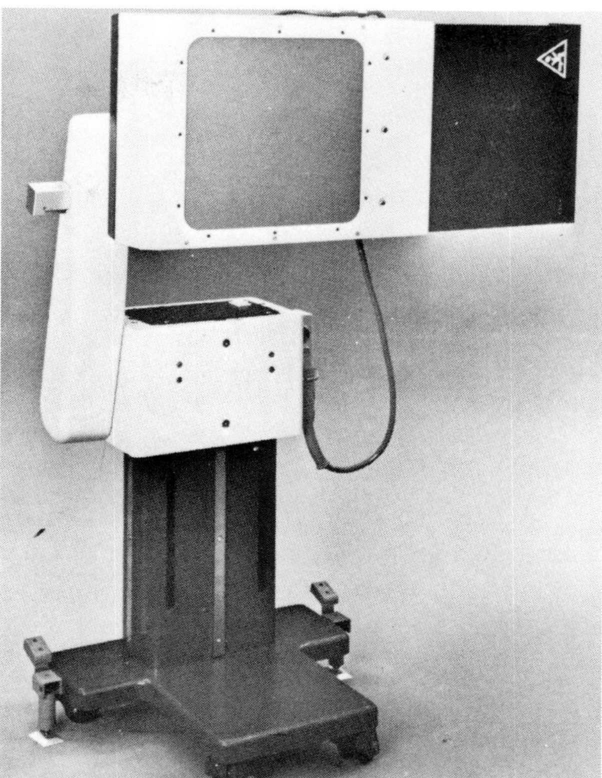

Figure 6-13. Puck film changer mounted vertically on a hydraulic stand.

20 cut films.* The films are pulled, one by one, by a transport finger over the transport roller *B,* which delivers each film to the exposure area. The intensifying screens are mounted on the two compression plates *C,* which are intermittently opened and closed, compressing the film firmly for good screen contact. As with other modern film changers, the front compression plate consists of carbon fiber–reinforced plastic (CFRP); this has high strength and a lower x-ray absorption than aluminum. After the x-ray exposure, the film, transported over the roller system *D,* is delivered to the receiving magazine *E.*

Figure 6-12. Puck film changer mounted horizontally on a hydraulic stand.

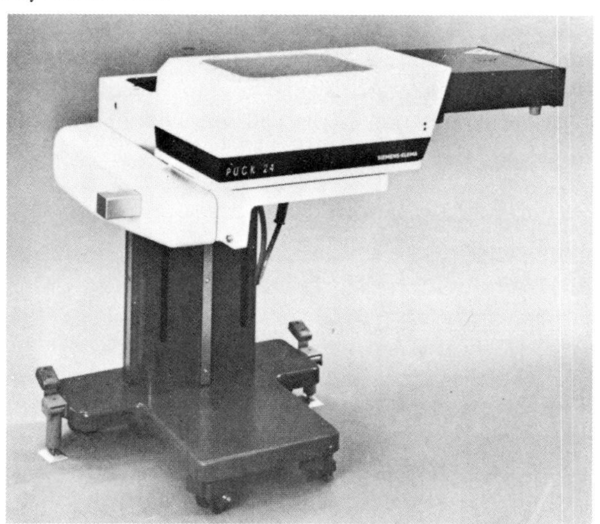

The punch-card control system lends itself to integration of injector, exposure sequence, and tabletop motion for long-leg angiography.

The Elema Roll-Film Changer

The Elema roll-film changer allows the highest exposure rate, 12 per second. For practical purposes this high exposure rate is not necessary, but it may be useful in research and in angiocardiography of infants. The horizontal and vertical changers are tied permanently together, so this apparatus is exclusively a biplane unit. The vertical exposure area is 12 × 12 inches

*The films are separated by an air space to prevent transport of two films simultaneously.

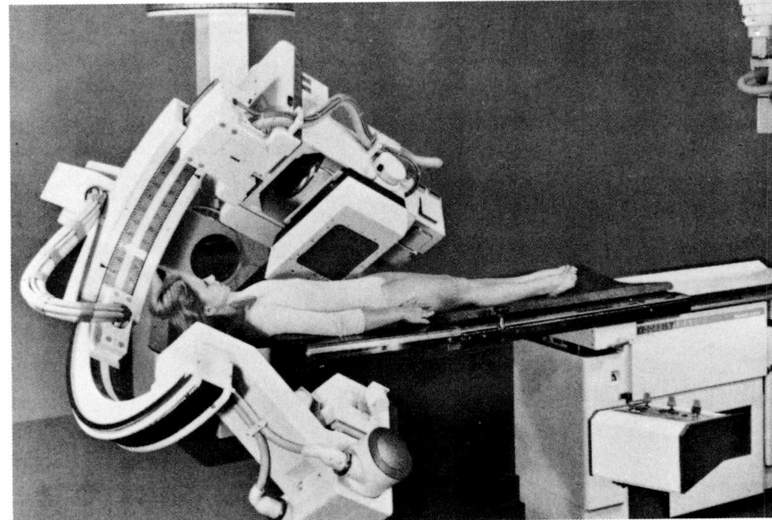

Figure 6-14. Puck film changer mounted on a C arm.

(30 × 30 cm), the horizontal field is 12 × 14 inches (30 × 35 cm), and both changers use 12-inch roll film (Fig. 6-16). The unit can be raised and lowered on a chain-operated mount and can be tilted to various positions on a pivot.

The attractive features of this apparatus are its simple construction and, consequently, more trouble-free operation (Fig. 6-17). Roll film is placed on the supply spool *A* and threaded through the separated intensifying screens and transport rollers to take-up spool *B*. Contact between intensifying screens and x-ray film is accomplished by the compression plates *C*. To ensure smooth transport, the spools are power-driven with an electromagnetic clutch system that may need occasional adjustment. The transport of the film is accomplished by serrated cam-rollers *D* and pinch-rollers *E*, which engage the film at both margins and cause characteristic serrations.

The unit, although mechanically simple and relatively trouble-free, must be loaded and unloaded in a darkened room. There is no footage indicator, so it is difficult to estimate the amount of film used. This unit is no longer in production.

The Franklin Roll-Film Changer

The Franklin changer is an American-made apparatus that has become popular, particularly for cerebral angiography. It is the commercial version of the apparatus described by Rigler and Watson.[12] The maximal exposure rate is six per second, and the 14-inch roll film offers an adequate exposure area of 11 × 14 inches (Fig. 6-18). The apparatus can be rotated easily in the vertical position and raised and lowered by a motor drive. Changers are not permanently connected to each other. As with the original design, intermittent transport of roll film is accomplished by a Geneva drive piercing the film edges by phonograph needles. Major advantages over the Elema roll-film changer are ease

Figure 6-15. Diagram of a Puck film changer. *A,* magazine; *B,* transport roller; *C,* compression plates; *D,* roller system; *E,* receiving magazine.

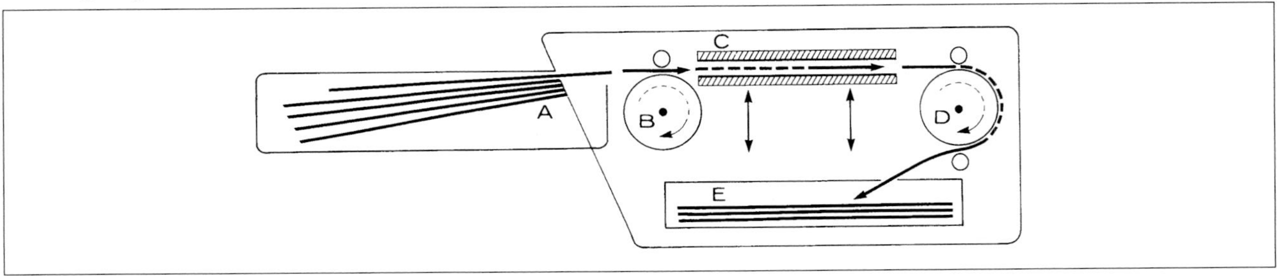

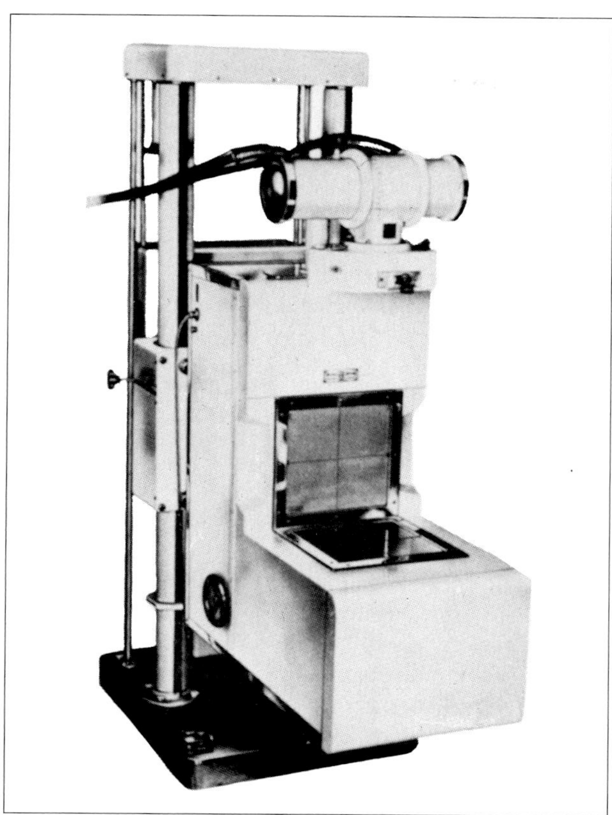

Figure 6-16. Elema roll-film changer.

of handling and daylight loading. The main disadvantage is the rather short exposure time suggested by the manufacturer, which limits its usefulness for rapid abdominal angiography. Very powerful generators should be used in conjunction with this versatile, practical apparatus, which has been superseded by the Puck film changer.

The Amplatz See-Through Changer

With the Amplatz roll-film changer it is possible to observe the radiographic image on the television screen. The apparatus combines the high resolution of rapid film changers with the convenience of cine recording to allow observation on the television screen.[23]

The radiolucency of the compression mechanism is accomplished by mounting the intensifying screens on prestretched Mylar membranes. These membranes contact the film in the center first and allow air to escape in uniform fashion toward the periphery* (see Fig. 6-4). Compressed gas is used to approximate the

*In its newest version, only one Mylar diaphragm is used for compression.

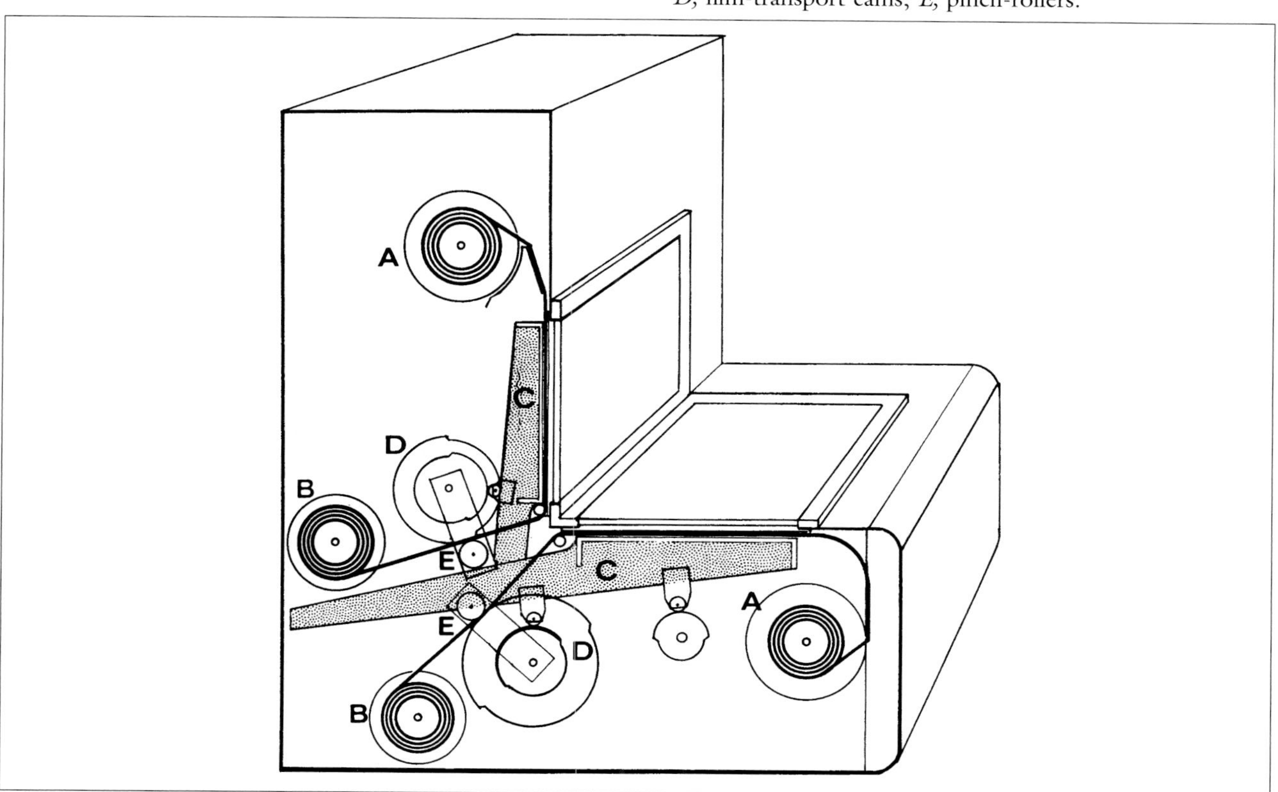

Figure 6-17. Simplified diagram of Elema roll-film changer. *A*, feeding spool; *B*, take-up spool; *C*, compression plates; *D*, film-transport cams; *E*, pinch-rollers.

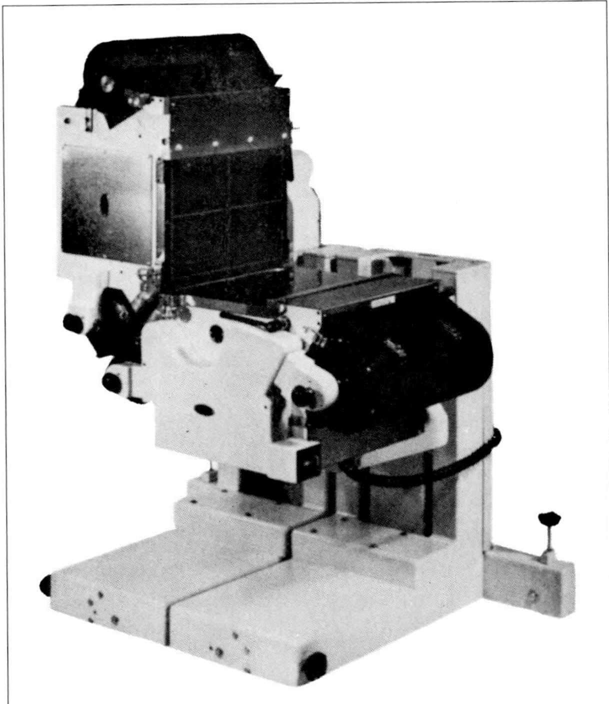

Figure 6-18. Franklin roll-film changer in biplane arrangement.

two round Mylar membranes by intermittent activation of large-bore solenoid air valves.

Twelve-inch roll film is simply transported by intermittent rotation of the take-up spool by an electromagnetic clutch and brake combination. To eliminate any waste of film, the exact amount of film can be inserted in the apparatus, just as is done in the cut-film changer. A supply of unexposed x-ray film, kept in the x-ray room in a storage bin, allows loading of the feeding magazine in daylight in the same room and cuts down trips to the darkroom.

The program can be preselected at six, five, four, three, two, and one exposures per second or it can be continuously changed, depending on the angiographic appearance on the television screen.

The intensifying screens absorb approximately 50 percent of the radiation, which is not objectionable for fluoroscopy (Fig. 6-19). The arrangement is not, however, desirable for cine recording, which by itself may represent a radiation hazard to the patient. A second arrangement is better for radiographic and cine recording. The apparatus is mounted on a hydraulic C-shaped frame with rollers and moves over the image intensifier when needed (Fig. 6-20). The patient does not have to be moved, and the radiographic image can again be observed on the television screen. The unit can be manually tilted into the vertical position, even with a permanently mounted image intensifier behind the changer.

The round exposure field allows the use of a rotating Bucky diaphragm and eliminates grid lines, even at the short exposure time of 1/120 second. Because the diaphragm is in continuous rapid motion, operation is vibration-free in horizontal and vertical positions and synchronization with the x-ray exposures is not necessary. If a round grid is rotated at slow speed, a broad band of visible grid lines can still be observed (Fig. 6-21B). If the speed of rotation is increased, the band of visible grid lines gets smaller (Fig. 6-21C), and at higher speeds of 800 to 1000 rpm, grid lines completely disappear (Fig. 6-21D).

Theoretically there should be demonstration of a stationary point in the true center of the grid, but this cannot be observed even with a magnifying glass. It is probably caused by imperfection of the rotation, which is not perfectly circular but also has lateral play. Ideally the grid should be supported around its circumference or it should rotate on invisible air bearings. The latter is a rather difficult engineering problem, so it was decided to support the grid in its center by a plastic bearing (Fig. 6-22). The round hole in the center of the aluminum cover for bearing support creates a radiolucency on the radiographs that is compensated for by the increase in density caused by the plastic-bearing material. Therefore, the radiographic image of the bearing is hardly visible on the actual radiograph.

In most cases, however, high-speed rotation of the grid is simply accomplished by an air jet, similar to that in an air turbine, directed against small veins. The rotation of the grid can be stopped by closing the air inlet, and the grid lines can be oriented parallel to the long axis of the table. Tube angulation in the direction of the grid lines is allowed, as is desirable for cerebral angiography. This unit was never produced commercially.

The CGR Roll-Film Changer

The rapid film changer CR835 combines the advantages of roll and cut film (Fig. 6-23). Fourteen-inch roll film is used because of the transport advantages of roll film, and cut film is delivered because of the advantages of handling, storing, and more rapid developing. A guillotine cuts the roll film at the same rate as the films are taken (up to eight exposures per second).

The film changer can be operated in biplane fashion up to six frames per second and up to three frames per second in the alternate mode.* As with other roll-film

*In single-plane operations, eight exposures per second can be made.

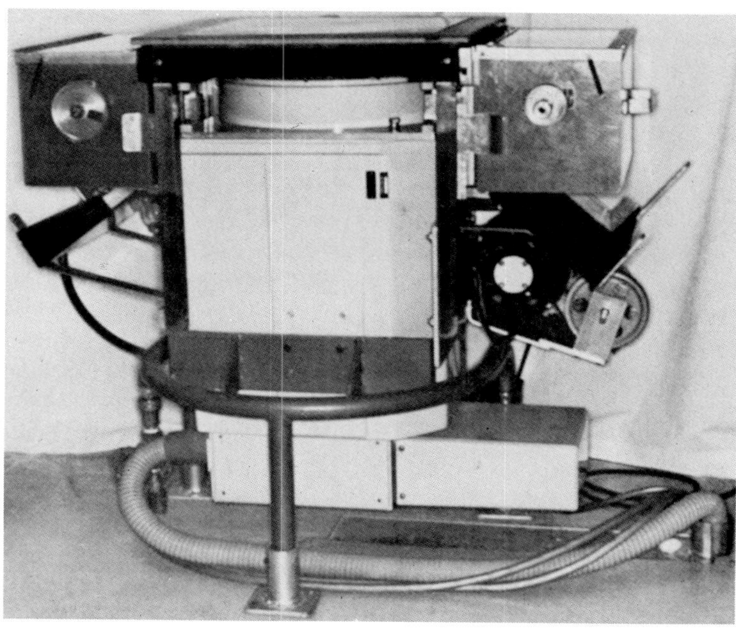

Figure 6-19. See-through changer permanently mounted over 9-inch image intensifier.

changers, cross-fogging can be eliminated by alternate firing, but every other frame is wasted.

The fact that the film changer can be loaded and unloaded in daytime is a distinct advantage over the Elema roll-film changer. The film is compressed intermittently between the intensifying screens. The lower plate is slightly curved, allowing escape of air. The compression or dwell time is longer than that in all other film changers. Most existing machines allow only one-third of the total cycle time for exposures. With the CGR changer, one-half of the cycle can be used as exposure time. The maximal exposure rate, for example, at two exposures per second is therefore 0.25 second, compared to 0.16 second with other film

Figure 6-20. Amplatz see-through changer, movable over image intensifier.

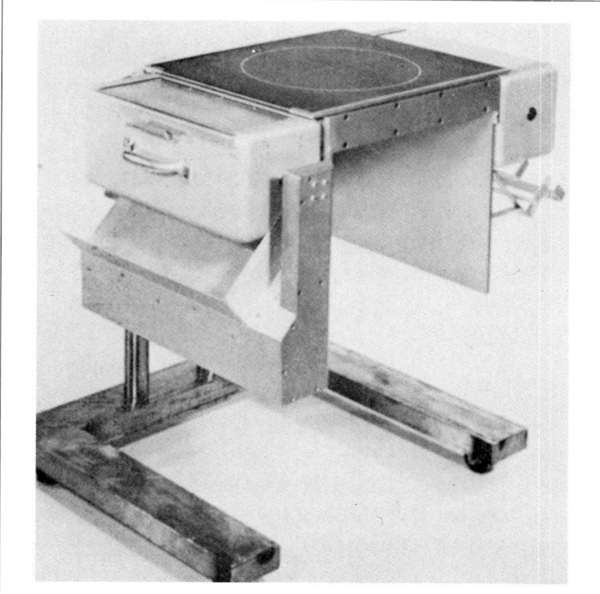

Figure 6-21. Rotating grid of see-through changer. (A) Stationary. (B) Slowly rotating. (C) Faster rotation. (D) 800 rpm.

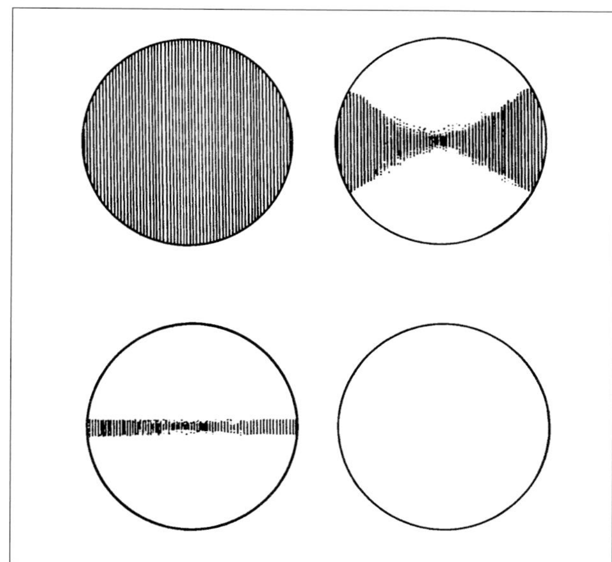

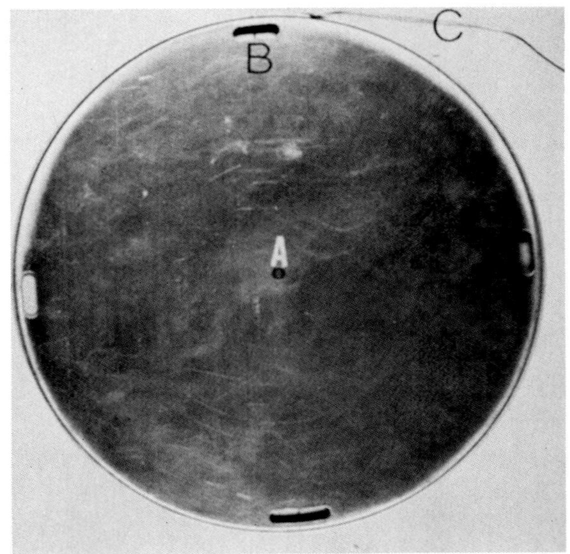

Figure 6-22. Stationary grid of see-through changer. *A,* plastic pivot; *B,* window for grid alignment; *C,* tubing for compressed gas.

changers. The lower kilovolt-peak level that can be used with this changer increases contrast.

The mechanical operation is similar to that of other devices. A full roll of 14-inch film is placed in the feeding magazine *A* (Fig. 6-24). The film is fed by rollers *B* through the intermittently closing intensifying screens *C.* The film is transported by a large-diameter drum *D,* which is rotated intermittently by a Geneva drive. During the exposure when the film transport is stationary, the roll film is cut into 14-inch-long films by the guillotine *E* and transported into the receiving magazine *G* by the rollers *F.*

The single-plane unit can be operated in horizontal or vertical position, or two changers can be arranged in biplane fashion.

Figure 6-23. CR835 rapid film changer.

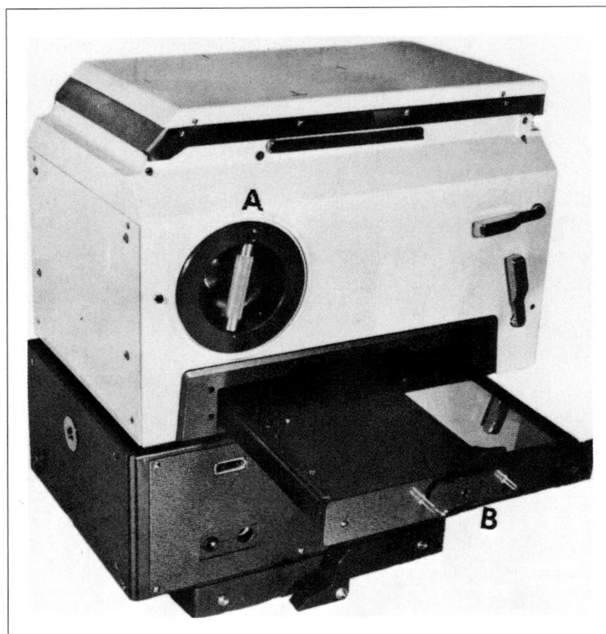

Large-Field Angiography

Technical Considerations

For visualization of the femoral-popliteal arterial system, the best results are obtained if the contrast medium is injected in the direction of the bloodstream either via a catheter introduced from the left axillary artery or by translumbar catheterization. This so-called downstream arteriography causes less dilution of contrast medium during diastole and consequently yields a much better contrast visualization of the leg arteries. The injection of contrast medium above the renal arteries and particularly against the bloodstream yields fainter visualization of the femoral-popliteal system in spite of a contrast volume as high as 60 to 80 ml.

An unusually slow, delayed blood flow due to the presence of obstructive disease also causes poor visualization of the vasculature below the knee. Sometimes a delayed film made 16 seconds after the injection may not be late enough to visualize the lower system. It is therefore advisable to speed up the blood flow either

Figure 6-24. Diagram of CR835 film changer. *A,* feeding magazine; *B,* rollers; *C,* intensifying screens; *D,* drum; *E,* guillotine; *F,* roller; *G,* receiving magazine.

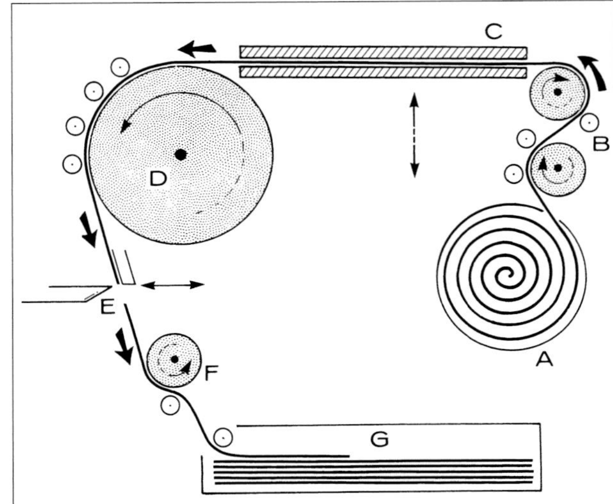

by exercise or, more conveniently, by reactive hyperemia.[24] For the latter, tourniquets are placed below the knees and inflated above arterial pressure for approximately 8 minutes. The contrast medium is injected immediately after removal of the tourniquets.

Basic Principles

With this system the problem involved is not rapid film transport (an exposure rate of one film every 1 to 3 seconds is usually adequate), but rather achievement of uniform radiographic density through the varying diameter of the abdomen and lower extremities. An even density can be obtained in various ways:

1. Use of wedge filters. Placement of an aluminum wedge filter in the primary beam allows the beam to be attenuated toward the patient's feet and thus creates comparatively uniform radiographic density. With this technique the x-ray beam tends to harden because of the interposed aluminum infiltration, causing some deterioration of the angiographic image.
2. Use of a combination of screens with various intensification factors such as high-speed, par-speed, and detail-intensifying screens. This approach is commonly used with 14 × 17 inch cassettes. With this technique the density gradient is not as uniform as with the wedge filters.
3. Use of a combination of high- and low-ratio grids.
4. Use of the heel effect of the x-ray tube.
5. Use of intensifying screens with a gradual change from high speed to low speed. This undoubtedly is the most satisfactory solution because the hardening of the x-ray beam by the aluminum wedge filter is eliminated and there is a gradual change in radiographic density without disturbing, abrupt density gradients.
6. Use of x-ray film of various speeds.

Long-Leg Film Changers

For certain applications of femoral arteriography and translumbar aortography, a much larger film size is desirable for demonstration of the abdominal aorta and leg arteries on the same film. Ideally, the entire vascular system from the abdominal aorta to the toes should be angiographically demonstrated with one injection. This visualization can be accomplished by using a 14 × 14 inch changer and moving the patient cranially at the same rate at which the contrast medium progresses in the vascular system. Motion of the radiographic table can be programmed as well as the change in exposure factors.

At first glance this solution appears to be satisfactory, although the main technical difficulty is estimation of the speed of blood flow, which may vary drastically with the disease process. Furthermore, there may be a considerable difference between the speed of blood flow through one leg and the other. This system is difficult, particularly for the novice, but it is said to be practical for experienced angiographers even though a repeat injection may be required to correct errors in timing. The speed of blood flow can be estimated by the injection of an isotope tracer or more simply by fluoroscopic observation and timing of a small contrast bolus. If a small amount of contrast medium is injected into the abdominal aorta, its arrival at the femoral artery and popliteal artery levels can be timed with a stopwatch.[9] It is not surprising that this complicated system has been unable to replace large-field angiography, which is much simpler to use and more foolproof.

Large-field angiography is satisfactorily carried out by various homemade stratagems, such as pushing 14 × 17 inch cassettes through a tunnel, pulling lead-protected cassettes manually according to the principle of a single-stage cassette changer, or changing cassettes by use of a spring, gravity, or other means.

With the extra-large-field angioseriograph,[25] three 14 × 17 inch films in a 51-inch cassette allow demonstration of the arterial tree from the pelvis to the toes (Fig. 6-25). Uniform density on each film is achieved by using all the previously mentioned means of obtaining uniform film density of different ratios: the heel effect of the anode, stationary grids, intensifying screens of different speeds, and wedge filters. Four 51-inch cassettes, each one protected by lead, are changed in a single-stage cassette changer with heavy weights as a simple transport mechanism. The system is simple to use and foolproof, but a target-to-film distance of 76 inches is required. This ceiling height is not available in most institutions. Fluoroscopy is not feasible with this apparatus, and the special-procedure room must be large because the apparatus is rather bulky.

The alternative to shifting oversized, heavy radiographic cassettes is intermittent closure of one single pair of graduated intensifying screens. The apparatus can then be much smaller, and the regular sliding tabletop of the examining table can be used. Also, fluoroscopy can be performed if the injection is made into the abdominal aorta by either transfemoral or translumbar catheterization. The intermittent closure of 14 × 36 inch intensifying screens similar to that in the film-changer principle cannot be satisfactorily accomplished by mechanical means because of the large forces required. In a new large-film changer, closure of the intensifying screens is accomplished by in-

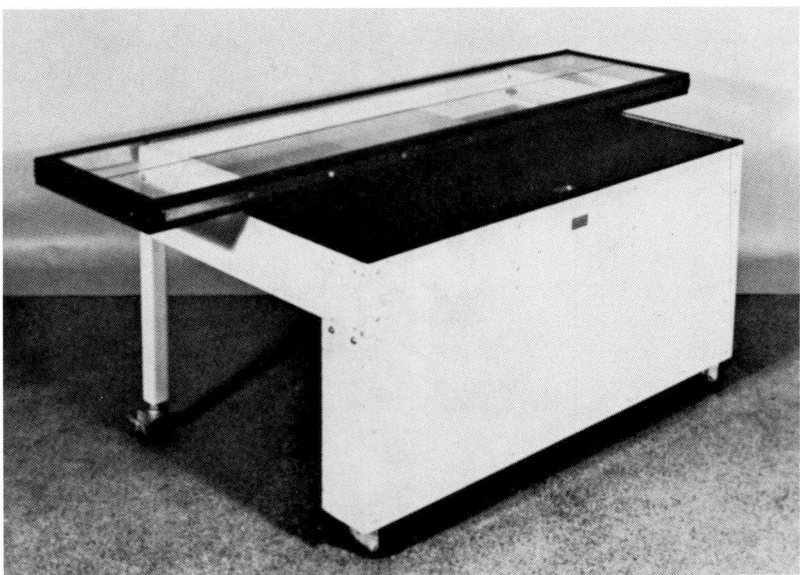

Figure 6-25. Large-field film changer, 14 × 51 inches.

termittent negative pressure. The basic principle of this machine is simple (Fig. 6-26). A 50-foot roll of 14-inch film is placed in supply magazine *A*. The roll film is pulled between the two intensifying screens and wound up intermittently on the spool in receiving magazine *B*. Film contact is achieved in intermittent fashion by a vacuum pump *C* and a large-bore solenoid valve. The maximal exposure rate is one film every 1.2 seconds. Injector and film changer are triggered automatically from a program selector (Fig. 6-27).

With the 36-inch field size it is possible to visualize the arterial tree only from the level of the renal arteries to the popliteal artery. If visualization of the smaller leg arteries is desirable, the patient is shifted on the angiographic table manually or by a motor drive over a distance of 20 inches.[26] In shifting the patient there is considerable overlap of both radiographic images so that timing is much less critical than it is with the use of a 14 × 14 inch cut-film changer. The unit is comparatively compact, but it is noisy because a vacuum-cleaner motor is used to achieve screen closure by negative pressure.

Figure 6-26. Schematic diagram of 14-inch roll-film changer. *A*, supply magazine; *B*, receiving magazine; *C*, vacuum pump.

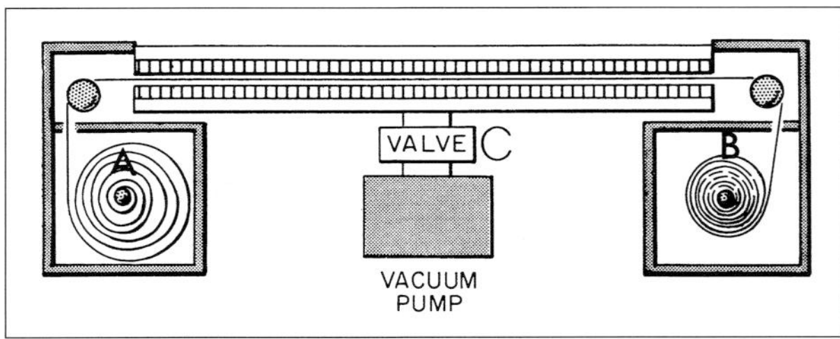

Figure 6-27. Amplatz large-field film changer for film size 14 × 36 inches. *A*, feeding magazine; *B*, exposure area; *C*, vacuum pump.

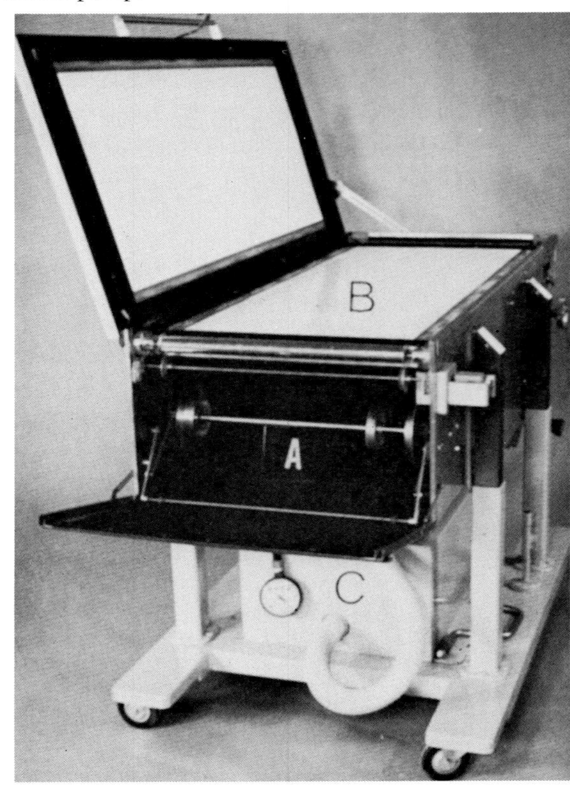

Peripheral Angiography Without a Film Changer

This concept was introduced at the University of Minnesota, where angiographic runoff studies are performed on a single 50-inch radiographic film without a film changer. The entire vascular system from the level of the abdominal aorta to the ankles can be visualized on a single film in most cases; radiation and radiographic film are thus saved.

This task could be accomplished by combining several principles: (1) a protracted injection of a large volume of contrast medium, (2) reactive hyperemia, (3) rotational scanography, (4) moving-slot radiography, and (5) occlusion angiography.

Protracted Injection of Contrast Material

Because the stepwise patient motion is eliminated with this technique, an attempt has to be made to fill the entire vascular system over a prolonged period of time. The delivery rate of contrast medium is estimated by fluoroscopic observation of a test injection into the abdominal aorta. In patients with peripheral vascular disease, a flow rate of 5 to 8 ml per second yields an excellent contrast visualization of the vascular system. Routinely, 80 ml of nonionic contrast medium is injected into the abdominal aorta, providing 8 to 10 seconds' duration for filling of the vascular system. Despite the protracted injection, the peripheral vascular system will not be filled, particularly in patients with severe vascular disease, unless the blood flow is speeded up by reactive hyperemia.

Reactive Hyperemia

Because there is a large variation in the speed of blood flow in patients with peripheral vascular disease, correct timing becomes difficult unless the blood flow is speeded up. This acceleration is routinely carried out by applying tourniquets[24] or pneumatic boots[27] inflated 20 mm above the arterial blood pressure for 8 to 10 minutes. The compression device is released, and the injection of contrast medium is started immediately thereafter.

Rotational Scanography

To cover a 50-inch radiographic cassette, a 17-degree target tube has to be mounted especially high, on the ceiling of the catheterization laboratory. With the new principle of rotational scanography,[28] adequate field coverage is achieved by a 6-degree target tube mounted at standard ceiling height. The x-ray tube pivots exactly through the center of the focal spot, thus using only a narrow scanning beam.

Because rotation occurs through the center of the focal spot, there is no blurring. Scanning speed for the 50-inch cassette can be adjusted between 5 and 10 seconds. A total elapse time after the beginning of the injection of 20 seconds (10 seconds exposure time and 10 seconds scanning time) is therefore available to allow filling of the arteries below the knee. With the use of reactive hyperemia, such a long delay invariably results in good vascular filling, even in patients with gangrene.

Moving-Slit Radiography

One of the major drawbacks of large-field radiography is the formation of a large amount of scatter degrading the quality of the radiographic image. Because only a 1-inch-wide x-ray beam is used to scan the object, secondary radiation can be more efficiently absorbed by means of the slit radiography principle (Fig. 6-28).[29–31] In slit radiography, secondary radiation formed by a narrow beam is absorbed by a secondary slit and a stationary grid. Slit radiography can be advantageously combined with the principle of scanography, resulting in marked improvement of contrast. Furthermore, variation in patient size can be compensated for by varying the scan speed.

Figure 6-28. Diagram illustrating the principle of slit radiography. The x-ray tube (*1*) rotates exactly through the center of the focal spot (*2*). The scan is rollimetered by a fixed rollimeter. A set of primary (*3*) and secondary (*4*) slits travels synchronously with the rotating x-ray tube slit. The small amount of secondary radiation formed by such a narrow beam is efficiently absorbed by the secondary slit (*4*) and the stationary grid (*5*). The image is recorded on a 50-inch vacuum cassette (*6*) with graduated screens.

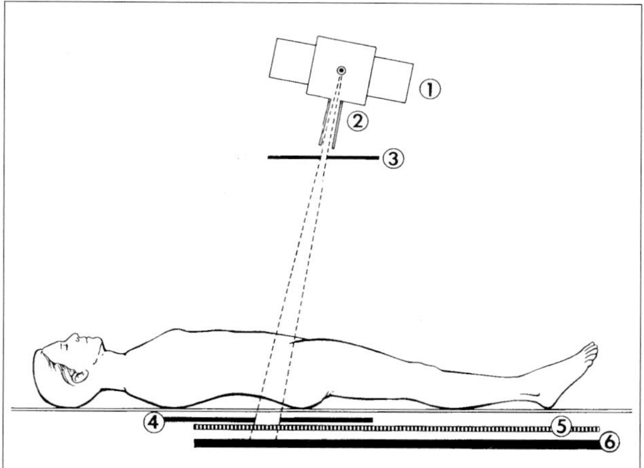

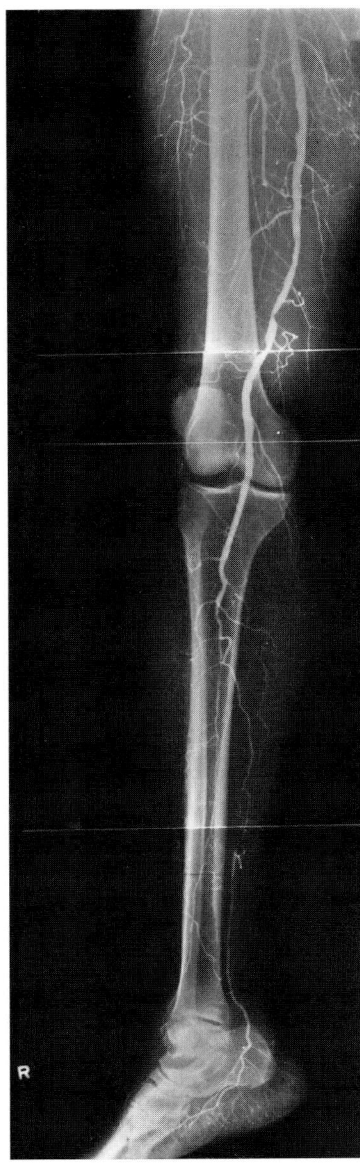

Figure 6-29. Long-leg angiogram in a diabetic patient made with balloon occlusion, reactive hyperemia, and slit radiography. The entire vascular tree is demonstrated to the level of the foot on one single film.

This technique is believed to be the most efficient way to perform long-leg angiography. It is hoped that electronic digital recording will make further progress to eliminate even the single film.

Occlusion Angiography

Balloon occlusion angiography has substantially improved the evaluation of patients with peripheral vascular disease. A pelvic arteriogram is carried out first. A Berman balloon catheter is inflated in the external iliac artery and 60 to 70 ml of nonionic contrast medium is injected after reactive hyperemia for 6 to 8 minutes.

This results in complete filling of the arterial tree, even in patients with gangrene. One single film is required for visualization in most cases (Fig. 6-29).

Acknowledgments

The author is grateful to representatives of various x-ray manufacturers, and particularly to Mr. Don O'Handley of General Electric X-ray Division, for supplying technical data and photographs of various changers.

References

1. Ruggles HE. X-ray motion pictures of the thorax. A motion picture presented at the 11th Annual Meeting of the Radiological Society of North America, Cleveland, Ohio, December 7–11, 1925.
2. Chamberlain WE, Dock W. The study of the heart action with the roentgen cinematograph. Radiology 1926;7:185.
3. Jarre HA. Roentgenologic studies of physiologic motor phenomena (with the aid of the cinex-camera). Radiology 1930; 15:377.
4. Jarre HA. The cinex camera. Grace Hosp Bull 1929;13:3.
5. Caldas JP. Artériographies en série avec l'appareil radio-carrousel. J Radiol Electrol Med Nucl 1934;18:34.
6. Van de Maele M. Direct radiocinematography. Radiology 1938;30:750.
7. Sussman ML, Steinberg MF, Grishman, A. A rapid film changer for use in contrast angiography. Radiology 1942;38:232.
8. Fredzell G, Lind J, Ohlson E, Wegelius C. Direct serial roentgenography in two planes simultaneously at 0.08 second intervals: physiological aspects of roentgen diagnosis; apparatus and its application to angiocardiography. AJR 1950;63:548.
9. Hanafee WN. Personal communication, 1969.
10. Sanchez-Perez JM. The cranial seriograph and its utility in neurologic radiology for cerebral angiography. Surgery 1943;13: 661.
11. Gidlund AS. A new apparatus for direct cineroentgenology. Acta Radiol (Stockh) 1949;32:81.
12. Rigler LG, Watson JC. A combination film changer for rapid or conventional radiography. Radiology 1953;61:77.
13. Axén O, Lind J. Table for routine angiocardiography: synchronous serial roentgenography in two planes at right angles. JAMA 1950;143:540.
14. Campbell JA, Lockhard PB. Improved vertical and horizontal multiple cassette changers for contrast angiography. Radiology 1950;54:559.
15. Schwarzschild MM. Multiple cassette changer for angiocardiography; device for rapid serial radiography. Radiology 1943; 40:72.
16. Scott WG, Moore S. Rapid automatic serialization of x-ray exposures by the rapidograph, utilizing roll film nine and one-half inches wide. Radiology 1949;58:846.
17. Sisson MA. A rapid cassette changer for angiocardiography. Radiology 1949;52:419.
18. Taylor HK. An apparatus for automatic multiple exposures. Radiology 1949;52:107.
19. Thompson WH, Figley MM, Hodges FJ. Full cycle angiography. Radiology 1949;53:729.
20. Scott WG. The development of angiocardiography and aortography. Radiology 1951;56:485.

21. Crummy AB. Digital subtraction angiography. In: Taveras JM, Ferucci JT, eds. Radiology: diagnosis–imaging–intervention. Philadelphia: Lippincott, 1992:1–7.
22. Amplatz K. Automatic injection syringe and cassette changer for cerebral angiography. JAMA 1963;183:430.
23. Amplatz K. New rapid roll-film changer. Radiology 1968;90: 130.
24. Kahn PC, Boyer DN, Moran JM, Callow AD. Reactive hyperemia in lower extremity arteriography: an evaluation. Radiology 1968;90:975.
25. Roy P, Jutras A, Longtin M. Extra-large field angiography: technique and results. J Can Assoc Radiol 1961;12:27.
26. Williams JDF. A special x-ray table for angiocardiography and cerebral angiography. Br J Radiol 1949;22:666.
27. D'Souza V, Formanek A, Castaneda W, Knight L, Amplatz K. Peripheral angiographic enhancement by long-leg pneumatic boots. Radiology 1976;120:209.
28. Amplatz K, Moore R, Korbuly D, Cross J, Kotula F, Castaneda W, Formanek A. Changerless peripheral angiography: a new concept. Radiology 1980;137:213.
29. Amplatz K, Moore R, Korbuly D. The swinging tube: a new concept. Radiology 1978;128:783.
30. Moore R, Korbuly D, Amplatz K. A method to absorb scattered radiation without attenuation of the primary beam. Radiology 1976;120:713.
31. Moore R, Korbuly D, Amplatz K. Removal of scattered radiation by moving slot radiography. Appl Radiol 1977;166:85.

7

Angiographic Equipment

MELVIN P. JUDKINS
BARRY T. KATZEN
MICHAEL S. VAN LYSEL

The major changes that have occurred in angiographic equipment and facilities design, since the third volume of this work, have been in noncardiac angiographic facility and digital angiography. The equipment used for noncardiac angiography is also used for general interventional procedures and therefore tends to be less procedure-specific.

Melvin Judkins's description of the optimal cardiac catheterization laboratory, the necessary patient support areas, the equipment needed to monitor the patient, emergency equipment and radiation, and electrical safety has withstood the test of time and remains the definitive work in this area. The sections on noncardiac angiographic equipment and digital angiography have been completely rewritten by Drs. Katzen and Van Lysel, respectively.

This chapter on angiographic equipment is dedicated to the memory of Melvin P. Judkins, M.D., who authored the first part of the chapter for the third edition of this book.

I. The Cardiac Catheterization Angiography Laboratory

MELVIN P. JUDKINS

The history and background of the development of cinefluorographic equipment were thoroughly described in Chapter 6 of the second edition of this work. In that chapter, which was written by Herbert L. Abrams, M.D., a pioneer in this field,[1] various methods of imaging by photographic means, television image display, stereo imaging, and methods of image amplification were discussed.

Time has done much to concentrate development of equipment on a relatively few designs, while broadening vistas of potential development. Comments in this chapter will be directed to the current state of the art, including equipment that is desirable for the present and forms the basis for laboratories of the future.

Most of the chapter will be devoted to a discussion of equipment used for cardiac angiography, which probably represents the most complex and technically demanding utilization of angiographic equipment. The same basic principles of equipment design and function generally also apply in abdominal, peripheral, and interventional angiography. The differences between the cardiac and the noncardiac applications of angiographic equipment will be considered in the second section of the chapter. Additional technical material pertaining to film changers and power injectors can be found in Chapters 6 and 8 of this edition.

In considering equipment for cardiac angiography one must first answer the question, "What studies are to be done in the facility to be designed?" Multipurpose facilities are necessarily a compromise with the ideal. For the purpose of this chapter, the facilities described pertain to three categories of investigation: (1) coronary arteriography and studies of other forms of heart disease in which cardiomegaly is not a characteristic; (2) a broad spectrum of cardiac examinations including but not limited to coronary arteriography and studies of valvular and other forms of acquired heart disease in which cardiomegaly is a characteristic; and (3) studies of congenital heart disease.

In most regions of the United States, the vast majority of cardiac studies are undertaken in patients whose primary problem is coronary artery disease and associated left ventricular dysfunction or in patients suspected of having coronary artery disease. The rest of the studies are divided between acquired and congenital valvular disease and congenital heart disease. There are certain diseases whose symptoms masquerade as ischemic heart disease, such as idiopathic hypertrophic subaortic stenosis and congestive cardiomyopathy. These are frequently studied in conjunction with or are discovered at the time of investigation of suspected ischemic heart disease.

The primary imaging modality for radiographic examination of the heart is cineradiography. All other forms of imaging are supplementary or complementary, with a few exceptions. The introduction of the cesium iodide input phosphor and of associated improvements in other components of the imaging system has provided a single modality that when properly designed, used, and maintained can supply the anatomic and dynamic information required for complete cardiac examination.

Serial film coronary arteriography, properly performed, provides exquisite anatomic detail and resolution. This detail cannot be obtained, however, unless suitably trained team personnel are actively involved in the examination and appropriate image-production equipment is available. Cineangiography affords optimal dynamic studies. Either method can and does provide both types of information when correctly performed and interpreted. Nevertheless, because the real world is not optimal, limited degrees of compromise may prove desirable. Cine equipment, properly operated and maintained by one adequately trained in the use of this modality, can yield excellent anatomic studies of the heart and coronary arteries.

Space Requirements

After determining what studies are to be done, one faces the question, "What space is required for an adequate facility in which to perform these studies?" The configuration of the laboratory and its auxiliary components will vary a great deal, usually depending on available space. Nevertheless, certain modules are mandated for procedural efficacy and safety of the patient and of laboratory personnel.

Patient safety and efficient time use require adequate space for rapid adjustment of patient and equipment supports during procedures, for smooth performance of personnel, and for unobstructed access to the patient for immediate team attendance. At least 700 sq ft (65 sq m) should be available for a modern catheterization laboratory, its controls and equipment; additional space is required for necessary support facilities. Equipment manufacturer brochures often suggest by drawing and photograph that a relatively small amount of procedure-room space is required for a particular primary imaging system. Commonly omitted in the room arrangement is all the secondary equipment necessary to support the function of the primary equipment that is featured.

Procedure Room

The optimal size is at least 500 sq ft (47 sq m). The minimum size should be 450 sq ft (42 sq m), with a ceiling height of at least 10 ft (3 m). In some settings this space requirement may have to be increased, depending on the equipment components selected.

A rectangular space in which the dimensions have a ratio of 1.25:1.0 is usually satisfactory. The exact shape of the room may have to be modified on the basis of the equipment selected and the internal structure of the building in which it is housed. Space on upper floors of a relatively narrow building with a central corridor presents difficult problems in design and space utilization. A space with a greater width and length than one structural span is desirable.

Control Room

There should be adequate space for the radiologic controls and the physiologic recording and monitoring equipment, positioned so that it is not exposed to direct radiation and is sufficiently protected from scatter. The equipment operator should have ready access to all instruments from a central location. A cockpit configuration permits the most effective use of personnel, equipment, and space (Fig. 7-1).

Radiation protection should extend from floor to a minimum height of 7 ft. However, the radiation barrier should *not* obscure full vision of the patient by personnel operating the radiologic controls and physiologic monitoring equipment. This requirement precludes using a barrier with a small peephole. The trans-

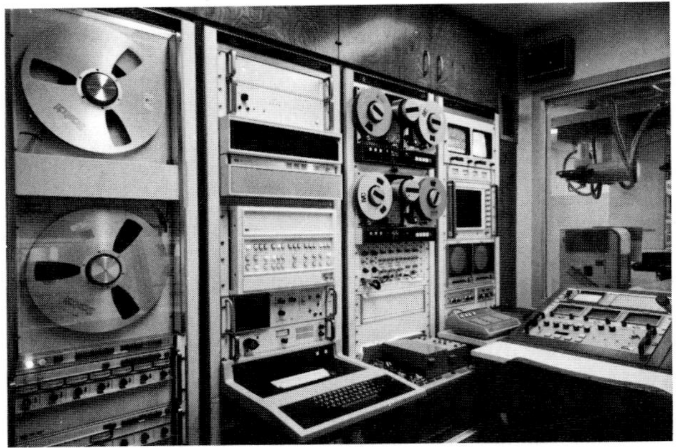

A

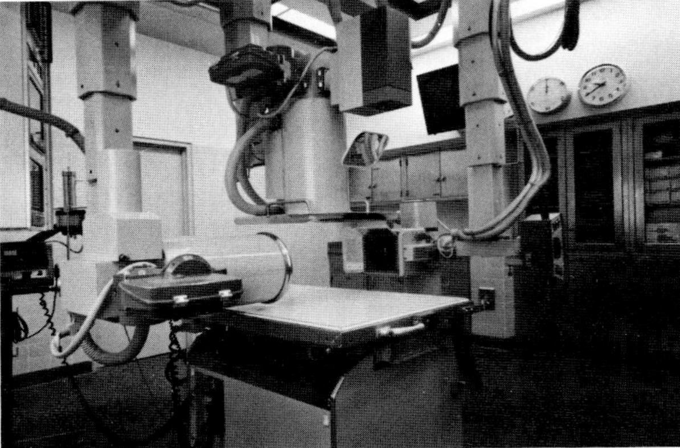

B

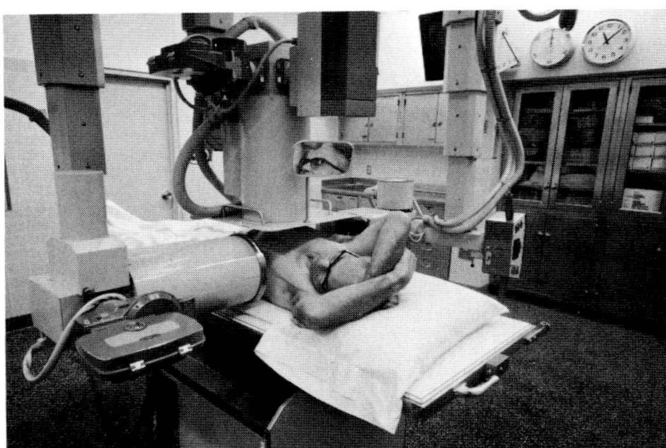

C

Figure 7-1. (A) Cockpit-type control room with x-ray, physiologic, and monitoring controls conveniently arranged for one-technologist operation in full view and communication with all procedure room functions. (B and C) Conventional patient support with Siemens radiologic equipment for biplane cineradiography. (Courtesy of Robert Rearick, Loma Linda University, Loma Linda, Calif.)

parent radiation shield may be of lead glass or plate glass with appropriate radiation attenuation. Lead-impregnated plastic is suitable for such a barrier. This material has the advantage of being lighter in weight for equivalent attenuation. Adequacy of radiation protection should be determined by a qualified physicist.

Because of the multitude of angles of radiation projection that are possible when using C-, U-, or Z-arm equipment, the design of radiation protection is more complex in these installations than in more conventional room designs. Some of the supermaneuverable C-, U-, and Z-arm devices may need to have their range of motion limited to protect personnel from impingement of the direct beam. If direct impingement is possible, attenuation of the barrier may have to be greater than is usually required and will be more expensive to provide. It is preferable to devise some method of mechanically preventing direct radiation in the direction of the barrier.

Equipment Room

An equipment room should be of sufficient size to contain the x-ray transformer(s), power module(s), cine pulse unit(s), and associated electronic and electric apparatus. It should be positioned to ensure that high-voltage cables are short—not more than 60 ft (20 m). Constant-potential equipment should have cables less than 40 ft (12 m) in length.

There should be adequate usable wall space in the equipment room for installation of all components. Wall space of the procedure room is more effectively used for nonradiographic equipment. Serial filming capability will require more space than a cine-only installation.

Placement of components in the room should provide easy access for maintenance and service. An adequate cooling and ventilation system is mandatory to dissipate generated heat. It is feasible to have the equipment in an enclosure along one wall that opens into the procedure room. However, an equipment enclosure does not provide as desirable sound, temperature, and grime separation as an equipment room. The x-ray control unit, transformers, power module, cine pulse unit, and associated electronic and electrical apparatus should not be installed in the procedure room. On occasion, it may be advantageous for a laboratory to have a common control-equipment room, but separate rooms are preferable.

Computer flooring in the control and equipment room provides space for and ready access to the cabling necessary for radiologic and physiologic equipment. This type of flooring permits future replacement or addition of components without major physical change. The structural loading capability of both floor and ceiling should be adequate.

Clean Supply and Workroom

Space is needed for the preparation and storage of clean and sterile supplies, catheters, guides, surgical packs, etc. This area should be separate from the facility for cleanup of items used during procedures.

Additional Space

The procedure, control, equipment, utility, and workrooms do not of themselves constitute a total functioning laboratory unit. Small-volume laboratories may share support facilities with other departments. Provision should be made for the following functions and services: reception, secretarial, and transcribing; waiting or holding area for patients; preparation room, recovery and observation area; darkroom and radiographic film processing; blood gas chemistry; film viewing and report; film file and storage; conference room; library and study room; teaching aid and file storage; office space for staff, trainees, and allied health personnel; doctors' and nurses' dressing rooms; storage for general supplies, linen, and chemicals; and a vented area for radioactive material and gases.

Components

When properly orchestrated, a complex of radiographic and associated equipment will produce a cardiac angiographic image and provide physiologic information that will assist the clinician in the care of the patient. In discussing radiologic components, we will not consider the advisability of using a given imaging modality for a given medical problem, but rather the suitability and requirements for each type of imaging.

An angiographic image is formed by absorption of x-ray photons in the input phosphor of an image intensifier or an intensifying screen of a film changer. An acceptable image must contain a minimum number of statistical events regardless of recording method (Fig. 7-2). X-ray quanta insufficient to produce an even distribution of "data points" result in a grainy image; this "noise" is termed *quantum mottle* and degrades image clarity. Quantum mottle is the most frequent cause of poor-quality cine and spot-film fluorographic studies.

The improved intrinsic contrast ratio and quantum detection efficiency of image intensifiers will produce an acceptable 16- to 35-mm cine-frame image with a 25- to 35-microroentgen (μR) radiation input level for a 15- to 17-cm field size and 15 μR per frame for a 22- to 25-cm field size when the cine frames are viewed at least 24 frames per second. A 70- to 105-mm fluorogram requires 150 μR per frame for the 15- to 17-cm field size and approximately 100 μR input per frame for the 22- to 25-cm field size. This refers to image brightness and should not be interpreted to mean that equal image quality per unit of patient area is obtained when using less radiation with a large format intensifier. In other words, 15 μR per frame using a 22-cm intensifier does not equal the image quality of 25 μR per frame using a 15-cm image intensifier. Manufacturers' literature implies that less radiation is required to produce an image if a large format intensifier is used. This is deceptive. Images of equal quality per unit of patient area require the same amount of radiation. If imaging detail is required for diagnosis, there is no difference in the microroentgen-per-frame requirement for large- and small-format intensifiers; an equal or slightly higher radiation level is required for a large-format intensifier to produce equal image quality.

For serial imaging, input to the intensifying screen should be 300 μR to 1 mR; the exact requirements vary widely depending on the screen and film used. The advent of high-efficiency rare-earth screens for serial imaging permits an input radiation dose reduction to the intensifying screens of two to three times for equivalent image quality. There is an approximately 400-μR input radiation requirement to maintain the quantum mottle performance level of the image.

Once the need for sufficient quanta to produce an acceptable image is satisfied, there are at least four other major factors that influence image sharpness: motion unsharpness, geometric unsharpness, system unsharpness, and absorption unsharpness. The total unsharpness of an image is not less than the greatest of the several factors. The first three unsharpness factors, along with quantum mottle and factors that influence contrast, must be considered in the selection of equipment for cardioangiography.

Generators

The x-ray generator, including the transformer and the control unit, and the radiographic tube are the power train for the production of the roentgen ray. A generator with stable output and precise control is indispensable for an angiographic laboratory. The purchase of an optimal generator for anticipated imaging methods should take financial preference over all other consid-

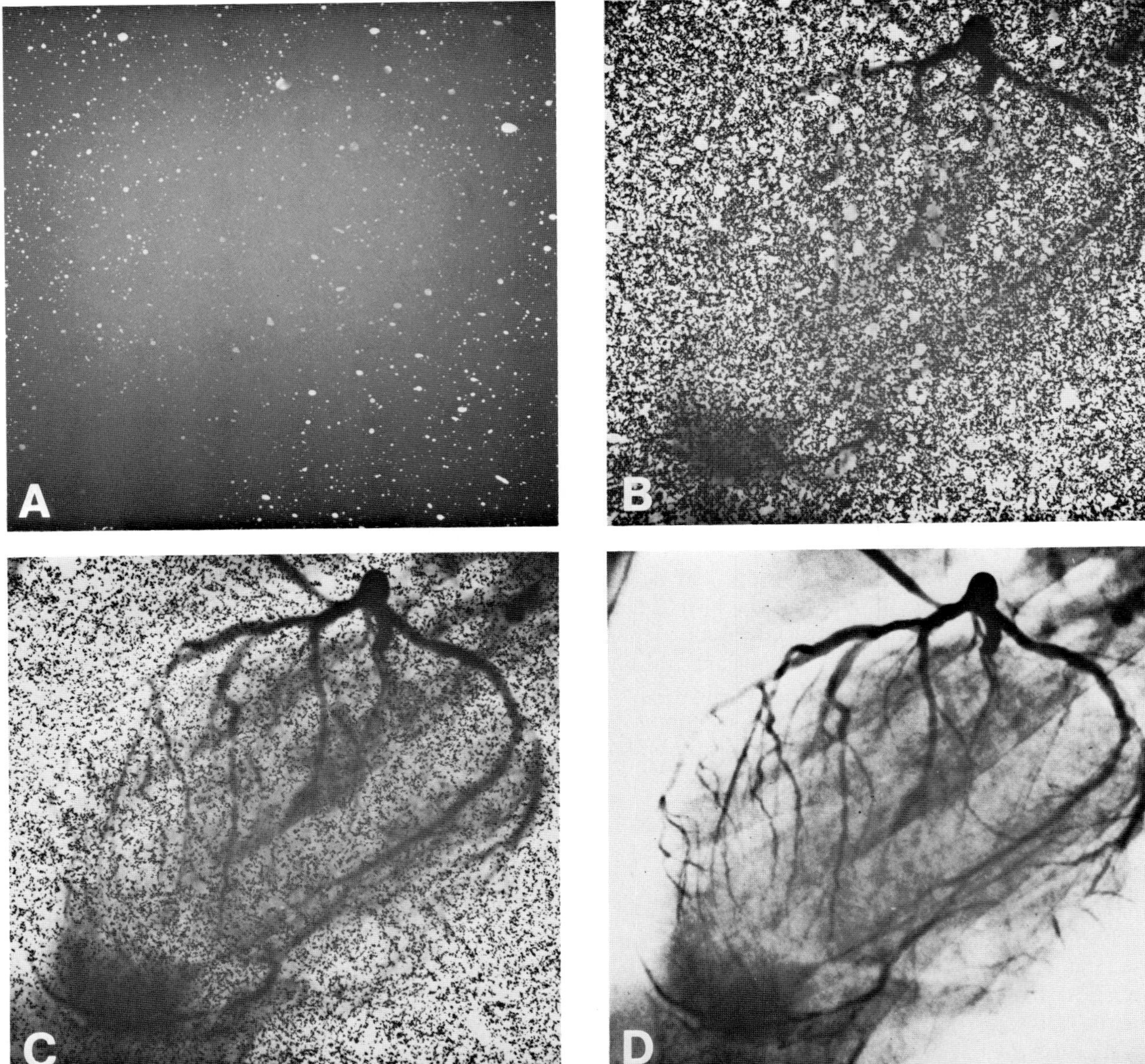

Figure 7-2. Cineangiograms showing that there must be sufficient photons to produce an adequate image to make a diagnosis with confidence. (A) If a very low radiation level is used, the result will be an image of the coronary arteries that is not recognizable and pathology within the vessels will not be recognizable. (B) If the level of radiation is increased, one can recognize proximal parts of the coronary tree. But one cannot be confident that the image obtained is a true likeness of even the more proximal parts of the coronary trunks. (C) If the radiation level is increased still further, one can visualize more of the coronary system and gain confidence that the image recorded depicts the anatomy of the more proximal portions of the system. (D) Further increase in the number of photons provides a truer image, one that reasonably portrays the anatomic detail important to diagnosis. The high-contrast images shown in this figure would be further improved by increasing latitude. When viewing a cineangiogram in motion, the eye integrates five successive frames so that the brain perceives an image similar to that shown in Figure 7-16.

erations. It is a fundamental error to couple an inadequate generator to sophisticated secondary components. It is also a needlessly expensive error to purchase an all-purpose, excessively sophisticated and high-power generator for a cine-only application. The key is to select the generator for the specific anticipated function.

There are two common methods of imaging recording, fluorography and rapid serial radiography. Fluorography may be cine or cine and spot film. Each may require a somewhat different power train. A generator that meets the most stringent requirement for cardiac serial radiography will meet the power needs for other imaging methods. A generator adequate for spot-film fluorography will fulfill the needs for cinefluorography. A generator for cinefluorography may be the least complex of the three. Cine generator controls can be simple, requiring a minimum of components in a generator of modular design (Fig. 7-3).

Cinefluorography

The basic generator for cinefluorography should have a current output one and a quarter to two times the cine pulse output. This will minimize voltage fluctuations during pulsing. The exact rating depends on transformer design, rectifiers employed, and contacting method. A 12-pulse generator with an output of 80 to 100 kW or a constant potential generator with an output of 100 or more kW at 100 kV is optimal. However, an economy system with a 12-pulse generator with an output of as low as 60 kW may be satisfactory if transformer design and contacting method ensure stable high-potential waveform and constant tube current output during pulsing.

Adapting a 12-pulse generator for cine usage requires the addition of a pulse system capable of an output of 40 to 75 kW, depending on the selection of radiographic tubes and other components. Constant-potential generators inherently include the circuitry for rapid pulsing and kV regulation. However, for cine-only applications, constant-potential generators do not have inherent superiority over silicon-controlled rectifier (SCR) contacting generators in the tube current range limits necessary for cineradiography. SCR contacting generators of comparatively low kW rating and simple design can provide equally satisfactory cine current and voltage output.

Future design improvements in cine systems are likely to be in areas other than increased power output. The heat generated in the x-ray tube, and its dissipation, is the prime limitation.

Spot-Film Fluorography

The generator should provide output of 80 kW at 100 kV. Twelve-pulse generators should have SCR contacting and SCR exposure termination or be of constant-potential design.

Automatic exposure control is essential; the contacting system and automatic exposure device should provide accurate exposure down to 2 milliseconds. The generator requirements for spot-film fluorography and cinefluorography are similar. Spot-film fluorography has the added requirement of a relatively expensive exposure termination system.

Rapid Serial Radiography

This imaging modality requires not less than 100 kW at 100 kV, provided by either a 3-phase, 12-pulse or a constant-potential generator. If a 12-pulse generator is used it should have SCR contacting and SCR inversion exposure termination. The contacting system and automatic exposure control should provide accurate exposures down to 2 milliseconds. Reaction time should be 2 milliseconds or less. Random variations of exposure triggering should be 8 milliseconds or less for high-speed serial radiography or spot-film fluorography. The timer and contacting system should provide exposure control in increments of 25 percent above 3 milliseconds. Tube current (mA) or mAs selection should be automatic or in steps of 25 percent. High tension (kV) should be continuously variable or have 25 percent density-equivalent step indications.

Constant-potential generators inherently have the possibility of more rapid response in the serial radiography mode than that of 12-pulse generators (all responses less than 1 millisecond) and have complete flexibility of control. Alternate firing of biplane equipment from the same transformer at different high-potential (kV) settings is possible. The output of a constant-potential generator for short motion-stopping exposure is square wave in form, increasing the effective film blackening per unit of time. The sophistication of a constant-potential generator with its attendant added expense is needed only for short (10 milliseconds or less) serial exposures or spot-film fluorography. Although constant-potential capability is desirable, in a given laboratory the benefits should be weighed against the additional cost. If the laboratory is designed for biplane serial radiography, generator costs may be similar for constant-potential or 12-pulse radiography because of component sharing of constant potential systems. Most cardiac laboratories do not require biplane serial radiography capability,

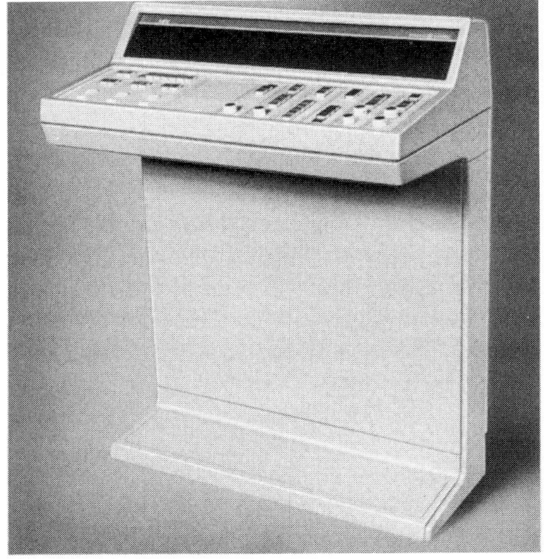

A

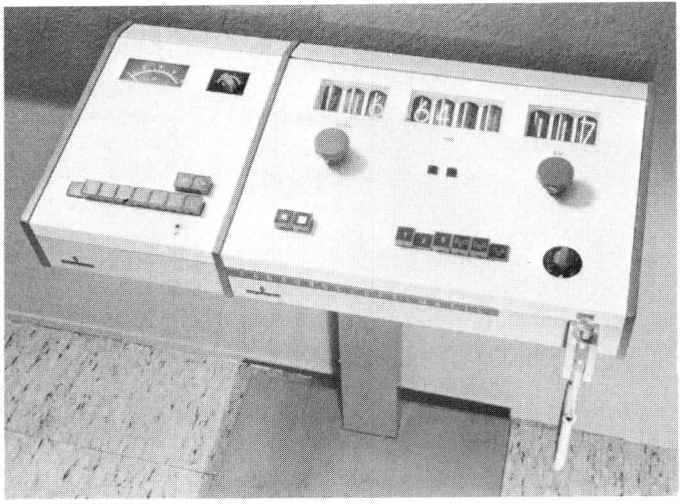

B

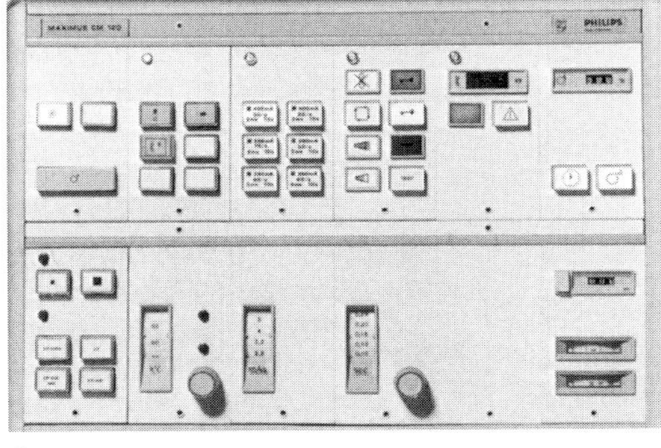

C

Figure 7-3. Modular generator controls. (A) General Electric, (B) Siemens, (C) Philips. Modular generators facilitate the selection of components necessary for the application. Generator controls for cine need not be complex. Elimination of unnecessary modules can considerably reduce generator cost without impairing function. (Courtesy of General Electric Co., Medical Systems Division, Milwaukee, Wisc.; Siemens Aktiengesellschaft, Bereich Medizinische Technik, Erlangen, Germany; Philips Gloeilampenfabrieken, Medical Systems Division, Eindhoven, Holland.)

nor is it cost-effective. Single-plane serial radiography powered by a 12-pulse generator is a satisfactory option. If a 12-pulse generator has been elected to power the cine system, it can satisfactorily provide the power requirements for serial cardiopulmonary radiography.

Cine Pulsing Systems

The cine pulse system is needed for each cineangiographic plane to control the length of exposure and to regulate x-ray photon flow from the radiographic tube to the image intensifier when the cine camera shutter is open. Exposure time should be sufficient to provide the quanta necessary to form a good image within the output limits of the pulse system (Fig. 7-4). An ultrashort exposure setting (2 milliseconds or less) may reduce image quality by reducing available total x-ray quanta, thereby increasing quantum mottle, or by requiring a high kV setting with resulting loss of image contrast. Motion-stopping exposures of 4 to 6 milliseconds usually provide a good balance between quantum mottle and motion unsharpness when a 40- to 60-kW or higher input is used. Constant-current, nonpulsed systems should be avoided; exposure control is inadequate, and radiation dosages to patient and operator are excessive.

Cine pulsing is best accomplished by secondary switching. Two satisfactory devices are commonly used: a grid-controlled x-ray tube and a high-potential

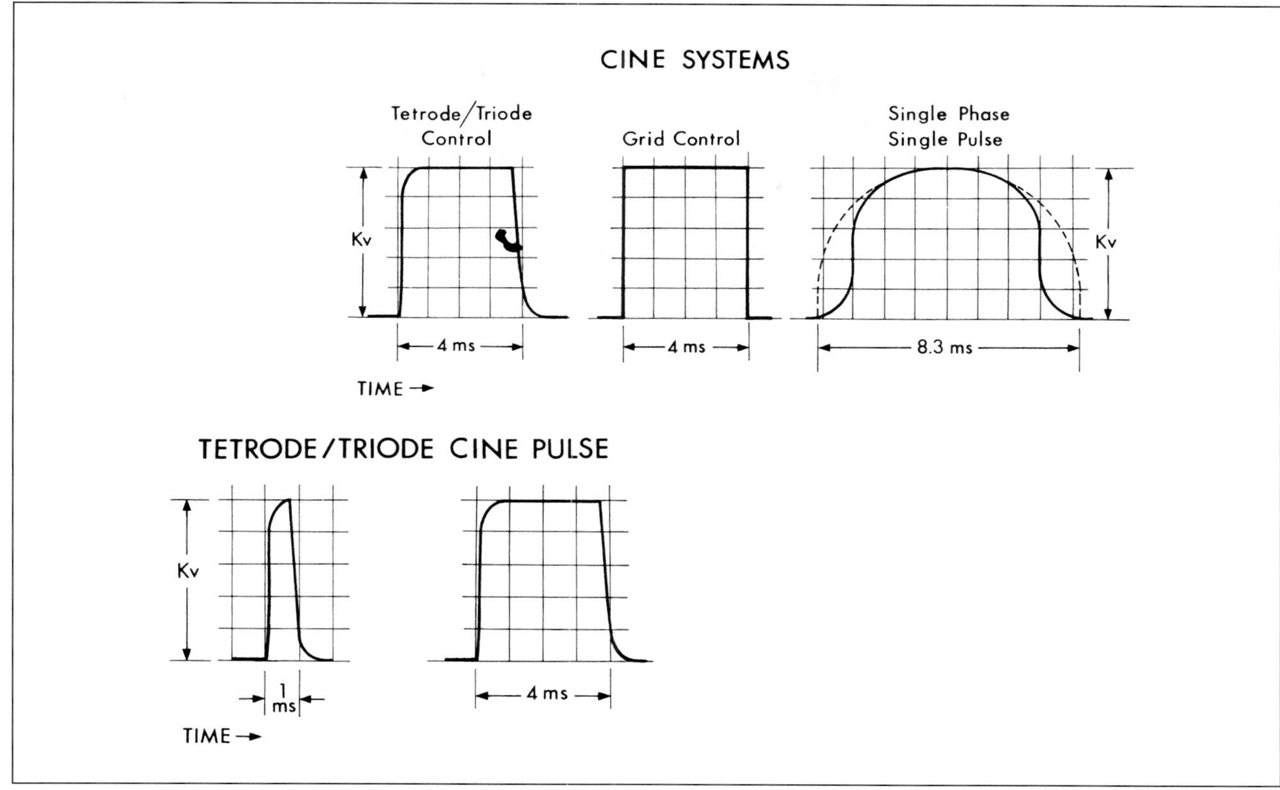

Figure 7-4. Cine pulse systems. Tetrode/triode switching has the advantage of more effective control of tube currents over 600 mA. Grid control has a square waveform with maximum film blackening per unit of time. Either grid or tetrode switching provides better waveform and control of a wide range of exposure times than primary switching. Single phase is normally limited to effective exposures of 6 milliseconds.

(kV), high-vacuum switching tube (triode or tetrode). In the first, a grid controls the flow of current in the radiographic tube when an appropriate bias voltage is applied. The second device employs a similar principle for controlling current flow, applied in a high-vacuum switching tube located in the x-ray generator. Either method is acceptable. When a cine-only system is employed, grid pulsing is the simplest and usually most economical of the two basic systems.

Optimal cine imaging can be obtained if high potential (kV) is kept in the range of 70 to 90 (pediatric, 60–80), thus providing good radiation contrast; exposure times of 4 to 6 milliseconds are employed for adult and 2 to 4 milliseconds for pediatric patients; motion unsharpness is controlled; good filming geometry is maintained, minimizing geometric unsharpness; and the radiation input dose is at a level that will minimize quantum noise.

A cine pulse system with a working output of 40 kW or more is advised. An important secondary part of pulsing is an automatic exposure control for both cine and television systems.

Automatic Exposure Control

It is essential to have an automatic brightness stabilization system for control of cine exposure and for fluorographics. The purpose of this system is to set proper x-ray factors rapidly at the start of a cineangiographic run and to compensate rapidly for changes in beam attenuation as "panning" is carried out during the run. There are four basic types: variable tube potential, variable tube current, pulsewidth variation, and combination systems. The signal to automatically increase or decrease x-ray factors is based on measurement of either current flowing through the image intensifier or brightness at the output phosphor.

Variable Tube Potential

Because of its simplicity, this was an early method of automatic brightness stabilization, and it is still used. A motor-driven variac or autotransformer in the primary circuit is used to vary high potential in response to brightness-sensing electronics.

Modern systems use pulsing units capable of handling 40 to 60 kW and have preselectable pulse time and tube current. If the proper control factors are selected, and the tube potential is kept at near-optimal levels during the cine run, this system has the advantage of a broad range of control, but it is relatively slow in response.

A kV-control system, if combined with a constant-potential generator, provides very rapid response. Because generators of this type have the capability of multiple-factor variability, they will be discussed under Combination Systems.

Variable Tube Current

A popular cine brightness control of the past used a pulsing system that varied tube current (mA). Preselection of exposure time and high potential (kV) are possible. In practice, the system frequently does not operate within optimal kV and time limits. Considerable control expertise is essential for maintenance of adequate photon input and usable kV levels. In actual practice, optimal mA levels are seldom achieved in the desirable kV range. Other modes of control have therefore gained favor. By today's standards this system is not adequate.

Pulsewidth Variation

Because of the narrow usable range of control (1–6 milliseconds) this method is seldom used as an independent exposure control. This system has the same range of control deficiency as the variable tube current method. Pulsewidth variation systems are combined with some method of predetermining desired kV or mA range and are therefore used as a form of combination system.

Combination Systems

There are two main combination systems employed by different manufacturers. One uses kV for the primary control and a secondary automatic mA level to maintain adequate photon flux. The other uses primary mA control and kV variability to extend system range.

In the first, optimal kV (contrast) is preset and mA used to vary film blackening. The weakness of this system is its limitation of film-blackening range at a given kV setting and its relatively slow response time.

In the second system, optimal mA setting is preselected for the radiographic components being used, and kV varied to regulate film blackening. Because of the wide range in film blackening obtainable with small changes in kV, there is little effect on contrast.

The second system has the wider range of instantaneous control, but either system is acceptable when used by an operator familiar with its characteristics. Both combination systems require knowledgeable presetting of exposure factors. They should have a capacity of 40 to 60 kW. These systems are limited by x-ray tube output.

Electrical Power

A well-engineered power source is essential to providing the voltage and current stability required for full generator output. For serial radiography the recommended generator should be supplied from 480-V lines originating from a 3-phase transformer rated at 300 kVA. This transformer should be reserved exclusively for supplying power to x-ray generators. Momentary line voltage fluctuation should not be more than 3 percent at the disconnect box. The line transformer secondary should be Y-wound, having a temperature rise of no more than 10°C (50°F) at full load and 0.08-ohm maximum impedance per phase. The line transformer should be located not more than 200 ft (60 m) from the generators it serves. Several generators of similar design can usually be supplied from the same power transformer. The mathematical chance of simultaneous serial exposure at full power is remote and at most would result in a single underexposed film. There should be no elevator, fluorescent light, or computer connections to these lines. It is prudent to make frequent checks to ascertain tapping of the x-ray power source. Power lines should transmit the three phases of electrical power plus a neutral and ground line.

If imaging is limited to cine and spot-film fluorography, a line transformer rated at 150 to 225 kVA is adequate (Fig. 7-5). An emergency electrical generator should be capable of supplying sufficient power to the x-ray generator and physiologic monitors to complete an examination in progress. This backup power source can be the medical facility emergency generator.

Radiographic Tubes

Electrical energy conversion to roentgen rays is very inefficient; less than 0.2 percent of the electrical energy is converted to x-ray photons. The remainder becomes heat, most of which is generated in the anode of the x-ray tube. In the selection of tubes for the laboratory,

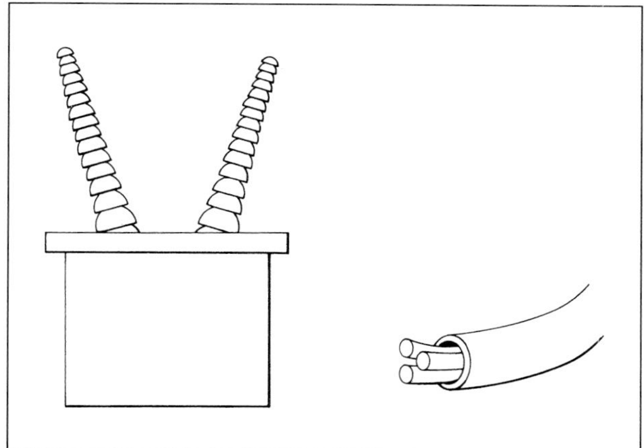

Figure 7-5. The average cine system will require a 150- to 225-kVA transformer and wire of appropriate size to transmit the load over the distance to be covered. Total voltage regulation, transformer and wire, should be 3 percent.

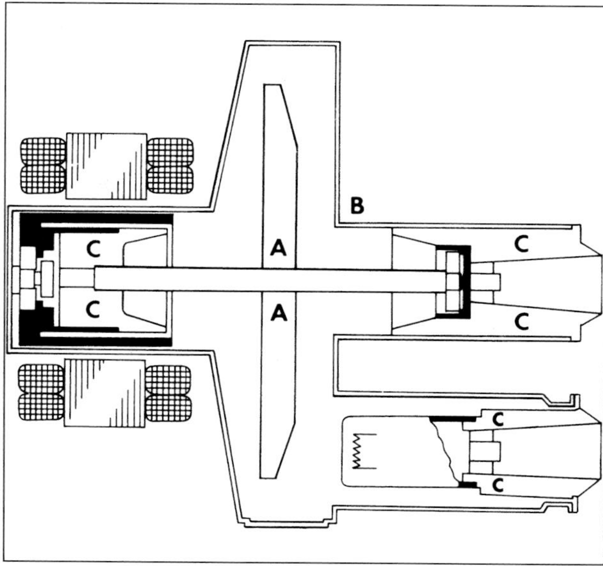

Figure 7-6. Super ROTALIX Ceramic (SRC 120) tube. Rotating anode (A) has dual bearing support inside an all-metal insert (B) with ceramic insulation (C). Drawing of tube insert without housing after Philips. (Adapted from Philips Medical Systems, Inc., Shelton, Conn., and Philips, Eindhoven, Holland.)

therefore, the production and dissipation of heat must be considered for each form of imaging. Tubes mounted in the angiographic table base or other form of enclosure and/or used for multiple sequential cine runs in a relatively short period of time must be cooled, preferably with circulated liquid and a heat exchanger. A similar cooling device is desirable for all heavy-duty tube applications. Regardless of cooling method, a heat indicator is desirable to give the user the exact thermal status of the anode before initiating additional exposures. Tubes mounted in C-, U-, or Z-arms may be incorporated in an orbiting enclosure and are not easily cooled. Forced-air cooling is helpful. Liquid cooling requires on-site engineering but is highly advisable if multiple cine runs in a short time are anticipated; for example, as in coronary arteriography. An adequate cooling system improves tube life.

Recent developments include replacement of the conventional glass tube with a metal envelope. One tube design has ceramic rotor insulation and a 120-mm target supported by bearings on both ends of a central shaft (Fig. 7-6). Other efforts are being directed toward improving focal-spot geometry and providing near-true gaussian distribution. When tubes with these capabilities are commercially available, image resolution can be expected to improve dramatically.

An electronic method of control of focal-spot size is available and desirable for tubes used for cine magnification angiography. At least one manufacturer has developed a triple focal-spot tube of high capacity suitable for cardiac cineangiography; the microfocal spot is electronically variable from 0.1 to 0.3 mm.

The instantaneous-output capability of a focal spot varies with the anode diameter, anode angle, rotational speed, and immediate-past-exposure heating. The maximum output over a period of time is influenced by the heat storage and dissipation of both the anode and the housing.

Tubes should have 100-mm or larger black-coated rhenium tungsten molybdenum (RTM) or laminated anodes, or have rhenium tungsten targets and graphite heat sinks capable of being rotated at high speed (10,000 rpm). Conventional x-ray tubes have a target angle of 15 to 17 degrees. For some time angiographic tubes have been available with target angles of 10 to 12 degrees. The ratings of these tubes are about 60 percent higher than for tubes with a 15- to 17-degree target angle—12 kW for a 0.3-mm focal spot, 40 kW for a 0.6-mm, 75 kW for a 1.0-mm, and 100 kW for a 1.3-mm. These tubes have limited but adequate field coverage for film changers and image intensifiers. They will cover a field of 35 × 35 cm at a distance of 1 m.

Special angiographic and cine tubes with target angles of 6 to 8 degrees are available. Their output is about 2.2 times that of an x-ray tube with a conventional 15- to 17-degree target angle. Field coverage is more limited than with tubes having 12-degree angles but is adequate for most cardiac examinations by cinefluorographic techniques with image intensifiers up to 17 cm in diameter and for use with small-size Schönander or Puck film changers.

Tubes made commercially available with an intermediate anode angle of 9 to 10 degrees and a 125-mm target may have advantages in an equipment configuration in which the focal-receptor distance is variable and exceeds 85 cm.

Target angles of 6 to 12 degrees may be used, depending on intensifier size and the distance between focal spot and receptor. The principal advantage of tubes with small target angles is their ability to maintain adequate x-ray quanta output during short exposures while using focal spots of very small size, thus reducing geometric unsharpness. They are recommended for use in a system devoted to the study of ischemic and congenital heart disease. Cranially and caudally angled views also increase the demand for high tube loading.

As already indicated, the disadvantages of tubes with smaller target angles are marked heel effect and limited useful field size. Care must be taken to orient the anode heel toward the less dense portion of the anatomic part (heel toward lung). In practice, the heel effect can be used to advantage to flatten the effective radiation distribution. At the usual working distance—70- to 100-cm source-to-image-receptor distance (SID)—the 6- to 8-degree target angle design is preferable for an intensifier 17 cm in diameter. These tubes do not exhibit any disadvantages in performance or undesirable quality of radiation if field coverage is limited within the tube's target angle capability.

Focal-spot size, shape, and intensity distribution are important to image quality. The original focal-spot measuring standard was published by the Internal Commission on Radiation Units and Measurements (ICRU) and was based on fluoroscopic tube current levels. Since under a higher load the focal spot can bloom or enlarge, the manufacturers developed the National Electrical Manufacturers Association (NEMA) focal-spot standards,[2] which were based on loading the tube to one-half of maximum rated load at 75 kW. The current NEMA self-imposed industry standards permit focal spots to be as much as 100 percent larger than the stated size in one direction and 50 percent larger in the other. The focal-spot tolerances are always positive and are at the upper end of the tolerance range to permit the high nominal load ratings required to stop motion. (A 0.6-mm focal spot typically measures 0.9 by 1.2 mm.)

Radiographic tubes for angiography should not be designed for voltages over 125 kV. The practice of building most high-output tubes for 150 kV places unnecessary limitations on tube design. This is the result of uninformed user demand for the higher kV rating. Lower kV rating, 120 to 125 kV, permits the placement of the filament closer to the anode, thus reducing electron saturation at low kV.

The number of radiographic tubes required will vary with the functions of the laboratory. Usually there will be a tube for fluoroscopy, cinefluorography, and/or spot-film fluorography (either undertable or mounted on a support arm); a second tube similar to the first will be mounted on a suitable support if biplane cinefluorography is employed. Up to two additional tubes will be mounted on overtable and lateral table supports if biplane serial filming is required. A minimum of 55 cm between the focal spot of an undertable fluoroscopic tube and the patient support is recommended for satisfactory geometry and reduction of patient skin radiation dose, except when magnification techniques are employed. The focal spot of the radiographic tube should be as small as possible, commensurate with the tube loading necessary to produce a satisfactory balance between motion unsharpness and geometric unsharpness within the angiographically acceptable kV range.

Cinefluorography

The facility primarily for the investigation of ischemic heart disease should have a radiographic tube with a target angle of 6 to 8 degrees and a diameter of 100 mm or larger with a (nominal) 0.3- to 0.6-mm, 20- to 50-kW small focal spot and a 0.8- to 1.0-mm, 50- to 100-kW large focal spot coupled with a 15- to 17-cm image intensifier. Focal spots of 0.3 mm (nominal) or less can be used for special magnification techniques.

Tubes should be capable of rotation at 10,000 to 20,000 rpm. Cinefluorographic tubes should have circulated liquid cooling; all tubes should have some form of anode-protecting device that will automatically provide a warning if there is anode overheating.

A nominal NEMA 0.8- to 1.0-mm focal spot, 50- to 80-kW, 100- to 125-mm, 6- to 8-degree target is recommended for C-, U-, or Z-arm applications for investigating ischemic disease. This focal-spot size is optimal for the long SIDs (95–120 cm) experienced with isocentric positioning and increased penetration requirements for the extreme-view angles. This focal-spot size provides an image quality performance balance in terms of penetration capability and modulation transfer function of system components with the required 4- to 5-millisecond exposure times to maximize motion stoppage. It will maintain radiation contrast at 90 kVp maximum while allowing for sufficient penetration of large patients in extreme view angles. A nominal 0.5- to 0.6-mm focal spot, 30- to 40-kW, 100- to 125-mm target is recommended for short SIDs (75–90 cm) to handle less-extreme-view angles with minimized patient attenuation. The 0.5- to 0.6-mm focal spot increases modulation transfer function.

The facility primarily designed for cardiac disease in which cardiomegaly is a prime factor should have a radiographic tube with a wider anode angle and therefore wider field of coverage. Such a laboratory should have a radiographic tube with a target angle of 9 to 12 degrees and a diameter of 100 to 125 mm with a (nominal) 0.5- to 0.6-mm, 30- to 50-kW small focal spot, and a 0.8- to 1.0-mm, 40- to 80-kW large focal spot coupled with a 22- to 25-cm intensifier. The use of a dual-mode intensifier requires a radiographic tube with an anode angle of 9 to 12 degrees to cover the intensifier input field size. Because it is necessary to use a wider anode angle, there is a coincident loss of radiographic kW tube loading capability and lower radiation output of the radiographic tube.

Spot-Film Fluorography

The tube requirements for spot-film fluorography are similar to those for cine. If both modalities are employed, it is especially important that the operator allow for sufficient tube cooling between cine and spot-film runs. Use of liquid cooling is urged.

Rapid Serial Radiography

The tube rating should be 100 to 150 kW at 100 kV, and the focal spot should be not larger than 1.3 mm (nominal). The anode angle need not be greater than 12 degrees for a 14 × 14 inch changer or 8 degrees for a 10 × 12 inch changer. A focal-film distance of not less than 1 m should be used. When special techniques are employed, a variety of focal spots, target angles, and distances may be elected. Image contrast may be improved and patient radiation exposure dose reduced if the field of radiation is kept to the absolute minimum size required for examination.

Magnification Cardioangiography

Rapid organ motion and loading limitations of tubes restrict the usefulness of cardiac magnification angiography. The principal practical applications are pediatric angiocardiography and pediatric and adult special and experimental techniques. In all types of magnification angiography there is a trade-off between focal-spot size and loading capacity. For the necessarily brief exposures of 8 milliseconds or less, the limited instantaneous-loading capacity usually precludes the use of a fine-focal-spot radiographic tube. The loading limitations may make these very low output tubes (2–4 kW) clinically unusable for most cardiac applications. The cinefluorographic frame rate is also limited by the tube capacity.

Focal spots for magnification work should be 0.1 to 0.3 mm; under no circumstances should focal-spot size exceed 0.3 mm. When choice of a microfocal-spot tube is being made, it is wise to select one in which the small size has been achieved by biasing or other techniques that limit focal-spot size and provide near-homogeneous distribution. Focal spots with pronounced or eccentric edge bands must be avoided.

Ultra-high-speed-rotation microfocal-spot x-ray tubes with a rating of 12 kW, a nominal focal-spot size of 0.2 mm, and anode rotation speed of about 20,000 rpm are available. The development of ultra-high-speed rotation increases the loading capacity of fine-focal-spot tubes and has extended the application of cardiac magnification techniques.

It is necessary to use rare-earth screens for magnification serial filming in pulmonary or cardiac angiography.

Collimation

A triple-leaf collimator fixed to the field size of the intensifier should be used to minimize off-focus radiation and scatter. A collimator that extends into a recess in the tube housing to reduce the distance between anode and collimator is particularly efficient in reducing off-focus radiation. For all types of filming a lead diaphragm should restrict the tube port opening to the maximum field size that will be used (not the maximum usable field area).

Cine- and spot-film fluorography requires coning to the round intensifier input. For this purpose, cones with a circular-field or a collimator with an iris-type diaphragm (Fig. 7-7) are preferred to rectangular collimators, unless near-total overframing of television and cine image is being used. Coning is more convenient (a single-shutter control) and tends to be tighter when circular collimators are used.

Dual-shaped (so-called heart-shaped) collimators are available. These incorporate both circular and elliptical shutters. In addition to the iris diaphragm, there are independently adjustable sickle-shaped leaves that can be rotated 360 degrees to modify the circular field for exact cardiac contour collimation (Fig. 7-8).

For serial filming, an additional circular or cardiac-

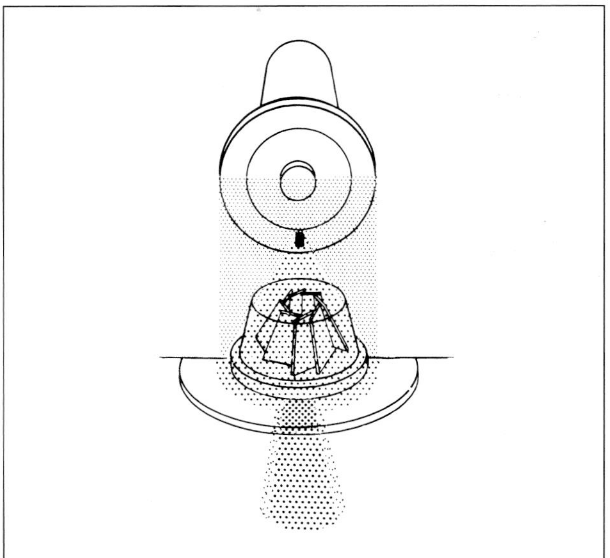

Figure 7-7. Iris-type collimator beam-shaping system useful for cineangiography. This is preferable to the usual square format "box" collimator. (Drawing after Machlett's Collimaster M., The Machlett Laboratories, Inc., Stamford, Conn.)

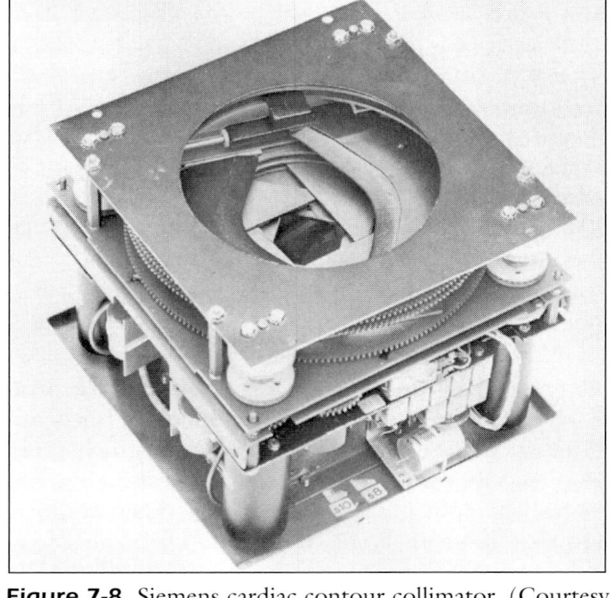

Figure 7-8. Siemens cardiac contour collimator. (Courtesy of Günther Theil, Siemens Aktiengesellschaft, Geschäftsbereich Röntgen, Erlangen, Germany.)

form extension cone can be used to simplify patient positioning and further reduce scattered radiation, thus enhancing image clarity.

Image Intensifiers

One of the most important advances in radiographic imaging since the introduction of the image intensifier has been the development of the cesium iodide input phosphor. Dramatic improvement of the cine image is not solely the result of this better input phosphor, however. There have been additional improvements in the photocathode, the electron optics, the output phosphor, tube geometry, construction of the tube housing, and the optical coupling. The advantage of the new intensifiers lies in their increase in QDE, conversion factor, resolution, and contrast ratio when compared with intensifiers of the past.

Image intensifiers are available in a number of sizes from 5 to 35 cm and in single, dual, and triple modes. The selection of an intensifier will depend on the specific function of the laboratory. In general, small-diameter, single-mode image intensifiers provide better image clarity in the clinical setting than do large, multiple-mode tubes.

The image intensifier for coronary arteriography should ideally be a single-mode cesium iodide, 15- to 17-cm instrument with high resolution. The 15- to 17-cm intensifiers combine high intensification and excellent resolution; they are ideal for coronary arteriography and pediatric angiocardiography. One advantage of a small-field intensifier (15–17 cm) is that it permits the use of a radiographic tube with a more shallow angle, thus giving a greater output than is possible with a large-format intensifier. Larger-size or dual-mode intensifiers may be needed for study of adults with large hearts. One should select the smallest intensifier that will do the job.

Within a given image intensifier design there is a trade-off between gain and resolution. Most manufacturers will supply a selected tube for a modest price premium. A selected intensifier tube should have maximum resolution and adequate gain. Selection of the highest gain tube available of a given design will ensure mediocrity in terms of resolution.

The resolution and contrast ratio of each intensifier in the laboratory should be validated individually and periodically every 3 months.

Cesium iodide intensifiers have a useful life of about 5 years. Because of technical improvements, most intensifiers more than 5 years old should be moved to less demanding use than angiocardiography or to a secondary laboratory where high performance and resolution are not critical. Recalibration and alignment

$$\frac{\text{Focal length of collimator lens (mm)}}{\text{Intensifier output phosphor diameter (mm)}} = \frac{\text{focal length of camera lens (mm)}}{\text{desired image diameter on film (mm)}}$$

of the entire system are essential whenever an intensifier tube is replaced.

Image intensifiers of 15- to 17-cm input diameter for cinefluorography or spot-film fluorography should provide on-site resolution through the optical system of not less than 4 line pairs per millimeter (LP/mm). Large multiple mode intensifiers of 22 to 25 cm should provide on-site resolution of 3 line pairs per millimeter. Under normal working distance and conditions, measurements should be calculated with a 0.05- to 0.2-mm lead line pair test object situated on the intensifier face without phantom at 50 kV. This simple on-site evaluation should be done regularly and consistently and results should be kept on file. Test results can then be compared for detection of image system changes or possible new equipment deficiencies. Any detected deficiency should be verified by a diagnostic radiophysicist.

The contrast ratio should be not less than 12:1 with QDE of not less than 50 percent. A single-mode 15- to 17-cm tube should have a conversion factor of at least 75 cd/m^2 per mR/s. Dual-mode intensifiers should have a conversion factor of 100 or more for the large field and 50 or more for the small field. A high conversion factor is not necessarily indicative of optimum performance.

Because of their crystalline structure, the relative thickness of the new input phosphors does not compromise resolution. Dyes used in the crystalline binder accomplish optical separation. Variables of resolution and QDE are affected by crystal density, size, and isolation. Current-generation phosphors, although relatively thick, do not restrict resolution capability in coronary artery imaging. If properly selected, they have the dual advantages of the desired resolution coupled with increased QDE.

Optics

High-quality matched optics are vital to image clarity. The modulation transfer function of the intensifier and its optics influences the total system resolution. The mixing of "off the shelf" components is discouraged. The entire optical system should be system-engineered for the application to maximize optical information transfer. The collimator lens and the camera lenses should be designed for tandem operation. This will ensure minimum optical aberrations and will maximize modulation transfer of the spatial frequency range of the intensifier tube over the spectral emission band of the output phosphor. The diameter of the camera lens should usually be less than half the diameter of the collimating lens when an image distributor is used.[3] All lens element surfaces should be coated to ensure high contrast and high transmission efficiency and should be dirt- and fingerprint-free. There should be *no smoking* in any areas where sophisticated optical systems are used. Residual smoke buildup will guarantee optical degradation.

The contrast ratio of the optical system should exceed 5 percent when subjected to a 10 percent area opacity test similar to the image tube contrast ratio test. The optical system MTF should exceed the image tube modulation transfer function. Focal length should be chosen to optimize film area utilization for the application. See box at top of page.

Image system usage requires careful weighing of trade-offs that influence the image for the particular type of examination to be employed (light input, film speed, f-stop of lens, image contrast). In general, it is best to avoid using f-stops larger than f/4 (e.g., f/2.8); contrast and resolution tend to be degraded if the lens aperture is too large. The best films available for cardiac cinefluorography have a relatively slow speed, so good light input is essential. Light output of the intensifier tube is influenced by several factors; the most important are radiation input, quantum gain, and light gain of the image tube. It has been indicated that the minimum radiation to produce an adequate cine image is 25 to 35 μR per frame. Because radiation input to provide brightness is fairly limited, adequate image conversion factor is important to the overall utility and quality of the image as viewed in the clinical setting. Nevertheless, tube gain is only one of several factors to be considered in image tube selection. Resolution and contrast ratio are at least of equal importance.

Cine Camera

The cine camera records sequential images that are formed on the output phosphor of the image intensifier by pulsed radiation provided by the x-ray power train—generator, cine pulse system, and x-ray tube. The eye has a persistence of about 0.2 second; thus when cine films are viewed at a rate of 24 frames per

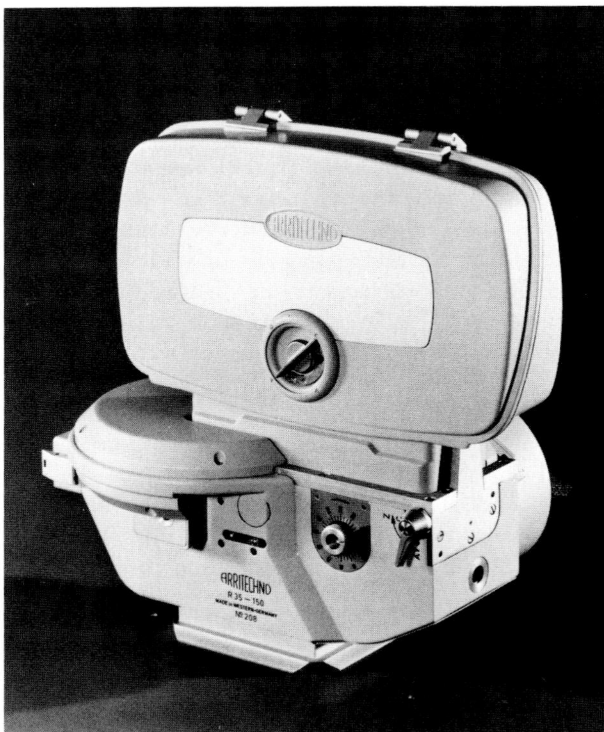

Figure 7-9. Arritechno 35 camera (Arnold and Richter, Cine Technik, 89 Türkenstrasse, D-8000 Munich 40, Germany). The Arritechno is the only satisfactory camera on the commercial market for 35-mm cardiac cineangiography. Other available cameras either require considerable adaptation, are even more expensive, or in some way have deficiencies for cineangiographic application. (The Arriflex camera, made by the same manufacturer, is no longer available. This is a nonsynchronous camera and less satisfactory than the Arritechno when used in today's equipment configurations.) (Courtesy of the manufacturer and Arriflex Corporation of America, Blauvelt, N.Y.)

second, the eye integrates the data presented in five frames. Images thus obtained can provide sharp anatomic detail and precise dynamic data.

For clinical imaging a synchronous 35-mm camera is recommended (Fig. 7-9). Sixteen-millimeter imaging may be useful in high-speed motion studies. The cine camera should be capable of smooth, vibration-free operation at 60 frames per second and electively should be able to operate at a variety of synchronous speeds: 60, 30, 15 frames per second, etc. Speeds other than 30 and 60 frames per second are seldom used for routine clinical work. Cine frame rates over 60 frames per second are rarely needed; rates of 90 to 180 frames per second may occasionally be useful in complex congenital abnormality studies or for research.

Framing rates of 60 frames per second are ideal to reduce cardiac motion during viewing. Cine images should be viewed while the image is in motion, forward and reverse being used to provide longer periods of time for image analysis. Single-frame sequential cine viewing can give a false impression of anatomic detail. Because of equipment limitations and/or for the purpose of decreasing film cost and radiation exposure, some clinicians have chosen to use 30 frames per second, electing to accept the attendant reduction of image viewing quality. This is an acceptable cost reduction trade-off in the hands of an experienced angiographer.

Precise frame registration, film pulldown, and maintenance of a flat film plane are essential. In the biplane mode, cine cameras and film changers should operate synchronously—180 degrees out of phase; such operation increases image quality and contrast by reducing scattered radiation to the image receptor. The camera must run smoothly at the selected frame rates, for vibration degrades the image.

With the imaging systems currently available, image clarity tends to decrease with frame rates above 60 frames per second, in part because of tube radiation input limitations (shutter time and tube output) and because of light lag in the output screen of the intensifier.

Measured resolution of a line pair test phantom of 0.1-mm lead equivalent placed in the entrance plane of the intensifier should be 4 line pairs per millimeter for a 15- to 17-cm image intensifier and 3 line pairs per millimeter for a 22- to 25-cm intensifier.

Cine Framing

The image presented at the output phosphor of an intensifier is circular. Most commonly employed 35-mm cine cameras have a rectangular usable film area of 18 × 24 mm. There are five common framing formats: exact framing, mean-diameter overframing, maximum horizontal overframing, subtotal overframing, and total overframing.

In *exact framing* the entire circular portion of the image intensifier appears on the cine frame. In *mean-diameter overframing* the diameter of the circle equals the mean of the vertical and horizontal frame measurements. This uses an additional 15 percent of the film frame over that used for exact framing. In *maximum horizontal overframing* the diameter of the circle equals the horizontal diameter of the rectangular film area. The area of the circle is approximately equal to the area of the rectangle. All but about 12 percent of available film is used for image display. In *subtotal overframing* the diameter of the circle is midway between the circle diameters of maximum horizontal overframing and total overframing. All but 4 percent of the available film is used. In *total overframing* the diameter of the circle is equal to the diagonal measurement of the rectangular film area. There is total use of the film area.

Exact framing is not recommended for angiocardiography. For many angiocardiographic studies, mean-diameter overframing will provide moderate magnification with only modest loss of field size. Maximum horizontal overframing provides additional magnification without loss of horizontal field and adapts well to cardiac shape and size; it is desirable for coronary arteriography and useful for most cardiac imaging. More severe overframing can be used with large intensifiers to produce intermediate formats; it can be used with small intensifiers for coronary arteriography when marked magnification is desired and panning is not objectionable. With each increase in overframing there is substantial loss of patient viewing area.

When multiple-mode intensifiers are used, consideration must be given to the effect overframing will have on each mode.

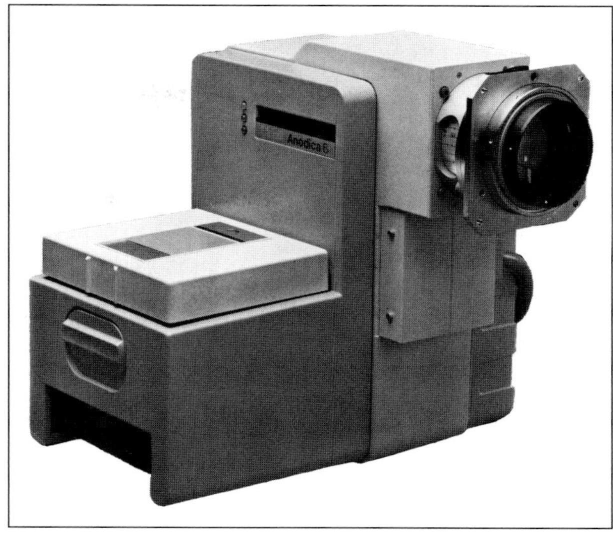

Figure 7-10. Anodica 6. The Anodica 2 and Anodica 6 are 100-mm sheet film cameras. The Anodica 2 is suitable for the majority of adult cardiac applications. The Anodica 6 (Oldelft, 260 Delft, Holland) provides more rapid sequencing if required, as in some pediatric applications. (Courtesy of Oldelft Corp. of America, Fairfax, Va.)

Spot-Film Cameras for Fluorography

Cameras for 100-mm cut film or 105-mm roll film have been designed to obtain rapid-sequence spot films from the output phosphor of an image intensifier (Fig. 7-10). Frame rates in excess of 6 per second are not required. More rapid sequencing is best accomplished with cine techniques.

Image informational transfer through the spot-film camera does not usually exceed that obtained by cinefluorography when normal viewing methods are used. Thirty-five-millimeter cine is superior to rapid-sequence spot filming from an overall diagnostic standpoint, in part because of the advantage of noise averaging and eye persistence. Also, the mobility patterns of tightly grouped overlapping coronary branches often serve to alert one to disease sites seen very transiently. Spot films provide a convenient supplementary method of viewing and reviewing the pathology present. The 100- and 105-mm films are of suitable size for direct viewing in the operating suite. This method of imaging does not replace cinefluorography.

Viewing during filming is limited by frequency of exposure and persistence of image. This blackout can be avoided by the use of specially designed electronics in conjunction with a video tape or video disk recorder that will replay each spot image on the video screen until the next image is recorded.

Spot-film cameras are normally coupled with an automatic exposure device. The automatic exposure control and generator control must be capable of accurate exposures down to 2 milliseconds. Minimum adequate radiation exposure is 150 μR per frame at the input plane of a 15- to 17-cm intensifier.

Measured resolution of a line pair test phantom of a 0.1-mm lead equivalent placed in the entrance plane of the image intensifier should be 3.8 line pairs per millimeter for the 15- to 17-cm field size and 3.3 line pairs per millimeter with the 22- to 25-cm field size.

Cardiac Serial Radiography

Serial film radiography can provide optimal and exquisite anatomic detail, but it requires considerable training, expertise, and experience in serial radiographic imaging not widely possessed by either cardiologists or radiologists. Successful coronary serial imaging also requires dedicated daily quality control by both the angiographer and the entire technical staff. Teams willing to expend the necessary time and effort will be richly rewarded by the excellence of depiction of the coronary vasculature.

A basic cine system is moderate in cost. Addition of the capability for either spot filming or rapid serial radiography will depend on individual laboratory needs and objectives and institutional budgetary constraints. The addition of other imaging methods, either spot filming or serial radiography, requires an equipment expenditure considerably higher than that needed for a cine-only installation. The user should be trained to employ these more sophisticated imaging modalities for them to be cost-effective.

Rapid serial imaging is based on the conventional screen-film combination. Film is exposed by intensifying screens that fluoresce as a result of direct impingement of x-ray photons. A film changer mechanically transports sheet or roll film to the exposure area at a predetermined rate. Large-film serial radiography provides maximum resolution of some vascular structures. Serial imaging and cine filming are complementary rather than competitive providers of anatomic and dynamic cardiac data.

For angiocardiography, the changer should provide a minimum of 3 frames per second; a rate of 6 frames per second is in reality a 35 × 35 cm cine technique without cine viewing capability. Film sizes range from 20 × 35 cm to 35 × 35 cm; the size selected for a given installation will vary with the intended function. The program selector should operate one or two changers. In the biplane mode, electrical synchronization should make provision for synchronous or 180-degree out-of-phase exposures.

Changer design should afford an optimum screen-film contact over the entire filming area, at the same time minimizing the absorption of the front pressure plate. Filtration of the front compression plate should not exceed 1 mm aluminum. Use of changers with carbon-fiber compression plates will minimize filtration and exposure and will improve image content.

Rapid shifting from the cinefluorography mode to serial film imaging may be desirable. The near equivalent of the see-through changer function is available on what are called integrated film changer beam positioning units. In these units, the image intensifier used for viewing is transferred out of the exposure field and the changer shifted into the field when serial recording is desired. The interchange time from viewing to recording is less than 10 seconds. Primary limitation is the 3-per-second rate currently available. Three per second is rapid enough for many cardiopulmonary examinations.

Rapid serial coronary arteriography can be performed without significant increase in risk to the patient, provided unaltered or undamped pressures can be maintained while the catheter tip is not in actual fluoroscopic view. If there is primary radiologic expertise in the day-to-day laboratory operation, it is likely that additional anatomic information will be obtained with supplemental serial film imaging. However, using this supplemental imaging method entails using additional contrast injections, which can be hazardous in patients with marginal left ventricular function and/or severe myocardial ischemia.

Video System

Viewing of the image during catheterization and angiography should be accomplished by the use of a television display chain. This viewing modality is used primarily for catheter placement, patient positioning, and image viewing during cine or spot filming and has no primary recording function. The video system must be adequate to permit instant recognition of significant anatomic findings and function changes—such as congenital defects, spasm in an arterial trunk, critical stenoses, subintimal dissection, or filling of major occluded coronary branches by intercoronary collateral channels. Moving objects must not fade from sight.

A high-quality video system that has excellent image clarity, signal regulation, and minimal lag is needed. The television system should have a rapidly responding automatic gain control that will prevent "blooming" and provide good image viewability through a field high in contrast in either view or cine mode. Image stabilization circuitry should provide center-to-edge image brightness uniformity. Circular blanking will improve contrast. If a disk recorder or network application is used, provision for external synchronization is advisable.

It is desirable to have a well-designed 525-line, 10- to 15-MHz bandwidth television camera system and monitor to take advantage of the resolution of the cesium iodide intensifier. The signal-to-noise ratio should be not less than 45 dB.

Measured resolution of a line pair test phantom of 0.1-mm lead equivalent placed in the entrance plane of the image intensifier should be not less than 1.8 line pairs per millimeter for a 15- to 17-cm field size and 1.4 line pairs per millimeter in the horizontal direction for a 22- to 25-cm field size when the limiting resolution of the image intensifier is not less than 4 line pairs per millimeter under the following test conditions: quantum density corresponding to 40 μR per second at 50 kV without additional filtration, without significant magnification, and with on-site focal-spot and distance geometry.

"High-resolution" television viewing systems with line scan rates of 800 or more are useful and cost-effective if the television chain is used for image recording. A high-line-rate system does not in itself provide a superior fluoroscopic television image. Total application must be considered.

Grids

X-ray grids increase image contrast and quality by reducing scattered radiation. Recommended for angiocardiographic serial film imaging is an 8:1 to 10:1, 40 lines/cm fiber-spaced focused grid. Grids with ratios below 8:1 are usually inadequate for scatter cleanup. Cross-hatch grids have little value except in specialized situations. Grids with fiber spacers generally require less radiation exposure than those with aluminum spacers. Choosing a proper grid represents another area in which a trade-off must be made. As the grid ratio increases, the absorption of scattered radiation increases, but so does the required radiographic exposure. Increasing the grid ratio beyond 10:1 provides relatively little improvement in scatter cleanup. Image intensifiers should be equipped with not less than an 8:1, 40 lines/cm focused grid. Focused grids should be used at the distance for which they were designed.

Patient and Equipment Supports

There have been rapid developments in supports for both patient and equipment. These have various functional goals, but in general they provide some method of triaxial movement of radiographic equipment around the patient for compound views (Fig. 7-11).

Ideally, primary imaging equipment movements should be readily accomplished by manual manipulation in preference to motor drive. This ideal would mandate the use of relatively lightweight, accurately counterbalanced equipment and the avoidance of unnecessarily heavy components. Procedural angulation and obliquity are most expeditiously and efficiently accomplished by manual adjustment. Skills for operating heavy motor-driven equipment can be developed. However, considerable practice and experience and a substantial laboratory case load are required to gain and maintain this expertise. I believe that when motor drive is imposed, procedural examination time is lengthened and there is a tendency for the operator to limit views, perhaps to the detriment of accomplishing a thoroughly diagnostic study. A readily overridden power-assist control is a viable alternative and may be mandated by heavy components.

An equipment and patient support configuration that one experienced angiographer finds near ideal may seem almost unusable to another experienced angiographer. Individual preference will vary depending on procedural protocol, technique, and the types of laboratory examinations performed.

The primary requirements for patient and equipment support devices are that they facilitate the rapid performance of the majority of procedures for which they are used, provide free access to the patient and to the entry site (brachial or femoral), facilitate both positioning of the patient and the modes of imaging to be used, and provide adequate radiation protection for the operator.

Before purchasing such specialized equipment, the laboratory director should carefully evaluate it using these criteria and preferably make on-site visits to several institutions that use the equipment for functions similar to those of the proposed new facility. Although individually designed laboratories may have certain desirable features, this individualism may be quite costly. Standardized laboratories properly designed and engineered by the manufacturer using the principles just described may provide significant cost reduction without loss of functional flexibility.

In general, the devices in the C-, U-, or Z-arm category, as usually supplied by the manufacturer, lack adequate operator radiation protection. Most have either no protective device or one that is unsatisfactory in design or ease of use. Some manufacturers have engineered protection for some of their models that is satisfactory if proper use is not thwarted by the operator. It is the responsibility of the operator and the manufacturer of the equipment to provide suitable radiation protection for use with either the femoral or brachial approach, or both.

Adult and pediatric angiographers and various manufacturers have developed techniques and equipment that facilitate the imaging of cardiac chambers and the coronary vessels and better depict the anatomic structures to be visualized. Of particular importance in angiocardiography and coronary arteriography are the craniocaudal and caudocranial views. Although views angled to 45 degrees in the sagittal plane are occasionally useful, angulation to 30 degrees is generally adequate and should be within the capability of any C-, U-, or Z-arm system being considered for purchase. Compound angled views that align the axes of the heart with the x-ray beam in three projections are particularly important in the study of congenital and valvular heart disease. The laboratory designer should keep in mind that generator and tube output requirements for angled views tax the capability of conventional tubes and pulse systems. The cine pulse system should provide an output of 40 to 60 kW.

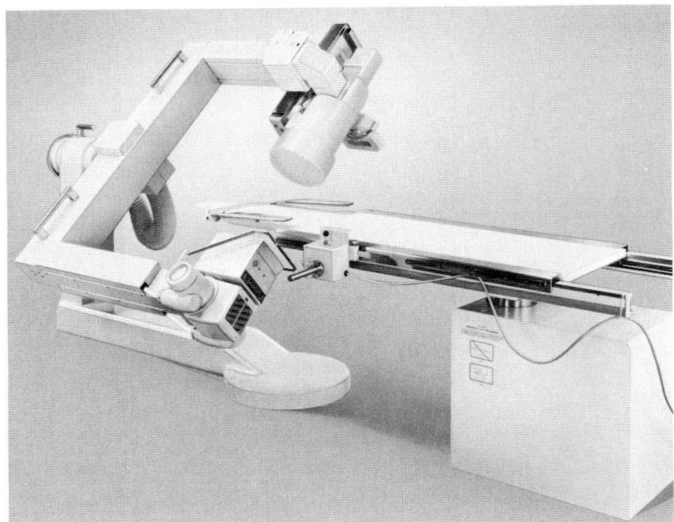

A

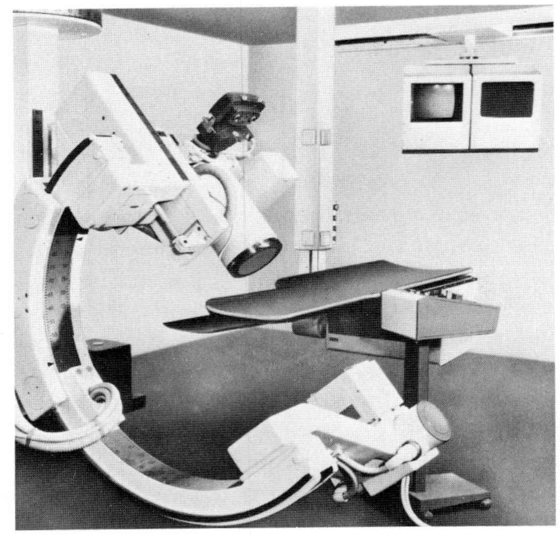

B

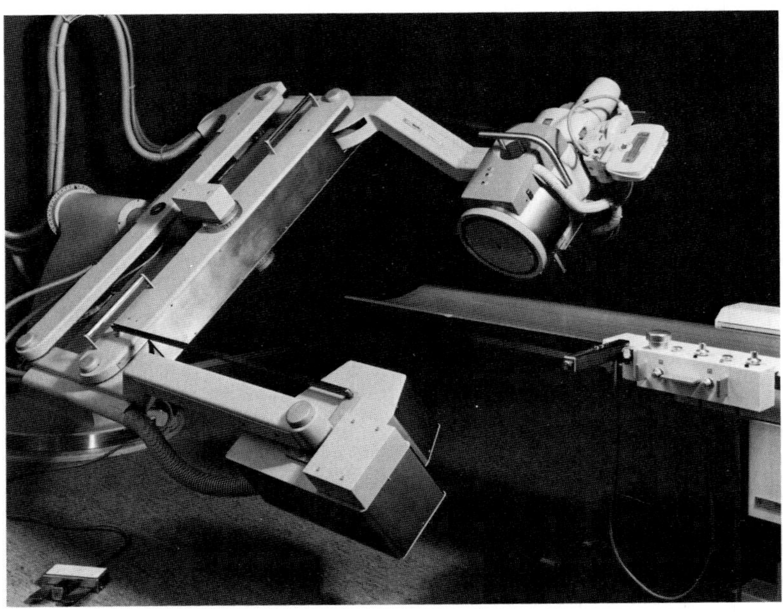

C

Figure 7-11. Equipment and patient supports with triaxial motion capability. This equipment facilitates multiangular projections. (A) General Electric L/U Cardio system. Third motion produces an image that is angled on the film but not on the television screen. The Philips Sones unit (Cardio Diagnost), not shown, angles the image on film and television. (B) Siemens Angioskop C system. Third motion produces image angulation on film one-half that produced by the equipment shown in (A). (C) Philips Poly Diagnost C system. The third motion does not angulate the image on film. However, the third-motion angulation increases the focal spot to intensifier distance. There is no perfect equipment-patient support. As is commonly true, certain trade-offs must be elected. Operator coordination is facilitated when there is the same type of equipment in multiple laboratories used by the same operator. (Courtesy of General Electric Co., Medical Systems Division, Milwaukee, Wisc.; Siemens-Elema AB, Solna, Sweden; Philips Gloeilampenfabrieken, Medical Systems Division, Eindhoven, Holland.)

The patient support or catheterization tabletop should be as radiolucent as possible to combine adequate strength with minimal but homogeneous radiation absorption. Tapered carbon-fiber tops integrated with C-arm, U-arm, or Z-arm supports reduce patient and operator radiation factors and improve imaging. Conventional table-edge image artifacts associated with angled projections are virtually eliminated with carbon-fiber tops. The support design should facilitate ready access for patient emergency. The patient support should incorporate a method of adjusting working height to the operator's height.

In older facilities or those in which there is shared performance of multiple types of examinations, including the noncardiac, there may be a conventional catheterization table having a free-floating top with longitudinal and lateral movement that may be incorporated with a patient-rotating device or cradle. If a patient-rotating device is used, it should permit rapid positioning of the patient during fluoroscopy and imaging and provide rotation of 180 degrees, thus facilitating the often neglected but extremely valuable lateral projection. Existing laboratories with laminated catheterization tabletops can improve their radiographic image and reduce patient and operator radiation factors by replacing them with tops made of carbon fiber.

Overhead supports for the lateral intensifier and radiographic tube of a biplane system should have positive, accurate manual or motor-driven alignment. A ceiling-mounted device is inherently more costly, but the cost is somewhat counterbalanced by the attendant clear floor space around the patient support.

When serial radiography is to be used, tabletop and film changers should be arranged so the patient-to-film distance is kept to a minimum. Because it is desirable to have the floor space around the patient as clear as possible, ceiling suspension of tubes, intensifiers, ancillary equipment, and even the patient support is recommended (Fig. 7-12). Such supports should be capable of carrying the weight of the x-ray equipment without vibration and providing smooth operation with a minimum of effort.

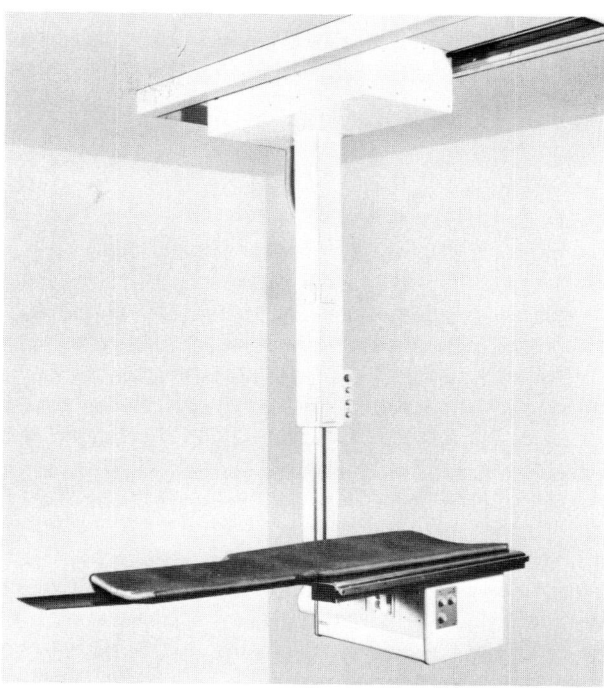

Figure 7-12. Koordinat 3D ceiling-mounted patient support. (Courtesy of Siemens-Elema AB, Solna, Sweden.)

Radiographic Film for Angiocardiography

The film and the parameters used in its processing must have the capability of recording a wide range of radiodensities, from air to bone and contrast agents. Angiographic contrast can be provided by using an adequate concentration of the contrast agent, optimum selection of kV (Fig. 7-13), reduction of scatter, selection of film and processing that produces a wide latitude image recording (Fig. 7-14), and use of the proper film density.

For cardiac cinefluorography the use of a wide-latitude, low-contrast, low-base-fog film processed to a relatively low average gradient of 1.2 to 1.5 has the potential for recording the greatest amount of anatomic information (Fig. 7-15). The use of a medium- to high-contrast film limits the anatomic information obtainable (Fig. 7-16). For serial radiography, film should be processed to an average gradient of 1.8 to 2.6.

For cine and spot-film fluorography, the color response of the film needs to be matched to the wavelength of the emitted light from the P20 output phosphor of the image intensifier. The International Standards Organization photographic ratings for natural light do not reflect the response to the green light from the intensifier. Film speed is no longer a limiting factor. Camera lens aperture can be varied to accommodate for the film speed, provided the chosen aperture is within the critical resolution of the lens.

Figure 7-13. Effect of kilovoltage on subject contrast.

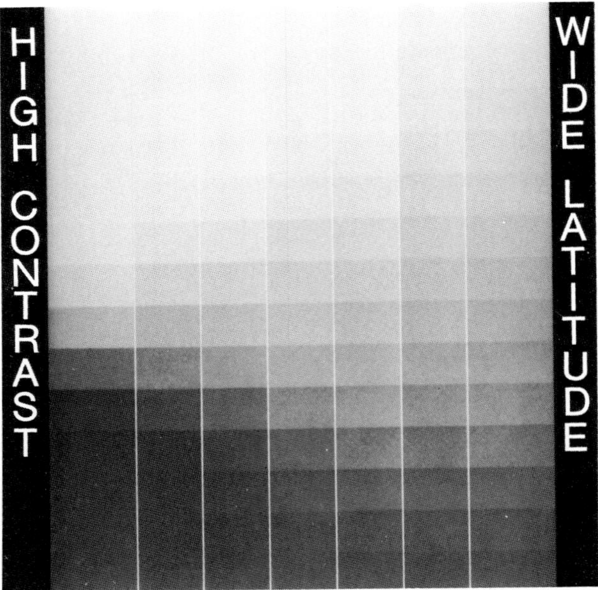

Figure 7-14. Contrast ⟷ Latitude.

Cine Processing

Improper cine processing and excessive quantum mottle are the two most important factors that degrade cine film image clarity.

Successful cine processing is a meticulous, professional endeavor, often neglected in the angiocardiographic laboratory. It is very common for the entire imaging output of a $600,000-plus laboratory to be relegated for processing to the laboratory's lowest-paid employee in an inadequate processor purchased as an afterthought. Expenditure of only 2 to 3 percent of the total laboratory cost will provide an adequate professional cine processor.

The processor should perform its function exactly and reproducibly and provide uniform quality throughout each film's width and length. To this end, *all* mechanical and chemical factors must be under control at all times.

The basic steps of developing, fixing, washing, and drying are similar to those of other forms of film processing. The eye has a persistence of vision of about 0.2 second. When cine film is viewed, the eye integrates five or more successively exposed frames of nearly identical images in about 0.2 second. Therefore, any frame with a processing artifact will be integrated with the properly processed frames and will degrade the retained image. In addition, in cinefluorography these frames are viewed at a magnification of 8 to 10 times on most projectors. Under these critical viewing conditions, it is easy to detect minute changes in tonal values from frame to frame. Physical defects such as streaks, dirt, and scratches of very small size can significantly degrade image quality.

Most angiographers are unaware that the actual surface area in a 250-ft roll of 35-mm cine film is about 27 sq ft. Obviously processing such a large area of film rapidly exhausts the solutions and requires stringent replenishment procedures. Furthermore, carryover of solutions from one tank to another results in dilution and contamination.

There is no standard cine processor. Rather, the types of processors available vary in respect to tank volume, film path length, film speed range, degree of agitation and recirculation, temperature control, and replenishment capability. These variables affect the results obtained in each processor. There is no guarantee that identical results will be obtained in all processors with the same film-processing chemicals and processing parameters. If all chemical and mechanical factors for an individual processor are carefully controlled, it should perform in a reproducible manner.

The key concept in processing control is that photography is a branch of practical chemistry. The materials used in photography and the changes wrought in them are subject to chemical laws. The film-processing

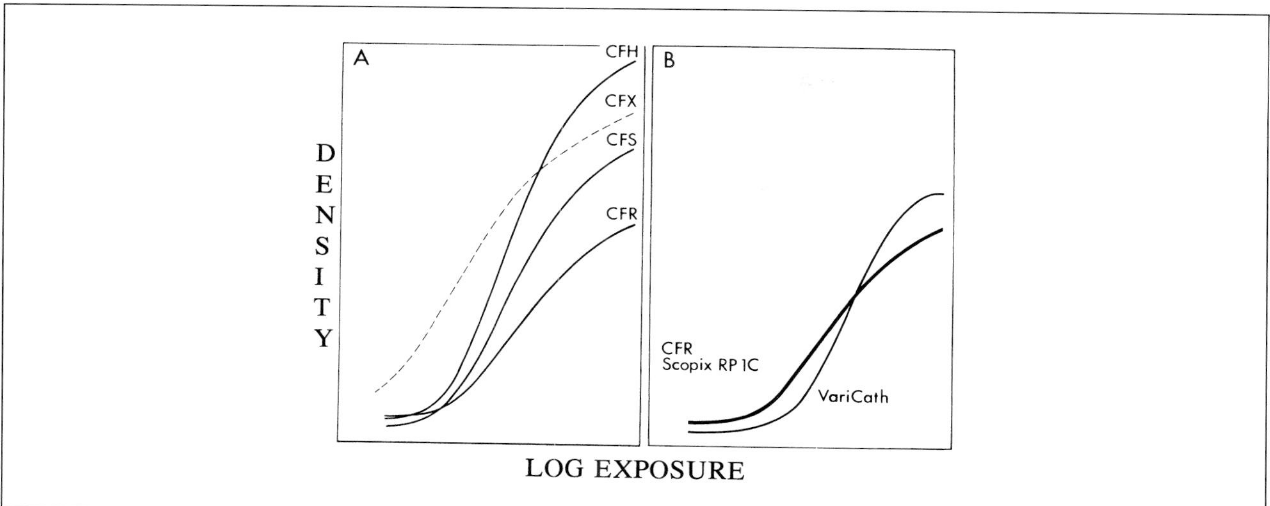

Figure 7-15. (A) Part of the Kodak family of cine films available for cardiac angiography. These curves depict film characteristics when fully developed (85% or more) as prescribed by the manufacturer. The steepest curve, CFH, is the film with the highest contrast. CFS, medium contrast; CFR, wide latitude (low contrast). CFX has a high-base fog, a contrast between CFR and CFS, and the speed is greater than CFR and CFS. (For comparison, CFX is indicated by the dashed line.) CFX is not a desirable film for coronary angiography except where equipment deficiencies require the use of a high-speed film, such as with an image intensifier with low light output. CFH is a high-contrast, medium-speed film whose only cardiac cineangiographic use is with old, very-low-contrast intensifiers. (B) When Kodak CFR and Agfa-Gevaert Scopix RP 1C are developed and processed at the same temperature with the manufacturer's recommended developer (KLX for CFR and C 138 for Scopix RP 1C), they have similar characteristics. One difference is that CFR has an acetate base and Scopix RP 1C has a polyester base. CFR has a blue-gray tint. Acetate film will tear before it damages the gears of the cine camera. Polyester film can cause expensive-to-repair camera damage. If used properly, either film may be satisfactory. Scopix RP 1C may be useful when the light output of the intensifier is limited. VariCath, an acetate base film, has a lower base fog than either Kodak or Agfa films. When fully developed, VariCath film has somewhat more contrast than CFS and less contrast than CFH film. When fully developed, the average gradient of VariCath is equivalent to CFX but does not have the high-base fog inherent in the high-speed CFX film. Kodak CFS, an ESTAR base film, is similar to Scopix RP 1C film processed at 33.9°C (93°F). Selection of film by characteristics is preferable to varying development time and temperature to obtain desired level of contrast ⟷ latitude.

Kodak provides a choice of films, Agfa provides a choice of temperatures, and VariCath provides a choice of temperatures and developers to modify film characteristics by underdeveloping and/or changing chemistry. Varying temperature and developer reduces manufacturer's inventory. Contrast of Agfa Scopix RP 1 film is relatively high and somewhat greater than CFS. It is not a satisfactory film for coronary arteriography except for use with an older intensifier lacking a desirable level of contrast. Comments in this section are directed to iodine contrast examinations. From this recitation it is obvious that there are several variables to consider when selecting a film for cardiac cineangiography, including age and condition of equipment and user preference concerning contrast versus latitude. (Courtesy of Robert Knabenbauer, Loma Linda University, Loma Linda, Calif.)

cycle, particularly the development of the image, is a series of complex chemical reactions whose mechanisms are not completely understood. The proper function of a cine processor is to control the chemical reactions in a repeatable manner; hence the mechanical devices that control temperature, processing time, agitation, solution recirculation, washing, and drying.

Temperature is one of the most critical variables because it affects the rate of the chemical reaction. Lowering the temperature decreases the rate of reaction; increasing temperature increases the rate. Fluctuations in temperature will cause variations of film density and contrast from roll to roll. Experience has shown that the developer temperature should be automatically regulated by a push-pull system with control to ±0.3°C (0.5°F) unless incoming water temperature remains at least 10° below developer temperature throughout the year. Some processors can maintain temperatures to ±1.8°C (0.1°F). In general, variations of developer temperature greater than ±0.3°C (0.5°F) produce a significant density variation that will degrade the film.

The *development time,* like temperature, is a critical variable. A chemical reaction occurs in a specific time for a given temperature for a given concentration of chemicals. Time and temperature are interrelated and

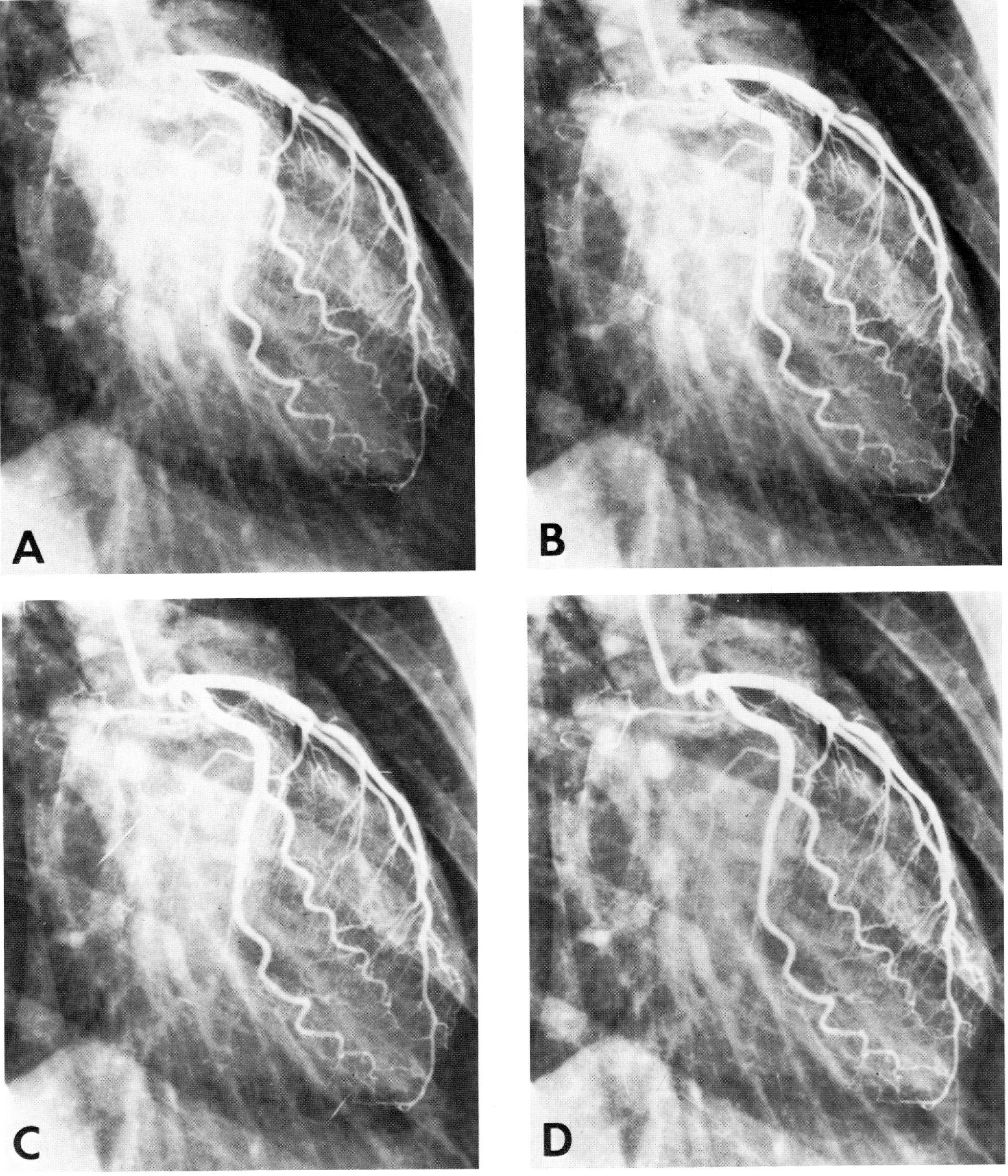

Figure 7-16. The difference between contrast and latitude. It should be recognized that contrast and latitude are opposites. These two terms are frequently misunderstood and misused. The untrained novice will usually select a high-contrast result over a wide-latitude result if shown two cine films to compare. Many physicians ask for increased contrast when what they really want is a wide-latitude cineangiogram such as portrayed in (D) rather than high contrast as portrayed in (A). (B) shows moderately high contrast; (C) shows medium latitude. Using Kodak cine film nomenclature, (D) is equivalent to CFR. (C) is equivalent to CFX in contrast, but (C) does not exhibit the high-base fog level inherent in this film. (B) is equivalent to CFS; (A) is equivalent to CFH. (Courtesy of James Simmons, Loma Linda University, Loma Linda, Calif.)

must be carefully controlled. In a cine processor, time is controlled by the speed at which the film travels. In general, the geometry of a given processor, and hence the number of feet of cine film in a specific solution, is relatively fixed. It is the speed of the travel of the film that must be controlled, not the speed of the film-driving device. It is wise to establish this by direct time measurement and then to recheck regularly as part of processor care, maintenance, and operation. Film transport speed should be maintained within ±5 percent by a stable drive mechanism.

Agitation is of vital importance in obtaining optimum uniformity of processing. Film surfaces should be constantly bathed with recirculated, replenished, and temperature-controlled developer. For any given development time and temperature, the degree of agitation will significantly affect these factors. Some agitation is provided by film motion through the solutions. This motion in itself is not adequate agitation. As agitation is increased by adequate recirculation, a point is reached beyond which no further increase in photographic effect will occur. An important requirement of agitation is to supply fresh developer solution continuously to the emulsion surface as it enters the tank. This is essential during the early stage to prevent uneven development, irregular streaks, and mottle.

Replenishment is necessary to maintain the concentration of the processing chemicals. The replenishment system should be designed to replace individual constituents in proper proportion because of rapid solution exhaustion and solution carryover. During processing, individual chemical constituents of the solutions are consumed at different rates. In addition, reaction products accumulate that affect film quality. There is also carryover of solution from one tank to another and potential dilution by water carryover from a washing stage. Replenishment must be established to (1) replace the individual constituents to their proper proportion, (2) dilute the tank solution to prevent excessive reaction product buildup, and (3) keep the tank solution at the proper level.

Replenishment is commonly and traditionally done by replacing exhausted chemical components. There is an alternative and sometimes preferable method of replenishment known as "flood" replenishment. Flood replenishment is particularly suitable for the small-volume laboratory but may also be useful in a large-volume laboratory, especially if the processor employed has tanks smaller than 5 gallons (19 liters).

Flood replenishment is designed to maintain start-up sensitometry by maintaining a level of developer and fixer rejuvenation slightly in excess of deterioration of chemicals. Chemical deterioration may be caused by such factors as evaporation, excessive variation in film density, use of films that have marked variation in silver content, and oxidation.

The flood method is intended to wash out the exhausted chemistry by flooding the tanks with a relatively large volume of fresh developer, thereby providing constant chemical activity. In this system, standard replenisher is not used. The solution used is new developer and starter. This method does require a larger quantity of developer and hence an increase in cost. If there is not the expertise to maintain strict quality control, this method may be the one of choice.

Recirculation and *filtration* assist in agitation and replenishment, and remove particulate matter.

The *developer solution* used for cine processing should be "hand tank" developer such as Kodak Liquid X-ray Developer (KLX). The *fixing* and *replenishing solutions* used for cine processing should be standard automatic processor chemicals such as Kodak RP X-Omat Fixer and Replenisher. The film should be fully developed (80–100 percent). Processing (underdeveloping) should not be used to vary film speed.

Continuous filtration of the wash *water* with a filter that can remove particles down to 25 μ is recommended. Sheet film processors are rarely installed without filters; cine processors often are. A similar filter should screen the water used to mix the photographic solutions, in order to prevent fine particles from settling on the film surface and contributing to degradation of film quality.

Film drying is an important phase of cine processing. Ability to control the drying process will vary with different processors. Generally, insufficient drying causes tackiness; overdrying may cause excessive curl and brittleness (particularly with acetate-base film).

Each of these processing factors, along with the film material and the developer formula, influences the average gradient to which the film is processed and the quality and density of the film. Proper processing of films for cinefluorography is too often the least understood and the most poorly controlled aspect of cinefluorography. It is possible to apply the principles of professional motion picture production in routine angiographic laboratory practice. The nature and importance of the procedures in this discipline require that this standard of excellence be achieved.

Features to Consider When Purchasing a Cine Processor

1. Complete, convenient operating controls for processing temperature, immersion time, agitation, recirculation, and replenishment.

2. Daylight operation. Most processors designed for daylight operation must have darkroom loading of the feeding magazine from the camera reel. Once magazine loading is accomplished, the processing is completed in daylight. One recommended processor has an accessory that permits total light room loading (Fig. 7-17).
3. Thermostatic control of chemical temperatures. This should allow regulation of ±0.3°C (0.5°F). There should be push-pull thermostatic control of chemical temperature if ambient incoming water is above 27°C (80°F)—10° less than working temperature—at any time during the year. Under these conditions a refrigeration water-chilling unit is necessary.
4. Accurate external reading thermometer for developer, fixer, and dryer sections.
5. Accurate variable film transport speed control.
6. Large-volume chemical tanks—5 to 20 gallons (19–76 liters). Smaller-volume tanks can be used in limited-volume laboratories. Small-volume tanks can be used quite satisfactorily in large-volume laboratories if flood replenishment is employed.
7. Replenishment system with floating-ball flowmeters. There are two methods of replenishment. One replaces exhausted constituents by using replenishing solution. The amount of replenisher is determined by the number of feet of film processed. The second method replaces exhausted constituents in the developer by flooding through the tanks an amount of developer about 20 percent greater than that needed for replacement of exhausted constituents. The latter method is less exacting and is best employed when tank volume is small or the volume of film processed is low or control for any reason is inexact. Conventional replenishment may be converted to the flood method by the use of developer instead of replenisher with an appropriate adjustment of flow rate. Any processor with developer tanks smaller than 5 gallons (19 liters) should be operated with the flood replenishment technique.
8. Recirculating pumps for developer and fixer with individual 25-μ filters.
9. Wipers to strip excess solution from surface of film as it moves from developer to fixer. A film path directly from developer through wipers to fixer is quite satisfactory. It is preferable for the film to travel through an abbreviated intermediate rinse or short stop bath. A film path directly from developer into fixer is preferable to a relatively long water rinse. A water bath abbreviates the developing but it does not completely stop the process. Processing that uses conventional photographic fixer should be done in a machine that has an intermediate water bath to avoid exhaustion of the relatively low acid content of photographic fixer. This is *not* the preferred processing chemistry.
10. Combination spray-wash followed by immersion wash. This is preferable; however, a wash system with a turbulent flow of fairly high volume is acceptable.
11. Wash water flowmeter.
12. Twenty-five-micron filters used in the water supply.
13. Air knife film squeegee or buffer to remove water from film prior to entry into the dryer section.
14. Air filter.
15. Variable dryer temperature.
16. Film guides or racks that can easily be removed for cleaning.
17. Built-in water rinse hose for maintenance.

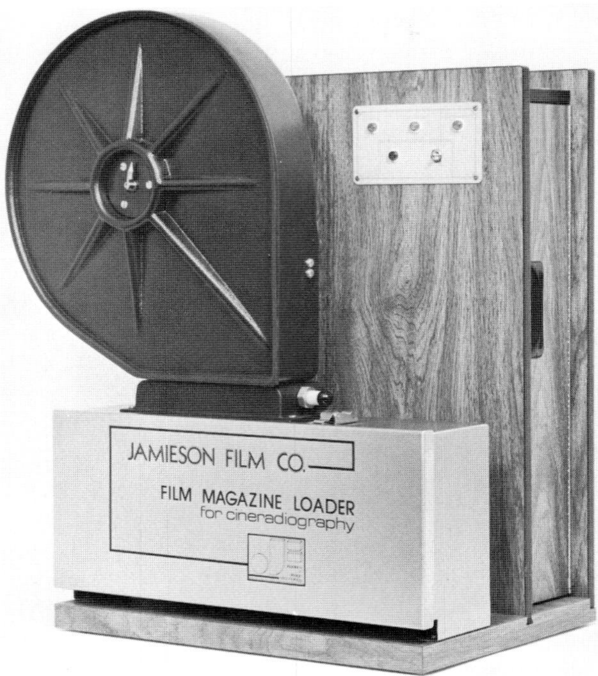

Figure 7-17. Jamieson Film Magazine Loader. Daylight film loading accessory permits operation without a darkroom. (Courtesy of Jamieson Film Co., 6901 Forest Park Rd., Dallas, Tex.)

Budgetary considerations for initial processor investment should include current and projected future film volume and the image product goal of the laboratory.

In selecting a cine processor it is wise to have the sophistication of the processor match the sophistication of the laboratory director and the technical ability of the processing technologist. The laboratory director who does not have the technical ability and background to train and supervise the processing technologist would be best advised to select a processor that is relatively simple to operate with control parameters that are not the most exacting.

Aside from budgetary considerations of initial processor investment, the laboratory director should carefully investigate the availability of an *established* service organization for the product under consideration. The laboratory director should be skeptical of promised service unless such service is guaranteed in writing by someone other than the local or regional sales organization (Figs. 7-18, 7-19).

Cine Viewers

Motion picture photography relies on the viewing of sequential images of an object. The eye integrates five or more successive images into a composite; the resultant depiction has an information content far greater than a single stationary image.

In cineradiography, because of radiation constraints a single image has limited information content. Cine frames viewed individually lose the advantage of image integration and have significantly less information content than the film viewed in motion. In general, cine images should be viewed in motion and not as single frames. Visual information integration becomes vital to adequate image production. The viewing of a single cine frame can give spurious information. If a lesion is seen only on a single frame, the existence of the "lesion" must be in doubt. The more radiation used (within limits) to produce an image, the less likelihood that false images will be encountered.

The quality of a projected cine image is influenced by both the capabilities of the projector and the method of viewing. The surface on which the image is projected can be critical if the high-level resolution capability of a projector is to be used to full advantage. Projecting on a wall or other makeshift "screen" will degrade an otherwise satisfactory image.

An often neglected item that has a *significant* influence on image quality, screen brightness, and projector downtime is preventive projector maintenance. The first step in a preventive maintenance program is a strict *no-smoking* rule in all areas of projector use and storage. Residuals of tobacco smoke deposited on the optics build an obscuring fog. The second step is keeping the projector optics free from dust, dirt, food, and fingerprints. The third step is frequent, careful periodic cleaning of the optical system, film gates, and film transport mechanism; this is greatly facilitated by adhering faithfully to the first two steps. If smoking is permitted, there should be a weekly optics cleaning program.

A cine film projector for the viewing of sequential cardiac images has two primary functioning components—the image optics and a film transport mechanism. Design problems revolve around the interface of these two systems in a manner that best meets the user's need. The resolution of the problems of these interfaces distinguish one piece of equipment from its competitor counterpart.

There are two basic types of cine projectors. The optical system of the traditional projector employs a rotating prism for image interruption between frames. The film is constantly in motion (except for stop framing mode) and the projector has the capability of continuously variable speed in forward and reverse. Because the film is constantly moving, image sharpness is degraded.

In the second type of projector, film is "pulled down" to the next frame and motion is completely stopped while each individual image is projected. A projector of this type requires greater precision of film handling, but has the potential of producing sharper images when they are viewed in motion. Available projectors of this type have a brilliant light source. One has a choice of a halogen lamp or an arc lamp for individual viewing versus classroom viewing. One projector has a wide range of framing speeds and automatic framing and looping. Another is limited to two framing speeds. The available ground glass, backlighted screen on one model degrades the image quality when compared to the potential of the basic projector.

Image Optics

The following are desirable features in the image optical system of a cine projector:

1. High-intensity illumination with continuously variable brightness control.
2. High-quality, high-resolution optics that faithfully reproduce the cine image across the entire field, corner to corner.
3. Critical focus control.
4. Heat control that will prevent film damage in the stop-frame mode.

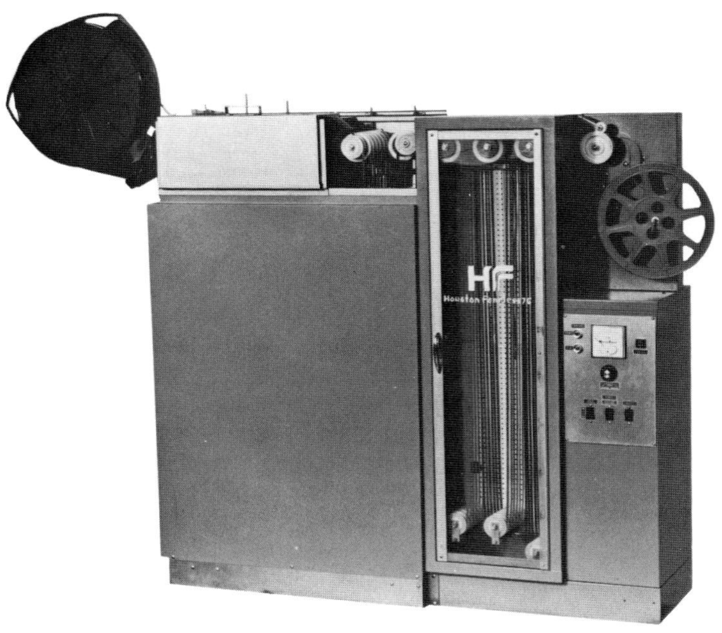

A

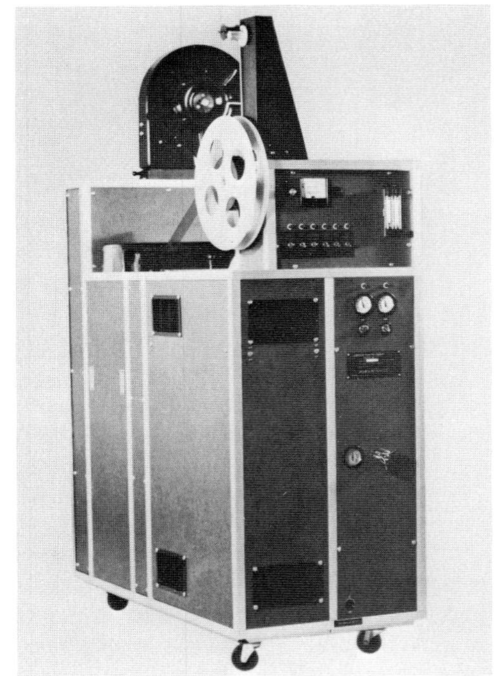

B

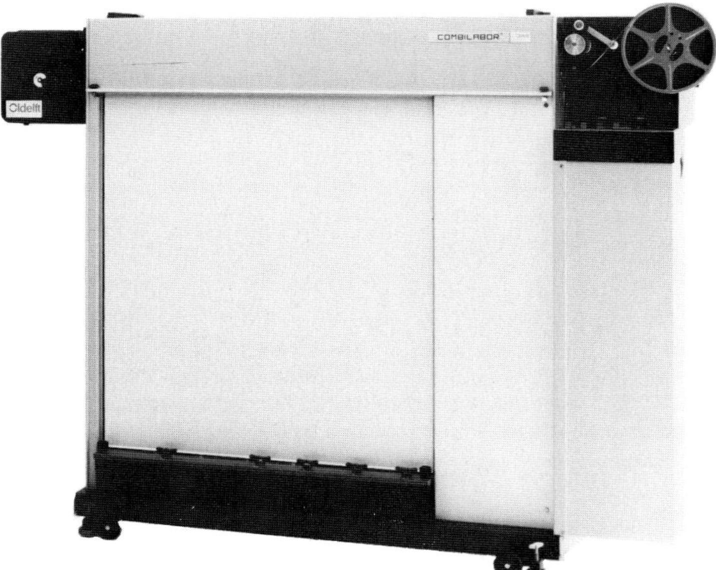

C

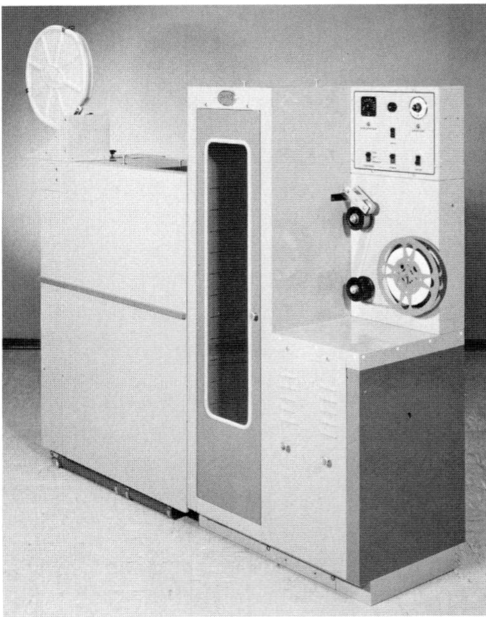

D

Figure 7-18. Automatic cine film processors. (A) Houston Fearless (833 E. Walnut St., Carson, Calif.). (B) Jamieson (6901 Forest Park Rd., Dallas, Tex.). (C) Combilabor (Oldelft, 260 Delft, Holland). (D) Pako (Pako Corp., 6300 Oldson Memorial Highway, Minneapolis, Minn.). (Photographs courtesy of Houston Fearless, Jamieson, Oldelft, and Pako.)

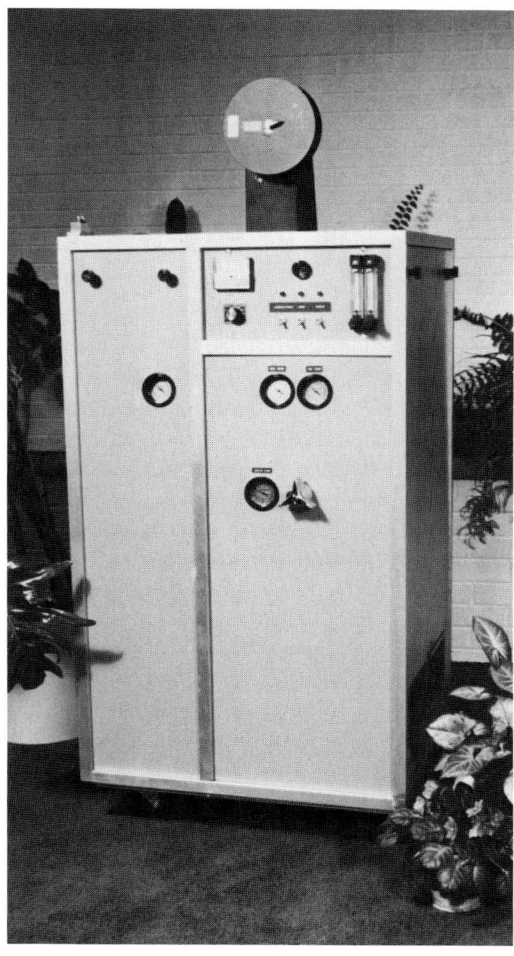

A

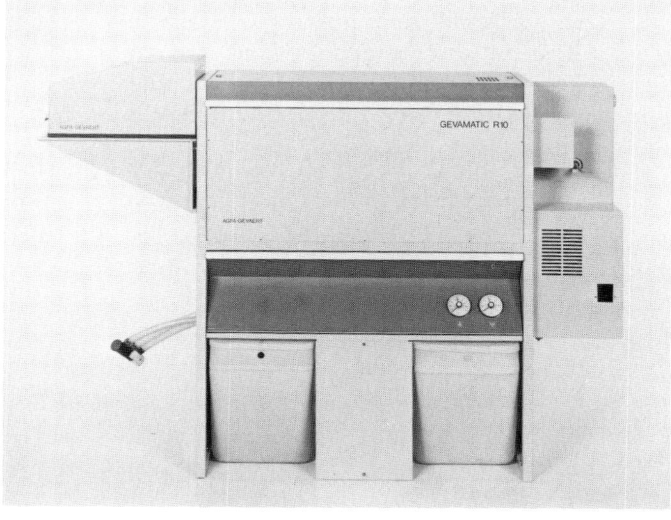

B

Figure 7-19. Automatic cine film processors. There is a need for a professional processor, designed for the small- to medium-volume laboratory, that occupies less space than many of the regular models yet has a full range of controls. Production of such models indicates manufacturer recognition that the daily processing requirements of many cineangiographic laboratories are less than 1000 ft of film. (A) The Jamieson Model 52 is one such processor. (Courtesy of Jamieson Film Co., 6901 Forest Park Rd., Dallas, Tex.) (B) Gevamatic R10 film processor. (Courtesy of Agfa-Gevaert N.V., B-2510 Mortsel, Belgium.) It has the advantage in the catheterization laboratory of the ability to process both 100-ml and cine film. Wash water is used to cool dryer exhaust air so that room heat is reduced. An accessory is available to permit total daylight operation. Gevamatic is not a "professional"-type processor. A serious disadvantage is the roller-type feed that produces artifacts on the film. The transport speed is relatively slow.

5. Easy access to the optical system that will facilitate periodic cleaning.
6. Image reversal capability to facilitate correct orientation.
7. Easy access for lamp replacement and accurate positioning of filament.
8. Large-field capability. Projection lamp wattage determines in part how large a projection screen can be used. However, lamp wattage is not the only factor; optical design and maintenance play a major role in screen brightness.

Film Transport

These are desirable features of a projector film transport mechanism:

1. Flickerless, shutter-closed transport and motionless film stop.
2. Ability to accept any standard film, spool, or reel.
3. Ability to accept 400-ft (120-m) acetate or 500-ft (150-m) ESTAR film lengths.
4. Precision transport mechanism capable of hand-

ling cine film without damage even after multiple runs.

5. Single-frame and continuous automatic operation capability without film damage.
6. Variable forward and reverse transport at frame rates of 1 to 60 frames per second.
7. Noise level should not preclude normal conversation during film review.
8. Remote control of appropriate functions (useful for lectures and teaching).

Ideally a cine projector should provide a flickerless, high-intensity, high-resolution reproduction of the cine film image. The angiographer must understand his or her own needs and the capability of available projectors. There are three primary competitors. A fourth projector now being marketed uses the rotating prism principle, a backlighted screen, and a bright halogen lamp light source (Fig. 7-20).

The purchaser should be acquainted with the product of the major competitors and their advantages and disadvantages as they relate to the particular operation. Ease of maintenance of both the optical and transport systems is an important consideration in projector selection.

The laboratory director will have to select the projector or projectors that will best satisfy needs within budgetary constraints. The density to which the cine film of a particular laboratory is processed should be varied and matched to the projector on which it is to be viewed.

Physiologic Studies and Equipment

An extensive range of physiologic information can be obtained by cardiac catheterization techniques. Much of the physiologic data traditionally obtained were valuable and useful and indeed essential in early studies of valvular heart disease for evaluating complex cardiac problems or for research. Some information that was routinely obtained in the past is of little value in today's decision-making process (particularly as applied to coronary artery disease) and increases the length of catheterization time and morbidity of the procedure. The incidence of thromboembolic complications is directly related to catheter time. Routine time-consuming collection of such data can no longer be justified. The laboratory physician must weigh both the cost effectiveness and the risk-benefit ratio in terms of procedure time.

In angiographic procedures both radiographic and physiologic data are obtained. The relative importance of the physiologic information will vary with the clinical problem, but rarely will one type of information suffice. Each study should be individualized so that only relevant diagnostic information is gathered while maximum patient safety is ensured and unnecessary cost avoided. The evaluation of ischemic heart disease entails excellent quality coronary arteriograms plus the collection of basic physiologic data that can usually be obtained in 30 minutes of catheter time. We cannot justify complete right and left heart catheterization for evaluation of uncomplicated ischemic heart disease. The addition of up to an hour or even more of physiologic evaluation to coronary arteriography materially increases the hazard of the procedure without a concomitant benefit to the patient from the information gained.

Monitoring for Patient Safety

Electrocardiography

Every patient should have a complete multilead electrocardiogram within 24 hours of catheterization. This tracing may reveal previously unsuspected abnormalities and is a baseline for later comparison in the event of procedural complications. Unstable angina or any clinical change is an indication for an additional complete electrocardiogram immediately before angiography.

Before catheterization begins, it is essential to establish a high-fidelity electrocardiographic display and recording; the display should be in full view of both angiographer and any assistants. It may be desirable to have more than one oscilloscopic display so the entire team can observe and monitor during the procedure. Patient respiration and/or movement should not produce obscuring artifacts of the electrocardiographic tracing. Frequency response should be maintained in accordance with American Heart Association standards.[4] Adequate skin preparation before electrode placement and common electrical ground of all laboratory equipment will eliminate two frequent causes of an erratic, noisy baseline. No interference in the tracing should be introduced when cine cameras, pressure injectors, densitometers, and transducers are in use. One of the most crucial times to interpret the electrocardiographic display is during angiographic contrast injections. If function of any angiographic equipment components creates tracing artifacts, vital information may be obscured; such artifacts may also signal potentially lethal currents that may be introduced into the patient.

All components of the electrocardiographic complex should be displayed and observed for significant change. Early recognition of arrhythmias is especially

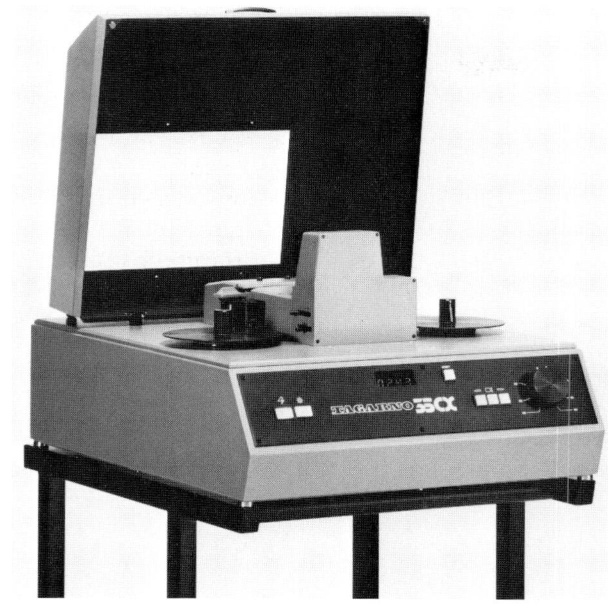

A

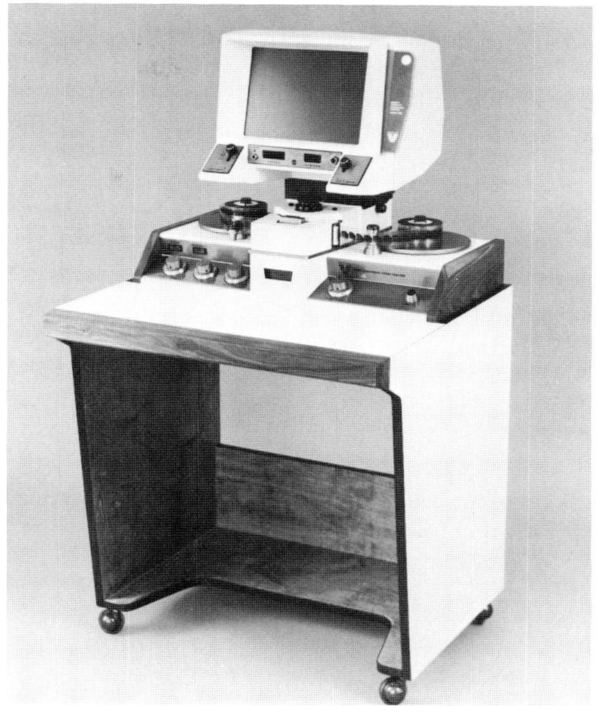

B

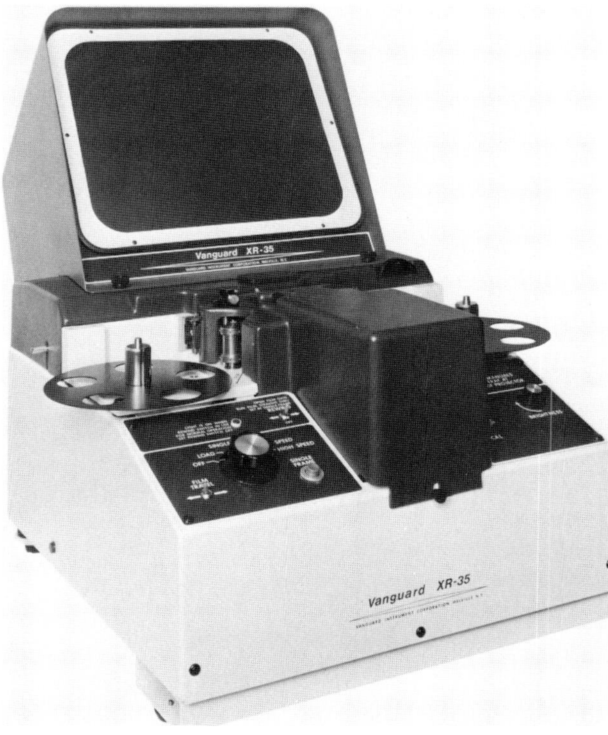

C

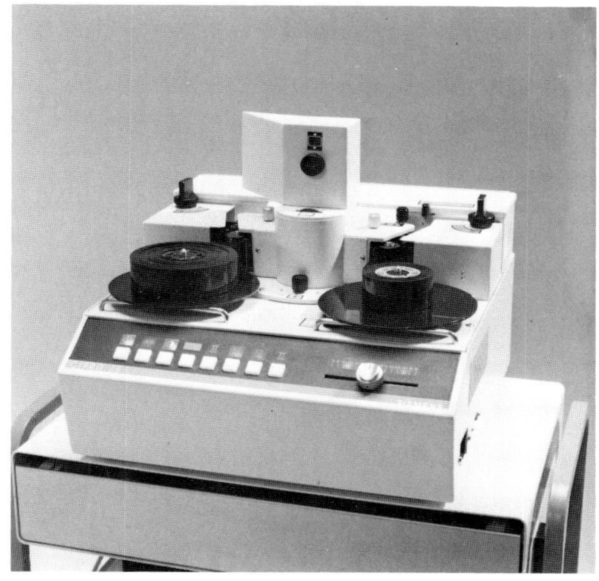

D

Figure 7-20. Cine viewers. (A) Tagarno (P.O. Box 276, DK 8700 Horsens, Denmark). (B) Birtcher (Birtcher Corp., P.O. Box 4399, El Monte, Calif.). (C) Vanguard (Vanguard Instrument Corp., 1860 Walt Whitman Rd., Melville, N.Y.). (D) Cipro 35 (Siemens Aktiengesellschaft, Medical Engineering Group, Erlangen, Germany). The Tagarno and Birtcher projectors are the rotating prism type. In the Vanguard and Cipro projectors, the rotating shutter is "closed" while the film is "pulled down" to the next frame. During shutter open phase of rotation, the stationary image is projected. (All photographs courtesy of Tagarno, Birtcher, Vanguard, and Siemens.)

important in patients with intraventricular conduction defects. The lead with the most easily discernible P waves is best selected for oscilloscopic display.

The electrocardiogram serves as a timing guide for repeat injections into the coronary circulation. Before repeat coronary artery injections are made, the T-wave changes that usually follow contrast injections should be allowed to revert to the control configuration.

Pressure

Systemic blood pressure can be almost continuously monitored by direct measurement through the catheter with a strain gauge transducer since most cardiac catheterization procedures involve entry into a systemic artery or the left ventricle. In examining patients with some forms of congenital heart disease and those in whom pulmonary disease or pulmonary embolism is the principal consideration, only right catheterization may be indicated. Continuous accurate intraarterial pressure readings are extremely valuable in the event of procedural complications. Direct monitoring of systemic artery pressure in high-risk patients is preferable to indirect measurement with a cuff and stethoscope or Doppler equipment. Procedural constraints limit the frequency and effectiveness of indirect measurements.

Other pressure data, obtained primarily for diagnosis, may often serve to alert the angiographer to a change in patient status and indicate a need to modify the examination. A transient fall in systolic pressure or a rising pulmonary arterial wedge pressure or left ventricular end-diastolic pressure may be a response to contrast material. Such changes persisting more than 2 or 3 minutes or a profound change in intravascular pressure may signal impending myocardial failure and indicate the need either to terminate the examination or at least to delay repeat contrast injection until the pressures are stabilized. The angiographer has to understand the hemodynamic response to radiographic contrast material, especially in patients with mitral valve or left ventricular disease. It must be recognized that different contrast agents affect these parameters to varying degrees. New nonionic agents have a lesser hemodynamic effect than the more commonly available ionic agents. The hyperosmolality of contrast materials may cause increases in blood volume and in left ventricular end-diastolic and pulmonary capillary pressure. The potential for complications increases when large cumulative amounts, greater than 3 ml/kg, are given.

Continuous monitoring of catheter tip pressure, particularly during coronary catheterization, will guide catheter placement and help avoid lumen obstruction or vessel injury. It is important to recognize immediately damping of catheter tip pressure that occurs in any vessel, since this may be the first indication of obstruction of the ostium or of dissection of the arterial wall by the catheter.

Standard equipment for each angiocardiographic laboratory should include a standby external pacemaker and an electrode catheter, both ready for instant use. This equipment should be periodically tested for functional capability.

For personnel radiation safety, the physiologic monitors and recorders should be located behind a radiation barrier or in the x-ray control room but with full vision of and in communication with the procedure participants. An intercom unit should provide two-way communication between angiographer and technician when equipment is located in separate rooms.

Measurements During Cardiac Catheterization

Electrocardiography

Not less than two electrocardiographic channels should have the capability of selecting chest or limb leads. Usually only one channel is required as a heart rate and rhythm indicator and a time reference for pressure records. The second channel provides backup in the event of procedural complications. Occasionally a second channel will be needed for intracardiac electrocardiography.

Pressure

Every angiocardiography laboratory needs the equipment to measure simultaneously, when required, two intravascular pressures with two sterile strain gauges of equal sensitivity. There should always be a spare gauge in reserve. Two pressure channels provide the capability to assess valve pressure gradients, to monitor systemic pressure during right heart catheterization, and to monitor catheter tip and intraaortic pressure simultaneously.

Proper calibration and zeroing of the strain gauge transducers require a constant reference point such as the midchest level. If two pressures are recorded simultaneously for measuring a valvular gradient, the two gauges must be at identical height and at equal calibration against a reference manometer, preferably a mercury column. A reference manometer should be used for frequent checking of the "electrical calibration" signal in physiologic recorders.

Distortions of the pressure waveform can provide misleading data. Faulty manometer systems and improper or inadequate flushing of catheters, connecting tube, or strain gauge transducers contribute to distorted pressure readings. Short of using fragile, expensive, inconvenient catheter tip manometers, the best way to obtain high-fidelity pressure records is with a fluid-filled system. Meticulously purging bubbles and avoiding excessive tubing between catheter hub and transducer will assure a satisfactory fluid-filled pressure transmission system. Any required connecting tubing should be noncompliant but also flexible.

Cardiac Output

Determination of cardiac output is of particular importance in evaluation of valvular heart disease. Two commonly employed methods of measuring cardiac output are dye dilution and thermodilution. In dye dilution, the indicator usually employed is indocyanine green. Cardiac output is measured from determining the amount of dilution of this indicator during its pass through the circulation. Careful calibration of the system with multiple concentrations of the indicator is required. Output can be determined from a dye-dilution curve either directly or with the aid of a small computer.

In thermodilution, the indicator is usually cold saline solution. Cardiac output is determined by the degree of temperature dilution of the indicator injected in the right atrium as sensed by a catheter thermistor in the pulmonary artery. The primary measurement is cardiac output; however, catheters currently available make it possible to assess other parameters such as right atrial, right ventricular, pulmonary artery, and pulmonary wedge pressures. The advantages of thermodilution include simplicity, ready repeatability, and no need for blood sampling. This method does not provide information about shunts, and the catheter cost also must be considered.

The dye-dilution and thermodilution methods of measuring cardiac output are now well developed and clinically reliable. If calibration is properly maintained, either method requires only an occasional comparison against one of the traditional, more time-consuming methods.

Small dedicated computers in use in several systems have proved to be accurate, reliable, and timesaving in the collection and interpretation of laboratory data.

Quantitative Ventriculography

By visual inspection of cineangiographic films, an experienced observer can make clinically useful conclusions about ventricular performance. For more accurate evaluation of ventricular function and for comparable interfacility and intrafacility or observer evaluation, there must be quantitative analysis of ventriculograms.

Quantitative ventricular measurements should be obtained from cineangiograms. An essential part of evaluation of cardiac function is the determination of global left ventricular function and segmental wall motion. Single-plane cineangiographic systems are currently most easily available and widely used. Quantitative measurement of ventricular function from a single-plane study is reasonably accurate and useful. However, in patients with localized or extensive dysfunction, visualization of only a portion of the recognized 10 contractile segments of the ellipsoid left ventricle may not give a true picture of contractility. Two-plane or biplane ventriculography better visualizes the 10 segments, 5 best seen in the right anterior oblique and 5 in the left anterior oblique projection. Several methods employing computers have been devised to reduce the laborious data collection and provide a reasonable and clinically useful estimate of left ventricular ejection fraction and global function. With the aid of suitable programming and computer reconstruction, the ventricle can be rotated in space, allowing the observer to view contractility in a given segment from any perspective.

Cmparison of segmental contraction before and after administration of cardioactive drugs (such as epinephrine or nitroglycerin) requires quantitative left ventriculography; this evaluation may aid in estimating valvular insufficiency and shunts. The effect of cardioactive drugs on ventricular function is used to help identify reversible ischemia of ventricular segments.

Equipment for Measurement During Cardiac Catheterization

A multiple-receptacle terminal box should be located on the patient support; it and the necessary cables should not interfere with the smooth functioning of the equipment. This precaution is more easily advised than accomplished. Thoughtful provision for cabling will eliminate the tangle of wires that will otherwise result from connecting multiple transducer and electrode cables directly into a recorder. Electrocardiographic and transducer leads strung across the procedure room to physiologic recorders create an unsatisfactory situation. Some patient/equipment supports lend themselves more readily to placement of terminals. This vital function should be carefully considered when one is selecting patient and equipment supports; manufacturers should, but frequently neglect to, engineer this capability into the system for factory or on-site installation. The mechanics of terminating the cable on the support will vary with the design.

There should be at least two high-fidelity amplifiers for electrocardiography. The physiologic monitoring equipment should be able to produce and record a standard 12-lead electrocardiogram when required. If this capability is not inherent in the data-recording system, a separate mobile electrocardiograph should be immediately available. A separate mobile electrocardiograph also provides backup in case of a patient emergency or equipment failure. Because of the possibility of equipment or power failure, each laboratory unit should have available for its immediate use a portable battery-operated defibrillator that has the capability of monitoring an electrocardiographic lead.

Pressures should be recorded with low-displacement strain gauge transducers. The frequency response should be linear in the 0- to 300-mmHg range at frequencies up to five times the cardiac rate.

For recording physiologic data it is necessary to have a multichannel display and recording system with a minimum of two pressure and two electrocardiographic channels. The system should combine signal conditioning, visual display, and graphic recording capabilities (Fig. 7-21). Additional channels are desirable for convenience, specialized functions, and backup. State-of-the-art signal conditioning requires fewer channels than has been traditional for processing a variety of information. Oscilloscopic recorders that use ultraviolet-sensitive paper produce an instantaneous archival tracing and are preferable to traditional recorders. A hard-copy recorder that is a direct slave to the display will produce recorded data identical to those displayed.

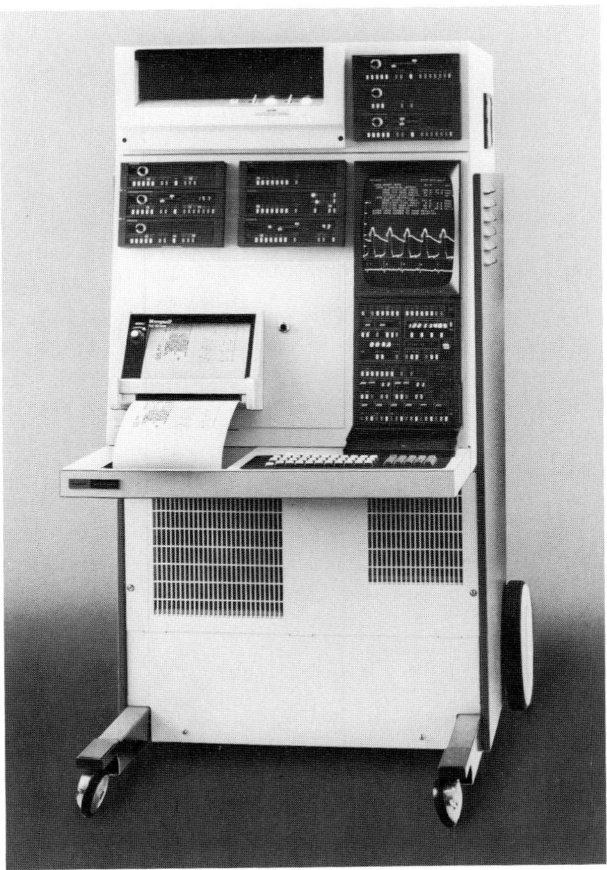

Figure 7-21. Honeywell MEDDARS physiologic display, analysis, and recording system. Physiologic monitoring equipment of modular design provides for the incorporation of electronics that facilitate the recording and processing of a wide range of parameters. (Courtesy of Electronics for Medicine/Honeywell, Inc., P.O. Box 5527, Denver, Colo.)

A slave oscilloscope mounted as near as possible to the fluoroscopy video monitor in the procedure room makes it possible for the angiographic team to observe catheter manipulation and the physiologic monitor scope within a narrow visual angle. Coordination of team function will also be enhanced if the operator of the physiologic recorder has a video monitor in his field of view.

An intercommunication system should provide efficient two-way voice contact between angiographer and the recorder operator when equipment is located in separate rooms.

Sophisticated microcomputer-controlled data analysis systems have been developed to assist in data collection, manipulation, processing, recording, and storage in the laboratory. This type of equipment is useful and can shorten information processing and improve the quality of data. However, because the capability exists, there is sometimes a tendency to collect a multitude of useless data. The angiographer must function as a logical, rational thinker, not as a slave to the equipment. The collection of some data that do not contribute to differential diagnosis may be of value for teaching, provided the student is simultaneously taught what is useful and the procedure time is not significantly increased. Although a variety of specialized computer instrumentation is available, physiological data collection in most laboratories should be an uncomplicated process requiring only a modest expenditure for equipment.

Emergency Equipment

A D.C. defibrillator should be on hand in each procedure room during any vascular procedure. To have a defibrillator in proximity to the laboratory is not sufficient. It is preferable to have the defibrillator fixed in place near the patient support and hard-wired to the electrical system. For emergencies, including a power failure, there should be a second, battery-operated or so-called portable defibrillator available within the physical vicinity of the procedure room; this unit should have the capability of monitoring an electrocardiographic lead. Defibrillators should be tested at frequent intervals to determine the adequacy of output.

When ventricular fibrillation or prolonged ventricular tachycardia occurs during a procedure, in a well-run laboratory, D.C. countershock should be instituted at once to convert the patient to sinus rhythm. If it is done expeditiously, little if any resuscitative effort will be necessary other than the cardioversion. Asystole of 10 seconds or either of the arrhythmias mentioned can frequently be converted to sinus rhythm by a sharp but moderate blow to the sternal area. This maneuver should not delay prompt electrical defibrillation but may be preferable if executed before consciousness is lost.

Once ventricular fibrillation, ventricular tachycardia, or asystole is established, the length of elapsed time to conversion will be inversely related to the rate of successful conversion. Resuscitative efforts should continue, if not immediately successful, until all electrical activity is lost. If fibrillation or asystole lasts more than 1 to 2 minutes, complete resuscitative efforts should be initiated with the assistance of a trained team including cardiologist, anesthesiologist, and respiratory therapist; the team should include a standby cardiothoracic surgeon. Vascular procedures should not be performed in the absence of such a trained resuscitative team. All cardiovascular laboratory personnel should maintain certification in closed-chest cardiopulmonary resuscitation.

Specific Laboratory Requirements

The equipment to be described is that which is desirable for a cardiac laboratory of moderate or high volume. It is presumed that the laboratory under discussion is one being planned as a new installation. However, in rebuilding an existing laboratory many of the equipment requirements are the same. Difference in equipment support will be the prime variation between new and rebuilt laboratories.

When considering whether to renovate an existing laboratory or install an entirely new facility, one must recognize that the useful life of most of the electronic components is relatively short because they become obsolete by the standards of the day. Some mechanical components will tend to have a little longer useful life—if not in the cardiac laboratory, then elsewhere within the institution or on the used-equipment market.

A laboratory designed purely for high-quality cineangiography can be installed at considerably less cost than one having multimodality recording capability. Such a high-quality cine laboratory is near optimal for the study of the coronary arteries and of adult acquired and congenital heart disease. However, a laboratory designed to provide optimal-quality serial arteriography does depict more precisely the coronary anatomy. Unless an angiographer has acquired and maintains the expertise essential for effective serial imaging, this modality is not recommended for either routine or occasional use. Readers with a strong radiologic background may find it more desirable to use multiple imaging modes than will those who have had less orientation and background in imaging.

Laboratory for Ischemic Heart Disease

Approximately 80 percent of adults undergoing cardiac angiographic procedures are studied because of the clinical suspicion of coronary artery disease. There are two basic essentials of complete diagnosis and decision making in this disease—accurate radiographic anatomic display of the coronary circulation and ventriculographic and physiologic assessment of global and segmental left ventricular function.

Coronary Anatomy

The anatomy of the coronary arteries as they course over the epicardial surface of the heart must be clearly depicted by selective arteriography in multiple planes without obscuring overlap. Contrast material should completely replace the blood for 3 to 4 seconds while high-resolution images are recorded in multiple projections, tailored to depict individual anatomy.

It is desirable to have equipment that will facilitate both cranial and caudal angulation of up to 45 degrees in the 30-degree right anterior oblique through various left anterior oblique projections to the left lateral. The most useful and commonly employed projections for coronary arteriography are the right anterior oblique, the shallow left anterior oblique with cranial angulation, the 70-degree left anterior oblique with cranial angulation, and the lateral. When equipment is not available to angle the x-ray beam along the long axis of the patient support, the patient can be propped and rotated.

Equipment for coronary arteriography must be capable of accurately and reproducibly portraying the anatomy of the coronary tree and the physiology of flow of all primary, secondary, and tertiary vessels down to 100 μ in diameter. It is true that vessels of this diameter are not in themselves therapeutically important, but the ability to visualize and recognize change in luminal character is important in the evaluation and treatment of disease, and particularly in assessing a patient's suitability for a specific therapy.

It is also imperative to assess the presence of collateral circulation consistently and accurately. Collateral flow is generally present when a vessel has been occluded and flow can be assessed when quality imaging is available and a suitable contrast injection has been made in the primary patent coronary vessels. If collateral circulation has failed to develop properly, myocardial fibrosis is more likely to be present than it is when well-developed collaterals exist. Failure to visualize collaterals adequately may occur if a high-quality imaging system is lacking or if the angiographer has failed to make an adequate contrast injection. In addition to portraying the anatomic features of the coronary tree, it is important to assess the dynamics of flow.

Left Ventricular Function and Anatomy

Depicting ventricular function includes the ability to assess both global and segmental wall motion. Depicting ventricular anatomy includes the ability to detect anbormalities within the ventricular cavity (such as thrombi or tumors) and abnormalities of the cardiac valves.

To assess ventricular function optimally, one should visualize the ventricle in two planes during normal sinus rhythm. It can be useful, but is not essential, to visualize ventricular motion during a premature contraction. It is important for the coronary arteriographer to learn to position the ventriculography catheter so that premature ventricular contractions do not result from contrast injection. For ventriculography a slow injection of a relatively large contrast bolus is desirable (10–12 ml per second for 3–4 seconds). Good ventricular opacification and visualization are obtained if the loop of a pigtail catheter[5] is placed in the inflow tract of the left ventricle.

When a pigtail catheter is used, "quiet" ventriculography is best accomplished by withdrawing the coiled tip to a midcavity position and simultaneously rotating the catheter 70 to 90 degrees counterclockwise (Fig. 7-22). When a Sones or straight catheter is used, similarly placing the tip near the mitral valve will reduce the frequency of premature ventricular contraction; however, catheter motion or whipping reduces the success rate. Ventriculography following nitroglycerin or postextrasystolic potentiation may be useful in

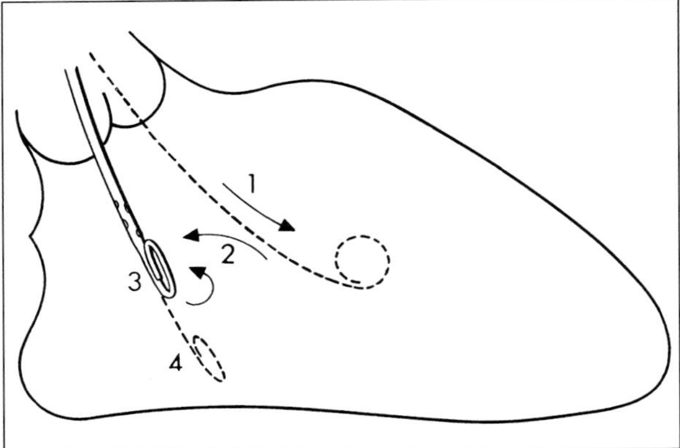

Figure 7-22. Positioning a pigtail catheter for "quiet" ventriculography. (Courtesy of Robert Knabenbauer, Loma Linda University, Loma Linda, Calif.)

evaluating contractile reserve. One can develop the skill, when using a pigtail catheter, of obtaining a "quiet" ventriculogram during the first few contractions after ventricular filling and then stimulating a premature contraction by manipulating the catheter against the left ventricular wall while the injection progresses.

In ischemic heart disease we commonly recognize at least 10 primary ventricular segments of contractility. Dysfunction of these segments represents corresponding ischemia if there is vascular obstruction. On the other hand, primary muscle disease does not follow patterns of vascular obstruction, and dysfunction tends to be generalized. In most patients ventricular function can be optimally assessed with two-plane ventriculography, preferably biplane ventriculography. Full and complete evaluation of ventricular function has been accomplished by computer reconstruction of ventricular function. By this method, the heart in motion can be visualized much as one would view an isolated contracting heart that the observer could completely "walk" around.[6]

Equipment

Equipment for ventricular visualization is similar to that needed for the study of coronary arteries. Visualization of fine detail is not as critical as in coronary arteriography. Therefore, equipment for coronary arteriography is usually adequate for ventriculography. For ventriculography, however, it is desirable, but not necessary, to have the capability of performing biplane studies. Ideally the planes should not be tied to a fixed 90-degree relationship to each other or to the long axis of the patient support. It is desirable to be able to position the long axis of the heart at or near right angles to the imaging plane. This technique was originally developed for the study of congenital cardiac abnormalities, but it is also desirable for the study of ischemic heart disease.[7]

Imaging modalities available for the study of ischemic heart disease include cineangiography, spot-film fluorography (100 and 105 mm), and serial-film radiography. Thirty-five-mm cineangiography should be considered the primary imaging modality for angiocardiography. Spot films do not provide additional information not provided by 35-mm cineangiography. However, they do provide films for immediate (and subsequent) viewing and can conveniently be viewed in the operating room during a coronary bypass operation. Serial-film radiography can provide films of the highest anatomic detail when performed by individuals who have developed expertise in this type of imaging. Serial radiography should not be done as a substitute for cineangiography, only as a supplement.

Those who establish laboratories primarily for coronary arteriography should give serious consideration to the imaging modalities needed in relation to the economics involved. Although biplane imaging facilities are desirable, the additional cost of fluoroscopic and cineangiographic capability in the second plane is significant. The most economically feasible high-quality laboratory handling a moderate volume of studies is the single-plane cineangiographic laboratory. It is my opinion that most cardiac laboratories should be primarily single-plane cine imaging facilities. Such a laboratory should be designed to use high-quality components; the equipment requirements can be relatively economical compared to those of a multipurpose laboratory.

The image intensifier for coronary arteriography should be a single-mode cesium iodide 15- to 17-cm instrument having moderate gain and high resolution. The intensifier tube should be selected for its resolution rather than primarily for gain. In general, there is a trade-off between resolution and gain. The laboratory director will be richly rewarded in image product if he or she pays the modest price premium for a selected tube that has maximum resolution and adequate gain.

Ideally, left ventricular function is studied by means of alternately firing biplane imaging equipment, thus avoiding two contrast injections and the consequent contrast load in patients with marginal ventricular function. Biplane imaging is useful only for ventriculography. It has no role in imaging of coronary vessels except for special research projects. The biplane system also provides a second imaging system that can be a backup in case of failure of a single plane.

Although somewhat less desirable, a single-plane system is adequate for most laboratories, is less complex, and may be technically less difficult to operate and maintain. For this reason, the end product may be more satisfactory than can be routinely obtained from a more sophisticated system requiring a higher level of maintenance. There is a considerable cost saving. A biplane system will cost at least 50 percent more than a single-plane system.

The designer of a laboratory for coronary arteriography should make no compromise with quality. However, the highest price does not necessarily signify maximum quality of the imaging product. The equipment requirements for cine coronary arteriography need not be as versatile as those called for by spot-film fluorography or serial-film studies, nor is it necessary to have as high a power rating.

Laboratory for a Broad Spectrum of Cardiac Disease

Ideally, a facility should have two angiocardiographic laboratories, one equipped primarily for coronary arteriography and the study of cardiac disease without cardiomegaly, and another equipped primarily for the study of cardiac disease with cardiomegaly. Equipment optimal for coronary arteriography is suitable for the study of all heart disease except that characterized by considerable cardiac enlargement. More than 95 percent of patients can be studied in a laboratory designed for coronary arteriography equipped with a single-mode, small intensifier (15–17 cm). This is true except in regions where there is a high incidence of rheumatic heart disease with cardiomegaly.

A laboratory designed primarily for the study of heart disease in which cardiomegaly is a predominant feature should have a 22- to 25-cm image intensifier to visualize the enlarged cardiac structure. The instrument most readily available is the dual-mode or so-called triple-mode intensifier. Intensifiers with a 35-cm field have become available, but I do not recommend them for cardiac angiography.

Certain equipment compromises must be accepted when both coronary artery disease and adult cardiac disease with cardiomegaly are to be studied in the same laboratory. A cost-saving compromise is to equip the laboratory with both a single-mode, small intensifier (15–17 cm) and a dual-mode intensifier. The equipment can be designed to function in single- or biplane configuration. A laboratory for the study of congenital heart disease should have biplane capability. Therefore, it is useful to have a dual-mode intensifier in a single-plane configuration when one laboratory needs the capability to study all forms of heart disease. Such a situation is common in limited-volume tertiary facilities.

Laboratory for Pediatric Angiocardiography

The angiographic study of complex congenital heart disease requires the capability to view the heart from two different angles during a single contrast injection. Biplane cinefluorography is thus the primary imaging modality for pediatric angiocardiography. This capability reduces the amount of contrast necessary for a complete examination, thereby lessening the potential for complications due to volume overload and toxicity. The concept of contrast dose reduction by the use of biplane angiocardiography is almost universally accepted in pediatric centers.

Video recording of the fluoroscopic image with provision for instant replay is essential; the angiographer should have this capability for procedural view, review, and assessment of completeness of study. The laboratory should have the capability for the procedural team to readily and simply position both the patient and the equipment in a biplane triaxial configuration. This combination of patient and equipment positioning places the area of suspected cardiac pathology in profile with the x-ray beam, rather than in an artificial axis dictated by procedure table or traditional equipment configuration.

Imaging should be accomplished by use of magnification angiographic principles. The degree of magnification should be such that the image of the infant's or child's heart completely fills the frame, with maximal use of the available film.

For the highest-quality images, a single-mode 15- to 17-cm intensifier should be used. If existing conditions require a compromise, a large-format intensifier (22–25 cm) with lenses designed for total overframing should be employed. Large-format image intensifiers are undesirable because they tend to obscure the infant from sight and interfere with positioning. It is my opinion that a large-format or dual-mode intensifier is undesirable and a needless additional expense for pediatric cardioangiography. Large children with large hearts are best examined in a laboratory designed for the study of adults with cardiomegaly.

Serial angiography can be useful and can offer an additional dimension in the study of the anatomy of complex congenital problems. It is a cost-effective modality if the angiographer and laboratory personnel have been fully trained in its use.

When infants and children must be examined in the same laboratory as adults, certain equipment compromises must be made. The radiographic equipment required in a laboratory for examination of ischemic heart disease can be adapted for acceptable joint use for pediatric angiocardiography. Further, less desirable compromises must be made in a laboratory used for general angiocardiography.

The major modifications for pediatric needs are not radiographic. Appropriate smaller-size ancillary equipment that must be available includes defibrillator paddles, electrocardiographic leads, catheters, resuscitation equipment, a microsample oximeter, and anything that is called for to meet the particular needs of the local pediatric staff. Monitoring and maintenance of body temperature are fundamental to the survival of the infant. The mechanism used must not compromise fluoroscopy or imaging.

Specially designed immobilization devices are required to deter patient motion during catheterization and filming. The device with as low a visual "fright" factor and as high a comfort factor as possible will maximize the "cooperation" of the tiny patient. Appropriate personnel should be present in the laboratory to monitor and attend to the needs of the infant.

Quality Control of the Cardiac Angiography Facility

The most sophisticated laboratory hardware and software will not produce an acceptable image product without the combined imaging expertise of the laboratory director, the x-ray technologist, and the darkroom technician. An ongoing, organized, periodic imaging equipment surveillance and maintenance program is essential for laboratory quality control regardless of the imaging modality to be employed. Such a program, involving all systems, is vital to obtaining the optimum amount of information with the least amount of radiation.

Routine evaluation of each facet of system performance should be made. Because of the complexity of the many components of the imaging systems—from generators to ultimate viewing—it is not feasible to check each component every day. But the two major areas that are most subject to variation can be evaluated daily: the conglomerate aspects of the exposure phase (x-ray source, image intensifier, automatic brightness system, cine cameras, and optical chain) and the film-processing phase.

The results of the quality-control studies must be

conscientiously recorded and reviewed at frequent intervals. Only in this way will it be possible to identify the source of a problem as it is developing. Otherwise there will be only a beautiful record of a degenerating system. If the films are too light and the cine processor is within control limits, one should immediately suspect technique. If the controls were set properly, one should suspect variation in the calibration of the x-ray generators. If the x-ray generators are checked and found to be properly calibrated relative to previous records, one should suspect the image intensifier. If previous measurements have been made on the conversion efficiency of the intensifier, this factor can readily be checked to determine whether this component is operating properly. When the operating parameters are known in advance and monitored, it will be easy to define precisely and correct problems. A small investment in an adequate quality-assurance program will result in savings of time and in the maintenance of a quality operating system.

Daily quality-assurance inspections should include calibration of the automatic brightness systems. At least every 3 months (more frequently when indicated) inspections should include measurement of resolution of image intensifiers, measurement of focal-spot size, and checks of calibration for kV, mA, and time. In a laboratory using serial film radiography, 3-month inspection will include measurement of resolution of the film changers and evaluation of film-screen contact during operation and not in a static mode. These should be done by a properly trained radiologic technologist working under the supervision of a physicist.

A test of imaging operation should be made at the start of each laboratory day. It includes exposure of two strips of cine film—one filmstrip exposed to x-ray of a suitable test object and the second filmstrip exposed with a regulated light sensitometer. Variation in the x-ray–exposed strip will reveal problems in either the cine exposure system or the film-development phase. Variation in the sensitometer-exposed strip can be isolated to cine processing problems. Details of daily quality-control testing of the cine processing system before the start of the laboratory day are presented in the following paragraphs. A test phantom should be included in the cine identification frames exposed to identify each patient's cine film. This provides an examination-by-examination index of system operation useful in evaluating the equipment's long-term operational status.

Cine magazines should be cleaned each time they are reloaded. "Blowing out" the magazine with compressed air is the most efficient way to remove film chips, dust, and other debris. Static artifacts on film can be minimized by the use of silicone on the runners of the cine camera. This is best accomplished by application of silicone with a Q-tip to the runners where the film touches. The runners need to be polished with a dry Q-tip after the initial application to remove all but a very thin layer. An antistatic aerosol sprayed in the camera magazine will also cut down on static artifacts. Only a small amount of spray is needed, otherwise it will coat unnecessarily. The interiors of the cameras, particularly the film gates, should be cleaned after every two or three rolls of film because of emulsion buildup. With some brands of film, cleaning may be needed after each cine run.

The objective of a quality control program for the cine processor is to measure the inherent variability of an operation so that any variation from the norm can be assumed to be caused by some out-of-control parameter of the process. Automatic film processors provide rapid access to finished radiographic images for immediate review and evaluation. Even though a good-quality automatic processor is available, it will not produce films of high diagnostic quality without a daily control program. To ensure film of high diagnostic caliber, an effective method of processor control is mandatory.[8]

Changes that affect film quality, whether due to processing or other factors, may come on insidiously and go undetected until there is a major degeneration. Detection and correction of problems are important, whether they are occurring in processing, improper film storage, degradation of image intensifier and/or the x-ray focal spot, etc. It is obviously preferable to be able to detect isolated deficiencies before they become far advanced and multiple.

A general awareness on the part of all angiocardiographic personnel that there is a quality-control program for film processing often has a very noticeable effect on quality. More care and attention are given to film handling, monitoring of developer temperature and replenishment rates, and processor maintenance; all these measures contribute to excellence in photographic imaging.

Some of the processor quality-control tasks can be performed by the darkroom technician, but the program must be carried out under the supervision of a physician. If the physician directing the angiocardiographic laboratory does not have the background and training, he or she should either acquire that knowledge or become associated with another physician who *is* familiar with quality-control techniques.

Unless the laboratory director carefully monitors the entire quality-control process, it will soon degenerate into a sporadic program that is worse than no program; there will be no standard for comparison. If film-processing quality is meticulously monitored and found to be optimal, any subsequent degradation of image quality can be presumed to be an equipment operational deficiency.

Quality control requires daily use of a sensitometer and a densitometer to produce and optically measure cine film control strips. A sensitometer exposes a filmstrip to a light source of precisely controlled steps of increasing density. A densitometer optically measures the relative densities produced on the processed sensitometric filmstrip. The densities measured on this sensitometric control filmstrip are expressed in numerical values, which, when plotted on a graph, will give the characteristic density versus log-exposure (D–log E) curve of a particular film as obtained through a particular processor.

In cine film processing, this operation involves exposing and processing sensitometric strips from a roll of film that has been set aside as control film. It is wise to eliminate as many variables as possible in the procedures for doing quality-control work, so that any variation in film density on the strip is a result of variation of film processing and not densitometry or human error. The basis of any quality-control program, then, must be a period of data collection to establish the "normal" or baseline of processing operations. These guidelines are intended to aid the physician and technologist in quantifying parameters that affect film processing and to help in plotting day-to-day results against the period of normal data collection.

Exposing, processing, and evaluating sensitometric strips should be done daily at regularly scheduled times and whenever there is reason to suspect an operational deficiency of the processor or solutions. Generally, if a processed sensitometric strip is within control limits at the beginning of the day, one can be satisfied that processing is proper. If repair or maintenance is performed, a strip should be run immediately thereafter to verify that the processor is operating normally. If the processor is idle for more than a few days, the solutions should be replaced.

Densitometric data can quickly and easily be used to ascertain the exact speed, contrast, and gross fog values necessary to produce excellent quality cine films on a continuing basis. The speed, contrast, and gross fog values should be determined each day, plotted on a processor control chart, and compared to the approved standard of accepted quality before any film is processed through that processor. Variances in densitometric data will detect changes in chemical temperature, film travel speed, replenishment rates, and/or chemical contamination that must be corrected.

The darkroom technician should be familiar with a suitable technique of daily processor control, be able to evaluate the information obtained, determine when corrections in the processing technique are necessary, and maintain a daily, weekly, and monthly log of the densitometric data acquired.

Radiation Protection in the Angiocardiographic Laboratory

No known ionizing radiation level can be characterized as completely safe. Despite expertise in x-ray imaging and data retrieval in catheterization laboratories, control of radiation dosage and radiation protection for patients and personnel have been neglected.

The precautions recommended by the National Council on Radiation Protection and Measurements (NCRP) and the International Commission on Radiological Protection (ICRP) are familiar to many radiologists, radiologic technologists, and persons teaching them. Knowledge of these precautions does not apply equally to all members of these professions; the situation is likely to be less satisfactory outside the discipline of radiology. While many radiologists do not understand the peculiar needs of the angiocardiographic laboratory, in general, radiologists have the background upon which they can readily build the expertise required in the catheterization laboratory.

An increasing number of cardiac examinations involve the use of C-, U-, and Z-arm x-ray support systems that have not been equipped with adequate operator and patient radiation protection devices for the examinations being performed. For the most part, the basic equipment unit does not provide for more than minimal protection for the operator. Additional protection is needed to complement the operator's examination techniques. Because of the relative recency of development of these supports, radiation protection systems are not fully established.

Infants with complex congenital heart disease often undergo several catheterizations in a relatively short time. Special effort must be made, therefore, to reduce their radiation exposure.

The x-ray equipment and procedure room must be designed and maintained according to accepted current national radiation protection standards. In addition to the basic standards, certain criteria are particularly applicable to angiocardiographic laboratories.

Beam Limitation

During fluorography and cinefluorography the radiologic equipment should permit production of radiation only when the primary beam is aligned with and completely intercepted by the image intensifier. The *primary beam* should never intercept any body portion of laboratory personnel. The major source of radiation exposure to personnel is secondary or scatter radiation.

Primary beam limitation should be accomplished by adjustable triple-leaf collimators, with or without additional coning to limit the field. If the angiographer requires visualization of the entire circular intensifier image, there should be a circular beam-limiting device. The system designed should limit the primary beam to dimensions no greater than those of the visible image. If equipment design permits independent movement of the intensifier and/or x-ray tube, unit design should limit the field size at the intensifier input plane to dimensions no greater than those of its visible image. Units equipped with multiple-mode intensifiers should have automatic beam limitation to the dimensions of the mode in use.

The structure of the C-, U-, and Z-arm type of unit has the advantage of automatically aligning the central ray of the x-ray beam with the intensifier. However, this type of unit must have automatic coning to the field size of the image intensifier as the focal-spot-to-intensifier distance changes.

Scatter

Every effort should be made to reduce scattered radiation to as low a level as possible.

Units with an undertable tube and overtable intensifier need shielding that extends up along the sides of the table to the edge of the tabletop. When there is an add-on cradle that positions the patient above the table surface, shielding should extend up to the cradle edge. Most laboratories with add-on or portable cradles do not use this form of shielding. In such a configuration, the increased distance from tabletop to patient is a plus because it usually mandates a longer focal-spot-to-intensifier distance. But this is undesirable because the operator is not usually adequately shielded from scatter from the tabletop and associated table components. The elevated add-on cradle creates an exit port allowing back or side scatter radiation to strike the hands and midbody of anyone adjacent to the table. The use of a wood or carbon-fiber top reduces this form of scatter. Scatter can be further reduced with appropriate shielding along the lateral edge of the tabletop. The floating tabletop, unused for patient support, not only increases scatter but also reduces image quality. This configuration must be considered unsatisfactory from an operator radiation exposure standpoint and because of the added absorption of the x-ray beam by the tabletop. To maintain the rotational cradle concept and reduce scatter, the user should have a table with interchangeable tops that mount flush with the edges of the table. A cradle built into the tabletop virtually eliminates scatter production from the tabletop itself but is undesirable from a geometric standpoint because of the reduced focal-spot-to-intensifier distance.

C-, U-, and Z-arm equipment configurations require modified applications of the classic methods of radiation protection. The x-ray tube and intensifier have the capability of triaxial motion about the horizontal patient support. Primary design thrust has been efficient mechanical function rather than maximal radiation protection. The design of protection devices is not well established because of the relatively limited usage of these supports for a short period of time. The shielding should be designed and engineered to be appropriate for the laboratory equipment configuration and its procedural use by the operator. Protection design has to be modified depending on whether the procedural approach is brachial or femoral; adequate protection becomes even more complex if both approaches are used in the same laboratory.

An installation with overtable tube and undertable intensifier creates many radiation protection problems for which there is no adequate solution. Exposures to the upper body have been shown to be 2 to 10 times higher for this configuration compared with an undertable source.[9] The overtable tube and undertable intensifier design results in increased scatter from the primary x-ray beam. In most instances the economic or technical advantages associated with an overtable source are outweighed by the inherent radiologic hazards.

There should be a detailed determination of isoexposure levels around the x-ray unit to establish the optimal procedural positions for laboratory personnel. When a C-, U-, or Z-arm unit is used, multiple measurements need to be made in each of the commonly employed equipment configurations. A complete evaluation may involve 30 to 50 separate measurements by a qualified radiation physicist. Scattered-radiation measurements should be determined by means of a phantom, exposed in all procedural geometric configurations. These data will also establish areas of minimum exposure for personnel who must remain in the procedure room during radiation. Monitoring and physiologic data-retrieval systems requiring the presence of an operator should be in an area screened from radiation. There is no valid reason to have the monitoring technician in the procedure room unless he or she is protected from radiation by a barrier of at least 0.25-mm lead equivalent. Actual protection requirements will vary with radiologic equipment and may be greater, as determined by a qualified physicist. The practice of requiring recording and monitoring personnel to perform their duties in the procedure room protected only by lead aprons is decried.

A shielded control room should be a basic part of the installation. It should house the main x-ray controls, physiologic monitoring equipment, and any other supplementary equipment that is not required in the room for the performance of the procedure.

Fluoroscopic Timer

The fluoroscopic control is equipped with an elapsed-time indicator that can be easily monitored by the angiographer and operating personnel. The indicator should record the total cumulative time for an entire procedure. There should be an audible automatic indication of elapsed time at 5-minute intervals; the audible indicator should have a variable sound or tone for each 5-minute interval.

Radiation Quality Control

All catheterization facilities should be evaluated by a qualified physicist experienced and knowledgeable in the peculiarities of the catheterization laboratory.

New Facility

The physicist should be involved during the planning stage of a new facility. Following the installation, a complete radiologic evaluation should precede any patient studies. This evaluation should include but not necessarily be limited to calibration of equipment. There should be measurements in milliroentgens per frame, made behind the grid at the plane of the image receptor (film or input phosphor). A grid should be used whether the image receptor is an intensifier or a film, from the standpoint of both image quality and patient protection. Nongrid techniques are not suitable for angiocardiographic examinations except in infants when magnification technique (air gap technique) is being used. Even in this situation, a low-ratio grid usually improves the image significantly. Paper-spaced grids are preferable to aluminum-spaced grids. The scatter radiation pattern should be mapped and appropriate measurements made at multiple sites with a chest phantom. The sites of measurement of scatter will depend on the type of radiographic equipment employed and the configuration of its installation—C arm versus U arm, versus Z arm, versus conventional table with undertable tube, versus overtable tube, etc. Sites of measurement of scattered radiation need to correspond with normal personnel locations during a variety of the most common types of angiographic procedures. The adequacy of radiation protection devices must be evaluated by a qualified radiation physicist who can determine whether the devices adequately screen physicians, technicians, nurses, and other ancillary personnel from as much radiation as possible. It is the responsibility of the laboratory director to design usable radiation protection devices for the laboratory in consultation with a qualified radiation physicist. There is no acceptable level of radiation, although there are limits that should not be exceeded. Radiation levels should be reduced to an absolute minimum in accomplishing the necessary examination. That is, all personnel should be "behind" suitable radiation shields throughout the examination. It is recognized that a suitable radiation shield for a limited number of personnel may be a simple device such as a lead apron plus eye and thyroid protection. The latter may be a lead-glass shield or some similar device that gives protection without significantly interfering with the examination (Fig. 7-23). The requirement, then, is adequate protection of personnel without significant interference with the examination.

Personnel not absolutely necessary at tableside should be outside the area of radiation and scatter. In control space that is provided with full visual and verbal contact with the angiographer during procedures, the shields are preferably stationary but may be movable if required by the physical space involved. If they are movable, the adequacy must be questioned until it has been fully determined and attested to by a qualified radiation physicist. The accomplishing of this level of radiation protection suggests that there should be a separate area, screened from radiation, in which personnel not required in the procedure room can satisfactorily function.

Established Laboratory

The established angiocardiographic laboratory should have a biannual evaluation of its imaging facilities by a qualified radiologic physicist experienced and knowledgeable in the idiosyncrasies of such a facility. In addition, a number of equipment functions should be evaluated routinely. The interlocking between the x-ray tube and the image intensifier should be checked. When a C-, U-, or Z-arm type of installation is used, the relationship between the x-ray tube and the image receptor is fixed. Most units provide for varying the focal-spot-to-image-intensifier distance. This variable feature is very useful, and essential to high-quality imaging. The 28- to 30-inch focal-spot-to-intensifier distance used in the Sones unit is a carryover from the past when tubes were of low capacity and intensifiers had low conversion efficiency. The power train of current imaging equipment permits the use of desirable

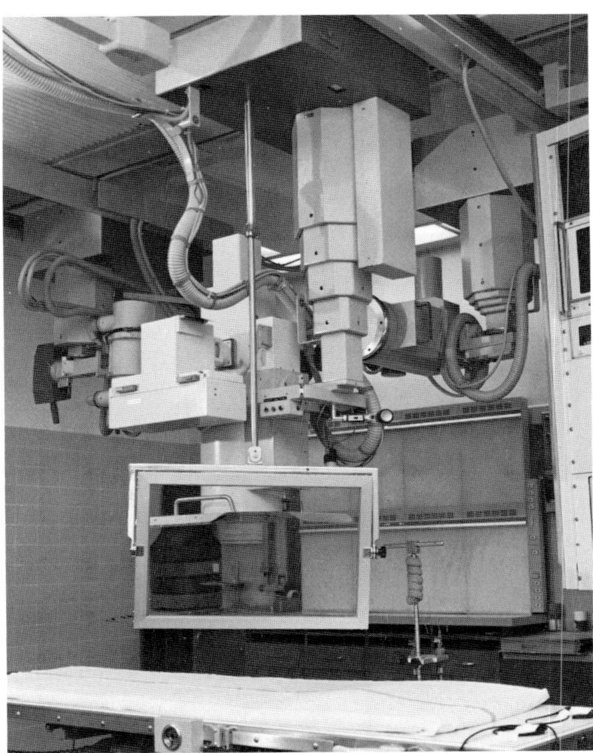

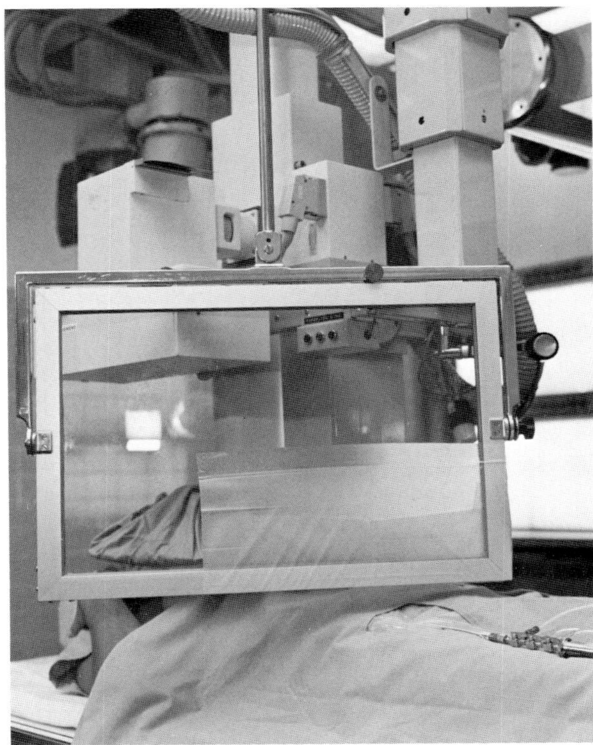

Figure 7-23. Radiation protection individualized for equipment and catheterization technique. This lead glass screen is used with the femoral technique. It is equally adaptable for conventional or C-, U-, or Z-arm configurations and is designed to be suspended and counterbalanced independent of the intensifier support. The transparent screen can be made of leaded glass or lead-impregnated plastic. The latter has the advantage of ease of counterbalancing because of reduced weight. (Courtesy of Robert Rearick, Loma Linda University, Loma Linda, Calif.)

geometry if a 36-inch focal-spot-to-intensifier distance is employed; there is an associated decrease in personnel radiation exposure.

If a traditional equipment configuration is employed, there should be an interlocking mechanism to ensure alignment of the x-ray beam with the intensifier regardless of whether there is an undertable or overtable intensifier or whether the intensifier can be angulated in relation to the patient support.

There are radiation protection problems peculiar to every type of patient and equipment support. Hence the necessity of close cooperation among equipment manufacturer, angiographer, and physicist in establishing and maintaining laboratory radiation safety. The traditional flat-top catheterization table with a wood or carbon-fiber top and overtable intensifier is the easiest configuration for which to provide radiation protection; it affords a level of radiation safety for which all other configurations should strive and a "gold standard" to which they must be compared.

Slow deterioration of the image-intensifier system may go undetected. This may result from a decrease in quantum conversion efficiency, requiring a higher incident x-ray level to achieve the necessary output brightness (more radiation), and/or a reduction of image resolution capabilities, which reduces the quality of diagnostic information available; that is, radiation may be adequate but there is an intrinsic defect in the system's imaging capability. Only periodic testing will identify these gradual, sometimes subtle changes.

The quality of image intensifiers is constantly improving. The average intensifier now has a longer useful life; nevertheless, intensifiers may insidiously deteriorate. The deterioration may be partially "covered" by automatic brightness systems—systems that hide the degradation from the operator.

There is another form of deterioration that is not true deterioration but rather obsolescence. The obsolescence created by improving technology plus the natural deterioration of the intensifier is currently limiting the useful life in vascular applications to about 5 years. Many intensifiers that have become obsolescent in vascular applications still have useful life if they can be rotated to less critical use within the institution, placed in a backup laboratory, used for the placement of pacemakers, or used in some other way. Following manufacturer service adjustment or replacement of components such as tubes and intensifiers, the entire system's performance should be evaluated.

Exposure Reduction

Minimum exposure to personnel and patient requires not only properly designed, engineered, and installed x-ray equipment but meticulous, consistent adherence to procedural and operational safety precautions (see box following). Maximum reduction of radiation exposure to personnel and patient does not mean minimum dosage to the patient per frame. Optimal dosage per frame may permit reduction in the number of frames required for accurate diagnosis.

Radiation Exposure Reduction

Smallest possible field size
Distance between source and operator
Reduction of fluoro/cine time
Appropriate shield between source and operator

Personnel Exposure

Radiation Monitoring

Yearly limits on occupational exposure for various parts of the body are already established (Table 7-1). (Background levels of radiation range from 0.05 to 0.1 rem/yr.) The lens of the eye, gonads, and red bone marrow are considered the critical organs for the whole-body limit of 5 rem/yr. A lead protective apron shields the gonads and major portions of red bone marrow. The eyes are the critical limiting organ not covered by the apron. The next most sensitive exposed area is the thyroid, with a yearly limit of 15 rem (Fig. 7-24).

A monitoring device, film badge, or thermoluminescent dosimeter (TLD) should be worn by all personnel. This monitor should be located at the head or neck level outside the protective lead apron. Periodically the laboratory director should obtain readings at selected other body locations chosen because of possible hazard related to specific equipment design. The angiographer and assisting personnel working "hands on" with the patient should wear an additional wrist

Table 7-1. Occupational Dose Limitation Recommendations Suggested by the National Council on Radiation Protection (Prospective Annual Limits)

Portion of Body Exposed	Rem/Yr
Whole body (including lens of eye, gonads, and red bone marrow)	5
Skin (unlimited areas other than hands and forearms)	15
Hands	75
Forearms	30
Other organs, tissues, and organ systems (i.e., thyroid)	15

From National Council on Radiation Protection and Measurements, Basic Radiation Protection Criteria, Report No. 39, Washington, D.C., 1971.

monitor since proximity of hands and arms to the patient and primary x-ray beam can result in high exposure. Measurements obtained at these sites should be evaluated, it being remembered that permissible tolerance is somewhat higher than for the eyes and thyroid, but not in excess of 75 rem/yr. If exposure levels for hand-position monitors are consistently low, their day-to-day use may not be necessary. However, techniques and habit patterns change, so measurements at these sites should be rechecked every 6 months.

A permanent log of personnel exposure levels should include sites of measurement as well as total levels.

Lead Apron

Work habits and procedure-related tasks of laboratory personnel will influence the selection of apron type. An individual more than occasionally positioned with his or her back to the patient should wear a full wraparound apron. "Shortie" designs should be discouraged. Lead aprons should be of multilayer fabrication. All personnel working in the procedure room should wear a 0.5-mm-equivalent lead apron.

Care of aprons directly relates to their useful life. When not in use they should be kept on a specially designed rack, not thrown in a pile on furniture or folded. Protective aprons need to be inspected for damage periodically.

Position During Radiation

During procedural radiation all personnel should be protected from scattered radiation by a suitable barrier; it may take one of several forms. Body parts that require special attention include but are not limited to the eyes, thyroid, and bone marrow. A lead apron itself is not an adequate protection barrier for eyes and thyroid (see Fig. 7-24). The cardiac angiographer cannot, for reasons of procedural safety, retire behind a remote

the basic support functions be performed by adequately trained personnel who maintain their skills. Although the required functions are well defined, it is not necessary or desirable for one person to qualify in only one job category. For example, with adequate cross-training a second radiologic technologist or a cardiopulmonary technician may assume monitoring and recording duties; the cardiopulmonary technician's role may be included in the duties of the nurse or the radiologic technologist. Cross-training for other personnel classifications is desirable so that 24-hour coverage of all essential team functions is possible.

Cross-training between radiologic technologists working in cardiac procedures and those working in general angiography and neuroangiography is practical and efficient. When these types of procedures are performed in contiguous areas, there can be optimal use of the radiologic technologist, especially in an emergency. Cross-training also provides for night and weekend coverage if there are limited facilities and personnel.

Some individuals have developed their skills by on-the-job training and observation and are very good at what they do. As new staff members are acquired, an effort should be made to bring in people who have basic skills and subtraining in laboratory-related functions.

II. Noncardiac Angiographic Equipment: Optimal Resources for Vascular Intervention

BARRY T. KATZEN

The scope and complexity of diagnostic and therapeutic procedures have increased significantly since the original description of the Seldinger technique for obtaining vascular access. Diagnostic angiography facilities increased through the 1960s and mid-1970s, and with the emergence of interventional radiology have contributed to further growth and change in the angiographic environment. Documents addressing optimal guidelines were developed for cardiac catheterization, but no specific documents existed for vascular and interventional procedures, although they had been mentioned.[12] The orientation of this section is predominantly clinical and emphasizes *optimal resources*. In the early years of the development of angiographic procedures, facilities for combined use in barium and vascular work were widely used in clinical practice. The complexity and clinical demands of these procedures today require the use of equipment dedicated to vascular and interventional procedures.

There are many facets to developing an optimal environment, including room size, radiographic equipment, and staffing. The development of endovascular procedures, which combine interventional and surgical techniques, make it reasonable to consider some of the issues or details necessary to perform surgery in the interventional environment.

Recently, a multidisciplinary task force to develop guidelines for peripheral and visceral angiographic and interventional laboratories was formed by the American Heart Association. The task force consisted of representatives from cardiovascular radiology, clinical cardiology, thoracic and vascular surgery, and renovascular medicine. This section draws heavily from the document written by that task force.[13] Before this document there had been significant efforts to define guidelines and optimal resources beginning in 1971.[14] These guidelines were updated periodically,[15,16] most recently in 1991.[17]

This section discusses the radiographic environment and radiation safety, the sterile environment, staffing, space, and quality improvement issues.

The Radiographic Environment

Significant advances in imaging equipment have occurred in the past 10 to 15 years as computer technology and minification have been incorporated into interventional equipment. Design teams from all major manufacturers have developed x-ray stands based on the changing needs of interventionalists, with integration of modern computerized imaging techniques derived initially from aerospace and military applications. These have given the interventionalist improved access to the patient and real-time availability of information critical to on-line decision making.

The *x-ray platform* should be of the C, U, or parallelogram design, allowing rotation in both axial and sagittal planes around the patient. The C arm should be of a sufficient size to allow easy access to the patient, and should be easily movable to allow procedures from the femoral, axillary, jugular, and transabdominal approaches. In addition, the stand should be freely movable away from the patient in the event urgent cardiovascular support is required. The movements of the stand should be motorized, but manual override is mandatory for patient safety. The position of the C arm should be lockable, with digital display of various angulations. Collision avoidance devices should be integrated to prevent inadvertent significant contact with the patient by the image intensifier and stand. The stand should be optimally equipped with an image intensifier of 14 inches or larger, with video camera and display. Older units have had 100- to 105-mm spot-film cameras, but these have been replaced by digital imaging in recent years.

The *table* should be able to allow stepping, either of the table itself or the entire stand, unless a long-leg film changer is used. At the time of this writing, film changers, both integrated and long-leg, are gradually diminishing in use as digital imaging continually improves as a stand-alone modality. At the Miami Vascular Institute and other major institutions, this change has already occurred, with virtually no film screen imaging being performed. The table should be easily movable to allow complete access to the patient. Modern tables are best made of carbon fiber materials, which allow reduced weight, high fluoroscopic translucency, and great flexibility in design. Weight limits should be at least 300 lb (140 kg).

The *generator* should be either a three-phase, 12-pulse generator or a high-frequency inverter type of generator with power ratings of 80 to 100 kW. In recent years these generators have become compact, and modern types have self-diagnostic capabilities. The generator should be capable of performing pulsed fluoroscopy at 30 frames per second (fps) with imaging display at 60 fps, allowing significant reduction in radiation exposure.

Modern intervention and vascular imaging have created new needs in *x-ray tubes.* In film screen imaging, the focal spot was frequently the limiting factor in ultimate resolution. In digital imaging, relatively little gain is acquired below 0.5 to 0.6 mm. Because of the high instantaneous tube loading during digital vascular imaging and the shorter examination times due to the availability of real-time information, heat capacity and heat dissipation have become more critical parameters. The minimum heat capacity should be 1.7 million heat units, with dissipation of at least 100 kHu per minute and a focal spot of 0.6 and 1.0 mm. X-ray tube indicators should be in place to avoid tube overload. Adequate anode angles should exist to accommodate large-field-of-view image intensifiers. Smaller focal spots may be of additional value, particularly if conventional film screen imaging is used.

Appropriate filtration of the x-ray beam to comply with regulatory specifications may be enhanced by additional aluminum up to 3 mm, which can further reduce dose without a significant reduction in image quality. Collimators should be visible at the edge of the fluoroscopic field and should be supplemented with rectangular or iris-shaped devices. Movable filters are of particular value in digital subtraction angiography (DSA) acquisition, in which severe density changes may exist, particularly in the chest and lower extremities.

The *image intensifier* should have a large field of view with three to four modes of electronic magnification. Intensifier technology has greatly improved over earlier versions, and high levels of gain and high contrast and spatial resolution are available. State-of-the-art intensifiers should include cesium-iodide phosphors and a titanium window, which allows high levels of radiation detection, thereby allowing a reduction in x-ray dose. Optimum specifications include a gain of greater than 250 cd/m^2 per milliroentgen (mR) per second measured at 80 kVP; a spatial resolution of at least 2.5 line pairs (lp)/mm in the 14-inch field of view, 3.3 lp/mm in the 9-inch field of view, and 4.6 lp/mm in the 6-inch field of view; and a contrast ratio of at least 20:1, with greater than 85 percent veiling glare. Integrated automatic brightness control should be present.

The image intensifier should be linked to a high-quality *video chain,* which provides the final output in the interventional suite. The TV camera and monitors should display 1000 raster liners per frame with flicker-free refresh rates. Greatly improved video cameras are available using conventional or charged coupled devices (CCD) technology. These should have signal-to-noise ratios of greater than 1000:1, with a frequency band pass of at least 20 MHz, with limited lag. Optimal viewing is obtained by monitors of at least 17-inch diagonal, with antiglare coatings. The spatial resolution of the TV and monitor should be 1.2 lp/mm in the 14-inch mode, 1.8 lp/mm in the 9-inch mode, and 2.6 lp/mm in the 6-inch mode. Numerous other functions are important to reduce lag, reduce flaring when varying body thickness, and reduce noise in the displayed image.

Imaging Modalities

In modern angiographic suites, digital subtraction angiography (and digital imaging in general) has become the standard for day-to-day operation. The advantages of real-time acquisition, high-contrast resolution, versatility, and simplicity of use (in newer designs) have made DSA the principal imaging modality. The high resolution of contemporary systems, their ease of use, and their flexibility of display have led to a significant reduction in conventional film screen imaging in many institutions. Specifications are based on both clinical needs and technologic standards.

The system should have a 1024 × 1024 image matrix with monitors capable of similar display. The system should be able to provide image acquisition in the 1024 × 1024 mode with a frame rate of at least five frames per second, and display at similar rates. Both fluoroscopic and pulsed radiographic modes should be available with "last image hold."

Optimally, operation should be tabletop to facilitate hands-on operation by the interventionalist. The tabletop operation should allow the interventionalist to perform basic acquisition and display functions with or without ancillary postprocessing functions. Easy review of the most recent acquisition as well as previous runs and the ability to store images into a "scrapbook" file should be available. Operator-controlled road-mapping should also be at the tabletop.

Adequate data storage should be available to allow 2 to 3 days' worth of image storage based on the site's normal operating load. Both linear and logarithmic format storage should have a minimum of 10 bits per pixel from the analog-to-digital converter.

The analysis console should allow text and image display on different monitors. The analysis console should have at minimum window level and width, region of interest, and image management functions. Additional important features in vascular intervention include vessel measurement functions. A second control console should be present in the procedure room. This console should have limited functions dedicated to technical operation of the equipment, and should allow the performance of common operations needed during procedures: changing acquisition frame rates, radiographic techniques, and other functions not performed by the operator at the table side.

The DSA system should have high-contrast sensitivity and be capable of resolving a 0.4-mm vessel with 1 percent iodine contrast. Similarly, spatial resolution at high contrast should be comparable to the video system spatial resolution and at least 2.4 lp/mm in the 6-inch field of view. A wide dynamic range is important and should be at least 1000:1. The final image output should have minimal lag and mottle and should be tailored to the operating physician's preferences.

Some investigators have found significant benefit to intravascular ultrasound for both diagnostic and therapeutic applications (adjunctive), and angioscopy may have a place in the future.

Physiologic monitoring capabilities should be available and provide information on cardiac conduction (ECG), pressure monitoring (preferably from two sites), hard copy capabilities, and pulse oximetry information.

Optimal Staffing

Optimal patient care will be most easily achieved by developing a specially trained staff of professionals, enhanced by ongoing education and quality improvement. The author's experience has shown that ideal results can be achieved by bringing together the particular talents and interests of physicians, nurses, and technologists.

The *medical director* should be a physician with the training, experience, and leadership ability required to provide control and direction to the laboratory environment. The medical director should be board certified in his or her specialty with training in cardiovascular and interventional radiologic procedures. Fellowship training should be necessary for recent appointments. The director should be responsible for developing and maintaining standards of care and ongoing quality assurance, for providing regular continuing education for both physicians and other professional staff, and in general for maintaining standards of the lab.

All physicians working in the facility should have met training standards that have been recently developed by various specialty organizations and have sufficient ongoing activity to maintain competence.[18–20]

If fellows and residents are part of the overall program, the appropriate credentialing guidelines and activity levels must be followed. Activity levels should be sufficient to allow ongoing competence of physician staff.

Technologists working in the vascular and interventional environment should be registered and certified radiologic technologists. They should have additional specialty training in this field as well as ongoing continuing education. The technologists should have working knowledge of the radiographic equipment and radiation safety, be familiar with the inventory, and be well integrated into the laboratory operations. When technologists are assisting physicians in the performance of procedures, they should have a working knowledge of sterile technique.

Interventional facilities should be staffed with a minimum of one full-time *registered nurse* per room. It is preferable for nurses to have critical care or cardiac catheterization experience. It is only in recent years that nurses have become a more integral part of the interventional radiology environment, and they have contributed greatly to quality of care and patient education. Nursing staff should be responsible for monitoring and assisting in the maintenance of the patient's physiologic state, maintaining a record of vital signs and medications administered, assisting in the use of conscious sedation, and keeping a written documentation of events.

Space Considerations

Considerable experience has been gained in developing optimal space for contemporary vascular and interventional facilities. The needs of these facilities have changed significantly as interventional medicine has evolved and equipment has changed. Ideal space planning comes only after adequate time is spent in specifying functional needs and equipment and personnel space requirements, and in addressing specific patient care issues. In designing new facilities, it would also be advisable to consider certain issues relating to the performance of some surgical procedures in the interventional environment. Unique concerns include air handling, sterile scrub facilities, and washable ceilings.

Space in the procedure room should be sufficient to house a C arm with a full range of direction, a table with an extended longitudinal range, physiologic equipment, injectors, additional imaging equipment such as intravascular or conventional ultrasound, an additional C arm, and three to six additional personnel. Space should be allowed for anesthesia and equipment that may be useful in pediatric patients, as well as in neurointervention, transjugular intrahepatic portosystemic shunt (TIPS), and some biliary procedures. Generally 700 sq ft, exclusive of the control room, is adequate, but given the direction of intervention, 900 sq ft would be more flexible. A ceiling of 12 ft will accommodate most types of equipment.

A scrub sink should be in or directly adjacent to the room, with a waste sink in close proximity. Suction and oxygen should be in the room, as well as other gases depending on anesthesia needs.

Heavy equipment such as generators and transformers should be housed in a separate room or space that can be isolated from the procedural rooms. This reduces heat and provides aesthetic advantages.

The *control room* houses the operation console and allows viewing into the room, if desired, through leaded glass. With newer digital systems, the function of the control room has changed somewhat, with more operation actually occurring in the procedure room. Nonetheless, 120 sq ft is generally sufficient, with computer flooring raising the floor over the interventional suite. A large viewing area into the procedural room is desirable, but blinds should be available for patient privacy when needed. The control room should have sufficient space to allow for review of images with consulting physicians.

Changes in the types of procedures and the greater use of outpatient procedures have increased the need for patient care before and after procedures. Although a room for these needs is frequently called a *recovery* or *prep room,* we have elected to call it a *procedural care room.* Space is needed to allow placement of IV lines, preparation of patients before procedures, and removal of lines after procedures. Longer-term "holding" may occur in this type of facility, or longer-term observation may be performed elsewhere, allowing more efficient patient movement through the interventional area. The amount of space depends on the room's function and the number of procedural rooms it is supporting. This space should have cardiac and life support equipment in addition to personnel specially trained and capable of providing pre- and postprocedural care.

Radiation Safety Considerations

The ionizing radiation used during vascular and interventional procedures provides both benefits and hazards. The National Council on Radiation Protection and Measurements (NCRP) established guidelines for clinical and occupational exposure and proposed the phrase *as low as reasonably achievable*[21] to describe safety and exposure goals. It is incumbent on the directors and users of the interventional suites to adopt this philosophy into operational policy.

Three variables can be addressed in reducing dose: *time of exposure, distance* from the x-ray source, and the use of appropriate *shielding*. Interventional procedures involve both patient and operator proximity, meaning that most efforts at protection are directed at reducing the time of fluoroscopy and maximizing shielding.

Significant reduction in fluoroscopic time and dose can be accomplished by greater awareness of the operator and attention to detail during procedures. With a little training increased cognitive information can be obtained during pulsed DSA, and one should avoid "staring" at the fluoroscopic image during procedures. One can also develop a pattern of intermittent fluoroscopy, although this is somewhat more difficult in training environments. Use of freeze frames and "last image hold" functions can also be helpful in making on-line decisions.

The NCRP has made specific rcommendations relating to structural shielding[22] and equipment[23] that should be incorporated into every installation. Recent technical improvements include pulsed progressive fluoroscopy, which can reduce the dose up to 50 percent compared to conventional fluoroscopic modes, and rotating and vertical collimators that are easily controlled by the operator at table side.

Overall fluoroscopic time should be recorded and made part of the procedural record, in addition to dose if available. Where high-dose fluoroscopy is available, it should be limited in time and activated by a system independent from the more commonly used foot pedal. The dose should be limited to 20 R/min and indicated to the operator by an audible signal during its use.

Radiation exposure to personnel is predominantly due to fluoroscopy and can be significantly reduced by using appropriate body, thyroid, and eye protection. The operator is the primary recipient of this radiation and has the responsibility of ensuring appropriate levels of protection for all personnel in the room.

Aprons of at least 0.5-mm lead equivalent should be worn by all personnel, and wraparound aprons should be used by circulating personnel who may periodically have their backs to the field during procedures. Shielding can be supplemented by ceiling-suspended glass shields, thyroid shields, and eyeglasses, and should be used by the primary operator, who by virtue of his or her position in relation to the x-ray beam and subject may exceed the maximum permissible dose of 50 mSv/yr or 10 mSv/yr averaged over a lifetime.[24] Leaded glasses may be of particular value to the radiation sensitivity of the eye's lens, which has a maximum yearly recommended dose of 150 mSv (15 rem).[25] Practicing interventionalists can lower their total body, cervical, and ocular radiation dose by employing lead converings (thyroid shields and glasses) in addition to lead aprons.[26] Radiation exposure to anesthesia personnel can be significantly higher[27] and the primary operator should provide appropriate protection, particularly as anesthesia is becoming more widely used for procedures such as TIPS and embolization.

Continuous Quality Improvement

Interventional procedures and the facilities in which they are performed have evolved dramatically since the birth of modern-day angiography with Seldinger's description of arterial access. Although initially performed in rooms used for general fluoroscopic procedures such as upper gastrointestinal studies and barium enemas, they are now performed in sophisticated suites, with dedicated fluoroscopic and computerized imaging equipment and sophisticated patient-monitoring capabilities.

A similar evolution has occurred in the regulatory aspects of health care. The Joint Commission of the Accreditation of Healthcare Organizations (JCAHO) mandates that each institution have an ongoing quality improvement program to "objectively and systematically monitor and evaluate the quality and appropriateness of patient care, pursue opportunities to improve patient care and clinical performance and resolve identified problems."[28] These principles have been increasingly applied to interventional suites, with much success.[29,30]

Future Developments

Rapid advancements in vascular intervention are leading to the need to combine interventional procedures with surgical access. Procedures such as treatment of aortic aneurysms and various other types of aneurysms and new approaches to aortic occlusive disease may require devices too large for percutaneous access, at least in current stages of development. Although some have advocated placing sophisticated imaging equipment in the operating room, for most institutions the expenses are redundant, and utilization may be minimal and certainly insufficient to justify the cost in the current economic environment of health care. High levels of economic investment in the operating room environment may not be warranted because the ultimate goal is to develop devices that can benefit from percutaneous introduction.

Because these new procedures depend heavily on the highest-quality imaging and interventional skills, at the Miami Vascular Institute appropriate modifications have been made to the interventional suite to allow surgical access and emergency open operation if necessary. We have chosen something short of making the facility into an operating room, but, in conjunction with staff and physicians from infection control, surgical services, interventional services, risk management, and anesthesia, have addressed many of the practical issues to implement this change. At the time of this writing, 10 procedures have been performed with surgical access (femoral arteriotomy) for the introduction of stent grafts of various types. In one patient, severe disruption of the iliac artery required emergency ileofemoral bypass, which was performed uneventfully and with a normal postoperative course. Initial evaluation demonstrates no increased infection rates in these patients.

A detailed discussion of this subject is beyond the scope of this chapter, but institutions considering the development of new facilities should be aware of this issue.

III. Digital Angiography

MICHAEL S. VAN LYSEL

Both the technology and applications of digital subtraction angiography (DSA) have evolved significantly since DSA was commercially introduced in the early 1980s. Major technical advances include refinements in video cameras, signal processing, and storage devices. Clinically, digital angiography originated as a subtraction modality. However, digital systems now also incorporate nonsubtraction acquisition for cases, such as cardiac, peripheral bolus-chase, and rotational angiography, where artifact-free subtraction imaging can be difficult to achieve. Fluoroscopic enhancement has also become a very important digital tool. As a consequence, the more general term *digital angiography* better describes this new technology.

The major advantages of digital angiography, the high-contrast resolution of DSA and the flexibility with which images can be managed and manipulated, are a result of the digital data format. The contrast resolution of film angiography is limited by the superposition of overlying anatomic structures, as well as by inhomogeneities in the film, screen, and development processes.[31] A second limiting factor is the inability to modify the display contrast of film. Even with subtraction, low-contrast detectability of film is limited to an exposure contrast of about 1 percent.[32] By comparison, the contrast resolution of DSA is limited, in many cases, only by the radiation exposure that can be appropriately used.

Digital imaging greatly facilitates the angiographic examination. Digital image processors provide a subtraction method of vastly greater ease than film subtraction. Images are reviewed immediately after acquisition, shortening procedure time. Specific images and sequences of images are conveniently accessed and displayed. The actual generation of films is limited, producing a substantial decrease in operating cost, although capital costs increase with the purchase of a digital system.[33,34] Interventional procedures are significantly enhanced by the application of digital processing techniques to fluoroscopic imaging, providing advantages such as noise reduction, dose reduction, edge enhancement, and road-mapping.

Digital angiography does present some disadvantages with respect to film. The spatial resolution limit of digital angiography is in the neighborhood of 2 lp/mm, versus 5 or more lp/mm for film. In addition, the field of view is limited by the circular input phosphor of the image intensifier, the largest available size being about 16 inches in diameter. Many laboratories include both a digital system and an integrated film changer so that both modalities are available in the same laboratory.

DSA was originally introduced as a method of performing angiographic studies using intravenous (IV) injections of contrast. Although it was demonstrated that this is feasible, practical limitations have reduced the attractiveness of this approach. A primary limitation is motion artifacts. Swallowing, coughing, bowel peristalsis, cardiac motion, respiratory motion, and gross patient motion all produce misregistration artifacts that can interfere with the diagnosis. Motion artifacts, coupled with poor opacification in patients with low cardiac output, decrease the reliability of IV DSA. Additional disadvantages include superposition of opacified vessels and higher volumes of contrast media. However, IV DSA remains an alternative for selected patients and procedures.[35]

Intraarterial DSA has gained favor over IV DSA because of its higher image quality and consistency of results. Problems related to motion artifacts are reduced, although not eliminated, with intraarterial injections. With a shorter delay between mask and vessel image acquisition, the period during which motion can occur is reduced. In addition, higher vessel contrast reduces the degree to which artifacts interfere with vessel visualization. The high contrast sensitivity of intraarterial DSA can provide good image quality with smaller amounts of injected iodine, lower injection rates, and less selective catheterization than are required with film, as well as providing real-time monitoring of the procedure.[34-36]

Video Systems

The introduction of digital angiography was greatly facilitated by the prior existence of fluoroscopic systems. DSA stimulated further development of these systems. For example, large-field-of-view image intensifiers appeared to assist in the performance of large-format studies, such as peripheral angiography. However, the component that has undergone the greatest development is the video system.

Camera Aperture

The peak x-ray exposure to the face of the image intensifier (II) varies from a few μR per frame during fluoroscopy to greater than 1 mR per frame during some DSA applications. Whereas the light output of the II is linear over several decades of input x-ray exposure, the useful range of the video camera is more restricted. The video camera aperture is used to present the camera with the proper light level. The aperture, an adjustable diaphragm between the image intensifier output phosphor and the video camera target, establishes the relationship between the x-ray exposure incident on the II face and the image brightness seen by the video camera (Fig. 7-25).

An optical distributor couples the II output to the cameras. Figure 7-26 shows the components of an optical distributor designed for use with both video and film cameras (either cine or photospot). A beam-splitting mirror directs light to both cameras simultaneously. "Cineless" catheterization laboratories have appeared in which image recording is performed using an analog optical disk rather than cine film. The beam splitter is removed. The claim is sometimes made that cineless laboratories require less x-ray exposure because it is not necessary to produce light to send to the cine camera. This argument ignores the fact that the image intensifier produces an excess level of light, which is then reduced by the camera apertures. X-ray exposure levels are set not by the need to produce a given light level but rather by the need to maintain a given level of quantum noise in the image.

The peak detected x-ray exposure during an angiographic examination is fixed by the diameter of the camera aperture. It is selected on the basis of the competing goals of high signal-to-noise ratio versus low patient exposure and x-ray tube load. Because of the low iodine contrast, intravenous studies require the highest x-ray exposures. Intraarterial studies can be performed at an equal, or perhaps somewhat lower, exposure than that required of film. Subtraction in-

Figure 7-25. X-ray exposure versus aperture size. The aperture provides the video camera with a fixed brightness level over several decades of x-ray exposure.

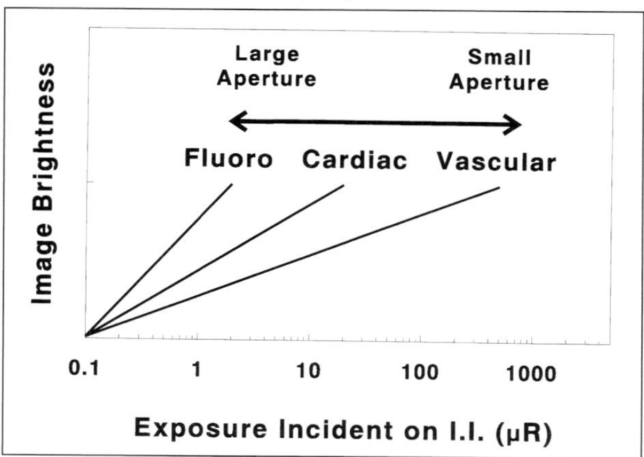

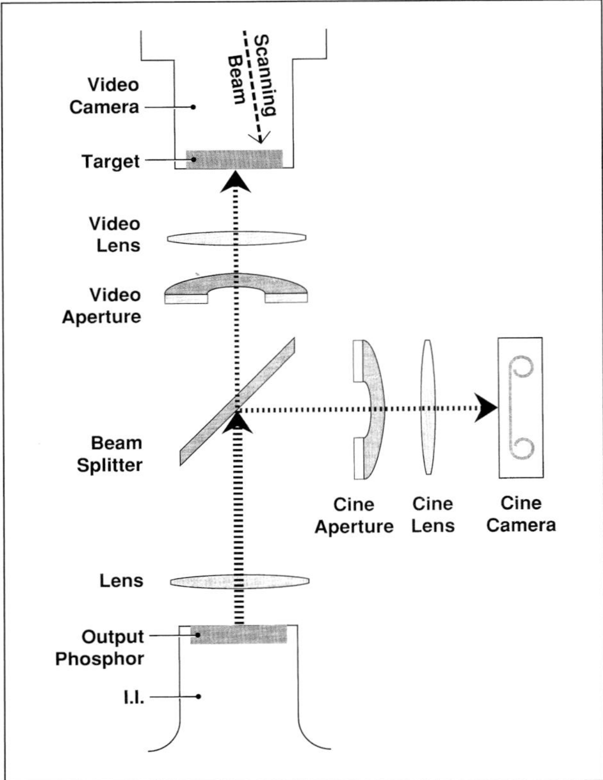

Figure 7-26. Components of an optical distributor. The optical distributor couples the image intensifier (II) output with the video and cine cameras.

creases image noise, but this is offset by an increase in display contrast and signal conspicuity.

Once the aperture diameter has been set, the x-ray exposure factors must be determined empirically before the imaging sequence is initiated. A "test shot" procedure, analogous to a scout film, is performed to adjust the factors (kVP, mAs) so that the brightest portion of the image is mapped to the maximum digital level. An image that is too bright saturates the video camera, whereas an underexposed image contains an excessive level of noise. Some early digital systems required a laborious manual test shot procedure. Other systems dispensed with this test shot procedure by adjusting the aperture diameter, rather than the exposure factors, to provide the proper light level for the camera. This approach, however, improves ease of use at the expense of poor image quality or excessive patient exposure. Newer equipment, designed as an integrated system, greatly reduces the operator interaction required to obtain a proper exposure.

Pickup Tube

Digital angiographic images are formed by digitizing the output of the video camera. The camera output, a voltage proportional to image brightness, is produced by the pickup tube of the video camera. Light from the output phosphor of the image intensifier is focused onto the photoconductive "target" of the pickup tube, which converts the light image into a charge distribution. The charge then resides on the surface of the target until it is read by a scanning electron beam.

The first photoconductive tube developed, the vidicon, used a target material of antimony trisulfide. Antimony trisulfide vidicons are useful for fluoroscopy, but the high degree of lag (image retention) makes this tube inappropriate for digital angiographic applications. In cardiac applications the major concern is decay lag, which results in a blurring of rapidly moving objects. At lower frame rates the primary concern is buildup lag, which slows the response of the camera to a sudden increase in brightness. Buildup lag can result in shading artifacts in a subtraction image. Vidicon-style tubes with different target materials, such as the Plumbicon, Saticon, and Primicon, are used in DSA systems because of their lower degree of lag. Light biasing of the target is also used to reduce lag.

Another important property for DSA applications is the signal-to-noise ratio (SNR) of the video system. The primary sources of noise in a DSA image, quantum and electronic noise, add in quadrature to produce the total noise level present in the image. It is desirable that quantum noise exceed electronic noise so that the x-ray dose delivered to the patient is not "wasted." Quantum noise dominates in the brightest portion of the image, but as the brightness decreases electronic noise becomes more significant. At some point in the dark regions of the image, electronic noise becomes the dominant contributor to total image noise.[37] The analysis is complicated, however, by the fact that the quantum and electronic noise power spectra have significantly different frequency characteristics.[38]

Electronic noise primarily originates in the video camera. Fluoroscopic video systems operated in an environment of low x-ray exposure and, consequently, high quantum noise levels. As a result, video SNRs in the neighborhood of 200:1 were acceptable. When early DSA systems attempted to produce high-quality angiographic images, x-ray exposure levels were substantially increased. However, camera noise prevented the higher exposures from improving the image quality in the dark portions of the image. Improvements in camera design, especially an increase in tube signal currents up to 2 to 3 μA, have resulted in SNRs in excess of 1000:1 (60 dB).

The relationship between the light intensity (I) incident on the camera target and the voltage output (V) of the camera is $(V/V_o) = (I/I_o)^{\gamma}$. A property shared by the pickup tubes used for angiographic applications is that $\gamma = 1$, so the signal output of the video camera exhibits a linear relationship with the light input. This limits the ability of the camera to accept a wide dynamic range in the light levels presented to it. As a result, good image quality requires that the dynamic range of the image be limited. Because the noise amplitude increases dramatically in the more attenuating regions of the patient, mechanical filters are often used to decrease the x-ray level reaching the II in regions of low attenuation, allowing the signal in the darker regions to be increased. Filter mechanisms include "semitransparent wedges" built into the x-ray collimator and other bolus materials (saline bags, flour, etc.) that are placed under or on the patient. Recently, systems have been introduced in which the transfer function of the analog circuitry between the video camera and the image processor has been modified so that bright spots in the image are suppressed. Although the details of this transfer function modification vary among vendors, the effect is similar to a pickup tube with $\gamma < 1$. This γ-mapping technique improves the display characteristics of high-dynamic-range images. However, unlike bolusing, γ-mapping does not improve the degrading effects that noise and x-ray scatter impose in the dark portions of the image. Therefore, even with γ-mapping, the highest image quality is obtained if mechanical bolusing is also used.

Many years of design experience have resulted in pickup tubes with a high degree of signal fidelity. However, there are limitations to the technology. A promising new technology is the charge coupled device (CCD) video camera, in which the pickup tube is replaced with a solid-state sensor. CCD cameras promise improvements in lag, contrast, linearity, spatial distortion, and scanning flexibility. CCD cameras are already appearing in fluoroscopic applications. However, they are not yet of sufficient quality to replace vacuum tubes in the demanding application of digital angiography. The current limitations of CCD cameras include fixed pattern noise and the inability to perform high-resolution imaging ($\geq 1000 \times 1000$ pixels per frame) at frame rates of 30 frames per second using single channel readout. However, CCD cameras are expected to eventually replace vacuum-based pickup tubes.

Target Scanning

Each region of the camera target integrates the light incident upon it until the scanning electron beam passes over ("reads") that region of the target. Starting at the top of the image, the scanning of the electron beam is performed in a raster fashion, dissecting the image into a series of horizontal lines. When the scanning beam reaches the bottom of the image, the beam quickly retraces back to the top of the target to begin scanning the next image. This process is controlled by the sweep generator of the camera control unit (CCU), which produces a series of "synchronization" pulses. The most important of these is the vertical synchronization (V SYNC) pulse. Having reached the bottom of the target, V SYNC instructs the scanning beam to return to the top to begin the next scan.

Raster scanning converts the two-dimensional image on the target to a one-dimensional voltage waveform suitable for digitization. Two scanning modes are used: interlaced and progressive scanning. With interlaced scanning, only half of the target area is read as the camera beam traverses from the top of the image to the bottom. This first "field" consists of the odd horizontal lines (line 1, line 3, line 5, . . .). A second top-to-bottom scan is required to scan the even field (line 2, line 4, line 6, . . .). The two fields taken together constitute the complete image, referred to as a "frame." This cumbersome technique is inherited from the broadcast industry, where it was developed to meet the 60-Hz refresh rate required to diminish the brightness flicker perceived by the human observer, yet limit the video bandwidth to 5 MHz. Although interlaced scanning is often used to digitize fluoroscopic images, it has generally been replaced in DSA applications by progressive scanning.

Progressive scanning (also referred to as sequential scanning) is noninterlaced. The electron beam simply scans the target in a sequential fashion (line 1, line 2, line 3, . . .). The advantages of progressive scanning include improved x-ray exposure use and higher spatial resolution of moving objects.[39] The problem with progressive scanning is that almost all video monitors, on which the image will be displayed, require an interlaced scan. Therefore, progressive scan acquisition requires a digital system to perform "scan conversion," converting the progressive scan desirable for image acquisition to the interlaced scan required for display.

Because light is integrated by all regions of the target simultaneously, yet is read off only where the scanning beam is sweeping across it, image artifacts result if the x-ray exposure and scanning beam are not synchronized. The most common synchronization

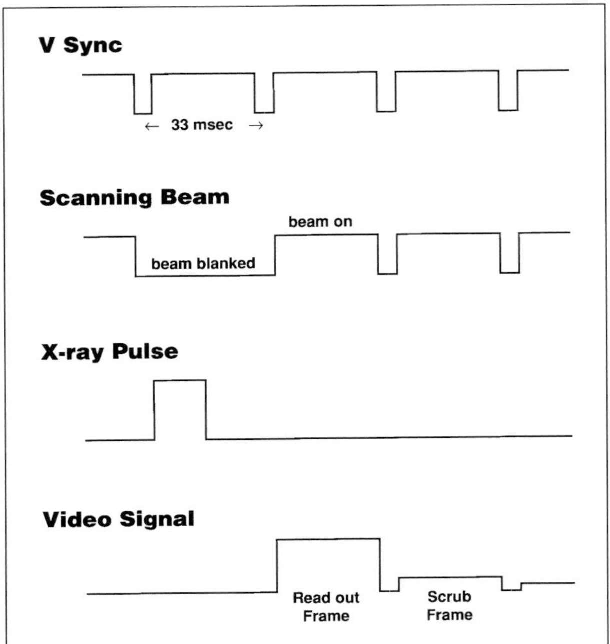

Figure 7-27. Timing diagram for pulsed-progressive image acquisition.

method is "pulsed-progressive" acquisition (Fig. 7-27). In the pulsed-progressive mode, the scanning beam is turned off, or "blanked," during the x-ray pulse. As a result, all of the light incident on the target during the x-ray pulse is integrated. After the x-ray pulse is terminated, the scanning beam is turned back on, synchronous with V SYNC, to read out the image frame. After completion of the readout frame, scanning continues to reduce the residual signal (lag) still residing on the camera target. These additional frames, which are not digitized or stored by the digital processor, are referred to as "scrub" frames.

Slow-scan mode is a variation of the pulsed-progressive technique in which the time period allotted for scanning a video frame is increased. A system designer can, for example, increase the digitization matrix from 512^2 to 1024^2 without increasing either the video bandwidth or the sampling rate of the analog-to-digital converter (ADC) by increasing the readout frame period from 33 to 132 milliseconds (4× slow scan).

Pulsed-progressive acquisition makes use of a high exposure rate to produce a short x-ray pulse. A less common method of image acquisition is to increase the pulsewidth (reducing the exposure rate so that the total exposure in the image remains unchanged) in order to extend the x-ray pulse over several video frames (Fig. 7-28). Target scanning continues during the x-ray pulse. These frames (typically four) are then integrated by the image processor to produce a single image. The shading artifacts that occur during the first video frames(s) in this mode are ignored by not including the first frame(s) in the image summation. The advantages of integrated acquisition are that (1) a lower SNR video camera is acceptable because electronic noise is averaged, and (2) the method is more forgiving with respect to system stability because brightness fluctuations and other artifacts tend to be averaged. The disadvantages of the integrated method are that (1) discarding video frame(s) increases patient exposure, and (2) the longer x-ray pulse can increase motion blurring.

Digital Systems

Digitization

An ADC digitizes the output of the video camera, converting the continuous analog voltage into discrete digital levels that the image processor can manipulate. The digitization process results in a digital value that is an approximation of the original analog value. The difference between the two, called the *quantization error,* can be an additional source of image noise. Proper system design can limit the noise increase to an insignificant amount by providing a sufficient number of levels to characterize the brightness range of the image. Digitizing the analog image too finely, however, is disadvantageous because of the subsequent need to provide increased storage for the insignificant bits. In addition, there is a limit to the number of levels that current ADCs can provide at the required sampling rates (e.g., 40-MHz for a 1024^2 matrix at 30 frames per second). The required number of levels is simply the range of signals to be digitized divided by the gray-level spacing. To choose a gray-level spacing smaller than the amplitude of the noise in the analog signal imparts no advantage with respect to image quality.[37] Using this criterion, the appropriate number of digital levels can be calculated.[40] The primary determinant of the number of levels required is the x-ray exposure incident on the image intensifier; higher x-ray exposures require a greater number of levels.

An ADC is specified by the number of output "bits," rather than the number of levels, which are used to characterize the digital result. The number of levels encoded by a given number of bits is given by levels = 2^{bits}. The most common ADCs used in digital angiographic systems are either 8- or 10-bit devices, producing 256 and 1024 levels, respectively. A 10-bit

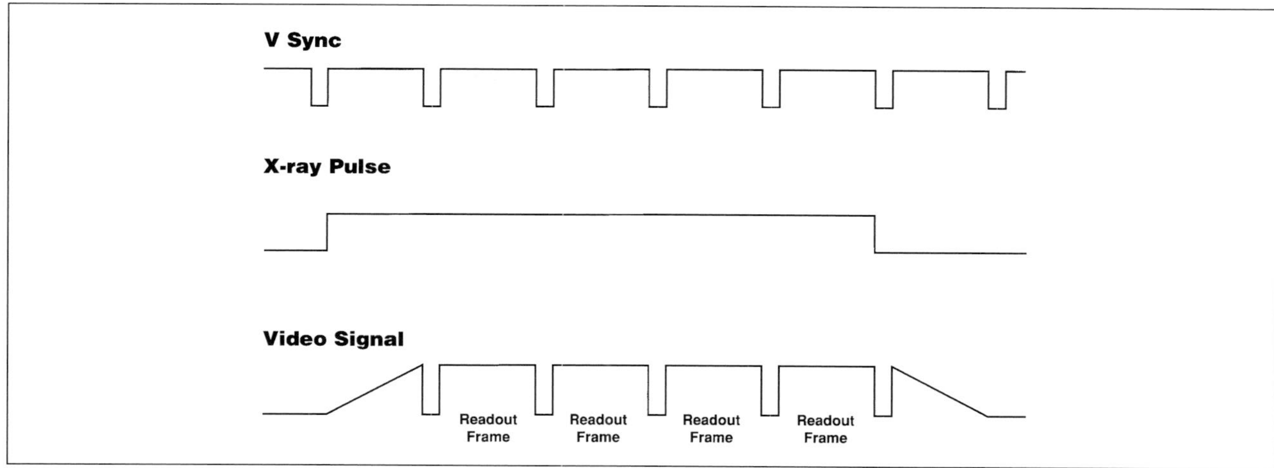

Figure 7-28. Timing diagram for image acquisition using frame integration.

ADC is required for most angiographic applications. Cardiac systems limit themselves to an 8-bit ADC because it is sufficient at the lower exposure levels used, and because of the extreme data storage demands of cardiac procedures. Fluoroscopic applications also require only 8 bits.

Pixel Matrix

The digitization process produces an image described by a matrix of digital values. Most systems use a matrix size of either 512 × 512 (512^2) or 1024 × 1024 (1024^2) pixels. Early DSA systems were limited to a 512^2 image matrix because conventional video cameras provided 525 horizontal lines per frame and because ADCs were limited to a 10-MHz digitization rate (producing 512 pixels along a line). Improving ADC performance and high-line video cameras (approximately 1000 lines per frame) have allowed the development of 1024^2 systems, which are becoming the norm for noncardiac applications. For cardiac systems, however, the high cost of image storage cannot be ignored and 512^2 matrices are still common.

It would seem that a 1024^2 matrix would double the spatial resolution for high-contrast objects, and indeed, resolution measurements of lead line pair phantoms with high x-ray exposure and no geometric magnification demonstrate this increased spatial resolution. However, under clinically relevant situations, several factors can prevent this improvement from being fully realized. These include image noise, focal-spot blur, and the modulation transfer function (MTF) of other system components.

Focal-spot blur can limit the actual resolution increase obtained from a larger pixel matrix. For example, the observed difference in limiting resolution between a 512^2 and a 1024^2 matrix in the 6.5-inch mode is minimal above a geometric magnification of about 1.3 or 1.4 due to focal-spot blurring.[40] With a 1.2-mm (nominal) focal spot, over the normal range of geometric magnification (1.1–1.5), focal-spot blur limits the resolution obtained with a 512^2 matrix only in the small II modes. However, focal-spot limitations become more significant with a 1024^2 matrix, especially with large focal spots and small II modes. A larger pixel matrix does significantly extend the limiting resolution for smaller focal spots and larger II modes. Table 7-2 gives the geometric magnification above which focal-spot blur is the predominant limitation to spatial resolution.

Another factor limiting spatial resolution is the performance of the other system components. Although the MTFs of the image intensifier, optical lenses, and video camera demonstrate tails that extend to high frequencies, the contrast loss at more moderate frequen-

Table 7-2. Geometric Magnification Above Which Focal-Spot Blur Exceeds the Pixel Matrix as a Limitation to Spatial Resolution*

	Magnification			
	1.2-mm Focal Spot		0.6-mm Focal Spot	
II Mode	512^2	1024^2	512^2	1024^2
6.5″	1.4	1.2	1.7	1.4
10″	1.6	1.3	2.1	1.6
14″	1.8	1.4	2.5	1.8

*Actual focal spot widths are assumed to be 1.7 mm and 0.9 mm for nominal widths of 1.2 mm and 0.6 mm, respectively, as per NEMA standards.[41]

cies (e.g., 1 lp/mm) from these components is substantial. As a result, the total system MTFs of 512^2 and 1024^2 systems differ little at these spatial frequencies.[40,42] Observable resolution improvement for a 1024^2 system, therefore, requires an object with significant energy in the high spatial frequency regions of the signal spectrum.

Image-Processing Hardware

For a digital angiographic system to be clinically useful, images must be processed in real time so that one video frame is completed before the next frame is acquired. During the 33-millisecond frame period the digital value of up to 1 million pixels, each one of which may depend on several operations, must be calculated. To accomplish this task, the pixel data are processed by a "pipeline" of specialized hardware modules that perform their function and then pass the data to the succeeding stage in time to receive the next pixel (Fig. 7-29).[43] The image processor is controlled by a much slower, but more flexible, "host" computer, which configures the processor to perform selected algorithms. The host also controls the process of image acquisition and responds to operator instructions.

Images are stored in solid-state random access memory (RAM). RAM is volatile, retaining data only while it is powered. RAM is used for the temporary storage of images that are currently being acquired, manipulated, or displayed.

The arithmetic logic unit (ALU) consists of extensive digital circuitry that can perform arithmetic operations on one or more images. Arithmetic operations commonly available within the ALU include image subtraction, image addition (for frame integration), image multiplication (e.g., for recursive filtering), and pixel-by-pixel comparisons of images (e.g., for motion detection algorithms).

Intensity transformations are generally performed with a *look-up table* (LUT), also referred to as an *intensity transformation table* (ITT). A LUT is a solid-state memory device that replaces the input value of the pixel with a new value. The pixel value is applied to the address lines of the LUT. The new value is stored at that memory location and is therefore output from the LUT. Because LUTs are RAM devices, the intensity transformation function may be changed as needed. LUTs are generally found at several locations along the image pathway. Typical intensity transformation functions include logarithmic transformations before subtraction, gamma correction to compensate for nonlinear processing of the video signal, and window and level (contrast and brightness) transformations for contrast enhancement.

One processing operation that has become essential for digital angiographic systems is spatial convolution. Spatial convolution is a filtering operation in which the value of a given pixel is replaced by a linear combination of its neighbors. Low-pass filtration decreases noise and spatial resolution. High-pass filtration is used to provide edge enhancement (Fig. 7-30). A convolution "kernel" defines the spatial extent over which the averaging process extends. For example, a 3×3 kernel averages the 9 pixels within a 3-pixel-high by 3-pixel-wide box centered on the pixel destined to receive the calculated value. Larger kernels (e.g., up to 15×15 pixels) produce higher degrees of image smoothing and high-frequency peaking. The weighting applied to a given pixel is often not constant, but rather is a function of the pixel's distance from the center of the kernel. For example, a gaussian kernel gives the greatest weight to the center pixel and decreases the weight, in a gaussian manner, with increasing distance from the center. Digital systems often allow the user to define kernels so that the degree of frequency manipulation can be tailored to the user's preference. Each pixel in a spatially filtered image may be the result of many arithmetic operations extending over several

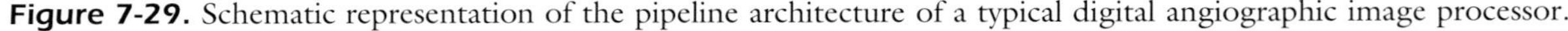

Figure 7-29. Schematic representation of the pipeline architecture of a typical digital angiographic image processor.

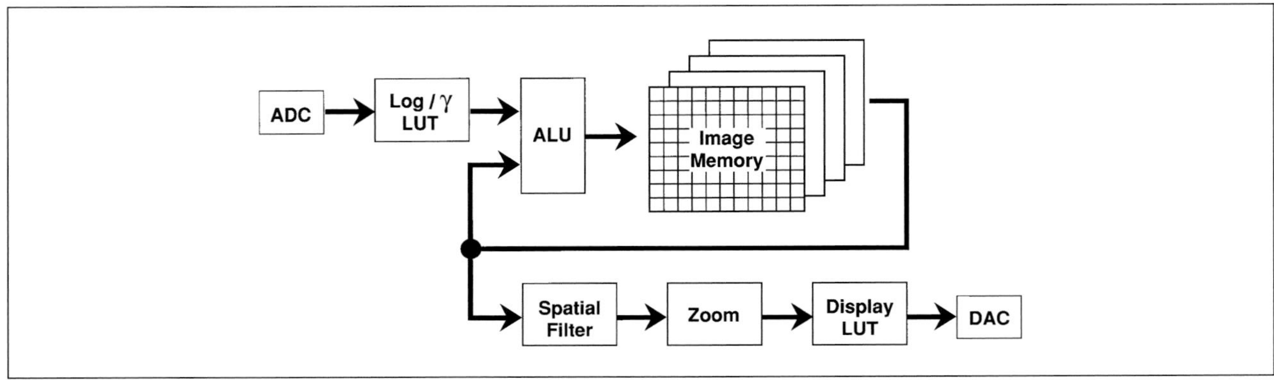

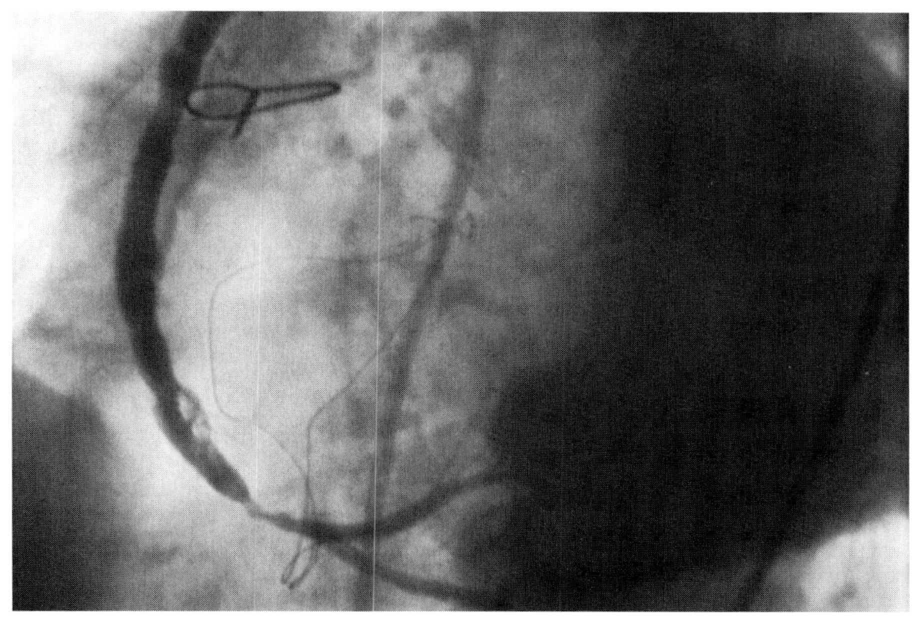

A

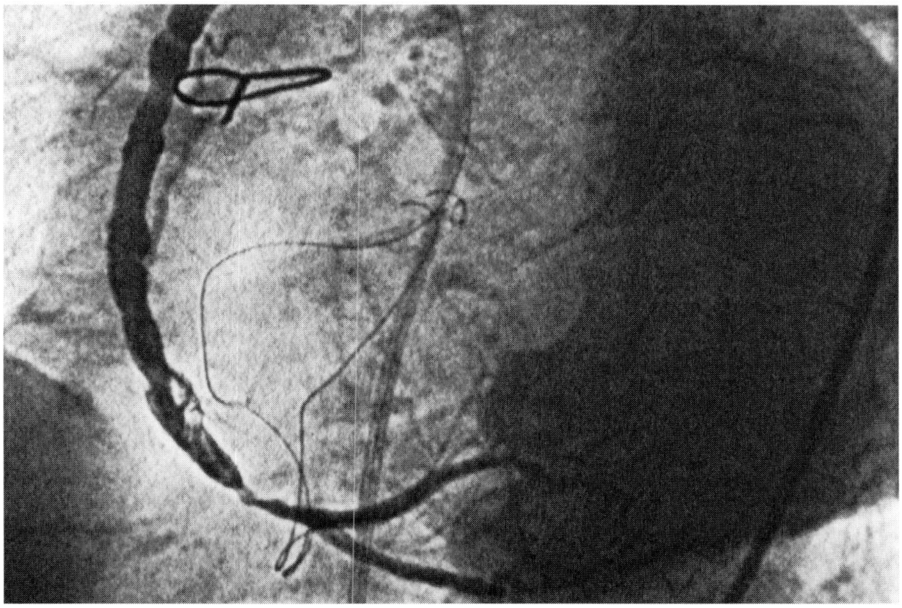

B

Figure 7-30. Original (A) and edge-enhanced (B) coronary angiographic frames. (Courtesy of Camtronics Medical Systems, 900 Walnut Ridge Dr., Hartland, Wisc.)

video lines. The real-time implementation of spatial filtering has been aided by the recent availability of specialized digital filters available as integrated circuits.

Image Display

Several commonly performed algorithms are primarily image display operations. Progressive-acquisition-to-interlaced-display scan conversion is one example. Another scan conversion operation is "upscanning." Upscanning usually entails displaying an image acquired with 512 lines as a 1024-line image by interleaving lines of calculated data between the actual image data. The calculated data are obtained by either replication or interpolation of the data on adjacent lines. Interpolation, resulting in a smoother display, is the preferred method. Interpolation may be a linear average or a spline fit to the actual data above and below the interpolated value.

Upscanning is generally not found on noncardiac systems because of the popularity of true 1000-line systems. For cardiac systems, however, where storage capacity is a concern, upscanning is an attractive compromise because, although the image acquisition chain limits the improvement in resolution available with 1000-line acquisition, 1000-line displays are definitely superior to conventional 525-line displays. This improvement is seen as an increase in display contrast and a reduction in the perceived raster pattern, especially at the interface between a bright and a dark region.

A related display operation is the ability to digitally magnify, or "zoom," the displayed image. The ability to pan the zoomed image is also provided. Again, zoom can be implemented by simple pixel replication or, more desirably, by bidirectional interpolation of the actual image data. Zooming provides no real increase in spatial resolution but is valuable during interventional procedures when the physician must stand at some distance from the monitor.

Processing functions at the output of the image processor enhance both the perception and cosmetic appearance of the displayed information. It is at this point that window and level (contrast and brightness) operations are performed on the image. "Video invert" allows the display of black iodine on a white background or vice versa. Electronic shutters may be applied, masking off extraneous information at the periphery of the image. Annotation is added to provide textual information.

The digital image must be converted back to an analog voltage waveform in order to be displayed on a video monitor. This conversion is performed by a digital-to-analog convertor (DAC). Eight bits is sufficient resolution for the DAC. Display monitors are characterized by a "line rate" specification. Standard-line monitors conform to the EIA RS-170 standard, displaying 525-line, 2:1 interlaced video at a 60-Hz field rate (30-Hz frame rate). Thousand-line systems (either true or upscanned) require a high-line monitor, typically 1023- or 1049-line, 2:1 interlaced video at a 60-Hz field rate. The high-line display provides a substantial improvement in image quality. However, each line is still presented below the flicker-fusion frequency of the human observer, which can result in both interline flicker and resolution loss under close scrutiny. One current system provides a 2:1 interlaced display with a 120-Hz field rate, eliminating perceived flicker.

Depending on the system architecture, it is often desirable that the video monitors be line-rate switchable, detecting whether a video source is using standard or high-line video and automatically providing the proper display format. This allows trouble-free display of both high-line digital outputs and standard-line sources such as an S-VHS videotape recorder. Another important ergonomic consideration of system design is how easily the display of multiple sources is handled. Typically, two monitors per plane are provided to display reference and live images simultaneously. Alternate methods include "picture-in-picture" display or a video switcher, which automatically switches from reference to live images as required.

On-line Disk Storage

During the procedure, images are displayed in real time using RAM memory. The images are also simultaneously transferred to an on-line digital disk. The term *on-line* refers to the fact that the disk is permanently mounted on the system (i.e., it is not removable). After completion of the run, the results are assessed by playing back the images recorded on the disk. Although large RAM storage devices are available (>1 gigabyte), disk storage is generally more economical above 100 to 200 megabytes. Another advantage of disk storage is that it is nonvolatile.

A notable feature of digital angiographic systems is the ease with which images are stored and displayed. Images are presented in sequential order, providing viewing characteristics similar to roll film. Image management software can provide specialized viewing modes for rapid review of the procedure, such as a single-screen display of all images acquired during a run (Fig. 7-31) or the middle image of each injection on a given patient. This expedites the selection of im-

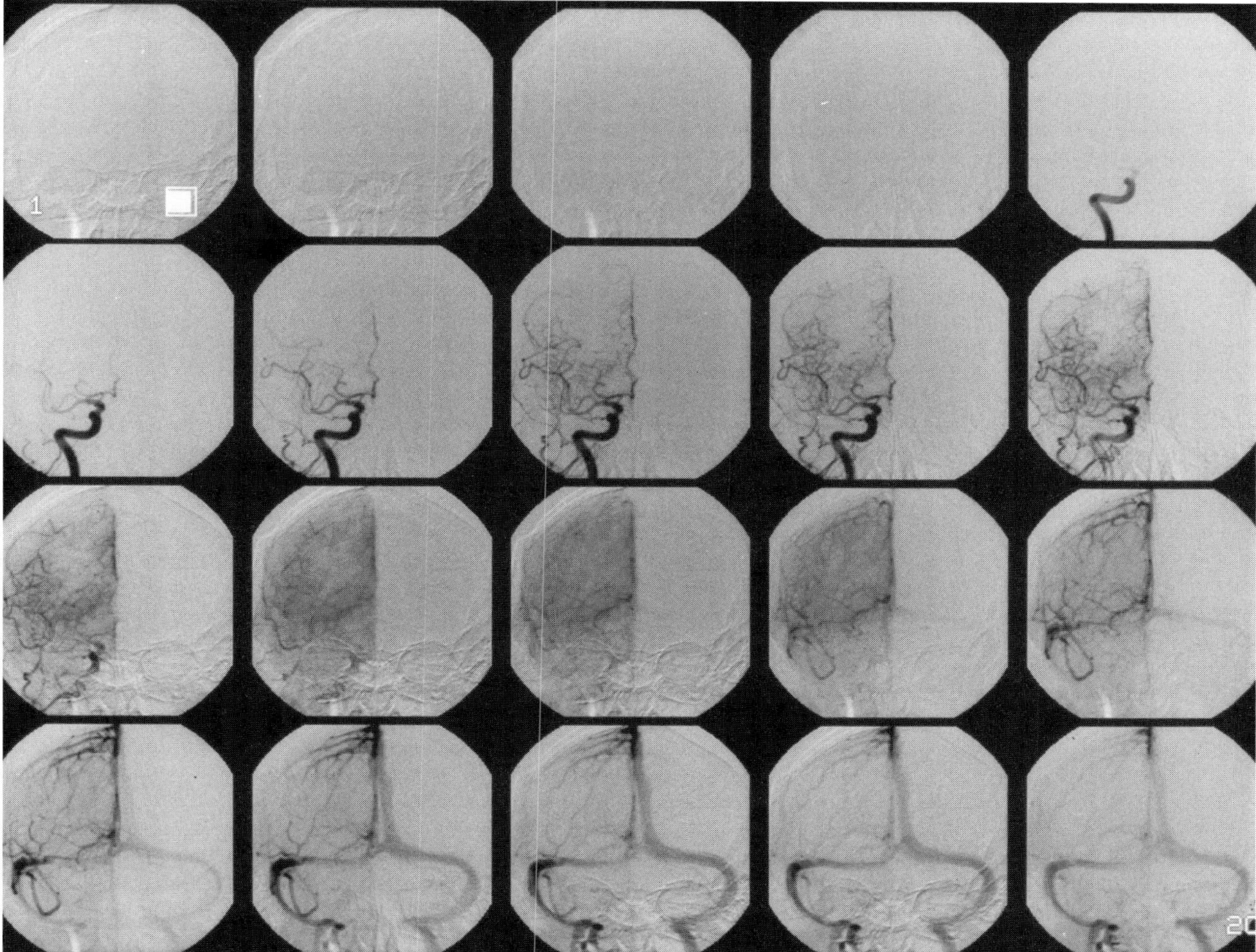

Figure 7-31. Image mosaic displaying all the images in a single injection. (Courtesy of Philips Medical Systems, 710 Bridgeport Ave., Shelton, Conn.)

ages, which can then be stored, short term, in a partitioned section of the disk for rapid referral. Many systems allow this process to be controlled tableside with an infrared remote control.

When DSA was first introduced, the slow recording rates of digital storage devices restricted their use to frame rates of less than one frame per second. Higher rates required analog magnetic disk or tape (videotape). A complication of analog storage is the need to redigitize images before postprocessing. Analog storage devices also have signal-to-noise ratios of only 100 to 200:1. As a result, storage significantly increases total image noise unless storage is limited to subtracted, contrast-enhanced images or images with an inherently high noise level (e.g., cardiac images).

The development of fast digital magnetic disks has made on-line digital recording standard. Speed has been increased through the use of parallel head drives, multiple disks configured as a single system, and data compression. Vendors often provide the ability to select the number of disk drives purchased with a system, allowing the user to tailor both storage capacity and maximum frame rate to their individual needs. The storage capacity of these devices is easily estimated. Each pixel in an image is described by either an 8-bit or a 10-bit word, depending on the bit depth of the ADC. Eight bits make up a unit of data storage called a byte. The value of a pixel is therefore described by approximately 1 byte of data. The amount of storage required to store one image is given in units of megabytes. One $512^2 \times 8$-bit image requires 1/4 megabyte of storage. One $1024^2 \times 8$-bit image requires 1 megabyte. Storage capacities of currently available disks are in the neighborhood of hundreds of megabytes to 1 or more gigabytes (1 gigabyte = 1024 megabytes). A 1-gigabyte disk should store approximately 1000 1024^2 images, or 4000 512^2 images. Actual disks store either somewhat less than or a fair amount more than this ballpark figure. Storage of 10 bits, rather than 8, reduces the number of images that can be stored, as does overhead needed for formatting and image management data.

Data compression algorithms encode the digital data in a more compact form, increasing both storage capacity and recording rate. An algorithm is specified by its compression ratio. For example, a compression ratio of 2:1 reduces the amount of data actually recorded by a factor of 2. Compression algorithms are characterized as to whether, upon playback, the original data are restored exactly. If they are, the algorithm is referred to as lossless or error-free. If the restored data are not identical to the original data, the algorithm is referred to as lossy or irreversible. Lossless compression is limited to compression ratios of about 3:1 or less. Lossy compression algorithms in the range of 3:1 to 10:1 are sometimes referred to as "visually lossless," and the claim is made that the difference between the original and restored data is insignificant. The acceptability of lossy algorithms is currently a matter of investigation.

Flexible disk systems are available that support digital recording at any frame rate required. A typical disk system may use one disk drive to record up to 15 frames per second. The addition of a second drive would increase the recording rate to 30 frames per second. Drives can often be configured to record both 512^2 and 1024^2 images. A system capable of 30-frames-per-second storage of a 512^2 matrix will also record a 1024^2 matrix at 7.5 frames per second. Some systems support biplane recording at half the frame rate of single-plane recording. A disk system capable of 30-frames-per-second recording is often referred to as a real-time digital disk. The fastest real-time disks available can store a 1024^2 matrix at 30 frames per second. The need for real-time digital recording is primarily restricted to cardiac procedures, although high-flow vascular lesions and procedures such as gantry rotation during image acquisition also benefit from high frame rates.

Archival Storage

When DSA was introduced in the early 1980s, on-line digital storage constituted a recording bottleneck. Now that on-line storage limitations no longer exist, a new storage bottleneck has appeared with the long-term, off-line archival storage of digital images. This limitation is felt most acutely for cardiac systems.

Archival needs in a vascular laboratory are usually met by storing hard copy films of selected images. Hardware for the generation of hard copy output includes multiformat cameras (laser or video) and video printers. Early systems made use of multiformat video cameras in which a video monitor exposed a film cassette. These early cameras used the conventional 525-line video format and suffered from obvious raster line structure and the resulting inability to produce a dark black gray scale. Modern multiformat video cameras use techniques such as digital interpolation and low-angle deflection monitors to produce high-contrast, high-resolution films. However, in most applications, multiformat laser cameras, which directly expose the film with a laser scanner, have supplanted video cameras. Laser cameras also produce high-contrast, high-resolution films and have the added advantage of being capable of producing the large-format images desirable for surgical suite viewing. Video thermal printers can conveniently produce images for chart documentation, report generation, and distribution to referring physicians.

Digital archives are primarily in demand in teaching environments, cardiac laboratories, and large institutions implementing Picture Archiving and Communication Systems (PACS). The American College of Radiology and National Electrical Manufacturers Association (ACR-NEMA) communications protocol establishes an interface standard for the network transfer of images (DICOM v3.0).[44] Digital archiving can be provided by optical disks and magnetic tape. Digital optical disks, currently limited to non-real-time rates, are available in both write-once-read-many (WORM) and erasable formats.

Archiving of cardiac images is an area of intense development pressure. Limitations include insufficient recording rates and a lack of standards to support the interchange of image data. Real-time (or near-real-time) digital archival recording can be provided by magnetic tape. Several archival tape devices are offered by vendors, including digital video recording using the SMPTE D-2 format, 8-mm tape cassettes, and other devices generally referred to as digital "streamer tapes." Systems capable of near-real-time recording can be designed so that image archiving occurs in the background, with the acquisition system acting as a buffer. Equivalent buffering capability must then also be provided at the review station. Review stations are under development in which non-real-time archives are temporarily loaded into RAM or a real-time digital disk to provide cinelike review capabilities.

The largest obstacle confronting digital archiving of cardiac images is the portability of image data.[45] Cine film is the model of portability. Everyone's 35-mm film can be reviewed on the ubiquitous cine projector. Most cardiac laboratories now record angiographic data on both digital and cine formats simultaneously, a technique referred to as "parallel cine." This provides the image enhancement and short-term review features of digital angiography while providing the archival properties of film. This situation is viewed by many as a bridge to the fully digital catheterization laboratory. However, an increasing number of new installations are "cineless," lending urgency to the establishment of a data-exchange standard. Typically, cineless laboratories use S-VHS videocassette tape as the means of sharing image data with colleagues. However, the image quality of S-VHS tape is insufficient for diagnostic purposes. An apparent resolution to this problem is the recordable compact disk (CD-R) interchange medium standard recently endorsed by a group working under the aegis of the ACR, NEMA, and the American College of Cardiology (ACC).[46]

Image-Processing Algorithms

Temporal Subtraction

The subtraction algorithm used by DSA systems is temporal (or time) subtraction.[47] This algorithm subtracts a preopacification mask from serially acquired images of the opacified vessels. Because this operation removes the fixed anatomy, contrast enhancement can be performed on the difference image to fill the dynamic range of the display device. Unlike film subtraction, DSA provides a real-time display of the subtraction result. This ability to view subtractions in real time spurred the initial interest in IV angiography, because without it timing image acquisition to coincide with the contrast bolus is difficult.

When subtraction is to be performed on angiographic images, a logarithmic transformation is first performed on the image data. The log transform compensates for the fact that the absolute attenuation signal decreases with decreasing x-ray fluence (increasing patient attenuation). The attenuation produced by a low-contrast vessel is given by

$$\Delta N = -\mu_I N x_I$$

where N is the photon fluence, ΔN is the change in fluence due to the opacified vessel, μ_I is the linear attenuation coefficient of iodine, and x_I is the thickness of the vessel. Because the vessel signal, ΔN, decreases as N decreases, vessel contrast is reduced in strongly attenuating regions of the image even though the vessel thickness remains constant.

Most systems use a look-up table to log the image. The value of a pixel at the input to the log LUT is converted to a new value according to the relationship $y = a[ln(x - s)]$, where s is a correction for the effects of scatter (see below). Figure 7-32 shows this relationship for $s = 0$. Signals in the bright regions of the image are compressed, whereas those in the dark regions of the image are greatly expanded. After logarithmic amplification, the difference signal, D, is given by

$$D \propto (\mu/\rho)_I \rho_I x_I$$

where $(\mu/\rho)_I$ is the mass attenuation coefficient of iodine, ρ_I is the concentration of iodine in the blood, and x_I is the vessel thickness. Because of the logarithmic transformation, the iodine signal is directly proportional to the product $\rho_I x_I$ and, assuming uniform iodine concentration, to the thickness of the vessel.

The linearity portrayed above is an idealization of the actual imaging situation. Signal linearity can be lost because of the effects of x-ray scatter and veiling glare (SVG).[48] As in general radiographic applications, SVG reduces the radiographic contrast of the signal. SVG can also result in an error in the logarithmic transformation by placing signals too high up on the log curve. This is compensated for by subtracting off the constant, s, mentioned in the preceding paragraph. However, this is only a first-order correction, because the value of SVG varies greatly from point to point in the image. Vessel contrast is especially reduced in dark

Figure 7-32. Logarithmic transformation applied to the image data by the log look-up table prior to subtraction. For comparison a linear transformation, in which the input level is unchanged, is also shown.

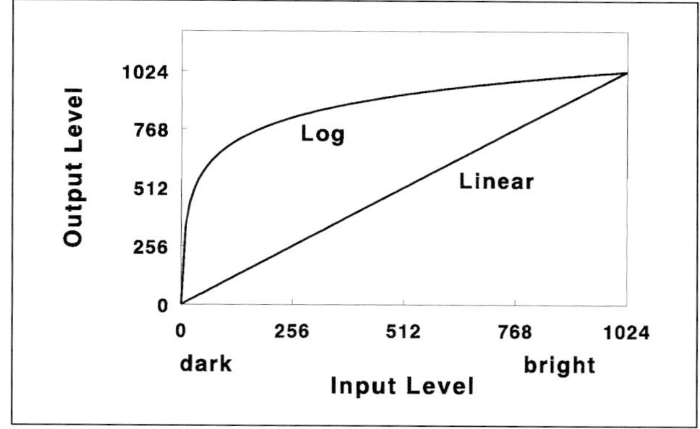

portions of the image in close proximity to a bright region. Proper radiographic technique, including collimation and bolusing to decrease bright spots, is important in reducing this problem. It should be noted that the often encountered statement that the degradation due to scatter is reduced by the subtraction operation is incorrect.

Loss of contrast can also occur if the log transform is not set aggressively. Because the log curve is very steep in the dark regions of the image, noise fluctuations in the dark regions are greatly enhanced. In addition, if the log transform is performed in the digital domain, large steps between populated levels can result in a contoured appearance to the digital data. To diminish the perception of these fluctuations, the gain at low signal level is often reduced from that required of a true log transform. In this case, amplification of the dark signals is less than is required and a reduction in the iodine signal occurs where, for example, the artery crosses a dense bone. An extreme example of this phenomenon is observed when, as is occasionally seen in DSA images, no logarithmic transformation at all is used.

Contrast enhancement of DSA images markedly increases the perceptibility of image noise. Subtraction also increases the absolute noise amplitude. If the rms noise amplitude in the mask image is given by σ_M, and in the iodine image by σ_I, the rms amplitude of the noise in the subtraction image, σ_S, is given by

$$\sigma_S = \sqrt{\sigma_M^2 + \sigma_I^2}$$

If the noise in the mask and iodine images are of equal amplitude ($\sigma_M = \sigma_I$), then the noise in the subtraction image is increased by $\sqrt{2}$ (40 percent). This is the usual case, in which the mask and iodine images are both single images. It is possible to decrease the noise level of subtraction images by summing several images together. For example, integration of preopacification images to form an integrated mask can be used to reduce image noise without reducing vessel detail. If M frames are integrated to form a mask, the noise amplitude in the subtraction image is given by

$$\sigma_S = \sqrt{1 + \frac{1}{M}}\,\sigma_I$$

It is also possible to integrate contrast images so that several images from the run produce a single composite image. This can be used to demonstrate arteriovenous relationships on one image or to compensate for slow flow such as is often observed in peripheral runoff studies. Integration of contrast images can also be used to increase the signal-to-noise ratio when iodine contrast is low. The optimum method of image integration with respect to signal-to-noise ratio improvement is the matched-filter subtraction algorithm.[49] This postprocessing technique weights the individual images, before summation, to cancel the background anatomy while optimizing the signal-to-noise ratio in the final image. Practical limitations to image integration include a potential loss in vessel resolution due to pulsatile motion and, more importantly, misregistration artifacts. Images included in a summation must be well registered with the other images in the sequence.

The primary technical problem with image subtraction is the artifacts that result from misregistration of the mask and opacification images. The principal strategy for dealing with misregistration artifacts is "remasking." If the initially formed subtraction image is marred by misregistration artifacts, the operator searches for a different mask image that registers with the opacified image. This interactive process is frequently required, so it is important that the processor software handle it smoothly. It is not uncommon for the best registration to be obtained by using an image acquired after the peak of the contrast bolus as the mask (this is termed a *late mask*). Another strategy employed to clean up an artifact-marred subtraction is "pixel shifting." The operator interactively shifts the mask to try to produce better registration. Images may be shifted a distance shorter than the width of a pixel by using an interpolation technique. Sophisticated hardware allows interpolated pixel shifting to be performed in real time, guided by the operator with a mouse or trackball. Unfortunately, the complex nature of patient motion is often not correctable by simple image translation or rotation. An area where pixel shifting may make a significant impact is in the recent application of subtraction imaging to peripheral angiography with automated stepping[50] and to rotational angiography.[51]

Cardiac DSA is limited by motion artifacts to such a degree that most cardiac digital imaging is performed without subtraction. Artifacts arise from cardiac, respiratory, and general patient motion. Respiratory motion can produce significant artifacts, covering the entire image. Several methods exist for forming cardiac masks. Integrated-mask mode sums the individual frames spanning one cardiac cycle. Motion artifacts are muted because cardiac structures in the mask are blurred by the summation. Phase-matched-mask mode stores individual mask images spanning the cardiac cycle. These masks are matched in phase with the opacified images. Phase-matched masking effectively

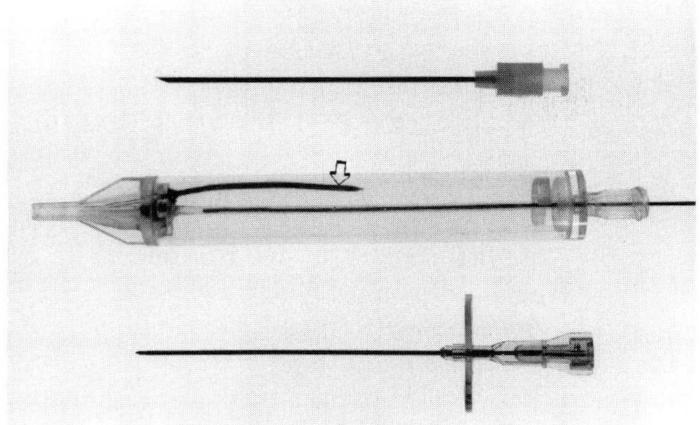

Figure 8-3. Arterial blood containment device (Arrow International). This device permits intermittent monitoring of the strength of the arterial jet for guidance during back-and-forth probing of the vessel lumen with the guidewire. A valve in the distal guidewire channel prevents backflow of blood. Simple or coaxial arterial needles may be used with this device. The *arrow* points to the internal cannula jet nozzle.

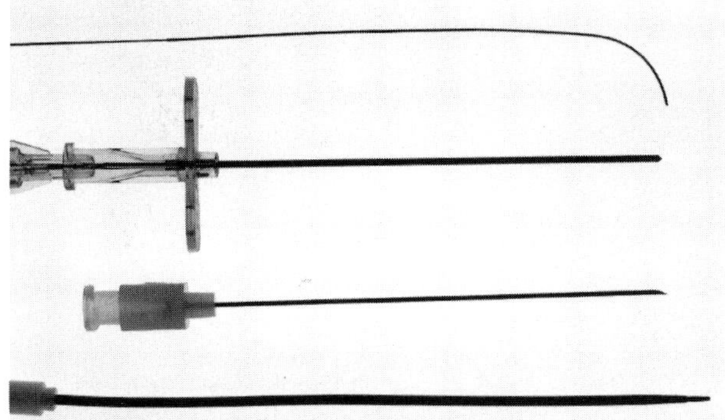

Figure 8-4. The Cook micropuncture introducing set. This set consists of a 0.018-inch guidewire, a 7-cm 21-gauge needle, and a 3 French or 5 French coaxial catheter dilator. Note the significant difference in diameter between a standard 18-gauge arterial needle (*second from top*) and the micropuncture needle.

are available that allow the guidewire to be introduced into the vessel through a valve system after blood return is seen to fill a connecting tube[7] or a bag (Angiodynamics Sos bloodless entry needle).

The arterial needle sizes most commonly used are thin-walled 18 gauge or 19 gauge, which allow insertion of standard 0.038-inch or 0.035-inch stainless steel helical spring guidewires. One should remember not to use plastic-coated nitinol guidewires through an introducing metal needle because the coating may be sheared off by the sharp edge and embolize downstream. These wires should therefore only be introduced through a catheter or through the plastic dilator used to predilate the tract to prevent the catheter tip from fraying during its introduction through the soft tissues.

Although 18-gauge needles are very reliable for puncturing easily palpable large vessels such as the femoral artery, the operator should also be familiar with the use of 21-gauge micropuncture needles.[8] These needles are very useful for decreasing the trauma to vessel walls and perivascular vital structures associated with repeated attempts to puncture poorly palpable arteries and grafts; for facilitating puncture of vessels that are slippery or prone to spasm, such as the axillary and brachial arteries; and for decreasing the potential for developing significant hematomas in patients with coagulopathies. The micropuncture needle, by virtue of its smaller diameter and resulting reduced tissue resistance to penetration, is less painful, provides a better feel of the transmitted arterial pulse, and has a sharper bite for the vessel wall. It is available in an introducer set (Cook, Inc.) (Fig. 8-4) that permits the needle to be exchanged for a 5 French plastic cannula over a 0.018-inch guidewire, which then allows standard-sized guidewires to be used.

Introduction Sheaths

Introduction sheaths are important safeguards used to protect the vascular or graft puncture site from trauma during long and complex diagnostic or interventional procedures, which can otherwise lead to laceration or irregular overdilatation of the transmural tract. This is especially prone to occur when exchanging for multiple catheters and guidewires, inserting stiff atherectomy devices, and removing completely deflated balloon catheters. These sheaths are also very valuable for introducing nontapered catheters, a combined aortic catheter and a visceral selective safety guidewire to check angioplasty results,[9] foreign-body retrieval devices, biopsy forceps, and so forth. Introducing sheaths, also available in longer lengths from 20 cm to over 50 cm, are commonly used to shield the wall of severely atherosclerotic iliac arteries and the lower abdominal aorta (Fig. 8-5) from guidewire and selective catheter trauma, which might result in severe atheroembolic disease. Recently, more flexible curved catheter introducers less given to kinking have been introduced and are found to be extremely convenient for coaxially passing thrombolytic or angioplasty balloon catheters[10] across the aortic bifurcation to the contralateral iliofemoral arterial tree.

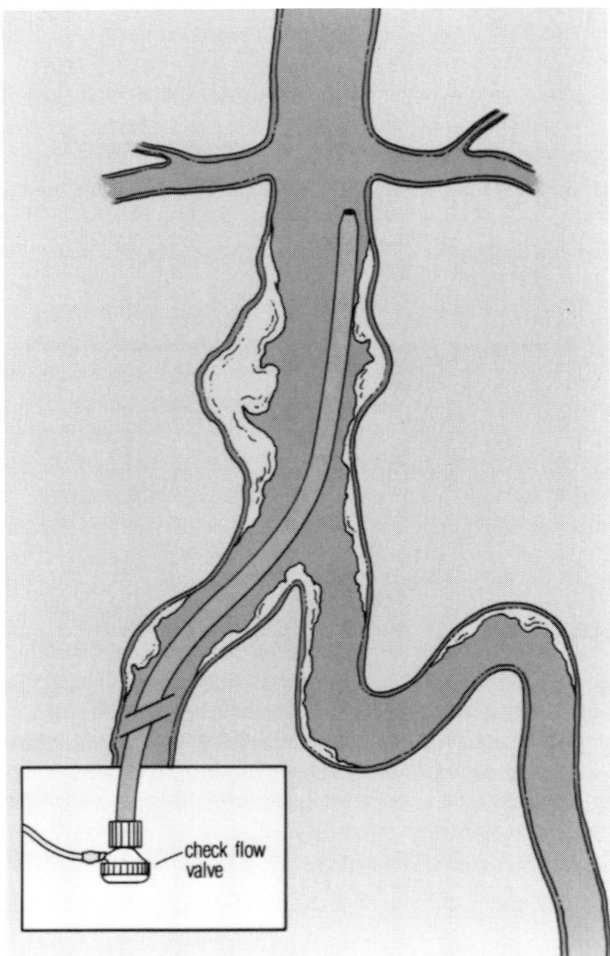

Figure 8-5. A long 7 French catheter-introducing sheath has been advanced past the aortic aneurysm to minimize dislodgment of atheroemboli during selective visceral catheterization. (From Cope C, Burke DR, Meranze SG, eds. Atlas of interventional radiology. St. Louis: Mosby, 1990. Used with permission.)

Abdominal Aortography

Aortography is usually performed from the femoral artery. Catheterization of the aorta is normally feasible even in the presence of aneurysms or severe atherosclerotic disease by maneuvering an angled Glidewire (Medi-tech) to the level of the diaphragm and then threading over it a 5 French pigtail catheter with a tightly coiled tip.

Although often bypassed in favor of immediate visceral catheterization, midstream aortography can be a useful step for obtaining a vascular road map before selective studies. Despite the slightly increased load of contrast medium involved, aortography may save catheterization time and lessen later confusion by alerting the angiographer to the presence of anomalous takeoff of primary branches and accessory vessels as well as to unsuspected aneurysms and arteriosclerotic stenoses. Aortograms are also very useful in displaying branching vessels in the natural state, an important diagnostic baseline study that allows the operator to distinguish vasospasm secondary to selective catheterization from vascular encasement due to tumor.

In the presence of complete obstruction of both iliac arteries or of the lower aorta, aortography can be performed either from the high brachial or axillary route or otherwise by translumbar aortic puncture (Fig. 8-6). The left brachial or axillary route is more flexible and generally preferred because it allows the angiographer to do selective visceral catheterization and interventional procedures. However, if the subclavian artery and the thoracic aorta are very tortuous and atherosclerotic, access to the abdominal aorta from this site can be lengthy, complex, and hazardous because of potential dislodgment of atheroemboli to brachiocephalic vessels, brachial plexus injury, and the development of pseudoaneurysms. Under these circumstances, translumbar aortography can be a better approach because it is a quicker, simpler procedure that is very safe as long as the patient does not have a coagulopathy or severe hypertension.[11] Even selective vessel catheterization can be performed from this approach through a 5 French catheter introducer.

Figure 8-6. Illustration of translumbar aortography performed with 5 French or 6 French over-the-needle catheters introduced at T12 or L3 levels. These can be replaced over a stiff guidewire with an introducing sheath or with longer pigtail or selective catheters. (From Cope C, Burke DR, Meranze SG, eds. Atlas of interventional radiology. St. Louis: Mosby, 1990. Used with permission.)

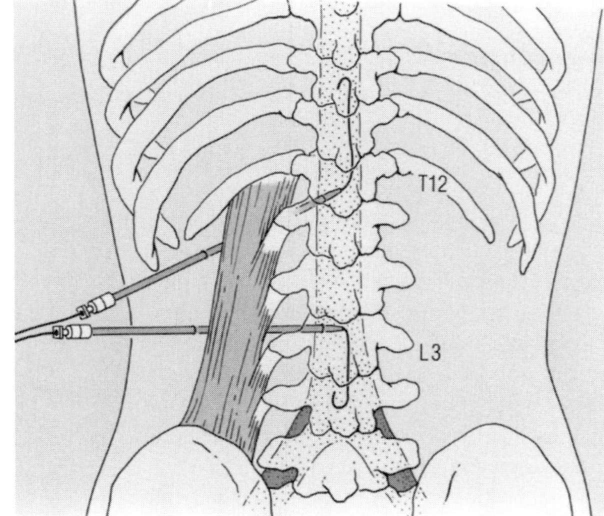

Superselective Catheterization with Simple Catheters

Preshaped Catheters

Because most interventional studies begin with the use of a conventional selective catheter, it is always tempting (and less expensive) to see whether this primary catheter can be successfully advanced superselectively, especially in patients with classic vascular anatomy.[12] This, in fact, can usually be done with a high degree of success on the arterial side for the control of bleeding or for tumor embolization in the bronchial,[13] gastric,[14] hepatic,[12] renal,[15] pelvic,[16] and extremity[17] circulations; and on the venous side these catheters are important for sampling of parathyroid,[18] adrenal and gonadal,[19] and pancreatic hormones,[20] and for embolization of esophageal varices[21] and gonadal varicoceles.[22]

The preferred site of entry for most studies of the chest and abdomen is the femoral artery or vein. The brachial or axillary artery route is used for difficult branch vessel angulation or for long-term infusion chemotherapy.

Six or 7 French introduction sheaths are usually first inserted as a safety precaution to prevent vascular trauma from repetitive guidewire and catheter exchanges. The same standard catheters chosen for catheterization of thoracic and abdominal aortic branches are also used for superselective work; the most commonly used preshaped catheters include those with a C, shepherd's crook, or cobra curve. For catheterizing acutely angled vessels, the author prefers using a 5 or 5.5 French Simmons catheter type 1 or 2, or a cobra catheter formed into a "Waltman loop" (Fig. 8-7).[23] Simmons catheters can be quickly reformed in the proximal abdominal aorta by simple traction on a 4ō plastic suture friction-fitted between the catheter tip and the guidewire (Fig. 8-8).[24] If the operator is unable to make the catheter follow the guidewire superselectively because of complex angulation, it should be exchanged for a straight or hockey stick curved catheter, preferably with a more flexible and slippery surface, such as the Venuela catheter (Cook, Inc.) or a hydromer-coated Anthron catheter (Toray Industries, Tokyo, Japan). When the inlying spring guidewire is too short for catheter exchange, the working length of the guidewire can be easily extended by tying a 100-cm length of fine stainless steel suture to its proximal stiff end.[25]

Figure 8-7. The Waltman loop. Following selective catheterization of the splenic artery (or other convenient aortic branches), the Waltman loop is formed by further advancing the guidewire and catheter up the thoracic aorta. The new configuration is convenient for subselective catheterization of the hepatic or left gastric artery. (From Cope C, Burke DR, Meranze SG, eds. Atlas of interventional radiology. St. Louis: Mosby, 1990. Used with permission.)

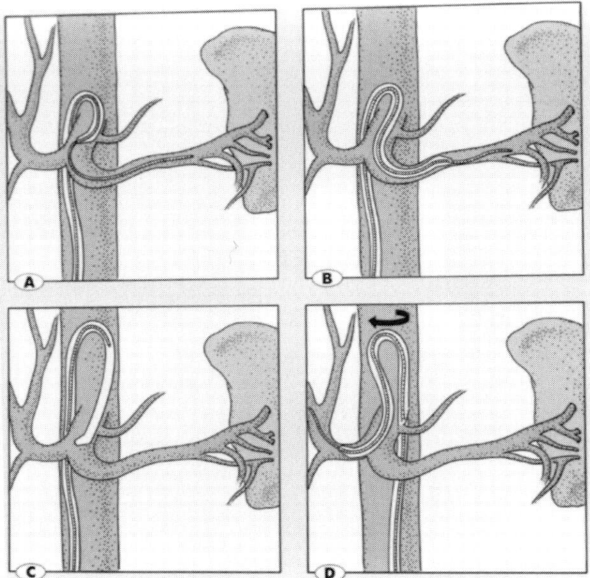

The Toposcopic Catheter

This is a compound catheter consisting of a 5 or 6 French polyurethane catheter and an inner thin-walled catheter sleeve that can be advanced only when the annular sealed space separating the catheter and sleeve is pressurized.[26] The inner catheter deploys itself by eversion and moves forward by unrolling itself within the vessel lumen with minimal friction (Fig. 8-9). As it is propelled forward, it is able to negotiate atraumatically multiple complex arterial twists and curves with little operator guidance. Thus catheter buckling, kinking, and torquing problems are essentially eliminated and potential endothelial damage is minimized. Its major disadvantage is its lack of directional control, although this can be partially remedied by inserting an angled torqueable guidewire through its lumen before pressurization; the everting tube will then carry the wire forward in the direction to which it is pointing. Because of manufacturing problems, marketing of this potentially useful catheter delivery system has been delayed.

Use of Balloon Catheters

A quick and easy method for catheterizing high-flow lesions such as arteriovenous fistulas or vascular tumors is to insert a two-lumen occlusion balloon catheter in

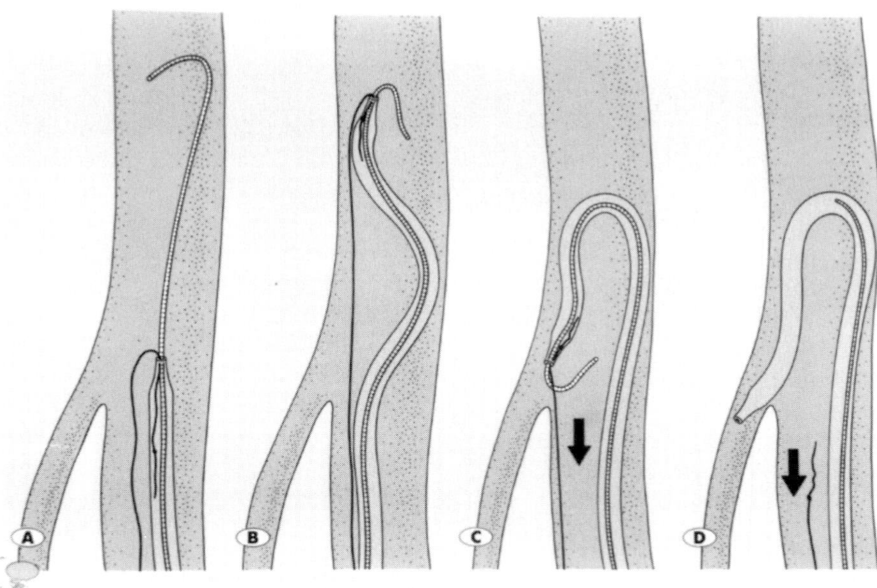

Figure 8-8. Suture technique to reform a Simmons catheter. (A) A catheter preloaded with a 4ō knotted plastic suture is threaded over a standard guidewire to the lower thoracic aorta. (B) The guidewire is pulled back to within 1 to 2 cm of the catheter tip. (C) The proximal free end of the suture is pulled while the catheter is slowly advanced until the sidewinder curve is reformed. (D) Withdrawal of the floppy-tipped guidewire frees the knotted suture and allows selective catheterization. The same technique can be used to form Waltman loops with hockey stick or cobra-shaped catheters. (From Cope C, Burke DR, Meranze SG, eds. Atlas of interventional radiology. St. Louis: Mosby, 1990. Used with permission.)

the major proximal aortic branch feeding the lesion. Once the catheter is sufficiently inflated with carbon dioxide or dilute contrast medium, it will be carried into the lesion by the more rapid blood flow and end well positioned for embolization. Alternatively, a 2 or 3 French single-lumen latex balloon catheter can be threaded through the selective catheter, inflated, and

Figure 8-9. Toposcopic catheter. The clear catheter sleeve is being advanced by eversion after the sealed annular space (containing air bubbles) has been pressurized.

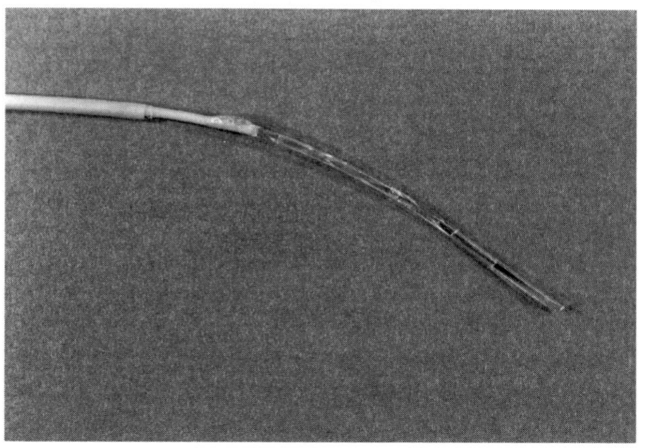

allowed to be carried to the vascular lesion (Fig. 8-10).[27] Once in place, the balloon is deflated, and a fine mandrel guidewire is then inserted within its lumen to allow the outer catheter to track over it more easily without kinking. Balloon catheters can also be redirected at bifurcations by infusing a vasoconstricting drug selectively in the unwanted vascular limb to allow the balloon to free-float to the other patent limb.[28]

Another useful function of small nondetachable balloons is to divert blood flow toward the vessel to be embolized. For example, an occasional patient may present with a bleeding duodenal lesion and, because of severe tortuosity or atherosclerotic disease, the operator may find it impossible to selectively catheterize the gastroduodenal artery from the proper hepatic artery. Under these conditions, a 2 French Fogarty balloon catheter can be released from the guiding catheter, and the balloon can be inflated to occlude the common hepatic artery just distal to the gastroduodenal artery. If a contrast test injection shows good antegrade flow into the gastroduodenal artery, the operator may then safely inject embolic particles through the side arm of the guiding catheter adapter to occlude pancreaticoduodenal branches. A similar principle was used by Nakamura[29] to redirect blood flow through periportal collaterals for hepatic chemoembolization

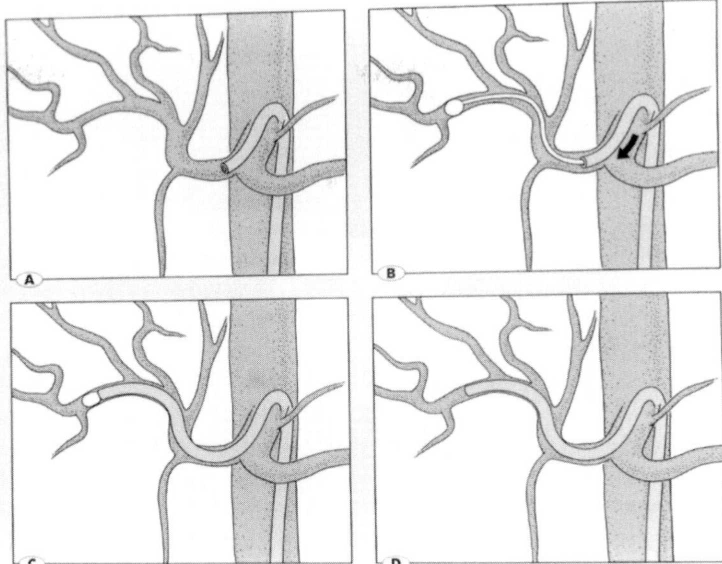

Figure 8-10. Balloon catheter guidewire. A partially inflated 3 French Fogarty balloon catheter has been carried by blood flow through a selective celiac catheter (A) to a hepatic artery branch (B). The coaxial catheter can then be advanced over it (C), especially if it is stiffened with a fine mandrel wire. (D) Final catheter position.

when the common hepatic artery distal to the gastroduodenal artery was occluded.

Superselective Catheterization with Coaxial Technique

Because the human body has a great variety of arterial curves and branching patterns further complicated by disease states, the interventionist needs a wide variety of catheter systems to be able to navigate freely through the vascular tree. Five to 7 French preshaped catheters are very practical for superselective catheterization of third- or fourth-order vessels as long as their lumen is of adequate caliber and the branching vascular path is fairly simple. As the tortuosities of the feeding vessels leading to the area of interest increase in number and complexity, these selective catheters become not only less effective because of loss of torque control but also more traumatic to vascular endothelium because of increasing friction between the relatively stiff catheter and the vessel wall, especially at branching points and tight curves. When the diameter of the advancing catheter tip begins to approximate that of the vessel, there is increased friction against the intima and reduction in blood flow, which can lead to spasm, blood stasis, ischemia of normal adjacent tissue, and occasionally even difficulty in withdrawing the catheter. For these reasons, superselective catheterization is performed with as fine and as flexible a catheter as possible that will still retain some operator control, possess adequate radiopacity, and have a lumen large enough to allow injection of embolization glues or particles.

Guidewire-Controlled Superselective Catheterization

Early attempts to reach peripheral lesions superselectively with coaxial catheter systems were stymied by the lack of small radiopaque catheters and suitable torqueable guiding wires. In the late 1960s Eisenberg[30] devised the first commercially available steerable guidewire-catheter combination for coaxial use (Fig. 8-11). The set consisted of a 3.5 French thin-walled Teflon catheter with a flexible, shapeable tip connected to a hemostatic irrigation adapter, through which could be fitted a 0.025-inch torqueable guidewire. The guidewire consisted of a relatively stiff, 65-cm-long, spring stainless steel cannula that ended in a very floppy but torqueable 15-cm spring segment with a shapeable tip. The system was used through a 6 French C-shaped thin-walled polyethylene guiding catheter that could be introduced selectively into primary or secondary aortic branches with a special torque guide.[31] It was successfully used for many years for superselective catheterization of abdominal visceral arteries[32] and of thyrocervical arteries and for sampling

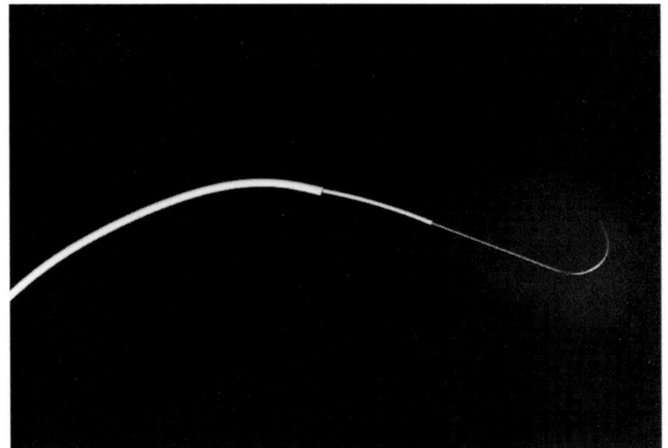

Figure 8-11. Eisenberg coaxial set. The distal floppy segment of the 0.025-inch torqueable guidewire is protruding from the 3.5 French Teflon catheter, which has been inserted through a 6 French nontapered polyethylene preshaded guiding catheter.

thyroid veins for possible functioning parathyroid tumors.[18] A decade later, Cope introduced a simpler steerable 0.018-inch guidewire initially designed for transhepatic catheterization[33] but subsequently also used for vascular catheterization. It consisted of a core guidewire tapered distally to a very fine flexible tip wrapped with either a stainless steel or a platinum helical spring for improved radiopacity. The tip configuration could be easily reshaped manually.

Today's sophisticated wires, which are based on the same design principles, can vary in diameter from 0.010 to 0.018 inch, and in length from 65 cm to exchange lengths. Steerable guidewires are commercially available in a wide array of configurations designed to better fit the needs of a variety of anatomical circulatory patterns. A number of variable factors can change the torque characteristics, the flexibility, the pushability, and the tip shape of these fine steerable guidewires, such as shaft diameter, length and smoothness of taper, direct connection of core taper to the coil tip versus its attachment through an intermediary safety ribbon, slipperiness of surface coating, thrombogenicity, and degree of tip shape memory (Fig. 8-12).

As a result of the increasing clinical success of percutaneous coronary artery transluminal angioplasty, microwires quickly became a crucial part of the armamentarium of cardiologists for safely guiding balloon catheters through tortuous diseased coronary arteries.[34] Steerable wires also began to play a key role in passing microcatheters into the cerebral, hepatic, and peripheral circulation for diagnosis, thrombolysis, or embolization (Fig. 8-13). The first 3 French catheters

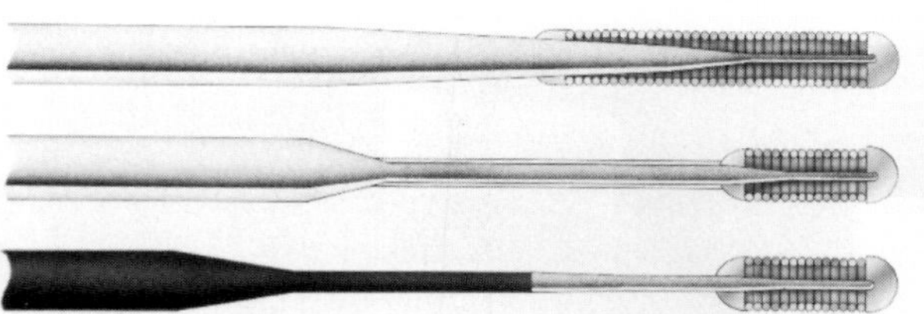

Figure 8-12. Steerable microguidewires (Target). Guidewire characteristics are varied by altering the taper length and thickness of the distal inner core.

to be tried in conjunction with these specialized wires were made of Teflon for their inherent lubricity, but they were found to be too stiff to negotiate complex curves. More flexible, open-ended, coated, coiled spring guidewires, introduced by Sos,[35] were found to

Figure 8-13. Coaxial superselective catheterization requires a 6 French or 7 French introducing catheter through which 3 French or 4 French catheters can be advanced over a fine torqueable guidewire. Continuous irrigation between the two catheters is important to prevent clotting. (From Cope C, Burke DR, Meranze SG, eds. Atlas of interventional radiology. St. Louis: Mosby, 1990. Used with permission.)

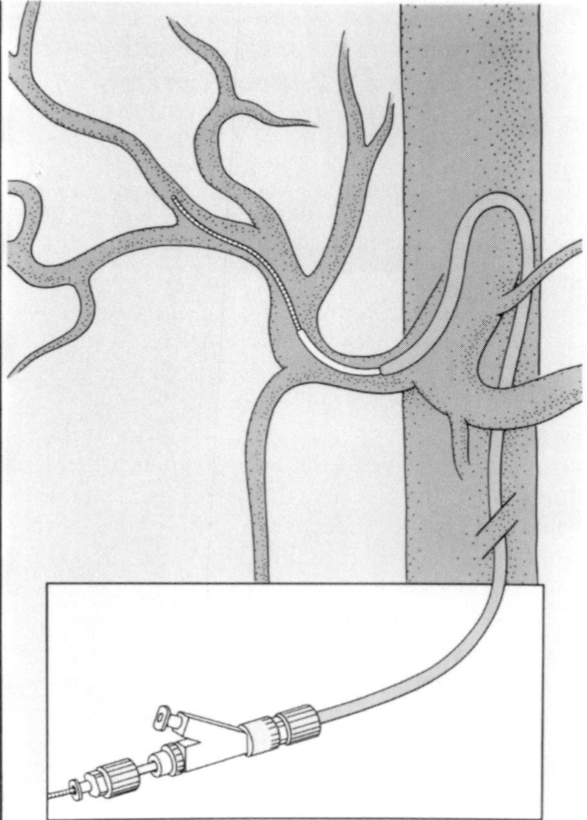

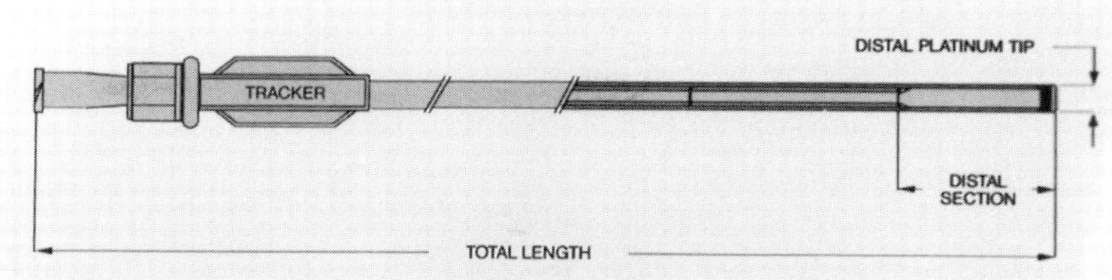

Figure 8-14. Typical microcatheter (Target) made with three increasingly flexible segments.

be useful in conjunction with steerable guidewires for superselective thrombolysis and embolization, especially in the abdomen[36] and extremities. Although these spring-sheathed catheters have excellent radiopacity, high pressure tolerance, good pushability, and the ability to accept relatively large particulate emboli, they are often not flexible enough to follow a fine guidewire through multiple tight vascular curves.

The modern plastic microcatheter for superselective catheterization is designed with a progressive stiffness profile and consists of a relatively rigid body to provide some torqueability and pushability, a middle segment of intermediate flexibility, and a floppy distal segment with a radiopaque metal marker at the tip (Fig. 8-14). The catheter body wall is made more rigid by using a stiffer plastic, two plastic layers, or incorporating a wire mesh. The distal floppy tail can be made of polyethylene, polyurethane, or Pursil (Balt Extrusion, Montmorency, France) catheter tubing, all of which have a sufficiently low coefficient of friction to allow the free insertion of a matching steerable guidewire. Microcatheter systems currently in use are available from Target Therapeutics, Balt, and Terumo (Tokyo, Japan). Although these catheters are primarily designed for treating neurovascular lesions, they have been eagerly adopted by general interventional radiologists for use throughout the body. Representative of microcatheter systems available in this country is the popular Tracker 18 high-flow infusion catheter from Target Therapeutics. Extruded from a composite of stiffer polypropylene core and an outer clear polyethylene coat over its proximal and middle sections, the catheter tapers from a 3.2 French body to a floppy, nonradiopaque, polyethylene 2.2 French distal segment through two smooth transition zones with a corresponding diminution in internal diameter from 0.039 to 0.021 inch.[37] The platinum radiopaque marker enlarges the catheter tip slightly to 2.7 French (Fig. 8-15). Because its wall surface has a low coefficient of friction, this catheter can be readily threaded through any standard preshaped selective guiding catheter with a 0.038-inch tip opening and will freely track over a 0.018- or 0.016-inch steerable guidewire. Its tip can be manually preshaped to any desirable curve with steam. Despite its limited lumen, it will allow the injection of 60 percent contrast medium at a rate of 0.4 to 1.0 ml per second and will accept particulate microemboli up to 600 to 700 μ. In addition, it is capable of allowing a variety of fibered platinum coils (Fig. 8-16) to be threaded through it with a special pusher stylet. As with any coaxial system, it is important to prevent possible backup of blood, microemboli, and binding of the guidewire by using a continuous pressurized flushing system with heparinized saline through both the guidewire and the superselective catheter (Fig. 8-17).

Superselective catheterization is usually performed by a series of steps, consisting first of advancing both the microcatheter and the steerable wire through the guiding catheter to the second- or third-order branch, then further manipulating the angled-tip guidewire to the vessel feeding the lesion under study, and finally sliding the catheter over the wire to its tip. The guidewire and the catheter should be advanced in slow, measured steps with frequent back-and-forth maneu-

Figure 8-15. Floppy tip of Tracker catheter (Target) with protruding microguidewire (0.016 inch). Note the platinum radiopaque sleeve marker.

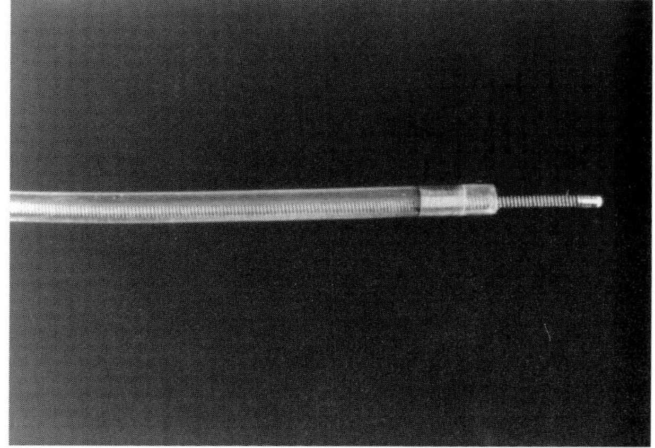

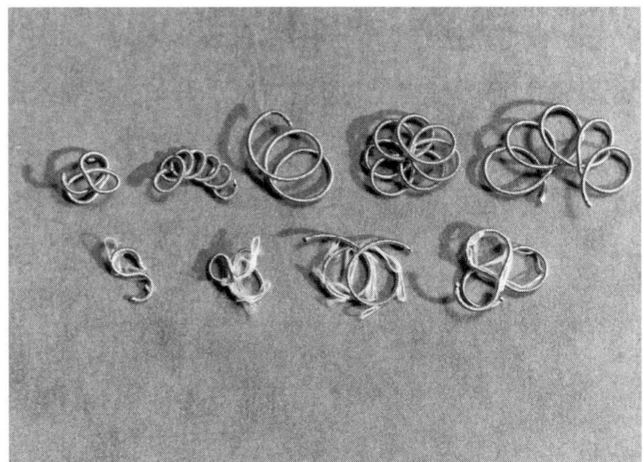

Figure 8-16. Assortment of embolization coils for the Tracker catheter (Target).

vers with the aid of fluoroscopic digital road-mapping or with frequent opacifications of the vascular bed to ensure that these devices are following the proper course. In difficult cases, the operator should strongly consider preshaping the tip of the catheter with steam to allow it to track better over the guidewire. This can also allow the operator to use the softer bent tip for primary guidance while the guidewire is partially withdrawn within the catheter.

Flow-Sensitive Microcatheters

The catheter that is potentially ideally suited to negotiate very complex vascular branching patterns with minimal trauma should be superflexible and flow-directable and should not require a steerable guide past the tip of the catheter. Such a catheter, which is used by neuroradiologists, is usually made of very floppy, rubbery Silastic-type material that can be launched from a fluid-filled propulsion chamber through a nontapered guiding catheter toward a high-flow lesion, such as an arteriovenous malformation or a very vascular tumor. So that these catheters can be more efficiently drawn toward the lesion by the higher blood flow, they can be fitted with either a detachable balloon or a calibrated leak balloon that can be partially inflated.[38] Because this technique is cumbersome and sometimes unreliable, flow-guided catheters with more directional control have been devised. Typical of this construction is the progressive-suppleness Pursil Magic catheter (Balt), which consists of a stiff 3 French polyurethane shaft to which is bonded a 25-cm length of floppy Pursil catheter that tapers from 2.5 to 1.8 French and has a radiopaque platinum marker at its tip.[39] At a pressure of 80 psi, this catheter can deliver 60 percent contrast at a rate of 10 ml per minute and permits the use of a wide variety of liquid and particulate agents for embolization. The floppy tip can not only be curved by heat but can also be flared into a bulbous tip so that it can be freely carried by the bloodstream (Fig. 8-18). Because of its stiffer shaft, there is also some torque transmission to the delicate, whiplike extremity. The direction of this catheter can also be controlled by rapidly injecting small amounts of saline or contrast, which causes recoil and realignment of the curved floppy tip. Some increased degree of control may be gained by inserting a fine torque guidewire (Dasher 10, Target Therapeutics) partially

Figure 8-17. Tracker catheter assembly (Target). Note the double irrigation system for the guiding catheter and the inner catheter.

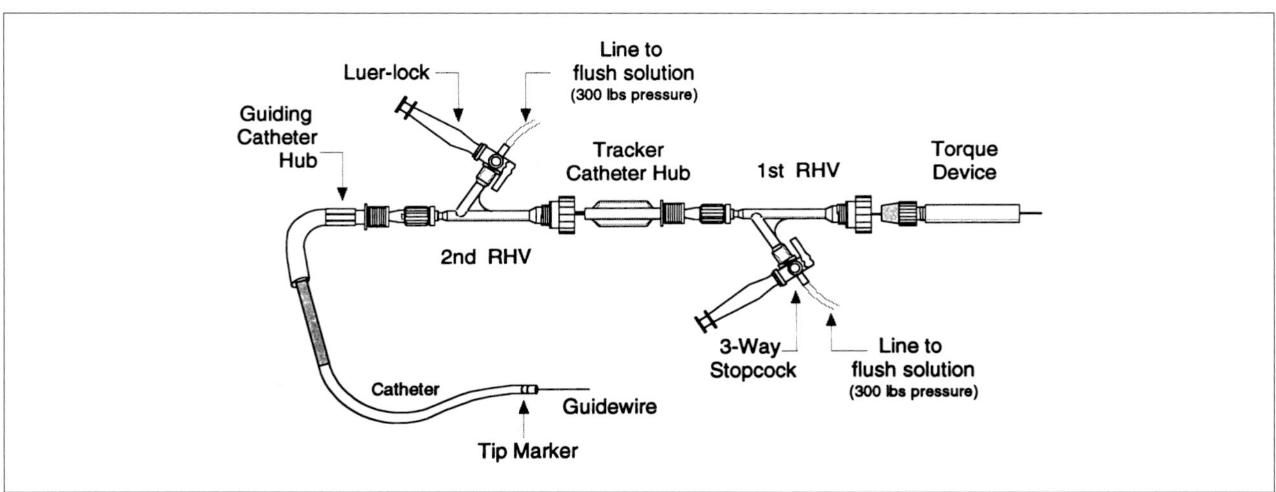

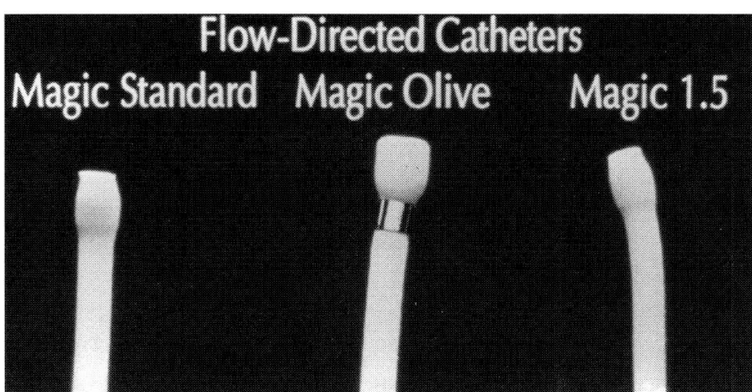

Figure 8-18. Floppy bulbous-tipped Magic microcatheters (Balt). These microcatheters are propelled forward by the bloodstream.

or completely within it. This catheter is inserted with a special stiffening mandrel through a standard 5 French guiding catheter. Because of the small caliber and remarkable floppiness of these flow-guided microcatheters, they are associated with the least risk for compromise of blood flow, vascular spasm, or perforation and the greatest potential for navigating through very peripheral vascular branches. Despite the small lumen of these catheters, they can be used for microembolization and injection of liquid glue and can be fitted with detachable balloons. A larger, less flexible 4.5 French Pursil catheter with a 1-mm lumen is available and is more suitable for use in the abdomen.[40] It is inserted by exchanging it over a guidewire that has been previously placed subselectively with a standard preshaped catheter. Because of its larger caliber, it can also be directed with a slippery hydromer-coated guidewire. The value of this catheter system outside the study of the head and neck will be better evaluated as soon as it is approved in this country. It would appear to have great potential for reaching peripheral hepatic and renal lesions as well as bleeding points in distal small bowel arcades when the guidewire-driven technique proves to be unsatisfactory.

Problems Associated with Superselective Catheterization

Although there are definite advantages to using standard-size catheters and guidewires for superselective catheterization whenever possible because of their sturdiness, good radiopacity, torqueability, and large lumen, there is always a very real risk of their inducing vascular spasm, dissection, or occlusion, especially when excessive zeal is used during the procedure (Fig. 8-19). Although the use of supple microcatheters and

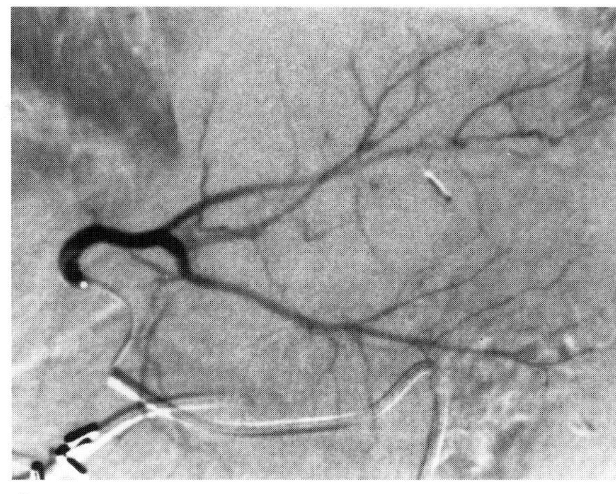

A

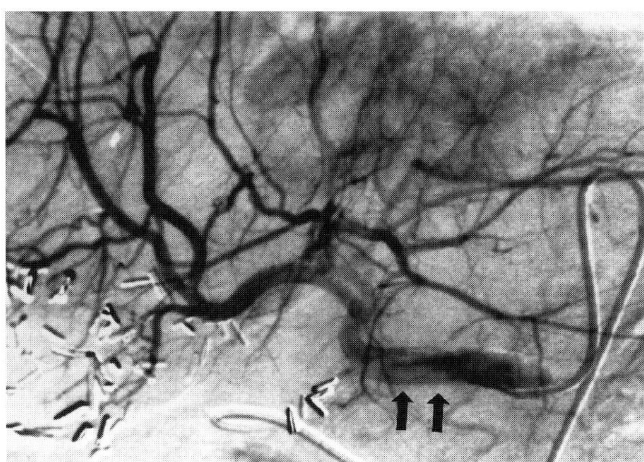

B

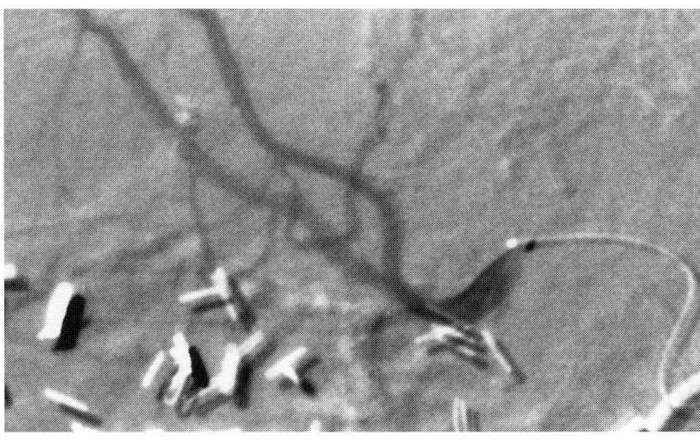

C

Figure 8-19. Superselective chemoembolization of colonic metastatic disease to the liver. (A) The Simmons introduction catheter has been successfully advanced to the distal common hepatic artery for introducing a Tracker catheter superselectively in the left hepatic lobe. (B) On a subsequent visit, the distal common hepatic artery was dissected (*arrows*) by the Simmons introducing catheter and guidewire. (C) Despite the fresh dissection, it was still possible to pass a Target catheter superselectively through the damaged vessel to the right lobe for continued chemoembolization.

steerable guidewires greatly diminishes the chance of serious vascular trauma, problems inherent in the miniaturization of the system can nevertheless still occur.

Catheter and Guidewire Fragility

Because both microcatheters and guidewires are extremely delicate, they must be inspected for defects before use and be handled as carefully as possible to prevent kinking, tearing, or separation. Microcatheters should be inserted with a stylet or a splinting guidewire through the valve of the pressurized directing catheter, and their tips should be followed fluoroscopically until they are in the target artery. A microcatheter should always be advanced or rotated slowly in measured steps to prevent excessive coiling or kinking. The matching guidewires can have exceedingly fine spring tips that can be easily damaged when they are improperly passed through the irrigating valve or when they are being reshaped by hand. The safety wire or distal weld of these guidewires should always be repeatedly checked for integrity during the course of the procedure. If the tip of the catheter or the guidewire is immobilized by small vessels in spasm, it is possible for the tip of the wire[41] or the catheter to separate if the operator tries to withdraw the devices too rapidly.

Radiopacity

Because of the difficulty in visualizing the full length of these microcatheters, the angiography suite should be equipped, in addition to standard screen film changers, with a state-of-the-art digital fluoroscopy system with road-mapping compatibility and with a 1024-line matrix that can provide a resolution of at least three line pairs per mm. The image intensifier should be mounted on a multidirectional C-arm, which can enable the angiographer to easily open up confusing coils of overlapping vessels.

The microcatheter is usually furnished with a platinum or gold ring marker at its tip because the floppy terminal segment is too fine to be rendered adequately radiopaque. This relatively invisible part of the catheter is best monitored by leaving the platinum-tipped steerable guidewire within it whenever possible. If the catheter has to be advanced without the guidewire supporting the terminal segment, it may unknowingly be made to buckle or kink within the larger proximal arterial branches. This may then lead to difficulty in injecting contrast medium or emboli or in reinserting the guidewire or rupture.

The 30 to 42 percent contrast medium used when performing superselective arteriography can be well seen with digital subtraction techniques. It can be safely injected by hand at a rate of 1 ml per second.

Microcatheter Perforation, Rupture, and Separation

Although the static burst pressure of a Tracker Unibody 18 catheter is in the range of 250 to 350 psi, it can withstand slowly increasing infusion rates at higher pressures. The distal floppy segment of the catheter has the thinnest wall and is the most likely to burst. In the author's experience a flow rate of dilute contrast at 1 ml per second or more can be safely achieved as long as the operator does not use a rapid bolus injection technique. If that thin-walled segment is twisted too quickly or allowed to become redundant by advancing it without a guidewire, it may partially collapse or kink, especially around tight turns. When the operator is unaware that the catheter lumen is thus restricted, the tubing may then rupture at the point of narrowing when he or she subsequently injects contrast medium or embolic particles. If the catheter is unknowingly kinked, reinsertion of the guidewire can easily lead to perforation of the wall. When using coaxial catheters, it is extremely important to ensure that both catheters are continuously irrigated. If for some reason the pressurized system is not functioning, a fibrin coating from refluxing blood can build up very quickly and cause increasing friction either between the two catheters or between the microcatheter and the steerable guidewire.[31] If the operator continues to advance the guidewire tip when the wire is bound to the distal catheter, there is a potential risk that the floppy elastic tip may separate from its body.

Catheter Reflux and Whipping

Rapid bolus injection through a small very floppy endhole catheter leads to uncontrolled whipping of the tip. This can cause significant problems such as displacement of the catheter tip from its intended position into a different side branch or else trauma to small peripheral vessels, which can be manifested by spasm or thrombosis or even perforation. If the catheter is being used for fluid sclerosis or particulate embolization, then again excessive pressure and flow through it may lead to dislodgment of the tip and accidental infarction of adjacent normal tissue.[42] On the other hand, careful, purposeful, and controlled rapid injections of small volumes of contrast medium can be a useful maneuver to redirect angled-tip floppy catheters into target vessels.

Clinical Usefulness of Superselective Catheterization

Although superselective catheterization dates back to the mid-1960s, it was not widely used clinically over the next 10 to 15 years because of the lack of well-trained angiographers with sufficient skill and judgment to perform these procedures consistently and safely. Because the simple catheters and guidewires that were used at that time were relatively stiff and had poor maneuverability and trackability, it often proved difficult even for highly experienced angiographers to catheterize branch vessels superselectively with predictable success. The gradual development of a wide variety of specialized 5 to 6 French preshaped catheters and more torqueable guidewires greatly facilitated the practice of these demanding procedures. As a result, the catheterization of second- to fourth-order aortic branches from the thyrocervical through the bronchial, hepatic, gastroduodenal, pancreatic, renal, pelvic, and large limb arteries eventually became fairly routine in many centers.

The more recent introduction of coaxial microcatheter systems has led to a virtual explosion of superselective procedures for lesions that had previously been technically out of reach or too hazardous to catheterize. The peripheral vessels of virtually any organ of the body down to 1-mm branches can today be catheterized with a great chance of success in a rapid and efficacious manner with a markedly diminished chance of causing vascular spasm and dissection.

The following clinical examples typically seen in a busy angiographic practice will demonstrate the value of coaxial microcatheterization in reaching complex lesions for diagnosis or embolization (Fig. 8-20).

Occult Parathyroid Adenoma

The microcatheter system is very useful in sampling for parathormone, not only from the thyroid veins but also from the small cervical and upper mediastinal veins.[18] When an angiographic study demonstrates an adenoma, it can often be defunctionalized with an injection of hypertonic contrast medium[43] if its feeding vessel can be catheterized superselectively.

Hemoptysis

In the evaluation of patients with massive hemoptysis for embolization, the operator needs to be concerned

Figure 8-20. Chemoembolization of hepatoma omental metastases. (A) Selective splenic arteriogram demonstrates the course of the gastroepiploic artery (*arrows*) before superselective catheterization. (B) Tracker catheter positioned in the distal gastroepiploic artery for chemoembolization.

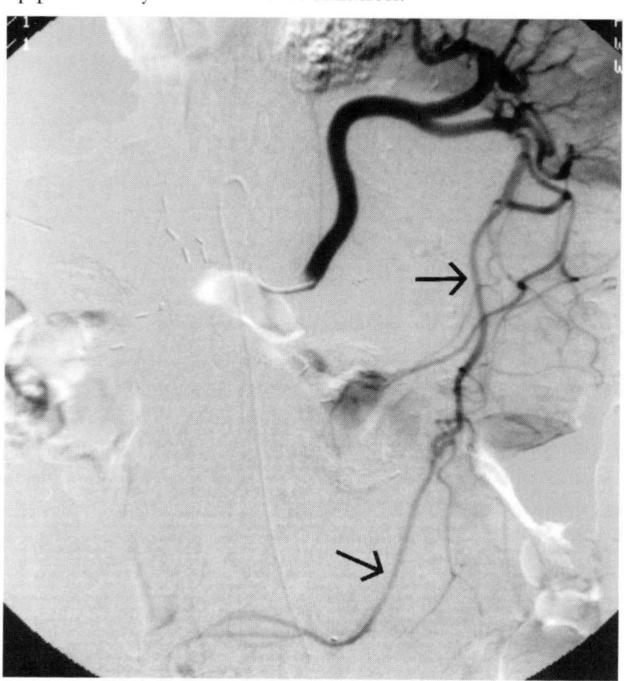

A

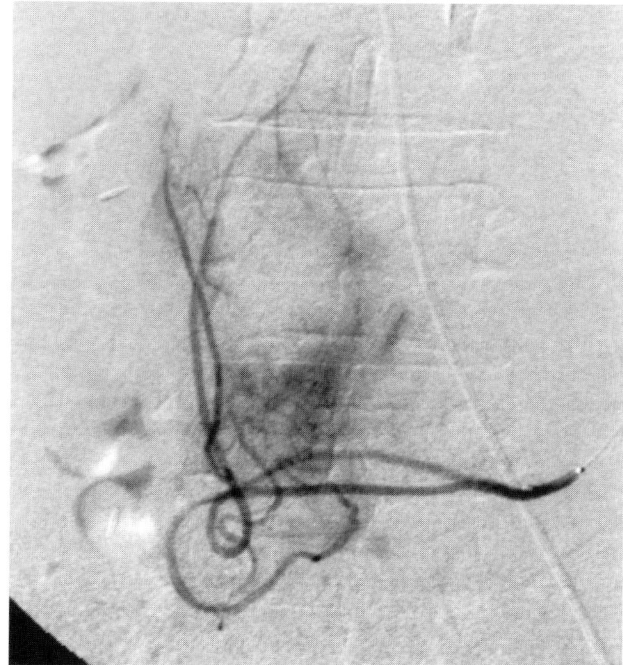

B

with the exact identification of the bleeding vessel and the prevention of spinal cord ischemia.[44]

Because of the small diameter of the microcatheter in relation to the intercostal-bronchial arteries, there is less chance of impairing spinal cord blood supply. In addition, the chances of infarcting the spinal cord are much diminished because the embolization catheter can be advanced past spinal feeders to a safer superselective position. This coaxial system is also very efficacious for catheterizing aberrant bronchial and parasitic vessels arising from subclavian artery branches.

Pancreatic and Gastrointestinal Hemorrhage

The microcatheter system allows very selective embolization of pancreatic and bowel bleeding points or vascular lesions.[45] Embolization of the peripheral arcades of the small[46] and large bowel can be performed to arrest bleeding in some cases without requiring subsequent surgery for possible infarction.

Patients who are hypotensive from gastrointestinal hemorrhage often have marked vasoconstriction of visceral vessels, a condition that can render subselective catheterization difficult or impossible. Because microcatheters do not usually exacerbate visceral artery spasm, they can often be used very successfully to reach and embolize the vascular bleeding point of these shocky patients.

Liver Trauma and Tumor

Although superselective catheterization of the hepatic artery and its branches can often be performed with preshaped 5 French catheters and Terumo guidewires (Medi-tech), the coaxial technique is far more dependable for reaching deeply into the liver. By using superselective embolization[47] or chemoembolization,[48] more normal tissue parenchyma is spared, and one minimizes ischemic damage to the duodenum, gallbladder, and central bile ducts from possible reflux embolization. The coaxial system is especially useful for catheterizing accessory hepatic branches from the su-

Figure 8-21. Superselective embolization of renal metastatic lesion (A) with alcohol (B) in a patient with contralateral nephrectomy.

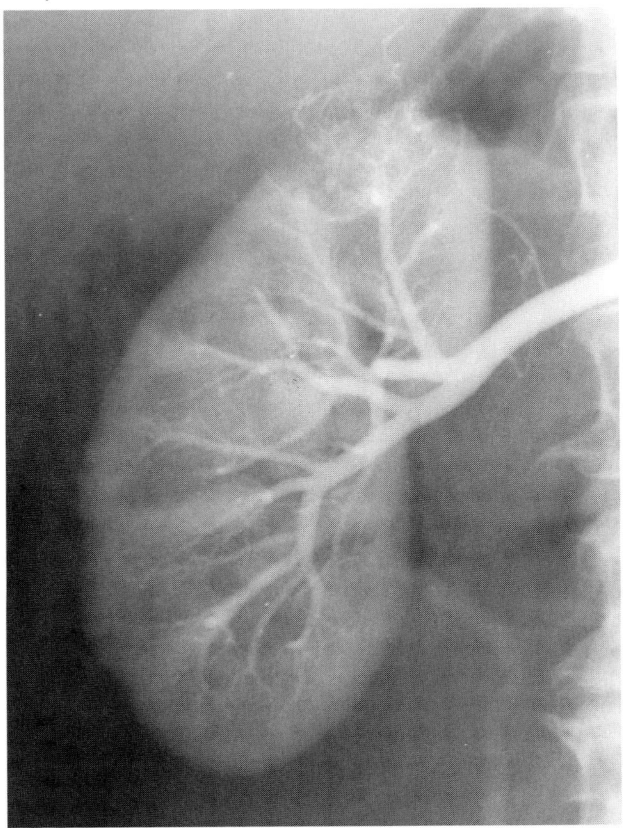

A

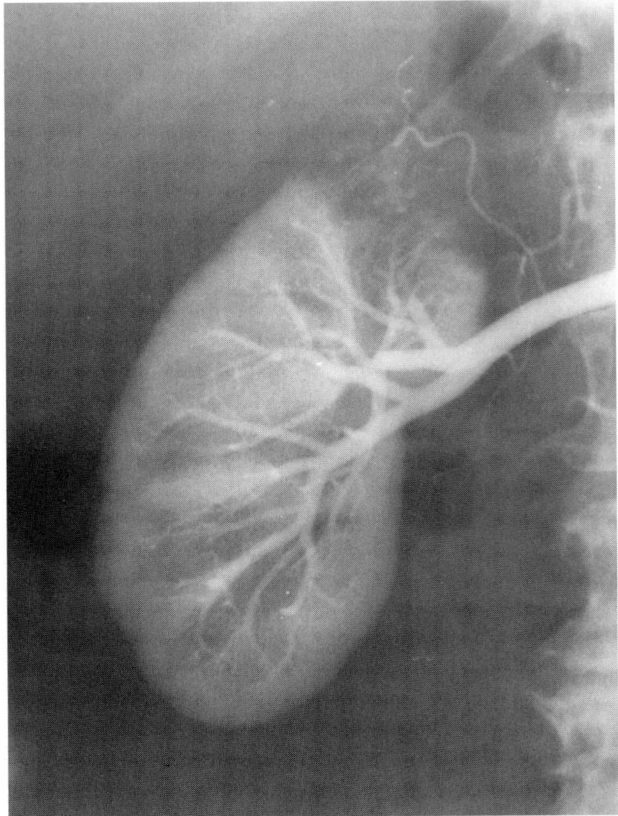

B

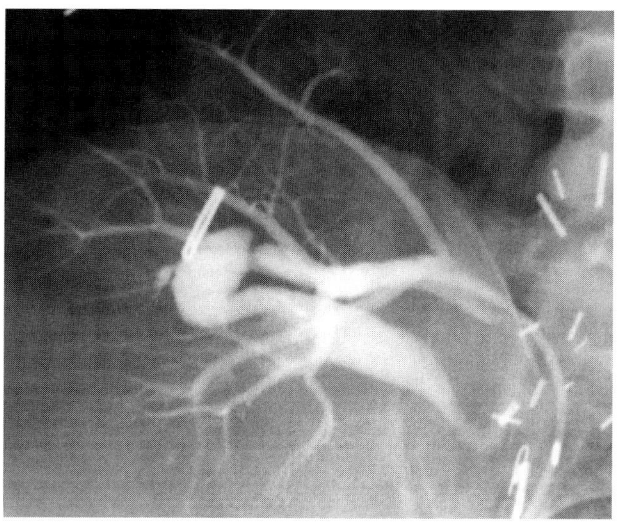
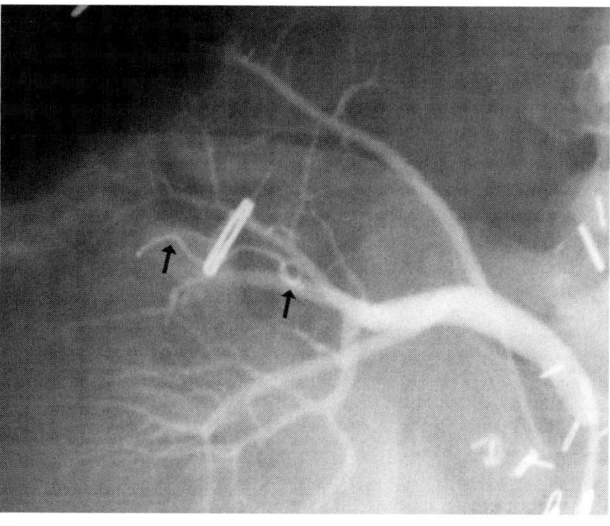

A B

Figure 8-22. Use of microcatheter for renal trauma. (A) Arteriovenous fistula in renal transplant. (B) Tissue-sparing superselective occlusion of the fistula with a coil placed across the feeding artery (*arrows*).

perior mesenteric or the left gastric artery. When the celiac axis or proximal hepatic artery is occluded, a skillful angiographer can use the microcatheter and guidewire to navigate successfully through dilated pancreatic-duodenal-biliary collateral vessels, phrenic, or internal mammary arteries to reach the reconstituted hepatic branches.

Renal Trauma and Tumor

Because renal arteries branch very early into small-caliber radicals and are very prone to go into spasm, the microcatheter is ideally suited for embolization of third- and fifth-order arterial branches for minimizing loss of functioning parenchyma (Fig. 8-21).[49] This is an especially important consideration in the renal allograft, which lacks the potential for collateral flow (Fig. 8-22).[50]

Pelvic Trauma, Tumors, and Impotence

Because of the danger of causing spinal cord and major nerve damage, gluteal muscle infarction, and impotence, embolization of pelvic vessels for traumatic arterial bleeding should be as selective as possible to prevent nontarget ischemia.[51]

In the evaluation of vasculogenic impotence, pudendal artery catheterization may require the use of microcatheters and microangioplasty balloon catheters.[52]

Upper and Lower Extremity Trauma

Microcatheters are ideally suited for reaching wrist and ankle arteries atraumatically without inciting spasm for diagnosis, embolization, or thrombolysis.[53]

Because it is possible to seat these microcatheters deeply into 1- to 2-mm branch arteries, one can successfully embolize small traumatic vascular lesions with little danger of refluxing particles to the hand or foot (Fig. 8-23).

Concluding Remarks on Superselective Catheterization

The skilled angiographer and vascular interventionist can reach almost any vessel in the body with relative ease and safety as a result of ongoing technological improvements in the material and design of catheter-guidewire systems. Superselective catheterization is vital to the proper evaluation and management of remote lesions amenable to embolization or chemotherapy. By allowing an operator to bypass branch vessels that potentially feed major nerves, the spinal cord, or other susceptible tissues, microcatheters are indispensable for preventing catastrophic complications.

Superselective catheterization is a very powerful method for sampling hormonal blood levels to detect functioning endocrine tumors. In the future, when more sensitive, specific tumor markers are developed,

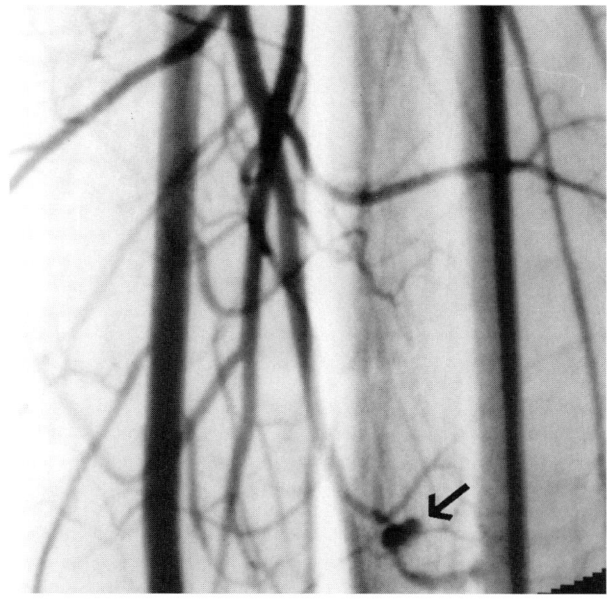

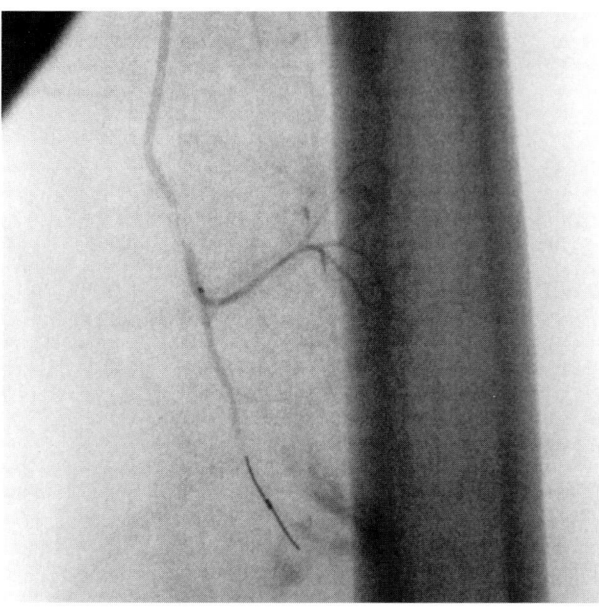

A B

Figure 8-23. Proximity bullet wound in thigh. (A) Bleeding point (*arrow*) from the superficial femoral artery appears at first glance to arise from the deep femoral artery. (B) Coaxial superembolization of the pseudoaneurysm arising from a small side branch of the superficial femoral artery.

it may play an even more important role for localizing and destroying nascent malignancies of all types.

Mechanical Injectors

A great deal of dilution occurs when contrast material is injected into the vascular system. The amount of dilution depends on the velocity of blood flow in the vessel or chamber as well as on the rate and amount of contrast material being injected. Selective coronary arteriography can be performed at injection rates of 4 ml per second, and very satisfactory studies can be obtained with hand injections. Aortography or angiocardiography requires injection rates up to 40 to 50 ml per second. Obviously, these rates can be accomplished only with a mechanical injector.

The factors controlling flow through nondistensible catheters can be expressed as Poiseuille's law:

$$Q = \frac{\pi P r^4}{8 n l}$$

in which

Q = cubic centimeters of contrast material delivered per second
P = hydraulic pressure in dynes per cubic centimeter
r = radius of the catheter lumen in centimeters
n = viscosity coefficient of the contrast material in poises
l = length of catheter in centimeters

This formula assumes that laminar flow is maintained throughout the injection. The viscosities of frequently used contrast materials, measured at 38°C (95°F) and expressed in centipoises, are as follows:

Hypaque 50%	2.5
Renovist II	3.4
Renografin 60%	4.0
Conray 60%	4.0
Isopaque 280	4.1
Hypaque 60%	4.2
Conray 400	4.4
Renovist	5.3
Hypaque—M 75%	8.3
Angio—Conray 80%	8.4
Renografin 76%	8.4
Isopaque 440	10.4
Cardiografin	14.0
Hypaque—M 90%	18.7

One can draw the following conclusions from this information:

1. The speed of injection can be increased by using contrast material with low viscosity. Because the viscosity decreases as the temperature rises, it is important that the contrast be at body temperature at the time of injection.
2. The speed of injection can be increased by using short, thin-walled catheters. As the ratio of lumen to wall thickness increases, there is a corresponding increase in flow rate through the catheter. A short catheter decreases the peripheral resistance and thereby increases the speed of injection. Side holes have a similar effect.
3. Increasing the pressure of injection will increase the delivery rate. The rupture pressure of the specific catheter is an obvious limiting factor.

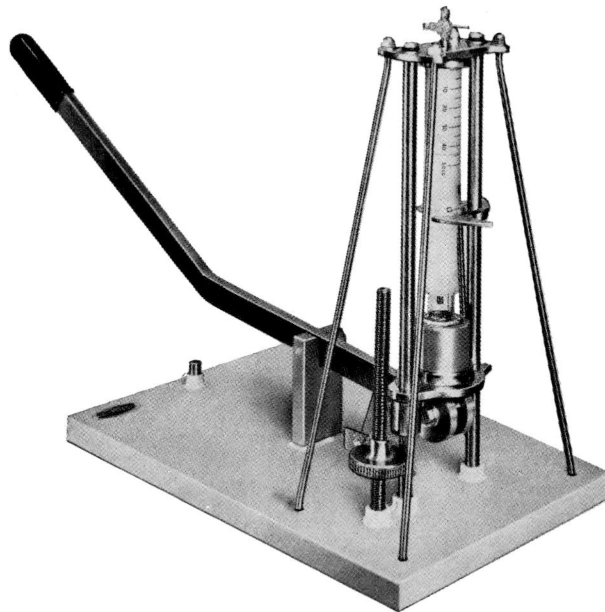

Figure 8-24. Lehman manual injector (Hogan X-Ray Co.).

Basic Types of Pressure Injectors

Hand Injectors

Usually, hand injectors incorporate movable levers that transmit force to a steel or reinforced-glass syringe. These are simple instruments: the force they deliver is inconstant and therefore difficult to reproduce on multiple injections. The maximum pressure is generally inadequate for injections through small catheters (Fig. 8-24).

Pneumatic Power Injectors

These devices use compressed gases to transmit pressure directly to a cylinder, which is connected to the injector syringe. They operate under basic pneumatic and hydraulic principles. In keeping with Pascal's law that pressure applied to a liquid at any point is transmitted equally in all directions, if the area of the pressure cylinder is larger than that of the syringe, a mechanical advantage or power factor is obtained. Thus a power factor of 5 means that the area of the pressure cylinder is five times the area of the syringe.

Because of the very high pressures that such a system generates, it is necessary to use specially designed stainless steel syringes that tolerate high pressures. Because these syringes are not transparent, special features have to be built in to avoid the inadvertent injection of any air that may enter the syringe while it is being filled with contrast material.

Many injectors have been described that work on the principle of compressed gases. In 1956 Gidlund[54] described a compressed-air injector with a stainless steel syringe that could be placed in a vertical position. This position facilitated the addition of a valve for air removal at the top of the syringe. The contrast material was kept at body temperature by a thermostatically controlled water bath that surrounded the injector syringe. Injection pressure could be varied.

In 1960 Amplatz[55] described a cardiovascular injector powered by carbon dioxide cartridges such as those commonly used for the preparation of carbonated beverages (Fig. 8-25). The syringe was bathed by a thermostatically controlled water bath so that the contrast material could be kept at 38°C (95°F). The major advantage of this system was that the injector weighed only 5 kg.

Mechanical Injector Powered by a Series of Springs

The hydraulic system of the Taveras injector (Picker X-Ray Co.) is powered by a series of springs, and the speed of injection can be controlled by an adjustable valve. The syringe is made of stainless steel, and contrast material can be kept at body temperature by a thermostatically controlled water bath. The syringe is pointed downward so that air bubbles in the system will rise to the surface and will not be injected. As an additional assurance against the inadvertent injection of air, the unit retains approximately 3 to 6 ml of con-

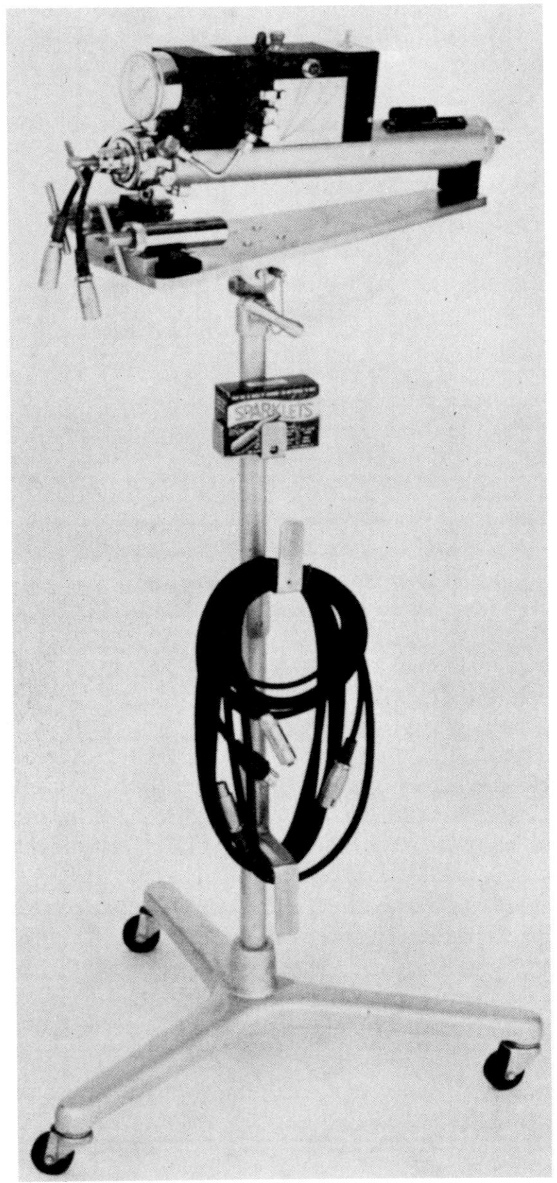

Figure 8-25. Amplatz injector (Nedmac Inc.).

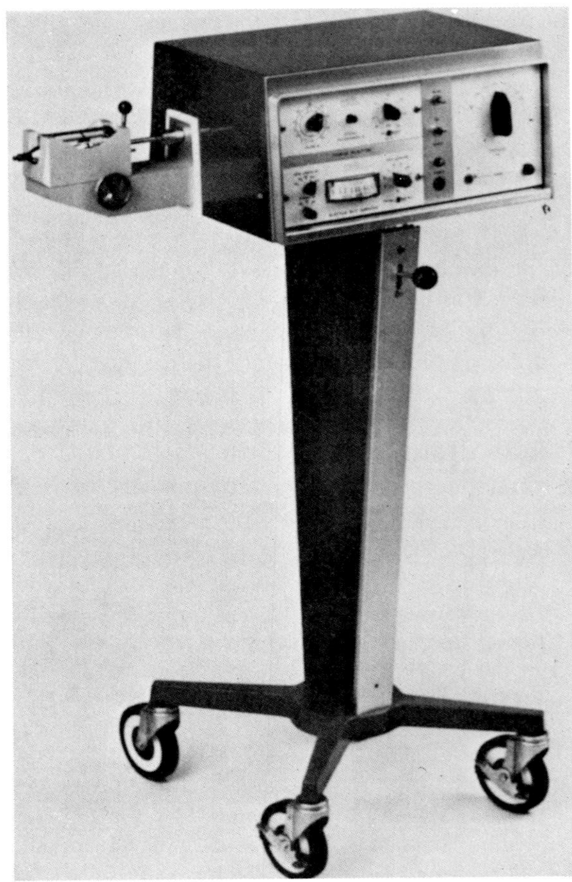

Figure 8-26. Cordis injector (Cordis Corp.).

trast material within the syringe. The injector has been very popular in retrograde brachial arteriography for the visualization of the carotid and vertebral circulation. Because the plunger of the syringe moves from top to bottom, saline may be layered on top of the contrast, thus reducing the volume of contrast material usually required. During injection, the physiologic saline follows the contrast and fills the brachial artery. This method makes the procedure much less painful for the patient.

Electrically Powered Mechanical-Drive Injectors

Most injectors in use today are mechanical-drive injectors that are electrically powered. They are portable, and the only source of power necessary is an electric outlet. They can be programmed with the electrocardiogram so that multiple small injections can be made during very specific phases of the cardiac cycle. The Cordis injector was one of the earliest such units available, and it has remained very popular in the United States (Fig. 8-26).

More recently introduced automatic injectors incorporated built-in safeguards against the hazards of ventricular fibrillation resulting from inadequate grounding of an electric injector at the time the patient's catheter is connected to the syringe (Figs. 8-27 through 8-29). An incorporated ground-safe detector detects malfunction of any of the electric circuits in which the preferential voltage ground would be conducted from the patient via the catheter to the injector

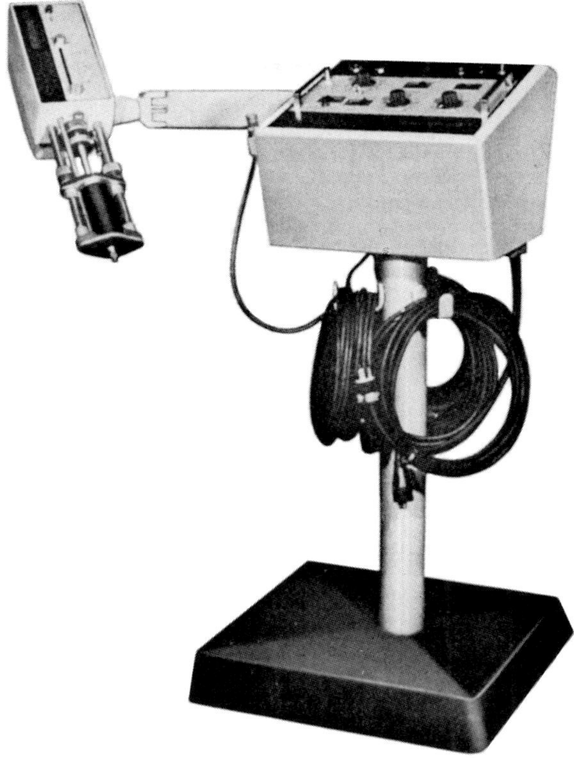

Figure 8-27. Viamonte-Hobbs injector (Barber-Colman Electro-Mechanical Products).

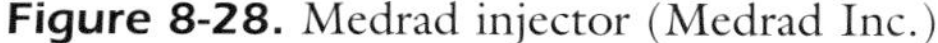

Figure 8-28. Medrad injector (Medrad Inc.).

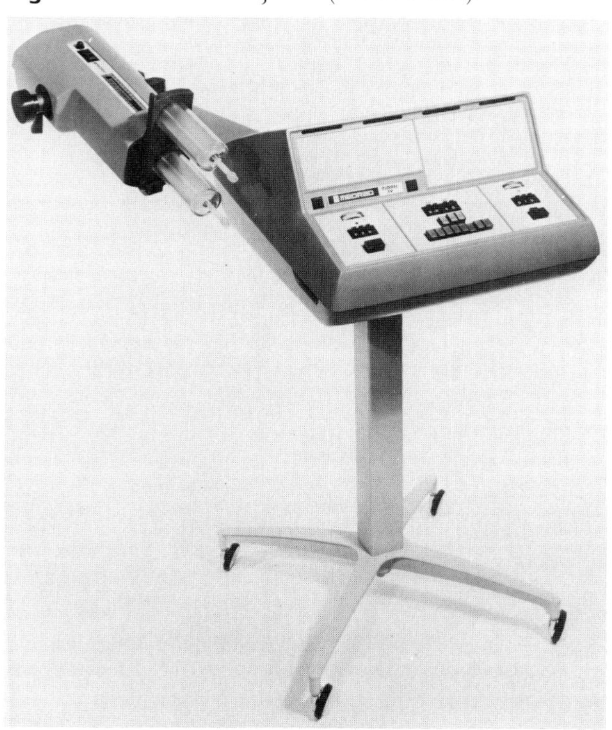

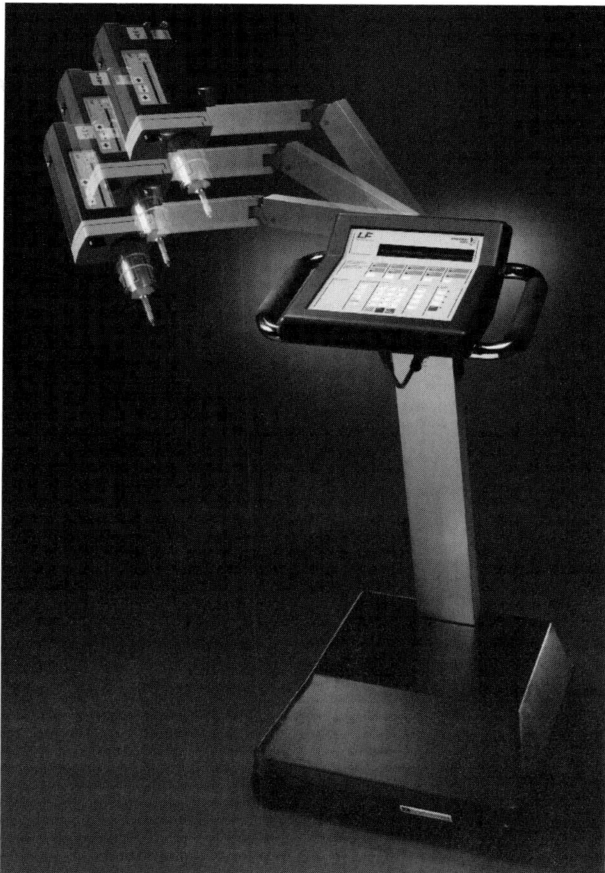

Figure 8-29. Liebel-Florsheim injector.

and to the building ground. The detector has a sensitive sensing circuit that can detect the potential difference of 40 mV or higher; the injector then automatically breaks its ground circuit, the procedure stops, and an audible alarm sounds. Because a catheterization laboratory uses so much electric equipment that comes in contact with the patient (e.g., electrocardiograph, electric catheterization tables, pressure transducers, pressure injectors), unsafe grounding is potentially hazardous. Currents as low as 20 μA (60 cycles per second A.C.) with voltages as low as 60 mVA can induce ventricular fibrillation in dogs. Currents of 1 to 4 μA (60 cycles per second A.C.) have fibrillated the human heart during surgery.

These injectors also operate on the principle of metered delivery rate, which not only provides an automatic control of flow rate by compensating for injection variables but also eliminates time-consuming charts. One dial on the control panel selects the duration of the injection (1–4 seconds), and a second dial selects the delivery rate (2–60 ml per second).

References

1. Seldinger SI. Catheter placement of needles in percutaneous arteriography: a new technique. Acta Radiol 1953;39:368–376.
2. Ödman P. Percutaneous selective angiography of the main branches of the aorta. Acta Radiol 1956;45:1–14.
3. Boijsen E. Selective hepatic angiography in primary and secondary tumors of the liver. Rev Int Hepat 1965;15:385–395.
4. Paul RE, Miller HH, Kahn PC, et al. Pancreatic angiography with application of subselective angiography of the celiac and superior mesenteric artery for the diagnosis of carcinoma of the pancreas. N Engl J Med 1964;272:283–287.
5. Takayasu K, Muramatsu Y, Moriyama N, et al. Plastic-coated guide wire for hepatic arteriography. Radiology 1988;166: 545–546.
6. Cope C, Machan L. Method to control spraying of high-velocity infected blood droplets during arterial catheterization. Radiology 1990;174:1055.
7. Olsen LW, Jeffrey RB, Tolentius CB. Closed system for arterial puncture in patients at risk for AIDS. Radiology 1988;166: 551–552.
8. Cope C. Minipuncture angiography. Radiol Clin North Am 1986;24:359–367.
9. Frink NC, Paolella LP, Dorfman GS. Angioplasty sites: assessment with the dual access technique. Radiology 1990;174:264.
10. Kaufman SL. Angioplasty from the contralateral approach: use of a guiding catheter and coaxial angioplasty balloons. Radiology 1990;177:577.
11. Cope C, Burke DR, Meranze SG, eds. Atlas of interventional radiology. St. Louis: Mosby, 1990.
12. Chuang VP, Soo C-S, Carrasco CH, et al. Superselective catheterization technique in hepatic angiography. AJR 1983;41: 803–811.
13. Remy J, Arnaud A, Fardou H, et al. Treatment of hemoptysis by embolization of bronchial arteries. Radiology 1977;122: 33–37.
14. Carsen GM, Casarella WJ, Spiegel RM. Transcatheter embolization for treatment of Mallory-Weiss tears of the esophagogastric function. Radiology 1978;128:309–313.
15. Richman SD, Green WM, Kroll R, et al. Superselective transcatheter embolization of traumatic renal hemorrhage. AJR 1977;128:843–844.
16. Matalon T, Athanasoulis CA, Margolies MN, et al. Hemorrhage with pelvic fractures: efficacy of transcatheter embolization. AJR 1979;133:859–867.
17. Fisher RG, Ben Menachem Y. Embolization procedures in trauma: the extremities—acute lesions. Semin Intervent Radiol 1985;2:118–124.
18. Eisenberg H, Palotta J, Sherwood LM. Selective arteriography, venography and venous hormone assay in diagnosis and localization of parathyroid lesions. Am J Med 1974;56:816–820.
19. Kirschner MA, Jacobs JB. Combined ovarian and adrenal vein catheterization to determine the site(s) of androgen overproduction in hirsute women. J Clin Endocrinol 1971;33:199–209.
20. Roche A, Raisonnier A, Gillon-Sauouret MC. Pancreatic venous sampling and arteriography in localizing insulinomas and gastrinomas: procedure and results in 55 cases. Radiology 1982;145:621–627.
21. Lunderquist A, Borvesson B, Owman T, et al. Isobutyl II cyanocrylate (Bucrylate) on obliteration of gastric coronary vein in esophageal varices. AJR 1978;130:1–6.
22. Formanek A, Rusnak B, Zollikofer C, et al. Embolization of the spermatic vein for treatment of infertility: a new approach. Radiology 1981;139:315–321.
23. Waltman AC, Courey WR, Athanasoulis CA, et al. Technique for left gastric artery catheterization. Radiology 1973;109: 732–734.
24. Cope C. Suture technique to reshape the sidewinder catheter curve. J Intervent Radiol 1986;1:63–64.
25. Cope C. Guidewire extension. Radiology 1985;157:163.
26. Doppman JL, Goldstein SR, Jones RE, et al. The toposcopic catheter: a catheter design for maneuvering through tortuous vessels. Radiology 1979;132:735–737.
27. Sawada C. Selective hepatic angiography using a balloon catheter guide. Radiology 1985;156:545–546.
28. Okasaki M, Nakamura T, Higashihara H, et al. Successful transcatheter arterial embolization for the replaced right hepatic artery: a new technique using a balloon catheter and norepinephrine infusion. AJR 1989;152:204.
29. Nakamura H, Hashimoto T, Oi H, et al. Hepatic embolization through periportal collaterals: balloon occlusion technique. AJR 1987;148:626–628.
30. Eisenberg H. Angiography of the pancreas. In: Hilal S, ed. Small vessel angiography. St. Louis: Mosby, 1983:405–409.
31. Cope C. A new one-catheter torque-guide system for percutaneous exploratory abdominal angiography. Radiology 1969; 92:174–175.
32. Eisenberg H, Steer HL. The nonoperative treatment of massive pyloroduodenal hemorrhage by retracted autologous clot embolization. Surgery 1976;79:414–420.
33. Cope C. Conversion from small (0.018 in) to large (0.038 in) guidewires in percutaneous drainage procedures. AJR 1982; 138:974–976.
34. Simpson JB, Baim DS, Robert EW, et al. A new catheter system for coronary angioplasty. Am J Cardiol 1982;49:1216–1222.
35. Sos TA, Cohn DJ, Srur M, et al. A new open-ended guidewire catheter. Radiology 1985;154:817–818.
36. Bilbao JI, Aqueretta JD, Longo JM, et al. The open-ended guidewire as superselective catheter for intraarterial chemotherapy: experience in 190 procedures. Cardiovasc Intervent Radiol 1990;13:375–377.
37. Rüfenacht DA, Latchaus RE. Principles and methodology of intracranial endovascular access. Neuroimag Clin North Am 1992;2:251–268.
38. Kerber CW, Bank WJ, Cromwell LO. Calibrated leak balloon microcatheter: a device for arterial exploration and occlusive therapy. AJR 1979;132:207–212.
39. Dion JE, Duckwiler GR, Lylyk P, et al. Progressive suppleness. Pursil catheter: a new tool for superselective angiography and embolization. AJNR 1989;10:1068–1070.
40. Hori S, Matsushita M, Narumi Y, et al. Hepatic arterial catheterization with use of a supply catheter with a ball tip. Radiology 1989;171:860–861.
41. Wolpert SM, Kwan ESK, Heros D, et al. Selective delivery of chemotherapeutic agents with a new catheter system. Radiology 1980;166:547–549.
42. Encarnacion CE, Kadir S, Malone RB. Subselective embolization with gelatin sponge through an open-ended guidewire. Radiology 1990;174:265–267.
43. Miller DL, Doppman JL, Change R, et al. Angiographic ablation of parathyroid adenomas: lessons from a 10-year experience. Radiology 1987;165:601–657.
44. Mauro MA, Jaques PF, Morris S. Bronchial artery embolization for control of hemoptysis. Semin Intervent Radiol 1982;9:45–51.
45. Encarnacion CE, Kadir S, Beam CA, et al. Gastrointestinal bleeding: treatment with gastrointestinal arterial embolization. Radiology 1992;183:545–548.
46. Okazaki M, Higashihara H, Koganemaru F, et al. A coaxial catheter and steerable guidewire used to embolize branches of the splanchnic arteries. AJR 1990;155:405–406.
47. Savader SJ, Trerotola SO, Merine DS, et al. Hemobilia after percutaneous transhepatic biliary drainage: treatment for transcatheter embolotherapy. J Vasc Intervent Radiol 1992;3:345–352.
48. Pentecost MJ, Teitelbaum GP, Katz MD, et al. Chemoembolization in hepatic malignancy. Semin Intervent Radiol 1992;9: 28–37.

49. Kaufman SL, Martin LG, Zuckerman AM, et al. Peripheral transcatheter embolization with platinum microcoils. Radiology 1992;184:369–372.
50. Sousa NM, Reidy JF, Kuffman CG. Arteriovenous fistulas complicating biopsy of renal allografts: treatment of bleeding with superselective embolization. AJR 1991;156:507–510.
51. Quinn SF, Frau DM, Saff GN, et al. Neurologic complications of pelvic intraarterial chemoembolization performed with collagen material and cisplatin. Radiology 1988;167:55–57.
52. Fellmeth BD, Bookstein JJ, Valji K. Treatment of arteriogenic impotence with transluminal angioplasty. Semin Intervent Radiol 1989;6:212–219.
53. Hanks SE, Pentecost MJ. Angiography and transcatheter treatment of extremity trauma. Semin Intervent Radiol 1992;9:19–27.
54. Gidlund A. Development of apparatus and methods for roentgen studies in haemodynamics. Acta Radiol (Stockh) 1956; 130(Suppl):1.
55. Amplatz K. A vascular injector with program selector. Radiology 1960;75:955.

9

Magnification Angiography

RICHARD H. GREENSPAN
STANLEY BAUM

Alternative angiographic imaging modalities such as ultrasound, computed tomography, and magnetic resonance angiography have diminished the indications for "scout" angiography in which only major vessels are visualized. These vessels can be seen less invasively by these newer techniques. When angiography is performed, the study is frequently carried out using digital techniques because larger image intensifier tubes make it possible to examine large vascular beds such as the pulmonary and mesenteric circulation. However, if fine vascular detail is demanded, this can only be accomplished with techniques that use a film-screen combination coupled with direct geometric magnification. Improvements in x-ray tube design and materials as well as the availability of rare-earth screens have widened the clinical applicability of magnification angiography and allowed for considerably greater detail than was previously possible.

Three methods have been used to produce a magnified x-ray image: (1) photographic or optical magnification, (2) direct geometric magnification, and (3) electronic magnification.

Photographic or Optical Magnification

This method is applicable only to examination of injected specimens (microangiography) or to very selected experimental and clinical in vivo studies. Basically it consists of obtaining an ultrafine detailed contact angiogram, which is then magnified with either a photographic enlarger or a microscope.[1,2] The specimen must be extremely thin, because the penumbra (edge unsharpness) is subject to the same magnification as the vessel or vessels being studied. To avoid artifacts, attention must be paid to the pressure used for injection and to the particle size and viscosity of the injectate.[3] Good microangiograms can be made from specimens varying in thickness from 1 cm down to a few microns. In examining thin sections, low kilovoltage is essential to preserve contrast. The energy of the beam commonly used is between 10 and 20 kV, and a sealed-off diffraction-type x-ray tube with a beryllium window and a 0.5- to 1.0-mm focal spot is available for use in this examination. Fine-grain film or fine-emulsion glass plates are used to record the image.[4] The time involved in obtaining a proper exposure usually lasts from several minutes up to an hour. Therefore, the specimen must be motionless. Radiographs made by this method may be enlarged up to several hundred times with preservation of fine vascular detail.[5]

Under certain circumstances, microangiography can be accomplished in the living animal. Bellman and coworkers[6–8] and Harrington and Wiedeman[9] studied small vessels in the rabbit's ear and the bat's wing, respectively. It must be emphasized that these are, in general, specific research applications and are not clinically applicable.

Photographic enlargements of contact angiograms made in living animals have been used to study small vessels. The special requirement for any such study is that the tissue or organ being radiographed must be thin and must be in immediate apposition to the film. If deep-lying visceral structures are examined, they must be exposed by surgery, immobilized, and then placed as close as possible to the x-ray film. In the studies reported, fine-grain film in cardboard cassettes was used. With this technique, the angiogram obtained can be photographically magnified up to approximately 10 times with maintenance of reasonable image clarity.[4,10–13]

The aforementioned techniques, although useful in certain limited clinical situations, are not applicable to angiography of visceral vessels in intact larger animals and humans. Photographic enlargement of in vivo standard angiograms in humans made with commercially available equipment is, in general, unsatisfactory.[14] Edge unsharpness due to the penumbra secondary to the use of large focal spots (used to shorten exposure time), magnification of grid lines, and poor contrast due to secondary radiation all degrade the image.[15]

Direct Geometric Magnification

In direct geometric magnification, the x-ray source acts as the enlarging device. The focal spot-to-object distance is short, and the object-to-film distance is long. The divergence of the x-ray beam magnifies the image of the object being filmed (Fig. 9-1). Magnification is in proportion to the ratio of focus-to-object distance to total focus-to-film distance.

X-ray Tubes

The critical element in the system is the x-ray tube. The focal-spot size must be as small as possible (0.3 mm or less).[16] Larger focal spots cannot be used for direct geometric magnification, because the penumbra (edge unsharpness) is magnified as well as the image, and the magnified penumbra destroys detail (see Fig. 9-1).[14,17–19] The tube must also have sufficient power capacity to permit relatively short exposures, thus minimizing motion blurring. X-ray tube technology has advanced to the point that tubes adequate for magnification angiography are commercially available. These tubes have large anodes with the target material specifically designed to withstand the currents necessary for serial magnification techniques. They also possess increased capacity to store and dissipate heat. The anode target angles have been diminished to permit accentuated use of the line-focus principle, permitting a larger area of the target to be bombarded with electrons. This increases the capacity of the tube while retaining a small effective focal spot. The anode rotates rapidly (10,000 rpm) and should be powered by a three-phase generator, which increases the efficiency of production of x-rays. The tubes currently available include a bias control, which can alter the size of the effective focal spot from approximately 0.3 mm down to 0.1 mm. At 0.3 mm the power rating is approximately 30 kW. This diminishes as the selected focal-spot size becomes smaller. It is necessary, therefore, to increase the exposure time when using the smallest possible focal spot. The choice of focal-spot size must be individualized depending on depth of vessel, body part thickness, and anticipated motion of vessels and the body part being radiographed.

Figure 9-1. (A) X-ray film made by standard geometry. (B) Photographic or optical enlargement of x-ray film made by standard geometry. The image itself and the penumbra are both larger, accentuating image unsharpness. (C) Geometric magnification using broad focal spot. The image unsharpness is markedly accentuated, destroying edge detail visibility. (D) Geometric magnification using a theoretical "point source." The image is magnified but retains its edge sharpness.

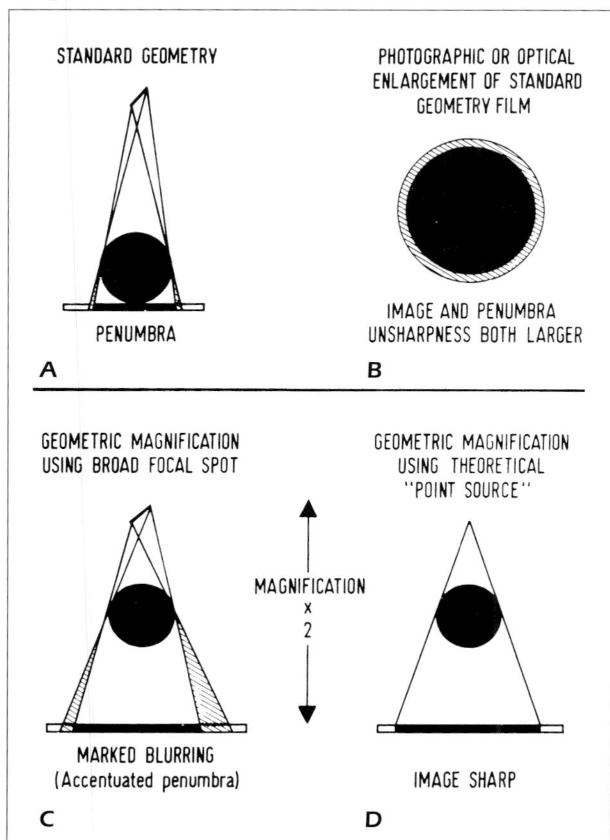

Grids, Screens, and Film

In performing magnification angiography, no grid or Bucky diaphragm is used. The air gap between the object being radiographed and the film dissipates the nonparallel secondary radiation, so that very little of it reaches the film (Fig. 9-2).[14] This is a significant advantage because the use of a grid necessitates longer exposure times to obtain adequate film blackening[20] and increases motion blurring.

The advent of rare-earth screens has been a great aid to magnification angiography. These screens are between four and eight times as efficient as calcium tungstate in capturing x-ray photons and converting them to light. Considerable reduction in exposure duration can be obtained, thus diminishing image blurring due to motion. In the examination of vessels in thin parts of the body, where exposure duration is not a critical factor, the current (mA) can be reduced. This has the effect of reducing the size of the focal spot, because it eliminates the "blooming" effect that high

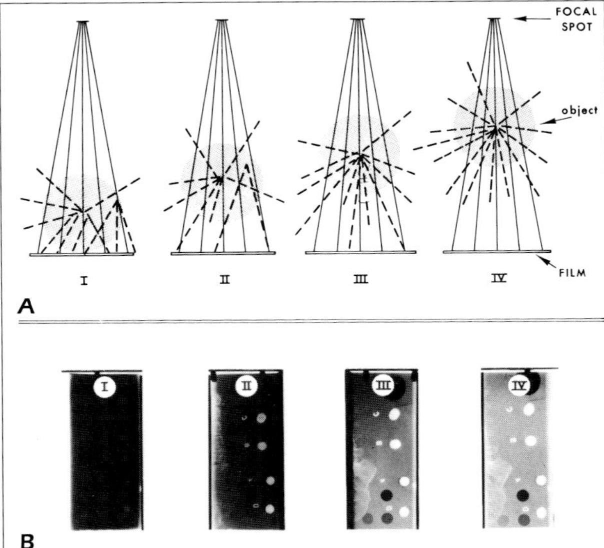

Figure 9-2. (A) Geometric arrangement of experiment. (B) X-ray films of a phantom to demonstrate reduction of scattered radiation by the air gap. All films made with a 0.27-mm focal spot. Identical x-ray technique and focal spot-to-film distance used for all four films. No grid was used. Film *I,* phantom directly on cassette containing x-ray film. Film *II,* phantom moved 4 inches toward tube and away from film. Film *III,* phantom moved 8 inches toward tube and away from film. Film *IV,* phantom moved 12 inches toward tube and away from film. Note that secondary radiation is very intense and obscures detail in film *I.* As phantom is moved away from the film, contrast increases, detail becomes more visible, and magnification can be appreciated.

mA has on the x-ray tube. The result is less edge unsharpness, along with increased detail visibility. Rare-earth screens, however, present a disadvantage in that they possess double the conversion efficiency of standard par-speed screens. Each photon interacting with the screen produces twice as much light, adding radiographic mottle to the image and diminishing the contrast difference between the vessel and the surrounding medium, therefore decreasing the ability to visualize detail.[18,21,22] The mottle can be eliminated by the use of relatively slow film (matched to the spectral output of the screens). Although using slower film diminishes the speed of the system, this factor in most instances is outweighed by the increased contrast and detail visibility provided by the slow film. A rare-earth system using slow- or medium-speed film at approximately 80 kV is up to four times faster than a standard par-speed system and provides greater detail than either high-speed calcium tungstate screens and film or rare-earth screens with fast film.[23] The choice of film, however, should be individualized. In performing angiography through a very thick part, the fastest system (rare-earth screens and fast film) might be preferable, because reduction of motion blur could be a more important factor than eliminating radiographic mottle.

It is not the purpose of this chapter to delve deeply into the theories of visual perception, nor will a detailed discussion of the theoretical lower limits of visibility in magnification angiography be presented. Several theories and equations have been used to define the threshold of detailed perceptibility for x-ray images and screen-film systems. The important factors in these theories are (1) the contrast between the radiographic image and the surrounding medium and (2) the area of the perceived image.[14,22,24,25] Radiographic perceptibility of an object is proportional to its image area and its contrast. Magnification angiography has a distinct advantage over standard angiograms in that scattered radiation is more effectively limited because of the air gap provided by the magnification geometry. This increase in contrast affords better visualization of *large* vessels than one obtains using standard geometry.[14,26]

Figure 9-3. Late arterial phase of normal magnification pulmonary angiogram.

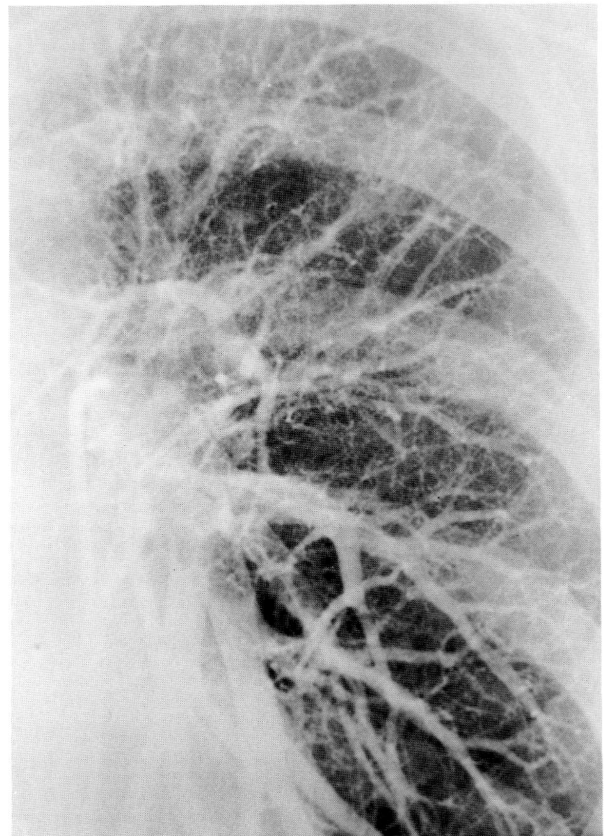

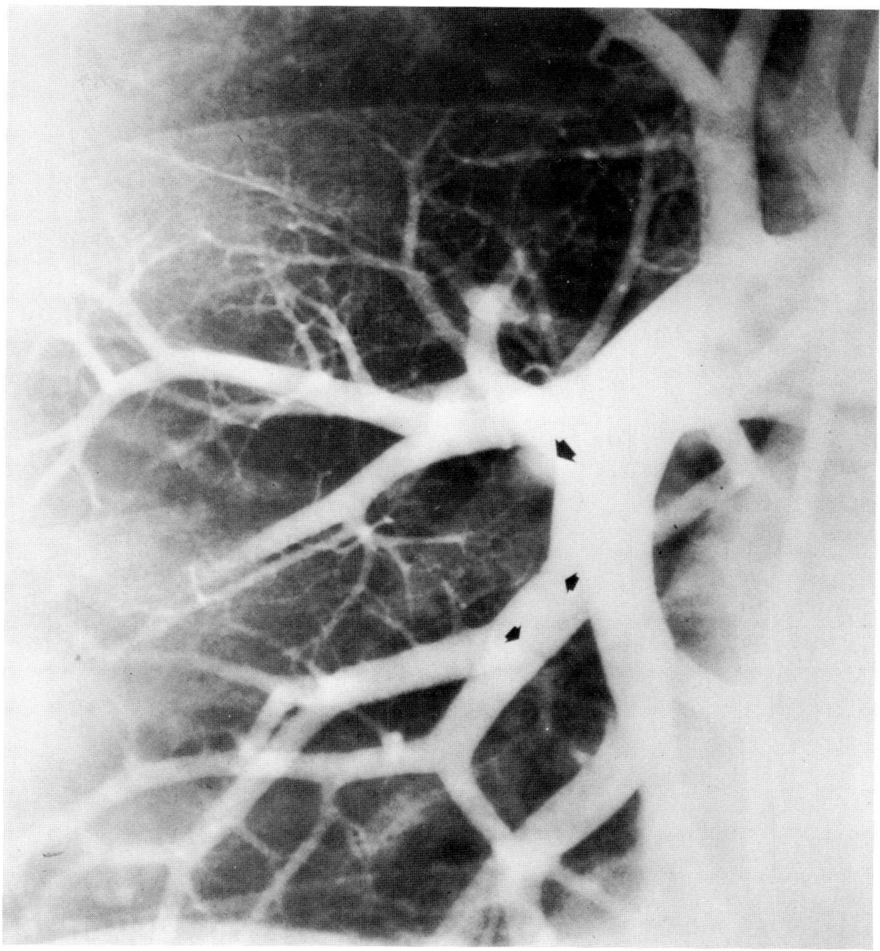

Figure 9-4. Transverse webs (*arrows*) in patient with resolving pulmonary emboli. (Magnification approximately ×3.) The vessels containing the webs are large and could easily be seen on a standard nonmagnified angiogram. The detail on the standard study, however, was not sufficient to visualize these webs.

The area on the intensifying screen and the film over which the vessel is projected are also increased, permitting *smaller* vessels to be seen.[23] A larger number of screen crystals (and film grains) are exposed per object radiographed, thus reducing loss of detail perceptibility secondary to screen grain.[15,18,24,27,28] The resolving power of the screen-film system thus becomes less critical.[26]

Several factors enter into the final resolving power of a magnification system: (1) the size and shape of the effective focal spot, (2) the distribution of radiation across the focal spot, (3) the magnification geometry used, and (4) the screen-film combination chosen. Using the system in vivo for angiography brings into play two other very important factors: (1) the contrast of the vessel or object being studied in relation to the surrounding medium, and (2) the degree of motion blurring that may be present. Choice of focal-spot size (where variable bias tubes are being used), x-ray exposure factors, geometry, and film-screen combinations should be individualized for each type of examination. A combination that may appear best on a theoretical basis and on model testing may not be the best in studying a pulsating vessel in a thick part of the body. Selective injection of contrast material is very important, because a high concentration will permit more vascular detail to be visualized.

Formulas and mathematical models designed to predict magnification and penumbra unsharpness are frequently misleading if the x-ray focal spot is considered a homogeneous source. In most x-ray tubes radiation from the focal spot is nonuniform, and a variable band of decreased radiation intensity in the center of the focal spot may exist.[29,30] As a result, very small ob-

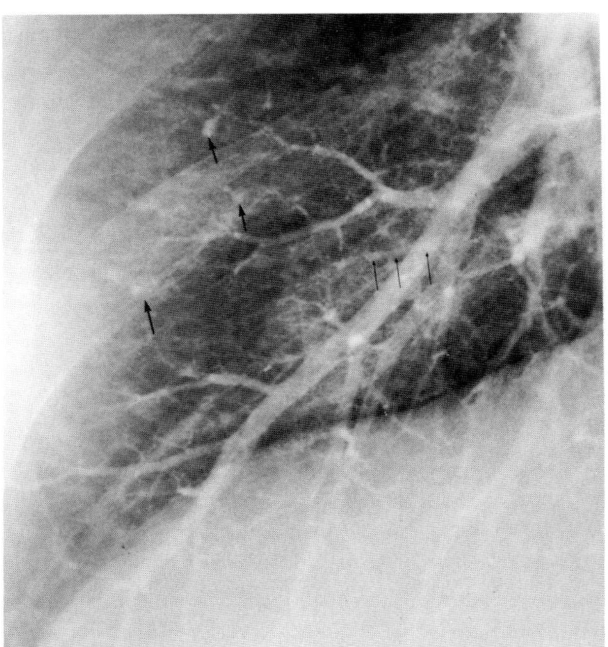

Figure 9-5. Magnification pulmonary angiogram (×3) demonstrating multiple small arteriovenous malformations in the lung (*large arrows*). The *fine arrows* point to an early-filling vein. The standard geometry angiogram was normal.

jects filmed at high magnification may produce a distinct double image, with each part of the image reflecting a much smaller effective focal spot than the overall size of the spot. In some tubes there is considerable discrepancy between the effective focal-spot size parallel to the anode-cathode axis and that perpendicular to the axis.[29]

Objects smaller than the focal-spot size can be recorded on the radiograph. However, the x-ray image of an object slightly larger than, equal to, or less than the focal-spot dimensions does not accurately reflect the true object size.[29,31-33] When the object being x-rayed is sufficiently small, the size of the x-ray image is more closely related to the size of the x-ray focal spot, the degree of magnification, and the orientation of the focal spot to the object than it is to the actual object size.[29,34] These factors must be taken into account when angiography is used to detect and study changes in size of small vessels resulting from physiologic or pharmacologic stimuli.[14,29,30]

Clinical Applicability

Clinically, magnification angiography is used to study all areas of the body. In many departments it is an inte-

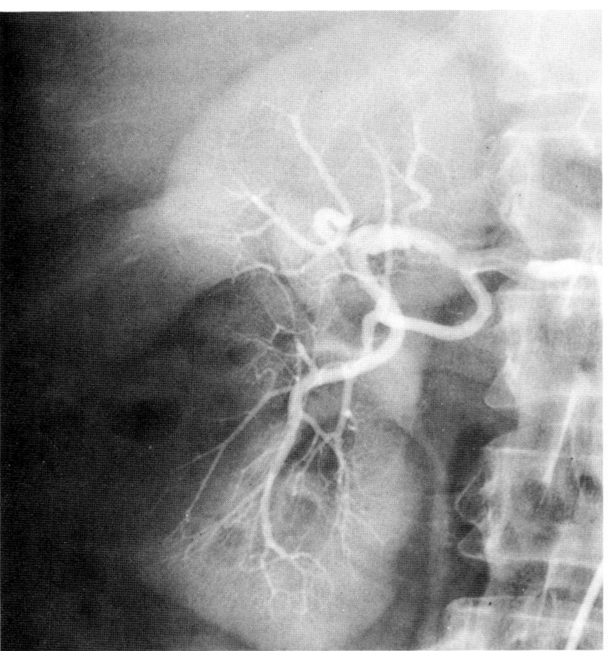

A

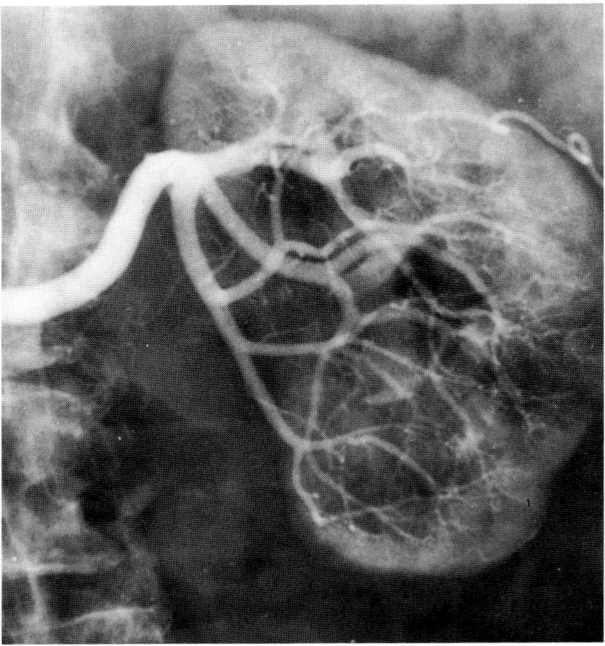

B

Figure 9-6. Magnified renal angiograms (×3). (A) A large avascular renal cyst is present in the right lateral aspect of the right kidney. Note the arcuate and interlobular arteries and the normal thickness of the cortex in the other areas of the kidney. (B) Inflammatory disease of the right lower pole, of long standing. Note the narrowing of the cortex and a small scar at the lower lateral pole of the left kidney.

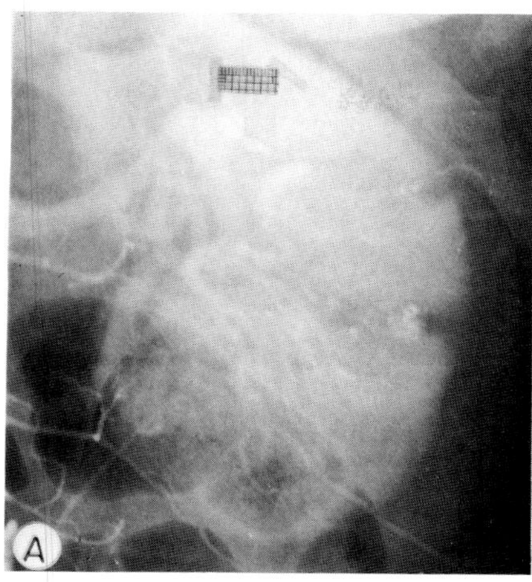

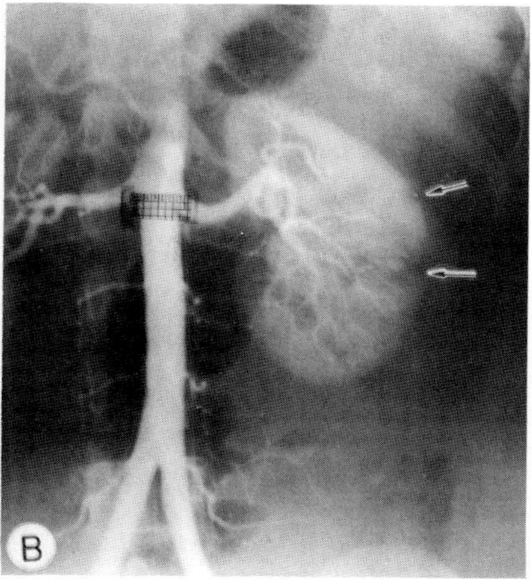

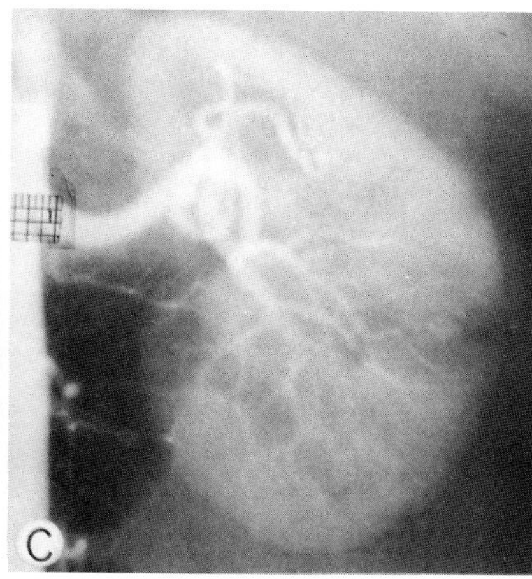

Figure 9-7. Two small arteriovenous malformations in the left kidney of a patient with recurrent hematuria. (A) Magnification (×2.5) arteriogram. The arteriovenous malformations are clearly seen and a zone of diminished perfusion is present distal to both lesions. (B) Standard renal arteriogram shows the zone of diminished perfusion (*arrows*), but the arteriovenous malformations are poorly seen. (C) Photographic magnification of the standard arteriogram. Note the unsharpness of the vessels and the fuzziness of the general kidney outline. (From Greenspan RH, Simon AL, Ricketts HJ, Rojas RH, Watson JC. In vivo magnification angiography. Invest Radiol 1967;2:419. Used with permission.)

gral part of most angiographic examinations.[35] Two basic advantages are apparent when a magnification angiogram is compared to a conventional study: (1) small vessels, poorly visualized or not seen at all with conventional angiograms, can be clearly demonstrated on the magnification study[36,37] (Fig. 9-3) and (2) the detail in arteries large enough to be visible by conventional angiography is significantly enhanced on the magnification study[14,17,26] (Fig. 9-4).

Magnification pulmonary angiography is routinely used in many institutions to detect the possible presence of small pulmonary emboli.[14,17,38] If emboli are not visualized on a standard angiogram, a selective lobar, segmental, or subsegmental angiogram is obtained, using a magnification of approximately 3:1. Selective injection is essential, because the contrast differential between the small vessels and the surrounding lung is a major determinant of the visibility of these vessels. A recently introduced technique involves the use of a double-lumen flow-guided balloon catheter. The catheter is guided into a segmental artery. The balloon is inflated to cut off blood flow, and the contrast material is injected distal to the inflated balloon. Excellent visualization of vessels down to approximately 100 μ can be obtained.[39–42] Characteristic changes have been observed in the vessels of patients with pulmonary hypertension[43] or emphysema, and smaller vascular malformations have been detected (Fig. 9-5). In animals, magnification angiography has been used to study hypoxic vasoconstriction,[44] pulmonary arteritis (in the presence of a normal chest film),[45] and drug effects on the pulmonary circulation.[14] Although the technique is not routinely used in coronary arteriography, it has been used experimentally in normal individuals as well as to demonstrate artificially produced coronary lesions.[46–48]

In the kidney, the arcuate and interlobular arteries are well visualized by this technique[14,36,37] (Fig. 9-6). Small vessels formed within tumors, arteriovenous malformations (Fig. 9-7), and inflammatory conditions are more clearly identified.[49,50] Changes thought to be characteristic of nephrosclerosis have also been identified. The technique has been employed to correlate alterations in the caliber of fine vessels with renal blood flow under experimental conditions, and the response of the renovasculature to pharmacologic stimulation has also been studied.

The tubes initially available for magnification angiography were deficient in power and were not very effective for studying the celiac and mesenteric vessels in large patients because of motion blurring. Current equipment used with rare-earth film-screen systems, however, is adequate for magnification studies of deep-seated abdominal vessels and has proved useful in

Text continues on page 186

Figure 9-8 (overleaf). (A) Standard geometry celiac angiogram. (B) Same patient. Direct geometric magnification (×3). Slightly different timing. Note the vascular detail, in particular the small pancreatic vessels. (Courtesy of Morton Glickman, M.D.)

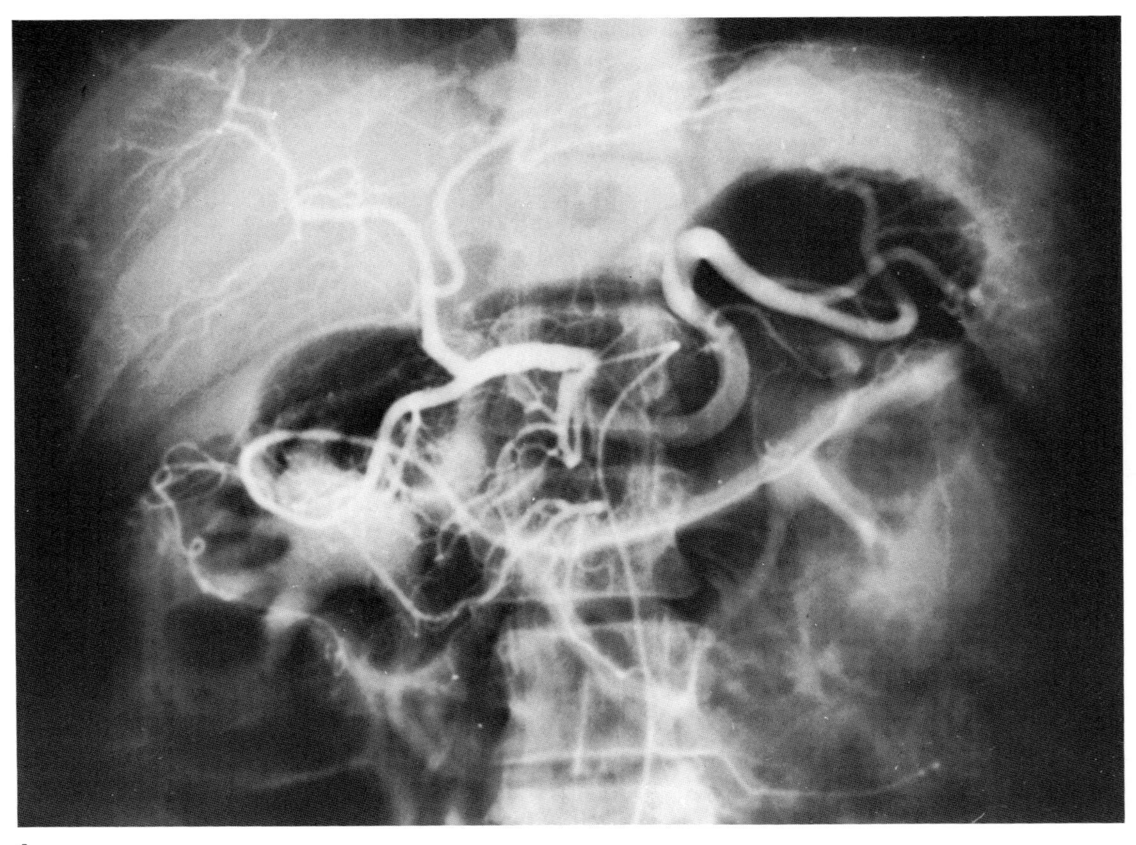
A

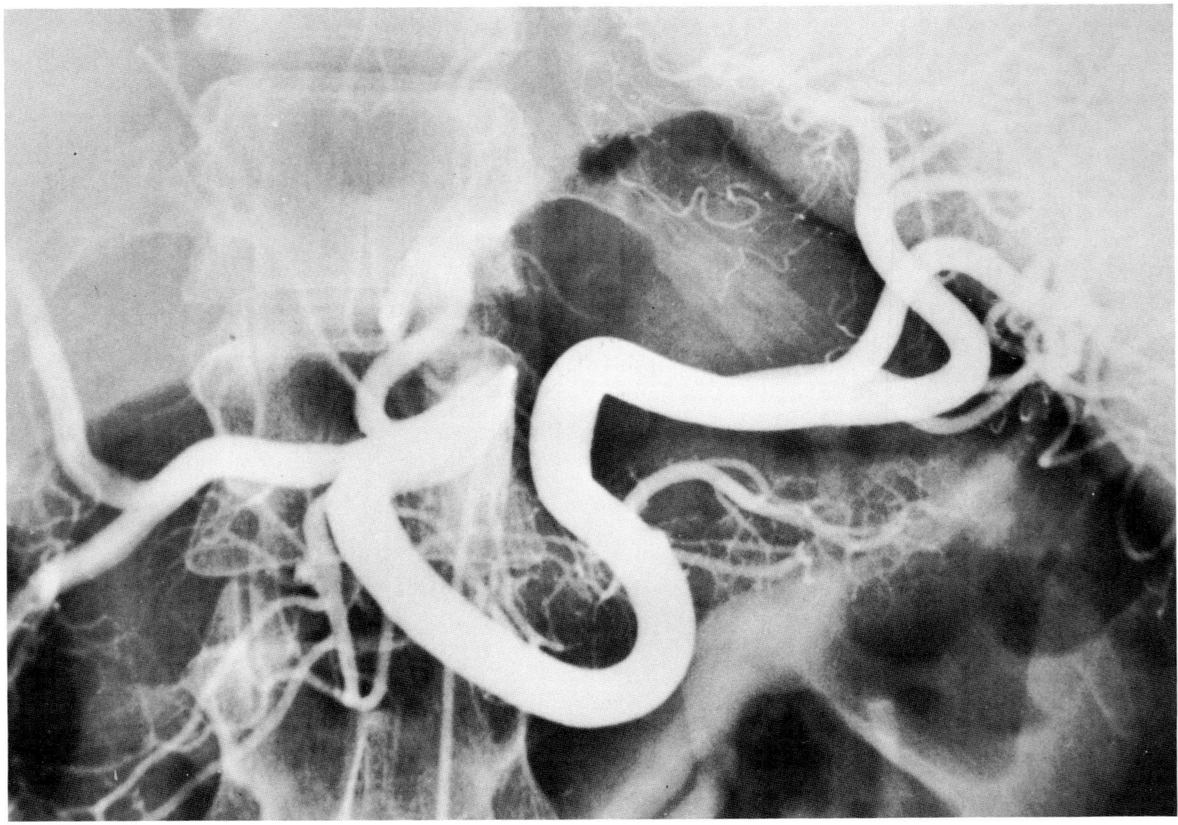
B

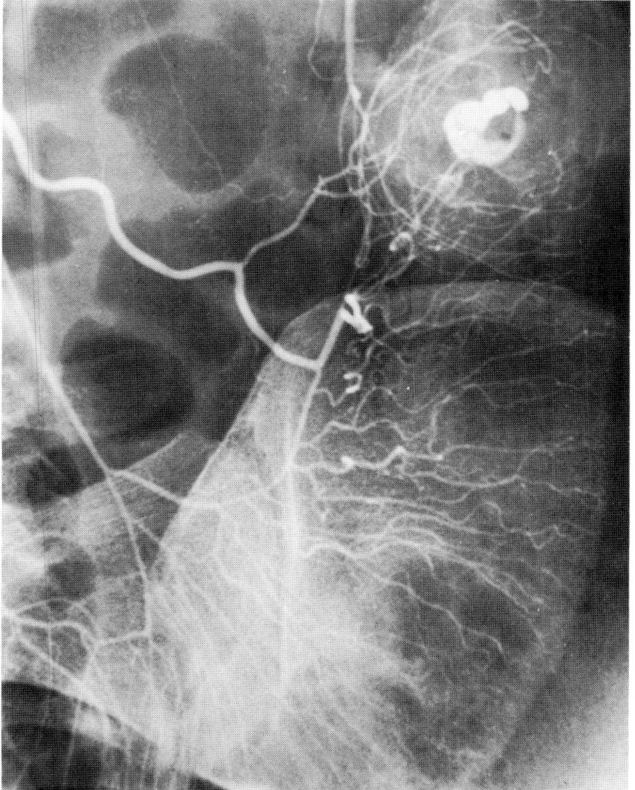

A

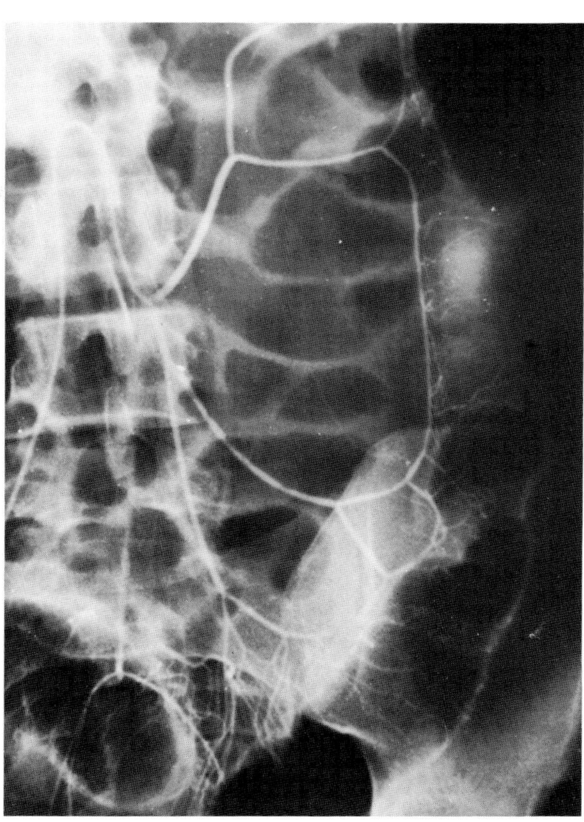

B

Figure 9-9. (A) Mesenteric arteriogram in a patient with a bleeding diverticulum. Note the exquisite detail of the small vascular radicles to the bowel. (Magnification ×3.) (B) Angiogram done by standard technique following cessation of bleeding. Small-vessel detail is not nearly as well seen as in (A). (Courtesy of Morton Glickman, M.D.)

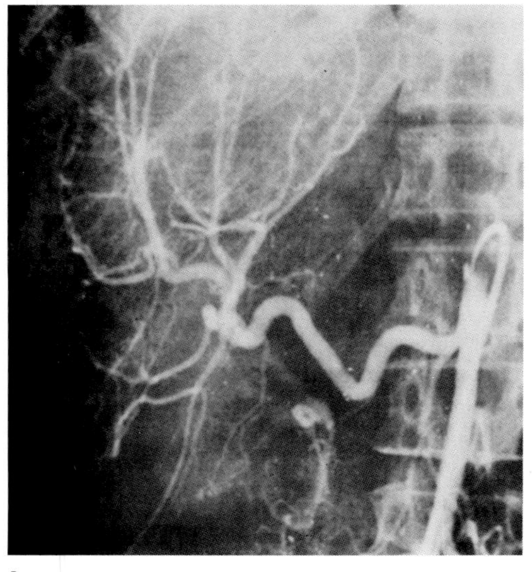

A

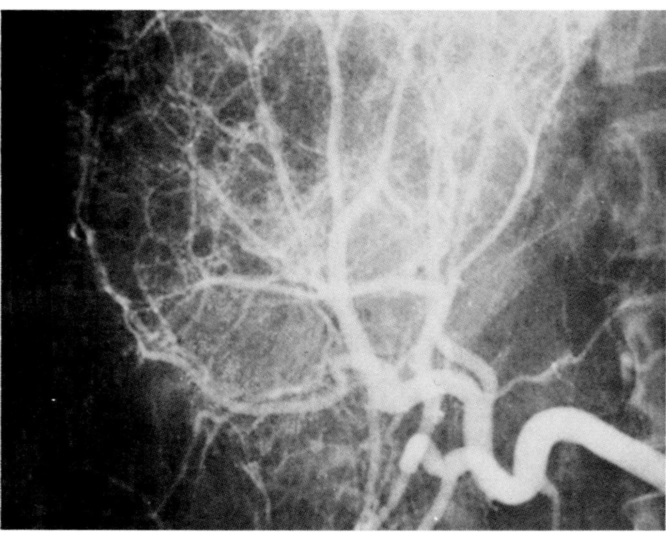

B

Figure 9-10. Adenocarcinoma of the colon metastatic to the liver. (A) The hepatic artery arises from the superior mesenteric artery. Selective superior mesenteric arteriography demonstrates displaced intrahepatic branches associated with a mottled appearance of the finer intrahepatic radicles. (B) Direct serial magnification arteriography demonstrates small tumor vessels as well as displacement of the intrahepatic branches to much greater advantage. Vessels of approximately 100 μ in diameter can be visualized with direct radiographic magnification using a fractional focal-spot x-ray tube.

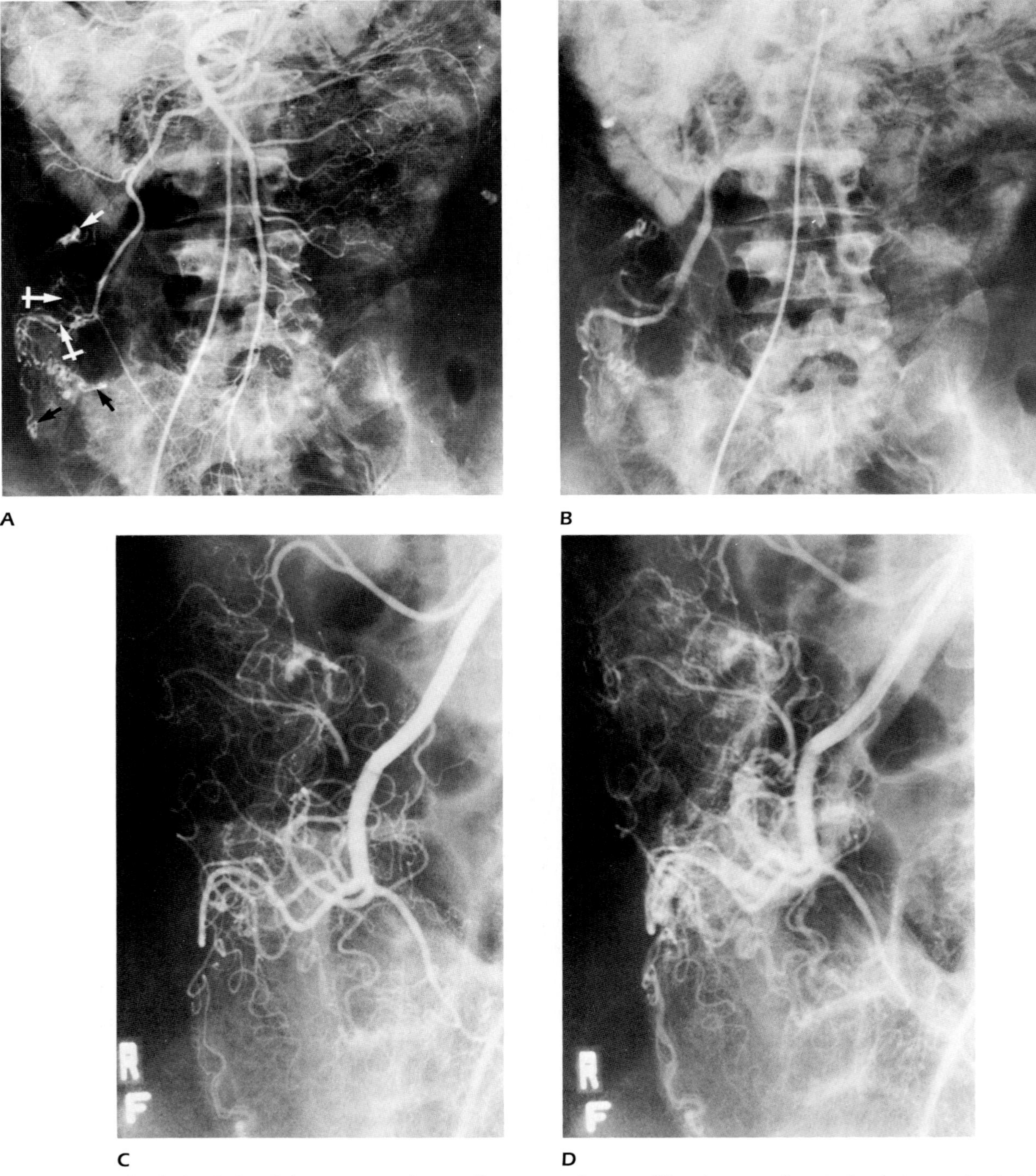

Figure 9-11. Angiodysplasia of the cecum and ascending colon. (A) During the arterial phase of a selective superior mesenteric arteriogram, abnormal clusters of small arteries can be identified in the cecum and ascending colon (*solid arrows*) associated with early-draining veins (*barred arrows*). (B) During the capillary phase of the examination, densely opacified colonic veins are seen draining the right colon. (C, D, and E) Direct serial magnification studies of the cecum and ascending colon with a catheter positioned in the ileocecal artery. The changes of angiodysplasia are clearly identified, with most of the increased vascularity and early-draining veins appearing on the antemesenteric border of the colon. The patient underwent a right colectomy, which extended from the cecum to the distal transverse colon. Pathologically, multiple areas of angiodysplasia were identified with large, thin-walled vascular channels in the colonic wall, predominantly in the submucosa and associated with ulceration and thinning of the overlying mucosa.

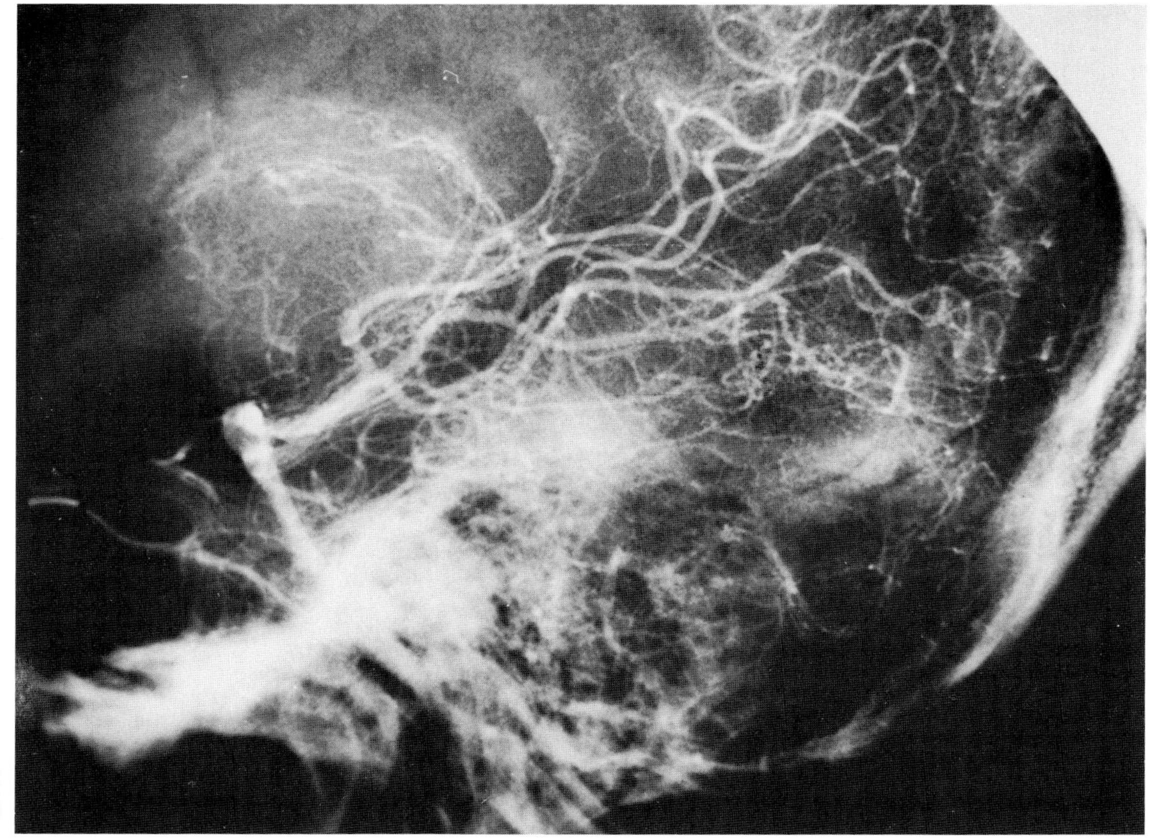

A

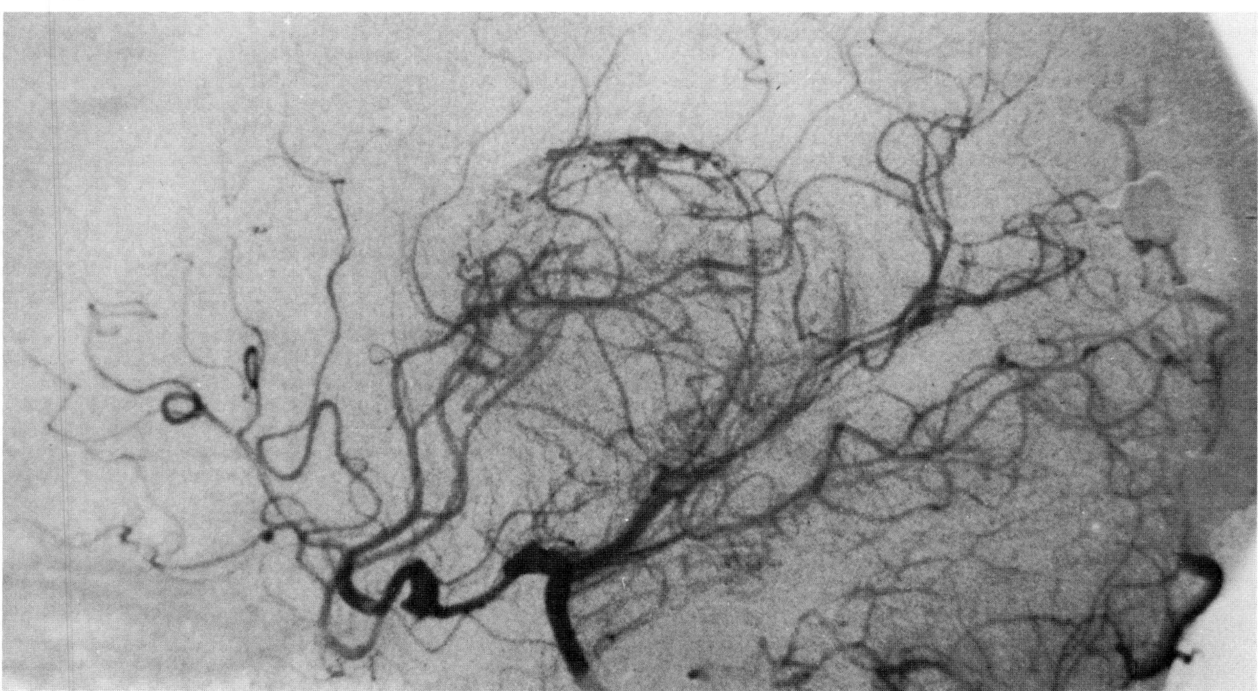

B

Figure 9-12. (A) Magnified cerebral angiogram (×2 plus). Note the vascular detail visible in the region of the thalamus. (B) Subtraction angiogram in the same patient using magnification ×2 plus (different injection phase). This type of vascular detail cannot be obtained with standard geometry. (Courtesy of E. Leon Kier, M.D.)

the detection of abnormal vascularity associated with tumors, benign pathologic processes, and bleeding sites in the gastrointestinal tract[51–53] (Figs. 9-8 through 9-11). Organs with very small vessels, hitherto poorly visualized angiographically, are now frequently studied with magnification techniques. These include the spine and spinal cord,[54] adrenal glands, testes,[55,56] thyroid and parathyroid glands, and skin.[57]

Routine use of magnification angiography in studying the intracerebral circulation has aided in the visualization of fine vessels with the consequent detection of abnormalities not seen in conventional angiograms (Fig. 9-12).[58–61] In many institutions the magnification study has replaced the routine cerebral angiogram in the study of intracerebral vessels.

Electronic Magnification

The profusion of image-processing techniques that has occurred in the past two decades, although altering the full field of imaging dramatically, has not yet provided a practical method for obtaining magnified angiograms. The resolution of systems currently available does not approach that obtainable with film-screen systems.[62] The limiting factor is the quality and the detail of the initial image produced, regardless of the method of its production.[63] Edge-enhancement techniques have been attempted, and subtraction techniques in association with scan-projection radiography or digital fluoroscopy would appear to have enormous potential for use with angiography. However, in their current state of development, neither provides the detail necessary to visualize the size of vessel that can be studied with direct geometric magnification angiography.

References

1. Barclay AE. Micro-arteriography. Br J Radiol 1947;20:394.
2. Goby P. New application of the x-rays: microradiography. J R Micr Soc 1913;33:373.
3. Rubin P. Microangiography: facts and artifacts. Radiol Clin North Am 1964;2:499.
4. McAlister WH, Margulis AR. Angiography of malignant tumors in mice following irradiation. Radiology 1963;81:664.
5. Engström A. Contrast microradiography: a general survey. In: Cosslett VE, Engström A, Pattee HH, eds. X-ray microscopy and microradiography. New York: Academic, 1957.
6. Bellman S. Microangiography. Acta Radiol Suppl (Stockh) 1953;102:1.
7. Bellman S, Block E, Odeblad E. A microangiographic study of the minute ovarian blood vessels in albino rats. Br J Radiol 1953;26:584.
8. Bellman S, Engström A. Microangiography. Acta Radiol (Stockh) 1952;38:98.
9. Harrington GJ, Wiedeman MP. The effect of contrast media on endothelial permeability. Radiology 1965;84:1108.
10. Bosniak MA. In vivo magnification arteriography of the bowel wall. Am J Surg 1967;114:359.
11. Bosniak MA, Farmelant MH, Bakos C, Hasiotis CA, Williams LF Jr. Experimental in vivo photographic magnification angiography of the canine kidney and bowel. Invest Radiol 1968; 3:120.
12. Margulis AR. Arteriography of tumors: difficulties in interpretation and the need for magnification. Radiol Clin North Am 1964;2:543.
13. Margulis AR, Carlsson E, McAlister WH. Angiography of malignant tumors in mice. Acta Radiol (Stockh) 1961;56:179.
14. Greenspan RH, Simon AL, Ricketts HJ, Rojas RH, Watson JC. In vivo magnification angiography. Invest Radiol 1967; 2:419.
15. Morgan RH. An analysis of the physical factors controlling the diagnostic quality of roentgen images: Part V. Unsharpness. AJR 1949;62:870.
16. Wood EH. Preliminary observations regarding value of a very fine focus tube in radiologic diagnosis. Radiology 1953;61: 382.
17. Greenspan RH. Magnification angiography. In: Abrams HL, ed. Angiography. 2nd ed. Boston: Little, Brown, 1971.
18. Morgan RH, Bates LM, Gopalarao VV, Marinaro A. The frequency response characteristics of x-ray films and screens. AJR 1964;92:426.
19. Baum S, Nusbaum M, Kuroda K, Blakemore WS. Direct serial magnification arteriography as an adjuvant in the diagnosis of surgical lesions in the alimentary tract. Am J Surg 1969;117: 170–176.
20. Ter-Pogossian MM. The physical aspects of diagnostic radiology. New York: Hoeber Med. Div., Harper & Row, 1967.
21. Nemet A, Cox WF. The improvement of definition by x-ray image magnification. Br J Radiol 1956;29:335.
22. Sturm RE, Morgan RH. Screen intensification systems and their limitations. AJR 1949;62:617.
23. Sandor T, Adams DF. Minimum blood vessel diameter measured by magnification angiography. AJR 1979;132:433.
24. Morgan RH. Visual perception in fluoroscopy and radiography. Radiology 1966;86:403.
25. Rose A. Sensitivity performance of human eye on an absolute scale. J Opt Soc Am 1948;38:196.
26. Sandor T, Nott P. Effect of radiographic magnification on image contrast of blood vessels. AJR 1980;134:159.
27. Rossman K. Image forming quality of radiographic screen-film systems: linespread function. J Opt Soc Am 1963;90:178.
28. Warren SR Jr. Roentgenographic unsharpness of the shadow of a moving object. Radiology 1937;28:450.
29. Friedman PJ, Greenspan RH. Observations on magnification radiography: visualization of small blood vessels and determination of focal spot size. Radiology 1969;92:549.
30. Takenaka E, Kinoshita K, Nakajima R. Modulation transfer function of the intensity distribution of the roentgen focal spot. Acta Radiol Oncol Radiat Phys Biol 1968;7:263.
31. Bookstein JJ. Angiographic resolution of small vessels. Presented at the Meeting of the Association of University Radiologists, Columbus, Ohio, May 9, 1968.
32. Maloney JE, Wexler L. Measurement of the dimensions of small structures with magnification radiography. Presented at the Meeting of the Association of University Radiologists, San Francisco, May 9, 1969.
33. Takahashi S, Yoshida M. Roentgenography in high magnification: reliability and limitation of enlargement. Acta Radiol (Stockh) 1957;48:280.
34. Milne ENC. Circulation of primary and metastatic pulmonary neoplasms: a postmortem microarteriographic study. AJR 1967;100:603.
35. Takahashi S, Sakuma S, Kaneko M, Koga S. Angiography at fourfold magnification with special reference to examination of tumors. Acta Radiol (Stockh) 1966;4:206.

36. Takaro T, Scott SM. Angiography using direct roentgenographic magnification in man. AJR 1964;91:448.
37. Takaro T, Scott SM, Sewell WH. Arteriography utilizing radiographic magnification techniques. Surg Forum 1961;12:143.
38. Takaro T, Scott SM. Angiography of the minute vessels of the lung. Dis Chest 1964;45:28.
39. Bynum LJ, Wilson JE III, Christensen EE, Sorensen C. Radiographic techniques for balloon occlusion pulmonary angiography. Radiology 1979;133:518.
40. McIntyre KM, Sharma GVRK. Subselective pulmonary arteriography with balloon occlusion for the detection of pulmonary embolism. Am J Cardiol 1974;33:154.
41. Orta DA Jr, Eisen S, Yergin BM, Olsen GN. Segmental pulmonary angiography in the critically ill patient using a flow directed catheter. Chest 1979;76:269.
42. Wilson JE, Bynum LJ. An improved pulmonary angiographic technique using a balloon-tipped catheter. Am Rev Respir Dis 1976;114:1137.
43. Nihill MR, McNamara DG. Magnification pulmonary wedge angiography in the evaluation of children with congenital heart disease and pulmonary hypertension. Circulation 1978;58: 1094.
44. Allison DJ, Stanbrook HS. A radiologic and physiologic investigation into hypoxic pulmonary vasoconstriction in the dog. Invest Radiol 1980;15:178.
45. Hicken P, Hogg JC, Pare PD. Experimental pulmonary arteritis. Invest Radiol 1980;15:299.
46. Simon AL, Greenspan RH. Magnification coronary arteriography: Part I. Normal. Clin Radiol 1965;16:414.
47. Simon AL, Greenspan RH. Magnification coronary arteriography: Part II. Experimental pathology. Clin Radiol 1966;17:89.
48. Takaro T, Scott SM, Sewell WH. Experimental coronary arteriography using roentgenographic magnification. AJR 1962;87: 258.
49. Chew QT, Nouri MS, Woo BH. Small renal pelvic carcinomas: value of epinephrine magnification angiography. J Urol 1978; 120:243.
50. Wixson D, Baltaxe HA, Balter S, Rothenberg LN. Comparative diagnostic accuracy of 105 mm versus conventional and magnification radiographic techniques in the arteriographic diagnosis of renal and perirenal masses. Invest Radiol 1977;12:527.
51. Rösch J, Mayer BS, Campbell JR, Campbell TJ. "Vascular" benign liver cyst in children: report of two cases. Radiology 1978;126:747.
52. Seo KW, Bookstein JJ, Brown HS. Angiography of intussusception of the small bowel. Radiology 1979;132:603.
53. Velasquez G, Katkov H, Formanek A. Primary liver tumors in the pediatric age group: an angiographic challenge. Rofo Fortschr Geb Rontgenstr Neuen Bildgeb Verfahr 1979;130: 408.
54. Shiozawa Z, Tanaka Y, Makino N, Sugita K. Spinal cord angiography using 4× magnification. Radiology 1978;127:181.
55. Kormano M, Nordmark L. Angiography of the testicular artery: III. Testis and epididymis analyzed with a magnification technique. Acta Radiol (Stockh) 1977;18:625.
56. Nordmark L, Nyberg G. Angiography of the testicular artery: IV. Magnification angiography in intrascrotal abnormalities. Acta Radiol (Stockh) 1979;20:353.
57. May JW Jr, Athanasoulis CA, Donelan MB. Preoperative magnification angiography of donor and recipient sites for clinical free transfer of flaps or digits. Plast Reconstr Surg 1979;64: 483.
58. Nakayama N, Wallenfang T. Magnification angiography of the posterior cranial fossa in pediatry. Mod Probl Paediatr 1976; 18:106.
59. Rosa M, Michelozzi G, Donati PT, Schiavoni S, Borzone M. Magnification angiography of the small vessels in cerebrovascular disease in advanced age. Neuroradiology 1978;16:101.
60. Sato O, Kanazawa I, Kokunai T, Kobayashi M. Seven intracranial aneurysms of the internal carotid arteries: diagnosis by magnification angioautotomography. Neuroradiology 1978;15: 189.
61. Shiozawa Z, Ohya M, Tanaka Y, Maekoshi H. Direct serial magnification angiography applied to cerebral aneurysms. Radiology 1978;126:263.
62. Ter-Pogossian MM. The physico-mathematical era of radiology—the impact of modern technology on radiology—the big machines. New Horizons for Radiologists Lecture. Radiology 1968;90:857.
63. Chase NE, Hass WK, Kricheff II. New instrumentation for cerebral microangiography. Radiology 1965;85:736.

10

Principles of Magnetic Resonance Angiography

FELIX W. WEHRLI

One of the remarkable features of magnetic resonance imaging (MRI) is the sensitivity of amplitude and phase of its signal to moving spins, a situation that applies to flowing blood. The first documented observation of blood flow in human MR images presumably is the one by Hinshaw et al., who observed a signal increase in a cross-sectional image of the vessels in the wrist.[1] Although blood flow had first been studied by nonimaging MR at least two decades earlier, the pioneering imaging work that led to magnetic resonance angiography (MRA) dates back to the mid-1980s.[2–4] Shortly thereafter, the first projection angiograms were reported.[5–8]

Although initially limited, compared with conventional angiography, and marred by artifacts resulting from a plethora of technical difficulties, MRA has, during recent years, evolved from an experimental technique to a method approaching clinical practicality. Reflecting this evolution is an exponential increase in clinical MRA literature.[9,10] Although there is still no consensus on MRA's current role in clinical practice, its potential in vascular radiology is now being explored intensely for determining its effectiveness relative to x-ray contrast angiography and color Doppler scanning.

Initially, clinical evaluations of the technology focused on neurovascular applications,[11–13] but more recently they proliferated into other vascular territories, including the pulmonary vascular system,[14–16] the vessels of the abdomen (e.g., portal and renal system),[17–19] the peripheral vessels,[20–22] and even the coronary arteries.[23,24]

This chapter discusses the principles of MRA, beginning with a review of the fundamental blood flow manifestations—time-of-flight and phase effects—that constitute the basis of MRA. This is followed by a discussion of the two major families of MRA techniques: time-of-flight (TOF) or inflow angiography, and phase contrast (PC) angiography. Of particular practical importance to the user is the understanding of the dependence of the vascular signal on pulse sequence parameters such as pulse repetition time, radiofrequency pulse flip angle, imaging slab thickness, and the characteristics of the flow-encoding gradients, as well as intrinsic quantities, notably blood flow velocity and its spatial and temporal distribution. Which of the various techniques is most appropriate for imaging a particular vascular territory is addressed as well, although this subject continues to evoke debate. In the following, the author assumes the reader to be familiar with the basic principles of MRI.

Paralleling methods for vessel visualization have been efforts to quantitate blood flow, including flow velocities and flow rates, by combining spatial and velocity encoding. Although the basic methodology for velocity measurement draws upon the same principles as the techniques used for vessel visualization, the field is too diverse and complex to be included in this chapter.

Effects of Blood Flow on the MR Signal

Time-of-Flight Effects

The relative signal amplitude of vascular structures is usually dominated by a combination of two effects. The first, conceptionally simpler effect, exploited in the early nonimaging work mentioned in the previous section, is often referred to as the *time-of-flight effect,* and has been reviewed by Axel.[25] In order to be present, this effect demands that spins that have not previously been excited enter the imaging slice between two successive radiofrequency (RF) pulses.

The effect is readily understood when considering proton spins of blood flowing in a direction perpendicular to the imaging slab. These protons are excited repetitively every pulse repetition time (TR) such that TR is less than T_1 of the protons in blood (about 1 second at typical imaging field strengths). Under these conditions, spins entering the imaging slice may not previously have sensed an RF pulse, and thus carry full magnetization. By contrast, spins that remain in the

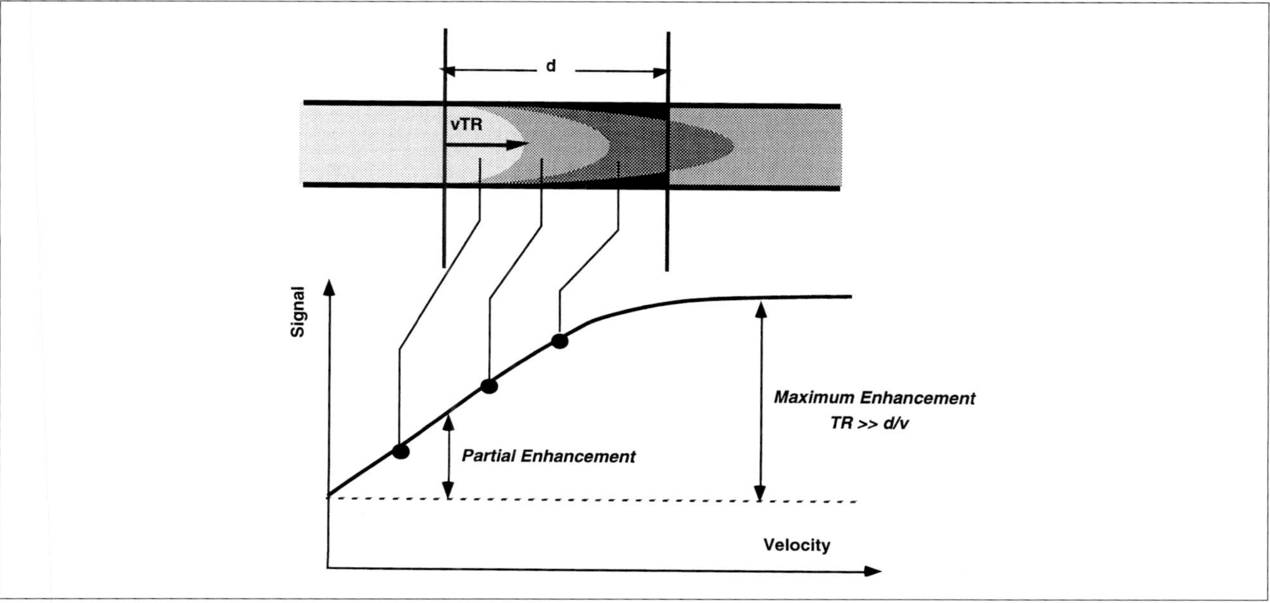

Figure 10-1. Inflow of spins between successive excitations leads to vascular signal enhancement because the freshly entering spins carry full magnetization (as opposed to those that have remained in the slice between excitations). The length of the bolus of "fresh" blood within the slice is the product of centerline velocity (the velocity at the center of the vessel, assuming laminar flow) and TR. An equal amount of blood is displaced from the vessel downstream (not shown). The flow enhancement is given by the difference in signal amplitude between the one observed in the presence and absence of flow and is related to the slice thickness *d,* the pulse repetition time *TR,* and the blood flow velocity *v.* Maximum enhancement occurs when the pulse repetition time is greater than the transit time ($TR >> d/v$).

slice between excitations will have their signal attenuated. The degree of enhancement of the vascular signal depends on the extent of spin replacement, which is related to the transit time of the moving spins across the slice. Suppose laminar flow with a centerline velocity *v,* as depicted in Figure 10-1. It then is obvious that washing of "fresh" spins increases with either increasing pulse repetition time or velocity. The signal is a composite of contributions from spins that have entered the slice between successive excitations and those that have remained in the slice. It is further seen from Figure 10-1 that the signal should increase with increasing blood flow velocity. Of course, once complete replacement of spins within the imaging slice has occurred, the signal cannot further rise. The relative increase in the signal (also termed *flow-related enhancement, time-of-flight enhancement*) is the difference in signal amplitude between moving and stationary spins. It is evident from Figure 10-1 that the extent of inflow of fresh spins depends on three parameters: the thickness *d* of the imaging slice, the velocity *v,* and the pulse repetition time *TR.* The first two quantities determine the transit time, $T_t = d/v$, that is, the time it takes for the blood to traverse the slice, which increases with increasing slice thickness and decreasing blood flow velocity. Maximum enhancement occurs if the transit time is shorter than the pulse repetition time.

The above situation applies in gradient-echo imaging,[26] in which the signal is derived from a single RF pulse, followed by gradient-echo readout. This technique is the basis of one of the most common MRA projection techniques, denoted *time-of-flight* or *inflow* angiography.[13] Figure 10-2 illustrates these effects with a transverse gradient-echo image of the base of the skull showing enhancement for vascular structures.

Phase Shifts and Intravoxel Phase Dispersion

The second effect exploited for the generation of vascular images is related to the phase of the magnetic resonance signal. To understand this effect, we first need to remember that the MR signal has vector properties, that is, it has both a magnitude and a direction. The latter is usually expressed in terms of the angle the magnetization makes relative to some fiducial direction.

Let us assume that spins at some spatial location r_o are exposed to a gradient magnetic field, as shown in

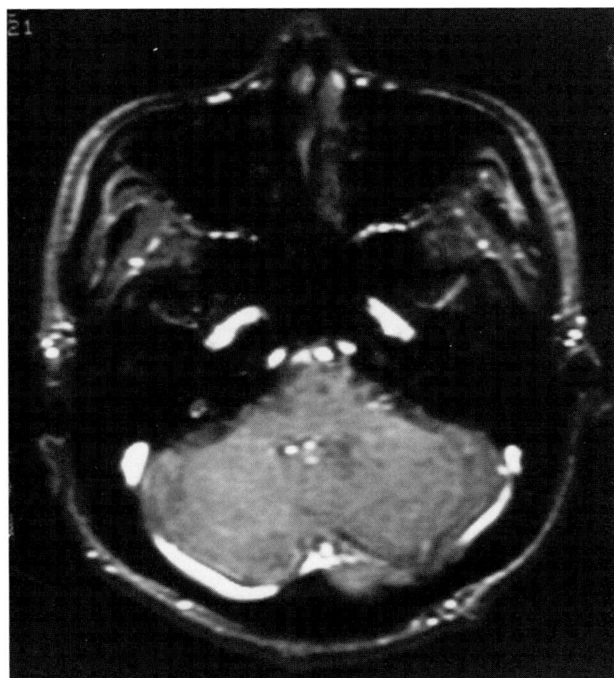

Figure 10-2. Transverse gradient-echo images acquired at the base of the head, showing enhancement of vascular structures.

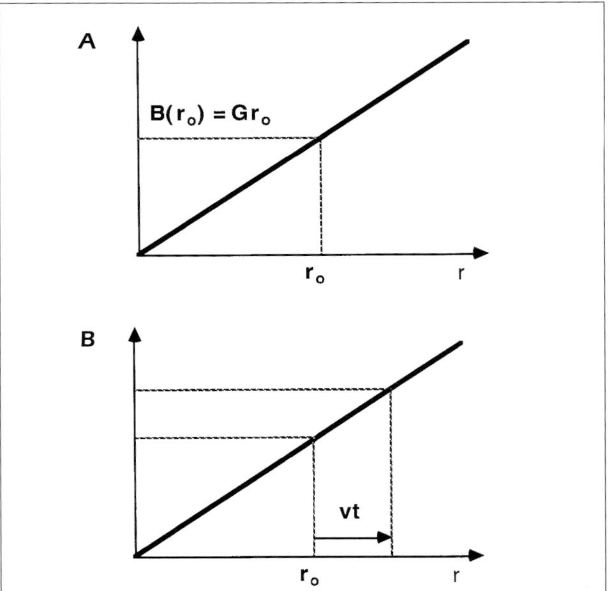

Figure 10-3. (A) Spins located at position r_o along some magnetic field gradient G are subjected to a field $B = Gr_o$ and thus precess at a frequency $\omega = \gamma Gr_o$. (B) If the spins move for a period t at constant velocity v, it becomes obvious that the field they experience increases linearly, and so does the resonance frequency, which becomes $\omega(t) = \gamma G(r_o + vt)$.

Figure 10-3A. These spins then will experience a magnetic field $B = Gr_o$, and will thus precess at a frequency

$$\omega = \gamma Gr_o, \quad (1)$$

where γ is the gyromagnetic ratio. Their phase at some time t after precession started becomes

$$\phi = \omega t = \gamma Gr_o t \quad (2)$$

Phase is the total angle the magnetization has made on its precessional path. Phase may thus be regarded the counterpart of distance for circular motion. Just as distance is proportional to the speed at which an object moves and to time, phase is the product of angular frequency and time.*

A complication arises when the frequency of precession varies during the period of precession. This is precisely the situation for spins moving in the direction of a magnetic field gradient, such as with flowing blood. Suppose spins move at constant velocity v in a field gradient G. It then becomes obvious that their resonance frequency is no longer constant but instead increases linearly (see Fig. 10-3B). Although motion does not affect the magnitude of the transverse of the signal, it causes a shift in the phase of the magnetization. Figure 10-4A shows the transverse magnetization after having been rotated onto the y axis by an RF pulse applied around the x axis and after precession by slightly over one revolution (Fig. 10-4B). In Figure 10-4C and D we assume that during the time period t the spins travel at constant velocity v, as shown in Figure 10-3B. Consequently, their frequency increases linearly with time. Although the initial frequency was the same as in Figure 10-4A and B, the transverse magnetization has processed by an additional half-revolution (see Fig. 10-4C). Hence, although the magnitude of the magnetization, and thus of the MR signal, remains unaltered, in this example the two have different, nearly opposite, phase. It can readily be shown that although the phase for stationary spins increases linearly with time, it evolves quadratically for spins that move at constant velocity in the direction of a field gradient.

In general, the pixel value of an MR image is proportional to the magnitude of the signal, and the phase

*In the more general case in which the frequency is a function of time, the phase is the integral of frequency over time, that is, $\phi = \int \omega(t)\,dt$.

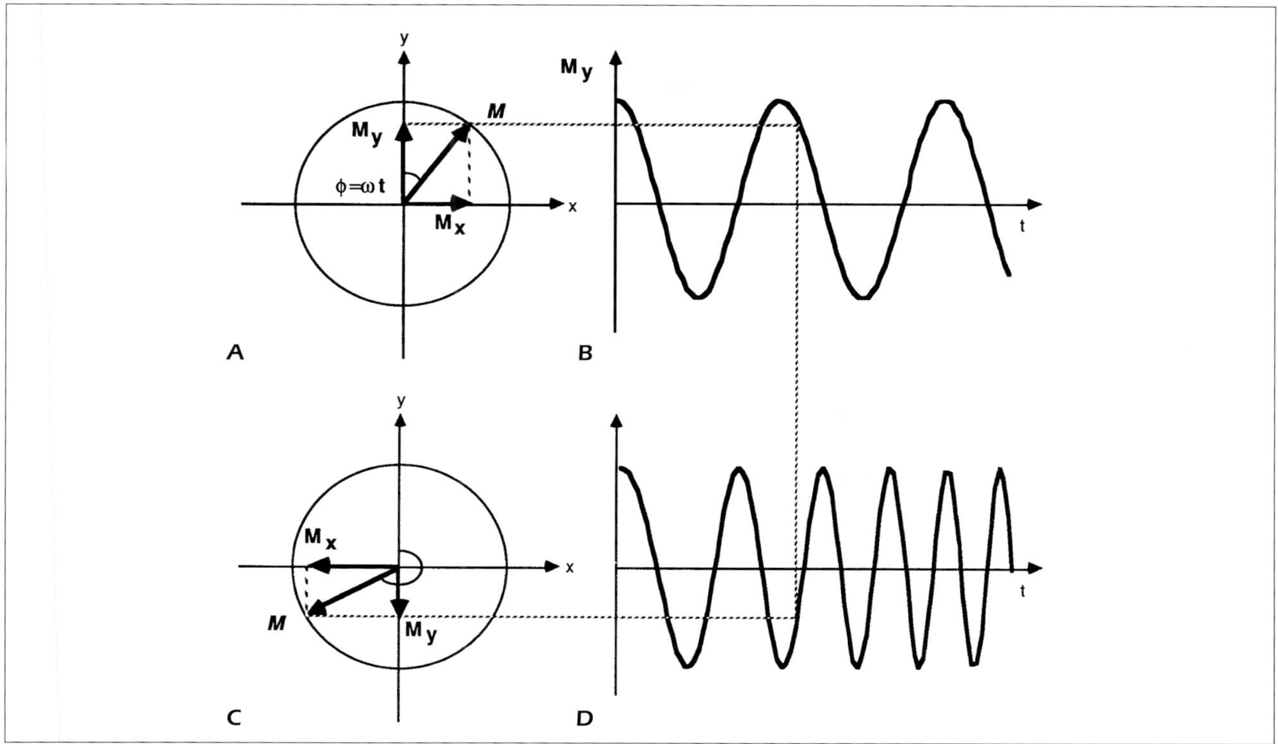

Figure 10-4. (A) Transverse magnetization at time *t* and (B) plot of *y* component for precession in constant magnetic field. (C and D) Motion of spins at constant velocity along a field gradient leads to a phase advance. Note in the example shown that in the presence of motion (D) the magnetization has advanced an additional half-cycle (C).

information—although readily available—is discarded after reconstruction. However, it is possible to display the phase of the signal instead of the magnitude.

By assigning gray scale to the phase angle, one can display phase images. For example, it is convenient to display signals from stationary material in intermediate gray. By contrast, spins that have moved along the direction of the gradient have acquired an additional phase rotation and are thus displayed in lighter gray values, and those that result from motion in the opposite direction—that is, those that have lost phase relative to their stationary counterparts—are displayed in darker gray values. Figure 10-5 illustrates this concept. Any phase shift greater than 180 degrees will lead to what is referred to as *aliasing*. For example, a phase shift of 200 degrees resulting from fast forward motion will appear like much slower motion in reverse direction, resulting from a phase shift. Figure 10-6 shows a transverse spin-echo image of the thighs in both magnitude (see Fig. 10-6A) and phase reconstruction (see Fig. 10-6B,C).

Phase effects caused by flow motion can also occur in magnitude images, typically in the form of reduced signal or complete signal void. The attenuation of magnitude signal is caused by phase shifts resulting from spatial distributions of flow velocities. Shear resulting from laminar flow or turbulence (caused by very rapid flow in stenotic vessel segments) causes a distribution of flow velocities across the voxel and therefore phase scrambling, with a net reduction in the signal and eventual signal loss due to the destructive effects of adding the individual vector components.[27] This effect is the principal cause of the vascular flow void typically encountered in spin-echo imaging.

From Transverse Images to Projection Angiograms: Time-of-Flight Angiography

Inflow effects, as described above, can be exploited for the generation of angiographic images. The principle of the method is the acquisition of a stack of images in such a manner that the direction of the flow is essentially orthogonal to the imaging plane. Inflow of

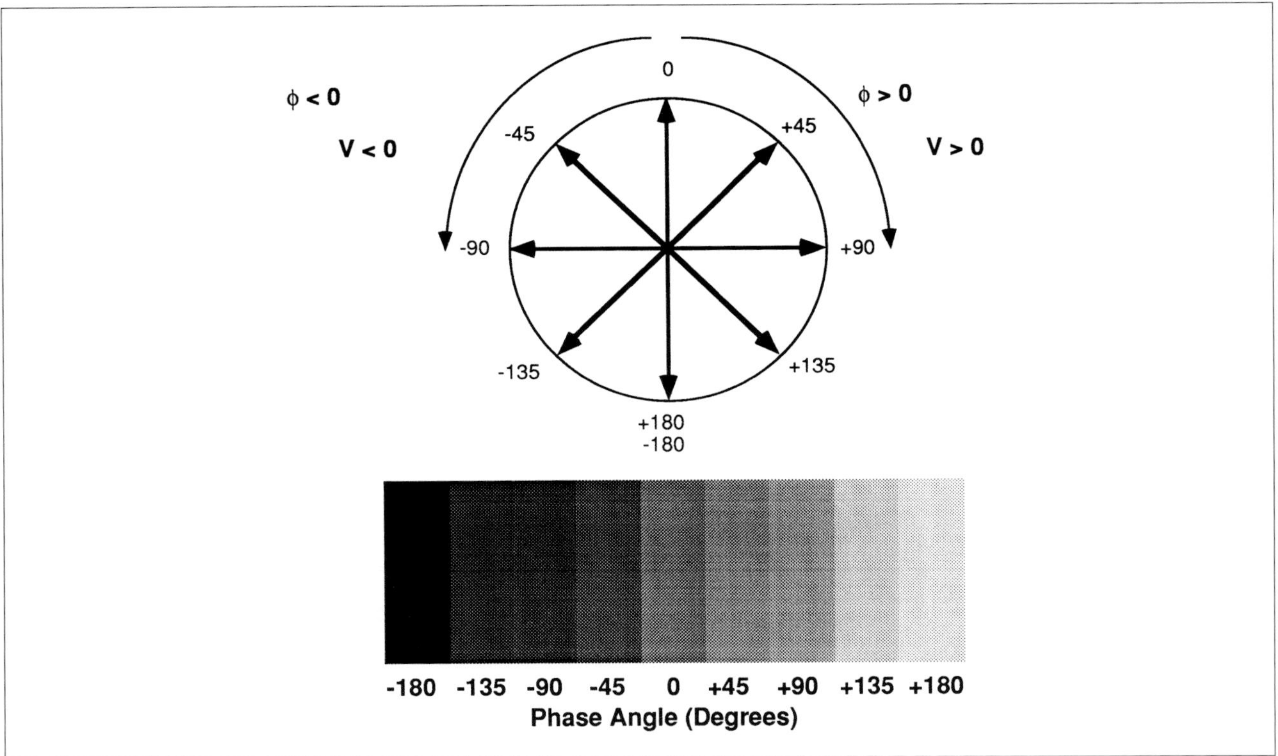

Figure 10-5. Gray scale for the display of phase images. The phase angle $\phi = \text{atan}\,(I/R)$ is defined such that for stationary spins $\phi = 0$, which is displayed in intermediate gray. Phase angles $\phi > 0$ correspond to forward flow (flow in the direction of the gradient), which is displayed in brighter shades of gray, and reverse flow, corresponding to $\phi < 0$, is displayed in darker shades of gray.

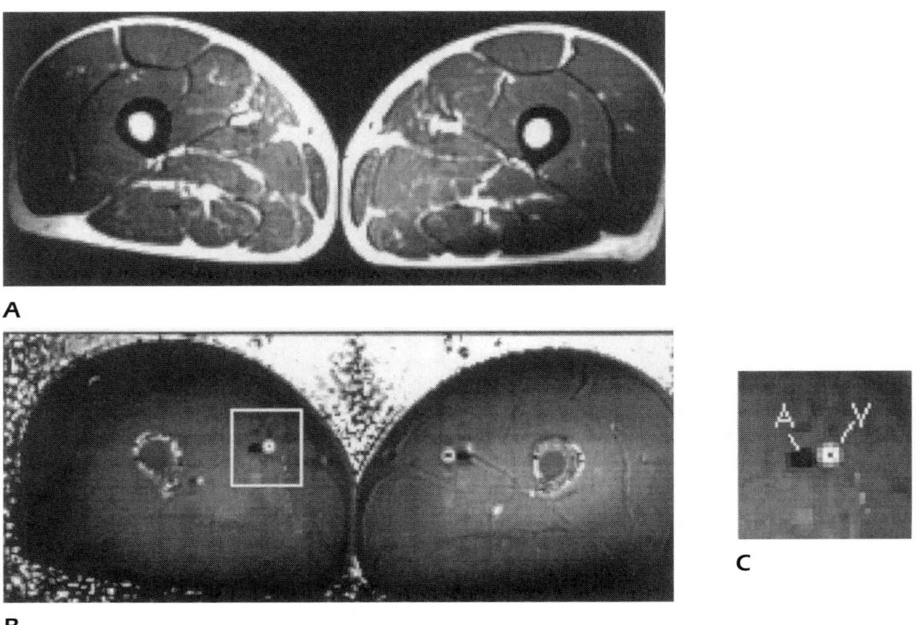

Figure 10-6. Spin-echo image of the thighs showing femoral artery and vein. (A) Magnitude image. (B) Phase image. Both data sets were obtained from the same acquisition. In (B) phase shifts induced by blood flow motion in the presence of the slice-selection gradient modulate the signal (see Fig. 10-5 for details). Note that the femoral vein appears with increased intensity, the artery with decreased intensity, relative to stationary background signal, consistent with a phase advance and retardation, respectively, due to flow parallel and opposite to the gradient. (C) Magnification of the ROI in (B): the black dot in the center of the femoral vein results from aliasing due to higher velocity at the center of the vessel, causing a phase shift greater than 180°.

"fresh" blood between successive excitations causes enhanced signal intensity, as discussed earlier and illustrated in Figure 10-1. Ideally, one would like to completely suppress signal from stationary tissue components. In practice, this is not possible, and one of the features of TOF angiograms is some residual background. Fortunately, however, as discussed later, undesirable background can be attenuated in various ways.

There are multiple embodiments of TOF angiography. First, a distinction needs to be made between techniques that are based on either two-dimensional (2D) or three-dimensional (3D) image acquisition. In 2D TOF angiography a stack of thin (approximately 1.5-mm) gradient-echo images is acquired sequentially. This acquisition mode, in particular when combined with a short pulse repetition time, provides effective flow-related enhancement and background attenuation. At a pulse repetition time of 50 milliseconds and a slice thickness of 1.5 mm, for example, a flow velocity of 3 cm per second (0.15 cm/0.05 sec) suffices for complete washout of saturated spins between successive excitations, and thus optimum flow-related enhancement. In fact, the relative insensitivity to signal loss from slow flow is one of the significant strengths of 2D TOF angiography.[8,13]

Without any special precautions, an angiogram obtained in the manner described would display both veins and arteries alike. To generate an arteriogram, the signal from veins has to be suppressed. In practice, this is achieved by making use of the directional properties of arterial and venous flow. The predominant direction of flow for the vessels of the neck is cranial–caudad for veins and caudad–cranial for arteries. Application of a spatially selective presaturation pulse encompassing a slab superior to the imaging slice immediately preceding slice selection thus ensures suppression of the signals from jugular veins since the spins entering the imaging slice are saturated and thus carry low magnetization. To be effective, the saturation slab needs to follow the imaging slice as the scan proceeds. For this reason the saturation region is sometimes referred to as a *walking saturation band* (Fig. 10-7). Figure 10-8 shows a series of axial images derived from 1.5-mm slices, obtained with spatial presaturation superiorly for suppressing signals from veins along with a projection arteriogram. Note the low signal level of the stationary tissues due to partial saturation, which is achieved by a combination of high flip angle and short pulse repetition time.

Instead of creating a stack of 2D slices, it may be advantageous to derive angiograms from 3D volume data sets.[28] The latter offers the usual benefits of 3D volume imaging in that it allows for the generation of thinner slices, which is important because, upon projection into images orthogonal to the initial scan plane (e.g., anteroposterior [AP] and lateral), the slice thickness determines the pixel size and thus the resolution in inferior–superior direction. Therefore, 3D MRA is preferred over 2D TOF techniques for intracranial applications, in which resolution is critical.

Saturation Effects

Besides spatial resolution, however, the most significant difference between 2D and 3D TOF angiography concerns vessel-to-background contrast, which in some instances can be inferior in 3D acquisitions. This is apparent from the fact that in 3D imaging the spins are excited within a slab of several centimeters' thickness. Hence the blood's transit time across the

Figure 10-7. Suppression of venous signal, achieved by saturating spins upstream relative to the venous flow direction.

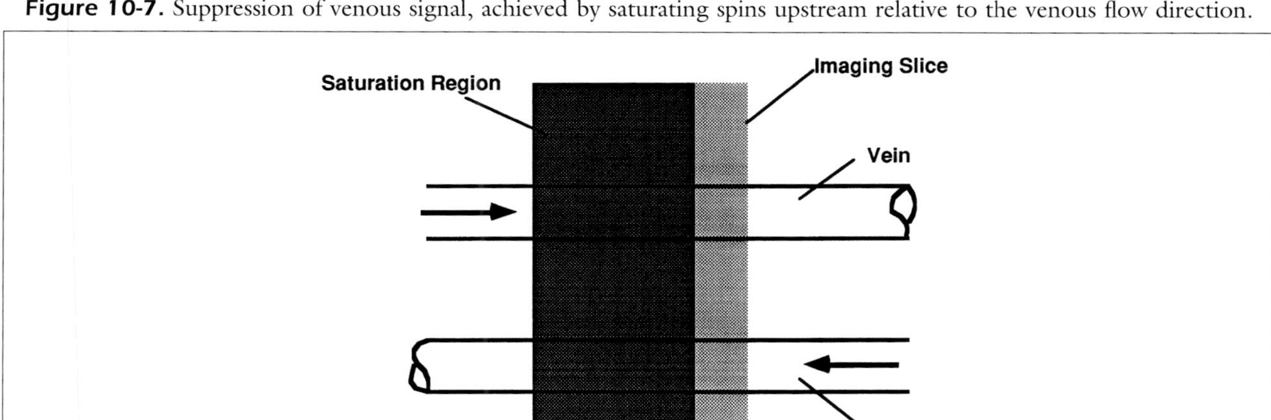

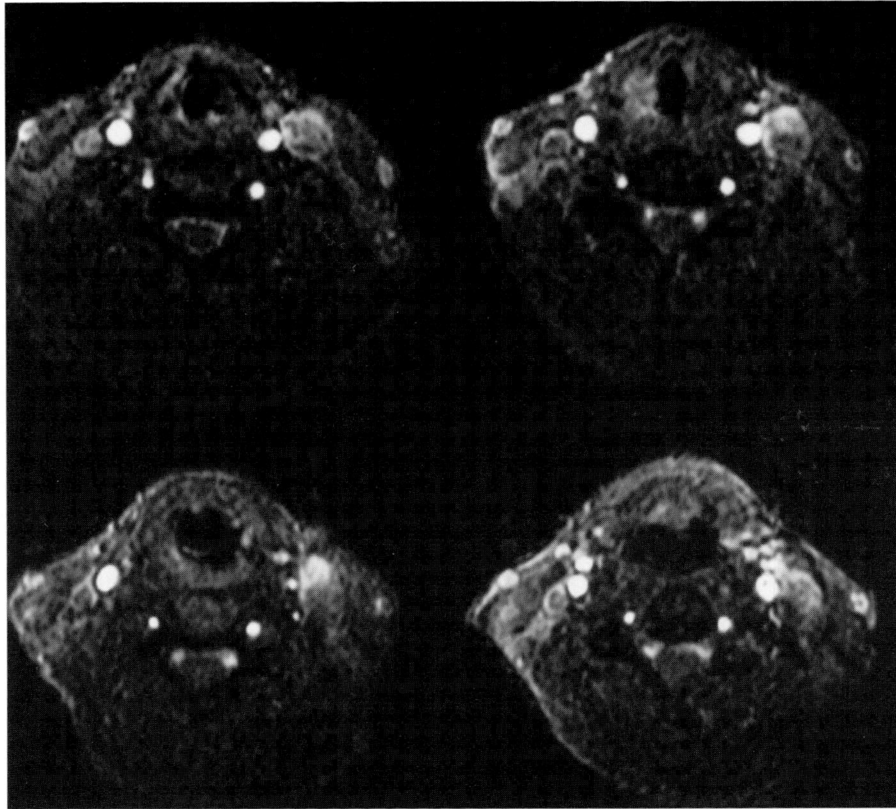

A–D

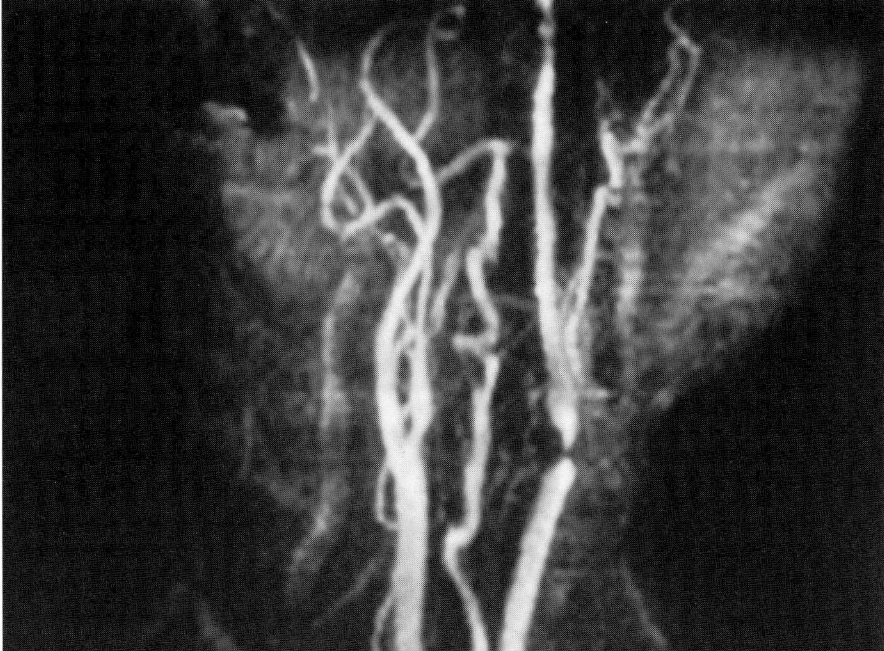

E

Figure 10-8. (A to D) Axial gradient-echo images obtained from 1.5-mm slices obtained with spatial presaturation superiorly for suppressing signals from veins. (E) Projection arteriogram derived from 60 contiguous images like the ones shown in (A) to (D). Note the tight stenosis of the left common carotid artery, also noticeable in (C).

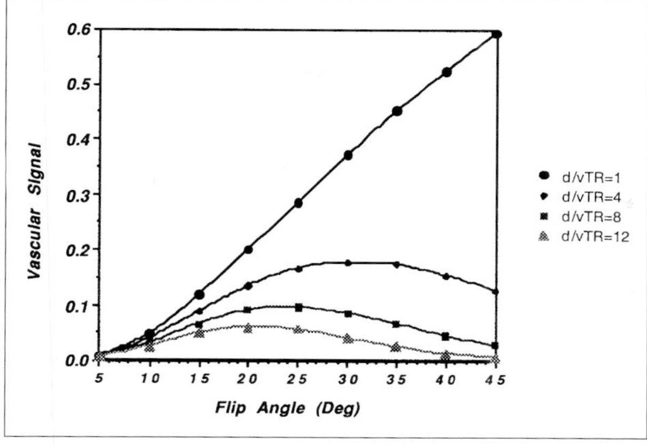

A

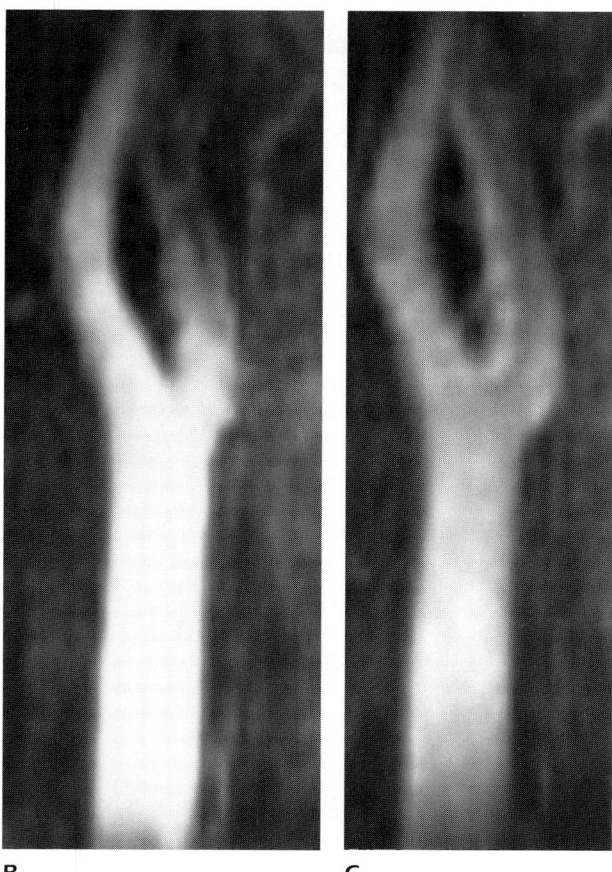

B C

Figure 10-9. (A) Calculated vascular signal as a function of the pulse flip angle for various values of the parameter $n = z/vTR$, that is, the ratio of the slab thickness z divided by the bolus advancement during a pulse repetition time period. Note the decrease in signal with decreasing n due to increased saturation. Further, there is an optimum flip angle that decreases with increasing values of n. (B and C) 3D TOF angiograms of carotid bifurcation, obtained from 64 1-mm sections, at a pulse repetition time of 50 msec, showing saturation signal losses and apparent vessel narrowing distally at $\alpha = 45°$, but less so at 30°.

slice is far longer. Assuming, for example, a slab thickness of 5 cm and a mean flow velocity of 10 cm per second, the transit time is

$$\frac{5 \text{ cm}}{10 \text{ cm/sec}} = 0.5 \text{ sec}$$

At a pulse repetition time of 50 milliseconds, for example, the same spins will thus "see" 10 RF pulses while traveling across the slab and consequently may be significantly saturated. If we denote the slab thickness d, the flow velocity v, and the pulse repetition time TR, the vascular signal can readily be computed as a function of a parameter $n = d/(vTR)$, with n expressing the number of excitations the spins experience on their transit across the slice.[29,30] An increased number of RF pulses applied to the same spins leads to progressive saturation and therefore attenuation of the vascular signal. Figure 10-9A shows the computed vascular signal as a function of flip angle for various values of the parameter n. It is therefore not surprising that the more distal portions of a vessel are often suppressed in 3D TOF angiography. These adverse effects on vascular contrast can be minimized by judicious choice of the pulse flip angle. Intuition would tell us that increasing n would demand lower values of the pulse flip angle α, which is quantitatively predicted by the curves in Figure 10-9A. The effect of flip angle on signal loss and apparent vessel narrowing for the more distal locations is illustrated in Figure 10-9B and C.

Methods for Improved Background Suppression

One of the hallmarks of the TOF MRA technique is the relatively intense background from stationary tissue. This problem is exacerbated in 3D imaging because of the requirements of a low RF-pulse flip angle as a means of minimizing saturation of the protons in blood caused by multiple excitation during transit of the blood across the slab of tissue.

In 1992 Pike et al.[31] showed that a substantial reduction in background signal can be achieved in neurologic MRA by exploiting the magnetization transfer principle.[32] In brief, irradiation off-resonance of the (unobservable) protons in the protein matrix causes saturation of the (observable) tissue water protons via a cross-relaxation process. The protein protons do not give rise to a signal because of their very short T_2 relaxation times ($T_2 << 1$ msec). This principle can be used for suppression of the signal from gray and white matter. Of course, blood also contains proteins. Therefore, if not properly implemented, the method could lead to a reduction in the vascular signal as well. However, if the saturation pulse is constructed in such a

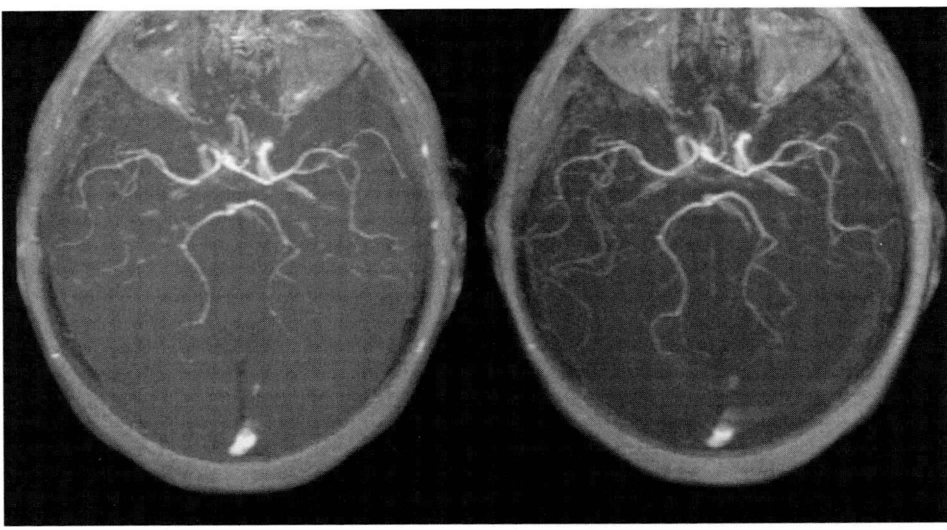

Figure 10-10. 3D TOF images of the circle of Willis (TR = 50 msec, TE = 5 msec, NEX = 1, 64 1-mm partitions), without (A) and with (B) magnetization transfer. Note the reduced background in image (B) and visualization of the tertiary branches of the posterior and middle cerebral arteries.

manner that it has zero net rotation of the magnetization (a so-called 0 pulse), the magnetization of the observable protons will be restored, whereas protons with very short T_2, that is, those pertaining to proteins, will be saturated because their transverse magnetization does not persist long enough to be rotated back onto the z axis. Pike et al. showed that in this manner vessel-to-background contrast for small vessels can be doubled. Figure 10-10 compares images obtained with and without magnetization transfer background suppression, demonstrating the effectiveness of the method for improved vessel visualization.

We have seen that the 2D approach consisting of sequential acquisition of a stack of these slices is advantageous from the point of view of minimizing saturation of slow-moving protons. On the other hand, resolution is limited by the finite slice thickness achievable in the 2D imaging mode. This mode is also more prone to section-to-section misregistration from subject motion because the data are acquired sequentially. An approach that minimizes saturation while retaining the features inherent to 3D imaging is acquiring multiple, relatively thin, 3D slabs that partially overlap one another. The technique has been termed MOTSA (*m*ultiple *o*verlapping *t*hin *s*lab *a*cquisitions).[33] Its efficiency can further be enhanced by interleaving data acquisition in such a manner that during one TR period several slabs can be excited (analogous to multislice imaging). Of course, this requires increased TR and thus increased stationary signal.

Another, more recently proposed technique focuses on enhancing the vascular signal by minimizing saturation losses in the distal portions of vessels (see Fig. 10-9B and C) without reducing slab thickness. The idea is to spatially vary the flip angle across the slab in such a manner that the flip angle is lower at the entry point, increasing toward the distal sections. In this manner the magnetization is retained for spins that see a larger number of RF pulses (those near the distal edge of the slab). The desired effect can be achieved in various ways, for example, by combining a gaussian slice profile with saturation of the leading-edge profile[34] or by creating a spatially varying excitation profile in such a manner that the RF pulse flip angle increases from the inflow to the exit edge of the slab[35–37] created by Fourier synthesis of the desired profile. At typical pulse repetition times (about 50 msec) and slab thicknesses (about 5 cm), doubling of the flip angle between entry and exit point and a mean flip angle of about 20 degrees were found to be a good compromise, yielding uniform vessel signal intensity.[36] The principle is illustrated schematically in Figure 10-11A, and a comparison of constant versus linearly increasing flip angle in a 3D TOF arteriogram of the neck is displayed in Figure 10-11B and C.

A very different approach aims at minimizing saturation signal loss and thus improving vessel delineation by shortening blood water proton relaxation times via gadolinium injection.[38,39] From measurements of the signal enhancement in the sagittal sinus upon adminis-

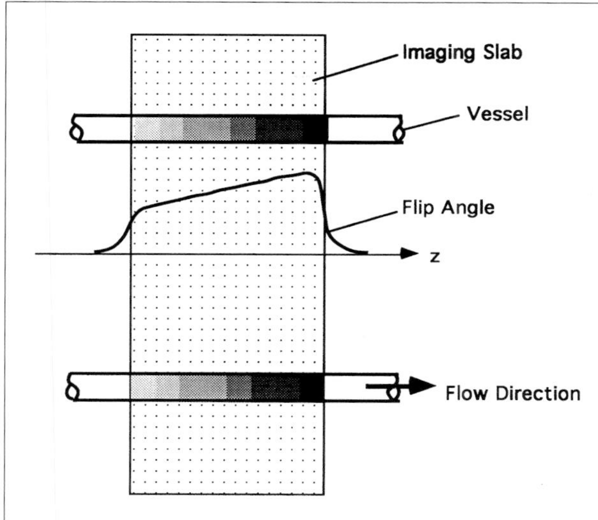

A

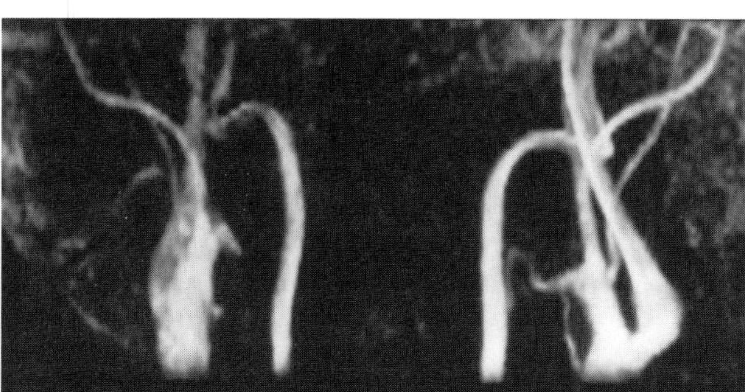

B

C

Figure 10-11. (A) A pulse designed so that its Fourier transform results in a ramp with the flip angle increasing between the vessel's inflow and exit point minimizes saturation of the more distal vessel locations. The flip angle increases linearly along the z axis so that the spins initially will experience little saturation, thus ensuring that more magnetization will be available downstream when experiencing further excitation. (B and C) 3D TOF angiograms of the neck with constant excitation (B) and ramped excitation (C), the latter showing improved visualization of distal vessels.

tration of 0.1 mmol/kg Gd(DTPA), Lin et al.[39] estimate that at 1.5 T field strength T_1 is reduced from its native value of 1.2 seconds to about 600 milliseconds. They show that for slowly flowing blood in the brain, small-vessels contrast is nearly doubled and that aneurysms (where spin saturation is particularly prominent due to recirculation) are better depicted with Gd(DTPA). Among the major problems with this approach are leakage of contrast material into background tissues (e.g., meninges) and enhancement of veins, which, because of the shortened T_1, are more difficult to saturate.

Physiologic Motion

For many applications of MRA in the body, notably in the thorax and abdomen, physiologic motion is a formidable problem that has been dealt with in different ways, including by suspended respiration and gating.

Various approaches are currently being practiced for pulmonary imaging,[14–16] an application of great clinical importance for the evaluation of patients with pulmonary emboli.[16] Two-dimensional techniques, in conjunction with high-speed gradient-echo imaging, permit sequential acquisition of multiple slices within a single breath-hold period of 10 to 15 seconds. Alternatively, a single slice of several centimeters' thickness can be acquired, and the additional time available can be used for increased signal averaging. The multiple thin slice technique is advantageous in achievable spatial resolution and maximizing inflow. If data acquisition is triggered to the R wave, a gating delay can be selected so that the low-spatial-frequency data (which provide most of the signal) are acquired during diastole, thus minimizing signal loss from flow dephasing.[15] The critical role of the trigger delay is demonstrated with the images in Figure 10-12.

Three-dimensional pulmonary MRA has also been reported, offering the usual advantages in terms of spatial resolution. Wielopolski et al. generated excellent pulmonary angiograms by means of a high-speed TOF, 3D gradient-echo pulse sequence in conjunction with cardiac gating.[14] It is designed in such a manner that during the RR interval 64 to 128 slice encodings can be applied, and thus one K-space plane is scanned during each heartbeat. This process is repeated N_y times, with N_y representing the number of phase-encoding increments. To maximize inflow of fresh spins, a waiting period of an additional heartbeat is inserted between phase encodings. One of the drawbacks of 3D techniques is their relatively long scan times, which can cause substantial blurring of vascular structures arising from respiratory motion.

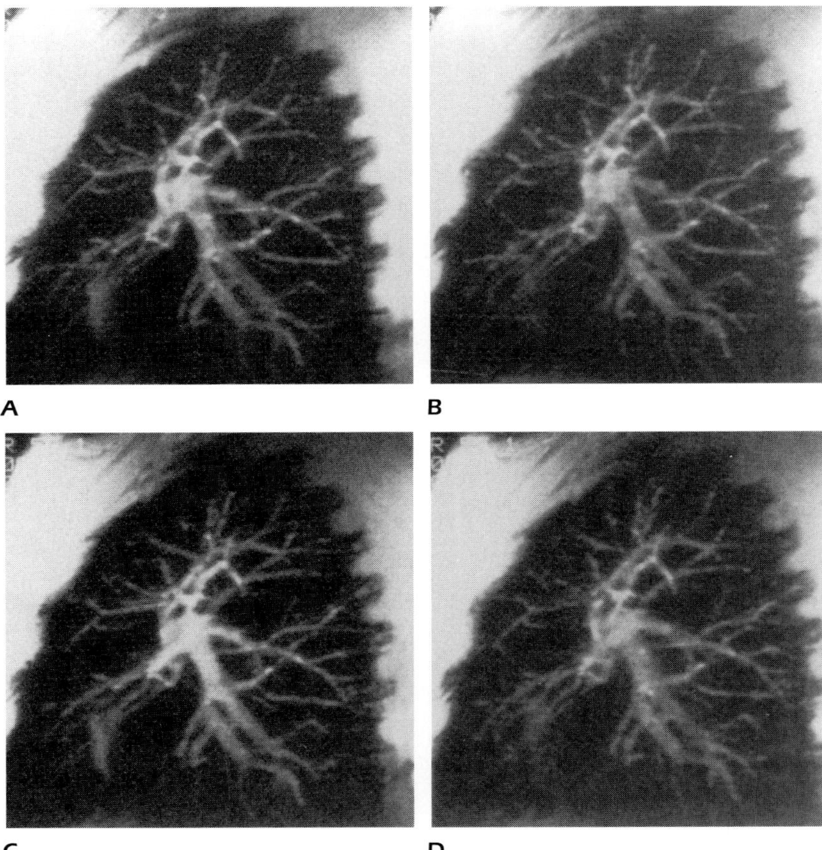

Figure 10-12. Peripherally triggered images of the right lung, obtained by MIP reconstruction of a set of 2D high-speed gradient-echo images (TR/TE 6.8/2.2 msec) in a single 14-sec breath-hold period. The images were collected with trigger delays of 50 msec (A), 200 msec (B), 400 msec (C), and 600 msec (D). (From Foo T, et al. Pulmonary vasculature; single breath-hold imaging with phased-array coils. Radiology 1992;183:473–477. Used with permission.)

A similar technique has recently been reported for imaging the renal arteries.[19] The method is a variant of the magnetization-prepared rapid acquisition gradient-echo (MP-RAGE) technique.[40] Background suppression is achieved by means of an inversion pulse followed by a delay such that the stationary signal is minimum at the time the low-flip-angle RF pulses are played out. The pulse sequence is ECG-triggered to systole in such a manner that during the T_1 interval inflow of fresh blood into the imaging slab is maximized, and data collection during diastole ensures minimal signal loss through intravoxel phase dispersion. Further, the signal from fat is suppressed by applying a frequency-selective RF pulse before data acquisition.

MRA of the coronary arteries poses a particular challenge in that it requires dealing with both respiratory and cardiac motion. If the total scan time can be reduced to 10 to 20 seconds, the motion degradation from breathing can be eliminated by suspending respiration. One such TOF approach makes use of what has been termed *segmented k-space* acquisition[24,41] in conjunction with cardiac gating. In brief, the cardiac cycle is divided into segments of 50 to 100 milllisec-onds' duration, during which cardiac motion can be regarded as relatively insignificant. However, instead of collecting only a single data line per cardiac phase as in conventional cine imaging, 4 to 8 lines are acquired per segment. Therefore, if 8 data lines were to be scanned per segment (and thus during one particular RR interval), 128 data lines could be sampled in 16 heartbeats, which can be effected in a single breath-hold period.

Projection Techniques

Once the stack of images has been acquired, an angiogram is produced by generating projection images. Typically, this is achieved by reprojecting the image data along the desired projection direction. Simple summing of the signal from all voxels along the projection direction would give rise to excessive background, which is readily seen by considering a situation in which the vascular signal is 10 times more intense than the signal from parenchymal tissue and, further, that the signal from a particular vessel to be displayed occupies two voxels. Suppose further that the projection ray encounters 128 voxels on its path across the imaging volume. The total signal then is $2 \times 10 + 126 \times 1 = 146$. The signal from an adjacent ray involving background only would be $128 \times 1 = 128$, and thus the vessel signal would be only about 14 percent more intense than background. A common algorithm that circumvents this problem is called *maximum intensity projection* (MIP) ray tracing.[42] It consists of casting parallel rays in a projection direction in such a manner that only the voxel of maximum intensity is retained and the signal from all other voxels is discarded. Hence the algorithm entails a very significant data reduction. Returning to the previous example, under these conditions a much more favorable vessel-to-background signal intensity ratio of 10:1 is obtained. The principle is illustrated in Figure 10-13.

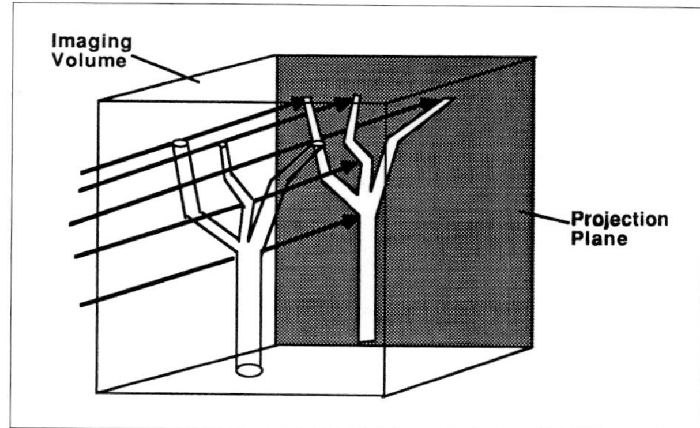

Figure 10-13. Principle of ray-tracing algorithm. Parallel rays are cast through the imaging volume at a user-specified angle to create a projection image. In the MIP version of the algorithm, the maximum signal intercepted by each ray is retained and displayed, and the signal from all other voxels is discarded.

Many more possible projection algorithms exist, although MIP ray tracing is by far most commonly used. For a review the interested reader is referred to Siebert and Rosenbaum.[43] One approach that is advantageous for singling out specific vessels makes use of connectivity criteria.[39,44,45] After an intensity threshold is set, all voxels with intensities below the threshold are discarded. The remaining voxels are classified into discrete objects by means of a region growing from a seed point, which is chosen within a region unambiguously assignable to a vessel. One of the problems with region-growing algorithms is their need for frequent operator intervention.

Phase Contrast Angiography

Basic Principle

A radically different approach to MRA makes use of the motion dependence of the signal phase. As already mentioned, precessing transverse magnetization acquires phase, which in the presence of magnetic field gradients is position-dependent (see Fig. 10-3). The position-dependent phase shift can be reversed by applying a second gradient pulse of opposite polarity because the positive phase shift ϕ_+ is exactly balanced by a phase shift of equal magnitude but opposite sign such that $\phi_+ = -\phi_-$ (Fig. 10-14). However, if the spins move as in the case for flowing blood, it becomes evident that the two opposing phase rotations do not cancel and a residual phase shift occurs that is proportional to the displacement vT, where v is the blood flow velocity and T the time interval between the two gradient pulses. A more detailed analysis shows that the flow-induced phase shift for two gradient pulses of area A_g and opposite polarity, spaced T seconds apart, is given by*

$$\phi(v) = \gamma v A_g T \tag{3}$$

To produce an angiogram, that is, an image displaying vessels only, one needs to isolate the signal from flowing blood, which can be achieved in various ways. The first that comes to mind is to assign gray levels to the flow-induced phase shift, as discussed earlier. To do so, however, one needs to subtract the data obtained with the bipolar flow-encoding gradient from a second data set that could be acquired without application of a flow-encoding gradient. In this manner the phase for all stationary protons would be zero, and the one for moving spins is given by equation 3. A more efficient method consists of acquiring the second data set with a bipolar flow-encoding gradient altered in such a manner that the polarity of the two gradient lobes is reversed (minus/plus instead of plus/minus). The magnitude of the resulting flow-induced phase shift remains the same in this case, but the sign is reversed. Hence the phase difference becomes $2\phi_+ = -2\phi_-$.

Depending on the direction of flow (forward or re-

*The product A_gT is also called the first moment (M_1) of the encoding gradient. For the bipolar gradient the first moment can assume values of $+A_gT$ or $-A_gT$, depending on whether the gradient polarities are $-/+$ or $+/-$.

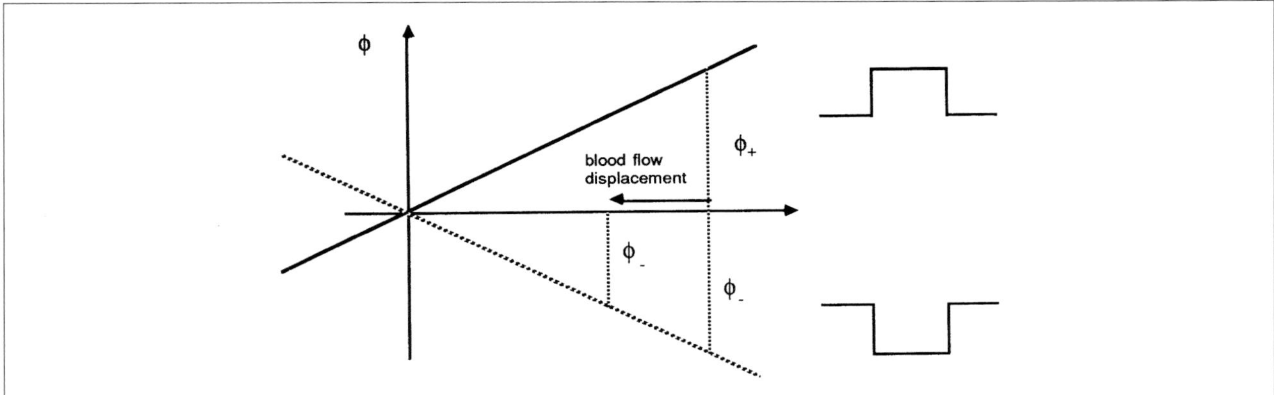

Figure 10-14. Effect of gradient reversal on spin phase. A first gradient pulse of positive polarity (*top right*) causes a phase shift ϕ_+ that is exactly compensated by a phase shift ϕ_- of equal magnitude but opposite sign caused by a gradient of opposite polarity (*bottom right*). Hence the two gradient pulses have no net effect on the phase of stationary tissue protons. However, in the presence of blood flow the protons change position, and in this case $\phi_+ \neq \phi_-$. The resulting residual phase shift is proportional to flow velocity.

verse), the phase difference is positive or negative, and some vessels would therefore appear bright, others dark. For these reasons it is more common to display the magnitude of the difference signal, obtained from a vector (complex) subtraction. Recall that two vectors $\vec{a}$ and $\vec{b}$ are subtracted from one another by the addition $\vec{a} + (-\vec{b})$. Complex subtraction of the two signals S_+ and S_- results in a signal that is proportional to $2\sin|\phi|$ with the phase angle $|\phi|$ being the absolute value of the phase shift imparted by the bipolar flow-encoding gradient Fig. 10-15). Since the phase angle ϕ is proportional to flow velocity, one recognizes from Figure 10-15 that there must be a critical flow velocity that leads to maximum signal. This condition corresponds to $2|\phi| = 180$ degrees. Both faster and slower flow thus will reduce the vascular signal. According to the relationship expressed by equation 3, the phase angle is also related to the properties of the gradient (area and spacing between the two lobes). As will be discussed, selection of this parameter, called v_{enc} (the maximum encoding velocity), is a critical user-selectable parameter that has significant implications for the quality of the resulting phase contrast angiograms.

Multidirectional Phase Contrast Angiography

It was noted previously that the phase contrast signal depends on the direction of flow relative to the orientation of the flow-encoding gradient. If a vessel altered its course to become orthogonal to the orientation of the flow-encoding gradient, its signal would be exactly nulled because it would behave like stationary tissue. In practice, vessels are tortuous, and thus encoding in a single direction is not sufficient. One obvious solution to this problem is to repeat the procedure described three times to obtain three sets of data corresponding to encoding along the *x, y,* and *z* direction and to combine the three data sets into multidirectional phase contrast images with equal sensitization

Figure 10-15. Effect of bipolar gradient on MR signal. Depending on gradient polarity and direction of flow, a positive or negative phase shift ensues ($-\phi$, $+\phi$). Vector subtraction of two data sets, $S^+ - S_-$, results in a signal of magnitude $2S\sin(\phi)$ from flowing spins only. Axis labels *I* and *R* stand for imaginary and real components of the complex signal.

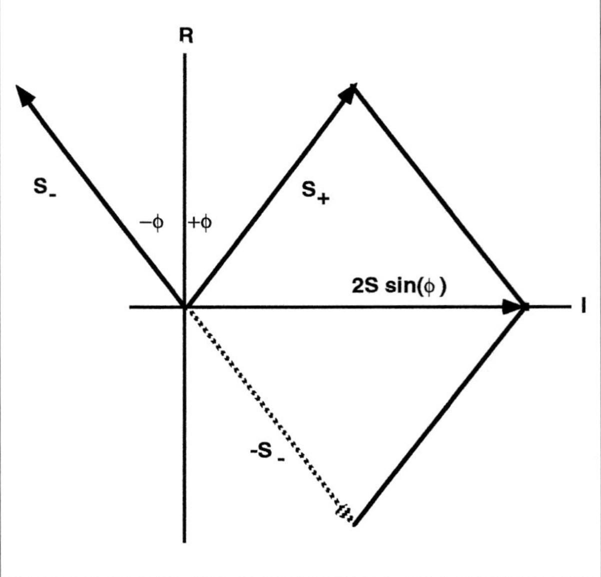

along all three spatial axes.[46] It is readily seen that this is equivalent to an acquisition corresponding to NEX = 6, which would imply that phase contrast angiograms require excessively long scan times and thus do not seem to be competitive with their faster TOF counterparts. Fortunately, the constraints imposed by the technique are not quite so severe. First, the increased number of signal averages entails a signal-to-noise benefit, which means that some of the increased SNR can be traded for shorter pulse repetition times. In fact, phase contrast angiography should be performed at the minimum TR admissible by the scan software. In practice, this reduces scan time by about a factor of 2, which suggests that it is still three times less efficient than TOF MRA.

It has more recently been shown that four independent acquisitions suffice for the reconstruction of images with multidirectional flow sensitivity because there are only four different components, stationary protons and protons with motion along *x*, *y*, and *z* direction. The simplest among these more efficient approaches consists of acquiring three data sets, each with sensitization in the three orthogonal directions, and a phase reference data set without motion sensitization.[47] Alternatively, one can acquire the data in such a manner that bipolar flow-encoding gradients are applied in all four acquisitions, which is the most commonly used phase contrast method.[48] The data are decoded by taking sums and differences to yield S_x, S_y, and S_z, the magnitude signal pertaining to flow in the three orthogonal directions, from which images are computed as

$$S = \sqrt{S_x^2 + S_y^2 + S_z^2} \tag{4}$$

The signal in these images is proportional to blood flow speed.[48] Figure 10-16 shows projection angiograms pertaining to flow sensitization in an anterior–posterior direction (*a*), as opposed to encoding in all three spatial directions (*b*).

An alternative processing strategy consists of computing the phase difference

$$\Delta\phi = \phi_+ - \phi_- = 2 \text{ atan } (R/I) \tag{5}$$

where *R* and *I* denote the real and imaginary component of the signal (see Fig. 10-15). One can then assign gray scale to the phase as illustrated in Figure 10-5. This approach, although less desirable for anatomic vessel display, provides quantitative flow information because the gray value is directly related to velocity and direction of blood flow. Further, in contrast to simple phase display, the phase shifts are due to blood flow motion only as all other phase shifts (e.g., from magnetic field inhomogeneity) are eliminated by the subtraction procedure.

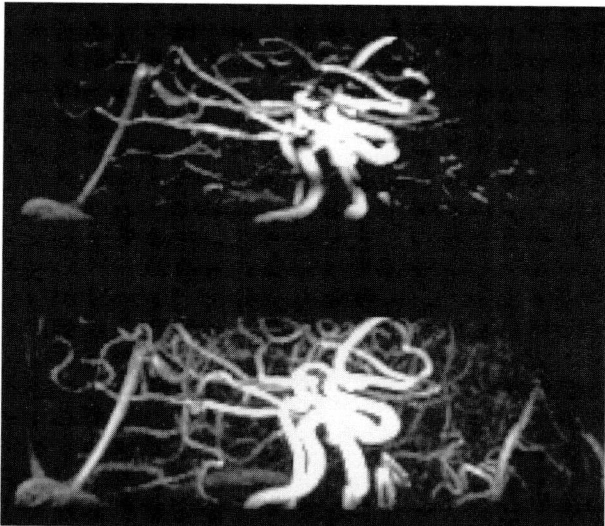

Figure 10-16. Effect of motion sensitization. (*Top*) Single projection from 3D phase contrast data set obtained by processing unidirectional sensitization (anterior–posterior), emphasizing vessel segments with an anterior–posterior orientation. (*Bottom*) Multidirectional angiogram showing uniform vessel signal irrespective of direction.

Maximum Encoding Velocity (v_{enc}) Parameter

For encoding in a single direction, there is a maximum velocity without causing aliasing. From Figure 10-15 it is evident that the maximum flow signal is obtained for a phase difference $\Delta\phi$ = 180 degrees (π radians). The maximum encoding velocity (v_{enc}) is thus defined as the velocity which, for a given encoding gradient (defined by gradient area A_g and lobe spacing T (see equation 3), produces a 180-degree phase shift, that is,

$$v_{enc} = \frac{\pi}{2\gamma A_g T} \tag{6}$$

Equation 6 shows that the maximum encoding velocity is inversely proportional to the gradient area A_g and the time interval T between the two lobes. Hence, if the signal from small vessels (slow flow) is to be emphasized, lower values of v_{enc} should be selected (achieved by increasing either A_g or T.

The choice of v_{enc} is important for yet another reason. Since the flow velocity varies across the lumen—it is slower near the vessel wall than at the center—the vascular signal is spatially variant as well. In the case of laminar flow, the flow velocity is exactly zero

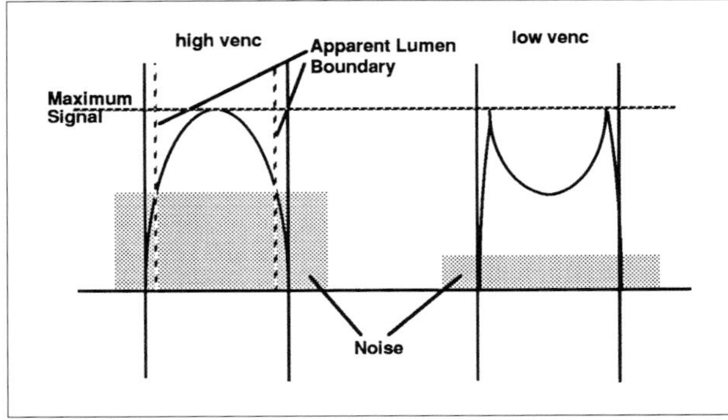

A

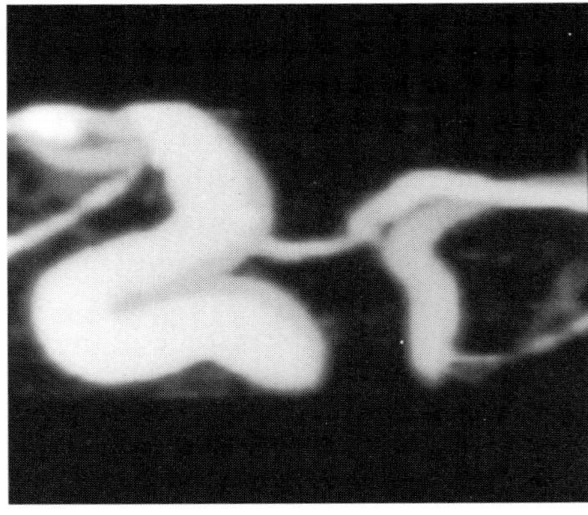

B

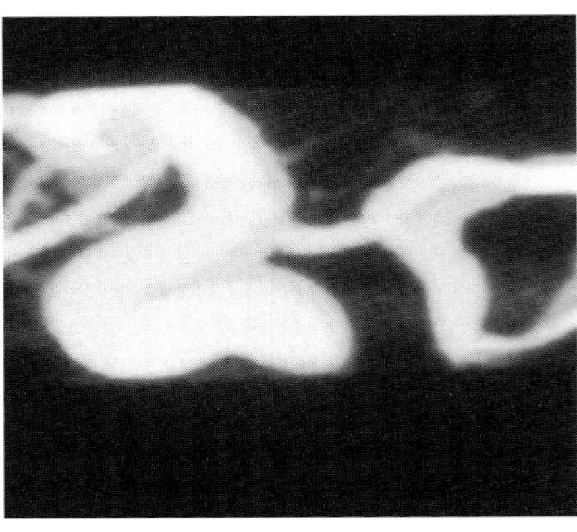

C

Figure 10-17. (A) Because of the distribution of flow velocities across the vessel lumen, the lower velocities near the vessel wall may fall below the noise threshold, leading to an apparent lumen narrowing (*left*). Reducing v_{enc} so that the maximum velocity in the vessel (corresponding to the more central locations) is aliased enhances the signal from slow peripheral flow while lowering the noise floor, to yield luminal diameters closer to reality (*right*). (B) Phase contrast angiogram obtained with v_{enc} = 90 cm/sec exhibiting artifactually reduced vessel lumina when compared to an underencoded image (C) in which v_{enc} = 30 cm/sec was selected. (Images courtesy Dr. Scott Atlas, Department of Radiology, University of Pennsylvania Medical Center.)

at the vessel wall and maximum at the center. If one were to select v_{enc} to match the centerline flow velocity, one would lose signal peripherally and the lumen would appear narrower than in reality. Since the noise is proportional to v_{enc},[48] the weak peripheral signal near the vessel wall would fall below the noise floor and thus not be detected. By contrast, the choice of a lower value of the v_{enc} parameter ensures that the apparent lumen diameter is closer to the true one. In this case, of course, the central signal corresponding to velocities higher than v_{enc} will be aliased to lead to reduced signal (Fig. 10-17A). However, in a MIP reconstructed image the central reduction in signal intensity caused by this phenomenon will not be visible. It is thus advantageous to "underencode," that is, to select a value of v_{enc} that is significantly less than the maximum velocity to be encountered. Figure 10-17B and C displays two phase contrast projection angiograms from the same subject, differing only in the choice of v_{enc}. The apparent lumen diameter is reduced in the image obtained with the higher value of v_{enc} (90 cm/sec versus 30 cm/sec).

Conclusions

In summary, most MRA techniques practiced today make use of either the TOF-principle, based on inflow of unsaturated spins combined with relative saturation of background protons by rapid pulsing, or flow-encoding gradients causing a velocity-dependent phase shift (phase contrast MRA). In both classes of techniques the vascular signal depends on the direction and velocity of the blood, and the parameters (pulse repetition time, RF pulse flip angle, slab thickness, imaging plane, direction) have to be selected as a compromise to cover the wide range of blood flow velocities present. The most common artifacts are signal losses due to spin dephasing as a result of disturbed flow at the site of a constriction and distal to it.[49] These artifacts can be minimized by shortening echo times,[50] using fractional echoes to minimize the gradient moments,[51] and using velocity-compensating gradient waveforms.[30,52]

TOF techniques are more efficient by permitting shorter scan times, typically on the order of 5 to 10 minutes for 64 to 128 sections, but they suffer from stationary background signals, which may interfere with the vascular structures. Phase contrast methods, on the other hand, in order to ensure vessel display independent of flow direction, require more complex acquisition schemes corresponding to at least four excitations, resulting in scan times of 10 to 20 minutes for a comparable scan volume and resolution. They are also more sensitive to gradient imperfections such as eddy currents and thus, in general, demand actively shielded gradients.[53] On the other hand, given appropriate hardware, phase contrast angiograms are virtually free of background and thus often better depict small vessels. This advantage, however, is somewhat mitigated by the recent advances in background suppression such as magnetization transfer[31,54] and fat suppression.

Acknowledgments

The author is grateful to Carolyn Kaut-Watson for her assistance in acquiring some of the images and to Dr. Atlas for the images in Figures 10-9 and 10-16.

References

1. Hinshaw WS, Bottomley PA, Holland GN. Radiographic thin-section imaging of the human wrist by nuclear magnetic resonance imaging. Nature 1977;270:722–723.
2. Singer JR, Crooks LE. Nuclear magnetic resonance blood flow measurements in the human brain. Science 1983;221:654–656.
3. Wehrli FW, MacFall JR, Axel L, et al. Approaches to in-plane and out-of-plane flow imaging. Noninvasive Med Imaging 1984;1:127–136.
4. Feinberg DA, Crooks L, Hoenninger III J, Arakawa M, Watts J. Pulsatile blood flow velocity in the human arteries displayed by magnetic resonance imaging. Radiology 1984;153:177–180.
5. Wedeen VJ, Meuli RA, Edelman RR, et al. Projective imaging of pulsatile flow with magnetic resonance. Science 1985;230:946–948.
6. Meuli RA, van Wedeen J, Geller SC, et al. MR gated subtraction angiography: evaluation of lower extremities. Radiology 1986;159:411–418.
7. Dumoulin CL, Hart HR. Magnetic resonance angiography. Radiology 1986;161:717–720.
8. Gullberg GT, Wehrli FW, Shimakawa A, Simons MA. MR vascular imaging with a fast gradient refocusing pulse sequence and reformatted images from transaxial sections. Radiology 1987;165:241–246.
9. Potchen E, Haacke E, Siebert J, Gottschalk E. Magnetic resonance angiography. Philadelphia: Mosby, 1993.
10. Anderson CM, Edelman RR, Turski PA. Clinical magnetic resonance angiography. New York: Raven Press, 1993.
11. Masaryk TJ, Modic MT, Ruggieri PM, et al. Three-dimensional (volume) gradient-echo imaging of the carotid bifurcation: preliminary clinical experience. Radiology 1989;171:801–806.
12. Masaryk TJ, Modic MT, and Ross JS. Intracranial circulation: preliminary clinical results with three-dimensional (volume) MR angiography. Radiology 1989;171:793–799.
13. Keller PJ, Drayer BP, Fram EK, et al. MR angiography with two-dimensional acquisition and three-dimensional display. Radiology 1989;173:527–532.
14. Wielopolski P, Haacke E, Adler A. Three-dimensional MR imaging of pulmonary vasculature: preliminary experience. Radiology 1992;183:465–472.
15. Foo T, MacFall J, Hayes C, Sostman H, Slayman B. Pulmonary vasculature: single breath-hold MR imaging with phased-array coils. Radiology 1992;183:473–477.
16. Grist T, Sostman H, MacFall J, et al. Pulmonary angiography with MR imaging: preliminary clinical experience. Radiology 1993;189:523–530.
17. Vock P, Terrier F, Wegmüller H, et al. Magnetic resonance of abdominal vessels: early experience using the three-dimensional phase contrast technique. Br J Radiol 1991;64:10–16.
18. Kent K, Edelman R, Kim D, et al. Magnetic resonance imaging: a reliable test for the evaluation of proximal atherosclerotic renal arterial stenosis. J Vasc Surg 1991;13:311–318.
19. Li D, Haacke E, Mugler III J, Berr S, Brookeman J, Hutton M. Three-dimensional time-of-flight MR angiography using selective inversion-recovery RAGE with fat saturation and ECG triggering: application to renal arteries. Magn Reson Med 1994;31:414–422.
20. Owen R, Carpenter J, Baum R, Perloff L, Cope C. Magnetic resonance imaging of angiographically occult runoff vessels in peripheral arterial occlusive disease. N Engl J Med 1992;326:1577–1581.
21. Owen R, Baum R, Carpenter J, Holland G, Cope C. Symptomatic peripheral vascular disease: selection of imaging parameters and clinical evaluation with MR angiography. Radiology 1993;187:627–635.
22. Yucel E, Kaufman J, Geller S, Waltman A. Atherosclerotic occlusive disease of the lower extremity: prospective evaluation with two-dimensional time-of-flight MR angiography. Radiology 1993;187:637–641.
23. Cho Z, Mun C, Friedenberg R. NMR angiography of coronary vessels with 2D planar image scanning. Magn Reson Med 1991;20:134–143.
24. Edelman RR, Manning WJ, Burstein D, Paulin S. Coronary arteries: breath-hold MR angiography. Radiology 1991;181:641–643.
25. Axel L. Blood flow effects in magnetic resonance imaging. AJR 1984;143:1157–1166.
26. Wehrli FW. Fast-scan magnetic resonance: principles and applications. New York: Raven, 1991.
27. Moran PR, Moran RA, Karstaedt N. Verification and evaluation of internal flow and motion: true magnetic resonance imaging by the phase gradient modulation method. Radiology 1985;154:433–441.
28. Ruggieri PM, Laub GA, Masaryk TJ, Modic MT. Intracranial circulation: pulse sequence considerations in three-dimensional (volume) MR angiography. Radiology 1989;171:785–791.
29. Cline HE, Lorenson WE, Herfkens RJ, et al. Vascular morphology by three-dimensional magnetic resonance imaging. Magn Reson Imaging 1989;7:45–54.
30. Haacke EM, Masaryk TJ, Wielopolski PA, et al. Optimizing blood vessel contrast in fast three-dimensional MRI. Magn Reson Med 1990;14:202–221.
31. Pike GB, Hu BS, Glover GH, Enzmann DR. Magnetization transfer magnetic resonance angiography. Magn Reson Med 1992;25:372–379.
32. Wolff SD, Balaban RS. Magnetization transfer contrast (MTC) and tissue water proton relaxation in vivo. Magn Reson Med 1989;10:135–144.
33. Parker DL, Yuan C, Blatter DD. MR angiography by multiple thin slab 3D acquisition. Magn Reson Med 1991;17:434–451.
34. Matsuda T, Morii I, Kohno F, et al. An asymmetric slice profile: spatial alteration of flow signal response in 3D time-of-flight NMR. Magn Reson Med 1993;29:783–789.
35. Laub G, Purdy D. Use of tilted optimized nonsaturating excitation (TONE) RF pulses and MTC to improve the quality of MR angiograms of the carotid bifurcation. Proc Soc Magn Reson Med 1992;2:3905.
36. Purdy D, Cadena G, Laub G. The design of variable tip angle slab selection (TONE) pulses for improved 3D angiography. Proc Annu Meet Soc Magn Reson Med 1992;1:882.
37. Nägele T, Klose U, Grodd W, Petersen D, Tintera J. The effects of linearly increasing flip angles on 3D inflow MR angiography. Magn Reson Med 1994;31:561–566.
38. Marchal G, Bosmans H, van Freyenhoven L, et al. Intracranial vascular lesions: optimization and clinical evaluation of three-

dimensional time-of-flight MR angiography. Radiology 1990; 175:443–448.
39. Lin W, Haacke E, Smith A, Clampitt M. Gadolinium-enhanced high-resolution MR angiography with adaptive vessel tracking: preliminary results in the intracranial circulation. J Magn Reson Imaging 1992;2:277–284.
40. Mugler JP III, Brookeman JR. Three-dimensional magnetization-prepared rapid gradient-echo imaging (3D MP RAGE). Magn Reson Med 1990;15:152–157.
41. Edelman RR, Wallner B, Singer A, Atkinson DJ, Saini S. Segmented turboFLASH: method for breath-hold MR imaging of the liver with flexible contrast. Radiology 1990;177:515–521.
42. Laub G, Kaiser W. MR angiography with gradient motion refocusing. J Comput Assist Tomogr 1988;12:377–382.
43. Siebert J, Rosenbaum T. Image presentation and post-processing. In: Potchen EJ, Haacke, Siebert, Gottschalk, eds. Magnetic resonance angiography. Philadelphia: Mosby, 1993.
44. Cline H, Lorensen WE, Kikinis R, Jolesz F. Three-dimensional segmentation of MR images of the head using probability and connectivity. J Comput Assist Tomogr 1990;14:1037–1045.
45. Saloner D, Hanson WA, Tsuruda JS, van Tyen R, Anderson CM, Lee RE. Application of a connected voxel algorithm to MR angiographic data. J Magn Reson Imaging 1991;1:423–430.
46. Dumoulin CL, Souza SP, Walker MF, Wagle W. Three-dimensional phase contrast angiography. Magn Reson Med 1989;9: 139–149.
47. Hausmann R, Lewin JS, Laub G. Phase contrast MR angiography with reduced acquisition time: new concepts in sequence design. J Magn Reson Imaging 1991;1:415–422.
48. Pelc NJ, Bernstein MA, Shimakawa A, Glover GH. Encoding strategies for three-direction phase-contrast MR imaging of flow. J Magn Reson Imaging 1991;1:405–413.
49. Urchuk SN, Plewes DB. Mechanisms of flow-induced signal loss in MR angiography. J Magn Reson Imaging 1992;2:453–462.
50. Schmalbrock P, Yuan C, Chakeres DW, Kohli J, Pelc NJ. Volume MR angiography: methods to achieve very short echoes. Radiology 1990;175:861–865.
51. Listerud J. First principles of magnetic resonance angiography. Magn Reson Q 1991;7:136–170.
52. Pattany PM, Phillips JJ, Chiu LC, et al. Motion artifact suppression technique (MAST) for MR imaging. J Comput Assist Tomogr 1987;11:369–377.
53. Roemer PB, Edelstein WA, Hickey JS. Self-shielded gradient coils. Proc Annu Meet Soc Magn Reson Med 1986;13:1067.
54. Lin W, Tkach JA, Haacke EM, Masaryk TJ. Intracranial MR angiography: application of magnetization transfer contrast and fat saturation to short gradient-echo velocity-compensated sequences. Radiology 1993;186:753–761.

11

Vascular Sonography

JOSEPH F. POLAK

This chapter discusses the role of ultrasound in noninvasive imaging of the arterial and venous systems. The major emphasis is on the use of this technology for evaluating the peripheral arteries and veins as well as for abdominal and small parts imaging.

Imaging Physics

Gray Scale Imaging

Principles of Image Formation[1]

The sonographic image is created in two steps. In the first, a series of short pulses of radiofrequency signals is applied to piezoelectric crystals. Displacement of the piezoelectric crystals causes a pressure wave and transmission of a sound signal in the soft tissues in contact with the crystals. The second step of image formation is the acquisition of the returning echoes. These echoes are created when the sound pulse interacts with the underlying soft tissues. Three types of physical interactions are at play. The first, and less common, is straightforward reflection. This reflection normally occurs perpendicular to sharp interfaces between tissues of different acoustic impedance, for example, between blood and the intimal lining of an artery. The second type, the major component of the returning signals, is caused by smaller scatterers that cause returning echoes in various directions. The heterogeneity of these small scatterers accounts for the background texture seen on sonographic images of the soft tissues. In the third type of interaction, signals arising from blood are caused by the scattering of sound against the cellular components of blood, principally red blood cells. The red blood cell, being much smaller than the wavelength of the applied sound signal, sends back a very weak signal. This is called *Rayleigh scattering*. In order of magnitude, the strength of the signal from blood is one-ten-thousandth to one-millionth that of the surrounding soft tissues. This explains why the vessel lumen appears black with respect to the surrounding soft tissues (Fig. 11-1A).

Transducer and Frequency Selection

Most imaging of the lower extremity arteries and veins can be conducted with a carrier frequency of 5 MHz. This permits a clear delineation of vessels that range in size from 1 mm to slightly over 1 cm. It also permits the identification of plaques and thrombi within these vessels.

The actual resolution of a transducer improves as frequency increases. For example, a standard frequency pulse of two cycles at a 5-MHz carrier frequency would result in a minimum spatial resolution of 0.3 mm. Increasing the frequency to 10 MHz, for the same length of two cycles, will improve the resolution to 0.15 mm. Conversely, decreasing the frequency to 2.5 MHz decreases the resolution to 0.6 mm.

Transducer frequency is also responsible for penetration of the ultrasound signal in the soft tissues and the strength of the returning echoes. An ultrasound beam of 5 MHz can easily penetrate distances up to 6 cm. On occasion, with a larger body habitus, this may not be sufficient to reach the more deeply lying artery and vein; this is often the case when imaging the popliteal artery and vein, since they lie in the adductor or Hunter canal. Better penetration can be achieved by selecting a lower carrier frequency, for example, a 2.5- or 3.75-MHz transducer. In the pelvis and abdomen, the 5-MHz transducer can, in very thin individuals, be used to image the aorta, the vena cava, and the major visceral arteries and veins. However, in general, either a 2.5- or 3.75-MHz transducer is preferred.

Transducer shape also affects the way imaging is performed. In the lower extremities, the neck, and the distal upper extremities, the linear array transducer permits a rapid evaluation of long segments of arteries and veins. This transducer shape is less well suited for investigating the abdomen and pelvis. These areas are better evaluated with a curved array or sector scanner capable of better visualizing the deep-lying vessels (Fig. 11-2). These transducer shapes are also useful when interrogating the more central portions of the neck vessels, such as the

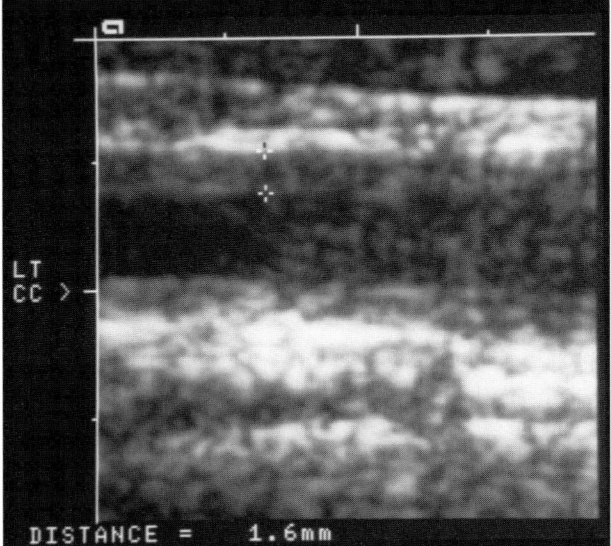

A

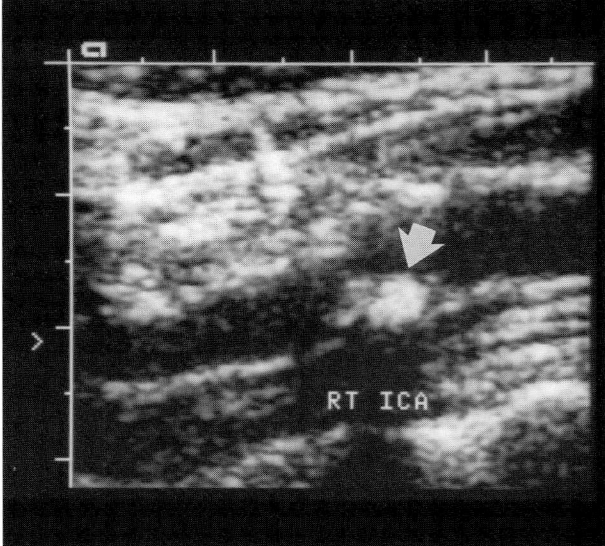

B

Figure 11-1. (A) This gray scale image shows, on the *left*, a clearly demarcated thickened wall of the common carotid artery. This is obscured on the portion of the carotid artery to the *right* because of noise. Such noise can be caused by reverberation of echoes and down-ringing of signals from the surrounding soft tissues. (B) This gray scale image shows a hyperechoic lesion (*arrow*) in the proximal internal carotid artery. The black areas on a gray scale image correspond to areas where there are few scatterers. These can be in the lumen of an artery or vein, in cysts, and in collections such as seromas, abscesses, and hematomas. Atherosclerotic plaque and thrombus are better visualized when the target vessel is closer to the skin. In general, the resolution of the image decreases with depth while the noise levels in the image increase in importance.

brachiocephalic veins. In addition, transducers with smaller footprints can be used to directly image the intracranial vasculature and profit from a smaller imaging window through the temporal bone.

Appearance of Vessels

The lumens of both arteries and veins appear dark with respect to the surrounding soft tissues because of the low intensity of the scattering interaction between sound waves and the red blood cells and smaller cellular components within blood. Because of this relative paucity of signal, atherosclerotic plaque and occasionally thrombi are often clearly outlined in the vessel lumen (Fig. 11-3). Similarly, orienting the ultrasound beam perpendicular to the interface between artery wall and blood will normally cause a very strong returning echo at the interface. This interface line can then be used to measure the relative thickness of the arterial wall as the combined thickness of the intima-media complex, since the intima itself cannot be discerned.[2] This may be difficult in certain circumstances because the wall interfaces can easily be lost with very tortuous arteries, partly because of their course outside the imaging plane defined by the transducer, but also because of the relative angle between the artery wall and the ultrasound beam.

Doppler Sonography[3,4]

Principles of Velocity Measurements

The Doppler principle can be summarized as follows. The returning frequency of a signal with a given carrier frequency changes as a function of the relative speed of the scatterer with respect to the receiver. For example, red blood cells flowing toward a transducer will cause a relative increase in the frequency of the returning signals as compared to the carrier signal. This change in frequency is normally small when compared to the carrier frequency. A carrier frequency of 4 MHz, for example, will have a frequency shift of 5000 Hz when the velocity of blood reaches 1.25 m per second. The returning frequency would then be 4,005,000 Hz. Conversely, motion away from the transducer causes a relative decrease in the frequency of the signal returning to the transducer. In this case, the same 5000-Hz frequency shift shows up as an absolute decrease in the frequency of the returning signal (3,995,000 Hz). Typically, the highest velocities of flowing blood that can be generated at stenoses are below 5 to 6 m per second.

By keeping the relative position of transducer and moving blood fixed with respect to each other, the velocity of flowing blood can be calculated from the fre-

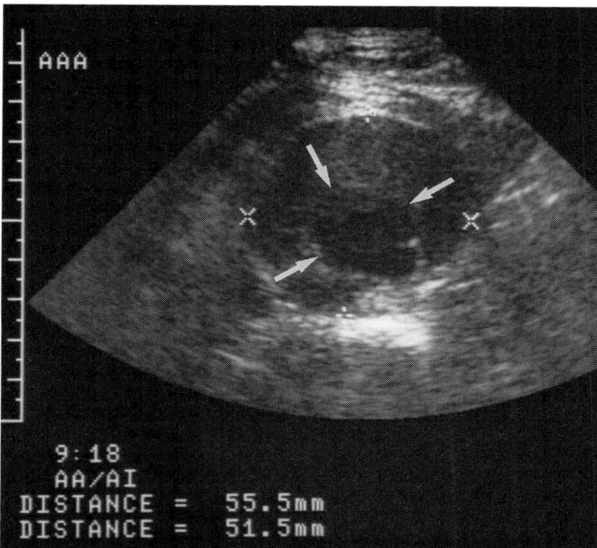

Figure 11-2. Transverse image of the abdominal aorta showing a well-defined aneurysm. The central lumen (*arrows*) is surrounded by thrombus that has deposited along the wall of the aneurysm. The outer wall is marked by the two sets of calipers (X and +).

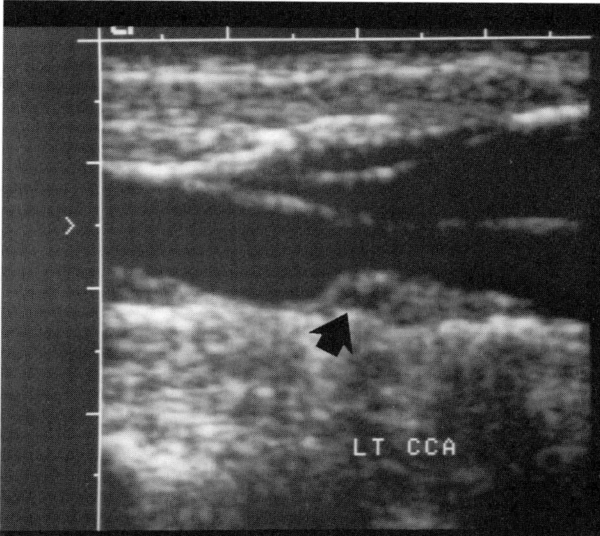

Figure 11-3. Sonogram showing a heterogeneous plaque in the common carotid artery. The zone of hypoechoic signal (*arrow*) probably represents an area of intraplaque hemorrhage.

quency shift. For example, assuming an arbitrary 60 degrees between the sonographic beam and motion of blood, one can directly relate velocity to the measured frequency shift. This is the basis for the early use of nonimaging Doppler devices and the derived Doppler shift measurements for the detection of arterial stenosis.

Waveform Analysis

Doppler waveform analysis is a method of retrieving the frequency shift information returning to the transducer and displaying it in a semiquantitative fashion. The waveform is created as follows (Fig. 11-4). Over a very short time interval, approximately 1 to 5 milliseconds, the sonographic transducer receives signals. This short segment of signal is then submitted to a signal-processing device and undergoes Fourier transformation. This process breaks down the information within the returning echoes and displays it as a map on which the amplitude corresponds roughly to the number of red blood cells or scatterers and the x axis corresponds to their frequency. This information, obtained every 1 to 5 milliseconds, is then further processed and displayed in a more complex manner. The number, or intensity, of scatterers then corresponds to the intensity or brightness on display, which shows the relative frequency shifts presented along the y axis. The x axis is the time axis and is used to sequentially display this information, as it is being processed, in time increments of 1 to 5 milliseconds.

The resultant display is a semiquantitative map of the number of red blood cells that have a given velocity relative to the direction of the ultrasound beam.

Pulsed Doppler Applications

The pulsed Doppler technique is used to specifically locate the origin of returning frequency shifted signals. With pulsed Doppler sonography, a relatively short ultrasound pulse (10–20 cycles in duration, for example) is sent out. A receiver then listens for the return of these echoes. By adjusting the time delay and picking the specific time point when the receiver acquires the returning signals, one can accurately determine their depth. The location of the Doppler gate defines this depth and corresponds to the time interval between pulse transmission and pulse reception. In addition, because the angle of the sound beam can often be selected, any location on the image can be selected and be subjected to this type of analysis.

Doppler Gate Location

The position of the Doppler gate can be used to selectively image an artery or vein within the boundaries of the gray scale image. By decreasing the size of the gate, one can selectively image a small portion of the vessel gate. This approach is referred to as *duplex imaging*.[5] In the normal flow pattern of an artery, slowly moving blood is located near the artery wall. Velocities near the center of the vessel are larger. Selective place-

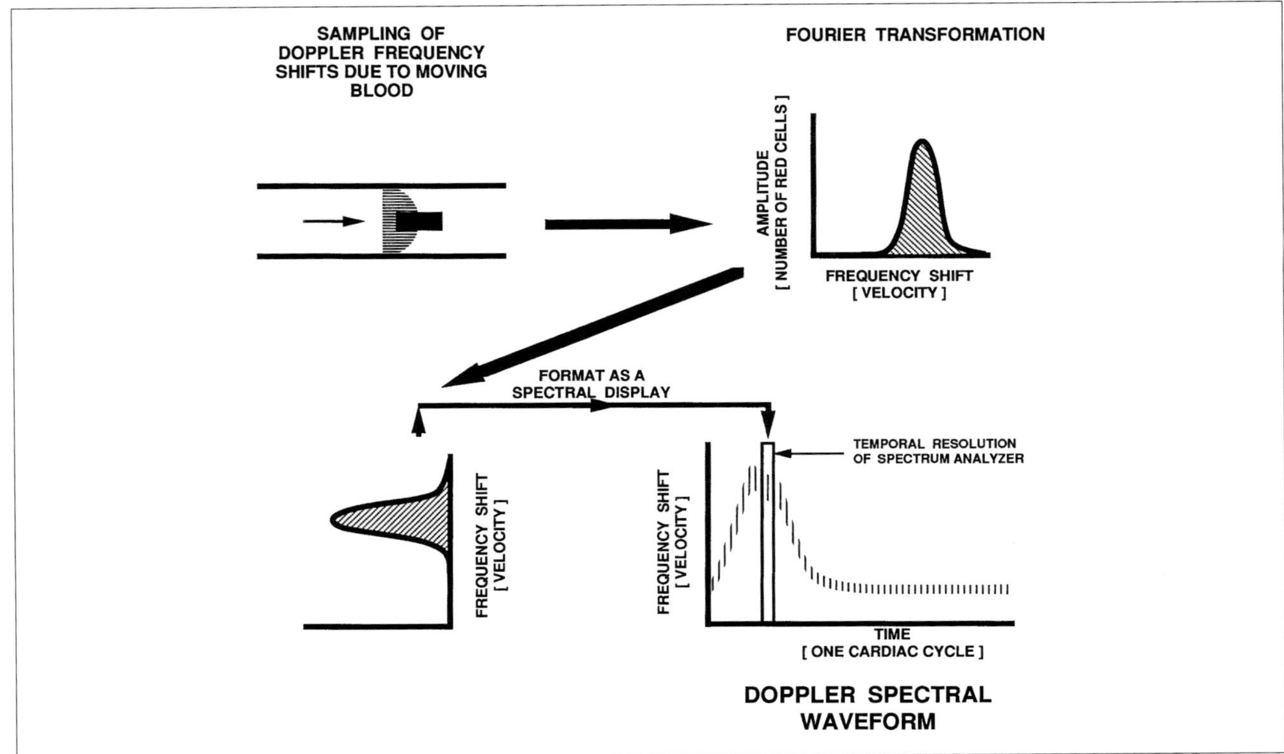

Figure 11-4. Diagram summarizing the steps in the creation of the Doppler waveform. Frequency shift information is decoded and presented in the form of a frequency shift histogram (often with the aid of a Fourier transform). This histogram is created for each time increment of 1 to 5 msec and then rendered in the form of a waveform in which the intensity of the trace is roughly proportional to the number of red cells and the *y* axis is a reflection of the Doppler peak frequency shifts (velocities).

ment of a small Doppler gate in these portions of the artery can readily demonstrate the typical pattern of laminar flow. Conversely, opening up the Doppler gate will acquire signals from a larger volume and therefore cause the resultant waveform to represent the broader distribution of red blood cell velocities across the artery lumen (Fig. 11-5).

A stenosis can be detected and its severity graded with the aid of Doppler sonography. Starting from the Doppler spectrum, acquired from different portions of the artery, it is easy to estimate the peak frequency shift of flowing blood. This has been shown to correlate directly with the velocity of the red blood cells.[6] Because areas of relative narrowing in the artery cause an increase in the velocity of flowing blood, these stenotic lesions are identifiable whenever areas of increased frequency shifts are detected. In vitro experiments have shown that the frequency shift measured on the Doppler waveform is roughly proportional to the severity of the stenosis. This basic principle was first investigated and proved for carotid artery stenosis.[6] It is the basis for grading stenosis severity throughout the arterial system.

Angle Correction

The relative angle formed between the direction of the Doppler beam and the direction of the moving red blood cells is critical to the accurate determination of their velocity. There are two basic principles to remember in placing the Doppler gate. The first is the basic concept behind the Doppler principle. Under ideal circumstances, the beam should be as parallel as possible with the motion of blood. Conversely, the worst scenario is to sample Doppler signals when the beam is perpendicular. In addition, because of the physical constraints of in vivo imaging, all of the red blood cells flowing into the volume defined by the Doppler gate need not share the same relative angle with respect to the transducer. This can cause a markedly distorted signal sometimes referred to as *mirroring* of the spectrum. Under ideal circumstances, the angle between the beam used to interrogate the vessel and flow within the vessel should be kept at 60 degrees or lower to minimize this effect. The second reason for variability in the determination of a velocity estimate is the need to achieve an accurate determination of the angle made between the sound beam used to measure

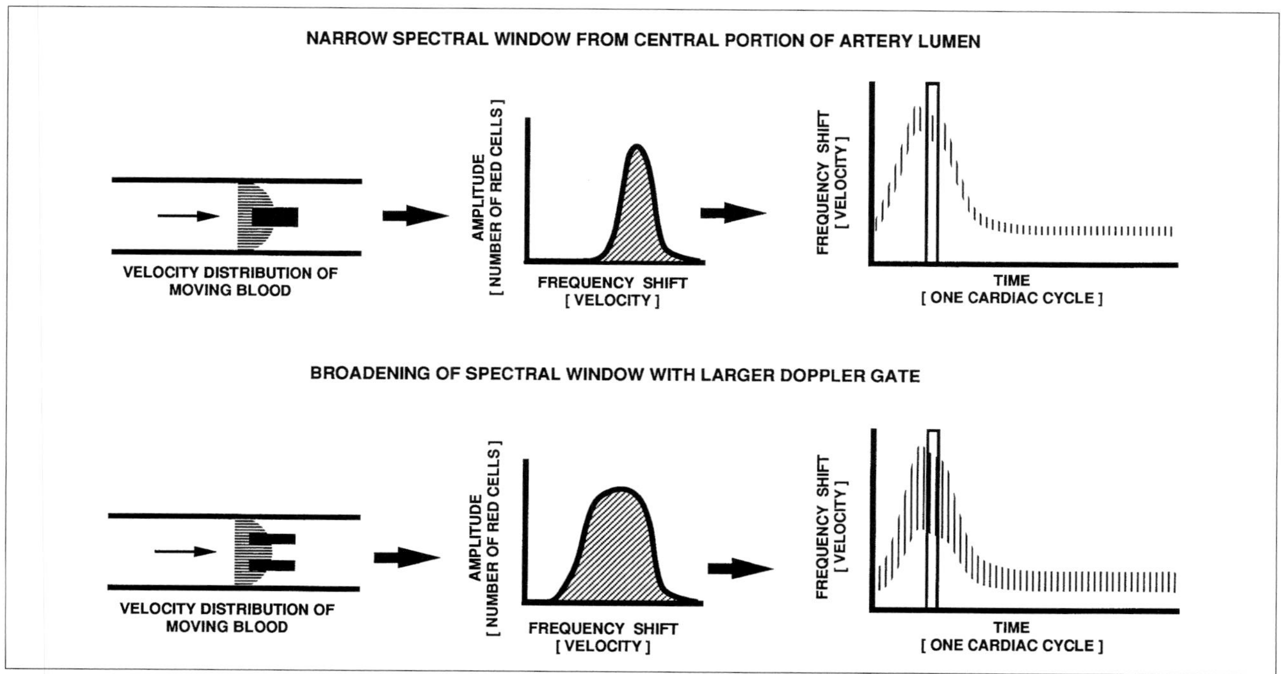

Figure 11-5. Diagram showing the effect of increasing the size of the Doppler gate in an artery with laminar flow. The red blood cells at the center of the artery are moving more quickly, and the red blood cells close to the walls are moving more slowly. Opening the Doppler gate can cause spectral broadening, that is, filling in of signal below the envelope of the Doppler waveform, because lower-velocity signals are now detected by the ultrasound device.

the Doppler shift and the vessel. This principle can be summarized by the Doppler equation. If the ultrasound beam and moving blood are in the same direction, the frequency shift is maximal. This frequency shift is affected by the angle between moving blood and the ultrasound beam (theta = θ). The Doppler equation is given by

$$\Delta\nu = 2\ \nu_o \left[\frac{V \times \cos\theta}{c} \right]$$

where $\Delta\nu$ is the frequency change, ν_o is the original frequency, c is the velocity of sound in the body, V is the blood velocity, and θ is the angle between the direction of blood flow and the direction of the sound beam. This equation makes the Doppler angle crucial to relating a frequency shift to the velocity of flowing blood. The operator is responsible for placing the Doppler gate and determining this relative angle. Any error will have a significant effect on the measured velocities. For example, the operator typically corrects the frequency shift information by moving a key that helps measure the angle in 1-degree increments. A 1-degree error, when the angle beam to the vessel is 30 degrees, causes less than 5 percent uncertainty. This same 1-degree error, when the beam vessel relationship is 60 degrees, causes an 8 percent error. This error quickly increases with larger angles, reaching 20 percent at 70 degrees and more than 40 percent at 80 degrees.

Aliasing

As discussed earlier, acquisition of the sonographic signals takes place during a fixed small time interval, usually 1 to 5 milliseconds. This is equivalent to opening an electronic door for a fixed amount of time and then closing it. The rate at which this electronic door can be opened limits the maximum information that can be processed and then displayed. This basic restriction in information content is commonly referred to as the *Nyquist frequency limit* or the sampling theorem. A simple rule follows: the higher the rate of sampling or peak repetition frequency, the higher the velocities or frequency shifts that can be displayed without ambiguity. Once the frequency shifts of the returning echoes reach twice the sampling rate, the ability to determine the frequency content of these acquired signals becomes ambiguous. This creates an artifactual folding over of the frequency content from the higher frequencies to the lower ones and is referred to as *aliasing*. If the peak repetition frequency cannot be further increased, it may not be possible to directly measure peak velocities. One strategy, in the carotid

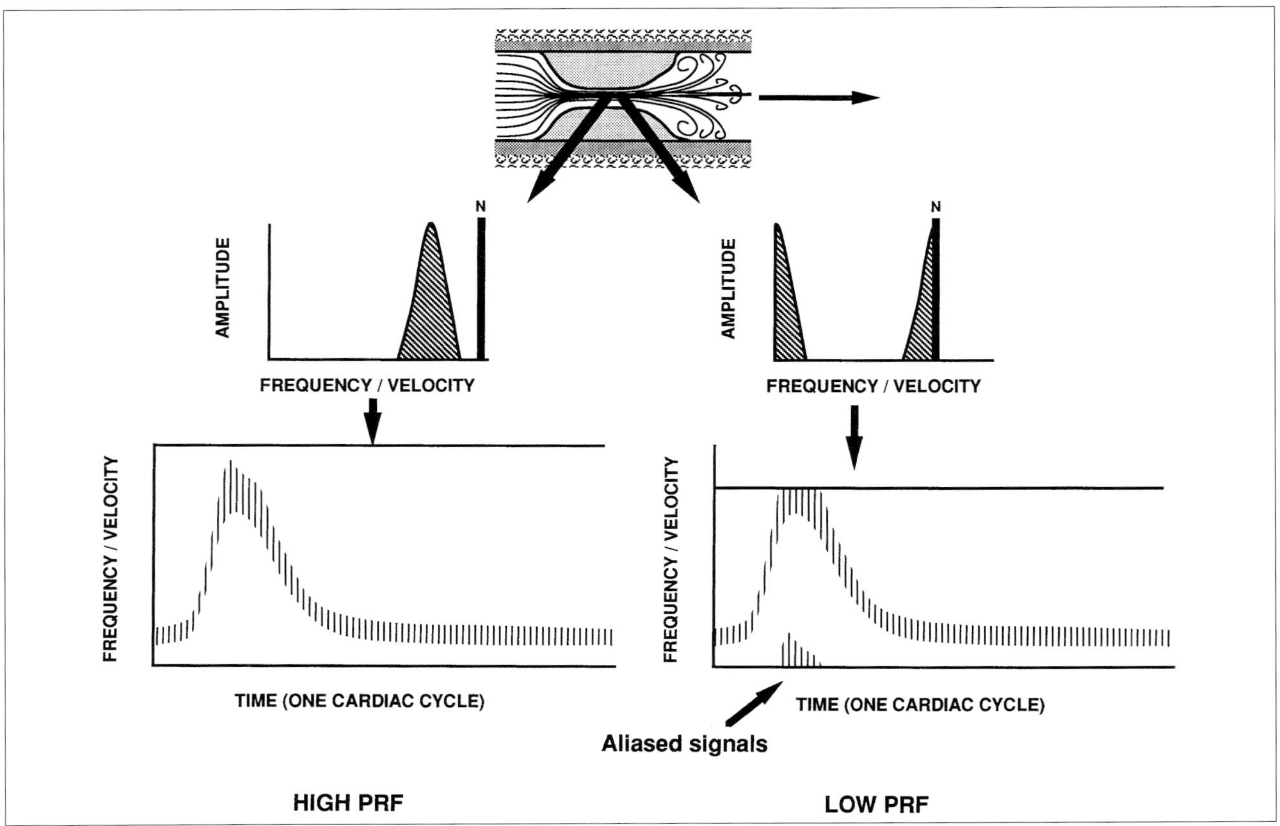

Figure 11-6. Diagram showing a folding over of the frequency shift information as the velocity of moving blood exceeds the processing limits of the ultrasound device, or the Nyquist limit (N). High velocities are inappropriately represented as low-velocity signals once they exceed the Nyquist limit. This is more likely to occur for high-grade stenoses when the velocities are markedly elevated, when the velocity scale (peak repetition frequency, or PRF) is too low, or when the chosen Doppler carrier frequency is too high.

arteries, is to measure diastolic flow, which is typically much lower than the peak systolic values (Fig. 11-6). Other approaches include lowering the transducer Doppler carrier frequency or decreasing the distance between the transducer face and the vessel being sampled. The latter approach will increase the peak repetition frequency and decrease aliasing.

Color Flow Imaging[7]

Color flow imaging generally uses a series of small gates distributed throughout the physical volume being imaged. Returning ultrasound signals are processed in such a way that the average Doppler shift is calculated.[8] In general, the process relies on a specialized algorithm commonly referred to as an *autocorrelator*. The final product is the creation of a "flow" image. Further superposition of this Doppler information on top of the gray scale image creates the final image. In general, the peak repetition frequencies of the color flow image component are much lower than those of pulsed Doppler. In effect, the color flow image is a large series of pulsed Doppler gates simultaneously being sampled over the volume of the image. The color flow image will therefore alias earlier than the pulsed Doppler waveform. It also contains flow information proportional to the mean velocity of flowing blood and cannot display the various frequency components, as is possible with pulsed Doppler waveform analysis.

A great advantage of the color flow image is that it permits direct visualization of various flow patterns within arteries and veins. It can easily show the arterial flow fluctuations between systole and diastole and the sharp reversal of flow during early diastole. It can also easily demonstrate the relatively constant or slowly varying flow pattern within the different venous channels.

The clear depiction of flowing blood on a color flow image serves as a guide for the sonographer, who can then further investigate selected areas with pulsed

Doppler analysis. For example, small vessels that may not be visualized in a transplant kidney can be seen with color flow imaging. The Doppler gate can then be positioned over the sites identified on the color flow image and the Doppler waveform analysis performed. In cases of suspected stenosis, the relative increase in the velocity of flowing blood can create areas of increased frequency shift that are easily displayed as a shift on the color map. In fact, these velocity increases are often so high that they cause aliasing of the color flow signals (Color Plates 1 and 2). These sites where aliasing occurs, especially when the Doppler device is operating at the maximal peak repetition frequency or maximal velocity scale, must be further interrogated by Doppler waveform analysis. They probably correspond to areas of high-grade stenosis.

The general limitations of color flow imaging are mostly related to limitations in the ability to display high velocities while respecting the constraints of performing simultaneous gray scale imaging. Processing of the image for both gray scale and color flow imaging is normally shared by the imaging device. Other strategies have separated much of these competing tasks to improve the relative frame rates and more accurately display both the real-time image and the color flow information.[9]

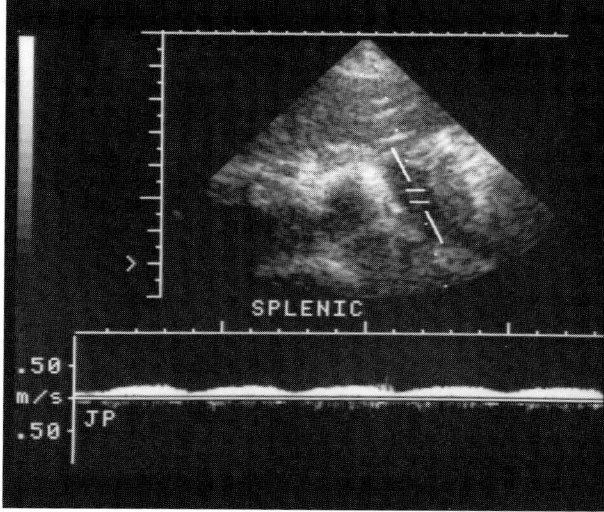

Figure 11-7. Doppler waveform sampled in the splenic vein showing a typical low-amplitude variation due to breathing. A similar pattern can be seen in the proximal leg veins.

Patterns of Interest

Normal Flow Patterns

Doppler waveform analysis is used to identify and characterize the flow patterns within the arteries and veins in different portions of the body. Although various pathologies can be identified whenever the expected waveform is perturbed, there is poor specificity in determining the actual pathophysiologic process responsible for the alteration in flow pattern.

Leg Veins

The deep as well as the superficial veins of the lower extremities show a relatively continuous pattern of flow on which is superimposed slowly varying patterns caused by respiration (Fig. 11-7). Typically, during inspiration, flow decreases because of the increase of intraabdominal pressure. At end-expiration, there is release of this pressure and a return to higher velocity flows. This pattern is typically seen in the common femoral and proximal femoral veins. It is also apparent in the popliteal vein and, with proper settings of the Doppler analyzer, can be seen in the more peripheral posterior tibial veins as well. This respiratory phasicity is less pronounced in the superficial and perforating veins.

Leg Arteries

Typically, flow in the peripheral arteries shows a triphasic pattern (Fig. 11-8). This consists, during systole, of a rapid acceleration of the velocity of blood flow. During early diastole, there is reversal of flow. This is followed by varying amounts of antegrade diastolic flow, which typically has a low amplitude. On occasion, diastolic flow may be absent in normal subjects with vasoconstricted arteries. In patients with very compliant arteries and distal vasoconstriction, retrograde flow can occur during late diastole (Fig. 11-9). With migration toward the peripherally located arterial branches, the amplitude of antegrade systolic relative to retrograde diastolic flow changes slightly and shows a decrease. Peak velocity also typically decreases from an average of 1.2 m per second in the iliac and common femoral arteries to an average of 0.7 m per second at the level of the popliteal artery.

Two indices are used to quantitate the information on the Doppler waveform (Fig. 11-10). The first is the pulsatility index. It is defined as the peak systolic flow velocity minus the peak end-diastolic flow velocity divided by the "mean velocity." The second is the resistive or Pourcelot index. It is defined as the peak systolic velocity minus the peak end-diastolic velocity divided by the peak systolic velocity. Both indices are relatively independent of the angle between vessel and ultrasound beam.

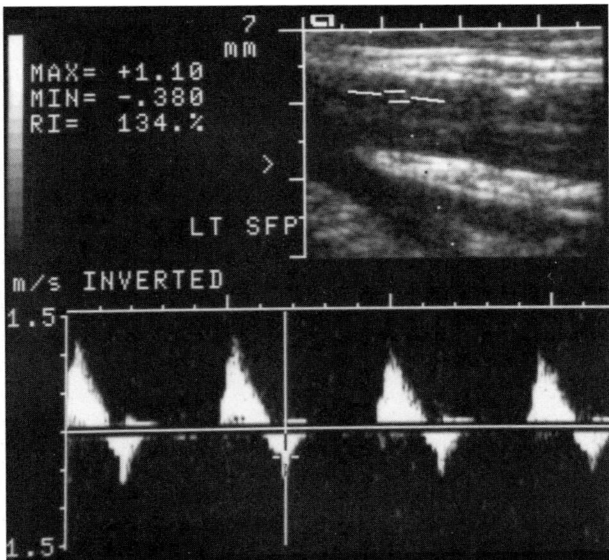

Figure 11-8. Image of a typical normal triphasic waveform in the proximal superficial femoral artery. Peak systolic velocity is within normal limits.

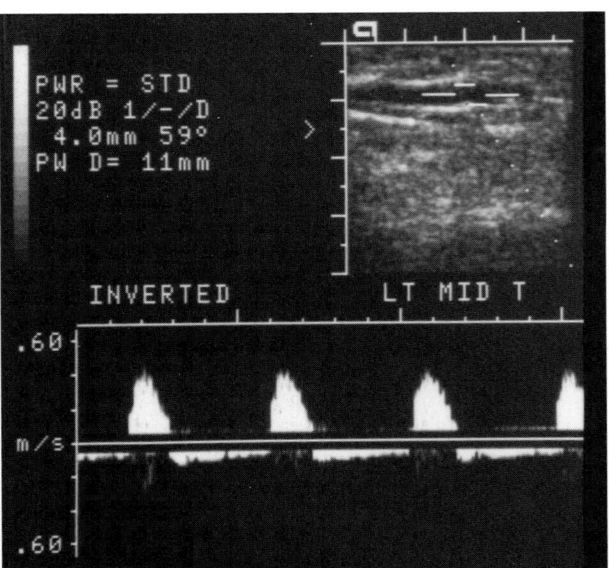

Figure 11-9. Doppler waveform that is encountered when a relatively compliant arterial segment is interposed between the sampling site and a high-grade occlusion. Reversal of flow occurs during diastole as the blood within the segment is pushed back into the lower-pressure proximal bed. A similar waveform can be seen in the proximal arteries of a kidney transplant when there is renal vein occlusion.

Arm Veins, Including Those on the Thorax

Flow within the arm veins is distinct from what is seen in the peripheral veins of the leg. Respiratory phasicity is less pronounced. The more centrally located axillary and subclavian veins typically show a pronounced pulsatility not normally seen in the leg veins. The cardiac A and V waves are transmitted and are the basic components of the waveforms within these veins. These are more marked within the jugular, proximal, and middle subclavian vein segments and the brachiocephalic branches. They are sometimes seen in the more distal subclavian and axillary veins.

Figure 11-10. Diagram summarizing the two quantitative indices used to quantify the appearance of the Doppler waveform. The resistive index is useful for quantifying renal dysfunction after transplantation. (Values above 0.9 are typical of rejection, and values below 0.7 are normal.) The pulsatility index has occasionally been substituted for the resistive index but is more difficult to determine because the peak velocity envelope of the Doppler spectrum must be traced.

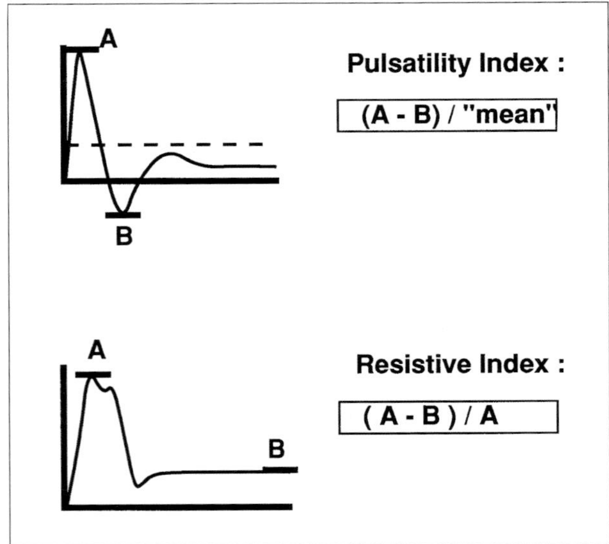

Arm Arteries

The peripheral arteries of the arm show the same triphasic pattern as the lower extremity arteries. In amplitude, the peak systolic velocity varies between 1.0 and 1.2 m per second in the proximal subclavian artery and decreases to approximately 0.8 or 0.9 m per second in the axillary artery.

Extracranial Arteries

The extracranial artery branches are the carotid and vertebral arteries. The internal carotid artery feeds a low-resistance bed and has antegrade flow during systole and diastole (Fig. 11-11). The amplitude is greater in systole. The external carotid artery feeds a high-resistance bed (Fig. 11-12); however, there is no significant early diastolic flow reversal. The spectral contour is somewhat irregular because of the reflec-

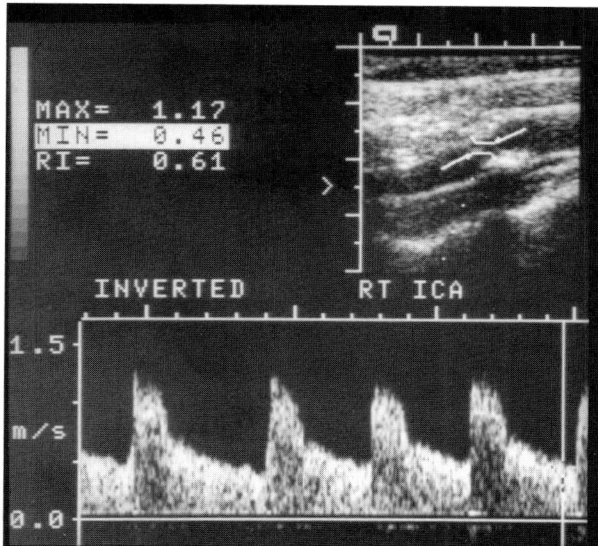

Figure 11-11. Doppler velocity waveform obtained in the proximal internal carotid artery. It is a low-resistance waveform with a strong component of forward flow during diastole. This typical appearance is explained by the low resistance to flow offered by the intracerebral vessels. The peak systolic velocities are at the upper limits of normal because of a plaque.

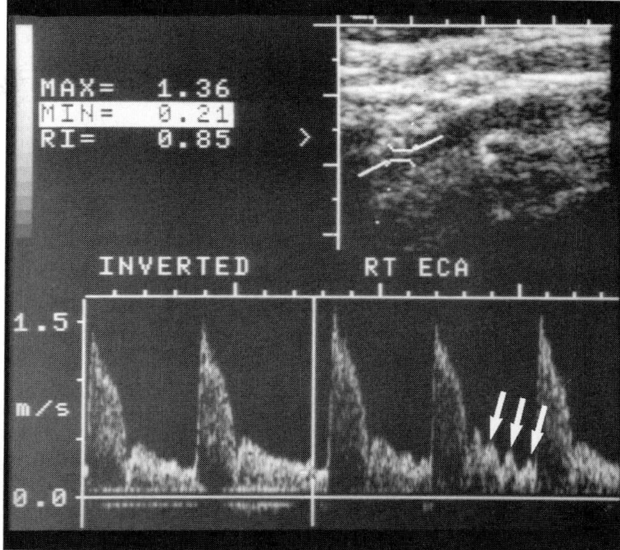

Figure 11-12. Doppler waveform in the external carotid artery showing a somewhat lower diastolic velocity than in the internal carotid artery (see Fig. 11-11). The systolic pulsations are also somewhat prominent. The oscillations during diastole in the tracings to the right (*arrows*) have been induced by applying pressure on the ipsilateral temporal artery (temporal tap maneuver).

tions from the multiple branches of the external carotid artery. The common carotid artery waveform shares the characteristics of both the internal and the external waveforms (Fig. 11-13). The vertebral artery also feeds a low-resistance bed and has a waveform similar to that of the internal carotid artery. Its peak systolic velocity is lower, averaging 0.4 millisecond, than the 0.6 to 0.8 millisecond seen in the carotid artery.

The Aorta and Its Intraabdominal Branches

Flow within the proximal aorta is antegrade during early systole and is of lower amplitude during diastole. This pattern holds to the level of the renal arteries, below which the typical triphasic pattern with diastolic reversal starts to emerge and finally becomes prominent at the level of the common iliac arteries (Fig. 11-14).

Flow patterns at rest in the major visceral branches in the superior mesenteric and inferior mesenteric arteries have a high-resistance pattern (Fig. 11-15A). The effects of a meal on flow dynamics can be dramatic in the superior mesenteric artery: after a meal, the flow pattern changes from a triphasic waveform to a low-impedance monophasic pattern. Peak velocities also typically increase by at least 50 percent (see Fig. 11-

Figure 11-13. Doppler waveform sampled in the common carotid artery proximal to the carotid bulb. This waveform typically shows a mixture of the characteristics from the external carotid (increased pulsatility during diastole) and internal carotid (low-resistance waveform) artery branches. In this example, the waveform resembles the internal carotid artery waveform.

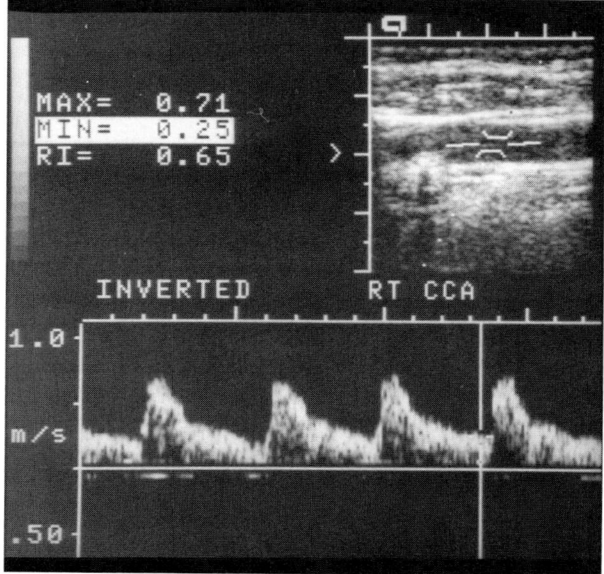

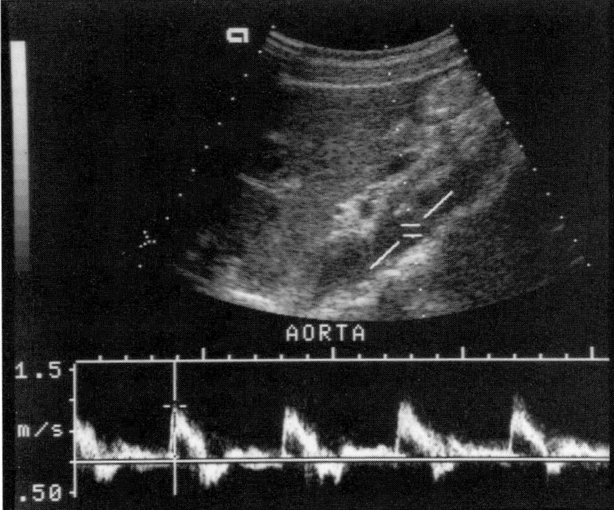

Figure 11-14. Sonogram showing the typical waveform obtained in the proximal abdominal aorta. There is a strong pulsatile component of blood flow. Diastolic flow is mostly due to flow through the celiac axis and both renal arteries.

15B). The inferior mesenteric artery waveform behaves like the superior mesenteric artery. The celiac trunk and renal artery waveforms typically have a low-resistance monophasic waveform.

The Inferior Vena Cava and Its Intraabdominal Branches

Flow patterns within the inferior vena cava are variable and are modulated by intraabdominal and transthoracic pressures. In general, the pulsations from the heart are transmitted into the inferior vena cava and are somewhat dampened. Respiratory changes are pronounced. There is also a tendency for the inferior vena cava to collapse during inspiration and during the Valsalva maneuver. These changes in the flow pattern are also noted in the hepatic veins and are similar to what can be detected on occasion within the renal veins.

The Portal Venous System

The flow pattern of the portal venous system is mostly continuous and antegrade toward the liver and shows some respiratory phasicity. It can increase following a meal or decrease as the resistance within the hepatic parenchyma increases (Fig. 11-16).

Abnormal Flow Patterns

Arterial Occlusion and Stenosis

The principal reason for using Doppler sonography in the arterial system is to detect stenosis or occlusion. Arterial occlusion is easily identified by the obvious absence of flow signals during either color flow imaging or Doppler waveform analysis. Confirming the presence of the occlusion depends on technical factors such as the overall sensitivity of the Doppler device

Figure 11-15. (A) Doppler waveform obtained in the proximal superior mesenteric artery. It shows a strong pulsatile appearance with early diastolic flow reversal. (B) Doppler waveforms obtained in the same subject after a fatty meal. Diastolic reversal has been lost and forward diastolic flow has increased. There is also an increase in peak systolic flow velocity caused by the increased flow requirement during digestion.

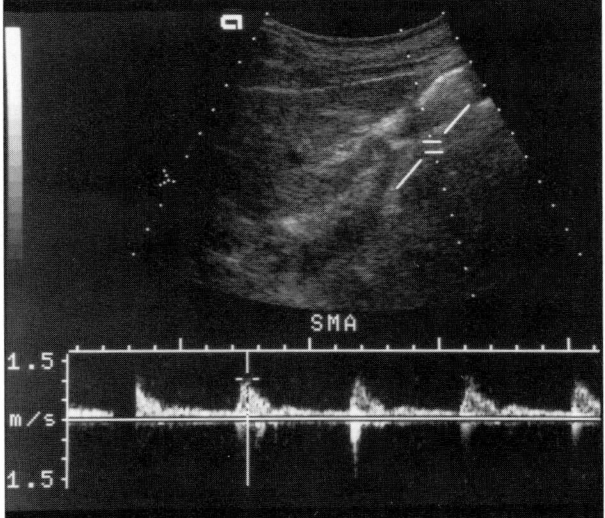

A

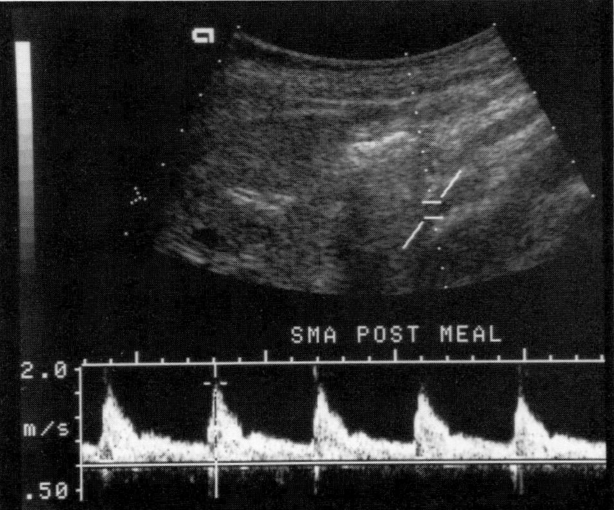

B

and the range of velocity display (peak repetition frequency, or PRF). A simple rule is to normalize the signal being acquired to the signals from within adjacent vessels. This ensures that the proper gain settings are being used.

As stenotic lesions evolve and increase in significance, they perturb normal arterial flow patterns. A diameter narrowing of more than 50 percent is considered to be the point of hemodynamic significance when a pressure drop develops across the stenosis. Alterations in the arterial waveform consist of a loss of the normal laminar flow pattern and the emergence of small disturbances in the waveform. These disturbances are detectable as spectral broadening of the Doppler waveform. Higher-grade (above 50 percent diameter narrowing) stenoses will cause an area of increased peak systolic velocity and a more homogeneous flow profile—plug flow instead of laminar flow—with loss of the spectral broadening effect at the throat of the stenosis (narrowest point). A distinct jet often emerges distal to the stenosis and can be seen on color flow imaging. Peak systolic velocities are maintained within this jet for varying distances, which, in the peripheral arterial system, typically extend for 2 to 4 cm beyond the narrowing. Within this zone, an area of flow reversal forms beside the jet (Color Plate 3 and Fig. 11-17). The boundary between the jet and the zone of flow reversal, if sampled, will show evidence of turbulence with a filling in of the spectral window and an alteration in the contour of the spectral envelope (see Color Plate 3).

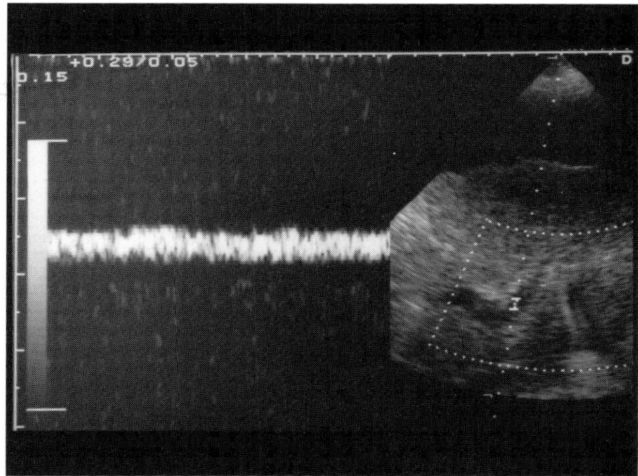

Figure 11-16. Doppler waveform obtained in the portal vein showing blunting of the normal respiratory phasicity. In this patient with cirrhosis and ascites, flow direction has not yet reversed.

Venous Occlusion and Stenosis

Absence of flow signals within a vein is one of the diagnostic criteria used for determining the presence of occlusion. This absence of flow may occur at the level of the abnormality or upstream from the actual physical obstruction. In such cases, it is impossible to distinguish intrinsic or extrinsic compression of the more proximal vein. A venous stenosis manifests itself in a fashion similar to that seen in the arteries: as an eleva-

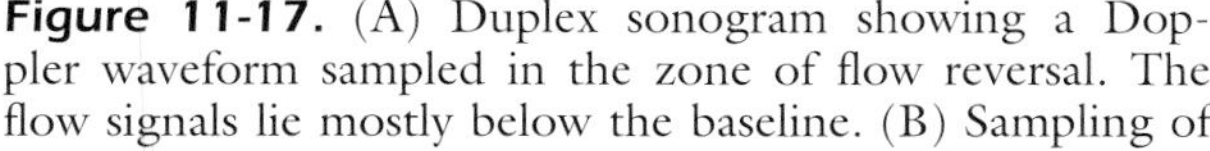

Figure 11-17. (A) Duplex sonogram showing a Doppler waveform sampled in the zone of flow reversal. The flow signals lie mostly below the baseline. (B) Sampling of the Doppler waveform at the site of maximal narrowing. The sampling shows a dramatic increase in the peak systolic velocities to 3.0 m/sec.

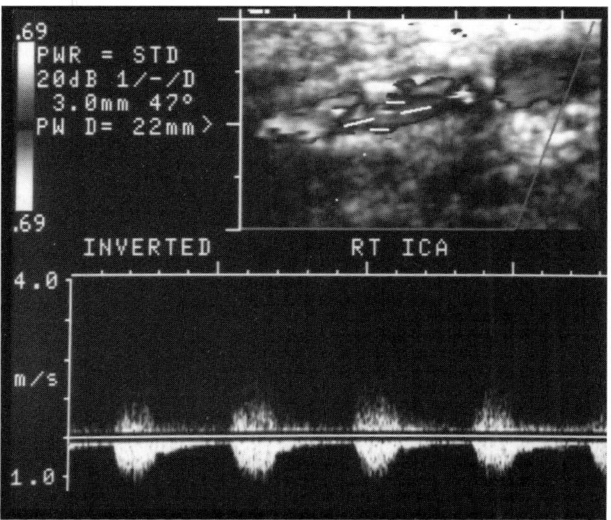

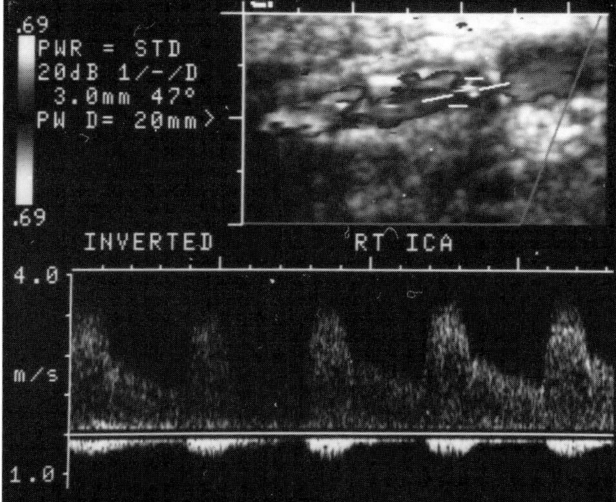

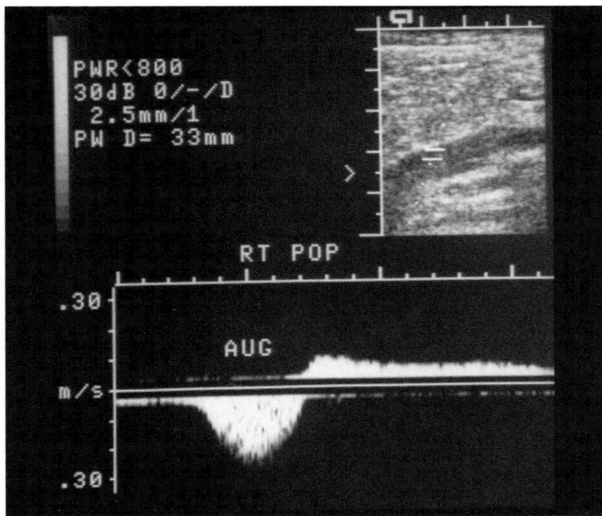

Figure 11-18. Doppler waveform showing the typical appearance of an incompetent vein. After augmentation, there is a prolonged reversal of blood flow down the leg.

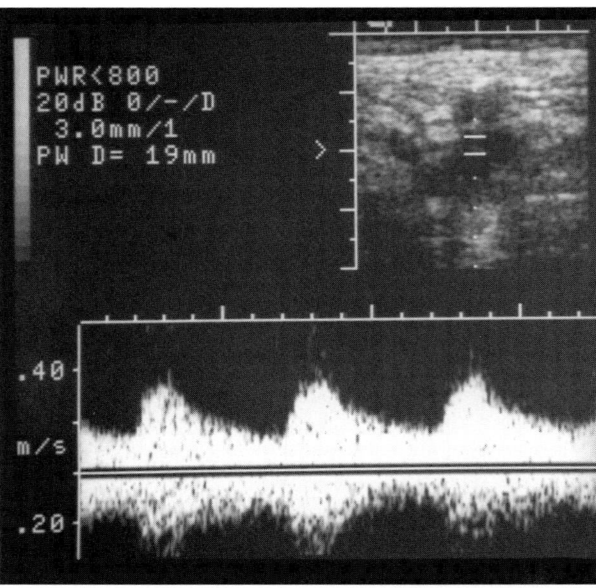

Figure 11-19. Duplex sonogram showing an arterial signal in the common femoral vein. This finding is typical of an iatrogenic AV fistula.

tion of flow velocities. The respiratory phasicity normally seen typically disappears when a significant stenosis is present.

The actual diagnosis of intrinsic venous thrombosis is, however, more reliably achieved by gray scale imaging or color flow imaging (Color Plate 4). The typical changes used to establish the diagnosis are an echogenic structure within the vein lumen and, more importantly, loss of compressibility when external pressure is applied to the skin overlying the vein.

Miscellaneous Patterns

Venous flow in an incompetent segment is reversed from the normal direction after augmentation or during a Valsalva maneuver (Fig. 11-18). Such changes are typically seen in the lower extremity where vein valve dysfunction is present. Upper extremity vein insufficiency is more difficult to document and has not been the subject of any large studies.

Arteriovenous malformations (AVMs) show multiple channels containing flow signals. The velocities and magnitude of these signals are variable. More extensive congenital malformations can show low-velocity flow signals and can be difficult to detect. Iatrogenic AVMs cause a direct shunt between artery and vein. Flow velocities tend to be high and show an arterialized component in the vein (Fig. 11-19 and Color Plate 5). Sites of iatrogenic-induced shunting can be clearly visualized and detected by color flow imaging (see Fig. 11-19B).

Peripheral masses are likely to be evaluated when there is a clinical suspicion of aneurysm or pseudoaneurysm formation. Pseudoaneurysms are caused by a localized rupture of the arterial wall: a communicating channel is typically seen. The pseudoaneurysm shows a mixture of forward and backward flow, often called a "swirling motion."[10] This pattern is variable because of the presence of partial thrombosis within the collection (Color Plate 6). However, the communicating channel between the artery and pseudoaneurysm will show a typical to-and-fro pattern (Color Plate 7). Aneurysms tend to be continuous with the artery walls and typically show layering of the thrombus along the walls (see Fig. 11-2).

In general, hematomas, abscesses, and other masses do not contain flow signals. Flow signals can, however, be detected at their periphery. On occasion, hyperplastic or malignant lymph nodes show areas of velocity signals within the central region close to the hilum.[11]

Neoplastic masses, if they are vascular, may tend to show areas of increased flow velocities toward the periphery of the abnormality.[12]

Real-Time Gray Scale Patterns

Atherosclerotic Plaque

The gray scale image can detect interesting variations in the appearance of atherosclerotic plaque. Plaque is characterized on the sonogram with respect to texture, surface characteristics, and density or structure.[13] *Calcification* is considered an adjunctive descriptive term.

Echogenicity or *density* refers to the intensity of the echoes within the plaque as compared to the surrounding soft tissues. Although iso- or hypoechoic components within the plaque are thought to correspond to areas of hemorrhage (see Fig. 11-3), lipid accumulation within the plaque and fibrointimal hyperplasia share a similar appearance.[14–16] Therefore, there is no specificity to this appearance. Nevertheless, areas of increased density are thought to correspond to fibroatheroma and the presence of dense fibrous tissue (see Fig. 11-1B).

The surface characteristics of the plaque vary from mild irregularities less than 1 mm in extent to frank ulceration, which is defined as a gap of more than 2 mm within the plaque.[17] *Texture* is described as the relative proportion of tissue within the plaque that is of a homogeneous nature.[18] In general, this varies from homogeneous to markedly heterogeneous. Most plaques, however, have a mixture of different components. In general, as atherosclerotic plaque increases in size and as the severity of the stenosis increases, the overall echogenicity and heterogeneity increase and the surface of the plaque becomes more irregular.[16,19]

Arterial Thrombosis

Thrombus within an artery can vary in appearance from mildly echogenic to isoechoic with respect to the background echoes of the lumen (Color Plate 8 and Fig. 11-20). Therefore, it is impossible to quantitate its extent by gray scale imaging alone.

More chronic arterial thrombosis can be identified by indirect signs, such as a decrease in arterial diameter and as an increase in echogenic signals as part or all of the contents of the arterial lumen are transformed into fibrous tissue (Color Plate 9).

Venous Thrombosis

Venous thrombosis, although it can appear as echogenic material within the lumen, is often not visualized on the gray scale because it is isoechoic with respect to the lumen.[20,21] The echogenic appearance is thought to have a diagnostic sensitivity of approximately 50 percent for deep vein thrombosis.[22]

If care is taken to carefully image the full length of the thrombosis, scattered zones with increased echoes

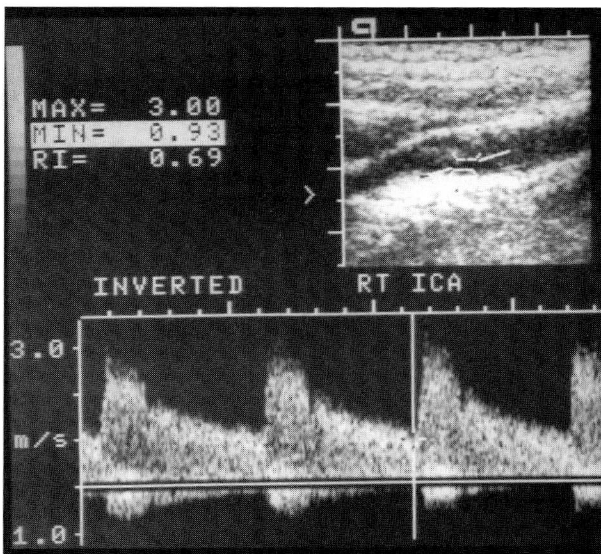

Figure 11-20. The Doppler waveform sampled at this site of increased velocity has a peak systolic velocity of 3.0 m/sec, corresponding to an 80 percent diameter stenosis.

will often be noted within the thrombus. The administration of thrombolytic therapy will often give a markedly heterogeneous appearance to the thrombus.

Intimal Hyperplasia

Fibrointimal hyperplasia typically appears as a hypo- or isoechoic lesion along the periphery of the arterial or venous wall. These may be difficult to detect, and their extent may be difficult to determine on gray scale imaging alone.

Venous Thrombosis (Extremities)

Lower Extremity

Technique and Diagnostic Criteria

Three complementary diagnostic criteria are used to determine the presence of peripheral venous thrombosis. Loss of compressibility of the vein wall when external pressure is applied is considered the principal diagnostic criterion.[23,24] In general, compression is applied in the transverse plane along the full length of the vein that is being studied (Fig. 11-21). The compression ultrasound examination typically starts at the level of the groin. The transducer is displayed in increments of 1 to 2 cm, compression is applied and then released, and the transducer is displaced again. This is repeated

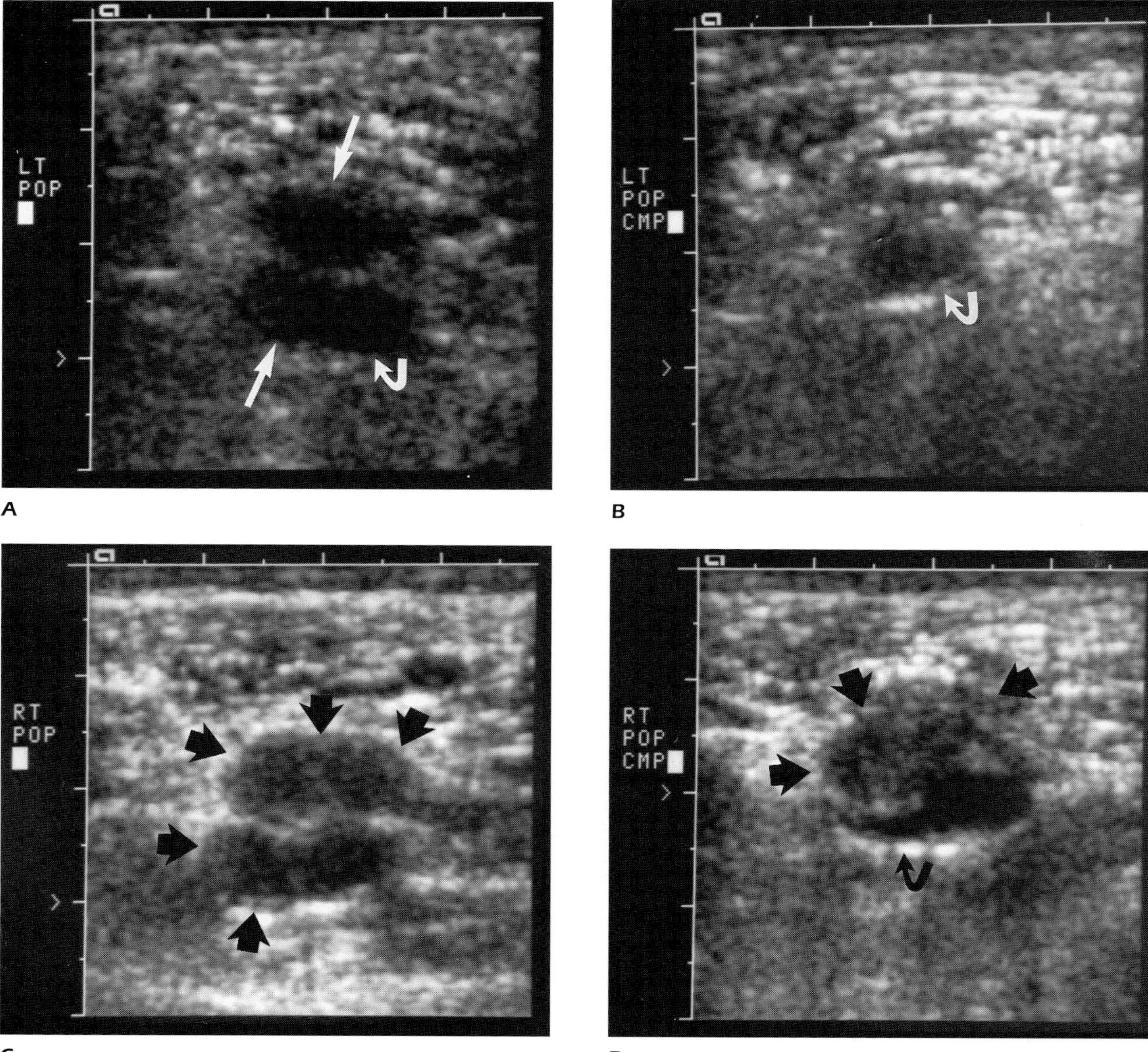

Figure 11-21. (A) Transverse image showing duplicated popliteal veins (*arrows*) and one artery (*curved arrow*) before pressure is applied to the skin. (B) Image showing the effect of pressure applied to the overlying skin. The veins collapse and the artery does not (*curved arrow*). (C) The popliteal veins in the contralateral leg contain echogenic material (*arrows*) consistent with thrombus. (D) One of the duplicated veins does not collapse when pressure is applied to the overlying skin (*arrows*). This is consistent with a deep vein thrombosis. The other vein partly collapses (*curved arrow*), either because of the partly obstructing thrombus or because of the inability to transmit sufficient pressure at the location of the vein.

along the course of the femoral and popliteal veins. A similar approach can be used to study the calf veins using both medial and posterolateral approaches.

Disturbances in flow dynamics can assist in the diagnosis of venous thrombosis. First, the presence of respiratory phasicity is easily confirmed with Doppler waveform analysis and color flow imaging. Loss of flow signals within the vein is seen in all instances of a complete thrombosis.[22] False positives may occur when a more proximal obstruction decreases venous return. In addition, there may be flow at the periphery of a partly obstructing thrombus. This diagnosis may be missed by Doppler waveform analysis but is identifiable with the aid of color flow imaging.[25,26]

Specific maneuvers are used in addition to simply observing the spontaneous flow noted during respiration or augmented respiration. Compressing the calf veins by applying external pressure to squeeze the calf or by having the patient dorsiflex and plantar flex the toes will augment blood flow within the more proximal vein. This phenomenon is caused by the emptying of some of the blood volume stored within the muscular vein sinuses of the calf. Normal flow augmentation excludes the presence of a significant obstruction in the proximal veins. A potential pitfall to the diagnostic criterion is flow through collateral pathways or duplicated segments not involved with venous thrombosis.

Echogenicity is the least reliable of the three diagnostic criteria.[20,22] The presence of echogenic signals within a vein segment that is noncompressible supports the diagnosis of vein thrombosis. Unfortunately, the full length of the thrombus is rarely echogenic. Loss of compressibility remains the most reliable diagnostic criterion.

Diagnostic Accuracy

Obstructive venous thrombosis predominates in symptomatic patients, more typically in the outpatient population. For this clinical scenario, the accuracy of venous ultrasound is above 97 percent for the diagnosis of femoral and popliteal vein thrombosis.[24]

There is some controversy over the accuracy of this technique for the calf veins. Some studies have noted that the sensitivity and the specificity are close to 90 percent, whereas others have noted much lower accuracy. This issue can be further addressed by clarifying whether isolated calf vein thrombosis is present[27] or whether it is part of a more extensive involvement of the deep veins.[26,28] The sensitivity and specificity for evaluating the extent of calf vein thrombosis are decreased when proximal venous thrombosis is also present. This is likely secondary to the edema caused by the more proximal venous obstruction.[26] In cases of isolated calf vein thrombosis, although the numbers are small, it appears that the diagnostic accuracy is close to 90 percent[27] and possibly more.[29]

Venous thrombi tend to be predominantly nonobstructive in postoperative patients.[30,31] These thrombi can arise, as they do in symptomatic patients, in the calf veins or more typically at valve sites within the femoral and popliteal veins. For these patients, the imaging protocol must be modified so that every segment of the veins is fully visualized with compression ultrasound. Despite this, the diagnostic sensitivity and specificity of the examination are decreased. Although some reports suggest that the sensitivity and specificity are between 80 and 90 percent for the femoral and popliteal veins,[28] others suggest that the sensitivity is much lower—63 percent.[32] This low sensitivity may be due to incomplete visualization of all of the venous segments because the sensitivity increased to 80 percent in 81 of 119 patients in whom a complete ultrasound examination was obtained.[32] Small thrombi are typically missed (less than 1 cm in size).[33,34] There is, however, a learning curve, because the same group reporting a sensitivity of 54 percent and a specificity of 91 percent[33] later reported an improvement in diagnostic performance in a similar patient group, with a sensitivity for ultrasound of 71 percent and a specificity of 94 percent.[34] For this reason, the accuracy probably ranges between 70 and 90 percent.[35] Large-outcome studies are needed to evaluate the implications of the smaller thrombi that may be missed by venous imaging.

Vena Cava Filters

Ultrasound serves as the diagnostic end point for making the diagnosis of deep vein thrombosis before filter placement. After filter placement, sonography has shown that iatrogenic thrombi develop at the access sites used for filter placement.[36,37] The incidence of these thrombi can be decreased by using balloon dilation instead of dilators for tract preparation[36] and by adopting small-diameter filters.[38]

Upper Extremity

Technique and Diagnostic Criteria

The diagnostic criteria used for the upper extremity veins are similar to those used in the lower extremity. However, arm vein anatomy and the presence of the clavicle force necessitate some modifications. For example, the jugular vein, the more lateral subclavian vein, the axillary vein, and the more peripherally located veins can be evaluated with compression ultrasound.

Color flow imaging and the gray scale image are more heavily used for evaluating the proximal subclavian vein because compression cannot be applied to these venous segments.[39] The innominate and brachiocephalic veins are evaluated in the same fashion by relying on the use of gray scale changes and by evaluating the flow pattern within the vein lumen with color flow signals. Pulsed Doppler ultrasound can document the presence of a total occlusion but lacks diagnostic accuracy for detecting partly obstructing thrombus.[40] Flow augmentation is often difficult to elicit in the upper extremity veins.

Diagnostic Accuracy

For symptomatic patients, the diagnostic accuracy is probably close to 90 percent because, by definition, the process is obstructive. The technique, when it shows obstruction to venous flow, cannot distinguish a more central thrombus or an extrinsic process. Partly obstructive catheter thrombi may manifest themselves by nonspecific signs and symptoms such as fever or possible septic emboli. The presence of the catheter should not affect blood flow in the venous channels.[41] The diagnostic accuracy of venous ultrasound has yet to be evaluated in any systematic fashion but appears to be poor for nonobstructing thrombi.[42] Partly obstructing thrombi often adhere to these catheters while the patients remain completely asymptomatic.[42]

Venous Insufficiency

Technique and Diagnostic Criteria

The principal diagnostic criterion used to confirm the presence of venous insufficiency is reflux of blood down the lower extremity veins. This reflux can be induced by asking the patient to perform a Valsalva maneuver or by applying compression to the limb above the area being evaluated. For example, popliteal vein insufficiency can be achieved by compressing the thigh. Venous reflux is defined as a reversal of the typical pattern of blood returning toward the heart. A transient reversal of short duration can be seen at the level of the common femoral vein because the vein can distend early before valve closure occurs. This can be seen at the level of the popliteal vein but is less pronounced.

More recently, systematic methods of evaluating venous insufficiency have been proposed. The simplest—standing vein compression—consists of inducing venous augmentation by squeezing the calf with the patient standing and then observing the venous response.[43,44] For example, venous augmentation causes a rapid increase in flow velocity. A normal, transient reversal of blood flow lasting less than 0.5 second can be seen in the proximal common femoral vein and profunda femoral vein as well as in the popliteal vein. Prolonged reversal of blood flow that lasts longer than 0.5 second suggests venous insufficiency (see Fig. 11-18). The author uses the range of 0.5 to 1.0 second as suggestive of venous insufficiency and values above 1.0 second as definite for its presence. By sampling different sites in the femoral and popliteal venous systems, it is possible to evaluate the level of venous reflux and to document whether the deep and/or superficial systems are involved. In addition, it is possible to image the location of the perforating veins.

Diagnostic Accuracy

Evaluation of the accuracy of this technique has been hampered by lack of a sufficient gold standard. Reflux venography is useful in evaluating more severe proximal involvement of the venous valves. Doppler sonography is now being evaluated with respect to outcome after selective ligation of incompetent segments and of involved superficial veins in patients with venous ulceration. It appears that the technique offers a new approach for evaluating venous insufficiency and may become the new "gold standard."[43]

The Doppler technique has been used to study the incidence of deep venous reflux following episodes of acute venous thrombosis. It appears that the time to recanalization following an episode of acute deep vein thrombosis is related to the likelihood of venous insufficiency.[45] In addition, it appears that the likelihood of ulceration is linked to the magnitude of the reflux detected by sonography.[46]

Extracranial Neck Arteries

Doppler Evaluation

Diagnostic Criteria

The common carotid, internal carotid, and external carotid peak systolic velocities normally range between 0.6 to 0.8 m per second. The amount of diastolic flow varies. It is low in the high-resistance external carotid artery and larger in the internal carotid artery. In general, elevations in the peak systolic velocity are used to detect hemodynamically significant stenoses.[6,47–50] The normal cutoff value for the presence of the hemodynamic significant stenosis (≥ 50 percent diameter narrowing) is considered to be 1.25 m per second.[50] This criterion performs with an accuracy of close to 90 percent for the detection of hemodynamically significant stenosis.[49,50] Abnormal flow patterns can be seen following carotid endarterectomy. In these cases, the increase in blood flow velocity is accompanied by a loss of the smooth outline of the Doppler waveform.[51] This irregular Doppler waveform contour is normally explained by the presence of turbulence.[51,52]

Diagnostic Accuracy

The Doppler evaluation of suspected carotid stenosis can be viewed from two points of view. First, in the detection of *hemodynamically significant* stenosis, the test performs with an accuracy of approximately 90 percent when a threshold peak systolic velocity of 1.25 m per second is used.[49,50,53] The efficacy of this screening approach for detecting carotid stenosis is obvious when one looks at the fraction of patients shown to have significant stenosis in their carotid arteries at arteriography. This rate currently reaches 90 percent as compared to less than 30 percent in the era before carotid screening with Doppler ultrasound.[50,54] More recently, new thresholds for surgical intervention, specifically a 70 percent diameter stenosis threshold proposed in 1991 and 1992 following the North American Carotid Endarterectomy Trial Collaborators study,[55] have led to the recognition that a peak systolic velocity of 2.3 to 2.5 m per second can serve as a discriminating point for *clinically significant* stenosis.[56,57]

Doppler sonography is still limited for distinguishing a total from a subtotal internal carotid occlusion.[6,58] A small residual lumen can sometimes be missed because of difficulties in sampling the full length of the severely stenosed vessel.[59] This problem may be helped by color flow imaging.[60] Cases of subtotal occlusion are also difficult to establish by angiography and require a special arteriographic approach with prolonged injection of contrast and delayed filming over the suspected subtotal occlusion.[61]

Evaluation of Plaque

Diagnostic Criteria

As discussed above, the different characteristics of the atherosclerotic plaque include plaque density (iso-, hypo-, and hyperechoic), plaque structure (homogeneous and heterogeneous), and plaque surface characteristics (smooth, irregular, and ulcerated). Greater emphasis is given to the evaluation of atherosclerotic plaque when lesions are not hemodynamically significant. Measurement, with Doppler velocity estimates, of the actual degree of stenosis appears to be a better predictor for both prevalent and incident stroke and transient ischemic attack (TIA) than a simple evaluation of plaque characteristics.[19,62] On occasion, plaque characteristics can help in the diagnosis of persistent TIAs when a hemodynamically significant stenosis is absent. For example, chronic ulceration of a borderline hemodynamically atherosclerotic plaque may explain persistent symptoms and the failure of more conservative therapies.[63] This may then justify a more aggressive investigation[64] and possibly intervention.

Diagnostic Accuracy

In general, there has been some difficulty in establishing the overall diagnostic accuracy of gray scale sonography for evaluating atherosclerotic plaque. Most of the studies have looked at plaques obtained during endarterectomy and are therefore biased toward more significantly stenotic atherosclerotic plaques. In general, the severity of the stenosis correlates with the extent of heterogeneity and the presence of hypoechoic areas.[65] These hypoechoic areas (see Fig. 11-3) are thought to represent areas of intraplaque hemorrhage.[14,16,66,67] There is also evidence that there is a preponderance of chronic hemorrhagic zones in the majority of these hemodynamically significant plaques.[68]

The detection of ulceration remains a topic of great controversy. Early reports described an accuracy of between 80 and 90 percent for determining the presence of ulceration.[14] More critical evaluations suggest that this accuracy is much lower, closer to 50 percent.[69]

The Vertebral Artery

In general, the vertebral artery is evaluated for the presence and the direction of flow.[70] Technically, the imaging transducer must be positioned more laterally and posteriorly to image the segments of the vertebral artery lying in between the transverse processes of the cervical spine. Waveform analysis consists of confirming persistent antegrade flow during systole and diastole (Fig. 11-22). Changes in this waveform pattern suggests the likelihood of a more proximal subclavian stenosis and possible subclavian steal syndrome.[71]

Figure 11-22. Typical waveform in the vertebral artery, showing the same appearance as the internal carotid artery waveform. Peak velocities are lower, typically 0.3 to 0.7 m/sec, whereas the internal carotid peak systolic velocities average 0.8 m/sec.

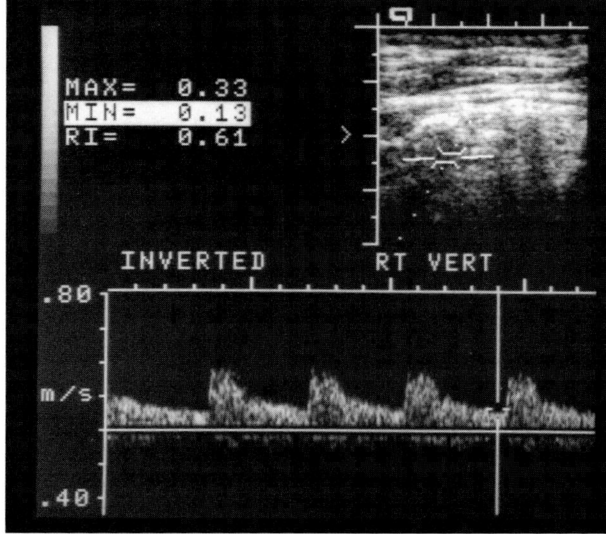

Some authors have suggested sampling the length of the vertebral artery to determine the presence of focal stenosis.[72,73] This diagnostic strategy, however, has only been verified in small series.[74]

Peripheral Arterial Disease

Since the introduction of color flow imaging, Doppler sonography has played an increasing role in the evaluation of the peripheral arterial system. Over the past few years, this technique has been adopted as the most sensitive and specific noninvasive approach for monitoring postoperative vein graft stenosis.[75,76] It is also being evaluated as a screening method for detecting femoral and popliteal segment disease[77] and for discriminating between those lesions suitable for angioplasty and those suitable for more traditional surgical approaches.[78]

The diagnosis of aneurysms is reliably made by vascular sonography. In fact, this technique is considered the best approach for evaluating more peripherally located aneurysms.[79]

Lower Extremity

Diagnostic Criteria

The approach used to detect an arterial stenosis within the femoral, popliteal, or more peripherally located arteries is similar to what is done in the carotid system. However, normal velocities vary with arterial diameter, location in the leg, and cardiac output. It is difficult to ascribe a fixed velocity threshold above which a significant stenosis is present. Instead, the ratio of the peak systolic velocities is used.[80] This consists of measuring the highest peak systolic velocity at the site of a suspected stenosis. A stenosis is increasingly being identified with color flow mapping and typically shows up as a region of aliasing on a color flow image.[81] The peak systolic velocity is then also measured at a point proximal to this lesion, normally 4 cm, and the velocity ratio is calculated. Elevations of 100 percent or doubling of the peak systolic velocity is considered to represent hemodynamically significant stenosis with above 50 percent diameter narrowing (Figs. 11-8 and 11-23).

A proximal arterial lesion can affect the waveform and velocities in the more distal arterial segments. For example, the peak systolic velocity in the distal segment decreases (parvus), whereas the time to reach this peak velocity is delayed (tardus).[82] In general, this occurs when the proximal lesion is more severe and is notable when a proximal occlusion is present. The normal triphasic pattern is lost and a relatively monophasic pattern with relative increase and importance of the diastolic flow can be seen in the peripheral branches (Fig. 11-24). Unfortunately, there is marked variability in the changes seen for the diastolic velocities. This portion of the Doppler waveform is not as useful for grading stenosis severity.[83]

A common pitfall is seen following the development of collateral branches.[81,84] Inadvertent sampling of a collateral branch, likely to occur in the region of the adductor canal, can falsely lead to the diagnosis of a high-grade or subtotal occlusion of the artery when the arterial segment is in fact occluded.

Diagnostic Accuracy

The sensitivity and specificity for the detection of arterial lesions, more than half of which are stenoses and occlusions, are approximately 80 to 90 percent.[80,81,85–87] A sonographic approach relying on color flow mapping tends to show a very high diagnostic sensitivity (over 90 percent) for detecting the presence of a total occlusion. In general, the Doppler velocity estimates tend to overestimate the severity of focal lesions when compared to arteriography.[77]

Upper Extremity

Diagnostic criteria for the presence of focal stenosis are similar to criteria for stenosis localized in the lower extremity. More central lesions at the origin of the subclavian artery can be missed, and care must be taken to evaluate the region of the clavicle for the presence of aneurysm or stenoses associated with the thoracic outlet syndrome.

Postoperative Changes and Complications

Synthetic Vascular Bypass Grafts

In general, synthetic vascular bypass grafts are easily evaluated by sonography. In the early postoperative period, the presence of gas within the wall of the synthetic material may obscure imaging of the lumen. However, a few days following surgery, sound waves can normally penetrate the synthetic bypass grafts and permit a full evaluation. In the early postoperative period, sonography is useful for evaluating masses adjacent to the bypass graft, such as hematomas or possible pseudoaneurysm formations.[88]

In the later follow-up period, sonography is used to confirm the presence of occlusions and to detect stenoses. The latter are more likely to occur at anastomotic sites.[89] These lesions are typically due to fibrointimal hyperplasia and manifest themselves within the first 2 years following surgery. Imaging of older grafts

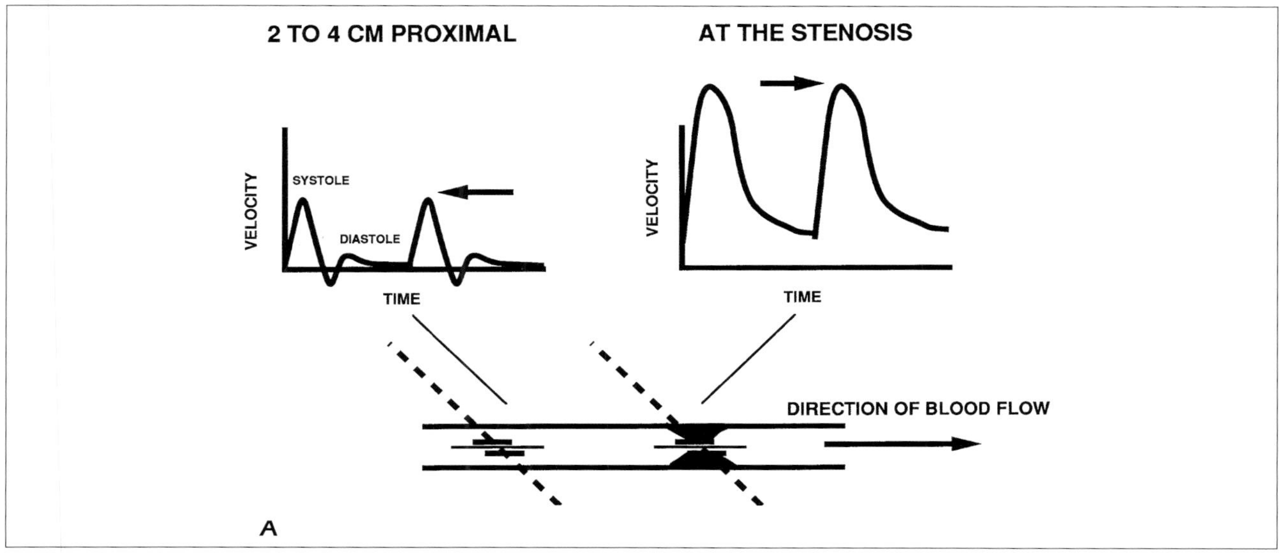

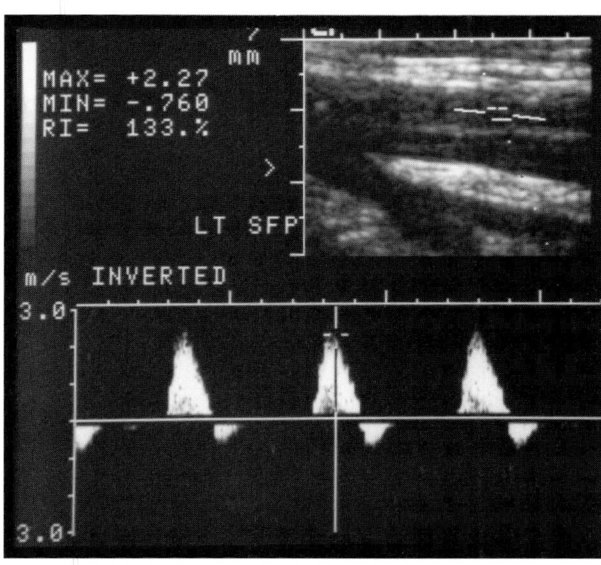

Figure 11-23. (A) Diagram summarizing the principle of the Doppler velocity ratio. A stenosis in the artery causes an increase in the peak systolic velocity. This is then compared to the velocity in a normal segment, typically 2 to 4 cm upstream to the lesion. The velocity ratio is constructed by dividing the velocity at the stenosis by that measured at a point 2 to 4 cm proximal to the stenosis. (B) Two centimeters downstream from the sampling site shown in Figure 11-8, the peak systolic velocity has doubled. This was shown to be a 50 percent diameter stenosis by arteriography. The presence of such a stenosis may not affect the flow dynamics in the involved artery at rest. With exercise, this patient had symptoms of claudication.

often shows a more diffuse deposition of thrombus and fibrointimal reaction within the graft conduit.

Autologous Vein Grafts

In general, the vein graft conduit shows variations in caliber as it progresses from the more proximal to the more distal arterial anastomosis. In the case of a reversed bypass graft, the proximal portion of the graft tends to have a smaller diameter than the distal portion. In situ bypass graft diameters more closely match artery diameter at the proximal and distal anastomoses.

Flow velocities within the bypass graft should resemble those seen within the native arterial tree. In general, however, the early diastolic reversal can be quite short and barely perceptible.[90]

The principal utility of sonography for the postoperative monitoring of vein bypass grafts is in the detection of stenosis and confirmation of possible occlusion.[91] The development of bypass graft stenosis appears to follow a specific pattern. In the first month after surgery, technical defects can cause lesions responsible for early bypass graft failures.[92,93] In addition to focal stenosis, a small communicating AV fistula can be detected and diagnosed for in situ veins. Following this critical month, the process of fibrointimal hyperplasia is responsible for the development of stenoses

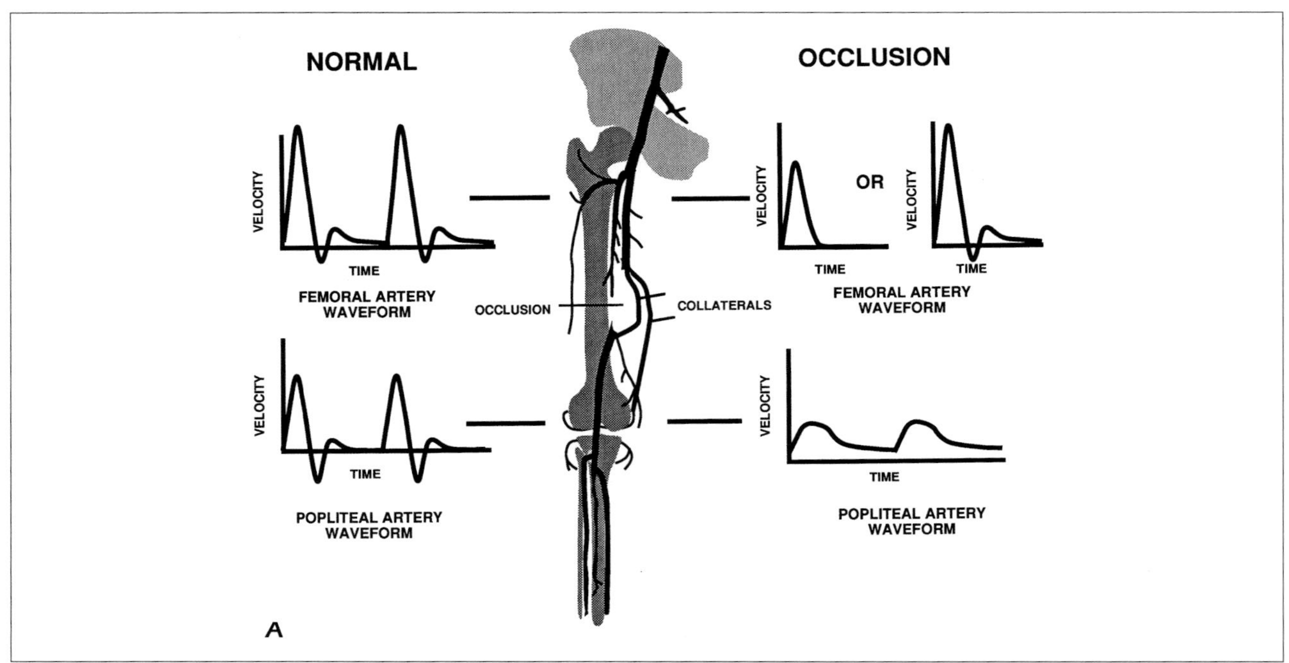

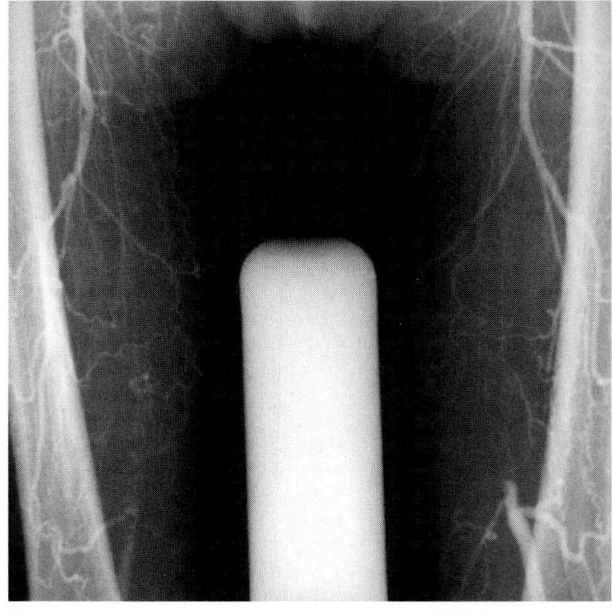

Figure 11-24. (A) Diagram showing the effect of a proximal arterial obstruction on the Doppler waveform sampled downstream. There is loss of early diastolic flow reversal with persistent forward flow during diastole. The peak systolic velocity is typically reduced. (B) Arteriogram showing bilateral femoral artery occlusions. (C) This Doppler waveform measured in the occluded right femoral artery shows absent flow signals. The velocity scale (PRF) has been set to a low level to detect low-velocity signals. The signal gain has been set to a high sensitivity and shows some baseline noise. (D) Doppler waveform sampled in the popliteal artery where flow reconstitutes shows a low-amplitude pattern with persistent monophasic flow during diastole. In this specific instance, the systolic rise time is greater than expected (decreased acceleration), a pattern commonly referred to as the *tardus waveform*. The decreased systolic amplitude is referred to as the *parvus waveform*.

located at different sites along the graft conduit, most likely at the site of lysed valves, or at the anastomoses. Early stenotic lesions normally manifest themselves as an area of increased flow velocity.[94,95] With time, as the lesions become more severe, the velocity at the stenosis increases. With higher-grade lesions, the velocity in the proximal conduit of the bypass graft can decrease below a threshold value of 0.45 m per second. Velocities below this threshold, in normal-diameter bypass grafts of approximately 3.0 mm, suggest a dysfunctional bypass graft with inflow and outflow difficulties or intrinsic focal lesions.[90] This last stage precedes complete failure and thrombosis (Color Plate 10 and Fig. 11-25) of the bypass graft.[75]

The diagnostic accuracy of color flow mapping and Doppler sonography for postoperative graft surveillance is now well accepted (Color Plate 11 and Fig. 11-26). The diagnostic sensitivity and specificity are

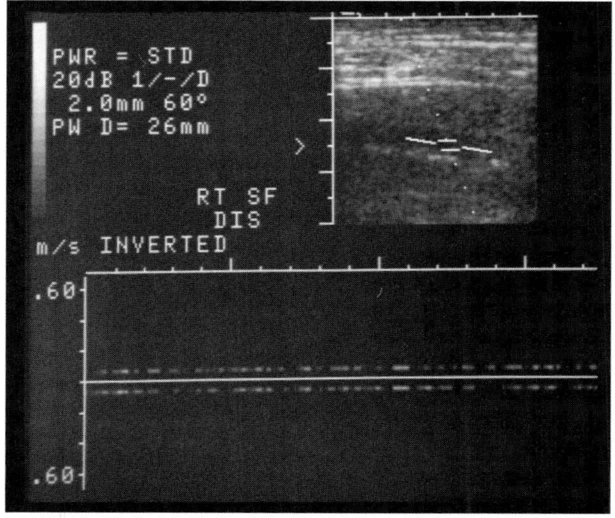

C

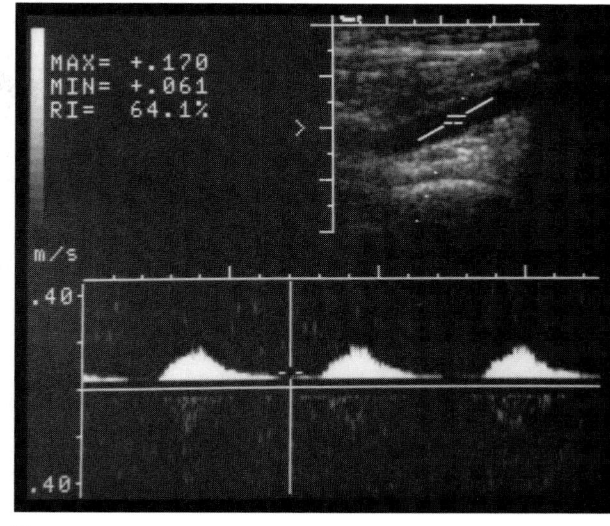

D

Figure 11-24 (continued).

much higher than for serial monitoring with ankle-brachial indices or segmental pressures.[75,96] Case control studies looking at the natural history of bypass grafts with early lesions have shown that lesions above 70 percent diameter narrowing are almost always associated with total occlusion of the bypass graft within 3 to 6 months following detection.[76] A stenosis in the 50 to 70 percent range has a 30 percent likelihood of occluding within 3 to 6 months and probably warrants more careful monitoring. Once lesions reach hemodynamic significance, they should be repaired. Doing so will improve graft patency rates to above 80 percent.[97]

Figure 11-25. Color flow imaging can be used to detect the site of focal stenoses before they progress to cause a total occlusion of a bypass graft. Simply sampling a velocity in the graft conduit (*middle panel*) only detects the more severe stenoses. The less severe stenoses (*upper panel*) are missed.

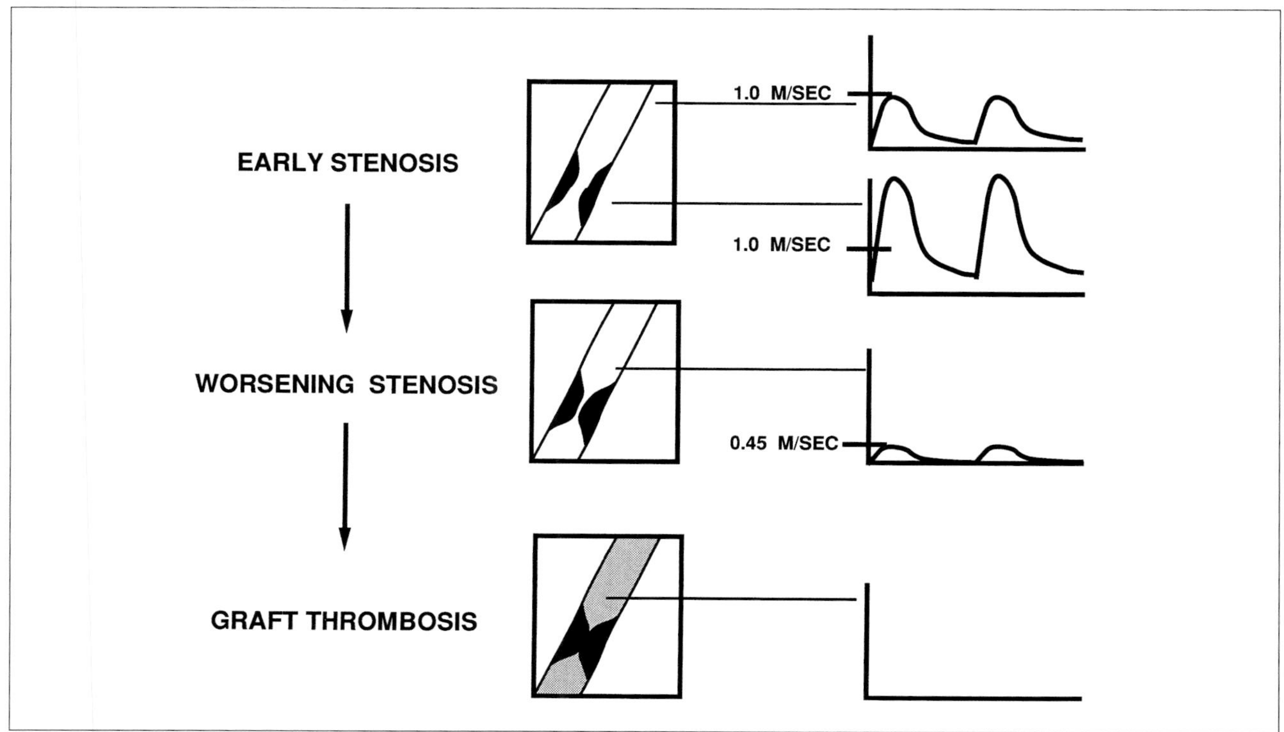

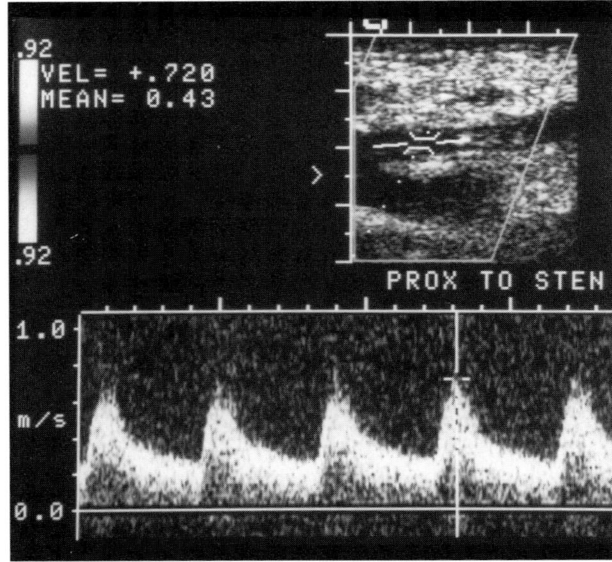

A

B

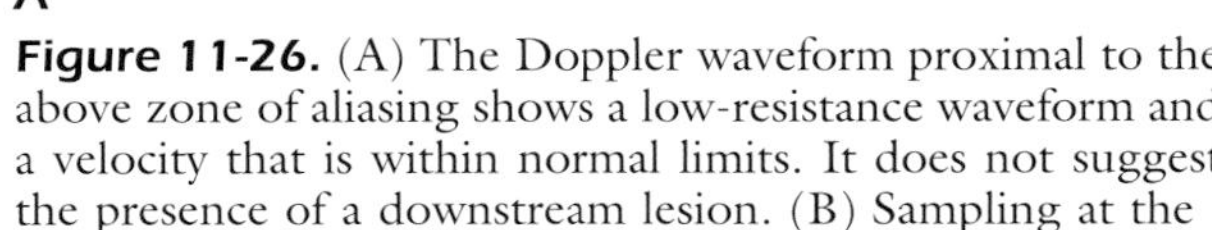

Figure 11-26. (A) The Doppler waveform proximal to the above zone of aliasing shows a low-resistance waveform and a velocity that is within normal limits. It does not suggest the presence of a downstream lesion. (B) Sampling at the site of aliasing shown in Color Plate 11 confirms a high-grade stenosis with a flow velocity above 5 m/sec, consistent with a 90 percent diameter stenosis.

Hemodialysis Shunts

There are three types of hemodialysis shunts: the Braescia-Cimino, the loop graft, and the straight interposition graft. The first is a direct communication between an artery in the forearm to a vein; in the others, a conduit is interposed between artery and vein. The material used for the conduit is more often synthetic polytetrafluoroethylene (PTFE). Color flow mapping and Doppler sonography typically show, in the inflow artery, a low-resistance waveform. Within the dialysis shunt, turbulent flow is normally present. At the outflow, velocities within the vein are typically in the range of 1 m per second or greater.

The presence of a stenosis is manifested, as it is in other arterial sites, by the development of zones of increased peak systolic velocity and diastolic velocity. These zones of increased velocity can be graded with the use of a velocity ratio, more often established with respect to the inflow artery.[98]

Most stenoses develop in the venous outflow of the graft. Peak systolic velocities are normally used to grade stenosis severity.[99,100] Color flow mapping and association with gray scale imaging can also detect the presence of aneurysms or pseudoaneurysms.[101,102] These are more likely to occur on the Braescia-Cimino shunts. The failure to detect stenoses of the more central subclavian and brachiocephalic veins remains a limitation of color Doppler evaluations, as is the tendency to overestimate the severity of stenotic lesions.[103] Despite these limitations, Doppler evaluation of hemodialysis fistulas appears to play a role in the monitoring of these patients[104] and may be used to identify subsets of patients in whom the graft is more likely to occlude in the near future.[105]

Percutaneous Angioplasty and Atherectomy

The role of vascular ultrasound for triaging patients for a vascular surgery procedure versus a percutaneous approach is increasing. In general, short focal lesions and occlusions or high-grade stenoses are treated by percutaneous angioplasty, since long-term results show that this strategy has reasonable patency rates.[106] The ankle-brachial index or segmental pressures are often not able to distinguish between longer segmental occlusions and shorter focal stenoses. Doppler sonography offers high sensitivity and specificity for the detection of stenotic lesions[107] and has been proposed as both a screening technique and a means of triaging patients.[77,78]

Doppler sonography can be used to monitor the success of the vascular intervention. Persistent elevations of velocity (100 percent or doubling of the peak systolic velocity) are associated with significant focal lesions (Color Plates 1 and 2 and Figs. 11-27 and 11-28). These warrant more careful monitoring because they may signify lesion recurrence. It appears that early

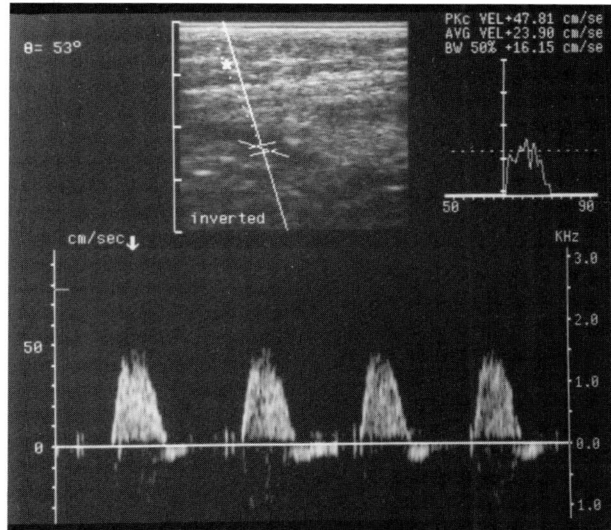

A

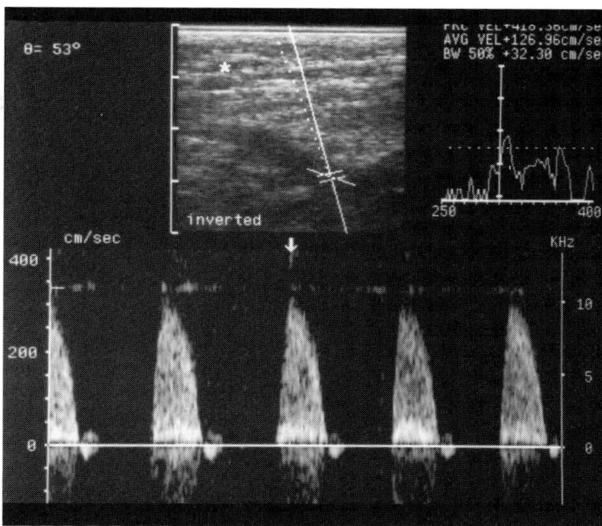

B

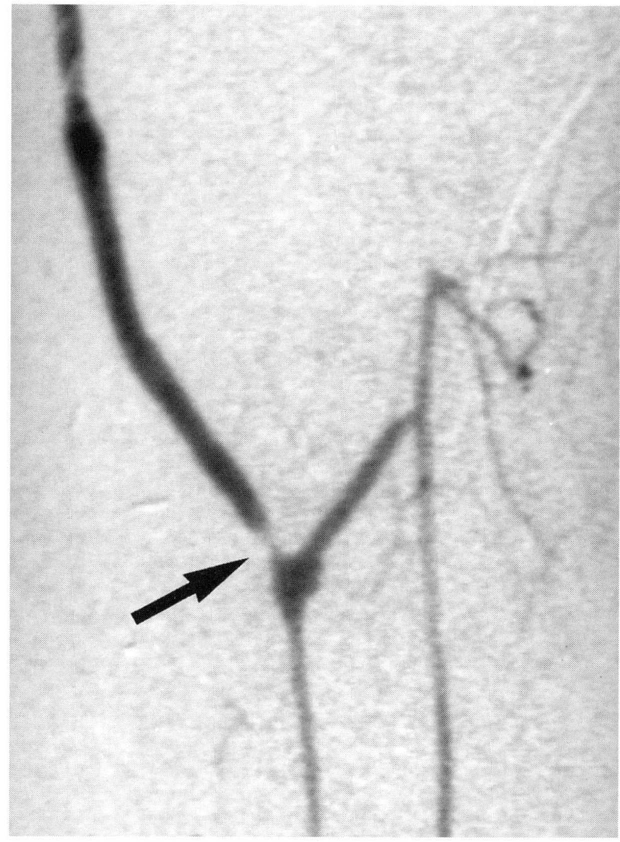

C

Figure 11-27. (A) Doppler waveform sampled in a bypass graft proximal to the anastomosis. Peak systolic velocities are somewhat depressed (48 cm/sec). (B) Second Doppler waveform sampled in the zone of maximal flow disturbance shown on the color flow image above. The peak velocity is markedly elevated, to above 300 cm/sec. This elevation corresponds to a greater than 75 percent diameter stenosis and is more consistent with the arteriogram (C) than the color flow image. (C) Corresponding arteriogram showing a high-grade stenosis (*arrow*).

appearance of a flow abnormality may predict long-term patency better than an evaluation made from the postprocedure arteriogram.[108] This observation has yet to be confirmed.[109]

Complications

Color flow mapping, in combination with gray scale imaging, can be used to detect specific complications. The presence of AV fistulas is shown by a zone of increased velocity between an artery and the adjacent vein.[110,111] Pseudoaneurysm formation at a surgical anastomosis[88] or at the site of previous percutaneous entry of a catheter is readily confirmed.[112–114] Pseudoaneurysms arising after catheterization may be treated with the help of sonography as a guide to the application of transcutaneous pressure to occlude the collection and the communicating channel.[114] The success rate of percutaneous ablation of pseudoaneurysms is high if patients are seen within a week of the inciting event. Sonography has also been used to confirm the high rate of spontaneous thrombosis of these same pseudoaneurysms.[115,116]

Vascular dissections are readily identified by the appearance of a free flap seen on color flow imaging.[117] Transverse imaging is useful in confirming their presence. Doppler velocity measurements can confirm whether both channels are patent and can identify the true lumen of the dissection.[118]

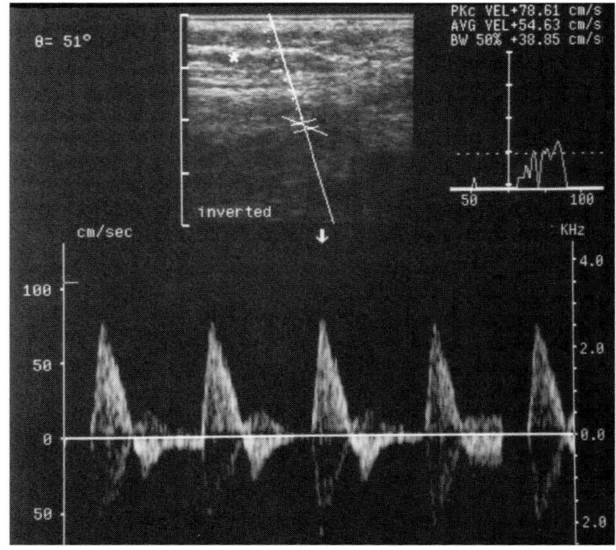

A

B

C

Figure 11-28. (A) Doppler waveform proximal to the distal anastomosis. The waveform shows an increase in the peak systolic velocity from 48 cm/sec before angioplasty to 78 cm/sec. (B) Doppler waveform at the distal anastomosis showing a residual flow abnormality to 180 cm/sec. This would be consistent with a 50 percent diameter stenosis. (C) Arteriogram showing the site of angioplasty (*arrow*) and an apparent 40 percent diameter residual stenosis.

The Abdominal Aorta and Its Branches

The uses of Doppler sonography in the abdomen have increased dramatically. The traditional evaluation of abdominal aneurysms has been complemented by a more aggressive use of sonography for detecting renal arterial disease and evaluating the mesenteric vessels.

Abdominal Aneurysms

The more traditional use of sonography for evaluating the abdominal aorta relies on gray scale imaging. This is primarily used to detect and size aortic aneurysms. The technique has significant advantages when compared to angiography because sonography is capable of documenting the extent of the lumen enlargement as well as of estimating the presence of mural thrombus (see Fig. 11-3), which is not detectable by contrast arteriography. Although computed tomography is also a noninvasive approach to evaluating the aorta, the low cost of sonography permits a cost-effective protocol for the serial monitoring of aneurysm growth.[119] In addition, sonography can be used for population surveys to detect the presence of asymptomatic aneurysms.[120–122] Physical examination lacks sensitivity[120] and specificity.[121] The technique has been shown to be reproducible, with reproducible measurements possible to within 3 mm.[123]

Presurgical planning for treatment of these lesions does, however, require a more anatomically precise technique such as aortography. Other techniques—spiral computed tomography or magnetic resonance angiography—may play a more important role in the near future.

Aneurysms are traditionally defined as having a diameter enlargement of more than 3.0 cm. A full evaluation of the abdominal aorta should include imaging from the level of the distal thoracic aorta, near the diaphragm, to the level of and including the common iliac artery bifurcations.

On occasion, the presence of iliac artery aneurysms can be detected by sonography. However, there is some discussion as to the reliability of imaging in the abdominal and iliac arteries. Many imaging protocols require overnight fasting and the administration of an oral agent to minimize bowel gas during imaging.

Aortic Occlusion and Stenosis

Isolated abdominal aortic stenosis is uncommon. There are no specific series addressing the reliability of Doppler sonography in establishing this diagnosis. Since gray scale imaging of the aorta can be conducted in most subjects, however, it appears that Doppler sonography should be capable of making this diagnosis. There are no specific diagnostic criteria available for grading the severity of stenosis within the abdominal aorta.

The normal aortic flow profile varies for the different levels being imaged. Proximal to the major mesenteric vessels and the renal arteries, there is a strong unilateral component of blood flow. Distal to the origins of the renal arteries, the Doppler waveform develops a more pulsatile appearance because of an increase in outflow impedance. Outflow impedance above the renal arteries, because of the low-impedance renal arterial bed, gives the Doppler waveform a slightly prominent diastolic component.

Renal Artery Stenosis

There has been much interest in the use and application of Doppler sonography for the detection, grading, and monitoring of renal artery stenosis (Fig. 11-29). Early reports suggested an accuracy of 90 percent for the detection of renal artery stenosis.[124,125] A ratio of the peak systolic velocity in the proximal renal artery with respect to the peak systolic velocity in the abdominal aorta above 3.5 suggests the presence of a high-grade (>60 percent diameter stenosis) of the renal artery.[125]

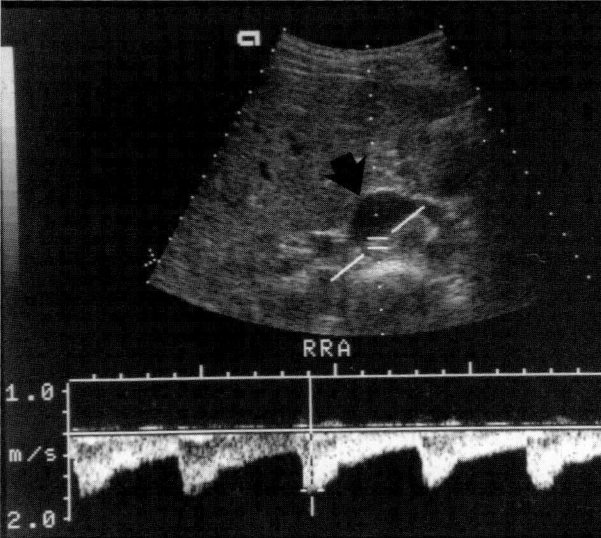

Figure 11-29. Flow signals obtained from within the right renal artery showing a typical low-resistance waveform. The proximal renal artery can normally be visualized over its proximal few centimeters. The right renal artery typically lies below the inferior vena cava (*arrow*) on this image.

This technique has a significant limitation: accessory renal artery branches are often missed. Recent reviews that evaluate the technique have distinguished between time-intensive and time-limited examinations.[126,127] In general, time-limited examinations are not capable of screening the renal arteries appropriately and fail to detect the presence of all significant lesions within the 1-hour interval. Time-intensive surveys, conducted for a length of 1 to 2 hours, appear to perform better.

It has recently been suggested that high-grade stenosis can compromise renal hemodynamics and can affect the waveform sampled within the renal parenchyma.[128] Waveforms from the segmental, subsegmental, and arcuate renal branches show a decrease in peak amplitude (parvus) as well as a relative delay in the upstroke during early systole (tardus).[129] This appearance, although specific for the presence of a proximal high-grade stenosis of 80 percent or more, lacks diagnostic sensitivity as a screening test.[130]

Mesenteric Branch Occlusion and Stenosis

The normal resting waveform within the mesenteric artery is typical of a high-resistance arterial bed.[131] After the ingestion of a meal, there is relatively increased flow to the abdominal vasculature and vasodilatation, causing a typical low-resistance waveform to appear (see Fig. 11-15). The peak systolic velocity also increases. The normal range of peak systolic velocities in the mesenteric artery has recently been defined to be less than 2.0 m per second. Increases beyond this threshold suggest the presence of a hemodynamically significant stenosis.[132] The diagnostic criteria have not proven themselves in large series of patients.[133,134] Their application for monitoring the presence of recurrent stenosis following an intervention may prove cost-effective.

Although the main mesenteric artery trunk can be imaged and quite accurately identified, the major branches cannot be reliably evaluated by Doppler sonography because of limitations in resolution and penetration. The inferior mesenteric branch can also be identified.

The accuracy of the technique may be compromised in patients with chronic mesenteric lesions when large collateral pathways have developed.

The celiac artery has typically a low-resistance waveform because both the hepatic artery and splenic artery supply low-resistance arterial beds.

Postoperative and Postintervention Follow-up

The major application of Doppler sonography in the abdomen is for monitoring known arterial lesions. For example, after renal artery angioplasty, the number of accessory renal arteries and the location of previous stenoses are clearly known.[135,136] Image-directed evaluation of the site of angioplasty or stent placement in the renal artery can then be performed with Doppler sonography. Lesion progression can be detected early.

Although no large series have addressed the issue of monitoring therapeutic treatment of the abdominal aorta and iliac arteries following angioplasty or stent placement, the feasibility of this approach has been clearly demonstrated.

Renal Transplantation

Doppler sonography was earlier thought to be capable of detecting early rejection of renal transplants.[137,138] The primary criterion was the development of either a resistive index of 0.9 or above[137] or a pulsatility index of 1.5 or more.[138] It appears, however, that the arterial branches within the transplanted kidney can develop a high-resistance waveform because of other pathologic entities such as chronic rejection, urinary obstruction, or acute tubular necrosis.[139,140] This obviously compromises the utility of Doppler sonography for monitoring the postoperative transplant for evidence of developing rejection.

A diagnostic sign with poor prognostic significance is the development of reversed flow in the renal artery segments during diastole.[141] One of the more important causes for this finding is the presence of renal vein thrombosis.[141,142]

Masses

The major application of Doppler sonography is for the identification of suspected abdominal masses. Once the presence of an abdominal aneurysm has been ruled out, other etiologies such as pseudoaneurysms or masses in close proximity to the aorta can be evaluated. Once the mass has been clearly identified and shown to be relatively avascular, an ultrasound-guided biopsy is more easily justified.

The Vena Cava and Its Branches

Gray scale imaging and Doppler ultrasound of the vena cava and its major branches have increased over the past few years. The more specific application is for the evaluation of venous thrombosis, either extending from lower extremity veins or spreading into the vena cava from branches such as the renal and hepatic veins.

Inferior Vena Cava Filters, Thrombosis, and Occlusion

Gray scale imaging of the inferior vena cava can be readily performed in most patients. The position of filter prongs and filter orientation can be readily assessed.[143] Obstructing thromboses within the inferior vena cava, the iliac and femoral veins are readily detected by flow imaging.[144,145] Vena cava patency can also be shown following placement of inferior vena cava filters. Sonography is limited in evaluating partial thrombosis within the filter proper, but large free-floating thrombi can readily be detected. The actual size threshold for detecting thrombi within the inferior vena cava has yet to be determined.[146] In general, however, the diagnosis requires an unequivocal gray scale image of the thrombus.

Renal Vein Thrombosis

Renal vein thrombosis is more often detected when tumor thrombus arises from the kidney in association with renal cell carcinoma. The actual extension of the tumor thrombus from the renal vein into the inferior vena cava is readily documented.[147-149] Direct imaging

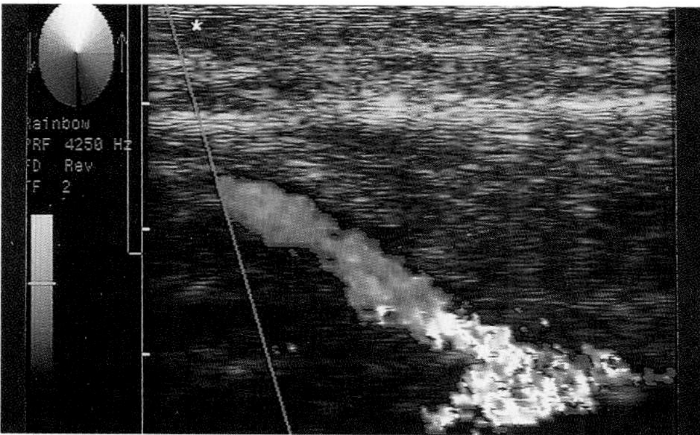

Plate 1. Color flow image showing a pattern referred to as a *color mosaic*. This pattern corresponds to the site of a high-grade stenosis at the distal anastomosis of a bypass graft (see Fig. 11-27). The actual lumen delineated by the color flow image does not appear to be narrowed. The color flow signals overflow beyond the normal physical limits of the arterial segment.

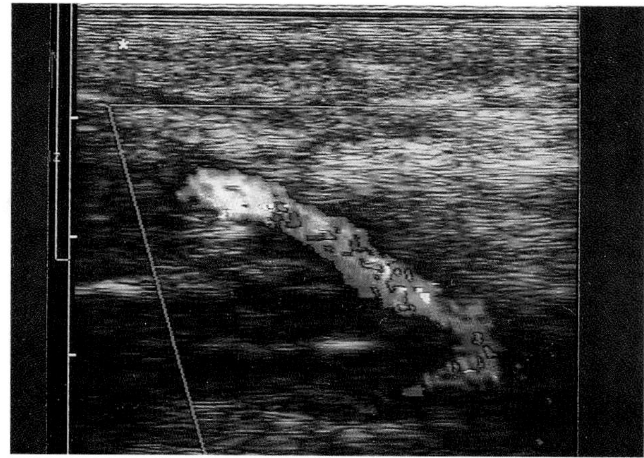

Plate 2. Color flow image obtained at the same location as Plate 1 after an angioplasty. There is aliasing of the color flow image, but the color "mosaic" pattern is now absent. A residual stenosis, shown on Figure 11-28, is not clearly seen as a zone of narrowing on the color flow image.

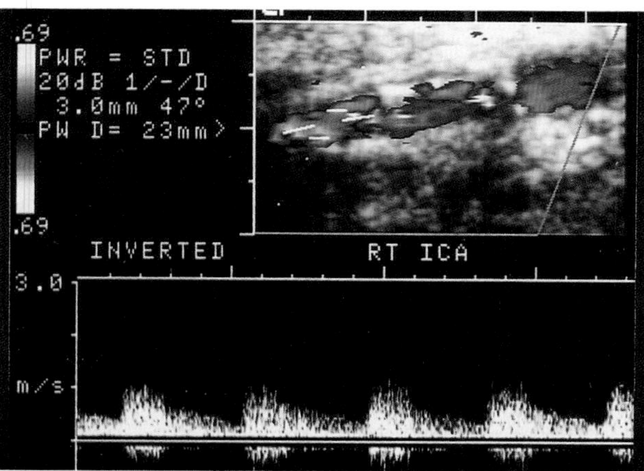

Plate 3. Color flow image showing a typical stenotic lesion, flow reversal (in *blue*) generated downstream to the lesion, and turbulent flow where the Doppler gate is located. The flow disturbance can extend for more than 2 cm distal to the stenosis. The jagged appearance of the spectral envelope and the filling in of the spectral window are evidence of turbulent flow.

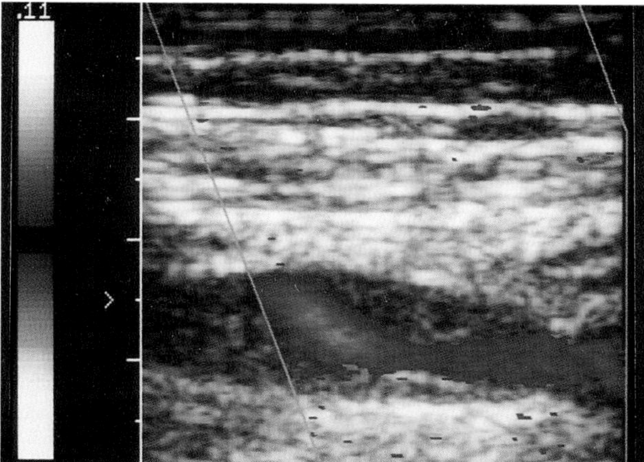

Plate 4. Color flow image showing a *blue* flow channel outlining a nonobstructing venous thrombus at a valve site in the proximal femoral vein. This type of thrombus is typically seen in the postoperative patient.

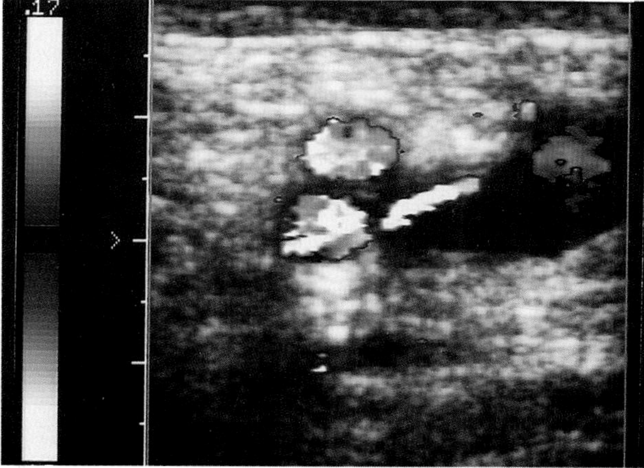

Plate 5. Color flow image showing a signal jet between the deep femoral artery (*left side* of image) directed into the common femoral vein (*right side*). This patient had undergone a cardiac catheterization the preceding day.

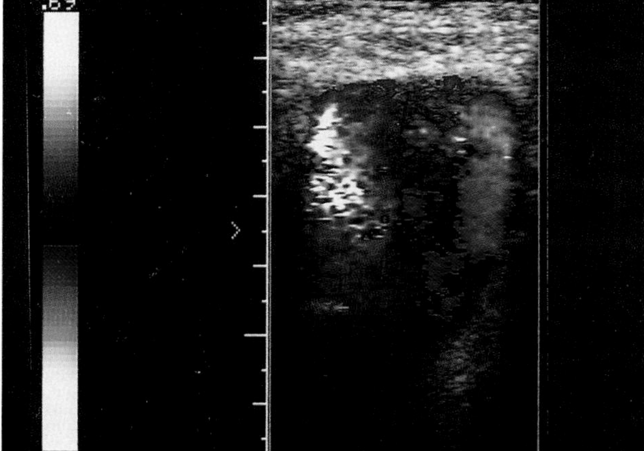

Plate 6. Color flow image showing a typical mixture of forward and reversed flow in a large collection outside the confines of an artery. This pattern is typical of a pseudoaneurysm.

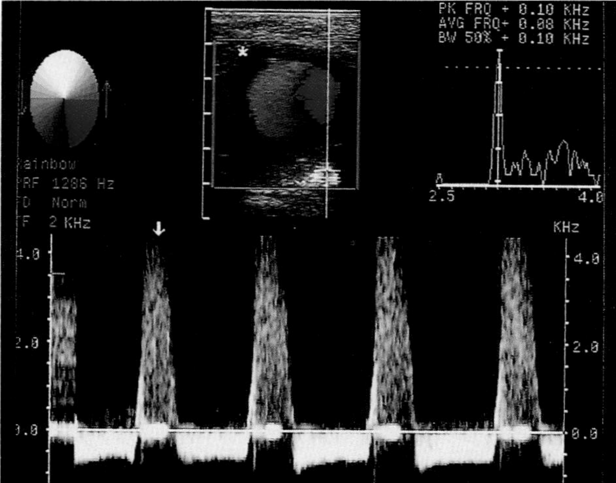

Plate 7. Doppler waveform sampled in the communicating channel of the pseudoaneurysm showing a typical mixture of forward and backward (to-and-fro) flow. The high-amplitude portion represents flow into the collection during systole. The low-amplitude reversed flow during diastole is due to flow outward from the collection.

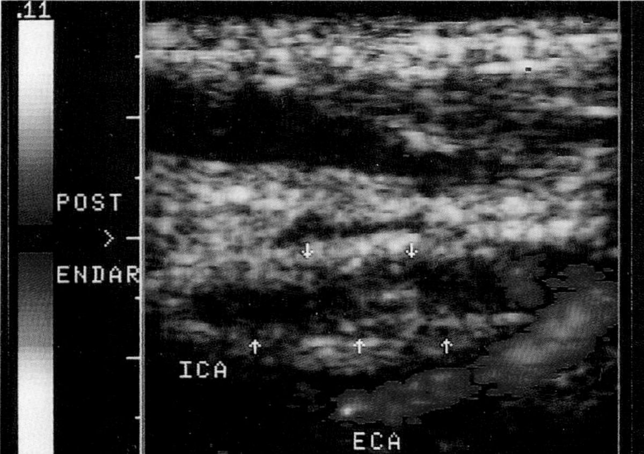

Plate 9. Color flow image showing an obstruction of the proximal internal carotid artery. Flow reversal at the proximal portion of the obstruction (*right*) is outlined by the *arrows.*

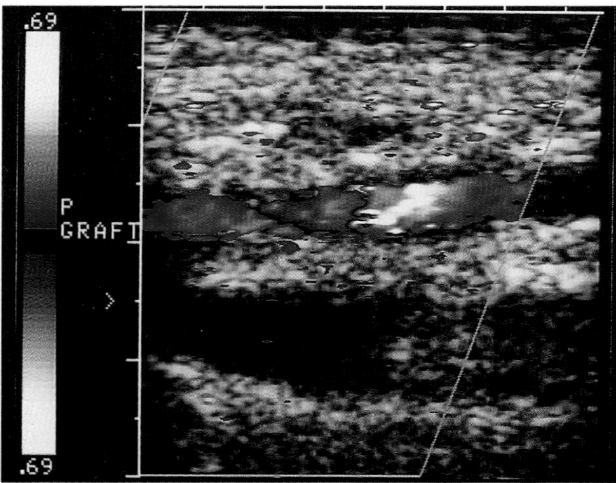

Plate 11. Color flow image showing a zone of aliasing in the conduit of a bypass graft.

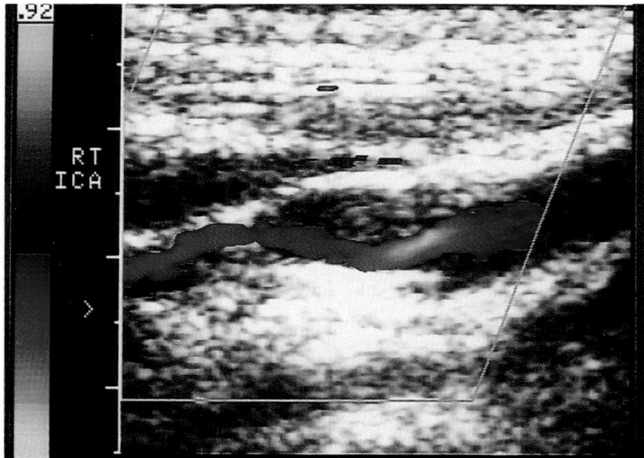

Plate 8. Color flow image showing an isoechoic plaque causing a zone of increased velocity in the proximal internal carotid artery.

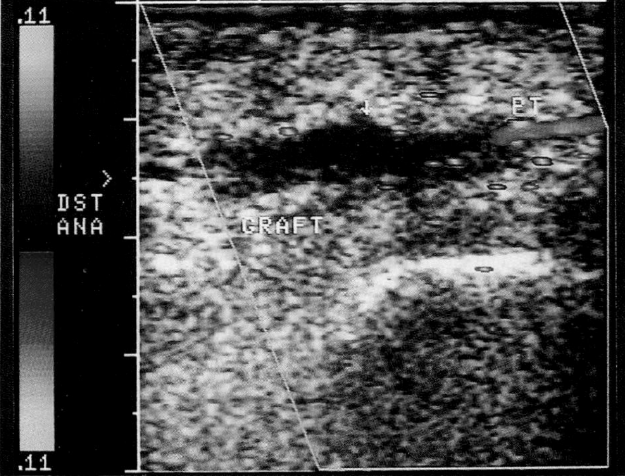

Plate 10. Occlusion of a femorotibial bypass graft (*arrow*) is easily confirmed with color flow imaging. The posterior tibial artery distal to the thrombosed graft has flow (*orange*) because of flow reconstitution through a collateral (zone of *blue/yellow* located below the letters *PT*).

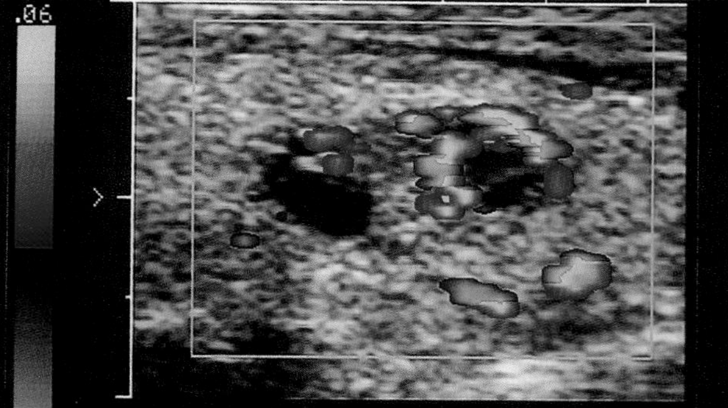

Plate 12. Color flow image showing a thyroid adenoma outlined by color flow signals. This is a nonspecific finding that cannot be used to distinguish benign from malignant lesions.

of the extent of the thrombus within the renal vein is probably not as accurate as that reported with other modalities such as computed tomography[149] and magnetic resonance imaging.

A suggestive diagnostic criterion is, after identification of the renal vein at its junction with the inferior vena cava, the absence of flow signals within the renal vein. An unequivocal diagnostic criterion is the presence of an echogenic mass in the vein lumen. Thrombus, unfortunately, may be difficult to visualize since it is often hypoechoic.[150,151] An effect on the arterial waveform—reversed diastolic flow—has been described in renal vein thrombosis of the transplant kidney[142] but does not seem to apply to the native kidney.[152]

The accuracy of sonography for renal vein thrombosis associated with the presence of nephrotic syndrome or relative entrapment of the renal veins by extrinsic compression has not been systematically studied.

Mesenteric Vein Thrombosis and Occlusion

In general, Doppler sonography can be used to monitor the patency of surgically placed shunts[153] between the portal or mesenteric veins and the systematic circulation, such as the inferior vena cava or the renal vein. There are isolated case reports but no systematic study on the overall accuracy of sonographic techniques when they are used for this purpose.

Hepatic Vein Thrombosis and Occlusion

Hepatic vein thrombosis can be diagnosed with the aid of pulsed Doppler sonography[154] and, more dramatically, with color flow imaging. Absence of flow within the hepatic veins is clearly documentable and has been studied in patients with the Budd-Chiari syndrome.[155,156]

The traditional diagnostic criteria include the loss of flow signals within the hepatic veins, dilatation, abnormal course, and changes in vein wall appearance.[157]

The Portal Vein

Doppler sonography of the portal venous system is used principally in patients with portal venous hypertension, patients following hepatic transplantation, and more recently, patients following transjugular placement of portosystemic shunts.

Thrombosis and Occlusion

The portal vein normally shows a phasic variation with respiration. Loss of flow signals, although consistent with the diagnosis of occlusion, may be due to technical factors. Thrombosis is normally diagnosed when echogenic material is seen within the portal venous system, although enlargement to a diameter of more than 13 mm is suggestive of either thrombosis or portal venous hypertension.[158] This diagnosis is presumed when the portal vein is not visualized. In cases of chronic occlusions, the presence of cavernous transformation supports the diagnosis. Partial thrombosis, easily missed before the introduction of color flow imaging, may now be more easily detected. Correlative studies remain small in number.

Portal Venous Hypertension

Portal venous hypertension is suspected whenever the diameter is more than 13 mm or when portal vein flow signals are altered. These signals lose their normal respiratory phasicity.[159,160] With more severe portal venous pressure elevations, signals may be decreased and the direction of blood flow reversed, favoring the hepatofugal direction. The amplitude and shape of the portal venous waveform cannot, however, be used to quantitate the severity of portal hypertension or to grade the severity of the pressure gradients between the portal and systemic venous systems.[161] The development of collaterals is indirect evidence of portal venous hypertension. Specific enlargement of one of these, the coronary vein, has also been used to indicate portal venous hypertension.[162] Doppler analysis of splanchnic and portal vein flow dynamics also correlate with the results of arteriography in 80 percent of instances.[163]

In cases of congestive right heart failure, the portal vein can develop a pulsatile pattern that emphasizes the A and V waves seen in the internal vena cava and hepatic veins.[164]

Procedure Follow-up

Sonographic monitoring of mesocaval and portal caval shunt patency can be easily done.[153] Although direct visualization of the shunt is often not possible,[165] changes in flow dynamics are readily documented. Mesocaval shunts appear to establish normal hepatopetal flow less often than splenorenal shunts.[161] Although shunt patency can be documented, stenoses are likely to be missed.[166] It also appears that the effectiveness of therapeutic interventions can be more

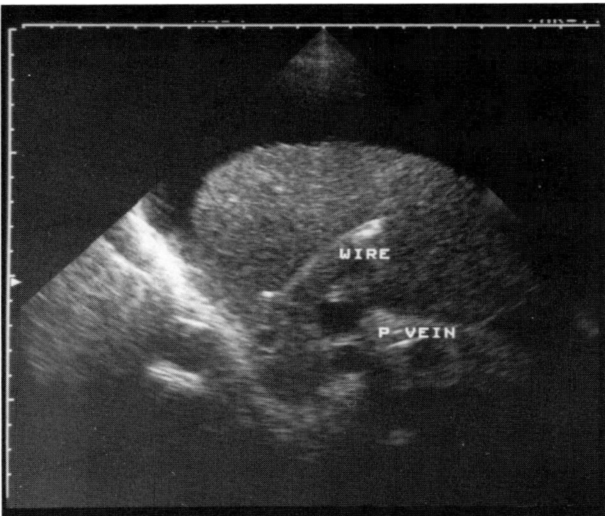

Figure 11-30. Gray scale image taken during a TIPS procedure. A guidewire is clearly outlined in a hepatic vein just anterior to the portal vein.

readily evaluated with sonography. For example, sclerotherapy to control variceal bleeding seems to cause a lower incidence of portal vein thrombosis and to return portal vein flow dynamics to normal faster than surgical shunting.[167]

Follow-up is increasingly obtained with Doppler sonography in cases of an intrahepatic portosystemic shunt placed via the transjugular approach (Fig. 11-30). The stent that ensures shunt patency is readily identified on the gray scale image. Color flow imaging and pulsed Doppler sonography can be done because the wide spacing of the wire mesh used for stent construction does not obstruct the sound signals. Shunt patency is readily confirmed,[168] as is the development of stenoses, partial thromboses, and kinks.

Liver Transplantation

The role of Doppler sonography in the preoperative period has been superseded by that of arteriography. Although sonography can document additional pathologies such as hepatic neoplasms, it cannot establish an adequate road map for the operating surgeon. In addition, it consistently misses hepatic artery aneurysms.[169]

The detection of liver rejection by means of Doppler sonography is unreliable. The hepatic artery waveforms are not consistently altered by acute rejection and are therefore unreliable for monitoring transplants.[170] The presence of hepatic artery thrombosis appears to be reliably detectable by sonography.[171] Finally, loss of hepatic vein pulsations have been suggested as a useful parameter for monitoring the appearance of rejection in patients with normal venous signals in the early postoperative period.[172]

Small Parts

Penis

Doppler sonography has been used to evaluate male impotence and to detect evidence of arterial insufficiency in the cavernosal branches of the penis. The evaluation is performed following the intracavernosal injection of papaverine or of a prostaglandin analogue to induce an erection. The changes in hemodynamics then follow a typical time course.[173] Doppler evaluation is performed during the erection, and peak systolic velocities typically reach a maximum within 2 to 5 minutes after the injection. Peak flow velocities within the cavernosal branches are measured, and peak systolic velocities of less than 0.25 m per second are normally associated with significant arterial insufficiency.[174] An asymmetry of 10 cm per second can also indicate insufficiency.[175]

Persistent low-resistance flow in the artery is suggestive of a venous leak, especially if the end-diastolic velocity is above 5 cm per second.[176]

Varicocele and Testis

Gray scale imaging and color flow imaging can be used to confirm the presence of a varicocele. The sensitivity of ultrasound is greater than that of the physical examination for detecting a varicocele.[177] A varicocele can also be seen on sonography but not be detected by clinical examination following embolotherapy or ligation of the gonadal vein. The presence of such a varicocele does not seem to correlate with clinical outcome and improved sperm counts.[178]

The diagnosis of testicular torsion is readily made with Doppler sonography.[179-182] Although the absence of flow signals can confirm this emergent diagnosis, cases of partial torsion can be missed.[183,184] In addition, flow patterns within the testis can be used to make the diagnosis of inflammatory problems such as orchitis or epididymitis.[185]

Lymph Nodes

Superficial lymph nodes can easily be imaged with high-resolution gray scale sonography. Malignancy is suggested by a change in the shape of the lymph node from an elongated ovoid shape to a more circular heterogeneous contour.

Blood flow increases in hyperplastic[11] or malignant[186,187] lymph nodes can be readily detected by Doppler sonography. Increased flow velocities and distinct flow channels are seen in the hilum and stalk of hyperplastic nodes and are altered with the morphologic changes seen with malignancies.[187]

A recent color Doppler evaluation of cervical lymph nodes used a rigorous protocol that looked at the resistive index within the node and the pattern of flow. This showed overlap in the findings for malignant and nonmalignant lymph nodes.[188] When used to detect lymph node involvement in breast malignancy, color flow imaging also appears to only have a sensitivity of 70 percent but a high specificity.[189]

Thyroid

The role of color flow imaging and Doppler sonography for the evaluation of various thyroid pathologies remains somewhat limited. The increased flow signals seen in Graves disease can cause marked alterations in the Doppler signals.[190]

Most adenomas show a capsule (Color Plate 12) with increased vascularity surrounding the nodule.[12] Unfortunately, papillary carcinomas cannot be reliably distinguished from thyroid adenomas.[12,191] Sampling within the vessel surrounding the actual adenoma or malignancy will typically show, in both cases, a low-resistance flow profile. A further limitation of this approach is its failure to detect flow signals in small thyroid nodules, whether they are benign or malignant.[192]

Breast

Gray scale imaging has traditionally been used to confirm the cystic nature of a mass that is detected during clinical or mammography evaluation of the breast. The addition of Doppler flow imaging has been suggested to be an accurate approach to help differentiate benign from malignant, solid, noncystic breast masses.[193] Typically, malignant lesions show low-resistance flow signals and high-frequency shifts (velocities). More recently, the sensitivity of Doppler sonography has been shown to be lower than this early result and closer to 80 percent.[194] However, it does appear that the presence of flow signals by color flow imaging should prompt a biopsy.[195] In addition, other factors such as lesion morphology, patient age, and size of lesions should complement Doppler waveform analysis and therefore improve accuracy.[196]

The measurement of lesion flow signals and density of flow channels, in addition to being useful for improving the diagnostic specificity of sonography,[195] can also be used to monitor therapeutic responses in large lesions that are not operated on. Decreases in flow signal intensity and amplitude will typically precede, by up to 4 weeks, morphologic changes indicating a positive response to therapy.[197]

Ocular Vessels

The evaluation of the ocular vessels may be conducted as part of the extracranial carotid artery evaluation. In such cases, altered flow within the ophthalmic artery and retinal branches is used to confirm the presence of occlusive arterial disease.[198,199]

An additional pathologic entity that can be detected by this approach is a carotid-cavernous fistula.[199] Doppler sonography can also document the fact that the surgical treatment of glaucoma patients results in improved flow dynamics to the eye.[200]

Ovaries

The recognition that there is a high likelihood of malignancy developing in offspring of women with ovarian carcinoma has motivated an investigation of the use of gray scale imaging and, more importantly, color flow mapping, as a screening test.

In general, malignant lesions have a pattern of low-resistance flow. This observation appears to be related to the extent of angiogenesis.[201] The vascular signals in the ovary also show a decrease in vascular resistance during the luteal phase of the menstrual cycle, thereby introducing more variability in this segment of the female population. Nevertheless, a low-resistance index seems to correlate with the presence of a malignancy, especially if used as part of a scoring system.[202] This finding is disputed by groups that emphasize that Doppler analysis does not contribute much information beyond that available by gray scale imaging alone.[203,204] This lack of diagnostic accuracy also seems to apply to postmenopausal women.[205]

Conclusion

The use of color flow imaging and Doppler sonography has dramatically increased for evaluating the most accessible vascular beds in the body. Use of sonography continues to grow, in part because of its portability and noninvasive nature. However, it remains operator-dependent and requires great technical skill.

Although it plays an important role for screening

patients with suspected vascular pathologies, one of the major advantages it offers is the opportunity of performing serial examinations. This has important implications for establishing outcome analysis of the effectiveness of vascular interventions.

References

1. Kremkau FW. Diagnostic ultrasound: principles, instrumentation, and exercises. 2nd ed. Orlando: Grune & Stratton, 1984.
2. Pignoli P, Tremoli E, Poli A, et al. Intimal plus medial thickness of the arterial wall: a direct measurement with ultrasound imaging. *Circulation* 1986;74:1399–1406.
3. Kremkau FW. Doppler ultrasound: principles and instruments. Philadelphia: Saunders, 1990.
4. Burns PN, Jaffe CC. Quantitative flow measurements with Doppler ultrasound: techniques, accuracy, and limitations. Radiol Clin North Am 1985;23:641–657.
5. Barber FE, Baker DW, Nation AWC, et al. Ultrasonic duplex echo Doppler scanner. IEEE Trans Biomed Eng 1974;21: 109–113.
6. Spencer MP, Reid JM. Quantitation of carotid stenosis with continuous-wave (C-W) Doppler ultrasound. Stroke 1979; 10:326–330.
7. Mitchell DG. Color Doppler imaging: principles, limitations, and artifacts. Radiology 1990;177:1–10.
8. Kasai C, Namekawa K, Koyano A, et al. Real-time two-dimensional blood flow imaging using an autocorrelation technique. IEEE Trans Sonics Ultrasound 1985;S32:458–463.
9. Bonnefous O, Pesque P. Time domain formulation of pulse-Doppler ultrasound and blood velocity estimation by cross-correlation. Ultrason Imaging 1986;8:73–85.
10. Wilkinson DL, Polak JF, Grassi CJ, et al. Pseudoaneurysm of the vertebral artery: appearance on color-flow Doppler sonography. AJR 1988;151:1051–1052.
11. Bjork L, Leven H. Intra-arterial DSA and duplex-Doppler ultrasonography in detection of vascularized inguinal lymph node. Acta Radiol 1990;31:106–107.
12. Shimamoto K, Endo T, Ishigaki T, et al. Thyroid nodules: evaluation with color Doppler sonography. J Ultrasound Med 1993;12:673–678.
13. Bluth EI, Stavros AT, Marich KW, et al. Carotid duplex sonography: a multicenter recommendation for standardized imaging and Doppler criteria. Radiographics 1988;8:487–506.
14. O'Donnell TF, Erdoes L, Mackey WC, et al. Correlation of B-mode ultrasound imaging and arteriography with pathologic findings at carotid endarterectomy. Arch Surg 1985; 120:443–449.
15. Weinberger J, Marks SJ, Gaul JJ, et al. Atherosclerotic plaque at the carotid artery bifurcation: correlation of ultrasonographic imaging with morphology. J Ultrasound Med 1987; 6:363–366.
16. Bassiouny HS, Davis H, Massawa N, et al. Critical carotid stenoses: morphologic and chemical similarity between symptomatic and asymptomatic plaques. J Vasc Surg 1989;9:202–212.
17. Bluth EI, McVay LV, Merritt CRB, et al. The identification of ulcerative plaque with high-resolution duplex carotid scanning. J Ultrasound Med 1988;7:73–76.
18. Gray-Weale AC, Graham JC, Burnett JR, et al. Carotid artery atheroma: comparison of preoperative B-mode ultrasound appearance with carotid endarterectomy specimen pathology. J Cardiovasc Surg 1988;29:676–681.
19. Lennihan L, Kupsky WJ, Mohr JP, et al. Lack of association between carotid plaque hematoma and ischemic cerebral symptoms. Stroke 1987;18:879–881.
20. Coelho JCU, Sigel B, Ryva JC, et al. B-mode sonography of blood clots. JCU 1982;10:323–327.
21. Alanen A, Kormano M. Correlation of the echogenicity and structure of clotted blood. J Ultrasound Med 1985;4:421–425.
22. Killewich LA, Bedford GR, Beach KW, et al. Diagnosis of deep venous thrombosis: a prospective study comparing duplex scanning to contrast venography. Circulation 1989;79: 810–814.
23. Cronan JJ, Dorfman GS, Scola FH, et al. Deep venous thrombosis: US assessment using vein compression. Radiology 1987;162:191–194.
24. White RH, McGahan JP, Daschbach MM, et al. Diagnosis of deep-vein thrombosis using duplex ultrasound. Ann Intern Med 1989;111:297–304.
25. Foley WD, Middleton WD, Lawson TL, et al. Color Doppler ultrasound imaging of lower-extremity venous disease. AJR 1989;152:371–376.
26. Rose SC, Zwiebel WJ, Nelson BD, et al. Symptomatic lower extremity deep venous thrombosis: accuracy, limitations, and role of color duplex flow imaging in diagnosis. Radiology 1990;175:639–644.
27. Yucel EK, Fisher JS, Egglin TK, et al. Isolated calf venous thrombosis: diagnosis with compression US. Radiology 1991; 179:443–446.
28. Mattos MA, Londrey GL, Leutz DW, et al. Color-flow duplex scanning for the surveillance and diagnosis of acute deep venous thrombosis. J Vasc Surg 1992;15:366–376.
29. Bradley MJ, Spencer PA, Alexander L, et al. Colour flow mapping in the diagnosis of the calf vein thrombosis. Clin Radiol 1993;47:399–402.
30. Comerota AJ, Katz ML, Grossi RJ, et al. The comparative value of noninvasive testing for diagnosis and surveillance of deep vein thrombosis. J Vasc Surg 1988;7:40–49.
31. Barnes RW, Nix ML, Barnes CL, et al. Perioperative asymptomatic venous thrombosis: role of duplex scanning versus venography. J Vasc Surg 1989;9:251–260.
32. Elliott CG, Suchyta M, Rose SC, et al. Duplex ultrasonography for the detection of deep venous thrombi after total hip or knee arthroplasty. Angiology 1993;44:26–33.
33. Borris LC, Christiansen HM, Lassen MR, et al. Comparison of real-time B-mode ultrasonography and bilateral ascending phlebography for detection of postoperative deep vein thrombosis following elective hip surgery. The Venous Thrombosis Group. Thromb Haemost 1989;30:363–365.
34. Borris LC, Christiansen HM, Lassen MR, et al. Real-time B-mode ultrasonography in the diagnosis of postoperative deep vein thrombosis in non-symptomatic high-risk patients. The Venous Thrombosis Group. Eur J Vasc Surg 1990;4:473–475.
35. Vanninen R, Manninen H, Soimakallio S, et al. Asymptomatic deep venous thrombosis in the calf: accuracy and limitations of ultrasonography as a screening test after total knee replacement. Br J Radiol 1993;66:199–202.
36. Mewissen MW, Erickson SJ, Foley WD, et al. Thrombosis at venous insertion sites after inferior vena caval filter placement. Radiology 1989;173:155–157.
37. Dorfman GS, Cronan JJ, Paolella JP, et al. Iatrogenic changes at the venotomy site after percutaneous placement of the Greenfield filter. Radiology 1989;173:159–162.
38. Molgaard CP, Yucel EK, Geller SC, et al. Access-site thrombosis after filter placement of inferior vena cava filters with 12-14-F delivery sheaths. Radiology 1992;185:257–261.
39. Knudson GJ, Wiedmeyer DA, Erickson SJ, et al. Color Doppler sonographic imaging in the assessment of upper-extremity deep venous thrombosis. AJR 1990;154:399–403.
40. Grassi CJ, Polak JF. Axillary and subclavian venous thrombosis: follow-up evaluation with color Doppler flow US and venography. Radiology 1990;175:651–654.

41. Burbridge SJ, Finlay DE, Letourneau JG, et al. Effects of central venous catheter placement on upper extremity duplex US findings. J Vasc Intervent Radiol 1993;4:399–404.
42. Haire WD, Lynch TG, Lieberman RP, et al. Utility of duplex ultrasound in the diagnosis of asymptomatic catheter-induced subclavian vein thrombosis. J Ultrasound Med 1991;10:493–496.
43. Araki CT, Back TL, Padberg FT Jr, et al. Refinements in the ultrasonic detection of popliteal vein reflux. J Vasc Surg 1993; 18:742–748.
44. Polak JF. Peripheral vascular sonography: a practical guide. Baltimore: Williams & Wilkins, 1992.
45. Meissner MH, Manzo RA, Bergelin RO, et al. Deep venous insufficiency: the relationship between lysis and subsequent reflux. J Vasc Surg 1993;18:596–608.
46. Weingarten MS, Branas CC, Czeredarczuk M, et al. Distribution and quantification of venous reflux in lower extremity chronic venous stasis disease with duplex scanning. J Vasc Surg 1993;18:753–759.
47. Blackshear WM Jr, Phillips DJ, Chikos PM, et al. Carotid artery velocity patterns in normal and stenotic vessels. Stroke 1980;11:67–71.
48. Dreisbach JN, Seibert CE, Smazal SF, et al. Duplex sonography in the evaluation of carotid artery disease. AJNR 1983; 4:678–680.
49. Robinson ML, Sacks D, Perlmutter GS, et al. Diagnostic criteria for carotid duplex sonography. AJR 1988;151:1045–1049.
50. Polak JF, Dobkin GR, O'Leary DH, et al. Internal carotid artery stenosis: accuracy and reproducibility of color-Doppler-assisted duplex imaging. Radiology 1989;173:793–798.
51. Russell D, Bakke SJ, Wiberg J, et al. Patency and flow velocity profiles in the internal carotid artery assessed by digital subtraction angiography and Doppler studies three months following endarterectomy. J Neurol Neurosurg Psychiatry 1986; 49:183–186.
52. Glover JL, Bendick PJ, Dilley RS, et al. Restenosis following carotid endarterectomy: evaluation by duplex ultrasonography. Arch Surg 1985;120:678–684.
53. Withers CE, Gosink BB, Keightley AM, et al. Duplex carotid sonography: peak systolic velocity in quantifying internal carotid artery stenosis. J Ultrasound Med 1990;9:345–349.
54. O'Leary DH, Clouse ME, Potter JE, et al. The influence of non-invasive tests on the selection of patients for carotid angiography. Stroke 1985;16:264–267.
55. North American Carotid Endarterectomy Trial Collaborators. Beneficial effect of carotid endarterectomy in symptomatic patients with high-grade stenosis. N Engl J Med 1991;325: 445–453.
56. Moneta GL, Edwards JM, Chitwood RW, et al. Correlation of North American Symptomatic Carotid Endarterectomy Trial (NASCET) angiographic definition of 70% to 99% internal carotid stenosis with duplex scanning. J Vasc Surg 1993; 17:152–159.
57. Hunink MGM, Polak JF, Barlan MM, et al. Detection and quantification of carotid artery stenosis: efficacy of various Doppler velocity parameters. AJR 1993;160:619–625.
58. Zwiebel WJ, Crummy AB. Sources of error in Doppler diagnosis of carotid occlusive disease. AJR 1981;137:1–12.
59. Farmilo RW, Scott DJA, Cole SEA, et al. Role of duplex scanning in the selection of patients for carotid endarterectomy. Br J Surg 1990;77:388–390.
60. Steinke W, Kloetzsch C, Hennerici M. Carotid artery disease assessed by color Doppler flow imaging: correlation with standard Doppler sonography and angiography. AJNR 1990;11: 259–266.
61. Blaisdell WF, Clauss RH, Galbraith JG, et al. Joint study of extracranial occlusion IV: a review of surgical considerations. JAMA 1969;209:1889–1895.
62. Langsfield M, Gray-Weale AC, Lusby RJ. The role of plaque morphology and diameter reduction in the development of new symptoms in asymptomatic carotid arteries. J Vasc Surg 1989;9:548–557.
63. Thiele BL, Young JV, Chikos PM, et al. Correlation of arteriographic findings and symptoms in cerebrovascular disease. Neurology 1980;30:1041–1046.
64. Kricheff II. Arteriosclerotic ischemic cerebrovascular disease. Radiology 1987;162:101–109.
65. Polak JF, O'Leary DH, Kronmal RA, et al. Sonographic evaluation of carotid artery atherosclerosis in the elderly: relationship of disease severity to stroke and transient ischemic attack. Radiology 1993;188:363–370.
66. Reilly LM, Lusby RJ, Hughes L, et al. Carotid plaque histology using real-time ultrasonography: clinical and therapeutic implications. Am J Surg 1983;146:188–193.
67. Bluth EI, Kay D, Merritt CRB, et al. Sonographic characterization of carotid plaque: detection of hemorrhage. AJR 1986;146:1061–1065.
68. Lusby RJ, Ferrell LD, Ehrenfeld WK, et al. Carotid plaque hemorrhage: its role in production of cerebral ischemia. Arch Surg 1982;117:1479–1488.
69. O'Leary DH, Holen J, Ricotta JJ, et al. Carotid bifurcation disease: prediction of ulceration with B-mode US. Radiology 1987;162:523–525.
70. Walker DW, Acker JD, Cole CA. Subclavian steal syndrome detected with duplex pulsed Doppler sonography. AJNR 1982;3:615–618.
71. Kotval PS, Babu SC, Shah PM. Doppler diagnosis of partial vertebral/subclavian steals convertible to full steals with physiologic maneuvers. J Ultrasound Med 1990;9:207–213.
72. Davis PC, Nilsen B, Braun IF, et al. A prospective comparison of duplex sonography vs angiography of the vertebral arteries. AJNR 1986;7:1059–1064.
73. Bluth EI, Merritt CRB, Sullivan MA, et al. Usefulness of duplex ultrasound in evaluating vertebral arteries. J Ultrasound Med 1989;8:229–235.
74. Visona A, Lusiana L, Castellani V, et al. The echo-Doppler (duplex) system for the detection of vertebral artery occlusive disease: comparison with angiography. J Ultrasound Med 1986;5:247–250.
75. Mills JL, Harris EJ, Taylor LM Jr, et al. The importance of routine surveillance of distal bypass grafts with duplex scanning: a study of 379 reversed vein grafts. J Vasc Surg 1990; 12:379–389.
76. Idu MM, Blankestein JD, de Gier P, et al. Impact of a color-flow duplex surveillance program on infrainguinal vein graft patency: a five-year experience. J Vasc Surg 1993;17:42–53.
77. Polak JF, Karmel MI, Meyerovitz MF. Accuracy of color Doppler flow mapping for evaluation of the severity of femoropopliteal arterial disease: a prospective study. J Vasc Intervent Radiol 1991;2:471–479.
78. Edwards JM, Goldwell DM, Goldman ML, et al. The role of duplex scanning in the selection of patients for transluminal angioplasty. J Vasc Surg 1991;13:69–74.
79. MacGowan SW, Saif MF, O'Neil G, et al. Ultrasound examination in the diagnosis of popliteal artery aneurysms. Br J Surg 1985;72:528–529.
80. Kohler TR, Nance DR, Cramer MM, et al. Duplex scanning for diagnosis of aortoiliac and femoropopliteal disease: a prospective study. Circulation 1987;76:1074–1080.
81. Polak JF, Karmel MI, Mannick JA, et al. Determination of the extent of lower-extremity peripheral arterial disease with color-assisted duplex sonography: comparison with angiography. AJR 1990;155:1085–1089.
82. Kotval PS. Doppler waveform parvus and tardus: a sign of proximal flow obstruction. J Ultrasound Med 1989;8:435–440.
83. Hutchison KJ, Karpinski E. Stability of flow patterns in the in vivo post-stenotic velocity field. Ultrasound Med Biol 1988;14:269–275.
84. Sacks D, Robinson ML, Marinelli DL, et al. Peripheral arterial Doppler ultrasonography: diagnostic criteria. J Ultrasound Med 1992;11:95–103.

85. Cossman DV, Ellison JE, Wagner WH, et al. Comparison of contrast arteriography to arterial mapping with color-flow duplex imaging in the lower extremities. J Vasc Surg 1989;10:522–529.
86. Whelan FF, Barry MH, Moir JD. Color flow Doppler ultrasonography: comparison with peripheral arteriography for the investigation of peripheral arterial disease. J Clin Ultrasound 1992;20:369–374.
87. Ranke C, Creutzig A, Alexander K. Duplex scanning of the peripheral arteries: correlation of the peak velocity ratio with angiographic diameter reduction. Ultrasound Med Biol 1992;18:433–440.
88. Polak JF, Donaldson MC, Whittemore AD, et al. Pulsatile masses surrounding vascular prostheses: real-time US color flow imaging. Radiology 1989;170:363–366.
89. Sanchez LA, Suggs WD, Veith FJ, et al. Is surveillance to detect failing polytetrafluoroethylene bypasses worthwhile? Twelve-year experience with 91 grafts. J Vasc Surg 1993;18:981–990.
90. Bandyk DF, Seabrook GR, Moldenhauer P, et al. Hemodynamics of vein graft stenosis. J Vasc Surg 1988;8:688–695.
91. Bandyk DF, Schmitt DD, Seabrook GR, et al. Monitoring functional patency of in situ saphenous vein bypasses: the impact of a surveillance protocol and elective revision. J Vasc Surg 1989;9:286–296.
92. Whittemore AD, Clowes AW, Couch NP, et al. Secondary femoropopliteal reconstruction. Ann Surg 1981;193:35–42.
93. Bandyk DF, Jorgensen RA, Towne JB. Intraoperative assessment of in situ saphenous vein arterial bypass grafts using pulsed Doppler spectral analysis. Arch Surg 1986;121:292–299.
94. Grigg MJ, Nicolaides AN, Wolfe JH. Detection and grading of femorodistal vein grafts stenoses: duplex velocity measurements compared with angiography. J Vasc Surg 1988;8:661–666.
95. Polak JF, Donaldson MC, Dobkin GR, et al. Early detection of saphenous vein arterial bypass graft stenosis by color-assisted duplex sonography: a prospective study. AJR 1990;154:857–861.
96. Berkowitz HD, Greenstein SM. Improved patency in reversed femoral-infrapopliteal autogenous vein grafts by early detection and treatment of the failing graft. J Vasc Surg 1987;5:755–761.
97. Cohen JR, Mannick JA, Couch NP, et al. Recognition and management of impending vein-graft failure: importance for long-term patency. Arch Surg 1986;121:758–759.
98. Tordoir JH, de Bruin HG, Hoeneveld H, et al. Duplex ultrasound scanning in the assessment of arteriovenous fistulas created for hemodialysis access: comparison with digital subtraction angiography. J Vasc Surg 1989;10:122–128.
99. Schwab SJ, Quarles LD, Middleton JP, et al. Haemodialysis-associated subclavian vein stenosis. Kidney Int 1988;33:1156–1159.
100. Barrett N, Spencer S, McIvor J, et al. Subclavian stenosis: a major complication of subclavian dialysis catheters. Nephrol Dial Transplant 1988;3:423–425.
101. Scheible W, Skram C, Leopold GR. High resolution real-time sonography of hemodialysis vascular access complications. AJR 1980;134:1173–1176.
102. Middleton WD, Picus DD, Marx MV, et al. Color Doppler sonography of hemodialysis vascular access: comparison with angiography. AJR 1989;152:633–639.
103. Dousset V, Grenier N, Douws C, et al. Hemodialysis grafts: color Doppler flow imaging correlated with digital subtraction angiography and functional status. Radiology 1991;181:89–94.
104. Nonnast-Daniel B, Martin RP, Lindert O, et al. Colour Doppler ultrasound assessment of arteriovenous hemodialysis fistulas. Lancet 1992;339:143–145.
105. Strauch BS, O'Connell RS, Geoly KL, et al. Forecasting thrombosis of vascular access with Doppler color flow imaging. Am J Kidney Dis 1992;19:554–557.
106. Hunink MGM, Donaldson MC, Meyerovitz MF, et al. Risks and benefits of femoropopliteal percutaneous balloon angioplasty. J Vasc Surg 1993;17:183–194.
107. Moneta GL, Yeager RA, Lee RW, et al. Noninvasive localization of arterial occlusive disease: a comparison of segmental pressures and arterial duplex mapping. J Vasc Surg 1993;17:578–582.
108. Mewissen MW, Kinney EV, Bandyk DF, et al. The role of duplex scanning versus angiography in predicting outcome after balloon angioplasty in the femoropopliteal artery. J Vasc Surg 1992;15:860–866.
109. Sacks D, Robinson ML, Summers TA, et al. The value of duplex sonography after peripheral artery angioplasty in predicting subacute stenosis. AJR 1994;162:179–183.
110. Helvie MA, Rubin J. Evaluation of traumatic groin arteriovenous fistulas with duplex Doppler sonography. J Ultrasound Med 1989;8:21–24.
111. Roubidoux MA, Hertzberg BS, Carroll BA, et al. Color flow and image-directed Doppler ultrasound evaluation of iatrogenic arteriovenous fistulas in the groin. JCU 1990;18:463–469.
112. Coughlin BF, Paushter DM. Peripheral pseudoaneurysms: evaluation with duplex US. Radiology 1988;168:339–342.
113. Helvie MA, Rubin JM, Silver TM, et al. The distinction between femoral artery pseudoaneurysms and other causes of groin masses: value of duplex Doppler sonography. AJR 1988;150:1177–1180.
114. Fellmeth BD, Baron SB, Brown PR, et al. Repair of postcatheterization femoral pseudoaneurysms by color flow ultrasound guided compression. Am Heart J 1992;123:547–551.
115. Kresowik TF, Khoury MD, Miller BV, et al. A prospective study of the incidence and natural history of femoral vascular complications after percutaneous transluminal coronary angioplasty. J Vasc Surg 1991;13:328–335.
116. DiPrete DA, Cronan JJ. Compression ultrasonography: treatment for acute femoral artery pseudoaneurysms in selected cases. J Ultrasound Med 1992;11:489–492.
117. Bluth EI, Shyn PB, Sullivan MA, et al. Doppler color flow imaging of carotid artery dissection. J Ultrasound Med 1989;8:149–153.
118. Kotval PS, Babu SC, Fakhry J, et al. Role of the intimal flap in arterial dissection: sonographic demonstration. AJR 1988;150:1181–1182.
119. Nevitt MP, Ballard DJ, Hallett JW. Prognosis of abdominal aortic aneurysms. N Engl J Med 1989;321:1009–1014.
120. Cabellon SJ, Moncrief CL, Pierre DR, et al. Incidence of abdominal aortic aneurysms in patients with atheromatous disease. Am J Surg 1983;146:575–576.
121. Beede SD, Ballard DJ, James EM, et al. Positive predictive value of clinical suspicion of abdominal aortic aneurysm: implications for efficient use of abdominal sonography. Arch Intern Med 1990;150:549–551.
122. Carty GA, Nachtigal T, Magyar R, et al. Abdominal duplex ultrasound screening for occult aortic aneurysm during carotid arterial evaluation. J Vasc Surg 1993;17:696–702.
123. Yucel EK, Fillmore DJ, Knox TA, et al. Sonographic measurement of abdominal aortic diameter: interobserver variability. J Ultrasound Med 1991;10:681–683.
124. Kohler TR, Zierler RE, Martin BS, et al. Noninvasive diagnosis of renal artery stenosis by ultrasonic duplex scanning. J Vasc Surg 1986;4:450–456.
125. Taylor TC, Kettler MD, Moneta GL, et al. Duplex ultrasound in the diagnosis of renal artery stenosis: a prospective evaluation. J Vasc Surg 1988;7:363–369.
126. Berland LL, Koslin DB, Routh WD, et al. Renal artery stenosis: prospective evaluation of diagnosis with color duplex US compared with angiography: work in progress. Radiology 1990;174:421–423.
127. Desberg AL, Paushter DM, Lammert GK, et al. Renal artery stenosis: evaluation with color Doppler flow imaging. Radiology 1990;177:749–753.
128. Patriquin HB, Lafortune M, Jéquier J-C, et al. Stenosis of the

renal artery: assessment of slowed systole in the downstream circulation with Doppler sonography. Radiology 1992;184: 479–485.
129. Stavros AT, Parker SH, Yakes WF, et al. Segmental stenosis of the renal artery: pattern recognition of tardus and parvus abnormalities with duplex sonography. Radiology 1992;184: 487–492.
130. Kliewer MA, Tupler RH, Carroll BA, et al. Renal artery stenosis: analysis of Doppler waveform parameters and tardus-parvus pattern. Radiology 1993;189:779–787.
131. Moneta GL, Yeager RA, Dalman R, et al. Duplex ultrasound criteria for diagnosis of splanchnic artery stenosis or occlusion. J Vasc Surg 1991;14:511–520.
132. Bowersox JC, Zwolak RM, Walsh DB, et al. Duplex ultrasonography in the diagnosis of celiac and mesenteric artery occlusive disease. J Vasc Surg 1991;14:780–788.
133. Moneta GL, Lee RW, Yeager RA, et al. Mesenteric duplex scanning: a blinded prospective study. J Vasc Surg 1993;17: 79–86.
134. Harward TRS, Smith S, Seeger JM. Detection of celiac axis and superior mesenteric artery occlusive disease with use of abdominal duplex scanning. J Vasc Surg 1993;17:738–745.
135. Soulen MC, Benenati JF, Sheth S, et al. Changes in renal artery Doppler indexes following renal angioplasty. J Vasc Intervent Radiol 1991;2:457–461.
136. Hudspeth DA, Hansen KJ, Reavis SW, et al. Renal duplex sonography after treatment of renovascular disease. J Vasc Surg 1993;18:381–390.
137. Rifkin MD, Needleman L, Pasto ME, et al. Evaluation of renal transplant rejection by duplex Doppler examination: value of the resistive index. AJR 1987;148:759–762.
138. Rigsby CM, Burns PN, Weltin GG, et al. Doppler signal quantitation in renal allografts: comparison in normal and rejecting transplants, with pathological correlation. Radiology 1987;162:39–42.
139. Don S, Kopecky KK, Filo RS, et al. Duplex Doppler US of renal allografts: causes of elevated resistive index. Radiology 1989;171:709–712.
140. Drake DG, Day DL, Letourneau JG, et al. Doppler evaluation of renal transplants in children: a prospective analysis with histopathologic correlation. AJR 1990;154:785–787.
141. Kaveggia LP, Perrella RR, Grant EG, et al. Duplex Doppler sonography in renal allografts: the significance of reversed flow in diastole. AJR 1990;155:295–298.
142. Reuther G, Wanjura D, Bauer H. Acute renal vein thrombosis in renal allografts: detection with duplex Doppler US. Radiology 1989;170:557–558.
143. Liu GC, Angtuaco TL, Ferris EJ, et al. Inferior vena caval filters: noninvasive evaluation. Radiology 1986;160:521–524.
144. Park JH, Lee JB, Han MC, et al. Sonographic evaluation of inferior vena caval obstruction: correlative study with venography. AJR 1985;145:757–762.
145. Pasto ME, Kurtz AB, Jarrell BE, et al. The Kimray-Greenfield filter: evaluation by duplex real-time/pulsed Doppler ultrasound. Radiology 1983;148:223–226.
146. Vorwerk D, Hollman J, Gunther R. Long-term follow-up of vena-caval filters: real-time sonography and the native x-ray image. Rofo Fortschr Geb Rontgenstr Neuen Bildgeb Verfahr 1987;146:558–562.
147. Goldstein HM, Green B, Weaver RM Jr. Ultrasonic detection of renal tumor extension into the inferior vena cava. AJR 1978;130:1083–1085.
148. Schwerk WB, Schwerk WN, Rodeck G. Venous renal tumor extension: a prospective US evaluation. Radiology 1985;156: 491–495.
149. Didier D, Racle A, Etievent JP, et al. Tumor thrombus of the inferior vena cava secondary to malignant abdominal neoplasms: US and CT evaluation. Radiology 1987;162:83–89.
150. Rosenfield AT, Zeman RK, Cronan JJ, et al. Ultrasound in experimental and clinical renal vein thrombosis. Radiology 1980;137:735–741.
151. Braun B, Weilemann LS, Weigand W. Ultrasonographic demonstration of renal vein thrombosis. Radiology 1981;138: 157–158.
152. Platt JF, Ellis JH, Rubin JM. Intrarenal arterial Doppler sonography in the detection of renal vein thrombosis of the native kidney. AJR 1994;162:1367–1370.
153. Lafortune M, Patriquin H, Pomier G, et al. Hemodynamic changes in portal circulation after portosystemic shunts: use of duplex sonography in 43 patients. AJR 1987;149:701–706.
154. Hosoki T, Koroda C, Tokunaga A, et al. Hepatic venous outflow obstruction: evaluation with pulsed duplex sonography. Radiology 1989;170:733–737.
155. Grant EG, Perella R, Tessler FN, et al. Budd-Chiari syndrome: the results of duplex and color Doppler imaging. AJR 1989;152:377–381.
156. Brown BP, Abu-Yousef M, Farner R, et al. Doppler sonography: a noninvasive method for evaluation of venoocclusive disease. AJR 1990;154:721–724.
157. Menu Y, Alison D, Lorphelin JM, et al. Budd-Chiari syndrome: US evaluation. Radiology 1985;157:761–764.
158. Weinreb J, Kumari S, Phillips G, et al. Portal vein measurements by real-time sonography. AJR 1982;139:497–499.
159. Bolondi L, Gandolfi L, Arienti V, et al. Ultrasonography in the diagnosis of portal hypertension: diminished response of portal vessels to respiration. Radiology 1982;142:167–172.
160. Koslin DB, Berland LL. Duplex Doppler examination of the liver and portal venous system. JCU 1987;15:675–686.
161. Kawasaki T, Moriyasu F, Nishida O, et al. Analysis of hepatofugal flow in the portal venous system using ultrasonic Doppler duplex system. Am J Gastroenterol 1989;84:937–941.
162. Subramanyam BR, Balthazar EJ, Madamba MR, et al. Sonography of portosystemic venous collaterals in portal hypertension. Radiology 1983;146:161–166.
163. Nelson RC, Lovett KE, Chezmar JL, et al. Comparison of pulsed Doppler sonography and angiography in patients with portal hypertension. AJR 1987;149:393–397.
164. Hosoki T, Arisawa J, Marukawa T, et al. Portal blood flow in congestive heart failure: pulsed duplex sonographic findings. Radiology 1990;174:733–736.
165. Bolondi L, Gaiani S, Mazziotti A, et al. Morphological and hemodynamic changes in the portal venous system after distal splenorenal shunt: an ultrasound and pulsed Doppler study. Hepatology 1988;8:652–657.
166. Hederstrom E, Forsberg L, Ivancev K, et al. Ultrasonography and Doppler duplex compared with angiography in follow-up of mesocaval shunt patency. Acta Radiol 1990;31:341–345.
167. Rice S, Lee KP, Johnson MB, et al. Portal venous system after portosystemic shunts or endoscopic sclerotherapy: evaluation with Doppler sonography. AJR 1991;156:85–89.
168. Longo JM, Bilbao JI, Garcia-Villarreal L, et al. Transjugular intrahepatic portosystemic shunt: evaluation with Doppler sonography. Radiology 1993;186:529–534.
169. Kolmannskog F, Jakobsen JA, Schrumpf E, et al. Duplex Doppler sonography and angiography in the evaluation for liver transplantation. Acta Radiol 1994;35:1–5.
170. Marder DM, Demarino GB, Sumkin JH, et al. Liver transplant rejection: value of the resistive index in Doppler US of hepatic arteries. Radiology 1989;173:127–129.
171. Kubota K, Billing H, Ericzon BG, et al. Duplex Doppler ultrasonography for monitoring liver transplantation. Acta Radiol 1990;31:279–283.
172. Britton PD, Lomas DJ, Coulden RA, et al. The role of hepatic vein Doppler in diagnosing acute rejection following pediatric liver transplantation. Clin Radiol 1992;45:228–232.
173. Schwartz AN, Wang KY, Mack LA, et al. Evaluation of normal erectile function with color flow Doppler sonography. AJR 1989;153:1155–1160.
174. Lue TF, Hricak H, Marich KW, et al. Vasculogenic impotence evaluation by high resolution ultrasonography and pulsed Doppler spectrum analysis. Radiology 1985;155:777–781.
175. Benson CB, Vickers MA. Sexual impotence caused by vascular

disease: diagnosis with duplex sonography. AJR 1989;153: 1149–1153.

176. Quam JP, King BF, James EM, et al. Duplex and color Doppler sonographic evaluation of vasculogenic impotence. AJR 1989;153:1141–1147.
177. Petros JA, Andriole GL, Middleton WD, et al. Correlation of testicular color Doppler ultrasonography, physical examination and venography in the detection of left varicoceles in men with infertility. J Urol 1991;145:785–788.
178. Cvitanic OA, Cronan JJ, Sigman M, et al. Varicoceles: postoperative prevalence—a prospective study with color Doppler US. Radiology 1993;187:711–714.
179. Middleton WD, Siegel BA, Melson GL, et al. Acute scrotal disorders: prospective comparison of color Doppler US and testicular scintigraphy. Radiology 1990;177:177–181.
180. Burks DD, Markey BJ, Burkhard TK, et al. Suspected testicular torsion and ischemia: evaluation with color Doppler sonography. Radiology 1990;175:815–821.
181. Atkinson GO Jr, Patrick LE, Ball TI Jr, et al. The normal and abnormal scrotum in children: evaluation with color Doppler sonography. AJR 1992;158:613–617.
182. Lerner RM, Merorach RA, Hulbert WC, et al. Color Doppler US in the evaluation of acute scrotal disease. Radiology 1990; 176:355–358.
183. Wilbert DM, Schaerfe CW, Stern WD, et al. Evaluation of the acute scrotum by color-coded Doppler ultrasonography. J Urol 1993;149:1475–1477.
184. Hollman AS, Ingram S, Carachi R, et al. Colour Doppler imaging of the acute pediatric scrotum. Pediatr Radiol 1993;23: 83–87.
185. Horstman WG, Middleton WD, Melson GL. Scrotal inflammatory disease: color Doppler US findings. Radiology 1991;179:55–59.
186. Mountford RA, Atkinson P. Doppler ultrasound examination of pathologically enlarged lymph nodes. Br J Radiol 1979;52: 464–467.
187. Swischuk LE, Desai PB, John SD. Exuberant blood flow in enlarged lymph nodes: findings on color flow Doppler. Pediatr Radiol 1992;22:419–421.
188. Chuang VP. Radiation-induced arteritis. Semin Roentgenol 1994;29:64–69.
189. Walsh JS, Dixon JM, Chetty U, et al. Colour Doppler studies of axillary node metastases in breast carcinoma. Clin Radiol 1994;49:189–191.
190. Ralls PW, Mayekawa DS, Lee KP, et al. Color-flow Doppler sonography in Graves disease: "thyroid inferno." AJR 1988; 150:781–784.
191. Hubsch P, Niederle B, Barton P, et al. Color-coded Doppler sonography of the thyroid: an advance in carcinoma diagnosis? Rofo Fortschr Geb Rontgenstr Neuen Bildgeb Verfahr 1992;156:125–129.
192. Gooding GA, Clark OH. Use of color Doppler imaging in the distinction between thyroid and parathyroid lesions. Am J Surg 1992;164:51–56.
193. Britton PD, Coulden RA. The use of duplex Doppler ultrasound in the diagnosis of breast cancer. Clin Radiol 1990;42: 399–401.
194. Dixon JM, Walsh J, Paterson D, et al. Colour Doppler ultrasonography studies of benign and malignant breast lesions. Br J Surg 1992;79:259–260.
195. Cosgrove DO, Kedar RP, Bamber JC, et al. Breast diseases: color Doppler US in differential diagnosis. Radiology 1993; 189:99–104.
196. McNicholas MM, Mercer PM, Miller JC, et al. Color Doppler sonography in the evaluation of palpable breast masses. AJR 1993;161:765–771.
197. Kedar RP, Cosgrove DO, Smith IE, et al. Breast carcinoma: measurement of tumor response to primary medical therapy with color Doppler flow imaging. Radiology 1994;190:825–830.
198. Lieb WE, Flaharty PM, Ho A, et al. Color Doppler imaging of the eye and orbit. A synopsis of a 400 case experience. Acta Ophthalmol Suppl 1992;204:50–54.
199. Munk P, Downey D, Nicolle D, et al. The role of colour flow Doppler ultrasonography in the investigation of disease in the eye and orbit. Can J Ophthalmol 1993;28:171–176.
200. Trible JR, Sergott RC, Spaeth GL, et al. Trabeculectomy is associated with retrobulbar hemodynamic changes: a color Doppler analysis. Ophthalmology 1994;101:340–351.
201. Wu CC, Lee CN, Chen TM, et al. Incremental angiogenesis assessed by color Doppler ultrasound in the tumorigenesis of ovarian neoplasms. Cancer 1994;73:1251–1256.
202. Timor-Tritsch LE, Lerner JP, Monteagudo A, et al. Transvaginal ultrasonographic characterization of ovarian masses by means of color flow-directed Doppler measurements and a morphologic scoring system. Am J Obstet Gynecol 1993;168: 909–913.
203. Hata K, Hata T, Manabe A, et al. A critical evaluation of transvaginal Doppler studies, transvaginal sonography, magnetic resonance imaging, and CA 125 in detecting ovarian cancer. Obstet Gynecol 1992;80:922–926.
204. Levine D, Feldstein VA, Babcock CJ, et al. Sonography of ovarian masses: poor sensitivity of resistive index for identifying malignant lesions. AJR 1994;162:1355–1359.
205. Bromley B, Goodman H, Benacerraf BR. Comparison between sonographic morphology and Doppler waveform for the diagnosis of ovarian malignancy. Obstet Gynecol 1994; 83:434–437.

II

The Central Nervous System

12

Cerebral Vascular Angiography: Indications, Technique, and Normal Anatomy of the Head

CHRISTOPHER J. MORAN
DANIEL K. KIDO
DEWITTE T. CROSS III

History

Cerebral vascular angiography began in 1927 with Moniz, who localized brain tumors by directly injecting contrast into exposed carotid arteries.[1] Modern vascular angiography began in 1953 when Seldinger was able to replace the needle with a catheter.[2]

Cerebral angiography was further advanced by the development of less toxic contrast agents, rapid film changers, and mechanical contrast injectors. Meanwhile, changes in catheter construction allowed for the development of smaller, thinner-walled catheters. These new materials improved catheter maneuverability and stability while preserving adequate flow rates. Guidewire advances included the development of a safety core, which ensured that broken guidewires would not be left behind in a patient; heparin coating of guidewires, which reduced the incidence of thrombus formation[3]; and hydrophilic coating of guidewires, which decreased friction between the catheter and the guidewire, making difficult catheter placements possible.

High-resolution (1024 × 1024) digital subtraction angiography (DSA) is replacing standard film screen systems because it allows for instant availability of high-quality images. In addition, the incorporation of road-mapping capabilities with DSA systems permits the rapid placement of guidewires and catheters without the need for repeated injections of contrast media. Patient monitoring during angiography has also evolved. Besides the neurologic examination, advances in physiologic monitoring allow routine monitoring of blood pressure, cardiac rhythm, and blood oxygenation. Quality has improved through the development of standards for operators and equipment by several organizations, including the American College of Radiology (ACR) and the Society of Cardiovascular and Interventional Radiology (SCVIR).[4]

Indications

The indications for cerebral angiography have changed since it was first developed. Initially, angiography was used not only to examine the cerebral vascular system but also to indirectly screen the central nervous system (CNS) for lesions. The development of computed tomography (CT) and magnetic resonance imaging (MRI) has eliminated the need to use cerebral angiography as a screening tool.

The extracranial carotid and vertebral arteries are examined to detect the presence of atherosclerotic disease, dissections, intimal tears due to trauma, the vascularity of head and neck tumors, and arteritis. Extracranial tumors such as glomus tumors (jugulare, vagale, tympanicum), carotid body tumors, and angiofibromas are studied as a prelude to embolization. Although meningiomas usually are intracranial, a significant portion of their blood supply frequently arises from the extracranial circulation. The intracranial circulation is examined for atherosclerotic disease, aneurysms, arteriovenous malformations, vasospasm, and arteritis. To avoid bleeding, intracranial tumors such as gliomas are examined before possible percutaneous biopsy to determine their vascularity.

Materials

Supplies

Prepackaged angiography trays containing sterile gauze, syringes, needles, lidocaine for local anesthesia, syringes for flushing and contrast injections, connecting tubing for the injector, and a manifold system for flushing saline, contrast, and a closed waste system are available in a variety of configurations. A scalpel blade, hemostat, stopcock, basin, sponge sticks, small basin for povidone-iodine (Betadine), Band-Aid dressing, and sterile towels, drapes, and gowns may be added to the tray.

Contrast Media

The decision as to whether low-osmolar (nonionic) or high-osmolar (ionic) contrast media should be used for angiography is important because nonionic agents cost approximately 10 times more than ionic agents. Katayama et al. found that the incidence of nausea, vomiting, sensation of heat, itching, urticaria, flushing, and sneezing was 12.7 percent after the intravenous injection of ionic contrast media and was 3.1 percent for nonionic contrast media.[5] Severe reactions that require treatment of dyspnea, blood pressure changes, cardiac arrest, or loss of consciousness had an incidence of 0.22 percent with ionic and 0.04 percent with nonionic contrast media. The very severe reactions that required hospitalization and emergent treatment had the same incidence of 0.04 percent with each agent. One death occurred after the intravenous administration of contrast with each class of agent. Fewer adverse reactions in patients perceived to be at high risk were observed in those receiving nonionic contrast.[6]

Arterial administration of ionic contrast media produces fewer systemic reactions than intravenous administration.[7] No comparison of reactions following intraarterial injection of ionic and nonionic contrast agents has been performed. Animal data suggest lower neuronal toxicity with nonionic contrast agents in the brain, but this benefit has been difficult to document in humans.[8] Human studies have not shown statistically significant differences in neurologic effects between ionic and nonionic contrast in cerebral angiography. However, slight changes in heart rate have been observed with ionic contrast during cerebral angiography.

Low-osmolar contrast seems to cause less nephrotoxicity in patients with preexisting renal insufficiency. In patients with normal renal function, the risks of nephrotoxicity are similar with both groups.[9] Risk factors that increase the incidence of contrast-induced nephropathy include preexisting renal disease, dehydration, diabetes, advanced age, and large amounts of contrast.

There is some debate regarding the thrombogenicity of both groups of agents. Some investigators feel that nonionic contrast agents do not inhibit thrombin formation, as do the ionic contrast agents.[10,11] Others feel that the increased thrombogenicity associated with nonionic agents is a theoretic rather than a clinical problem.[12–14] These researchers believe that it is difficult to cause clotting in vitro in contrast-blood mixtures and that many other factors, such as platelet activation, blood-catheter-syringe interactions, and endothelial damage (procedural trauma), need to be considered in the clotting of blood-contrast media mixtures.

How then does one determine who will receive a nonionic or ionic contrast agent? The authors use the ACR guidelines to select patients who will receive nonionic contrast agents. These are (1) patients with a prior history of contrast reactions (not just a sensation of heat and flushing, or a single episode of nausea or vomiting), asthma, or other significant allergy; (2) patients in whom a history cannot be obtained; (3) patients who have systemic diseases such as atherosclerotic heart disease, congestive heart failure, arrhythmias, recent myocardial infarction, pulmonary hypertension, or renal insufficiency; (4) severely debilitated patients; (5) patients who are to undergo angiography of the external carotid artery or selective branches of the subclavian artery because nonionic agents cause less pain, and thus less motion; (6) patients who are undergoing spinal angiography; and (7) patients undergoing interventional procedures.[15]

Needles

For adults and children who weigh more than 20 kg, 18-gauge needles are used for double-wall punctures. These needles accept guidewires up to .038 inch in diameter. For children between 10 and 20 kg in weight, a 19-gauge needle is used with a .025-inch guidewire. For children under 10 kg, a 21-gauge needle is used with a .018-inch guidewire.

Guidewires and Catheters

The maneuverability of guidewire-catheter systems results from the combination of their stiffness and torqueability. The proper balance between these characteristics is important when selecting a catheter or guidewire for a procedure.

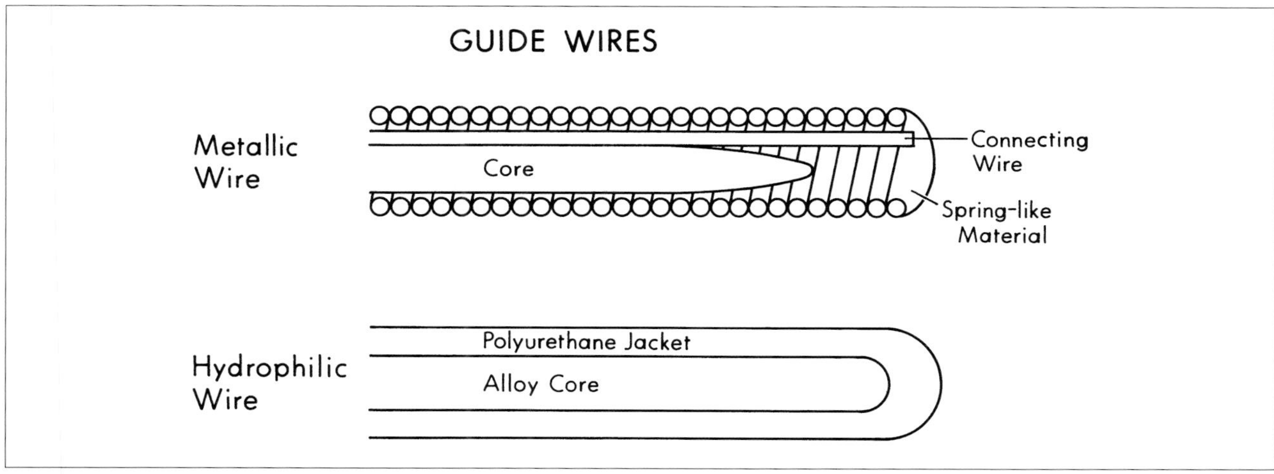

Figure 12-1. Sagittal midline drawing of a straight metallic and hydrophilic guidewire. The springlike material of the metallic wire usually is coated with Teflon and may also be coated with heparin. The hydrophilic coating is applied to the polyurethane jacket of the hydrophilic wire.

Guidewires

Guidewires were developed to increase the ease and safety of catheter placement in the vascular system. Metallic guidewire design incorporates several different features that make this possible. The outer shell is a very flexible springlike material. This feature, combined with curving of the tip, helps to lessen intimal damage and enhance passage within the vascular lumen. A central core stiffens the guidewire to provide a track for the catheter to follow. Between the flexible outer shell of the guidewire and the stiff central core is a smaller wire that is welded to both (Fig. 12-1). This joins the three components so that the guidewire is flexible (springlike outer shell), maneuverable and trackable (stiff central core), and nonseparable (joining wire). Movable core guidewires maximize these features. The addition of heparin and Teflon outer coatings decreases the thrombogenicity of the guidewire and increases the trackability of the catheter over the positioned guidewire.

A major advance in guidewire technology has been the development of hydrophilic coatings. In this design, the central core is a very flexible alloy enveloped with polyurethane to which a hydrophilic polymer has been bonded (see Fig. 12-1). This results in a guidewire that is very flexible and maneuverable. The addition of the hydrophilic polymer decreases friction so the catheter will more easily follow the guidewire. The decrease in surface friction also decreases the need for stiffness in the catheter. The hydrophilic wire must be kept moist and free of contrast or the surface may become "tacky" and the desired trackability feature lost. The detachable torque device enclosed in the guidewire package helps manipulate the guidewires. Some hydrophilic wires are so flexible that the catheter will not follow the guidewire. Recently, some of these wires have been modified so that only the tip and distal 10 cm are very flexible while the more proximal portions are relatively stiff. This modification eases passage of the catheter over the wire.

Occasionally the catheter (most are 100 cm in length) will not follow over a positioned guidewire (most are 145 cm in length). In this instance, one catheter may be used to select the vessel and a longer exchange wire (200–260 cm) can be placed through it and left in place while the catheter is withdrawn. Then another, more flexible catheter (such as nonbraided polyethylene) can be advanced over the exchange wire and placed in the desired vessel.

Catheters

Many of the current 4 or 5 French catheters used for cerebral angiography contain wire braid in the shaft, which increases their maneuverability. This braid usually does not continue into the tip, which therefore is more flexible. There are numerous catheter shapes with or without wire braiding that can be used to perform cerebral angiography. Most catheter materials are radiopaque, and some catheter tips have radiopaque markers.

Aortic arch injections are performed with pigtail-shaped catheters that have multiple side holes. This design allows for rapid injection of large volumes of con-

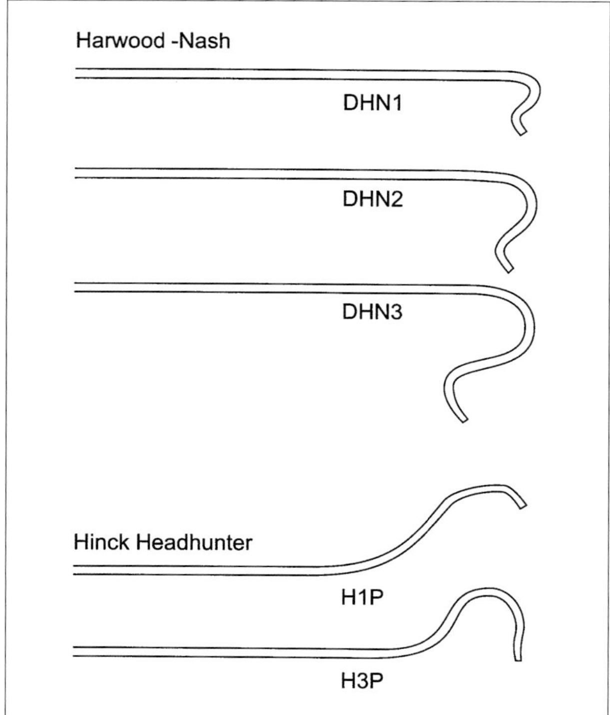

Figure 12-2. Pediatric angiography catheters.

trast in a bolus and reduces catheter recoil during injection.

Pediatric catheters include the Derek Harwood-Nash series of catheters (DHN1, 2, or 3) (Fig. 12-2). The DHN1, which is used for infants up to 10 kg in weight, is 3 French and 40 cm long and is used with a .018-inch guidewire. The DHN2, which is used for children weighing 10 to 20 kg, is 4.1 French and 40 cm in length and is used with a .025-inch wire. For larger children, the 5 French, 70-cm-long DHN3 may be used with a 0.35-inch guidewire. The pediatric version of the Hinck Headhunters (H1P and H3P) (see Fig. 12-2) range from 4.5 to 6 French, are up to 80 cm long, and are used with .028- to .035-inch guidewires.

For teenagers and young adults, 100-cm catheters with only a slight bend, such as a Hinck Headhunter (H1), a Bentson-Hanafee-Wilson (JB1), a Newton (HN1), or a Weinberg (WNBG) can be used to select the neck vessels (Fig. 12-3). The distal portions of these catheters are pliable and may be carefully advanced without a guidewire. However, if any resistance is encountered, a guidewire should be used to place the catheter.

For patients with an elongated aortic arch or common origins of the innominate or left common carotid artery, a catheter with a more complex curve is usually necessary to engage the orifice of the vessel. Examples of these catheters include the Bentson-Hanafee-Wilson (JB2 or JB3), Kerber (CK1), Mani (MAN), Simmons (SIM1), and Newton (HN2, 3, 4, or 5) (Fig. 12-4). These catheters cannot be advanced without placement of a guidewire.

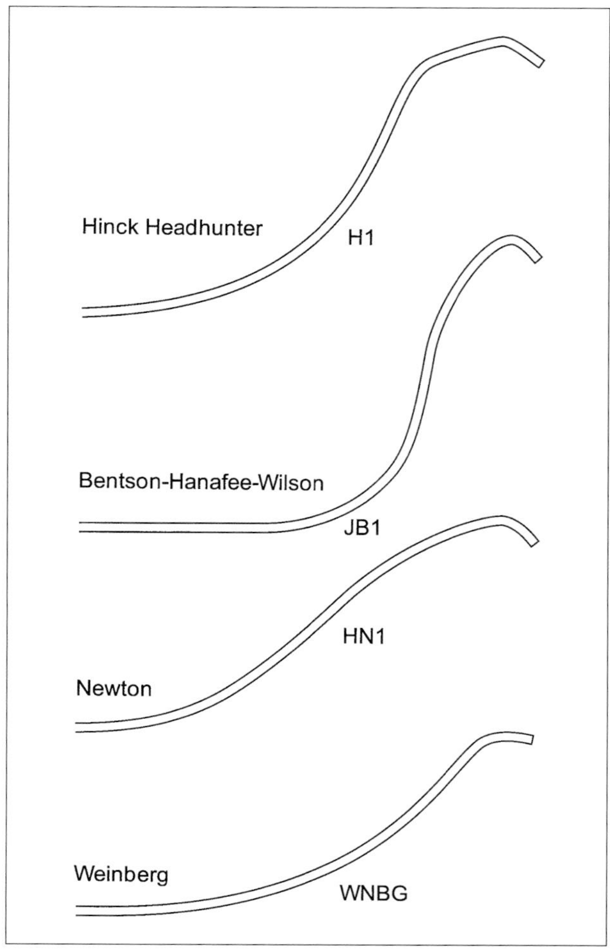

Figure 12-3. Simple catheter curves used in young adults.

For even more tortuous and elongated aortic arches, catheters such as the Hinck Headhunter (H3), the Simmons (SIM2), and the Hilal Modified Headhunters (H3H, H5H, and H6H) may be necessary (Fig. 12-5). The Hinck Headhunter H3 and the Hilal Modified Headhunter H3H are similar in shape. Originally these catheters were constructed of 6.5 French material with the distal 10 cm tapering to 5 French material. These complex curved catheters usually are reformed in the abdominal aorta, iliac artery, renal arteries, left subclavian artery, and ascending aorta. The operator positions their tips at the orifice of the desired vessel and then advances them by withdrawing the catheter. In contrast, when the examination is finished, the operator disengages the catheter from the vessel by advancing the hub of the catheter.

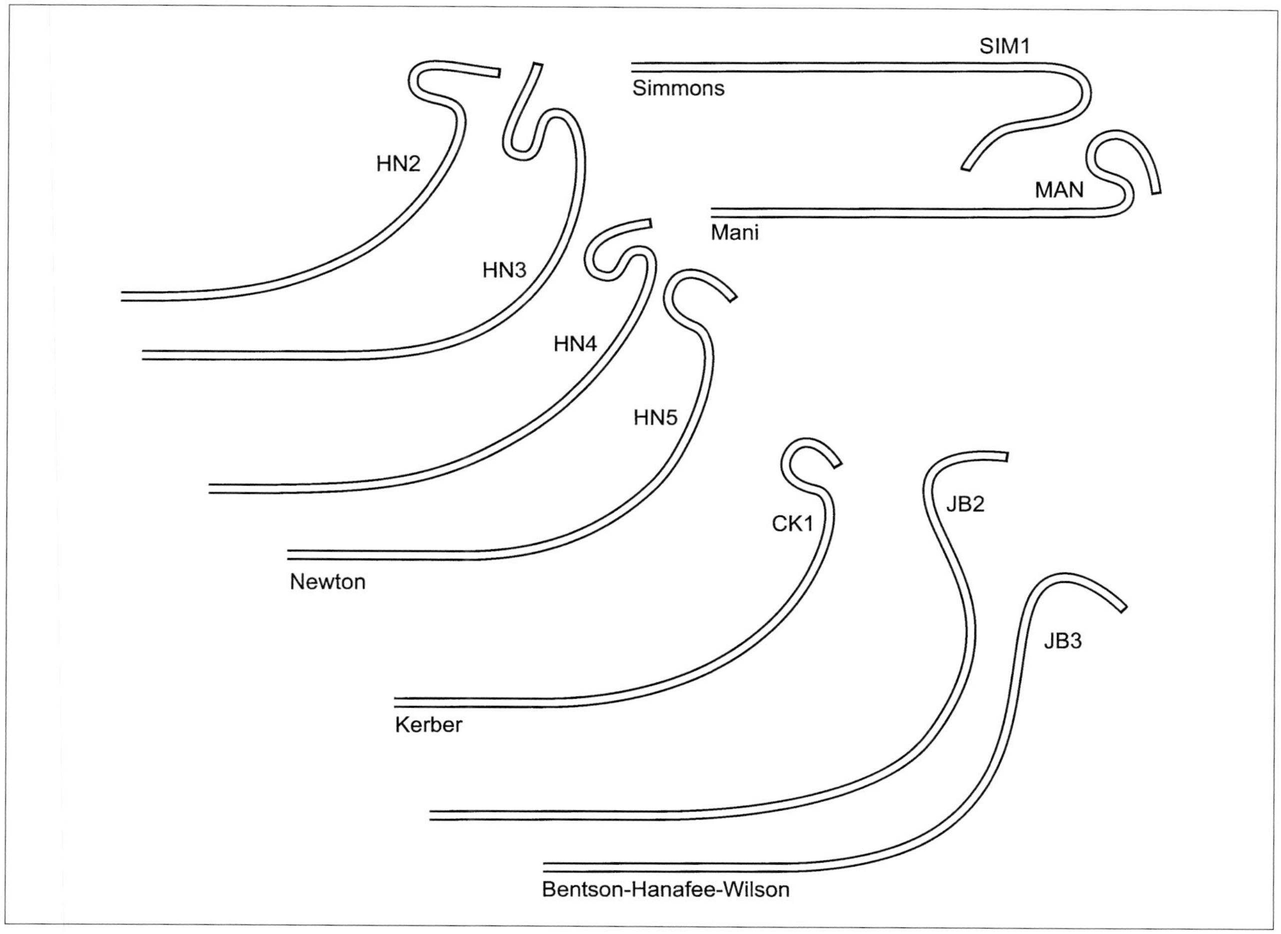

Figure 12-4. Moderately curved catheters used as the aorta elongates.

These catheters are used to examine the carotid, innominate, and left subclavian arteries. Although all of the catheters may be used in a selective fashion, severe tortuosity may preclude safe placement. In these instances, subclavian or innominate injections are prudent. Vertebral catheterization may also be performed with a Davis or Bernstein catheter. For studies performed through the brachial or axillary approach, a catheter with a relatively tight curve such as a Simmons 1 (SIM1) is useful (see Fig. 12-4).

Technique for Performing a Cerebral Angiogram

When a request for cerebral angiography is received, the patient's prior imaging examinations should be reviewed and the case should be discussed with the referring physician. If these two steps are followed, the risks and benefits can be clearly discussed with the patient and his or her family when the consent is obtained. The indication for angiography should be discussed with the patient and explained in the context of the patient's previous diagnostic tests. The risks of complications should also be discussed. Rapport can be established at this time if care is taken to thoroughly explain the procedure and allay the patient's concerns. During this process, important information regarding the patient's basic health as well as possible allergies is obtained. If the patient is reluctant to undergo the procedure, further discussion with family members and the referring physician may be necessary. Ideally, the patient is interviewed the evening before the examination. Unfortunately, many patients are admitted on the day of examination.

Complications

The most important complication of cerebral angiography is stroke. This usually is the result of emboli dislodged from atherosclerotic plaque, clots that have formed on the catheter or guidewire, or the injection

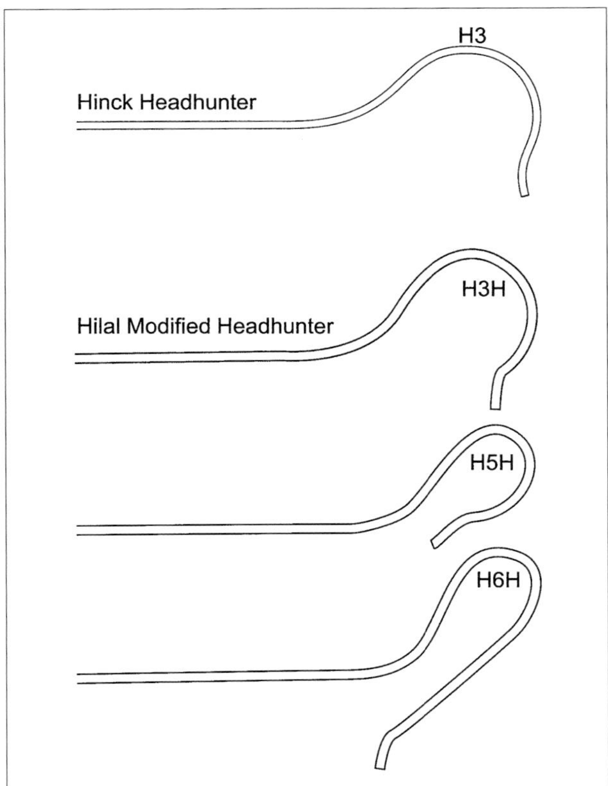

Figure 12-5. Complex curved catheters used in patients with elongated or tortuous aortas.

of clots, particulate matter, or air during contrast injections and catheter flushing. In addition, catheter or contrast injection trauma may raise an intimal flap, which may cause emboli or occlusion of the vessel. The incidence of temporary neurologic complications with conventional film screen cerebral angiography ranges from 1.9 to 4.1 percent. The incidence of permanent complications is less, ranging from 0.6 to 1 percent.[16] The rate of complications using DSA is also less, with transient ischemic attacks (TIA) occurring in 0.6 percent and stroke in 0.3 percent of patients.[17] In an analysis of 5000 catheter angiograms, Mani found that angiographic proficiency leads to fewer complications. In this study, trainees had an overall complication rate of 3.9 percent, radiologists and angiographers 1.8 percent, and fully trained neuroradiologists 0.7 percent.[18]

Another type of complication is related to the puncture site (femoral, brachial, axillary) or catheter manipulation and includes hemorrhage, arterial obstruction, pseudoaneurysm, arteriovenous fistula, or limb amputation. Hessel reported that 0.47 percent of patients having the transfemoral approach and 1.7 percent of patients undergoing the transaxillary approach required surgery.[19] A recent series of brachial arteriograms using 4 French catheters found that 0.3 percent needed surgery for laceration or thrombosis.[20] Hematoma formation is the most frequent puncture site complication and occurs in up to 10 percent of patients. Significant hematomas, defined as needing transfusion or evacuation or delaying discharge, occur in 0.5 to 2.0 percent of patients.[4] Most hematomas are not of clinical significance, but the patient and family should be forewarned that the groin and upper thigh may become "bruised" after the procedure and that this will resolve like other bruises over several weeks. Nerve damage is infrequent but is most severe when involving the brachial plexus and usually less severe when involving the median nerve. Femoral nerve involvement is rare. The injury can result from the anesthetic injection, arteriotomy needle, or hematoma formation. So rare are infections related to percutaneous punctures that prophylactic antibiotics are not administered.

Sedation

An intravenous line should be inserted before the angiogram to permit the administration of medications if necessary. Mild intravenous sedation is given to lessen anxiety and may be titrated for the desired effect. The authors usually give 25 μg fentanyl and 1 mg Versed. Fentanyl may be reversed with Narcan and Versed with Romazicon. Occasionally droperidol may be added for its tranquilizing effects. This is particularly true if the patient has an adverse response to Versed by becoming agitated or confused. All patients should be monitored with pulse oximetry, electrocardiographically, and by intermittent blood pressure readings.

Puncture Site

Most cerebral vascular evaluations are performed after the femoral artery is punctured. Because most people are right-handed, most angiographic rooms are designed for puncture of the right femoral artery. The femoral, dorsalis pedis, and posterior tibial arteries should be palpated and marked and the strength of these pulses recorded. The nurse who monitors the patient should also palpate the prepuncture pulses because that nurse will help monitor the patient's pulses after the procedure. Conditions that may preclude puncturing of the right femoral artery include a nonpalpable pulse, previous right herniorrhaphy, groin infection, preexisting hematoma, and a unilateral graft. In these situations it would be preferable to use the left femoral artery. However, previous groin surgery or graft insertions are not absolute contraindications. The dilation of a tract for a catheter may be more difficult in these latter instances but not impossible. A femoral puncture site should be selected, if at all possible, before a brachial approach is selected.

The next favored approach is the brachial artery. Since this artery is smaller than the femoral artery, thrombosis of the artery can occur more readily. The complications associated with brachial arteriography are higher than with femoral arteriography but are lower than with axillary arteriography. The axillary artery is the last choice because it carries the additional risk of brachial plexus injury, either from needle insertion or from hematoma formation. When the upper extremity is chosen as the access site, the axillary, brachial, and radial pulses are palpated and marked. Direct carotid or vertebral punctures are now uncommonly performed.

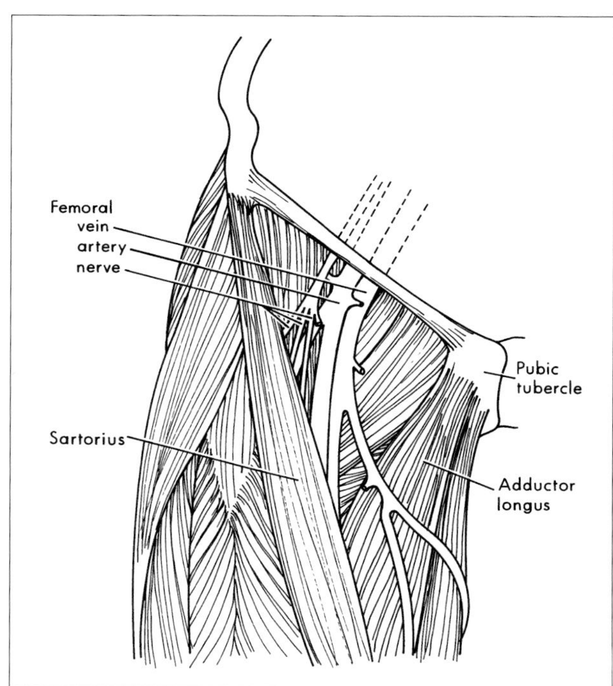

Figure 12-6. Frontal view of the right femoral triangle. The femoral vein, femoral artery, and femoral nerve are located from medial to lateral in the femoral triangle.

Clothing

Occupational Health and Safety Administration (OSHA) guidelines mandate that individuals who may be exposed to blood-borne pathogens such as hepatitis and AIDS wear protective clothing. This includes nonpermeable gowns, gloves, a surgical mask, and eye protection. Surgical caps and shoe covers should also be worn.

Figure 12-7. Frontal view of the right femoral triangle without the surrounding muscles. Note the relationship of the femoral artery and femoral head to the inguinal ligament at the selected puncture site. The needle has been inserted into the femoral artery over the femoral head.

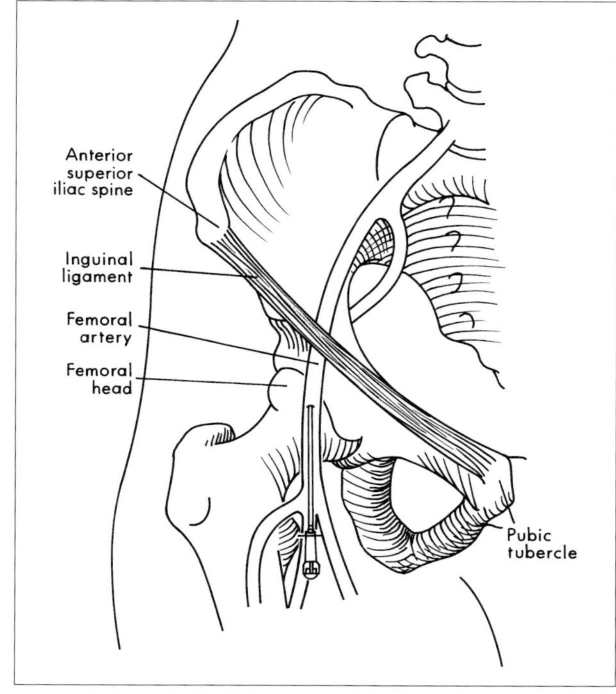

Preparation

After the hair at the puncture site has been shaven, the skin is cleansed with Betadine and sterile towels are placed about the puncture site. Next, a large sterile aperture drape is placed over the patient. A sterile manifold is placed at the foot of the drape and connected to the saline flush, contrast, and waste bag. If nonionic contrast material is used, 1000 units of heparin may be added to the contrast. Two thousand units of heparin are added to the 1000-ml saline flush bag.

Puncture

Femoral Artery

The groin is palpated for the femoral pulse (Fig. 12-6), and a hemostat is placed at the proposed puncture site. The tip of the hemostat is observed fluoroscopically and positioned so it overlies the femoral head (Fig. 12-7).[21] A puncture above the femoral head makes compression difficult, particularly if it is above the inguinal ligament.

The skin at the puncture site is anesthetized with

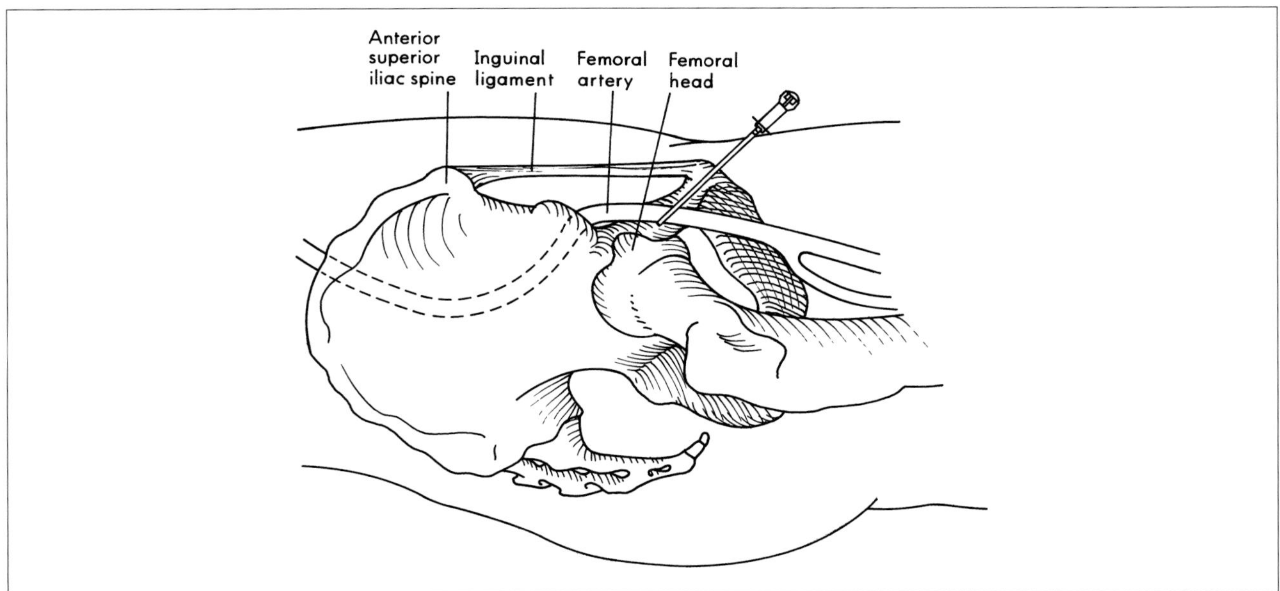

Figure 12-8. Lateral drawing of a double-wall femoral puncture showing the relationship of the needle to the femoral head and inguinal ligament.

1 percent lidocaine using a 25-gauge needle. Deeper anesthesia above, lateral, and deep to the femoral artery is administered using a 21-gauge needle. Before the injection of the lidocaine, the plunger on the syringe should be withdrawn to check for arterial blood. If the artery has been punctured, the needle should be removed and the artery compressed. Next, a small incision is made in the skin overlying the puncture site. The incision is made horizontally so that the skin and immediate subcutaneous tissues are incised rather than the femoral artery. The subcutaneous tissues are spread with the hemostat.

There are two types of arterial puncture: single wall and double wall. The single-wall technique requires a needle with a hollow stylet so blood will exit when the anterior wall of the artery has been punctured and the lumen entered. Although the arterial needle with a hollow stylet can be used for a double-wall puncture, most arterial needles used in this technique have a solid stylet. For trainees, the single-wall puncture seems to result in more intimal dissections and difficulty in cannulation of the artery. Conversely, single-wall puncture seems to cause fewer hematomas.

The needle is inserted through the incision site in a line along the course of the artery (see Fig. 12-7) at an angle of approximately 45 to 60 degrees (Fig. 12-8). Both walls of the artery are punctured (see Fig. 12-8). The inner stylet is withdrawn and the cannula is withdrawn slowly at a more horizontal angle until arterial blood returns from the needle. A guidewire is introduced through the cannula of the needle into the iliac artery to at least the level of the aortic bifurcation. After the guidewire is stabilized, the cannula is withdrawn, the guidewire cleansed with moist gauze, and the vessel dilator sheath system introduced over the guidewire. After the vessel dilator is removed, the sheath system is continuously flushed with heparinized saline under pressure.

Brachial Artery

The patient's arm is extended on an armboard and abducted approximately 45 degrees. The wrist is turned in a vertical position with the radius uppermost to facilitate palpation of the brachial artery in the antecubital fossa. The wrist is then fixed in this position on the armboard with adhesive tape. The proposed puncture site is cleansed with Betadine, draped, and anesthetized with 1 percent lidocaine. Since the brachial artery is superficial, deep anesthesia is usually unnecessary. A superficial incision is performed at the puncture site. The needle is inserted along the course of the palpated brachial artery using the same technique as for femoral punctures. Because of the smaller size of the brachial artery, 4 French sheaths and catheters are usually used, but 5 French systems may also be used.

Axillary Artery

The patient's arm is placed behind the head with the upper arm horizontal to the table. After the axillary pulse is localized, the proposed puncture site is prepared and draped in the usual fashion. The puncture site is usually located high in the axilla over the humeral head. The technique for the incision and arterial puncture is identical to that used for both femoral and brachial puncture.

Sheaths

Placement of an arterial sheath has both advantages and disadvantages. Among the many advantages is patient comfort. After the sheath has been placed, catheter manipulation and exchange do not cause patient discomfort. In addition, the incidence and extent of oozing and hematoma formation are lessened. Trauma at the puncture site is reduced because the sheath is manipulated only on insertion. The sheath may also make catheter manipulation easier by partially straightening the vessels. When catheter replacement is necessary, additional arterial trauma does not occur because arterial access is maintained with the sheath. Finally, indwelling sheaths allow access for repeat angiograms when necessary and may also be used as interim arterial lines. These advantages come with relatively few disadvantages. One is that the hole in the artery is slightly larger than that of the angiographic catheter. Another slight disadvantage is the need for an additional heparinized saline flush solution, which must be monitored during the procedure.

Contrast Injection

Once the angiographic catheter has been introduced, test injections to determine catheter position are performed by hand. For the angiograms, machines reliably inject rates and volumes of contrast; this consistency makes angiograms reproducible. Machine injection also reduces the radiation exposure to the angiographer, who can step back from the x-ray equipment.

Catheterizing Arteries Arising from the Aortic Arch

Arch Aortography

Biplane DSA of the aortic arch and its major arterial branches with a pigtail-type catheter optimizes catheter selection for carotid and vertebral arteriography. The catheter is introduced over a guidewire and positioned in the abdominal aorta. The guidewire is withdrawn and the catheter contents are aspirated with a syringe and then flushed with heparinized saline. The guidewire is again introduced into the catheter, and both the catheter and the guidewire are advanced across the aortic arch proximal to the origins of the great vessels. The shaft of the catheter should approximate the outer wall of the aorta to prevent catheter movement during the arteriogram.

The positions of the great vessels are best demonstrated in the left anterior oblique (LAO) and right anterior oblique (RAO) projections. The optimal filming rate is two frames per second in each plane. Contrast is injected at a rate of approximately 20 ml per second for a total volume of 25 ml. The patient is positioned so that the aortic arch (origins of the great vessels) is at the lower edge of the field.

Immediately after the angiogram, the catheter should be withdrawn from the ascending aorta into the descending aorta. While the arch images are being reviewed, frequent, brisk flushes of the catheter should be performed to maintain patency of the side holes and to prevent clot formation. If difficulty was encountered in traversing the abdominal aorta or iliac systems, the catheter should be withdrawn over a guidewire.

Innominate or Subclavian Arteries

For imaging the innominate and subclavian arteries, the selective catheter is introduced with a guidewire and flushed proximal to the aortic arch. This selective catheter is then positioned in the innominate or subclavian artery proximal to the disease process or the branching vessel. A test injection of contrast material is performed to confirm the position of the catheter and to test its stability. An injection of 5 ml per second for a total of 10 ml is adequate for DSA images. Frontal and oblique images should be filmed at a rate of two frames per second. The field of view should place the innominate or subclavian artery at the bottom of the image.

Vertebral Arteries

To observe the vertebral artery, the tip of the catheter is placed in the subclavian artery proximal to the origin of the vertebral artery so that a test injection of contrast material can be performed. If the artery appears normal, the catheter is advanced over a guidewire to the desired location in the vertebral artery. Once the catheter is positioned, another test injection of contrast should be performed to determine the artery's flow characteristics. If the catheter is difficult to flush or stasis of the contrast media occurs in the vertebral artery, or if the tip of the catheter indents the vertebral arterial wall, the catheter should be repositioned or withdrawn. If the vertebral artery is the dominant supply to the basilar artery, 10 ml of contrast may be injected at a rate up to 7 ml per second. This injection rate usually results in reflux of contrast into the opposite vertebral artery and filling of its posterior inferior cerebellar artery (PICA) branch. If adequate filling of the contralateral PICA is not obtained, catheterization of the opposite vertebral artery may be necessary. Images should be obtained in both the Towne and lateral projections. If the basilar artery is to be studied, a direct anteroposterior (AP) or even a Water projection may be desirable. Oblique images at 45 degrees are useful to evaluate the origins of the PICA, the anterior inferior cerebellar arteries (AICA), and the superior cerebellar arteries (SCA).

Carotid Arteries

For the carotid arteries, the tip of the catheter should be placed in the common carotid artery proximal to the bifurcation. Contrast material is injected to assess the position of the catheter and flow. The catheter tip should parallel the course of the vessel and not be directed at the wall. A total volume of 7 ml of contrast should be injected at a rate of 5 ml per second. Images should be obtained in the frontal and lateral planes at two frames per second. An oblique series may be obtained if vessels overlap or a lesion is not imaged in profile. Next, the intracranial circulation is evaluated in the frontal and lateral projection at two frames per second. The frontal view is obtained by superimposing the orbital roof with the petrous bones. The contrast injection rate is increased to 7 ml per second for a total volume of 10 ml.

If the carotid bifurcation is free of significant atherosclerotic disease, selective external and internal carotid injections can be performed without increased risk. With the catheter tip in the common carotid artery, a small amount of contrast media is injected for road-mapping. If catheterization of the external carotid artery is desired, the tip of the guidewire or catheter should be advanced into the road-mapped image of the proximal external carotid artery. This catheter manipulation should be performed gently to prevent spasm of the external carotid artery. Contrast can be injected at a rate of 2 ml per second for a total volume of 4 ml while filming in the AP and lateral planes at a rate of two frames per second. Too vigorous an injection of contrast material will cause unwanted movement of the catheter tip or reflux of contrast into the internal carotid artery.

The catheter can be safely maneuvered into the internal carotid artery if it appears normal after the images of the common carotid bifurcation are reviewed. If a small plaque is imaged at the origin of the internal carotid artery, a soft guidewire and catheter can be advanced safely beyond the plaque by using road-mapping. The position of the catheter tip in relation to the arterial wall is ascertained with a test injection of contrast. Usually 5 ml of contrast per second for a total volume of 8 ml are injected with biplane DSA filming of the head at two frames per second performed in a similar fashion as in the common carotid intracranial injection.

Techniques for Specific Clinical Indications

Atherosclerotic Disease

Patients who have had a stroke, transient ischemic attack (TIA), carotid bruit, or severe sonographic stenosis frequently undergo arch aortography and common carotid bifurcation evaluation of the neck as well as the head. The vertebral arteries are selectively examined if severe stenosis or occlusion is encountered in other cranial vascular distributions. A patient with an apparently occluded internal carotid artery should also receive a prolonged injection of contrast (2 ml per second for a total volume of 15 ml). Biplane filming is prolonged at one frame per second for a total of 15 seconds. This injection technique attempts to demonstrate the "string sign" of a very severe stenosis and also to evaluate collateral flow. The carotid siphon is placed at the top of the field and the common carotid bifurcation at the bottom of the field.

Subarachnoid Hemorrhage

With subarachnoid hemorrhage, the intracranial carotid circulation should be initially examined by common carotid injections because this technique will permit diagnosis of aneurysms as well as dural malformations. If the patient does not have significant atherosclerotic disease, additional oblique images may be obtained with the catheter advanced into the internal carotid artery to examine the anterior communicating artery for aneurysms. Compression of the opposite common carotid artery in the neck is occasionally necessary if the anterior communicating artery does not fill spontaneously. A base view is performed when the standard projections cannot optimally demonstrate the anterior communicating artery. The middle cerebral bifurcation is evaluated with a direct AP view through the orbit. A base view may also be useful in visualizing aneurysms in this region. The lateral projection is best for evaluating posterior communicating artery aneurysms. Angled lateral views help to separate the anterior choroidal artery from the posterior communicating artery. The vertebral arteries are examined with the frontal and lateral projections as well as with 45-degree oblique projections. Direct AP views may be helpful in separating aneurysms of the distal basilar artery from the posterior cerebral and the superior cerebellar arteries. Occasionally, it may be necessary to compress the carotid artery in the neck while injecting a vertebral artery to fill a posterior communicating artery on the side of carotid compression.

An angiogram searching for a source of subarachnoid hemorrhage is adequate when all of the intracranial vessels, including the communicating arteries, have been thoroughly examined.[22] Patient motion and vasospasm can compromise diagnostic accuracy and may necessitate a later study. The older literature indicates that an aneurysm will be found in approximately 10 to 23 percent of patients who have had an initially negative angiogram.[23] More recent but smaller studies suggest that if the initial angiogram is of good quality and vasospasm is not present, then less than 2 percent of patients will have an aneurysm on repeat cerebral angiography.[24,25] Although this detection rate is approaching that of the complication rate of angiography, the authors currently repeat angiography in 7 to 10 days if a bleeding source is not identified.

Parenchymal Hemorrhage

For parenchymal hemorrhage, the aortic arch and the vessels that supply the hemorrhagic region should be examined. For example, if the hemorrhage is in the anterior frontal region, both carotid arteries should be examined. If the hemorrhage is lateral in the frontoparietal region, only the respective carotid artery needs to be examined. Evaluation of a temporal lobe hemorrhage requires opacification of both the middle cerebral and posterior cerebral arteries. This may be accomplished by examination of the respective carotid artery alone, but injection of the vertebral artery to fill the posterior cerebral artery may also be necessary. If the hemorrhage is in the posterior fossa, examination of the vertebrobasilar system is required.

If an arteriovenous malformation (AVM) is encountered, supplemental oblique images and rapid-sequence filming of the supplying vessels are frequently necessary. These rapid-sequence angiograms are performed at a rate of eight frames per second in each plane. A study for aneurysms should also be part of the evaluation because aneurysms occur in about 10 percent of patients with an AVM. If an avascular mass or tumor vascularity is present in the region of the hemorrhage, additional angiography is not necessary.

Arteritis

An examination for arteritis is similar to that for atherosclerotic disease. In addition, magnification oblique frontal and lateral projections are helpful. Magnification Towne and direct AP views of the posterior fossa are useful in evaluating the posterior cerebral and vertebrobasilar arteries.

Trauma

Arteriography performed for trauma is similar to that performed for atherosclerotic disease. If the site of the penetrating injury is in the neck, it should be evaluated with arch aortography and ipsilateral common carotid and vertebral arteriography of the neck and head. If both sides of the neck have been injured, both sides need to be selectively injected. The head is examined to assess collateral flow if the vessel requires repair.

Tumors

The vessels supplying the tumor are selectively injected after arch aortography. In suspected meningiomas and tumors with external carotid arterial supply, the internal and external carotid arteries are evaluated after a common carotid bifurcation arteriogram. Meningiomas are frequently supplied by arteries from the contralateral side.

Summary

Before the conclusion of the procedure, the angiograms should be reviewed to ensure that an adequate examination has been performed. The questions that were to be answered by the angiogram and any questions arising during the angiogram should also have been answered. Appropriate postprocessing (filming) of the examination is the responsibility of the radiologist.

Sheath Removal and Hemostasis

The patient is transferred to a stretcher, two fingers are placed proximal to the puncture site with the index finger placed lightly over the catheter insertion site, and then the catheter is gently withdrawn and moderate pressure is applied to the puncture site. Compression should be adequate to prevent oozing or hematoma formation but not so strong that the distal pulses become nonpalpable. Compression must be continuous for at least 10 minutes to avoid a hematoma. If oozing occurs after compression has been released, an additional 10 minutes of compression should be undertaken. Patients who have been recently anticoagulated or who are taking aspirin require longer periods of compression.

If a peripheral pulse disappears after compression has been released, the possibility of an embolic complication must be considered. Doppler examination is helpful in evaluating the absent pulse. Surgical consultation should be obtained anytime questions arise regarding the adequacy of perfusion. In children and young adults, vasospasm may play a larger role than emboli. Warming a cold, pulseless extremity may relieve vasospasm.

Postprocedural Care

The patient is kept in bed with the punctured extremity extended. The puncture site, peripheral pulses, and vital signs are monitored frequently, for example, every 15 minutes times 4, every 30 minutes times 4, and finally every 60 minutes times 3. At the same time, the puncture site is observed for signs of bleeding and the extremity for signs of ischemia. If the patient can tolerate the encouraged oral fluids, the intravenous infusion of fluids is discontinued and a diet resumed. Heparin therapy can be reinstituted 6 hours after the procedure. If pain medications are necessary, consultation with the patient's physician is recommended to determine whether there is a contraindication to a medication that may cause CNS depression.

A note should be placed in the chart to report the type of examination that was performed, the medications that were used, the condition of the puncture site, the catheters and contrast media that were used, the patient's clinical condition at the end of the procedure, and the preliminary radiologic findings. On review of the angiogram, a final report should be written. Although this report should be similar to the preliminary chart note, it should also include a brief history or indication for the procedure, the procedural details, nonionic contrast indications, any problems or complications, the patient's condition upon release, and the radiologic findings. Finally, conclusions based on the correlation of the angiographic findings with the other examinations should be given.

Other Methods of Imaging the Neck and Head

Noninvasive Methods

Carotid duplex ultrasonography is a noninvasive method of evaluating the carotid bifurcations. Its accuracy in separating the normal carotid artery from those with significant stenosis is excellent.[26] Characterization of the plaque in the abnormal carotid artery as well as the ability to noninvasively monitor changes in the plaque are important advantages. Disadvantages of ultrasonography include difficulty in evaluating the high-bifurcation and tortuous vessels. A highly calcified plaque and a very high grade stenosis cause further difficulty. In addition, the carotid siphons and intracranial vasculature cannot be evaluated.

Magnetic resonance angiography (MRA) is another method of noninvasively evaluating the vasculature. MRA has an important advantage over ultrasound by being able to evaluate the carotid siphons as well as the major intracranial branches. In addition, it is not solely dependent on velocity measurements to produce an image. However, its ability to characterize plaque and depict ulceration is not yet known. Although its reliability in detecting flow alterations in the extracranial circulation is relatively high, its reliability in the carotid siphons and the major intracranial vessels has not yet been evaluated.[27] No prospective study evaluating intracranial aneurysms in patients with subarachnoid hemorrhage has been undertaken.

Another competing technology in the evaluation of the neck vessels is spiral or helical computed tomography (CT), which requires the intravenous injection of contrast material. Nonionic contrast material is favored because of fewer swallowing artifacts. In preliminary evaluations, the sensitivity and specificity of spiral carotid bifurcation evaluation are similar to that of ultrasound and MRA.[28-30] Heavily calcified plaques and noncooperative patients decrease the accuracy of this technique. In addition, vessels in the skull base and the cavernous sinus region are difficult to evaluate because of artifacts arising from bone and contrast within the cavernous sinus.

Intraoperative Angiography

In the past it has been difficult to monitor vascular therapy during surgery. Fluoroscopy offers only a fleeting glimpse of the operated vessels, and film changers are too bulky and cumbersome to use in the operating room. The combination of portable digital subtraction and fluoroscopy has made intraoperative angiography a practical procedure.

Indications for intraoperative angiography include AVM surgery, aneurysm clipping, carotid endarterectomy, vascular damage during surgery, and emergency surgery for intracranial hemorrhage. In AVM surgery, it is important to examine clipped vessels and complete the nidus resection. In aneurysm surgery, it is important to obliterate the aneurysm while preserving parent vessel patency and to also evaluate vasospasm. Postendarterectomy patency of the carotid artery and any intimal injury are easily assessed intraoperatively. Vessel damage during tumor resection, particularly meningiomas of the skull base, may occur during temporary clipping or as a result of the tumor resection. Occasionally a patient whose intracranial hemorrhage results in marked mass effect and herniation requires emergency surgery. Either as the patient is being prepared for surgery or after the hematoma has been evacuated, intraoperative angiography can be used to identify an aneurysm or AVM.

The authors use a C-arm fluoroscopic unit coupled to a DSA unit. The ability to remask and replay several angiographic sequences makes this arrangement convenient. Direct magnification after localization of the area of interest is also possible. Hard copy films are produced, reviewed, and stored after the procedure is concluded.

In elective operations, access is usually established by inserting a femoral sheath after the patient has been anesthetized. The standard 5 French sheath is connected to an electronic pump for continuous infusion with heparinized saline, which is monitored by anesthesia. The patient is positioned on a nonradiopaque table in a nonradiopaque head frame by the neurosurgeon. For most patients, the head position chosen for the surgery will result in a supine or slightly oblique torso position. A lateral decubitus position makes catheterization of vessels from the arch difficult because of overlapping structures. Even prone positioning allows angiography if bolsters are positioned so that access is possible. In this instance, the sheath is placed in the left femoral artery with the patient supine. Then, with the radiologist monitoring the sheath, the patient is turned prone and appropriate bolsters placed.

The radiology team leaves the operating room after placing the sheath and is recalled later when the angiogram is needed. The neurosurgeon removes the retractors and the operating microscope and covers the field with sterile drapes. The C arm is draped with a sterile plastic cover and appropriately positioned for the angiogram. Right–left orientation is determined fluoroscopically and a selective catheter is inserted into the appropriate vessel. After a test injection to ensure proper catheter position, DSA is performed while the anesthesiologist suspends respirations. Most angiographic runs last about 10 seconds. After the angiograms have been performed and reviewed, the catheter is withdrawn. However, the sheath is removed later after the patient has been taken to the recovery room or the intensive care unit. For carotid endarterectomy, direct needle puncture has been used instead of the femoral sheath approach.

In one series of 112 patients, intraoperative angiography changed surgical management in 9 percent of aneurysms, in 16 percent of AVMs, and in 11 percent of carotid endarterectomies.[31] Only one neurologic complication could be attributed to the intraoperative angiogram. Angiography could not be performed in two patients with very tortuous aorta-iliac systems. One patient developed three temporarily ischemic toes despite normal peripheral pulses 1 week after sheath removal. The sheath in this patient had been used as an arterial line for 5 days before it was removed. The authors now remove sheaths within 48 hours.

In a series of 50 consecutive intraoperative angiograms, the mean calculated cumulative skin dose to the patient from fluoroscopy was 6.24 R, and to the angiographer it was 66.1 mR. The intraoperative angiograms resulted in a total average dose of 2.7 R to the patient and 1 mR to the angiographer. The radiation exposure to the radiologic technologist and the anesthesiologist were similar to that of the angiographer and were well within National Commission on Radiation Protection (NCRP) guidelines for medical radiation. These doses are similar to those received during routine angiography.[32]

Venography

In the past, orbital venography and jugular venography were performed to evaluate structures within the orbit and cavernous sinus. Because of the development of CT and MRI, these screening examinations are no longer performed. However, one diagnostic indication for venography remains: inferior petrosal venous sampling for adrenocorticotropic hormone (ACTH) levels.

There are two approaches to the cavernous sinus. One is through the femoral vein and the other is through the neck, which is less commonly used. Standard preparation and draping of the groin are performed. The skin medial to the palpated femoral artery is anesthetized with 1 percent lidocaine and a dermatotomy performed. The femoral vein is reliably medial to the femoral artery, so venous access is not difficult (see Fig. 12-6). The common femoral vein is usually punctured with the patient performing a Valsalva maneuver while the other hand is palpating and protecting the femoral artery. After obtaining venous blood, a guidewire is advanced through the needle, which is then withdrawn. A standard 5 French sheath assembly is placed in the femoral vein. Since simultaneous bilateral sampling is necessary, the procedure is repeated in the opposite groin. If the femoral artery is punctured, the needle is withdrawn and pressure applied for approximately 10 minutes. Heparinized saline is slowly infused through the sheaths. A 5 French H1-type catheter is inserted and maneuvered through the inferior vena cava into the superior vena cava and one of the jugular veins. The catheter is placed in the jugular bulb, where injections of contrast material are performed to identify the inferior petrosal vein, which courses anteriorly and superiorly in the lateral projection and medially and superiorly in the frontal projection. Road-mapping techniques are very useful in positioning the catheter tip in the distal inferior petrosal sinus. Catheter position is confirmed with a gentle injection of contrast material, which should outline the respective inferior petrosal sinus and the cavernous sinus. Soft guidewires are used because the veins are fragile and easily perforated. If contrast extravasation is observed, the procedure is terminated and repeated in several days. After the first catheter is placed, the procedure is repeated on the opposite side. Simultaneous sampling is performed after bilateral catheter placement. Depending on the levels of the samples, the location of the side of increased ACTH secretion can be ascertained.

Normal Vascular Anatomy of the Head

The blood supply to the face and cerebrum (supratentorial region) originates from three large arteries located on the superior convexity of the aortic arch. In about two-thirds of individuals the innominate artery is the first vessel to originate from the aortic arch, the left carotid artery the second, and the subclavian artery the third. In this arrangement the right carotid and right vertebral arteries are supplied by the innominate artery, and the left vertebral artery is supplied by the left subclavian artery.[33,34]

In the remaining one-third of individuals, one of three variations may be displayed.[33–35] In the most usual variation, the left common carotid artery either forms a common origin with the innominate artery or originates from the proximal portion of the innominate artery itself. Less frequently, the left vertebral artery originates directly from the aortic arch between the left carotid and left subclavian arteries. The least frequent variation is the aberrant origin of the right subclavian artery from the aortic arch distal to the left subclavian artery. Selective catheterization of the carotid and vertebral arteries may be difficult if these variations are not recognized.

The posterior fossa (infratentorial region) is supplied by the vertebral arteries and its major extension, the basilar artery. Selective catheterization of the left vertebral artery is easier than the right because it is located along a more vertical axis and there is also one less arterial branch to traverse before reaching the vertebral orifice.

Common Carotid Artery

The carotid artery is enclosed within the carotid sheath with the vagus nerve and jugular vein. The left common carotid artery is usually longer than the right because it originates directly from the aortic arch. The common carotid arteries usually bifurcate opposite the superior border of the thyroid cartilage (C3-4 or C4-5). The bifurcation tends to be higher in short-necked individuals and lower in long-necked individuals and in children.[36]

External Carotid Artery

The external carotid artery usually arises medial and anterior to the internal carotid artery. However, in approximately 15 percent of individuals the external carotid artery originates lateral to the internal carotid artery (Fig. 12-9).[37] This external carotid artery variation tends to occur more frequently on the right (3:1).[37]

The branches of the external carotid artery are important because interventional radiologic procedures are frequently performed in this circulation.[38,39] The branches can be divided into those that are directed anteriorly and those that are directed posteriorly.[40] Anteriorly directed branches include the superior thyroid, lingual, facial, and internal maxillary arteries. Posteriorly directed arteries include the ascending pharyngeal, posterior auricular, and occipital arteries.

Anterior Branches. The superior thyroid artery is the first anterior branch to originate from the external carotid artery. The lingual and facial arteries are the second and third anterior branches. On lateral angiograms, the initial course of the lingual and facial arteries may be difficult to distinguish in the submental and oral regions because of their similar course and tortuosity (Fig. 12-10). The initial segments of both the lingual and facial arteries first form a tight concave curve inferiorly and then a second, wider convex curve inferiorly. During this part of their course the lingual artery supplies the tongue, sublingual gland, and muscles in the floor of the mouth; the facial artery supplies part of the pharynx, tongue, submandibular gland, and muscles in the floor of the mouth. More distally, the facial artery can be separated from the lingual artery because its terminal branch (angular artery) runs anterior and superior to the oral cavity to supply the lips, nose, and medial angle of the eye. On anteroposterior angiograms the course of these vessels in the submental region and floor of the mouth may again be difficult to differentiate until the facial artery courses superficially to the mandible and angles medially toward the corner of the eye.

Although the internal maxillary artery is one of two

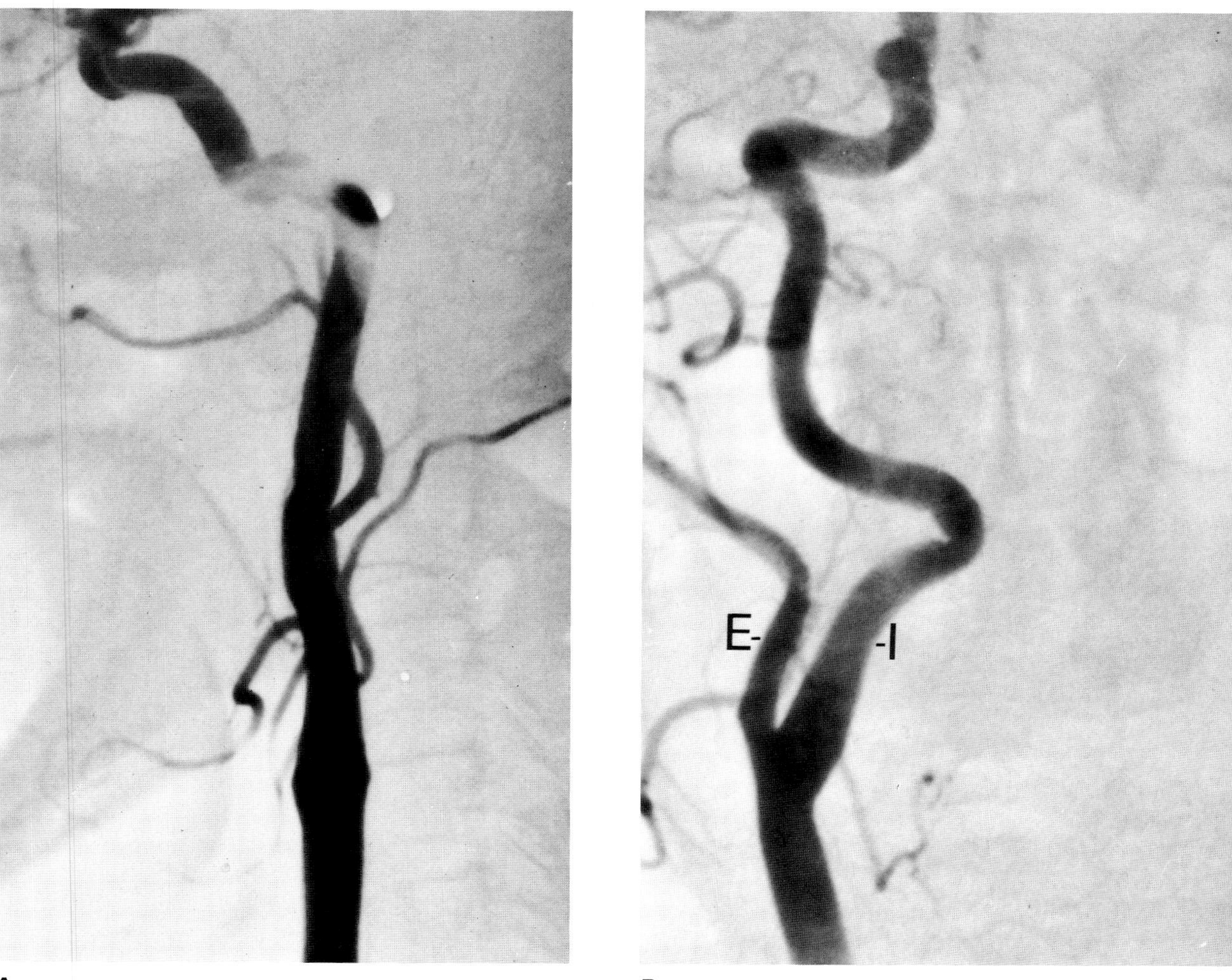

Figure 12-9. Lateral origin of the external carotid artery. (A) The internal and external carotid arteries overlap on the lateral arteriogram. (B) The external carotid (*E*) artery originates lateral to the internal carotid (*I*) artery. (A) Lateral projection; (B) anteroposterior (AP) projection.

terminal branches, it will be discussed along with the other anterior branches because its course is largely anterior. It can be divided into three segments: mandibular, pterygoid, and pterygopalatine.[41]

The mandibular segment, which is horizontal, is located behind the neck of the mandible. It gives off branches to the external auditory canal, tympanic cavity, mandible, and meninges. The meningeal branch (middle meningeal artery) enters the middle fossa through the foramen spinosum, courses laterally to the vault, and then divides into an anterior branch, which courses superiorly behind the coronal suture, and a posterior branch, which courses posteriorly along the superior border of the squamosa of the temporal bone (see Fig. 12-10). In traumatic epidural hematomas it is the posterior division that is usually injured. The accessory meningeal artery enters the middle cranial fossa through the foramen ovale and supplies the dura in the floor of the middle cranial fossa.[42]

The pterygopalatine segment enters the pterygopalatine fossa and terminates by dividing into several branches that can be categorized by the direction in which they exit from this fossa. Anterior exiting branches, from inferior to superior, are the posterior superior alveolar, greater palatine, and infraorbital arteries (see Fig. 12-10). The posterior superior alveolar

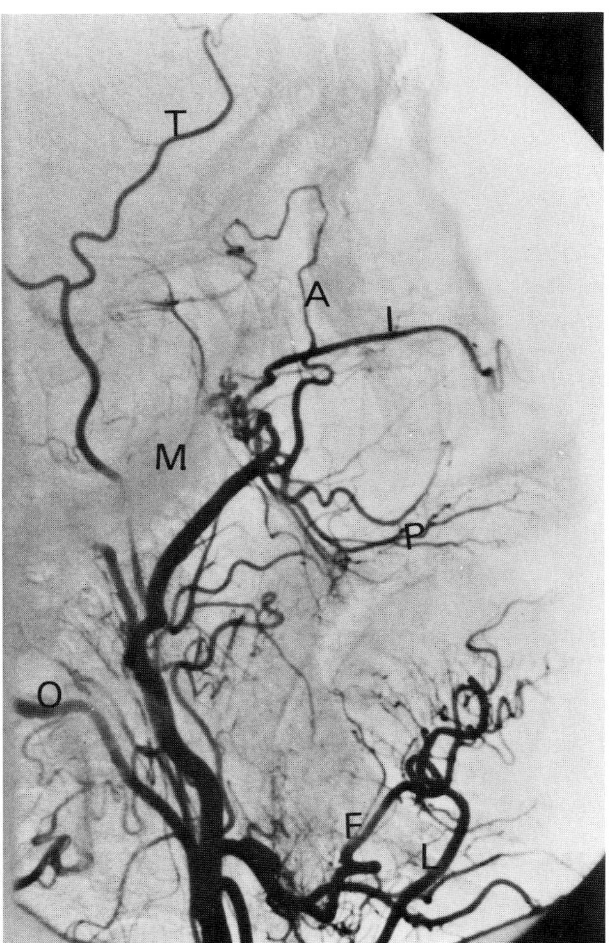

Figure 12-10. Branches of the external carotid artery. The lingual (*L*) and facial (*F*) arteries overlap in the oral region. The middle meningeal (*M*) artery originates from the first segment of the internal maxillary artery. The anterior deep temporal (*A*) artery originates from the second segment and is especially prominent in this patient since it is acting as a collateral channel because of the occlusion of the internal carotid artery. The infraorbital (*I*) and greater palatine (*P*) arteries originate from the third segment of the internal maxillary artery. Also shown are the superficial temporal (*T*) and the occipital (*O*) arteries. Lateral projection.

artery outlines the inferior lateral wall of the maxillary antrum and supplies the teeth and mucosa in the maxillary antrum. The greater palatine artery runs inferiorly along the posterior wall of the maxillary antrum before coursing anteriorly along the inferior surface of the hard palate. It supplies the hard palate, the soft palate, and adjacent bone and gingiva. The infraorbital artery courses anteriorly in the infraorbital canal and, upon exiting from the canal, supplies the cheek, lower eyelid, and upper lip. Posterior exiting branches, from inferior to superior, are the pharyngeal artery, vidian artery, and artery of the foramen rotundum. The pharyngeal artery passes through the pharyngeal canal before supplying the upper part of the nasopharynx and auditory canal. The vidian artery passes posteriorly through the vidian (pterygoid) canal before supplying the lateral pharyngeal recesses, the auditory tube, and the tympanic cavity. The artery of the foramen rotundum also passes posteriorly before anastomosing with the cavernous branches of the internal carotid artery. The medial exiting branch is the sphenopalatine artery; it is considered the terminal branch of the internal maxillary artery. This artery passes into the nasal cavity through the sphenopalatine foramen to supply the mucosa in the nasal cavity and ethmoid sinuses.

Posterior Branches. Of the three posterior branches of the external carotid artery, the occipital artery is the largest (see Fig. 12-10). It courses posteriorly to supply the muscles and skin in the suboccipital and occipital regions. Its muscular branches anastomose with similar muscular branches from the subclavian, vertebral, and other branches of the external carotid arteries. Its scalp branches anastomose with the posterior auricular and superficial temporal arteries. Its meningeal branches anastomose with the vertebral and other external carotid artery branches that supply the posterior fossa.

The ascending pharyngeal artery, another posterior branch, passes almost directly upward, giving off anterior branches to the pharynx and the prevertebral muscles. It terminates by supplying the meninges around the foramen magnum and jugular foramen. At times these meningeal branches may extend more laterally to supply the cerebellopontine angles, anteriorly to supply the clivus, and posteriorly to supply the occipital region. The meningeal branches, which supply the clivus and occipital region, are an important supply to tumors of the base of the skull. The posterior auricular artery, the last posterior branch, originates in the parotid gland and then courses upward and posteriorly. It supplies the parotid gland, the pinna, and the scalp posterior to the ear. A branch from the posterior auricular artery may enter the stylomastoid foramen to help supply the tympanic cavity and mastoid air cells.

Terminal Branches. The superficial temporal artery, a terminal branch of the external cerebral artery, arises within the parotid gland and continues upward as the natural extension of the external carotid artery (see Fig. 12-10).[43] It sends anterior branches to both the lateral, superior portion of the face (transverse facial artery) and the anterior portion of the pinna and external auditory canal (anterior auricular artery). Terminally, it supplies the skin over the anterior two-thirds of the scalp (anterior frontal and parietal branches). The internal maxillary artery, the other terminal branch, is discussed with the anterior branches.

Internal Carotid Artery

The internal carotid artery can be divided into five segments: cervical, petrous, precavernous, intracavernous, and supraclinoid. The cervical segment originates at the bifurcation of the common carotid artery and extends to the base of the skull. It usually lies lateral and posterior to the external carotid artery. The cervical segment is usually straight but may be curved (23 percent) or looped (9 percent), especially in older individuals.[44]

The petrous segment extends from the base of the skull to the apex of the petrous bone. The petrous segment consists of a vertical portion of about 1 cm and a horizontal portion of 3 to 4 cm. The horizontal portion passes forward and medially through the carotid canal, about 45 degrees to the midsagittal plane.[45] The petrous segment gives off a posterior branch to the tympanic cavity (caroticotympanic artery) and an anterior branch to the vidian canal. The artery to the vidian canal anastomoses with the internal maxillary artery. These two branches are not visible unless they become hypertrophied secondarily to vascular tumors or occlusion of the external carotid artery.

The precavernous segment begins at the apex of the petrous bone just above the foramen lacerum, where it exits from the carotid canal. The precavernous segment is short and runs upward until it ends just lateral to the lower border of the dorsum sellae. The meningohypophyseal trunk may originate from this segment.

The intracavernous segment begins at the lower border of the dorsum sellae, passes forward in the carotid sulcus along the lower border of the sella, and ends anteriorly by curving upward, medial to the anterior clinoid process. While passing forward along the carotid groove it gives off two major groups of vessels: (1) the meningohypophyseal trunk, which supplies the posterior pituitary lobe, the dura over the dorsum and clivus, and the dura along the margins of the tentorium; and (2) the inferior cavernous sinus artery, which supplies the structures within the inferior cavernous sinus, the adjacent dura, and the dura in the middle cranial fossa.[46,47] The dural branches of the meningohypophyseal trunk and the inferior cavernous sinus artery are not usually visible unless there is a lesion involving the dura.[48]

On lateral angiograms the cavernous segment is reversed S-shaped, the posterior knuckle is located adjacent to the dorsum sellae, and the anterior knuckle is below the anterior clinoids. On anteroposterior carotid angiograms, the posterior knuckle is projected medially and superiorly to the anterior knuckle.

The supraclinoid segment of the internal carotid artery begins after it passes through the dura and continues until it terminates by bifurcating into the anterior and middle cerebral arteries. The supraclinoid segment is the origin of three arteries: the ophthalmic, the posterior communicating, and the anterior choroidal arteries.

Supraclinoid Segment of the Internal Carotid Artery

Ophthalmic Artery. The first artery to originate from the supraclinoid segment of the internal carotid artery is the ophthalmic artery. It courses anteriorly through the optic foramen to supply the globe, extraocular muscles, lacrimal gland, ethmoid and nasal mucosa, and part of the dura above it in the anterior fossa (Fig. 12-11A). The ophthalmic artery's intraorbital course can be divided into three segments. The first segment begins at the optic canal and ends when the artery begins to loop laterally; the second segment loops around the optic nerve; and the third segment courses anteromedially along the medial wall of the orbit.[49,50]

The globe is supplied by the central retinal and ciliary arteries. The central retinal artery branches can be visualized directly by using an ophthalmoscope but cannot be imaged angiographically. The posterior ciliary arteries usually originate from the second segment, enter the sclera, and supply the choroid and ciliary processes. On lateral angiograms the choroid is visible as a thin crescentic concavity during the capillary and venous phases (see Fig. 12-11B). The crescent is usually projected 2 to 4 mm posterior to the anterior margin of the frontozygomatic bone.[51]

The extraocular, intraorbital structures are supplied by the muscular and lacrimal branches of the ophthalmic artery. The lacrimal artery originates from the second segment of the ophthalmic artery, courses along the lateral wall of the orbit to supply the lacrimal gland, and then terminates farther forward in the lateral palpebral area by anastomosing with the superficial temporal artery (Fig. 12-12). Soon after its origin, the lacrimal artery gives rise to a recurrent meningeal artery that passes backward through the superior orbital fissure to anastomose with the middle meningeal artery in the floor of the middle fossa. The muscular arteries divide into a superolateral group and an inferomedial group.

The extraorbital structures that receive their blood supply from the ophthalmic artery do so via its posterior ethmoid, anterior ethmoid, supraorbital, lacrimal,

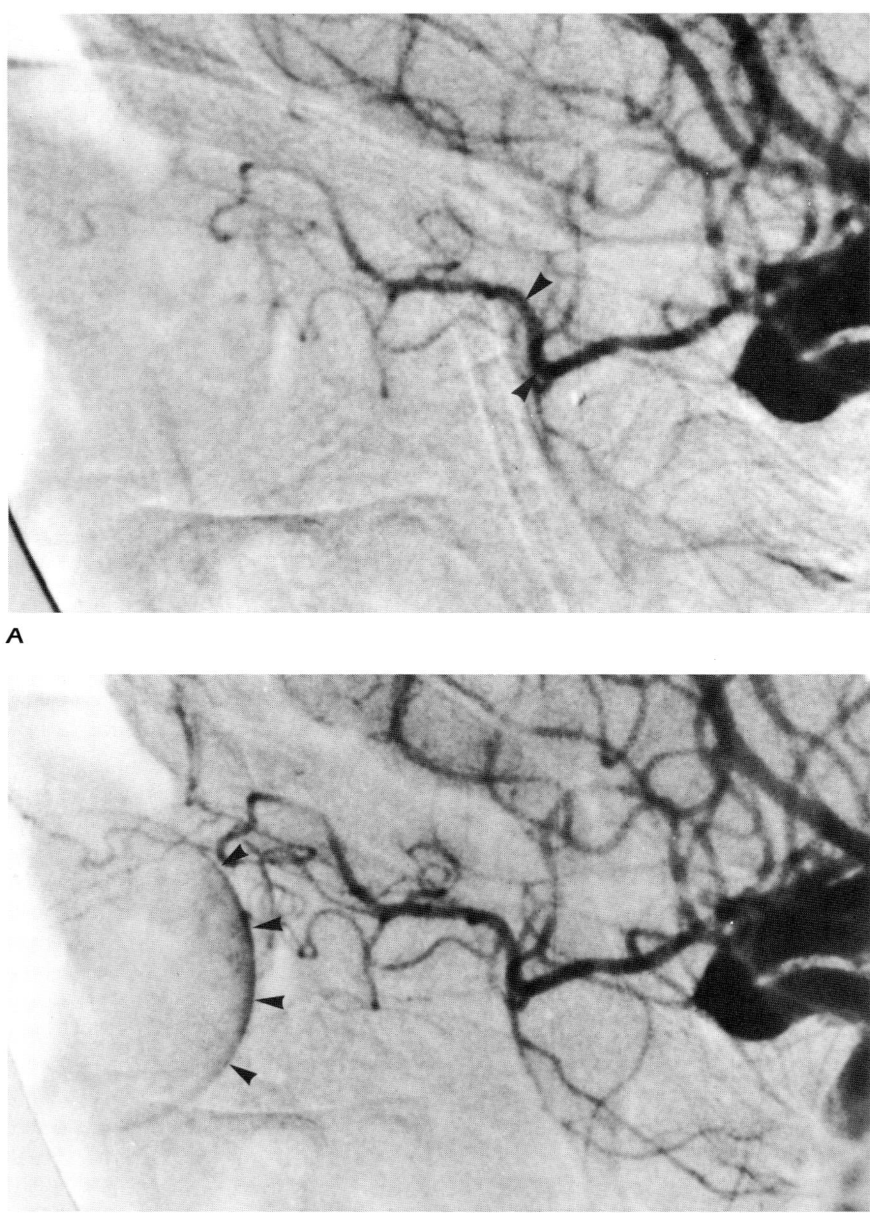

Figure 12-11. Ophthalmic artery. (A) On this lateral arteriogram the ophthalmic artery initially courses anteriorly below the optic nerve. The artery then loops over the optic nerve (*between the arrowheads*) before coursing further anteriorly along the medial surface of the orbit. (B) The choroid blush (*arrowheads*) appears slightly later in the arterial phase. The blush is projected over the zygomaticofrontal arch. The exact position of the blush may vary somewhat with eye position. (A and B) Lateral projection.

and terminal branches. The ethmoidal arteries, which originate from the second and third segments of the ophthalmic artery, supply the nasal and ethmoid mucosa as well as the overlying dura in the anterior fossa. A branch of the anterior ethmoid artery (anterior falx artery) supplies the anterior portion of the falx (Fig. 12-13).[52] The mucosal and ethmoid branches anastomose with the internal maxillary artery via the sphenopalatine artery, and the meningeal branches anastomose with the middle meningeal artery. The supraorbital artery, which originates from the second segment of the ophthalmic artery, courses along the superomedial wall and exits through the supraorbital foramen, where it anastomoses with the superficial

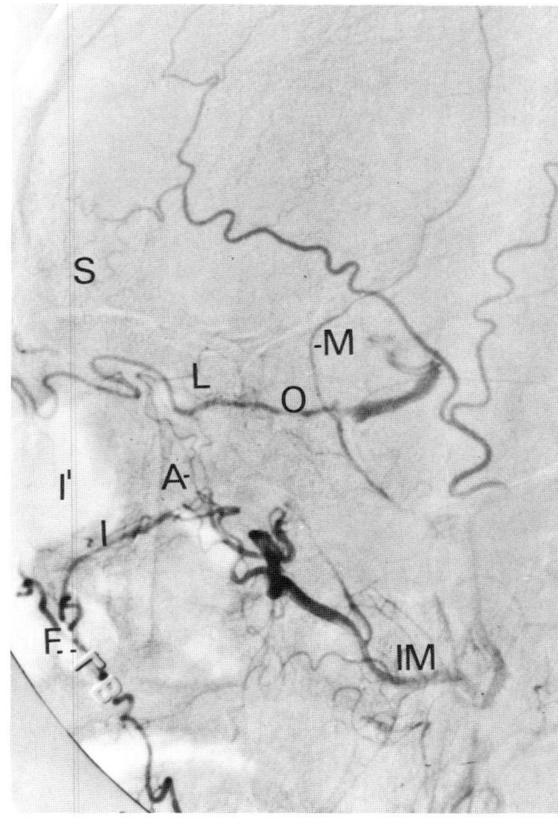

A

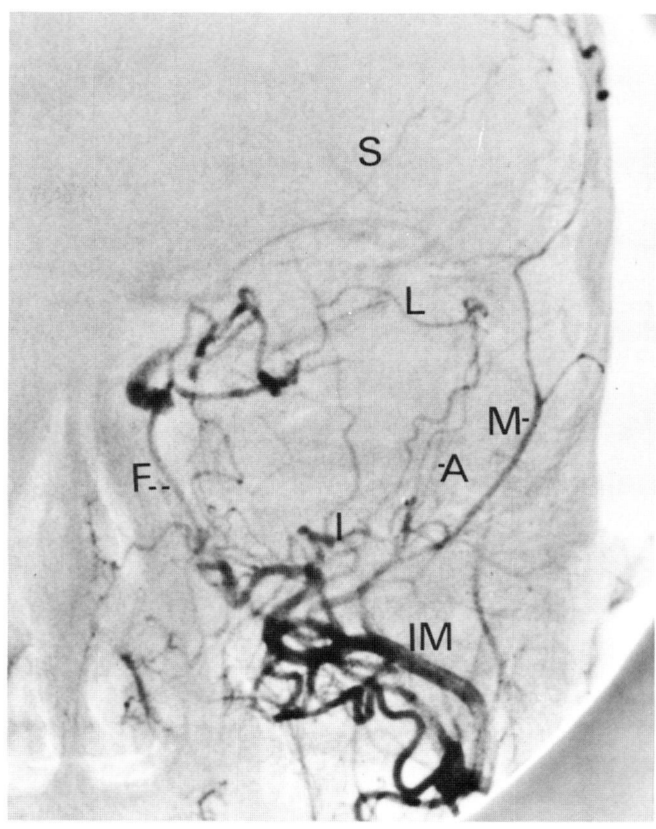

B

Figure 12-12. Retrograde opacification of the internal carotid artery via the ophthalmic artery. (A) The ophthalmic (*O*) artery is opacified by retrograde flow of contrast from the anterior deep temporal (*A*), infraorbital (*I*), branches of the infraorbital (*I′*), facial (*F*), supraorbital (*S*), and superficial temporal arteries. Middle meningeal (*M*), internal maxillary (*IM*), and lacrimal (*L*) arteries are also shown. (B) Collateral arteries that fill the ophthalmic artery retrograde come from an inferomedial (facial artery), inferolateral (anterior deep temporal and infraorbital arteries), and superior (superficial and temporal artery) directions. (A) Lateral projection; (B) AP projection.

Figure 12-13. Anterior falx artery. (A) The ophthalmic artery gives origin to the middle meningeal (*M*), anterior falx (*F*), and supraorbital (*S*) arteries. An anterior temporal (*T, arrowhead*) artery and a false anterior temporal (*FT, arrowhead*) artery originate from the middle cerebral artery. (B) The anterior falx (*F*) artery courses along the left surface of the falx. The middle meningeal (*M*) artery courses laterally toward the calvarial vault. An anterior temporal (*T*) artery is also shown. (A) Lateral projection; (B) AP projection.

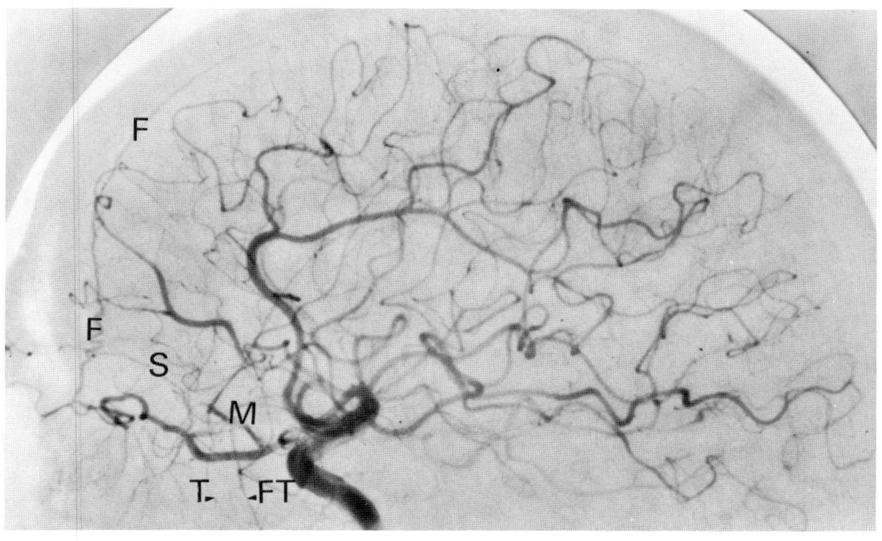

A

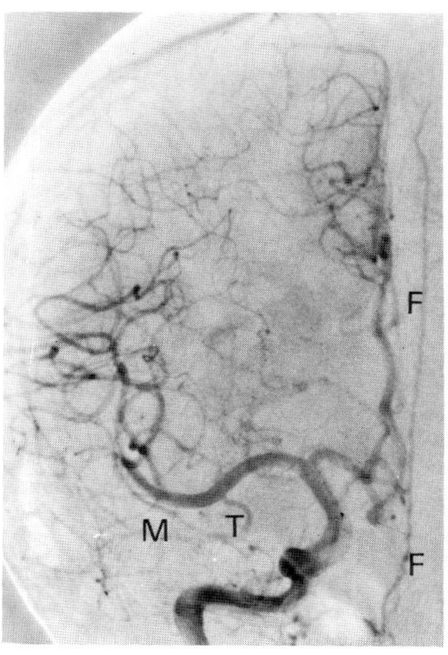

B

temporal artery. The ophthalmic artery terminates by dividing into a superior (supratrochlear) and an inferior (dorsal nasal) branch. The superior branch anastomoses with the superficial temporal artery and the inferior with the facial artery. These anastomoses become important as collateral channels when either the external or internal carotid arteries are occluded (see Fig. 12-12).

The middle meningeal artery occasionally originates from the ophthalmic artery (0.5 percent)[53] (see Fig. 12-13). This and other variations of the ophthalmic artery usually occur during development because of the ophthalmic artery's origin from the stapedial artery.[54,55]

Posterior Communicating Artery. The posterior communicating artery connects the internal carotid and posterior cerebral arteries and is variable in size. It may be as large as the posterior cerebral artery, in which case it is referred to as a *fetal* posterior cerebral artery. When small, it may be difficult to determine whether the posterior communicating artery exists. A slight dilatation may occur at the origin of the posterior communicating artery (Fig. 12-14). If this dilatation is less than 3 mm, it is normal and is referred to as an *infundibulum;* if larger, it is considered an *aneurysm*.[56] Several branches (anterior thalamoperforate arteries) arise from the superior surface of the posterior communicating artery and help supply the hypothalamus, the genu of the internal capsule, and the anterior pole of the thalamus.

Anterior Choroidal Artery. The last branch to originate from the internal carotid artery is the anterior choroidal artery. It, like the posterior communicating artery, can be used to diagnose transtentorial herniations. This artery is divided into a cisternal and a plexal segment.[57] The cisternal segment is located in the crural cistern, beneath the optic tract. It sends superior perforating branches into the posterior two-thirds of the optic tract, the posterior limb of the internal capsule, and the adjacent parts of the basal ganglia; medial branches to the midbrain; lateral branches to the uncus; and posterior branches to the lateral geniculate

Figure 12-14. Infundibulum of the posterior communicating artery. (A) A prominent infundibulum (*arrow*) is located beneath the origin of the anterior choroidal artery (*arrowheads*).

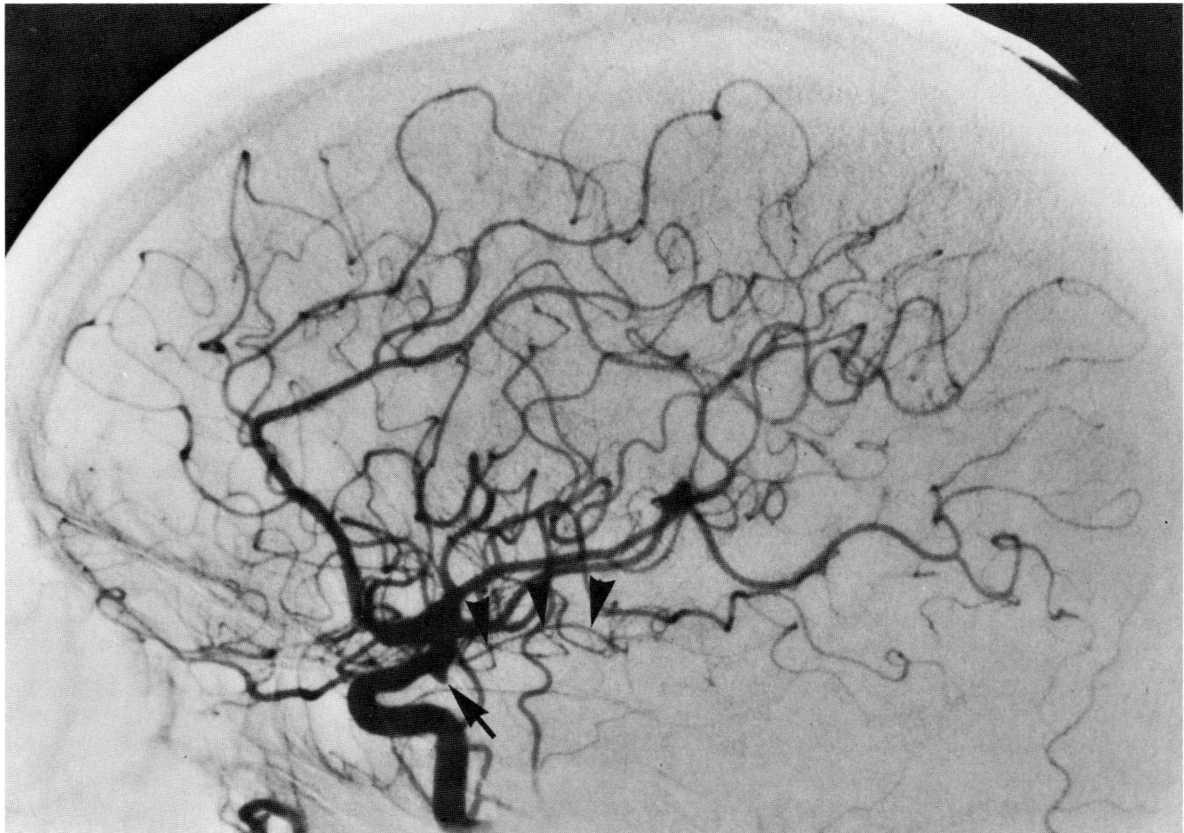

A

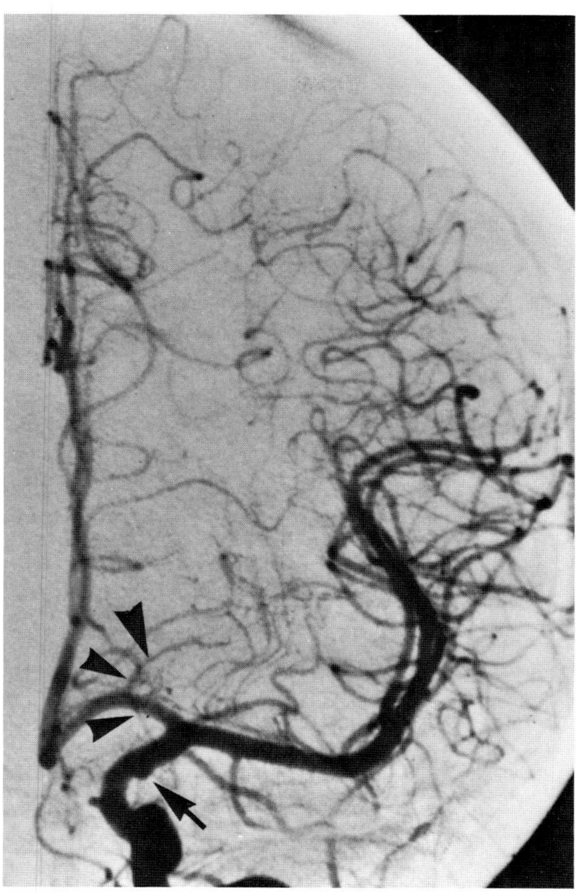

B

Figure 12-14 (continued). (B) The inferolateral surface of the infundibulum is seen on the anteroposterior angiogram (*arrow*). The crural segment of the anterior choroidal artery arcs gently above the infundibulum (*arrowheads*). The lateral lenticulostriate arteries are located lateral to the origin of the anterior choroidal artery. (A) Lateral projection; (B) AP projection.

body. The plexal segment begins as the anterior choroidal artery enters the choroid fissure and ends by supplying the choroid plexus in the anterior portion of the temporal horn.

On anteroposterior cerebral angiograms the right anterior choroidal artery appears S-shaped and the left is reversed S-shaped; the lower half of the S is the cisternal segment (Fig. 12-15). In the lateral projection the cisternal segment forms a superior convexity, and the subsequent plexal segment forms a downward convexity. These two segments roughly follow the course of the sylvian fissure.[45] Inferior displacement of the cisternal segment suggests uncal herniation, whereas a similar displacement of the plexal segment suggests hippocampal herniation. Large masses can displace both of these segments downward (Fig. 12-16; see Fig. 12-31). In the anteroposterior projection, if the cisternal segment extends more medially than the base of the posterior clinoids, it indicates uncal herniation.[45]

Anterior Cerebral Artery and Its Branches

The supraclinoid segment of the internal carotid artery bifurcates into the anterior cerebral artery and the middle cerebral artery. The anterior cerebral artery is divided into two segments: horizontal and pericallosal.

Horizontal (A_1) Segment

The horizontal (A_1) segment of the anterior cerebral artery extends from the bifurcation of the internal carotid artery to the midline.[58] The right and left A_1 segments are usually the same size, but one or both can be hypoplastic or aplastic.[59] Differentiation between hypoplastic and aplastic A_1 segments can be made by compressing the contralateral common carotid artery while injecting contrast into the ipsilateral carotid artery. Determining whether the A_1 segment is patent is important in patients undergoing surgery that may involve ligation of the A_1 segment.

In the frontal projection, the A_1 segment usually courses horizontally or downward (Fig. 12-17A and B).[60] However, in about 13 percent of normal individuals the A_1 segment is inclined upward, erroneously suggesting the presence of a sellar mass (see Fig. 12-17C). About three-quarters of these individuals are below the age of 20.[60]

The medial lenticulostriate arteries, the recurrent artery of Heubner, and the anterior communicating artery are branches of the A_1 segment. The six to nine medial lenticulostriate arteries that arise from the superior surface of the anterior cerebral artery supply the optic nerve and a small part of the globus pallidus. They form a gentle S-shaped configuration on anteroposterior angiograms on the right, whereas the left is reversed S-shaped.

The recurrent artery of Heubner usually originates medial to the medial lenticulostriate arteries but then courses laterally for 2 to 3 cm to enter the anterior perforated substance lateral to the medial lenticulostriate arteries. The recurrent artery of Heubner supplies the anterior medial portion of the head of the caudate nucleus, the adjacent putamen, and the inferior portion of the anterior limb of the internal capsule.[61,62]

The anterior communicating artery connects the A_1 segments in the midline and completes the anterior portion of the circle of Willis. When it is important to determine the patency of the anterior communicating artery, it may be necessary to cross-compress the con-

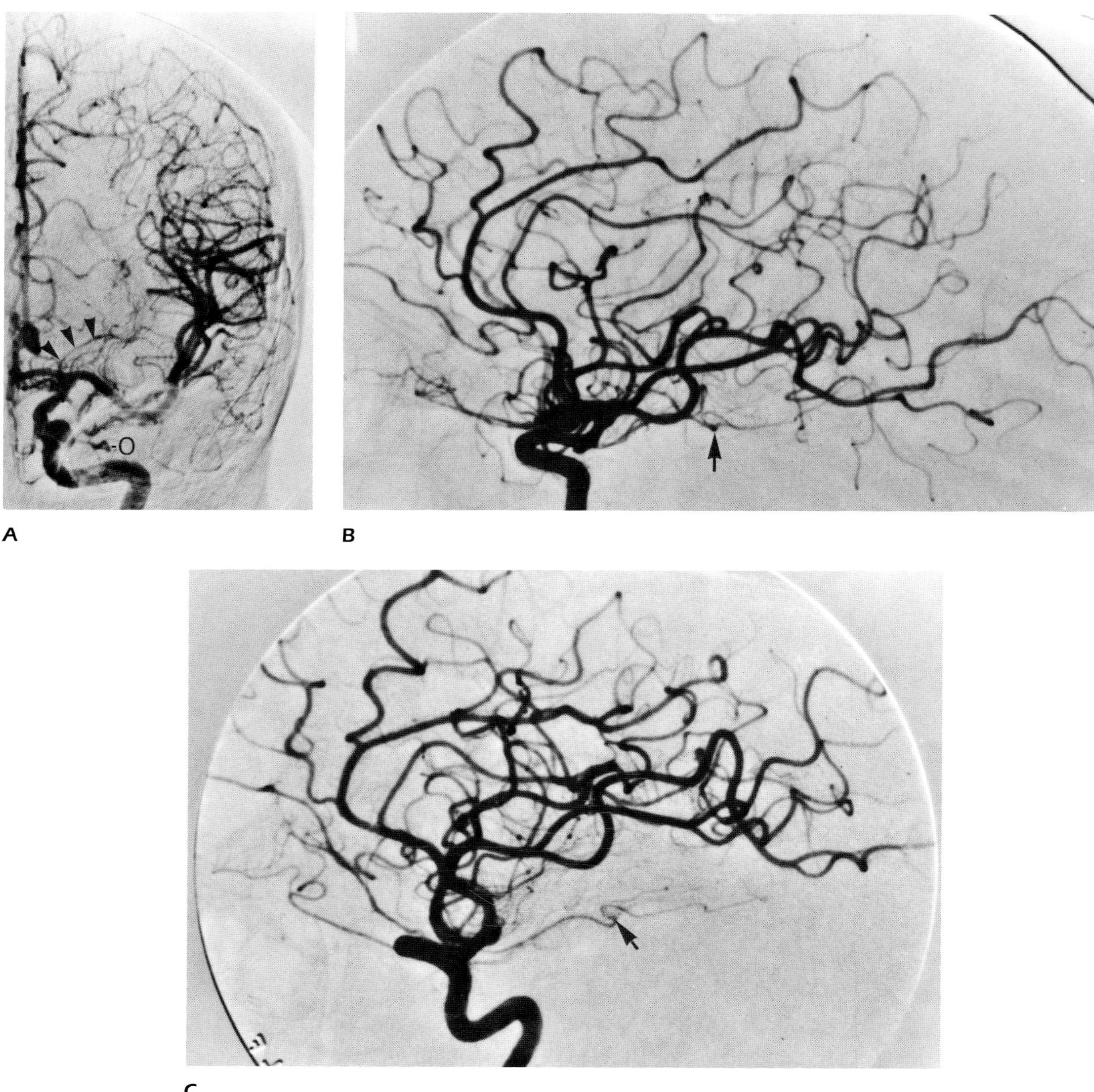

Figure 12-15. Anterior choroidal artery. (A) The crural segment (*arrowheads*) arcs around the uncus as it courses laterally to enter the choroidal fissure. The lateral lenticulostriate arteries are located lateral to the origin of the anterior choroidal artery. *O,* ophthalmic artery. (B) The junction between the crural and plexal segments of the anterior choroidal artery is denser than the remainder of the artery since it is seen on end (*arrow*). Note that the crural segment is convex upward and the plexal segment is convex downward. (C) The anterior choroidal artery has been thrown clear of the middle cerebral artery by caudal angulation of the x-ray tube. The junction between the crural and plexal segments of the anterior choroidal artery is marked by an *arrow*. (A) AP projection; (B) lateral projection; (C) lateral projection, caudal angulation.

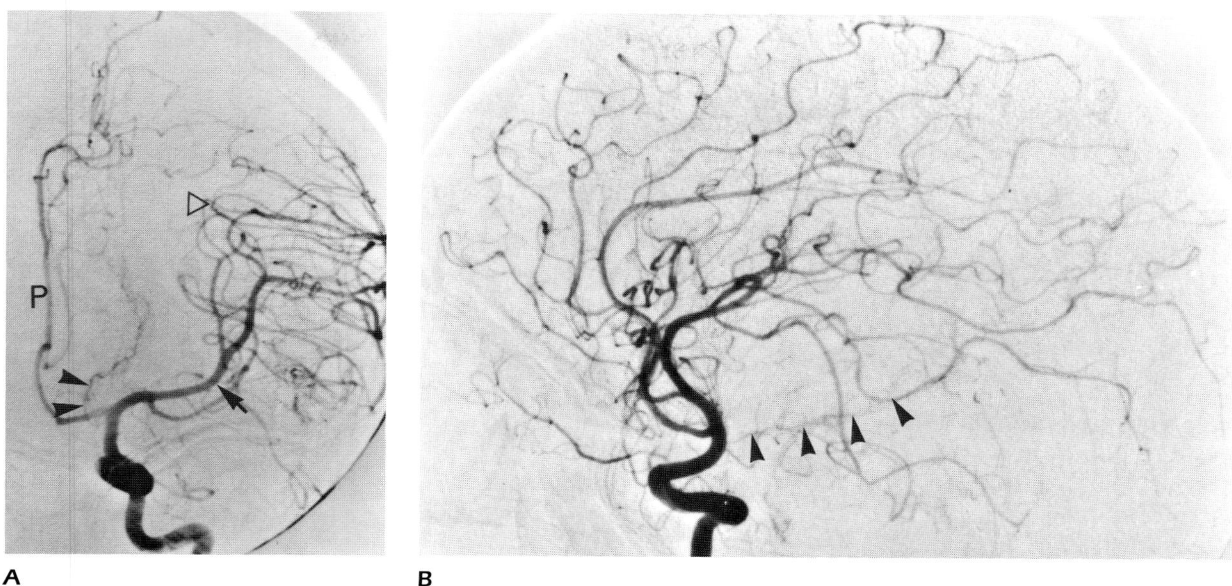

Figure 12-16. Glioblastoma multiforme of the temporal lobe. (A) The crural segment of the anterior choroidal artery (*arrowheads*) is displaced to the midline by a slightly vascular temporal lobe tumor. In addition, the tumor has elevated the M_1 segment and moved the "knee" of the middle cerebral artery superiorly and medially (*arrow*). The sylvian point is displaced upward and medially (*open arrowhead*). The pericallosal (*P*) artery demonstrates a square shift. (B) The anterior choroidal artery is displaced inferiorly (*arrowheads*). The inferior portion of the sylvian triangle is pushed upward. (A) AP projection; (B) lateral projection.

Figure 12-17. Major variations in the course of the A_1 segment (anterior cerebral artery). The darkened A_1 segment may course horizontally (A), downward (B), or upward (C). (A, B, and C) AP projection.

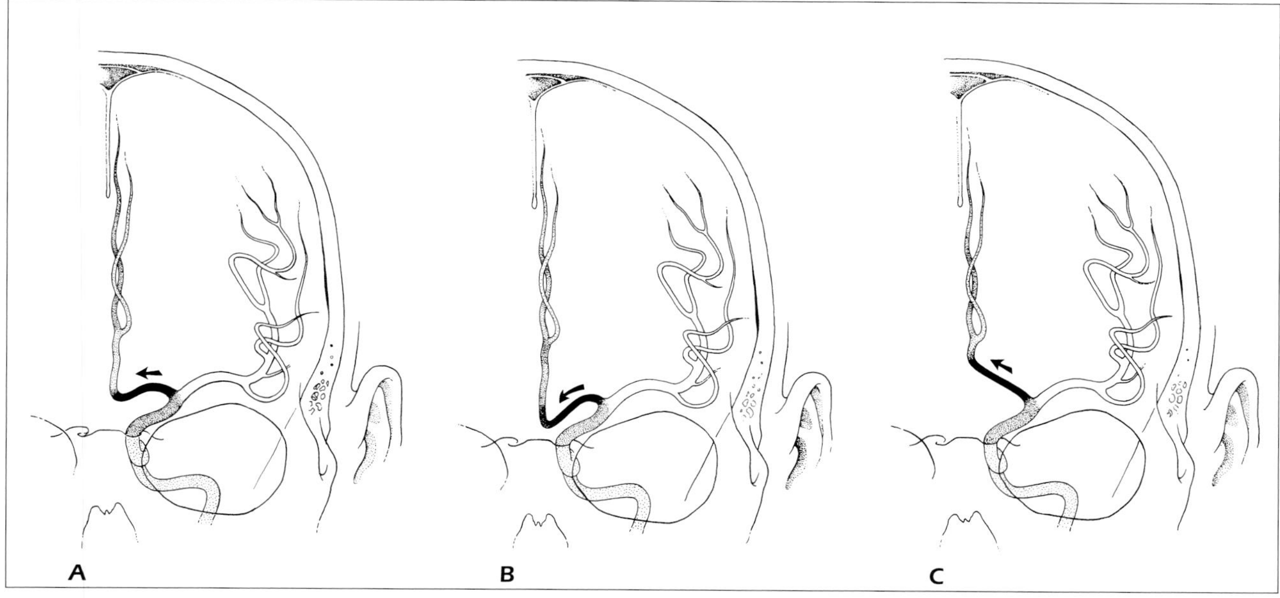

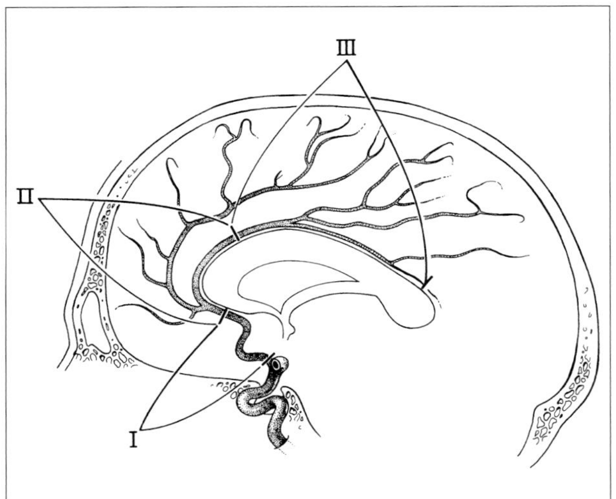

Figure 12-18. Major divisions of the pericallosal artery: *I*, infracallosal; *II*, precallosal; *III*, supracallosal. Lateral projection.

tralateral carotid artery during the injection of contrast media.

Pericallosal (A_2 Segment) Artery

The pericallosal (A_2 segment) artery begins at the origin of the anterior communicating artery, extends around the genu and body of the corpus callosum, and terminates by anastomosing with the posterior pericallosal artery near the splenium of the corpus callosum. On lateral angiograms the pericallosal artery can be divided into three segments based on its relationship to the corpus callosum: infracallosal, precallosal, and supracallosal (Fig. 12-18).

The infracallosal segment extends from the origin of the anterior communicating artery to the beginning of the genu of the corpus callosum. The proximal portion of the infracallosal segment usually has a convex downward curve and the distal segment a convex upward curve (82 percent) (see Fig. 12-18).[63] Less frequently, the infracallosal segment is either straight (parallel to the orbital plate) or semivertical (14 per-

Figure 12-19. Normal inferior concavity of the infracallosal segment of the pericallosal artery in four individuals. Note that the smaller arteries adjacent to the infracallosal segment do not appear stretched. Lateral projection.

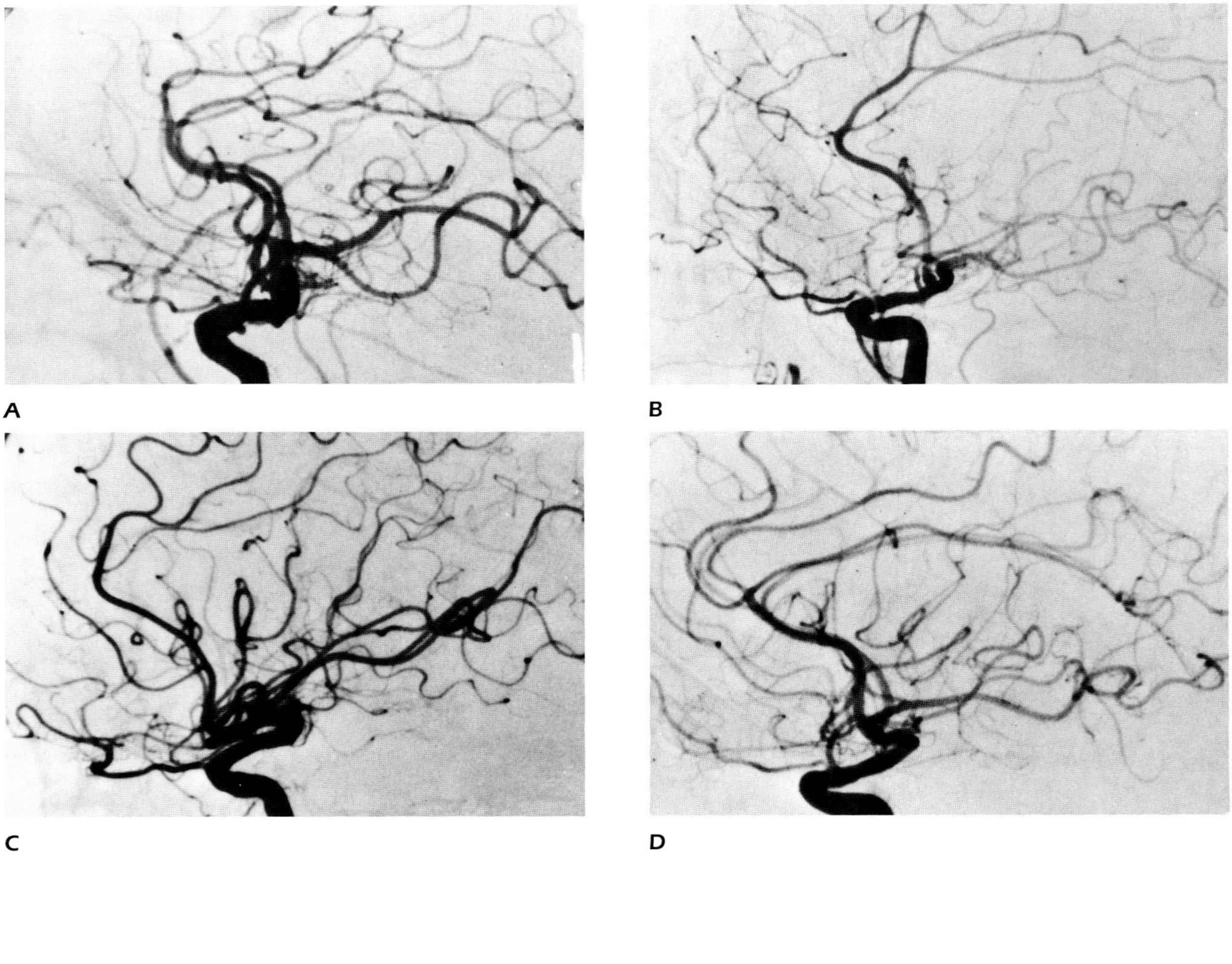

A

B

C

D

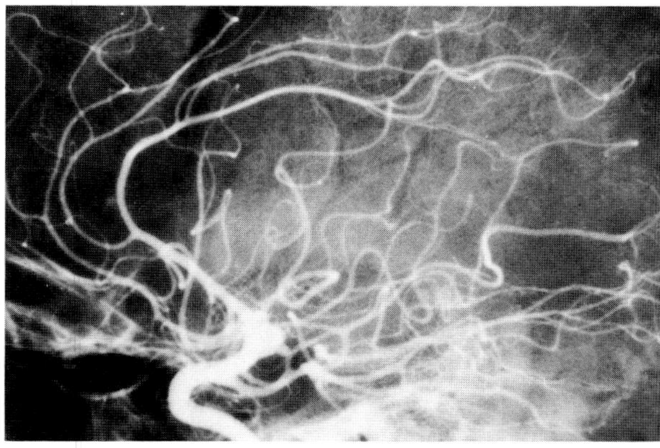

A

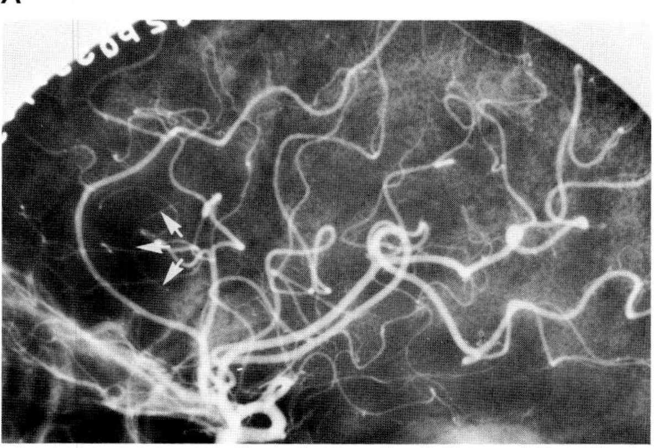

B

Figure 12-20. (A) Normal wide curve of the precallosal segment. (B) The dominant callosomarginal artery mimics the wide curve of the precallosal segment in (A). There is only flash filling of the pericallosal artery (*arrows*). (A and B) Lateral projection.

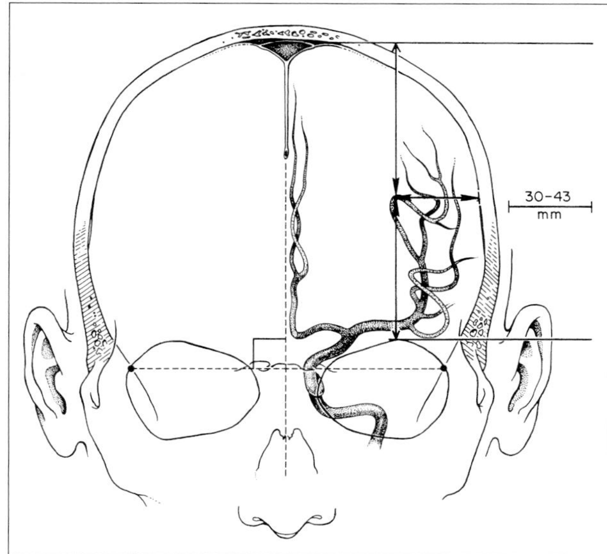

Figure 12-21. Diagram localizing the midline position of the pericallosal artery and the sylvian point. The midline is located by placing dots at the intersection of the orbital rims and the linea innominata, connecting the dots by a line, and finally drawing a line superiorly perpendicular to the midpoint of the horizontal line. The sylvian point is located 30 to 43 mm from the inner table of the skull. It is also located midway (±1 cm) along a vertical line whose superior border is formed by a line tangent to the highest point along the inner table of the skull and whose inferior border is formed by either the roof of the orbit or the upper border of the petrous ridge, whichever is lower. AP projection.

cent). Finally, this segment is occasionally concave inferiorly, suggesting the presence of an avascular low frontal or subfrontal mass (Fig. 12-19). The infracallosal segment of both pericallosal arteries may form a single trunk (azygous anterior cerebral artery) in about 2 percent of individuals.[64] This unusual variation is associated with aneurysms, arteriovenous malformations, and congenital midline defects.[65]

The precallosal segment usually forms about a 60-degree arch around the genu of the corpus callosum (see Fig. 12-18). More acute angulations between 30 and 60 degrees may occur normally (22 percent) but may also indicate a mass located above this segment, such as a parasagittal meningioma or a medial posterior frontal tumor.[63] Less frequently, the precallosal segment forms a wide curve (17 percent), which can appear angiographically similar to that in patients with hydrocephalus, corpus callosum tumors, and anterior intraventricular tumors (Fig. 12-20).

The supracallosal segment usually curves smoothly or undulates gently over the superior surface of the corpus callosum (84 percent). Less frequently, the midportion of the artery may be bowed upward (16 percent), suggesting the presence of a parasagittal corpus callosum tumor.[63] When the supracallosal segment extends as far posteriorly as the splenium of the corpus callosum, it usually anastomoses with the posterior cerebral artery.

Although the three segments of the pericallosal artery cannot be well differentiated on AP angiograms, they can be used to monitor midline shifts (subfalcine shifts) because they are located in or adjacent to the interhemispheric fissure (Fig. 12-21). The pericallosal artery usually lies close to the midline but may assume a wavy appearance if it becomes tortuous and courses into the pericallosal sulcus or if the interhemispheric fissure widens with atrophy. When this vessel courses deeply into the pericallosal sulcus, it may deviate up

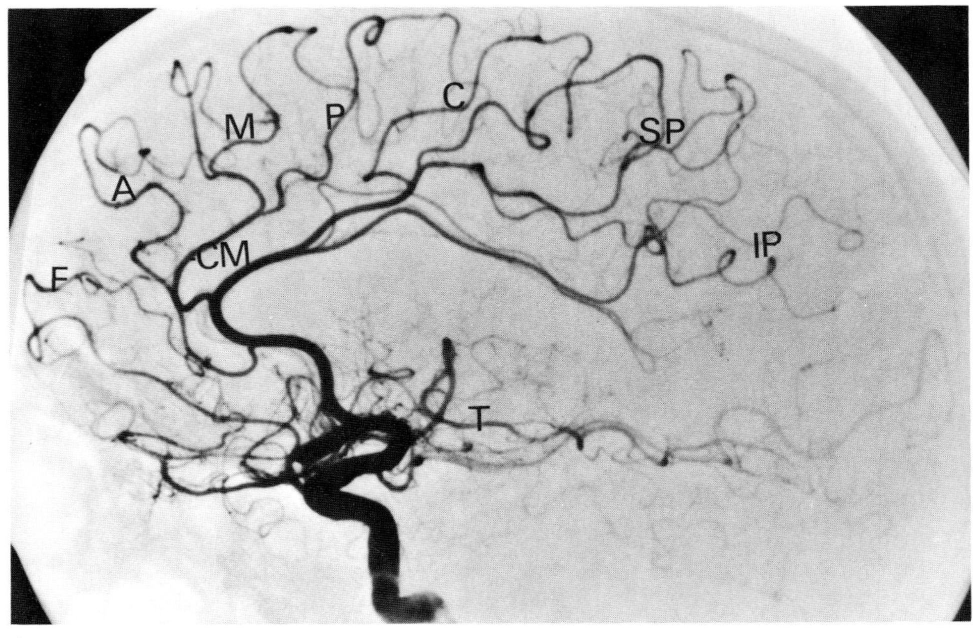

A

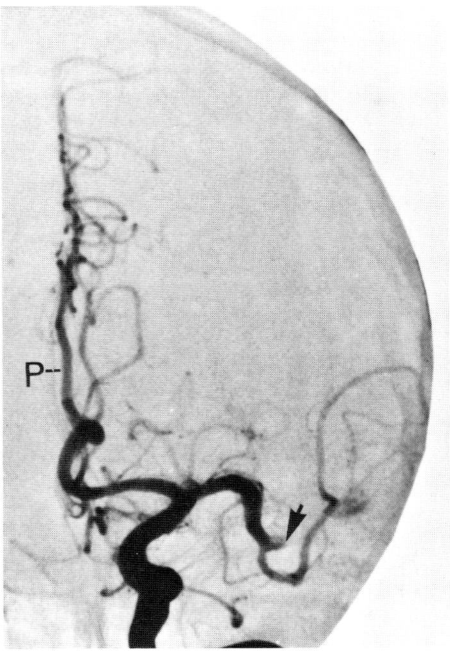

B

Figure 12-22. The pericallosal artery and its branches. These arteries are demonstrated without superimposition of the middle cerebral artery because the superior division of the middle cerebral artery has been occluded. (A) Pericallosal artery and its branches: frontopolar (*F*), callosomarginal (*CM*), anterior internal frontal (*A*), middle internal frontal (*M*), posterior internal frontal (*P*), paracentral (*C*), superior parietal (*SP*), and inferior parietal (*IP*) arteries. The posterior temporal artery (*T*) is the only remaining cortical branch of the middle cerebral artery. (B) The pericallosal (*P*) artery and its branches are located in the midline. Occlusion of the superior division of the middle cerebral artery is marked by an *arrow*. (A) Lateral projection; (B) AP projection.

to 10 mm from the midline; its lax appearance and its eventual return to the midline, however, suggest that it is normal.[60]

Cortical Branches of the Anterior Cerebral Artery

On lateral angiograms the cortical branches of the pericallosal artery have a variable course even though the three anatomic areas they supply are relatively constant. The anatomic areas are divided by surface sulci into the superior frontal gyrus, the paracentral lobule, and the precuneus.

The internal surface of the superior frontal gyrus anterior to the paracentral lobule is supplied by three arteries.[66] The most anteroinferior territory is supplied by the orbitofrontal artery. This artery, on lateral angiograms, approximates the course of the ophthalmic artery. The orbitofrontal artery may arise from either the pericallosal or the frontopolar artery. The frontal pole is supplied by the frontopolar artery and is located just above the territory supplied by the orbitofrontal artery (Fig. 12-22). This artery usually arises from the pericallosal artery but may also arise from the orbitofrontal or callosomarginal artery. The area superior and posterior to the frontal pole is supplied by the internal frontal branches, which arise from either the callosomarginal artery or from the pericallosal artery.

The callosomarginal artery is the largest branch of the pericallosal artery (see Fig. 12-22). Superior to the pericallosal artery it courses posteriorly in the cingulate sulcus. It leaves this sulcus to cross the anterior border of the paracentral lobule (coronal suture) and terminates in this lobule (80 percent). When the paracentral lobule is supplied by two vessels (20 percent), at least one vessel crosses the anterior border of the paracentral lobule.[67] In neither case does the paracentral lobule receive its blood supply from behind the marginal ramus. If a vessel does cross the marginal ramus to supply the paracentral lobule, it can be assumed that the normal routes have been occluded.[66] The callosomarginal artery usually originates from the precallosal segment of the pericallosal artery (72 percent); it may, however, originate from the infracallosal segment (19 percent) or the frontopolar artery (9 percent).[60] The callosomarginal artery is usually either the same size as (34 percent) or larger than the corresponding pericallosal artery (44 percent).[60] Occlusion of this vessel is demonstrated in Figure 12-23.

Middle Cerebral Artery and Its Branches

The middle cerebral artery is about 20 percent larger in diameter than the anterior cerebral artery.[68] The middle cerebral artery can be divided into three segments: horizontal, insular, and cortical. The horizontal segment helps supply the basal ganglia, the orbital surface of the frontal lobe, and the temporal pole; the insular segment supplies the insula; and the cortical branches supply the lateral convexity of the cerebrum.

Horizontal (M_1) Segment

The horizontal (M_1) segment begins at the carotid bifurcation, extends laterally in the lateral cerebral fissure, and ends by entering the sylvian fissure. The junction between the end of the M_1 segment and the beginning of the insular (M_2) segment is called the "knee" of the middle cerebral artery because of its appearance. The horizontal segment is not always horizontal, as its name suggests, but may course obliquely downward, especially in older adults (Fig. 12-24A and B).[60] The M_1 segment may even course upward, suggesting the presence of a temporal or subtemporal mass (see Fig. 12-24C). In these individuals the "knee" may also appear to be displaced medially. The normal upward course of the M_1 segment usually occurs in individuals below 20 years of age.

The M_1 segment gives origin to the lenticulostriate, orbitofrontal, and anterior temporal arteries. The six to nine lateral lenticulostriate arteries arise from the superior surface of the horizontal segment and enter the lateral two-thirds of the anterior perforated substance above it. These vessels, on lateral angiograms, spread out like a fan and supply most of the superolateral head of the caudate nucleus, the body of the cau-

Figure 12-23. Occlusion of the branches (*arrowheads*) that supply the paracentral lobule. Lateral projection.

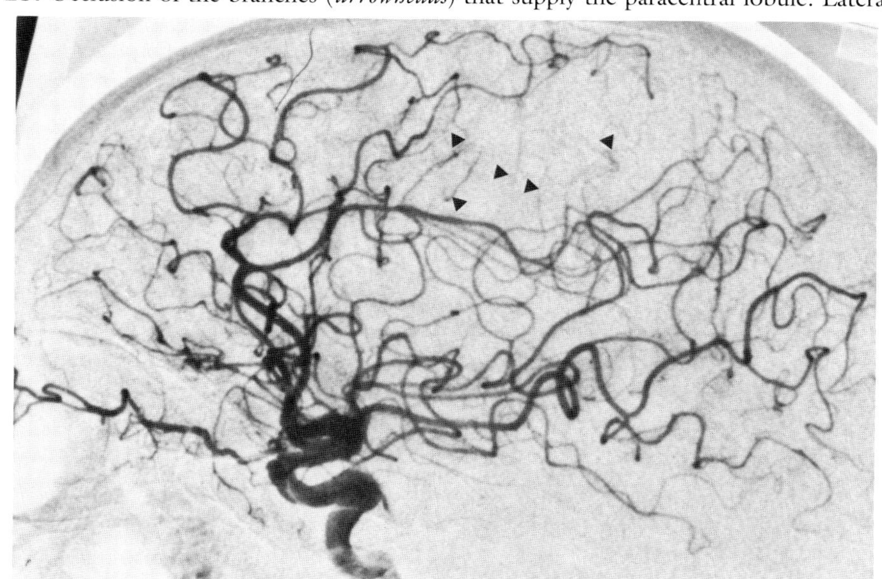

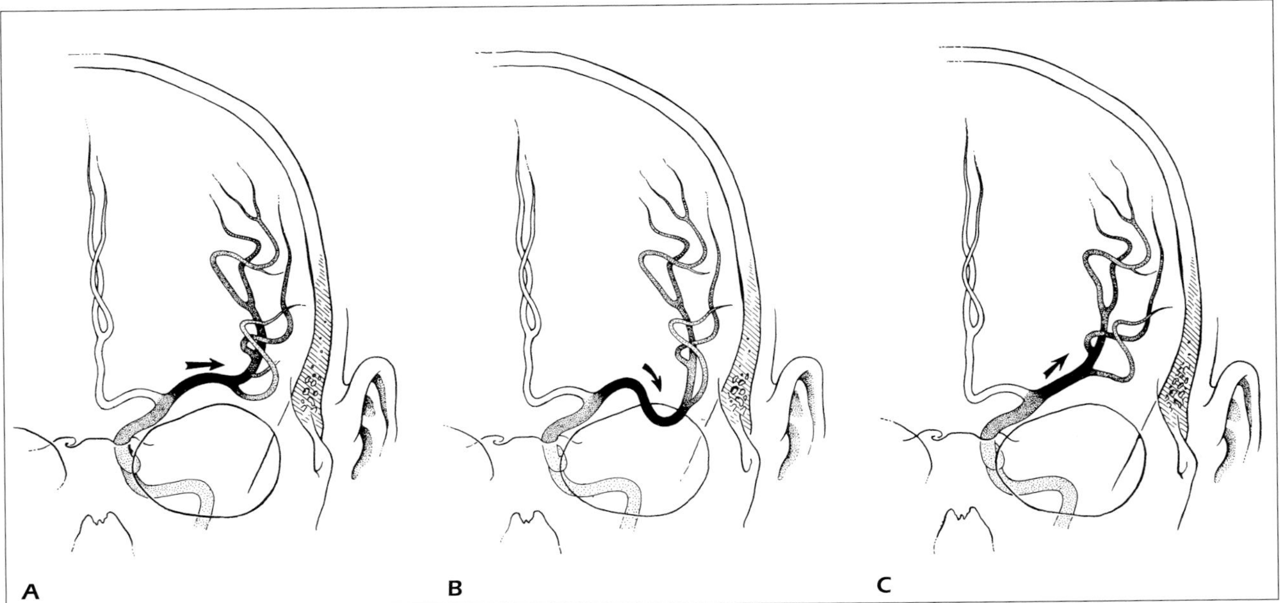

Figure 12-24. Major variations in the M_1 segment of the middle cerebral artery. (A) Horizontal. The darkened M_1 segment of the middle cerebral artery courses horizontally below the temporal lobe. (B) Downward. The M_1 segment courses downward in the lateral cerebral fissure before entering the sylvian fissure. (C) Upward. The M_1 segment courses upward before entering the sylvian fissure. (A, B, and C) AP projection.

date nucleus, most of the putamen, the lateral one-third of the globus pallidus, and the superior half of the anterior limb of the internal capsule. In the anteroposterior projection these vessels form a gentle S-shaped configuration on the right (see Figs. 12-14 and 12-15). Compression of the lenticulostriate arteries is caused by tumors located above them. Compression of the striate vessels can also be simulated by decreasing the caudal angulation. Localized straightening and separation of the striate arteries indicate a mass in the basal ganglia. The most lateral convex portions of these striate arteries are separated from the insular segment of the middle cerebral artery by 11 to 14 mm.[69]

The anterior temporal artery arises from the anterior surface of the M_1 segment and courses over the temporal pole. Lateral angiograms show that it lies close to the anterior border of the middle fossa (see Fig. 12-13). Intraaxial masses may push the anterior temporal artery forward against the anterior wall of the middle fossa, whereas extraaxial masses may push it posteriorly. The anterior temporal artery is not separated from the anterior border of the middle fossa by more than 7 mm unless there is an extra-axial mass.[70]

The orbitofrontal artery also arises from the anterior surface of the horizontal segment and passes forward to supply the inferior and lateral surface of the frontal lobe. The size of this artery is inversely proportional to the size of the frontopolar branch of the pericallosal artery.

Insular (M_2) Segment

The insula, an area of the cerebral cortex hidden by the operculum, is outlined by branches of the middle cerebral artery in the circular sulcus. They exit through the sylvian fissure to supply the cortex over the cerebral convexities. The arteries coursing over the insula are triangular in appearance when viewed laterally (Fig. 12-25). The inferior point of the triangle is formed by the horizontal segment of the middle cerebral artery, the anterior superior point is formed by the most anterior artery over the insula as it begins to loop inferiorly to leave through the sylvian fissure, and the posterior superior point is formed by the most posterior artery as it begins to loop inferiorly to leave the insula. The posterosuperior point is also referred to as the *sylvian point.*

The superior border of the triangle is drawn by connecting the arteries in the superior limiting sulcus before they loop inferiorly to leave through the sylvian fissure (see Fig. 12-25). If more than one consecutive artery is located below this line, it may suggest a mass above the insula (Fig. 12-26).[71] The inferior border of the sylvian triangle can be related to the clinoparietal line. In adults, the inferior border of the sylvian trian-

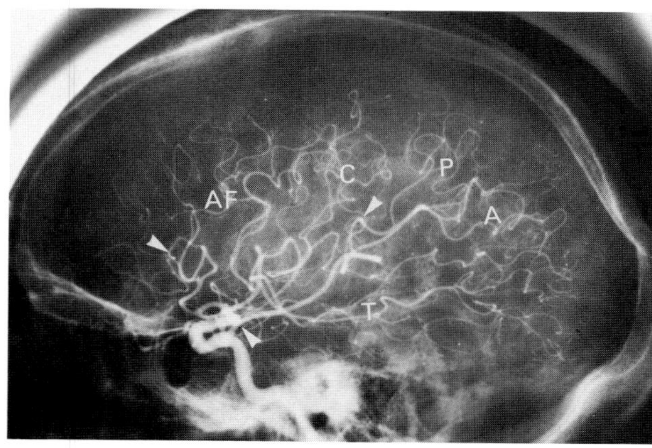

A

B

Figure 12-25. Middle cerebral artery branches without overlying anterior cerebral and posterior cerebral arteries. (A) The anterior superior, posterior superior, and inferior points of the insula are outlined by the branches of the middle cerebral artery as they course over its surface. These three points in the insula are marked by *arrowheads* and correspond to the corners of the sylvian triangle. The cortical branches of the middle cerebral artery consist of the ascending frontal (*AF*), posterior parietal (*P*), angular (*A*), and posterior temporal (*T*) arteries and the artery to the central sulcus (*C*). (B) A drawing that corresponds roughly to the arteriogram in (A) is drawn with the sylvian triangle in place. The cortical branches are marked with abbreviations from (A). (A and B) Lateral projection.

gle should not extend more than 1.0 cm above or 0.5 cm below the clinoparietal line.[56] In children, the inferior border is never more than 1.5 cm above this line and never below it.[72]

Because the sylvian triangle is located laterally, it is deformed more readily by masses located along the cerebral convexities. Masses adjacent to the sylvian triangle cause the following deformities: anterior masses push it posteriorly, posterior masses push it anteriorly, superior masses push it inferiorly, and inferior masses push it superiorly (Fig. 12-27).[73]

In the frontal projection the insular branches of the middle cerebral artery bow gently upward until they reach the superior limiting sulcus. These branches are located 20 to 30 mm from the inner table of the skull. The anterior portion of the insula is more medially located than the posterior portion. The sylvian point, the most medial point of the last branch to leave through the sylvian fissure, is projected as the most superior vessel over the insula because cerebral angiograms are taken with a 13-degree caudal angulation. The sylvian point is located 30 to 43 mm from the inner table of the skull and midway (±1 cm) along a vertical line tangent to the inner table of the vertex superiorly and the roof of the orbit or upper margin of the petrous ridge, whichever is lower inferiorly (see Fig. 12-21).[56] The sylvian point is usually lower on the left than on the right because the left operculum is better developed in most right-handed individuals.[74]

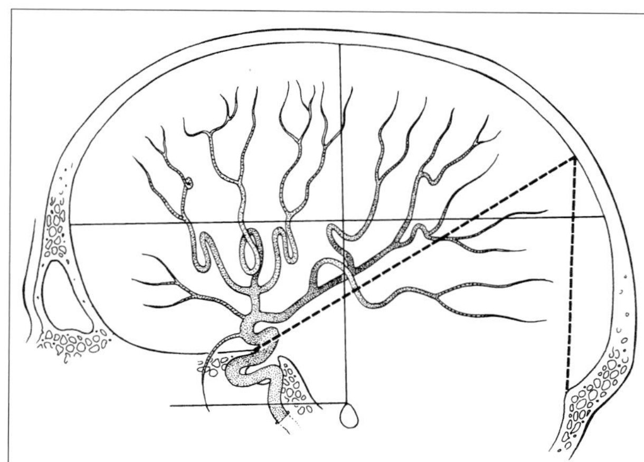

Figure 12-26. Measurements to localize the superior and inferior borders of the sylvian triangle. The superior border of the triangle is located close to the midpoint of a vertical line extending from the superior border of the external auditory canal to the inner table of the skull. The superior border is also roughly perpendicular to this line (±5 degrees). The inferior border of the triangle can be related to the clinoparietal line (a line connecting the anterior clinoid process to a point 9 cm above the internal occipital protuberance, a 40-cm target-film distance). In adults the inferior border should not be more than 1.0 cm above or 0.5 cm below this line. Lateral projection.

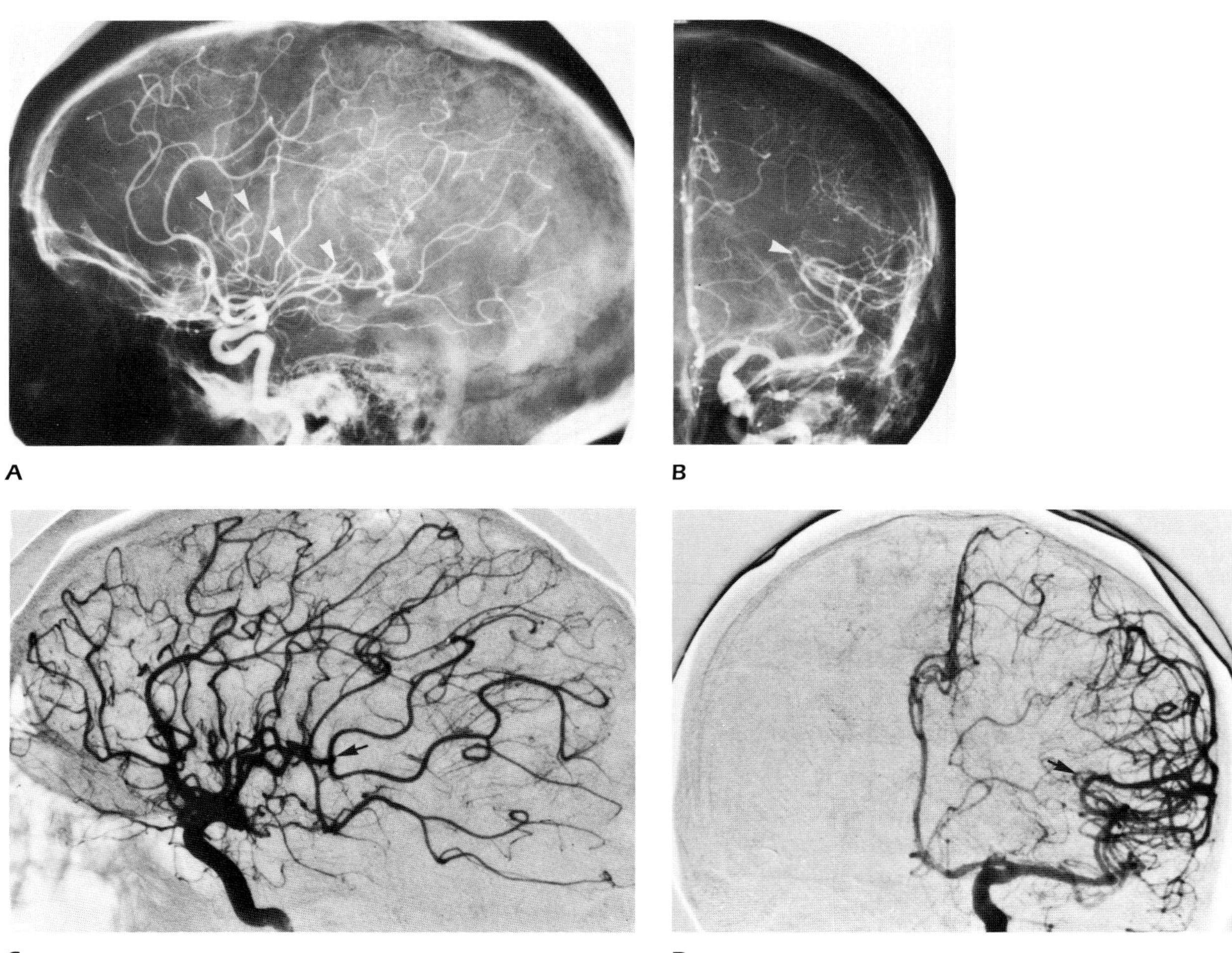

Figure 12-27. Displacement of the sylvian triangle. (A) A vascular glioblastoma multiforme displaces the posterior two-thirds of the sylvian triangle inferiorly. The vessels composing the superior border of the sylvian triangle are marked by *arrowheads*. (B) The anteroposterior arteriogram corresponding to (A) shows the sylvian point displaced inferiorly (*arrowhead*). In addition, the pericallosal artery shows a slight distal shift. (C) A glioma located predominately in the occipital region displaces the sylvian triangle forward. The sylvian point is marked with an *arrow*. (D) The anteroposterior arteriogram corresponding to (C) shows downward displacement of the sylvian point (*arrow*). The pericallosal artery demonstrates a square shift. (A and C) Lateral projection; (B and D) AP projection.

Cortical Branches of the Middle Cerebral Artery

Within the circular sulcus, the middle cerebral artery divides into a superior and inferior division in roughly 80 percent of individuals.[75] The superior division always supplies the lateral surface of the frontal lobe and the anteriormost portion of the parietal lobe (postcentral gyrus) through branches of the ascending frontal arteries and the artery to the central sulcus. The inferior division always supplies most of the lateral surface of the temporal lobe through the posterior temporal artery. The blood supply to the parietal lobe behind the posterior central gyrus and the angular region can come from either the superior or inferior division, depending on which is larger. These locations can be approximated on a lateral angiogram by a method suggested by Ring (Fig. 12-28).[76,77]

The ascending frontal arteries have been divided into three groups: orbitofrontal, candelabra, and the artery of the central sulcus.[67] The orbitofrontal arteries take an anterior course to supply the inferior surface of the frontal lobe, and the candelabra group behind it takes a vertical course to supply the lateral surface of the frontal lobe. The candelabra group received its name because its major branches bow downward be-

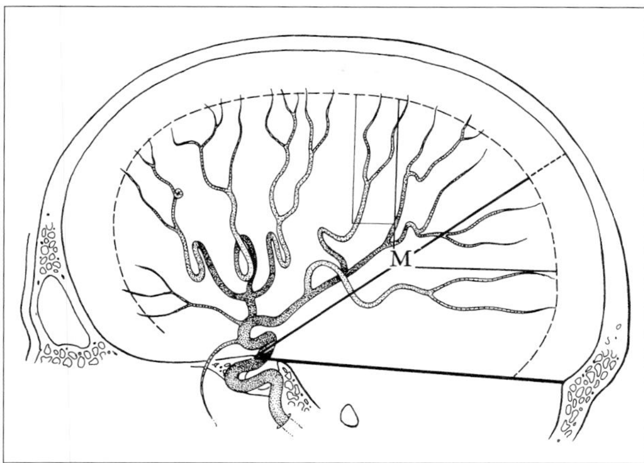

Figure 12-28. Ring's template to identify cortical branches of the middle cerebral artery. Lateral projection. (Adapted from Ring BA. The cerebral cortical arteries. In: Salamon G, ed. Advances in cerebral angiography. Berlin: Springer, 1975:25–32. Used with permission.)

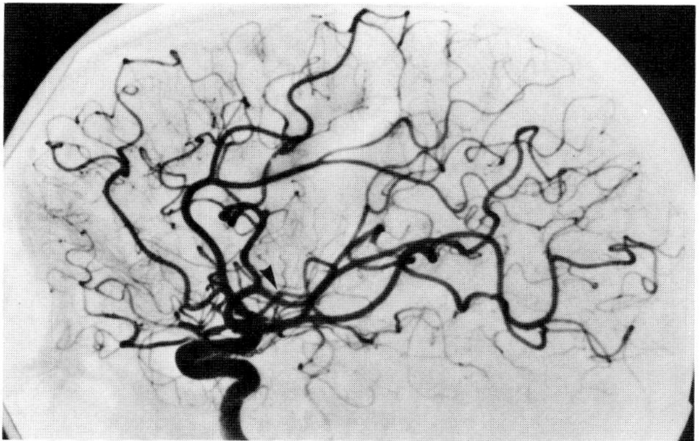

Figure 12-29. Occlusion of ascending frontal branches that supply the posterior frontal region. The occluded vessel is marked by an *arrowhead*. Lateral projection.

fore curving upward to bifurcate and trifurcate like a candelabrum. Occlusion of these vessels is demonstrated in Figure 12-29. The artery (or arteries) to the central sulcus supplies the motor and sensory areas.

The posterior temporal artery is the only vessel with a characteristic appearance on lateral angiograms. It rises to exit the sylvian fissure and then descends in a characteristic loop, concave inferiorly, over the posterosuperior border of the temporal lobe (see Figs. 12-22 and 12-25). The angular artery is the last artery to leave the sylvian fissure and forms the sylvian point. The angular artery takes a horizontal course parallel to the long axis of the skull. The posterior parietal artery frequently originates from the angular artery and then takes a posterior and superior course to supply most of the parietal lobe.

Posterior Cerebral Artery and Its Branches

The posterior cerebral arteries receive their blood supply mainly from the basilar artery. They are, however, included with the supratentorial arteries because they are located above the tentorium and originally derive all their blood supply from the internal carotid arteries. The posterior cerebral arteries supply structures related to ocular function and cerebrospinal fluid production.

The posterior cerebral arteries originate at the basilar artery bifurcation in the interpeduncular fossa. They nearly encircle the mesencephalon by coursing through the crural, ambient, and quadrigeminal cisterns. In the half-axial projection the arteries are maximally separated in the ambient cisterns (3.5–5.5 cm) and minimally separated in the quadrigeminal cisterns (1–3 cm).

The origin of the posterior cerebral arteries is variable: when low, because of a short basilar artery, they are on a level parallel to the floor of the sella; when high, because of an elongated basilar artery, they may be up to 2 cm above the dorum sellae.[36] In the half-axial projection, a low origin is associated with a Y-shaped bifurcation and a high origin with a T-shaped bifurcation (Fig. 12-30).

On lateral angiograms, the proximal portions of the posterior cerebral arteries take a caudal dip as they encircle the mesencephalon; this dip may be absent in individuals with low basilar artery bifurcation. Further downward displacement of the posterior cerebral artery indicates transtentorial herniation (Fig. 12-31).[78]

The major posterior cerebral artery branches are the thalamoperforating arteries, the medial and lateral posterior choroidal arteries, and the cortical branches to the temporal and occipital lobes. Three to five posterior thalamoperforating arteries arise from the posterior cerebral artery just after they originate from the basilar artery (Fig. 12-32). The arteries are located on either side of the midline and take a slightly posterior, superior course to supply the thalamus and lateral geniculate bodies.

The posterior medial choroidal artery originates in the ambient cistern. It courses posteriorly until it reaches the quadrigeminal cistern, where it passes medially and forward to supply the choroid plexus in the roof of the third ventricle. The posterior lateral choroidal artery also originates in the ambient cistern but courses laterally through the choroid fissure to supply the choroid plexus in the posterior portion of the tem-

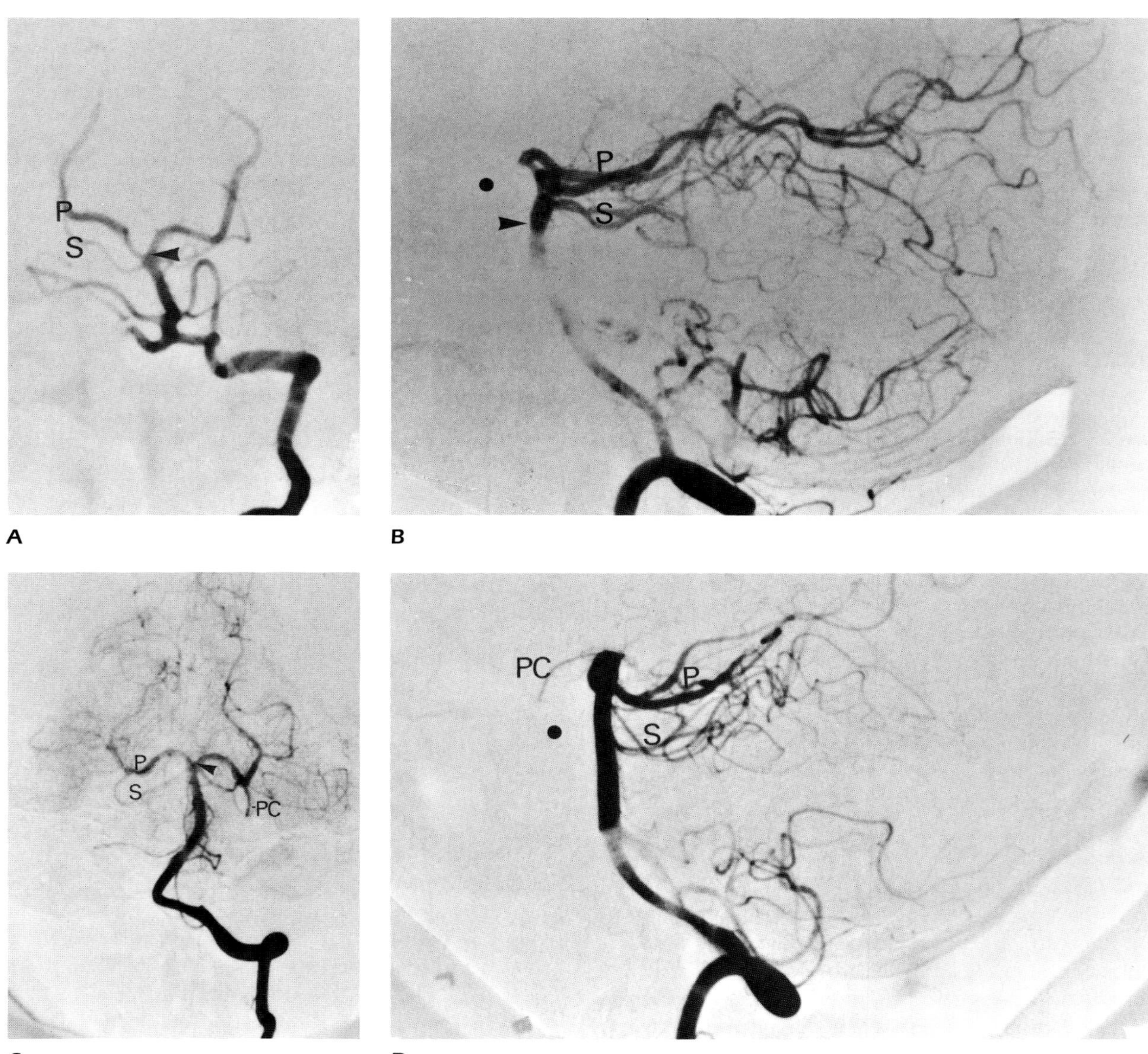

Figure 12-30. Bifurcations of the basilar artery. (A) Y-shaped bifurcation of the basilar artery (*arrowhead*). Also shown are the superior cerebellar (*S*) and posterior cerebral (*P*) arteries. (B) The bifurcation of (A) is marked with an *arrowhead*. The tip of the dorsum sellae is marked with a *dot*. The proximal portion of the posterior cerebral (*P*) artery does not show a prominent caudal dip. The superior cerebellar (*S*) artery is also shown. (C) T-shaped bifurcation of the basilar artery (*arrowhead*). Also shown are the posterior communicating (*PC*), posterior cerebral (*P*), and superior cerebellar (*S*) arteries. (D) The basilar bifurcation in (C) is located above the dorsum sellae (*dot*). The proximal portion of the posterior cerebral (*P*) artery shows a prominent caudal dip. The proximal portion of the posterior cerebral artery and the distal portion of the basilar artery overlap and cause a pseudoaneurysm. Posterior communicating (*PC*) and superior cerebellar (*S*) arteries are also shown. (A) AP half-axial projection; (B and D) lateral projection; (C) AP transfacial projection.

poral horn and the atrium and body of the lateral ventricle. The size of the posterior lateral choroidal artery is inversely proportional to the size of the anterior choroidal artery.

On a lateral angiogram the medial choroidal artery is located close to the pineal and is 3-shaped (see Fig. 12-32). Behind it the lateral choroidal artery forms a smooth arch that roughly parallels it and outlines the

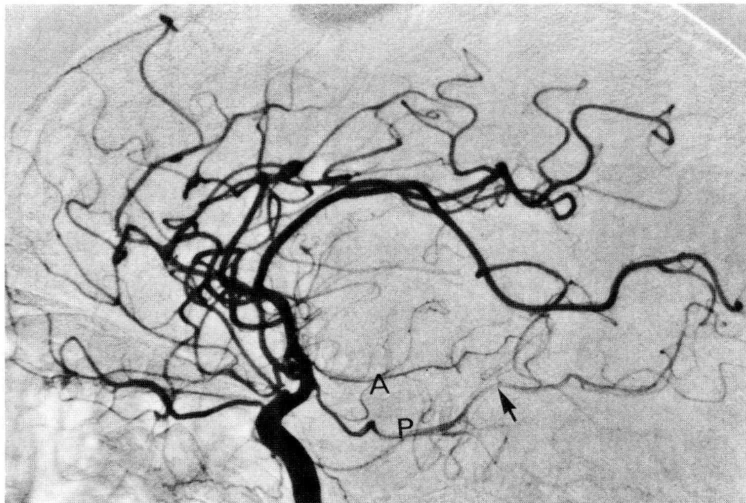

Figure 12-31. Vascular glioma. The glioma is producing downward transtentorial herniation that is reflected in inferior displacement of the anterior choroidal (*A*) and posterior cerebral (*P*) arteries. An *arrow* is placed where the posterior cerebral artery returns over the free edge of the tentorium. The tumor also displaces the sylvian triangle upward and anteriorly. The accompanying anteroposterior angiogram, which is not included, shows medial displacement of the posterior cerebral and anterior choroidal arteries. Lateral projection.

Figure 12-32. Cortical branches of the posterior cerebral artery. (A) The medial cortical branches (parietooccipital [*PO*] and calcarine [*C*] arteries) are located medial to the lateral group (posterior temporal [*PT*] artery). The thalamoperforating (*T*) arteries are located just to the right of the midline. The cranial loop (*arrowhead*) and inferior vermian segments (*arrow*) of the left posterior inferior cerebellar artery (PICA) are located to the left of the midline. The posterior communicating (*PC*) artery is also shown. (B) The calcarine (*C*) artery is located between the parietooccipital (*PO*) and posterior temporal (*PT*) arteries. Also identified are the thalamoperforating (*T*), medial posterior choroidal (*M*), lateral posterior choroidal (*L*), posterior pericallosal (*P*), and posterior communicating (*PC*) arteries. (A) AP half-axial projection; (B) lateral projection.

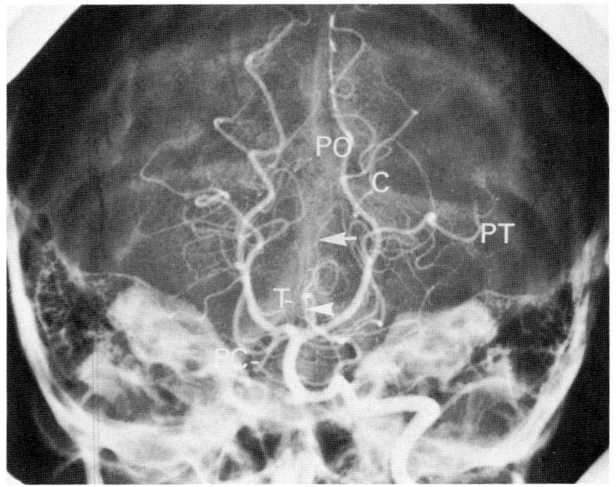

A

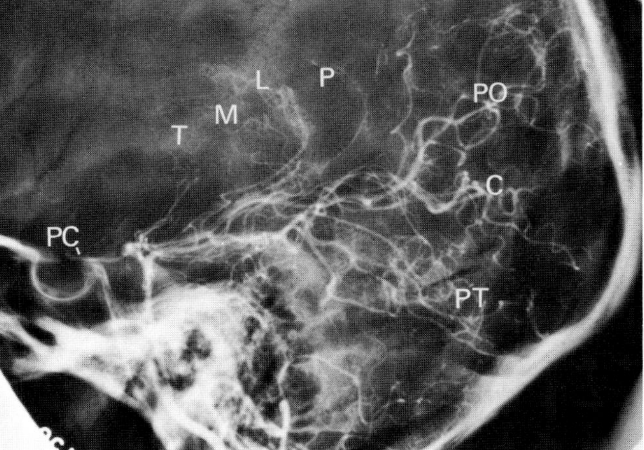

B

posterior border of the thalamus. Behind these two vessels the posterior pericallosal artery forms a third arch as it courses around the splenium of the corpus callosum. These three vessels are important when examining pineal region tumors.

The cortical branches of the posterior cerebral artery can be divided into a medial and a lateral group. The lateral group (the posterior temporal artery) supplies the medial border of the hippocampus as well as the inferior surface of the temporal lobe. On lateral angiograms the lateral group is located just above Twining's line (a line connecting the tuberculum sella and torcular Herophili), and it frequently overlaps the hemispheric branches of the superior cerebellar artery.

The medial group of cortical branches supplies the medial surface of the occipital lobe and consists of the calcarine and parietooccipital arteries. The calcarine artery takes a relatively straight course and is located between the parietooccipital and posterior temporal arteries (see Fig. 12-32). The medial vessels are therefore located above the lateral group. On anteroposterior angiograms the origin of the parietooccipital artery is usually more medial than that of the calcarine artery. Both these vessels are medial to the posterior temporal artery.

Supratentorial Venous System

The supratentorial venous system can be divided into a superficial and a deep group. These two groups of veins then drain into the dural sinuses.

Superficial System

The lateral cerebral convexity above the sylvian fissure is drained by anterior frontal, central, and parietal veins (Fig. 12-33). These lateral veins also receive venous blood from the medial surface of the cerebrum just before they drain into the superior sagittal sinus. The largest vein above the sylvian fissure is designated the *vein of Trolard.* This vein is usually located in the parietal region.

The superficial middle cerebral vein drains the lateral surface of the cerebrum adjacent to the sylvian fissure. The superficial middle cerebral vein usually drains posteriorly into the transverse sinus but may also drain

Figure 12-33. Supratentorial venous system. (A) The superficial veins above the sylvian fissure (anterior frontal [*AF*], posterior frontal [*PF*], and parietal [*P*] veins) drain into the superior sagittal sinus (*SSS*). The superficial veins beneath the sylvian fissure (vein of Labbé [*L*] and occipital veins) drain mainly into the transverse sinus (*T*). The vein of Labbé anastomoses with the anterior frontal vein. The subependymal veins drain into the deep system, which consists of the anterior caudate (*C*), thalamostriate (*TS*), and anterior septal (*S*) veins. The internal cerebral (*IC*) vein and the basal vein of Rosenthal (*B*) drain into the great vein of Galen (*G*), which in turn drains into the straight sinus (*SS*). (B) The internal cerebral vein is located in the midline. The distance between the medial border of the internal cerebral vein and the superolateral aspect of the thalamostriate vein corresponds to the width of the lateral ventricle (*arrows*). The distal portion of the superior sagittal sinus (*SSS*) deviates slightly to the left of the midline before entering the left transverse sinus. The right transverse sinus is reconstructed distal to the torcular by veins from the occipital and posterior temporal lobes. (A) Lateral projection; (B) AP projection.

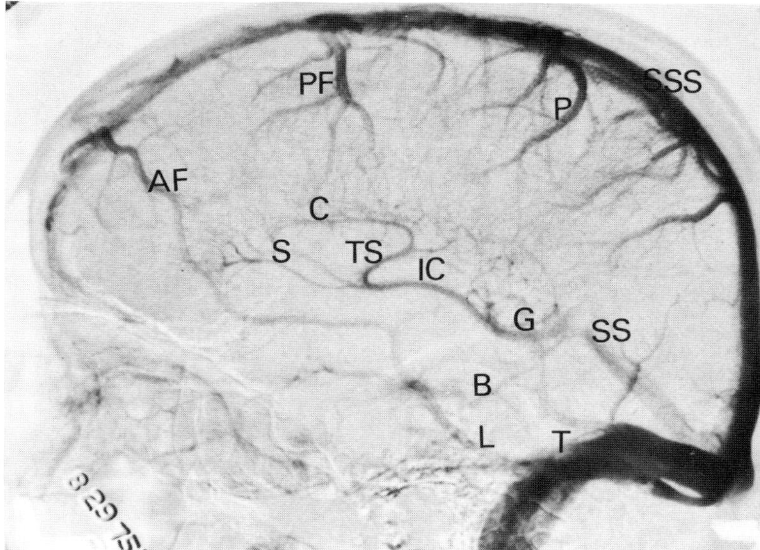

A

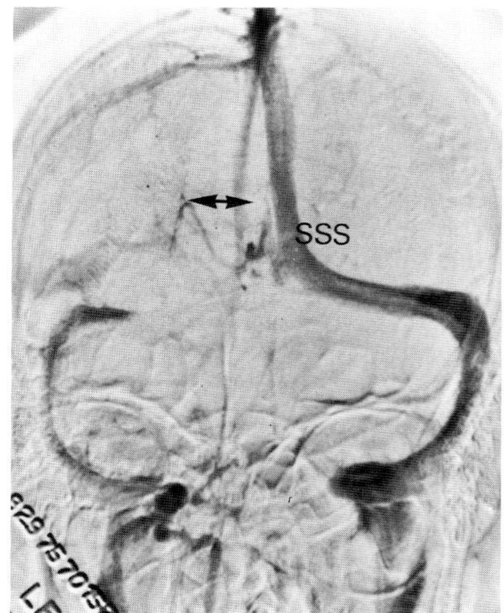

B

anteriorly into the sphenoparietal sinus or medially into the deep middle cerebral vein.

The lateral surface of the cerebrum beneath the sylvian fissure and the inferior surfaces of the temporal and occipital lobes drain directly into the transverse sinus. The largest lateral vein beneath the sylvian fissure is called the *vein of Labbé* (see Fig. 12-33).

Deep System

The deep venous system consists of the internal cerebral veins, the basal veins of Rosenthal, and the thalamic veins. These veins drain into the great vein of Galen and then into the straight sinus. The internal cerebral veins lie within 2 mm of the midline (see Fig. 12-33).[79]

The internal cerebral veins drain the deep white matter around the frontal horns and the body of the lateral ventricles via medial and lateral subependymal veins.[80] The largest lateral subependymal (thalamostriate) vein outlines the inferolateral wall of the body of the lateral ventricle (see Fig. 12-33). The junction of the thalamostriate vein and the internal cerebral vein is usually located at the foramen of Monro.

The anterior septal veins are medial subependymal veins that drain the white matter around the frontal horns and genu of the corpus callosum. On lateral angiograms the septal veins appear to be an anterior extension of the internal cerebral veins.

The medullary veins, which drain into the subependymal veins, are usually not well seen. When present, they are best developed along the superior surface of the ventricle (see Fig. 12-33). Their visualization, under normal conditions, appears to be related to the quantity of contrast injected and to the quality of the radiographic images.[81] When these veins appear early, are enlarged in caliber, or are increased in tortuosity and number, they may indicate the presence of an infiltrating glioma.[82] Less frequently, these findings may be associated with angiomas, metastases, multifocal leukoencephalopathies, or superior sagittal thrombosis.[81]

The basal veins of Rosenthal are formed in the medial portion of the lateral cerebral fissures by receiving lateral branches from the insulae (deep middle cerebral veins), superior branches from the anterior perforated substances, anterior branches from the undersurface of the frontal lobes, and medial branches from the interhemispheric fissures (Fig. 12-34).[83] After the basal veins leave the lateral cerebral fissures they course around the superior aspect of the uncus before passing posteriorly in the perimesencephalic cisterns to drain into the great vein of Galen. The basal veins are only a rough indicator of the position of the mesencephalon since they may be located laterally in the choroidal fissure. While circling the mesencephalon the basal veins also drain the inferior portion of the ventricles (inferior

Figure 12-34. The basal vein of Rosenthal. (A) The basal vein of Rosenthal (*B*) drains the deep middle cerebral vein (*M*). The deep middle cerebral vein in turn drains the insular (*I*) veins. The thalamostriate (*T*) vein is also shown. Air is present in the frontal and temporal horns. (B) The basal vein of Rosenthal (*B*) is marked on the corresponding lateral arteriogram. The thalamostriate (*T*) vein, great vein of Galen (*G*), and inferior sagittal (*I*) and straight (*SS*) sinuses are also shown. (A) AP half-axial projection; (B) lateral projection.

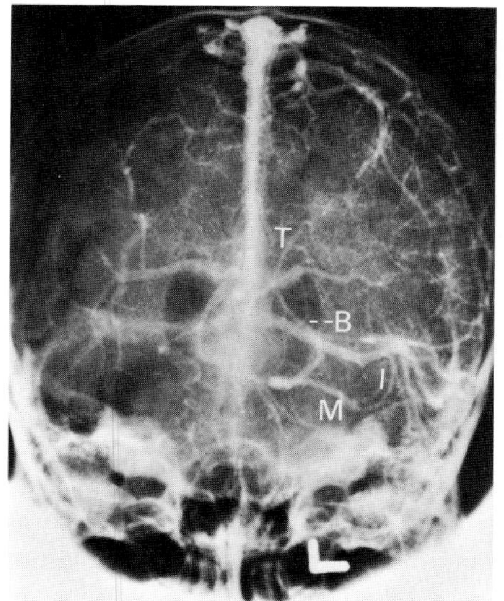

A

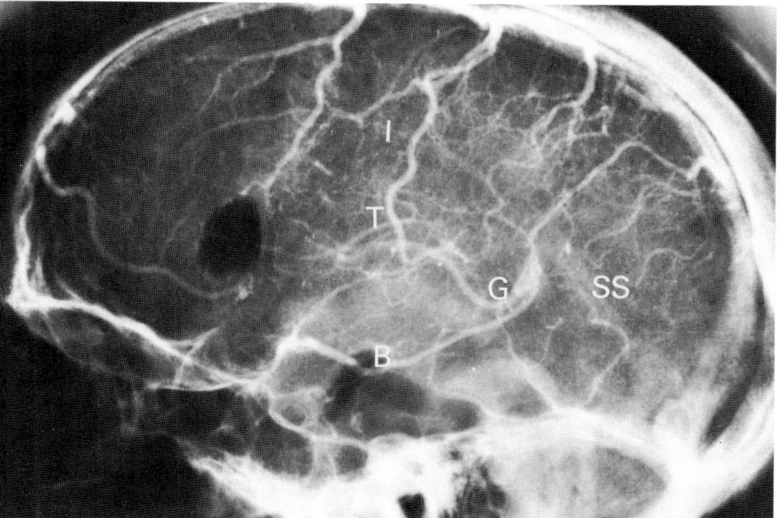

B

ventricular veins), the thalamus, and the hippocampus. A large inferior ventricular vein can be used to diagnose thalamic masses because it courses over the posterior surface of the thalamus.

The basal veins of Rosenthal usually drain posteriorly into the great vein of Galen but can drain anteriorly into the sphenoparietal sinus or the superior petrosal sinus, inferiorly into the lateral mesencephalic vein or anterior pontomesencephalic vein, or medially into the contralateral basal vein of Rosenthal via the posterior communicating vein. These variations, and others, occur when the mesencephalic portion of the vein fails to segment properly.

The thalamus is drained by a group of veins: the anterior supermedial portion (anterior thalamic vein) drains into the internal cerebral vein close to the foramen of Monro, the posterior supermedial portion drains into the posterior portion of the internal cerebral vein or great vein of Galen (superior thalamic vein), the anterior inferolateral surface drains downward into either the basal vein of Rosenthal or the posterior mesencephalic vein (inferior thalamic veins), and the posterior inferolateral portion drains into the posterior part of the basal vein of Rosenthal or the posterior mesencephalic vein (see Fig. 12-37).[84]

The internal cerebral veins, the basal veins of Rosenthal, and the veins that drain the superior aspect of the posterior fossa all drain into the great vein of Galen. The great vein courses beneath the splenium of the corpus callosum and then drains into the straight sinus. The posterior pericallosal vein, which also drains into the great vein of Galen, indicates the position of the splenium of the corpus callosum.

Dural Sinuses

The triangular-shaped superior sagittal sinus (SSS) is located within the dura at its junction with the falx cerebri, close to the midline (about 20 percent of SSSs are located more than 1 cm from the midline).[45] It is connected laterally with the venous lacunae into which arachnoid granulations drain.

The SSS may begin just behind the foramen cecum or as far posteriorly as the coronal suture.[85] In the latter situation the frontal veins run posteriorly, parallel to the midline, before draining into the superior sagittal sinus. The torcular Herophili, which drains the SSS, also receives blood from the straight and occipital sinuses before draining into the transverse sinuses.

In about one-third of individuals the SSS may diverge from the torcular Herophili and not drain into it (see Fig. 12-33). In this situation the SSS is three times more likely to drain into the right transverse sinus. The straight sinus, in turn, drains into the left transverse sinus.[60]

The cavernous sinus forms the lateral border of the sella turcica and receives blood anteriorly from the superior and inferior ophthalmic veins and anterolaterally from the sphenoparietal sinus. The cavernous sinus occasionally receives blood from the superficial sylvian veins and uncal veins. The cavernous sinus may drain posteriorly into the superior petrosal sinus (which subsequently drains into the transverse sinus), posteroinferiorly into the inferior petrosal sinus (which in turn drains into the sigmoid sinus), or inferiorly into the pterygoid plexus through the foramina of Vesalius, ovale, and lacerum.

Sequence of Venous Drainage

The sequence of venous filling is important in evaluating patients suspected of having either a venous occlusion or early venous drainage. Changes in venous drainage are detectable because the sequence of drainage in both the superficial and deep systems is relatively constant. The superficial venous system fills sequentially from anterior to posterior. The frontal and middle cerebral veins usually fill first. The posterior frontal veins may, however, fill before the anterior frontal veins.[86] The parietal veins almost always fill after the frontal veins.[87] Next, the occipital veins (which are located behind the parietal veins) and the veins of Labbé (which are located behind the superficial middle cerebral veins) fill almost simultaneously. The last superficial vein to fill is generally the vein of Trolard.[86]

The deep system usually begins to opacify later than the superficial system and continues to be opacified longer because blood flow is slower in the white matter, which the deep system largely drains.[88] The thalamostriate veins, the internal cerebral veins, and the basal veins of Rosenthal usually fill at about the same time as the parietal veins. The last deep vein to fill is the septal vein, possibly because this vein exclusively drains white matter.

Circulation Time

The average supratentorial circulation time is 3.43 ± 0.51 seconds.[89] The arterial phase lasts approximately 1.0 to 2.5 seconds, the capillary phase 0.25 to 1.00 second, and the venous phase 1.5 to 4.5 seconds.[60,87] The entire supratentorial venous phase is not included in the supratentorial circulation time because it is ordinarily defined as the time interval between maximal filling of the cavernous segment of the internal carotid artery and maximal filling of the parietal veins.

The circulation time can be affected by the type, rate, and volume of contrast that is injected. It can also be affected by PCO_2, pH, blood volume, and blood pressure. Finally, it can be affected by the patient's age, with younger individuals having shorter circulation time than older individuals. The variability of circulation time has limited its usefulness.

Posterior Fossa

The structures located in the posterior fossa are supplied by branches of both the vertebral and basilar arteries. The brain stem is supplied by end-arteries and thus has poor collateral flow. The arteries that supply the brain stem are usually not visible. In contrast, the vessels that supply the vermis and cerebellar hemispheres have good collateral circulation and are readily visible.

Vertebral Artery

After entering the cranium through the foramen magnum, the vertebral artery supplies the medulla and the inferior half of the cerebellum as well as the meninges. The arteries that supply the medulla, the tonsils, and the inferior half of the vermis and cerebellar hemispheres are paired, whereas the arteries that supply the meninges are not paired. The extracranial portion of the vertebral artery extends from its subclavian artery origin to the foramen magnum. This portion of the artery is well protected because it ascends through the transverse foramen of C6 to C1.

Anterior and Posterior Meningeal Arteries. The dura covering the occipital bone, as well as the adjacent falx and tentorium, is supplied by the posterior meningeal branch of the vertebral artery.[90] The anterior meningeal artery supplies the dura in the condylar area.[89] The two vertebral meningeal arteries may be augmented by the middle meningeal, ascending pharyngeal, and occipital branches of the external carotid artery.[91,92] In addition, the meningohypophyseal trunk of the internal carotid artery also supplies the clivus.

Posterior Inferior Cerebellar Arteries (PICAs). The PICAs are usually the last branches to originate from the vertebral artery and supply the medulla, the tonsils, and the inferior half of the vermis and cerebellar hemispheres. In approximately 25 percent of normal individuals, the PICAs may be absent. In this situation their territories are supplied by the anterior inferior cerebellar arteries.[93,94]

The course of the PICAs begins on the anterior surface of the medulla close to the olive and then proceeds laterally around the medulla, where the PICAs loop inferiorly (caudal loops)[95,96] (Fig. 12-35). The caudal loops course beneath the foramen magnum in approximately one-third of individuals.[97]

After the PICAs reach the back of the medulla, they usually run superiorly along the posterior medullary velum on either side of the midline (anteromedial aspect of the tonsils). They then course over the superior pole of the tonsils (cranial loops). The cranial loops

Figure 12-35. Termination of the right vertebral artery in the right PICA. (A) The caudal (*bottom arrow*) and cranial (*top arrow*) loops of the PICA are identified. The apex of the cranial loop is not as well rounded as that of the caudal loop. (B) The cranial loop (*left arrow*) can be used to evaluate midline shifts (±5 mm). The caudal loop (*right arrow*) is also identified. The contralateral left PICA is partially filled from the right PICA. The right inferior vermian artery (*arrowheads*) demonstrates a typical outward convexity, whereas the contralateral vermian artery is straight. The vermian arteries, although closely related to the midline, are a less reliable indicator than the cranial loop of the PICAs. (A) Lateral projection; (B) AP half-axial projection.

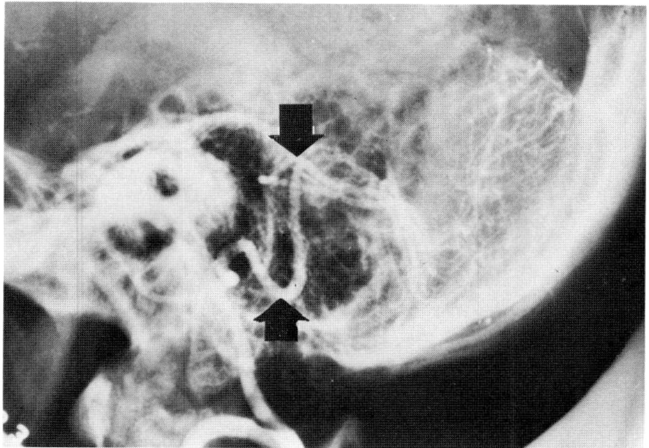

A

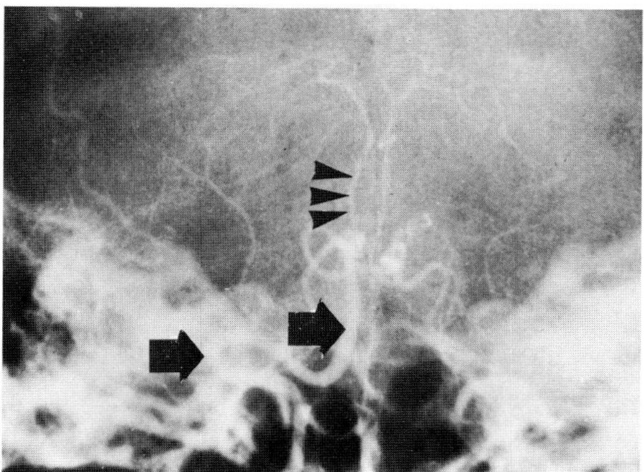

B

may be low or high depending on the attachment of the inferior medullary velum.[96,98]

After the PICAs have reached the posterior surface of the tonsils, they continue downward and then loop convex inferiorly around the vermis (inferior vermian arteries). As the PICAs begin to course posteriorly on the vermis, they give off tonsillar and hemispheric branches. On half-axial views the inferior vermian arteries are usually located on either side of the midline. However, they may be located up to 1 cm from the midline.[97]

Basilar Artery

The basilar artery, which is formed by a union of the vertebral arteries, frequently takes a tortuous course. Tortuosity is related to vertebral dominance, with the proximal portion of the basilar artery curving away from the dominant vertebral artery and the distal segment curving back toward the same artery (see Fig. 12-30).[99] The two major groups of branches of the basilar artery, the anterior inferior cerebellar arteries and the superior cerebellar arteries, are paired arteries.

Anterior Inferior Cerebellar Arteries (AICAs). The AICAs are the first large vessels to arise from the basilar artery. On anteroposterior angiograms they course horizontally toward the cerebellopontine angle and then bifurcate (Fig. 12-36). The lateral division curls around the flocculus, thereby giving the appearance of a loop, before continuing farther laterally to supply the anterior inferior surfaces of the cerebellum. The medial divisions course downward to anastomose with the PICAs.

On anteroposterior angiograms the AICAs are usually displaced superiorly by cerebellopontine angle masses but can also be displaced posteriorly and inferiorly by these masses. On lateral angiograms the AICAs frequently loop upward toward the porus acusticus internus. The arteries may form a second loop to create an M-shaped appearance if they course over the flocculus.[100]

Superior Cerebellar Arteries. The superior cerebellar arteries are useful in evaluating the midbrain because they almost encircle the mesencephalon (see Fig. 12-30). They usually originate in the interpeduncular cistern and then follow a slight downward direction as they begin to course around the mesencephalon. The medial continuation of the arteries outlines the superior surface of the vermis (superior vermian arteries). The lateral branches to the cerebellar hemispheres may project superiorly to the occipital branches of the posterior cerebral arteries on lateral angiograms because of the slope of the tentorium.

Outward displacement of the perimesencephalic portion of the superior cerebellar arteries on a half-axial projection indicates expansion of the brain stem. On a lateral angiogram the same mass causes the initial segments of the arteries to lose their downward arc and assume a straight line.[101] Inward displacement indicates an extra-axial mass anterior or anterolateral to the upper brain stem.

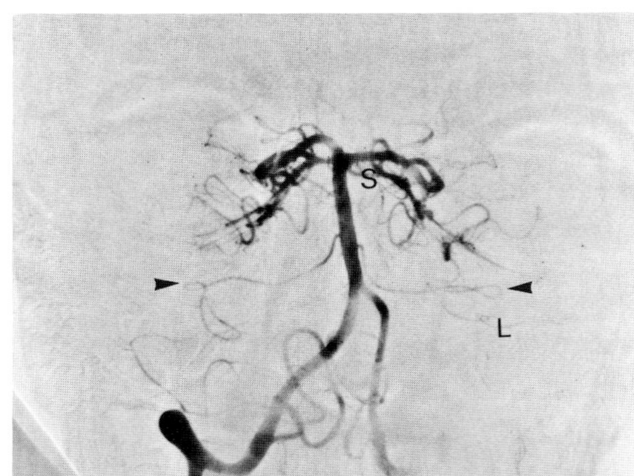

Figure 12-36. The anterior inferior cerebellar arteries. The arteries course laterally into the cerebellopontine angle cisterns, where they loop (*arrowheads*). A lateral branch (*L*) supplies the anteroinferior surface of the cerebellum. The superior cerebellar (*S*) artery is also shown. AP transfacial projection.

Posterior Fossa Veins

The three major groups of veins in the posterior fossa are identified according to their direction of flow. A superior group drains into the great vein of Galen, an anterior group drains into the petrosal sinuses, and a posterior group drains into the torcular Herophili and the transverse sinuses.[98] Dominance of one of these three groups of veins will usually result in decreased prominence of the other two groups of veins.

Superior Group. The superior group is perhaps the most important because it contains the precentral cerebellar vein (PCV). The PCV, which originates deep in the precentral cerebellar fissure, can be used on lateral angiograms to divide the superior portion of the posterior fossa into an anterior and a posterior compartment. The inferior colliculus, superior medullary velum, and lingula lie just anterior to the PCV, with the vermis posterior to it.[102] The inferior portion of this vein is located at the midpoint of Twining's line (±5 percent) (Fig. 12-37).[103] Lesions located anterior to this point push it backward whereas lesions posterior to it displace it forward.

The posterior mesencephalic veins drain the posterior perforated substance and the cerebral peduncles.

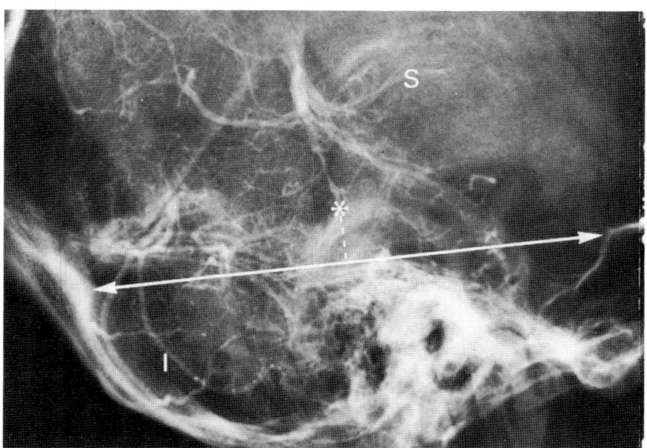

Figure 12-37. Precentral cerebellar vein. The colliculocentral point (*asterisk*) is located at the midpoint of Twining's line (*solid line*). The superior thalamic (*S*) and inferior vermian (*I*) veins are also shown. Lateral projection.

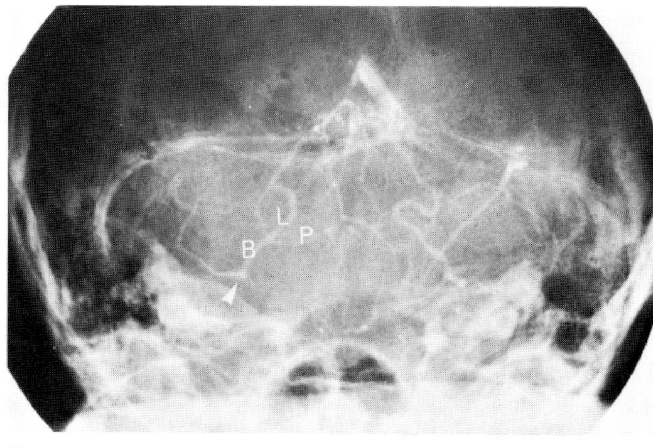

A

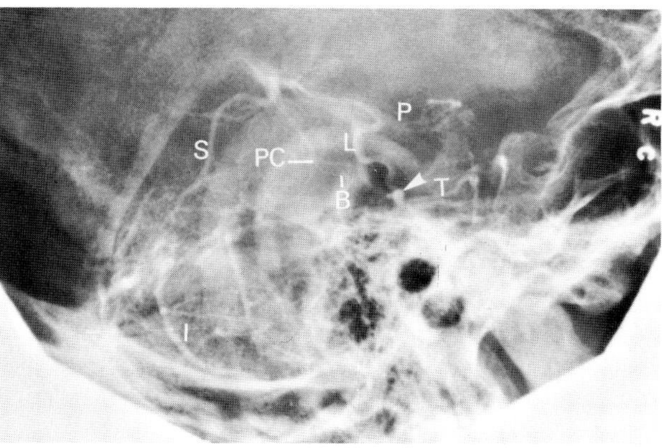

B

Figure 12-38. Superior posterior fossa veins. (A) The posterior mesencephalic (*P*) vein outlines the mesencephalon and drains into the great vein of Galen. The brachial (*B*) vein drains into the petrosal vein (*arrowhead*). The lateral mesencephalic (*L*) vein connects the posterior mesencephalic and brachial veins. (B) The corresponding posterior mesencephalic (*P*), lateral mesencephalic (*L*), brachial (*B*), and petrosal (*arrowhead*) veins are shown. In addition, the precentral cerebellar (*PC*), superior vermian (*S*), inferior vermian (*I*), and transverse pontine (*T*) veins are identified. (A) AP half-axial projection; (B) lateral projection.

They are usually closely related to the cerebral peduncles and on a half-axial projection frequently outline it (Figs. 12-38 and 12-39). The posterior mesencephalic veins usually take a more direct course to the great vein of Galen than do the basal veins of Rosenthal.

The superior vermian veins drain the superior surface of the vermis and adjacent cerebellum. These veins outline the superior surface of the vermis and occupy a position that roughly corresponds to the vermian branches of the superior cerebellar arteries.

Anterior Group. The anterior pontomesencephalic (APMC) vein drains the interpeduncular fossa, as well as the anterior surfaces of the pons and cerebellum. The APMC vein outlines the anterior surface of the pons and should be located just posterior to the basilar artery. It usually drains into the petrosal veins via the transverse pontine veins (see Fig. 12-39).

The petrosal veins are located in the cerebellopontine angles close to the porus acusticus internus. In the half-axial projection the petrosal veins resemble a star because they receive tributaries from various directions (see Fig. 12-39; Fig. 12-40). They receive medial branches from the pons (transverse pontine veins), lateral branches from the cerebellar hemispheres (superior hemispheric veins, veins of the greater horizontal fissure, and inferior hemispheric veins), supermedial branches from the wings of the precentral cerebellar fissure (brachial veins), and inferomedial branches from the cerebellar pontine fissure (inferior branches from the hemisphere and veins of the lateral recess). Displacement and nonfilling of a petrosal vein may suggest a cerebellopontine angle tumor, especially if the ipsilateral PICA is well filled.[104]

Posterior Group. The inferior vermian veins outline the inferior surface of the vermis and roughly correspond to the position occupied by the vermian branches of the PICA (see Fig. 12-39). They are formed by superior and inferior retrotonsillar tributaries, which outline the posterior border of the tonsils.

Collateral Circulation

Following the occlusion of a cerebral artery, the need for blood in the affected portion of the brain may be met if the collateral circulation is sufficiently well developed. Collateral flow may occur extracranially from the external carotid artery to the internal carotid artery

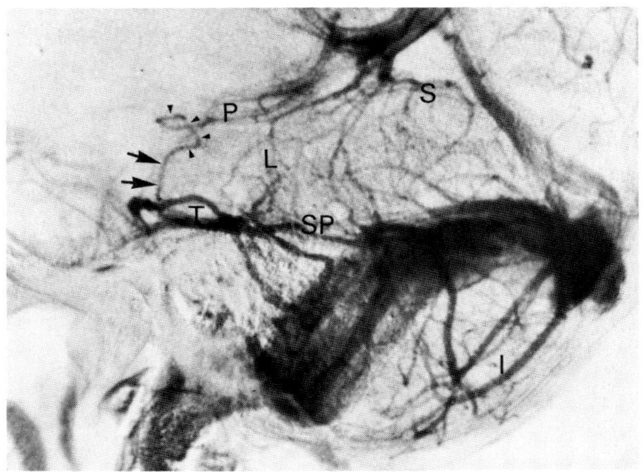

A

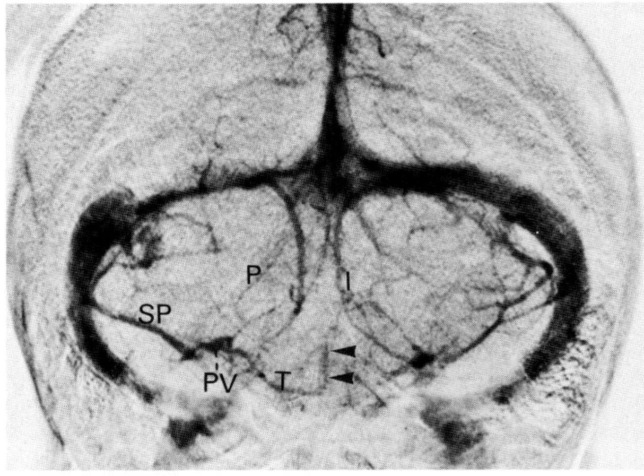

B

Figure 12-39. Anterior group of posterior fossa veins. (A) The anterior pontomesencephalic vein outlines the anterior border of the interpeduncular fossa (*arrowheads*) and the pons (*arrows*). Posterior mesencephalic (*P*), lateral mesencephalic (*L*), superior vermian (*S*), inferior vermian (*I*), and transverse pontine (*T*) veins are identified, as is the superior petrosal (*SP*) sinus. (B) The anterior pontomesencephalic veins (*arrowheads*) drain into the transverse pontine (*T*) vein, which subsequently drains into the petrosal vein (*PV*). The superior petrosal (*SP*) sinus and the posterior mesencephalic (*P*) and inferior vermian (*I*) veins are also shown. (A) Lateral projection; (B) AP half-axial projection.

or intracranially by anastomoses in the subarachnoid space and the leptomeninges. Intracranial subarachnoid shunts occur in the circle of Willis, in the terminal branches of the cerebral arteries, and in embryonic connections between the basilar and carotid arteries.

The best-known intracranial collateral system is the circle of Willis. It is made up anteriorly by a segment of the supraclinoid internal carotid arteries, the A_1 segments of the anterior cerebral arteries, and the anterior communicating artery; laterally by the posterior communicating arteries; and posteriorly by the proximal portion of the posterior cerebral arteries. When one of the major vessels in the circle is occluded, blood flows from the normal to the lower-pressure areas, thus minimizing neurologic complications.[105] Unfortunately, the circle is complete in about only 50 percent of individuals.[64]

Figure 12-40. Petrosal vein. The left petrosal vein (*PV*) drains the brachial (*B*) vein, vein of the great horizontal fissure (*H*), and vein of the lateral recess (*L*). The inferior vermian (*I*) vein is also shown. AP half-axial projection.

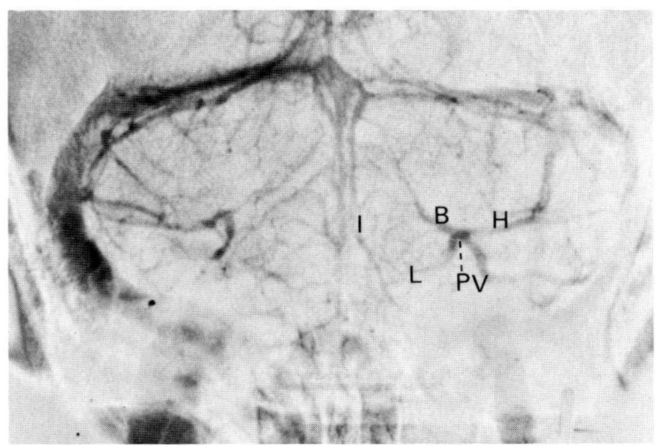

Anteriorly, the anterior communicating artery is anatomically hypoplastic in 3 percent of individuals and the A_1 segment is hypoplastic in another 2 percent.[64] Cross-compression, however, can exaggerate anatomic changes in the anterior segment of the circle; it has been shown that when this technique is used, the contralateral middle cerebral arteries are not visualized in 23 percent of patients.[106] Anterior cerebral artery hypoplasia of the A_1 segment is associated with aneurysms of the anterior communicating artery.[107] Posteriorly, anatomic variations are more frequent; the posterior communicating arteries are hypoplastic in 22 percent of individuals.[64]

When the circle of Willis is incomplete and the internal carotid artery is occluded, blood may be supplied by extracranial arteries. The most common route is antegrade flow through the external carotid artery and then retrograde flow through the ophthalmic artery to the internal carotid artery (see Fig. 12-12).[108] A small amount of additional blood may be supplied through the rete mirabile from the meningeal arteries to the cortical arteries on the surface of the cerebrum.[109] When the posterior communicating arteries are hypoplastic and the vertebral vascular system is oc-

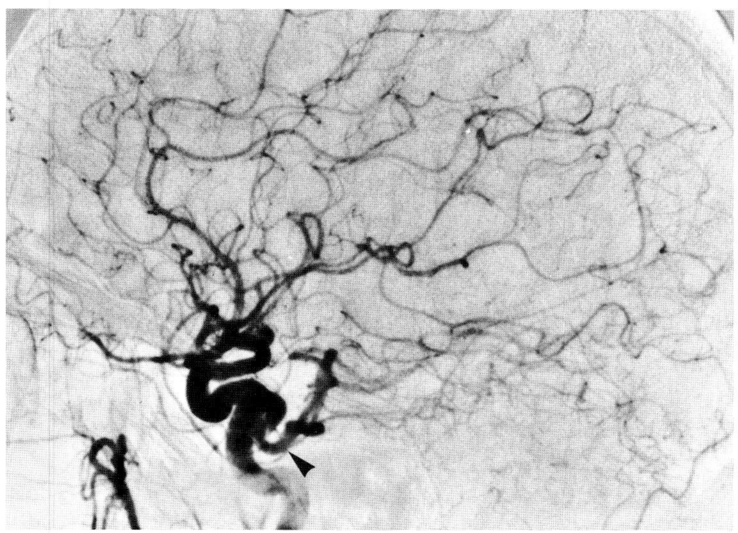

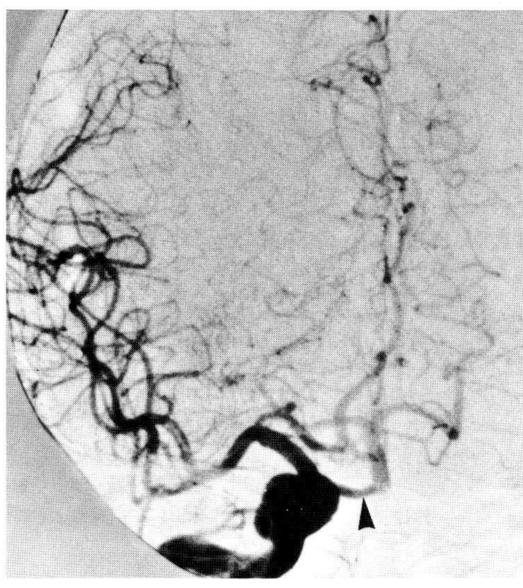

Figure 12-41. Views of the trigeminal artery (*arrowhead*) as it connects the precavernous segment of the internal carotid artery to the midportion of the basilar artery. (A) Lateral projection; (B) AP projection.

cluded, blood may flow through muscular branches to the distal vertebral artery.

The terminal cortical branches of the anterior, middle, and posterior cerebral arteries anastomose supratentorially on the surface of the cerebrum, and similar branches of the posterior inferior, anterior inferior, and superior cerebellar arteries communicate with one another infratentorially on the surface of the cerebellum.[110] The network formed by these vessels supplies blood whenever a pressure gradient arises or when local factors such as PCO_2, pH, and PO_2 change.[111] Unfortunately, the deep penetrating (medullary) arteries that arise from this network do not anastomose with one another, so occlusion of these vessels invariably results in infarctions.

Of the potential embryonic communications between the internal carotid artery and the basilar artery, the persistent trigeminal artery is the most common. It connects the precavernous segment of the internal carotid artery with the basilar artery (between the superior cerebellar and anterior inferior cerebellar arteries) (Fig. 12-41).[112] This anomaly has been associated with aneurysms, arteriovenous malformations, and both primary and metastatic brain tumors.[113,114] The hypoglossal artery, a less frequent connection, joins the cervical portion of the internal carotid artery with the lower end of the basilar artery after passing through the hypoglossal canal. The persistent hypoglossal artery has been associated with aneurysms, other anastomoses, primary brain tumors, and internal carotid occlusions.[115,116] The persistent otic artery connects the petrous segment of the internal carotid artery with the anterior inferior cerebellar artery after traversing the temporal bone and exits through the internal auditory canal.

References

1. Moniz E. L'encéphalographie artérielle, son importance dans la localisation des tumeurs cérébrales. Rev Neurol (Paris) 1927;2:72–90.
2. Seldinger SI. Catheter replacement of the needle in percutaneous arteriography. Acta Radiol (Stockh) 1953;39:368–376.
3. Geddes LA, Geddes LE. The catheter introducers. Chicago: Mobium, 1993.
4. American College of Radiology and Society of Cardiovascular and Interventional Radiology. Standard for diagnostic arteriography in adults. Reston, VA: ACR, 1993.
5. Katayama H, Yamaguchi K, Kozuka T, et al. Adverse reactions to ionic and nonionic contrast media. Radiology 1990;175: 621–628.
6. Barrett BJ, Parfrey PS, McDonald JR, et al. Nonionic low-osmolality versus ionic high-osmolality contrast material for intravenous use in patients perceived to be at high risk: randomized trial. Radiology 1992;183:105–110.
7. Shehadi WH, Toniolo G. Adverse reactions to contrast media. Radiology 1980;137:299–302.
8. Latchaw RE. The use of nonionic contrast agents in neuroangiography: a review of the literature and recommendations for clinical use. Invest Radiol 1993;28(Suppl 5):S55–S59.
9. Goldfarb S, Spinler S, Berns JS, et al. Low-osmolality contrast media and the risk of contrast-associated nephrotoxicity. Invest Radiol 1993;28(Suppl 5):S7–S10.
10. Fareed J, Walenga JM, Saravia GE, et al. Thrombogenic potential of nonionic contrast media? Radiology 1990;174: 321–325.

11. Kopko PM, Smith DC, Bull BS. Thrombin generation in nonclottable mixtures of blood and nonionic contrast agents. Radiology 1990;174:459–461.
12. Grabowski EF, Kaplan KL, Halpern EF. Anticoagulant effects of nonionic versus ionic contrast media in angiography syringes. Invest Radiol 1991;26:417–421.
13. Grabowski EF, Head C, Michelson AD. Nonionic contrast media: procoagulants or clotting innocents? Invest Radiol 1993;28(Suppl 5):S21–S24.
14. Dawson P, Cousins C, Bradshaw A. The clotting issue: etiologic factors in thromboembolism: II. Clinical considerations. Invest Radiol 1993;28(Suppl 5):S31–S36.
15. American College of Radiology. Manual on iodinated contrast media. Reston, VA: ACR, 1991.
16. Hankey GJ, Warlow CP, Sellar RJ. Cerebral angiographic risk in mild cerebrovascular disease. Stroke 1990;21:209–222.
17. Waugh JR, Sacharias N. Arteriographic complications in the DSA era. Radiology 1992;182:243–246.
18. Mani RL, Eisenberg RL, McDonald EJ, et al. Complications of catheter cerebral arteriography: analysis of 5,000 procedures: I. Criteria and incidence. AJR 1978;131:861–865.
19. Hessel SJ, Adams DF, Abrams HL. Complications of angiography. Radiology 1981;138:273–281.
20. Gritter KJ, Laidlaw WW, Peterson NT. Complications of outpatient transbrachial intraarterial digital subtraction angiography. Radiology 1987;162:125–127.
21. Rupp SB, Vogelzang RL, Nemcek AA, et al. Relationship of the inguinal ligament to pelvic radiographic landmarks: anatomic correlation and its role in femoral arteriography. J Vasc Intervent Radiol 1993;4:409–413.
22. Lin JP, Kricheff II. Angiographic investigation of cerebral aneurysms. Radiology 1972;105:69–76.
23. Perret G, Nishioka H. Cerebral angiography. In: Sahs AL, Perret GE, Locksley HB, Nishioka H, eds. Intracranial aneurysms and subarachnoid hemorrhage. Philadelphia: Lippincott, 1969:109–124.
24. Gilbert JW, Lee C, Young B. Repeat cerebral pan-angiography in subarachnoid hemorrhage of unknown etiology. Surg Neurol 1990;33:19–21.
25. Forster DMC, Steiner L, Hakanson S, et al. The value of repeat pan-angiography in cases of unexplained subarachnoid hemorrhage. J Neurosurg 1978;48:712–716.
26. Zweibel WJ. Duplex sonography of the cerebral arteries: efficacy, limitations and indications. AJR 1992;158:29–36.
27. Bowen BC, Quencer RM, Margosian P, et al. MR angiography of occlusive disease of the arteries in the head and neck: current concepts. AJR 1994;162:9–18.
28. Dillon EH, van Leeuwen MS, Fernandez MA, et al. CT angiography: application to the evaluation of carotid artery stenosis. Radiology 1993;189:211–219.
29. Schwartz RB, Jones KM, Chernoff DM, et al. Common carotid artery bifurcation: evaluation with spiral CT. Radiology 1992;185:513–519.
30. Marks MP, Napel S, Jordan JE, et al. Diagnosis of carotid artery disease: preliminary experience with maximum-intensity-projection spiral CT angiography. AJR 1993;160:1267–1271.
31. Derdeyn CP, Moran CJ, Cross DT, et al. Intraoperative digital subtraction angiography: a review of 112 consecutive examinations. Am J Neuroradiol;16:307–318.
32. Derdeyn CP, Moran CJ, Eichling J, Cross DT. Radiation exposure to patients and personnel during intraoperative neuroangiography. AJR 1994;162:S115.
33. Bosniak MA. An analysis of some anatomic-roentgenologic aspects of the brachiocephalic vessels. AJR 1964;91:1222–1231.
34. Williams GD, Edmonds HW. Variations in arrangement of the branches arising from aortic arch in American whites and negroes. Anat Rec 1935;62:139–146.
35. Sutton D, Davies ER. Arch aortography and cerebrovascular insufficiency. Clin Radiol 1966;17:330–345.
36. Wilson M. The anatomic foundation of neuroradiology of the brain. 2nd ed. Boston: Little, Brown, 1972.
37. Teal JS, Rumbaugh CL, Bergeron RT, et al. Lateral position of the external carotid artery: a rare anomaly? Radiology 1973;108:77–81.
38. Djindjian R, Merland JJ. Super-selective arteriography of the external carotid artery. Berlin: Springer, 1978:127–149.
39. Rosen L, Hanafee W, Nahum A. Nasopharyngeal angiofibroma, an angiographic evaluation. Radiology 1966;86:103–107.
40. Newton TH, Kramer RA. Clinical uses of selective external carotid arteriography. AJR 1966;97:458–472.
41. Allen WE III, Kier EL, Rothman SLG. Maxillary artery in craniofacial pathology. AJR 1974;121:124–138.
42. Baumel JJ, Beard DY. The accessory meningeal artery of man. J Anat 1961;95:386–402.
43. Elliot PD, Baker HL, Brown AL. The superficial temporal artery angiogram. Radiology 1972;102:635–638.
44. Moniz E, Lima PA, Caldas P. A filmogen da circulacão cerebral. Med Contemp 1933; No. 3.
45. Dilenge D, Heón M. The internal carotid artery. In: Newton TH, Potts DG, eds. Radiology of the skull and brain: Vol. 2. Angiography. Great Neck, NY: MediBooks, 1974:1202–1245.
46. Parkinson D. Collateral circulation of cavernous carotid artery: anatomy. Can J Surg 1964;7:251–268.
47. Wallace S, Goldberg HI, Leeds NE, et al. The cavernous branches of the internal carotid artery. AJR 1967;101:34–46.
48. Kramer R, Newton TH. Tentorial branches of internal carotid artery. AJR 1965;95:826–830.
49. Hayreh SS. The ophthalmic artery: III. Branches. Br J Ophthalmol 1962;46:212–247.
50. Hayreh SS, Dass R. The ophthalmic artery: II. Intra-orbital course. Br J Ophthalmol 1962;46:165–185.
51. DiChiro G. Angiographic topography of the choroid. Am J Ophthalmol 1962;54:232–237.
52. Pollock JA, Newton TH. The anterior falx artery: normal and pathologic anatomy. Radiology 1968;91:1089–1095.
53. Dilenge DD, Ascherl GF Jr. Variations of the ophthalmic and middle meningeal arteries: relation to the embryonic stapedial artery. AJNR 1980;1:45–54.
54. Gabriele OF, Bell D. Ophthalmic origin of the middle meningeal artery. Radiology 1967;89:841–844.
55. Vignaud J, Hasso AN, Lasjaunias P, et al. Orbital vascular anatomy and embryology. Radiology 1974;111:617–626.
56. Taveras JM, Wood EW. Diagnostic neuroradiology. Baltimore: Williams & Wilkins, 1964.
57. Sjögren SE. The anterior choroidal artery. Acta Radiol (Stockh) 1956;46:143–157.
58. Lindgren E. Röntgenologie. In: Olivecrona H, Tönnis W, eds. Handbuch der Neurochirurgie. Berlin: Springer, 1954; 2:1–295.
59. Riggs HE, Rupp C. Variation in form of circle of Willis. The relation of the variations to collateral circulation: anatomic analysis. Arch Neurol 1963;8:8–14.
60. Krayenbuhl HA, Yasargil MG. Cerebral angiography. 2nd ed. London: Butterworths, 1968.
61. Ostrowski A, Weber JE, Gurdjian ES. The proximal anterior cerebral artery: an anatomic study. Arch Neurol 1960;3:661–664.
62. Stephens RB, Stilwell DL. Arteries and veins of the human brain. Springfield, IL: Thomas, 1969.
63. Morris AA, Peck CM. Roentgenographic study of the variations in the normal anterior cerebral artery: one hundred case studies in the lateral plane. AJR 1955;74:818–826.
64. Alpers BJ, Barry RG, Paddison RM. Anatomical studies of the circle of Willis in normal brain. Arch Neurol 1959;81:409–418.
65. LeMay M, Gooding CA. The clinical significance of the azygous anterior cerebral artery (A.C.A.). AJR 1966;98:602–610.

66. Ring BA, Waddington MM. Roentgenographic anatomy of the pericallosal arteries. AJR 1968;104:109–118.
67. Ring BA, Waddington MM. Ascending frontal branch of middle cerebral artery. Acta Radiol (Stockh) 1967;6:209–219.
68. Gabrielsen TO, Greitz T. Normal size of the internal carotid, middle cerebral and anterior cerebral arteries. Acta Radiol (Stockh) 1970;10:1–16.
69. Leeds NE, Goldberg HI. Lenticulostriate artery abnormalities: value of direct serial magnification. Radiology 1970;97: 377–383.
70. Dahlstrom L, Fagerberg G, Lanner L, et al. Anatomical and angiographic studies of arteries supplying anterior part of temporal lobe: a preliminary report. Acta Radiol (Stockh) 1969; 9:257–263.
71. Vlahovitch B, Gros C, Adib-Yazdi IS, et al. Réparage du sillon insulaire supérieur sur l'angiographie carotidienne de profil. Neurochirurgie 1964;10:91–99.
72. Taveras JM, Poser CM. Roentgenologic aspects of cerebral angiography in children. AJR 1959;82:371–391.
73. Fernandez Serrats AA, Vlahovitch B, Parker SA. The arteriographic pattern of the insula: its normal appearance and variation in cases of tumor of the cerebral hemispheres. J Neurol Neurosurg Psychiatry 1968;31:379–390.
74. LeMay M, Culebras A. Human brain—morphologic differences in the hemisphere demonstrable by carotid arteriography. N Engl J Med 1972;287:168–170.
75. Gibo H, Carver CC, Rhoton AL, Len Koy C, Mitchell RJ. Microsurgical anatomy of middle cerebral artery. J Neurosurg 1981;54:151–159.
76. Ring BA. Middle cerebral artery: anatomical and radiographic study. Acta Radiol (Stockh) 1962;57:289–300.
77. Ring BA. The cerebral cortical arteries. In: Salamon G, ed. Advances in cerebral angiography. Berlin: Springer, 1975:25–32.
78. Azambuja N, Lindgren E, Sjögren SE. Tentorial herniations: III. Angiography. Acta Radiol (Stockh) 1956;46:232–241.
79. Wolf BS, Newman CM, Schlesinger B. The diagnostic value of the deep cerebral veins in cerebral angiography. Radiology 1955;64:161–177.
80. Wolf BS, Huang YP. The subependymal veins of the lateral ventricles. AJR 1964;91:406–426.
81. Hooshmand I, Rosenbaum AE, Stein RL. Radiographic anatomy of normal cerebral deep medullary veins: criteria for distinguishing them from their abnormal counterparts. Neuroradiology 1974;7:75–84.
82. Huang YP, Wolf BS. Veins of white matter of the cerebral hemisphere (the medullary veins): diagnostic importance in carotid angiography. AJR 1964;92:739–755.
83. Wolf BS, Huang YP, Newman CM. The superficial sylvian venous drainage system. AJR 1963;89:398–410.
84. Giudicelli G, Salomon G. The veins of the thalamus. Neuroradiology 1970;1:92–98.
85. Kaplan HA, Browder AA, Browder J. Atresia of the rostral superior sagittal sinus: associated cerebral venous patterns. Neuroradiology 1972;4:208–211.
86. Bub B, Ferris EJ, Levy PS, et al. The cerebral venogram: a statistical analysis of the sequence of venous filling in cerebral angiograms. Radiology 1968;91:1112–1118.
87. Leeds NE, Taveras JM. Dynamic factors in diagnosis of supratentorial brain tumors by cerebral angiography. Philadelphia: Saunders, 1969.
88. White E, Greitz T. Subependymal venous filling sequence at cerebral angiography: influence of grey and white matter distribution. Acta Radiol (Stockh) 1972;13:272–285.
89. Greitz T, Lauren T. Anterior meningeal branch of the vertebral artery. Acta Radiol (Stockh) 1968;7:219–223.
90. Newton TH. The anterior and posterior meningeal branches of the vertebral artery. Radiology 1968;91:271–279.
91. Levine HL, Ferris EJ, Spatz EL. External carotid blood supply to acoustic neurinomas: report of two cases. J Neurosurg 1973;38:516–520.
92. Théron J, Lasjaunias P. Participation of the external and internal carotid in the blood supply of acoustic neurinomas. Radiology 1976;118:83–88.
93. Stopford, JSB. The arteries of the pons and medulla oblongata. J Anat 1916;50:131–164.
94. Takahashi M, Wilson G, Hanafee W. The anterior inferior cerebellar artery: its radiographic anatomy and significance in the diagnosis of extra-axial tumors of the posterior fossa. Radiology 1968;90:281–287.
95. Greitz T, Sjögren SE. The posterior inferior cerebellar artery. Acta Radiol (Stockh) 1963;1:284–297.
96. Wolf BS, Newman CM, Khlilnani MT. The posterior inferior cerebellar artery on vertebral angiography. AJR 1962;87: 322–337.
97. Margolis MT, Newton TH. Borderlands of the normal and abnormal posterior inferior cerebellar artery. Acta Radiol (Stockh) 1972;13:163–176.
98. Huang YP, Wolf BS. Angiographic features of fourth ventricle tumors with special reference to the posterior inferior cerebellar artery. AJR 1969;107:543–564.
99. Haverline M. The tortuous basilar artery. Acta Radiol (Stockh) 1974;15:241–249.
100. Naidich TP, Kricheff II, George AE, et al. The anterior inferior cerebellar artery in mass lesions: preliminary findings with emphasis on the lateral projection. Radiology 1976;119:375–383.
101. Mani RL, Newton JH. The superior cerebellar artery: arteriographic changes in the diagnosis of posterior fossa lesions. Radiology 1969;92:1281–1287.
102. Huang YP, Wolf BS. The veins of the posterior fossa—superior or galenic draining group. AJR 1965;95:808–821.
103. Huang YP, Wolf BS. Precentral cerebellar vein in angiography. Acta Radiol (Stockh) 1966;5:250–262.
104. Takahashi M, Wilson G, Hanafee W. The significance of the petrosal vein in the diagnosis of the cerebellopontine angle tumors. Radiology 1967;89:834–840.
105. Kramer SP. On the function of the circle of Willis. J Exp Med 1912;15:348–357.
106. Sedzimir CB. An angiographic test of collateral circulation through the anterior segment of the circle of Willis. J Neurol Neurosurg Psychiatry 1959;22:64–68.
107. Allcock JM. Aneurysms. In: Newton TH, Potts DG, eds. Radiology of the skull and brain: Vol. 2. Angiography. Great Neck, NY: MediBooks, 1974;2435–2489.
108. Bossi R, Pisani C. Collateral cerebral circulation through the ophthalmic artery and its efficiency in internal carotid occlusion. Br J Radiol 1955;28:462–469.
109. Weidner W, Hanafee W, Markham CH. Intracranial collateral circulation via leptomeningeal and rete mirabile anastomoses. Neurology (Minneap) 1965;15:39–48.
110. Vander Eecken HM, Adams RD. The anatomy and functional significance of the meningeal arterial anastomoses of the human brain. J Neuropathol Exp Neurol 1953;12:132–156.
111. Meyer JS, Denny-Brown D. The cerebral collateral circulation: I. Factors influencing collateral blood flow. Neurology 1957;7:447–458.
112. Perryman CR, Gray GH, Brust RW Jr, et al. Interesting aspects of cerebral angiography with special emphasis on some unusual congenital variations. AJR 1963;89:372–383.
113. Gannon WE. Malformation of brain, persistent trigeminal artery and arteriovenous malformation. Arch Neurol 1962;6: 496–498.
114. Wolpert SM. The trigeminal artery and associated aneurysms. Neurology 1966;16:610–614.
115. Gilmartin D. Hypoglossal artery associated with internal carotid stenosis. Br J Radiol 1963;36:849–851.
116. Udvarhelyi GB, Lei M. Subarachnoid hemorrhage due to rupture of an aneurysm on a persistent left hypoglossal artery. Br J Radiol 1963;36:843–847.

13

Abnormalities of Cerebral Vessels

DEWITTE T. CROSS III
DANIEL K. KIDO
CHRISTOPHER J. MORAN

Indications for cerebral angiography have changed since computed tomographic (CT) and magnetic resonance imaging (MRI) have come into widespread use for diagnosing disorders of the central nervous system. When skull radiographs, pneumoencephalography, and angiography were the main diagnostic tools of the neuroradiologist, cerebral angiography was often requested as a screening examination to detect masses and extraaxial fluid collections. A thorough knowledge of vascular anatomy was the foundation for diagnosing what were sometimes subtle anatomic shifts, and diagnosing those abnormalities became an art that has, in many respects, been lost to the generation that grew up in neuroradiology after the advent of cross-sectional imaging. Whereas CT and MRI have greatly improved the ability of the physician to correctly diagnose tumors, infections, infarctions, hemorrhages, and extraaxial fluid collections beyond what would have been possible with angiography alone, conventional angiography has assumed a more important role in directing treatment because endovascular techniques such as embolization, fibrinolysis, and angioplasty are more commonly employed to improve patient outcome. Today cerebral angiography is frequently used to direct vascular or surgical intervention for a patient whose CT, MRI, or sonogram has already identified an abnormality that explains the clinical problem, or to simply identify and further characterize abnormalities of the vessels themselves.

Methods of performing cerebral angiography have also been modified with time. The standard cerebral angiogram of the past was an often lengthy procedure in which multiple rapid-sequence x-ray exposures were obtained on roll or cut film, development of the film was necessary to evaluate the images, and handmade subtractions were made after the examination was complete. Final analysis of the results on subtracted films after patient departure might have raised a question that led to repeat examination. Cut-film techniques are being replaced by digital methods of image acquisition in which image intensifiers take the place of film and electronic imaging chains take the place of manual development and subtraction methods. Final digital images can be recorded on film, but the time to perform and evaluate the examination is considerably shortened. Advances in imaging chains have led to digital images that are comparable to cut-film images in resolution, but which, compared to cut-film techniques, also offer a wider range of imaging rates, a greater variety of image manipulations, and a better chance for the physician to obtain adequate information from any one examination by virtue of the fact that final images are available for analysis immediately during and after contrast injection. If biplane digital capability exists, digital techniques can also lower contrast dose from that necessary for a comparable biplane cut-film examination.

Catheter and guidewire improvements have led to the use of smaller systems and improved vascular access. Selective examinations that would have been impossible in the past are less challenging now that hydrophilic materials are being used in manufacture. Microcatheters, some as small as 1.5 French, have been introduced and permit distal, superselective injections and intricate study of the vasculature in cases of arteriovenous malformations, aneurysms, thromboses, and tumors.

The cerebral angiogram of today, therefore, is likely to be ordered for different reasons and to be performed in a different manner than one ordered in the pre-CT, pre-MRI era. Noninvasive techniques such as MRA and MRV are now used for some indications. Findings on today's cerebral angiogram can lead to entirely different therapeutic interventions. Even though technology and therapy may have changed over the years, the underlying pathology and abnormalities evident on angiographic examinations have not changed, and these are the subject of this chapter.

Atherosclerotic Disease

Patients with a history of stroke or transient ischemic attack (TIA) are candidates for cerebral angiography. Angiography in most of these patients is performed to accurately assess the distribution and degree of atherosclerotic disease in order to direct patients to surgery, to angioplasty, or into medical treatment protocols (Fig. 13-1). Some patients with acute stroke symptoms are studied emergently for potential fibrinolytic therapy.[1] Some asymptomatic patients are studied because noninvasive imaging tests demonstrate high degrees of stenosis that might place them at increased risk for stroke.[2]

Extracranial carotid arteries can be imaged fairly reliably with ultrasound. Transcranial Doppler ultrasound, if available, may even provide limited information regarding intracranial vessels. Abnormally increased velocity in the middle cerebral artery, for example, suggests stenosis or spasm. Ultrasound, however, is more operator-dependent than other imaging methods[3] and has inherent technical limitations that limit accuracy and applicability. Heavily calcified arteries, for example, are difficult to assess, and stenosis may be overestimated. Ultrasound may indicate total occlusion of an internal carotid artery when, in fact, the artery is patent with a high-grade stenosis. Tandem stenotic lesions of the cervical and intracranial segments of the internal carotid arteries cannot be detected by ultrasound methods (Fig. 13-2).

Magnetic resonance angiography can be employed to evaluate both the extracranial and the intracranial cerebral vessels. Like ultrasound, the current methods have inherent technical limitations that do not allow foolproof distinctions between high-grade stenosis

Figure 13-1. Progressive carotid stenosis. A 59-year-old man was evaluated for transient ischemic attacks. (A) Initial left common carotid angiogram reveals 80 percent stenosis of the internal carotid artery origin (*arrow*). (B) Angiogram 2 years later reveals progression of the origin stenosis to 99 percent (*large arrow*). There is a "string sign" (*small arrows*) of the cervical internal carotid artery. (See Fig. 13-5.)

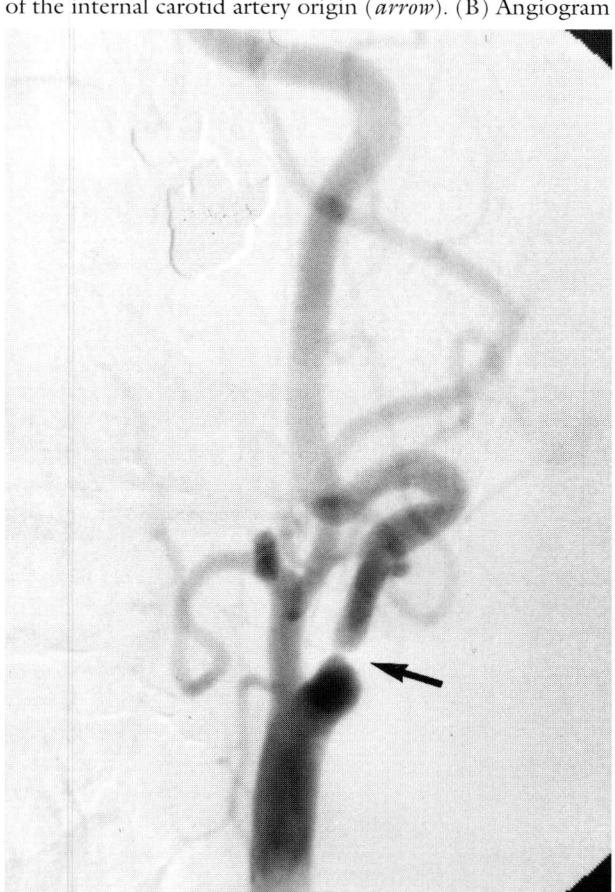

A

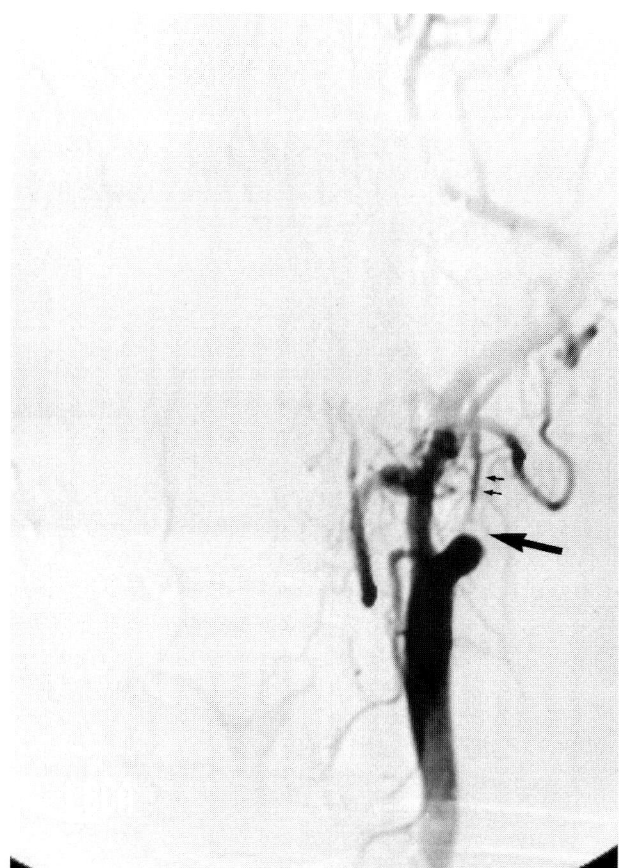

B

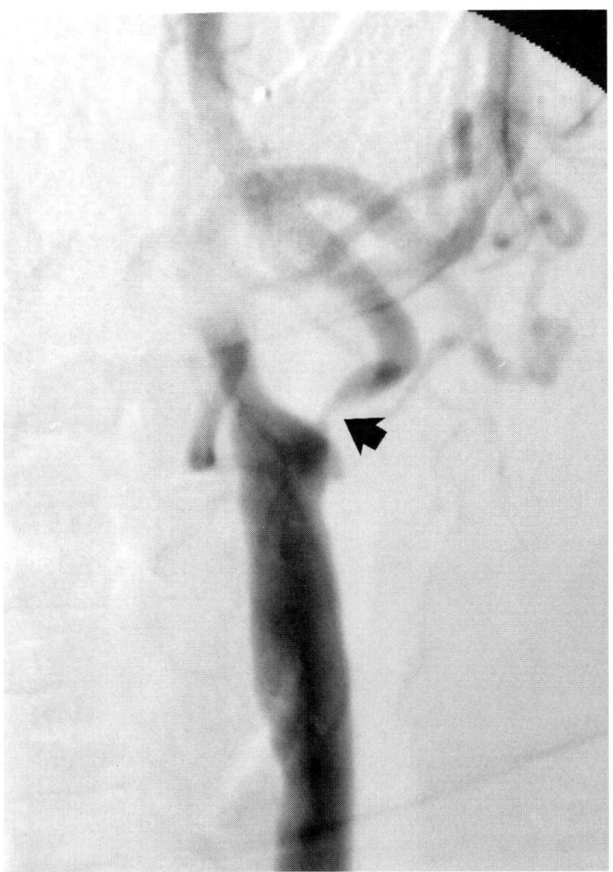

A

B

Figure 13-2. Tandem lesions. A 66-year-old woman experienced two episodes of right-hand weakness and aphasia. (A) Left common carotid angiogram demonstrates 85 percent stenosis of the internal carotid artery origin (*arrow*), but there is also disease distal to the carotid bifurcation. (B) Left common carotid angiogram shows 75 percent stenosis of the petrous segment of the internal carotid artery (*arrow*), and irregular atherosclerotic plaque is present just distal to the petrous stenosis.

and occlusion or provide accurate measurements of stenosis.[4,5] There have been proposals that ultrasonography and magnetic resonance angiography be employed together as a combined noninvasive screening method, and when abnormal or in disagreement, be followed by angiography for a definitive determination of disease. Adequate data are lacking, however, to permit replacement of conventional angiography by these less accurate noninvasive imaging tools, given current technology.[6–12]

The efficacy of surgical repair of carotid stenosis for the prevention of stroke was established by the North American Symptomatic Carotid Endarterectomy Trial (NASCET).[13] That multicenter trial of surgical versus medical therapy for patients with prior stroke or transient ischemic attack demonstrated a benefit from surgery if the degree of internal carotid stenosis was 70 percent or greater, specifically, a 17 percent reduction in the risk of ipsilateral stroke following endarterectomy in a 2-year follow-up period as compared to patients with similar stenoses who were treated medically. The surgical benefit occurred with a 2.1 percent incidence of perioperative major stroke and death and would have been eroded had surgical complications exceeded 10 percent. As a result of the study, there is continued interest in accurately evaluating the carotid artery in patients with TIA or stroke. The NASCET convention for measuring carotid stenosis is illustrated in Figure 13-3.[14]

Although the NASCET study answered some questions, others remain. The Asymptomatic Carotid Atherosclerosis Study showed a slight surgical benefit for asymptomatic carotid stenosis, given that surgical complications were kept low. For men with greater than 60 percent internal carotid artery stenosis who were asymptomatic, endarterectomy reduced the inci-

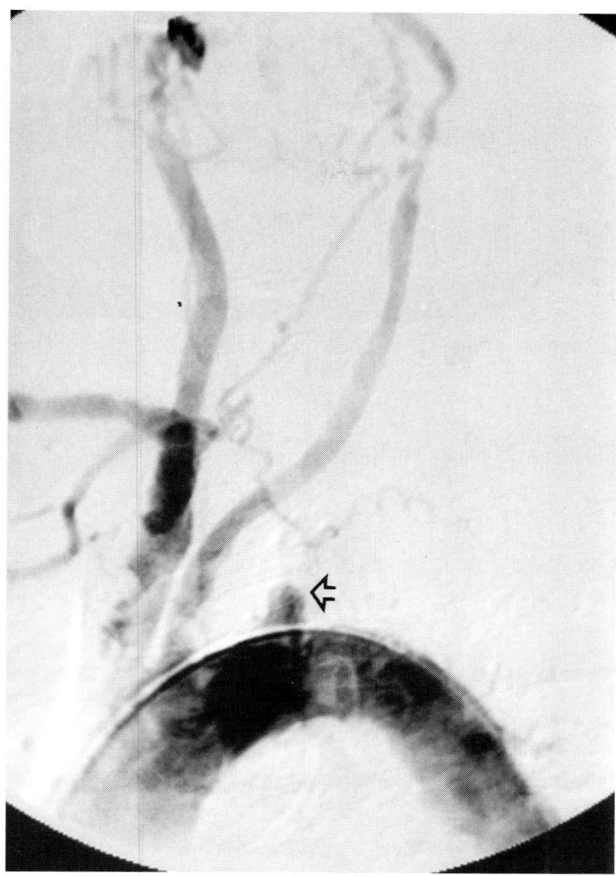

A

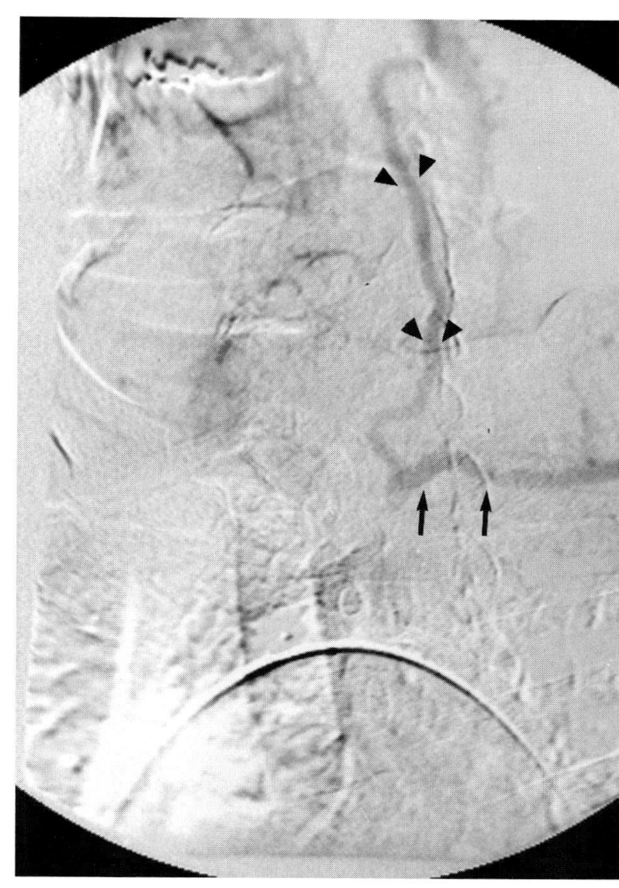

B

Figure 13-7. Subclavian steal. An 80-year-old man was evaluated for carotid artery disease. His aortic arch study reveals occlusion of the left subclavian artery at its origin (*open arrow,* A) and delayed filling of the distal subclavian artery (*solid arrows,* B). The distal subclavian artery is filled by retrograde flow from the left vertebral artery (*arrowheads,* B), so that there is a "steal" of flow from the cerebral circulation. In this case, the steal was asymptomatic.

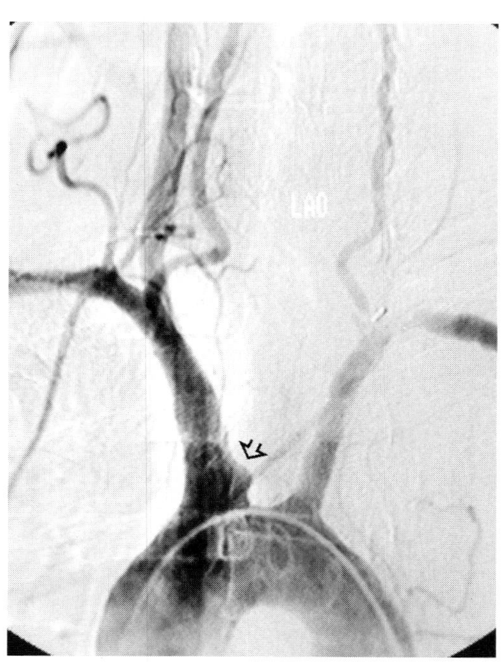

A

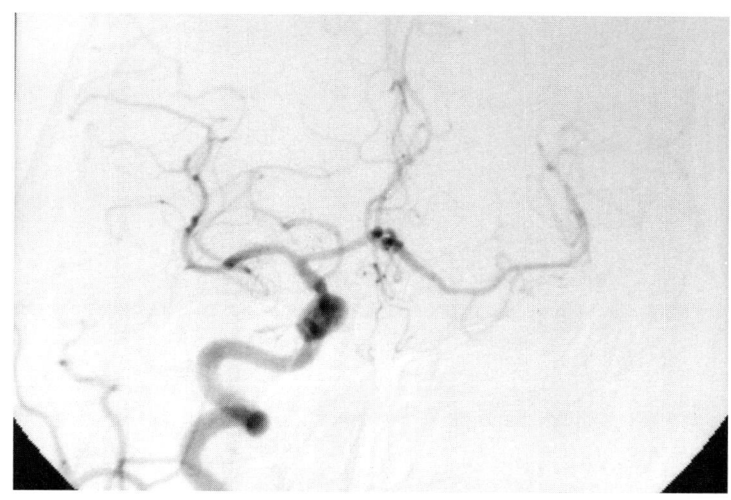

B

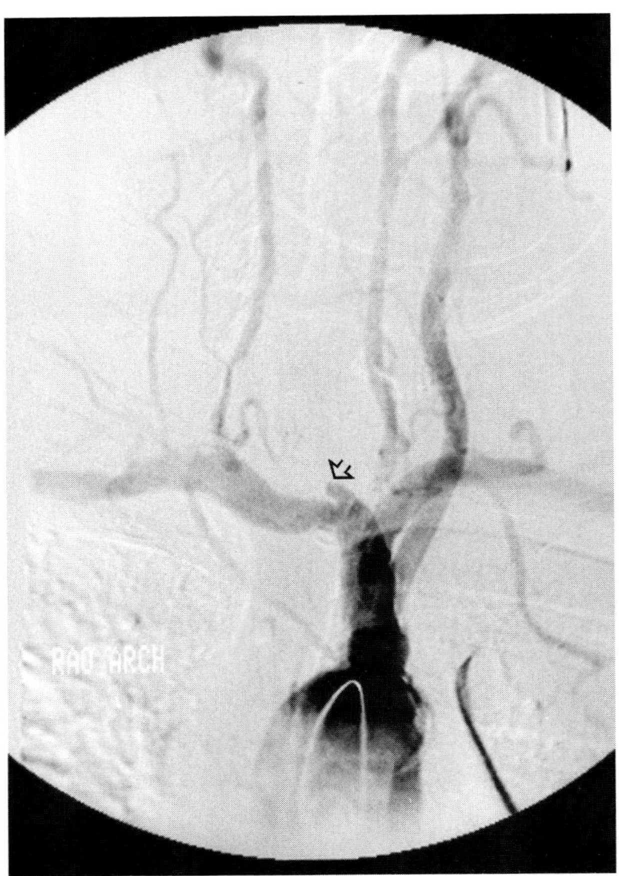

A

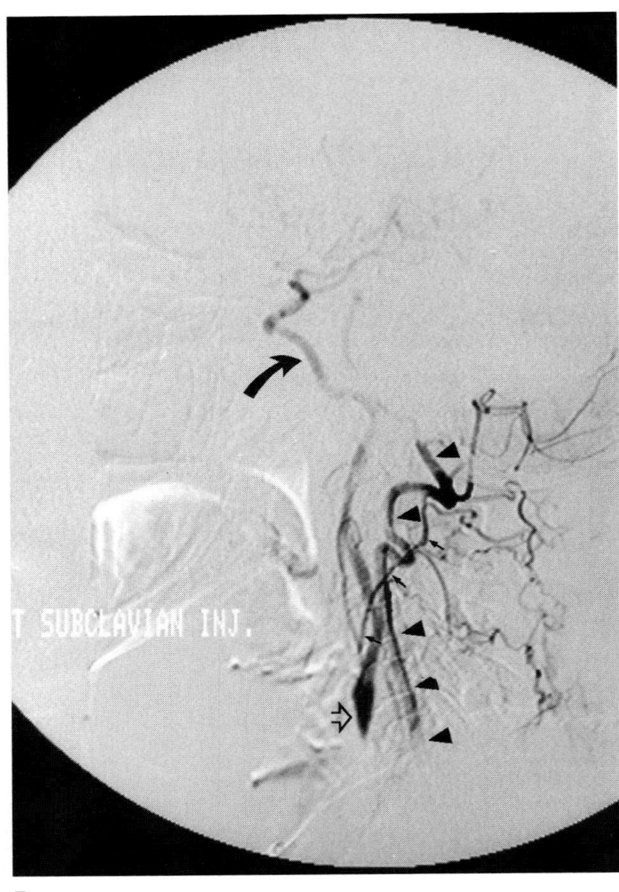

B

Figure 13-9. Muscular collaterals to the carotid artery. There is complete occlusion of the right common carotid artery at its origin (*open arrow,* A). A right subclavian injection fills the right vertebral artery (*arrowheads,* B), which in turn fills muscular branches of the neck. The muscular branch collaterals to the occipital artery (*small arrows,* B) result in retrograde flow to the right carotid birfurcation (*open arrow,* B). From the carotid bifurcation, flow progresses up the right internal carotid artery (*curved arrow,* B) to fill the anterior circulation. This is also a common pathway for collateral flow to reach an internal carotid artery following surgical ligation or clamping of a distal common carotid artery for the treatment of a giant cavernous internal carotid artery aneurysm.

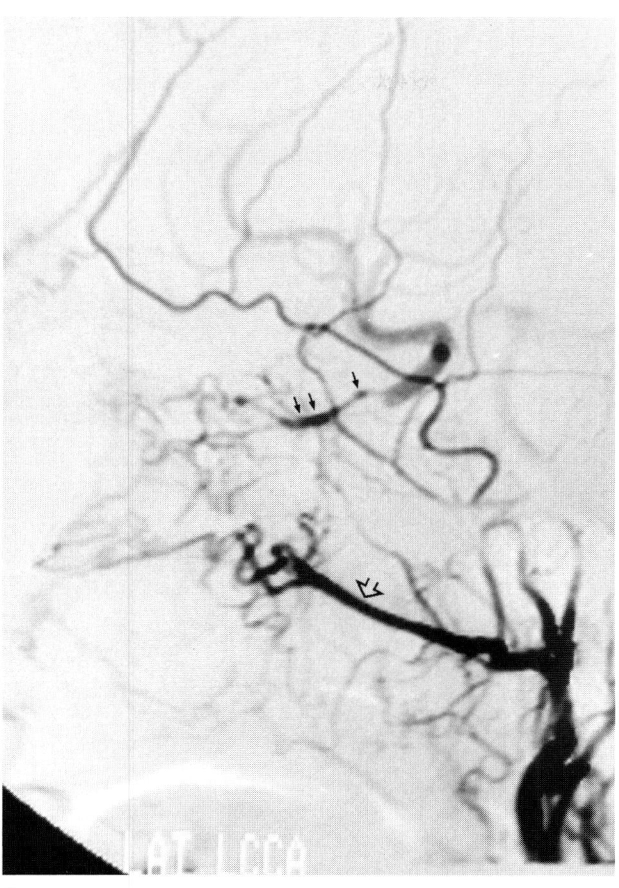

A

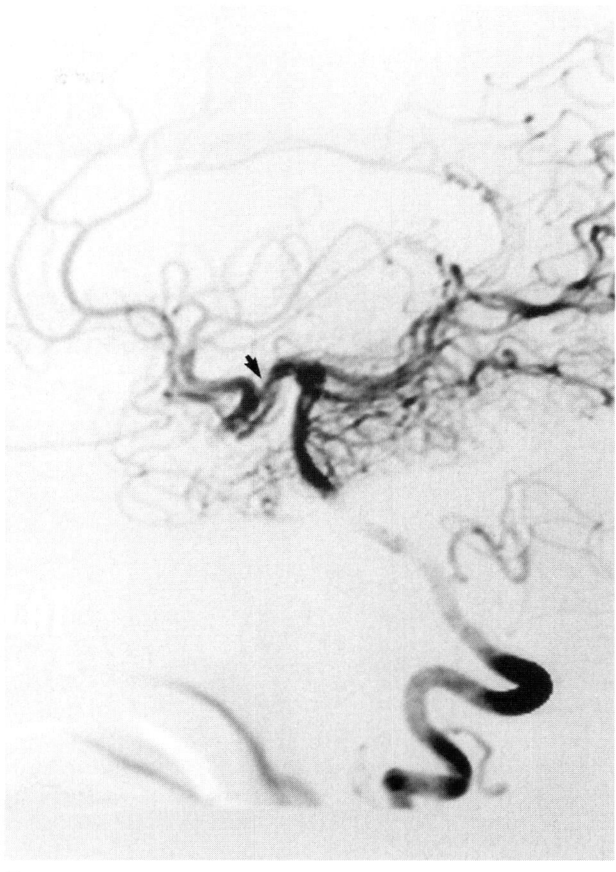

B

Figure 13-10. Combined external-to-internal carotid and circle of Willis collateral flow. A 62-year-old man was evaluated for transient ischemic attacks. His left internal carotid artery was occluded at its origin. On injection of the left common carotid artery, there is filling of the supraclinoid internal carotid artery by retrograde flow in the ophthalmic artery (*small arrows,* A). The ophthalmic artery fills via ethmoidal branches of the maxillary artery (*open arrow,* A), a branch of the external carotid artery. On injection of the left vertebral artery, flow from the posterior communicating artery (*arrow,* B) also fills the supraclinoid internal carotid artery.

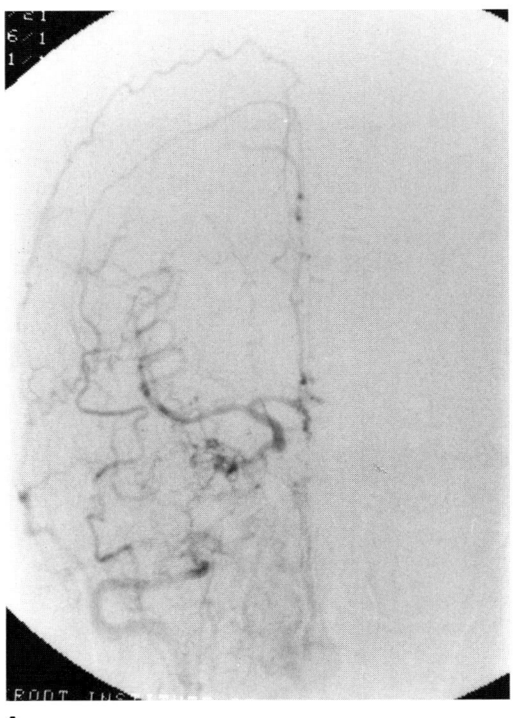

A

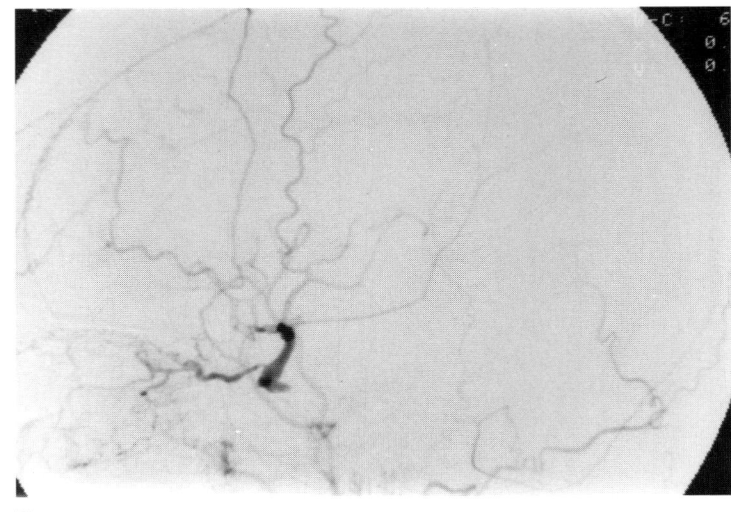

B

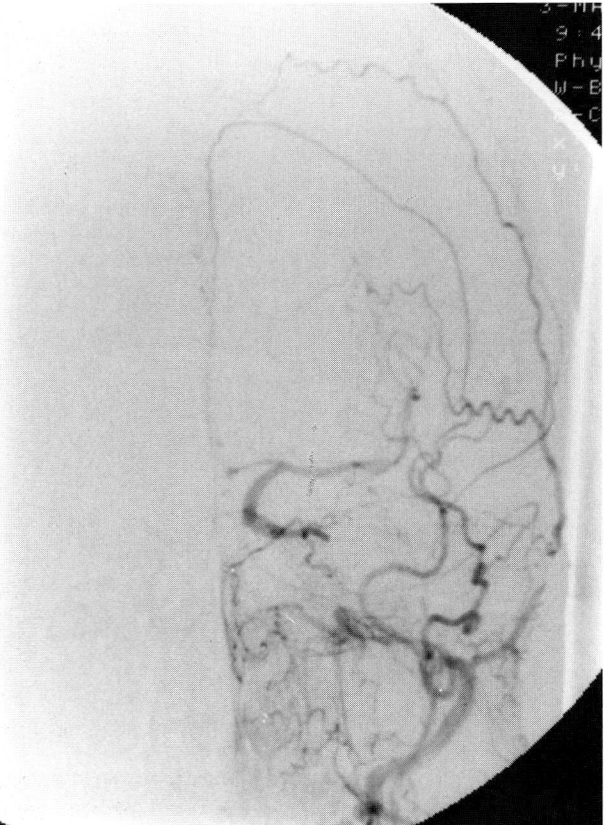

C

Figure 13-11. Combined external-to-internal carotid and pial collateral flow. This example shows bilateral internal carotid artery origin occlusions. The right common carotid injection (A and B) and left common carotid injection (C) demonstrate external-to-internal carotid artery collateral flow bilaterally via retrograde flow in the ophthalmic arteries. The left vertebral artery injection (D and E) reveals no circle of Willis collateral; no posterior communicating arteries are seen. There is, however, pial collateral flow to both hemispheres. The posterior cerebral arteries are seen to fill anterior and middle cerebral arteries by leptomeningeal connections.

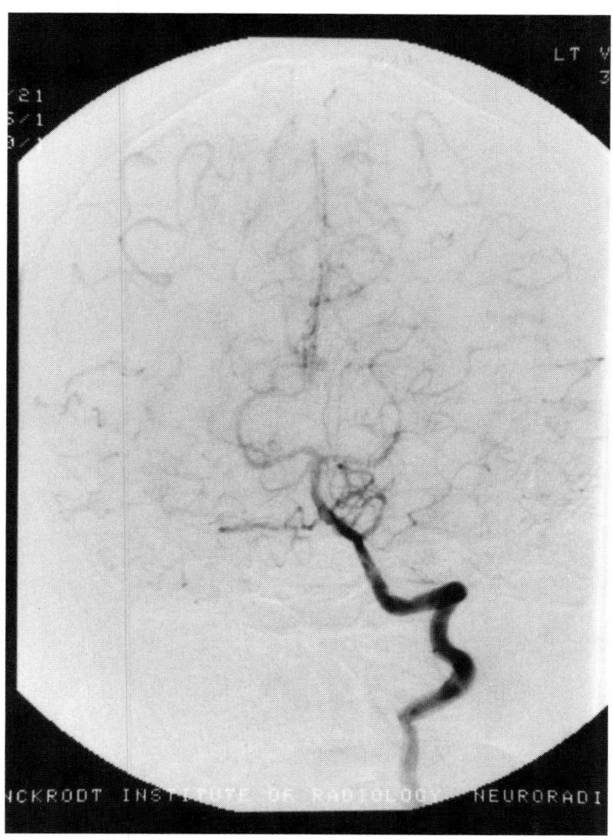

D

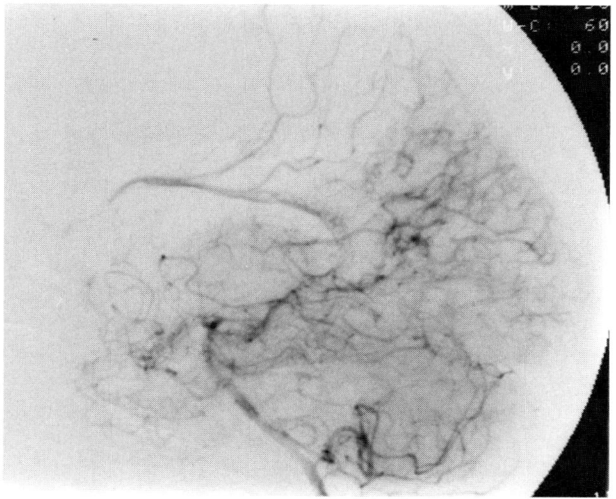

E

Figure 13-11 (continued).

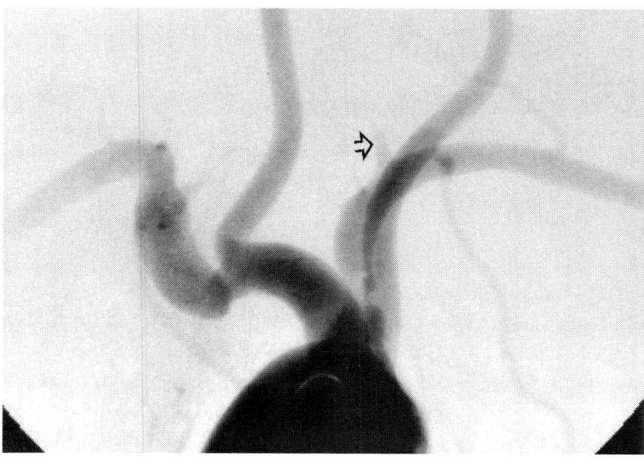

A

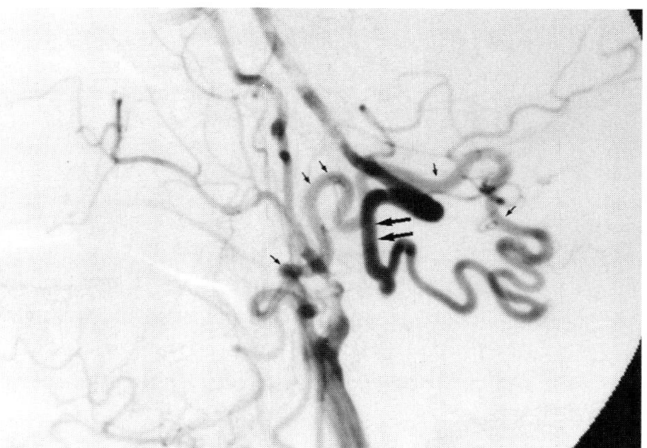

B

Figure 13-12. Muscular collaterals to the vertebral artery. There is an occlusion of the proximal left vertebral artery (*open arrow,* A). The left common carotid artery injection (B) reveals reconstitution of the distal left vertebral artery (*large arrows*) via muscular branch connections between the occipital artery (*small arrows*), a branch of the external carotid artery, and the vertebral artery. The communication in this example is quite large. Note that the direction of collateral flow in this case is the opposite of that in Figure 13-9.

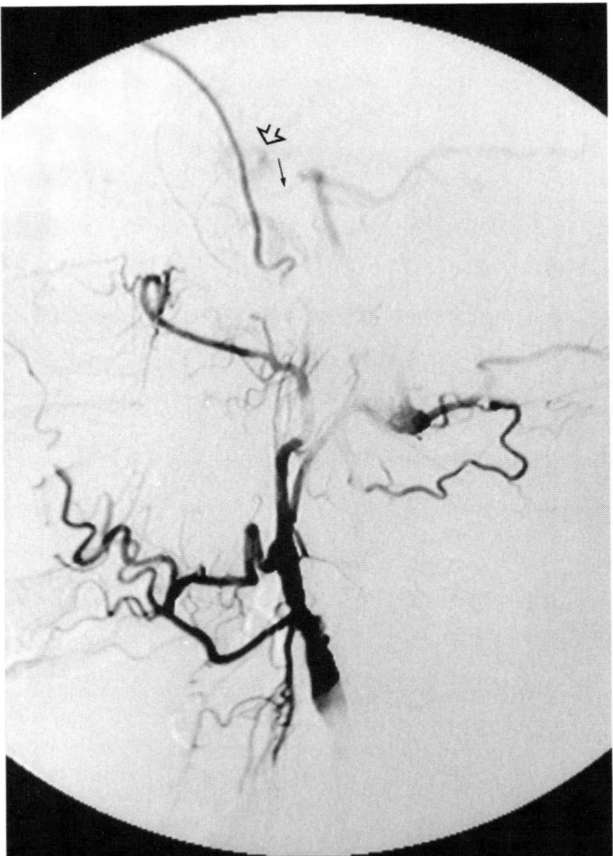

Figure 13-13. Carotid-to-vertebral-to-carotid collateral flow. The internal carotid artery and the ipsilateral vertebral artery are occluded at their origins. There is flow from the occipital branch of the external carotid artery via muscular collaterals to reconstitute the distal vertebral artery. The vertebral artery then fills the basilar and posterior cerebral arteries, resulting in filling of the posterior communicating artery. The posterior communicating artery (*small arrow*) is seen faintly opacifying the supraclinoid internal carotid artery and anterior circulation (*open arrow*).

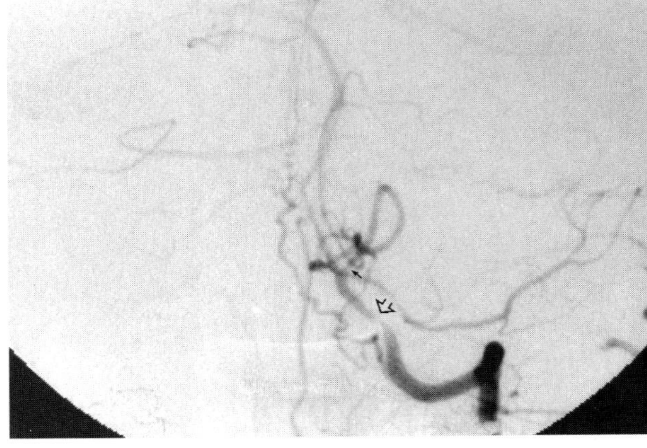

A

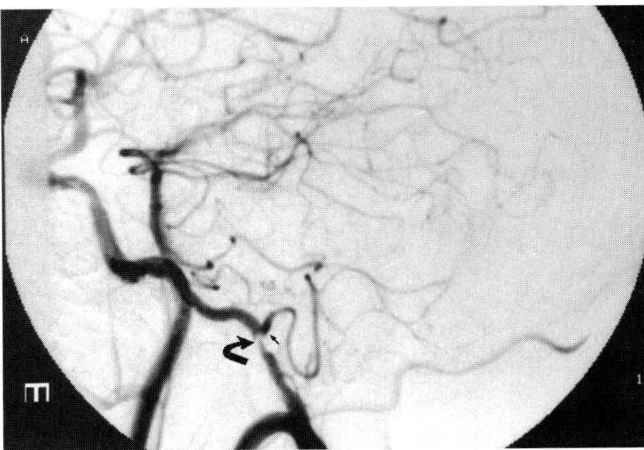

B

Figure 13-14. Bilateral distal vertebral artery disease. A 52-year-old man was evaluated following a left occipital infarction. The frontal view of the left vertebral injection (A) reveals very high grade stenosis of the distal left vertebral artery (*open arrow*) proximal to the posterior inferior cerebellar artery origin (*small arrow*). The lateral view of the innominate injection (B) reveals very high grade stenosis of the distal right vertebral artery (*curved arrow*) at the posterior inferior cerebellar artery origin (*small arrow*).

flow in the ophthalmic artery directs blood from maxillary artery branches to an occluded internal carotid artery. A third collateral route is via the pial or leptomeningeal system, for example, when branches of the anterior and posterior cerebral arteries provide flow to distal middle cerebral artery branches (MCA) in cases of proximal middle cerebral artery occlusion. There are collateral routes in muscular branches of the neck, for example, when an occipital branch of the external carotid artery provides flow to the distal vertebral artery in cases of proximal vertebral occlusion.

Some patients are asymptomatic with a single artery supplying the entire brain because of a highly developed network of collaterals, whereas other patients become symptomatic with disease in only one of four patent major cerebral arteries because of embolic events. It is always important to evaluate the angiogram in the context of the clinical presentation. What is angiographically abnormal may be of therapeutic significance to one patient and insignificant to another.

With regard to intracranial atherosclerotic disease, common sites of stenosis include the cavernous segments of the internal carotid arteries and the distal vertebral arteries (Fig. 13-14). Focal areas of stenosis in cerebral artery branches are not uncommonly seen in elderly and hypertensive patients (Fig. 13-15). Patients can develop atherosclerotic changes purely in the extracranial arteries, purely in the intracranial arteries, or in both areas. Racial or cultural factors may influence the distribution of lesions. In African Americans, stenoses of intracranial vessels predominate, whereas in Caucasians, stenoses of extracranial vessels predominate.[18]

Clinical symptoms of atherosclerotic disease result when collateral flow is inadequate or when emboli or thrombi form in atherosclerotic cerebral vessels and cause arterial occlusions. Thromboembolic events causing symptoms are discussed in detail in the following section.

Stroke

Neurologic deficits can result from thrombotic or embolic events within cerebral arteries or veins. Cerebral angiography may be indicated to detect and determine the extent and location of disease so that anticoagulant therapy may be initiated and an attempt made to prevent clot propagation, or so that fibrinolytic therapy may be initiated and an attempt made to dissolve the clot.

Arterial thrombi can form on plaque and cause occlusions of diseased vessels or produce emboli that occlude vessels remote from the sites of atherosclerotic disease. Emboli in cerebral vessels can also originate from the aorta, innominate artery, or subclavian arteries proximal to the origins of the cerebral vessels (Fig. 13-16) or from cardiac sources such as diseased valves or enlarged chambers.[19] Emboli in peripheral veins reaching the right atrium may travel through septal defects as "paradoxical emboli" and reach the cerebral arteries. Finally, in some conditions there is an increased frequency of thrombotic events, as when an anticardiolipin antibody disorder or sickle cell disease exists or when patients are taking oral contraceptives.[20–22]

Dissection of cerebral vessels, whether spontaneous or traumatic, may result in stroke (Fig. 13-17). The internal carotid artery tends to dissect at the junction between the upper cervical portion and petrous portions. The dissection occurs at the transition between

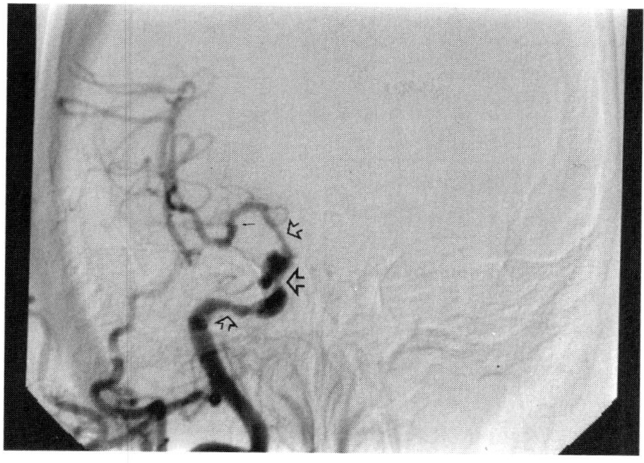

A

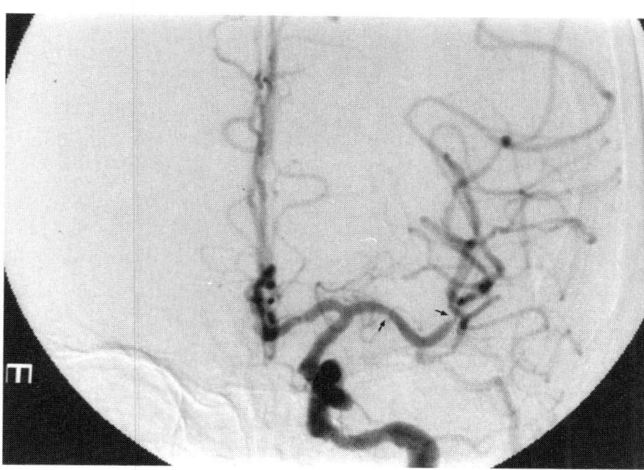

B

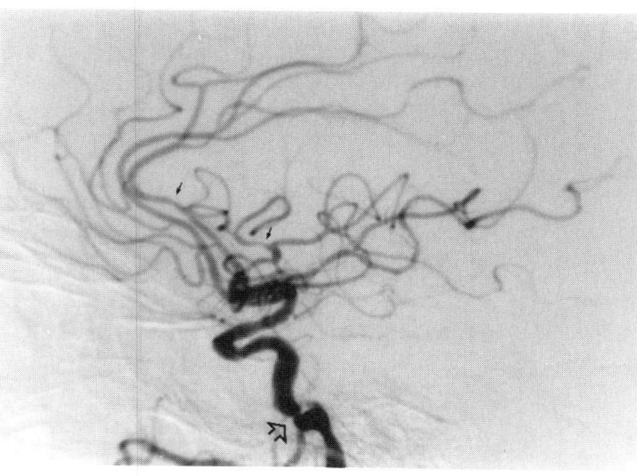

C

Figure 13-15. Intracranial atherosclerotic changes of the anterior circulation. A 71-year-old male was examined for complaints of right amaurosis fugax. In addition to carotid bifurcation disease (not shown), his angiogram disclosed intracranial atherosclerotic changes. The right common carotid injection (A) reveals moderate stenoses of the petrous, cavernous, and supraclinoid segments of the internal carotid artery (*open arrows*) and irregularity of the M_1 segment of the middle cerebral artery (*small arrow*). The left common carotid artery injection (B and C) discloses a stenosis of the petrous segment of the internal carotid artery (*open arrow*, C) as well as focal stenoses of the middle cerebral arteries (*small arrows*, B and C).

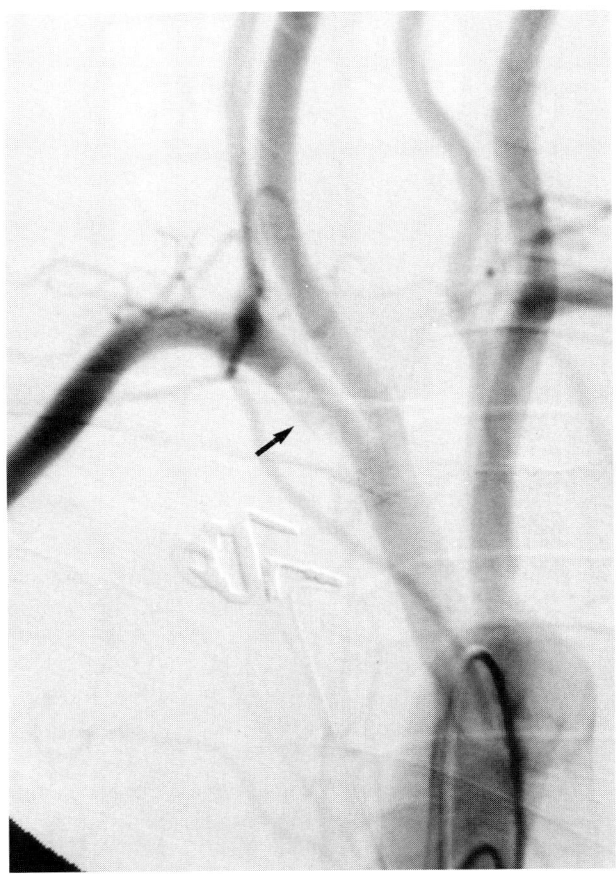
A

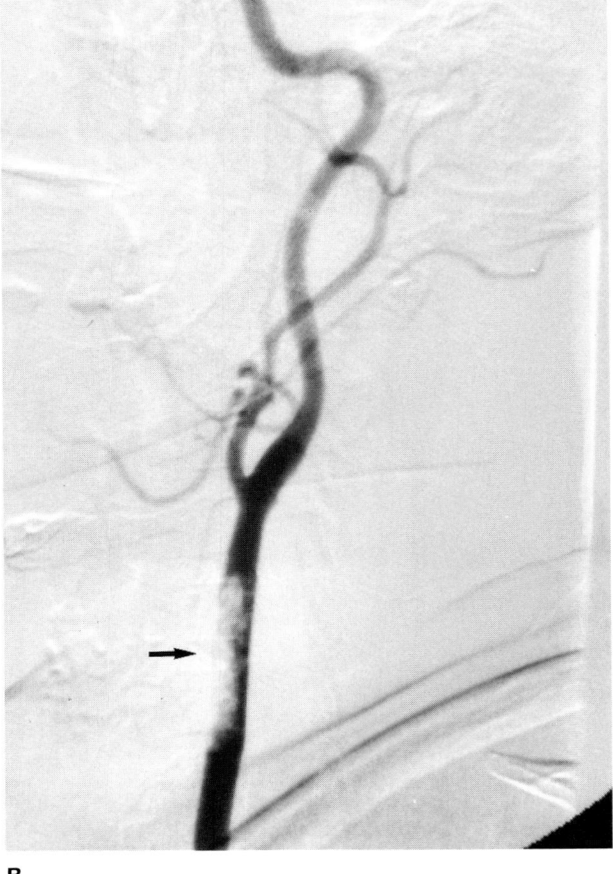
B

Figure 13-16. Clots in the great vessels. In the first case, a 38-year-old woman presented with an acute right cerebellar infarction in the distribution of the right posterior inferior cerebellar artery, a branch of the right vertebral artery. Her aortic arch angiogram (A) reveals an acute thrombus (*arrow*) in the right subclavian artery proximal to the origin of the vertebral artery. The thrombus was removed surgically. In the second case, a 40-year-old woman presented with right-hand weakness and dysarthria. Following admission, her neurologic deficits progressed to hemiplegia and aphasia. Her aortic arch study (not shown) and left common carotid angiogram (B) demonstrate acute thrombus within the left common carotid artery (*arrow*). The value of aortic arch injections in cases of transient ischemic attacks and strokes is obvious. Diagnostic catheters and guidewires are not advanced through acute thrombi or over heavily diseased atherosclerotic lesions of cerebral vessels.

where the artery is mobile and where it is fixed in its bony canal. Dissection may be evidenced on an angiogram by an actual intimal tear or flap, or by stenosis, irregularity, occlusion, or an associated pseudoaneurysm. The vertebral artery also tends to dissect just below the skull base, usually at the C1-C2 level. Carotid and vertebral dissections may be seen in association with emboli in distal branches.[23]

Angiographic findings with migraine headaches may include spasm or inappropriate stenosis of cerebral arteries. Drug abuse, also associated with cerebral infarction, may also lead to inappropriate caliber changes similar to vasculitis, a topic of a subsequent section. Both conditions can be associated with stroke.[24]

With regard to the actual findings in acute stroke, it is important to correlate the angiographic abnormalities with the clinical presentation. Some patients with acute neurologic deficits and cross-sectional imaging findings of acute stroke do, in fact, have abnormal angiographic findings to explain their deficits; however, other patients with acute deficits have negative angiograms. Some patients may have preexisting arterial occlusions that are unrelated to acute deficits.[21,22] Assuming that the angiographic abnormalities correlate with the acute clinical syndrome, the findings in acute

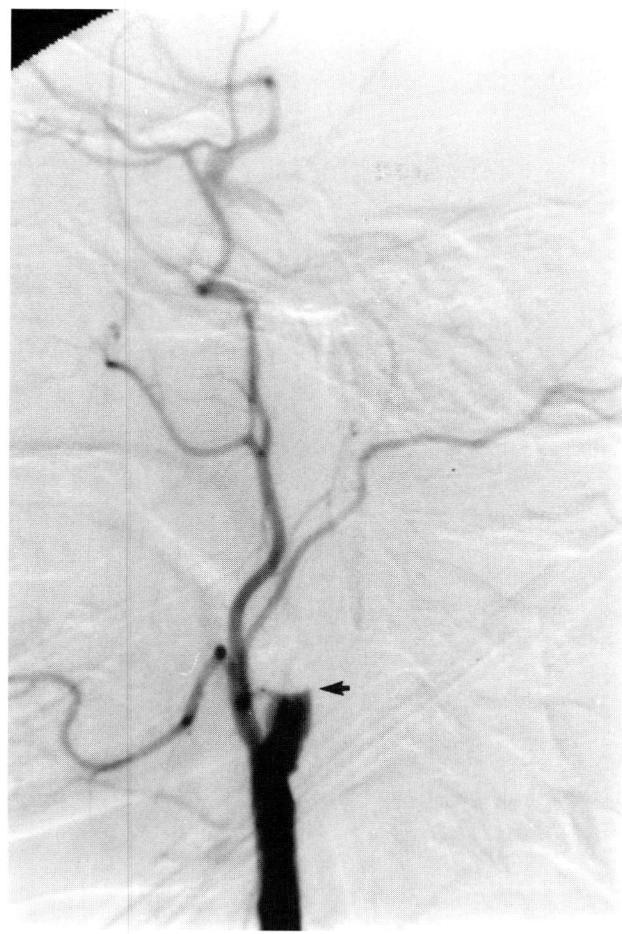

A

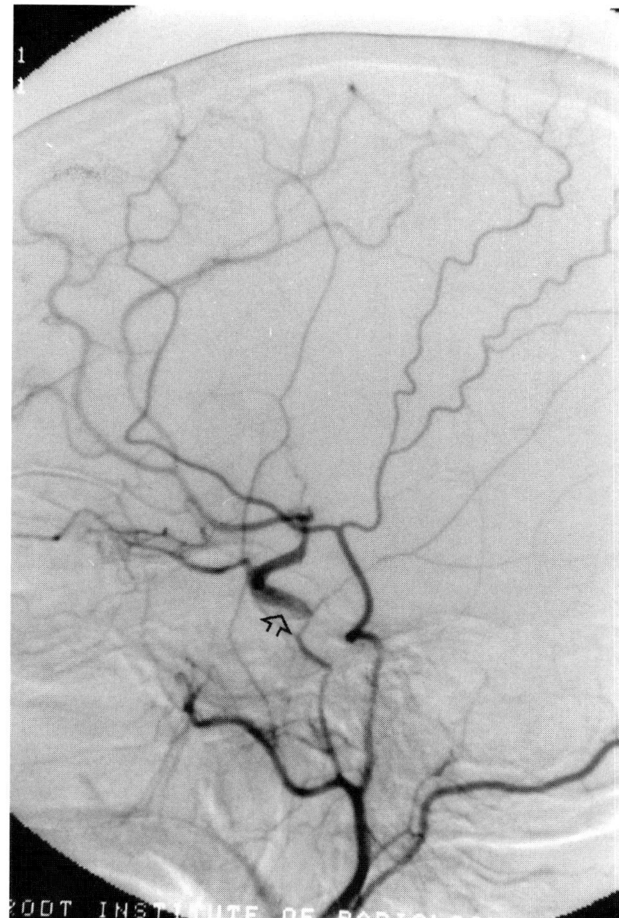

B

C

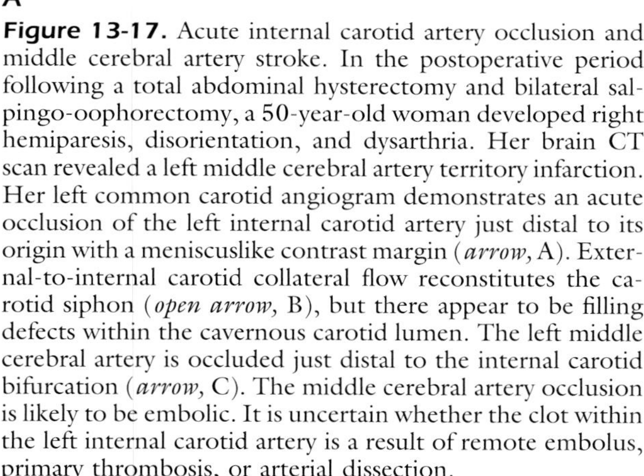

Figure 13-17. Acute internal carotid artery occlusion and middle cerebral artery stroke. In the postoperative period following a total abdominal hysterectomy and bilateral salpingo-oophorectomy, a 50-year-old woman developed right hemiparesis, disorientation, and dysarthria. Her brain CT scan revealed a left middle cerebral artery territory infarction. Her left common carotid angiogram demonstrates an acute occlusion of the left internal carotid artery just distal to its origin with a meniscuslike contrast margin (*arrow,* A). External-to-internal carotid collateral flow reconstitutes the carotid siphon (*open arrow,* B), but there appear to be filling defects within the cavernous carotid lumen. The left middle cerebral artery is occluded just distal to the internal carotid bifurcation (*arrow,* C). The middle cerebral artery occlusion is likely to be embolic. It is uncertain whether the clot within the left internal carotid artery is a result of remote embolus, primary thrombosis, or arterial dissection.

stroke may include intraluminal filling defects representing thrombus or embolus within cerebral arteries (Fig. 13-18), arterial trunk or branch occlusions (Figs. 13-19 and 13-20), regions of hypovascularity in the capillary phase corresponding to the ischemic zone, and mass effect if the infarction has had the time to develop edema. Edema is usually maximal at 3 to 4

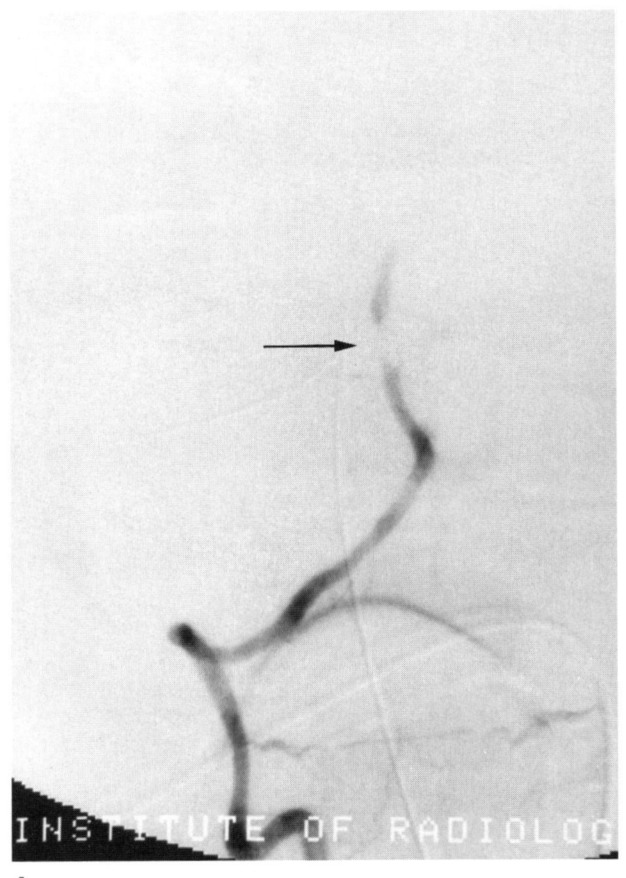
INSTITUTE OF RADIOLOG

A

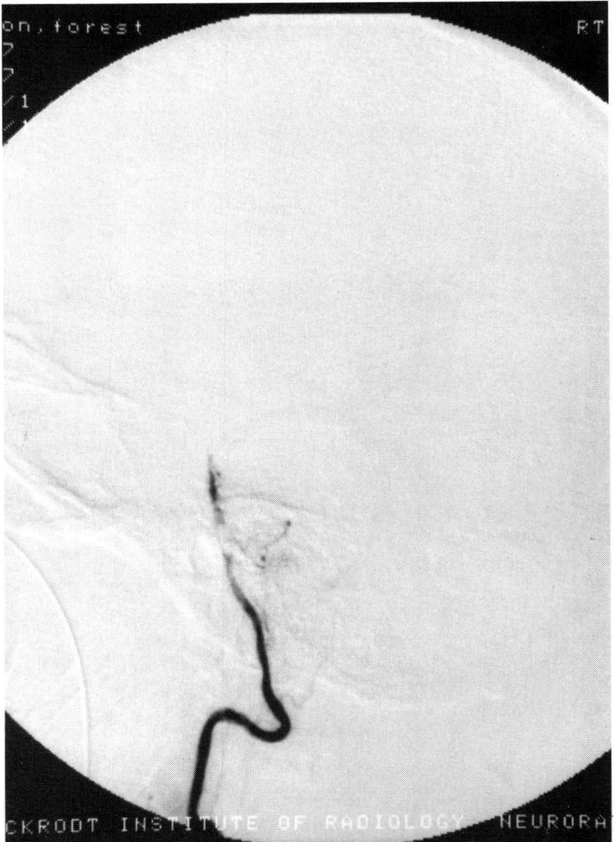
on,forest
RT
CKRODT INSTITUTE OF RADIOLOGY NEURORA

B

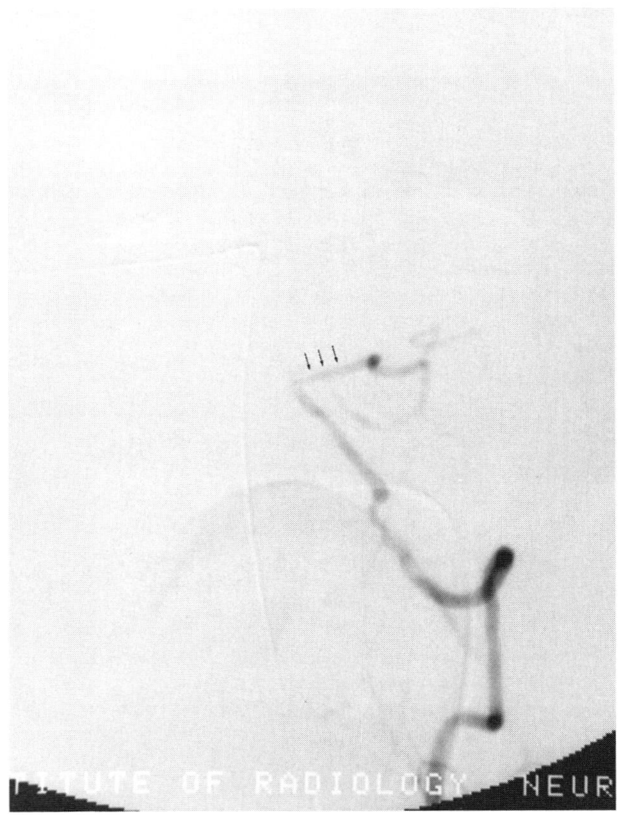
TITUTE OF RADIOLOGY NEUR

C

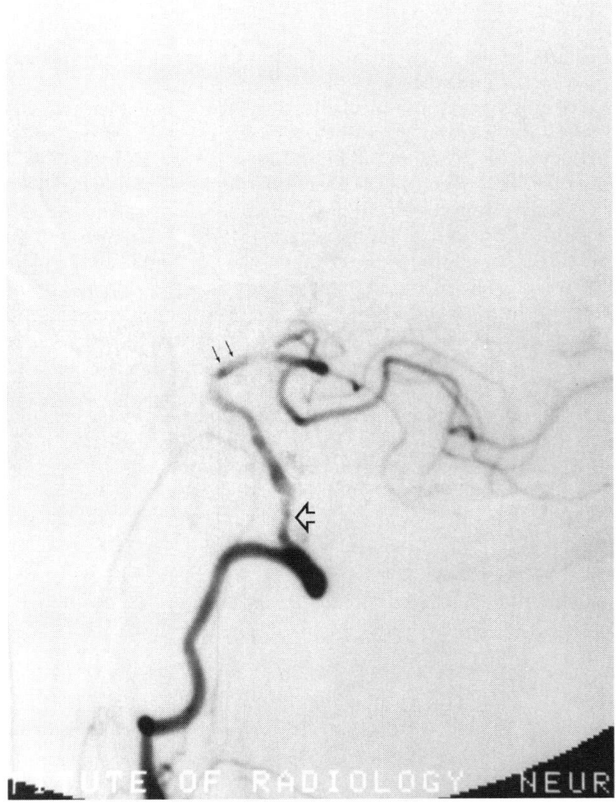
TITUTE OF RADIOLOGY NEUR

D

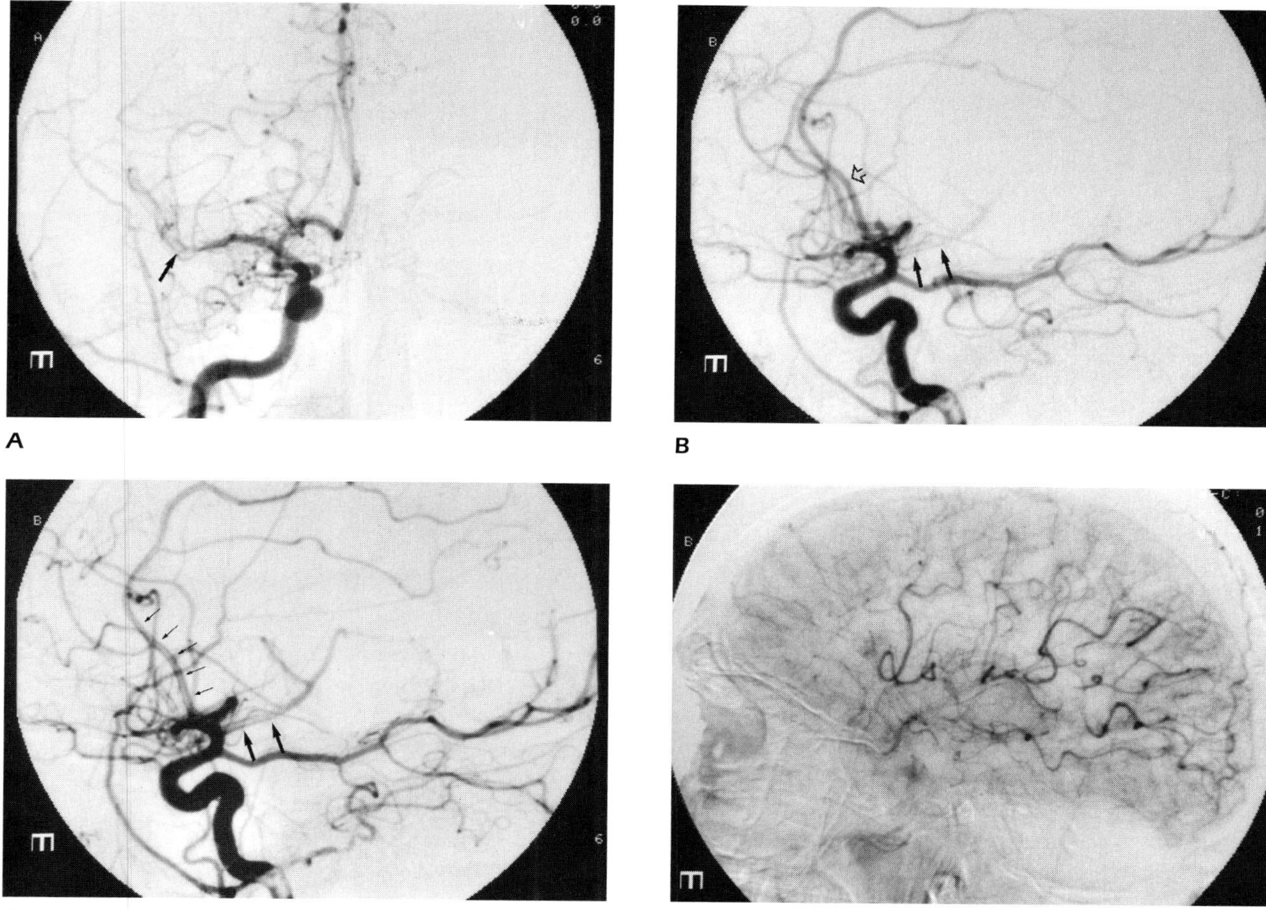

Figure 13-19. Acute right middle cerebral artery infarction, believed embolic. A 23-year-old man was examined for left hemiparesis of three days' duration. His right common carotid angiogram demonstrates filling defects within the posterior division of the right middle cerebral artery (*large arrows,* A, B, and C) representing clot. This appearance is not to be confused with streaming, inflow of unopacified blood, as is seen in this case in the right anterior cerebral artery (*small arrows,* C). Filling defects from intraluminal clot persist throughout the arterial phase in this right middle cerebral artery. Inflow of unopacified blood from the left carotid artery, crossing the anterior communicating artery, is not seen in this right anterior cerebral artery in the early arterial phase (*open arrow,* B). The defect only appears later, once contrast has begun to wash out of the vessel. Very late opacification of the proximally occluded right middle cerebral artery branches is seen in (D), a result of retrograde flow from pial collaterals.

◄ **Figure 13-18.** Basilar thrombosis. A 47-year-old man was treated with intravenous tissue plasminogen activator (tPA) for an acute myocardial infarction. On the night of his treatment, he developed left hemiparesis, bilateral third nerve palsies, and a decline in alertness. A brain CT scan excluded intracranial hemorrhage. Frontal and lateral views of his right vertebral angiogram (A and B) demonstrate a filling defect within the midbasilar artery (*arrow,* A) and nonvisualization of basilar branches. The frontal and lateral views of his left vertebral angiogram (C and D) demonstrate no opacification beyond the posterior inferior cerebellar artery (*small arrows,* C and D) and reveal irregularity of the distal vertebral artery (*open arrow,* D). It is possible that an embolus was thrown from the heart to the left vertebral and basilar arteries.

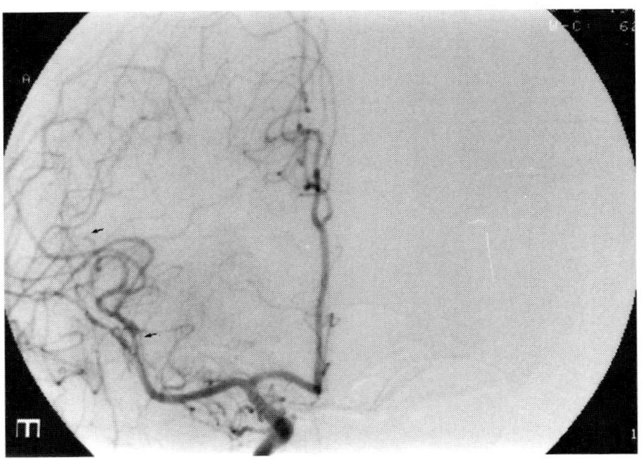

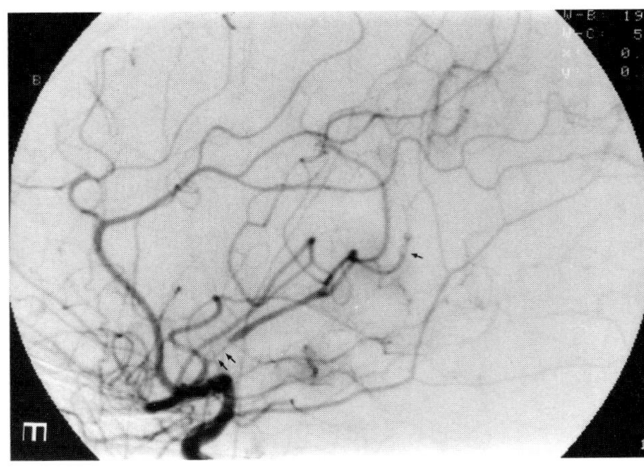

A B

Figure 13-20. Multiple emboli. Another example of right middle cerebral artery infarction shows separate filling defects probably representing emboli within both proximal and distal branches (*arrows,* A and B). The abnormalities are more easily seen on the lateral view, where there is less vessel overlap.

days after an infarction. Another associated finding may be evidence of collateral supply to the territory of the infarction. For example, the anterior and posterior cerebral arteries may be seen to fill middle cerebral branches in a retrograde fashion via pial collaterals following MCA occlusion by an embolus, or the MCA may provide collaterals to the PCA following PCA occlusion (Fig. 13-21).

In the subacute phase of infarction, there can be a period of hyperemia at the periphery of the infarction, termed *luxury perfusion*. This is a reactive vasodilatation and an attempt to reestablish flow to the ischemic tissue and can be as brisk as to be associated with arteriovenous shunting.[25] If interpreted without clinical history, a subacute infarction can be confused with a neoplasm. The edema, hyperemia, and shunting associated with an infarction should disappear within 2 to 4 weeks, whereas that associated with a tumor should persist or worsen. CT and MRI should also be useful in differentiating these lesions.

In those cases in which angiography is normal in acute infarction, it may be assumed that a thrombus or embolus was reabsorbed or recanalized before the angiogram was obtained. Unfortunately, the natural

Figure 13-21. Right occipital infarct. A 58-year-old woman developed a left visual field deficit. The frontal view of her right vertebral angiogram (A) demonstrates an occlusion, probably embolic, within the right posterior cerebral artery (*arrow*). The lateral view of her right carotid angiogram (B) shows evidence of some pial collateral supply from the anterior circulation to the posterior cerebral branches.

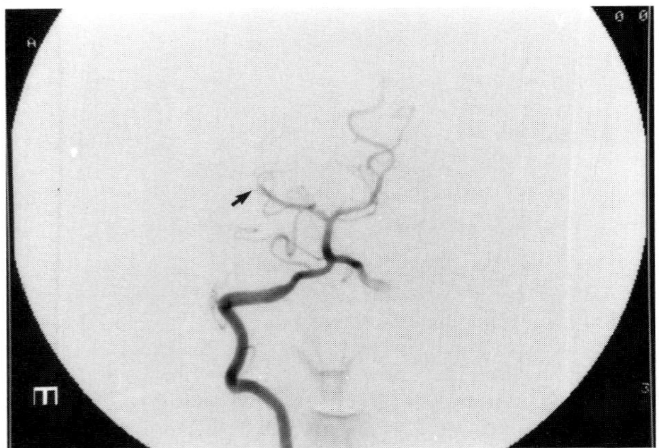

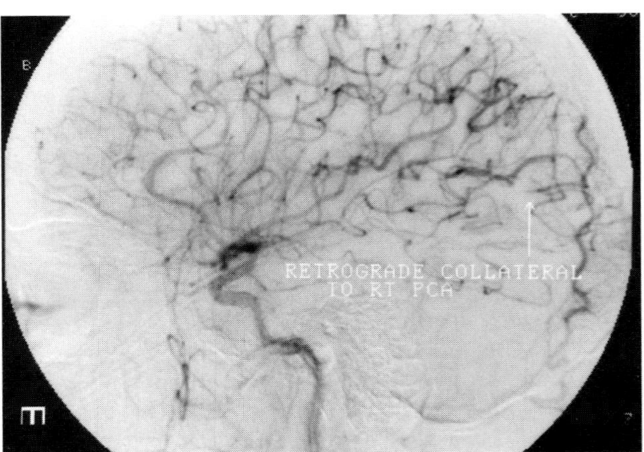

A B

recanalization time may be too long to preserve the viability of the brain affected by the ischemia resulting from such an occlusion.

If a filling defect or occlusion is found at angiography in acute stroke, a question that often arises is whether the occlusion resulted from thrombus forming at the site of an atherosclerotic lesion or whether the occlusion was the result of an embolus originating from a more proximal site. Clues from the study may be found to answer that question. For example, if an occluded vessel has evidence of atherosclerotic disease or if there are other sites of intracranial stenoses and the carotid and vertebral arteries and aortic arch are normal, one might deduce that the occlusion was local, whereas if the intracranial vessels generally appear smooth and the internal carotid origin is severely stenosed and ulcerated, one might conclude that the occlusion was the result of an embolus from the neck. If intracranial and extracranial arteries appear otherwise normal, the occlusion might be the result of an embolus from the heart or the result of a hypercoagulable state. Such determinations could help direct further evaluation or select treatment to prevent additional infarctions.

Venous thrombosis can be precipitated by a number of factors, including dehydration, infection, trauma, surgery, the use of oral contraceptives, and pregnancy. In some cases, no cause is evident.[26] It is frequently possible to identify or suspect venous thrombosis in the major cranial sinuses or larger cortical veins by MRI or magnetic resonance venography. A filling defect in the superior sagittal sinus or torcular on a postcontrast CT scan, termed the *delta sign,* can confirm the presence of venous sinus clot, but false negatives are not uncommon. MRI or CT scanning can reliably demonstrate some of the sequelae of venous thrombosis, such as cerebral edema or hemorrhage. It may also be possible to date the duration of thrombosis using signal characteristics of the clot on MR images. Conventional angiography is usually definitive for the diagnosis of venous thrombosis, and is used to guide therapy.

Angiographic findings in venous sinus thrombosis could include nonvisualization of a sinus, visualization of venous collaterals, or visualization of actual filling defects within the sinuses (Fig. 13-22). Extensive venous sinus thrombosis resulting in increased intracranial pressure can prolong circulation time. If venous sinus thrombosis has resulted in the development of edema or parenchymal hemorrhage, signs of mass effect on cerebral vessels might be seen. For example, superior sagittal sinus thrombosis can be associated with biparietal edema and hemorrhage. Further discussion of mass effects, as might be seen from swelling and edema in infarction, will follow in the section on tumors.

Vasculitis and Similar Disorders

Cerebral angiography may be helpful in the diagnosis of inflammatory disorders of vessels. Abnormalities in arterial caliber, arterial occlusions, and irregularities of vessel margins are seen with these disorders. Typically, vasculitis results in tapering of vessels over long segments; however, vasculitis can also cause focal stenoses and dilatations that result in a beaded appearance. Vasculitis can also cause focal stenoses without dilatations or promote microaneurysm formation. Because the reactions of arteries to diseases are rather limited in scope and the arteriographic findings are common to many inflammatory disorders and other disease processes, the distribution of vessel abnormalities and clinical presentation are used to suggest the presence of vasculitis. The usual problem is differentiating vasculitis from atherosclerotic disease in the elderly population. Inflammatory changes often affect vessels too small to visualize by angiography, and brain biopsy can be necessary for diagnosis.[27]

Infection of the neck may be associated with the development of mycotic pseudoaneurysms of extracranial cerebral arteries. Such aneurysms were more common before the advent of antibiotic therapy, but are occasionally seen today. Because infectious pseudoaneurysms are more prone to rupture than traumatic pseudoaneurysms and to result in rapid exsanguination and death, they are an important entity to recognize (Fig. 13-23).

Bacterial, tuberculous, and fungal inflammations cause characteristic intracranial changes. These infectious vasculitides have a predilection for causing visible arteriographic abnormalities of major arteries near the skull base. Bacterial disease is associated with shaggy, irregular-appearing vessel walls, a finding that is useful in distinguishing between infectious and noninfectious inflammation. The cavernous internal carotid artery may dilate as a result of adjacent cavernous sinus infection.[28] Bacterial infection, particularly infective endocarditis, may also be responsible for mycotic aneurysms and septic emboli. Mycotic aneurysms are typically found on middle cerebral artery branches distal to the MCA bifurcation, and can result in both subarachnoid and intraparenchymal bleeds,[29] discussed further in the section on intracranial aneurysms.

Tuberculosis has a preference for the subarachnoid space at the base of the skull and thus affects the supraclinoid carotid artery, the M_1 segment of the middle cerebral artery, the A_1 segment of the anterior cerebral

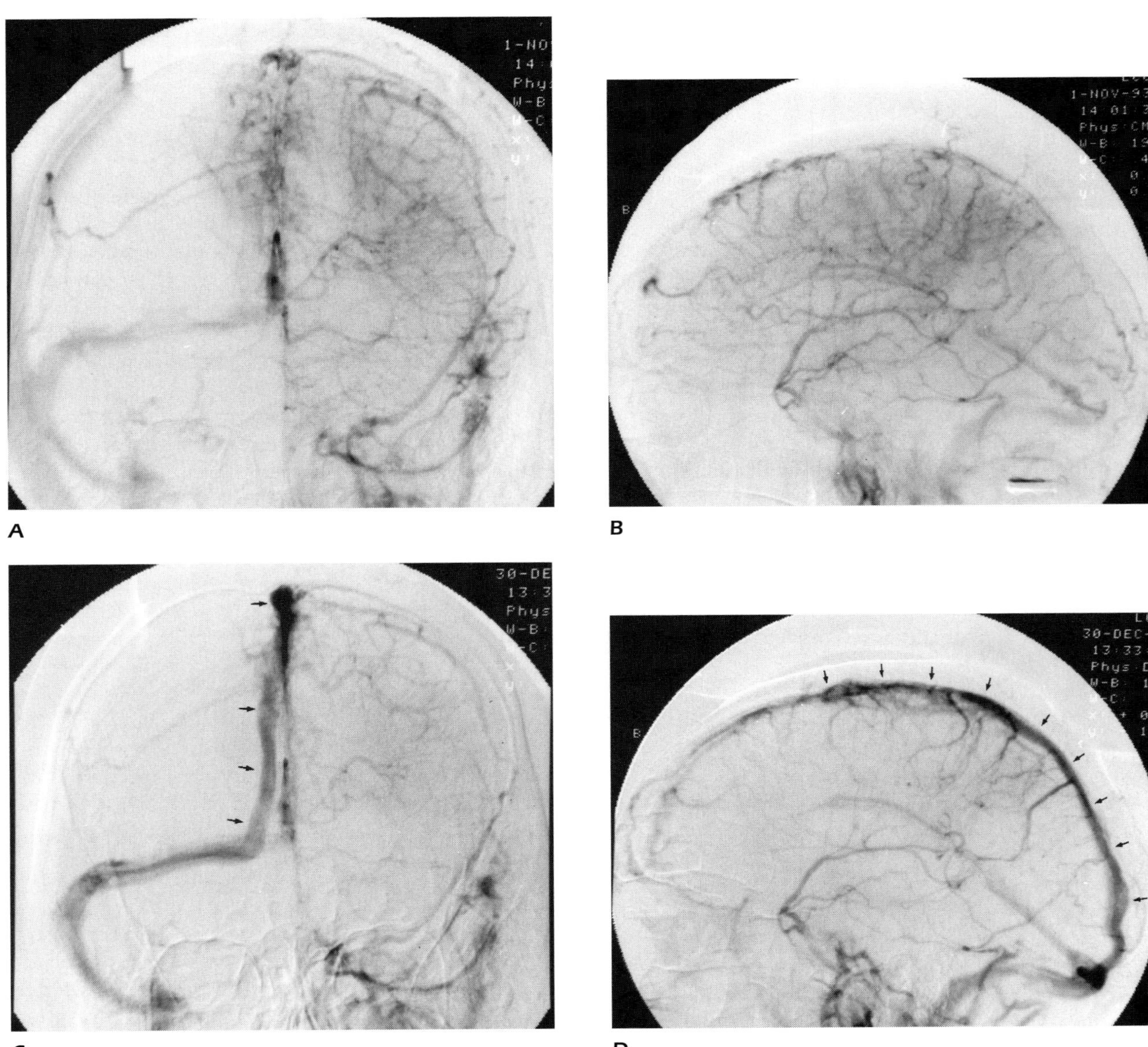

Figure 13-22. Superior sagittal sinus thrombosis. A 55-year-old man presented with a new onset of seizures and a headache. A brain CT scan demonstrated right frontal and left parietal hemorrhages. The venous phase of his left carotid angiogram (A and B) reveals nonfilling of most of the superior sagittal sinus as a result of thrombosis. The patient was treated with anticoagulants. A follow-up angiogram 2 months later (C and D) reveals that the superior sagittal sinus is recanalized (*arrows*).

artery, the basilar artery, and the proximal posterior cerebral arteries (Fig. 13-24). The most common finding is irregular narrowing of the inferior surface of the M_1 segment and smooth narrowing of the supraclinoid carotid.[28] Fungal infection can cause changes similar to those of tuberculosis and may be associated with septic emboli that lead to abscesses.[28]

With regard to noninfectious vasculitides, temporal arteritis, a giant-cell arteritis, rarely involves the branches of the carotid artery on angiography. The most likely sites for abnormalities on imaging studies are the distal subclavian, the proximal axillary, the brachial, the brachiocephalic, and the femoral arteries.[30] Associated atherosclerotic disease is likely to be present because temporal arteritis is usually seen in the elderly. One distinguishing point is that atherosclerotic

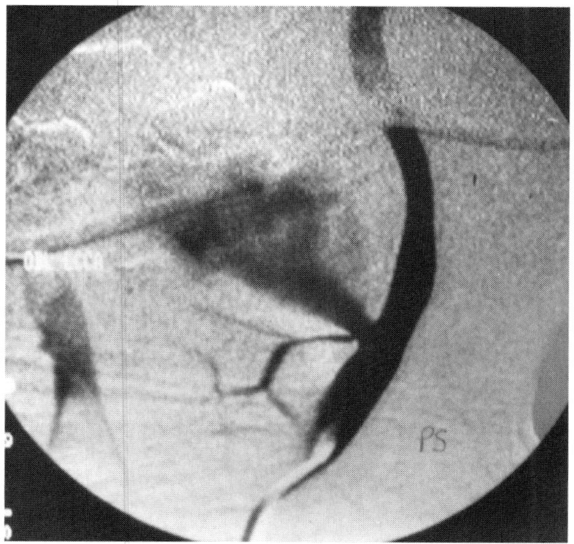

A

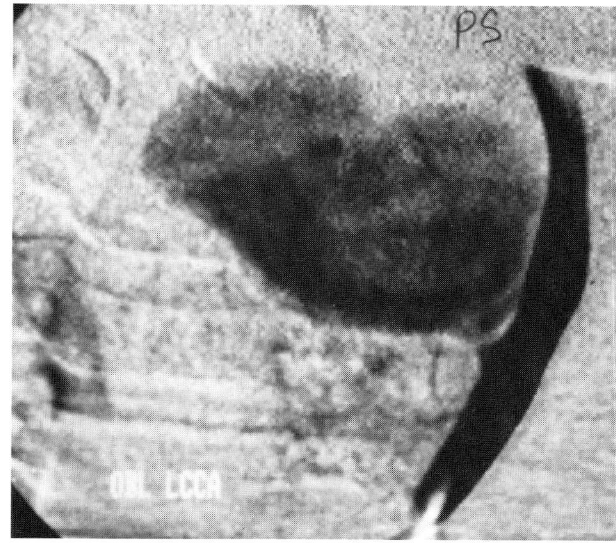

B

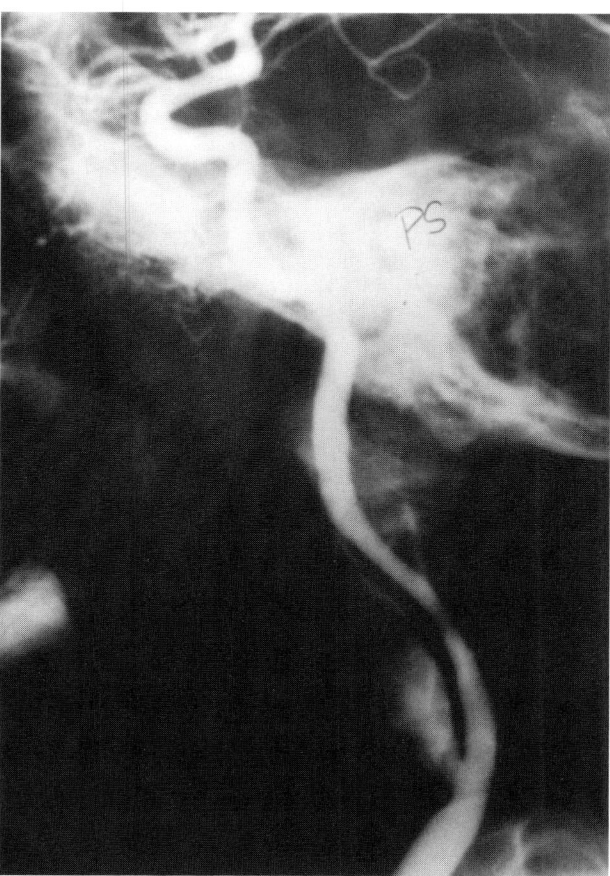

C

changes usually result in short segments of irregular stenosis in proximal subclavian locations whereas temporal arteritis is associated with smooth, long-segment, tapered stenoses in distal subclavian or axillary locations.[30] Even though visible temporal artery involvement is rare, when present it is fairly specific for temporal arteritis. Atherosclerotic involvement of the temporal artery is unusual. Temporal arteritis may result in microaneurysms, beading, and focal stenoses.[28] Intracranial involvement is rare in temporal arteritis, but when it occurs, it is manifested as focal areas of stenosis and dilatation.[31] The diagnosis of temporal arteritis is usually made by biopsy.

Takayasu arteritis is another giant-cell arteritis. Like temporal arteritis, it causes smooth, tapered stenoses, but the two disorders have different distributions. The arteries affected by Takayasu arteritis include the proximal and distal subclavian arteries, the common carotid arteries proximal to the carotid bifurcations, the innominate artery, the axillary artery, and the brachial artery (Fig. 13-25). There may be irregular ectatic change of the aorta. Visceral arteries are commonly involved. Unlike temporal arteritis, Takayasu arteritis affects a younger population and there is little confusion with atherosclerosis. The disease can usually be diagnosed by angiography.[30]

Polyarteritis nodosa, referred to as a necrotizing an-

Figure 13-23. Giant mycotic pseudoaneurysm. A 9-year-old girl was examined for a left neck mass that had been palpable for 3 weeks. In addition to the mass, she was found to have osteomyelitis of the left mandible. Her left common carotid angiogram (A, B, and C) reveals a large pseudoaneurysm originating at the carotid bifurcation near the external carotid artery origin. The aneurysm interferes with opacification of the external carotid artery. At surgery, a pseudoaneurysm of the external carotid artery was confirmed, and the carotid artery was sacrificed.

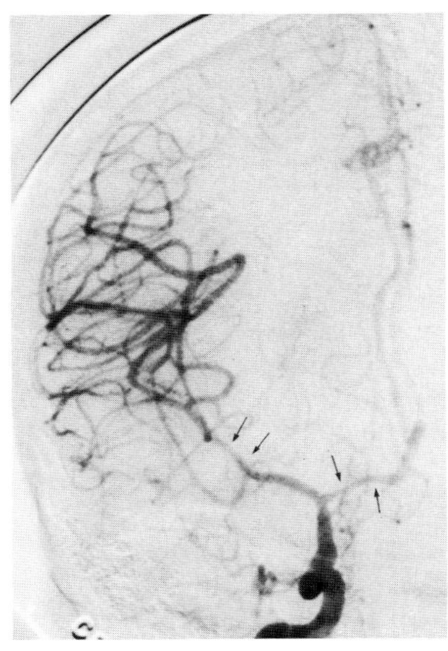

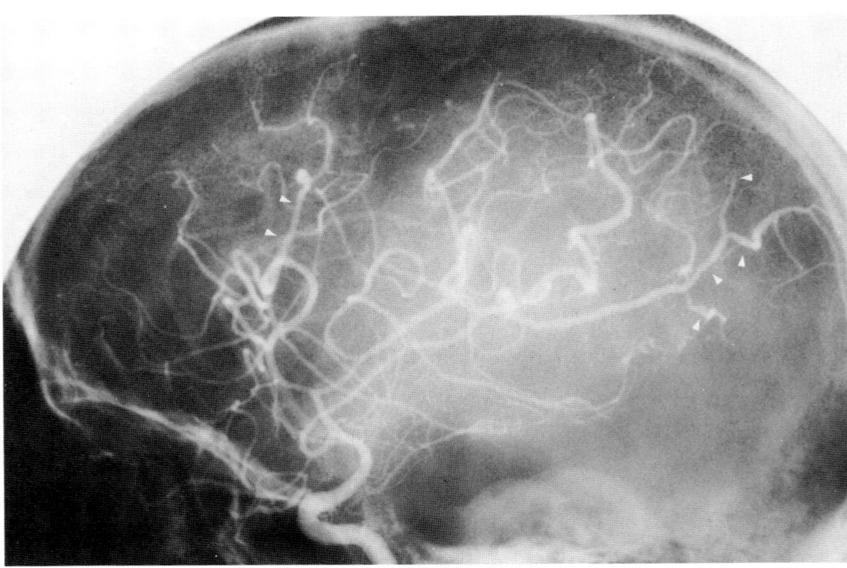

A B

Figure 13-24. Arteritis. A 27-year-old man with miliary tuberculosis and acid-fast bacilli on cerebrospinal fluid smear had episodic confusion, amnesia, ataxia, and blurred vision. (A and B) Right internal carotid angiogram. In addition to the right temporal expansion, the distal internal carotid and proximal middle cerebral arteries and the anterior cerebral artery are narrowed (*arrows*). The widespread vascular narrowing, irregularity, and occlusion (*arrowheads*) are best appreciated in (B). (A) AP projection; (B) lateral projection.

Figure 13-25. Takayasu arteritis. A young Caucasian woman had noticed tenderness in the right side of her neck for 1 year. Noninvasive studies demonstrated a diminished right carotid artery flow. (A and B) Innominate injection. An abrupt narrowing of the right common carotid artery occurs near its origin (*arrow*, A). The smooth long segment of stenosis continues to near the bifurcation (*white arrow*, B). The left common carotid artery (*arrowheads*), filled by reflux, appears normal. (C) Left internal carotid angiogram. The supratentorial circulation is well filled from the left carotid artery. (A and C) AP projection; (B) lateral projection.

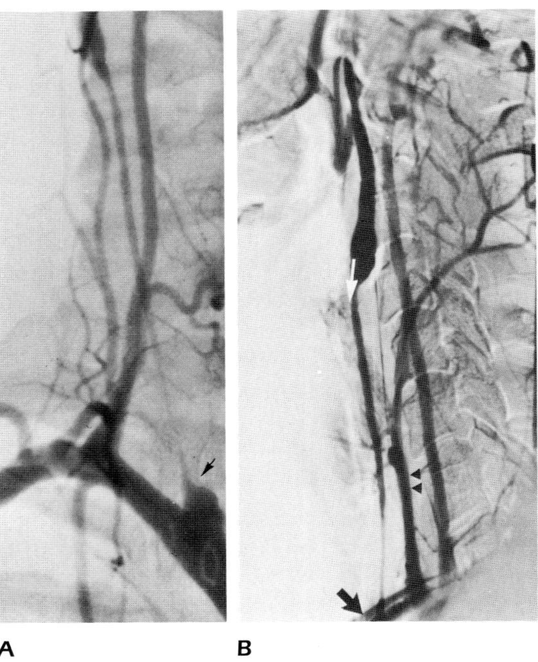

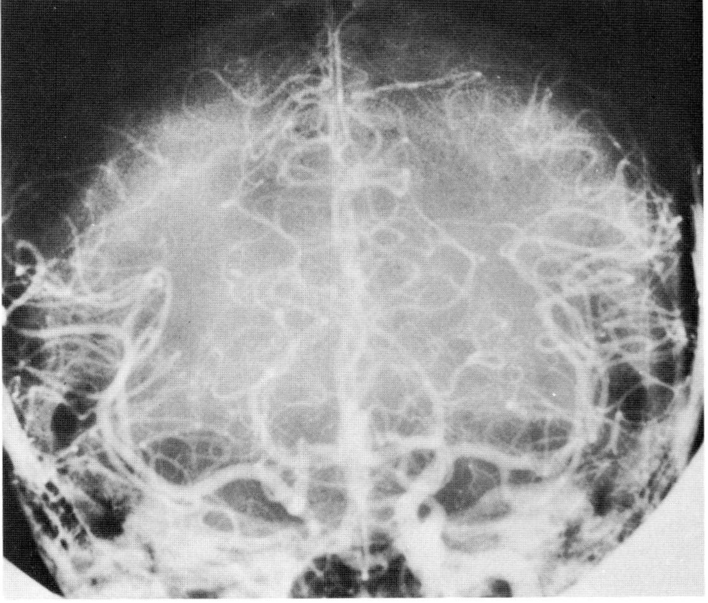

A B C

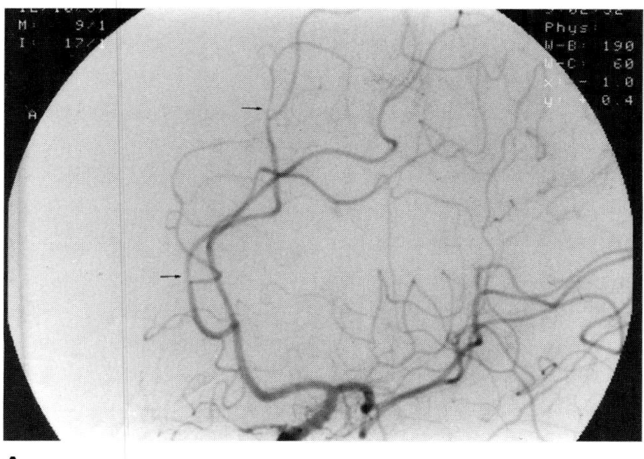

A B

Figure 13-26. Presumed CNS vasculitis. A 36-year-old woman presented with confusion and difficulty speaking. A brain MRI revealed infarcts of varying ages in multiple vascular territories, one of which was hemorrhagic. Her initial angiogram had only subtle caliber changes. A brain biopsy was done at that time, demonstrated evidence of infarction, but did not confirm vasculitis. A repeat angiogram was done 5 months later, and it revealed a progression of abnormal caliber changes. Her left carotid injection (A and B) reveals inappropriate narrowing of anterior cerebral branches (*arrows*). The biopsy was not repeated, and the patient was treated for vasculitis.

giitis, is a multisystem disorder. Arterial abnormalities are most common at bifurcations.[32] The disease results in focal arterial narrowing and dilatation, multiple occlusions, and characteristic microaneurysms. It especially affects small- to medium-size arteries.[28] There is a preference for abdominal involvement, and cerebral arteries rarely appear abnormal. Visceral arteries such as those to the liver, kidneys, and small bowel are the most commonly involved vessels.[30] Microaneurysm formation, common in visceral arteries, is uncommon in cerebral vessels.[32] Polyarteritis nodosa is similar to hypersensitivity angiitis.[28]

Isolated CNS vasculitis is rare (Figs. 13-26 and 13-27). Involvement is limited to cerebral vessels and has a mean age of onset of 43 years. Patients may present with headache, confusion, or other global CNS dysfunction, and one-third have associated cranial nerve deficits. Because angiography may be normal, diagnosis is usually established by biopsy.[33]

Carotid arteritis in infancy and childhood has been described as resulting in smooth narrowing of the supraclinoid carotid artery, with possible extension proximally into the internal carotid artery or distally into the anterior and middle cerebral arteries. It may also cause stenoses of the lenticulostriate arteries and of the anterior choroidal and posterior communicating arteries.[28]

Moyamoya disease (basal occlusive disease with telangiectasia) is a process that results in occlusions and stenoses of the distal internal carotid artery and the proximal middle and anterior cerebral arteries in children and young adults (Fig. 13-28). The disease may affect the distal basilar artery in some cases. There is often pronounced telangiectasia and pseudoangiomatous involvement of the lenticulostriate arteries and the anterior choroidal artery as they attempt to form collaterals around the diseased major arteries at the skull base. This lenticulostriate proliferation is what is referred to as the "puff of smoke" appearance that gives the disorder its name.[28,32]

In the category of collagen vascular diseases, systemic lupus erythematosus (SLE) can cause arteriographic abnormalities of small arteries, resulting in ectasia at bifurcations, stenoses, and occlusions. SLE may affect the branches of the internal or external carotid artery, and in some cases is associated with multiple aneurysms.[28,32] Rheumatoid arthritis can also be associated with arteritis; however, angiographic abnormalities are usually confined to the small arteries in the extremities.[30]

Fibromuscular dysplasia (FMD) is a disease of women, usually presenting between the ages of 40 and 70. Symptoms most often relate to ischemic events (56 percent of patients), although others come to attention because of cerebral aneurysms (present in 22 percent of patients). Typically, somewhat asymmetric alternating areas of stenosis and dilatation are seen in the upper cervical portions of both internal carotid arteries (Fig. 13-29). In a minority of patients, there is involvement of the vertebral arteries (15 percent) or intra-

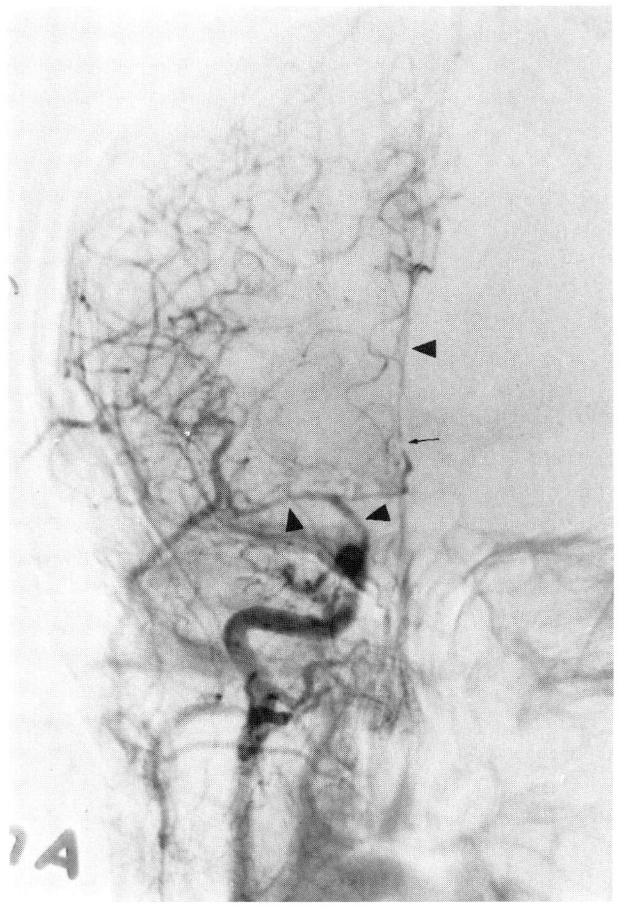

A

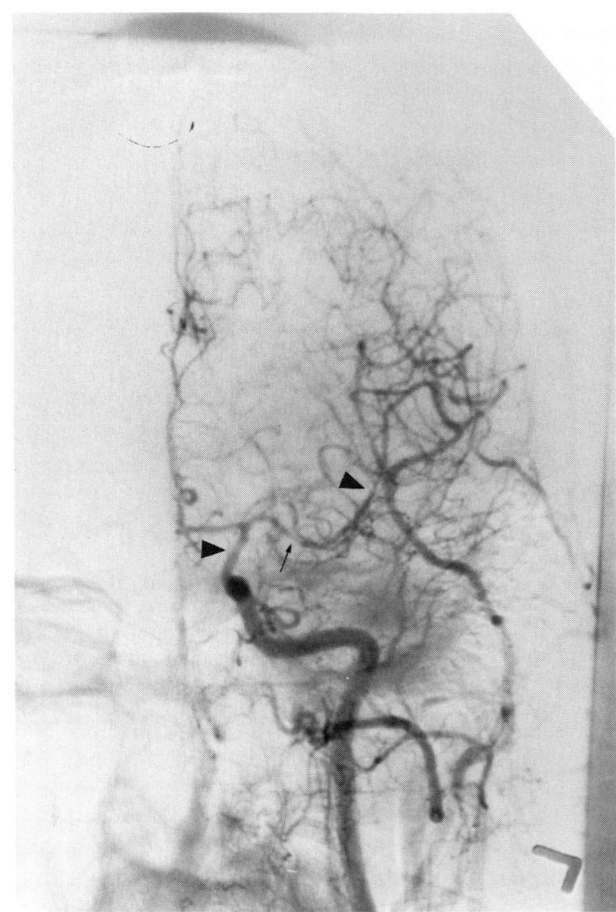

B

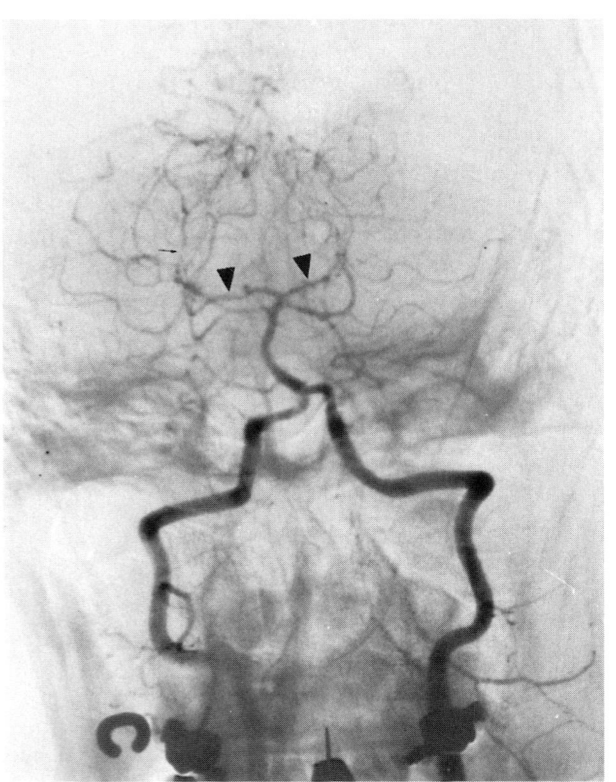

C

Figure 13-27. CNS vasculitis. A 38-year-old man initially presented with right hemiparesis, but over the course of several weeks he became disoriented and unable to follow commands. A brain MRI revealed focal hemorrhages in both lenticular nuclei and in the left thalamus, as well as nonhemorrhagic infarction in the left paraventricular white matter. He underwent two cerebral angiograms about 3 weeks apart. There was an interval progression of abnormal arterial caliber changes. (A to F) Final angiogram. Many long segments of arteries are narrowed (*arrowheads*). In addition, there are areas of focal stenosis (*arrows*) and dilatation (*open arrows*).

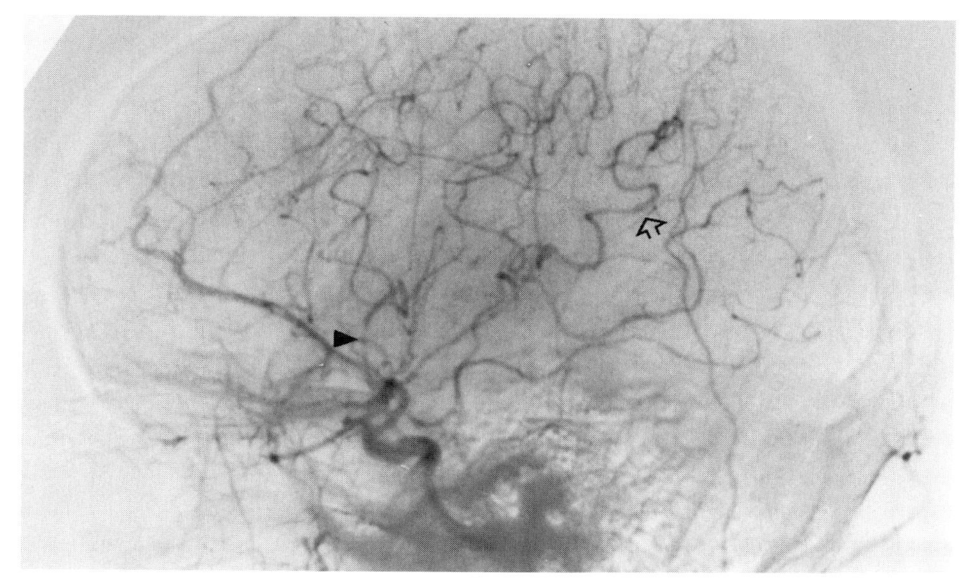

D

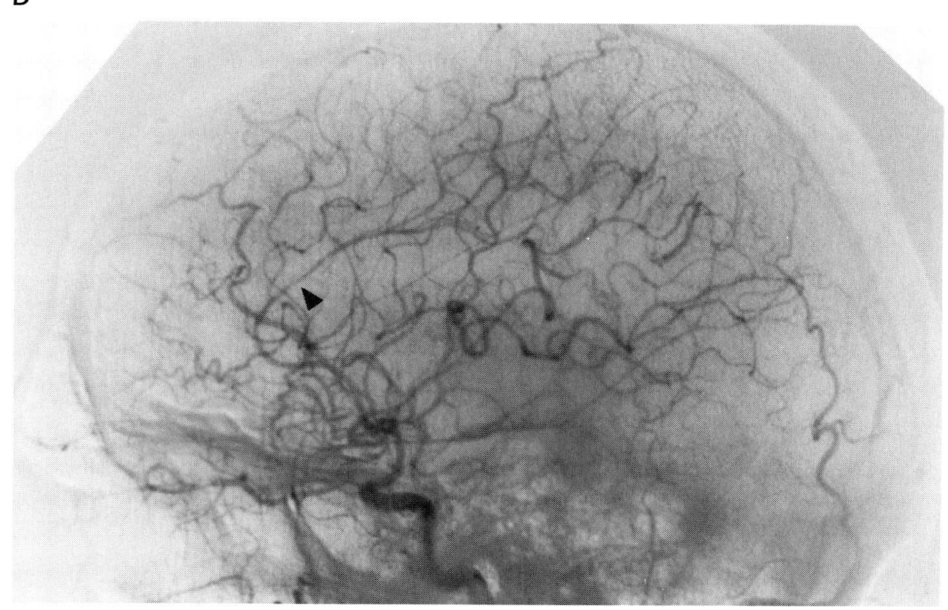

E

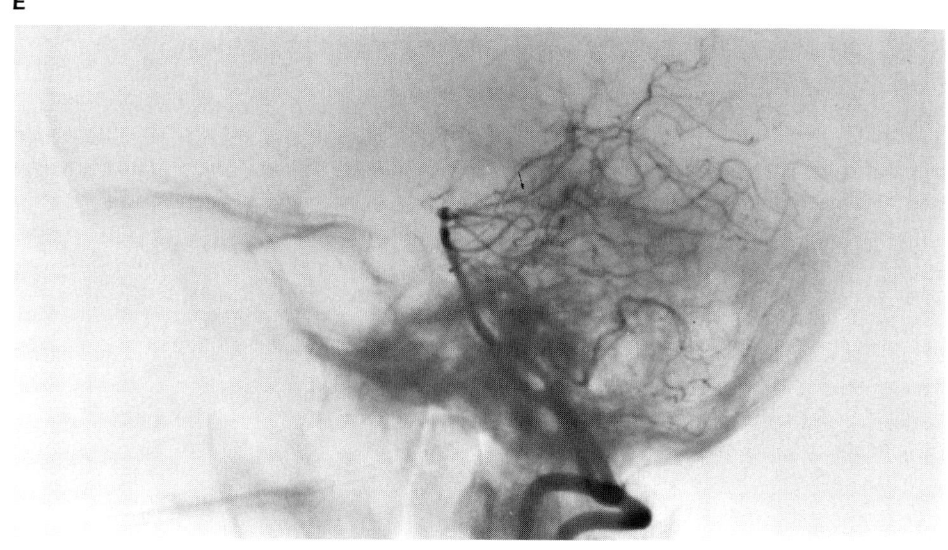

F

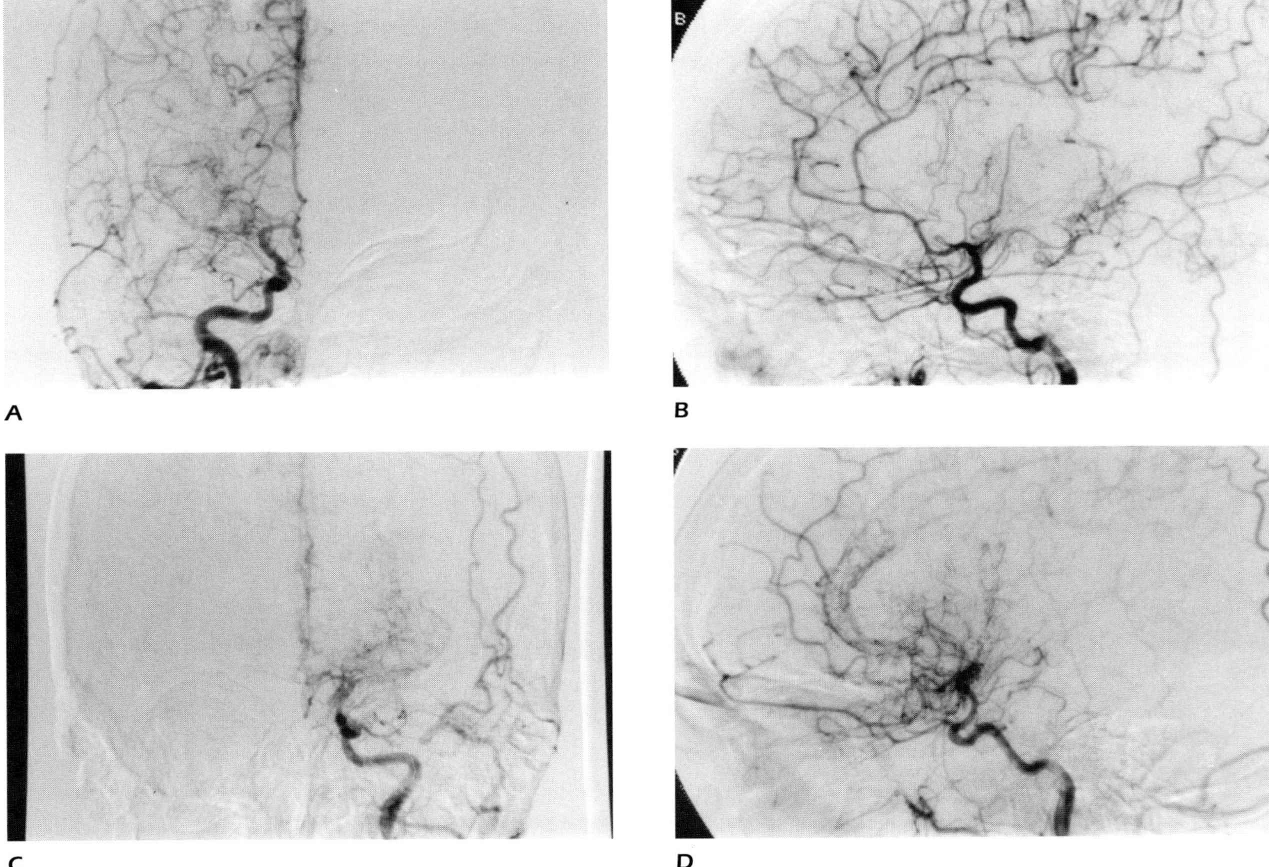

Figure 13-28. Moyamoya. A 34-year-old woman with neurofibromatosis presented with mental status changes and right lower extremity weakness. Her brain MRI revealed an old right temporoparietal infarct and a subacute left frontal infarct, atrophy, and paraventricular white matter signal abnormalities. Her angiogram (right carotid, A and B; left carotid, C and D) demonstrates near-total occlusions of both middle cerebral arteries, narrowing of the supraclinoid left internal carotid artery, and narrowing of the left anterior cerebral artery. There are proliferative angiomatous changes of the lenticulostriate arteries and along the left anterior cerebral artery.

cranial branches (10 percent). The appearance has been likened to a string of beads.[34] Fistulas, including carotid-cavernous fistulas, may develop as a complication of the disease.[35]

Ehlers-Danlos syndrome is another disorder of arteries that may lead to dissection and inappropriate caliber changes of cerebral vessels (Fig. 13-30). The syndrome may affect both extracranial and intracranial vessels, and has also been associated with an increased incidence of cerebral aneurysms and fistulas.[36,37]

In addition to the above diseases, many other processes may lead to arterial caliber changes. Radiation can result in arterial changes similar to those of vasculitis. Narrowed vessels or occlusions can be found within radiation ports.[28] Neurofibromatosis can produce similar findings, and migraine can result in caliber changes or occlusions.[28] Drugs, such as amphetamines, are known to be associated with cerebral artery branch narrowing and dilatation, and sickle cell disease has been known to cause distal internal carotid and proximal anterior and middle cerebral artery narrowing or occlusion.[28] Focal vasculitislike changes may be seen in association with intracerebral tumors.[28] Narrowed arteries have been described with coital headache[38] and are commonly seen as a result of vasospasm following subarachnoid hemorrhage. Transient acute hypertension can be associated with vasculitislike angiographic changes (Fig. 13-31) that resolve with reestablishment of a normotensive state.[39] Narrowed arteries have also been described in eclampsia (Fig. 13-32) and preeclampsia.[40]

As is evident from this discussion, there are many potential causes for caliber changes of cerebral arteries. When arterial caliber changes are present on angiog-

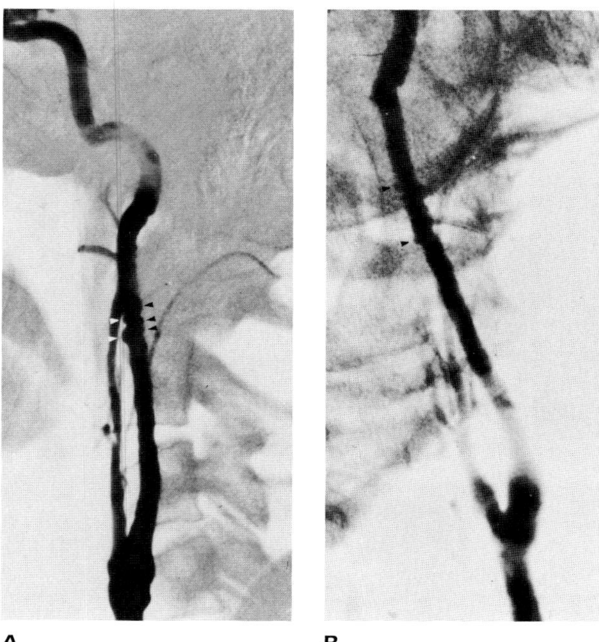

Figure 13-29. Fibromuscular dysplasia. (A and B) Left common carotid angiogram. There is incidental demonstration of nearly regular outpouching along the internal carotid artery, with several areas wider than the adjacent lumen (*arrowheads*). The presumptive diagnosis is fibromuscular dysplasia. (A) Lateral projection; (B) AP oblique projection.

Figure 13-30. Ehlers-Danlos syndrome. A 33-year-old woman presented with chemosis, proptosis, and loss of visual acuity in her right eye. She was found to have a recurrent right carotid-cavernous fistula. Her right carotid angiogram (A and B), in addition to showing the arteriovenous shunting from the fistula, reveals a very irregular appearance of the internal carotid artery with focal areas of abnormal dilatation. There are coils in the cavernous sinus from a previous embolization. Other examinations of the patient revealed aortic and coronary artery dissections, characteristic of this systemic arterial disease.

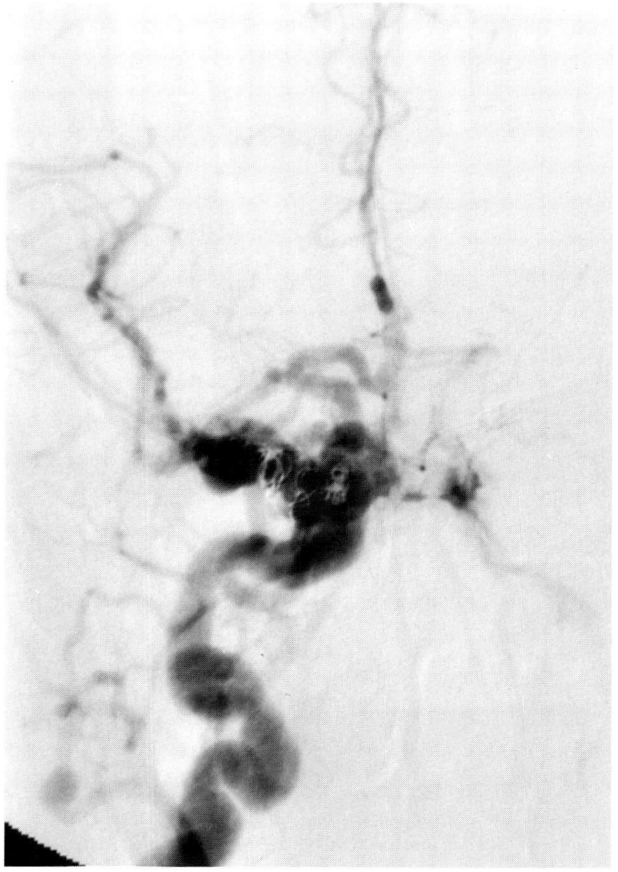

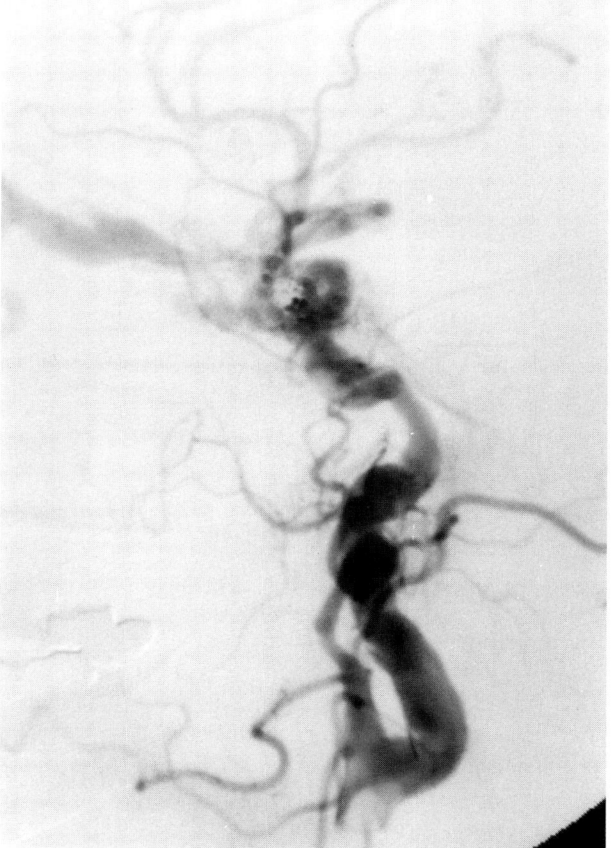

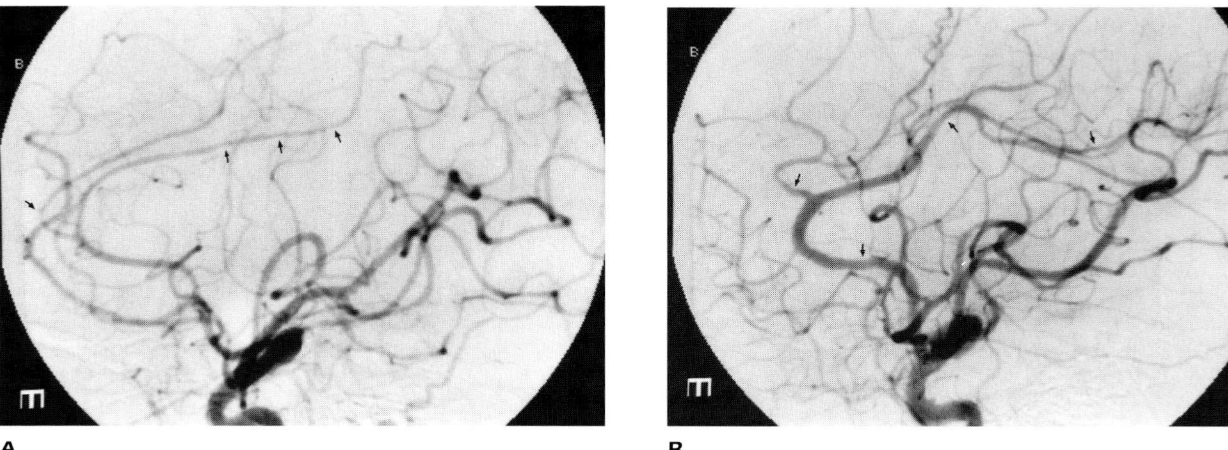

A B

Figure 13-31. Hypertension. A 46-year-old woman was admitted in hypertensive crisis and developed symptoms of a right hemispheric stroke. A brain MRI revealed multiple lacunar infarctions. Her angiogram (A and B) demonstrates focal areas of arterial stenosis (*arrows*).

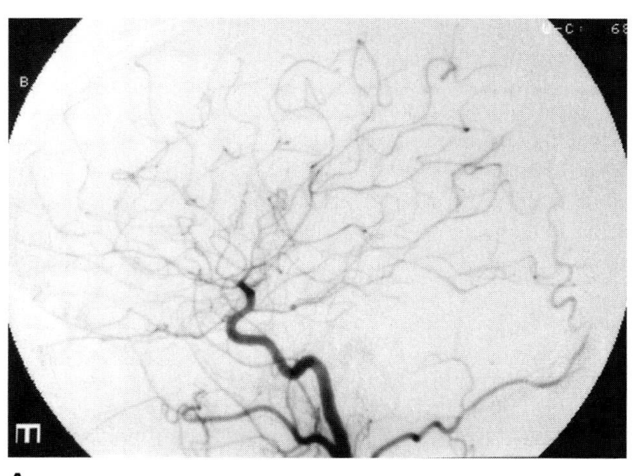

A B

Figure 13-32. Eclampsia. A 20-year-old woman developed seizures and difficulty walking postpartum. Her carotid (A) and vertebral (B) angiograms reveal diffuse narrowing of the anterior, middle, and posterior cerebral arteries, the cerebellar arteries, and the basilar artery. Serial MR angiograms showed a gradual improvement in arterial caliber over several weeks.

raphy, the problem becomes one of making a rather nonspecific vascular response specific for a particular diagnosis (Fig. 13-33). The diagnosis of vasculitis may be correct if other possible causes and conditions for the arteriographic abnormalities can be excluded by history, physical examination, and laboratory data. The further diagnosis of a particular form of vasculitis may be suggested by the type and distribution of the abnormalities, the age of the patient, and other available clinical information. Vasculitis can be present despite a normal cerebral angiogram, and biopsy may be necessary for diagnosis in these cases.

Aneurysms

Berry (saccular) aneurysm rupture is the most common cause of subarachnoid hemorrhage, and occurs in 75 percent of such cases. Berry aneurysms are abnormal, saclike outpouchings of cerebral arteries that typically have defined necks (Fig. 13-34). They are thought to arise at weak points in arterial walls and are most common at branch points. Giant aneurysms, those defined as 2.5 cm in size or larger, are a special class of cerebral aneurysms, and are often more difficult to treat than small aneurysms.[41] Other types of

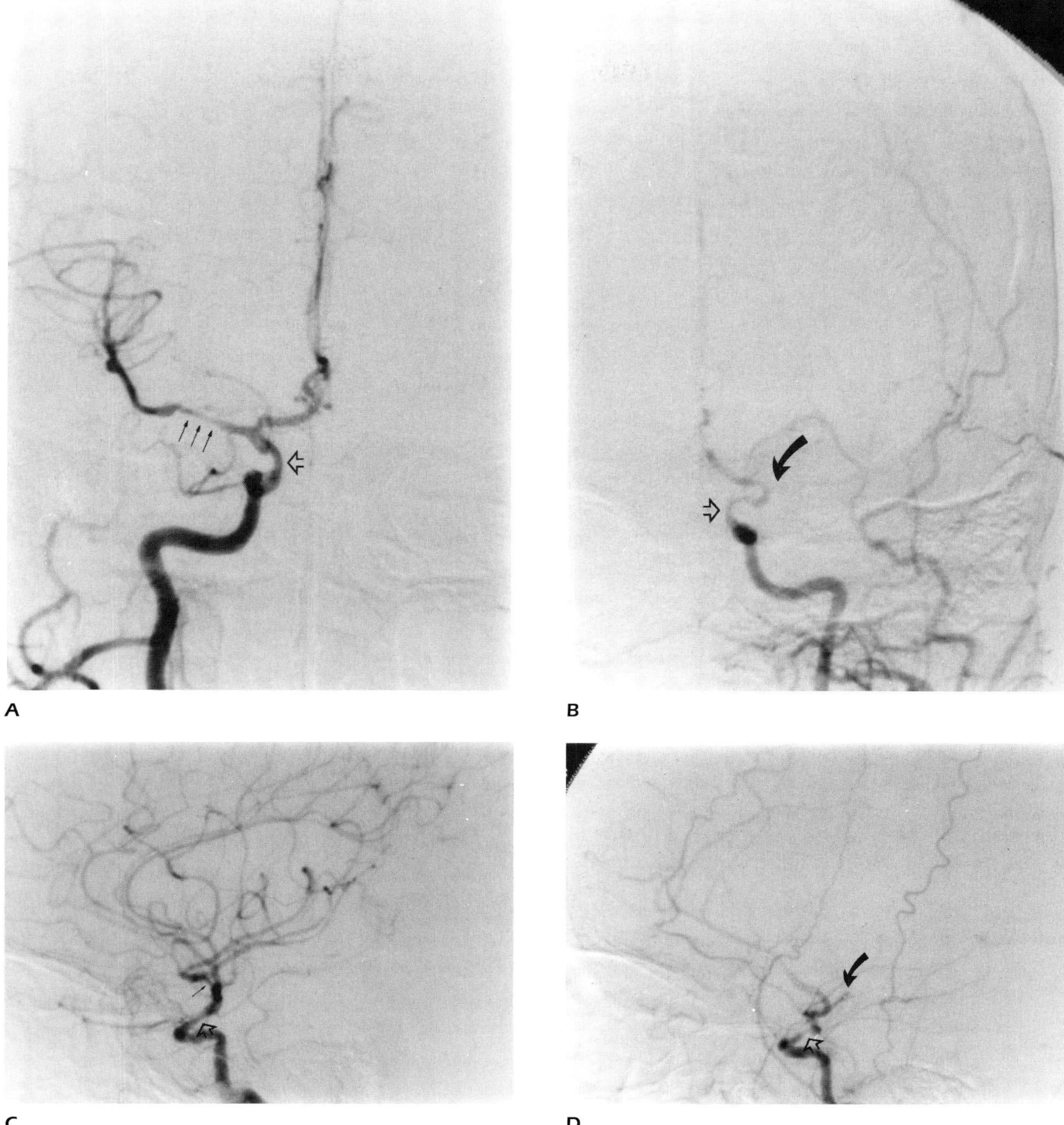

Figure 13-33. Basal occlusive disease, unknown etiology. A 46-year-old woman was evaluated because of a right parietooccipital hemorrhage. A bone marrow biopsy was suggestive of Waldenström macroglobulinemia, but there were no other medical illnesses. Her angiogram reveals narrowing of the supraclinoid right and left internal carotid arteries (*open arrows,* A to D), an occlusion of the left middle cerebral artery (*curved arrows,* B and D), and a long segment of narrowing in the right middle cerebral artery (*small arrows,* A and C). There is no angiomatous proliferation of small basal arteries, in contrast to Figure 13-28. The patient was asymptomatic with respect to the left middle cerebral artery occlusion.

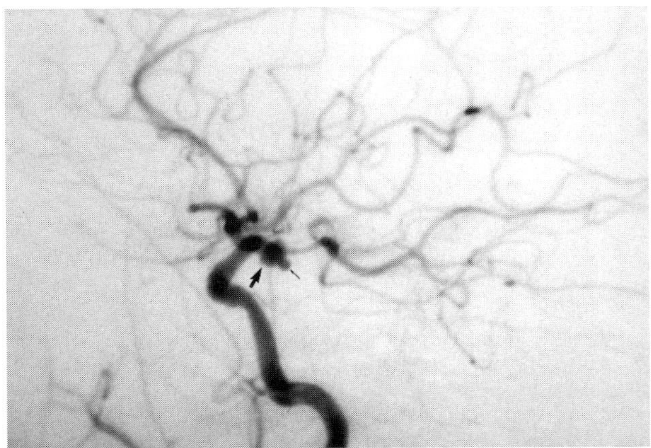

Figure 13-34. Posterior communicating artery aneurysm. A 49-year-old woman presented with an acute subarachnoid hemorrhage. A single aneurysm (*large arrow*) of the supraclinoid internal carotid artery was found at angiography at the level of the posterior communicating artery. The outpouching at the dome of the aneurysm (*small arrow*) is an irregularity of the aneurysm's lumen that is suggestive of rupture. These aneurysms typically point posteriorly.

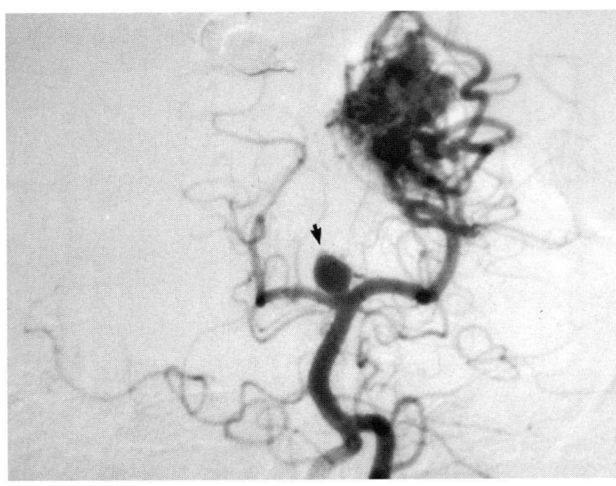

A

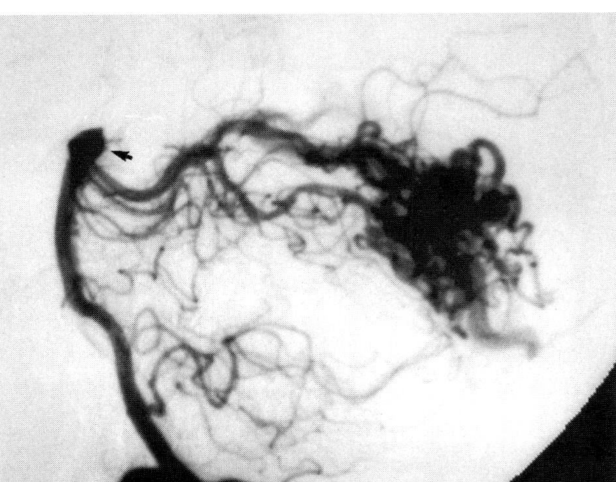

B

Figure 13-35. Basilar tip aneurysm in association with AVM. A 38-year-old man was involved in a motor vehicle accident. A brain CT scan disclosed subarachnoid and intraventricular hemorrhage, but no parenchymal blood. His left vertebral angiogram demonstrates a left occipital AVM and a basilar tip aneurysm (*arrows,* A and B). It was assumed that a spontaneous aneurysm rupture had occurred, leading to the patient's loss of consciousness and control of the vehicle.

aneurysms include mycotic aneurysms, atherosclerotic or fusiform aneurysms, and traumatic aneurysms.

The prevalence of cerebral aneurysms is estimated to be about 5 percent. Some data suggest a higher incidence of aneurysms, about 18 percent, in individuals with a positive family history of subarachnoid hemorrhage within the second degree of consanguinity.[42] Risk factors for berry aneurysms include a history of smoking, polycystic kidney disease, coarctation of the aorta, Ehlers-Danlos syndrome, and fibromuscular dysplasia, and there are associations with other vascular abnormalities or anomalies, such as arteriovenous malformations (AVMs) (Fig. 13-35), persistent trigeminal arteries, and azygous anterior cerebral arteries.[43–48] The bleeding rate for an incidentally discovered unruptured aneurysm is about 1 percent per year, whereas the rebleeding rate for an untreated ruptured aneurysm is about 3 to 4 percent per year, if the patient survives the initial month, in which the chance of rebleeding is 30 to 40 percent.[45,46] Only about 60 percent of patients with ruptured aneurysms who survive to reach the hospital return to normal, productive lives without deficits.[49] Aside from death and rebleeding, the complications of ruptured aneurysms include ischemic brain injury from cerebral vasospasm and hydrocephalus from impaired cerebral spinal fluid (CSF) absorption. Vasospasm is estimated to occur in up to 80 percent of patients with ruptured aneurysms, but is symptomatic in only 18 to 44 percent (Fig. 13-36). The incidence of symptomatic vasospasm may be lower in patients who receive early surgical repair of a bleeding aneurysm.[50]

Some sites are more common for berry aneurysms than others. The anterior communicating (ACOM) artery, the internal carotid artery (ICA) at the posterior communicating artery level, and the MCA bifurcation are usually the most frequent sites (Figs. 13-37 through 13-39). Other but less common locations include the internal carotid artery at the level of the oph-

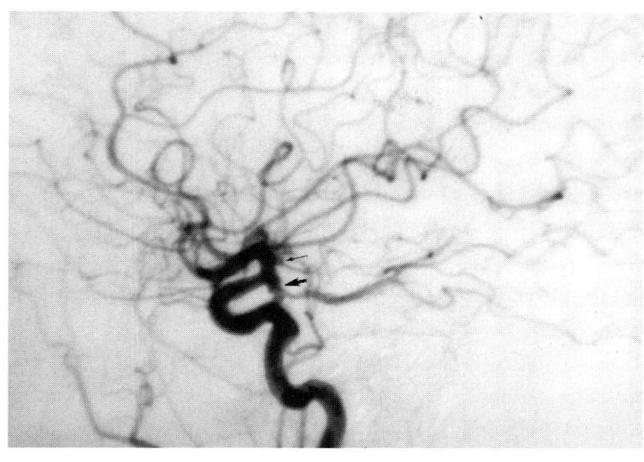

A

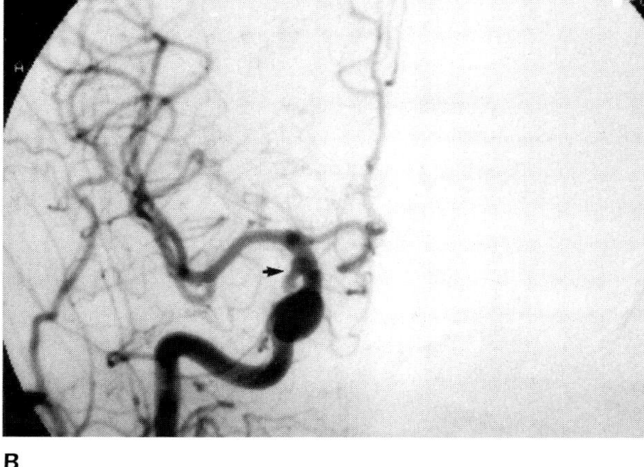

B

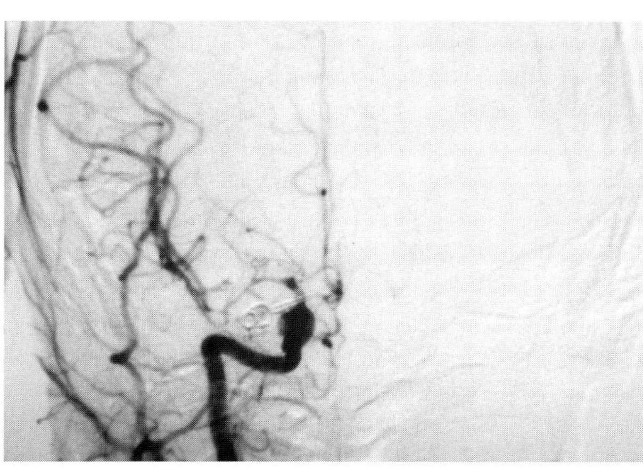

C

Figure 13-36. Symptomatic vasospasm. A 34-year-old woman presented with an acute subarachnoid hemorrhage. Her initial angiogram (A and B) demonstrates an irregular right posterior communicating artery aneurysm (*arrows*). A tiny, second aneurysm is also seen at the anterior choroidal artery origin (*small arrow*, A). The posterior communicating artery aneurysm was clipped and the patient made an uneventful recovery. She returned to the hospital following discharge, 9 days after the hemorrhage, with a left hemiparesis. Her second angiogram (C) demonstrates satisfactory clipping of the aneurysm, but the development of moderate to severe vasospasm. There is narrowing of the supraclinoid internal carotid artery as well as of the proximal middle and anterior cerebral arteries. The hemiparesis resolved immediately after balloon angioplasty and intraarterial papaverine infusion.

Figure 13-37. Anterior communicating artery aneurysm. A 46-year-old woman presented with an acute subarachnoid and intraventricular hemorrhage with associated mild hydrocephalus by CT. Her angiogram reveals a lobulated anterior communicating artery aneurysm (*arrows*, A and B).

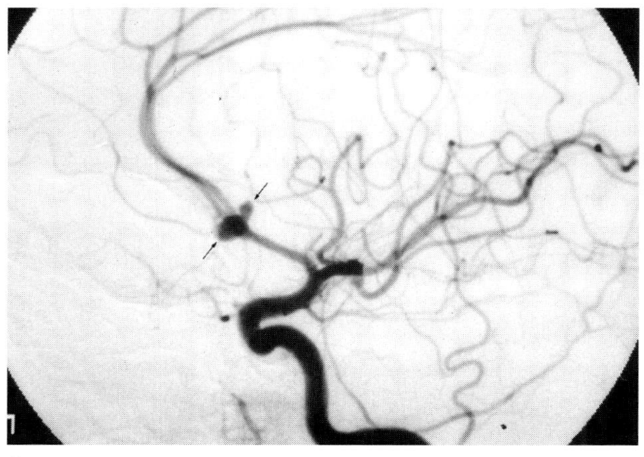

A

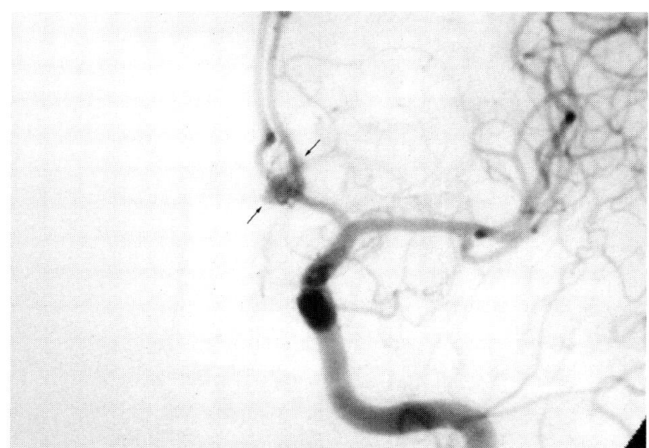

B

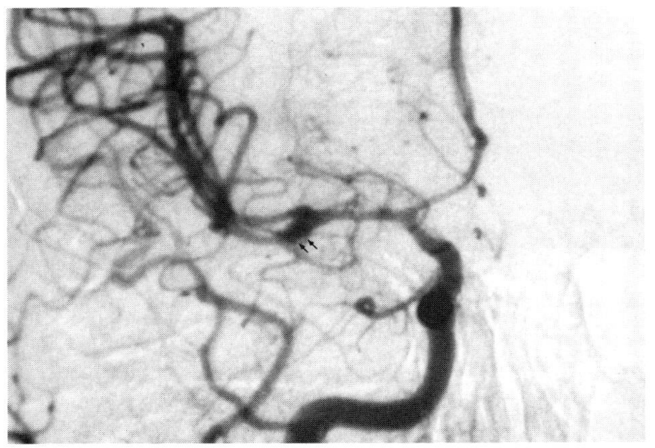

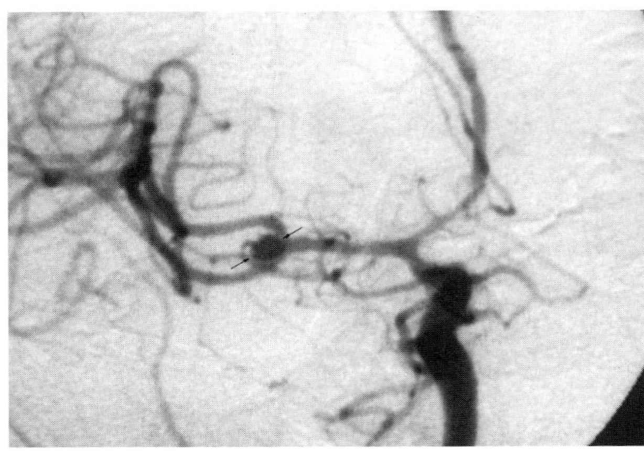

A B

Figure 13-38. MCA bifurcation aneurysm. A 38-year-old woman presented with an acute subarachnoid hemorrhage. Her CT scan demonstrated blood confined to the right sylvian fissure. The PA (A) and oblique (B) views of her right carotid angiogram reveal a small aneurysm at the bifurcation of the middle cerebral artery (*arrows*). The aneurysm is seen to better advantage on the magnified oblique view.

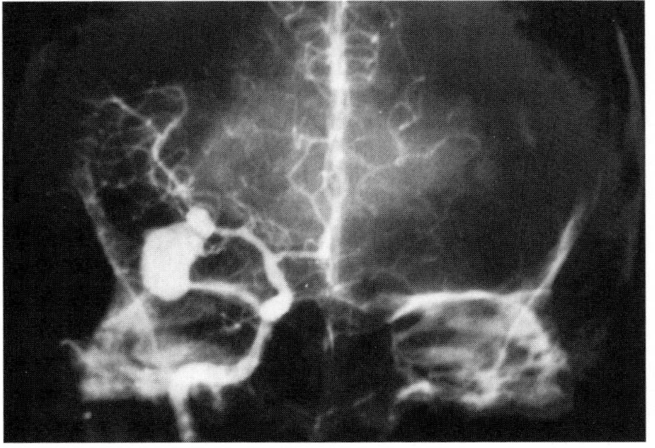

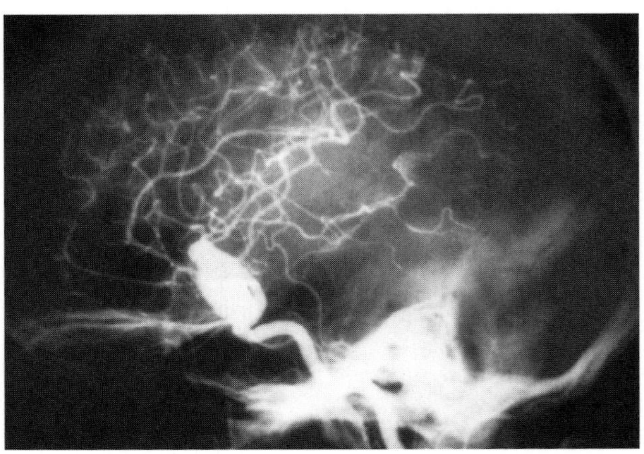

A B

Figure 13-39. Giant MCA aneurysm. A 48-year-old woman had been suspected of having a neoplasm or giant aneurysm in her right middle fossa on MRI. She had not experienced a subarachnoid bleed. Her right carotid angiogram (A and B) demonstrates a giant middle cerebral artery aneurysm.

thalmic artery and the basilar tip (Figs. 13-40 through 13-43). Table 13-1 lists the relative frequencies of aneurysms at these locations.[51,52] In the pediatric population, aneurysm type and location differ from the adult. Aneurysms are more often giant or related to infection in children.[53] Cerebral arterial aneurysms are seen in 10 percent of patients with cerebral AVMs; these may or may not be on the feeding arteries.[54]

The incidence of multiple aneurysms ranges from 8.6 to 33.5 percent.[43–46] Women are more likely than men to have multiple aneurysms.[43] A cooperative study found a 19 percent incidence of multiple aneurysms, but only 24 percent of registered cases included bilateral carotid and vertebral angiography (see Table 13-1).[52] The majority of examinations in the study were limited to bilateral carotid injections, so the actual incidence of multiple aneurysms might be higher. Regardless, there is a high enough incidence of multiple aneurysms to justify investigation of the entire cerebral circulation during an angiogram for subarachnoid hemorrhage.

If multiple aneurysms are found on cerebral angiography, certain characteristics can help identify the anl-eurysm responsible for the subarachnoid bleed. The

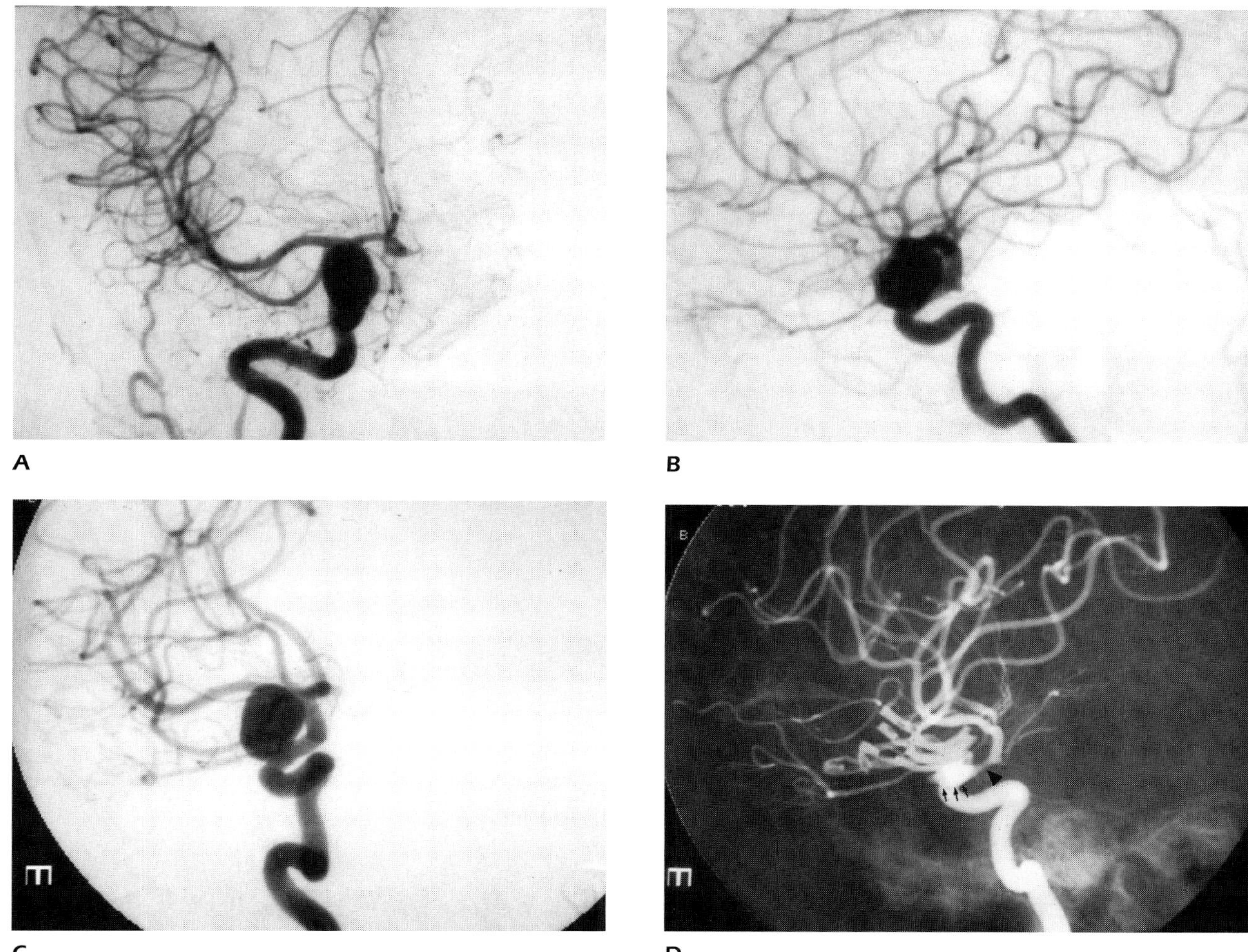

Figure 13-40. Ophthalmic aneurysm. A 45-year-old woman was referred for surgery of a previously diagnosed aneurysm. Her preoperative right carotid angiogram (A, B, and C) demonstrates a large supraclinoid carotid aneurysm at the level of the ophthalmic artery. Ophthalmic aneurysms typically point superiorly. The oblique view (C) provides the best view of the aneurysm neck. The aneurysm was clipped, but surgery was made difficult by the size of the aneurysm and the calcification within its walls. The postoperative angiogram (D) demonstrates multiple aneurysm clips but a residual aneurysm neck (*small arrows*). There is mild spasm of the supraclinoid carotid artery (*arrowhead*).

Table 13-1. Frequency of Cerebral Aneurysms at Common Sites

	All Cases (%)	Bleeding Aneurysms (%)	Unruptured Symptomatic Aneurysms (%)	Incidental Aneurysms (%)
Supracavernous internal carotid	32	36	80	37
Anterior communicating	23	31	2.4	23
Middle cerebral	16	21	9.1	27
Vertebrobasilar	4.5	5.5	5.5	9.6
Multiple aneurysms	19			

Data from the Cooperative Study of Intracranial Aneurysms and Subarachnoid Hemorrhage.[51,52]

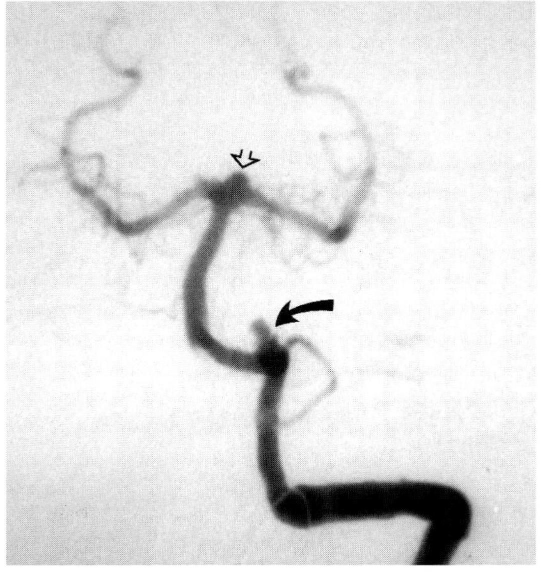

A

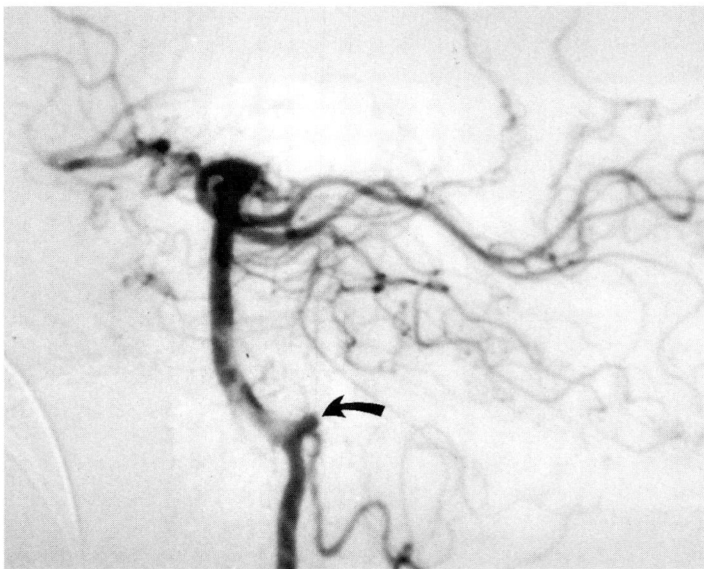

B

C

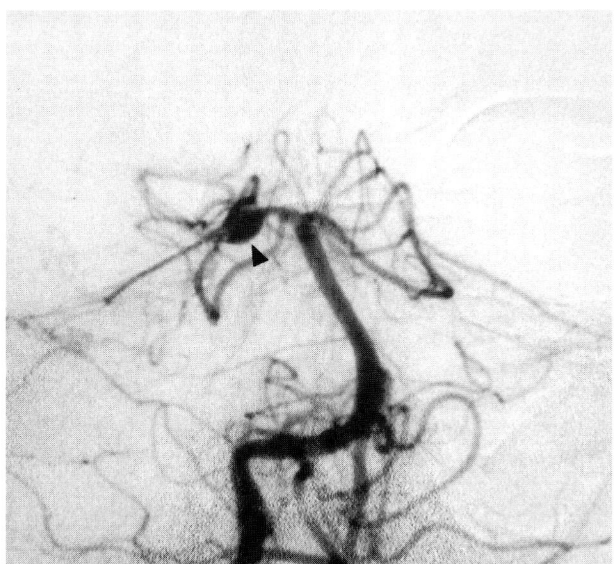

D

Figure 13-41. Posterior circulation aneurysms. A 70-year-old woman lost consciousness and suffered a respiratory arrest. Her CT scan showed subarachnoid and intraventricular hemorrhage with mild hydrocephalus. Her carotid angiograms (not shown) revealed bilateral internal carotid artery occlusions. Her left vertebral angiogram demonstrates a small posterior inferior cerebellar artery (PICA) aneurysm (*curved arrows,* A and B) as well as a tiny basilar tip aneurysm (*open arrow,* A). In another patient, a tiny aneurysm of the basilar artery at the left superior cerebellar artery origin is demonstrated by left vertebral angiography (*arrow,* C). In a third example, the right vertebral angiogram of a 54-year-old woman with fibromuscular dysplasia and a previous subarachnoid hemorrhage demonstrates an aneurysm of the right posterior cerebral artery at the P1-P2 junction, where the posterior communicating artery joins the posterior cerebral artery (*arrowhead,* D).

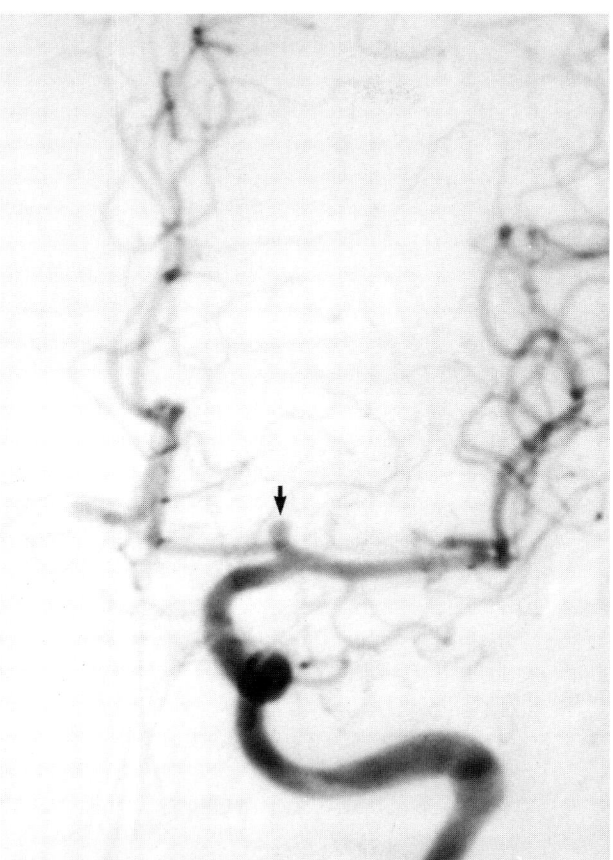

Figure 13-42. Internal carotid artery bifurcation aneurysm. A 58-year-old woman was evaluated for a dural AVF involving the right orbit. Her left carotid angiogram reveals an incidental aneurysm at the bifurcation of the left internal carotid artery (*arrow*).

localization of the hemorrhage on CT scanning of the brain may be useful. Wherever subarachnoid blood is greatest may be the appropriate site, although subarachnoid blood, once present, may pool after time in the dependent portion of the head. A septal hematoma points to rupture of an anterior communicating artery aneurysm, just as parenchymal hemorrhage in the parasylvian region indicates rupture of a middle cerebral artery aneurysm. Localization of blood in the third ventricle may suggest a basilar tip aneurysm, just as blood in the fourth ventricle suggests a bleed from a posterior inferior cerebellar artery aneurysm. The appearance of the aneurysms themselves on angiography can also be helpful. Irregularity of an aneurysm may be the most important sign suggesting rupture. The larger an aneurysm, the more likely it is to have bled. The presence of vasospasm near an aneurysm may indicate that it was the source of hemorrhage, but vasospasm may not be seen initially. Vasospasm typically does not occur until 2 days after subarachnoid hemorrhage and peaks at about 2 weeks.[50]

Recent reports have tended to support the concept of early diagnosis and repair of cerebral aneurysms.[55] Early repair of ruptured aneurysms allows maximum therapy for prevention or treatment of vasospasm and subsequent ischemic injury. This typically includes treatment with induced hypertension, hypervolemia, and calcium channel blockers, and, in symptomatic cases, may include balloon angioplasty of cerebral vessels or intraarterial infusions of spasmolytic agents.

Not all subarachnoid hemorrhages are explained by angiographic findings, and some aneurysms can be missed on initial examination. In the cooperative study, there were 1251 initially unexplained subarachnoid hemorrhages in 5484 patients. Only 219 of the 1251 were subjected to repeat angiography or autopsy, and of those, 47 (22 percent of the 219) were found to have aneurysms that had been missed on initial angiography. This constituted 3.8 percent of the 1251 cases of initially negative angiograms in the 1966 study.[47] It is probably reasonable to estimate that 5 percent or less of aneurysms are missed on an initial comprehensive study today because of technical factors, misinterpretation, or spasm that interferes with filling of parent vessels or aneurysms. Repeat angiograms may be obtained in these cases after intervals of 1 to 2 weeks. If a repeat examination is negative, myelography or MRI to exclude the presence of a spinal AVM as a source of subarachnoid bleeding may be indicated.[56]

Mycotic aneurysms are most frequently associated with infective endocarditis and tend to arise in locations that are unusual for typical berry aneurysms (Fig. 13-44). They can also behave differently by rupturing into brain parenchyma without bleeding into the subarachnoid space. Mycotic aneurysms tend not to be saccular with necks that can be clipped with preservation of the parent vessels; rather, they tend to be fusiform dilatations of the branches of intracranial arteries. The parietal branches of the middle cerebral artery are the most frequent sites for the development of mycotic aneurysms in patients with endocarditis.[57] Fusiform mycotic aneurysms of the cavernous internal carotid artery can form as a result of infection in the cavernous sinus. Mycotic cerebral aneurysms may also result from CNS tuberculosis.[58] Treatment may include trapping (occluding the parent vessel proximal and distal to the aneurysm) and antibiotic therapy. It is worthy of note that, if a patient with a mycotic aneurysm is studied in the acute period of hemorrhage and is found to have a given number of mycotic aneurysms, that number

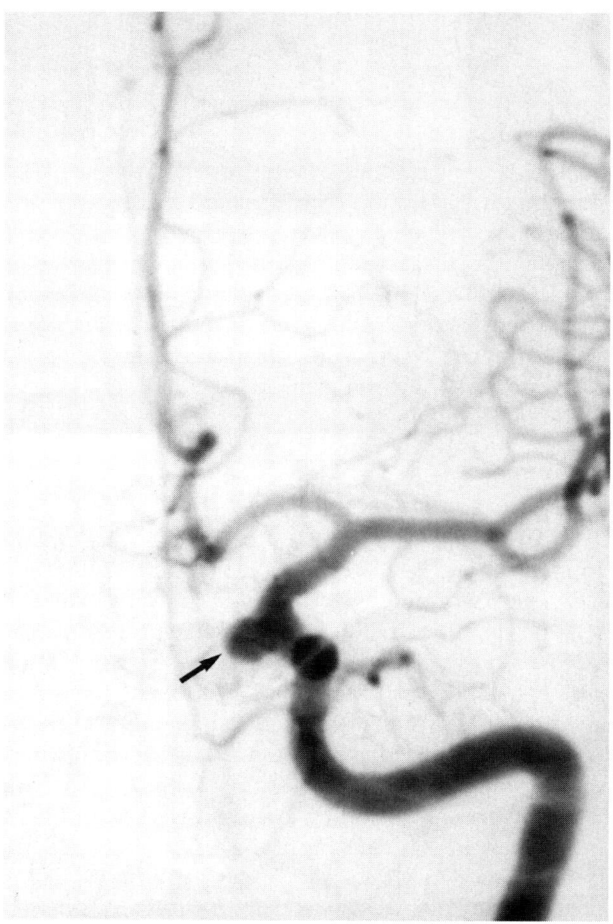

A

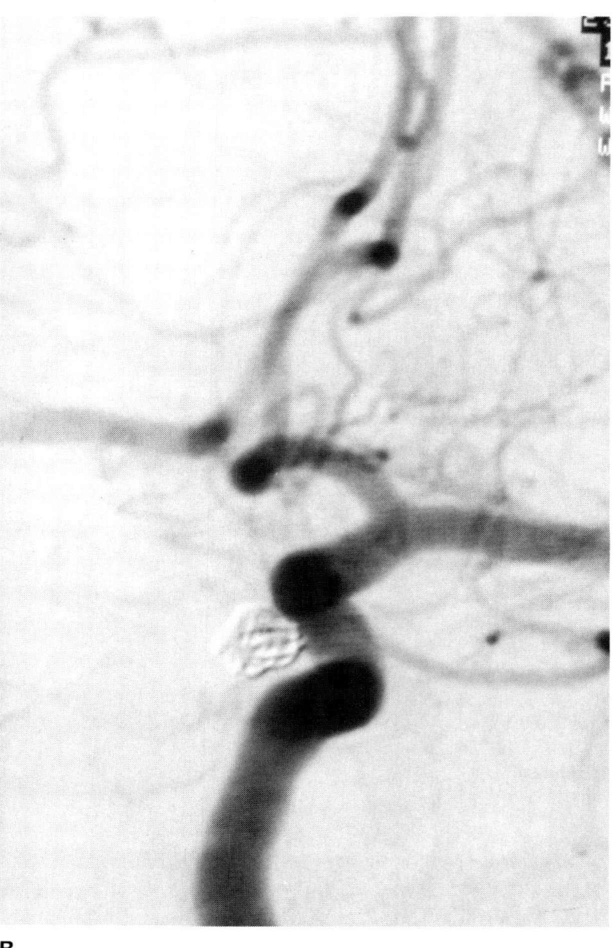

B

Figure 13-43. Superior hypophyseal aneurysm. A 47-year-old woman was evaluated for a left frontal mass, subsequently resected and proven to be a meningioma. Her angiogram reveals an incidental aneurysm of the left internal carotid artery (*arrow,* A) that arises opposite to the origin of the ophthalmic artery and points inferiorly and medially. A follow-up angiogram (B), obtained after outside referral for endovascular treatment, shows Guglielmi detachable coils (GDCs) within the aneurysm.

may be different on a subsequent examination regardless of antibiotic therapy. If more aneurysms are detected on repeat examination, therapy could be altered or lengthened.

Atherosclerotic aneurysms tend to be fusiform enlargements of the cavernous internal carotid artery or the basilar artery. These usually do not present with subarachnoid hemorrhage. They may be found incidentally or as a result of associated thromboembolic events (Fig. 13-45). Large carotid or basilar aneurysms may come to attention as a result of symptoms related to mass effect, such as headache, facial pain, seizures, cranial neuropathies, or other neurologic dysfunction. Ruptures of cavernous carotid aneurysms may result in signs and symptoms of carotid-cavernous fistulas. Acute severe headache can occur, unrelated to sub-

Figure 13-45. Cavernous carotid aneurysm. A 77-year-old woman had a brain MRI scan for a facial nerve palsy. In addition to the finding of a parotid gland tumor, the scan revealed an aneurysm at the level of the left cavernous sinus. Her left carotid angiogram (A and B) confirms the presence of a large cavernous carotid aneurysm. The base view (B) demonstrates the aneurysm lateral to the carotid artery. Although this patient was asymptomatic with respect to the aneurysm, others may present with compression palsies of cranial nerves that course through the cavernous sinus. ▶

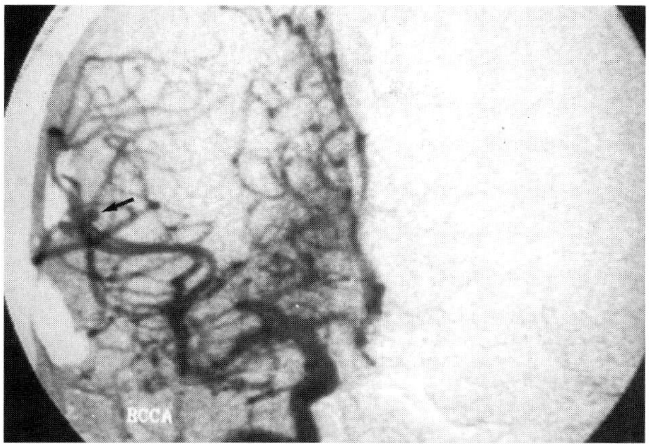

A

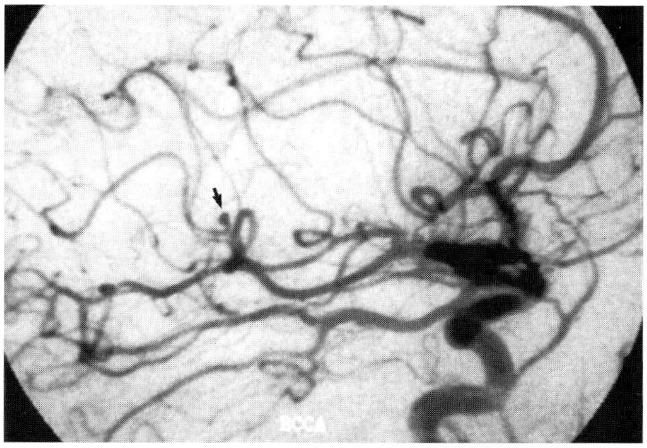

B

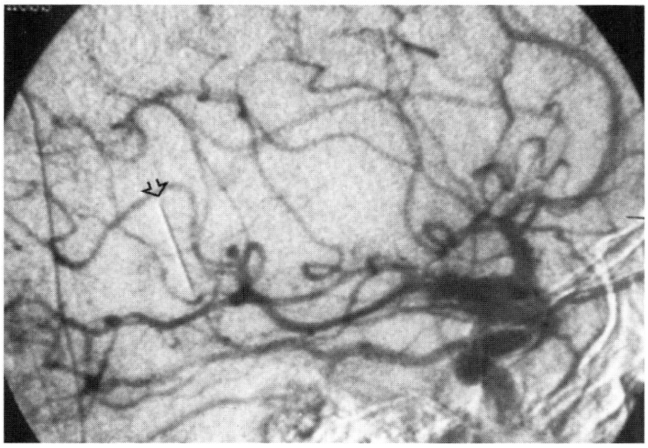

C

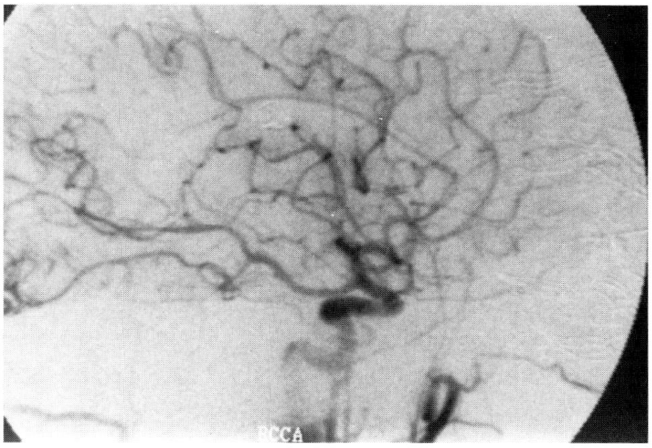

D

Figure 13-44. Mycotic aneurysm. A 34-year-old man with infective endocarditis and tricuspid valvular disease was evaluated for declining alertness and a left hemiparesis. His brain CT scan revealed a 5 × 4 cm right frontal and temporal parasylvian hemorrhage with transtentorial herniation. He was taken to the operating room for immediate decompression of the hematoma. An intraoperative angiogram was obtained just prior to skin incision. It demonstrates a small mycotic aneurysm of a branch of the right middle cerebral artery (*arrows,* A and B) in addition to mass effect from the hematoma that depresses the MCA branches. The location of the aneurysm was marked with a scalp needle for craniotomy (*open arrow,* C). The aneurysm is no longer seen on the angiogram following resection of the aneurysm (D), and there is resolution of the mass effect following hematoma evacuation.

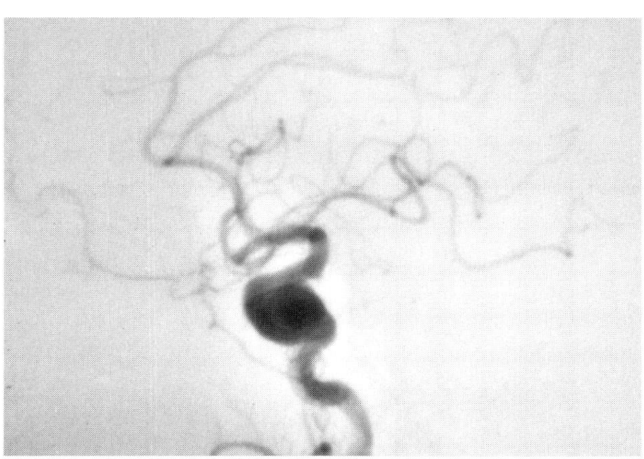

A

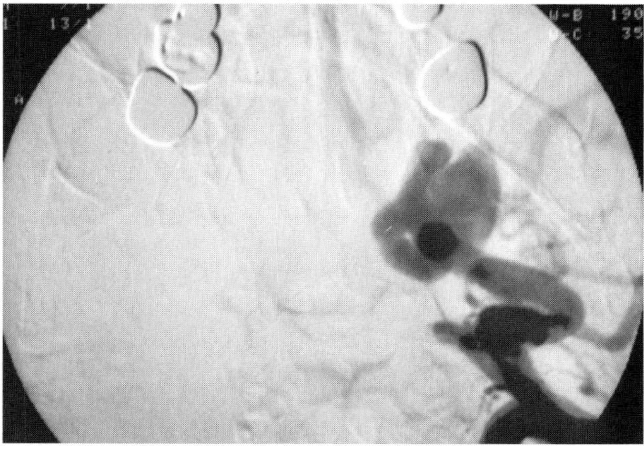

B

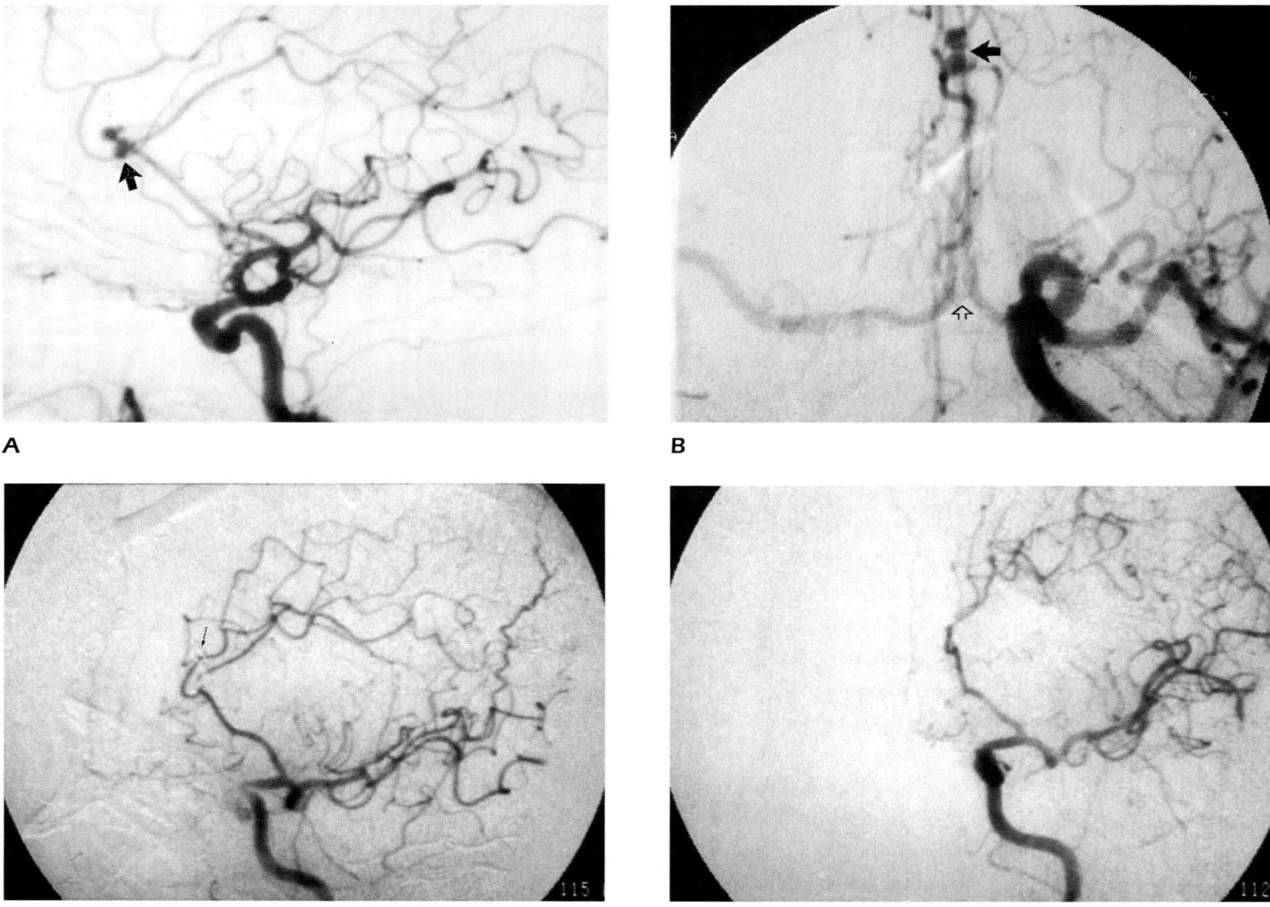

Figure 13-46. Intraoperative study of anterior cerebral artery aneurysm. A 47-year-old man was admitted with a severe occipital headache. His brain CT scan demonstrated subarachnoid hemorrhage. An irregular aneurysm of the left anterior cerebral artery at its division into pericallosal and callosomarginal branches is seen on his preoperative angiogram (*arrows,* A and B). The aneurysm is distal to the site of the anterior communicating artery (*open arrow* on base view, B), the more common site of anterior cerebral artery aneurysms. An intraoperative angiogram (C and D) was obtained after clip placement. It demonstrates no residual aneurysm and patency of the pericallosal and callosomarginal arteries. The clip is noted as a subtraction artifact (*small arrow,* C).

arachnoid hemorrhage, as a result of giant aneurysm thrombosis or localized meningeal inflammation.[59]

In the setting of subarachnoid hemorrhage or in the patient suspected of having an aneurysm responsible for symptoms related to its mass effect, cerebral angiography is used to identify the symptomatic aneurysm, exclude additional aneurysms, identify any associated vascular malformations, characterize potential collateral pathways, and define the extent of vasospasm. A CT scan is important to confirm the presence of subarachnoid blood and to evaluate for complications such as hydrocephalus, but noninvasive techniques have not yet been able to equal the sensitivity and accuracy of conventional angiography in detecting and characterizing aneurysms, except in the rare instances of completely thrombosed aneurysms.

In addition to the preoperative angiogram used to aid in planning treatment and the postoperative angiogram used to assess the repair and evaluate for vasospasm, intraoperative angiography can be employed during clip placement (Fig. 13-46). These examinations, performed with portable digital subtraction equipment in the operating room, can identify an unsuspected residual aneurysm neck or an unexpected

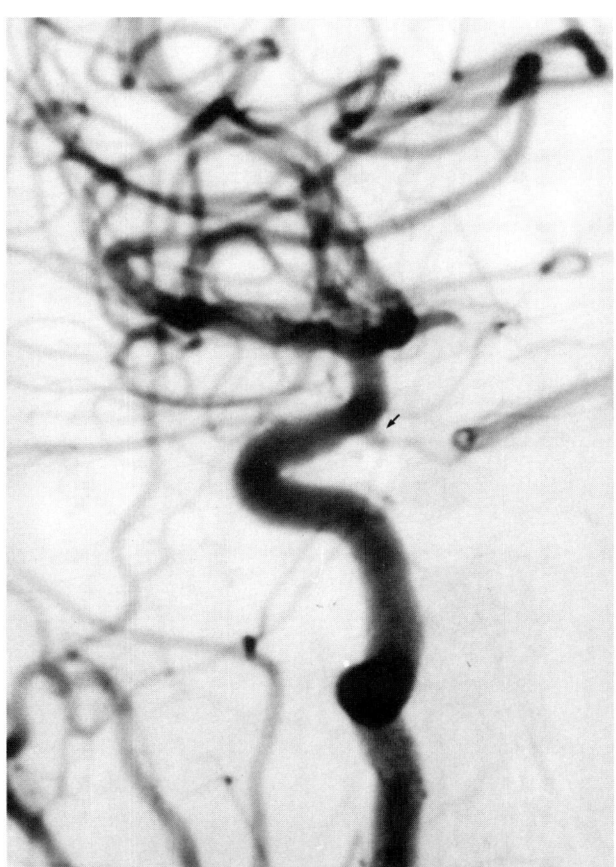

Figure 13-47. Infundibulum. On angiography obtained for unrelated disease, this lateral view of a carotid injection demonstrates a small infundibulum of the posterior communicating artery (*arrow*), seen in about 6 percent of the population.

parent vessel occlusion. An alteration in clip position could eliminate the need for a second operation or help prevent complications.[60]

A normal variant, termed an *infundibulum,* may sometimes be confused with an aneurysm. An infundibulum is a dilatation of an origin of a vessel that is not pathologic (Fig. 13-47). The most common site for an infundibulum, with an estimated incidence of 6.5 percent,[47] is the origin of the posterior communicating (PCOM) artery at the supraclinoid internal carotid artery. Here, the PCOM artery origin is considered normal if the dilatation is triangular in shape, the apex points posteriorly, the width is under 3 mm, and the PCOM artery arises from the apex of the triangle.[61,62] The basilar artery may also be slightly dilated at its bifurcation into the posterior cerebral arteries, termed a *junctional infundibulum.* There is some evidence that in rare cases an infundibulum enlarges to become an aneurysm.[63]

Vascular Malformations and Fistulas

Vascular malformations of the brain may be of the arterial, venous, or capillary type. Arteriovenous malformations (AVMs) are the most commonly encountered type angiographically. Pial AVMs typically consist of enlarged supplying arteries, a nidus of tangled arteriovenous communications, and dilated draining veins (Fig. 13-48). They lie within the brain parenchyma and derive their blood supply from cerebral arteries. There is rapid shunting of blood leading to early venous opacification, and there may be associated arterial, nidal, or venous aneurysms (Fig. 13-49).[48,64] Dural AVMs are common to the posterior fossa, involving the transverse and sigmoid sinuses (Fig. 13-50). They derive their blood supply from meningeal or extracranial vessels. Dural malformations may also involve other meningeal surfaces, and, if they involve the cavernous sinus, they can cause clinical syndromes similar to direct carotid-cavernous fistulas. Capillary telangiectases are dilated, thinned capillaries with intervening neural tissue that rarely bleed and may be difficult to identify angiographically. Cavernous malformations (cavernomas) are foci of dilated abnormal small vessels with slow flow and without intervening neural tissue. Although cavernomas may bleed, they are not often identified angiographically. They may appear as staining areas but are more easily diagnosed by MRI.[65] Venous angiomas are simply anomalous-appearing concentrations of veins that constitute the venous drainage for the underlying normal brain. These typically consist of a number of small, tortuous, deep veins converging in a spokelike fashion to join a single draining vein that courses to the surface and appears at the normal time in the venous phase of the study. Venous angiomas are rarely, if ever, symptomatic from hemorrhage.[66] Fistulas are direct arterial-to-venous connections without an intervening nidus, basically holes between arteries and veins. The best-known fistulas involve the cavernous portion of the internal carotid artery. These carotid-cavernous fistulas can produce proptosis, chemosis, and visual disturbances.[35] Pial AVMs, capillary telangiectases, venous angiomas, and cavernomas are believed to be congenital. Dural AVMs can be the result of venous thrombosis or trauma. Fistulas can be spontaneous or the result of trauma.

It is estimated from pathologic studies that the prevalence of cerebral AVMs is 0.6 percent to 0.8 percent. Of these, 90 percent are supratentorial and 10 percent are infratentorial. About 70 percent of supratentorial AVMs are purely pial, whereas about half of

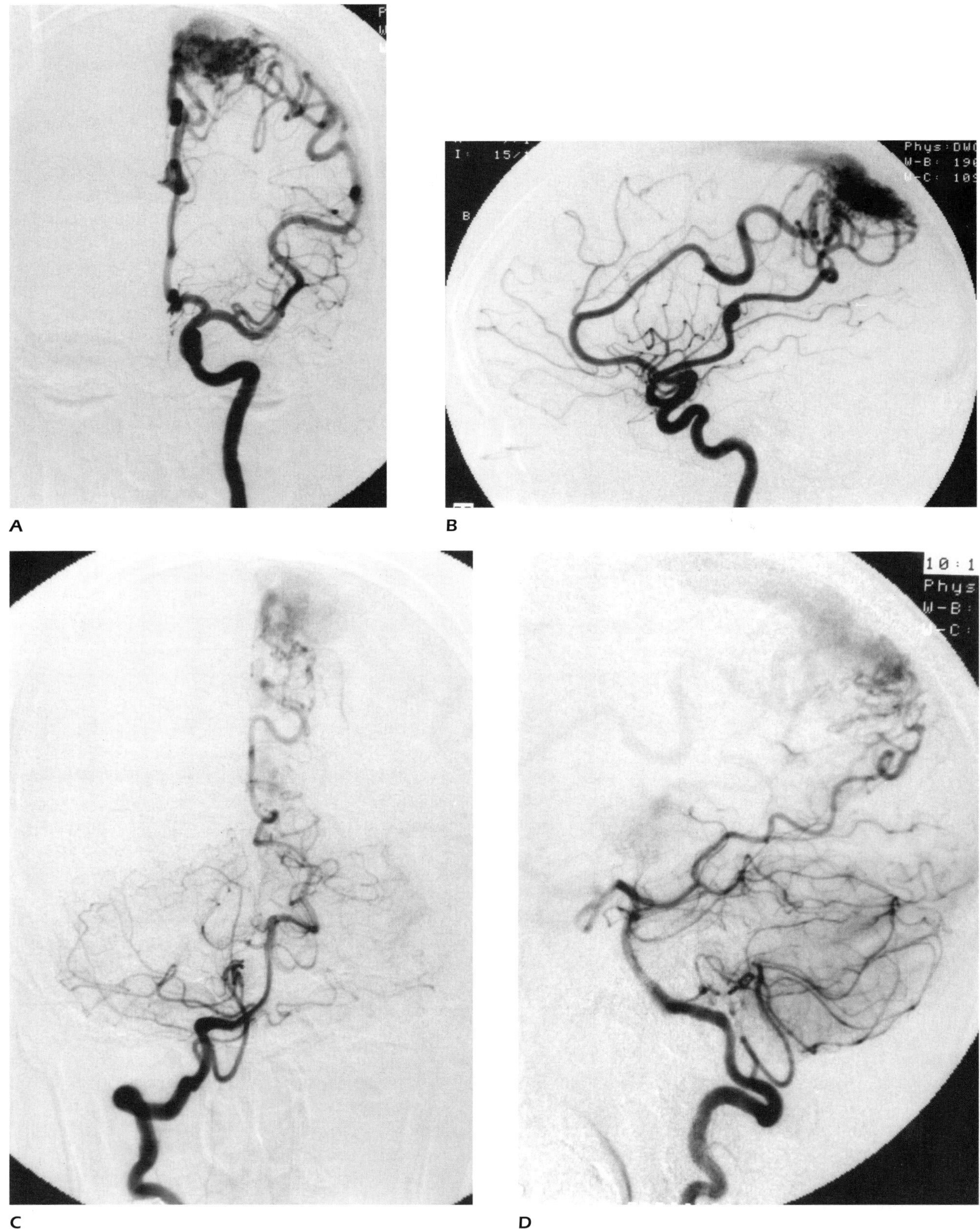

Figure 13-48. Parietal AVM. A 40-year-old woman developed a headache and had the first seizure of her life. CT and MR examinations of the brain revealed a small left parietal hemorrhage from an AVM. Her left carotid angiogram (A and B) demonstrates enlarged anterior and middle cerebral branches supplying a pial AVM in the left parietal lobe. Venous drainage is superficial, to the superior sagittal sinus. Her right vertebral angiogram (C and D) demonstrates some additional arterial supply to the AVM from the parietooccipital branches of the left posterior cerebral artery.

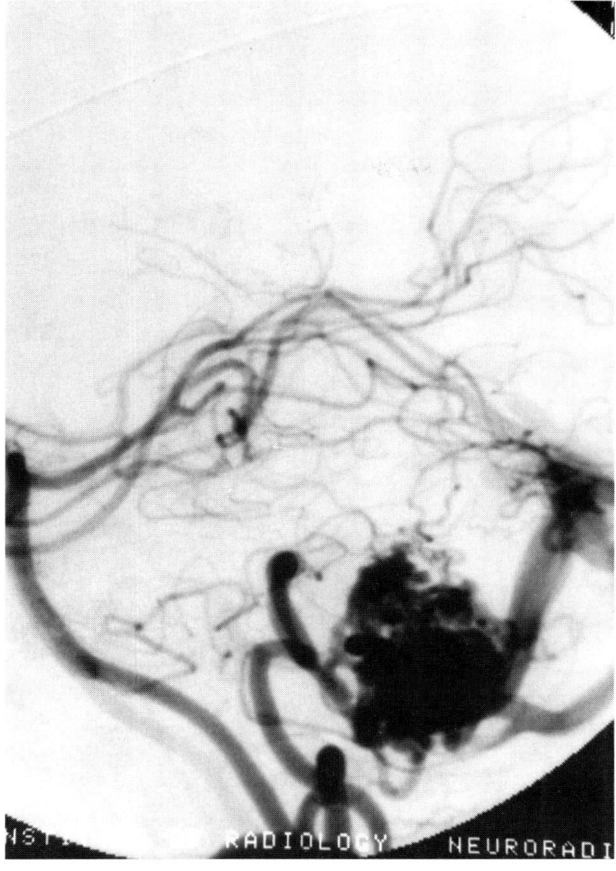

A

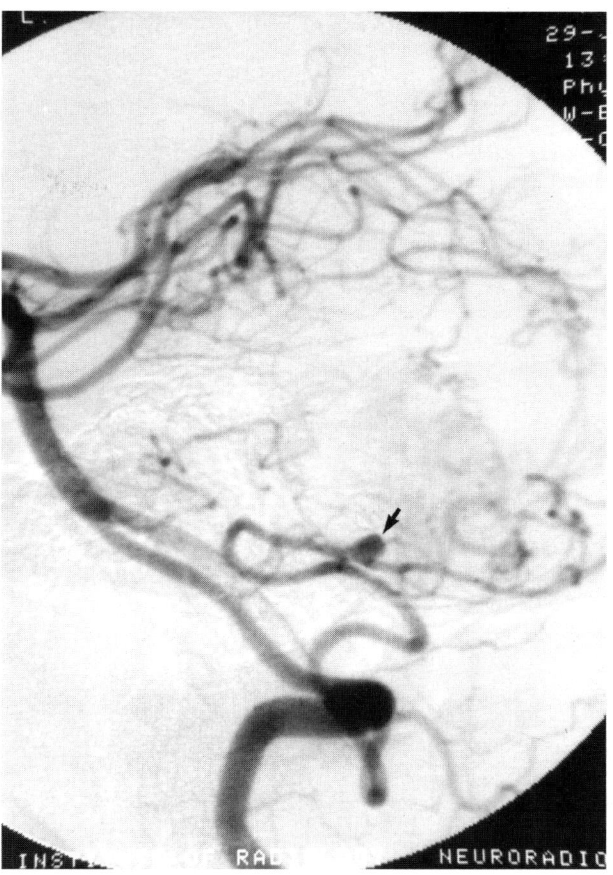

B

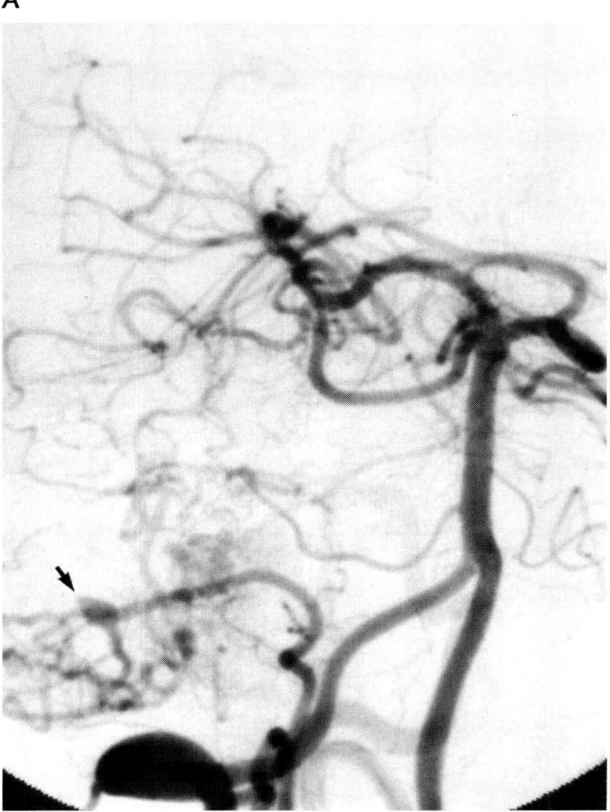

C

Figure 13-49. Cerebellar AVM with distal PICA aneurysm. A 45-year-old woman was admitted with a subarachnoid hemorrhage and a small amount of intraventricular hemorrhage by brain CT. There was no parenchymal hematoma. Her left vertebral angiogram (A) demonstrates a cerebellar AVM supplied by a greatly enlarged left posterior inferior cerebellar artery and small superior cerebellar artery branches. Her right vertebral angiogram (B and C) reveals a right PICA contribution to the AVM as well as a distal PICA aneurysm (*arrows*). The hemorrhage was believed to have been from a rupture of the aneurysm.

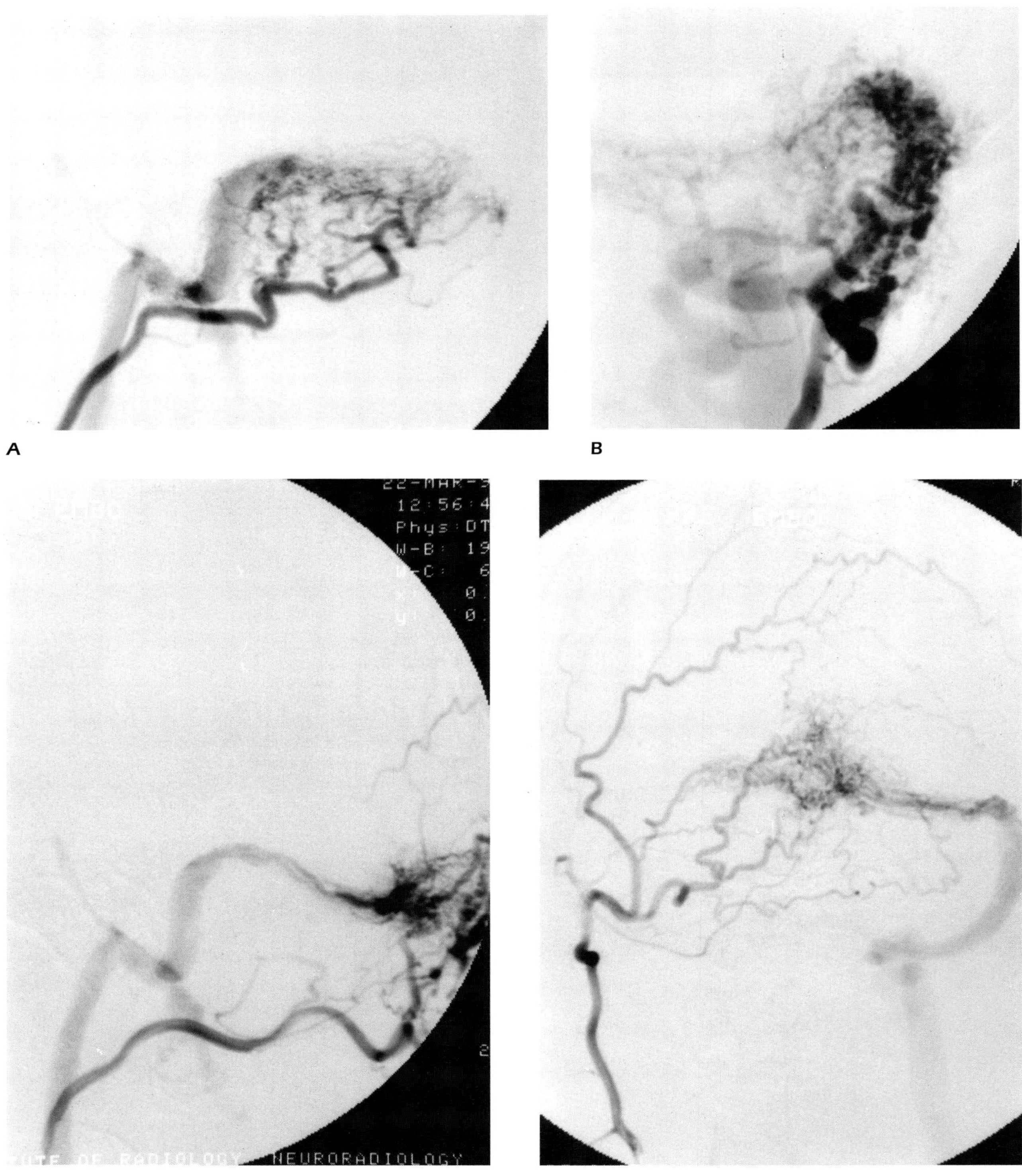
A
B
Phys:DT
NEURORADIOLOGY
C
D

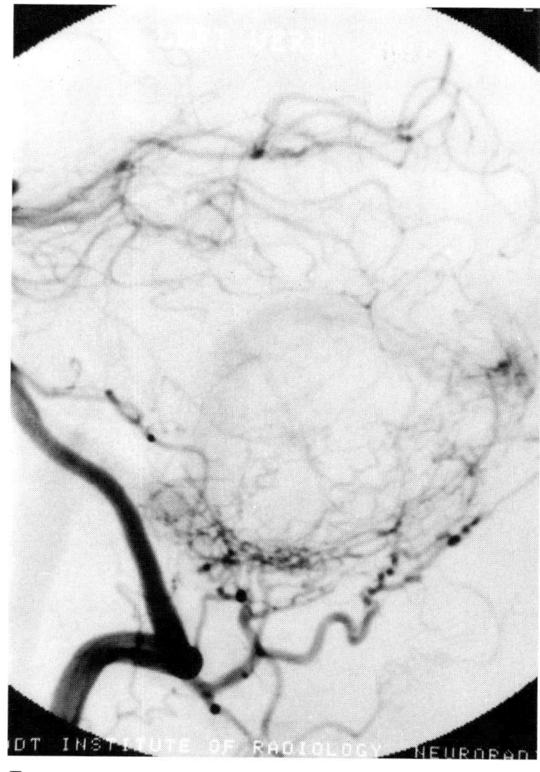

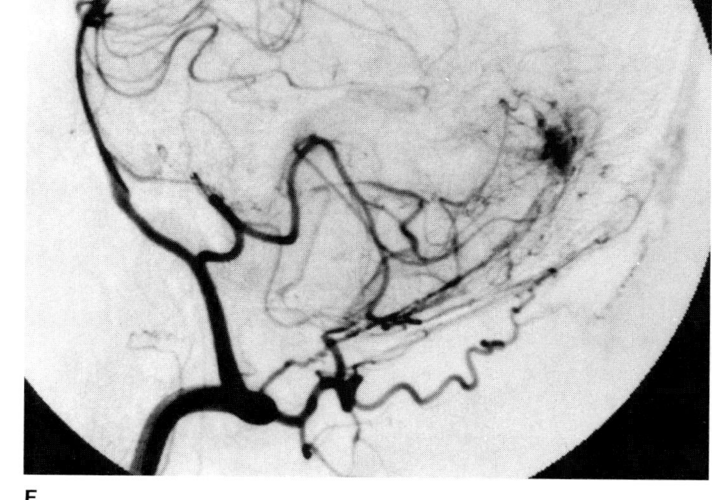

E F

Figure 13-50. Dural AVM. A 58-year-old man complained of a loud bruit in his left ear and frequent, severe headaches. There had been a history of head trauma several years earlier. His left occipital artery injection (A and B), right occipital artery injection (C and D), left vertebral injection (E), and right vertebral injection (F) demonstrate an extensive dural malformation of the posterior fossa that drains into the torcular and left transverse and sigmoid sinuses. The arterial supply is via right and left occipital and right and left vertebral meningeal branches.

the posterior fossa AVMs are either purely dural or mixed pial-dural. Not all AVMs come to clinical attention, although the majority eventually produce symptoms. Most AVMs fall into the small (under 3 cm) to moderate (3 to 6 cm) size range, with the minority being large (over 6 cm) (Fig. 13-51).[67,68]

The presenting symptom for about 50 percent of cerebral AVMs is hemorrhage. Hemorrhage is most likely to occur in the third decade of life. Large AVMs are less frequently associated with hemorrhage than the small- and moderate-size AVMs. Intranidal aneurysms, deep venous drainage, and close proximity to a ventricle may increase the risk of hemorrhage, and angiomatous change may decrease the risk.[69] A dural malformation that drains into cortical veins or is associated with large venous aneurysms is more likely to hemorrhage than one that drains directly into a venous sinus.[70,71] Hemorrhage is parenchymal in about two of three AVM ruptures and subarachnoid in the remainder. For unruptured AVMs, the incidence of hemorrhage is estimated to be about 2 to 3 percent per year, whereas for ruptured AVMs, the incidence of hemorrhage is estimated to be 6 percent in the first year after hemorrhage and 2 percent per year thereafter. The mortality for the first hemorrhage is about 10 percent, but higher rates are reported for successive hemorrhages. Of the hemorrhage survivors, about 30 percent have permanent morbidity.[67]

Another common presenting symptom of AVMs is seizure. The peak incidence of first seizure falls later in the third decade of life than that of first hemorrhage, but about 50 percent of AVM patients who come to clinical attention have had a seizure by the age of 30. Other associated symptoms may include headache, neurologic deficits from arterial steal, or venous congestion, and, in the very young, hydrocephalus and cardiac failure. Symptoms of steal appear to be more common in large AVMs with angiomatous change.[72]

Angiography may be requested in patients who present with subarachnoid or intraparenchymal hem-

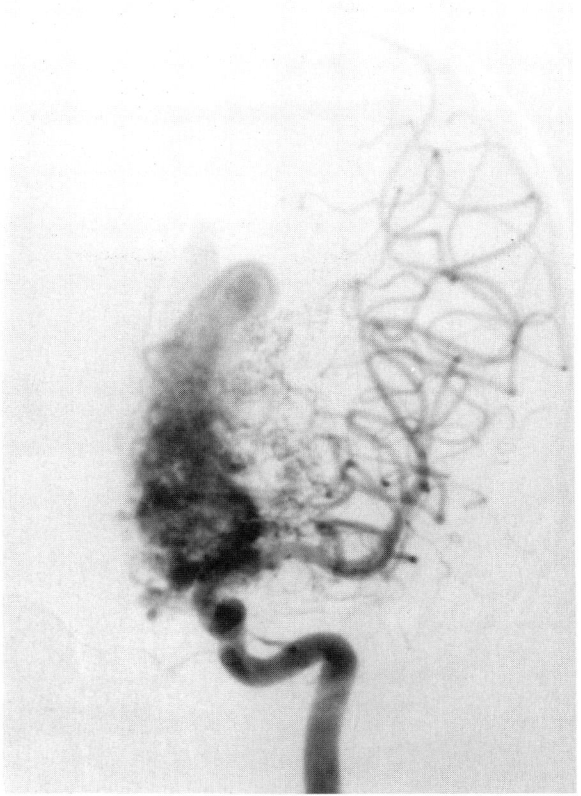

A

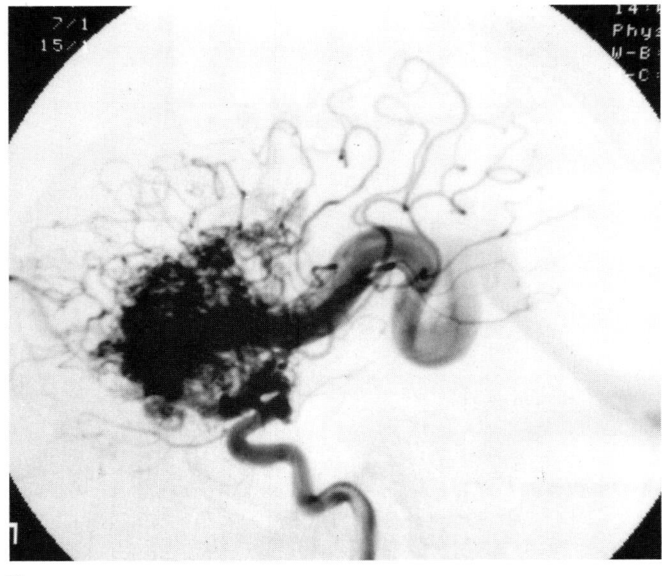

B

Figure 13-51. Large frontal AVM. A 19-year-old man had recurrent intraventricular hemorrhages. A large corpus callosal AVM is seen on his left carotid angiogram (A and B). Although difficult to determine from these images, the arterial supply is predominantly from the left and right pericallosal arteries. There is angiomatous change of perforating branches, which also contribute to the malformation. Venous drainage is via a greatly enlarged left internal cerebral vein.

orrhage to identify a vascular malformation. Angiography also serves to document the size and location of the malformation, the location and number of feeding arteries and draining veins, and the presence of associated arterial, nidal, or venous aneurysms. This information is crucial for treatment planning, whether treatment is to consist of conservative management, embolization, radiation, surgery, or a combination of these modalities. MRI can be helpful in localizing the pial and parenchymal malformations with respect to the surrounding brain anatomy and in accurately measuring the size of the malformation. CT or MRI may also be important in identifying hemorrhage or hydrocephalus.[73,74] Dural malformations, however, may be missed by CT and MRI.[75]

Fistulas are discussed in further detail in the section on trauma. Chapter 12 discusses endovascular techniques used in the treatment of these disorders.

Tumors and Mass Effects

Today, angiography is requested in patients with intracranial masses to help narrow the differential diagnosis of a particular lesion based on its vascular characteristics, to help decide on the particular approach to biopsy or operation, or increasingly to serve as a preliminary step to endovascular intervention.[76] Some questions regarding the vascularity of a particular lesion may be answered with magnetic resonance angiography, but frequently more detail is needed.[77] Neoplasms range from appearing avascular to appearing hypervascular. In some instances tumor location and vascularity are very specific for a particular diagnosis, and in others a particular angiographic appearance of a neoplasm might be mistaken for infarction, inflammation, or vascular malformation. Correlation with

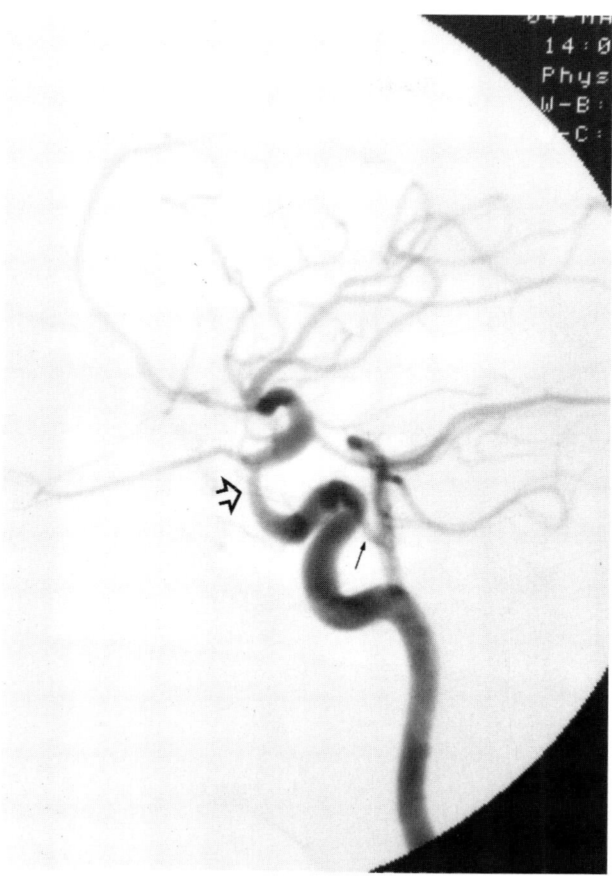

A

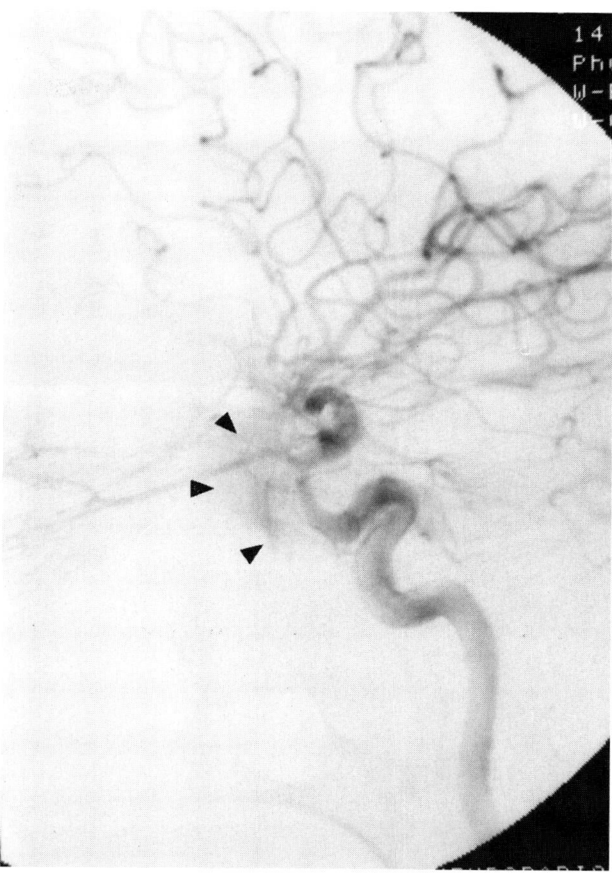

B

Figure 13-52. Carotid encasement by tumor. A 47-year-old woman presented with right proptosis. Her MRI and CT scans demonstrated hyperostosis of the right orbit, sphenoid wing, and middle fossa with enhancing meningioma en plaque. The imaging also indicated that the tumor surrounded the cavernous carotid artery. Her right carotid angiogram (A and B) reveals internal carotid artery narrowing as a result of tumor encasement (*open arrow,* A). There is an anatomic variant present. A small trigeminal artery is noted (*small arrow,* A) connecting the carotid artery to the basilar artery. Later in the arterial phase of the injection, mild tumor staining is identified (*arrowheads,* B).

cross-sectional imaging and the clinical presentation can provide useful clues in such circumstances.

Without regard to tumor vascularity, one may identify stretching and displacement of arteries or veins by masses, and in some cases, there are pathologic caliber changes of the vessels encased (Fig. 13-52) or invaded by neoplasms.[78,79] The mass effect may be as a result of the neoplasm, but frequently there is associated edema that is contributory, and occasionally there is additional mass effect from associated hemorrhage. Typical shifts of the anterior cerebral arteries have been described with masses in certain locations (Figs. 13-53 through 13-56). The round shift is associated with frontal masses adjacent to the anterior cerebral vessels, whereas the proximal shift is associated with anterior temporal masses with more remote mass effects from the vessels. The distal shift is associated with more posterior masses in the frontal, parietal, temporal, and occipital lobes. The square shift is associated with posterior masses that are large or have considerable edema. Shifts of the sylvian point or internal cerebral vein may be useful for analysis. Masses in the posterior fossa may affect the basilar artery or central cerebellar vein, and extraaxial masses may be distinguished from intraaxial masses by effects on adjacent vessels.[80]

Tumors may also be identified by either a decreased or increased amount of tissue staining on angiography as compared to normal brain, or as a result of arterial hypovascularity or hypervascularity. The phase of the angiogram in which an abnormal stain appears may have implications for diagnosis. Neovascularity, or abnormal-appearing vessels, can also be seen with

Text continues on page 334

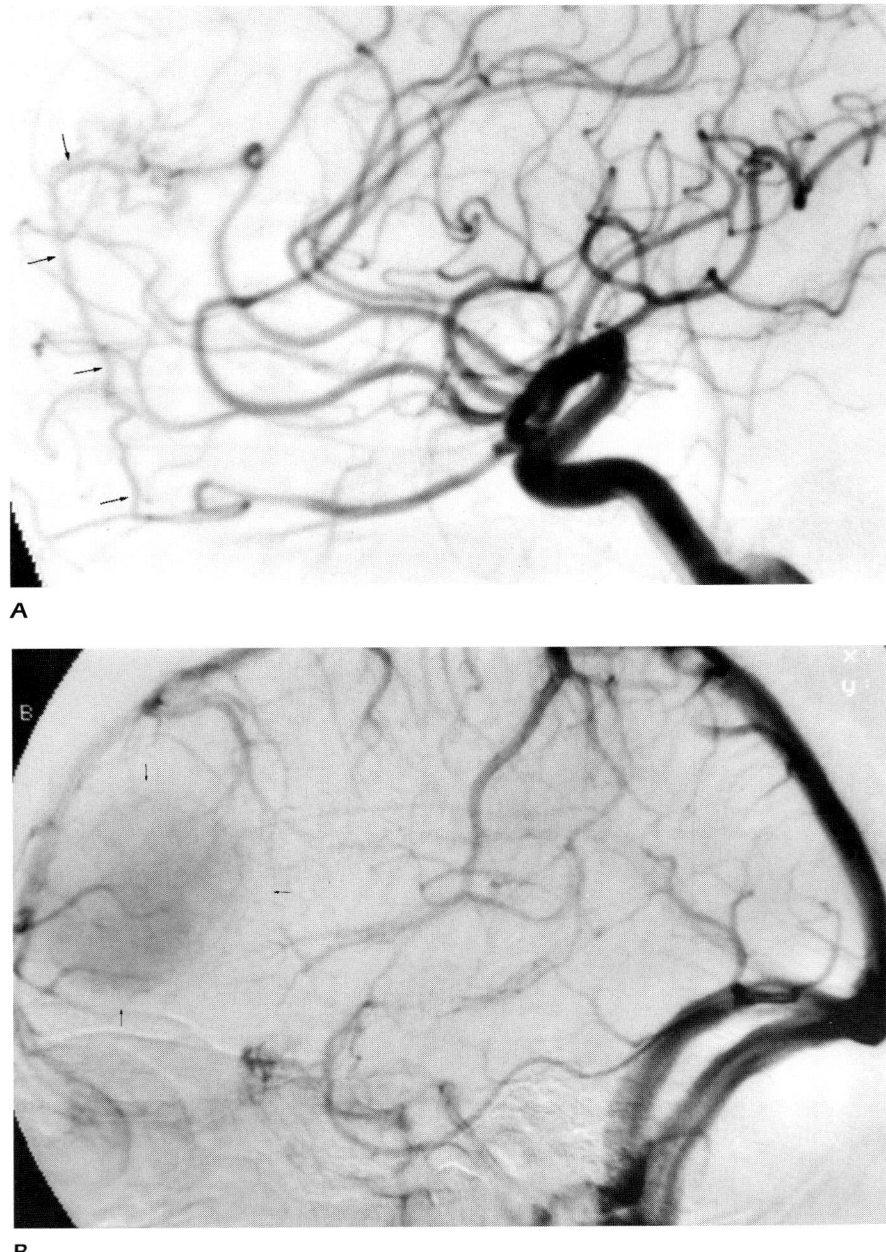

Figure 13-53. Round shift. A 72-year-old man was imaged for head trauma and an incidental 4 × 3 × 2 cm left frontal mass was discovered adjacent to the falx. The imaging characteristics were typical for meningioma. The lateral view of his left carotid angiogram demonstrates no external carotid supply to the mass, but reveals an enlarged anterior falx artery (*arrows,* A), a branch of the ophthalmic artery, feeding the tumor. In the venous phase of the injection (B and D), a persisting tumor stain is evident (*small arrows*). A frontal view of the angiogram in the arterial phase (C) demonstrates a round shift of the anterior cerebral arteries (*arrowhead*).

Figure 13-54. Distal shift. In this case, frontal views from a right carotid injection reveal a distal shift of the anterior cerebral artery (*arrows,* A), an inferior displacement of the sylvian point (*arrowhead,* A), and a leftward shift of the internal cerebral vein (*open arrow,* B), indicative of a right parietal mass. ▶

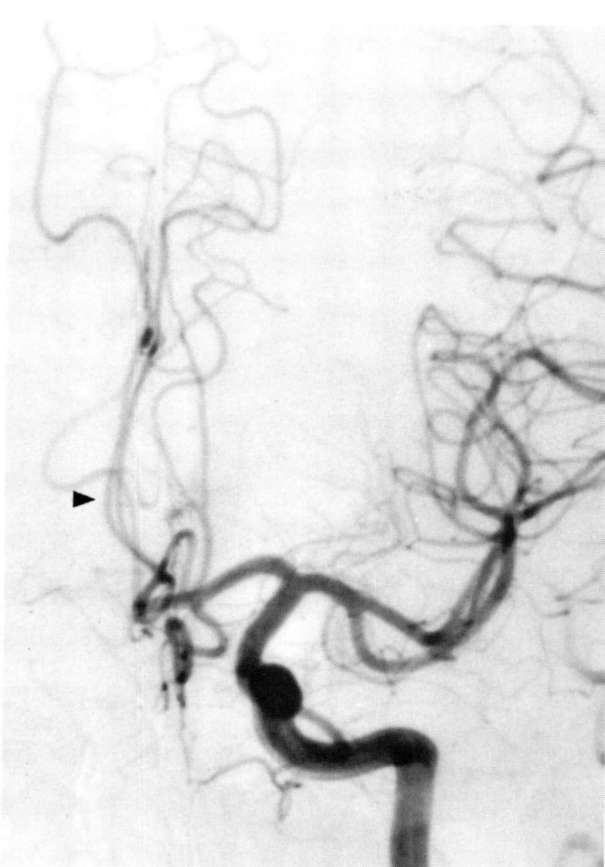

C

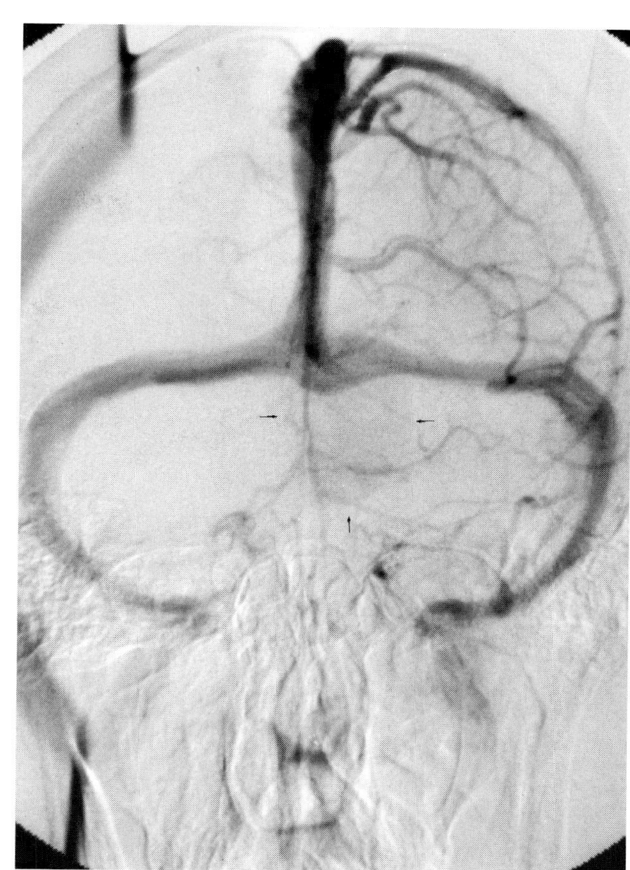

D

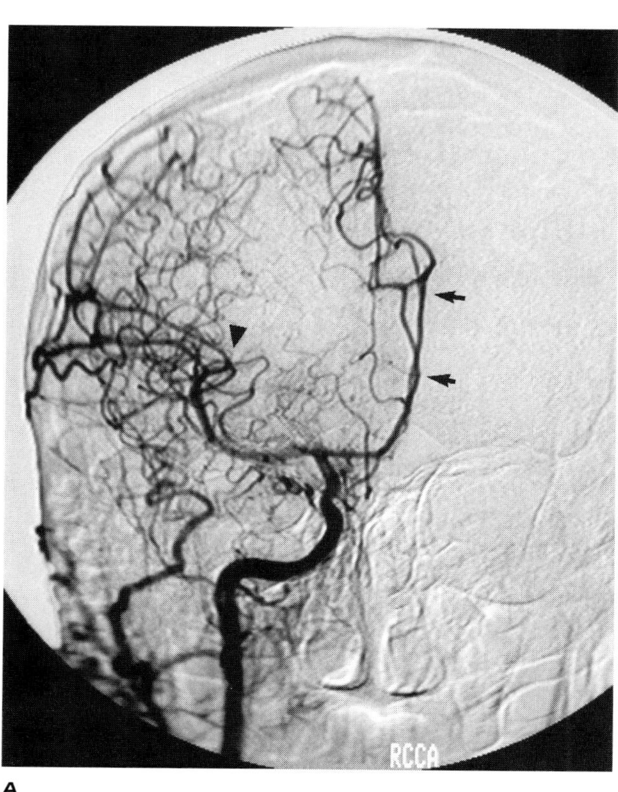

A

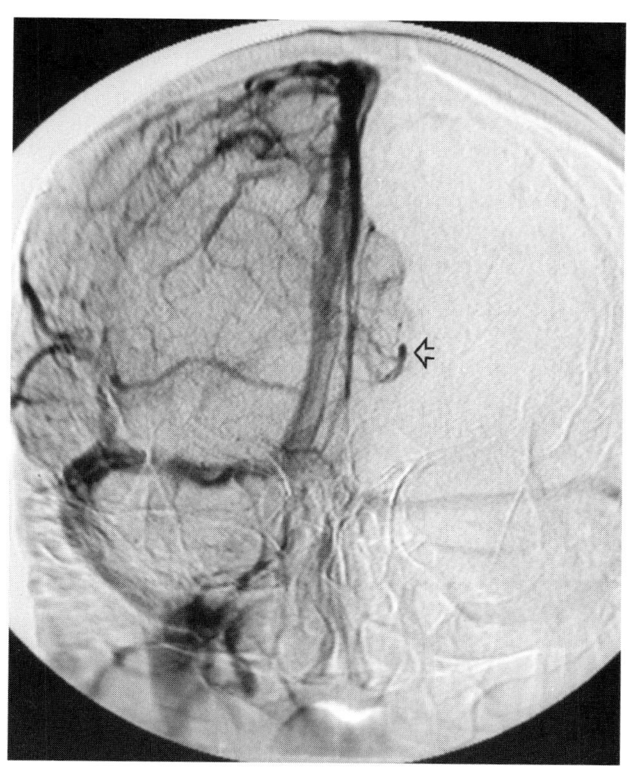

B

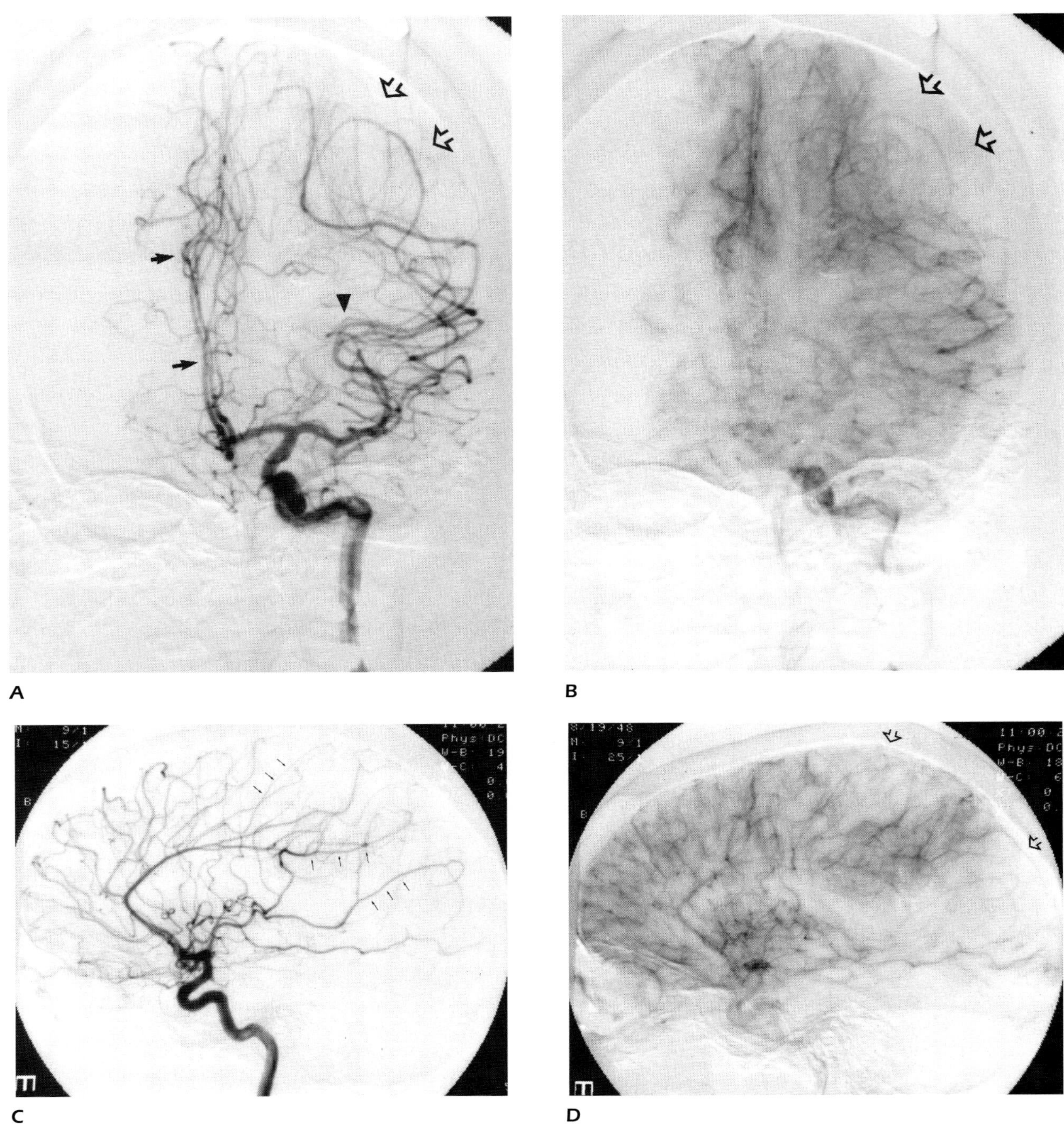

A B C D

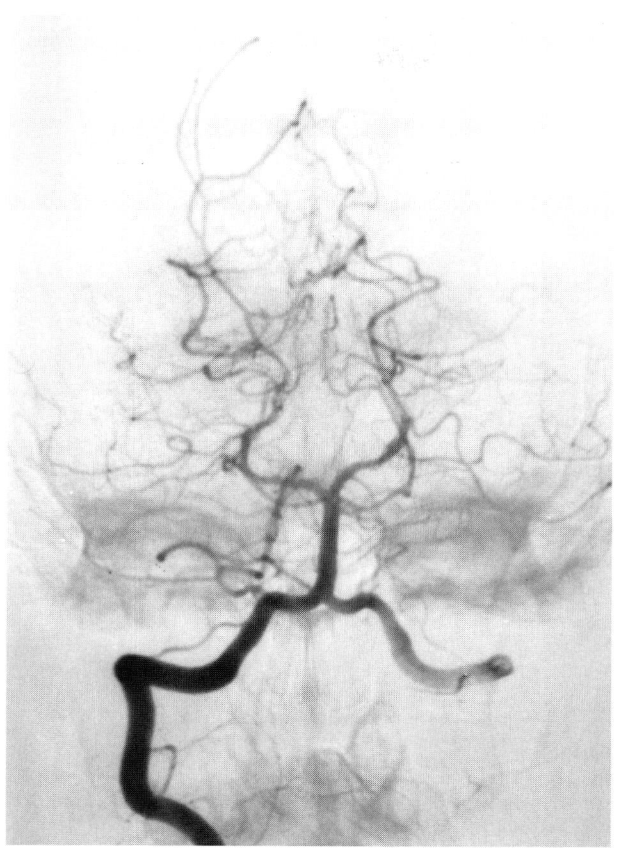

E

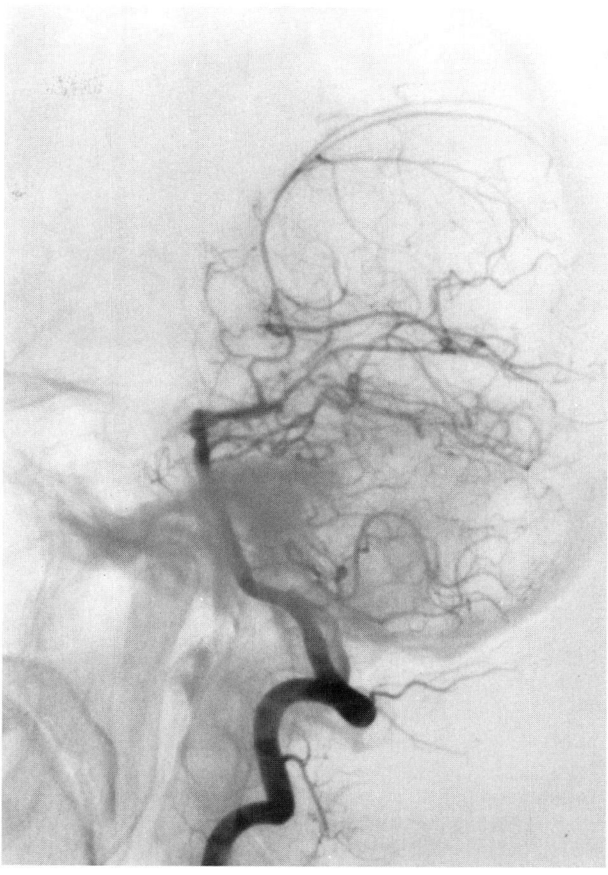

F

Figure 13-55. Distal shift, draping of vessels. A 45-year-old woman with minimal symptoms was found to have a 7-cm calcified left parietal mass on a brain CT scan. Frontal views of her left carotid angiogram show a distal shift of the anterior cerebral arteries (*arrows,* A), an inferior displacement of the sylvian point (*arrowhead,* A), and draping of middle cerebral artery branches around an avascular area in the left parietal lobe (*open arrows,* A and B). Lateral views also show draping of arterial branches (*small arrows,* C) and an avascular zone (*open arrows,* D) corresponding to the mass. The diagnosis of anaplastic glial neoplasm, probably of oligodendroglial origin, was obtained at surgery. In another case, a 43-year-old woman presented with a 2-month history of headaches and bumping into things as a result of a left visual field deficit. Her brain MRI disclosed a 5 × 7 × 8 cm right occipital mass. Frontal (E) and lateral (F) views of her right vertebral angiogram demonstrate draping of right posterior cerebral artery branches about the mass. The diagnosis of glioblastoma multiforme was made at surgery.

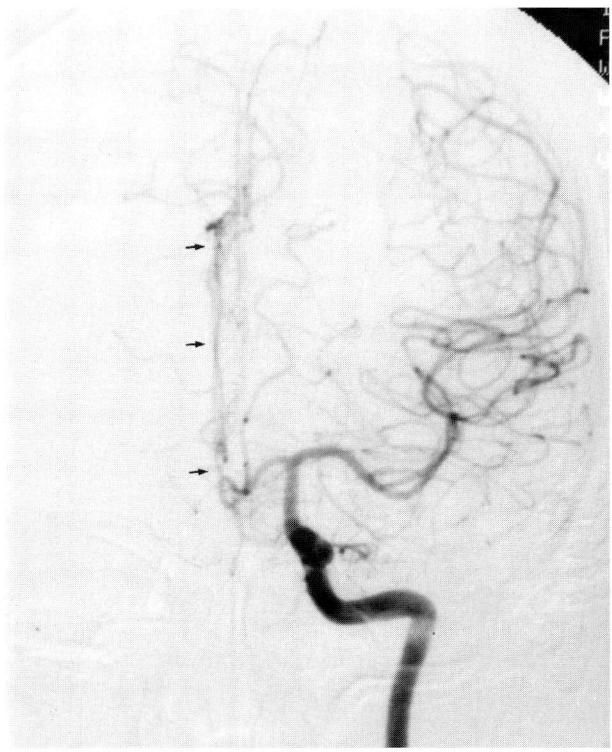

A

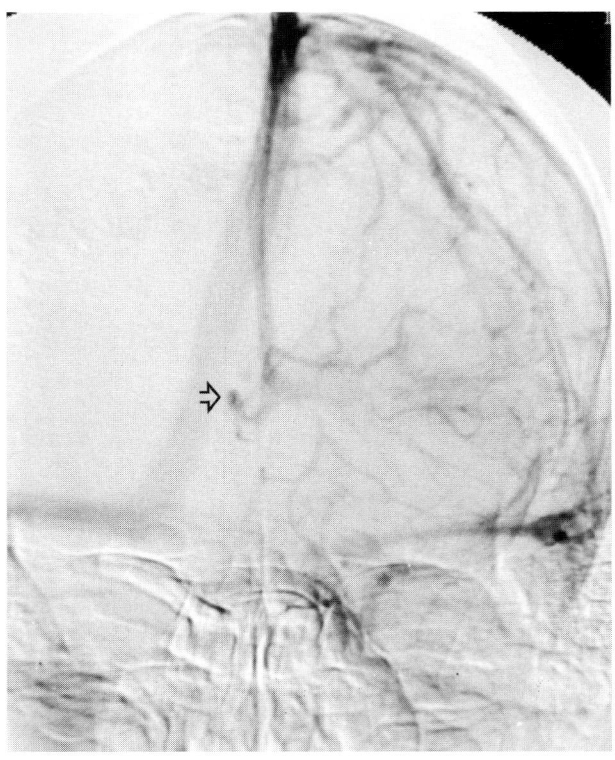

B

Figure 13-56. Square shift. A 39-year-old man was found to have a left parietooccipital mass. An angiogram was performed in conjunction with a Wada test. Frontal views from the left carotid injection demonstrate a square shift of the anterior cerebral arteries (*arrows,* A) and a rightward shift of the internal cerebral vein (*open arrow,* B).

neoplasms, and the arterial supply to a tumor may help with diagnosis. Flow changes may accompany a cerebral tumor. Early venous opacification is seen with tumors in which there is arteriovenous shunting. Shunting is often associated with malignant lesions but may also be seen with benign neoplasms such as hemangioblastomas and even with nonneoplastic lesions such as infarctions. Another angiographic finding seen with some tumors is puddling of contrast in dilated, slowly emptying vascular spaces.

In general, mass effect, location, staining characteristics, vascularity, arterial supply, and effects on flow and adjacent vessels are used as criteria to diagnose and describe cerebral neoplasms.[81] The differential diagnosis is usually aided considerably by cross-sectional imaging. Characteristic angiographic appearances of specific tumors will be described in text following.

Meningiomas, in terms of location, are extraaxial or intraventricular. They can be avascular, hypervascular, or anywhere in between in the degree of staining. If a stain is present, it tends to appear late in the arterial phase relative to other tumor stains and to persist into the venous phase. Many meningiomas have a characteristic "spokewheel" pattern of neovascularity (Fig. 13-57). There is usually no shunting, although slightly early venous filling can be seen in a few of these tumors. Because most meningiomas originate from dural surfaces, arterial supply tends to be, at least in part, meningeal. The middle meningeal artery supplies convexity and sphenoid meningiomas, whereas the anterior falx artery, a branch of the ophthalmic artery, supplies falx meningiomas. Tentorial meningiomas may be fed by marginal tentorial arteries, branches of the internal carotid arteries.[82] Large meningiomas can outgrow their meningeal blood supply and recruit tumor vessels from pial branches of the cerebral arteries. Meningiomas at the skull base may encase major arteries and create stenoses, whereas meningiomas at the convexity or in the posterior fossa can compress, invade, or occlude venous sinuses (Fig. 13-58).[79] Because these tumors have usually been diagnosed by MRI or CT before angiography, the questions to be answered by an angiogram are most often for surgical or embolization treatment planning purposes. It is thus more im-

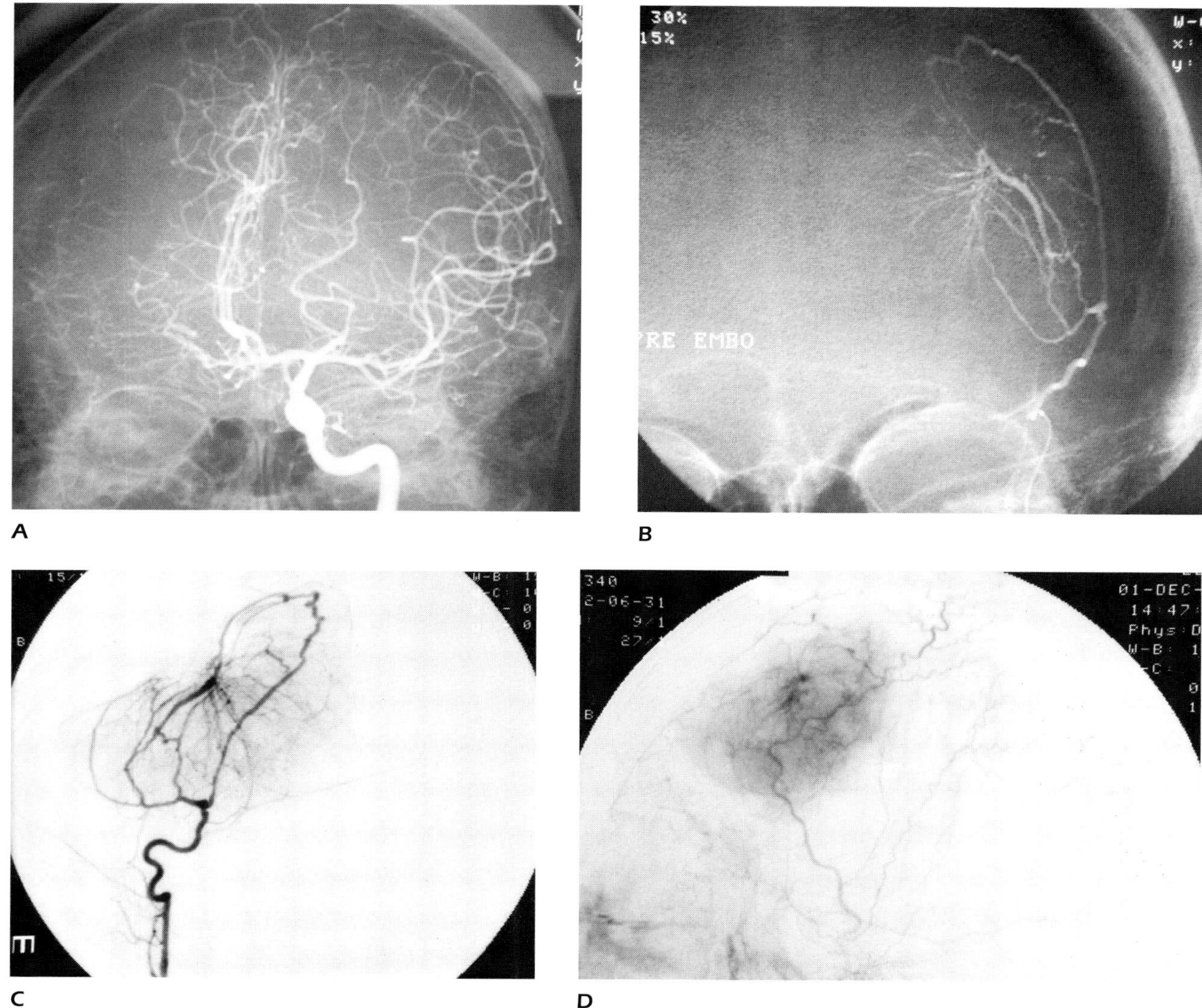

Figure 13-57. Vascular meningioma. A 62-year-old woman presented with a progressive aphasia of subacute onset over several weeks. Her CT and MRI studies demonstrated a 6 × 4 × 6 cm lateral left frontal mass containing calcification and associated with hyperostosis of adjacent bone and frontal lobe edema. The frontal view of her left internal carotid injection (A) reveals a round shift of the anterior cerebral arteries. The frontal view of her left middle meningeal artery injection (B) demonstrates the spokewheel pattern of tumor vessels typical for a meningioma and shows the relationship of the tumor to the arterial shift in (A). The lateral views of the middle meningeal injection show the tumor vessels (C) and stain (D).

portant to determine the degree of vascularity, arterial supply, and effect on adjacent arteries and venous sinuses than to determine the location of the tumor or amount of mass effect. Occasionally, the meningeal origin of the blood supply and staining characteristics may strengthen the diagnosis of meningioma if the diagnosis is uncertain from noninvasive imaging methods. Balloon occlusion testing may be a relevant part of the examination if vessel sacrifice is anticipated during resection.[83]

Schwannomas, other extraaxial masses, may also derive their blood supply from external carotid artery branches. The ascending pharyngeal and occipital arteries are typical feeders from the external carotid artery, whereas the anterior inferior and posterior inferior cerebellar arteries from the vertebrobasilar system

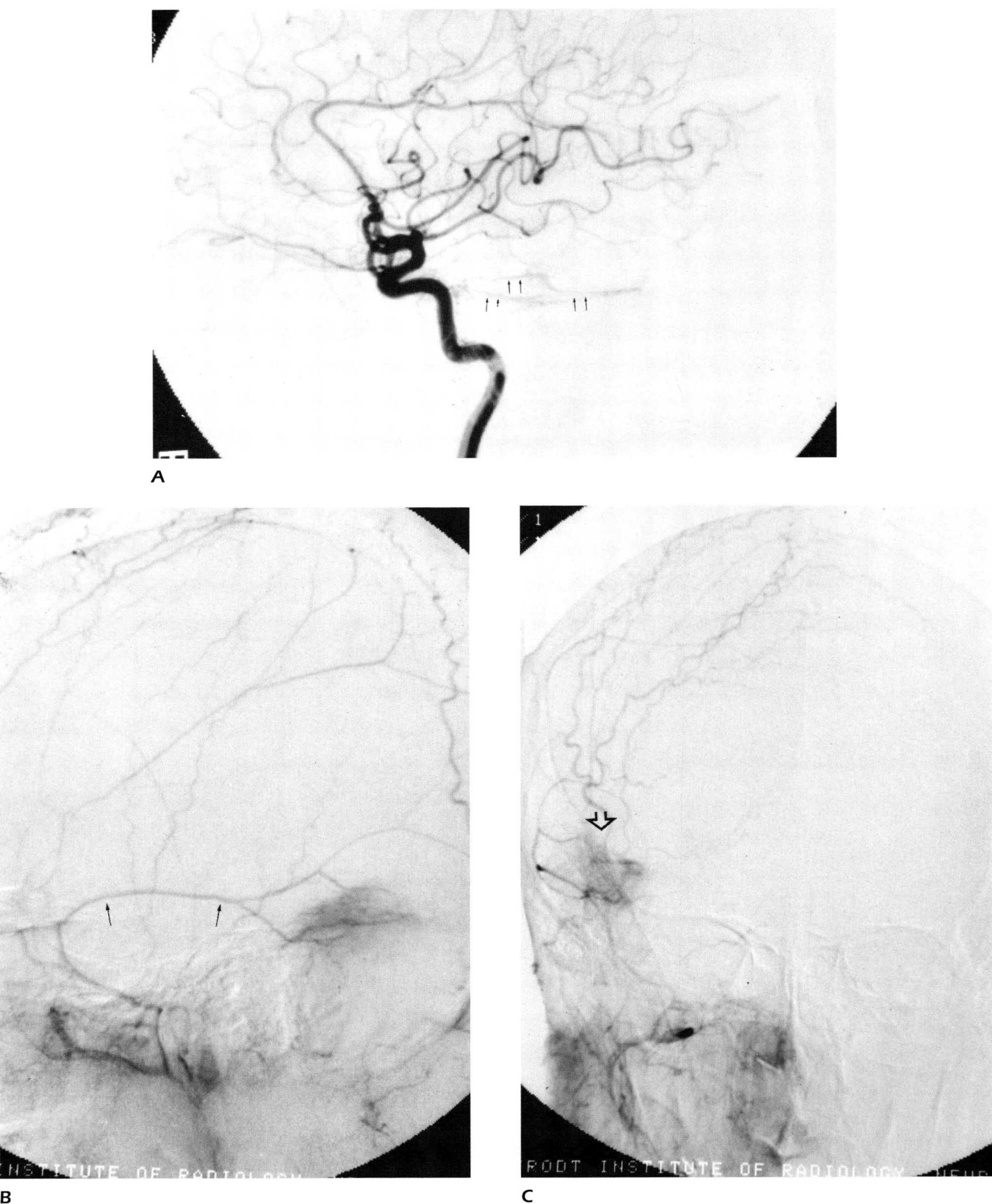
A
INSTITUTE OF RADIOLOGY
B
1
RODT INSTITUTE OF RADIOLOGY
C

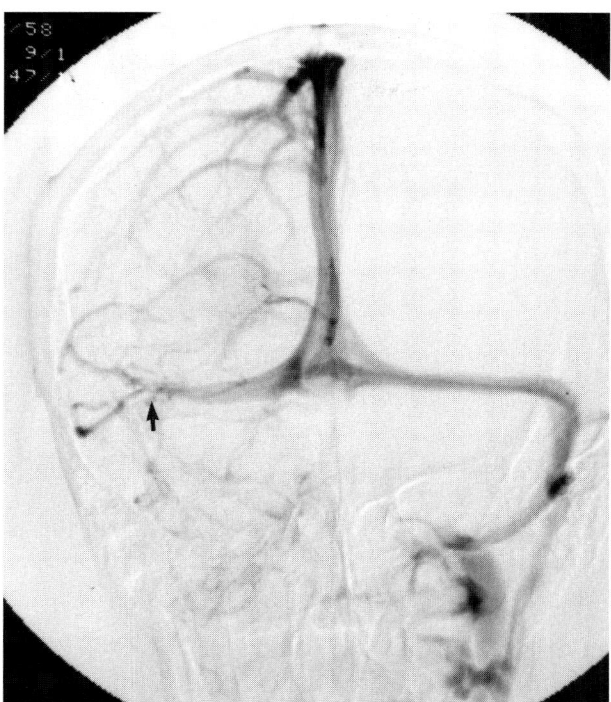

D

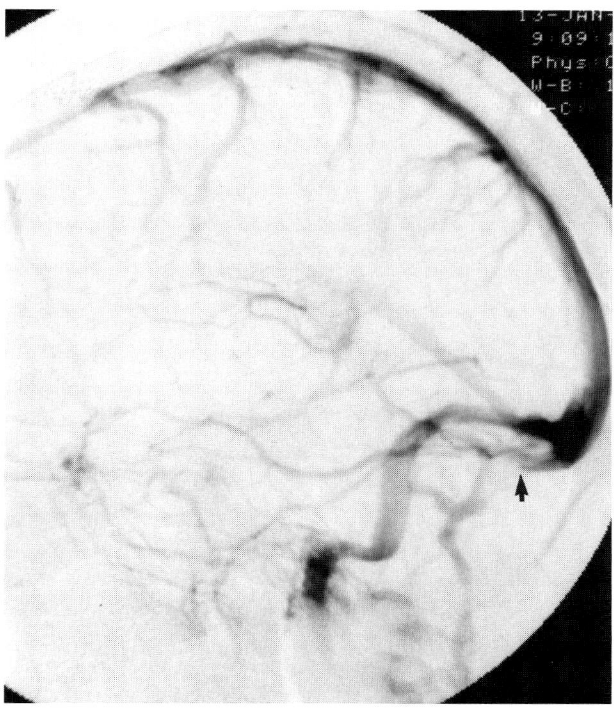

E

Figure 13-58. Venous sinus occlusion from meningioma. A 35-year-old woman developed cranial neuropathies. Her brain MRI revealed a mass based at the tentorium. The lateral view of the right internal carotid injection demonstrates enlarged marginal tentorial arteries (*arrows,* A). The lateral view of the right external carotid injection demonstrates a tumor stain, with additional arterial supply from the middle meningeal artery (*arrows,* B). The frontal view of the external carotid injection shows the location of the tumor stain (*open arrow,* C) in relationship to an occlusion of the right transverse sinus on the venous phase of the internal carotid injection (*arrow,* D). This is also evident on the lateral view in the venous phase (*arrow,* E). The diagnosis of meningioma was confirmed at surgery. Meningiomas may compress, invade, or occlude venous sinuses, and sinus invasion can make resection difficult.

and the meningohypophyseal trunk from the carotid system may supply these tumors, depending upon their location. Most are hypervascular with tortuous tumor vessels, multiple feeding arteries, and areas of puddling of contrast within them. Shunting is not typically seen.[84,85] These tumors may also be found in the spine (Fig. 13-59).

Glomus tumors, such as glomus jugulare, glomus vagale, and carotid body tumors, are angiographically markedly hypervascular neoplasms. Their typical locations and MRI appearances usually result in a diagnosis before the time of angiography, but angiography can

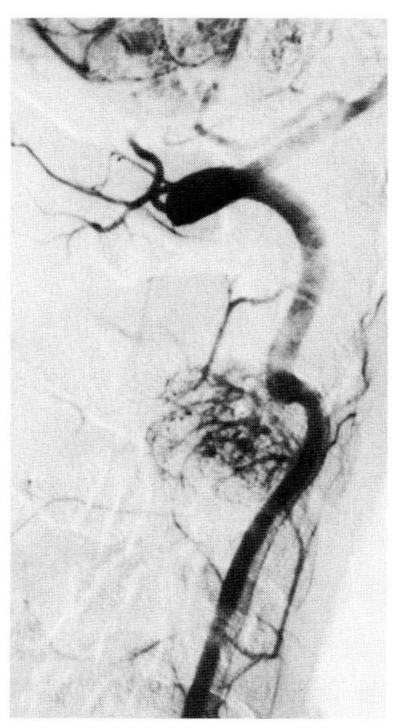

A

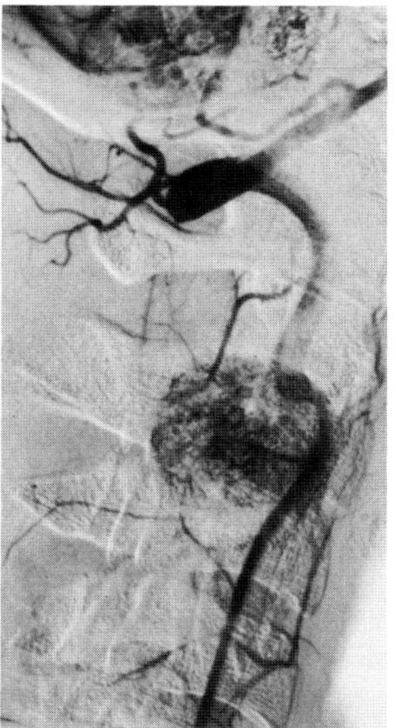

B

Figure 13-59. Neurofibroma. A young athlete had progressive right hemiparesis and right hemisensory changes. (A) Right vertebral angiography. A profusion of vessels varying in caliber and regularity terminates from the cervical portion of the vertebral artery. (B) The blush is more homogeneous and intense 0.5 second later. (A and B) Lateral projection.

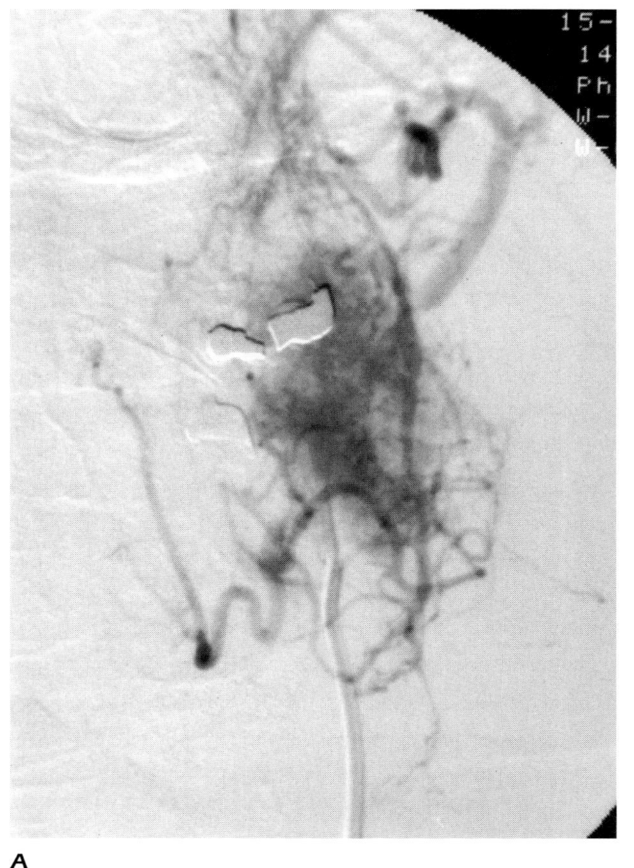

A

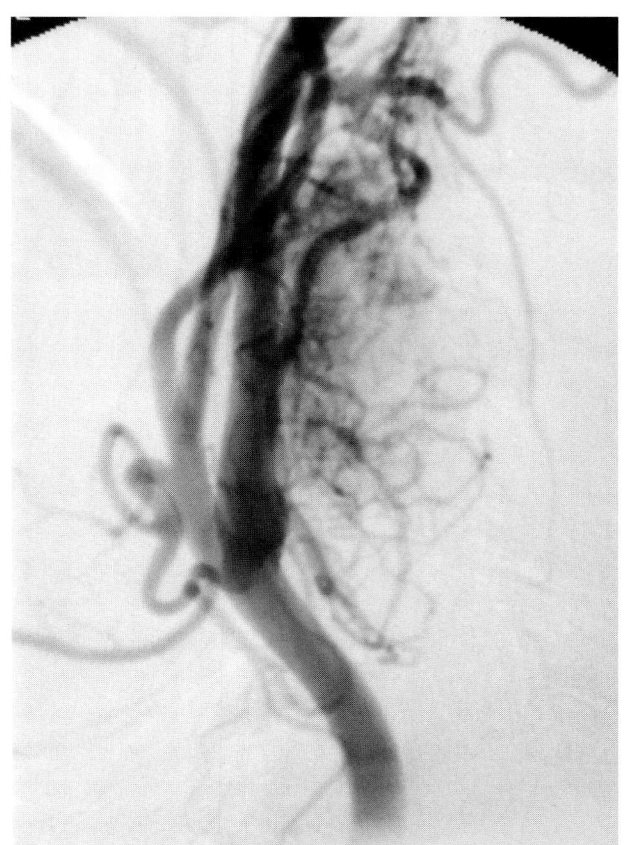

B

C

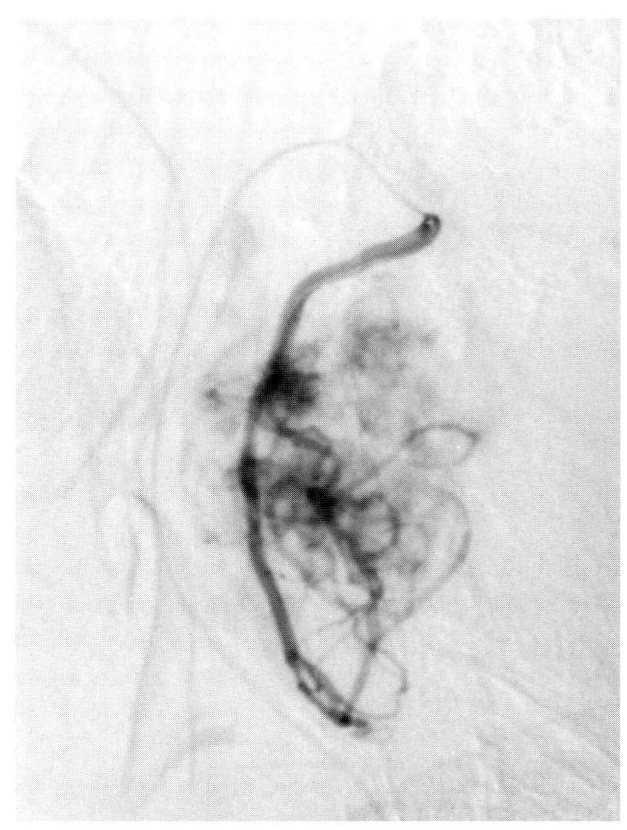

D

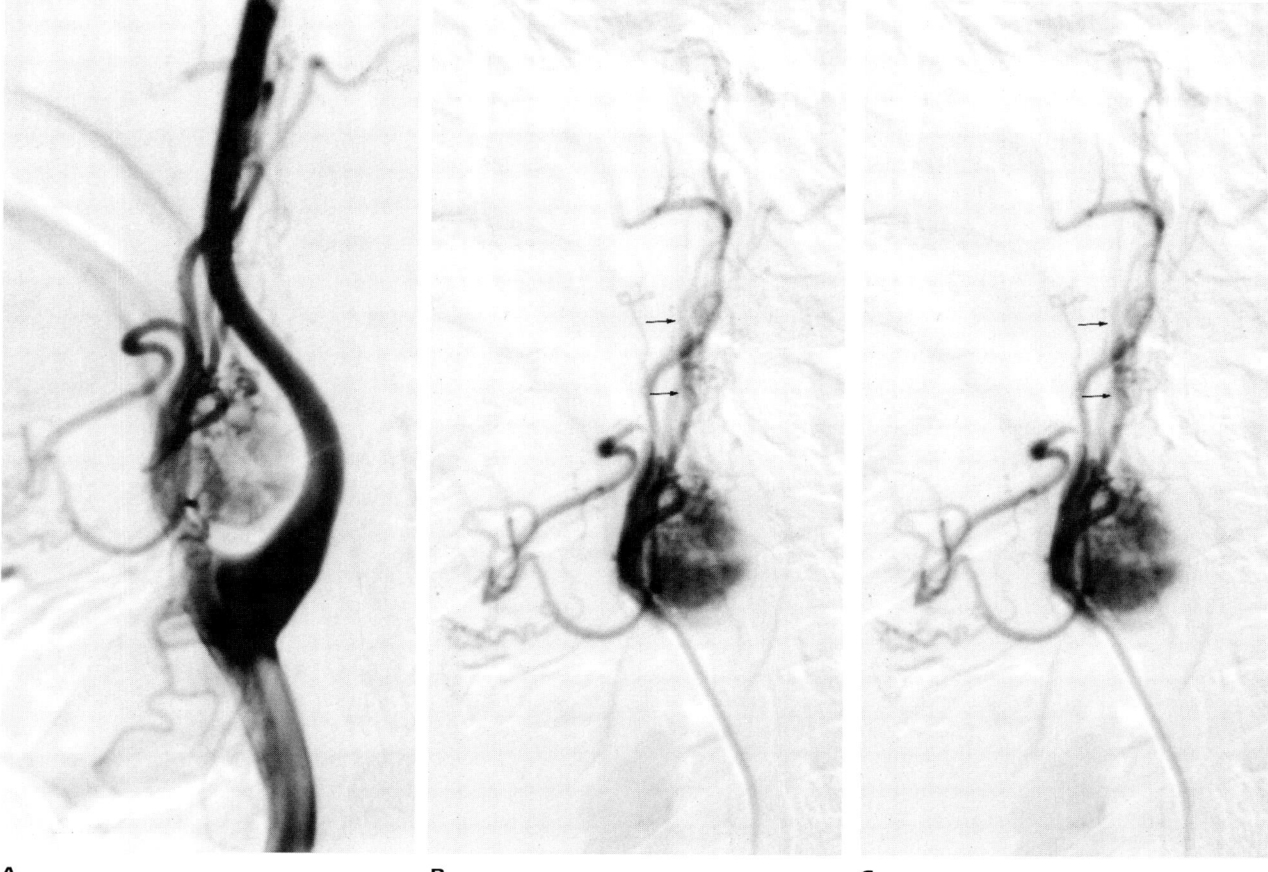

Figure 13-61. Carotid body tumor. A 68-year-old man was found to have a new left neck mass. He had had a right carotid body tumor resected and a right glomus vagale partially resected 2 years earlier. The lateral view of the left common carotid angiogram (A) demonstrates a hypervascular mass situated between the internal and external carotid arteries, splaying them apart. The lateral (B) and frontal (C) views of the left external carotid angiogram demonstrate an enlarged ascending pharyngeal artery (*arrows*) supplying the mass, which also derived some of its blood supply from smaller external carotid branches. This carotid body tumor was resected following embolization.

confirm the hypervascularity and examine the arterial supply for potential embolization. Glomus jugulare tumors are known for their involvement of the jugular foramen at the skull base. They, along with the other glomus tumors, appear early in the arterial phase as intensely staining masses with arteriovenous shunting. Glomus jugulare tumors may also be seen as a filling defect of the jugular vein in the venous phases of cerebral angiograms, provided the tumors have not already obstructed the vein entirely. The arterial supply of a glomus jugulare tumor can arise from the ascending pharyngeal artery, the occipital artery, or the vertebral artery. The glomus vagale tumor (Fig. 13-60) tends to be more inferior in location than the glomus jugulare tumor. A large glomus vagale tumor in the upper neck tends to displace both the internal and external carotid arteries anteriorly, a distinction from the carotid body tumor (Fig. 13-61), which tends to lie between and splay apart the internal and external carotid arteries.[86,87]

Juvenile angiofibromas are nasopharyngeal tumors typically seen in adolescent males.[88] These hyper-

◀ **Figure 13-60.** Glomus vagale. A 55-year-old woman presented with a left neck mass. The frontal view of her left external carotid injection (A) reveals a large, markedly hypervascular mass. The lateral view of her left common carotid injection (B) demonstrates anterior displacement of the internal and external carotid arteries by the staining tumor. Lateral views of superselective injections into the left ascending pharyngeal artery (C) and a branch of the left occipital artery (D) show contributions of these external carotid branches to the neoplasm. This glomus vagale was embolized and resected.

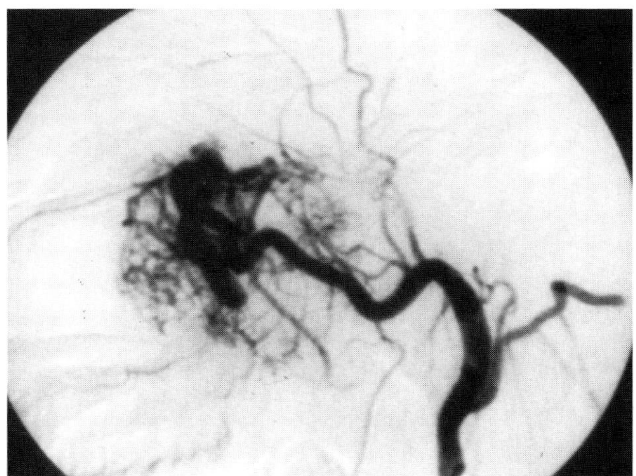
A

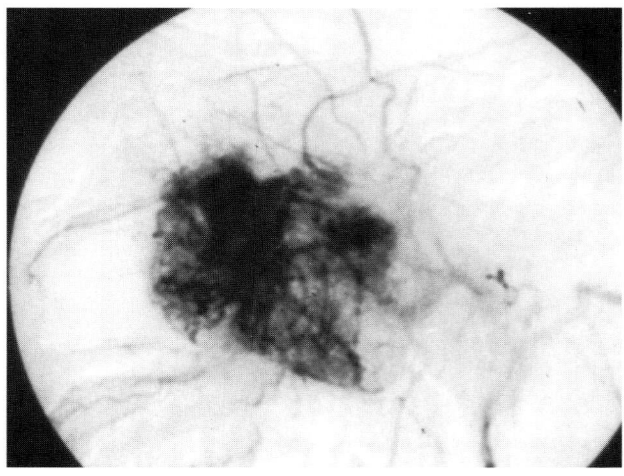
B

Figure 13-62. Juvenile angiofibroma. Lateral views of an external carotid angiogram in an adolescent male with a nasopharyngeal mass demonstrate the tumor to be hypervascular, with arterial supply from the maxillary artery (A) and an intense stain (B). This juvenile angiofibroma was resected following embolization.

vascular masses may be associated with airway obstruction or bleeding and are most often supplied by the ascending pharyngeal artery and branches of the maxillary artery (Fig. 13-62). If these tumors enlarge into the sphenoid sinus, there may be additional supply from the internal carotid artery. Angiographic evaluation is usually for confirmation of diagnosis and potential embolization before resection. Angiography demonstrates a homogeneous blush persisting into the venous phase, reticulated vessels, and a lack of shunting, although these angiographic findings may be seen with other nasopharyngeal masses.[89]

Gliomas, which are intraaxial tumors, often involve locations deep in the white matter, but may be seen subcortically or in the basal ganglia or brainstem. Mass effect depends on the size of the tumor and associated edema, and glioblastomas may initially present as hemorrhages. Vascularity may range from avascular in the benign or lower-grade tumors to hypervascular with shunting in the higher-grade, malignant lesions, although tumor grading by angiography is not necessarily accurate (Fig. 13-63).[90,91] The arterial supply is pial, although invasion of the dura may result in recruitment of some meningeal vessels.[92] These tumors may be heterogeneous, with varying grades and areas of necrosis within the mass, and this heterogeneity may be reflected in the angiographic stain. The stain usually appears earlier in the arterial phase than in the meningiomas referred to above and tends to wash out by the late venous phase, unlike meningiomas. There can be inappropriate caliber changes of tumor vessels or of encased cerebral branches, as well as enlargement of draining veins.

Lymphomas, also typically deep intraaxial tumors, tend to be avascular masses angiographically. Staining is rare, so although these tumors may appear similar to high-grade gliomas on CT and MRI, they tend to behave differently on angiographic evaluation.[93]

Hemangioblastomas, common to the posterior

Figure 13-63. Glioblastoma. A 71-year-old left-handed man was evaluated because of drooling and was found to have a facial droop on neurologic examination. His brain CT scan revealed a 7-cm right temporal mass, which on a brain MR image was seen to be a ring-enhancing structure. An angiogram and Wada test were performed preoperatively. The frontal view of his right internal carotid injection in the arterial phase (A) demonstrates a proximal shift of the anterior cerebral artery (*curved arrow*), elevation of the M_1 segment of the middle cerebral artery and the sylvian point (*open arrows*), medial displacement of the anterior choroidal artery (*small arrows*), and stretching of the supraclinoid internal carotid artery (*arrowhead*). The lateral view (B) demonstrates draping of the anterior choroidal artery over the mass (*small arrows*) and elevation of middle cerebral artery branches (*open arrows*). In the venous phase of the examination, there is leftward displacement of the internal cerebral vein on the frontal view (*arrow,* C) and elevation of the internal cerebral vein (*arrow,* D) and basal vein of Rosenthal on the lateral view (*u-shaped arrow,* D). The mass was confirmed to be a glioblastoma multiforme at surgery. This particular tumor was not hypervascular. Glioblastomas may be much more vascular than this, with accompanying arteriovenous shunting. ▶

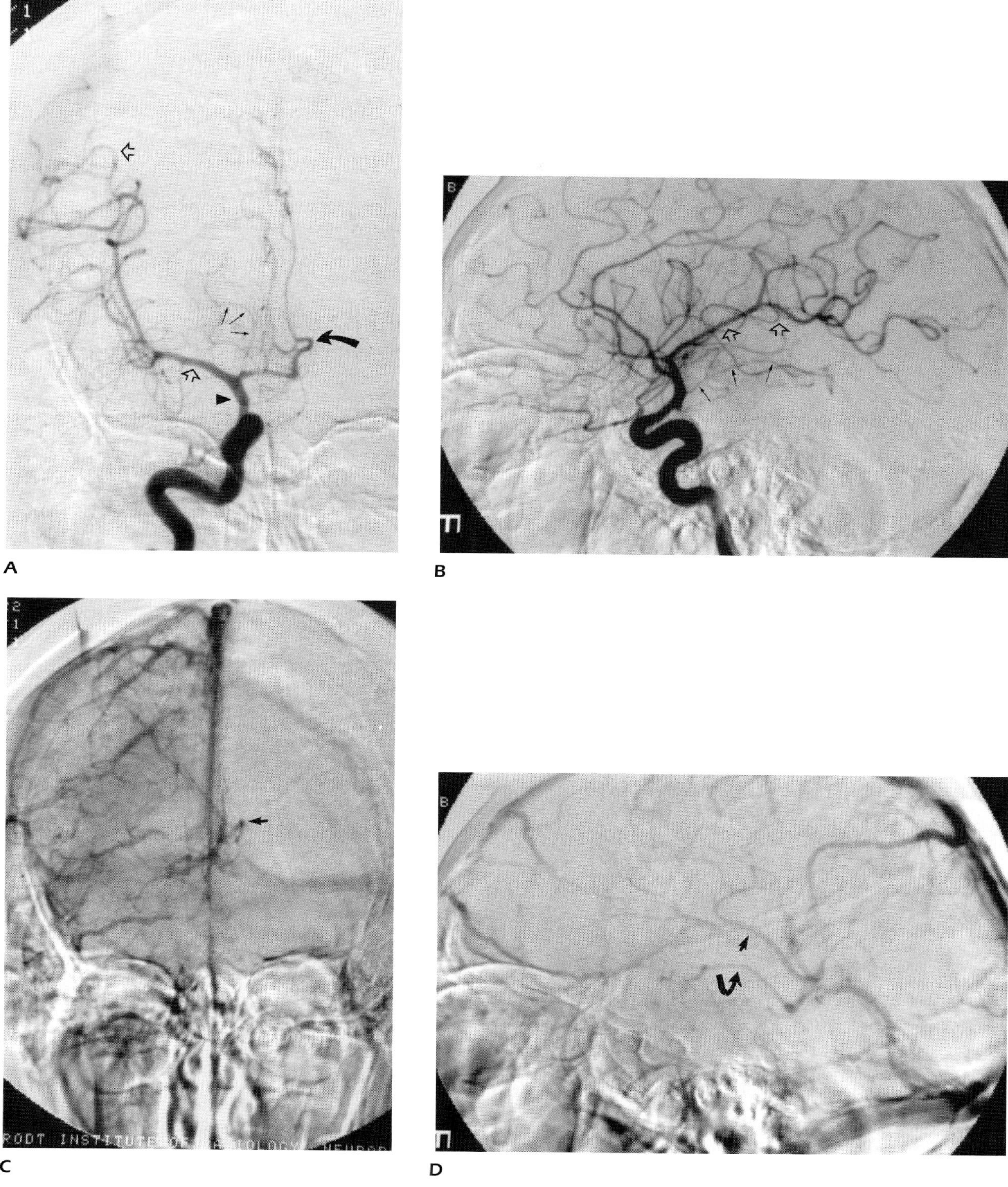
A
B
C
D

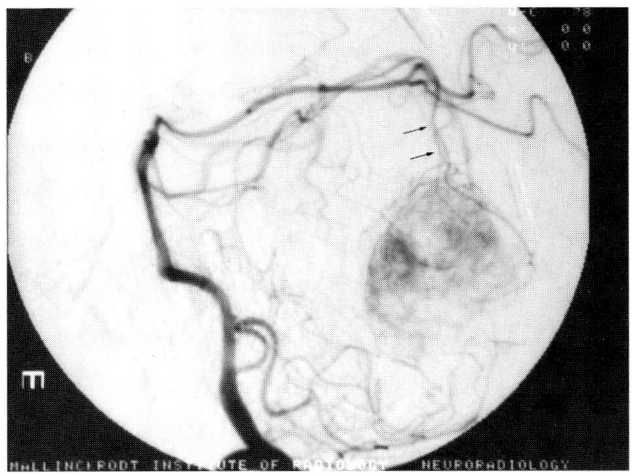

A

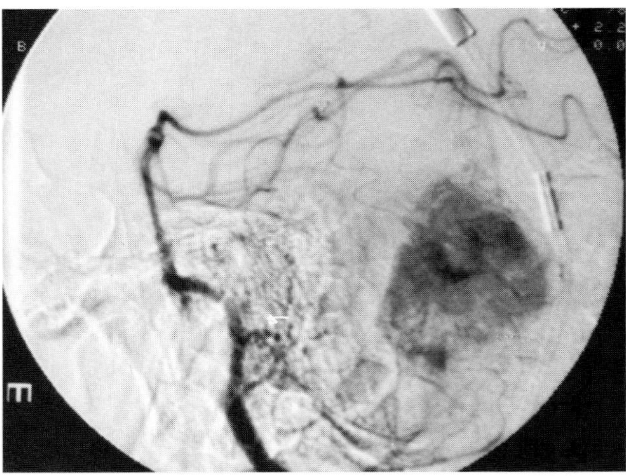

B

Figure 13-64. Hemangioblastoma. A 45-year-old man was found to have a cerebellar neoplasm. At initial biopsy, there was profuse bleeding from the mass. Lateral views of his vertebral angiogram demonstrate it to be markedly hypervascular, with arterial supply from the superior cerebellar arteries (*arrows,* A) and a dense stain (B). Following embolization, the tumor was resected and confirmed to be a hemangioblastoma.

fossa and rare above the tentorium, are usually highly vascular intraaxial neoplasms.[94] They may be seen in association with von Hippel–Lindau syndrome, may be multiple under those circumstances, and may be seen in the spinal cord as well.[95] Hemangioblastomas may be cystic or solid.[96] The cystic neoplasms typically have a nodule at a border that may be seen as an enhancing structure on CT and MRI examinations and as an intensely staining lesion on angiography. The solid neoplasms typically appear as hypervascular masses on angiography (Fig. 13-64). At times, there can be such a degree of early-phase neovascularity and shunting that hemangioblastomas may be confused with arteriovenous malformations.

Metastases to the brain may be hypervascular, especially in cases of metastatic renal cell carcinoma and melanoma. The multiplicity of lesions on CT or MRI or association with disease elsewhere in the body usually suggests the diagnosis, but a single lesion could be confused with another disease process, such as a high-grade glial neoplasm.[97,98]

Radiation necrosis may be indistinguishable from recurrent tumor on CT and MRI. Angiographically, radiation necrosis has been described as having an avascular mass effect, abnormally narrowed or occluded arteries in the radiation field, and slowing of circulation.[99] Aside from radiation necrosis, radiation injury has also been associated with direct effects on vessels, including generalized narrowing, stroke, and the development of multiple aneurysms.[100–104]

Intraparenchymal hemorrhages and edema from infarctions may also cause mass effects on cerebral vessels. Draping of arteries, stretching of vessels, and shifts of arteries and veins may be seen, just as when tumors are responsible for mass effects. In cases of cerebral intraaxial hematomas, there may be associated arterial abnormalities that indicate the underlying cause for the bleed, such as a vascular malformation, a mycotic aneurysm, or a hypervascular neoplasm, or there may be atherosclerotic changes that correlate with a hypertensive history. The hematoma itself should be avascular, so unless an underlying abnormality is evident, findings are often limited to the avascular mass effect. It is possible to see a hypervascular rim and even a slight degree of shunting from bleeds and infarctions in the subacute stage.

Trauma

Cerebral angiography may be necessary in the evaluation of trauma patients to identify sites of vessel injury that could be responsible for immediate or delayed neurologic events. This is particularly true for gunshot and knife wounds to the head and neck and for cases of cervical spine fractures involving the vertebral artery foramina. Dissections or occlusions can occur in the carotid and vertebral arteries as a result of blunt or penetrating trauma, and pseudoaneurysms can complicate dissections (Figs. 13-65 through 13-67). Dis-

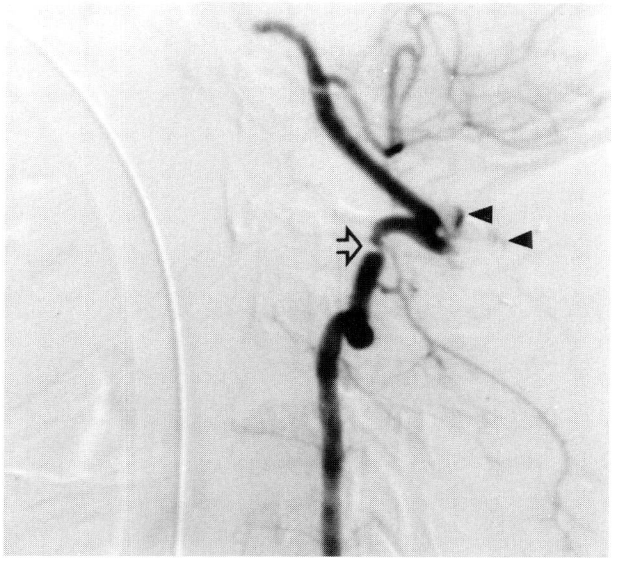

A

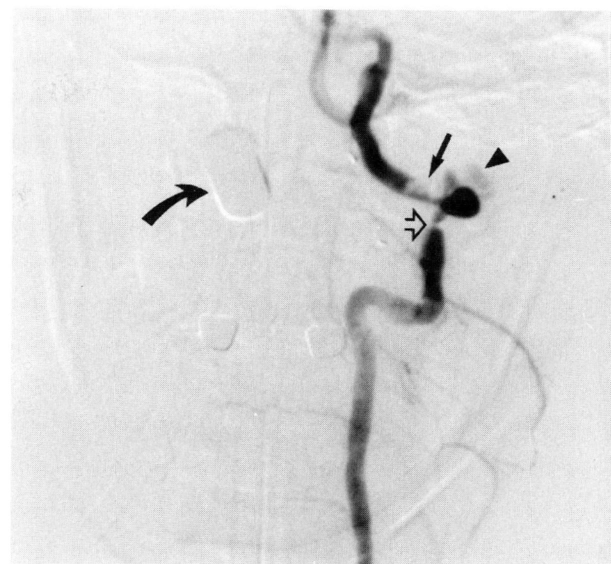

B

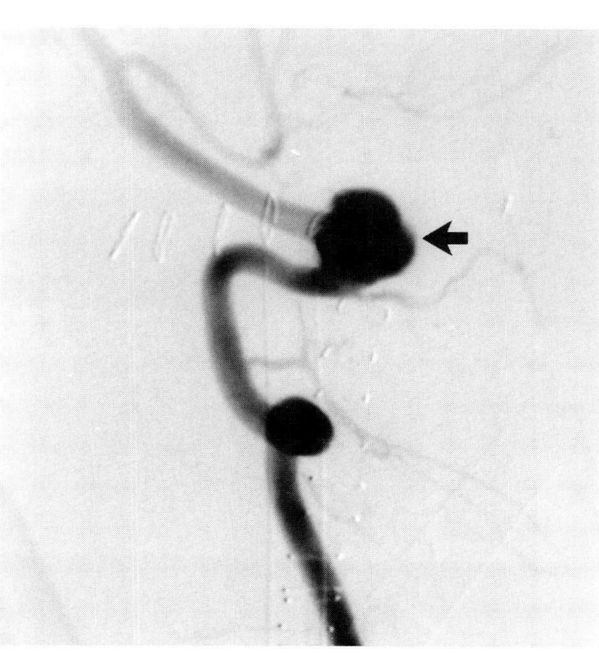

C

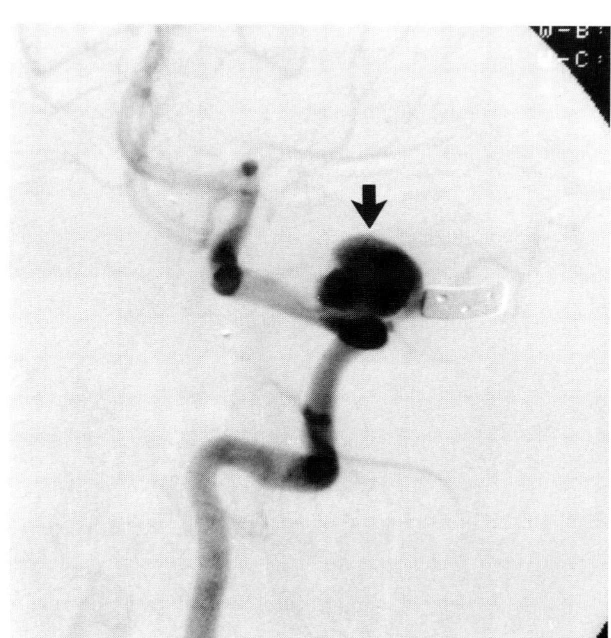

D

Figure 13-65. Gunshot wound with vertebral dissection and pseudoaneurysm. A 16-year-old man was shot in the neck. His left vertebral angiogram on admission reveals tight spasm of the vertebral artery (*open arrows,* A and B) and a small amount of extraluminal contrast at the C1 level (*arrowheads,* A and B). In addition, filling defects, possibly secondary to thrombus, are noted within the vertebral artery just distal to the site of presumed extravasation (*arrow,* B). The bullet is seen as a subtraction artifact (*curved arrow,* B). On follow-up left vertebral angiography after a 2-day interval, the area of spasm has resolved, but at the site of extraluminal contrast on the initial examination there is now a large pseudoaneurysm (*thick arrows,* C and D). The pseudoaneurysm was trapped by embolization, and the patient was discharged neurologically intact. He returned 9 months later with another gunshot wound to the neck (not shown).

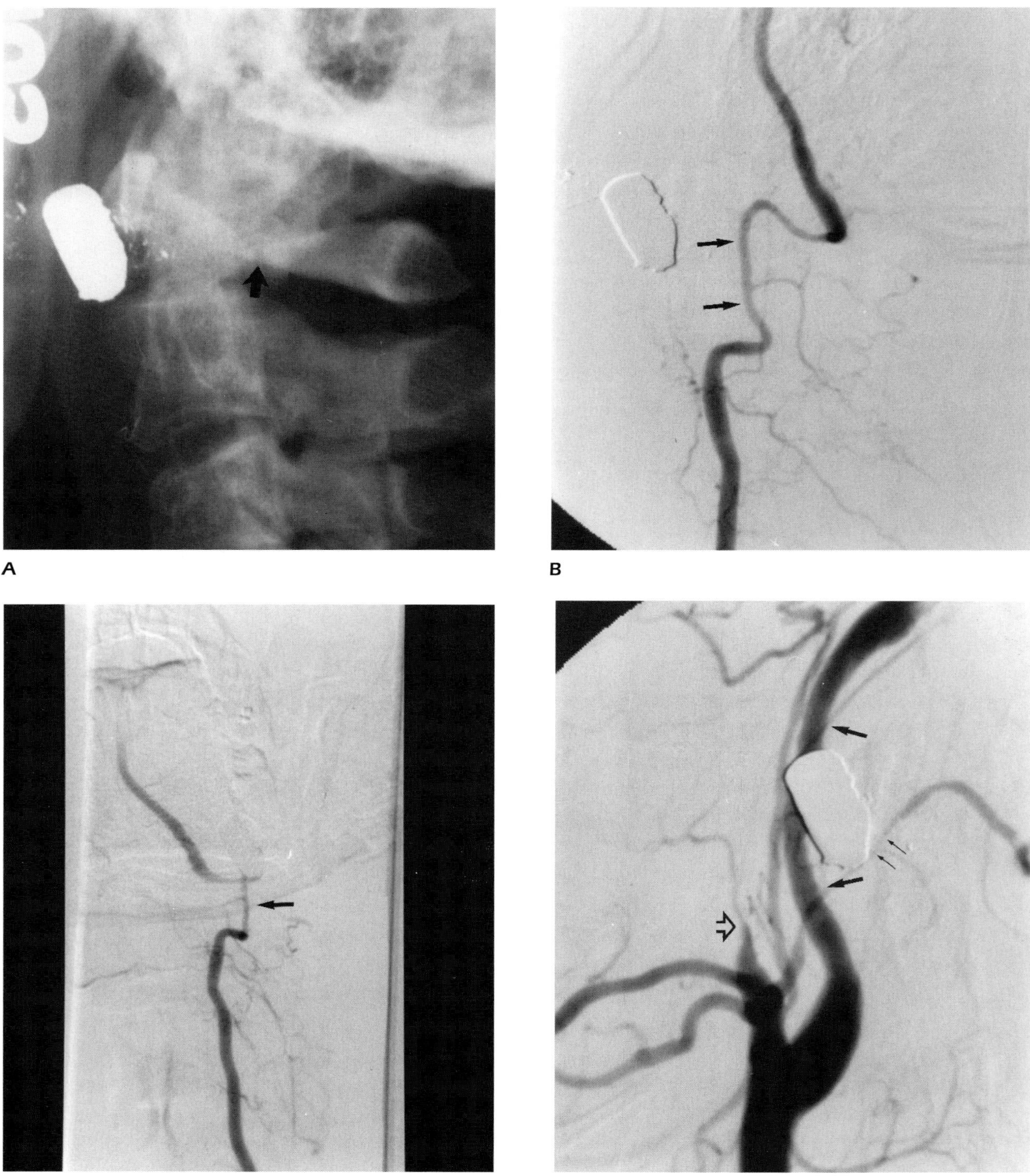

Figure 13-66. Gunshot wound with vertebral and carotid artery spasm. A 44-year-old man sustained a gunshot wound to the neck that resulted in a fracture of the C1 vertebral body (*arrow,* A). The fracture extended into the left lateral mass of C1 on CT scanning. His left vertebral angiogram demonstrates abnormal caliber narrowing of the vertebral artery of the C1 level (*arrows,* B and C) without an evident flap or extravasation. This was presumed to represent spasm; no follow-up angiogram was obtained. His left common carotid angiogram (D) reveals mild narrowing and anterior displacement of the internal carotid artery (*arrows*), probably on the basis of spasm and compression from an adjacent hematoma, an abrupt narrowing of the external carotid artery (*open arrow*), and spasm of the occipital artery (*small arrows*). The patient was treated conservatively and remained neurologically intact.

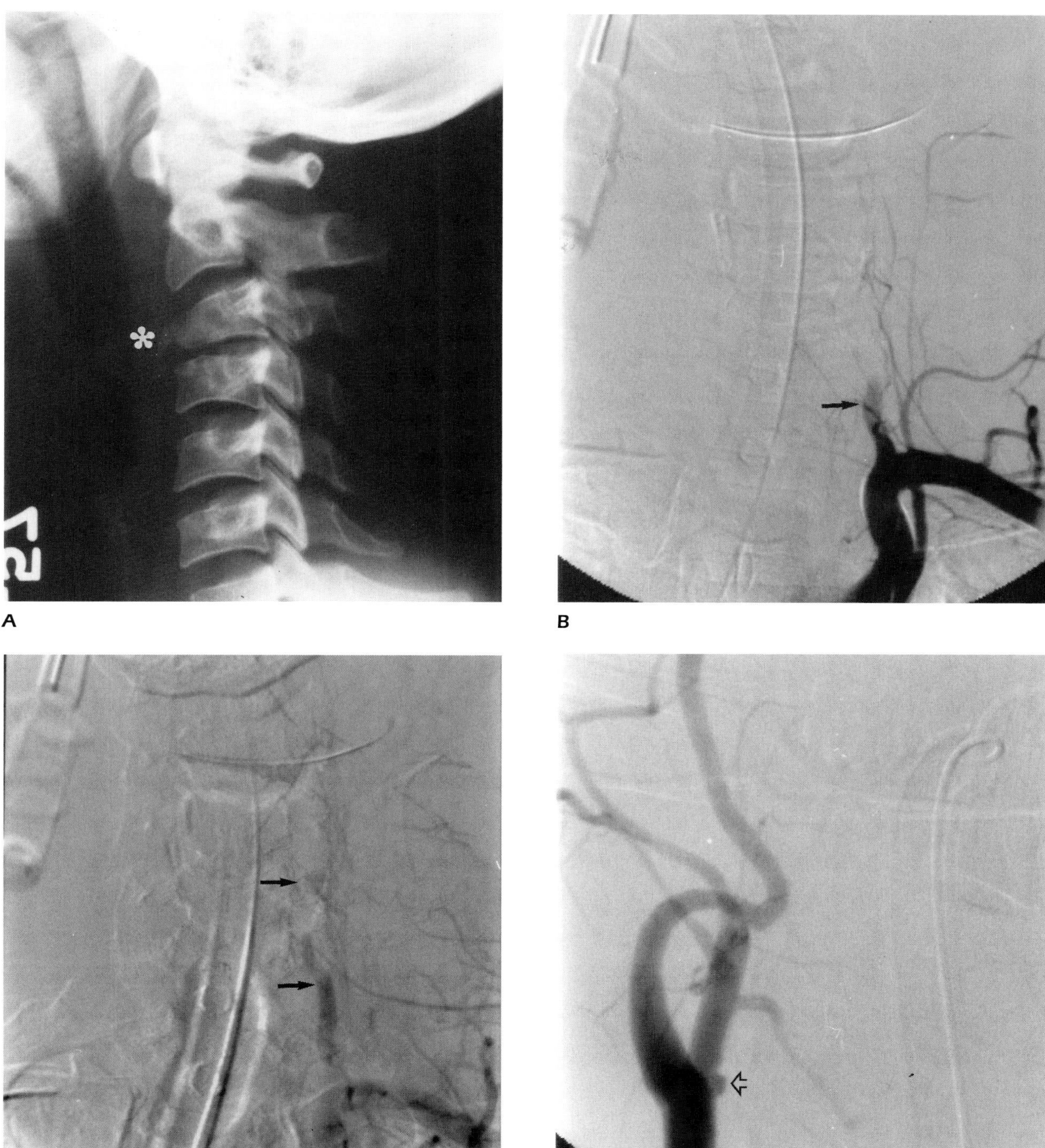

Figure 13-67. Gunshot wound with vertebral occlusion and carotid pseudoaneurysm. A 30-year-old man sustained a gunshot wound to the neck. On neurologic examination, the patient was found to have a cervical cord syndrome and mental status changes. His cervical (C)-spine film reveals a fracture of the C3 vertebral body (*asterisk*, A). A CT scan of the C-spine disclosed another fracture, one of the left lateral mass of C4 involving the vertebral artery foramen. His left subclavian angiogram reveals an occlusion of the left vertebral artery in the mid C-spine (*arrows*, B and C). His right carotid angiogram discloses a small pseudoaneurysm of the carotid bifurcation (*open arrow*, D).

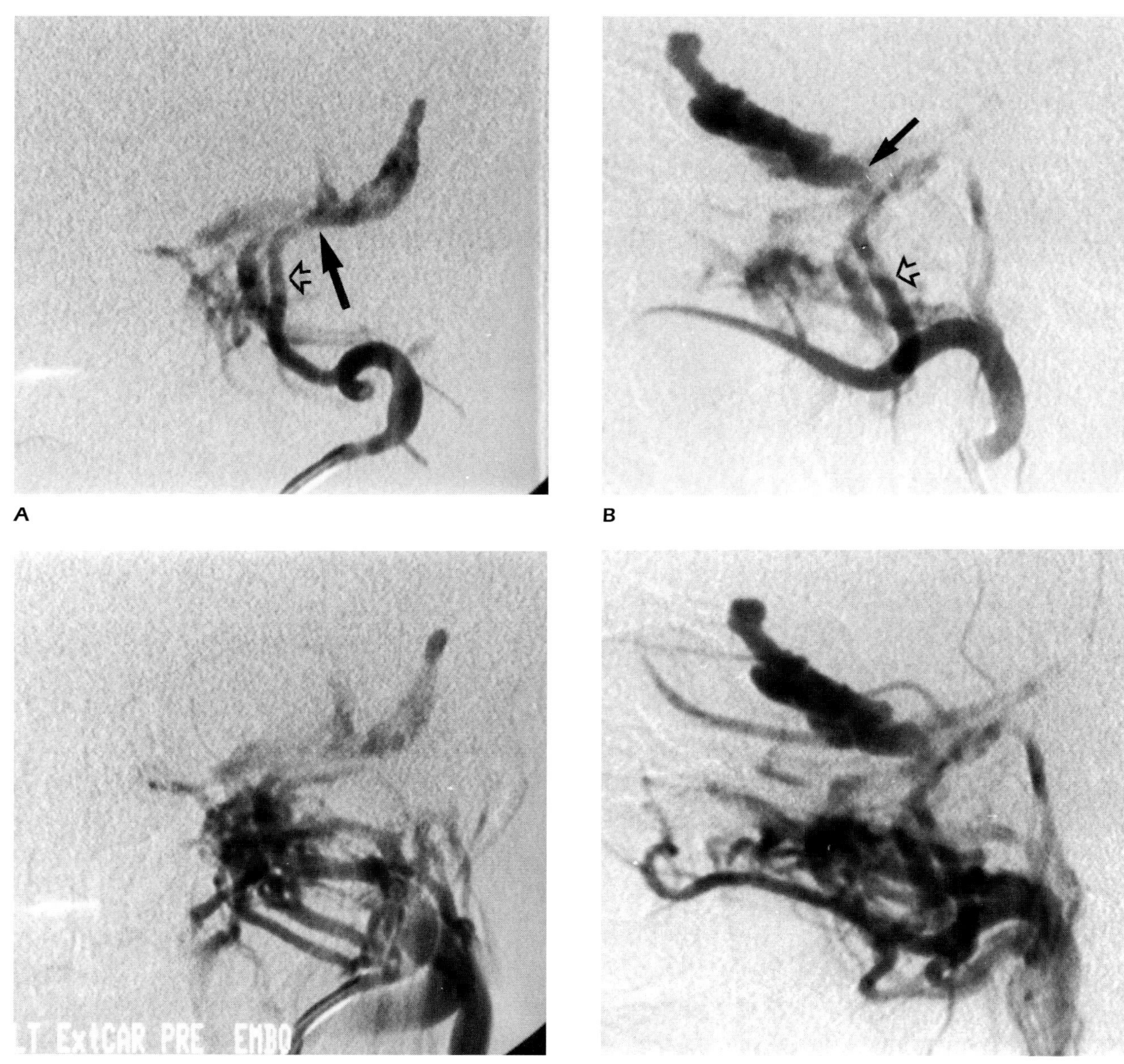

Figure 13-68. Traumatic fistula. A 27-year-old woman sustained a left skull fracture in a fall. At the time of the injury, there was an acute epidural hematoma at the fracture site, and the fracture extended through the foramen spinosum on her CT scan. Several weeks after the fall, the patient complained of a loud bruit in her left ear that interfered with sleep. Frontal (A) and lateral (B) views early in the arterial phase of her left external carotid angiogram demonstrate an enlarged left middle meningeal artery (*open arrows*) and a fistula (*solid arrows*) that results in arteriovenous shunting and venous opacification slightly later in the arterial phase of the study (C and D).

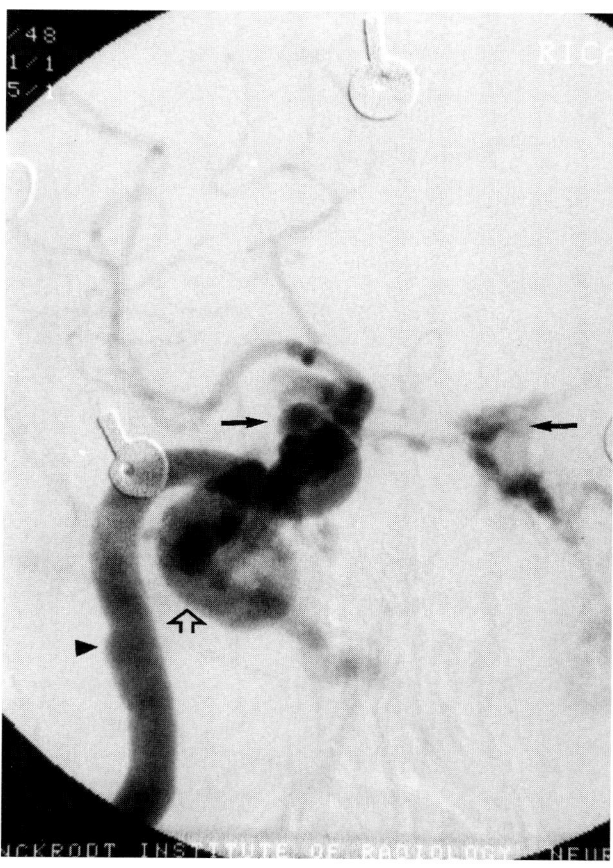

A

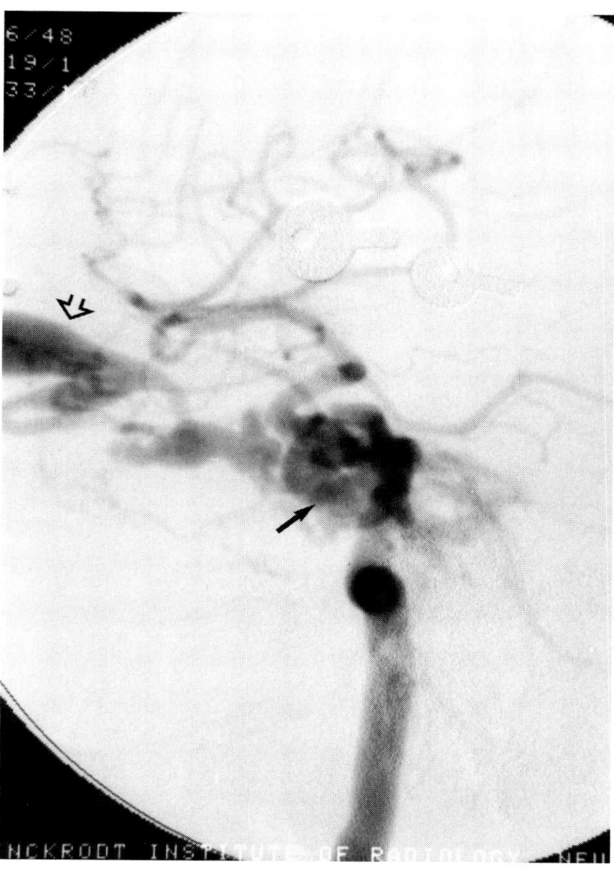

B

Figure 13-69. Carotid-cavernous fistula. A 45-year-old man presented with diplopia and right proptosis and chemosis. Frontal (A) and lateral (B) views in the arterial phase of his right internal carotid angiogram demonstrate immediate filling of the cavernous sinuses (*arrows*) and a greatly enlarged superior ophthalmic vein (*open arrows*) from a single-hole carotid-cavernous fistula. (The actual site and type of fistula were determined during a subsequent embolization.) A small focal dilatation of the right internal carotid artery below the skull base (*arrowhead,* A) may be the result of a healed dissection.

sections may even occur after seemingly insignificant trauma. Fistulas may develop between arteries and veins at sites of penetrating trauma or between the carotid artery and cavernous sinus after head injury (Figs. 13-68 and 13-69). Aside from its neurologic role, angiography can be used to identify the bleeding site in an expanding hematoma of the head or neck (Fig. 13-70)[105,106] or in cases of epistaxis (Fig. 13-71).

Symptoms associated with cerebrovascular injury vary. Patients can experience transient ischemic attacks or strokes as a result of dissections, occlusions, and pseudoaneurysms of cerebral vessels, and patients with internal carotid artery dissections can develop unilateral headache and Horner syndrome.[107,108] Dissections involving intracranial segments of cerebral arteries may result in subarachnoid bleeding.[109] Patients with fistulas may develop bruits or signs of increased venous pressure. Some initially asymptomatic patients develop delayed neurologic sequelae. These can be the result of delayed effects of abnormalities identified on angiograms at the time of initial injury, or the result of abnormalities not discovered until repeat angiography is performed, for example, when aneurysms arise at sites of occult arterial injury. These aneurysms, usually false, can rupture, creating symptoms of parenchymal or subarachnoid bleeding, depending on the aneurysm's location.[110] A pseudoaneurysm of the petrous internal carotid artery can rupture and cause massive epistaxis.[111]

The site of dissection from blunt trauma is usually the internal carotid artery (Figs. 13-72 and 13-73). Rotational injuries of the neck can result in vertebral

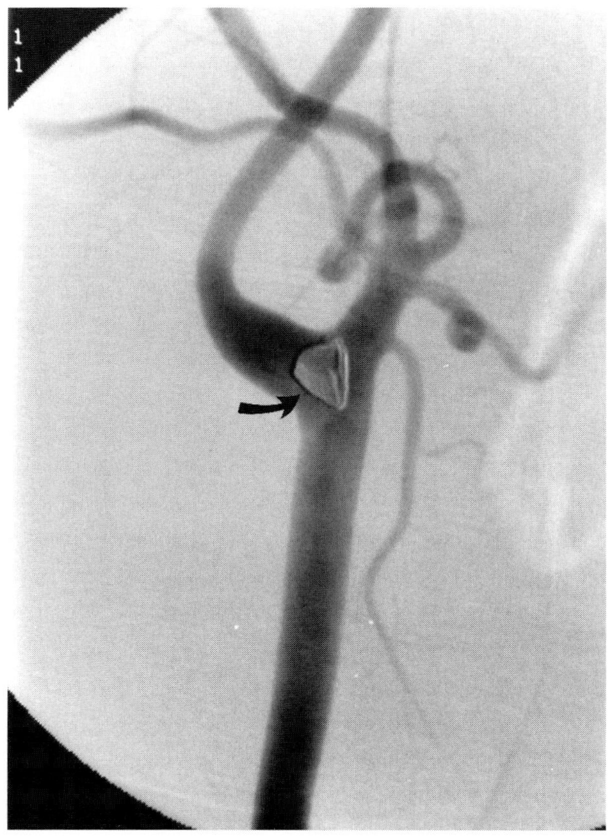

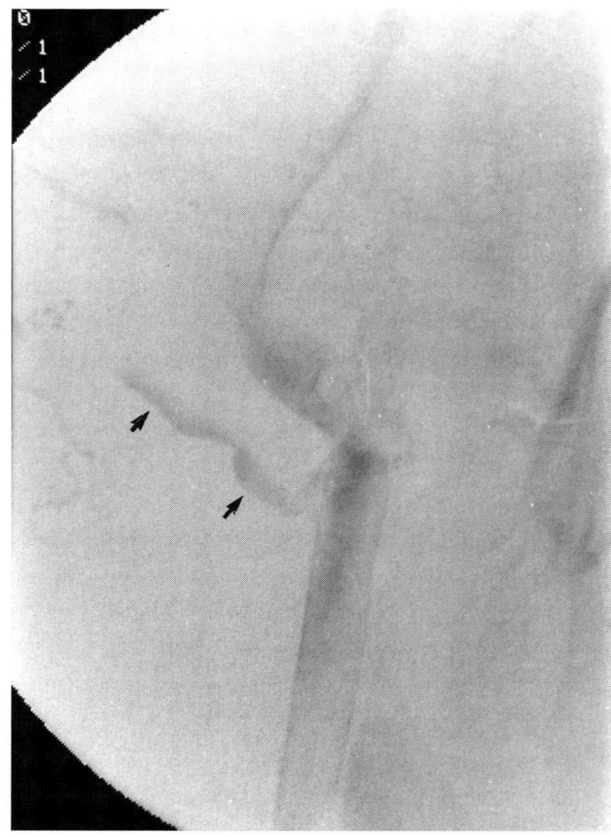

A B

Figure 13-70. Carotid extravasation. A 33-year-old man sustained a gunshot wound to the neck. Oblique views of his right common carotid angiogram demonstrate the bullet fragment overlying the carotid bifurcation (*curved arrow,* A) and subsequent extravasation of contrast (*arrows,* B). The specific site of vessel injury is not apparent.

artery dissections, usually at C1-C2. Internal carotid artery dissections are more common than vertebral dissections.[107] Penetrating injuries can affect other arterial locations. Iatrogenic dissections can also occur from angiography or interventional procedures (Fig. 13-74).

Traumatic intracranial aneurysms should be suspected when there is an intracerebral hematoma secondary to wartime missile injury. These are most often found on middle cerebral artery branches.[110,112] Whereas high-velocity missiles usually transect arteries, low-velocity missiles are associated with aneurysm development.[113]

With regard to clinical correlation, it is noteworthy that vertebral artery occlusions, fistulas, and dissections can be unilateral or bilateral and at any level as a result of penetrating gunshot or knife wounds or fractures, but unilateral injury seldom causes neurologic symptoms.[114] Neurologic deficits from trauma could be the result of epidural or subdural hematomas.

Figure 13-71. Epistaxis. A 45-year-old man had undergone transsphenoidal resection of a pituitary adenoma 3 years earlier. He presented with meningitis. CT scans demonstrated an expansive, destructive process in the sphenoid sinus, and MRI, in addition to showing meningeal enhancement, suggested the presence of a sphenoid sinus abscess. Sphenoid endoscopy 1 day prior to his angiogram confirmed the presence of pus in the sphenoid sinus. The patient underwent emergency angiography for massive epistaxis resulting in hypotension. The initial frontal view of his right maxillary artery injection reveals what appears to be a small pseudoaneurysm (*open arrow,* A). Later frontal (B) and lateral (C) images from the same injection demonstrate active extravasation of contrast into the nose and nasopharynx (*arrows*). The patient was embolized to stop the epistaxis. ▶

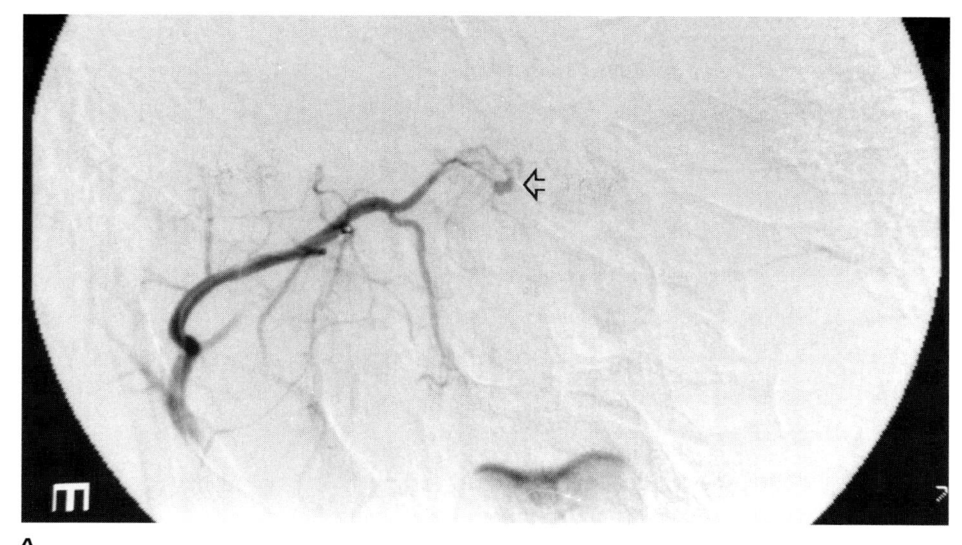

A

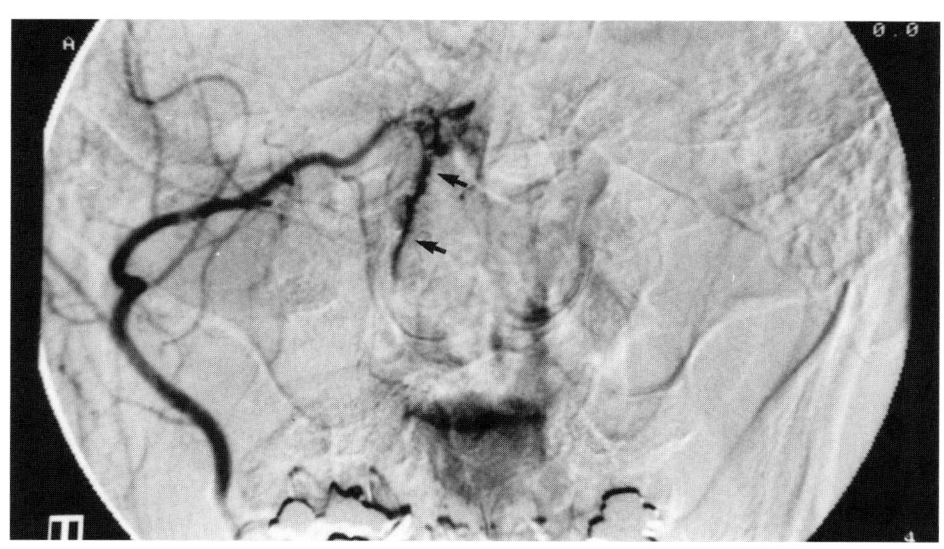

B

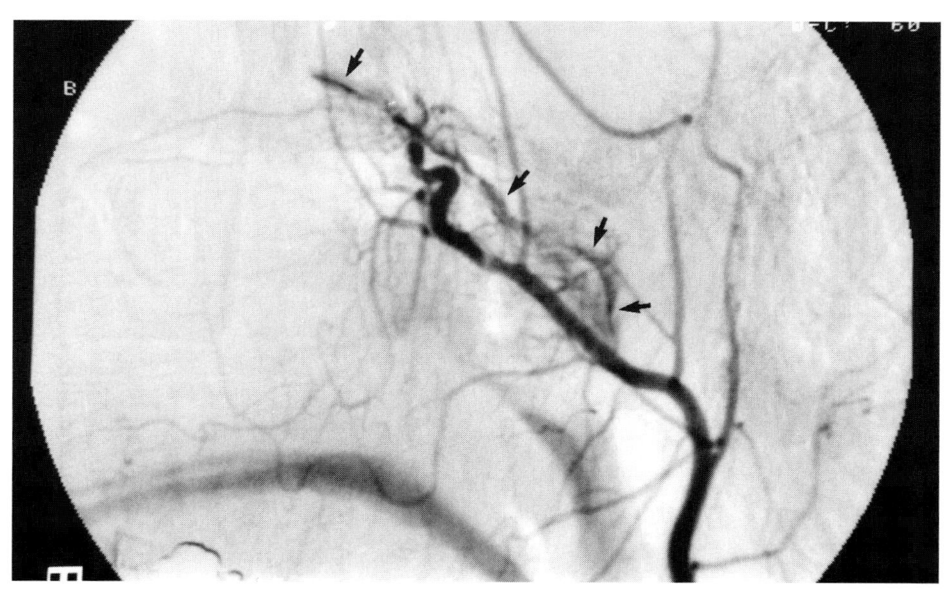

C

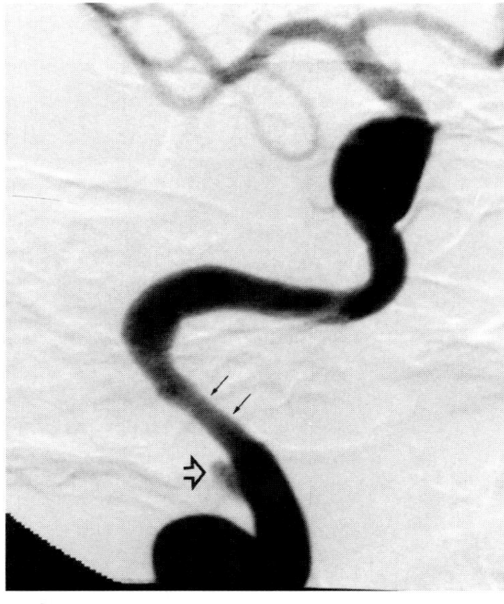

A

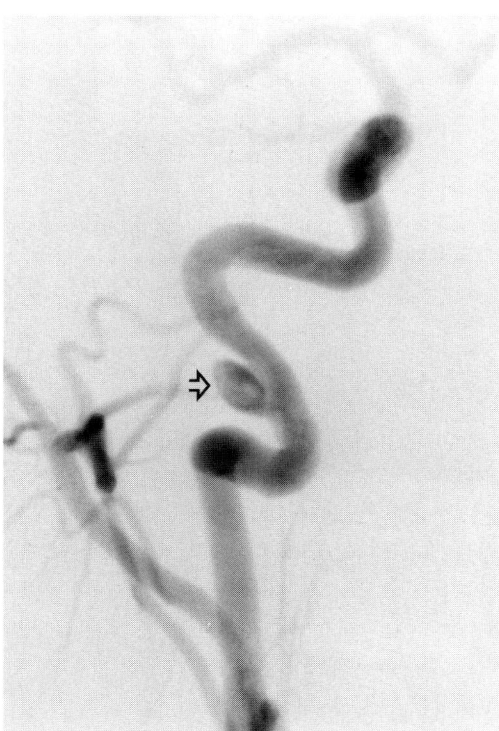

B

Figure 13-72. Mctor vehicle accident with carotid pseudoaneurysm. A 24-year-old woman was involved in a motor vehicle accident. She sustained a right frontal lobe contusion, developed bilateral subdural collections, and had a small amount of subarachnoid blood on brain CT imaging. An oblique view of her initial right carotid angiogram (A) reveals a small pseudoaneurysm of the right internal carotid artery (*open arrow*) just proximal to an area of spasm (*small arrows*). A follow-up angiogram 2 months later in the same projection (B) reveals resolution of the spasm but interval enlargement of the pseudoaneurysm (*open arrow*).

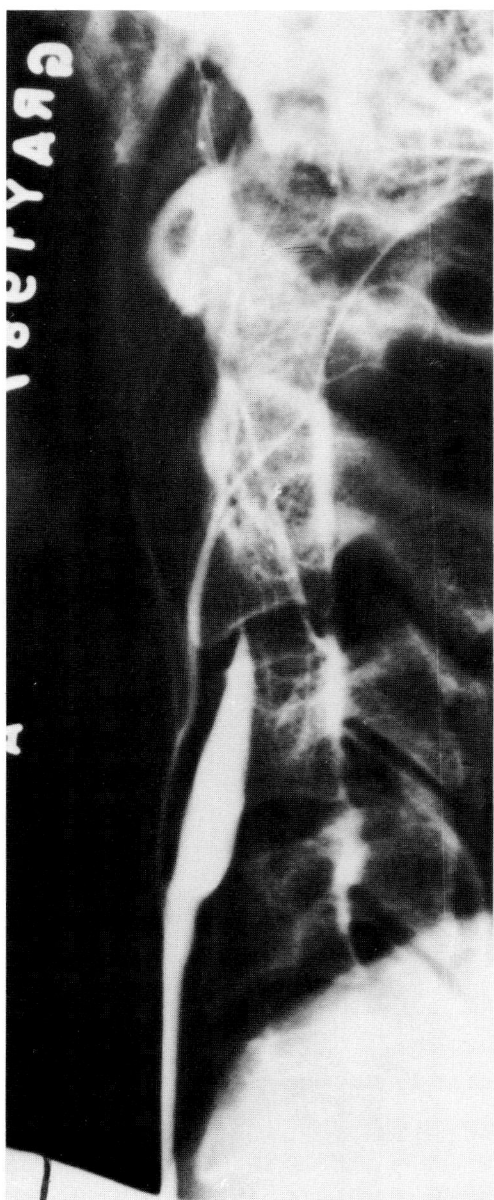

Figure 13-73. Traumatic occlusion of the internal carotid artery. A 30-year-old woman sustained blunt trauma to the neck. Subsequently she developed a headache, then aphasia with slow resolution. In this left common carotid angiogram, a long, tapered occlusion of the internal carotid artery is seen more than 2 cm beyond the bifurcation. The precise site of the occlusion is at the level of the second cervical vertebra or above. Lateral projection.

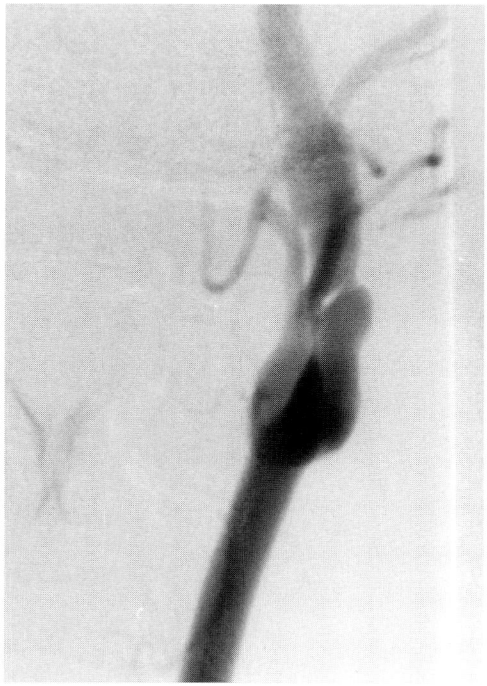

A

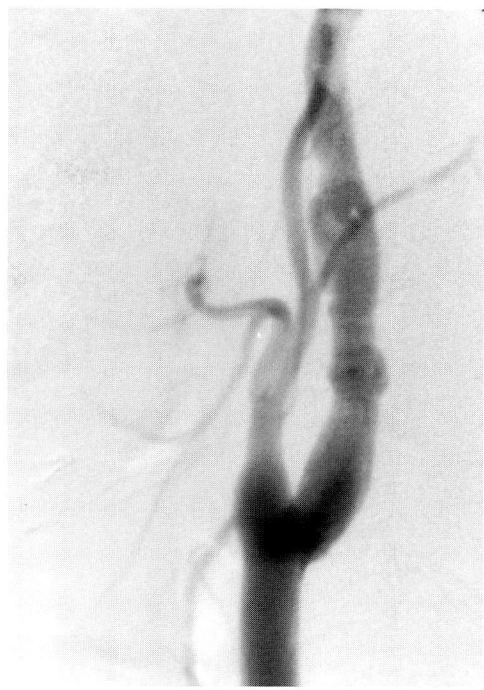

B

Figure 13-74. Iatrogenic dissection. The AVM of a 40-year-old woman was embolized using a left carotid approach. One week after the embolization, the patient complained of sudden left neck pain. Frontal (A) and lateral (B) views from her subsequent left common carotid angiogram demonstrate luminal irregularity and stenosis of the cervical internal carotid artery not present at the time of her previous procedure. The dissection was presumed secondary to microcatheter manipulation.

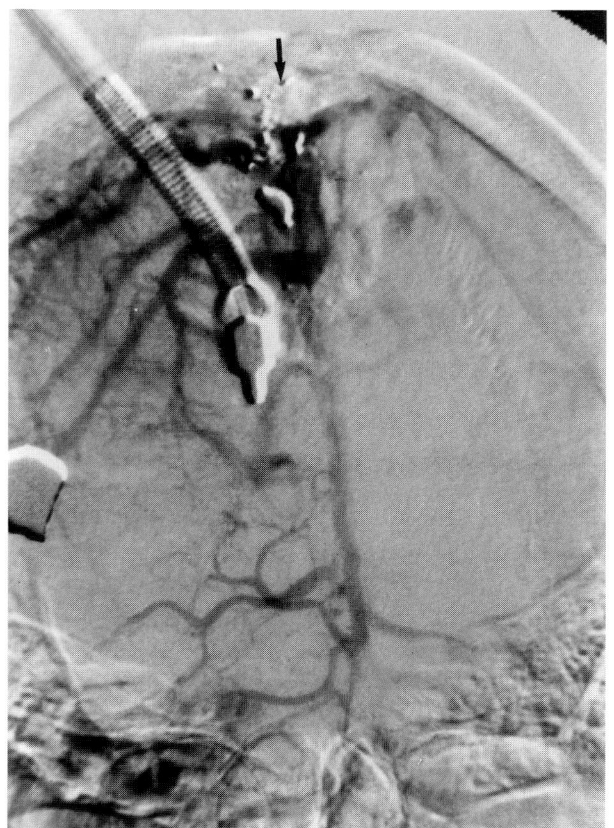

A

B

Figure 13-75. Gunshot wound with venous sinus occlusion. A 17-year-old woman sustained a gunshot wound to the head. In the neurologic intensive care unit, she was noted to have persisting, unexplained increased intracranial pressure. Frontal (A) and lateral (B) views of the venous phase of her cerebral angiogram demonstrate bullet fragments at the site of an occlusion of the superior sagittal sinus (*arrows*).

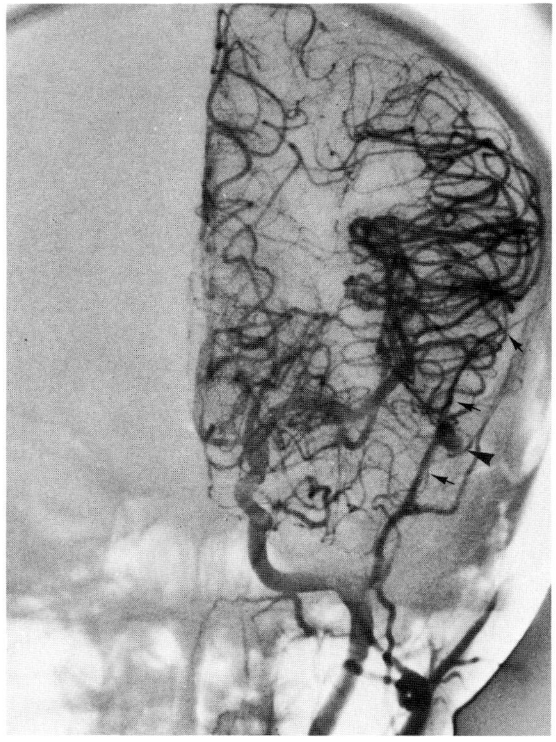

A B

Figure 13-76. Epidural hematoma and aneurysm of the middle meningeal artery in addition to fistulas. (A) Left common carotid angiogram shows medial displacement of the middle meningeal artery (*arrows*) by an epidural collection. Note the aneurysm of the middle meningeal artery (*arrowhead*). (B) The aneurysm (*large arrowhead*) and fistulas (meningeal artery–meningeal veins) (*small arrowheads*) are more graphically demonstrated in this view. (A) AP projection; (B) lateral projection.

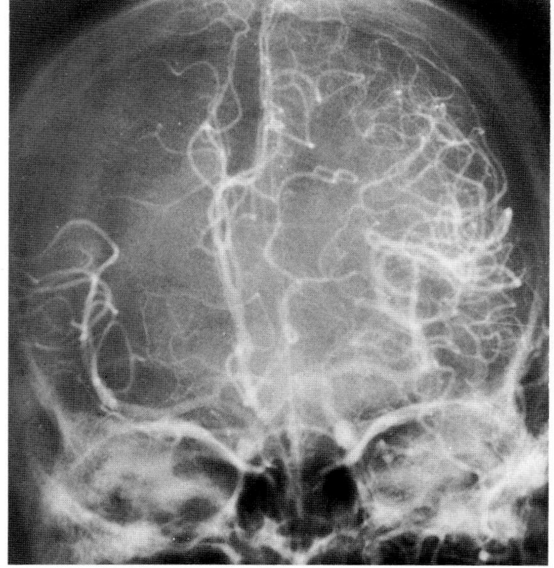

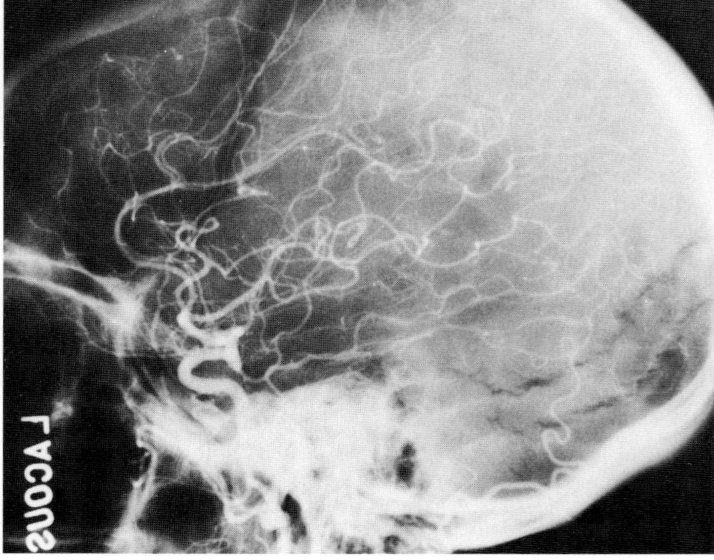

A B

Figure 13-77. Acute left convexity and right parasagittal subdural hematoma. (A) Left common carotid angiogram shows a large extracerebral collection displacing cortical vessels with no apparent involvement of meningeal arteries. A second separate collection is noted in the right parasagittal position. (B) This view is nearly normal in spite of a large subdural collection. There is only minimal distortion of perisylvian vessels. (A) AP projection; (B) lateral projection.

Although these are usually diagnosed and followed with CT scanning, extraaxial collections may be seen as incidental findings on angiography undertaken for trauma or other indications (Figs. 13-75 through 13-77).

Carotid-cavernous fistulas, which may develop as a result of head trauma or spontaneously, have been classified into four types, A through D. Type A is a direct, single-hole fistula between the internal carotid artery and the cavernous sinus. Type B is a dural fistula between the meningeal branches of the internal carotid artery and the cavernous sinus. Type C is a dural fistula between the meningeal branches of the external carotid artery and the cavernous sinus. Type D is a dural fistula with combined internal and external carotid meningeal branch supply.[115]

References

1. Zeumer H, Freitag HJ, Zanella F, Thie A, Arning C. Local intra-arterial fibrinolytic therapy in patients with stroke: urokinase versus recombinant tissue plasminogen activator (r-TPA). Neuroradiology 1993;35:159–162.
2. Pujia A, Rubba P, Spencer MD. Prevalence of extracranial carotid artery disease detectable by echo-Doppler in an elderly population. Stroke 1992;23:818–822.
3. Weinstein R. Noninvasive carotid duplex ultrasound imaging for the evaluation and management of carotid atherosclerotic disease. Hematol Oncol Clin North Am 1992;6:1131–1139.
4. Laster RE, Acker JD, Halford HH, Nauert TC. Assessment of MR angiography versus arteriography for evaluation of cervical carotid bifurcation disease. AJNR 1993;14:681–688.
5. Heiserman JE, Drayer BP, Keller PJ, Fram EK. Intracranial vascular stenosis and occlusion: evaluation with three-dimensional time-of-flight MR angiography. Radiology 1992;185: 667–673.
6. Anderson CM, et al. Assessment of carotid artery stenosis by MR angiography: comparison with X-ray angiography and color-coded Doppler ultrasound. AJNR 1992;13:989–1003.
7. Ackerman RH, Candia MR. Assessment of carotid artery stenosis by MR angiography. AJNR 1992;13:1005–1008.
8. Huston J, Lewis BD, Wiebers DO, Meyer FB, Riederer SJ, Weaver AL. Carotid artery: prospective blinded comparison of two-dimensional time-of-flight MR angiography with conventional angiography and duplex US. Radiology 1993;186: 339–344.
9. Polak JF, Kalina P, Donaldson MC, O'Leary DH, Whittemore AD, Mannick JA. Carotid endarterectomy: preoperative evaluation of candidates with combined Doppler sonography and MR angiography. Radiology 1993;186:333–338.
10. Masaryk TJ, Obuchowski NA. Noninvasive carotid imaging: caveat emptor. Radiology 1993;186:325–331.
11. Riles TS, Eidelman EM, Litt AW, Pinto RS, Oldford F, Schwartzenberg GW. Comparison of magnetic resonance angiography, conventional angiography, and duplex scanning. Stroke 1992;23:341–346.
12. Poindexter JM, Shah PM, Clauss RH, Babu SC. The clinical utility of carotid duplex scanning. J Cardiovasc Surg 1991; 32:64–68.
13. North American Symptomatic Carotid Endarterectomy Trial Collaborators. Beneficial effect of carotid endarterectomy in symptomatic patients with high-grade stenosis. N Engl J Med 1991;325:445–453.
14. Fox AJ. How to measure carotid stenosis. Radiology 1993; 186:316–318.

14a. Executive Committee of the Asymptomatic Carotid Atherosclerosis Study. Endarterectomy for asymptomatic carotid artery stenosis. JAMA 1995;273(18):1421–1428.

15. Eliasziw M, Streifler JY, Fox AJ, Hachinski VC, Ferguson GG, Barnett HJ. Significance of plaque ulceration in symptomatic patients with high-grade carotid stenosis. North American Symptomatic Carotid Endarterectomy Trial. Stroke 1994;25: 304–308.
16. Higashida R, Tsai F, Halbach V, Dowd C, Smith T, Frasier K, Hieshima G. Transluminal angioplasty for atherosclerotic disease of the vertebral and basilar arteries. J Neurosurgery 1993;78:192–198.
17. Kachel R, Basche S, Heerklotz I, Grossman K, Endler S. Percutaneous transluminal angioplasty (PTA) of supraaortic arteries, especially the internal carotid artery. Neuroradiology 1991;33:191–194.
18. Gorelick PB, Caplan LR, Hier DB, Parker SL, Patel D. Racial differences in the distribution of anterior circulation occlusive disease. Neurology 1984;34:54–59.
19. Broderick JP. Heart disease and stroke. Heart Disease and Stroke 1993;2:355–359.
20. Borgousslavsky J, Pierre P. Ischemic stroke in patients under age 45. Neurol Clin 1992;10:113–124.
21. Lanzino G, Andreoli A, DiPasquale G, Urbinati S, Limoni P, Serracchioli A, Lusa A, Pinelli G, Testa C, Tognetti F. Etiopathogenesis and prognosis of cerebral ischemia in young adults: a survey of 155 treated patients. Acta Neurol Scand 1991;84(4):321–325.
22. Lisovosky F, Rousseux P. Cerebral infarction in young people: a study of 148 patients with early cerebral angiography. J Neurol Neurosurg Psychiatry 1991;54(7):576–579.
23. Sue DE, Brandt-Zawadzki MN, Chance J. Dissection of cranial arteries in the neck: correlation of MRI and arteriography. Neuroradiology 1992;34(4):273–278.
24. Solomon S, Lipton RB, Harris PY. Arterial stenosis in migraine: spasm or arteriopathy? Headache 1990;30:52–61.
25. Hilal SK. Cerebral hemodynamics assessed by angiography. In: Newton TH, Potts DG, eds. Radiology of the skull and brain: Vol. 2. Angiography. Great Neck, NY: MediBooks, 1986:1049–1088.
26. Ameri A, Bousser MG. Cerebral venous thrombosis. Neurol Clin 1992;10:87–111.
27. Kendall B. Cerebral angiography in vasculitis affecting the nervous system. Eur Neurol 1984;23:400–406.
28. Ferris EJ, Levine HL. Cerebral arteritis: classification. Radiology 1973;109:327–342.
29. Salgado AV, Furlan AJ, Keys TF. Mycotic aneurysm, subarachnoid hemorrhage, and indications for cerebral angiography in infective endocarditis. Stroke 1987;18:1057–1060.
30. Stanson AW. Roentgenographic findings in major vasculitic syndromes. Rheum Dis Clin North Am 1990;16:293–308.
31. Hinck VC, Carter CC, Rippy JG. Giant cell (cranial) arteritis. Am J Roentgenol Radium Ther Nucl Med 1964;92:769–775.
32. Ferris EJ. Arteritis. In: Newton TH, Potts DG, eds. Radiology of the skull and brain: Book 4. Specific disease processes. Great Neck, NY: MediBooks, 1986:2566–2597.
33. Tervaert JWC, Kallenberg C. Neurologic manifestations of systemic vasculitides. Rheum Dis Clin North Am 1993;19: 913–940.
34. So EL, Toole JF, Dalal P, Moody DM. Cephalic fibromuscular dysplasia in 32 patients. Arch Neurol 1981;38:619–622.
35. Halbach VV, Hieshima GB, Higashida RT, Reicher M. Carotid cavernous fistulae: indications for urgent treatment. Am J Roentgenol 1987;149:587–593.
36. Halbach VV, Higashida RT, Dowd CF, Barnwell SL, Hieshima GB. Treatment of carotid-cavernous fistulas associated with Ehlers-Danlos syndrome. Neurosurgery 1990;26:1021–1027.
37. Schievink WI, Limburg M, Oorthuys JW, Fleury P, Pope FM.

Cerebrovascular disease in Ehlers-Danlos syndrome type IV. Stroke 1990;21:626–632.
38. Kapoor R, Kendall BE, Harrison MJ. Persistent segmental artery constrictions in coital cephalgia. J Neurol Neurosurg Psychiatry 1990;53:266–267.
39. Garner BF, Burns P, Bunning RD, Laureno R. Acute blood pressure elevation can mimic arteriographic appearance of cerebral vasculitis. J Rheumatol 1990;17:93–97.
40. Trommer BL, Homer D, Mikhael MA. Cerebral vasospasm and eclampsia. Stroke 1988;19:326–329.
41. Solomon RA, Smith CR, Raps EC, Young WL, Stone JG, Fink ME. Deep hypothermic circulatory arrest for the management of complex anterior and posterior circulation aneurysms. Neurosurgery 1991;29:732–738.
42. Nakagawa T, Hashi K. The incidence and treatment of asymptomatic, unruptured cerebral aneurysms. J Neurosurg 1994; 80:217–223.
43. Nihls DG, Flom RA, Carter LP, Spetzler RF. Multiple intracranial aneurysms: determining the site of rupture. J Neurosurg 1985;63(3):342–348.
44. Nakstad P, Nornes H, Hauge HN, Kjartansson O. Cerebral panangiography in spontaneous subarachnoid hemorrhage from intracranial aneurysms. Acta Radiol 1988;29(6):633–636.
45. Wirth FP, Laws ER, Piepgras D, Scott RM. Surgical management of incidental intracranial aneurysms. Neurosurgery 1983;12(5):507–511.
46. Wirth FP. Surgical management of incidental intracranial aneurysms. Clin Neurosurg 1986;33:125–135.
47. Perret G, Nishioka H. Report on the cooperative study of intracranial aneurysms and subarachnoid hemorrhage: IV. Cerebral angiography. An analysis of the diagnostic value and complications of carotid and vertebral angiography in 5,484 patients. J Neurosurg 1966;25:98–114.
48. Perret G, Nishioka H. Report on the cooperative study of intracranial aneurysms and subarachnoid hemorrhage: VI. Arteriovenous malformations. An analysis of 545 cases of craniocerebral arteriovenous malformations and fistulae reported to the cooperative study. J Neurosurg 1966;25:467–490.
49. Saveland H, Hillman J, Brandt L, Edner G, Jakobsson KE. Overall outcome in aneurysmal subarachnoid hemorrhage: a prospective study from neurosurgical units in Sweden during a 1-year period. J Neurosurg 1992;76:729–734.
50. Inagawa T. Effect of early operation on cerebral vasospasm. Surg Neurol 1990;33:239–246.
51. Locksley HB. Report on the cooperative study of intracranial aneurysms and subarachnoid hemorrhage: Section V, part II. Natural history of subarachnoid hemorrhage, intracranial aneurysms and arteriovenous malformations. J Neurosurg 1966; 25:321–368.
52. Locksley HB, Sahs AL, Knowler L. Report on the cooperative study of intracranial aneurysms and subarachnoid hemorrhage: II. General survey of cases in the central registry and characteristics of the sample population. J Neurosurg 1966; 24:922–932.
53. Amacher LA, Drake CG. Cerebral aneurysms in infancy, childhood and adolescence. Childs Brain 1975;1:72–80.
54. Cunha e Sa MJ, Stein BM, Solomon RA, McCormick PC. The treatment of associated intracranial aneurysms and arteriovenous malformations. J Neurosurg 1992;77:853–859.
55. Solomon RA, Onesti ST, Klebanoff L. Relationship between the timing of aneurysm surgery and the development of delayed cerebral ischemia. J Neurosurg 1991;75:56–61.
56. Nishioka H, Torner JC, Graf CJ, Kassall NF, Sahs AL, Goettler LC. Cooperative study of intracranial aneurysms and subarachnoid hemorrhage: a long-term prognostic study: III. Subarachnoid hemorrhage of undetermined etiology. Arch Neurol 1984;41:1147–1151.
57. Barrow DL, Prats AR. Infectious intracranial aneurysms: comparison of groups with and without endocarditis. Neurosurgery 1990;27:562–572.
58. Cross DT, Moran CJ, Brown AP, Oser AB, Goldberg DE, Diego J, Dacey RG. Endovascular treatment for epistaxis in a patient with tuberculosis and a giant petrous carotid pseudoaneurysm. AJNR; in press.
59. Raps EC, Rogers JD, Galetta SL, Solomon RA, Lennihan L, Klebanoff LM, Fink ME. The clinical spectrum of unruptured intracranial aneurysms. Arch Neurol 1993;50:265–268.
60. Derdeyn CP, Moran CJ, Cross DT, Grubb RL, Dacey RG. Intra-operative digital subtraction angiography: a review of 112 consecutive examinations. AJNR 1995;116:307–318.
61. Epstein F, Ransohoff J, Budzilovich GN. The clinical significance of the junctional dilatation of the posterior communicating artery. J Neurosurg 1970;33:529–531.
62. Fox JL, Baiz TC, Jakoby RK. Differentiation of aneurysm from infundibulum of the posterior communicating artery. J Neurosurg 1964;21:135–138.
63. Misra BK, Whittle IR, Steers AJ, Sellar RJ. De novo saccular aneurysms. Neurosurgery 1988;23:10–15.
64. Newton TH, Troost BT, Moseley I. Angiography of arteriovenous malformations and fistulas. In: Wilson CB, Stein BM, eds. Intracranial arteriovenous malformations. Baltimore: Williams & Wilkins, 1984:64–104.
65. Simard JM, Garcia-Bengochea F, Ballinger WE, Mickle JP, Quisling RG. Cavernous angioma: a review of 126 collected and 12 new clinical cases. Neurosurgery 1986;18:162–172.
66. Biller J, Toffol GJ, Shea JF, Fine M, Azar-Kia B. Cerebellar venous angiomas: a continuing controversy. Arch Neurol 1985;42:367–370.
67. Lussenhop AJ. Natural history of cerebral arteriovenous malformations. In: Wilson CB, Stein BM, eds. Intracranial arteriovenous malformations. Baltimore: Williams & Wilkins, 1984:12–23.
68. Mohr JP. Neurological manifestations and factors related to therapeutic decisions. In: Wilson CB, Stein BM, eds. Intracranial arteriovenous malformations. Baltimore: Williams & Wilkins, 1984:1–11.
69. Marks MP, Lane B, Steinberg GK, Chang PJ. Hemorrhage in intracerebral arteriovenous malformations: angiographic determinants. Radiology 1990;176:807–813.
70. Lasjaunias P, Chiu M, ter Brugge K, Tolia A, Hurth M, Bernstein M. Neurological manifestations of intracranial dural arteriovenous malformations. J Neurosurg 1986;64:724–730.
71. Gaston A, Chiras J, Bourbotte G, Leger JM, Guibert-Tranier F, Merland JJ. Meningeal arteriovenous fistulae draining into cortical veins: 31 cases. Neuroradiology 1984;11:161–177.
72. Marks MP, Lane B, Steinberg G, Chang P. Vascular characteristics of intracerebral arteriovenous malformations in patients with clinical steal. AJNR 1991;12:489–496.
73. Smith HJ, Strother CM, Kikuchi Y, Duff T, Ramirez L, Merless A, Toutant S. MR imaging in the management of supratentorial AVMs. Am J Roentgenol 1988;150:1143–1153.
74. Leblanc R, Levesque M, Comair Y, Ethier R. Magnetic resonance imaging of cerebral arteriovenous malformations. Neurosurgery 1987;21:15–20.
75. Kucharczyk W, Lemme-Pleghos L, Uske A, Brandt-Zawadzki M, Dooms G, Norman D. Intracranial vascular malformations: MR and CT imaging. Radiology 1985;156:383–389.
76. Cross DT. Interventional neuroradiology. Curr Opin Neurol Neurosurg 1993;6:891–899.
77. Ruggieri PM, Masaryk TJ, Ross JS, Modic MT. Intracranial magnetic resonance angiography. Cardiovasc Intervent Radiol 1992;15:71–81.
78. Lin JP, Kricheff II. Effect of masses on cerebral vessels. In: Newton TH, Potts DG, eds. Radiology of the skull and brain: Vol. 2. Angiography. Great Neck, NY: MediBooks, 1974: 1164–1170.
79. Launay M, Fredy D, Merland JJ, Bories J. Narrowing and occlusion of arteries by intracranial tumors: review of the literature and report of 25 cases. Neuroradiology 1977;14:117–126.
80. Peterson HO, Kieffer SA. Introduction to neuroradiology. Hagarstown, MD: Harper & Row, 1972:96–121.

81. Wickbom W. Tumor circulation. In: Newton TH, Potts DG, eds. Radiology of the skull and brain: Vol. 2. Angiography. Great Neck, NY: MediBooks, 1974:2257–2285.
82. Theron J, Bonafe A, Lasjaunias P, Clarisse J, Manelfe C. Tentorial meningiomas. J Neurosurg 1978;5:69–81.
83. De Vries EJ, Sekhar LN, Janecka IP, Schramm VL, Horton JA, Eibling DE. Elective resection of the internal carotid artery without reconstruction. Laryngoscope 1988;98:960–966.
84. Abramowicz J, Dion JE, Jensen ME, Lones M, Duckwiler GR, Vinuela F, Bentson JR. Angiographic diagnosis and management of head and neck schwannomas. AJNR 1991;12: 977–984.
85. McCormick PC, Bello JA, Post KD. Trigeminal schwannoma: surgical series of 14 cases with review of the literature. J Neurosurg 1988;69:850–860.
86. Carmody RF, Seeger JF, Horsley WW, Smith JR, Miller RW. Digital subtraction angiography of glomus tympanicum and jugulare tumors. AJNR 1983;4:263–265.
87. MacGillivray DC, Perry MO, Selfe RW, Nydick I. Carotid body tumor: atypical angiogram of a functional tumor. J Vasc Surg 1987;5:462–468.
88. Sinha PP, Aziz HI. Juvenile nasopharyngeal angiofibroma: a report of seven cases. Radiology 1978;127:501–503.
89. Shaffer K, Haughton V, Farley G, Friedman J. Pitfalls in the radiographic diagnosis of angiofibroma. Radiology 1978;127: 425–428.
90. Leeds NE, Elkin CM, Zimmerman RD. Gliomas of the brain. Sem Roentgenol 1984;19:27–43.
91. Joyce P, Bentson J, Takahashi M, Winter J, Wilson G, Byrd S. The accuracy of predicting histologic grades of supratentorial astrocytomas on the basis of computerized tomography and cerebral angiography. Neuroradiology 1978;16:346–348.
92. Hasuo K, Fukui M, Tamura S, Numaguchi Y, Kishikawa T, Uchino A, Kudo S, Kitamura K, Matsuura K. Gliomas with dural invasion: computed tomography and angiography. J Comput Tomogr 1988;12:100–107.
93. Jiddane M, Nicoli F, Diaz P, Bergvall U, Vincentelli F, Hassoun J, Salamon G. Intracranial malignant lymphoma: report of 30 cases and review of the literature. J Neurosurg 1986; 65:592–599.
94. Seeger JF, Burke DP, Knake JE, Gabrielsen TO. Computed tomographic and angiographic evaluation of hemangioblastomas. Radiology 1981;138:65–73.
95. Adair LB, Ropper AH, Davis KR. Cerebellar hemangioblastoma: computed tomographic, angiographic and clinical correlation in seven cases. J Comput Tomogr 1978;2:281–294.
96. Ho YS, Plets C, Goffin J, Dom R. Hemangioblastoma of the lateral ventricle. Surg Neurol 1990;33:407–412.
97. Davis JM, Zimmerman RA, Bilaniuk LT. Metastases to the central nervous system. Radiol Clin North Am 1982;20:417–435.
98. De Padua Bonatelli A. Carotid angiography in cerebral metastases. Acta Radiol Suppl 1976;347:193–197.
99. Mitomo M, Kawai R, Miura T, Kozuka T. Radiation necrosis of the brain and radiation-induced cerebrovasculopathy. Acta Radiol Suppl 1986;369:227–230.
100. Benson PJ, Sung JH. Cerebral aneurysms following radiotherapy for medulloblastoma. J Neurosurg 1989;70:545–550.
101. Montanera W, Chui M, Hudson A. Meningioma and occlusive vasculopathy: coexisting complications of past extracranial radiation. Surg Neurol 1985;24:35–39.
102. Hirata Y, Matsukado Y, Mihara Y, Kochi M, Sonoda H, Fukumura A. Occlusion of the internal carotid artery after radiation therapy for the chiasmal lesion. Acta Neurochir 1985;74: 141–147.
103. Kestle JR, Hoffman HJ, Mock AR. Moyamoya phenomenon after radiation for optic glioma. J Neurosurg 1993;79:32–35.
104. Bowen J, Paulsen CA. Stroke after pituitary irradiation. Stroke 1992;23:908–911.
105. Menawat SS, Dennis JW, Laneve LM, Frykberg ER. Are arteriograms necessary in penetrating zone II neck injuries? J Vasc Surg 1992;16:397–400.
106. Sclafani SJ, Panetta T, Goldstein AS, Phillips TF, Hotson G, Loh J, Shaftan GW. The management of arterial injuries caused by penetration of zone III of the neck. J Trauma 1985; 25:871–881.
107. O'Sullivan RM, Graeb DA, Nugent RA, Robertson WD, Lapointe JS. Carotid and vertebral artery trauma: clinical and angiographic features. Australas Radiol 1991;35(1):47–55.
108. Applegate LJ, Pritz MB, Pribram HF. Traumatic pseudoaneurysm of the cervical carotid artery: the value of arteriography. Neurosurgery 1990;26:312–315.
109. Halbach VV, Higashida RT, Dowd CF, Fraser KW, Smith TP, Teitelbaum GP, Wilson CB, Hieshima GB. Endovascular treatment of vertebral artery dissections and pseudoaneurysms. J Neurosurg 1993;79:183–191.
110. Aarabi B. Traumatic aneurysms of the brain due to high velocity missile wounds. Neurosurgery 1988;22:1056–1063.
111. Ghorayeb BY, Kopaniky DR, Yeakley JW. Massive posterior epistaxis: a manifestation of internal carotid injury at the skull base. Arch Otolaryngol Head Neck Surg 1988;114:1033–1037.
112. Haddad FS, Haddad GF, Taha J. Traumatic intracranial aneurysms caused by missiles: their presentation and management. Neurosurgery 1991;28:1–7.
113. Achram M, Rizk G, Haddad FS. Angiographic aspects of traumatic intracranial aneurysms following war injuries. Br J Radiol 1980;53:1144–1149.
114. Golueke P, Sclafani S, Phillips T, Goldstein A, Scalea T, Duncan A. Vertebral artery injury: diagnosis and management. J Trauma 1987;27(8):856–865.
115. Barrow DL, Spector RH, Braun IF, et al. Classification and treatment of spontaneous carotid-cavernous fistulas. J Neurosurg 1985;62:248–256.

14

Spinal Angiography

ROBERT W. HURST

Recent advances in radiologic imaging, especially the widespread use of magnetic resonance imaging (MRI), have made possible the noninvasive visualization of spinal cord anatomy and most common spinal pathologies. The investigation of many types of spinal vascular disease is still problematic with the use of noninvasive imaging methods, however, and angiography remains the best method for visualizing the spinal vasculature. Yet despite the limitations of noninvasive imaging and the significant numbers of patients afflicted with vascular disease involving the spine, spinal angiography is an infrequently performed procedure. This remains true even though the knowledge of spinal vascular anatomy, well described since the studies of Adamkiewicz and Kadyi in the late nineteenth century, has been extended by more recent neuroanatomic work, including that of Lazorthes and Thron.[1,2] In addition, improved application of this anatomic knowledge in the form of selective spinal angiographic techniques has long been available.[3–5]

The reasons for the infrequency of spinal angiography remain largely those delineated at the time of the last edition of this chapter.[6] Adequate spinal angiographic examination is often a technically demanding procedure requiring numerous selective catheterizations of segmental arteries. Despite advances in digital angiographic technology, magnification filming, and subtraction techniques, the visualization of small spinal vessels located within the vertebral canal is often suboptimal. The perception that the cord is particularly susceptible to damage from effects of contrast media remains prevalent from reports of accidental injury to the spinal cord during visceral angiography. These factors often discourage attempts to perform spinal angiography. Nevertheless, definite indications exist for the angiographic examination of spinal blood supply, and this examination is essential when specific information regarding the vascular supply of the spine, cord, or adjacent tissue is required.

Evaluation of possible spinal vascular malformations is the major indication for spinal angiographic examination. Less frequently the study is performed in the workup for suspected vascular spinal cord tumors such as hemangioblastomas. Management of vascular primary or metastatic lesions involving the vertebral bodies may also be aided by complete knowledge of the surrounding vasculature. However, spinal angiography usually provides little useful information in the evaluation of occlusive vascular disease involving the spine.

Early studies of aortography for visualization of the spinal vasculature suggested that there were significant risks of permanent neurologic damage associated with the procedure. However, paradoxically, selective injections of spinal vessels resulted in fewer reports of such complications. The availability of less toxic nonionic contrast material has further contributed to the safety of the procedure. Two recent series indicate that spinal angiography carries an incidence of approximately 2 to 4 percent associated neurologic complications, most of which will be transient. Although the exact risk remains in question, available data suggest that when performed by experienced personnel, the risks of spinal angiography are similar to those of cerebral angiography.[7–9]

Neurologic deficits referable to the spinal cord may occur during nonspinal angiographic studies. Spinal cord damage results most often during unintentional injection of a vessel that gives rise to a radiculomedullary contribution to the anterior spinal artery. The most important factor in preventing spinal cord injury during nonspinal angiography is thorough knowledge of the potential sources of spinal artery supply within the various regions of the spinal cord. Nevertheless, even with the utmost care, such injuries are not totally preventable. Angiographic evaluation of subclavian branches, including parathyroid angiography, bronchial angiography, and evaluation of retroperitoneal tumors, has the highest risk for potential spinal cord injury. Unintentional high-volume, high-pressure injection into a small spinal vessel may result in dissection of the vessel, thrombosis, and possible embolization to the spinal blood supply. Catheter wedging in vessels giving rise to spinal supply may also be a mechanism of injury. Most spinal cord injuries associated with angiography are believed to occur on an ischemic basis. The contribution of the direct effects of contrast material, particularly with the use of nonionic contrast agents, is less clear.

Any premonitory symptoms suggesting spinal cord dysfunction, including paresthesias or muscular spasms, should prompt immediate removal of the catheter from the involved vessel. Evidence of spinal cord damage necessitates immediate neurologic consultation. Therapeutic options are limited, although the use of high-dose steroids may be considered. Intravenous treatment with diazepam has been recommended for severe muscle spasms. Earlier recommendations regarding cerebral spinal fluid (CSF) exchange for saline via lumbar puncture remain of unknown efficacy.

Embryology

By 2 to 3 weeks of gestation, 31 pairs of segmental vessels originating from the dorsal aorta are growing along the developing nerve roots to reach the neural tube. The terminal capillary networks of these radicular vessels ramify on the surface of the neural tube, coalescing into two longitudinal vascular channels along the ventrolateral aspect of the developing spinal cord. By the second month of gestation, medial displacement and fusion of these paired channels has occurred to form the midline anterior spinal artery. Where fusion remains incomplete, the anterior spinal artery remains duplicated. Penetrating vessels, the sulcocommissural arteries, arise from the dorsal aspect of the anterior spinal artery to enter the cord in the midline.[10]

The terminal capillary networks of the radicular arteries also differentiate into a circumferential pial arterial plexus on the lateral and posterior surface of the cord. The two posterior spinal arteries develop as separate channels of longitudinal flow through the pial plexus. Although radially directed perforating vessels from the pial plexus later penetrate the cord, the anterior and posterior intrinsic arterial supplies to the cord remain functionally and anatomically separated.

Originally, both the anterior and posterior spinal arteries receive supply from each segmental vessel. In addition, the same segmental vessel initially supplies the cord segment, spinal root, dura, vertebral body, and paraspinal musculature at each level. Regression of most of the segmental branches to the cord itself, although not of the supply to extramedullary structures, is completed by about 4 months' gestation. By that time an average of six segmental branches of the radicular arteries, termed *radiculomedullary arteries,* remain to supply the entire anterior spinal artery axis. This regression is most pronounced in the thoracolumbar region, where usually only one radiculomedullary vessel remains to supply the anterior spinal artery. In contrast, 10 to 20 branches of the radicular arteries, termed *radiculopial arteries,* continue to supply the paired posterior spinal arteries.[11]

In the thoracolumbar region, the early segmental arterial arrangement persists as the intercostal and lumbar arteries. In the cervical and sacral regions, however, considerable modification of the segmental arrangement occurs. In the cervical region, extraspinal intersegmental anastomoses establish the vertebral artery as well as the ascending and deep cervical arteries. Any of these three longitudinal vessels can potentially provide supply to the cervical spinal cord.[12] In the sacral region, regression of the dorsal aorta to become the median sacral artery and acquisition of the sacral radicular arteries by the internal iliac vessels are prominent features. Like radicular arteries at other levels, sacral vessels accompany nerve roots and may participate in spinal vascular supply under both normal and pathologic conditions.

Normal Blood Supply

Embryologic events result in the formation of a relatively constant intrinsic cord angioarchitecture that directly supplies the neural tissue within the cord. The sulcocommissural arteries arising from the anterior spinal artery and the pial perforating vessels originating from the circumferential pial plexus represent the two components of the intrinsic cord supply. The superficial cord supply consists of the longitudinal anterior spinal artery and the two posterior spinal arteries. These three surface vessels of the cord receive major contributions from radicular branches at variable spinal levels. In the cervical and sacral regions the origins of the radicular arteries are also variable, whereas in the thoracolumbar region, the origin of radicular arteries from the intercostal and lumbar arteries is constant.

Radicular Arteries

Each spinal nerve root is accompanied by a radicular artery. In addition to supplying the root, the radicular vessel gives rise to a dural branch supplying the root sleeve and adjacent dura. Dural anastomoses, although normally sparse, connect adjacent levels both ventrally and dorsally. Each radicular artery, like its accompanying spinal root, demonstrates a characteristic obliquity in the frontal projection, the steepness of which depends on the spinal level.

The three types of radicular arteries are classified according to their contribution to the spinal cord. Simple radicular arteries give no supply to the spinal cord. Usually quite small, supplying only the nerve root and dura, they may be invisible angiographically. Radiculopial arteries supply the posterior spinal arteries, the major arterial channels of the pial plexus, but make no direct contribution to the anterior spinal artery axis. From 10 to 20 radiculopial arteries originate at variable levels of the spine. Radiculomedullary arteries are defined as those vessels that supply the anterior spinal artery, the major blood supply to the cord. Only 6 to 8 radiculomedullary arteries are present. Running along the ventral surface of the nerve root, each radiculomedullary artery bifurcates near the midline into ascending and descending branches that form the anterior spinal artery.[12]

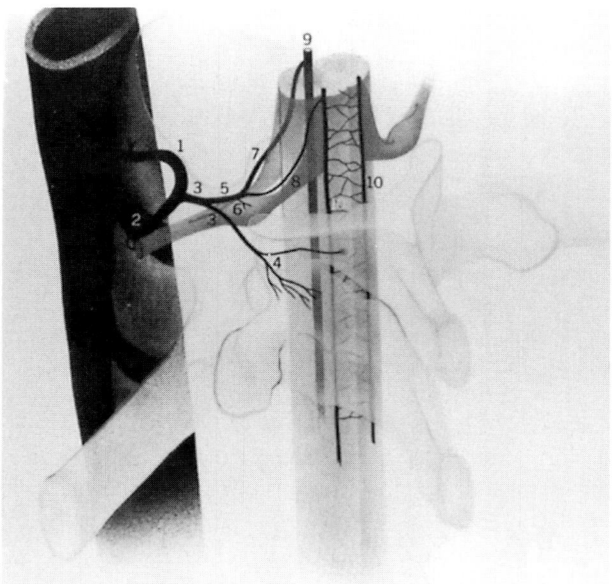

Figure 14-1. Superficial arteries of the spinal cord. *1,* Intercostal artery; *2,* ventral branch; *3,* dorsospinal branch; *4,* dorsal muscular branches; *5,* radicular branch; *6,* branch to dura and ganglion; *7,* radiomedullary branch; *8,* radiculopial branch; *9,* anterior spinal artery; *10,* posterior spinal artery. (From Doppman J, DiChiro G, Omaya A. Selective arteriography of the spinal cord. St. Louis: H Green, 1969. Used with permission.)

Superficial Spinal Cord Arterial System

Anterior Spinal Artery

Coursing in the anterior median fissure, the anterior spinal artery is a constant anatomic feature of the vascular supply to the cord. The longest artery in the body, the anterior spinal artery is usually continuous from the foramen magnum to the conus. This vessel provides the largest share of blood supply to the spinal cord at all levels (Fig. 14-1).

The anterior spinal artery actually represents an anastomotic channel between the ascending and descending branches of adjacent radiculomedullary arteries. It consists of contributions from radiculomedullary feeding vessels that characteristically divide into a larger caudal and smaller cranial branch. Paramedian Y-shaped bifurcations of the radiculomedullary arteries frequently occur at the junction with the anterior spinal artery. These intersections reflect incomplete fusion of the two primitive embryonic channels that formed the anterior spinal artery. The distinctive "hairpin" configuration, formed as the descending branch of the radiculomedullary artery joins the midline anterior spinal artery, is a characteristic feature to be identified on every spinal angiogram (Figs. 14-2 and 14-3).

Unlike most arteries, which narrow distally, the anterior spinal artery demonstrates a variable caliber throughout its length. The caliber of the anterior spinal artery at a particular level reflects not only its formation as a collection of longitudinal anastomoses and proximity to the nearest radiculomedullary feeding vessel, but also differences in the amount and metabolic demand of neural tissue at different cord levels. Because the metabolic demand of gray matter is three to four times that of white matter, those portions of the cord with relatively less gray matter require less blood flow. The amount of gray matter at each cord segment and its proportional requirement for blood supply therefore affects the size of the anterior spinal artery throughout the cord. In regions of smaller demand, smaller radicular contributions to the spinal arteries are present and the anterior spinal artery axis is often narrower, plexiform, or even interrupted.[2,3]

The most cranial extent of the anterior spinal artery originates from the intradural portion of one or both vertebral arteries. The most superior portion of the spinal cord is characterized by a relatively small proportion of gray to white matter. Accordingly, above C4, the anterior spinal artery is frequently diminutive or unfused, and occasionally discontinuous.

The lower four cervical and first thoracic segments constitute the cervical enlargement. This portion of the cord, in contrast to more superior levels, is characterized by a large proportion of gray matter that gives rise to the roots of the brachial plexus. The increased metabolic demand of the cervical enlargement ac-

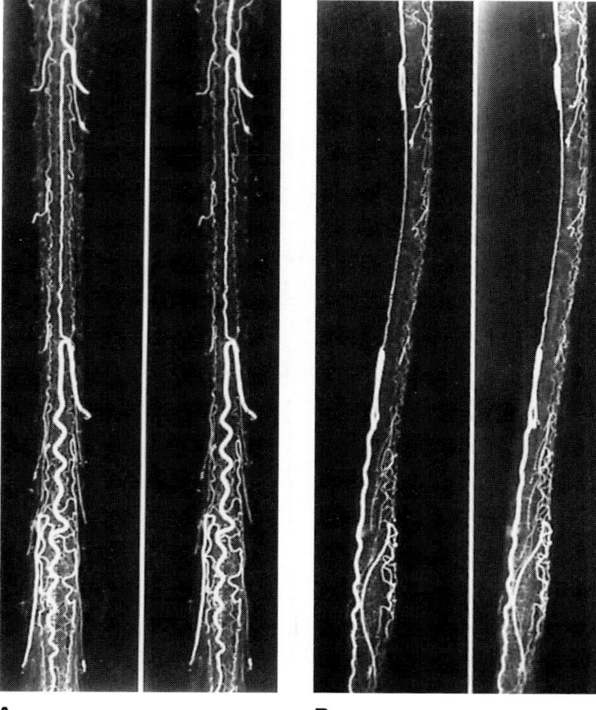

A B

Figure 14-2. Stereoscopic microradiology of an injected spinal cord in frontal (A) and lateral (B) projections. The continuity of the anterior spinal artery axis is well demonstrated despite its tortuosity at the lumbar level. Several sources of supply are clearly seen, as is the dorsolateral pial arterial plexus. Sulcocommissural perforators are visualized at the cervical and lumbar enlargements. Note that the supply to the filum terminale prolongs only the anterior spinal axis distal to the anastomosis with the posterior spinal arteries, and there is no contribution from the pial plexus. (From Lasjaunias P, Berenstein A. Surgical neuroangiography. Berlin: Springer-Verlag, 1990;3:55–60. Used with permission.)

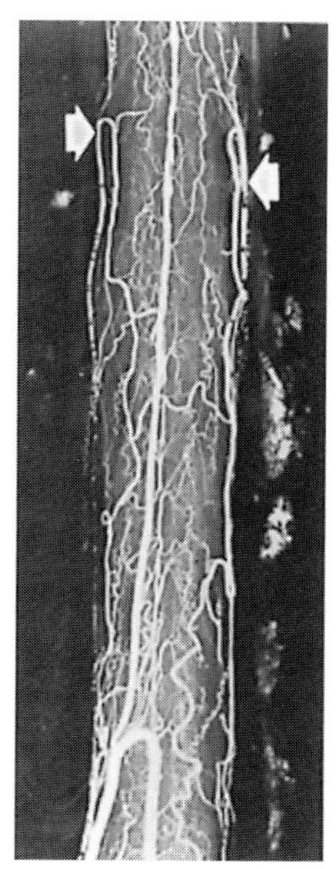

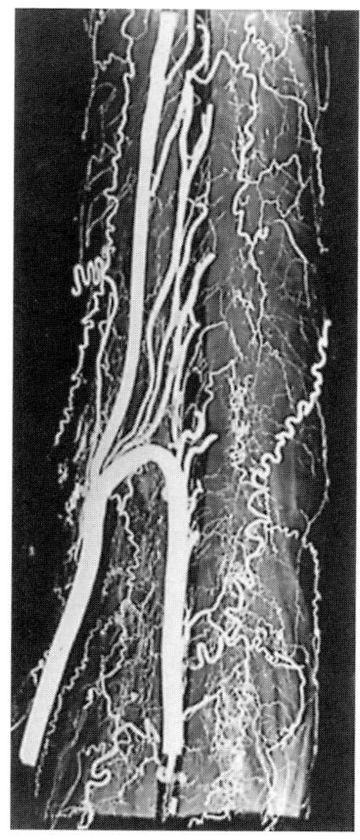

A B

Figure 14-3. Course and branching pattern of radiculomedullary and radiculopial arteries at thoracolumbar levels. (A) X-ray film in AP view. Radiculopial arteries of considerable size (*arrows*) continue as ascending or sharply descending branches of posterior spinal arteries. Numerous interconnections of the superficial pial arterial plexus form a densely meshed network. (B) Microangiogram of an anterior frontal section. Branching of radiculomedullary artery occurs just off the midline with the smaller ascending branch gradually approaching the anterior median fissure. The larger descending branch demonstrates the characteristic midline hairpin turn. Sulcocommissural arteries penetrate the anterior median fissure. (From Thron A. Vascular anatomy of the spinal cord. Vienna: Springer-Verlag, 1988:11–37. Used with permission.)

counts for the large size of the anterior spinal artery in this region.

The thoracic cord between T2 and T9, like upper cervical levels, is characterized by a relatively narrow anterior spinal artery, reflecting the paucity of gray matter throughout this region. The anterior spinal artery may even be occasionally interrupted in this region.

The lumbosacral region resembles the cervical enlargement because of the increased amount of gray matter related to lower extremity musculature. The relatively large size of the anterior spinal artery in the lumbosacral region corresponds to the increased demand at this level. Approximately 1 to 2 cm cephalad to the conus, the anterior spinal artery receives two constant circumferential contributions from the posterior spinal arteries. This anastomotic arcade at the conus level is the only cord location where the anterior spinal artery routinely receives well-developed anastomoses from the posterior spinal arteries.

The artery of the filum terminale runs caudally as the continuation of the anterior spinal artery at the conus medullaris. Coursing along the anterior aspect of the filum terminale, the caliber of this vessel rapidly diminishes caudally unless enlarged to supply pathologic processes in the region.

Regional Supply to the Anterior Spinal Artery

The best clinical evaluation of the normal vascular anatomy of the spine is based on an understanding of three major regions of supply to the anterior spinal artery axis: the cervicothoracic, the midthoracic, and the

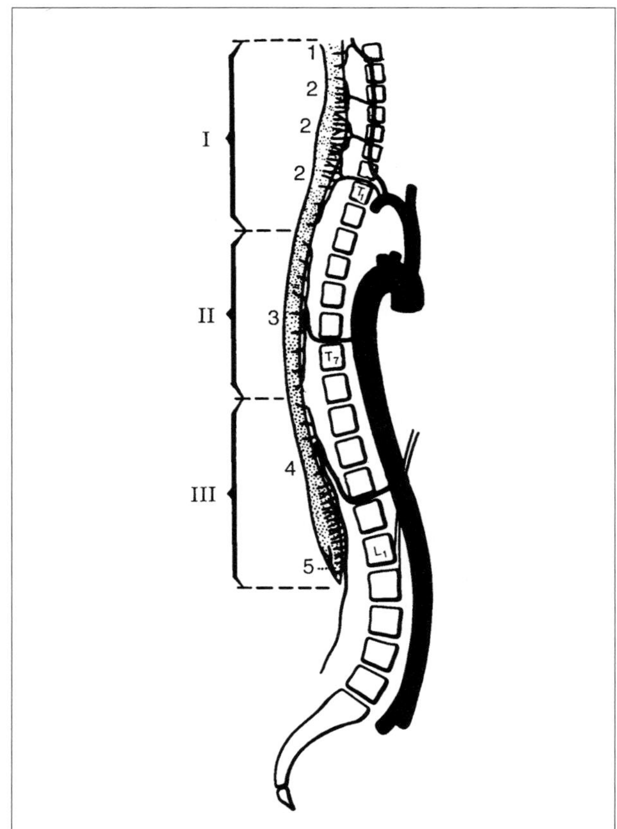

Figure 14-4. Diagram of the arterial regions of the spinal cord. *I,* Superior or cervicothoracic region; *II,* intermediate or midthoracic region; *III,* lower or thoracolumbar region. Also shown are *1,* anterior spinal artery; *2,* artery of the spinal enlargement (variable); *3,* posterior spinal artery; *4,* artery of the lumbar enlargement (artery of Adamkiewicz); *5,* anastomotic loop of the conus medullaris with continuation of the anterior spinal artery as the artery of the filum terminale. (From Lazorthes G, et al. Arterial vascularization of the spinal cord. J Neurosurg 1971;35:253–262. Used with permission.)

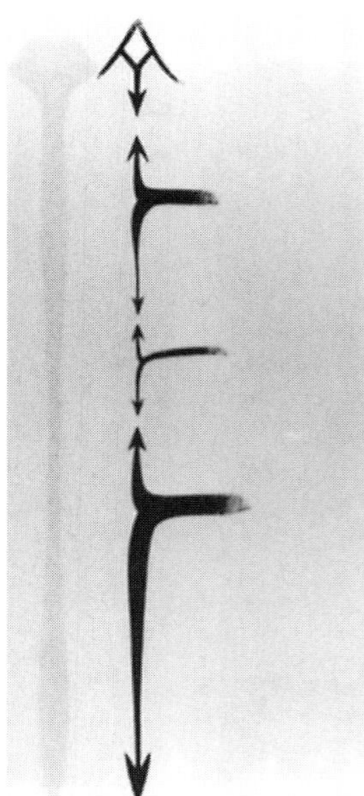

Figure 14-5. Bidirectional flow may occur along the anterior spinal artery. Note *small arrows* in the critical midthoracic region. (From Doppman J, DiChiro G, Omaya A. Selective arteriography of the spinal cord. St. Louis: H Green, 1969. Used with permission.)

thoracolumbar regions (Fig. 14-4).[1] Radiculopial supply to the less extensive posterior spinal artery territories is relatively uniform throughout the spine, with less variation from one region to another.

The margins of each of the three regions represent areas of relatively little net flow as opposing flows from the adjacent ascending and descending limbs of the anterior spinal artery axis encounter one another. This results in hemodynamic watershed areas at the borders of each region with relative isolation of the anterior spinal artery supply of each region from its neighbor. Although the anatomic continuity of the anterior spinal artery is usually maintained from one region to another throughout the length of the spinal cord, provision of adequate collateral flow is not always possible, particularly in the midthoracic region, where this vessel may be relatively small (Fig. 14-5). The spinal cord is therefore vulnerable to infarction in the event of compromise of a radiculomedullary feeding vessel.[13]

The cervicothoracic region extends from the foramen magnum caudally to include the first two thoracic segments. After originating intracranially, the anterior spinal artery usually receives an additional radiculomedullary branch from the vertebral artery at approximately the C3 level. The artery of the cervical enlargement, a relatively constant radiculomedullary vessel, usually accompanies the C6 nerve root after arising from the deep cervical artery. An additional radiculomedullary contribution from either the costocervical trunk or superior intercostal artery frequently joins the anterior spinal artery at lower cervical levels. Less often, a radiculomedullary feeding vessel may arise from the ascending cervical artery (Figs. 14-6 and 14-7).

In summary, the cervicothoracic region is characterized by multiple origins of potential spinal cord blood supply, which may provide an extensive network of extraspinal collaterals and anastomoses if called on to do so. Supply may originate from the vertebral artery as well as from branches of the costocervical or thyrocer-

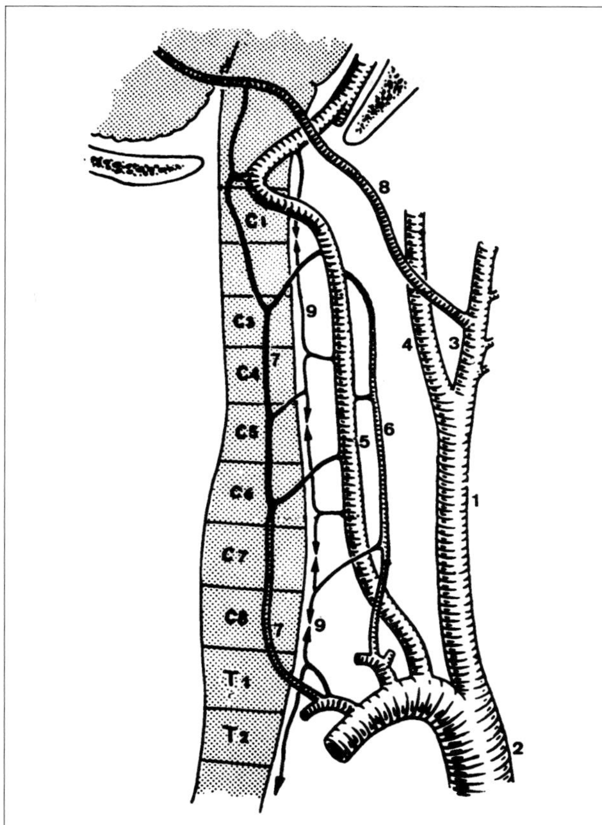

Figure 14-6. Diagram of vascularization and collateral pathways of the cervical spinal cord. *1,* Common carotid artery; *2,* innominate artery; *3,* external carotid artery; *4,* internal carotid artery; *5,* vertebral artery; *6,* ascending cervical artery; *7,* deep cervical artery; *8,* occipital artery; *9,* anterior spinal artery. Frequent anastomoses may occur between the vertebral (*5*), ascending cervical (*6*), deep cervical (*7*), and occipital arteries in the suboccipital area. (From Lazorthes G, et al. Arterial vascularization of the spinal cord. J Neurosurg 1971;35:253–262. Used with permission.)

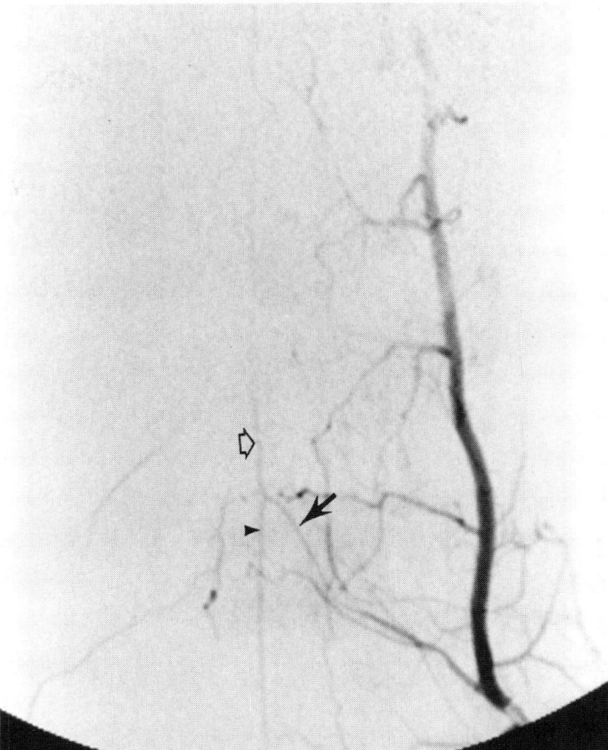

Figure 14-7. At the C6 level, the anterior spinal artery receives a frequent contribution from the deep cervical artery via the artery of the cervical enlargement (*arrow*). Note the midline hairpin loop and filling of both ascending (*open arrow*) and descending (*arrowhead*) branches of the anterior spinal artery. (Photo courtesy of A. Berenstein, M.D.)

vical trunks. The presence of multiple large radicular feeders to the anterior spinal artery in the region of the cervical enlargement is constant despite the potentially variable origins of these feeding vessels.

The midthoracic region, consisting of the next six or seven cord segments, with its lower metabolic demand, demonstrates a correspondingly small blood supply. Often only one radiculomedullary artery supplies the anterior spinal artery axis in this region, usually arising at the T4 or T5 level. The intercostal arteries represent the most likely source of both radiculomedullary and radiculopial supply throughout the thoracic cord. The segmental arrangement of the intercostal arteries provides relative uniformity for potential origins of midthoracic cord supply.

The inferior or thoracolumbar region extends from the T8 segment to the conus medullaris. The lumbar enlargement, encompassing spinal segments L3 through L5, is characterized by a relatively rich blood supply, usually provided by a single large radiculomedullary artery. This vessel, described by Adamkiewicz as the "arteria radicularis anterior magna," is also known as the *artery of the lumbar enlargement* or the *artery of Adamkiewicz* (Fig. 14-8).[13a] In 75 percent of cases, the artery of the lumbar enlargement enters the spinal canal at a level from T9 through T12, most commonly on the left, and in 10 percent of cases, the vessel accompanies the first or second lumbar nerves (Fig. 14-9). The artery has a high origin in 15 percent of cases, entering at levels from T5 through T8. When the higher origin is present, there is often an additional artery at a lower level, called the *artery of the conus medullaris.* The lumbar arteries usually arise from separate origins bilaterally from the aorta, but may, particularly at lower levels, arise bilaterally from a common midline lumbar trunk.

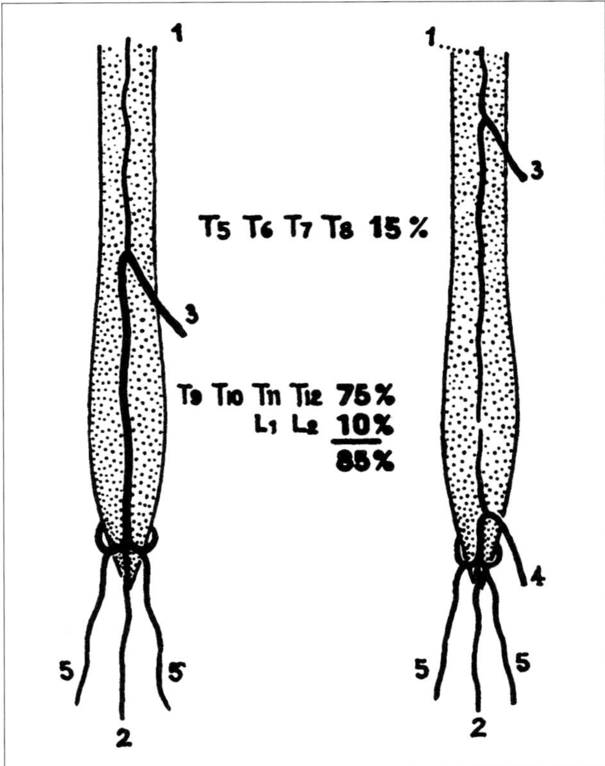

Figure 14-8. Variations in the location of the artery of the lumbar enlargement. *1,* Ascending branch of the anterior spinal artery; *2,* artery of the filum terminale; *3* and *4,* artery of the lumbar enlargement; *5,* sacral arteries. Percentages refer to the occurrence of the artery of the lumbar enlargement with specific spinal nerves in the vertebral canal. Note the anastomotic loop of the conus medullaris. (From Lazorthes G, et al. Arterial vascularization of the spinal cord. J Neurosurg 1971;35:253–262. Used with permission.)

Sacral arteries originate from the hypogastric artery or less frequently from the median sacral artery to accompany the sacral roots. Only uncommonly do the sacral arteries supply the anterior spinal artery directly, although they may give collateral supply via the anastomotic arcade of the conus medullaris.

Pial Plexus and Posterior Spinal Arteries

The surface of the spinal cord is covered by an extensive circumferential pial arterial plexus. The paired posterior spinal arteries represent the major channels of blood supply to the circumferential pial plexus, although the ventrolateral portions of the plexus receive contributions from the anterior spinal artery. The posterior spinal arteries run in parallel on the dorsal cord surface adjacent to the origins of the dorsal roots, with the most cephalad supply originating from the intradural vertebral arteries. Ten to 20 radiculopial arteries contribute to the posterior spinal arteries at individually variable levels throughout the spine. Like the radiculomedullary-anterior spinal artery junctions, the radiculopial arteries usually give rise to a larger descending contribution to the posterior spinal artery, forming a characteristic hairpin configuration. Always located off the midline, these distinctive junctions on the dorsal cord surface must be differentiated from the ventral paramedian bifurcations of the radiculomedullary arteries that form the anterior spinal artery. Usually smaller than the anterior spinal artery, the posterior spinal arteries may vary in caliber along the length of the cord.

Transverse connections across the dorsal cord surface provide intercommunication between the paired posterior spinal arteries, often permitting dominance of one or the other channel. In contrast, the pial plexus branches over the lateral cord surface are too attenuated to function reliably as anastomoses between the territories supplied by the anterior and posterior spinal arteries. The posterior spinal arteries terminate at the conus, and encircle the cord to join the anterior spinal artery.

Intrinsic Spinal Cord Supply

The arteries directly supplying the neural tissue of the spinal cord are divided into two distinct groups generally reflecting their origin from either the anterior or posterior spinal arteries (Fig. 14-10). The sulcocommissural arteries, a centrally directed system, originate from the anterior spinal artery. A separate system of innumerable small centripetally directed arteries, the rami perforantes, arises from the pial plexus to supply the periphery of the cord. The rami perforantes receive their supply mainly via the posterior spinal arteries, with contributions along the ventrolateral aspect from the anterior spinal artery.

The sulcocommissural arteries course in the anterior median fissure before turning left or right to enter the cord in the region of the anterior white commissure to give lateralized supply to the central portion of the cord (Fig. 14-11). Dense capillary networks from the sulcocommissural arteries supply the gray matter of the anterior, intermediate, and basal dorsal horns. Like the size of the anterior spinal artery, the density of sulcocommissural arteries has been related to metabolic demand, and therefore to the relative amounts of gray matter at different cord levels.

The second component of intrinsic cord supply consists of the radially directed rami perforantes, which supply the peripheral structures of the cord, including the posterior columns and the apices of the dorsal

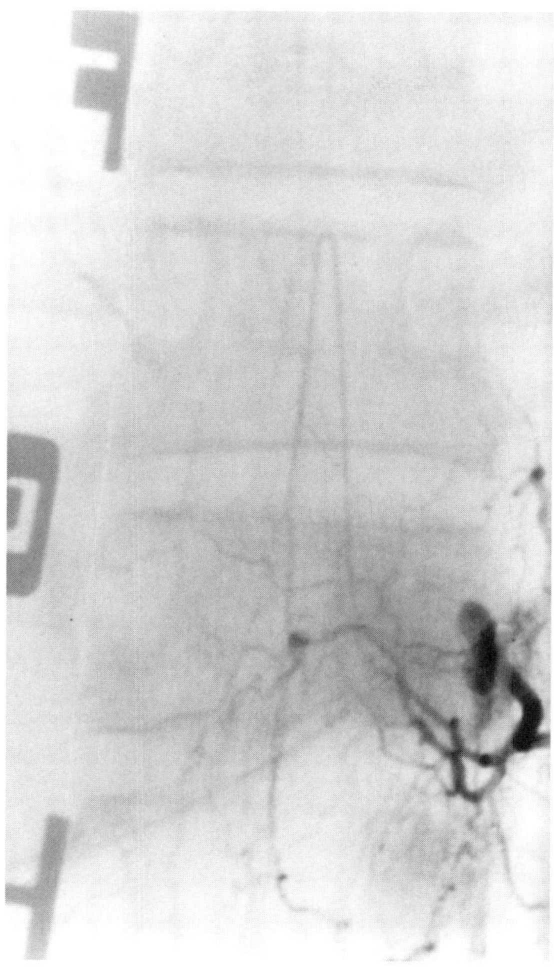

A

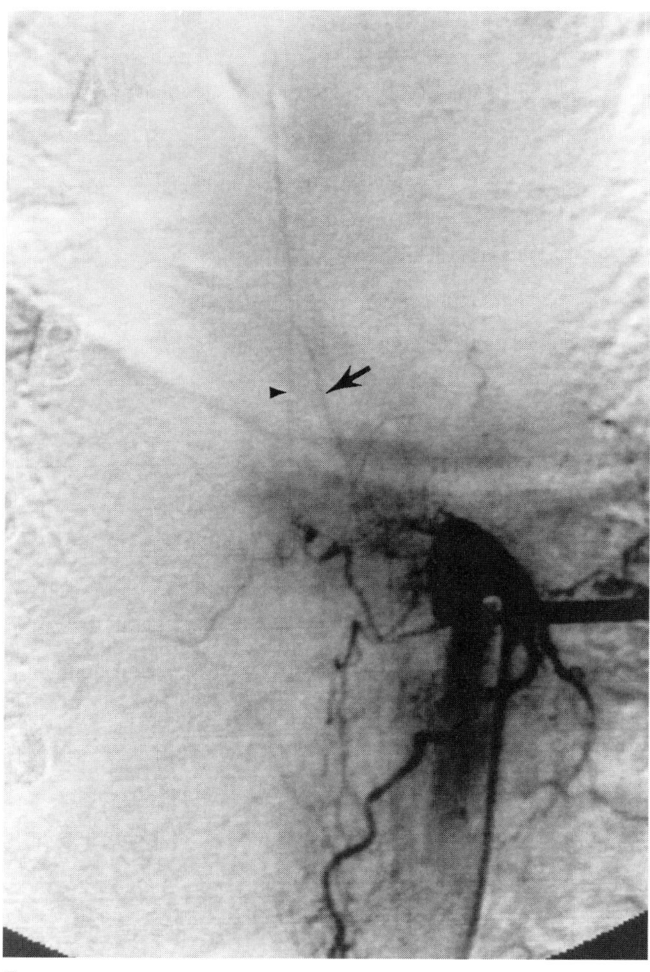

B

Figure 14-9. Injection of left T11 (A) and left T9 (B) intercostal artery in two different patients demonstrates the radiculomedullary contribution to the anterior spinal artery, the artery of Adamkiewicz (*arrow*, B). Note the midline hairpin loop with ascending and descending (*arrowhead*, B) limbs of the anterior spinal artery.

horns. A minimal amount of gray matter is supplied by the rami perforantes in comparison to that supplied by the sulcocommissural arteries.

The paucity of anastomoses between the anterior and posterior spinal artery territories results in a functional separation of the two intrinsic cord vascular distributions. Consequently, the anterior and central 60 to 80 percent of the cord, including most of the gray matter structures, is supplied exclusively by the anterior spinal artery (Fig. 14-12). The posterior columns and the majority of the cord periphery are supplied by perforating vessels originating from the posterior spinal arteries. A potential watershed area may arise at the gray–white matter junction of the cord where the centrifugal flow from the larger sulcocommissural artery distribution meets the centripetally directed flow from the rami perforantes.

Vertebral Supply

In addition to evaluating supply to the spinal cord, spinal angiography is often concerned with evaluating blood supply to the vertebrae. The angioarchitecture of the blood supply to each vertebra demonstrates similarities at all levels of the spine, with supply to each half usually originating from the ipsilateral side. Small branches perforate the anterior surface of the vertebral body deep to the anterior longitudinal ligament. Vessels in the epidural space supply both the anterior and posterior bony walls of the neural canal. At each verte-

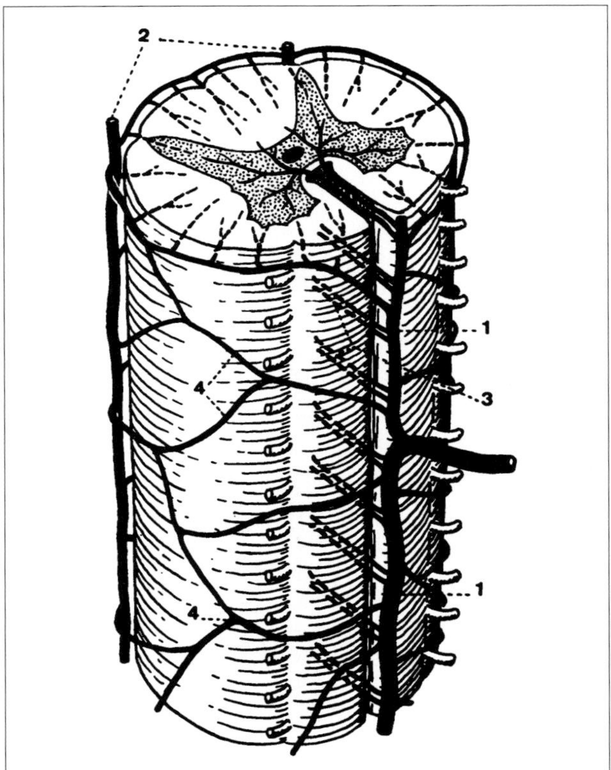

Figure 14-10. Superficial and intrinsic arteries of the spinal cord. *1,* Anterior spinal artery; *2,* posterior spinal arteries; *3,* sulcocommissural arteries; *4,* circumferential pial arterial plexus. (From Lazorthes G, et al. Arterial vascularization of the spinal cord. J Neurosurg 1971;35:253–262. Used with permission.)

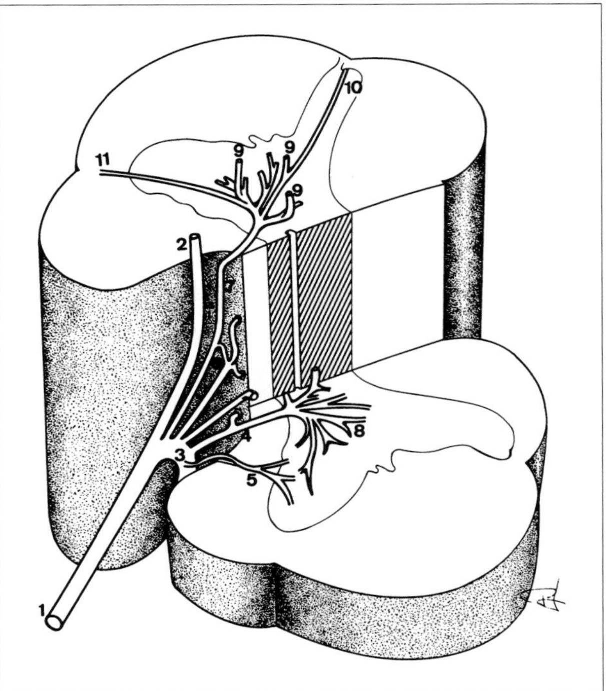

Figure 14-11. Sulcocommissural branches (*4,5,6,7*) of the descending branch of the anterior spinal artery (*3*) penetrate the cord in the anterior median fissure. Both the descending and ascending (*2*) branches of the anterior spinal artery are supplied by a radiculomedullary artery (*1*). The axial (*8,10,11*) and longitudinal (*9*) distribution of the sulcocommissural arteries is shown. (From Lasjaunias P, Berenstein A. Surgical neuroangiography. Berlin: Springer-Verlag, 1990;3:55–60. Used with permission.)

bral level, branches run posteriorly to supply the laminae, facets, and spinous processes. The origin of supply to the various territories of each vertebra varies with the different regions of the spine. In the cervical area, the ascending cervical, vertebral, and deep cervical arteries may each contribute vertebral supply. In the sacral spine, the lateral sacral arteries are the source of the majority of bony spinal supply. Throughout the thoracic and lumbar spine, however, the segmental arrangement persists, with each hemivertebrae receiving supply via an intercostal or lumbar artery, respectively (Fig. 14-13).

Branching at the lateral aspects of the neural foramina, each intercostal artery gives rise to a ventral branch to the transverse process and rib and a dorsospinal branch. From the dorsospinal branch the radicular artery or spinal branch enters the neural foramen. The radicular vessel provides branches to the anterior and posterior bony walls of the neural canal within the epidural space, and radiculomedullary and radiculopial vessels also originate at variable levels from the radicular branches. Intersegmental anastomoses along the anterolateral aspect of the vertebral body, adjacent to the transverse process, and within the neural canal connect each segmental vessel to neighboring levels (Figs. 14-14 and 14-15).[14,15]

Veins

The intrinsic veins of the spinal cord collect blood in a radially symmetric pattern. In certain regions, a slight dominance of flow toward the ventral or dorsal surface of the cord may be present, but the relatively equal division of venous drainage contrasts sharply with the significant differences in size of the anterior and posterior arterial distributions. Upon reaching the surface of the cord, venous blood collects into the longitudinal anterior and posterior spinal veins (Fig. 14-16).[16]

Multiple channels connect the anterior and posterior spinal venous systems. Superficial anastomoses

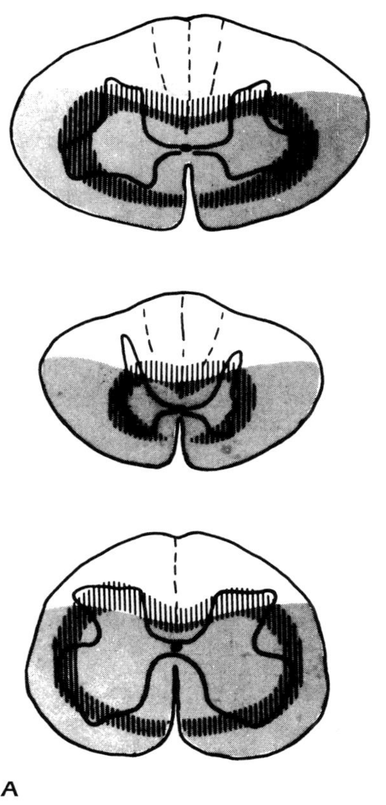

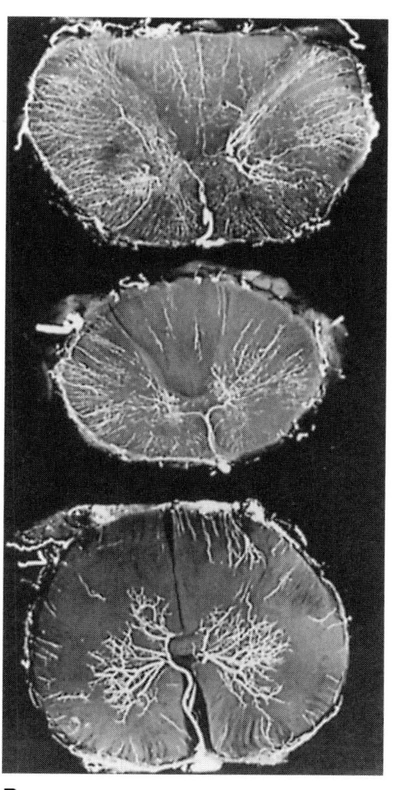

Figure 14-12. Territory of the supply to the intrinsic arterial systems of the spinal cord: (A) diagrams and (B) microangiograms of the cervical, thoracic, and lumbar cord segments. The gray zone corresponds to the area supplied by the anterior spinal artery (about two-thirds of the entire cross-sectional area), and the dorsal white zone is supplied by branches of the posterior spinal arteries. The cross-sectional area of the sulcocommissural branches of the anterior spinal arteries corresponds approximately to the volume and relative amount of gray matter, which is different at various levels. (From Thron A. Vascular anatomy of the spinal cord. Vienna: Springer-Verlag, 1988:11–37. Used with permission.)

Figure 14-13. Axial view of injected vertebra of a newborn. Note the radicular branches entering the spinal canal (*arrows*) as well as perforating branches to the dorsal and ventral aspects of the vertebral body. (From Lasjaunias P, Berenstein A. Surgical neuroangiography. Berlin: Springer-Verlag, 1990;3:55–60. Used with permission.)

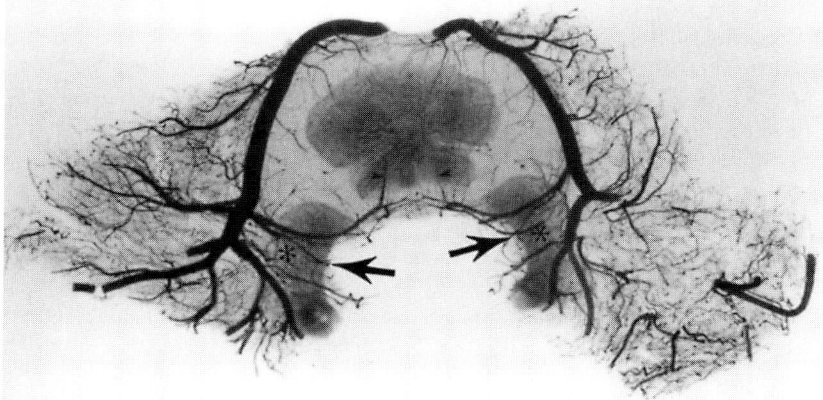

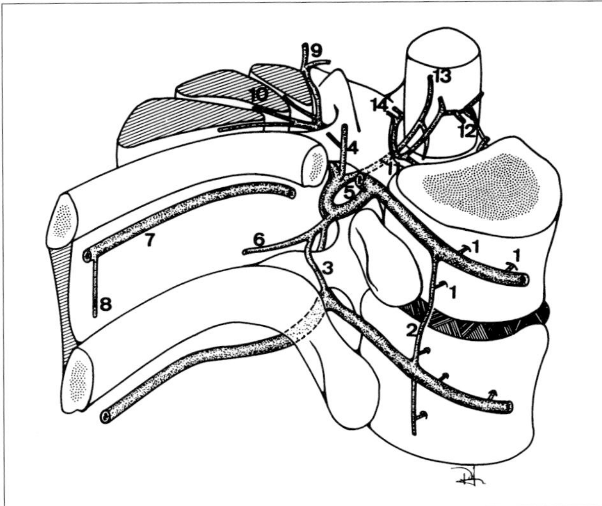

Figure 14-14. Diagram of the intercostal arterial system. *1,* Arteries to the vertebral body; *2,* anterolateral anastomotic artery; *3* and *4,* pretransverse anastomoses; *5,* dorsospinal artery; *6* and *8,* ventral muscular branches; *7,* ventral branch; *9* and *10,* dorsal muscular branches; *11,* radicular artery; *12* and *14,* epidural anastomoses; *13,* dural branch. (From Lasjaunias P, Berenstein A. Surgical neuroangiography. Berlin: Springer-Verlag, 1990;3:55–60. Used with permission.)

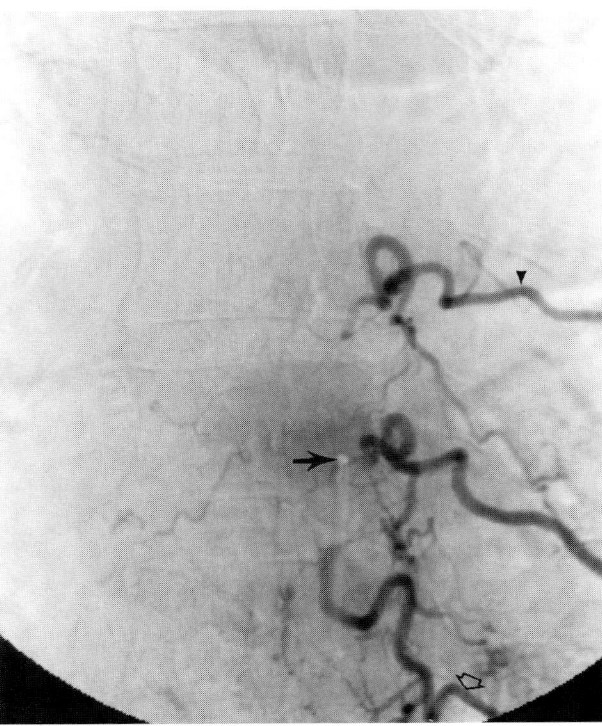

Figure 14-15. AP injection of left T11 intercostal artery (*arrow* at catheter tip) also fills T10 (*arrowhead*) and T12 (*open arrow*) intercostal arteries via intersegmental collaterals.

provide collateral routes along the lateral aspects of the cord, and transmedullary anastomotic veins connect the anterior and posterior spinal veins directly through the substance of the spinal cord. Transmedullary anastomoses are most prominent in the cervical and cervicothoracic regions, where the cord is most mobile. It is believed that these channels aid in equalizing pressure and flow between the anterior and posterior venous reservoirs. Should flexion or extension of the spine compress either venous tract, immediate diversion of flow into the other will occur.[12]

At multiple levels radicular veins drain the anterior and posterior spinal veins into the epidural venous plexus. A section of narrowing may be observed involving the transdural segment of the radicular vein. Although controversial, this region has received much attention as an antireflux mechanism protecting the pial veins of the cord from pressure alterations incident to respiration, postural changes, and movement.

Angiographic Technique

As with all angiographic examinations, the spinal angiogram must be tailored to each individual patient based on the region of the spine affected as well as the suspected pathologic process. Preangiographic imaging studies are invaluable for planning specific areas to be evaluated.

Local anesthesia is usually preferred to general anesthesia for diagnostic spinal angiography. This permits the close neurologic monitoring of the patient, which is essential throughout the study. For children or patients unable to remain still, general anesthesia may be necessary. If general anesthesia is used or embolization is contemplated, monitoring of somatosensory evoked potentials is necessary to disclose any evidence of neurologic dysfunction at the earliest possible time.

At the time of initial positioning, radiopaque letter markers are placed on the patient's back just lateral to the spine. Scout films are taken to correlate each marker with the corresponding vertebral level and to ensure that no relevant anatomy is obscured by the markers.

The use of nonionic contrast material in neuroangiography has been associated with a decreased incidence of neurologic complications. The potentially devastating effects of neurologic damage to the spinal cord dictate that nonionic contrast material should be used for spinal angiography.

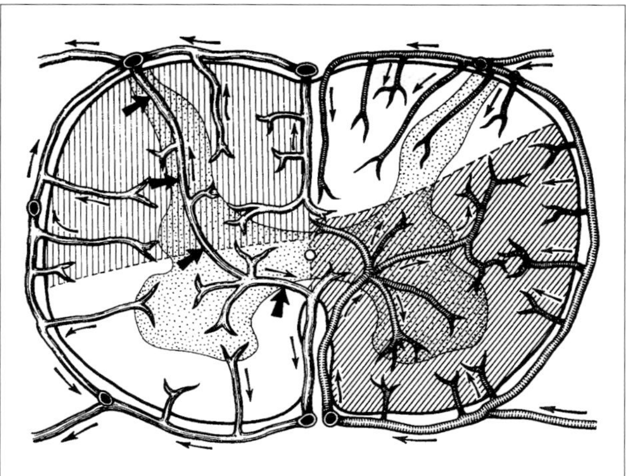

Figure 14-16. Cross-sectional diagram of the cord showing arterial supply (*right side* of diagram) and venous drainage (*left side* of diagram). Note the relatively equal size of the areas drained by the anterior and posterior pial veins (*left cross-hatched area*) and the transmedullary venous anastomosis (*large arrows*). (From Djindjian R, Hurth M, Houdart R. Angiography of the spinal cord. Baltimore: University Park Press, 1970. Used with permission.)

Spinal angiography may be performed using either cut film or high-quality digital subtraction angiography. The films are coned side to side, and magnification of the area of interest is routinely used.

An aortogram is not usually performed except for an initial overview of spinal intradural arteriovenous malformations (AVMs) or when selective catheterization of intercostal or lumbar vessels is not possible. Global aortic injections require increased contrast dosage and usually give relatively poor opacification of spinal vasculature. Safety considerations also dictate preferential use of selective injections for evaluating spinal feeding vessels.[4] A typical contrast injection for an intercostal artery is 2 ml per second for a total volume of 4 ml. Initial insertion of a sheath into the femoral artery facilitates catheter exchanges and permits more precise control of the catheter, particularly in the patient with atherosclerotic disease of the iliac arteries and aorta.

Filming is done at a rate of at least two films per second for the first 4 seconds. Filming is continued for at least 22 seconds to identify spinal veins, which normally are visualized by 14 to 18 seconds. The importance of dynamic information concerning spinal cord blood flow is often equivalent to that of anatomic findings in spinal angiography. Evaluation of the normal time of appearance as well as anatomy of the spinal veins should be sought on each injection and is essential to exclude venous hypertension secondary to pathologic processes such as spinal dural arteriovenous fistula (AVF).

Great attention to patient positioning is necessary to aid in the identification of the midline anterior spinal axis and to differentiate it from the more laterally placed posterior spinal supply. Apnea is essential during all filming, and high-quality subtracted films are necessary for the visualization of small spinal vessels. Glucagon (1 mg IV) may minimize bowel gas motion, which can cause subtraction artifacts.

With the exception of the cervical spine, lateral views may not be routinely performed. In specific cases, including spinal AVMs, however, lateral or oblique views are obtained as needed.

General protocols for the examination of various regions of the spine are followed to ensure complete evaluation of the spinal region in question. The three general regions considered are based on the sources of anterior spinal artery supply and include the cervicothoracic, the midthoracic, and the thoracolumbar (which may require evaluation of the sacral supply). Identification of radiculomedullary and radiculopial arteries supplying the spinal cord is an important goal regardless of the region under evaluation. This requires selective angiographic examination of all arteries that may supply the spinal cord.[1]

The origin of blood supply to the cervicothoracic region, from the foramen magnum to T2, encompasses the most variation. Because cervical spinal supply may arise from the vertebral arteries at any level, proximal vertebral artery injection is performed bilaterally with visualization to the level of the vertebrobasilar junction. The ascending cervical arteries, the deep cervical arteries, and the superior intercostals are also frequent contributors to spinal supply, and visualization of each may be required. Less frequently, supply to lesions of the cervical spine may arise from external carotid branches, including the ascending pharyngeal or occipital artery. Catheter selection for the vessels involved in cervicothoracic supply is based on well-known criteria for brachiocephalic artery catheterization.

The midthoracic spine from T2 through T7 represents the most poorly vascularized reigon of the cord. Most often only a single contribution to the anterior spinal axis is identified in this region, usually at T4 or T5. Evaluation of the region often requires selective injection of each intercostal artery supplying the region. Each intercostal artery is identified by the vertebral body supplied by the artery and the rib under which the artery courses. Careful accounting of each level injected is mandatory and is facilitated by the use of radiopaque letter markers, as noted above. Because

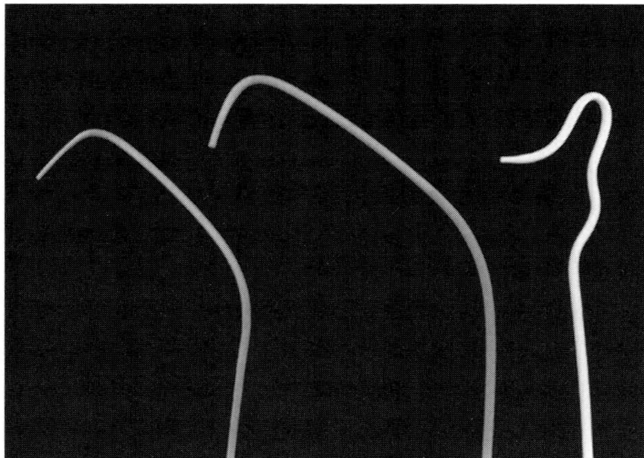

Figure 14-17. HS-1, HS-2, and Michelsson (*left to right*) catheters are most useful for selective catheterization of the lumbar and intercostal arteries.

the angulation of the intercostal origin from the aorta varies from thoracic to lumbar levels, several catheters may be useful. Frequently used catheters include HS-1 and HS-2 (Cook, Inc.), Cobra-1 (USCI), and Michelsson catheters (Fig. 14-17). Care is taken to prevent catheter wedging or spasm with resulting stagnation of flow in these small arteries. One to 2 ml per second for a total of 2 to 4 ml is usually injected into each intercostal artery.

The ostia of the intercostal arteries bear a relatively constant relationship to the pedicles of the vertebral bodies in each individual patient, although this relationship may vary among patients. It is most important to identify the relationship between the first intercostal artery catheterized and the adjacent vertebral body pedicle. After the most inferior vessel is injected, the catheter is gently withdrawn from the vessel and advanced cephalad until the next superior intercostal ostium is entered. The ostium of the adjacent intercostal artery is usually found to have a similar relationship to its vertebral pedicle as the vessel below. Several levels are sequentially evaluated in this fashion, and the catheter is then twisted slightly to enter the contralateral intercostal artery. After injection, the catheter is removed from the ostium and withdrawn inferiorly until the next inferior vessel is identified. This sequential evaluation of each level, first on one side, then the other, minimizes failing to evaluate a level in the area of interest. The use of live subtraction fluoroscopy to maintain a mask of the previously injected vessel aids in both keeping the proper catheter orientation and in identifying the ostium-pedicle relationship for the next vessel. The presence of two or three intercostals supplied by a single trunk is common and can explain the apparent absence of ostia at adjacent levels. More superior intercostal arteries tend to originate more closely together than vessels in the lower thoracic region. At the T5 or T6 levels, there is frequently a right-sided common intercostal-brachial trunk supplying the cord.

The third major region considered is the thoracolumbar region, located below the T8 level. The angioarchitecture of the superior portion of the thoracolumbar region involves intercostal arteries, and its evaluation is identical to that of the midthoracic region. Consequently, catheters with shapes similar to the HS-1 or Cobra are most useful. Careful catheter manipulation remains a paramount consideration, particularly in the face of atherosclerotic disease of the aorta. Identification of all vessels supplying the spinal axis, including the artery of the lumbar enlargement, is essential. The sequential procedure for catheterization of intercostal arteries noted above is also used in lumbar vessels. Bilateral lower lumbar vessels often arise from a single midline vessel and require a more medial catheter tip position (Fig. 14-18). Sacral supply may contribute to pathologic processes involving the lower spine and cord, making evaluation of medial and lateral sacral arteries necessary. The median sacral artery originates from the aortic bifurcation and may give rise to L5 lumbar arteries as well as to collaterals supplying spinal pathology. The origin of the lateral

Figure 14-18. AP injection of a common midline aortic trunk at the L4 level fills lumbar arteries bilaterally.

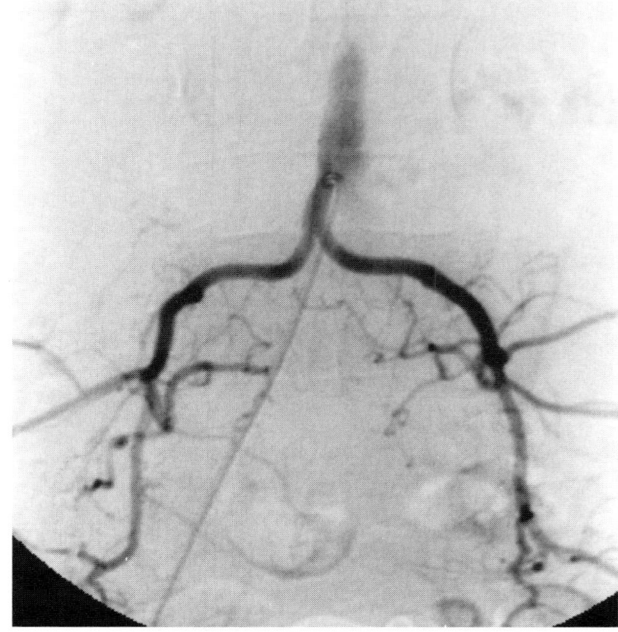

sacral arteries from the internal iliac arteries requires selective injection of these vessels if evaluation of sacral supply is necessary. A catheter with a reverse curve such as a Simmons 2 or shepherd's crook catheter is useful for both median sacral and internal iliac artery injections. The bladder should be empty during evaluation of sacral supply.

In summary, proper spinal angiography requires identification of a suspected region of interest followed by complete evaluation of all potential sources of blood supply. In particular, all contributions to the spinal cord blood supply must be identified in the region under evaluation. A complete knowledge of vascular anatomy and sequential evaluation of each vessel maximize the completeness of the evaluation. Attention to patient positioning and complete cessation of motion during filming are necessary for the visualization of these small vessels. As in all neuroangiography, meticulous technique and careful monitoring of the patient's neurologic status is essential to minimize potential complications.

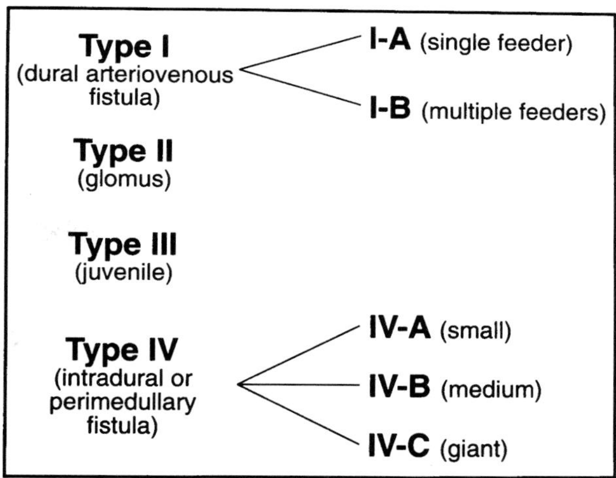

Figure 14-19. Classification schema for spinal AVMs. There are four major categories with subclassifications of types I and IV. Types II and III are both intradural spinal cord AVMs. (From Anson J, Spetzler R. Classification of spinal arteriovenous malformations. BNI Quarterly 1992; 8: 2–8. Used with permission.)

Classification of Spinal Vascular Malformations

Spinal vascular malformations represent a group of nonneoplastic vascular abnormalities that involve the spine. They were initially classified according to pathologic findings, but the use of selective spinal angiography has resulted in better understanding of the hemodynamics and anatomy of these uncommon lesions. Those most frequently requiring angiographic evaluation are characterized by arteriovenous shunting—the spinal AVMs. Multiple classification systems exist that include both spinal vascular malformations and the subgroup of spinal AVMs.

A frequently used classification delineates four major groups of spinal AVMs, numbered types I through IV. These include spinal dural arteriovenous fistulas, intradural spinal AVMs of both glomus and juvenile types, and intradural (perimedullary) arteriovenous fistulas (Fig. 14-19).[17]

The larger category of spinal vascular malformations includes not only the spinal AVMs but also vertebral hemangiomas, telangiectasias, and cavernous angiomas.[18] Complex vascular malformations, including metameric angiomatosis (Cobb syndrome) and spinal involvement by more widespread systemic disorders such as Osler-Weber-Rendu and Klippel-Trenaunay syndrome, may also be rarely encountered.[19,20]

Spinal Dural Arteriovenous Fistulas (Type I)

Spinal dural arteriovenous fistulas (SDAVFs) are diagnosed with increasing frequency, and a review of several large series indicates that they represent at least 35 percent of all spinal AVMs, although some estimates range as high as 80 percent (Fig. 14-20).[21,22]

Clinical Features

Predominantly a disease of men, who constitute 80 to 90 percent of cases, SDAVFs usually present in the sixth or seventh decade. The age range is broad, however, and patients from the third through the ninth decade have been reported. The most common initial symptom is back pain, which may be localized or radicular in distribution. Progressive development of lower extremity weakness and sensory symptoms follow so that, by the time of diagnosis, both are present in 90 to 95 percent of patients. The weakness is often characterized by both upper and lower motor neuron deficits. The development of disturbances of bowel, bladder, or sexual function occurs earlier in the course than is usually the case with cord neoplasms and is present in over 80 percent of patients by the time of diagnosis. Exacerbation of symptoms with straining, various positions, or exercise is commonly reported.

The slow progression of the clinical manifestations,

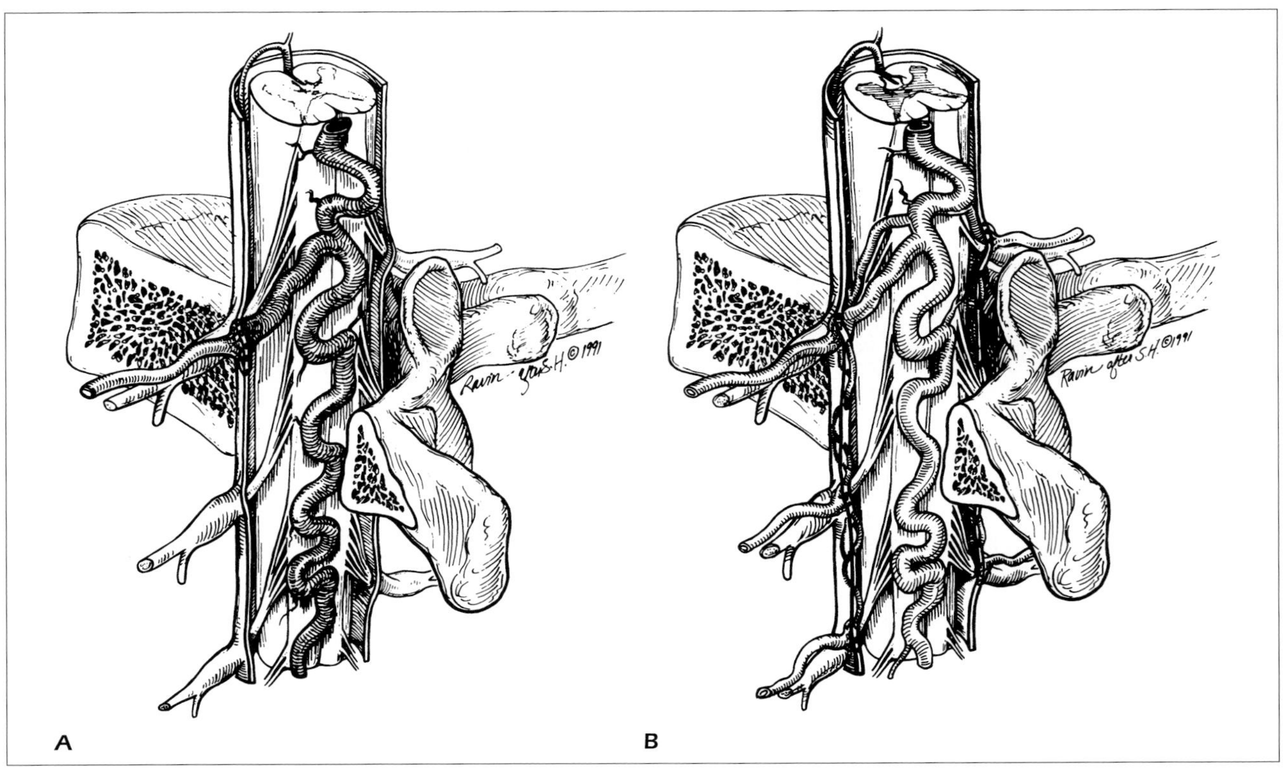

Figure 14-20. (A) Diagram of a type IA AVM illustrates the single dural feeder supplying the cluster of small vessels at the dural root sleeve that forms the fistula. The fistula flows into an enlarged efferent intradural vein that drains into the dilated coronal plexus of the spinal cord. (B) The type IB AVM has additional feeders at adjacent levels that communicate with the dural nidus via small vessels running within or beneath the dura. (From Anson J, Spetzler R. Classification of spinal arteriovenous malformations. BNI Quarterly 1992;8:2–8. Used with permission.)

representing an unusual course for most diseases of vascular etiology, often delays diagnosis. Nonetheless, such a slow progression is the rule in SDAVFs. SDAVFs may exhibit remissions or even improvements superimposed on deterioration during the clinical course. However, an apoplectic deterioration is uncommon, and hemorrhage from these lesions occurs rarely if at all. This is in marked contrast to the acute onset of symptoms, frequently heralded by hemorrhage, that often announces the presence of an intradural spinal AVM. A duration of symptoms exceeding 2 to 3 years at the time of diagnosis is not unusual in patients with SDAVFs.[23–28]

CSF examination may be normal in SDAVFs but often shows an increased protein content. Both red and white CSF cell counts are normal.

Most often SDAVFs are fed by a single feeding vessel and are categorized as type Ia. Those with multiple feeding vessels are referred to as type Ib.

The protracted development of clinical symptoms is also seen with more common clinical entities such as demyelinating disease involving the spinal cord, cervical spondylosis, and amyotrophic lateral sclerosis. Less common differential considerations include neoplasms, syringomyelia, degenerative processes, and infectious or inflammatory myelopathy such as that associated with AIDS.[29] Although other entities may often be clinically or radiologically differentiated from SDAVF, the nonspecific clinical picture raises the suspicion for the presence of SDAVF and is the most important factor in early diagnosis. Early identification and treatment of the shunt offer the best chance of halting progression or permitting recovery from neurologic deficits.

Anatomy and Pathophysiology

The actual shunt nidus of a SDAVF is usually located within the dura adjacent to the exiting nerve root, with drainage into intradural veins. The clinical picture is a result of this circumscribed area of arteriovenous shunting. The level of the shunt is variable but most commonly occurs at levels between T5 and L3 (Fig. 14-21).

SDAVFs arise from dural branches of radicular arteries, usually at levels with no associated supply to the

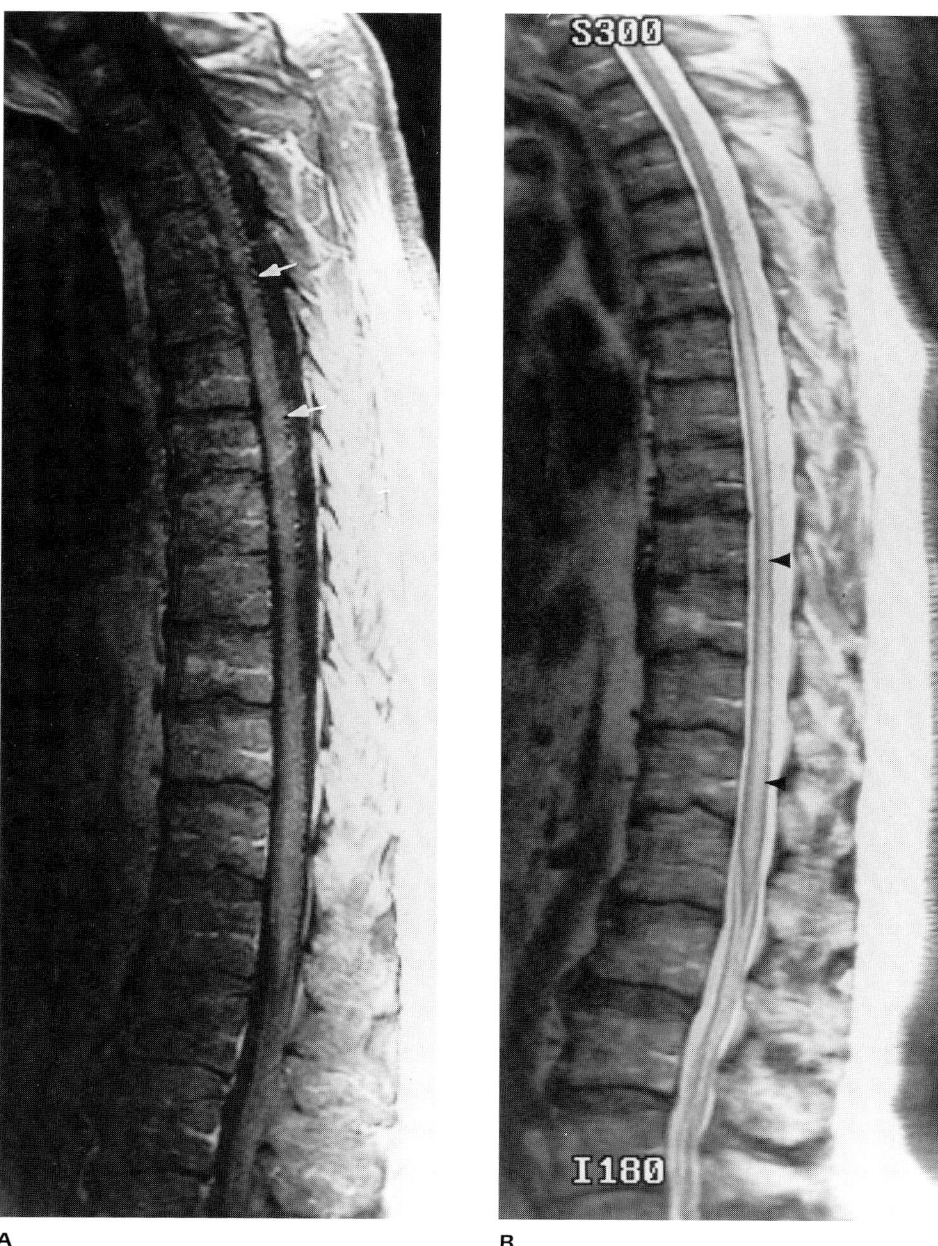

Figure 14-21. (A) Sagittal (700/11) T1- and (B) (4000/34) T2-weighted images show enlarged pial veins as areas of flow void on the dorsal surface of the cord (*arrows,* A). Intrinsic cord T2 signal abnormality extends from upper thoracic levels to the conus medullaris (*arrowheads,* B).

spinal cord. In 15 percent of cases, however, the lesions may arise at levels also giving rise to cord supply via radiculomedullary or radiculopial arteries.[30] Although the lesions are most often supplied by only one radicular artery, 10 percent of cases involve participation by radicular feeding vessels from two adjacent levels. The abnormal blood flow drains directly through tiny shunts within the dura, usually at a site within the neural foramen. An enlarged vein on the inner surface of the dura drains into the spinal cord venous system, most often along the posterior surface of the cord. Although usually a low-flow lesion, increased venous pressure from the shunt results in dilatation of the pial veins and is believed to be responsible for venous congestion and edema within the spinal cord. Stagnation of blood flow and hypoxia from perfusion impairment

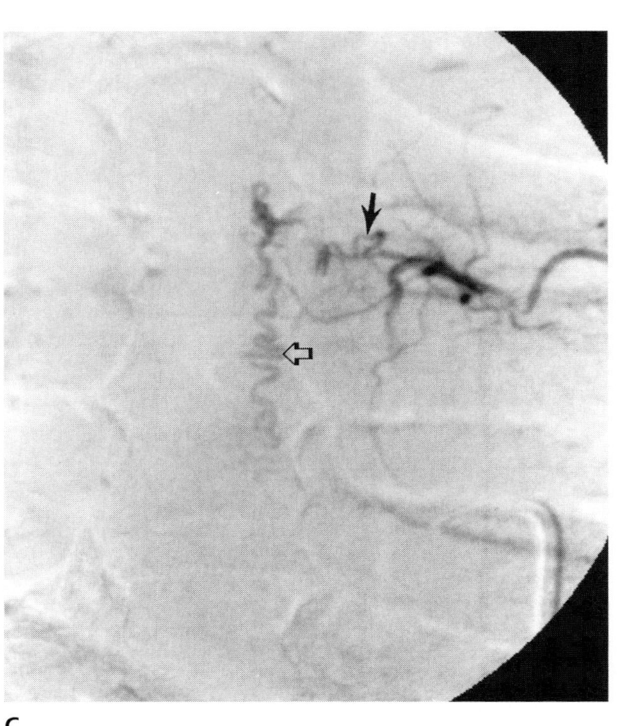

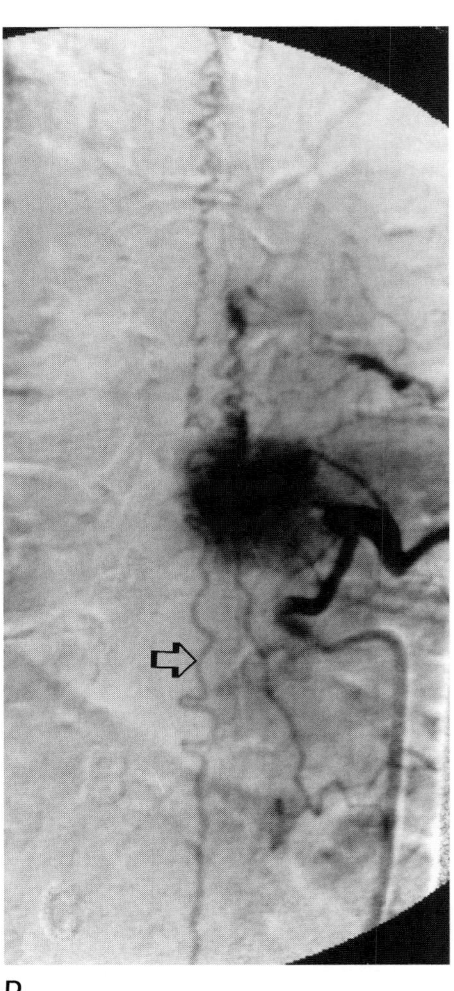

C D

Figure 14-21 (continued). (C and D) Early and late phase AP angiographic films after injection of left T6 intercostal artery demonstrate SDAVF (*arrow,* C) with early venous filling and extensive engorgement of pial spinal veins (*open arrow*). Note the hemivertebral blush.

lead to neurologic dysfunction. Pressure measurements at surgery have shown the mean spinal pial venous pressures in these lesions to be elevated to approximately 70 to 80 percent of the systemic arterial pressure. Increases of venous pressure associated with arterial pressure elevations may account for the clinical worsening seen with exercise.[31] The spread of venous involvement along the spine accounts for the poor correlation between the location of the shunt and the clinical level of spinal dysfunction. The uniform presence of weaknesss involving the lower extremities has been attributed to susceptibility of the venous drainage of the lumbar enlargement to compromise, possibly related to posture.[24] The lesions are believed to be acquired rather than congenital and are not associated with vascular malformations at other locations in the nervous system. However, the etiologic factors contributing to the genesis of SDAVF remain unknown.

Radiology

The pathophysiology of SDAVF, including the engorged venous system and abnormal cord tissue water content, is reflected in the MRI findings. These include decreased cord signal on T1-weighted images and increased signal intensity on proton density and T2-weighted images. The extent of the signal abnormality, which usually involves the thoracolumbar region, may be extensive. Generalized enlargement of the cord may be present. Enhancement of the cord has been observed after gadolinium administration. Areas of signal void representing the enlarged venous plexus are often seen over the posterior surface of the cord. Care must be taken to differentiate true areas of venous signal void from flow artifacts resulting from CSF motion. Areas of MR signal abnormality may or may not regress after interruption of the shunt.[32–34] MRI may, however, be normal or demonstrate only nonspecific cord signal abnormality in patients with SDAVF, and such patients require additional evaluation if warranted by the clinical picture.

Myelography, abnormal in over 90 percent of patients in some series, is useful to suggest the diagnosis of SDAVF before angiographic confirmation. Myelographic examination in the supine position is often necessary to demonstrate the enlarged, serpentine veins on the surface of the cord. The abnormal vessels most often are found in the thoracic region, but the location often correlates poorly with clinical levels of neurologic dysfunction. On occasion, a single dilated vein entering the dura in company with a nerve root may suggest the level of the shunt. The cord size is usually normal on myelographic examination. Postmyelographic CT scanning may show the dilated veins as filling defects in the contrast-filled subarachnoid space (Fig. 14-22).

Angiography

Angiographic examination for the diagnosis of SDAVF begins by selective injection of the lumbar arteries. The radicular afferent vessels to the shunt most often do not demonstrate significant enlargement. The small site of the shunt may result in the early opacification of the spinal venous system. The presence of early pial venous drainage is the most important diagnostic feature indicating the presence of the arteriovenous shunt. Later filming reveals the abnormally dilated venous system, which may course extensively over the surface of the cord (Fig. 14-23). Drainage most often is in a cranial direction.

A method for improving visualization of spinal

Figure 14-22. (A) Enlarged thoracic spinal cord pial veins on supine myelogram in a patient with an SDAVF (*arrows*). (B) Enlarged pial vessels appear as filling defects on postmyelogram CT scan (*arrow*).

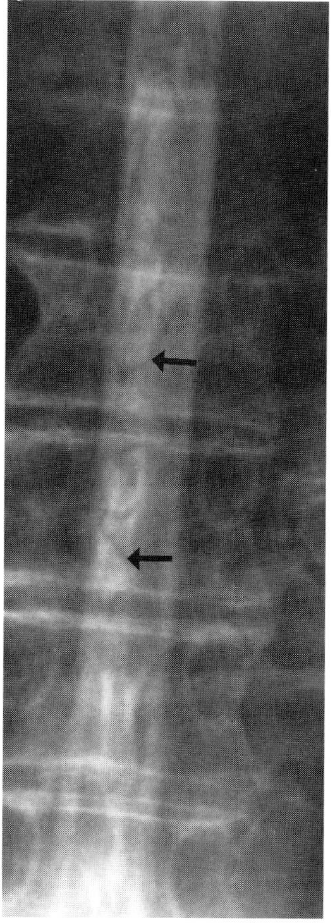

A

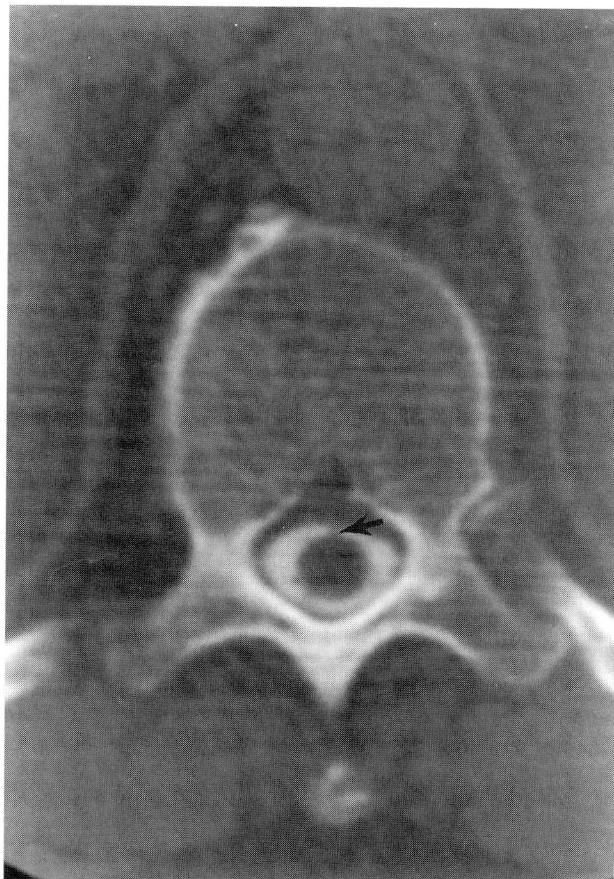

B

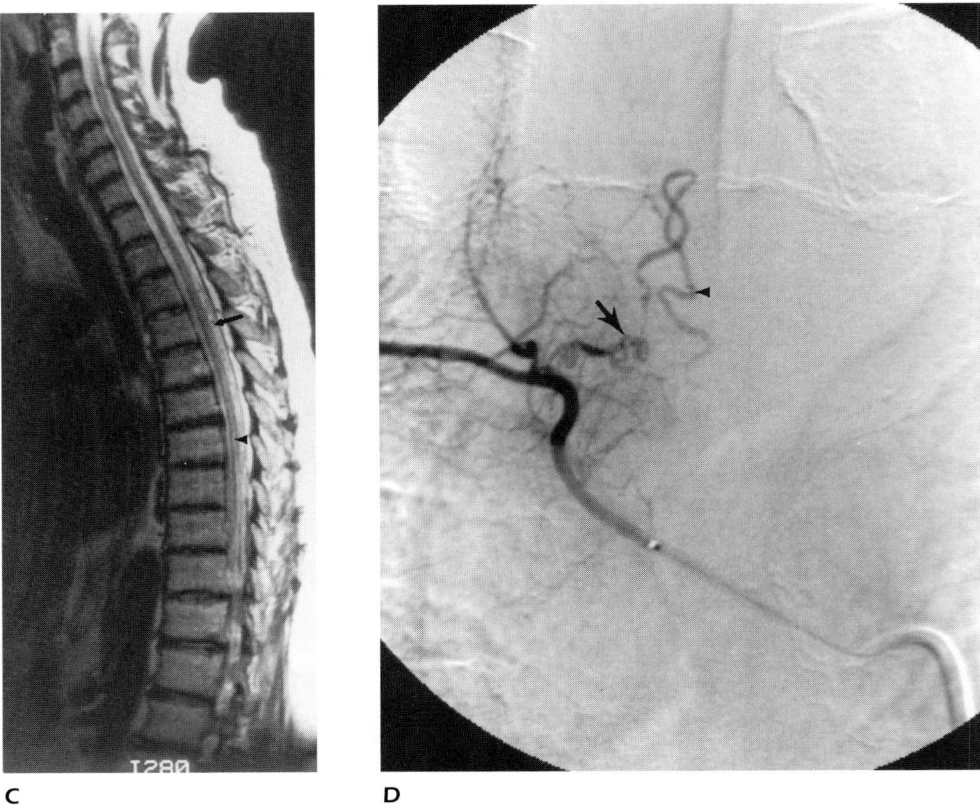

Figure 14-22 (continued). (C) Pial veins appear as flow voids on sagittal (3000/90) T2-weighted MR image (*arrow*). Diffusely increased intrinsic cord signal abnormality reflects venous hypertension (*arrowhead*). (D) AP injection of right T4 intercostal artery reveals SDAVF located in foramen of exiting nerve root (*arrow*) with early venous drainage into enlarged pial vein (*arrowhead*).

veins in suspected dural AVFs involves the injection of 1 ml per second for 9 ml into the segmental artery supplying the artery of the lumbar enlargement. Filming is continued for 24 seconds. A normal time of appearance of the spinal veins reportedly excludes venous hypertension secondary to dural AVF, whereas evidence of venous stasis suggests elevated venous pressure and requires additional spinal angiography to locate the shunt. Delayed visualization of spinal veins may also result from blockage of the artery by the catheter, arterial spasm, spinal stenosis, or spinal thrombophlebitis.[35]

Sequential evaluation of lumbar and intercostal arteries bilaterally will most often identify the location of the shunt. Selective angiographic examination of radicular vessels at levels above and below the site of the shunt is imperative to identify filling of the lesion via intersegmental anastomoses from neighboring levels. Radiculomedullary or radiculopial vessels originating at the level of the shunt must be identified because the presence of such vessels is a significant consideration in either surgical or endovascular therapy. Should the lesion not be found in the thoracic or lumbar regions, sacral and cervicoradicular vessels must be examined. In addition, drainage from intracranial pial or dural AVMs, most commonly located in the posterior fossa, may involve the pial veins of the spinal cord, resulting in spinal venous hypertensive myelopathy.[36-38] Evaluation for such lesions may reveal an otherwise occult source of engorgement of the spinal venous system (Fig. 14-24).

Treatment

Treatment of SDAVF requires permanent obliteration of the shunt nidus. Proximal occlusion of vessels is ineffective as a treatment because it permits continued shunting via collaterals. Elimination of shunting and reversal of venous hypertension has been reported to result in neurologic improvement in up to 80 percent of cases. Progression of symptoms is halted in virtually

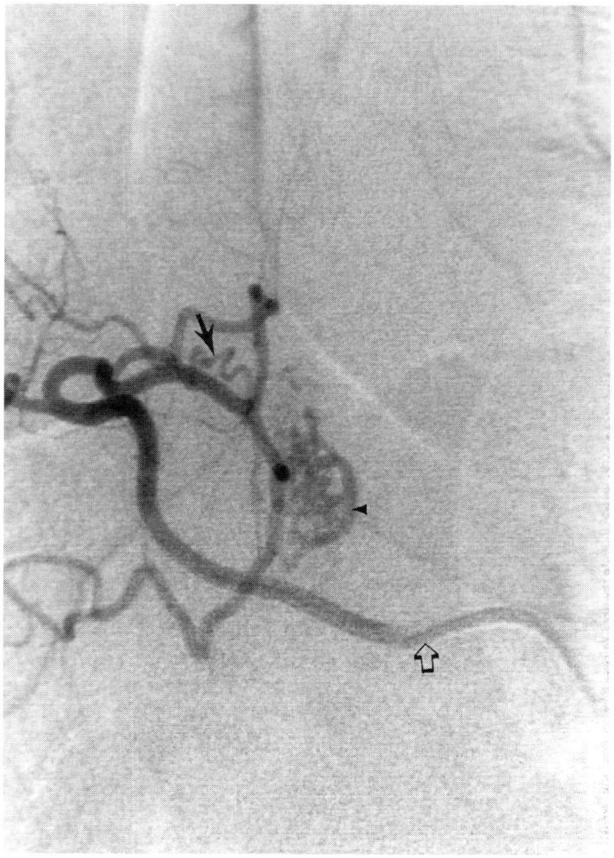

A 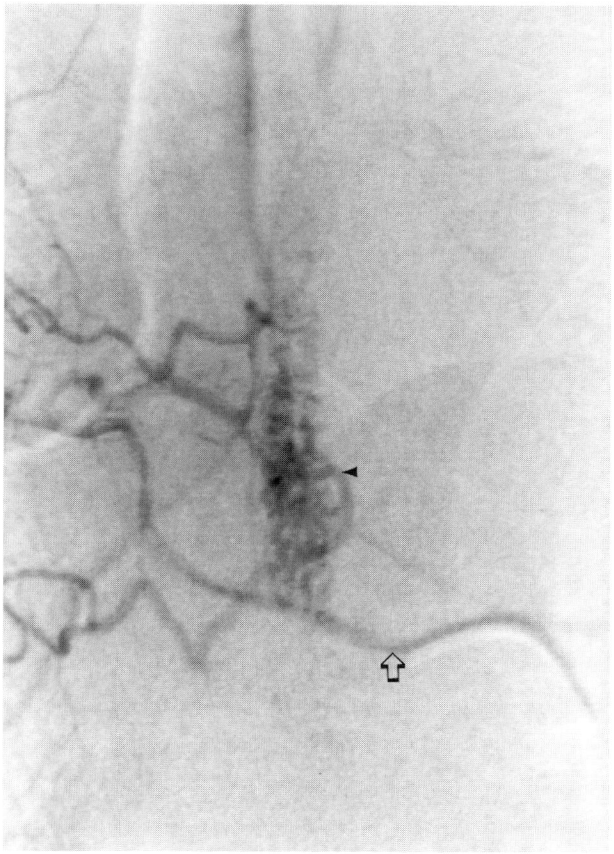 B

Figure 14-23. Early (A) and late (B) phase films following AP right T4 intercostal injection show SDAVF (*arrow*, A) with early filling of pial venous system (*arrowhead*). *Open arrow* is at catheter tip.

Figure 14-24. Early (A) and late (B) phases of selective ascending pharyngeal artery injection, lateral view, show filling of dural AV fistula of the jugular fossa with venous varix (*arrowhead*, A) and drainage into pial veins of the spinal cord (*arrow*, B). *Open arrow* is at catheter tip.

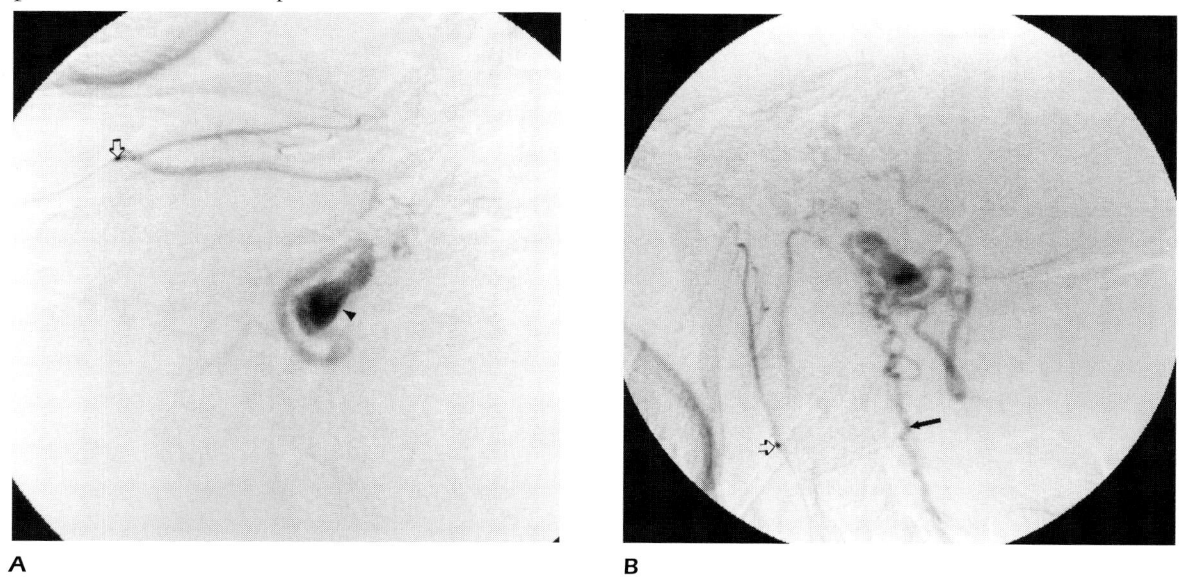

A B

all cases; an increased chance of neurologic improvement is correlated with less severe pretreatment deficits. Obliteration of the shunt may be performed using endovascular techniques or by surgical resection of the nidus. Embolization should be considered if available and if no vessels to the spinal cord originate from the afferent radicular vessel to the nidus. A common origin of the feeding vessel to the SDAVF and a radiculomedullary or radiculopial vessel to the spinal cord increases the risk of spinal cord damage and precludes safe endovascular treatment. Embolization is best accomplished with permanent liquid embolic agents such as *N*-butylcyanoacrylate. Recent studies evaluating the use of particulate emboli for occlusion of the SDAVF have revealed early recanalization and renewed progression of neurologic deficits.[28,39,40] The goal of embolization is complete occlusion of the nidus and the most proximal intradural portion of the vein. Surgical treatment of the lesion must always be considered because it is accompanied by very low morbidity and a high rate of success. Earlier techniques of stripping the dilated veins have been replaced with coagulation or resection of the site of the nidus and the surrounding dura to eliminate the shunt.[22]

Intradural Arteriovenous Malformations (Types II and III)

Intradural spinal AVMs are lesions in which the nidus of high-flow arteriovenous shunting is located on or within the substance of the spinal cord. Supplied by vessels that also supply the cord, intradural spinal AVMs display markedly differing demography, clinical presentation, pathophysiology, anatomy, and natural history in comparison to SDAVFs (Fig. 14-25).

Clinical Features

A slight male predominance may be present, but lesions are nearly equally divided between sexes. A relatively young age at presentation is characteristic, usually in the late second or third decade but often as early as the midteens. In nearly half of patients, an acute onset of back pain, paresis, and sensory deficits, frequently in association with subarachnoid hemorrhage, announces the clinical onset. Later, a progressive course with the development of motor and sensory deficits may be punctuated by acute worsening. More

Figure 14-25. (A) Diagram of a type II AVM with nidus located on and within the spinal cord. (B) A type III AVM demonstrates the extensive involvement of the diffuse juvenile AVM, which extends into the spinal cord, the intra- and extradural spaces, and even the bone. The AVM is supplied by all spinal arteries at multiple levels. (From Anson J, Spetzler R. Classification of spinal arteriovenous malformations. BNI Quarterly 1992;8:2–8. Used with permission.)

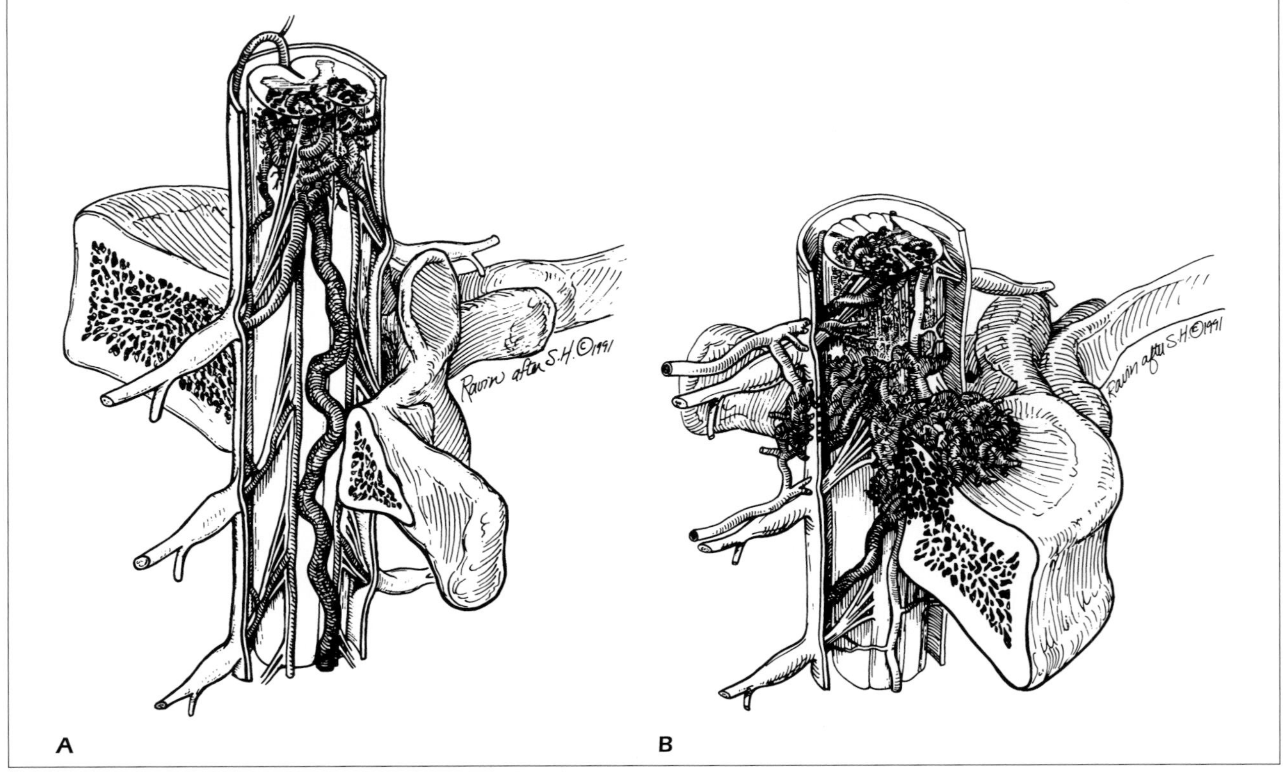

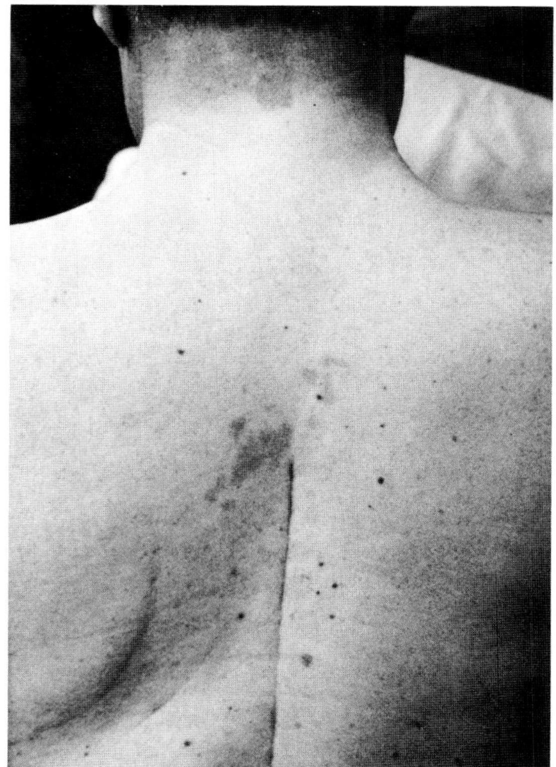

A

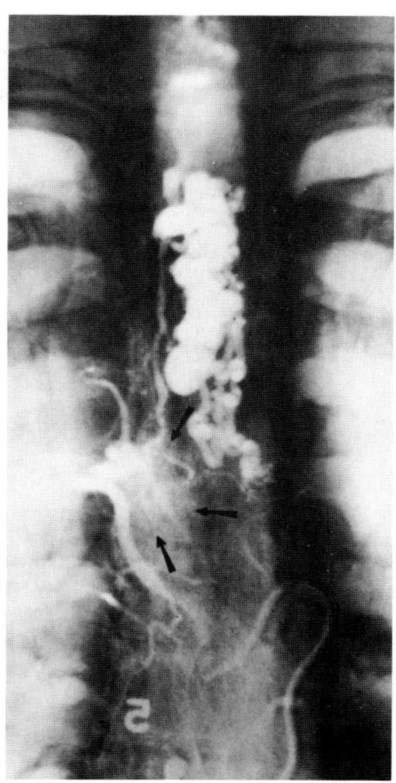

B

Figure 14-26. The cutaneous angioma just above the laminectomy scar (A) identifies the feeding vessel as a left-sided upper intercostal artery. Note in (B) not only the filling of the spinal AVM but also the faint staining (*arrows*) of the cutaneous lesion. (From Doppman JL, et al. Value of cutaneous angiomas in the arteriographic localization of spinal cord arteriovenous malformations. N Engl J Med 1969; 281:1440. Used with permission.)

than half of patients experience hemorrhage sometime during the course, with the incidence of hemorrhage even higher, almost 70 percent, in those AVMs involving the thoracic region. Mortality associated with acute hemorrhage may be as high as 30 percent.[41] Significant rebleeding rates have also been noted. By the time of diagnosis, significant compromise of bowel, bladder, and sensory functions is the rule. In untreated cases, an increasing number of severe deficits appear with time, with nearly half of patients confined to bed or wheelchair within 3 years of onset of symptoms.[42] The longer-term untreated prognosis is also poor, with nearly 60 percent of patients exhibiting significant neurologic deficits by 20 years, often with complete loss of spinal cord function.

A bruit over the location of the nidus is present in less than 10 percent of cases but, when found, suggests a high-flow lesion. A cutaneous angioma at the level of the nidus may be seen in 10 to 15 percent and should be sought in every patient (Fig. 14-26).

Intradural AVMs are believed to be congenital lesions, and their distribution is relatively uniform along the length of the spinal cord. Their potential to involve the cervical region permits the impairment of both upper and lower extremity function. The congenital origin also accounts for the occasional association with other vascular abnormalities involving the CNS or rarely with certain congenital disorders such as Rendu-Osler-Weber or Klippel-Trenaunay syndromes.

Anatomy and Pathophysiology

The nidus of intradural spinal AVMs is located within or on the surface of the spinal cord. Anterior spinal artery supply via sulcocommissural arteries indicates an intramedullary location, whereas exclusive involvement of the posterior spinal arteries, an uncommon condition, suggests a pial location. Most often, however, multiple sources of supply from both the anterior and posterior spinal arteries are present, providing high flow through the nidus. The AVM nidus is composed of multiple dysplastic arteriovenous shunt ves-

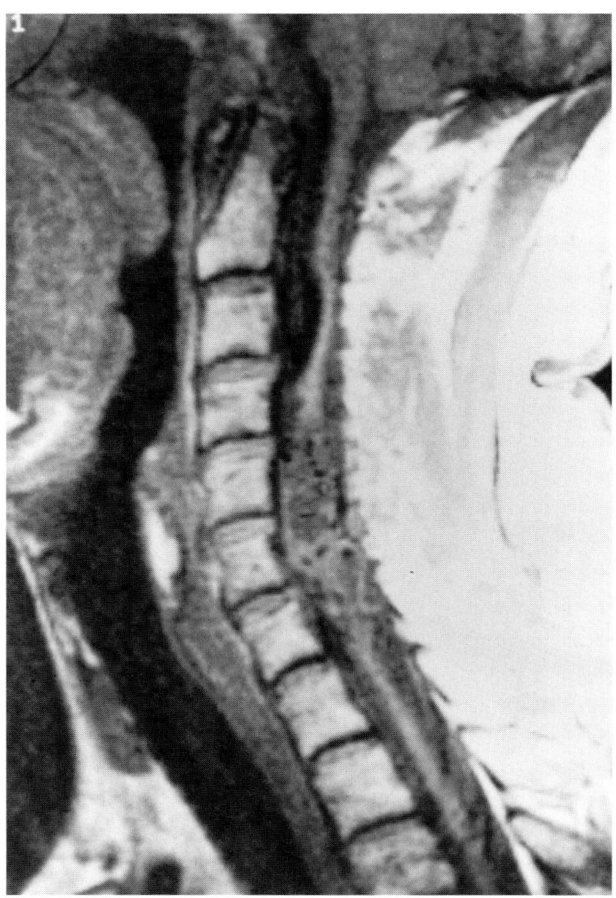

A

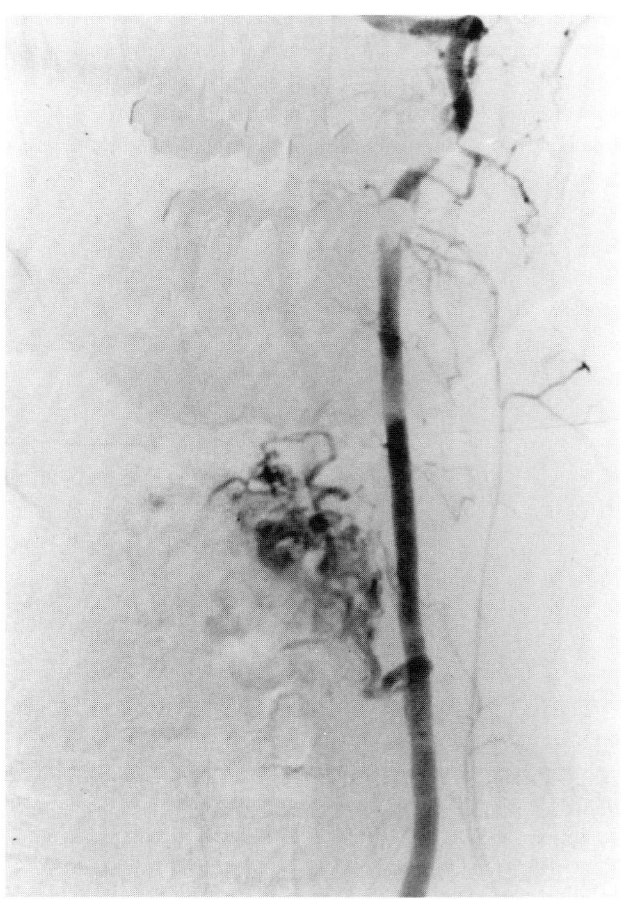

B

Figure 14-27. (A) Sagittal T1-weighted MR image (500/20) demonstrates intramedullary flow voids of AVM nidus and adjacent draining veins involving the lower cervical spinal cord. AP injection of the left vertebral artery (B) and right deep cervical artery (C) fills the AVM nidus from posterior spinal arteries. Note the nidus angioarchitecture and the early-draining veins (*arrow*, C). (Photo courtesy of A. Berenstein, M.D.)

sels. Both ascending and descending venous drainage occurs located both anterior and posterior to the cord. Usually tortuous and always dilated, the draining veins frequently leave the spinal canal at levels relatively close to the nidus. Two types of intradural AVMs are classified depending on the distribution of the nidus. Type II, or glomus types, have a relatively compact nidus located within the spinal cord (Fig. 14-27). Type III or juvenile types have a more extensive nidus that tends to be intramedullary but typically has extramedullary and even extraspinal extension.

The high-flow nature of the lesion and the common supply to both the cord and lesion permit the operation of multiple pathophysiologic mechanisms. Steal of blood from normal neural tissue may occur, resulting in ischemic symptoms. As with SDAVFs, venous hypertension secondary to the flow of high-pressure blood into the spinal venous system may develop followed by venous thrombosis and congestive symptoms. Associated venous varices or arterial aneurysms may compress spinal cord tissue or result in hemorrhage.[43,44] The clinical picture in an individual patient may arise from a combination of pathophysiologic mechanisms.

Radiology

Plain film radiographic changes may on occasion suggest the presence of an intradural spinal AVM. Widening of interpedicular distance, scalloping of the dorsal margins of the vertebral bodies, and enlargement of neural foramina have been described in association with these lesions. Kyphosis or scoliosis may be present.

Myelographic examination displays the enlarged feeding and draining vessels to the AVM and may be

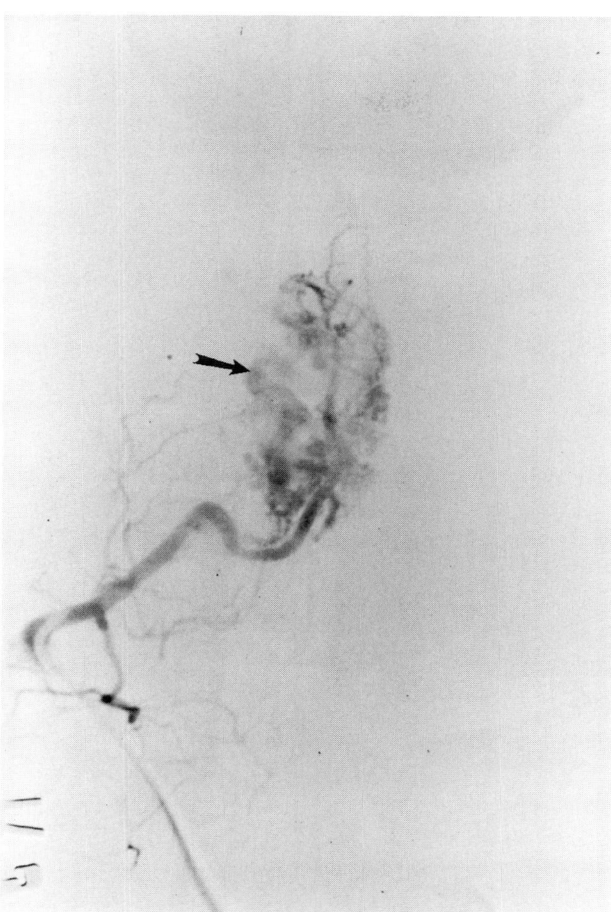

C
Figure 14-27 (continued).

remarkable for enlargement of the cord at the level of the lesion. Occasional block of contrast flow at the level of the lesion may be present. Reports of neurologic deterioration in patients with intradural spinal AVM after lumbar puncture suggest that MRI examination should replace myelography when this lesion is suspected.[45]

MRI examination usually provides the best imaging information regarding spinal intradural AVMs. The signal void associated with high-flow vessels and nidus is easily identified, although movement artifact from the high flow may create considerable interference with anatomic detail. Intramedullary hemorrhage may be visualized, although determining the presence of subarachnoid blood by MRI remains problematic. Nonhemorrhagic intramedullary signal abnormality may also be present, reflecting cord damage secondary to ischemia or other pathophysiologic mechanisms. Extension to extramedullary structures may also be evaluated by MRI (Fig. 14-28). MR angiography has not developed to the point where specific vessels can be reliably identified, although the presence of high flow in the region may aid in the differential diagnosis.

Angiography

Angiographic examination in intradural spinal AVMs is performed to delineate the complete angioarchitecture of the lesion, including feeding pedicles, nidus location, and draining veins. An aortogram may aid in the initial identification of enlarged feeding pedicles before selective injections. Unlike with SDAVFs, multiple intradural feeding pedicles from the anterior and/or posterior spinal arteries are often involved in supplying an intradural spinal AVM. Arterial supply may originate from either or both sides (Fig. 14-29). Arterial aneurysms must be identified if present and have been correlated with an increased risk of hemorrhage.

Venous drainage, although involving both the anterior and posterior spinal veins, is usually more prominent posteriorly. Frequent venous anastomoses connect the anterior and posterior spinal veins. Both ascending and descending drainage are usually observed with each lesion. Varicosities involving the venous system or evidence of outflow restriction may be present.

The normal spinal cord blood supply in the region must also be studied in these lesions. Angiographic examination is continued until both anterior and posterior spinal artery supply to uninvolved levels above and below the lesion are completely visualized. The potential for intradural AVMs to involve surrounding structures requires complete evaluation of blood supply to the vertebrae and paraspinous soft tissue as well.

Lateral films are necessary because of the complex angiographic anatomy of these lesions. The anterior or posterior location of the nidus is also an important feature for planning surgical or endovascular therapy. In addition, larger-volume injections and higher-speed filming are usually required for sufficient opacification of high-flow feeding vessels. Exact injection volumes vary markedly and must be determined on the basis of the size of individual vessels and flow through the AVM. The particular vessels studied depend on the region of the spine involved and on the anatomic considerations discussed earlier (see Fig. 14-29).

Treatment

Treatment of these lesions may involve considerable risk and is based on both the individual anatomy of the lesion and the clinical condition of the patient. Although complete removal of the nidus from the circu-

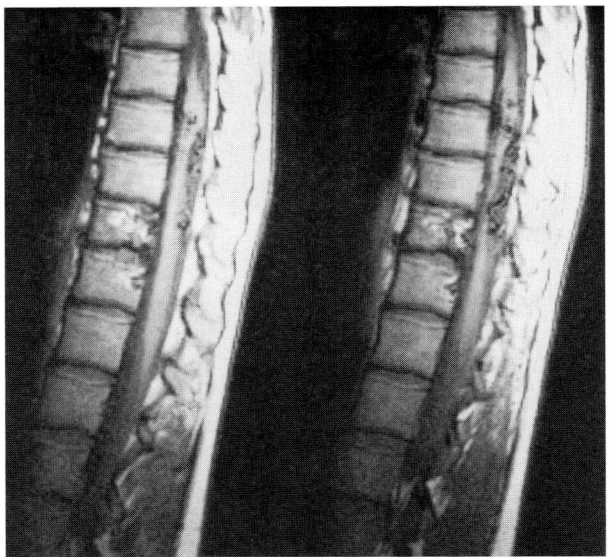
A

Figure 14-28. (A) Sagittal T1-weighted MR image (567/20) demonstrates a juvenile AVM nidus in both intramedullary and intervertebral locations. AP injection of left L2 lumbar (B) and right T12 intercostal (C) arteries fills feeding pedicles to the vertebral body component of the AVM with immediate arteriovenous shunting. (D) An enlarged anterior spinal artery fills from the left T6 intercostal artery and supplies the intramedullary AVM. Note the characteristic hairpin turn and the midline location of the anterior spinal artery (*arrow*). Supply from both left (E) and right (F) posterior spinal arteries (*open arrow*) also gives supply to the AVM nidus. The off-midline hairpin turn and course is characteristic of the posterior spinal arteries. (Photo courtesy of A. Berenstein, M.D.)

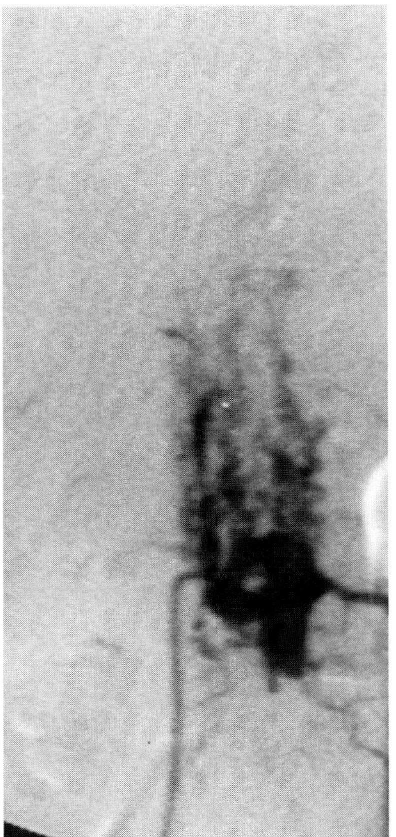
B

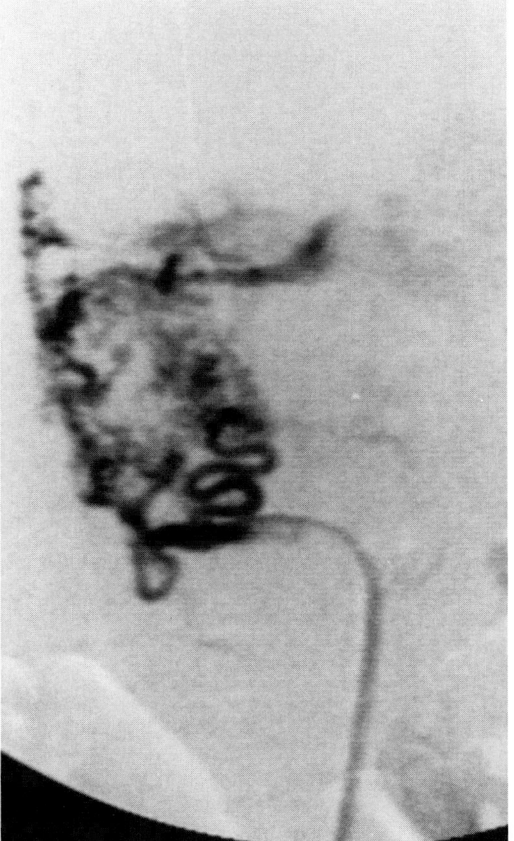
C

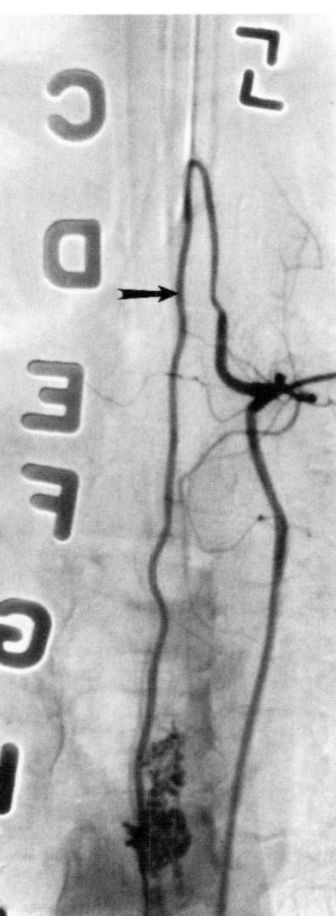
D

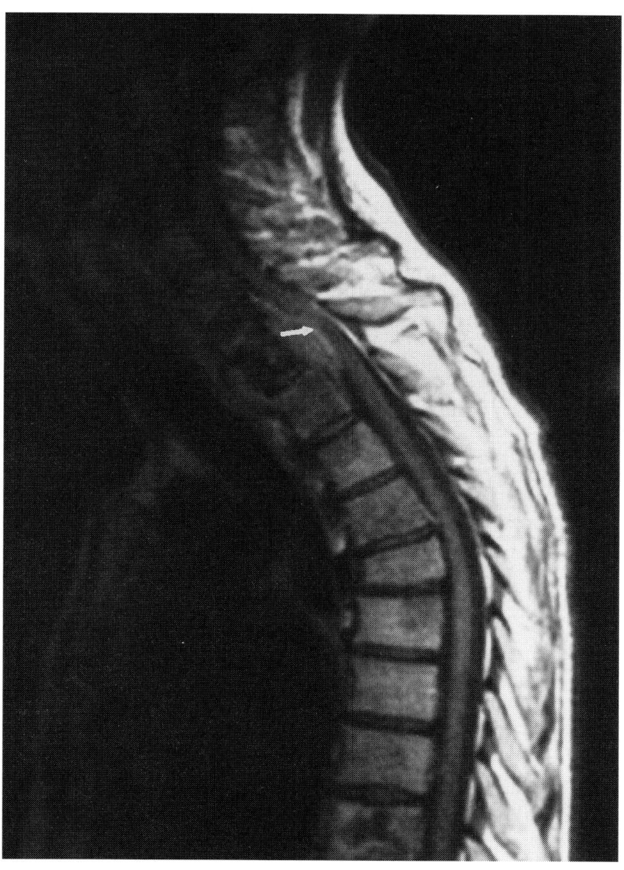

A

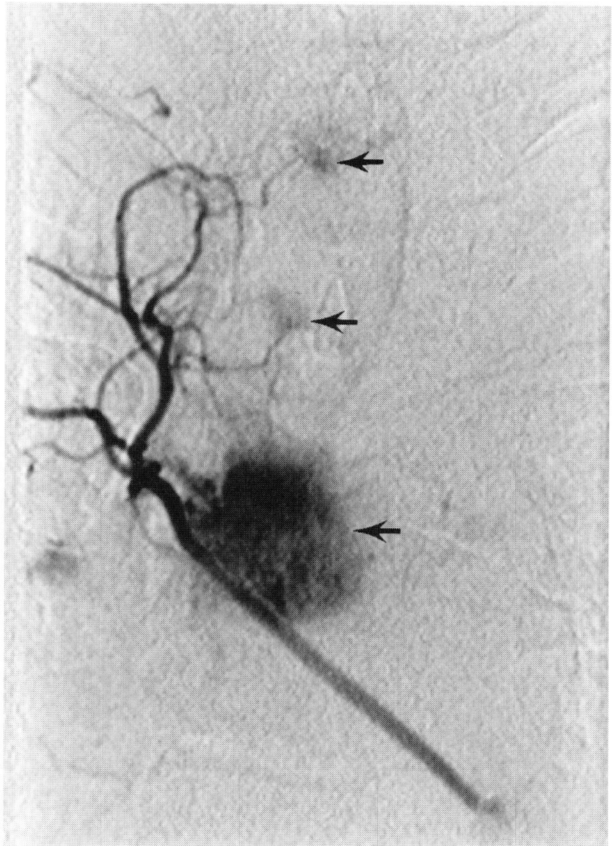

B

Figure 14-32. (A) Sagittal T1-weighted MR image (470/30) demonstrates vertebral metastasis from thyroid carcinoma with epidural component (*arrow*) causing spinal cord compression. Additional metastases are present at other levels. (B) AP injection of right superior intercostal artery shows tumor vascularity at three involved levels (*arrows*). (Photo courtesy of A. Berenstein, M.D.)

has been recommended in malignant lesions. Superselective catheterization of feeding vessels to the tumor is critical when using this agent to prevent serious necrosis of normal tissue.[70]

References

1. Lazorthes G, et al. Arterial vascularization of the spinal cord. J Neurosurg 1971;35:253–262.
2. Thron A. Vascular anatomy of the spinal cord. Vienna: Springer-Verlag, 1988:11–37.
3. Djindjian R, Hurth M, Houdart R. Angiography of the spinal cord. Baltimore: University Park Press, 1970.
4. DiChiro G, Wener L. Angiography of the spinal cord: a review of contemporary techniques and applications. J Neurosurg 1973;39(1):1–29.
5. Doppman J, DiChiro G, Omaya A. Selective arteriography of the spinal cord. St. Louis: H Green, 1969.
6. Doppman J. Spinal angiography. In: Abrams H, ed. Abrams' angiography. Boston: Little, Brown, 1983.
7. Kendall B. Spinal angiography with iohexol. Neuroradiology 1986;28:72–73.
8. Forbes G, et al. Complications of spinal cord arteriography: prospective assessment of risk for diagnostic procedures. Radiology 1988;169:479–484.
9. Hankey G, Warlow C, Sellar R. Cerebral angiographic risk in mild cerebrovascular disease. Stroke 1990;21:209–222.
10. Jellinger K. Pathology of spinal vascular malformations and vascular tumors. In: Pia H, Djindjian R, eds. Spinal angiomas: advances in diagnosis and therapy. Berlin: Springer-Verlag, 1978:18–44.
11. Turnbull I, ed. Blood supply of the spinal cord. In: Vinken P, Bruyn G, eds. Handbook of clinical neurology. Amsterdam: Elsevier, 1972;12.
12. Lasjaunias P, Berenstein A. Surgical neuroangiography. Berlin: Springer-Verlag, 1990;3:55–60.
13. Lazorthes G, ed. Pathology, classification, and clinical aspects of vascular diseases of the spinal cord. In: Vinken P, Bruyn G, eds. Handbook of clinical neurology. Amsterdam: Elsevier, 1972;12.

13a. Adamkiewicz, A. Die Blutgejäbe des Menschen Ruckenmarkes. S Ber Akad Wiss Wein Math Naturw Kl (Abt III) 1881;84:469–502.

14. Crock H, Yoshizawa H. The blood supply of the vertebral column and spinal cord in man. Vienna: Springer, 1977.
15. Chiras J, et al. Blood supply to the thoracic (dorsal) spine: normal angiographic appearances and comparative anatomy. Anat Clin 1982;4:23–31.

16. Gillian L. Veins of the spinal cord. Neurology 1970;20:860–868.
17. Anson J, Spetzler R. Classification of spinal arteriovenous malformations. BNI Quarterly 1992;8:2–8.
18. Vinuela F, Halbach V, Dion J, eds. Interventional neuroradiology: endovascular therapy of the central nervous system. New York: Raven, 1992.
19. Jessen R, Thompson S, Smith E. Cobb syndrome. Arch Dermatol 1977;113:1587–1590.
20. Miyatake S, et al. Cobb's syndrome and its treatment with embolization. J Neurosurg 1990;72:497–499.
21. Lasjaunias P, Berenstein A. Surgical neuroangiography. Berlin: Springer-Verlag, 1992;4.
22. Oldfield E, et al. Successful treatment of a group of spinal cord arteriovenous malformations by interruption of dural fistula. J Neurosurg 1983;59:1019–1030.
23. Rosenblum B, et al. Spinal arteriovenous malformations: a comparison of dural arteriovenous fistulas and intradural AVMs in 81 patients. J Neurosurg 1987;67:795–802.
24. Symon L, Kuyama H, Kendall B. Dural arteriovenous malformations of the spine: clinical features and surgical results in 55 cases. J Neurosurg 1984;60:238–247.
25. Zervas N, et al. Case records of the Massachusetts General Hospital. N Engl J Med 1992;326:816–824.
26. Aminoff M, Gutin P, Norman D. Unusual type of spinal arteriovenous malformation. Neurosurgery 1988;22(3):589–591.
27. Criscuolo G, Oldfield E, Doppman J. Reversible acute and subacute myelopathy in patients with dural arteriovenous fistulas. J Neurosurg 1989;70:354–359.
28. Muraszko K, Oldfield E. Vascular malformations of the spinal cord and dura. Neurosurg Clin North Am 1990;1(3):631–652.
29. Adams R, Salam-Adams M. Chronic nontraumatic diseases of the spinal cord. Neurol Clin 1991;9(3):605–623.
30. Doppman J, DiChiro G, Oldfield E. Origin of spinal arteriovenous malformation and normal cord vasculature from a common segmental artery: angiographic and therapeutic considerations. Radiology 1985;154:687–689.
31. Hassler W, Thron A, Grote E. Hemodynamics of spinal dural arteriovenous fistulas. J Neurosurg 1989;70:360–370.
32. Isu T, et al. Magnetic resonance imaging in cases of spinal dural arteriovenous fistula. Neurosurgery 1989;24:919–923.
33. Larsson E, et al. Venous infarction of the spinal cord resulting from dural arteriovenous fistula: MR imaging findings. AJNR 1991;12:739–743.
34. Masaryk T, et al. Radiculomeningeal vascular malformations of the spine: MR imaging. Radiology 1987;164:845–849.
35. Willinsky R, et al. Angiography in the investigation of spinal dural arteriovenous fistula. Neuroradiology 1990;32:114–116.
36. Wrobel C, et al. Myelopathy due to dural arteriovenous fistulas draining intrathecally into spinal medullary veins. J Neurosurg 1988;69:934–939.
37. Dickman C, et al. Myelopathy due to epidural varicose veins of the cervicothoracic junction. J Neurosurg 1988;69:940–941.
38. Partington M, et al. Cranial and sacral dural arteriovenous fistulas as a cause of myelopathy. J Neurosurg 1992;76:615–622.
39. Hall W, Oldfield E, Doppman J. Recanalization of spinal arteriovenous malformations following embolization. J Neurosurg 1989;70:714–720.
40. Morgan M, Marsh W. Management of spinal dural arteriovenous malformations. J Neurosurg 1989;70:832–836.
41. Casasco A, et al. Embolization of spinal vascular malformations. Neuroimag Clin 1992;2(2):337–358.
42. Aminoff M, Logue V. The prognosis of patients with spinal vascular malformations. Brain 1974;97:211–218.
43. Biondi A, et al. Aneurysms of the spinal arteries associated with intramedullary arteriovenous malformations: I. Angiographic and clinical aspects. AJNR 1992;13(3):912–923.
44. Biondi A, et al. Aneurysms of the spinal arteries associated with intramedullary arteriovenous malformations: II. Results of AVM endovascular treatment and hemodynamic considerations. AJNR 1992;13(3):923–933.
45. Awad I, Barnett G. Neurological deterioration in a patient with a spinal arteriovenous malformation following lumbar puncture. J Neurosurg 1990;72:650–653.
46. Oldfield E, Doppman J. Spinal arteriovenous malformations. Clin Neurosurg 1979;26:543.
47. Spetzler R, Zabramski J, Flom R. Management of juvenile spinal AVMs by embolization and operative excision. J Neurosurg 1989;70:628–632.
48. Tuoho H, et al. Successful excision of a juvenile type spinal arteriovenous malformation following intraoperative embolization. J Neurosurg 1991;75:647–651.
49. Biondi A, et al. Embolization with particles in thoracic intramedullary arteriovenous malformations: long term angiographic and clinical results. Radiology 1992;177(3):651–658.
50. Theron J, et al. Spinal arteriovenous malformations: advances in therapeutic embolization. Radiology 1986;158:163–169.
51. Djindjian M, et al. Intradural extramedullary spinal arteriovenous malformations fed by the anterior spinal artery. Surg Neurol 1977;8:85–93.
52. Gueguen B, et al. Vascular malformations of the spinal cord: intrathecal perimedullary arteriovenous fistulas fed by medullary arteries. Neurology 1987;37:969–979.
53. Heros R, et al. Direct spinal arteriovenous fistula: a new type of spinal AVM. J Neurosurg 1986;64:134–139.
54. Ueda S, et al. Cavernous angioma of the cauda equina producing subarachnoid hemorrhage. J Neurosurg 1987;66:134–136.
55. Cosgrove R, et al. Cavernous angiomas of the spinal cord. J Neurosurg 1988;68:31–36.
56. Bicknell J, et al. Familial cavernous angiomas. Arch Neurol 1978;35:746–749.
57. Ogilvy C, Louis D, Ojemann R. Intramedullary cavernous malformations of the spine. Neurosurgery 1992;31(2):219–230.
58. Barnwell S, et al. Cryptic vascular malformations of the spinal cord: diagnosis by magnetic resonance imaging and outcome of surgery. J Neurosurg 1990;72:403–407.
59. Ho V, et al. Radiologic-pathologic correlation: hemangioblastoma. AJNR 1992;13:1343–1352.
60. Sato Y, et al. Hippel-Lindau disease: MR imaging. Radiology 1988;166:241–246.
61. Yasargil M, Fiedeler R, Rankin T. Operative treatment of spinal angiomas. In: Pia H, Djindjian R, eds. Spinal angiomas: advances in diagnosis and therapy. Berlin: Springer-Verlag, 1978:171–188.
62. Ross J, et al. Vertebral hemangiomas: MR imaging. Radiology 1987;165:165–169.
63. Laredo J, et al. Vertebral hemangiomas: radiologic evaluation. Radiology 1986;161:183–189.
64. Mohan N, et al. Symptomatic vertebral hemangiomas. Clin Radiol 1980;31:575–579.
65. Dagi T, Schmidek H. Vascular tumors of the spine. In: Sundaresan N, et al, eds. Tumors of the spine: diagnosis and clinical management. Philadelphia: Saunders, 1990.
66. Sundaresan N, et al. Treatment of neoplastic epidural cord compression by vertebral body resection and stabilization. J Neurosurg 1985;63:676–684.
67. Voegeli E, Fuchs W. Arteriography in bone tumors. Clin Radiol 1976;49:407–415.
68. Gellad F, et al. Vascular metastatic lesions of the spine: preoperative embolization. Radiology 1990;176:683–686.
69. Choi I. Spinal angiography and embolization of tumors. In: Sundaresan N, et al, eds. Tumors of the spine: diagnosis and clinical management. Philadelphia: Saunders, 1990.
70. Choi I. Spinal dural arteriovenous fistula: the role of PVA embolization. AJNR 1992;13:941–943.

III

The Thorax

15

Technique, Indications, and Hazards of Thoracic Aortography and the Normal Thoracic Aorta

HERBERT L. ABRAMS
GUNNAR JÖNSSON

History of Thoracic Aortography

Thoracic aortography is a method of opacifying the thoracic aorta and recording radiographically the appearance of this vessel and its great branches as well as the route traversed by the injected contrast medium. Although contrast visualization of the abdominal aorta was accomplished in 1929,[1] it was not until 1936 that Nuvoli described thoracic aortography in humans.[2] Before that time, Rousthöi had demonstrated the aorta in animals.[3] It was perhaps natural that Nuvoli should have attempted direct puncture of the ascending aorta after dos Santos et al. had demonstrated that direct puncture of the abdominal aorta was a relatively safe procedure.[1] This method of visualizing the thoracic aorta was used successfully by others for about 2 decades.[4–8]

In 1939 Castellanos and Pereiras described a method of countercurrent aortography in infants[9] that they elaborated on in subsequent publications.[9–11] Although the method was ideal for infants, the aortic arch could not be adequately visualized in older children or adults. An indirect sign of coarctation of the aorta, namely, the dilated collateral vessels, was usually demonstrable in older patients.

A modification of the method of Castellanos, using retrograde injection of the carotid artery to opacify the aorta, was described in 1948 by a number of workers.[12–15] Subsequently, Jönsson used percutaneous insertion of a cannula through the carotid artery into the aortic arch, which he found useful in visualizing coarctation of the aorta.[16]

Finally, a third method of thoracic aortography was described in 1948 by Radner,[17] who introduced a catheter into the radial artery and advanced it by way of the brachial, axillary, and subclavian arteries into the aorta. Brodén, Hanson, Karnell, and Jönsson thoroughly explored the value of this method in the diagnosis of patent ductus arteriosus and coarctation of the aorta.[16,18–20] The monograph by Brodén, Jönsson, and Karnell on thoracic aortography constitutes a classic study, containing fine illustrations of patent ductus arteriosus and of many varieties of coarctation of the aorta.[21] Helmsworth et al., using the catheter technique, were able to study the coronary arteries in a number of patients.[22] Peirce modified the catheter technique by introducing percutaneous femoral artery puncture and catheter insertion through the needle.[23]

Technique of Thoracic Aortography

Premedication and Anesthesia

During the early experience with thoracic aortography, a general anesthetic was used in most patients. Now virtually all thoracic aortograms are performed using premedication and local anesthesia, with the patient responsive and cooperative. Atropine is commonly used in combination with diazepam for premedication.

The patient must always be forewarned of the kind of reaction that he or she will most commonly experience: a feeling of warmth in the face and frequently in much of the rest of the body. It is desirable to talk with the patient immediately after concluding the study to detect any incipient reactions.

Sensitivity Testing

In the past we subscribed to the notion that sensitivity testing might forewarn of a reaction and hence should be done routinely. It is our conviction at this time that there is no parallel between severe reactions to aortography and intravenous or intraarterial sensitivity testing. Sensitivity testing is therefore not warranted. For those who still believe in its efficacy, 0.5 ml of the medium to be used may be given either intravenously or intraarterially and followed by an observation period of 10 to 15 minutes (see Chap. 3).

Route of Injection

Direct Puncture

As noted above, the first attempt at thoracic aortography in humans used the method of direct puncture.[2] Later, in 1945, Radner reported studies in five patients using direct puncture,[7] and other reports have since appeared.[4–6,8] With the patient lying supine, a cannula such as is employed for sternal puncture may be passed through the manubrium, and thereafter a needle may be inserted through the orifice of the cannula directly into the aorta.[7] Alternatively, an intercostal approach may be employed,[6] with the needle directed dorsally and medially toward the aorta. Wickbom has described a method of puncture just above the right clavicle, lateral to the common carotid artery.[8] The needle is inserted parallel to the course of the common carotid artery, that is, downward and slightly to the left, and backward behind the first rib. The pulsations of the aorta are felt, and then the aorta is entered. A modified supraclavicular approach has also been advocated by others,[4,24] and transesophageal injection has been described. No matter where the direct puncture of the aorta is made, a free flow of blood from the aorta must be observed before injection. The exact position of the needle may be checked with a roentgenoscope or preliminary films.

Although direct puncture aortography can be performed successfully and yield good diagnostic studies, it has not received uniform acceptance throughout the world. The presumed risks of hemorrhage from the aorta and of lung puncture have been the major deterrents. In addition, relatively simple alternative techniques have been available.

Retrograde Brachial Aortography

This technique, as initially described by Castellanos and Pereiras,[11] was found to be useful in demonstrating coarctation of the aorta and patent ductus arteriosus in early life. A decade after the first report of its use, Keith and Forsyth reemphasized the value of this technique in studying infants with heart failure.[25] Subsequent studies confirmed its usefulness,[26–28] and certainly its simplicity is attractive. A recent report indicates that in some centers it remains an important method for clarifying the anatomy of the aortic arch in infants.[29] The skin and subcutaneous tissues in the antecubital fossa are infiltrated with 1 percent procaine hydrochloride solution. The left brachial artery, lying medial and deep to the vein, is palpated and exposed. A transverse incision is made in the arterial wall, and the largest possible Robb needle is inserted (Fig. 15-1). The artery is temporarily ligated distally, and the needle is anchored with a ligature. When the injection is made, the medium must be propelled against the normal current of blood flow. With a sufficiently forceful injection, however, this does not constitute a major problem, and the distal portion of the aortic arch is almost invariably opacified in infants and children up to the age of 4 years. Beyond that age, it is difficult to obtain a satisfactory examination of the aortic arch by this method.

Retrograde Carotid Aortography

Stephens and Freeman initially reported on the use of retrograde carotid aortography, injecting 70 percent Diodrast as the contrast medium.[13,15] Almost simultaneously, Burford and Carson used much the same method and obtained beautiful studies of patent duc-

Figure 15-1. Technique of retrograde brachial aortography. The filled syringe is attached to the Robb needle by way of a three-way stopcock and a short, flexible rubber tube.

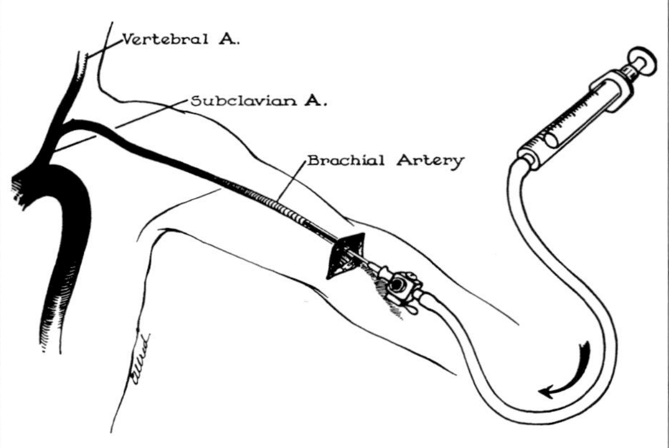

tus arteriosus, coarctation of the aorta, and the collateral system in coarctation.[30] A somewhat similar method was reported in 1949 by Jönsson, who introduced a cannula through the carotid artery into the aortic arch by employing percutaneous insertion.[16] He subsequently abandoned this method because of the "technical difficulties and risks" involved.[21]

Most patients studied by the carotid route received a general anesthetic. The incision was usually made in the left supraclavicular area over the left common carotid artery, and dissection was carried down to the carotid sheath. The vessel was dissected free for about 5 cm, and then a 16- or 18-gauge needle was inserted directly into the artery. The distal portion of the artery was temporarily occluded to prevent a large volume of the opaque medium from reaching the brain.

This method of thoracic aortography is no longer used except under very special circumstances.

Aortography Using Left Ventricular Puncture

Left ventricular puncture as a means of opacifying the aorta was first performed by Nuvoli[2] and later undertaken in a series of 30 patients by Ponsdomenech and Nunez.[31] Later, Smith et al.[32] and McCaughan and Pate[33] also advocated this method of "aortography." The technique involves placing the patient in a right posterior oblique projection and using a 4-inch large-bore, thin-walled, 18-gauge needle inserted near the xiphoid process and directed in a posterosuperior and slightly lateral direction.[33] When the point of the needle reaches a depth of 3 to 5 cm, movements of the heart usually can be felt. The needle is then inserted for an additional 3 cm, and after removal of the trocar, a free flow of blood is noted. McCaughan and Pate[33] used this procedure in 29 patients and found it satisfactory.

Angiocardiography

This technique has been used since 1938 for delineating the thoracic aorta. There is no need to describe the method in detail here, but it should be emphasized that the limitations of angiocardiography provided the impetus for elaborating better methods of opacifying the thoracic aorta. Nevertheless, there are definitely some instances in which lesions of the aorta may be demonstrated clearly by angiocardiography.[34] Occasionally the transseptal approach to left atrial angiography may be employed, and it has been shown to delineate left heart structures more clearly than does pulmonary artery injection.[35]

Balloon-directed angiography has proved successful in children with congenital heart disease. If the catheter is passed through the aortic valve and the balloon is inflated in the descending aorta, obstruction to the forward flow will result and the balloon-directed flow of contrast will fill any major arteriopulmonary anastomoses that are present.[36]

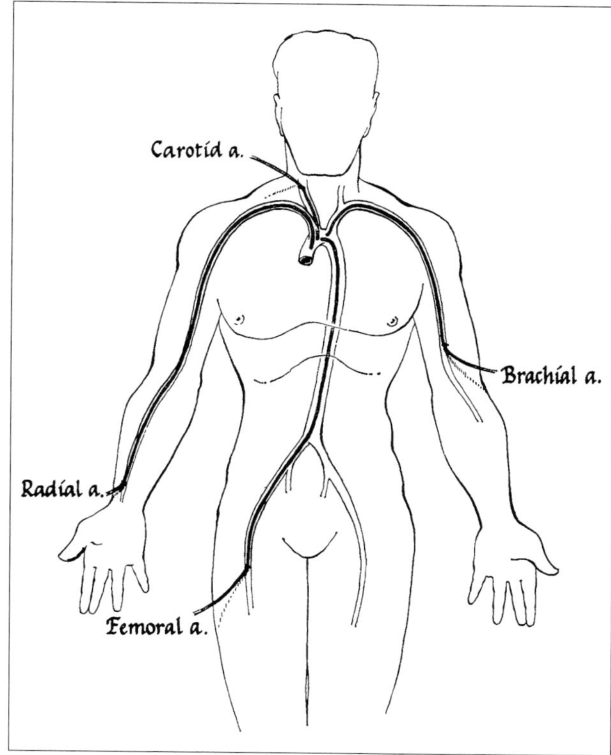

Figure 15-2. Catheter aortography of the thoracic aorta. The catheter may be inserted in a number of different sites, including the femoral artery, the radial artery, the brachial artery, and the carotid artery.

Catheter Aortography

Rousthöi, who used direct puncture of the aorta for thoracic aortography in animals, also employed catheter injection.[3] The application of the catheter technique to humans was described in 1941 by Fariñas, who inserted a catheter into the abdominal aorta through a cannula in the femoral artery.[37] His major interest was in supplanting the translumbar direct puncture technique of dos Santos et al.[1] in studying the abdominal aorta and its branches. Radner first applied the catheter method to thoracic aortography in clinical subjects[17] (Fig. 15-2). He exposed the radial artery on the right or left side and introduced a size 7 to 9 catheter into the artery. This was passed in retrograde direction and under fluoroscopic control via the brachial, axillary, and subclavian arteries into the ascending aorta. After the catheter tip was in the desired position, the injection was made. This method was used by Jönsson and his colleagues in the study of patent ductus arteriosus and coarctation of the aorta.[19,20,21,38] Helmsworth et al. used a similar technique for studying the aorta and the coronary vessels.[22] In 1951 Peirce[23] modified the method of Fariñas[37] to employ percutaneous femoral artery catheterization for thoracic aortography. This technique depends on initial arterial puncture and passage of the catheter through the artery for a distance of about 6 to 12 inches. The needle is then withdrawn, and the catheter, filled with an opaque medium, is passed to the desired point under fluoroscopic control. Ödman and Philipson[39] refined the percutaneous femoral catheter method by using the Seldinger technique[40] and the Ödman radiopaque polyethylene catheter. Their catheter has a distal hole smaller than the lumen and three side holes immediately behind the tip, directed obliquely backward. In addition, the distal 10 cm of the catheter is curved to fit into the aortic arch.

The right brachial artery is clearly a useful route to employ for catheterization of the ascending aorta and has been particularly applicable to the Sones method of selective coronary arteriography. At times it is difficult to pass the catheter beyond the junction of the subclavian artery and the carotid artery, but usually a little manipulation enables passage into the ascending aorta. Occasionally the catheter may enter the vertebral artery and thus require careful rotation for proper placement. A modified pigtail catheter has recently been described for use in transbrachial aortography.[41] Catheterization through the right carotid artery has also yielded satisfactory thoracic aortograms.[42]

The axillary artery has been enthusiastically supported as a superior route of entry to the aorta. Its use obviates the problems inherent in passing the catheter from below through the tortuous, arteriosclerotic aortas of some individuals in the older age group.[43–45]

The aorta has also become accessible via contrast injection through the umbilical artery. Technical improvements have increased the versatility of catheters, and various forms of guidewires (e.g., deflector, preformed curve, and variable stiffness types) have enhanced the ease of catheter aortography and selective catheter arteriography.[46] A double-catheter approach has proved useful for traversing the aortic arch, particularly when both thoracic and abdominal aortography are required. Carried out through the right axillary artery, this approach involves one exchange over a guidewire and is helpful when a deflector guidewire is not available or when other guidewires have not successfully traversed the aortic arch.[46]

During the past 4 decades, much experience has been accumulated with the transfemoral catheter approach to thoracic aortography.[47–49] The method has proved simple to learn and relatively easy to apply. Even in the presence of aortic dissection, it has presented no significant hazard as long as basic precautions are followed.[47,49] In most instances it is the method of choice.

In all studies the size of the catheter depends on the size of the artery; the catheter should be of adequate diameter to permit rapid injection of the required volume of contrast agent. Throughout the procedure continuous irrigation with saline containing a small amount of heparin is necessary.

The optimal position of the tip is at the midpoint of the ascending aorta. If aortic insufficiency is being evaluated, it may be desirable to have the tip just above the valve, but care must be taken not to insert it directly into a coronary artery. The use of a closed-end catheter prevents recoil, which may be a serious problem if the tip recoils into the carotid arteries and a quantity of the opaque medium reaches the brain without adequate dilution. A small amount of heparin may be injected to prevent clotting of the artery distally.

Among the foregoing methods of studying the thoracic aorta and its great branches, the retrograde transfemoral approach is now used most widely. In our experience it has been relatively safe, versatile, and simple to employ.

Preliminary Films

Before the arterial puncture, preliminary films of the chest are obtained. These should be obtained in both projections if a biplane study is to be performed. The shortest possible exposure time is desirable. We obtain three exposures in each projection at different kilovoltages. In general, it is desirable to use slight overpenetration. The films are reviewed not only for optimal exposure technique but also for the adequacy of the radiographic projections.

Radiographic Projections

The projections to be employed depend to some extent on the reason for the aortographic procedure. In general, the steep right posterior oblique projection unfolds the aortic arch and its great branches best. Thus, when biplane studies are available, a steep right posterior oblique projection and a left posterior oblique projection should be employed for the study of patent ductus arteriosus and coarctation of the aorta. When anomalies of the aortic arch are being investigated, however, the frontal and lateral projections often prove useful.

The Electrocardiogram

The electrocardiogram should be monitored throughout each study. A continuous direct-writing electrocardiographic tracing is satisfactory, although an oscilloscope clearly in view is perhaps the simplest approach to this problem. The electrocardiogram may furnish the first sign of a severe reaction.

The Injection

After the preliminary films have been reviewed and found satisfactory, the patency of the catheter must be ensured. The catheter is then attached to the syringe containing the opaque medium. A pressure injector should be employed. The catheter should be as thin-walled and as large as possible. Four side holes permit more rapid injection of the contrast agent with less catheter strain. The injection must be performed as rapidly as possible because the opaque medium is rapidly cleared from the aorta. If the injection is slow, the medium will be too diluted to delineate the anatomy of the area under investigation.

Number of Films

A minimum of two films per second in both projections for 3 to 5 seconds is required. The most significant information is usually present on the films obtained during the first 1½ seconds after injection. Therefore, if the film changer has a capacity for getting four or more films per second, it is desirable to program the study so that a larger number of films per second is obtained for the first 2 seconds of the study. Later films may give information about the collateral vessels or, in the case of patent ductus arteriosus, may show left atrial, left ventricular, and finally ascending aortic opacification. The use of digital subtraction in aortography has been popularized during the last decade.[50,51]

Postaortography Measures

Immediately after the procedure, the catheter is attached to a continuous drip or to a syringe containing heparinized saline. The patient is carefully observed, and the electrocardiogram is monitored. The films are processed as quickly as possible; immediate viewing of the films will reveal whether a satisfactory examination has been obtained. If the examination proves to have been adequate, the catheter should be removed and, if a cutdown has been performed, the arterial wall is repaired transversely with number 6-0 eyesilk sutures. Digital compression may be needed for hemostasis, and when percutaneous puncture has been employed, continuous pressure for at least 5 minutes is desirable. After arterial closure has been effected, the patient should be returned to his or her room. Careful palpation of the distal pulses is essential throughout and after compression of the puncture site, and continuous close observation for 4 hours is necessary. It is our policy to keep the patient under observation in the hospital for at least 24 hours after the procedure.

The Urogram

A conventional film of the abdomen obtained 10 to 15 minutes after the last injection usually furnishes a good urographic study. Particularly in patients in whom congenital anomalies are being studied, this film may render a surprisingly high yield of significant renal lesions.

Repeat Injections

We prefer to limit the number of injections during a single examination. If diagnostic information is not obtained at the initial injection, however, we have not hesitated to perform subsequent injections.

Medium Employed

Until the early 1980s, 60 percent or 76 percent Renografin (in adults), Hypaque, or Conray was the medium that we used. Below 40 pounds, the concentration was 60 percent; above 40 pounds, 76 percent. Since then, interest has grown in low-osmolality media such as Hexabrix (sodium meglumine ioxaglate), which offer greater patient tolerance but are considerably more expensive. Hexabrix 250 affords acceptable opacification with lower cost, smaller catheters, and slight diminution of patient discomfort as compared to Hexabrix 320.[52–54]

Volume of Medium

Body weight is the most useful criterion of volume of medium because chronologic and developmental age may differ widely, particularly in infants and children with heart disease. Table 15-1 gives the dosage schedule that we have adopted.

Table 15-1. Volume of Contrast Agent in Thoracic Aortography

Weight (pounds)	Volume (ml)
6–8	5
8–10	6
10–15	8
15–20	9
20–25	10
25–30	12
30–35	14
35–40	15
40–50	20
60–80	30
80–100	35
100–130	40
130+	45

Indications for Thoracic Aortography

Thoracic aortography is indicated when a diagnostic problem involving the aorta or its great branches cannot be clarified by conventional means. It is also useful when, in the presence of disease of the aorta or its branches, exact preoperative delineation of the deranged anatomy is required. To generalize about indications is unwarranted, however; each case must be individualized and dealt with on its own merits. In the chapters to follow, the usefulness of applying this technique to specific lesions will be described in detail. Briefly stated, thoracic aortography may be rewarding in the presence of the lesions described below.

Congenital Anomalies

Patent Ductus Arteriosus

In congestive heart failure in infants, retrograde brachial aortography may differentiate a patent ductus arteriosus from a large intracardiac shunt as the cause of failure. It is particularly helpful when the classic continuous murmur is absent.

Aortic Septal Defect

In the presence of a continuous murmur, the differentiation of a patent ductus arteriosus from an aortic window may depend on direct visualization of the communication.

Ruptured Aortic Sinus Aneurysm

A cardioaortic fistula can only be diagnosed conclusively by aortography.

Coarctation of the Aorta

In cases of coarctation, the clinical picture can be confusing, with a variety of lesions causing a lowered blood pressure in the left arm. Atypical forms of coarctation exist, involving atresia or stenosis of the left subclavian artery or a right subclavian artery rising distal to arch coarctation.[55] Aortography permits definitive diagnosis and indicates the location, degree, and length of the coarctation. The relationship of the great vessels to the narrowed zone is also shown. The effects of either surgery or balloon angioplasty may be depicted with precision.[56]

Pseudocoarctation

When the roentgenographic contours of coarctation are visible but the corresponding pressure changes are absent, the presence of pseudocoarctation may be ascertained.

Aortic Arch Anomalies

Most anomalies of the aortic arch are readily diagnosable by conventional roentgenologic techniques. In the rare instance in which the symptoms are severe and the nature of the anomaly is unclear, retrograde aortography may help elucidate the anatomy of the malformation.

Truncus Arteriosus

If a true truncus is present, with the pulmonary arteries arising from the aorta, the lesion is inoperable. In such a case, the exact origin of the pulmonary arteries may be clearly delineated.

Sequestration of the Lung

Branch vessels from the lower thoracic or upper abdominal aorta supplying a sequestrated portion of lung may be visualized preoperatively by aortography.

Study of the Blalock-Taussig Anastomosis

When a question arises as to the patency of the subclavian pulmonary artery anastomosis, thoracic aortography permits direct demonstration of patency or occlusion.

Acquired Disease

Aneurysm of the Aorta

The precise site of involvement of an aneurysm of the aortic arch is frequently important in determining the surgical approach to the lesion. At times it is necessary to distinguish aneurysm from tumor.

Aortic Dissection or Trauma

Aortography is of prime importance when dissection or rupture of the thoracic aorta is suspected. Especially after trauma, chest radiographs may show an increased width of the mediastinum or an abnormal aortic shadow, but these signs only indicate an increased likelihood of an abnormal, definitive aortogram.[57–59] Clinical signs in the absence of radiographic criteria may also warrant angiographic assessment,[60] but up to one-third of patients show no external evidence of trauma.[59] Aortography, as well as providing a definitive diagnosis, localizes the site and extent of the lesion and enables the surgeon to plan the approach. It is also valuable in showing the postoperative status of the ascending aorta.[48,61]

Aortic Insufficiency

Injection into the root of the aorta permits a rough estimation of the degree of regurgitation through the valve.

Aortic Stenosis

The anatomy of the valve may be visualized and the size of the orifice estimated by thoracic aortography.

Aortic Arch Syndrome

In the presence of so-called pulseless disease, aortography permits the demonstration of the precise site of stenoses of the great vessels arising from the aortic arch.

Buckling of the Brachiocephalic Arteries

At times a buckled innominate or carotid artery suggests the presence on plain films of a tumor at the thoracic inlet. Opacification of the aortic arch and its great branches permits ready differentiation of tumor from the relatively innocuous buckling of the vessels.

The foregoing, then, are some of the lesions in which aortography has proved a useful method of study in the past. Whether this kind of study is required must be determined in each case by the physicians responsible for the diagnosis and care of the patient's illness.

Hazards

The hazards of thoracic aortography have been incompletely explored in the past, although a number of deaths and serious reactions have been attributed to this technique.[22,62–72] An effort was made some years ago[73] to arrive at some reasonable estimate of the dangers of retrograde thoracic aortography as performed in many centers throughout the world in order to (1) provide a frame of reference in which the potential value of the information to be gained might be balanced against the risk and (2) to determine which technique seemed safest and what safeguards might be employed to minimize the risk. These data, obtained in the mid-1950s, are important in shedding light on the factors related to complications. Thoracic aortography clearly has a far larger margin of safety today, as will be noted later in this chapter.

Table 15-2. Thoracic Aortography: Concentration of Medium and Death

Concentration	No. of Cases	No. of Deaths	Mortality (%)
30–35%	370	1	0.027
50%	128	2	1.60
70% or higher	1162	24	2.07

Data from Abrams HL. Radiologic aspects of operable heart disease: III. The hazards of retrograde thoracic aortography: a survey. Radiology 1957;68:812.

Death in Thoracic Aortography

In the 1950s study,[73] 29 deaths were reported in a total of 1706 thoracic aortograms. This represented a mortality of 1.7 percent and included all types and concentrations of media and various sites of injection.

Contrast Agents

The concentration of the medium employed was found to be a significant factor (Table 15-2). There was only one death in 370 cases in which a 30 or 35 percent concentration of the medium was used,* contrasted with 24 deaths in 1162 cases in which a 70 percent concentration was employed. There was thus about eight times as high a death rate with the more highly concentrated media.

No conclusive statements can be made about the effect of total dosage. It is, however, of interest that in 11 of the 29 deaths, two or more injections of the opaque medium were employed. Many of the deaths followed the use of a high total dose, and this was also true of some of the severe nonfatal reactions. At the time of the survey, Urokon had been in general use and, together with Diodrast, accounted for most deaths. No deaths were recorded with Renografin, the agent most commonly used today, but the number of cases was small.

*The literature records an additional retrograde aortographic death purportedly associated with the use of a 35 percent medium.[70] This case was reviewed, and it was found that 70 percent Diodrast had been employed (WG Scott, personal communication, 1959).

Table 15-3. Thoracic Aortography: Route of Injection and Death

Route	No. of Cases	No. of Deaths	Mortality (%)
Brachial artery	521	4	0.71
Catheter in aorta	967	13	1.35
Carotid artery	210	11	5.24
Direct puncture	8	1	
Total	1706	29	1.70

Data from Abrams HL. Radiologic aspects of operable heart disease: III. The hazards of retrograde thoracic aortography: a survey. Radiology 1957;68:812.

Site of Injection

The data in Table 15-3 suggest that injection directly into the carotid artery increased the hazard. The mortality was higher than when brachial artery or catheter injections were used. The group of brachial artery injections was not entirely comparable with the group of carotid artery injections because the former included more studies with media of lower concentrations. When carotid and catheter injections of comparable media were compared, the mortality after carotid injection was significantly higher.

Premedication and Anesthesia

About three-fourths of the procedures were performed under general anesthesia. Open-drop ether or intravenous Pentothal were the preferred agents. Premedication given to those patients examined under local anesthesia usually included a combination of barbiturates and morphine or barbiturates and Demerol. A number of workers also routinely employed small doses of scopolamine or atropine.

The data failed to support the idea that the use of general anesthesia increases the danger of the procedure. On the other hand, a number of the comments suggested that death was due to the general anesthesia. Furthermore, the group of deaths associated with local anesthesia was weighted by two cases in which death preceded the injection of any medium, two instances in which the patients were moribund to begin with, and three instances in which most of the medium was injected by error into the innominate or common carotid artery. This factor is of little relevance today because aortography is generally performed under light sedation.

Age

A clear-cut influence of age on the risk involved was not apparent.

Condition of Patient

About two-thirds of the patients who died were in poor condition at the time of the procedure. A number of patients, however, were in relatively good health.

Certain factors are generally felt to increase the risk of aortography. Patients receiving anticoagulants and those having hypertension, arteriosclerosis, or aortic insufficiency are at greater risk from the procedure than are those with other medical problems.[74] The presence of aortic laceration also increases the risk.[75]

Mode of Death

Among those cases in which the factors responsible for death seemed most clear, brain damage and the complications thereof were noted in nine instances, the largest single group among the deaths.* In these cases, convulsions, hemiplegia, aphasia, and coma developed, and death occurred in hours to days. Among the pathologic findings described in these cases were cerebral edema, cerebral "damage," acute hemorrhagic foci in the brain, and cerebral necrosis. In the three instances in which a clear-cut respiratory death occurred, there seems a reasonable likelihood that this may have been due to medullary damage following the injection of the opaque medium. In these cases an initial respiratory apnea was sustained without subsequent recovery. In two cases death was attributed to heart failure, and in two cases death was due to renal failure. In three instances the question of an anesthetic death was raised, but the mode of death must be considered uncertain. In one case death certainly occurred from hemorrhage and in another from shock, and in four cases death was stated to be a combination of respiratory and cardiac failure.

Two of the catheter deaths occurred before injection. In 1 the catheter was thought to have lodged in a coronary artery, and in the second there was profuse hemorrhage about the site of insertion of the catheter, followed by the development of shock and death. The position of the catheter in the innominate or carotid artery was thought to contribute significantly to the death in four cases. Thus technical factors relating to the positioning of the catheter apparently contributed to at least 6 of the 13 catheter deaths.

Severe Nonfatal Reactions

Hemiplegia, with gradual return of function in a few days to a few months, developed in 13 patients. In 11 of these 13 patients, a 70 percent concentration of the

*Recommendations designed to forestall severe reactions are set forth in Chapters 3 and 4.

contrast agent was employed, and in 2 patients a 50 percent concentration. A large total dose was noted in a number of instances. The injection route was via a catheter in the aorta in 8 examinations and directly into the carotid artery in 4 examinations. In a few instances, some residual evidence of the hemiplegia remained over a long period of time.

Convulsions were noted after the procedure in six cases. In one of these cases, disorientation and blindness accompanied the convulsions, in another severe apnea and arrhythmias, and in a third, rather marked but temporary cyanosis. No permanent sequelae were observed.

A *severe renal reaction* with anuria or oliguria was observed in six cases. When recovery occurred, there was no evidence of residual renal damage. Although renal reactions are less common with the diatrizoate agents, they are still observed.[76–79]

Arterial thrombosis is among the most common and serious complications associated with aortography. It is diagnosed on the basis of decreased or absent pulsations distal to the site of arterial puncture and of other signs of impaired arterial circulation.[80] Depending on involvement, atheroembolizations can cause transient ischemic changes, monocular blindness, hemiparesis, and/or progressively fatal disease; the severity of the sequelae depends on the location of the organ obstructed by atheroemboli.[81] Postprocedure observation of aortography patients is critically important; in every case, diagnosis of arterial thrombosis should be possible within 4 hours of the procedure.[74] In one study of this complication, 7 of the 250 patients developed femoral artery thrombosis either (1) following arterial spasm, prolonged catheter manipulations in crossing the aortic valve, or prolonged local pressure to control hemorrhage from the puncture site or (2) as a result of cardiac failure and low cardiac output.[80] It was particularly common in the younger age group, and its frequency was thought to depend on catheter size (e.g., it was less common with polyethylene catheters and more common with Kifa or Gensini catheters).[80]

Diagnostic angiography has also resulted in atheroma embolization to the kidney, spleen, and pancreas.[17] Intimal damage with arterial dissection has occurred in arteriosclerotic patients with tortuous and atheromatous vessels; some authors feel that it is not worthwhile to struggle with negotiating a very tortuous and atheromatous aorta.[80]

Two other severe reactions deserve mention. In an adult patient with coarctation of the aorta, the tip of the catheter became lodged just above the site of the coarctation (at which time the patient complained of chest pain). When surgery for the coarctation was undertaken, a small dissection of the aorta was observed just above the site of coarctation; it was thought to have been initiated by the catheter tip. In one other patient, a Brown-Séquard syndrome developed with gradual recovery after a period of 2 weeks.

Other Reactions

Cardiovascular

Bradycardia was noted almost as frequently as tachycardia by most observers. Mild arrhythmias were observed in many cases, and among those who routinely employed continuous electrocardiography, electrocardiographic alterations of minor degree were not uncommon. Extrasystoles, T-wave changes, and nodal rhythm were recorded. Changes were prominent in patients with a large patent ductus arteriosus. Moderate lowering of blood pressure was described, and in a few instances a temporary shocklike state was reported.

Respiratory

Although short periods of apnea followed injection in some cases, hyperpnea was more commonly observed. In a small number of cases, Cheyne-Stokes respirations were reported. Cough was a common reaction, especially in the presence of patent ductus arteriosus.

Cerebral

Syncope and mental confusion, when they occurred, were usually associated with a major nonfatal reaction. Those instances in which convulsions and hemiplegia occurred are considered under the major nonfatal reactions.

Miscellaneous

Vomiting followed the aortogram in some cases but was usually associated with general anesthesia. Delayed allergic reactions with pruritus and fever were noted occasionally. In one case, a temporary brachial plexus palsy followed the procedure. In another, an inflammatory reaction occurred in an arteriovenous malformation about the shoulder. Gangrene of four fingers of the right hand after brachial artery catheterization was reported in one adult. There were two instances of ischemia of the hand after radial artery catheterization, both of which improved over a period of months. A single report of the appearance of the medium in the superior vena cava after brachial artery catheterization and injection indicated that a small rupture in the artery had occurred. This was substantiated by the appearance of a hematoma, but no permanent arteriovenous fistula resulted. One description of a postaortographic reaction resembling mesenteric thrombosis was included, and a case of rather severe laryngospasm was also noted.

Discussion

Because retrograde thoracic aortography, like all procedures involving the intravascular injection of contrast media,[82] has a significant complication rate, the risk must be weighed against the usefulness of the information to be derived in each instance. Unlike angiocardiography, a direct effect on the heart and the lungs is unlikely in thoracic aortography, except in the presence of patent ductus arteriosus or after injection into the coronary arteries. Unless the injection is through a catheter adjacent to the sinuses of Valsalva, the opaque medium seldom reaches the coronary circulation in significant amounts; indeed, in the retrograde brachial injection, the root of the aorta is rarely opacified.

The fact that electrocardiographic changes follow thoracic aortography does not constitute evidence of a direct effect on the heart in these cases; similar alterations are noted after encephalography,[83] electric shock,[84] or intracarotid Diodrast injection.[60] Although some of the opaque medium eventually reaches the lungs after transit through the brain and right heart, it is too diluted to produce significant or direct respiratory reactions. These reactions are probably mediated by the medullary respiratory centers. That the brain is a major center of postaortographic reactions is corroborated not only by study of the deaths but also by study of the severe nonfatal reactions—in which convulsions and hemiplegias predominate.

All the iodinated contrast media in general use are capable of producing profound cerebral damage. Broman and Olsson demonstrated that breakdown of the blood-brain barrier occurs after the injection of Diodrast into the carotid artery and that respiratory paralysis may develop.[85] They also noted that edema and punctate hemorrhages were visible histologically if the dosages of Diodrast were high enough.[85,86] They have pointed out that the severity of the disturbance of permeability is related to the concentration of the medium and to the duration of its action, that the injury is reversible if it is slight, and that preexisting cerebral tissue changes increase the risk of disturbing cerebrovascular permeability.[87] Their findings have been amply confirmed in subsequent investigations[66,88–90] and in clinical studies.[91,92] Nevertheless, the newer agents seem to be less noxious when they reach the cerebral circulation.

There were two deaths and a number of severe nonfatal reactions caused by renal injury, and certainly the effect on the kidney is another serious consideration. Probably preexisting renal damage with associated azotemia should be considered a relative contraindication to thoracic aortography. The risk of renal failure is particularly high in patients with long-standing diabetes and systemic complications.[77] Acute severe systemic illness, old age, and dehydration are predisposing factors, particularly when combined with preexisting renal failure.[77,79] Careful postangiographic monitoring—especially of high-risk patients—is essential for early detection and proper treatment.[93] Most cases respond to conservative management.

The role of general anesthesia as an additional hazard should be noted. In three instances, death was thought to be due to the general anesthetic. In spite of this, there is no objective evidence in the survey that general anesthesia augments the risk of thoracic aortography.

The technical errors attendant on catheter aortography have already been mentioned. The catheter should be in the midpoint of the ascending aorta at the time of injection.

The portion of our data on the complications of aortography that was collected during the mid-1950s was published initially in 1957.[73] Most deaths preceded the introduction of the diatrizoate agents. In 1959, data from a cooperative Swedish survey became available.[94] The mortality in our collected 1706 examinations was 1.7 percent, similar to that of the Swedish series, 1.5 percent in 340 examinations. Two of the five deaths in the Swedish series were related to the catheter procedure and preceded contrast injection; one other death was probably caused by vertebral artery thrombosis. In a subsequent series in which two deaths were associated with aortography, it was dubious whether the procedure itself accounted for the deaths.[95] What stands out in any review of the literature since 1959 is that the major complications seem to be related to the catheterization rather than to the contrast injection.[96–98] A few deaths have been reported[96,98] but no recent comprehensive survey of the complications of thoracic aortography is at hand. This is significant because the newer contrast media appear to be appreciably less hazardous and deaths from thoracic aortography less frequent.

The technical aspects of the catheterization deserve some comment. Manipulation of the catheter and prolonged procedure time have been found to greatly increase the risk of arterial hemorrhage and thrombosis. Thrombosis shares several predisposing factors with its forerunner, arterial spasm: (1) the size of the catheter used, (2) excessive compression of the artery after withdrawal of the catheter, (3) prolonged catheter manipulations, and (4) low cardiac output failure in the patient.[74,80]

Breakage of the catheter is an infrequent complication of aortography.[74]

As noted above, catheterization via both the brachial and femoral routes may be associated with occlusive manifestations.[97] In one study, 2 percent of patients undergoing axillary catheterization for thoracic aortography had a loss of pulse, and axillary thrombectomy was required in three patients.[43] Sutton and Davies reported one death in 330 patients and one patient with leg ischemia.[98] Others have recorded arterial dissection, major artery thrombosis, and pseudoaneurysm.[99] A death reported by Judkins and Dotter followed catheter embolism to the brain.[96] In one case cerebral ischemia developed in a patient with a dissecting aneurysm after injection into the false lumen; the entry was by brachial artery catheterization.[100]

Recent surveys of coronary arteriography (see Chap. 24) and of abdominal angiography (see Chap. 41) support the belief that the contrast agent no longer constitutes the major hazard of the procedure and that the mortality and morbidity have been sharply reduced in the past decade.[101,102] In a study of 118,000 examinations that included thoracic and abdominal aortography, the overall complication rate varied depending on the method of catheter entry. It was 1.73 percent for the femoral, 2.89 percent for the lumbar, and 3.29 percent for the axillary arteriographic approach. The mortality was an extraordinary 0.032 percent, compared to the 1.7 percent[73] and 1.5 percent[94] of earlier periods. There were 30 deaths, 8 of which were caused by aortic dissection or by aneurysm rupture. Among the three techniques, there was no difference in the incidence of cardiac complications. There were significantly more neurologic complications, including seizures, in the axillary group than in either the femoral or the lumbar group. Similarly, hemorrhage, arterial obstruction, and pseudoaneurysms were more common with the axillary technique than with either of the other approaches. Vessel perforation and extraluminal contrast were seen most frequently with the translumbar technique. There was an inverse relationship between the complication rate and the annual number of arteriograms, similar to that observed with coronary arteriography.[101]

Thus the evidence is strong that thoracic aortography requires continuous, careful attention to the details of the catheterization procedure by an experienced team. Procedure time should be kept as short as possible, arterial pressure monitored, vigorous flushing maintained, and careful femoral artery compression continued after catheter withdrawal with palpation of the distal pulse. Vascular occlusion or severe hemorrhage should be followed by prompt surgical intervention; and meticulous postangiographic observation and care will diminish the likelihood of both delayed hemorrhage and pseudoaneurysm formation.

The Normal Aorta in Infants

Contrast roentgenologic studies of the normal aorta in humans have been limited largely to older children and adults[38,103] although some material on infants is available.[25] Angiography and ultrasonography, both noninvasive techniques, have been used to measure and assess the mechanical properties of the normal aorta.[104] Attention has focused on (1) circumferential elasticity and pulse-wave velocity,[104] (2) wall distensibility and reflex hemodynamic responses,[105] (3) elastic stiffness and lumen volume,[106] and (4) the displacement of the aorta to the left of the spine that is common in old people and thought to result from arteriosclerotic elongation of the vessel.[107] To assess the appearance of the aorta in the first few years of life in detail, 40 normal aortographic studies were analyzed some years ago. Most of these studies were performed with the retrograde brachial technique, the method we employed at the time to define the aortic arch and its abnormalities in infants.[62] The number of examinations in each age group is noted in Table 15-4.

The Aortic Silhouette

When satisfactory opacification of the thoracic aorta is obtained, its radiographic appearance resembles an inverted J of variable configuration (Figs. 15-3 through 15-10).

The most proximal of the four segments of the thoracic aorta is the *aortic root,* or *aortic bulb.* It comprises the segment of the aorta from the valve cusps to the cephalad tip of the aortic sinuses (the sinuses of Valsalva) (see Fig. 15-8). Immediately above the aortic

Table 15-4. Age Distribution of 40 Patients with Normal Aortograms

Age	Number of Aortograms
Under 3 months	8
4–8 months	13
9–12 months	7
1–2 years	6
2–4 years	6

Data from Abrams HL. Radiologic aspects of operable heart disease: II. Retrograde brachial aortography. Circulation 1956;14:593.

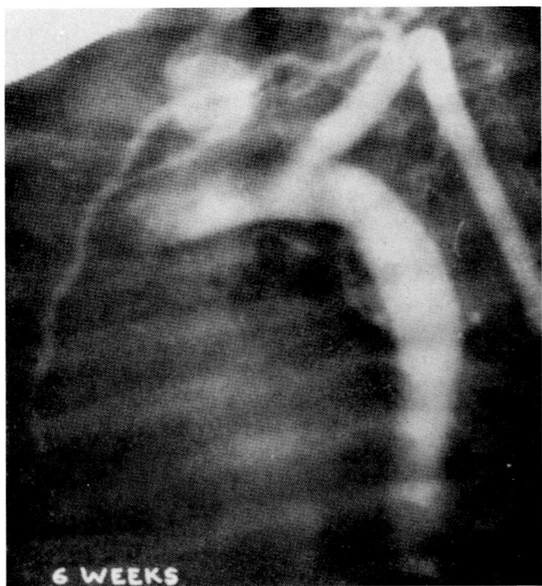

Figure 15-3. Normal aorta, 6 weeks. The left subclavian artery, internal mammary artery, much of the aortic arch, and the descending aorta are densely opacified. Distal to the origin of the left subclavian artery is an area of diffuse dilatation of the aortic arch that gradually merges with the descending aorta.

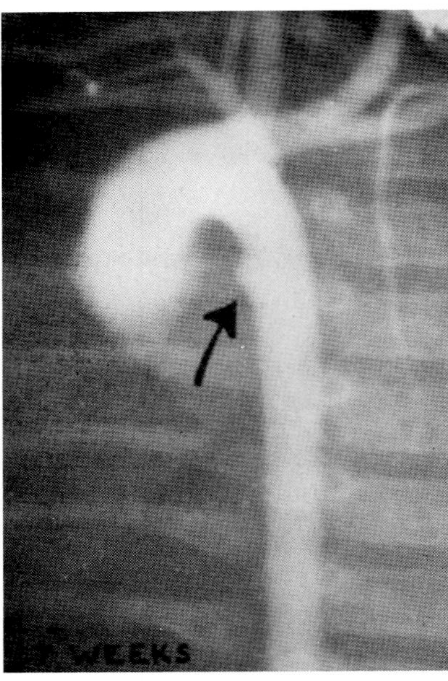

Figure 15-4. Normal aorta, 7 weeks. The aortic arch and its great branches are clearly defined. The silhouette of the arch and the descending aorta resembles an inverted J. A localized bulge at the site of the ligamentum arteriosum (*arrow*) corresponds to the "ductus diverticulum," or the "infundibulum" of the ductus.

Figure 15-5. Normal aorta, 7 weeks. Just opposite the origin of the left subclavian artery is a localized indentation or constriction, beyond which is a zone of dilatation (*arrow*). This dilatation is largely confined to the anterior wall and is probably related to the ligamentum arteriosum. The indentation is slight in degree and of no hemodynamic significance. Note the variable location of the origin of the left subclavian artery (compare with Figs. 15-3, 15-6, and 15-8). This probably reflects differing degrees of cephalad migration of the left subclavian artery in early development.

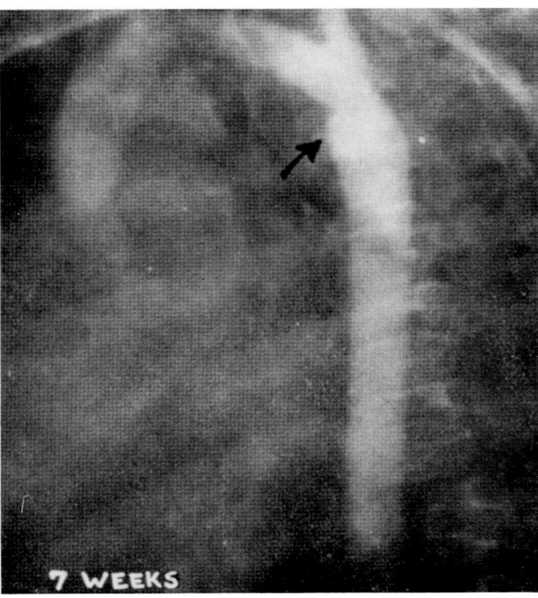

Figure 15-6. Normal aorta, 8 weeks. The entire aortic arch and the aortic sinuses are visible. A localized area of narrowing (*arrow*) in the isthmus of the aorta is followed by a rather diffuse area of dilatation. The narrowing was insufficient to produce a disparity between the blood pressures of the upper and lower limbs during life. At autopsy the zone of constriction was noted, but the aortic lumen seemed ample. This zone represents the residuum of the normal narrowing of the aortic isthmus present at birth.

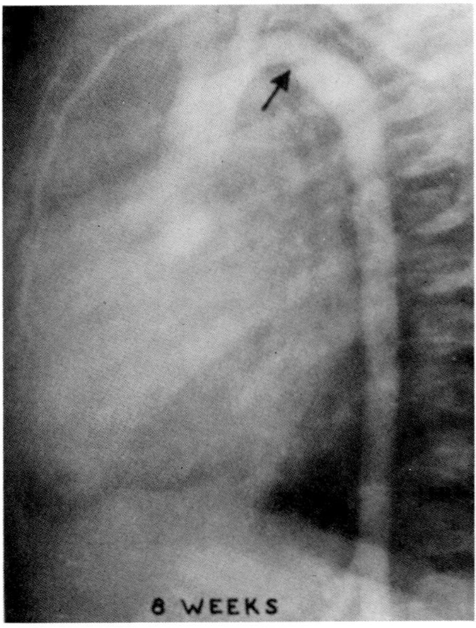

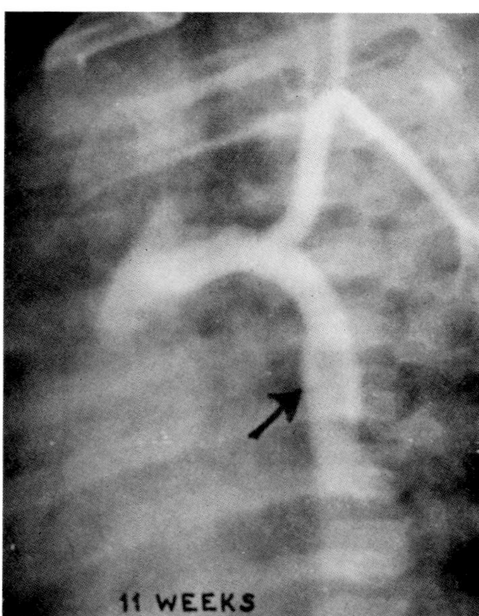

Figure 15-7. Normal aorta, 11 weeks. The aortic lumen distal to the origin of the left subclavian artery is narrower than the proximal portion of the arch. There is a relatively diffuse bulge (*arrow*) anteriorly at the junction of the aortic arch and descending aorta. Note the excellent visualization of the left vertebral artery.

sinuses, the ascending aorta extends almost to the level of origin of the innominate artery, to become the aortic arch. The ascending aorta joins the arch at the level of the second costal cartilage; the arch curves gently upward, backward, to the left, and finally downward to become continuous with the descending aorta at the lower border of the fourth thoracic vertebra (see Fig. 15-6). The ascending segment is the widest portion of the aorta (see Figs. 15-4 through 15-6) and arises from deep within the cardiac mass (see Fig. 15-6). The aortic arch normally narrows slightly beyond the origin of the innominate artery (see Fig. 15-8). Further narrowing occurs after the origin of the left common carotid and left subclavian arteries. A more striking narrowing may then be observed in the "isthmus" of the aorta, the segment between the origin of the left subclavian artery and the ligamentum arteriosum. At times this narrowing may be localized (see Figs. 15-5 and 15-6), and it is then followed by a distinctive dilatation of the aorta beyond. In other instances, the narrowing may be diffuse but relatively slight in degree. It then usually involves the entire isthmus and is followed by a definite widening of the aorta at the junction of the aortic arch and descending thoracic aorta (see Figs. 15-7 and 15-10). The descending aorta in the steep right posterior oblique projection

Figure 15-8. Normal aorta, 3½ months. (A) Left posterior oblique projection. (B) Right posterior oblique projection. A localized bulge at the site of the ligamentum arteriosum is clearly visible. The aortic valve is visible, and there is coronary artery filling. Note the relative size of the ascending and descending limbs of the aortic arch.

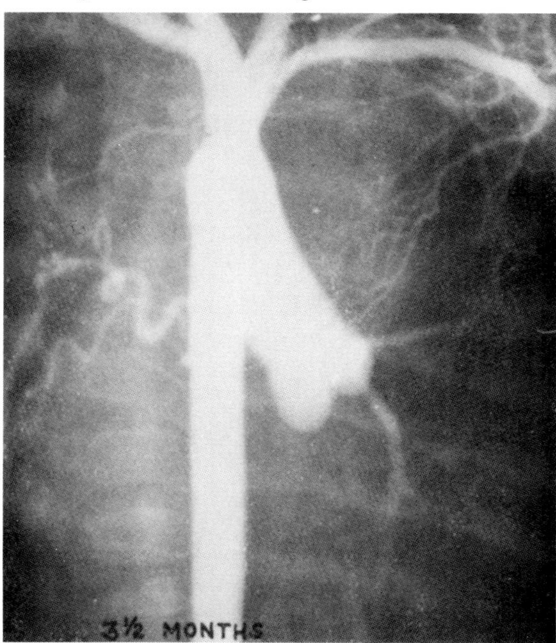

A

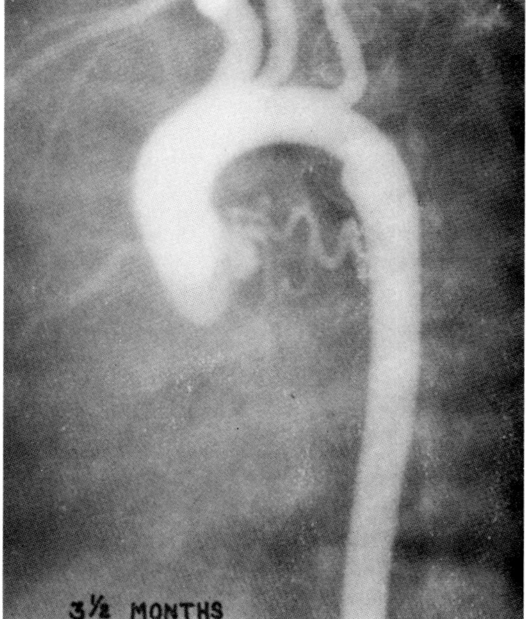

B

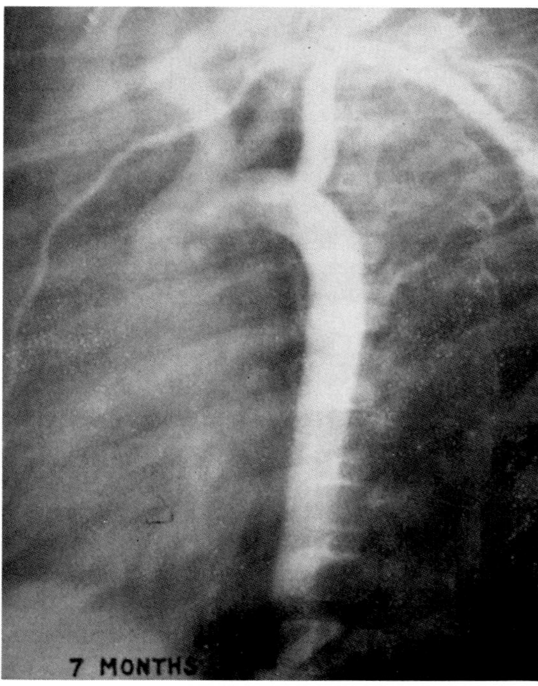

Figure 15-9. Normal aorta, 7 months. The aortic arch is smooth, with no evidence of local narrowing or dilatation. The origin of the innominate artery is clearly shown, and the internal mammary artery is well opacified.

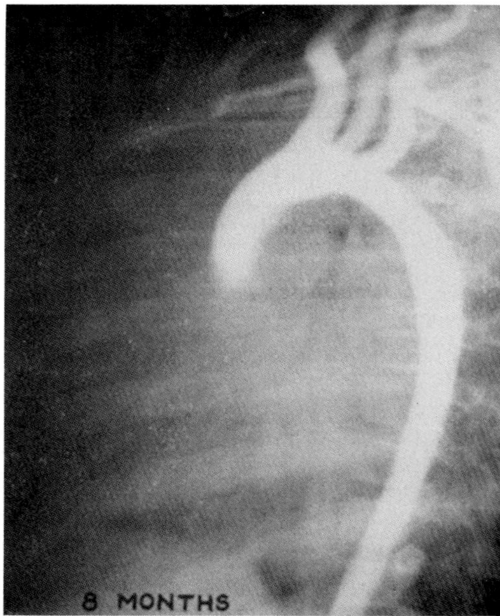

Figure 15-10. Normal aorta, 8 months. The aortic arch, its great branches, and the descending aorta are densely opacified. There is slight narrowing of the isthmus of the arch, followed by an area of diffuse dilatation at the junction of the arch and descending aorta. Note the inverted J configuration.

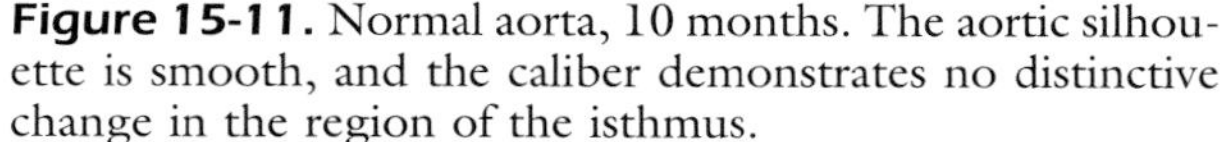

Figure 15-11. Normal aorta, 10 months. The aortic silhouette is smooth, and the caliber demonstrates no distinctive change in the region of the isthmus.

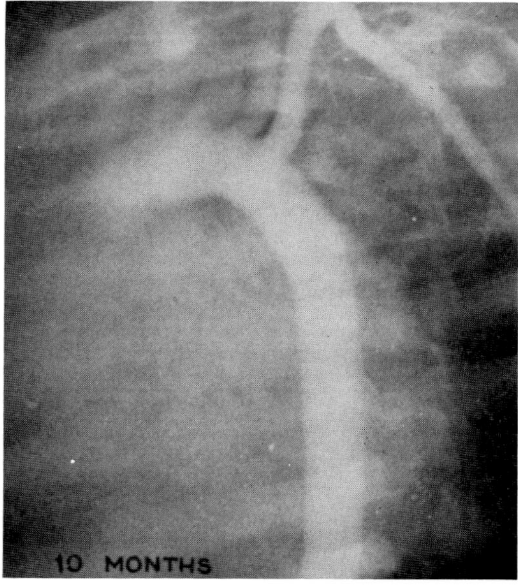

gradually crosses the spine and usually lies over the anterior portion of the spine when it reaches the diaphragm (see Fig. 15-10). As it descends, there is a slight but definite decrease in aortic caliber until, at the level of the diaphragm, it is about two-thirds of the diameter of the proximal descending aorta (Figs. 15-9 through 15-12).

The "Ductus Diverticulum"

Dilatation of the aorta distal to the origin of the left subclavian artery and in the region of the ligamentum arteriosum was noticed in 13 of the 40 patients (see Figs. 15-4, 15-5, 15-8, and 15-12). This bulge varied in size; was generally more pronounced in patients in the youngest age group; and usually, but not always, involved the anterior wall more than the posterior wall. In Figure 15-3, a diffuse dilatation of the aorta beyond the isthmus is apparent. In Figures 15-4 and 15-13, a localized bulge at the site of the ligamentum arteriosum may be observed.

The Effect of Increasing Age

According to the data presented in one analysis,[108] linear correlations exist between body length and the diameter of the aortic ostium. Although there is definite

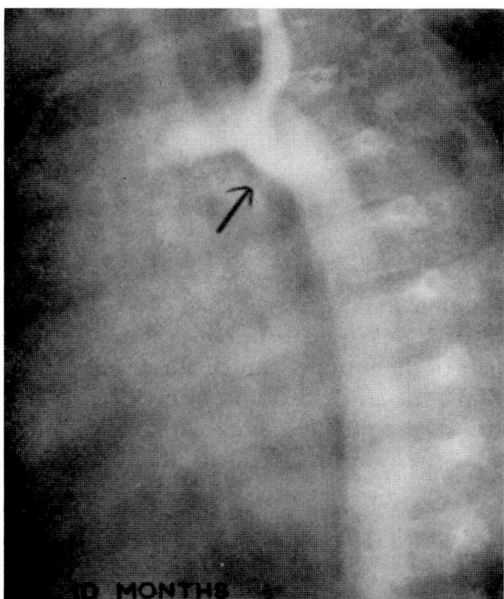

Figure 15-12. Normal aorta, 10 months. The bulge at the site of the ligamentum arteriosum is prominent (*arrow*), in contrast with the appearance in another 10-month-old infant (see Fig. 15-11).

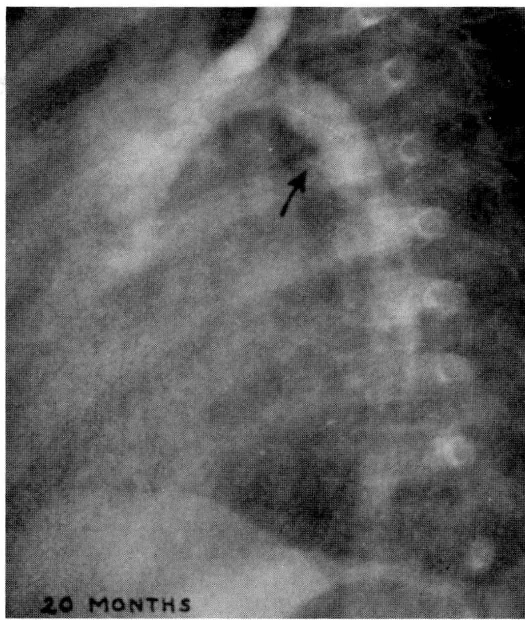

Figure 15-13. Normal aorta, 20 months. There is an outpouching in the region of the ligamentum arteriosum (*arrow*).

variation in the configuration of the arch, within the limits of our study no consistent age effect beyond the gradual loss of the narrowed isthmus was apparent. Even this finding was by no means constant, however. Thus, in Figures 15-9 and 15-11, there is no visible narrowing of the isthmus at the ages of 7 and 10 months, respectively; but in Figures 15-10 and 15-14, at the ages of 8 months and 4 years, respectively, some residual narrowing of the isthmus is present.

Next to the lateral or superior aspect of the arch, the left superior intercostal vein presents as a small mass that changes in size with alterations in posture and intrathoracic pressure. It is important to realize that this aortic "nipple" is a normal vascular shadow, not to be confused with tumor or with lymphadenopathy.[109]

In a general way, the semicircle described by the aortic arch in infancy is usually more shallow than that found in the adult aorta (the radius of which is approximately 1.5 cm, with a 4.5-cm radius of the curvature).[110] This probably is related to the relatively large transverse and anteroposterior diameters and somewhat short vertical height of the infant's chest.

The Vessels Opacified

Although with retrograde brachial aortography the left axillary, subclavian, and vertebral arteries are consistently visualized (see Figs. 15-3 through 15-5), the

Figure 15-14. Normal aorta, 4 years. The overall appearance of the aortic arch and the descending aorta is similar to that in the first year, except that the arc of the aortic arch is slightly steeper (compare with Figs. 15-3, 15-5, and 15-8).

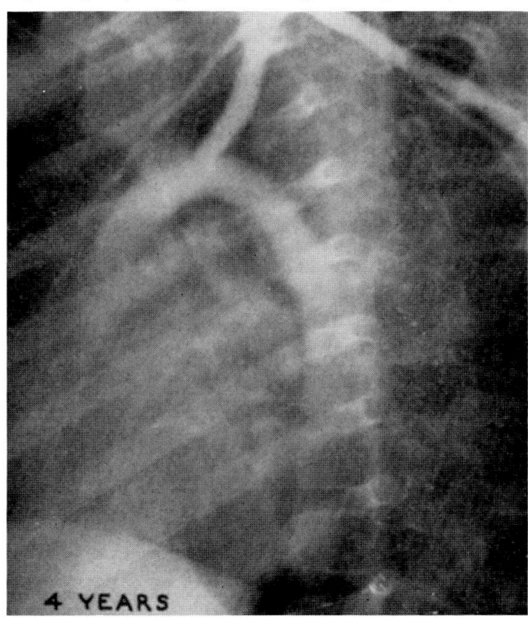

other branches of the aortic arch are not always opacified. Catheter aortography, with the tip in the ascending aorta above the aortic valve, generally ensures excellent delineation of all branches to the head, neck, and arms. Similarly, the ascending aorta, transverse portion of the aortic arch, descending thoracic aorta, and abdominal aorta may all be precisely defined. The intercostal and brachial arteries are frequently well opacified, particularly when they are enlarged and serve as collateral pathways. Although most anatomy books and classic descriptions state that the intercostal arteries, which vary in number from three to eight, arise from the dorsal aspect of the descending aorta, one study (based on examination of 600 cadavers) found that the upper right intercostal arteries arise instead from the ventral right aspect or right lateral aspect.[107] This observation may prove significant to the cardiovascular surgeon. (An interesting hypothesis arose from this study: namely, that during development, the heart rotates and the aorta rotates counterclockwise, which explains the position of the intercostal arteries.[107])

The normal internal mammary artery may be a vessel of considerable size in the infant aortogram. In comparing the size of the internal mammary artery in normal infants with that found in infants with coarctation, it becomes obvious that there is a wide range of overlap. Alone, the size of these vessels in infants is a poor index of their participation in a large collateral system designed to circumvent a constriction of the aorta. In addition, the gross tortuosity of the intercostal vessels visible in adults with coarctation of the aorta is not always present in infants. The demonstration of the collateral circulation in infants with coarctation is by no means as useful a sign as it has been considered to be in older children and adults.[111] Thus statements about the size of these arteries should be made with a clear realization of the range of normal variation.

Recirculation

A relatively large amount of opaque medium may reach the cerebral circulation. When this happens, its return via the jugular veins to the superior vena cava and right heart may be clearly observed in the later films in the series. Recirculation with opacification of the right atrium, right ventricle, and pulmonary artery was observed in 7 of the 40 normal aortograms. Maximal opacification of the right heart chambers and pulmonary arteries may be sufficient to suggest a misdiagnosis of patent ductus arteriosus. Careful observation of the sequence and foreknowledge of the amount of recirculation that may occur are useful safeguards against this possibility.

The Normal Aorta in Older Children and Adults

The adult thoracic aorta, like that of the infant, may conveniently be divided into four segments: the aortic bulb, the ascending aorta, the aortic arch, and the descending aorta (Figs. 15-15 and 15-16). It should be noted that the intrapericardial portion of the thoracic aorta is visible in perhaps one-half of adult chest films, possibly because of periaortic fat. Whenever this lowermost part of the intrapericardial aorta is discernible on chest films, the aortic ostium can be localized exactly; in addition, the phenomenon can be clinically useful for localizing intracardiac calcifications in relation to the aortic orifice and for evaluating the width and shape of the aortic root.[112]

As noted above, the *aortic root* is formed by the three sinuses of Valsalva. If the opaque substance has been correctly injected into the middle part of the ascending aorta, the sinuses of Valsalva and the semilunar valves will always be shown in the roentgenograms (see Figs. 15-15 and 15-16). The movements of the valves can be studied in detail with rapid serial large film aortography or, more commonly today, with cineangiocardiography. An idea of the valvular thickness can also be gained. To be regarded as normal, the valves should not appear thicker than roughly 1 mm on the aortogram. In posteroanterior views, the aortic bulb forms an angle of greater or lesser size (as a rule, 15–30 degrees) with the longitudinal axis of the body. The semilunar valves are nevertheless clearly seen in lateral views. In posteroanterior views, the aortic bulb overlies the vertebral column and consequently is not easily distinguished. Hence, if the aortic bulb is to be studied in more detail, the patient must be turned to the right 10 to 15 degrees around his or her longitudinal axis. If the aorta has been visualized by injecting the contrast agent into the pulmonary artery, the semilunar valves can be seen only in the lateral views (Fig. 15-17); in the posteroanterior view, the aortic bulb and all its details are obscured by superimposed opaque medium in the left atrium.

The *coronary arteries* are always more or less clearly distinguishable, and the first part of their course, at least, can be studied in detail after the injection of opaque medium into the ascending aorta (see Fig. 15-15). If the injection is into the pulmonary artery, the coronary vessels will not be as clearly shown.

The *ascending aorta* forms a tube of uniform width, 4 to 5 cm long. It curves backward and to the left and becomes continuous with the aortic arch at the level of the second right costal cartilage. If the ascending aorta is not of uniform width, it is not normal. When

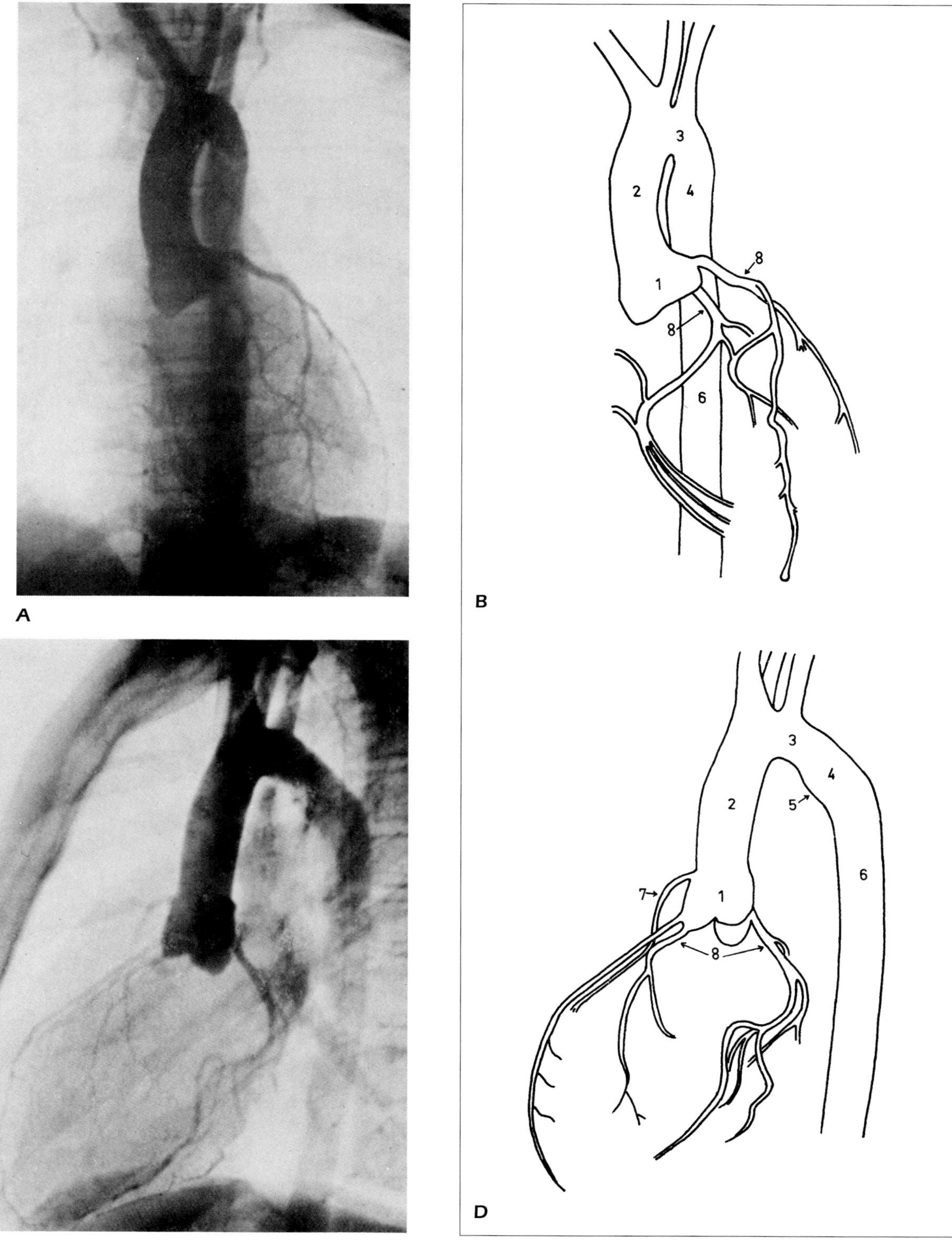

Figure 15-15. Normal thoracic aorta in a boy aged 15, anteroposterior (A and B) and lateral (C and D) views. The coronary arteries are well opacified. The left coronary artery is predominant and spreads out over the greater part of the heart. The right one is uncommonly small. The left originates from the left sinus of Valsalva, the right from the anterior sinus. All three sinuses of Valsalva are clearly visible in the lateral view. The valves are of normal thickness, and the aortic arch is semicircular. The left subclavian artery arises ventral to the vertex of the arch. A slight bulge distinguishable at the level of the isthmus is the remains of the infundibulum of the ductus arteriosus. *1,* Aortic bulb with sinuses of Valsalva; *2,* ascending aorta; *3,* aortic arch; *4,* isthmus of aorta; *5,* remains of infundibulum of ductus arteriosus; *6,* descending aorta; *7,* right coronary artery; *8,* branches of the left coronary artery.

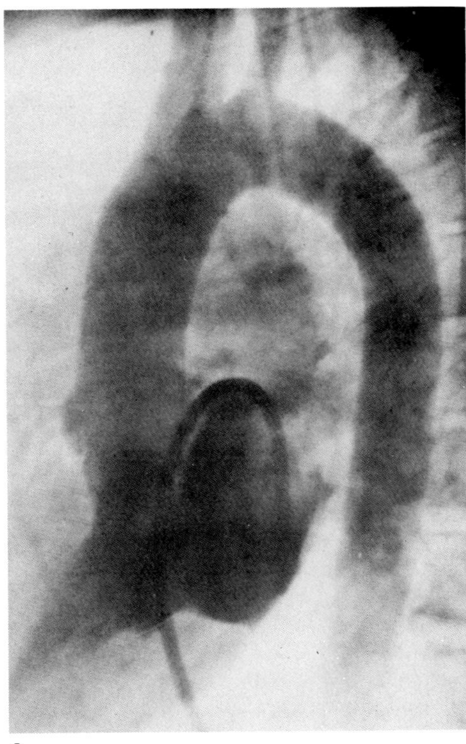

A

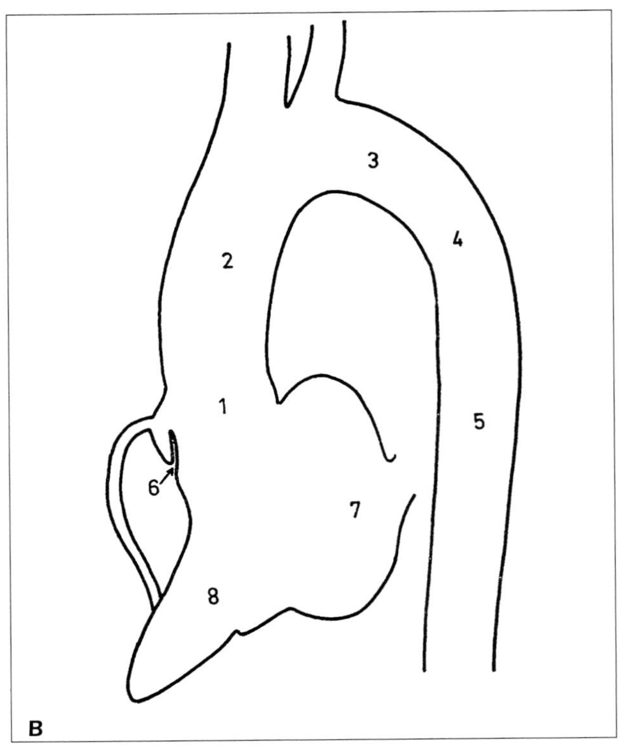

Figure 15-16. "Normal" thoracic aorta in a woman aged 25. (A and B) Lateral projection. There is a patent foramen ovale or a small atrial septal defect; nevertheless, the aorta can be regarded as normal. The contrast fluid was injected into the left atrium through a catheter, the tip of which had been maneuvered into that chamber from the right atrium. The outline of the aorta is consistently even, and at the level of the isthmus there are no signs either of indentation or of remains of the infundibulum of the ductus arteriosus. *1,* Aortic bulb; *2,* ascending aorta; *3,* aortic arch; *4,* isthmus of aorta; *5,* descending aorta; *6,* semilunar valve; *7,* left atrium; *8,* left ventricle.

measured in the lateral view and reduced to allow for the geometric magnification of the roentgenogram, the diameter in the middle part of the ascending aorta is usually 20 to 25 mm in juveniles between the ages of 7 and 16, and 25 and 30 mm in the 17- to 30-year age group.

The *aortic arch* has the shape of a semicircle with markedly longer arms than in infancy because of the more vertical orientation of the adult thorax. Slightly ventral to the vertex, it gives off the three large branches—the innominate, the left common carotid, and the left subclavian arteries. It is characteristic for the left subclavian artery normally to arise toward the ventral aspect of the arch. After the arch has given off the great vessels, its diameter is approximately two-thirds of the diameter of the ascending aorta. This means that the area of the arch is half as large.

The diameter of the aorta subsequently remains the same size as far as the transition into the descending aorta. The borderline between the arch and the descending aorta is marked by the isthmus, that is, the point at which the fourth left branchial arch artery unites with the dorsal aorta in the fetus. For the most part, there are no anatomic traces of this in adult life other than the insertion of the ligamentum arteriosum. The latter does not appear on the aortogram, but in some cases the anterior aortic wall is seen to be slightly irregular for a stretch of about 1 to 2 cm. The irregularity may be due to a slight indentation in the wall that causes a decrease in diameter of 1 to 2 mm. This is the isthmus. Shallow bulging of the anterior wall is found equally as often, however. This is a remnant of the infundibulum of the ductus arteriosus (see Fig. 15-15).

The *descending aorta* is situated at its upper end slightly to the left of the vertebral column. In its downward course it approaches the midline. It gives off numerous small branches, the majority of which consist of the intercostal arteries. In the normal individual these are of little aortographic interest. In pathologic cases, however, it is necessary to be familiar with their anatomy because they form collateral pathways in the stenosing processes.

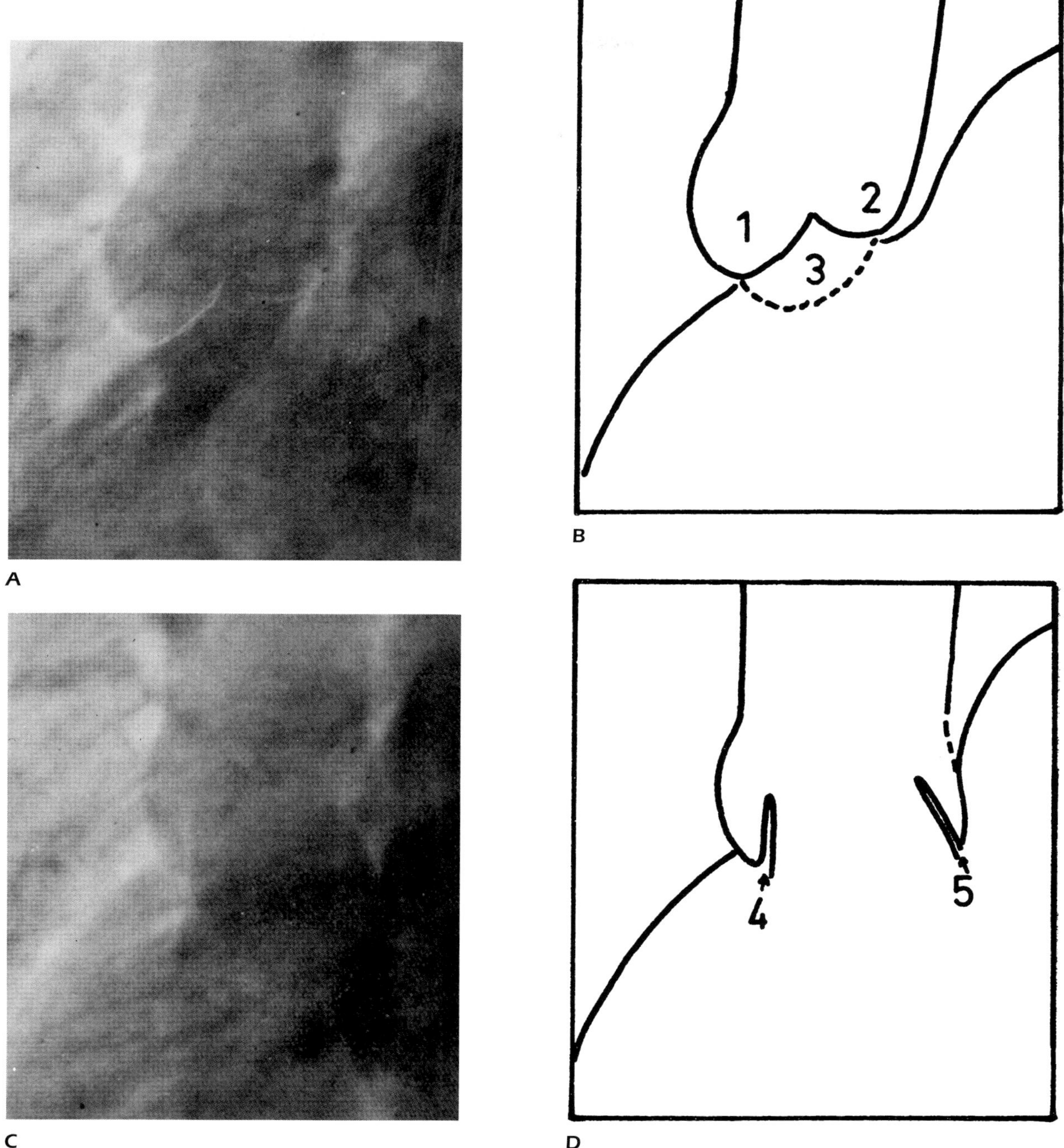

Figure 15-17. "Normal" aortic bulb in a woman aged 44. Lateral views in diastole and systole. Mitral stenosis, but no symptoms from the aortic valves. The sinuses of Valsalva are visible in diastole (A and B), and the semilunar valves open in systole (C and D). Two are distinguishable in the aortogram (C and D). They are thin, less than 1 mm thick. *1, 2, 3,* Sinuses of Valsalva; *4, 5,* semilunar valves.

General Observations

Dynamic Aspects

The mechanical properties of arteries, and of the thoracic aorta in particular, have been studied with increasing interest during the past few decades. Just as aortic diameter varies with distance from the aortic root, with tapering from the ascending to the descending portion below the brachiocephalic bifurcation, so pressure and distensibility are reduced along the aortic length.[113] Studies of bovine aortic tissue have sought information on the stress-transfer mechanism, in an effort to predict related properties in the human aorta. Removal of lipid and collagen from the bovine vessel has led to the observation that the response of elastin to tensile stress is linearly elastic over the entire deformation range.[114] The sympathetic reflexes within the ostia that modify the aortic pressure-diameter relationship have also been scrutinized, as has the relationship between diameter and diastolic pressure.[115] Experiments using the scanning electron microscope in rabbits have shown that the spiral ridged pattern on the luminal surface of the aorta disappears at pressures equivalent to those experienced at systole or diastole; such observations suggest that the pattern may not be present in a normally functioning artery.[116] It is also possible to study the mechanical properties of human arteries by such techniques as angiography and ultrasonography. Cineangiography has been employed to assess the thoracic aorta in humans, with stop-film cine projections employed to measure diameter at maximum and minimum points in the cardiac cycle.[104] Flow velocity has been studied in the thoracic aorta by means of the Doppler device and polygraph registration. Particular interest has focused on the effect of contrast medium on flow. Catheterization and subsequent infusion of the ascending aorta with 20 ml of contrast medium have been found to result in an increase in flow velocity in the right common carotid artery—an effect most probably due to diffuse vasodilatation.[117]

The Ductus Diverticulum Versus the "Aortic Spindle"

Anatomic studies have revealed that the portion of the aorta between the origin of the left subclavian artery and the site of entrance of the ductus arteriosus (the aortic isthmus) is narrowed in the newborn infant (Fig. 15-18).[118] The fetal narrowing at the isthmus takes at least 2 months to disappear, and it has been suggested that this process is related to the cessation of ductus contribution to aortic flow.[119] Beyond the ligamentum arteriosum, a fusiform dilatation may occur, which His has named the *aortic spindle* and which may persist in adult life.[120]

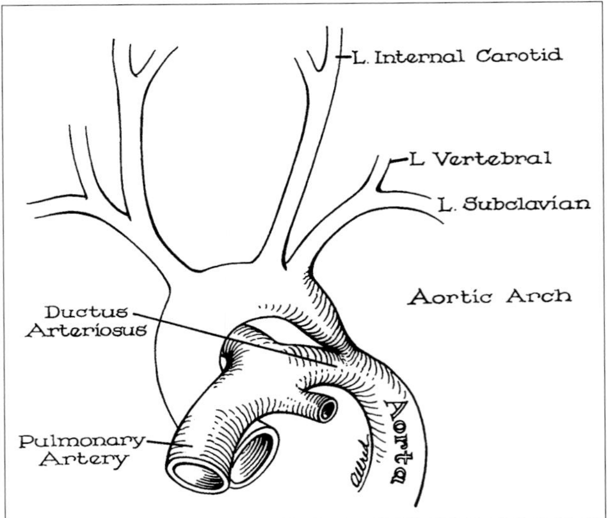

Figure 15-18. Normal aorta showing the aortic arch and its great branches at birth. The isthmus of the aorta (the segment between the origin of the left subclavian artery and the ductus arteriosus) is normally narrowed at birth. A residuum of this narrowing may be seen in the normal infant aortogram. (From Arey.[130])

Our own studies have clearly shown that the aortic bulge may be localized, involving predominantly the anterior aortic wall, or more generalized, involving most of the circumference of the aorta. An intermediate stage with a relatively long segment of the anterior wall affected has also been observed.

The localized bulge may properly be considered a remnant of the enlarged mouth of the ductus (the so-called ductus diverticulum) or a result of traction by the ligamentum arteriosum. The more diffuse dilatation probably represents the aortic spindle and seems more specifically related to the dynamics of the fetal circulation, in which blood to the abdomen and lower extremities flows largely from the pulmonary artery to the aorta via the ductus and the segment immediately proximal to the ductus is little used.

In 1943, Steinberg, Grishman, and Sussman,[121] in reporting the angiocardiographic findings in patent ductus arteriosus, described a localized dilatation of the descending aorta beyond the isthmus, which they considered characteristic of patent ductus arteriosus. Although they revised this concept subsequently, they reiterated the belief that the bulge was not encountered in normal individuals.[122] This view is not consonant with either earlier anatomic studies[123] or subsequent in vivo roentgenographic studies of the aortic arch.[38,103] Thus Jönsson and Saltzman,[38] in reporting their studies of the "infundibulum" of the ductus, noted its presence in 25 of 27 patients with patent ductus arteriosus. But they also observed a shallow bulge in the anterior wall at the site of the ligamentum arteriosum in three normal patients. They stated that this bulge was not greater than 1 mm in any of the cases. The studies summarized earlier in this chapter, in the section on The Normal Aorta in Infants, offer convincing evidence that a more or less localized dilatation may be present in the normal aortic arch, adjacent to the ligamentum arteriosum, in infants and children under the age of 4 years.

Normal Narrowing of the Isthmus Versus Coarctation of the Aorta

The narrowing of the isthmus of the aorta that is present in fetal life and at birth has already been noted (see Fig. 15-18). This segment, formed by the distal end of the left fourth branchial arch during the early weeks of development, performs a relatively minor function during intrauterine life, when aortic blood is delivered to the head and upper extremities above it and blood from the ductus arteriosus flows to the abdominal viscera and lower extremities below it. With the closure of the ductus, the isthmus becomes an essential avenue of transport of blood to the lower part of the body. Although the narrowing of the isthmus may bring its diameter down to that of the descending aorta, it is sometimes narrower than the aortic segment immediately beyond (see Fig. 15-10). Measurements on cadavers have shown (1) that narrowing of the isthmus is present most commonly under 10 weeks of age, and then usually when the ductus is patent; (2) that it may be severe; and (3) that after 10 weeks it generally disappears.[117]

The so-called infantile type of coarctation was thought to be a persistence of, or an extreme form of, the fetal isthmus; the etiology of the so-called adult type, juxtaductal in location, was a source of greater controversy. Analysis of the normal aorta at three points—proximal to, at the site of, and distal to the aortic isthmus—shows that, in normal individuals, the aorta at the isthmus has at least 80 percent of the cross-sectional area of the adjacent aorta. Significant coarctation, however, reduced the cross-sectional area of the aorta by at least 60 percent.[35] It has become increasingly clear that the distinction between the infantile and adult types of coarctation is by no means clear-cut. Because the distal left fourth branchial arch, which forms the aortic isthmus, may be distal to the ductus arteriosus,[124] it seems reasonable to conclude, as Blackford did many years ago,[125] that both types of coarctation are related to atrophy or to imperfect development of the left fourth arch and that this may at times originate in the dynamics of fetal blood flow. Furthermore, narrowing of the aortic isthmus is present in adult life as a normal finding, although it is usually not marked, and can be accounted for by the diversion of aortic flow to the great vessels of the head and upper extremities. The term *coarctation* then becomes a matter of degree, and narrowing of functional significance merges imperceptibly with narrowing that is only an anatomic curiosity.

An interesting recent hypothesis maintains that coarctation of the aorta has its basis in two components: a medial component that is congenital and an intimal component that is progressive. In 27 coarcted aortas, collected surgically and studied by light microscopy, a shaft of fibromuscular tissue covered by an intimal layer was found to protrude from the distal wall. The intimal layer, minimal in infancy but increasing with age, was laminated and often contained areas that stained for fibrin, giving rise to the notion that it is built up of fibrin and platelets over time.[126]

The wide spectrum of clinical disability present even among patients in whom a specific diagnosis of coarctation of the aorta has been made is well known. The marked variations in both systolic and diastolic pressures in upper and lower extremities in patients with coarctation are a further index of the range of gradation of the stenosis.[127] In addition, so-called pseudocoarctation of the aorta has been described as an anomaly in which there is demonstrable aortic narrowing and deformity in the absence of clinical symptoms or signs.[127] Obviously, the critical issue is the degree to which the deformity of the aortic lumen offers resistance to blood flow. Figures 15-5 and 15-6 clearly illustrate discrete deformities of the aortic lumen in infancy that resemble coarctation of the aorta but that were unaccompanied by either upper limb hypertension or lower limb hypotension. An autopsy performed on the child whose aortogram is shown in Figure 15-6 demonstrated a definite narrowing of the isthmus, but the lumen seemed ample.

These findings in the infant aortogram must therefore be interpreted as variations of normal anatomy without clinical significance. Furthermore, the narrowing of the isthmus commonly observed in early life should not be classified as hypoplasia of the aortic arch unless it is marked in degree.

Aortic Diameter and the Aortic Wall in Adults

The diameter of the thoracic aorta increases steadily from birth until death. In middle life, the aortic wall is twice as thick as it was at birth, and in old age it is nearly three times as thick. At the same time, in a process that begins during the prenatal life of the infant, its distensibility diminishes.[128] Diffuse intimal thickening (DIT) is considered by some to be a normal process of arterial growth and remodeling. Others maintain that it represents a form of atherosclerosis, while a third group believes that some of the factors involved in the pathogenesis of atherosclerosis might also influence the severity of DIT.[129] Although the process occurs alike in both sexes, and involves both the thoracic and abdominal aortas, the thoracic aorta increases in thickness much more extensively than does the abdominal aorta. At birth, their parameters are similar.[128]

References

1. dos Santos R, Lama AC, Pereira-Caldas J. Arteriografia da aorta e dos vasos abdominais. Med Contemp 1929;47:93.
2. Nuvoli I. Arteriografia dell'aorta toracica mediante puntura dell'aorta ascendente o del ventricolo. Policlinico (Prat) 1936; 43:227.
3. Rousthöi P. Über Angiokardiographie. Acta Radiol (Stockh) 1933;14:419.
4. Eiseman B, Rainer WG. A new technique for thoracic aortography using the right supraclavicular approach. Arch Surg 1955;71:859.
5. Gomez del Campo C, Meneses Hoyos J. Angiography of the aorta. Am Heart J 1947;33:729.
6. Meneses Hoyos J, Gomez del Campo C. Angiocardiography of thoracic aorta and coronary vessels, with direct injection of opaque solution into the aorta. Radiology 1948;50:211.
7. Radner S. Attempt at roentgenologic visualization of coronary blood vessels in man. Acta Radiol (Stockh) 1945;26:497.
8. Wickbom I. Death following contrast injection into the thoracic aorta. Acta Radiol (Stockh) 1952;38:350.
9. Castellanos A, Pereiras R. Counter-current aortography. Rev Cubana Cardiol 1939;2:187.
10. Castellanos A, García O, Pereiras R. On the value of retrograde aortography in the study of the congenital cardiac lesions operated. Rev Cubana Pediatr 1953;25:413.
11. Castellanos A, Pereiras R. Retrograde or counter-current aortography. AJR 1950;63:559.
12. Castellanos A, Pereiras R, Cazanas D. On the value of retrograde aortography for the diagnosis of coarctation of the aorta. Arch Med Inf 1942;11:9.
13. Freeman N. Discussion of R.E. Gross, Surgical treatment for coarctation of the aorta. JAMA 1949;139:291.
14. Freeman NE, Miller EA, Stephens HB, et al. Retrograde arteriography in the diagnosis of cardiovascular lesions: II. Coarctation of the aorta. Ann Intern Med 1950;32:827.
15. Stephens HB. Discussion of H.H. Bradshaw et al., Resection of coarctation of aorta. J Thorac Surg 1948;17:221.
16. Jönsson G. Thoracic aortography by means of a cannula inserted percutaneously into the common carotid artery. Acta Radiol (Stockh) 1949;31:376.
17. Radner S. Thoracic aortography by catheterization from the radial artery. Acta Radiol (Stockh) 1948;29:178.
18. Brodén B, Hanson HE, Karnell J. Thoracic aortography: preliminary report. Acta Radiol (Stockh) 1948;29:181.
19. Brodén B, Jönsson G, Karnell J. Thoracic aortography. Acta Radiol (Stockh) 1949;32:498.
20. Jönsson G, Brodén B, Hanson HE, et al. Visualization of patent ductus arteriosus Botalli by means of thoracic aortography. Acta Radiol (Stockh) 1948;30:81.
21. Brodén B, Jönsson G, Karnell J. Thoracic aortography with special reference to its value in patent ductus arteriosus and coarctation of the aorta. Acta Radiol (Stockh) 1951; 89(Suppl):1.
22. Helmsworth JA, McGuire J, Felson B. Arteriography of the aorta and its branches by means of the polyethylene catheter. AJR 1950;64:196.
23. Peirce EC. Percutaneous femoral artery catheterization in man with special reference to aortography. Surg Gynecol Obstet 1951;93:50.
24. Euler HE. Die periesophageale Aortenpunktion, ihre diagnostischen und therapeutischen Möglichkeiten. Arch Ohren Nasen Kehlkopfheikd 1949;155:536.
25. Keith JD, Forsyth C. Aortography in infants. Circulation 1950;2:907.
26. Abrams HL. Radiologic aspects of operable heart disease: I. Observations on the pre-operative approach to congenital anomalies. Radiology 1955;65:31.
27. Adams P Jr, Adams FH, Varco RL, et al. Diagnosis and treatment of patent ductus arteriosus in infancy. Pediatrics 1953; 12:644.
28. Singleton EB, McNamara DG, Colley DA. Retrograde aortography in the diagnosis of congenital heart disease in infants. J Pediatr 1955;47:720.
29. Anjos R, Kakadekar A, Murdoch I, et al. Countercurrent aortography: an alternative to cardiac catheterization in infancy. Pediatr Cardiol 1992;13:10.
30. Burford TH, Carson MJ. Visualization of the aorta and its branches by retro-arterial Diodrast injection. J Pediatr 1948; 33:675.
31. Ponsdomenech ER, Nunez VB. Heart puncture in man for Diodrast visualization of the ventricular chambers and great arteries: I. Its experimental and anatomophysiological bases and technique. Am Heart J 1951;41:643.
32. Smith PW, Wilson CW, Cregg HA, et al. Cardioangiography. J Thorac Surg 1954;28:273.
33. McCaughan JJ Jr, Pate JW. Aortography, utilizing percutaneous left ventricular puncture. Arch Surg 1957;75:746.
34. Steinberg I, Finby N. The importance of angiocardiography for visualizing the thoracic aorta. Arch Surg 1957;74: 29.
35. Winer HE, Kronzon I, Glassman E, et al. Pseudocoarctation and mid-arch aortic coarctation. Chest 1977;72:519.
36. Mulholland HC. Aortography in infantile coarctation. Br Med J 1978;2:57.
37. Fariñas PL. A new technique for the arteriographic examination of the abdominal aorta and its branches. AJR 1941;46: 641.
38. Jönsson G, Saltzman GF. Infundibulum of the patent ductus arteriosus studied by thoracic aortography. Acta Radiol (Stockh) 1952;37:445.
39. Ödman P, Philipson J. Aortic valvular diseases studied by percutaneous thoracic aortography. Acta Radiol (Stockh) 1958; 182(Suppl):1.
40. Seldinger SI. Catheter replacement of the needle in percutaneous arteriography: a new technique. Acta Radiol (Stockh) 1953;39:368.
41. Patel YD. Technical development: a modified pigtail catheter for transbrachial aortography. Clin Radiol 1990;41:128.
42. Crawford P, Molnar W, Klassen KP. Trans-carotid aortography. J Thorac Surg 1956;32:46.
43. Roy P. Percutaneous catheterization by the axillary artery. AJR 1965;94:1.
44. Sutton D. Thoracic aortography by percutaneous transcarotid catheterization. J Fac Radiol 1956;7:172.

45. Sutton D. Discussion on the clinical and radiological aspects of diseases of the major arteries. Proc R Soc Med 1956;49: 559.
46. Antoine JE, Middleton PJ, Carmody PW. Double-catheter technique in aortography. AJR 1974;121:634.
47. Kirschner LP, Twigg HL, Conrad PW, et al. Retrograde catheter aortography in dissecting aortic aneurysms. AJR 1968; 102:349.
48. Nath PH, Zollikofer C, Castaneda-Zuniga WR, et al. Radiological evaluation of composite aortic grafts. Radiology 1979; 131:43.
49. Stein HL, Steinberg I. Selective aortography, the definitive technique for diagnosis of dissecting aneurysm of the aorta. AJR 1968;102:333.
50. Sanders C. Current role of conventional and digital aortography in the diagnosis of aortic disease. J Thorac Imaging 1990; 5:48.
51. Grossman LB, Buonocore E, Modic MT, et al. Digital subtraction angiography of the thoracic aorta. Radiology 1984; 150:323.
52. Barth KH, Mertens MA. A double-blind comparative study of Hexabrix and Renografin-76 in aortography and visceral arteriography. Invest Radiol 1984;19:5323.
53. Grainger RG. The optimal concentration of contrast medium for aortography and femoral arteriography: a comparison of Hexabrix 320 and Hexabrix 250. Clin Radiol 1986;37:281.
54. Joyce PF, O'Neill M, Kweka E, et al. Comparison of Hexabrix 320 and Hexabrix 250 in aortoperipheral arteriography: towards cheaper low osmolar contrast media? Cardiovasc Intervent Radiol 1989;12:161.
55. Winer HE, Kronzon I, Glassman E, et al. Pseudocoarctation and mid-arch aortic coarctation. Chest 1977;72:519.
56. Suarez de Lezo J, Sancho M, Pan M, et al. Angiographic follow-up after balloon angioplasty for coarctation of the aorta. J Am Coll Cardiol 1989;13:689.
57. Pozzato C, Fedriga E, Donatelli F, et al. Acute posttraumatic rupture of the thoracic aorta: the role of angiography in a 7-year review. Cardiovasc Intervent Radiol 1991;14(6):338.
58. Barcia TC, Livoni JP. Indications for angiography in blunt thoracic trauma. Radiology 1983;147:15.
59. Mirvis SE, Bidwell JK, Buddemeyer EU, et al. Imaging diagnosis of traumatic aortic rupture: a review and experience at a major trauma center. Invest Radiol 1987;22:187.
60. Woodring JH, King JG. The potential effects of radiographic criteria to exclude aortography in patients with blunt chest trauma. J Thorac Cardiovasc Surg 1989;97:456.
61. Sturm JT, Hankins DG, Young G. Thoracic aortography following blunt chest trauma. Am J Emerg Med 1990;8:92.
62. Abrams HL. Radiologic aspects of operable heart disease: II. Retrograde brachial aortography. Circulation 1956;14:593.
63. Calodney MM, Carson MJ. Coarctation of the aorta in early infancy. J Pediatr 1950;37:46.
64. Chou SN, French LA, Peyton WT. Cerebral complications following cardioangiography. AJR 1955;73:208.
65. Deterling RA. Direct and retrograde aortography. Surgery 1952;31:88.
66. Freeman NE, Fullenlove TM, Wylie EJ, et al. The Valsalva maneuver: an aid for the contrast visualization of the aorta and great vessels. Ann Surg 1949;130:398.
67. Gasul BM, Weiss H, Fell EH, et al. Angiocardiography in congenital heart disease correlated with clinical and autopsy findings. Am J Dis Child 1953;85:404.
68. McAfee JG. Angiocardiography and thoracic aortography in congenital cardiovascular lesions. Am J Med Sci 1955;229: 549.
69. Peirce EC. Temporary hemiplegia from cerebral injection of Diodrast during catheter aortography. Circulation 1953;7: 385.
70. Scott WG. The development of angiocardiography and aortography. Radiology 1951;56:485.
71. Seaman WB, Goldring D. Coarctation of the aorta with patent ductus arteriosus. J Pediatr 1955;47:588.
72. Wickbom I. Death following contrast injection into the thoracic aorta. Acta Radiol (Stockh) 1952;38:350.
73. Abrams HL. Radiologic aspects of operable heart disease: III. The hazards of retrograde thoracic aortography: a survey. Radiology 1957;68:812.
74. Moore CH, Wolma FJ, Brown RW, et al. Complications of cardiovascular radiology: a review of 1204 cases. Am J Surg 1970;120:591.
75. LaBerge JM, Jeffrey RB. Aortic lacerations: fatal complications of thoracic aortography. Radiology 1987;165:367.
76. Borra S, Hawkins D, Duguid W, et al. Acute renal failure and nephrotic syndrome after angiocardiography with meglumine diatrizoate. N Engl J Med 1971;284:592.
77. Kamdar A, Weidmann P, Makoff DL, et al. Acute renal failure following intravenous use of radiographic contrast dyes in patients with diabetes mellitus. Diabetes 1977;25:643.
78. Krumlovsky FA, Simon N, Santhanam S, et al. Acute renal failure: association with administration of radiographic contrast material. JAMA 1978;239:125.
79. Stark FR, Coburn JW. Renal failure following methylglucamine diatrizoate (Renografin) aortography: report of a case with unilateral renal artery stenosis. J Urol 1966;96:848.
80. Kafkas P, Kontaxis A, Katsaros S. Complications of percutaneous aortic and left heart catheterizations performed with Gensini catheters. Acta Cardiol 1971;26:593.
81. Roscher AA, Endlich HL. Atheroembolization: a complication of vascular surgery and/or diagnostic angiography. Int Surg 1971;56:82.
82. Pendergrass EP, Hodes PJ, Tondreau RL, et al. Further consideration of deaths and unfavorable sequelae following the administration of contrast media in urography in the United States. AJR 1955;74:262.
83. Biorck G, Sylvan T, Lindblom-Tillman G. Electrocardiographic studies at angiocardiography. Acta Cardiol 1950;5: 509.
84. Hejtmancik MR, Bankhead AJ, Herrman GR. Electrocardiographic changes following electroshock therapy in curarized patients. Am Heart J 1949;37:790.
85. Broman T, Olsson O. Experimental study of contrast media for cerebral angiography with reference to possible injurious effects on the cerebral blood vessels. Acta Radiol (Stockh) 949;31:321.
86. Broman T, Forssman B, Olsson O. Further experimental investigations of injuries from contrast media in cerebral angiography. Acta Radiol (Stockh) 1950;34:135.
87. Olsson O. Contrast media in diagnosis and the attendant risks. In Proceedings of the 7th International Congress of Radiology, Copenhagen, 1953. Acta Radiol (Stockh) 1954; 116(Suppl):75.
88. Bassett RC, Rogers JS, Cherry GR, et al. The effect of contrast media on the blood-brain barrier. J Neurosurg 1953;10:38.
89. Bloor BM, Wrenn FR Jr, Margolis G. The experimental evaluation of certain contrast media used for cerebral angiography. J Neurosurg 1951;8:585.
90. Cotrim ES. Cardiac blood pressure, and respiratory effects of some contrast media. In Proceedings of the 7th International Congress of Radiology, Copenhagen, 1953. Acta Radiol (Stockh) 1954;116(Suppl):58.
91. Abbott KH, Gay JR, Goodall RJ. Clinical complications of cerebral angiography. J Neurosurg 1952;9:258.
92. Capurro FG, Francois RR, Azambuja N. Contrast media in radiology and their risks. In Proceedings of the 7th International Congress of Radiology, Copenhagen, 1953. Acta Radiol (Stockh) 1954;116(Suppl):49.
93. Bolasny BL, Killen DA. Surgical management of arterial injuries secondary to angiography. Ann Surg 1971;174:962.
94. Bagger M, et al. On methods in complications in catheterization of heart and large vessels, with and without contrast injection. Am Heart J 1959;54:766.
95. Davidsen HG, Gudbjerg CE, Thomsen G. Complications of selective angiocardiography and percutaneous transarterial aortography. Acta Chir Scand 1961;283(Suppl):168.

96. Judkins MP, Dotter CT. An uncommon complication of thoracic aortography. Radiology 1964;83:433.
97. Kottke BA, Fairbairn JF II, Davis GB. Complications of aortography. Circulation 1964;30:843.
98. Sutton D, Davies ER. Arch aortography and cerebral vascular insufficiency. Clin Radiol 1966;17:330.
99. Greenstone SM, Massell TB, Heringman EC. Hazards and complications of retrograde aortography and arteriography. Angiology 1965;16:93.
100. Hart WL, Berman EJ, LaCom RJ. Hazard of retrograde aortography in dissecting aneurysm. Circulation 1963;27:1140.
101. Adams DF, Abrams HL. Complications of coronary arteriography: a follow-up report. Cardiovasc Radiol 1979;2:89.
102. Hessel SJ, Adams DF, Abrams HL. Complications of angiography. Radiology 1981;138:273.
103. Dotter C, Steinberg I. Angiocardiography. New York: Hoeber, 1951.
104. Gozna ER, Marble AE, Shaw AJ, et al. Mechanical properties of the ascending thoracic aorta of man. Cardiovasc Res 1973; 7:261.
105. Lioy F, Malliani A, Pagani M, et al. Reflex hemodynamic responses initiated from the thoracic aorta. Circ Res 1974;34: 78.
106. Mirsky I, Janz RF. The effect of age on the wall stiffness of the human thoracic aorta: a large deformation "anisotropic" elastic analysis. J Theor Biol 1976;59:467.
107. Nathan H, Barkay M, Orda R. Anatomical observations on the origin and course of the aortic intercostal arteries. J Thorac Cardiovasc Surg 1970;59:372.
108. Van Meurs-Van Woezik H, Klein HW, Krediet P. Normal internal calibres of ostia of great arteries and of aortic isthmus in infants and children. Br Heart J 1977;39:860.
109. McDonald CJ, Castellino RA, Blank N. The aortic "nipple": the left superior intercostal vein. Radiology 1970;96:533.
110. Chandran KB, Yearwood TL, Wieting DW. An experimental study of pulsatile flow in a curved tube. J Biomech 1979;12: 793.
111. Pereiras R, Castellanos A. Retrograde aortography: its value in the diagnosis of coarctation of the aorta by means of a new indirect sign. Radiology 1949;53:859.
112. Bergstrand G, Szamosi A. Visibility of the intrapericardiac segment of the ascending aorta on conventional lateral chest films. Acta Radiol (Stockh) 1976;17:425.
113. Arndt JO, Stegall HF, Wicke HJ. Mechanics of the aorta in vivo: a radiographic approach. Circ Res 1971;28:693.
114. Lake LW, Armeniades CD. Structure-property relations of aortic tissue. Trans Am Soc Artif Intern Organs 1972;18:202.
115. Pagani M, Schwartz PJ, Bishop VS, et al. Reflex sympathetic changes in aortic diastolic pressure-diameter relationship. Am J Physiol 1975;229:286.
116. Swinehart PA, Bentley DL, Kardong KV. Scanning electron microscopic study of the effects of pressure on the luminal surface of the rabbit aorta. Am J Anat 1976;145:137.
117. Thijssen HOM, Colon E, Merx H. Changes in carotid flow velocity during catheterization of the aortic arch and common carotid artery. Neuroradiology 1976;12:171.
118. Schaefer JP, ed. Morris's human anatomy. 10th ed. Philadelphia: Blakiston, 1942.
119. Patten BM. The changes in circulation following birth. Am Heart J 1930;6:192.
120. Goss CM, ed. Gray's anatomy of the human body. 29th ed. Philadelphia: Lea & Febiger, 1973.
121. Steinberg MF, Grishman A, Sussman ML. Angiocardiography in congenital heart disease: III. Patent ductus arteriosus. AJR 1943;50:306.
122. Sussman ML, Grishman A. A discussion of angiocardiography and angiography. In: Dock W, Snapper I, eds. Advances in internal medicine. New York: Interscience, 1947;2.
123. Jönsson G, Saltzman GF. Infundibulum of patent ductus arteriosus: a diagnostic sign in conventional roentgenograms. Acta Radiol (Stockh) 1952;38:8.
124. Congdon ED. Transformation of the aortic arch system during the development of the human embryo. Contrib Embryol 1922;14:47.
125. Blackford LM. Coarctation of the aorta. Arch Intern Med 1928;41:702.
126. Kennedy A, Taylor DG, Durrant TE. Pathology of the intima in coarctation of the aorta: a study using light and scanning electron microscopy. Thorax 1979;34:366.
127. Brown GE Jr, Pollack AA, Clagett OT, et al. Intra-arterial blood pressure in patients with coarctation of the aorta. Mayo Clin Proc 1948;23:129.
128. Wolinsky H. Comparison of medial growth of human thoracic and abdominal aortas. Circ Res 1970;27:531.
129. Restrepo C, Strong JP, Guzman MA, et al. Geographic comparisons of diffuse intimal thickening of the aorta. Atherosclerosis 1979;32:177.
130. Arey LB. Developmental anatomy. 6th ed. Philadelphia: Saunders, 1954.

16

Patent Ductus Arteriosus

JOHN B. MAWSON
J. A. GORDON CULHAM

Patent ductus arteriosus (PDA) is one of the most common congenital heart lesions and among the simplest anatomically. It was the first lesion to be successfully corrected surgically and, more recently, among the first to be closed with interventional techniques.[1,2] However, despite half a century of active management of patients with PDA, there are still major gaps in our knowledge about this lesion, and controversies about how to manage it have come to the fore with the now widespread availability of interventional techniques.

This chapter discusses primarily the imaging of isolated PDA with comments about anatomy, embryology, and natural history where relevant. Current surgical and interventional techniques are discussed. Throughout, reference is made where appropriate to PDA associated with other cardiac anomalies, particularly those that are ductus-dependent.

Definition

Patent ductus arteriosus is a communication that is usually between the proximal left pulmonary artery (LPA) and the descending thoracic aorta immediately distal to the left subclavian artery (LSCA) origin. The communication results from persisting patency of the fetal ductus arteriosus. In 88 percent of normal individuals, PDA closes anatomically by 8 weeks of age.[3] When the process is delayed, prolonged patency of the ductus arteriosus results; when the process fails altogether, persisting patency of the ductus arteriosus results. There is debate about the time beyond which prolonged patency becomes persisting patency: Gittenberger-de Groot believes 3 months of age to be an appropriate time because this represents the upper limit for normal anatomic closure, whereas Ho and Anderson believe 12 months to be the changeover period.[4,5]

Incidence

Estimates of the incidence of PDA vary according to the population studied (premature infants, term infants, older children, and adults) and the assessment technique used (autopsy data, clinical findings, imaging). PDA has been quoted as occurring in 1:2500 to 1:5000 live births, representing approximately 9 to 12 percent of congenital heart disease in term infants with a 2:1 female-male preponderance.[6,7] Its incidence in the general population currently may well be higher, since more sensitive imaging techniques have shown trivial shunts not suspected clinically, and, because of the high incidence in premature infants, not all of these close spontaneously or are closed by medical or surgical means in the perinatal period. Musewe and Olley cite the incidence of delayed closure as approximately 20 percent in premature infants born beyond 32 weeks' gestation but about 60 percent in those born at less than 28 weeks.[8]

Embryology

Cassels has described in some detail the development of the fetal ductus arteriosus.[9] An appreciation of ductal development in conjunction with Edwards's concept of the double aortic arch is useful for understanding the anatomic variability of the ductus arteriosus (Figure 16-1).[10,11]

The sixth arch on each side is thought to arise from independent outgrowths from the dorsal aorta and the ventral aortic sac, joining the pulmonary plexus in the vicinity of the trachea. Ipsilateral ventral and dorsal roots communicate to form the sixth arch on each side, with the former forming branch pulmonary arteries (connected to the main pulmonary artery [MPA] after conotruncal division) and the latter forming the ductus arteriosus. The dorsal root of the sixth arch may arise from the aorta as a common origin with the

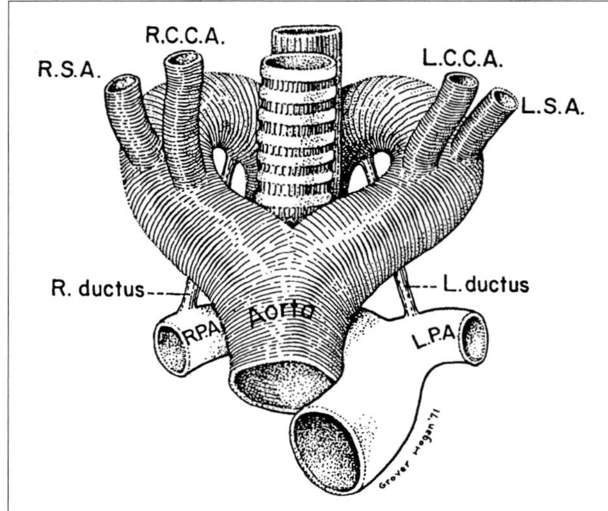

Figure 16-1. Edwards's hypothetical double aortic arch showing the position of both left and right ductus. (From Shuford WH and Sybers RG. The Aortic Arch and Its Malformation. Springfield, IL: Charles C. Thomas, 1974. Courtesy of Charles C. Thomas, Publisher, Springfield, Illinois.)

fourth arch or well distal to it. Thus the aortic end of the ductus shows marked variability, usually being just distal to the LSCA but rarely arising opposite the common carotid artery (CCA) or well distal to the subclavian.

In association with Edwards's theoretical double arch, possibilities for ductal situs and position can be worked out. In the isolated PDA lesion, the ductus is almost invariably in a left posterior position ("usual") despite the laterality of the arch.[12] The ipsilateral ductus is always posteriorly located. The contralateral ductus may be anterior or posterior, depending on whether the arch involutes anterior or posterior to the ductus insertion. If the ductus arises in common with the subclavian artery and involution of the dorsal aorta occurs both proximal and distal to these vessels, isolation of the subclavian artery results with ductal closure. Rarely the ductus may be absent or bilateral, usually in association with other cardiac lesions.

Anatomy

The typical left-sided ductus arises 2 to 10 mm beyond the origin of LSCA and travels centrally toward the origin of the LPA either directly or parallel to the undersurface of the aortic arch (Fig. 16-2).[3] The ductus is usually 5 to 10 mm in length but may be shorter or longer. The aortic end is usually wider than the pulmonary end, but both may be wide. Forty to 50 percent of cardiac output in utero is via the ductus from the right ventricle to the systemic circulation.[13] The caliber of the ductus equals that of the descending thoracic aorta at term.[14] A ductus on the contralateral side to the arch, whether anterior (arising from the brachiocephalic or subclavian artery) or posterior (arising from an aberrant vessel), still passes centrally toward the origin of its associated pulmonary artery, but it is usually longer, more craniocaudal in orientation, and may be tortuous (Fig. 16-3). At the aortic end, a posterior contralateral ductus may be bulbous as part of the diverticulum of Kommerell, the remnant of the involuted dorsal aortic root. Whereas the pulmonary end tends to mimic the usual appearance seen with the typical left-sided ductus, the systemic arterial end is usually different, being anything from restrictive, to the usual conical appearance, to bulbous as part of the diverticulum of Kommerell. The ductus may contribute to a vascular ring when associated with an aberrant vessel, a circumflex aorta, or a double arch. The ductus arteriosus sling represents a rare anomaly, with the patent ductus connecting the right pulmonary artery

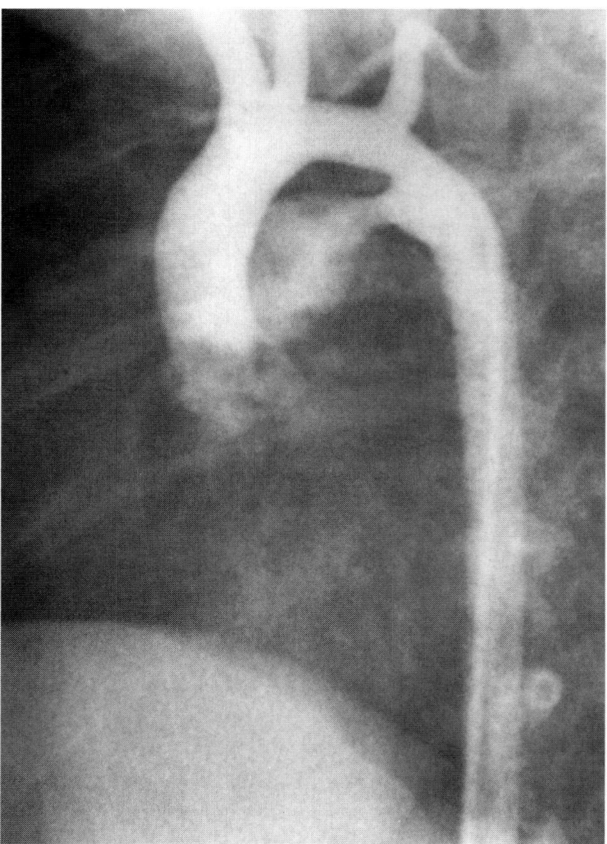

Figure 16-2. Aortogram in left anterior oblique (LAO) projection performed via retrograde arterial approach showing a left arch with left-to-right shunting through a "usual" left posterior PDA.

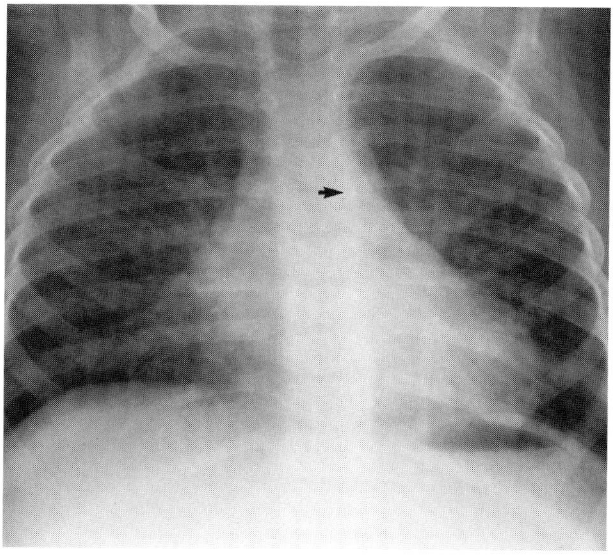

A

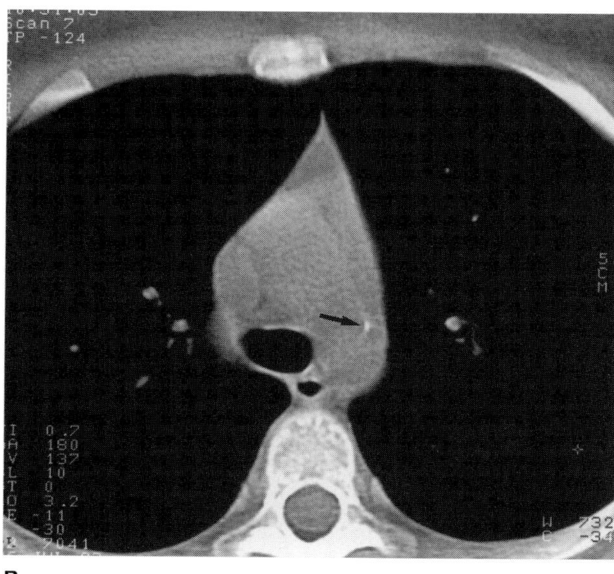

B

Figure 16-10. Two children with typical calcification in the left ligamentum arteriosum. (A) Frontal chest film shows calcification overlying the LPA (*arrow*) above the left main bronchus. (B) CT scan (noncontrast) shows calcification in the ligamentum adjacent to the proximal descending thoracic aorta (*arrow*).

Figure 16-11. Echocardiogram in a premature 2-kg neonate performed via an angled suprasternal approach ("ductal view"). (A) The right and left pulmonary arteries and the ductus are visible (*arrow*). (B) Shunting with turbulent flow from aorta to PA via the PDA is shown on the color Doppler image (shown here in black and white).

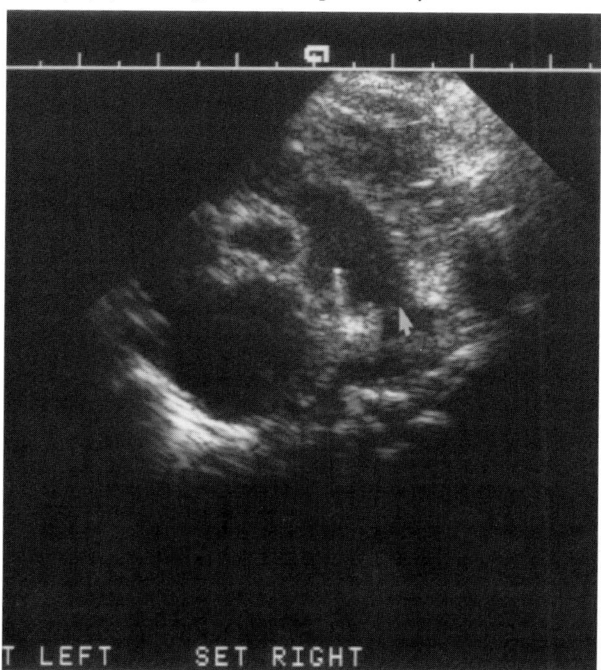

A

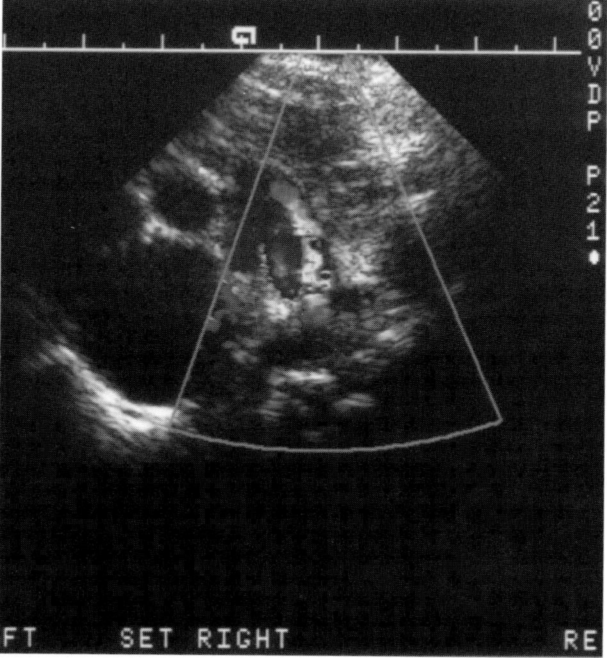

B

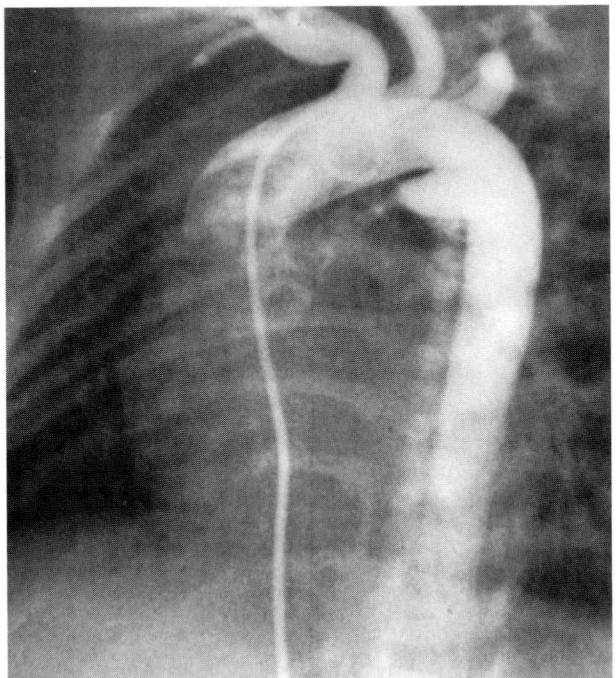

A

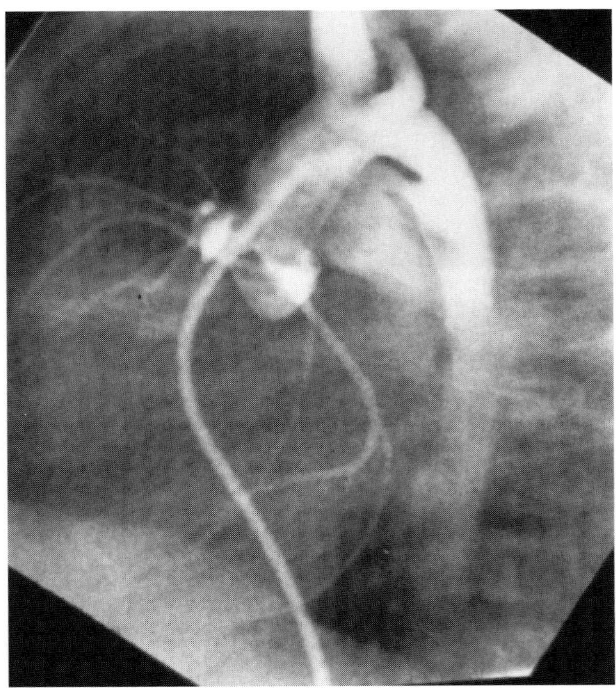

B

Figure 16-12. Aortograms in two patients performed antegrade. (A) Pigtail catheter from RV in complete TGA showing a left arch and PDA. The pulmonary end of the PDA is markedly narrowed and only a trivial shunt is present. (B) Typical PDA of moderate size. Note the acute proximal angle with the underside of the aortic arch and the obtuse distal angle. Compare with Fig. 16-4.

(Figs. 16-2, 16-4, and 16-12) or ventriculography (Figs. 16-3 and 16-13), the latter depending on whether ductal shunting is left to right or right to left, and what the ventriculoarterial connections are. The anatomy of the usual left-sided ductus between the LPA and aorta is best shown in a steep left anterior oblique (LAO) or lateral view, the latter routinely being used during ductal occlusion. Occasionally cranial tilt is needed to separate the ductus from the underside of the aortic arch. The PDA may not opacify with ventriculography in the presence of balanced ventricular pressures, although we have often been able to identify patency in this situation when favored by an ectopic beat. With balanced pressures, an aortogram usually confirms patency and often outlines the ductal anatomy well, but even this may occasionally fail.[67,68] Ductal patency may also be demonstrated by negative washout of the opacified pulmonary artery or aorta by unopacified blood (Fig. 16-14).

When an aortogram is performed to exclude a ductus in the presence of balanced ventricular pressures, the catheter is placed midway between valve level and the first aortic arch branch (usually just distal to the sinuses) to define arch anatomy and the branching sequence of arch vessels, to minimize regurgitation, and, if antegrade, to minimize the potential of trauma to coronary sinuses or valve leaflets. If retrograde, we advance the catheter to the desired position so it lies against the greater curve of the arch, thus reducing recoil during injection. A test injection (using approximately 10 percent of the calculated contrast volume) is performed to confirm a safe catheter position (especially important when antegrade, given the potential for the catheter tip to be in the orifice of LCA) and to confirm an appropriate contrast volume. For a full aortogram, we use approximately 1.0 to 1.5 ml/kg, depending on the strength of the nonionic contrast, and up to 50 ml in an adult, but will increase this volume up to 2 ml/kg in the presence of a large or torrential shunt or aortic regurgitation. The volume can concomitantly be reduced with digital imaging because of the greater contrast sensitivity of this modality.

If aortography is performed to confirm the presence of a PDA and to delineate the ductal anatomy and "size" the duct and shunt before possible umbrella closure, we position the retrograde multipurpose or NIH catheter (a pigtail may unwind into the ductus) in the distal arch and inject approximately 0.50 to 0.75 ml/kg up to 40 ml in an adult.

The ductus can provide a route for access to the

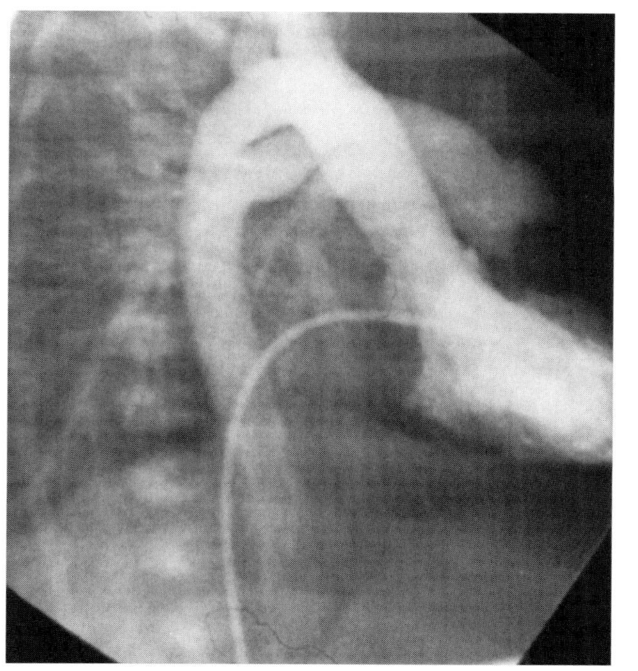

A

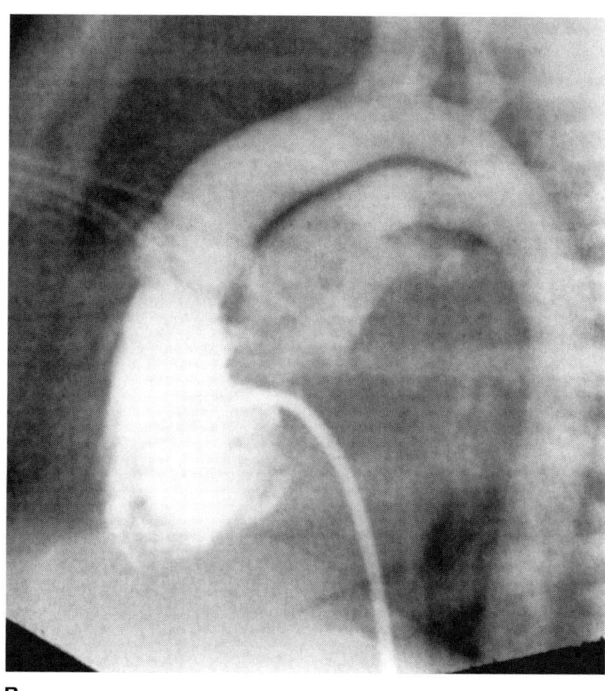

B

Figure 16-13. Left ventriculogram in a patient with isolated PDA. (A) RAO view. (B) Steep LAO view. Both views show a left arch and left-to-right shunting through a large PDA.

Figure 16-14. (A) Aortogram in steep LAO view showing momentary right-to-left shunting of unopacified blood from PA into aorta (*arrow*) late in systole. (B) Left ventriculogram in d-TGA. Cranially tilted LAO view showing left-to-right shunting of unopacified blood from aorta into pulmonary ductal diverticulum during systole (*arrow*).

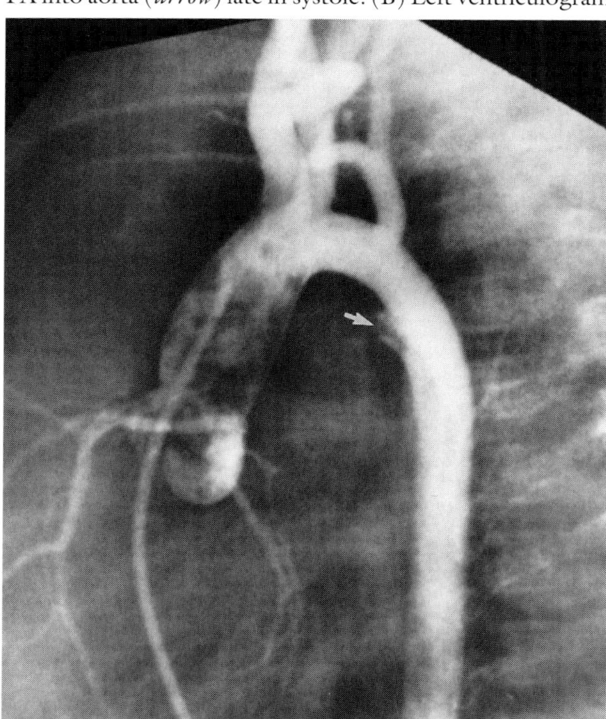

A

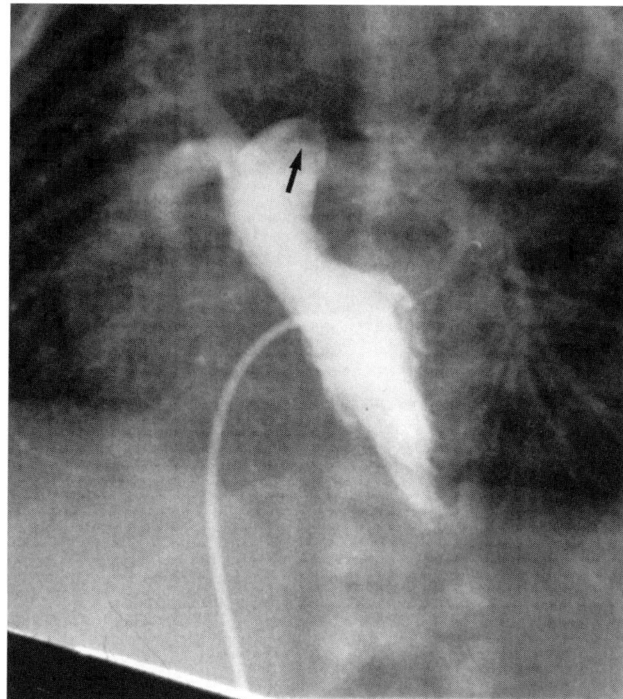

B

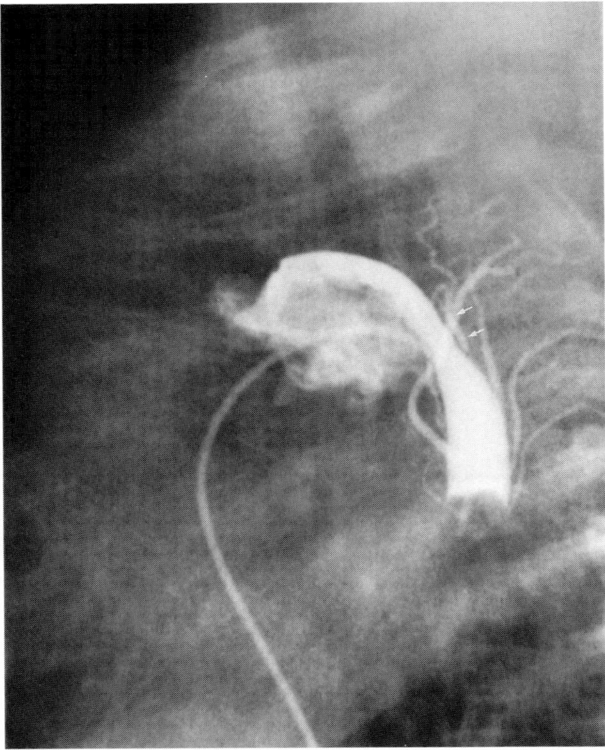

Figure 16-15. Balloon aortography in a patient with severe coarctation, essentially interruption. The catheter is positioned in the descending thoracic aorta via the PDA. Steep LAO view showing contrast outlining intercostal vessels, the severely hypoplastic isthmus proximal to the PDA (*arrows*), and spilling via the PDA into the pulmonary arteries.

descending thoracic aorta for balloon occlusion aortography to delineate coarctation, an interrupted arch (Fig. 16-15), or major aorticopulmonary collateral arteries (MAPCA) in tetralogy-type pulmonary atresia.[69] A ductal diverticulum is frequently identified in the aorta[70] but less frequently at the pulmonary end unless right ventricular outflow tract (RVOT) obstruction exists.[12] In the newborn, the diverticulum may be large and may represent a "ductus bump." Rarely, a ductus aneurysm is identified.

Magnetic Resonance Imaging

Magnetic resonance imaging (MRI) has had a limited application to the evaluation of the isolated PDA but has been used to evaluate complications.[71,72]

Management of PDA

Pharmacologic closure of the patent ductus in premature infants using indomethacin has been the subject of much discussion and controversy since the demonstration of its clinical efficacy and has been well summarized elsewhere.[8,73,74] Prostaglandins are widely used orally and parenterally to prolong ductal patency in duct-dependent congenital heart disease to stabilize the child until surgery.

Most asymptomatic, incidental murmurs require no acute medical treatment. Patients in congestive heart failure usually respond to digoxin and diuretic therapy until they become candidates for surgical or nonsurgical ductal closure. When there is failed acute medical management or failure to thrive, urgent surgical closure is indicated.

Surgical Closure

The indications for surgery have been reviewed elsewhere.[3] In the first month of life, surgical intervention is usually only necessary when symptoms of congestive cardiac failure are present. Beyond this, such intervention is regarded as appropriate at any time when congestive cardiac failure or failure to thrive is present despite appropriate courses of medical therapy. In term infants, children, and adults, persisting patency is an indication for surgical closure on the basis of the risk of infective endocarditis alone. However, there is some divergence of opinion as to the optimal age of closure of an asymptomatic PDA, with Kirklin and Barratt-Boyes advocating closure during the first year of life and Mullins suggesting 4 to 5 years as being more appropriate.[3,7] Severe pulmonary vascular disease is regarded as a contraindication to closure, with the criteria for inoperability being the same as for a ventricular septal defect (VSD), when closure will not decrease pulmonary arterial pressure or left arterial pressure and therefore will not lead to a fall in pulmonary vascular resistance. With severe pulmonary vascular disease, the early experience included a significant death rate of approximately 36 percent from both bleeding and unknown perioperative causes, and it is likely that the rate would be similar today.[3] There is no increased risk of death with mild or moderate pulmonary vascular disease even in the early operative era, but a slightly increased risk is present with older patients because of the technical problems associated with closure of often friable and calcified ducts, together with long-standing left ventricular volume overload leading to arrhythmias.

The division of the ductus without cardiopulmonary bypass is advocated as the definitive operation.[3,7] The technique involves exposure via a thoracotomy, usually at the left fourth interspace. The ends of the ductus are oversewn after division, and separation is maintained by Gelfoam to keep the suture lines from rubbing against each other. Duct ligation is also widely practiced. However, the technique of ligation is contraindicated in older patients in whom sutures may pull through a large, friable or calcified ductus. In preterm infants, the duct is usually large and may have a variable position relative to the aortic arch. It is often friable and composed of vascular tissue, which makes the usual complete dissection and division inadvisable. One hemoclip is usually placed at the aortic end and a second at the pulmonary end. More recently, a number of new techniques have been proposed, including a muscle-sparing thoracotomy and a thorascopic approach.[75,76]

In older patients between the fifth and sixth decades with a short ductus that may be friable and calcified, cardiopulmonary bypass is often used. The pulmonary artery is incised for access to the ductus, and closure is done with sutures.[3]

Postoperative measures include a chest tube for 24 hours, hospital convalescence for 6 to 7 days, and an additional 6 to 8 weeks to return to full unrestricted physical activity. Endocarditis prophylaxis is routinely used for 6 months after repair to allow cardiologic confirmation of closure and exclusion of other lesions that might have been masked by the PDA.

Complications of Surgical Closure

In addition to the obvious postthoracotomy complications of pain and a scar, a low but significant morbidity of approximately 6 to 10 percent and a mortality of approximately 0.4 to 1.0 percent (which includes patients with additional noncardiac anomalies) have been reported.[77,78] Increased risk is present in patients with severe pulmonary vascular disease and in older patients.[3,79] Bleeding, atelectasis, chylothorax, pneumothorax, and pneumomediastinum, together with temporary or permanent phrenic and recurrent laryngeal nerve palsy, do occur. Rarely, the wrong vessel is ligated or divided, with potentially disastrous results.[80,81]

At follow-up clinical assessment, persistent or recurrent patency has been infrequent, varying between 0.4 and 3.1 percent.[77,78] With the advent of echocardiography and color flow Doppler, however, clinically inapparent residual shunts have been detected in 6 to 23 percent of postoperative patients, with differences possibly due to the variability of patient groups, the type of operation performed, and the duration of follow-up.[82–85]

Occasionally, late ductal aneurysms are reported, usually after ligation rather than division.[38]

Nonsurgical Closure

A wide variety of techniques have been used both in animal models and clinical trials to close the patent ductus nonsurgically. These include detachable mechanical devices such as the Rashkind double-disk umbrella occluder, Porstmann's Ivalon plug, detachable balloons (Culham, personal communication, 1993), coil embolization,[86,87] a buttoned device,[88] a double balloon with a silicone filler,[89] and a heat labile polymer.[90] Two methods are in wide clinical use, Porstmann's Ivalon plug, used predominately in Japan and Germany, and Rashkind's umbrella device.

Porstmann's technique involves establishing a femoral artery–aorta–ductus–pulmonary artery–RV–RA–femoral vein guidewire loop, performing a femoral arteriotomy to introduce an appropriately sized and shaped conical plug (Ivalon foam plastic stabilized by an inner wire frame) via a 4.2- to 9.0-mm applicator sheath, and pushing the plug along the wire track into the aortic end of the patent ductus.[2,91–93] The plug is initially held in position by the pressure head and by thrombus formation, after which the guidewire and catheter are removed and an angiogram is performed to confirm closure. Because the femoral arteriotomy must be large enough to accept the plug, the technique is limited to children over 5 years of age. General anesthetic is required for children and occasionally for surgical exposure of the femoral artery (in total, approximately 22 percent of patients), and patients are mobilized on day 3 and discharged on day 5 or 6 after the procedure. More recently, the technique has been modified with duct dilatation via a venous approach before plug insertion via an arterial approach.[92] Further modifications involve tailoring the plug to duct shape and changes in the size of the stopper disk—smaller for children and larger for adults.[93]

Implantation rates of approximately 95 percent are reported.[92,93] There is a low but significant mortality, with some deaths due to anesthesia and ventricular perforation by a catheter, and early morbidity, including plug embolization, which may necessitate surgical removal and duct ligation. Arterial complications occur with femoral or iliac occlusion or stenosis and AVF formation, reflecting the size of the delivery system. Residual shunting is difficult to assess because reported follow-up involves clinical assessment rather than echocardiography. Mention should be made of a single case of low-grade fever, possibly endocarditis, that resolved with antibiotics and one late embolization to the pulmonary artery associated with infection and death.[2] These cases serve to emphasize that a foreign body is introduced.

Rashkind developed a completely different device for PDA closure via an arterial approach.[94] After modifications to the device and to the technique, it was introduced to clinical trials in 1981.[95] The technique of use is reported in detail elsewhere.[96] The device is composed of two small polyurethane fabric umbrellas on stainless steel frames (Fig. 16-16). The umbrellas are connected by a spring mechanism that holds them open in opposition to each other. The collapsed umbrella attached to a delivery wire is loaded into a "pod" and delivered through a long sheath. The device is available in 12- and 17-mm sizes requiring 8 and 11 French delivery systems, respectively.

The standard indication for PDA closure with this device is a duct of less than 9 mm diameter in a patient greater than 6 kg weight, normal atrial situs, and no arch abnormalities.[97] Because of the increased surgical risk in older patients, nonsurgical closure may be of benefit.[98] A second device has been recommended for residual leaks.[99]

The standard technique involves a venous approach from the right groin with heparinization, antibiotic prophylaxis, right heart catheterization, and passage of a 7 French catheter into the proximal descending thoracic aorta for angiography. Angiography is performed in anteroposterior (AP) and lateral projections to confirm the diagnosis, to determine the shape and size of the ductus, and to establish the relationship of the narrowest part of the ductus to the trachea. After it is determined that the duct is appropriate for closure, a 12- or 17-mm device is selected. For a duct 4 mm or less in diameter, a 12-mm device is used, and for ducts between 5 and 9 mm, a 17-mm device is chosen. A duct greater than 9 to 10 mm in diameter is too large for catheter closure. The distal arms of the device are opened in the aortic end of the ductus (Figs. 16-17 and 16-18); the position of the legs is confirmed by withdrawing slightly the whole system to flex the arms in the conical aortic end of the ductus; the dense hinge mechanism should then be at the narrowest point in the ductus. With the wire and catheter fixed, withdrawal of the delivery sheath allows the proximal limbs to open in the pulmonary artery. After confirmation of a satisfactory position, the device is released and the delivery system is removed. Patients are mobilized in the evening and discharged the next day. Antibiotic prophylaxis is continued for up to 1 year.

Figure 16-16. Rashkind ductal occluding device, 17 mm. Frontal view shows the four arms of the proximal disk, the two disks, and the suture through the distal arms before loading. (Device courtesy of Bard Canada, Inc.)

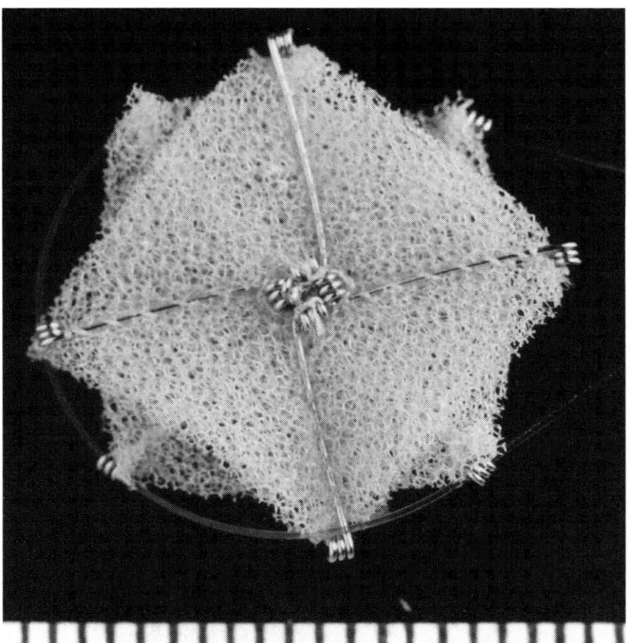

A number of modifications have been suggested. A clam shell device designed for atrial septal defect (ASD) closure has been used for ducts ranging from 4 to 14 mm diameter in 14 patients.[100] Four of these had pulmonary arterial hypertension and complex congenital heart disease. Three of 14 had residual shunts on Doppler at follow-up, and 1 embolized device was retrieved with a snare. Soaking the device in thrombin solution has been suggested, but one group showed no change in residual shunting at 24 hours after this procedure.[101,102]

Use of the procedure on an outpatient basis has been reported,[101] with the PDA anatomy and diagnosis being made with echocardiography before catheterization, no anticoagulation being used, and anesthesia modified. The same group reported use of a balloon catheter to temporarily occlude residual flow at the pulmonary end, but the success rate for this maneuver was not reported.

Small PDAs have been closed after dilatation or using a front-loading device.[97,103] The duct has been closed in association with other abnormalities, such as coarctation dilatation,[104–106] pulmonary valvuloplasty,[97,106] dilatation of Sennings,[106] and other congenital heart disease.[97,106]

Since the initial clinical experience was published 6 years ago, systematic reporting of results and complications has been the norm. This should continue in the United States where the Rashkind device is still under FDA supervision as an "investigative device" but may not continue in the Commonwealth or Europe, where it is now freely available.

Implantation rates of 95 percent with one or two attempts, sometimes in association with ductal dilatation, are reported.[97,106,107] A low but significant morbidity and mortality are apparent. The most significant immediate complication is device embolization of 0.5 to 2 percent, requiring surgical removal and duct ligation if catheter retrieval of the embolized device fails.[96,97,106,107] This complication clearly decreases as

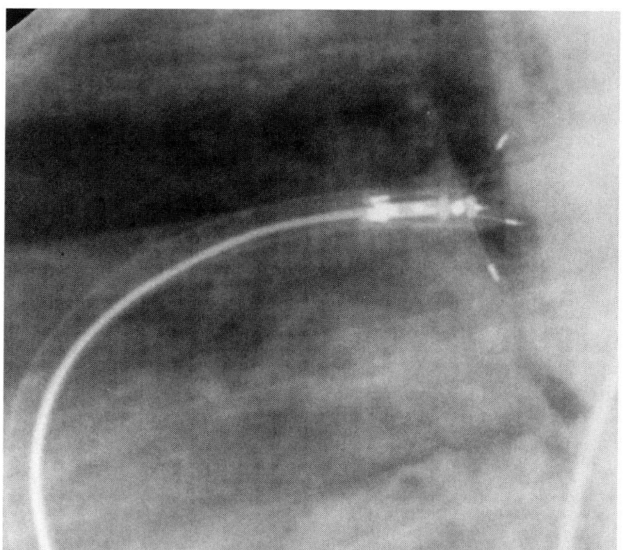

A

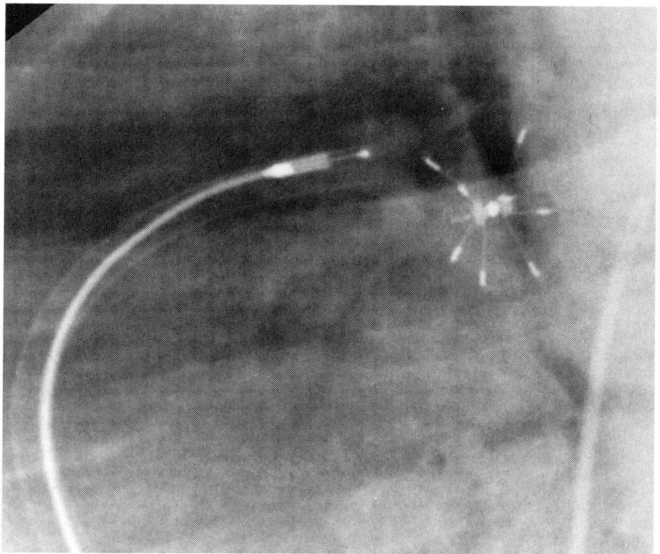

B

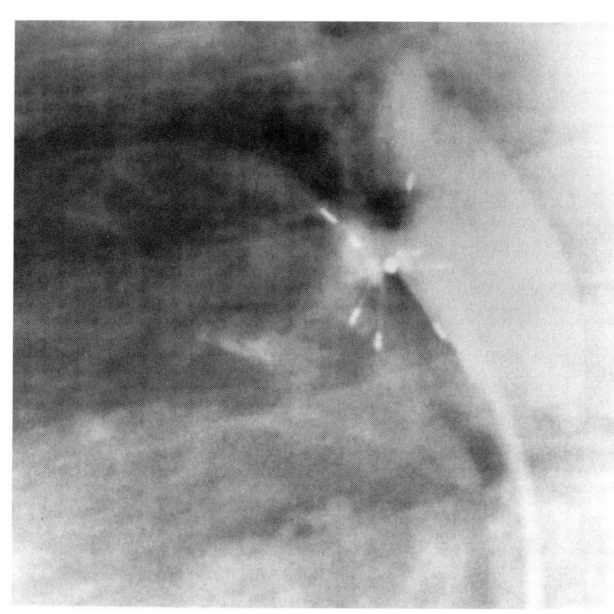

C

Figure 16-17. Placement of a 17-mm Rashkind device in a patient with a PDA and a moderate shunt. All views in lateral projection. (A) The distal limbs are open in the aortic end of the PDA. Note how this overlies the anterior margin of the trachea when under traction. The proximal limbs are retracted. (B) The proximal limbs are open in the pulmonary end of the PDA. The device has been released and the delivery catheter withdrawn into the Mullins sheath. (C) Aortography 15 minutes after device release shows a residual left-to-right shunt over the superior aspect of the device. (Courtesy of Dr. J. Ormiston, Dept. of Radiology, Greenlane Hospital, Auckland, New Zealand.)

operator experience increases. Hosking et al. report 200 procedures in 190 patients with four embolizations that required surgery, including one that became entangled in the tricuspid valve. Three of these were in the first 25 patients; only one was in the last 175.[97]

A small number of anesthetic complications and deaths are reported.[106] Other immediate complications include device entanglement in the tricuspid valve, transient hemolysis, and groin complications.[97,101,106] Two small studies suggest that systemic heparization during the implantation procedure reduces the incidence of femoral artery thrombosis.[101,108]

These procedures may be lengthy and have long fluoroscopy times, but radiation doses are rarely commented on. Average fluoroscopy times range from 17 to 29 minutes, with longer times required for placement of the second or third devices.[108–111]

Of the complications on follow-up, residual shunting detectable either clinically or with echocardiography is the most significant. Hosking et al. used color flow Doppler and reported 53 percent residual shunting at 24 hours, 34 percent at 12 months, 19 percent at 24 months, and 15 percent at 40 months after placement of a single device.[97] If patients with a second device placed for residual shunting are included in the series, a residual shunt was present in 8 percent at 40 months. Of 34 patients with the residual shunts at the time of reporting, all were asymptomatic, with 26 having no murmur, 6 a systolic murmur, and 2 a continuous murmur. A residual shunt is more likely with a 17-mm device. A second device was placed if a continuous murmur was present in patients with a residual shunt, and the authors noted that, if only a

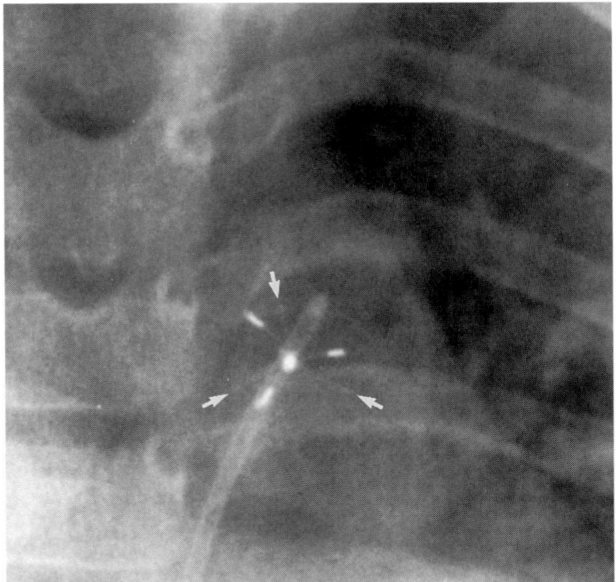

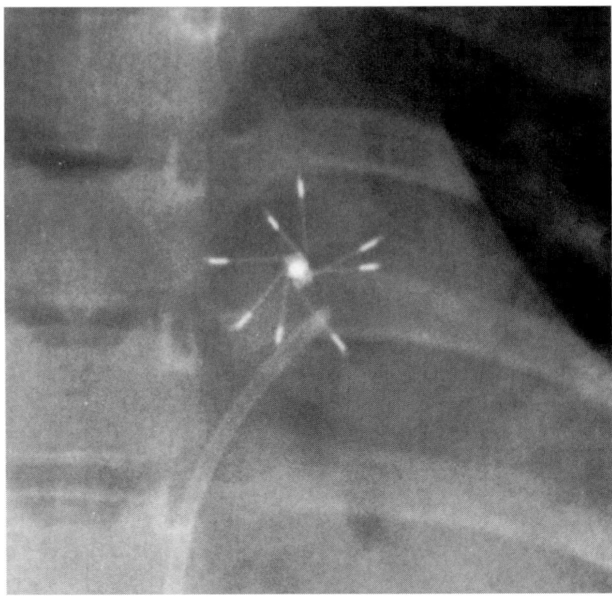

A

B

Figure 16-18. Frontal views in two patients showing Rashkind devices after placement in PDA. The NIH catheters remain in position before aortography to confirm duct closure. (A) 12-mm device. The three proximal limbs (*arrows*) are considerably harder to identify than the three distal limbs. The central density represents the core of the device seen in profile. (B) 17-mm device. Four proximal and four distal limbs are equally well seen. (Courtesy of Dr. J. Ormiston, Dept. of Radiology, Greenlane Hospital, Auckland, New Zealand.)

systolic murmur was present, they were unable to pass a guidewire in any of the patients. Hence a residual shunt with a systolic murmur would not be amenable to further catheter intervention, and the debate would then center around ongoing antibiotic prophylaxis or surgical intervention.

Ali Khan et al. reported a residual shunt in 22 percent of patients at 6 months (37 of 167 followed).[107] Twenty-one of the 37 had a continuous murmur at 6 months and received a second device, with 1 patient requiring a third device. At 6 months 10.5 percent (16 of 167) had a residual shunt after the last device was implanted.

The European Registry report on 652 patients showed 17.5 percent residual shunting at 12 months.[106] Of 108 patients who had a residual shunt at 1 year, 41 had attempted placement of a second device, with 37 reported to be occluded at follow-up. Thus 5.2 percent had residual shunts at 30 months after the last device was placed.

The significance of residual shunting is brought into sharp focus by two different late complications. First, a single episode of bacteremia has been identified that was managed with antibiotics.[97] Hosking et al. state that there have been "no reports of bacterial endocarditis in patients not known to have had a continuous murmur," although more recently a single case has been reported associated with a "silent ductus."[46] Although these data argue against a role for intervention in a patient with a "silent ductus," we do not believe that they necessarily apply to the patient in whom a residual shunt without a continuous murmur is present after device placement, since a foreign body has been introduced.[99] In this situation, it is unclear whether the whole of the device endothelializes or what the time course of this process is, but it is well known that after cardiac surgery the presence of a foreign body significantly increases the risk of infective endocarditis.[112]

The second late complication that highlights the significance of residual shunting is traumatic hemolysis. A number of recent reports have shown control of this complication by either placement of a second device or device removal.[106,113,114]

Other late complications include late embolization of devices,[106] device protrusion into the LPA with adherent clot,[115] fractured occluder arms (Mullins CE, personal communication, 1993), and encroachment of occluder arms into the LPA or aorta with narrowing or turbulence.[116,117]

Conclusion

There has been a resurgence of interest in this simple congenital heart lesion with interventional techniques now available for ductus closure. However, gaps remain in our knowledge of the natural history, particularly with respect to the ultrasound-detectable but clinically inapparent "silent ductus." Controversy exists about the efficacy and appropriateness of antibiotic prophylaxis for both PDA and congenital heart disease in general. The role of catheter closure relative to surgery has not been clearly defined, partly because data for surgical outcome are based on older surgical techniques and clinical follow-up, which cannot be fairly compared with ultrasound follow-up of catheter closure. Ultrasound data follow-up of current surgical cases is limited, and there are no prospective trials reported of patients who would technically be candidates for catheter closure, randomized to catheter or surgical closure. Current issues with catheter closure center around the significance of residual shunting, particularly whether this shunting constitute a risk for infective endocarditis because a foreign body has been introduced. Although catheter closure can clearly be recommended for high-risk surgical cases and for patients with complex congenital heart disease where ductus closure might delay the need for palliative surgery, its role in the closure of typical left-sided PDA in low-risk surgical candidates remains unclear.

Acknowledgments

We wish to thank Jane Rowlands for her artwork and Guili Farquharson for secretarial assistance in the preparation of this manuscript.

References

1. Gross RE, Hubbard JP. Surgical ligation of a patent ductus arteriosus. JAMA 1939;112:729–731.
2. Porstmann W, Wierny L, Warnke H, et al. Catheter closure of patent ductus arteriosus. Radiol Clin North Am 1971;9: 203–218.
3. Kirklin JW, Barratt-Boyes BG. Cardiac surgery. 2nd ed. New York: Churchill-Livingstone, 1992:841–859.
4. Gittenberger-de Groot AC. Persistent ductus arteriosus: most probably a primary congenital malformation. Br Heart J 1977;39:610–618.
5. Ho SY, Anderson RH. Anatomical closure of the ductus arteriosus: a study of 35 specimens. J Anat 1979;128:829–836.
6. Rowe RD. Patent ductus arteriosus. In: Keith JD, Rowe RD, Vlad P, eds. Heart disease in infancy and childhood. 3rd ed. New York: Macmillan, 1978:418–451.
7. Mullins CE. Patent ductus arteriosus. In: Garson A, Bricker JT, McNamara DG, eds. The science and practice of pediatric cardiology. Philadelphia: Lea & Febiger, 1990;2:1055–1069.
8. Musewe NN, Olley PM. Patent ductus arteriosus. In: Freedom RM, Benson LN, Smallhorn JF, eds. Neonatal heart disease. London: Springer-Verlag, 1992:593–609.
9. Cassels DE. The ductus arteriosus. Springfield, IL: Charles C Thomas, 1973:345.
10. Edwards JE. Anomalies of the derivatives of the aortic arch system. Med Clin North Am 1948;32:925–949.
11. Stewart JR, Kincaid OW, Edwards JE. An atlas of vascular rings and related malformations of the aortic arch system. Springfield, IL: Charles C Thomas, 1964:171.
12. Freedom RM, Culham JAG, Moes CAF. Angiocardiography of congenital heart disease. New York: Macmillan, 1984:691.
13. Elzenga NJ. The ductus arteriosus and stenoses of the adjacent great vessels (thesis). Leiden: University of Leiden, The Netherlands, 1986.
14. Heymann MA, Rudolph AM. Control of the ductus arteriosus. Physiol Rev 1975;55:62–78.
15. Binet JP, Conso JF, Losay J, et al. Ductus arteriosus sling: report of a newly recognized anomaly and its surgical correction. Thorax 1978;33:72–75.
16. Mancini AJ. A study of the angle formed by the ductus arteriosus with the descending thoracic aorta. Anat Rec 1951;109: 535–539.
17. Calder AL, Kirker JA, Neutze JM, et al. Pathology of the ductus arteriosus treated with prostaglandins: comparisons with untreated cases. Pediatr Cardiol 1984;5:85–92.
18. Rudolph AM, Heymann MA, Spitznas U. Hemodynamic considerations in the development of narrowing of the aorta. Am J Cardiol 1972;30:514–525.
19. Santos MA, Moll JN, Drumond C, et al. Development of the ductus arteriosus in right ventricular outflow tract obstruction. Circulation 1980;62:818–822.
20. Hiraishi S, Misawa H, Oguchi K, et al. Two-dimensional Doppler echocardiographic assessment of closure of the ductus arteriosus in normal newborn infants. J Pediatr 1987;111: 755–760.
21. Moss AJ, Emmanouilides G, Duffie ER. Closure of the ductus arteriosus in the newborn infant. Pediatrics 1963;32:25–30.
22. Daniels O, Hopman JCW, Stoelinga GBA, et al. Doppler flow characteristics in the main pulmonary artery and the LA/AO ratio before and after ductal closure in healthy newborns. Pediatr Cardiol 1982;3:99–104.
23. Lim MK, Hanretty K, Houston AB, et al. Intermittent ductal patency in healthy newborn infants: demonstration by color Doppler flow mapping. Arch Dis Child 1992;67:1217–1218.
24. Quiroga C. Partial persistence of the ductus arteriosus. Acta Radiol 1961;55:103–108.
25. Gittenberger-de Groot AC. Structural variation of the ductus arteriosus in congenital heart disease and in persistent fetal circulation. In: Godman MJ, ed. Pediatric cardiology. Edinburgh: Churchill-Livingstone, 1981;4.
26. Presbitero P, Bull C, Haworth SG, et al. Absent or occult pulmonary artery. Br Heart J 1984;52:178–185.
27. Elzenga NJ, Gittenberger-de Groot AC. The ductus arteriosus and stenoses of the pulmonary arteries in pulmonary atresia. Int J Cardiol 1986;11:195–208.
28. Campbell M. Natural history of patent ductus arteriosus. Br Heart J 1968;30:4–13.
29. Keys A, Shapiro MJ. Patency of the ductus arteriosus in adults. Am Heart J 1943;25:158–179.
30. Cosh JA. Patent ductus arteriosus. A follow-up study of 73 cases. Br Heart J 1957;19:13–22.
31. Sardesai SH, Marshall RJ, Farrow R, et al. Dissecting aneurysm of the pulmonary artery in a case of unoperated patent ductus arteriosus. Eur Heart J 1990;11:670–673.
32. Coard KCM, Martin MP. Ruptured saccular pulmonary artery aneurysm associated with persistent ductus arteriosus. Arch Pathol Lab Med 1992;116:159–161.
33. Jayakrishnan AG, Loftus B, Kelly P, et al. Spontaneous postpartum rupture of a patent ductus arteriosus. Histopathology 1992;21:383–384.

34. Green NJ, Rollason TP. Pulmonary artery rupture in pregnancy complicating patent ductus arteriosus. Br Heart J 1992; 68:616–618.
35. Higgins JC, O'Brien JK, Battle RW, et al. Left main coronary artery compression in patent ductus arteriosus. Am Heart J 1993;125:236–239.
36. Heikkinen ES, Simila S, Laitinen J, et al. Infantile aneurysm of the ductus arteriosus. Acta Paediatr Scand 1974;63:241–248.
37. Das JB, Chesterman JT. Aneurysms of the patent ductus arteriosus. Thorax 1956;11:295–302.
38. Lund JT, Jensen MB, Hjelms E. Aneurysm of the ductus arteriosus. Eur J Cardiothorac Surg 1991;5:566–570.
39. Falcone MW, Perloff JK, Roberts WC. Aneurysm of the nonpatent ductus arteriosus. Am J Cardiol 1972;29:422–426.
40. Malone PS, Cooper SG, Elliott M, et al. Aneurysm of the ductus arteriosus. Arch Dis Child 1989;64:1386–1388.
41. Baden B, Kirks DR. Transient dilatation of the ductus arteriosus—the "ductus bump." J Pediatr 1974;84:858–860.
42. Cruickshank B, Marquis RM. Spontaneous aneurysm of the ductus arteriosus. Am J Med 1958;25:140–149.
43. Tutassaura H, Goldman B, Moes CAF, et al. Spontaneous aneurysm of the ductus arteriosus. J Thorac Cardiovasc Surg 1969;57:180–184.
44. Taskar VS, John PJ, Mahashur AA. Ductal aneurysm presenting as acute lung collapse. J Assoc Physicians India 1992;40: 475–476.
45. Vargas-Barron J, Avila-Rosales L, Romero-Cardenas A, et al. Echocardiographic diagnosis of a mycotic aneurysm of the main pulmonary artery and patent ductus arteriosus. Am Heart J 1992;123:1707–1709.
46. Balzer DT, Spray TL, McMullin D, et al. Endarteritis associated with a clinically silent patent ductus arteriosus. Am Heart J 1993;125:1192–1193.
47. Bain RC, Edwards JE, Scheifley CH, et al. Right-sided bacterial endocarditis and endarteritis. Am J Med 1958;24:98–110.
48. Blumenthal S, Griffiths SP, Morgan BC. Bacterial endocarditis in children with heart disease. Pediatrics 1960;26:993–1017.
49. Rodbard S. Blood velocity and endocarditis. Circulation 1963;27:18–28.
50. Awadallah SM, Kavey RW, Byrum CJ, et al. The changing pattern of endocarditis in childhood. Am J Cardiol 1991;68: 90–94.
51. Chemoprophylaxis for infective endocarditis: faith, hope and charity challenged. Lancet 1992;339:525–526.
52. McGowan DA. A dental view of controversies in the prophylaxis of infective endocarditis. J Antimicrob Chemother 1987; 20:105–109.
53. Oakley CM. Controversies in the prophylaxis of infective endocarditis: a cardiological view. J Antimicrob Chemother 1987;20:99–104.
54. van der Meer JTM, van Wijk W, Thompson J, et al. Efficacy of antibiotic prophylaxis for prevention of native-valve endocarditis. Lancet 1992;339:135–139.
55. Houston AB, Gnanapragasam JP, Lim KM, et al. Doppler ultrasound and the silent ductus arteriosus. Br Heart J 1991; 65:97–99.
56. Brandt PWT, Clarkson PM, Barratt-Boyes BG, et al. An unusual oesophageal indentation caused by a long tortuous patent ductus arteriosus. Australas Radiol 1973;17:394–396.
57. Burney B, Smith WL, Franken EA, et al. Chest film diagnosis of patent ductus arteriosus in infants with hyaline membrane disease. AJR 1978;130:1149–1151.
58. Swischuk LE. Patent ductus arteriosus. Semin Roentgenol 1985;20:236–243.
59. Currarino G, Jackson JH. Calcification of the ductus arteriosus and ligamentum Botalli. Radiology 1970;94:139–142.
60. Reller MD, Ziegler ML, Rice MJ, et al. Duration of ductal shunting in healthy preterm infants: an echocardiographic color flow Doppler study. J Pediatr 1988;112:441–446.
61. Swensson RE, Valdes-Cruz LM, Sahn DJ, et al. Real-time Doppler color flow mapping for detection of patent ductus arteriosus. J Am Coll Cardiol 1986;8:1105–1112.
62. Szulc M, Ritter SB. Patent ductus arteriosus in the infant with atrioventricular septal defect and pulmonary hypertension: diagnosis by transesophageal color flow echocardiography. J Am Soc Echocardiogr 1991;4:194–198.
63. Stumper O, Witsenburg M, Sutherland GR, et al. Transesophageal echocardiographic monitoring of interventional cardiac catheterization in children. J Am Coll Cardiol 1991; 18:1506–1514.
64. Mugge A, Daniel WG, Lichtlen PR. Imaging of patent ductus arteriosus by transesophageal color-coded Doppler echocardiography. J Clin Ultrasound 1991;19:128–129.
65. Takenaka K, Sakamoto T, Shiota T, et al. Diagnosis of patent ductus arteriosus in adults by biplane transesophageal color Doppler flow mapping. Am J Cardiol 1991;68:691–693.
66. Dick C, Asinger RW. Contrast echocardiographic detection of a right-to-left shunting patent ductus arteriosus. J Am Soc Echocardiogr 1989;2:198–201.
67. Anand NK, Soloria M, Braudo JL, et al. Nonvisualization by aortography of patent ductus arteriosus associated with a large proximal left-to-right shunt. Chest 1971;60:156–160.
68. Rao PS, Thapar MK, Strong WB. Nonopacification of patent ductus arteriosus by aortography in patients with large ventricular septal defects. Angiology 1978;29:888–897.
69. Keane JF, McFaul R, Fellows K, et al. Balloon occlusion angiography in infancy: methods, uses and limitations. Am J Cardiol 1985;56:495–497.
70. Goodman PC, Jeffrey RB, Minagi H, et al. Angiographic evaluation of the ductus diverticulum. Cardiovasc Intervent Radiol 1982;5:1–4.
71. Chien C, Lin C, Hsu Y, et al. Potential diagnosis of hemodynamic abnormalities in patent ductus arteriosus by cine magnetic resonance imaging. Am Heart J 1991;122:1065–1073.
72. Friese KK, Dulce M, Higgins CB. Airway obstruction by right aortic arch with right-sided patent ductus arteriosus: demonstration by MRI. J Comput Assist Tomogr 1992;16:888–892.
73. Elliot RB, Starling MB, Neutze JM. Medical manipulation of the ductus arteriosus. Lancet 1975;1:140–142.
74. Clyman RI. Ductus arteriosus: current theories of prenatal and postnatal regulation. Semin Perinatol 1987;11:64–71.
75. Karwande SV, Rowles JR. Simplified muscle-sparing thoracotomy for patent ductus arteriosus ligation in neonates. Ann Thorac Surg 1992;54:164–165.
76. Laborde F, Noirhomme P, Karam J, et al. A new video-assisted thoracoscopic surgical technique for interruption of patent ductus arteriosus in infants and children. J Thoracic Cardiovasc Surg 1993;105:278–280.
77. Panagopoulos PG, Tatooles CJ, Aberdeen E, et al. Patent ductus arteriosus in infants and children. Thorax 1971;26: 137–144.
78. Trippestad A, Efskind L. Patent ductus arteriosus. Scand J Thorac Cardiovasc Surg 1972;6:38–42.
79. Morgan JM, Gray HH, Miller GAH, et al. The clinical features, management and outcome of persistence of the arterial duct presenting in adult life. Int J Cardiol 1990;27:193–199.
80. Pontius RG, Danielson GK, Noonan JA, et al. Illusions leading to surgical closure of the distal left pulmonary artery instead of the ductus arteriosus. J Thorac Cardiovasc Surg 1981;82:107–113.
81. Fleming WH, Sarafian LB, Kugler JD, et al. Ligation of patent ductus arteriosus in premature infants: importance of accurate anatomic definition. Pediatrics 1983;71:373–375.
82. Musewe N, Benson LN, Smallhorn JF, et al. Two-dimensional echocardiographic and color flow Doppler evaluation of ductal occlusion with the Rashkind prosthesis. Circulation 1989;80:1706–1710.
83. Sorensen KE, Kristensen BO, Hansen OK. Frequency of occurrence of residual ductal flow after surgical ligation by color-flow mapping. Am J Cardiol 1991;67:653–654.

84. Marantz P, Salgado G, Villa A, et al. Residual patent arterial duct after surgery. Cardiol Young 1993;3(Suppl 1):143.
85. Zucker N, Qureshi SA, Baker EJ, et al. Residual patency of the arterial duct subsequent to surgical ligation. Cardiol Young 1993;3:216–219.
86. Cambier PA, Kirby WC, Wortham DC, et al. Percutaneous closure of the small (<2.5 mm) patent ductus arteriosus using coil embolization. Am J Cardiol 1992;69:815–816.
87. Le TP, Neuss MB, Redel DA, et al. A new transcatheter occlusion technique with retrievable, double-disk shaped coils—first clinical results in occlusion of patent ductus arteriosus. Cardiol Young 1993;3(Suppl 1):38.
88. Rao PS, Wilson AD, Sideris EB, et al. Transcatheter closure of patent ductus arteriosus with buttoned device: first successful clinical application in a child. Am Heart J 1991;121:1799–1802.
89. Warnecke I, Frank J, Hohle R, et al. Transvenous double-balloon occlusion of the persistent ductus arteriosus: an experimental study. Pediatr Cardiol 1984;5:79–84.
90. Echigo S, Matsuda T, Kamiya T, et al. Development of a new transvenous patent ductus arteriosus occlusion technique using a shape memory polymer. ASAIO Trans 1990;36:M195–M198.
91. Wierny L, Plass R, Porstmann W. Transluminal closure of patent ductus arteriosus: long-term results of 208 cases treated without thoracotomy. Cardiovasc Intervent Radiol 1986;9: 279–285.
92. Wierny L, Plass R. Twenty-five years experience from transfemoral catheter closure of patent ductus arteriosus. J Intervent Cardiol 1991;4:301–310.
93. Sato K, Kawamoto S, Yoshida S, et al. Transfemoral plug closure of patent ductus arteriosus: experiences at Osaka Prefectural Hospital. J Intervent Cardiol 1991;4:295–300.
94. Rashkind WJ, Cuaso CC. Transcatheter closure of patent ductus arteriosus. Pediatr Cardiol 1979;1:3–7.
95. Bash SE, Mullins CE. Insertion of patent ductus arteriosus occluder by transvenous approach: a new technique. Circulation 1984;70:II–285.
96. Rashkind WJ, Mullins CE, Hellenbrand WE, et al. Nonsurgical closure of patent ductus arteriosus: clinical application of the Rashkind PDA Occluder System. Circulation 1987;75: 583–592.
97. Hosking MCK, Benson LN, Musewe N, et al. Transcatheter occlusion of the persistently patent ductus arteriosus: forty-month follow-up and prevalence of residual shunting. Circulation 1991;84:2313–2317.
98. Bonhoeffer P, Borghi A, Onorato E, et al. Transfemoral closure of patent ductus arteriosus in adult patients. Int J Cardiol 1993;39:181–186.
99. Huggon IC, Tabatabaei AH, Qureshi SA, et al. Use of a second transcatheter Rashkind arterial occluder for persistent flow after implantation of the first device: indications and results. Br Heart J 1993;69:544–550.
100. Bridges ND, Perry SB, Parness I, et al. Transcatheter closure of a large patent ductus arteriosus with the clamshell septal umbrella. J Am Coll Cardiol 1991;18:1297–1302.
101. Wessel DL, Keane JF, Parness I, et al. Outpatient closure of the patent ductus arteriosus. Circulation 1988;77:1068–1071.
102. Vitiello R, Benson L, Musewe N, et al. Factors influencing the persistence of shunting within 24 hours of catheter occlusion of the ductus arteriosus. Br Heart J 1991;65:211–212.
103. Perry SB, Lock JE. Front-loading of double-umbrella devices, a new technique for umbrella delivery for closing cardiovascular defects. Am J Cardiol 1992;70:917–920.
104. Pavlovic D, de Lezo JS, Medina A, et al. Sequential transcatheter treatment of combined coarctation of aorta and persistent ductus arteriosus. Am Heart J 1992;123:249–250.
105. Galal O, Al-Fadley F, Wilson N. Successful transcatheter closure of patent arterial duct six years after balloon dilatation of coarctation of the aorta. Int J Cardiol 1992;35:123–125.
106. Transcatheter occlusion of persistent arterial duct. Report of the European Registry. Lancet 1992;340:1062–1066.
107. Ali Khan MA, Al Yousef S, Mullins CE, et al. Experience with 205 procedures for transcatheter closure of ductus arteriosus in 182 patients, with special reference to residual shunts and long-term follow-up. J Thorac Cardiovasc Surg 1992;104: 1721–1727.
108. Latson LA, Hofschire PJ, Kugler JD, et al. Transcatheter closure of patent ductus arteriosus in pediatric patients. J Pediatr 1989;115:549–553.
109. Galal O, Wilson N, Al Fadley F, et al. Novice experience with transcatheter closure of the arterial duct in children, adolescents and adults. Cardiol Young 1992;2:285–290.
110. Dyck JD, Benson LN, Smallhorn JF, et al. Catheter occlusion of the persistently patent ductus arteriosus. Am J Cardiol 1988;62:1089–1092.
111. Al Yousef S, Ali Khan MA, Mullins CE, et al. Use in children of an additional umbrella for transcatheter occlusion of residual patency of the arterial duct following initial insertion of an umbrella device. Cardiol Young 1992;2:353–356.
112. Harris SL. Definitions and demographic characteristics. In: Kaye D, ed. Infective endocarditis. 2nd ed. New York: Raven, 1992.
113. Hayes AM, Redington AN, Rigby ML. Severe haemolysis after transcatheter duct occlusion: a non-surgical remedy. Br Heart J 1992;67:321–322.
114. Grifka RG, O'Laughlin MP, Mullins CE. Late transcatheter removal of a Rashkind PDA Occlusion Device for persistent hemolysis using a modified transseptal sheath. Cathet Cardiovasc Diagn 1992;25:140–143.
115. Ladusans EJ, Murdoch I, Franciosi J. Severe haemolysis after percutaneous closure of a ductus arteriosus (arterial duct). Br Heart J 1989;61:548–550.
116. Ottenkamp J, Hess J, Talsma MD, et al. Protrusion of the device: a complication of catheter closure of patent ductus arteriosus. Br Heart J 1992;68:301–303.
117. Fadley F, Al-Halees Z, Galal O, et al. Left pulmonary artery stenosis after transcatheter occlusion of persistent arterial duct. Lancet 1993;341:559–560.

17

Coarctation of the Aorta

RACHEL R. PHILLIPS
J. A. GORDON CULHAM

Definition

Coarctation of the aorta is a congenital obstructive anomaly of the aortic lumen characteristically localized near or at the junction of the aortic arch and descending aorta, adjacent to the ductus arteriosus and distal to the origin of the left subclavian artery. Rarely, coarctation of the intraabdominal aorta may occur, usually in isolation.

Hypoplasia of the transverse aortic arch proximal to the site of coarctation is frequently present in infants with coarctation. Arch atresia is the most severe expression of coarctation when the aortic lumen is not patent. A distinct entity is interruption of the aortic arch with discontinuity between the ascending and the descending aorta, with the classification based on the site of interruption. Interruption of the aorta is not discussed in this chapter.

Types of Aortic Coarctation

Traditionally, coarctation has been classified into infantile and adult types or into preductal and postductal forms. Both types of coarctation are recognized in the neonatal period, and relatively long segments of stenosis occur in a significant number of adults. The relationship of the coarctation to the ligamentum is difficult to define, does not appear to determine the presence and extent of a collateral circulation, and is not of proved prognostic significance and therefore not useful. It is our belief that both age groups have in common a discrete distal arch obstruction. In addition, there may be associated hypoplasia of the isthmus or arch.[1,2] The clinical presentation, associated anomalies, morphology, investigation, and treatment are different in infants than in older children and adults.

Coarctation in Infancy

In infants, coarctation consists of a discrete distal arch obstruction and proximal tubular hypoplasia (Fig. 17-1). There is an increased incidence of associated intracardiac lesions, including a high incidence of bicuspid aortic valve. Occasionally the hypoplasia is of such severity that extended repair is required; rarely, hypoplasia occurs alone. Growth of the arch is documented postoperatively, but some older children and adults have residual obstruction due to a small arch.[3]

Coarctation in the Older Child or Adult

A localized, short, juxtaductal narrowing is usually present in which there is an abrupt stenosis produced by a shelflike membrane extending from the posterior and lateral walls of the aorta (Fig. 17-2).[4] The circumferential narrowing is almost always just beyond the origin of the left subclavian artery near the ligamentum arteriosum. Associated intracardiac abnormalities are unusual except for bicuspid aortic valve.

Incidence

One percent of all live-born infants have congenital heart disease, and a further 1 percent have a bicuspid aortic valve. Five percent of infants with congenital heart disease have coarctation of the aorta.[5] Among children dying of heart disease in the first month of life, coarctation of the aorta previously accounted for between 13 and 17 percent of the autopsies and was the second most common cardiac anomaly.[6] Currently the mortality rate related to isolated coarctation is less than 3 percent.[7]

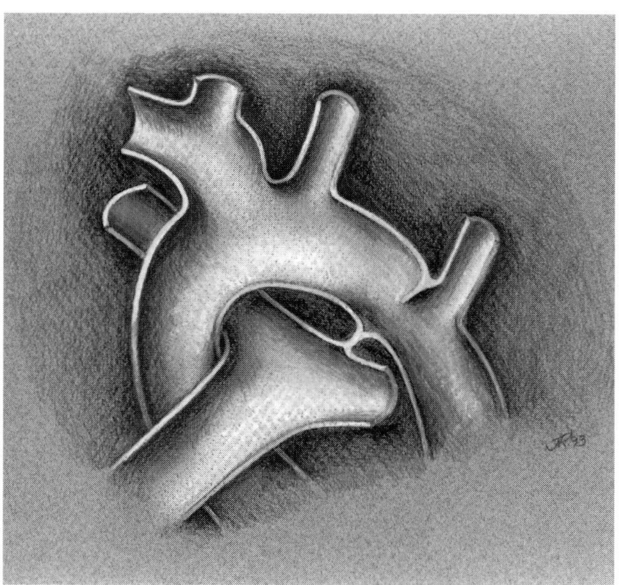

A

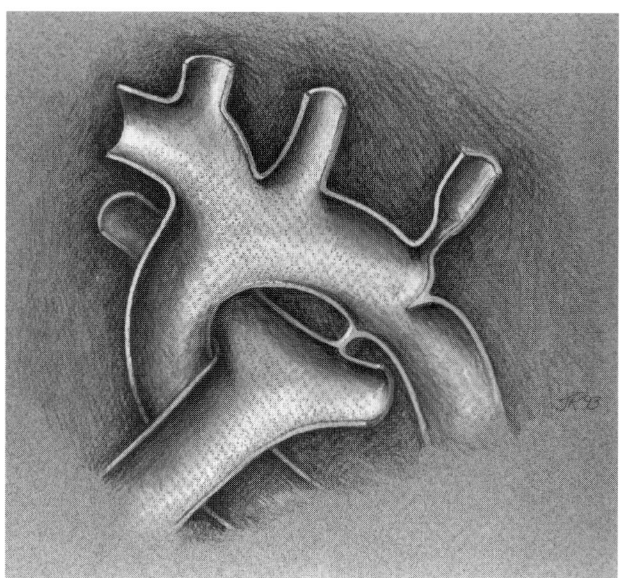

B

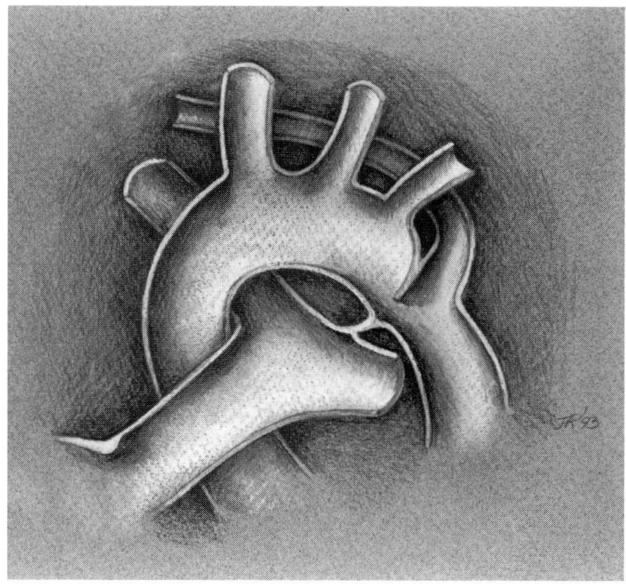

C

Figure 17-4. Diagrams illustrating coarctation angiograms proximal to the left subclavian artery (A), involving the left subclavian artery (B), and proximal to an aberrant right subclavian artery (C).

Clinical Variants

In cases with stenosis of the left subclavian artery or distal left subclavian artery, hypertension is only present in the right arm. If the right subclavian is aberrant, only the left upper limb is hypertensive. If both the subclavians are distal to the coarctation, then only the carotid arteries are hypertensive and there is no pulse or pressure discrepancy between the upper and lower limbs (Fig. 17-4).[25] Hypertension may be absent when severe aortic stenosis is associated with coarctation; however, the disparity in blood pressure is present, even though it may be relatively small in magnitude. The differential diagnosis in infants includes interrupted aortic arch and the hypoplastic left heart syndrome.

Older Children or Adults

The older child is often asymptomatic. The arch obstruction leads to increased left ventricular pressure and hypertension in the ascending aorta and branches proximal to the coarctation (i.e., hypertension in the arms, unless there is stenosis or an anomalous origin of the subclavian arteries) and decreased blood pressure in the legs. The brachial pulses are easily palpable, whereas the femoral pulses are usually delayed and weak or absent. Uncommonly there is lower limb claudication, epistaxis, or central nervous system hemorrhage (Fig. 17-5). A systolic murmur may be heard over the upper left chest and back. A thrill may be palpated over the back caused by collateral vessels. In adults the ECG is usually normal or shows a left ventricular hypertrophy pattern. Associated defects, apart from bicuspid aortic valve, are uncommon. The clinical picture of coarctation may be mimicked by vasculitis or peripheral vascular disease.

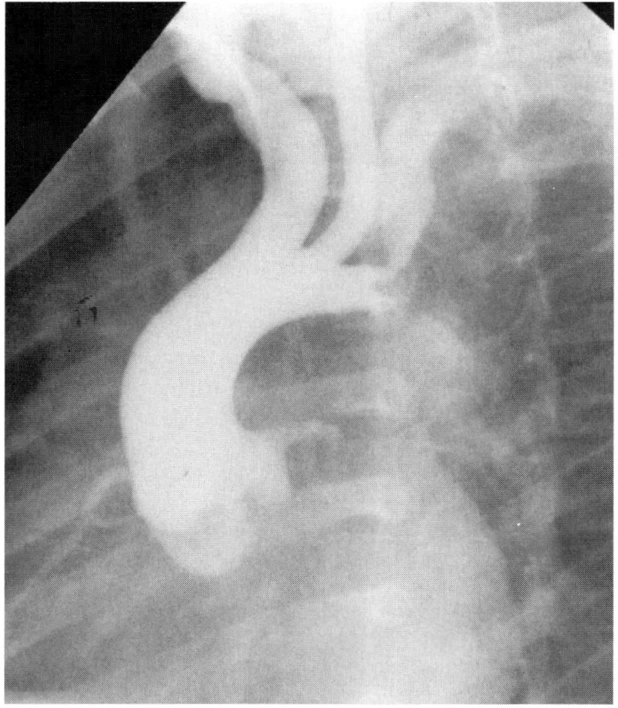

D

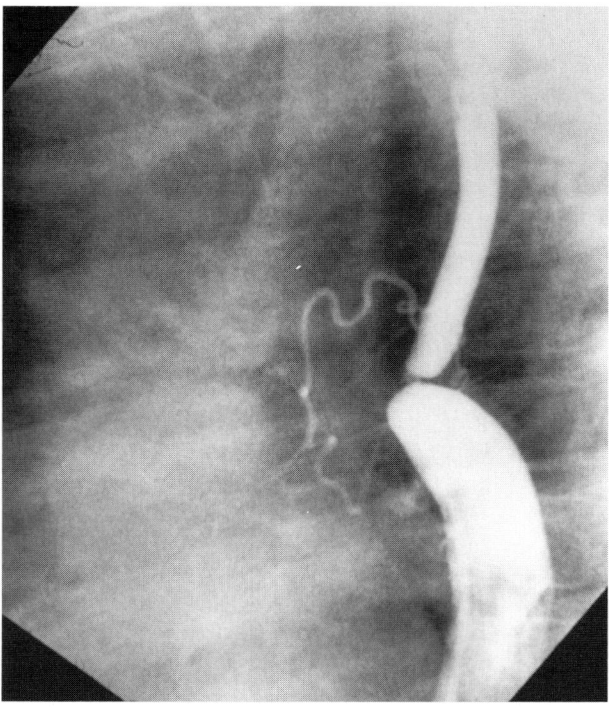

E

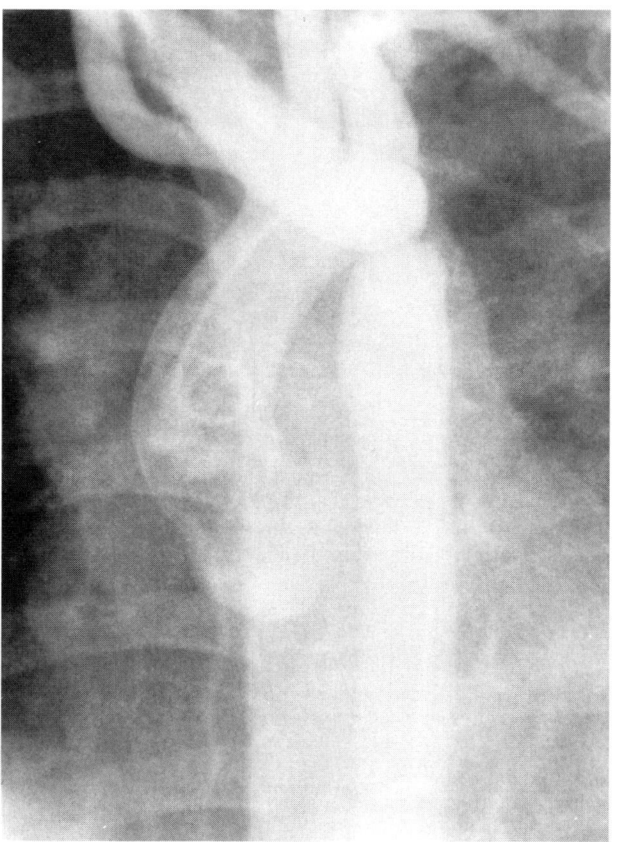

F

Figure 17-4 (continued). (D) Arch hypoplasia and severe coarctation are associated with stenosis of the origin of the left subclavian. (E) Another child shows a coarctation shelf involving the origin of the left subclavian artery. (F) Yet another patient has discrete coarctation with dilatation of the left and aberrant right subclavian arteries.

Complications of Aortic Coarctation

If the coarctation is untreated, life expectancy is shortened to 35 years, and there is morbidity associated with left ventricular failure, infective endocarditis, dissecting hematoma, mycotic or false aneurysm because of jet lesion on the wall of the aorta, aneurysm of the intercostal arteries, cerebrovascular events (rupture of aortic or cerebral aneurysm), and anterior spinal artery syndrome (the anterior spinal artery participates in collateral circulation below the site of coarctation and may become dilated, tortuous, and occluded). Older children and adolescents found to have coarctation often have elevated blood pressures early and later after adequate repair. Hypertension-related cardiovascular morbidity and mortality have been common in these patients on long-term follow-up.[26–28] The persistent systemic hypertension may be related to baroreceptor alteration, renin–angiotensin interaction, a neural crest origin of coarctation, decreased aortic compliance, or other factors.[28–30]

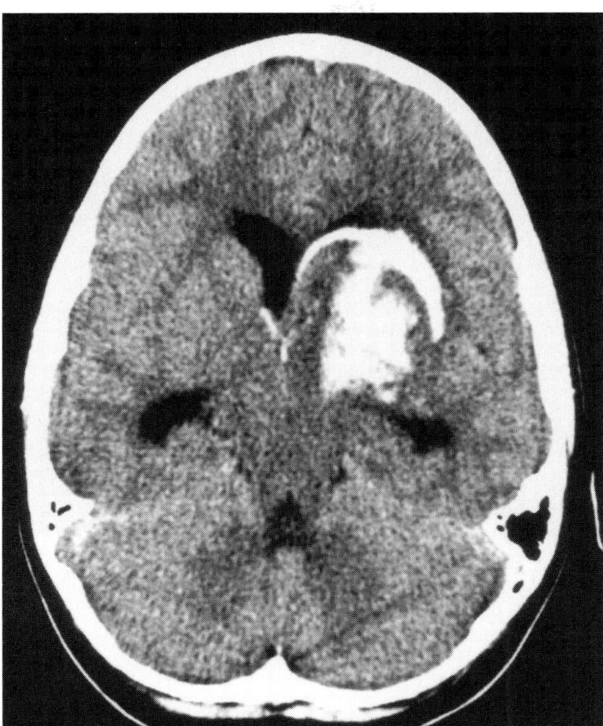

Figure 17-5. CT scan of the brain showing a hypertensive cerebral hemorrhage as the presenting feature of a teenage girl with coarctation.

Investigation

The goals of investigation in patients with coarctation are to assess the morphology of the aortic arch, to define the anatomy of the focal area of narrowing, to assess any associated lesions, to determine the most appropriate treatment, and to provide appropriate follow-up imaging.

The diagnosis of coarctation involves a combination of chest x-ray, echocardiography, angiography, and magnetic resonance imaging (MRI). Both computed tomography (CT) and digital subtraction angiography can be used to confirm the diagnosis.[31,32] Both modalities, however, use ionizing radiation, allow fewer planes of imaging than MRI, and require intravenous administration of contrast material. Digital subtraction angiography usually requires the placement of a central venous catheter.[33,34]

We suggest that the assessment of coarctation in infants should be made using a combination of chest x-ray, echocardiography, cardiac catheterization, and aortography, and that in older children and adults complete assessment should be made with a combination of echocardiography and MRI. In older children and adults, cardiac catheterization and aortography are not required unless angioplasty is to be performed.

Chest X-ray: Classical Roentgenographic Features

Imaging of coarctation of the aorta can in some instances be accomplished noninvasively by chest radiography, the appearances on plain film varying with the severity of the coarctation and the age of the child.[35,36] Conventional roentgenologic studies of infants with coarctation often demonstrate cardiomegaly due to heart failure with or without an intracardiac shunt (Fig. 17-6). In the young child, the chest x-ray most commonly demonstrates cardiomegaly and dilatation of the descending aorta distal to the coarctation (Fig. 17-7). In the older child or adult, the normal smooth curvilinear form of the arch is altered. Various deformities of the arch may occur: often a notch may be visualized and the classical number 3 sign may be seen, the upper portion of the 3 due to dilatation of the left subclavian artery and the lower portion due to poststenotic dilatation of the descending thoracic aorta. There is usually a normal heart size or slight left ventricular enlargement (Fig. 17-8). The administration of a small amount of barium before the chest radiograph may demonstrate an indentation on the esophagus at the level of the arch and another at the site of poststenotic dilatation of the descending thoracic aorta (reversed 3 sign). Dilatation of the ascending aorta may be present if there is a stenotic, usually bicuspid, aortic valve. Enlarged collateral vessels may often be seen in the adult as a retrosternal wavy opacity (due to enlarged internal thoracic arteries) or resulting in notching of the inferior surface of the third to ninth ribs. Rib notching below the age of 6 months is rare, whereas it is commonly present beyond the age of 5 years (see Fig. 17-8). The finding is usually bilateral, but unilateral rib notching may occur. Right-sided notching occurs if the coarctation is proximal to the left subclavian artery or if there is atresia or stenosis of the origin of the left subclavian artery (Fig. 17-9). Left-sided notching occurs if there is atresia or stenosis of the origin of the right subclavian artery or if there is an anomalous origin of the right subclavian artery distal to the site of coarctation.

Echocardiography

Two-dimensional echocardiography with simultaneous pulsed Doppler studies has been used as a noninvasive method to detect coarctation of the aorta and has been advocated by some as the sole preoperative im-

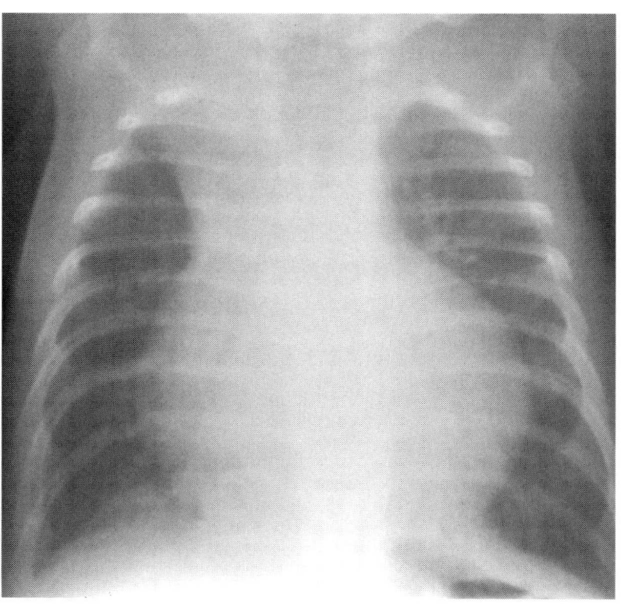
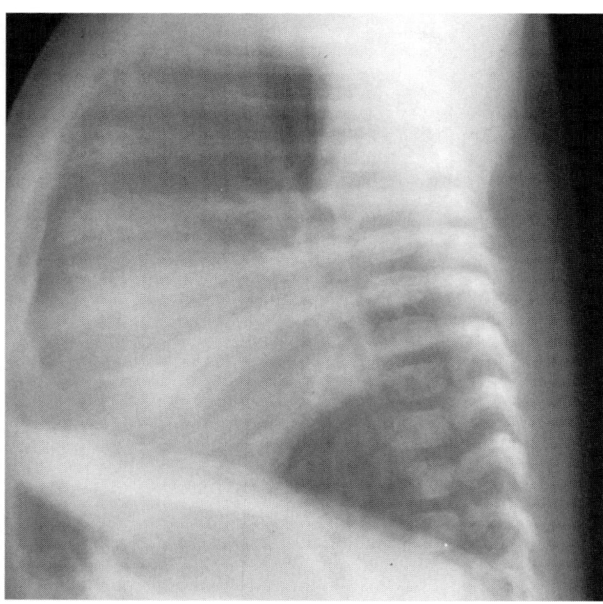

A B

Figure 17-6. Chest x-ray in frontal (A) and lateral projection (B) shows an infant with a large heart, normal vascularity, hyperinflation as a sign of failure, and dilatation of the descending thoracic aorta.

Figure 17-7. Chest x-ray in frontal projection in a child shows normal vascularity, a small arch, and marked dilatation of the descending thoracic aorta.

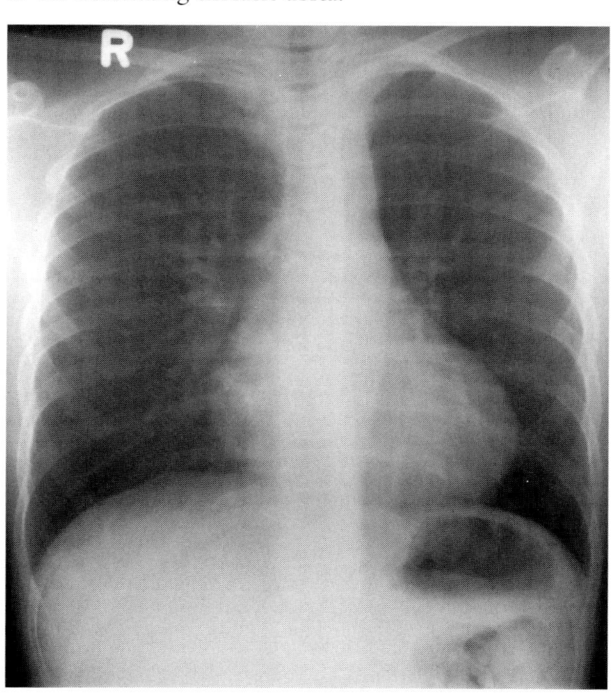

aging modality.[37,38] In infants, a combination of real-time cross-sectional echocardiography and Doppler echocardiographic methods makes reliable noninvasive diagnosis of coarctation of the aorta possible, as well as the evaluation of associated defects and indications for operation, without the application of invasive methods. The echocardiographic examination is easier in infants than in adults because the great vessels are better demonstrated using suprasternal or high right parasternal views, with a reported sensitivity for the detection of arch anomalies of 92 percent.[39] In infants, the suprasternal view uses the thymus as an acoustic window (Fig. 17-10). Tortuosity of the aorta at the level of the subclavian artery may cause the aorta to curve out of the beam path, creating the false appearance of a coarctation, and echocardiography may not be reliable in consistently depicting the proximal descending aorta.[40] In adults, the parasternal or apical window is used to visualize the thoracic aorta. The thymus is much smaller and the lung volumes are increased, and therefore the acoustic window is often lacking, the suprasternal view is not useful, and additional imaging may be required.

In patients with coarctation, two-dimensional echocardiography may reveal the following:

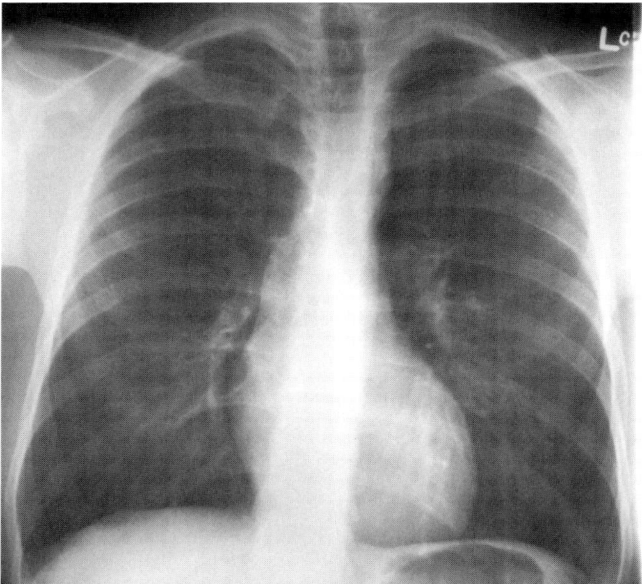

A

Figure 17-8. (A) Chest x-ray in frontal projection in an adult shows a normal heart, normal vascularity, a notch in the descending thoracic aorta (3 sign), and bilateral rib notching. (B) Detail view of the right chest of another patient shows notching of the undersurface of the fourth through eighth ribs.

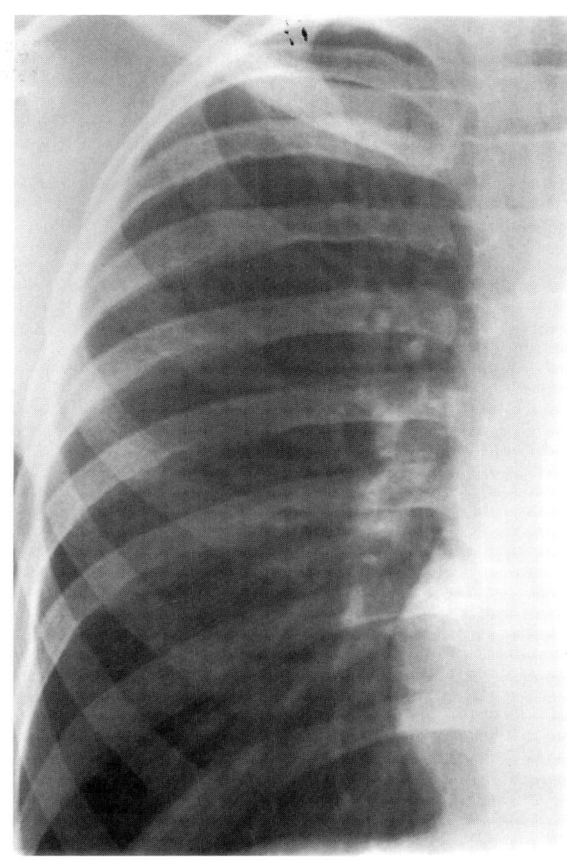

B

Figure 17-9. Chest film of an 8-month-old child shows unilateral right rib notching.

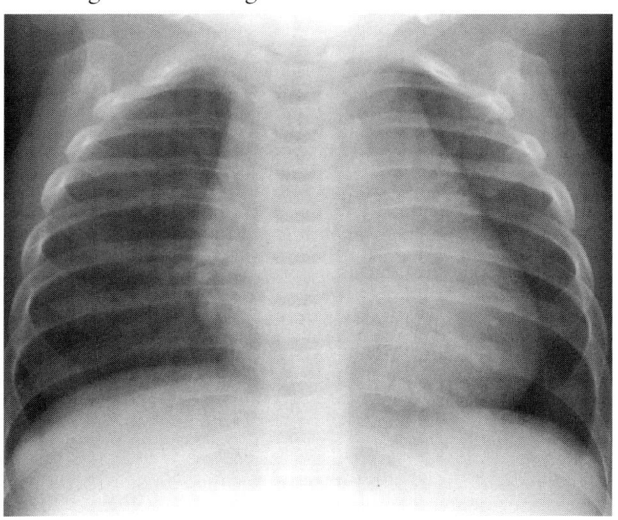

Figure 17-10. Echocardiographic examination from the suprasternal approach shows bright echos at the site of coarctation and arch hypoplasia.

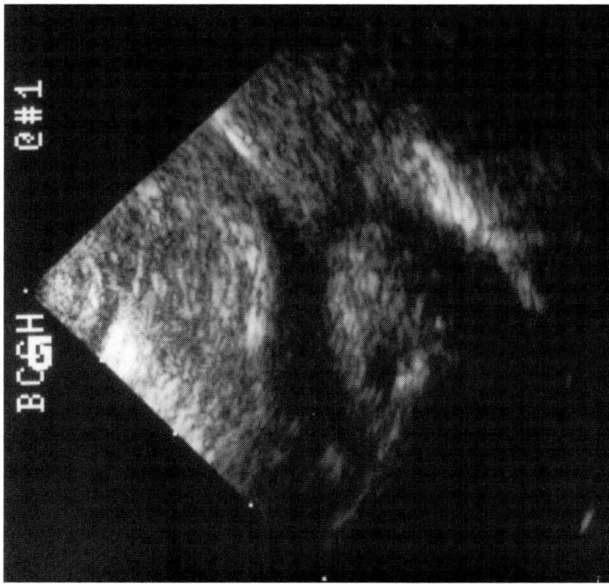

1. A shelf of echodense tissue obstructing the aortic lumen from its posterior aspect, arising just distal to the origin of the left subclavian artery, with poststenotic dilatation of the descending aorta distal to the site of coarctation.
2. Hypoplasia of the arch. The transverse arch and coarctation area are best visualized from the suprasternal notch (or subcostal approach in infancy) and may demonstrate mild to moderate arch hypoplasia.
3. Enlarged left carotid and left subclavian artery.
4. Abnormal flow pattern at the site of the coarctation with acceleration typical for the flow in a stenotic vessel.
5. Reduced pulsation of the descending thoracic and abdominal aorta, compared with the pulsation of the ascending aorta, which may be very pulsatile.
6. Presence or absence of a patent ductus arteriosus (PDA).
7. Bicuspid aortic valve and mitral valve anomaly.
8. Left ventricular outflow tract lesions, ventricular septal defects.
9. Left ventricular dysfunction and endocardial fibroelastosis.
10. In the neonatal period, pulmonary hypertension and increased right ventricular pressure and therefore right ventricular thickening and enlargement.

Overall, two-dimensional echocardiography has high sensitivity and specificity for detecting most aortic lesions in neonates and small infants. In older children, echocardiography and MRI are complementary. The use of both these modalities may produce an accurate diagnosis that obviates the need for angiography.

Examination by continuous-wave Doppler echocardiography is an effective noninvasive method of assessing the pressure drop across the coarctation, and pulsed Doppler shows altered flow in the ascending and descending aorta except in patients with an additional PDA.[25,41,42] There are a number of limitations of Doppler echocardiography, however, and, in the diagnosis of neonatal coarctation of the aorta, high-velocity jets (of 3 m per second or more in the descending aorta) are an infrequent finding. In addition, there may be poor agreement between the upper and lower limb blood pressure difference and the Doppler derived peak pressure drop. Doppler ultrasound may provide useful information on coexisting intracardiac abnormalities, but in the presence of ductal patency is of little value in the diagnosis of coarctation itself.[43] Occasionally normal flow velocities in the aortic arch may be recorded in patients with coarctation if there is an extensive collateral supply to the descending aorta.[44]

Angiocardiography and Aortography

Although the diagnosis of aortic coarctation can usually be made on clinical grounds, the assessment of the exact anatomy of the lesion is required to plan treatment. Cardiac catheterization and angiography are established techniques that have been regarded as the definitive preoperative diagnostic procedures essential to evaluating coarctation of the aorta presenting in infancy.[45,46] Left ventriculography provides satisfactory visualization of the ventricular septum, the subaortic region, the mitral and aortic valve, and left ventricular performance (which may be affected by endocardial sclerosis). In addition to the coarctation, aortography optimally defines the aortic valve, the coronary arteries, the branching pattern of the brachiocephalic vessels from the aortic arch, and the ductal status. However, it has some disadvantages. Cardiac catheterization is invasive, requires contrast media injection (with the added difficulty and risk imposed by the coarctation), and uses ionizing radiation.

In the older child and adult, angiography is essential if angioplasty is to be performed but has otherwise been superseded by the combination of echocardiography and MRI except in the unusual patients who are unable to be scanned by MRI (e.g., patients with pacemakers or other metallic implants).

Technique

In the infant, the left ventricle can often be entered via the foramen ovale from a venous approach. Alternatively, if there is a ventricular septal defect (VSD), the left ventricle may be entered from the right via the VSD. In the absence of shunting, a left ventriculogram will demonstrate the aortic arch well. If a shunt precludes good visualization, a selective aortic injection is needed. The angiogram should be recorded in biplane right anterior oblique projection and left anterior oblique projection with craniocaudal angulation. A good bolus of contrast (1 to 2 ml/kg) should be used, especially in the presence of a shunt.

Access to the ascending aorta may be difficult. A retrograde femoral approach is possible in mild coarctation, and a retrograde brachial approach may also be used. Axillary cutdown is not advocated, especially in babies, because it may compromise clinical follow-up, since the right arm may be the only reliable site to measure blood pressure after surgery. Denham reported floating a balloon angiocatheter from the pulmonary artery through a PDA to image the distal arch (Fig. 17-11).[47,48]

In the older child or adult, contrast is injected in the ascending aorta with a high-flow pigtail or NIH catheter using approximately 1 ml per kilogram body

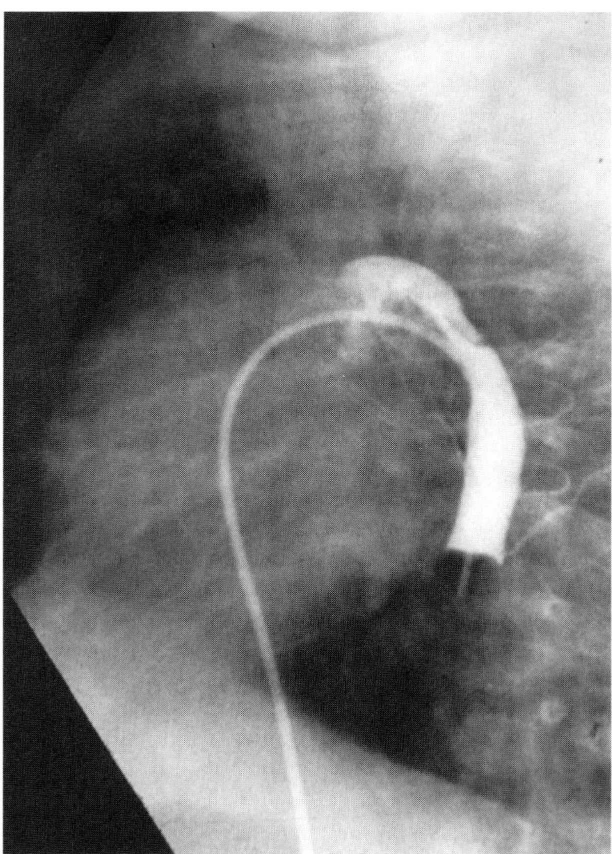

Figure 17-11. Angiogram performed via a PDA using a balloon to occlude the descending aorta.

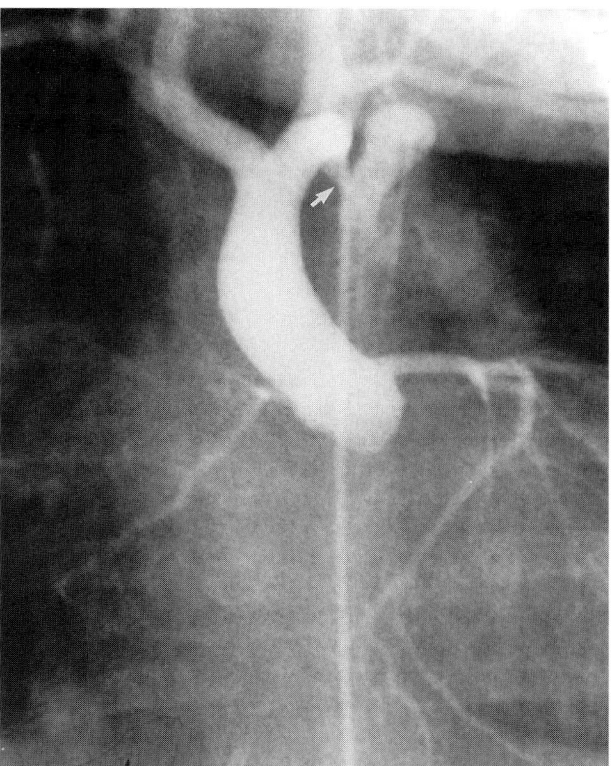

Figure 17-12. Aortic root injection in a frontal projection reveals an area of severe narrowing (*arrow*) that was obscured in LAO view by the dilated PDA.

weight. Filming is usually in the steep (65- to 75-degree) left anterior oblique (LAO) projection and in the 45- to 60-degree right anterior oblique (RAO) projection. Occasionally other views are needed (Fig. 17-12).

Angiographic Findings

Although all segments of the thoracic aorta show varying degrees of deformity in coarctation, the focal stenosis is the essential malformation. Aortography will provide information regarding the following:

1. The length, severity, and position of the stenosis.
2. The degree of forward displacement of the stenotic area at the level of the ligamentum arteriosum.
3. The appearance of the transverse aortic arch.
4. The presence of any associated malformations, including bicuspid aortic valve, dilatation of the aortic root, and any aberrant or stenosed vessels.
5. The collateral vessels.

In most neonates, the ductus arteriosus is patent. A discrete area of narrowing adjacent to the ductus or ligamentum arteriosum is present. In infants, focal narrowing at the classical site is seen, with or without arch hypoplasia (see Fig. 17-1). The hypoplasia of the aortic arch may begin at the origin of the innominate artery and extend to the insertion of the ligamentum arteriosum. The obstruction is of variable severity and may be so slight as to produce only a small gradient, or so severe as to virtually obstruct flow (Figs. 17-13 through 17-15).

In adults, the maximum stenosis is usually short and often resembles a diaphragm. The focal luminal narrowing may be associated with a posterior ridge and forward displacement (see Fig. 17-2). In approximately 2 to 3 percent of older patients a narrowing of the transverse arch and isthmus of the aorta is present in addition to the discrete stenosis. The left subclavian artery, if not stenotic at its origin, is often dilated and accounts for the soft tissue prominence seen in the left superior mediastinum. In half of all cases, the coarctation is well beyond the origin of the left subclavian

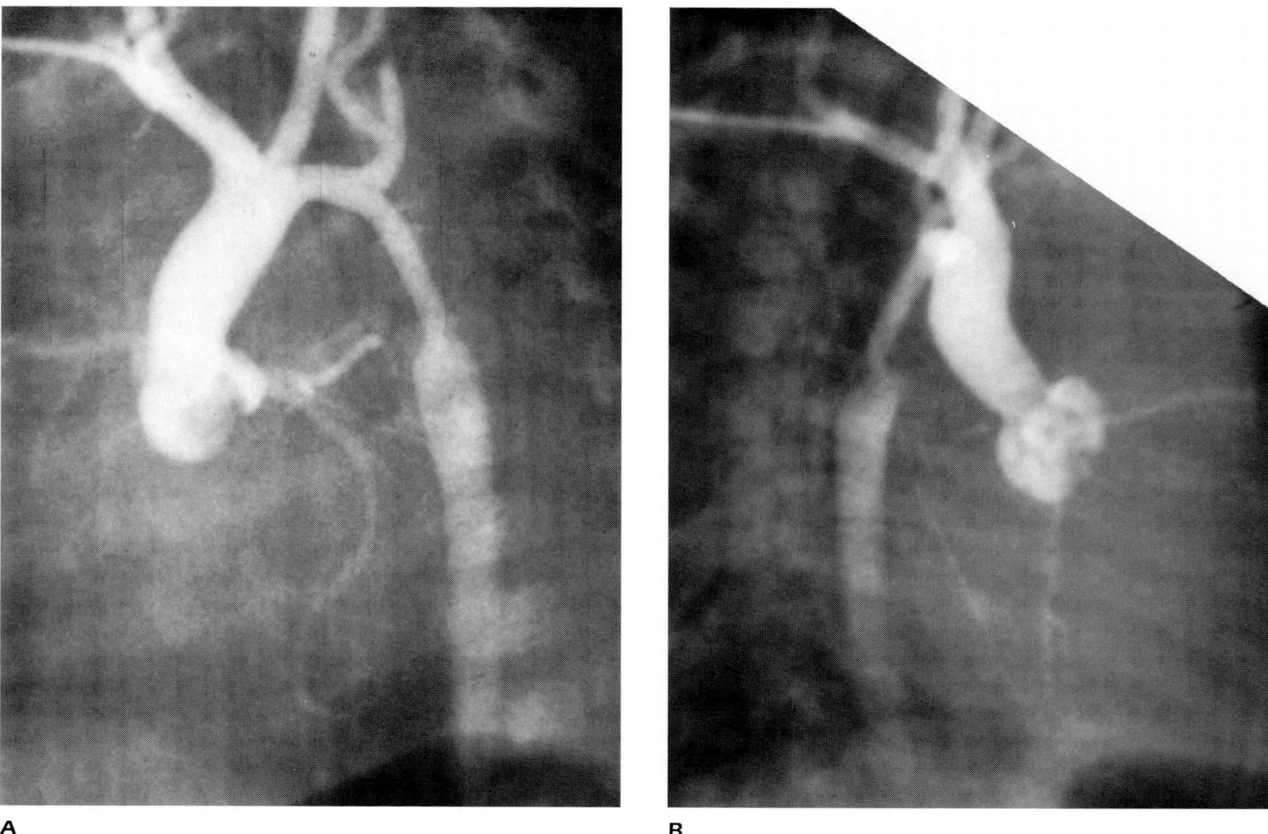

Figure 17-13. (A) Aortogram in LAO projection shows severe arch and isthmic hypoplasia. (B) The RAO view reveals the discrete coarctation. Note the long hypoplastic isthmus.

Figure 17-14. Retrograde catheter occluding the arch. Early (A) and later (B) images show severe obstruction proximal to the origin of the left subclavian artery.

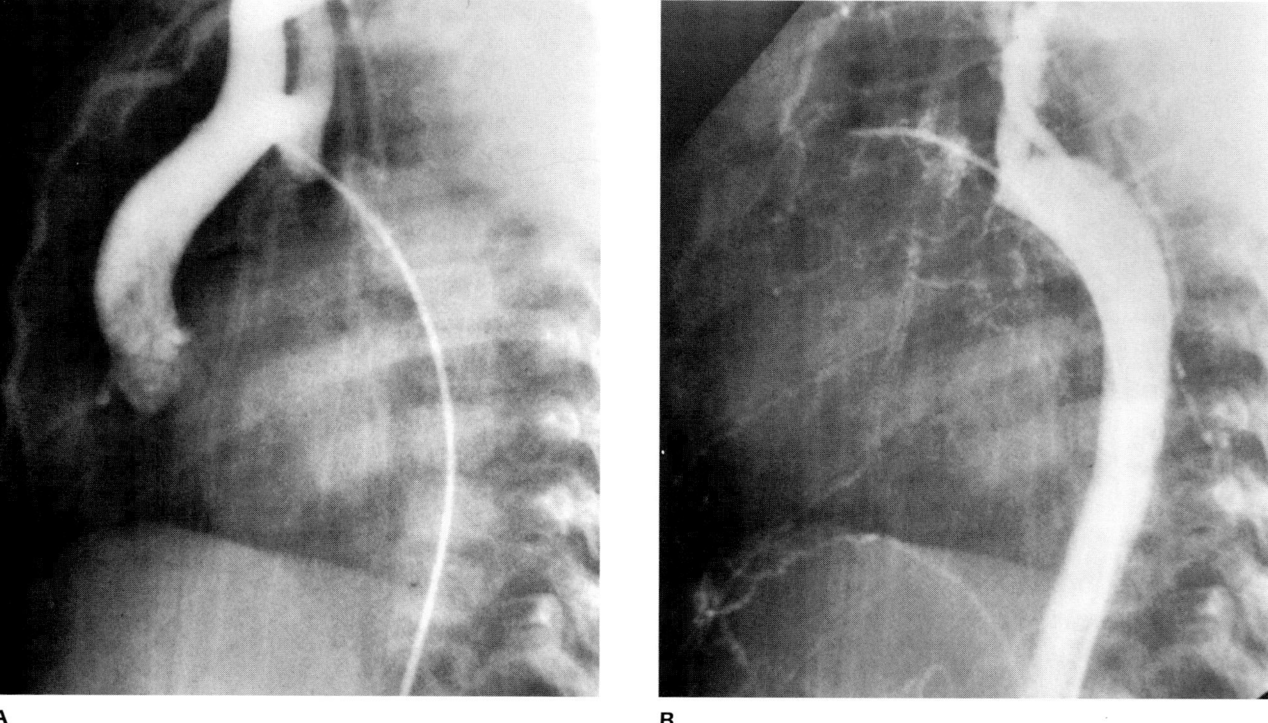

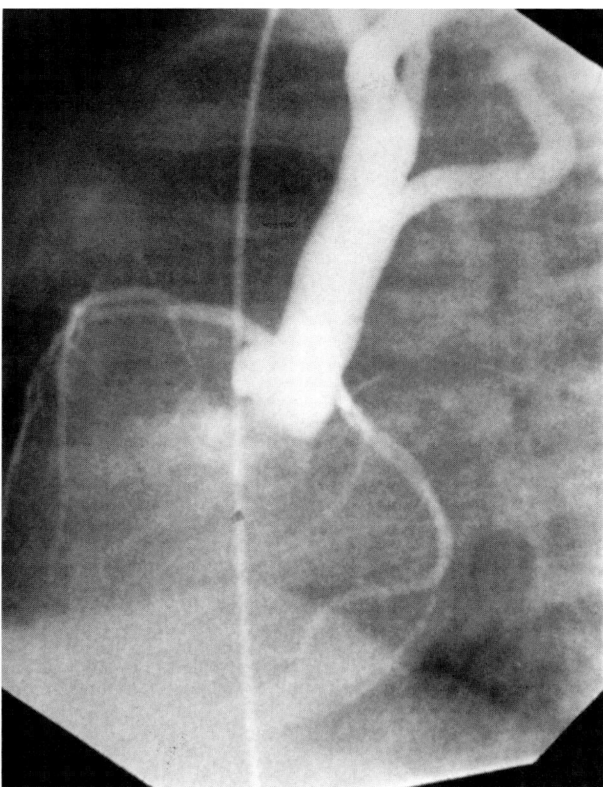

Figure 17-15. Aortogram from the right brachial approach showing arch atresia. The curve of the arch serves to distinguish arch atresia from interrupted aortic arch (see Fig. 18-2).

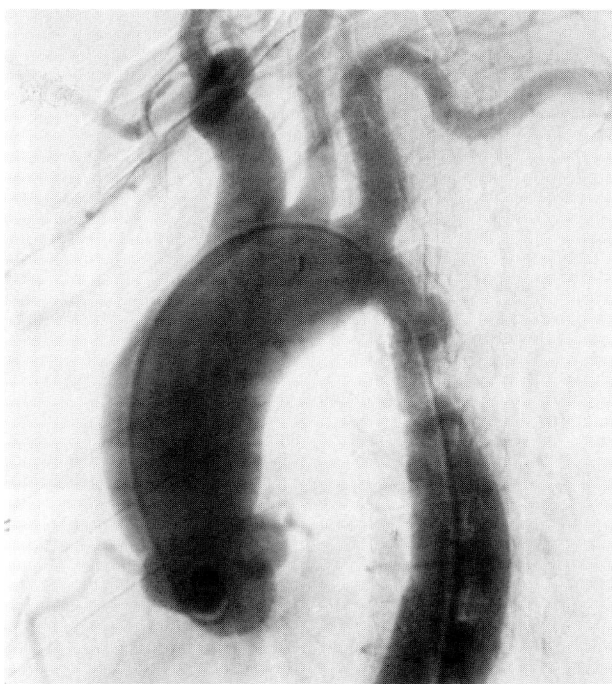

Figure 17-16. Aortogram in an adult shows an hourglass narrowing of the arch, marked dilatation of the ascending aorta, and an aneurysm. There has been no surgical or catheter intervention. (Courtesy of Drs. Ian Marsh and Jean Seely.)

artery (1–2 cm; see Fig. 17-13) and in slightly less than half the cases it is just distal to the origin (about 5 mm or less; see Figs. 17-1 and 17-2). Rarely, it is proximal to the origin of both subclavian arteries (see Fig. 17-14). The narrowing of the arch may involve the origin of the left subclavian, and the right subclavian may be aberrant (see Fig. 17-4). When localized juxtaductal coarctation is observed, poststenotic dilatation is present. Occasionally the narrowing has an hourglass shape (Fig. 17-16). Long segment narrowing may extend into the descending thoracic aorta, and coarctation can occur in the abdominal aorta (Figs. 17-17 and 17-18).

There is a frequent association of bicuspid aortic valve with aortic coarctation. The posterior cusp is enlarged and encompasses half of the circumference of the aortic root, forming one component of the bicuspid valve (see Fig. 17-2). The other half is made up by a cusp containing a rudimentary raphe. The bicuspid aortic valve may calcify and result in varying degrees of aortic stenosis and incompetence. Poststenotic dilatation of the ascending aorta may occur because of a jet of blood emanating through the bicuspid aortic valve, even if there is no gradient across the valve. Significant dilatation of the ascending aorta is present in about 50 percent of cases, usually in the most proximal portion of the ascending aorta (see Figs. 17-2 and 17-16). There is often a striking contrast between the dilated ascending aorta and the narrow middle segment of the arch, the mean cross section of the aortic arch distal to the left common carotid artery often only one-quarter of that of the ascending aorta, whereas the corresponding relationship in normal subjects is one-half or even more.[49] In long-standing severe coarctation, extensive collateral circulation develops involving chest wall vessels, mediastinal vessels, and even spinal arteries (Fig. 17-19). Aneurysms of the collaterals, especially of the posterior intercostal arteries, may develop.

Magnetic Resonance Imaging

The role of MRI in the diagnosis and follow-up of congenital cardiac abnormalities has expanded rapidly within the past decade. MRI has an advantage over

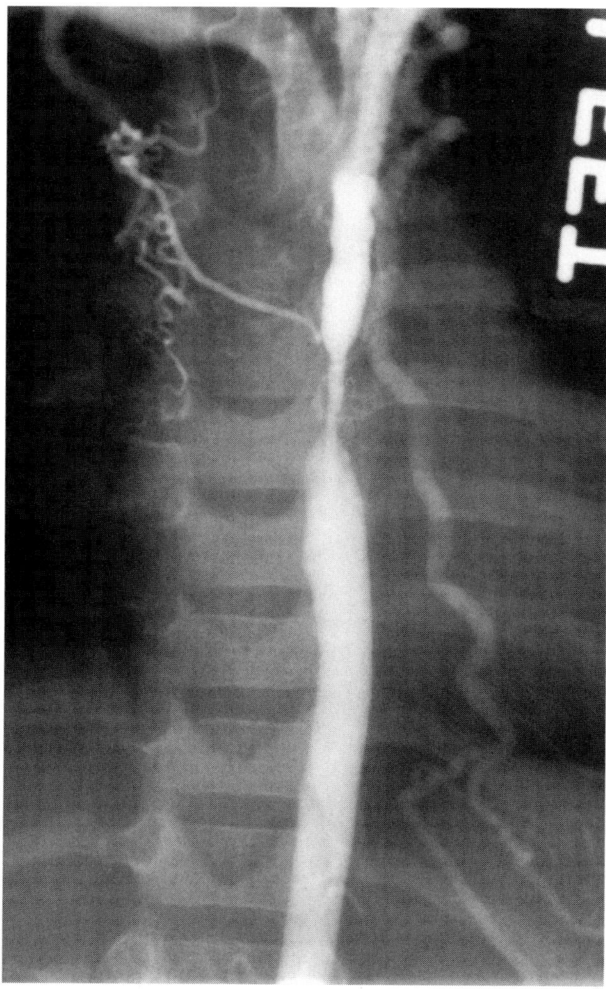

Figure 17-17. Narrowing of the distal arch persists after local coarctation repair. Severe narrowing is present in the descending thoracic aorta.

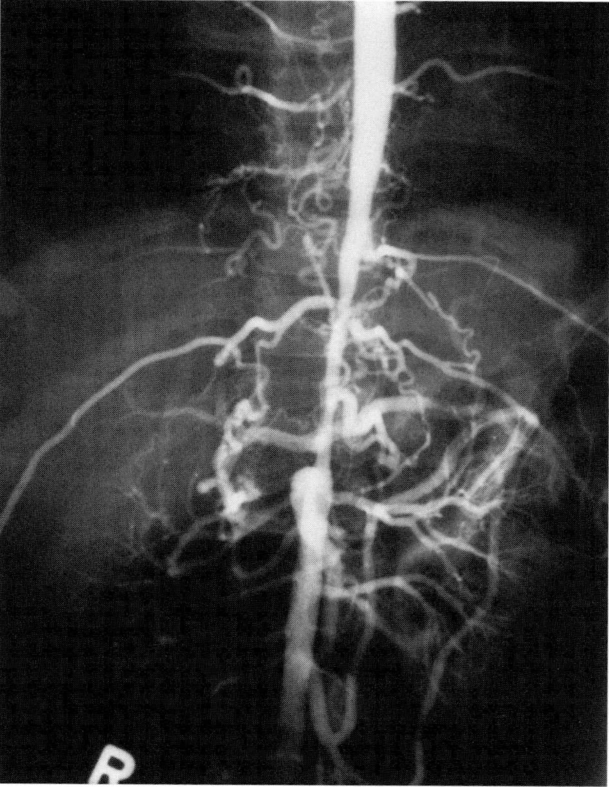

Figure 17-18. A long segment narrowing extends from the lower descending thoracic aorta to the upper abdominal aorta.

conventional or digital subtraction angiography because of its multiplanar capabilities and its noninvasive character, since it uses no ionizing radiation or iodinated contrast. It affords good spatial resolution and excellent contrast between blood vessels and soft tissues. Newer techniques such as cine MRI, MR angiography, flow quantification, stenosis evaluation, and echo-planar imaging all suggest that MRI will play an increasingly important role in the evaluation of cardiovascular disease, complimenting echocardiography. MRI is valuable during initial evaluation of the thoracic aorta and in documenting the response to treatment.[29,40,50–56] MRI is able to provide information on luminal dimensions, the status of the aortic wall, the longitudinal extent of the pathology, and the relation to and effect on branch blood vessels and paraaortic structures (Figs. 17-20 through 17-24). In addition, MRI is useful in assessing the anatomy and function of the aortic valve. The MRI diagnosis of aortic coarctation is very accurate, with a sensitivity of 94 percent.[56] A superior accuracy for diagnosis of coarctation using spin-echo MRI compared with echocardiography has been noted in older children.[52] MRI also compares well with angiography for evaluating both the site and the severity of the coarctation as well as the occurrence of collateral vessels and aortic dimensions.[57] It has been considered suitable to replace angiography in the pre- and postoperative assessment of coarctation even in infants.[58,59] MRI also accurately delineates the site and characteristics of the coarctation before balloon angioplasty. After balloon angioplasty, it demonstrates an increase in the diameter of the aorta at the coarctation in successfully treated cases and complications such as aneurysm formation, dissection, or hematoma.[40] A decrease in the number and size of collateral vessels has been identified in successfully treated patients.

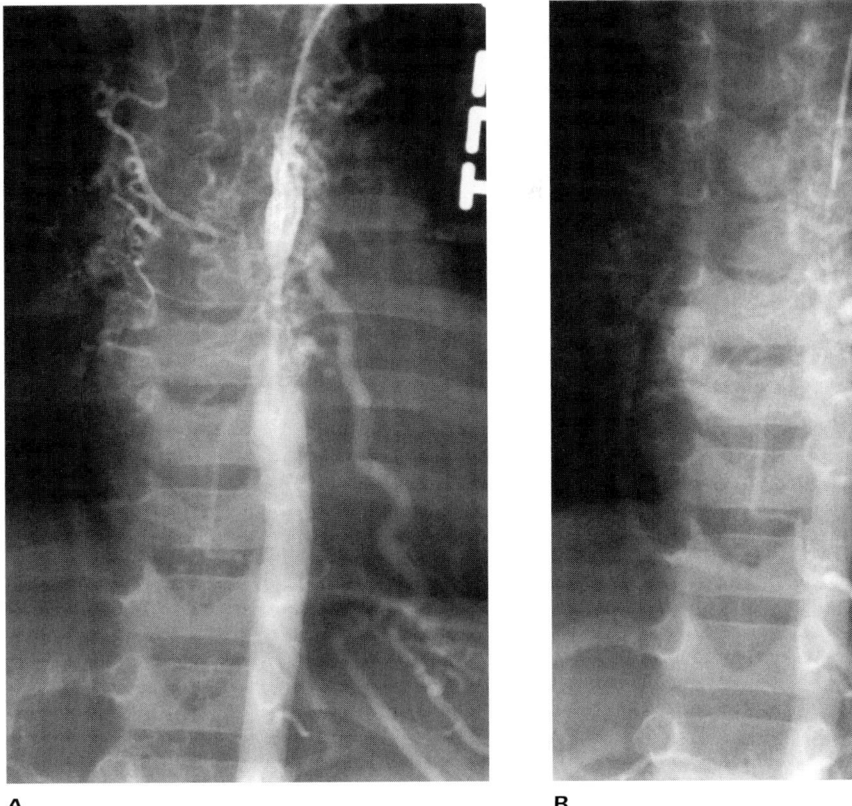

A B

Figure 17-19. Dilated collateral vessels include mediastinal, spinal, internal thoracic, and intercostal arteries (same patient as Fig. 17-17).

Rees et al. studied 36 patients with MRI 2 to 29 years after repair of coarctation of the aorta and compared clinical data, results of echocardiography, catheterization, angiography, and surgery. Satisfactory examination of the isthmus was achieved in 28 patients (78 percent) by echocardiography and in all MRI studies. Comparison with data from gradients measured at catheterization and Doppler ultrasound showed that the reduction in lumen diameter correlates well with the gradient and that restenosis at the site of repair can be suspected when the percentage of stenosis at the isthmus is greater than 50 percent. MRI showed a Dacron patch aneurysm in three patients.[29]

Cine MRI shows systolic signal loss in the ascending aorta that is presumed to be due, among other factors, to turbulent flow generated from a bicuspid valve. Similar signal loss is seen in the descending aorta distal to the site of the coarctation repair, not related to the presence or absence of a gradient (Fig. 17-25). Thus MRI is a reliable and accurate noninvasive method likely to supersede other methods of assessing the aorta and isthmus after coarctation repair.[29] Cine MRI can also be used to evaluate aortic stenosis. Images

Figure 17-20. Axial spin-echo MR image shows a dilated ascending aorta and narrowing of the descending aorta at the level of the carina (*arrow*).

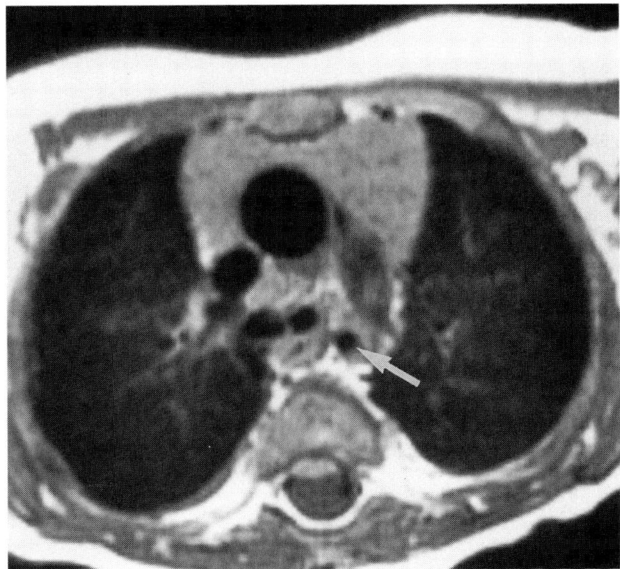

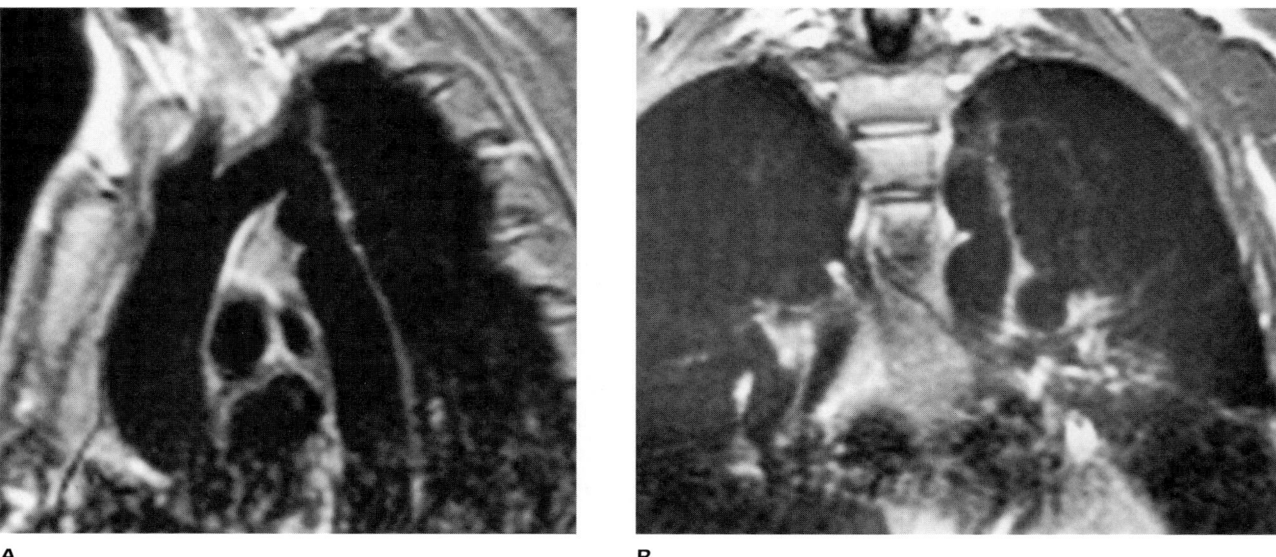

A B

Figure 17-21. Oblique (A) and coronal (B) spin-echo MR images after surgery show tortuosity, narrowing, and a residual anteromedial shelf.

Figure 17-22. (A) Oblique spin-echo MR image in an adult shows arch hypoplasia and discrete coarctation. (B) The adjacent slice shows dilated mediastinal collaterals.

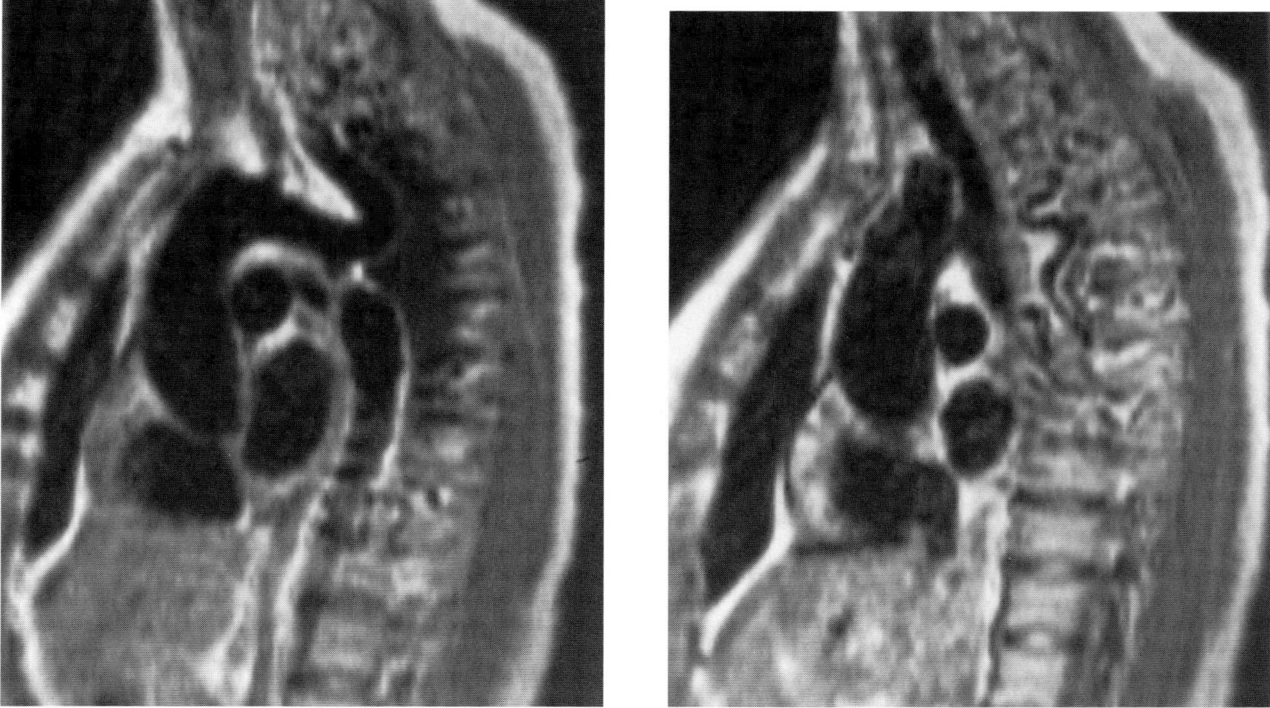

A B

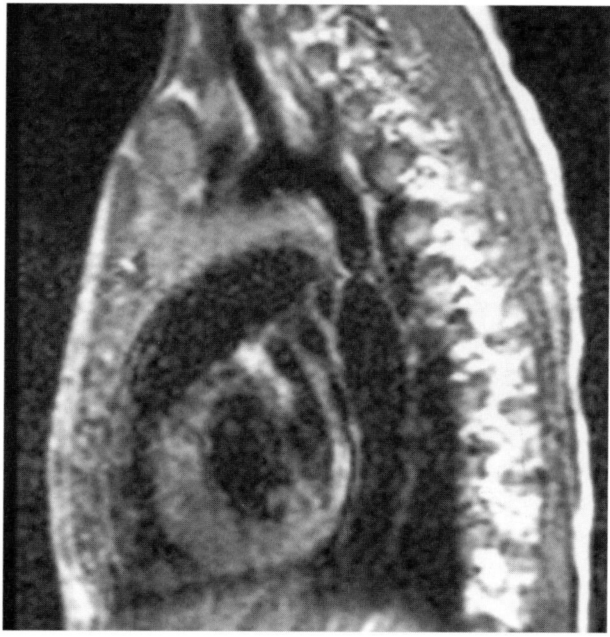

Figure 17-23. Oblique spin-echo MR image shows a long narrow isthmus, discrete narrowing, and poststenotic dilatation.

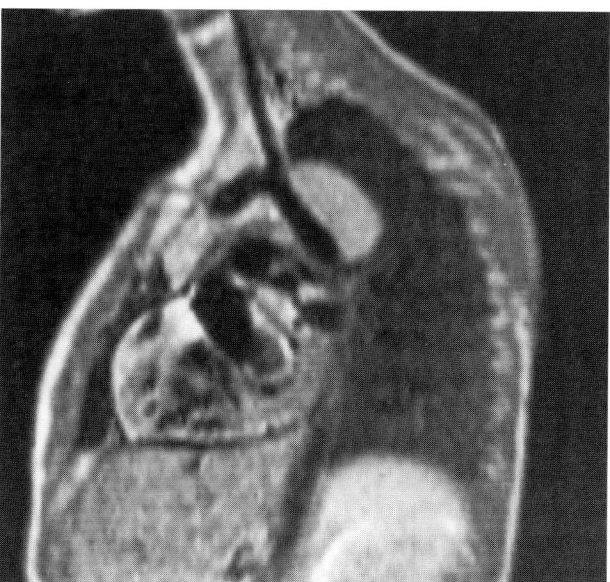

Figure 17-24. Oblique spin-echo MR image after patch repair shows residual narrowing due to arch hypoplasia and extrinsic compression by a high-signal-intensity serous fluid collection.

Figure 17-25. (A) Cine MR image shows high signal intensity in the aorta in diastole. (B) In systole there is signal loss in the ascending aorta, left subclavian artery, and descending aorta because of turbulent flow.

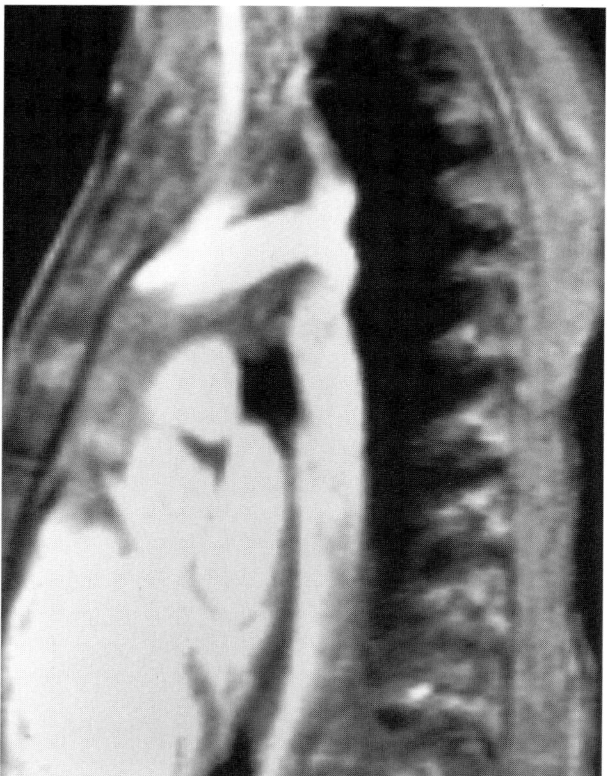

A

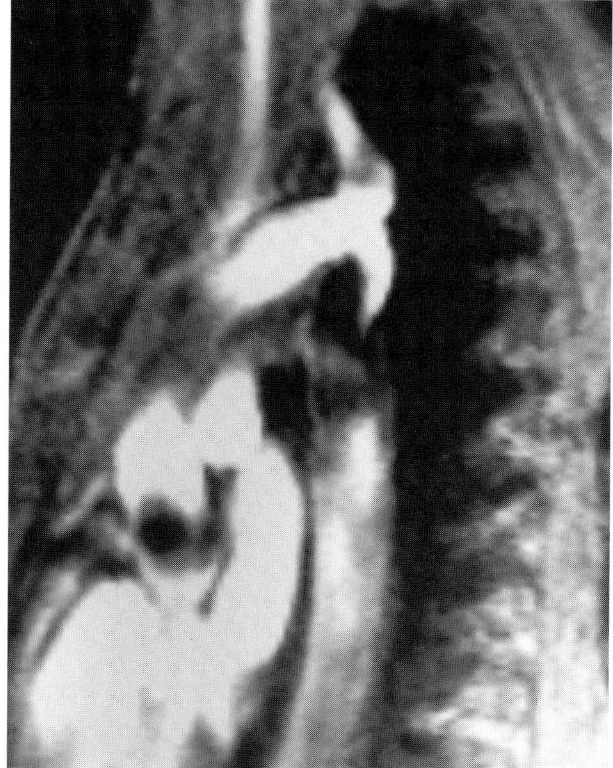

B

show a signal void in the ascending aorta due to turbulent flow, and velocity studies can quantify the transvalvular gradient.[60,61]

Unlike with echocardiography, the MRI signal is not impeded by the chest wall or intrathoracic air, and with the wider field of view MRI has the ability to define the structural relationships of the vascular structures airway. Thus it is capable of displaying the anatomic details of vascular malformations and their relationship to the airway. The wide field of view permits visualization of the entire aortic arch and descending thoracic aorta, which may occasionally be difficult using echocardiography. The isthmus is the least accessible part of the thoracic aorta to echocardiographic interrogation. The excellent anatomic detail provided with MRI, both at initial diagnosis and in the investigation of postoperative complications, suggests that this modality should replace conventional angiography. Functional assessment of pressure gradients and turbulent flow can also be provided, although echocardiography will probably remain the screening tool.

Limitations of MRI

There are also several limitations to MRI. Cardiac gated studies require a fairly regular rhythm for good quality, the acquisition time is longer than that of echocardiography, sedation is necessary for infants and children, and MRI is more expensive than echocardiography. As with echocardiography, tortuosity may impede visualization of coarctation on the sagittal oblique projection. The arch may swing out of the plane and therefore other planes and overlapping slices may be required to show the change in caliber (Fig. 17-26). Volume averaging within the image obtained may mean that a tight discrete shelf cannot be seen.

Surgical Treatment of Aortic Coarctation (Native or Recurrent)

Approximately half of all cases of coarctation of the aorta are diagnosed in infants, who usually present with severe congestive cardiac failure, particularly if associated anomalies are present.

Since the first report of successful infant repair, advances in surgery and anesthesia have led to great improvements and a reduction from an operative mortality of 30 to 40 percent in the 1960s to less than 15 percent in the 1980s and 4 percent currently for isolated coarctation.[62–69] Some authors suggest that the type of surgical repair influences the mortality rate.[64,67,68,70] Accurate diagnosis is imperative, and once the infant is stable, prompt operative repair should be performed.[71] Such operation, however, when performed in the first 3 months of life, still carries a mor-

Figure 17-26. (A) Oblique spin-echo MR image shows the ascending and descending aorta, but the transverse arch is out of plane. (B) View at right angles to the first one shows the transverse arch (*arrow*).

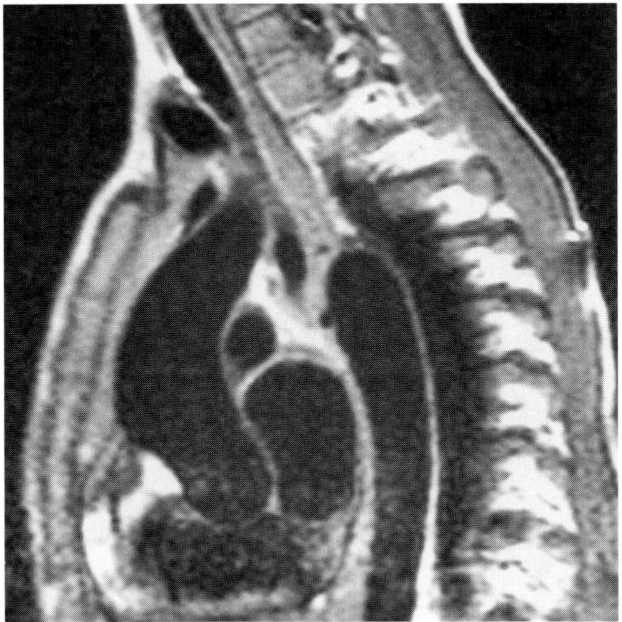

A

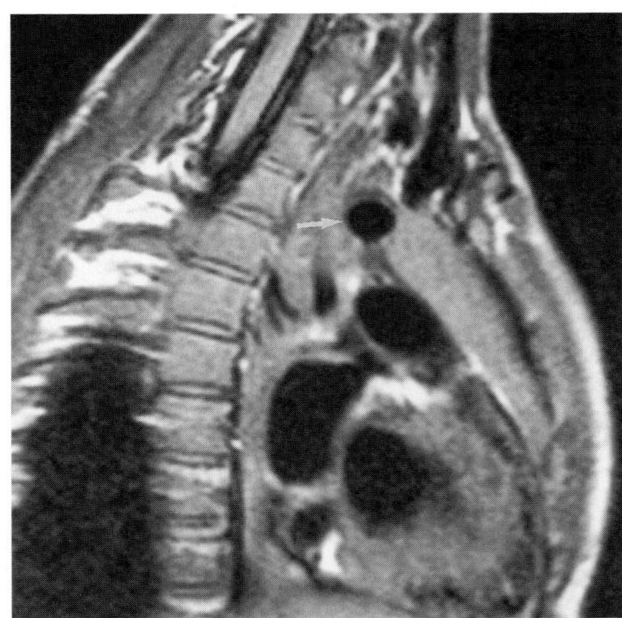

B

tality risk and an annoyingly high incidence of late recoarctation.[2,72] In older patients, surgical mortality rates are low.[73,74] The improvements in current survival can be attributed to the use of PGE_1 to stabilize the patient's condition before the operation, noninvasive diagnosis, improved perioperative care, adequate relief of the aortic obstruction, and appropriate palliation or repair of additional lesions.

Types of Repair

Much of the controversy surrounding the management of the newborn with coarctation has been rooted in the belief that modifying the surgical technique alone is the major determinant of the immediate and long-term outcome. The three commonly performed operations are resection and end-to-end anastomosis, patch enlargement, and subclavian flap aortoplasty (Waldhausen technique) (Fig. 17-27). All of the available surgical techniques have a high incidence of recurrence in infants (Fig. 17-28). The proponents of each procedure argue that it is important to remove all the abnormal tissue to prevent recurrence (resection and end-to-end anastomosis) or that it is important to preserve growth and eliminate a circumferential anastomosis.[66,71,75,76] Despite improved results, debate still exists about the optimal surgical procedure for repair of the coarctation, and with the improving survival rate of these infants, it is essential to continue to evaluate different techniques.

Results

The results of coarctation repair in early infancy probably depend on the morphology of the aortic arch and the presence or absence of associated cardiac lesions, which, in turn, largely determine the method of treatment.[1,2] In a study using standard techniques of repair, surgical technique did not influence the result.[77] The investigators used four different surgical techniques and reported a hospital mortality rate of 7.5 percent, which was limited to patients with additional complex intracardiac defects. Neither age nor surgical technique had an influence on the operative risk or predicted the likelihood of restenosis. The highest restenosis rates (42 percent) occurred in patients who underwent patch enlargement (who in general have less favorable anatomy) or the subclavian displacement technique (43 percent). Other studies suggest an increased mortality and restenosis rate in infants repaired by resection and end-to-end anastomosis.[78] The excellent results from the subclavian flap aortoplasty performed in infants are not compromised by the minor

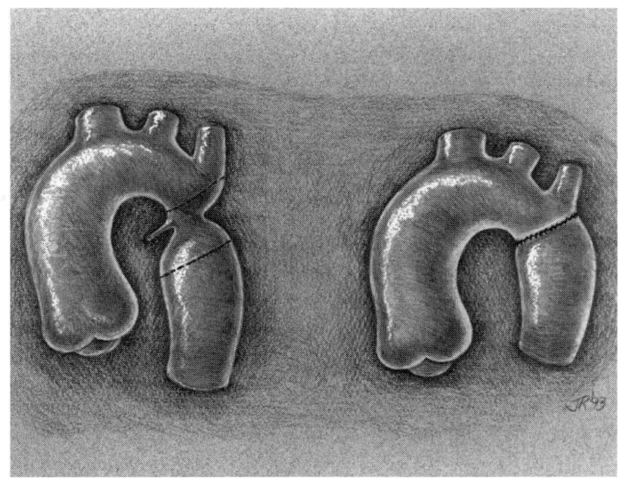

A

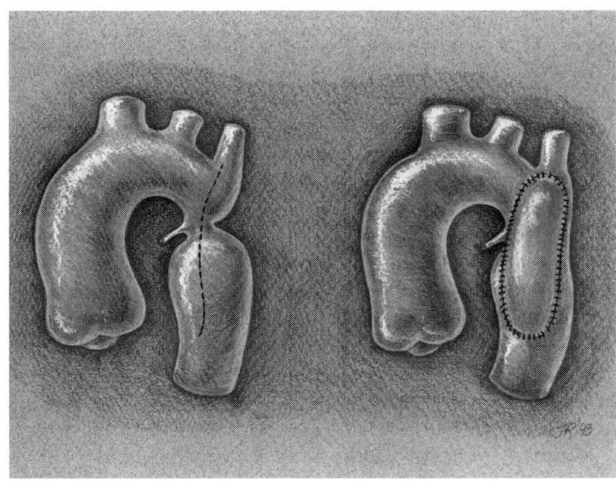

B

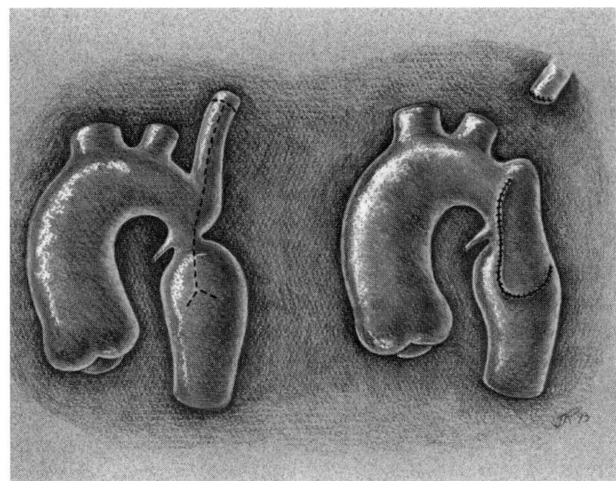

C

Figure 17-27. Diagrams illustrating resection and end-to-end anastomosis (A), patch repair (B), and the subclavian flap technique (C).

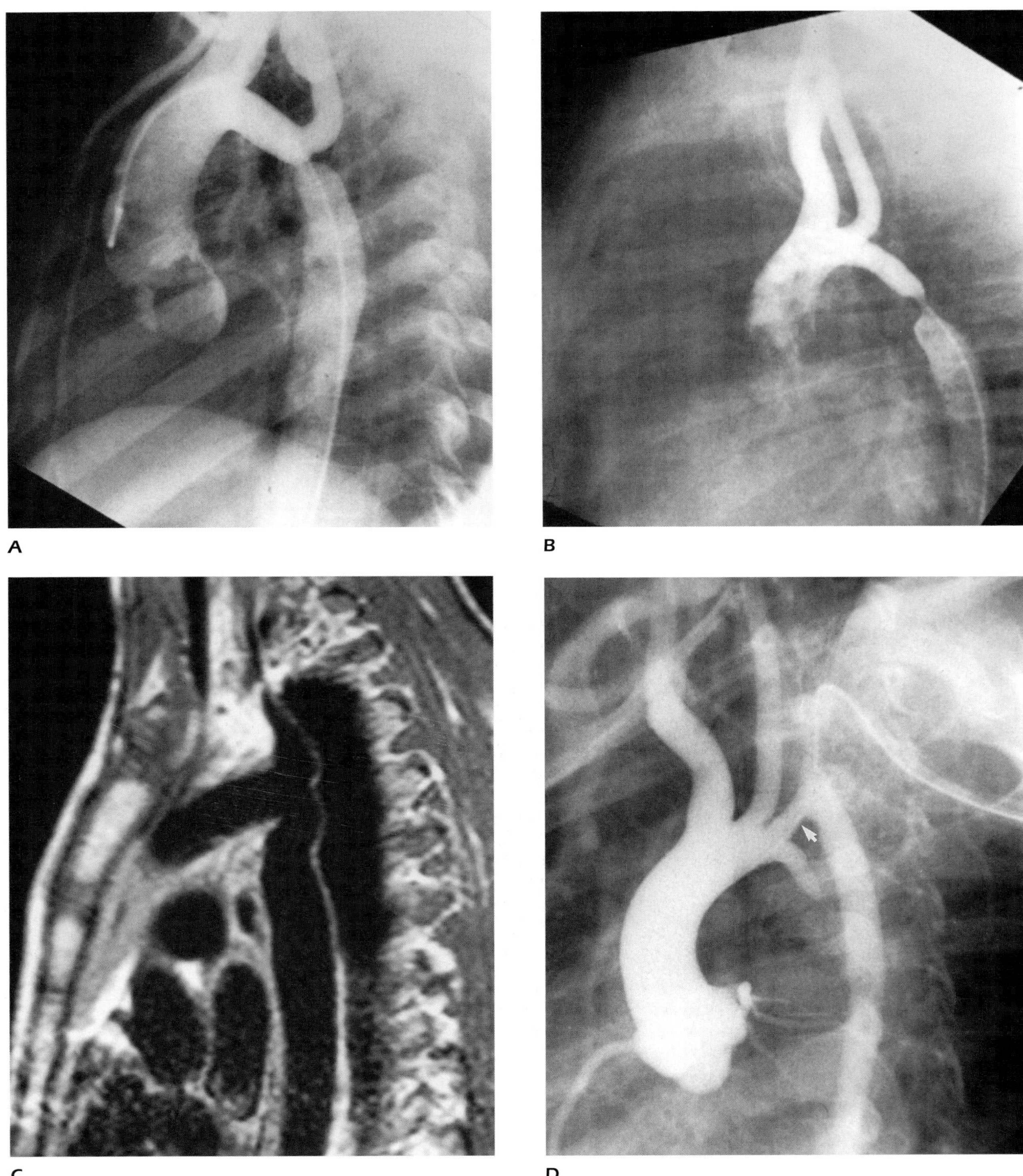

Figure 17-28. Recurrent obstruction is present after resection and end-to-end anastomosis (A), subclavian flap repair (B), patch repair (C), and in the subclavian artery (*arrow*, D) after a graft has been inserted to connect the subclavian to the descending aorta.

effects of ligating the left subclavian artery, and clinical sequelae are rare.[79,80]

Postoperative Complications

In the early postoperative period complications include anastomotic or patch leak, dissection, seroma, aneurysm, infection, and residual obstruction (see Figs. 17-24 and 17-28). Hypoperfusion during surgery can lead to paraplegia, renal failure, or necrotizing enterocolitis. Later obstruction due to restenosis or failure of arch growth is a major problem, particularly after infant repair. Aneurysm formation is common, and hypertension may persist with or without residual obstruction.

Recoarctation

Recoarctation after surgical repair is characterized by a resting peak pressure gradient across the arch. A persistent gradient (residual coarctation) noticed shortly after surgical repair may be related to inadequate relief of the obstruction or tubular hypoplasia of the transverse arch. More frequently, a true recurrent coarctation may be detected several months or even years after an initial successful repair (see Fig. 17-28).[64,81–85] The prevalence varies widely, from 7 to 60 percent after coarctation repair in infancy, depending on the definition used and the length of follow-up. The belief that the ductus arteriosus plays an important role in the anatomy and evolution of the coarctation lesion should influence the choice of the appropriate treatment.[2] It is likely that the ductal tissue (which is muscular tissue and a pathologic component of the aortic wall) should be removed at the time of operation because, if not removed, it may cause recurrence owing to retraction, fibrosis, and proliferation.[12] When only a small segment is excised, not only is ductal tissue left but the subsequent anastomosis may have an abnormal internal configuration leading to turbulent flow, which may contribute to recurrence or aneurysm.[86] Resection of the coarctation with excision of all pathologic tissue followed by end-to-end anastomosis may be preferred and the chance of recurrent coarctation reduced in older children, but in infants the circumferential anastomosis may not grow. Despite many studies, there is no clear superiority of one operation over the other, particularly in infants.[69,78,83–85,87–96] Long-term follow-up is important because the risk of recurrence increases with time.

Another area of controversy centers around the management of isthmic and arch hypoplasia. Resection or enlargement of the hypoplastic isthmic segment may relieve this component of the obstruction; however, this may not be necessary in the majority of patients, in whom this segment will increase in size after "simple" coarctation repair.[3,97] Even if the more radical repair of coarctation with isthmic enlargement is performed, the persistence of more proximal arch or intracardiac left ventricular outflow tract obstruction (LVOTO) may potentiate the development of recoarctation. Thus it is essential to look at coarctation and the other LVOTO obstructive lesions, from simple coarctation to hypoplastic left heart, as a spectrum, and immediate therapy should encompass an overall long-term plan for treating all these levels of obstruction.[70] The potential for growth of the transverse arch is still unpredictable, and a small number of older children and adults have a residual pressure gradient across the arch proximal to an effective repair of the discrete coarctation site (see Figs. 17-21, 17-25, 17-28, 17-30, and 17-31).

Aneurysms

Postoperative aneurysms are a serious late complication and have been reported after repair of coarctation of the aorta with synthetic patch materials, after subclavian flap arterioplasty, and after end-to-end anastomosis.[98–103] The reported incidence of aortic aneurysms after surgical repair or balloon angioplasty for aortic coarctation varies widely, and comparison with preoperative angiograms, especially for bulges at the ductus arteriosus, is essential before an aneurysm can be attributed to coarctation repair by any technique.[104] Many aneurysms are detected as enlarging mediastinal masses on follow-up chest radiographs (Fig. 17-29). Some have ruptured, with fatal consequences. Pinzon et al. reported 30 percent of patients followed postoperatively to have an "aneurysm," as defined by a ratio of repair site to diaphragmatic aorta greater than 1.5, with no relationship between the presence of an aneurysm and the time elapsed after repair or the type of surgery.[103] Fifty percent of subclavian flap repairs and 66 percent of synthetic patch repairs have a bulge at the repair site, which is a combination of ductal ampulla, oblique suture line, and poststenotic dilatation. Patch repairs and subclavian flaps may be "aneurysmal" at the time of surgery. The above definition may not predict those lesions that are at risk for progressive dilatation or rupture (Fig. 17-30). Follow-up imaging is necessary to identify lesions that are enlarging (Fig. 17-31). Bergdahl and Ljungqvist reported a 100 percent incidence of aneurysm formation in patients followed for 17 years after prosthetic patch angioplasty.[98] The inelasticity of the patch material, the lack of elastic lamina in the aortic wall opposite the patch, and the presence of a collagen scar may be contributing factors.[2,93,100,105] Cystic medial necrosis may also explain

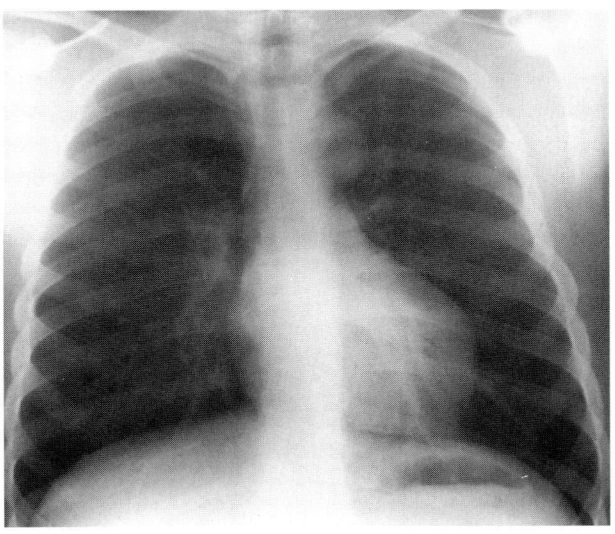

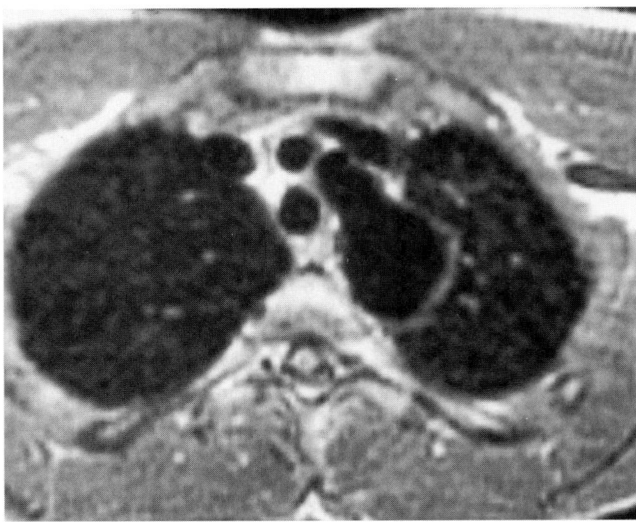

A B

Figure 17-29. (A) Frontal chest x-ray shows a bulge at the site of repair. (B) Axial MR image reveals an aneurysm of the distal arch.

the risk of aneurysm formation opposite the site of patch repair and after balloon angioplasty.[98] Extensive resection of a fibrous membrane of the aortic isthmus at the first surgical intervention may also be a predisposing factor for development of aneurysms.[74,101]

Figure 17-30. Oblique MR image after extensive patch repair shows residual narrowing in the transverse arch.

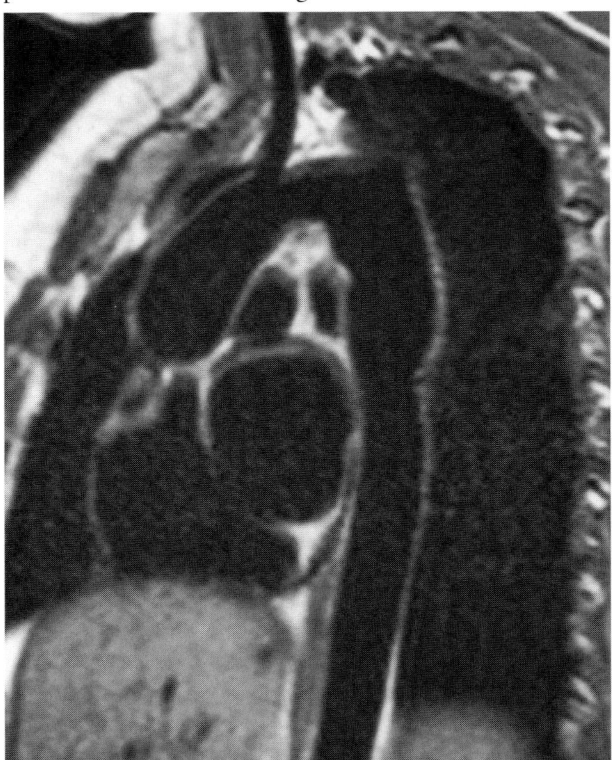

Figure 17-31. Aneurysm of the arch after subclavian flap repair that was enlarging on serial studies. Hypoplasia and stenosis are present in the transverse arch.

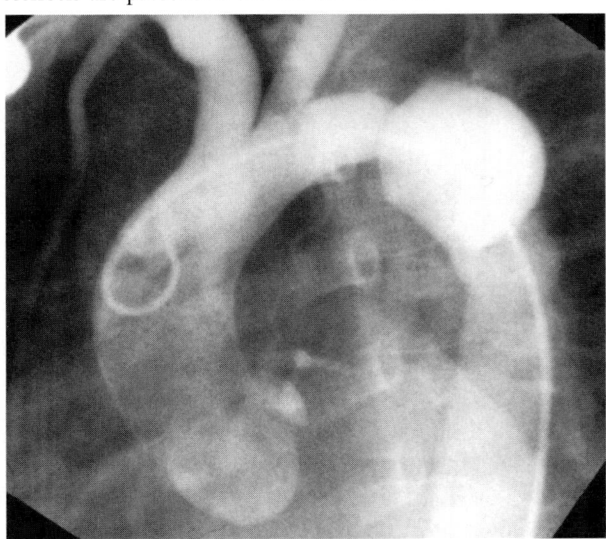

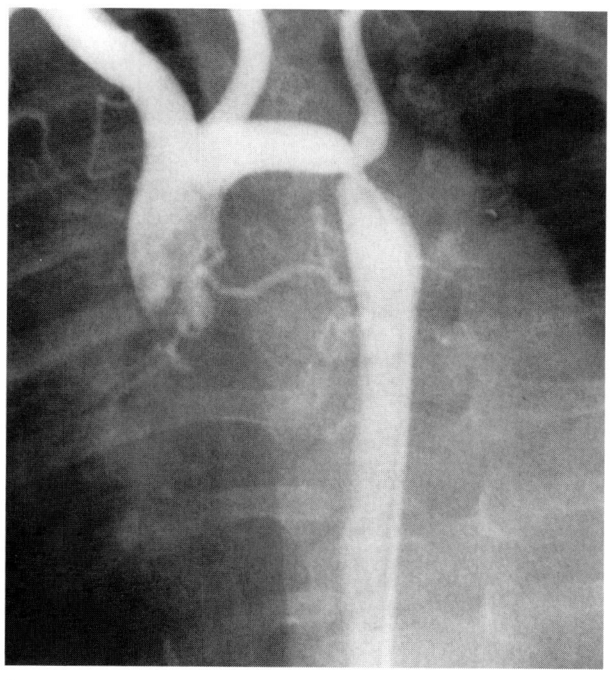

A

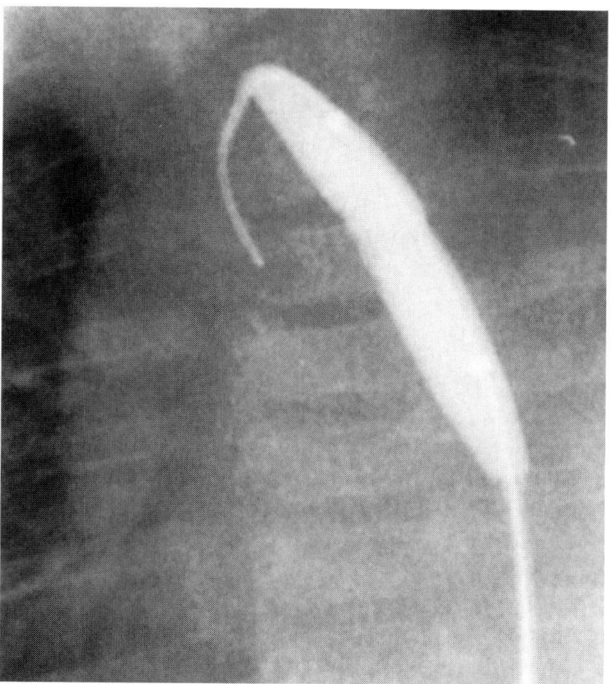

B

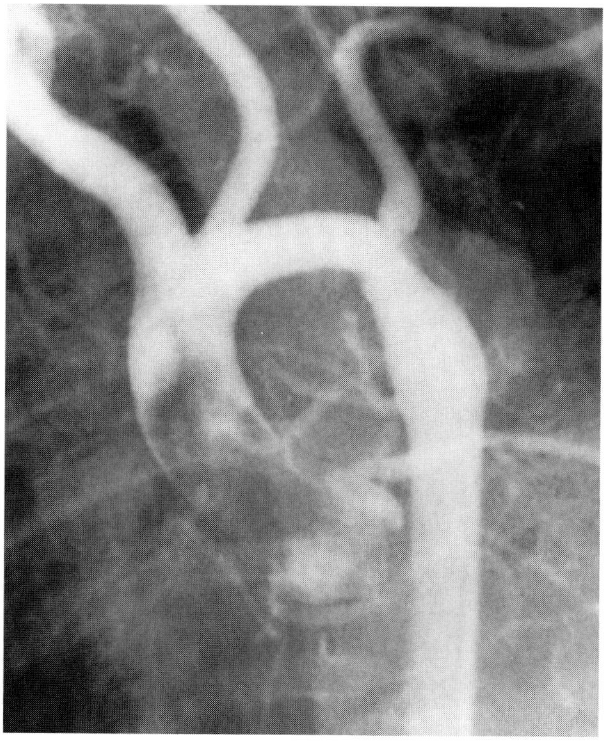

C

Figure 17-32. (A) Postoperative angiogram showing recurrent coarctation. Balloon dilatation (B) results in marked improvement (C).

Percutaneous Transluminal Angioplasty

An alternative to surgery is percutaneous transluminal angioplasty. This technique, based on the use of a catheter bearing an inflatable balloon, has been used with success in a wide variety of vascular and valvular lesions.[106] It can be performed for coarctation at all ages usually without general anesthesia, thus avoiding a thoracotomy (Fig. 17-32). The technique has been used both experimentally and clinically for the dilatation of aortic coarctation.[107–109] Its advantages are many, but they should be balanced against its risks. The most common serious complications have been in the central nervous system, at the site of coarctation, and at the peripheral site of catheter introduction.[110–112] Some deaths have been due to vessel rupture or arrhythmia.[113]

Indications

Many centers perform balloon dilatation for recurrent coarctation at the site of previous surgery. Reoperation is particularly difficult, with increased risk of bleeding and paraplegia, whereas angioplasty can be performed without blood loss and at low risk. The hospital stay is also shorter and there is less discomfort. Some centers perform angioplasty for unoperated coarctation. Many authors recognize that patients with long segments of hypoplasia are unlikely to benefit from balloon dilatation.[39,114]

In their initial report in 1983 Lock et al. found significant improvement after balloon dilatation of native coarctation and an incidence of recoarctation on follow-up of less than 30 percent.[109] In patients with recurrent coarctation, they reported an initial and late mortality and recoarctation rate lower than after surgical intervention. Rao and Chopra reviewed their experience as well as that published in the literature, including the Valvuloplasty and Angioplasty of Congenital Anomalies (VACA) Registry data, and have presented evidence in support of balloon angioplasty as a therapeutic procedure of choice for treating native and recurrent postoperative coarctations.[115] However, recommendations for the use of balloon angioplasty as a treatment procedure of choice are clouded by reports of aneurysm development at the site of coarctation.[116] Pelligrino et al. attempted to ascertain the anatomopathologic correlation of the thoracic aortic lesion to the surgical technique and the feasibility of angioplasty in individual cases.[2] They drew up guidelines for the treatment of coarctation in infancy based on autopsy evidence of infants with aortic coarctation who had died within the first 3 months of life and concluded that percutaneous transluminal angioplasty can be reasonably performed in the first few months of life when there is a shelf, irrespective of whether it is accompanied by a waist or isthmic narrowing. The procedure will only have a palliative effect, and a residual gradient should be expected and accepted, as should the likelihood of restenosis because of the unpredictable behavior of ductal tissue. Nonetheless, the procedure may resolve a critical situation such as severe cardiac failure or myocardial dysfunction without recourse to operation. Theoretically at least, this may allow the baby to grow until surgery can be performed more safely.

Technique

To yield optimal results, the choice of the catheter should take into consideration the size of the balloon, the type of shaft, and the shape of the balloon.[117] The size of the balloon chosen for angioplasty should be twice (or more) the size of the coarctate segment but no larger than the size of the descending aorta at the level of the diaphragm or the transverse arch. If the balloon is too small, little benefit may be accrued from the procedure; if it is too large, there is a risk of danger to adjacent normal vessels. A single, circular balloon has the advantage of distributing the dilating forces uniformly during inflation. More recently introduced alternative designs with two or three balloons mounted around the shaft have the advantage of allowing some blood flow to occur even at full inflation, but they also have the theoretical disadvantage of not ensuring an even distribution of circumferential force.

Results

The results of percutaneous transluminal angioplasty of aortic coarctation may be considered in three groups of patients: (1) native coarctation in the neonate and young infant less than 1 year old; (2) native coarctation in older children and adults; and (3) postoperative residual or recurrent recoarctation.

Native Coarctation in Infants

The role of angioplasty of native coarctation is unclear. Some authors report good success, others a very high recurrence rate, and still others a worrisome number of postprocedure aneurysms. Comparison with pooled surgical data has revealed that initial and late mortality rates were lower after balloon angioplasty and that rates of recoarctation and aneurysm formation were similar.[115] Recent histologic evidence has emerged showing cystic medial necrosis in all resected coarctation specimens and has suggested that the necrosis may explain the risk of aneurysm formation after balloon angioplasty.[118] At this time, this procedure needs to be performed in limited centers on an experimental basis and in other centers in occasional patients in whom surgery is very high risk.

The immediate results of the VACA Registry confirmed that native coarctations could be effectively dilated in both infants and older children, but the data do not support any conclusions concerning balloon size relative to results or complications. The VACA Registry data suggest that dilatation of the native coarctations can be performed effectively and relatively safely but do not answer whether this procedure should be performed.[117] Early restenosis is an important problem. Severe isthmic hypoplasia is a contraindication to balloon dilatation.

Angioplasty has a palliative role in symptomatic neonates with coarctation. There is a short-term beneficial effect in the treatment of critically ill neonates, who may successfully undergo surgical repair at an older age when surgical results are more favorable.[117,119]

Native Coarctation in Older Children and Adults

In a review of patients older than 1 year undergoing angioplasty, Mendelsohn et al. showed that 68 percent had a good initial outcome (i.e., a residual gradient less than 20 mmHg and no aneurysms), and longer clinical follow-up showed no late restenoses, hypertension, or late aneurysm formation.[120] Thirty-two percent had a poor initial outcome, defined as a residual gradient greater than or equal to 20 mmHg or aneurysm formation. There was no difference between the outcome groups with respect to age, balloon-isthmus ratio, or coarctation anatomy. Lababidi et al. concluded that balloon coarctation angioplasty is an alternative treatment for coarctation in adults, older children, and most infants. The long-term follow-up (with continuous-wave Doppler or cardiac catheterization) was up to 10 years, with no mortalities and minimal complications observed.[121]

Recoarctation

The term *recoarctation* fails to distinguish between residual obstruction due to a hypoplastic arch and incomplete repair from recurrent coarctation when there is evidence of a remaining discrete obstruction, often along with an anastomotic scar. Rao et al. treated nine patients with postoperative recurrent coarctation by balloon dilatation. The coarctation gradient was reduced immediately, and at a mean follow-up of 17 months there were no deaths, recurrent coarctations, or aneurysms. The balloon angioplasty group had a lower mortality rate compared with pooled data of repeat operation from the literature, but the recurrent coarctation rates were similar. The authors concluded that balloon angioplasty is the treatment of choice for symptomatic recoarctation, particularly in view of the high morbidity and mortality rates associated with repeat surgery for postoperative recoarctation.[122] Anjos et al. reported that in their patients undergoing angioplasty for recurrent coarctation a reduction of gradient occurred after the first dilation in 65 percent.[123] In follow-up, 58 percent of patients had a good result and 42 percent had a poor hemodynamic result. Aortic diameters at different levels of the aortic arch and at the reconstructed isthmus (normalized to the aorta at the level of the diaphragm) were significantly higher in the group with a good late result than in the group with a poor one, and the balloon-aortic diameter ratio at diaphragm level also had a significant effect on the late results. The investigators concluded that balloon angioplasty is the treatment of choice in recurrent coarctation regardless of the original surgery, whether end-to-end anastomosis, subclavian flap, or patch. In a multicenter prospective study, the VACA Registry reviewed the results of balloon angioplasty in 200 patients with recoarctation of the aorta. Using data on the decrease in the systolic pressure in the ascending aorta, the rise in the descending aortic systolic pressure, and the decrease in the peak systolic pressure differences along with the increase in the diameter of the recurrent coarctation site, the authors concluded that balloon angioplasty offers a satisfactory alternative to surgery for recurrent coarctation; both results and complications compared favorably with surgical therapy.[124]

Complications at the Coarctation Site

Although balloon angioplasty is an attractive alternative to surgical repair, restenosis in neonates and children is frequently reported because ductal tissue is left in situ. An early decrease in the peak systolic gradient and an increase in aortic diameter may not necessarily indicate successful coarctation dilatation.[109] Early restenosis at 6 to 8 weeks after balloon dilatation has been documented. The causes of recoarctation have been identified and include age less than 1 year, hypoplasia of the isthmus, and small coarctated aortic segment.[125]

Because the intima and part of the media are disrupted by controlled injury, there is a small chance of complete vascular disruption and of aneurysm formation at the dilatation site and a possible long-term risk of infective aortitis and aortic dissection at the site of dilatation. Despite good immediate and follow-up results, recommendations for balloon angioplasty as a treatment procedure of choice are clouded by the reports of aneurysm development at the site of dilatation.[113,126,127] Rupture of the aortic wall during angioplasty has also been reported.[111] Histologic changes of cystic medial necrosis and surgical findings of paper-thin aortic walls in some cases raise further concerns about the safety of balloon angioplasty for unoperated coarctation.

Postmortem examination of recently dilated native coarctation has been reported to show a lesion of the intima and media at the coarctation site with the adventitia alone preventing rupture of the vessel.[128] Intravascular ultrasound may reveal morphologic information not available by any other means and will allow a more precise definition of the results of intravascular procedures so that we can improve our understanding of lesion characteristics that predict a successful outcome. Intravascular ultrasound images used to evaluate aortic coarctation before and after balloon angioplasty have revealed dissection of the aortic wall and an intimal flap that was not appreciated on angiography.[129]

Complications at the Femoral Puncture

Vascular complications at the introduction site of the catheter have limited the use of this technique, particularly in neonates. Burrows et al. reviewed the medical and radiologic records of 64 consecutive infants and children who underwent transfemoral balloon dilatation of the aorta or aortic valve to determine the incidence, nature, and posttreatment outcome of acute iliofemoral complications. Forty-five percent had an acute iliofemoral complication, including thrombosis, complete disruption, incomplete disruption, and arterial tear.[112] The arterial pathology was confirmed by one or a combination of surgical exploration and repair, angiography, and MRI. A significant correlation was found between increased incidence of iliofemoral thrombosis or disruption (as well as abnormal pedal pulses at time of discharge) and low patient weight. A study from Boston revealed a 2.2 percent femoral artery complication rate after diagnostic catheterization and a 39 percent incidence after retrograde arterial balloon dilatation of the aortic valve or arch.[130]

Imaging Follow-up After Angioplasty

Chest x-ray, echocardiography, and MRI are the imaging modalities of choice. Aortic aneurysm and recoarctation are the most severe postinterventional complications after angioplasty of coarctation and require regular follow-up. MRI is an effective, noninvasive imaging method for the initial investigation and follow-up evaluation of coarctation.

Summary and Conclusions

Coarctation of the thoracic aorta is a lifelong disease with a variable presentation. It requires a different approach to investigation and treatment in the infant than in the older child or adult, and currently the results of treatment indicate a potential for further improvement. The surgical results depend on the underlying morphology and the associated lesions. Debate continues between those centers promoting the subclavian flap or patch repair and those in favor of resection and end-to-end anastomosis. The role of angioplasty in native coarctation is still investigational in most centers. Postrepair complications are relatively common, and long-term follow-up is required to identify complications and to continue the evaluation of the therapeutic alternatives.

Acknowledgments

We wish to thank Jane Rowlands for her artwork and Giuli Farquharson for secretarial assistance in the preparation of this manuscript.

References

1. Amato JJ, Galdieri RJ, Cotroneo JV. Role of extended aortoplasty related to the definition of coarctation of the aorta. Ann Thorac Surg 1991;52:615–620.
2. Pellegrino A, Deverall PB, Anderson RH, et al. Aortic coarctation in the first three months of life: an anatomopathological study with respect to treatment. J Thorac Cardiovasc Surg 1985;89:121–127.
3. Siewers RD, Ettedgui J, Pahl E, et al. Coarctation and hypoplasia of the aortic arch: will the arch grow? Ann Thorac Surg 1991;52:608–613.
4. Clagett OT, Kirklin JW, Edwards JE. Anatomic variations and pathologic changes in coarctation of the aorta: a study of 124 cases. Surg Gynaecol Obstet 1954;98:103–114.
5. Condon V, Jaffe R. The heart and great vessels. In: Caffey, ed. Pediatric x-ray diagnosis. 9th ed. St. Louis: Mosby, 1993:700.
6. Keith J, Rowe R, Vlad P. Heart disease in infancy and childhood. 3rd ed. New York: Macmillan, 1978:3–13.
7. LeBlanc JG, Williams WG. The operative and postoperative management of congenital heart defects. Mount Kisco, NY: Futura, 1993:7.
8. Gross RE. Coarctation of the aorta. Circulation 1953;7:757–768.
9. Bremer JL. Coarctation of the aorta and the aortic isthmuses. Arch Pathol 1948;45:425–434.
10. Abbott ME. Coarctation of the aorta of the adult type. Am Heart J 1928;3:381–421.
11. Elseed AM, Shinebourne EA, Paneth M. Manifestation of juxtaductal coarctation after surgical ligation of persistent ductus arteriosus in infancy. Br Heart J 1974;36:687–692.
12. Elzenga NJ, Gittenberger-de Groot AC. Localized coarctation of the aorta: an age dependent spectrum. Br Heart J 1983;49:317–323.
13. Kennedy A, Taylor DG, Durrant TE. Pathology of the intima in coarctation of the aorta: a study using light and scanning electron microscopy. Thorax 1979;34:366–374.
14. Elzenga NJ. The ductus arteriosus and stenosis of the adjacent great arteries. Doctoral thesis, University of Leiden, the Netherlands, 1986.
15. Sloan RD, Cooley RN. Coarctation of the aorta: the roentgenologic aspects of one hundred and twenty-five confirmed cases. Radiology 1953;61:701–721.
16. Soto B, Shin MS, Papapietro SE. Nonobstructive coarctation. Cardiovasc Radiol 1979;2:231–237.
17. Hynes DM, Grainger RG. The angiographic demonstration of coarctation of the aorta and similar anomalies. Clin Radiol 1968;19:438–456.
18. Janicek M, Hollmotz O. Interrenal type of abdominal aortic coarctation with unusual complications. Br Heart J 1971;33: 806–808.
19. Goldman S, Hernandez J, Pappas G. Results of surgical treatment of coarctation of the aorta in the critically ill neonate. J Thorac Cardiovasc Surg 1986;91:732–737.
20. Campbell DB, Waldhausen JA, Pierce WS, et al. Should elective repair of coarctation of the aorta be done in infancy? J Thorac Cardiovasc Surg 1984;88:929–938.
21. Olley PM, Coceani F, Bodach E. E-type prostaglandins: a new emergency therapy for certain cyanotic congenital heart malformations. Circulation 1976;53:728–731.
22. Heymann MA, Berman WJ, Rudolph AM, et al. Dilatation of the ductus arteriosus by prostaglandin E1 in aortic arch abnormalities. Circulation 1979;59:169–173.
23. Leanage R, Taylor JF, de Leval MR, et al. Surgical management of coarctation of aorta with ventricular septal defect: multivariate analysis. Br Heart J 1981;46:269–277.
24. Ward KE, Pryor RW, Matson JR, et al. Delayed detection of coarctation in infancy: implications for timing of newborn follow-up. Pediatrics 1990;86:972–976.

25. Sanders SP, MacPherson D, Yeager SB. Temporal flow velocity profile in the descending aorta in coarctation. J Am Coll Cardiol 1986;7:603–609.
26. Sorland SJ, Rostad H, Forfang K, et al. Coarctation of the aorta: a follow-up after surgical treatment in infancy and childhood. Acta Paediatr Scand 1980;69:113–118.
27. Cokkinos DV, Leachman RD, Cooley DA. Increased mortality rate from coronary artery disease following operation for coarctation of the aorta at a late age. J Thorac Cardiovasc Surg 1979;77:315–318.
28. Parker FBJ, Farrell B, Streeten DHP, et al. Hypertensive mechanisms in coarctation of the aorta: further studies of the renin-angiotensin system. J Thorac Cardiovasc Surg 1980;80: 568–573.
29. Rees S, Somerville J, Ward C, et al. Coarctation of the aorta: MR imaging in late postoperative assessment. Radiology 1989;173:499–502.
30. Sealy WC. Paradoxical hypertension after repair of coarctation of the aorta: a review of its causes. Ann Thorac Surg 1990; 50:323–329.
31. Godwin JD, Herfkens RJ, Brundage BH, et al. Evaluation of coarctation of the aorta by computed tomography. J Comput Assist Tomogr 1981;5:153–156.
32. Moodie DS, Yiannikas J, Gill CC, et al. Intravenous digital subtraction angiography in the evaluation of congenital abnormalities of the aorta and aortic arch. Am Heart J 1982; 104:628–634.
33. Amundson GM, Wesenberg RL, Mueller DL, et al. Pediatric digital subtraction angiography. Radiology 1984;153:649–654.
34. Tonkin ILD, Gold RE, Moser D, et al. Evaluation of vascular rings with digital subtraction angiography. AJR 1984;142: 1287–1291.
35. Figley MM. Accessory roentgen signs of coarctation of the aorta. Radiology 1954;62:671–687.
36. Martin EC, Strafford MA, Gersony WM. Initial detection of coarctation of the aorta: an opportunity for the radiologist. Am J Roentgenol 1981;137:1015–1017.
37. Sahn DJ, Allen HD, McDonald G, et al. Real-time cross-sectional echocardiographic diagnosis of coarctation of the aorta: a prospective study of echocardiographic-angiographic correlations. Circulation 1977;56:762–769.
38. Smallhorn JF, Huhta JC, Adams PA, et al. Cross-sectional echocardiographic assessment of coarctation in the sick neonate and infant. Br Heart J 1983;50:349–361.
39. Huhta JC, Gutgesell HP, Latson LA, et al. Two-dimensional echocardiographic assessment of the aorta in infants and children with congenital heart disease. Circulation 1984;70:417–424.
40. Bank ER, Aisen AM, Rocchini AP, et al. Coarctation of the aorta in children undergoing angioplasty: pretreatment and post-treatment MR imaging. Radiology 1987;162:235–240.
41. Shaddy RE, Snider AR, Silverman NH, et al. Pulsed Doppler findings in patients with coarctation of the aorta. Circulation 1986;73:82–88.
42. Marx GR, Allen HD. Accuracy and pitfalls of Doppler evaluation of the pressure gradient in aortic coarctation. J Am Coll Cardiol 1986;7:1379–1385.
43. Wilson N, Sutherland GR, Gibbs JL, et al. Limitations of Doppler ultrasound in the diagnosis of neonatal coarctation of the aorta. Int J Cardiol 1989;23:87–88.
44. Scott PJ, Wharton GA, Gibbs JL. Failure of Doppler ultrasound to detect coarctation of the aorta. Int J Cardiol 1990; 28:379–381.
45. Salen EF, Wiklund T. Angiocardiography in coarctation of the aorta. Acta Radiol 1948;30:299–315.
46. Dotter CT, Steinberg I. Angiocardiography in congenital heart disease. Am J Med 1952;12:219–237.
47. Denham B. Aortography in infantile coarctation [letter]. Br Med J 1978;1:1282–1283.
48. Denham B, Ward OC, McCann P, et al. Aortography in infantile coarctation: a simple and effective technique. Arch Dis Child 1979;54:717–719.
49. Broden B, Karnell J. Coarctation of the aorta: aortographic studies before and after operation. Acta Radiol 1958;165:1–61.
50. von Schulthess GK, Higashino SM, Higgins SS, et al. Coarctation of the aorta: MR imaging. Radiology 1986;158:169–174.
51. Didier D, Higgins CB, Fisher MR, et al. Congenital heart disease: gated MR imaging in 72 patients. Radiology 1986; 158:227–235.
52. Fletcher BD, Jacobstein MD. MRI of congenital abnormalities of the great arteries. AJR 1986;146:941–948.
53. Gomes AS, Lois JF, George B, et al. Congenital abnormalities of the aortic arch: MR imaging. Radiology 1987;165:691–695.
54. Boxer RA, LaCorte MA, Singh S, et al. Nuclear magnetic resonance imaging in the evaluation and follow-up of children treated for coarctation of the aorta. J Am Coll Cardiol 1986; 7:1095–1098.
55. Simpson IA, Chung KJ, Glass RF, et al. Cine magnetic resonance imaging for evaluation of anatomy and flow relations in infants and children with coarctation of the aorta. Circulation 1988;78:142–148.
56. Kersting-Sommerhoff BA, Diethelm L, Teitel DF, et al. Magnetic resonance imaging of congenital heart disease: sensitivity and specificity using receiver operating characteristic curve analysis. Am Heart J 1989;118:155–161.
57. Stern HC, Locher D, Wallnofer K, et al. Noninvasive assessment of coarctation of the aorta: comparative measurements by two-dimensional echocardiography, magnetic resonance, and angiography. Pediatr Control 1991;12:1–5.
58. Nyman R, Hallberg M, Sunnegardh J, et al. Magnetic resonance imaging and angiography for the assessment of coarctation of the aorta. Acta Radiol 1989;30:481–485.
59. Baker EJ, Ayton V, Smith MA, et al. Magnetic resonance imaging of coarctation of the aorta in infants: use of a high field strength. Br Heart J 1989;62:97–101.
60. Mitchell L, Jenkins JPR, Watson Y, et al. Diagnosis and assessment of mitral and aortic valve disease by cine-flow magnetic resonance imaging. Magn Reson Med 1989;12:181–197.
61. Kilner PJ, Manzara CC, Mohiaddin RH, et al. Magnetic resonance jet velocity mapping in mitral and aortic valve stenosis. Circulation 1993;87:1239–1248.
62. Sinha SN, Kardatazke ML, Cole RB, et al. Coarctation of the aorta in infancy. Circulation 1969;40:385–398.
63. Chen SC, Fagan LF, Mudd GJF, et al. Prognosis of infants with coarctation of aorta. Am Heart J 1977;94:557–561.
64. Williams WG, Shindo G, Trusler GA, et al. Results of repair of coarctation of the aorta during infancy. J Thorac Cardiovasc Surg 1980;79:603–608.
65. Nair UR, Jones O, Walker DR. Surgical management of severe coarctation of the aorta in the first month of life. J Thorac Cardiovasc Surg 1983;86:587–590.
66. Moulton AL, Brenner JI, Roberts G, et al. Subclavian flap repair of coarctation of the aorta in neonates: realization of growth potential? J Thorac Cardiovasc Surg 1984;87:220–235.
67. Bergdahl LAL, Blackstone EH, Kirklin JW, et al. Determinants of early success in repair of aortic coarctation in infants. J Thorac Cardiovasc Surg 1982;83:736–742.
68. Hammon JWJ, Graham TPJ, Boucek RJJ, et al. Operative repair of coarctation of the aorta in infancy: results with and without ventricular septal defect. Am J Cardiol 1985;55: 1555–1559.
69. Kamau P, Miles V, Toews W, et al. Surgical repair of coarctation of the aorta in infants less than six months of age: including the question of pulmonary artery banding. J Thorac Cardiovasc Surg 1981;81:171–179.
70. Moulton AL. Current controversies and techniques in congenital heart surgery. Ann Thorac Surg 1991;52:592–593.

71. Waldhausen JA, Whitman V, Werner JC, et al. Surgical intervention in infants with coarctation of the aorta. J Thorac Cardiovasc Surg 1981;81:323–325.
72. Shinebourne EA, Tam ASY, Elseed AM, et al. Coarctation of the aorta in infancy and childhood. Br Heart J 1976;38:375–380.
73. Hamilton DI, Medici D, Oyonarte M, et al. Aortoplasty with the left subclavian flap in older children. J Thorac Cardiovasc Surg 1981;82:103–106.
74. Hehrlein FW, Mulch J, Rautenburg HW, et al. Incidence and pathogenesis of late aneurysms after patch graft aortoplasty for coarctation. J Thorac Cardiovasc Surg 1986;92: 226–230.
75. Hamilton DI, Di Eusanio G, Sandrasagra FA, et al. Early and late results of aortoplasty with a left subclavian flap for coarctation of the aorta in infancy. J Thorac Cardiovasc Surg 1978; 75:699–704.
76. Harlan JL, Doty DB, Brandt BB III, et al. Coarctation of the aorta in infants. J Thorac Cardiovasc Surg 1984;88:1012–1019.
77. Messmer BJ, Minale C, Muhler E, et al. Surgical correction of coarctation in early infancy: does surgical technique influence the result? Ann Thorac Surg 1991;52:594–600.
78. Penkoske PA, Williams WG, Olley PM, et al. Subclavian arterioplasty: repair of coarctation of the aorta in the first year of life. J Thorac Cardiovasc Surg 1984;87:894–900.
79. Lodge FA, Lamberti JJ, Goodman AH, et al. Vascular consequences of subclavian artery transection for the treatment of congenital heart disease. J Thorac Cardiovasc Surg 1983;86: 18–23.
80. Todd PJ, Dangerfield PH, Hamilton DI, et al. Late effects on the left upper limb of subclavian flap aortoplasty. J Thorac Cardiovasc Surg 1983;85:678–681.
81. Waldman JD, Lamberti JJ, Goodman AH, et al. Coarctation in the first year of life: patterns of postoperative effect. J Thorac Cardiovasc Surg 1983;86:9–17.
82. Beekman RH, Rocchini AP, Behrendt DM, et al. Long-term outcome after repair of coarctation in infancy: subclavian angioplasty does not reduce the need for reoperation. J Am Coll Cardiol 1986;8:1406–1411.
83. Sanchez GR, Balsara RK, Dunn J, et al. Recurrent obstruction after subclavian flap repair of coarctation of the aorta in infants. J Thorac Cardiovasc Surg 1986;91:738–746.
84. Cobanoglu A, Teply JF, Grunkemeier GL, et al. Coarctation of the aorta in patients younger than three months: a critique of the subclavian flap operation. J Thorac Cardiovasc Surg 1985;89:128–135.
85. Ziemer G, Jonas RA, Perry SB, et al. Surgery for coarctation of the aorta in the neonate. Circulation 1986;74 (Suppl 1): 1–25.
86. Glancy DL, Morrow AG, Simon AL, et al. Juxtaductal aortic coarctation: analysis of 84 patients studied hemodynamically, angiographically, and morphologically after age 1 year. Am J Cardiol 1983;51:537–551.
87. Mayer JEJ. Invited letter concerning: coarctation [letter; comment]. J Thorac Cardiovasc Surg 1991;101:165–166.
88. Jonas RA. Coarctation: do we need to resect ductal tissue? Ann Thorac Surg 1991;52:604–607.
89. Sciolaro C, Copeland J, Cork R, et al. Long-term follow-up comparing subclavian flap angioplasty to resection with modified oblique end-to-end anastomosis. J Thorac Cardiovasc Surg 1991;101:1–13.
90. Korfer R, Meyer H, Kleikamp G, et al. Early and late results after resection and end-to-end anastomosis of coarctation of the aorta in early infancy. J Thorac Cardiovasc Surg 1985;89: 616–622.
91. van Son JA, Daniels O, Vincent JG, et al. Appraisal of resection and end-to-end anastomosis for repair of coarctation of the aorta in infancy: preference for resection. Ann Thorac Surg 1989;48:496–502.
92. Shrivastava CP, Monro JL, Shore DF, et al. The early and long-term results of surgery for coarctation of the aorta in the 1st year of life. Eur J Cardiothorac Surg 1991;5:61–66.
93. Kron IL, Flanagan TL, Rheuban KS, et al. Incidence and risk of reintervention after coarctation repair. Ann Thorac Surg 1990;49:920–925.
94. Palatianos GM, Thurer RJ, Kaiser GA. Comparison of operations for coarctation of the aorta in infants. J Cardiovasc Surg 1987;28:128–131.
95. Hesslein PS, McNamara DG, Morriss MJH, et al. Comparison of resection versus patch aortoplasty for repair of coarctation in infants and children. Circulation 1981;64:165–168.
96. Ehrhardt P, Walker DR. Coarctation of the aorta corrected during the first month of life. Arch Dis Child 1989;64:330–332.
97. Brouwer MHJ, Cromme-Dijkhuis AH, Ebels T, et al. Growth of the hypoplastic aortic arch after simple coarctation resection and end-to-end anastomosis. J Thorac Cardiovasc Surg 1992;104:426–433.
98. Bergdahl L, Ljungqvist A. Long-term results after repair of coarctation of the aorta by patch grafting. J Thorac Cardiovasc Surg 1980;80:177–181.
99. Kirsh MM, Perry B, Spooner E. Management of pseudoaneurysm following patch grafting for coarctation of the aorta. J Thorac Cardiovasc Surg 1977;74:636–639.
100. Clarkson PM, Brandt PWT, Barratt-Boyes BG, et al. Prosthetic repair of coarctation of the aorta with particular reference to Dacron onlay patch grafts and late aneurysm formation. Am J Cardiol 1985;56:342–346.
101. DeSanto A, Bills RG, King H, et al. Pathogenesis of aneurysm formation opposite prosthetic patches used for coarctation repair: an experimental study. J Thorac Cardiovasc Surg 1987; 94:720–723.
102. Martin MM, Beekman RH, Rocchini AP, et al. Aortic aneurysms after subclavian angioplasty repair of coarctation of the aorta. Am J Cardiol 1988;61:951–953.
103. Pinzon JL, Burrows PE, Benson LN, et al. Repair of coarctation of the aorta in children: postoperative morphology [see comments]. Radiology 1991;180:199–203.
104. Parikh SR, Hurwitz RA, Hubbard JE, et al. Preoperative and postoperative "aneurysm" associated with coarctation of the aorta. J Am Coll Cardiol 1991;17:1367–1372.
105. del Nido PJ, Williams WG, Wilson GJ, et al. Synthetic patch angioplasty for repair of coarctation of the aorta: experience with aneurysm formation. Circulation 1986;74 (Suppl 1): 1–32.
106. Gruntzig A, Kumpe DA. Technique of percutaneous transluminal angioplasty with the Gruntzig balloon catheter. AJR 1979;132:547–552.
107. Lock JE, Niemi T, Burke BA, et al. Transcutaneous angioplasty of experimental aortic coarctation. Circulation 1982; 66:1280–1286.
108. Lock JE, Castaneda-Zuniga WR, Bass JL, et al. Balloon dilatation of excised aortic coarctations. Radiology 1982;143:689–691.
109. Lock JE, Bass JL, Amplatz K, et al. Balloon dilation angioplasty of aortic coarctations in infants and children. Circulation 1983;68:109–116.
110. Rao PS. Aortic rupture after balloon angioplasty of aortic coarctation [editorial; comment]. Am Heart J 1993;125:1205–1206.
111. Roberts DH, Bellamy CM, Ramsdale DR. Fatal aortic rupture during balloon dilatation of recoarctation. Am Heart J 1993; 125:1181–1182.
112. Burrows PE, Benson LN, Williams WG, et al. Ileofemoral arterial complications of balloon angioplasty for systemic obstructions in infants and children. Circulation 1990;82:1697–1704.
113. Rao PS. Balloon angioplasty of aortic coarctation: a review. Clin Cardiol 1989;12:618–628.
114. Rocchini AP, Rosenthal A, Barger AC, et al. Pathogenesis of

paradoxical hypertension after coarctation resection. Circulation 1976;54:382–387.
115. Rao PS, Chopra PS. Role of balloon angioplasty in the treatment of aortic coarctation. Ann Thorac Surg 1991;52:621–631.
116. Radke W, Lock J. Balloon dilatation. Pediatr Clin North Am 1990;37:193–213.
117. Tynan M, Finley JP, Fontes V, et al. Balloon angioplasty for the treatment of native coarctation: results of Valvuloplasty and Angioplasty of Congenital Anomalies Registry. Am J Cardiol 1990;65:790–792.
118. Isner JM, Donaldson RF, Fulton D, et al. Cystic medial necrosis in coarctation of the aorta: a potential factor contributing to adverse consequences observed after percutaneous balloon angioplasty of coarctation sites. Circulation 1987;75:689–695.
119. Morrow WR, Vick GW III, Nihill MR, et al. Balloon dilation of unoperated coarctation of the aorta: short- and intermediate-term results. J Am Coll Cardiol 1988;11:133–138.
120. Mendelsohn AM, Crowley DC, Kocis KC, et al. Angioplasty of native coarctation of the aorta: eight year experience. Circulation 1992;86:I–633.
121. Lababidi Z, Madigan N, Wu JR, et al. Balloon coarctation angioplasty in an adult. Am J Cardiol 1984;53:350–351.
122. Rao PS, Wilson AD, Chopra PS. Immediate and follow-up results of balloon angioplasty of postoperative recoarctation in infants and children. Am Heart J 1990;120:1315–1320.
123. Anjos R, Qureshi SA, Rosenthal E, et al. Determinants of hemodynamic results of balloon dilation of aortic recoarctation. Am J Cardiol 1992;69:665–671.
124. Hellenbrand WE, Allen HD, Golinko RJ, et al. Balloon angioplasty for aortic recoarctation: results of Valvuloplasty and Angioplasty of Congenital Anomalies Registry. Am J Cardiol 1990;65:793–797.
125. Rao PS. Balloon angioplasty of aortic coarctation: a review. Clin Cardiol 1989;12:618–628.
126. Cooper RS, Ritter SB, Rothe WB, et al. Angioplasty for coarctation of the aorta: long-term results. Circulation 1987;75:600–604.
127. Beekman RH, Rocchini AP, Dick M II, et al. Percutaneous balloon angioplasty for native coarctation of the aorta. J Am Coll Cardiol 1987;10:1078–1084.
128. Hagemo PS, Bjornstad PG, Smevik B, et al. Aortic wall lesion in balloon dilatation of coarctation of the aorta. Eur Heart J 1988;9:1271–1273.
129. Harrison JK, Sheikh KH, Davidson CJ, et al. Balloon angioplasty of coarctation of the aorta evaluated with intravascular ultrasound imaging. J Am Coll Cardiol 1990;15:906–909.
130. Wessel DL, Keane JF, Fellows KE, et al. Fibrinolytic therapy for femoral arterial thrombosis after cardiac catheterization in infants and children. Am J Cardiol 1986;56:347–351.

18

Aorticopulmonary Window (Aortic Septal Defect)

J. A. GORDON CULHAM

An aorticopulmonary (AP) window is an uncommon circular or oval communication between the aorta and the pulmonary artery located above the level of the semilunar valves (Fig. 18-1). The defect may be proximal, immediately above the sinus ridges, or distal near the origin of the right pulmonary artery, or may involve the entire aortopulmonary septum.[1] A central defect has also been described.[2] The right pulmonary artery may arise from the aorta in association with the higher defects.[3,4] The defect may result from nonfusion, malalignment, or absence of the embryonic septum between the aorta and the pulmonary artery.[3] Approximately half of the cases have associated cardiovascular malformations (Fig. 18-2).[3,5] The first case was described in 1830, and the first repair was performed in 1948 by Gross.[6] The AP window has been linked embryologically to truncus arteriosus because of the similarity of the lesions in the great arteries, but recently it has been suggested that AP windows have a different basis due to a variation in the frequency of associated lesions.[2,3,7] Rarely, trauma may produce an AP communication, and recently an AP communication has been created surgically for the palliation of complex cardiac malformations (Fig. 18-3).

An AP window functions as an extracardiac left-to-right shunt, similar to a patent ductus arteriosus (PDA), and many reports include cases discovered at exploration for a PDA.[8,9] Distinguishing an aortic septal defect from PDA is difficult clinically but highly desirable for preoperative planning. A PDA is treated surgically through a left thoracotomy, whereas an AP window is treated through a sternotomy, usually under cardiopulmonary bypass. PDA is one of the more common associated lesions. Others include interrupted aortic arch, coarctation, ventricular septal defect (VSD), tetralogy of Fallot, coronary anomalies, and transposition of the great arteries.[3,10–13]

Clinically, most patients are acyanotic and present with signs of congestive heart failure, failure to thrive, and recurrent chest infections. A murmur is the most prominent physical finding. This may be a continuous murmur, indistinguishable from that of PDA, or simply a loud systolic murmur over the base. The electrocardiogram is variable, showing left ventricular hypertrophy, right ventricular hypertrophy, or biventricular hypertrophy.[5,14]

Radiologically, cardiac enlargement is present. The pulmonary artery segment is prominent and frequently huge. The pulmonary artery branches are enlarged as in any left-to-right shunt. The appearance of the heart may be similar to that found in PDA or atrial septal defect. With the development of pulmonary hypertension, right ventricular enlargement may be marked.

Cardiac catheterization shows a step-up in oxygen saturation from the right ventricle to the pulmonary artery. This finding is of no value, however, in distinguishing an aortic septal defect from a PDA in which there is also increased oxygen saturation in pulmonary artery blood. If a catheter enters the ascending aorta from the pulmonary artery, one may be reasonably certain of the diagnosis. Elevated pressures in the right ventricle and pulmonary artery are frequently found. In older patients, systemic desaturation may be found caused by the development of pulmonary vascular disease.[6,15]

Aortography has been the diagnostic method of choice. Injection of a large bolus of contrast material through a catheter whose tip lies in the proximal ascending aorta is desirable to establish the diagnosis. In the frontal projection the communication between the ascending aorta and the pulmonary artery may be sharply delineated (see Fig. 18-1). In more distal lesions the defect may be best shown on left anterior oblique projection or lateral projection. Cineaortography is particularly useful because of the high temporal resolution and in cases in which balanced shunts have developed because it clearly displays the bidirectional flow. PDA is easily differentiated with good angiography.[7] An important differential diagnostic consideration is that of truncus arteriosus. In truncus, a single

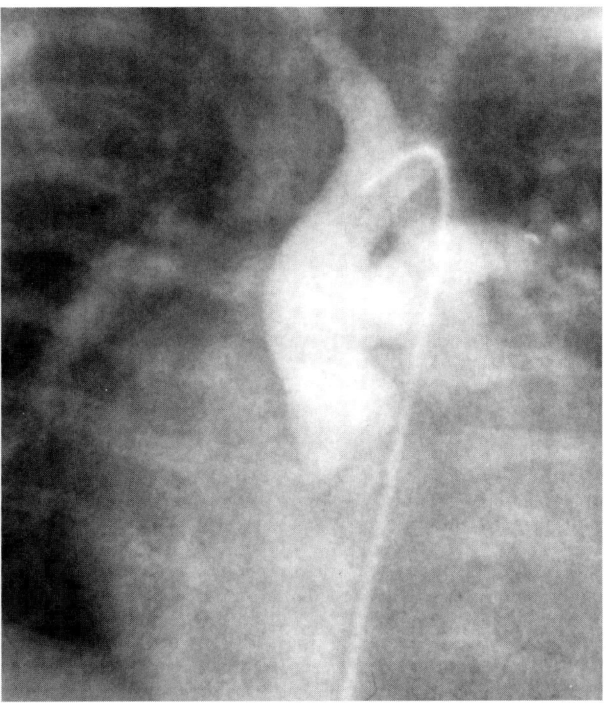

A

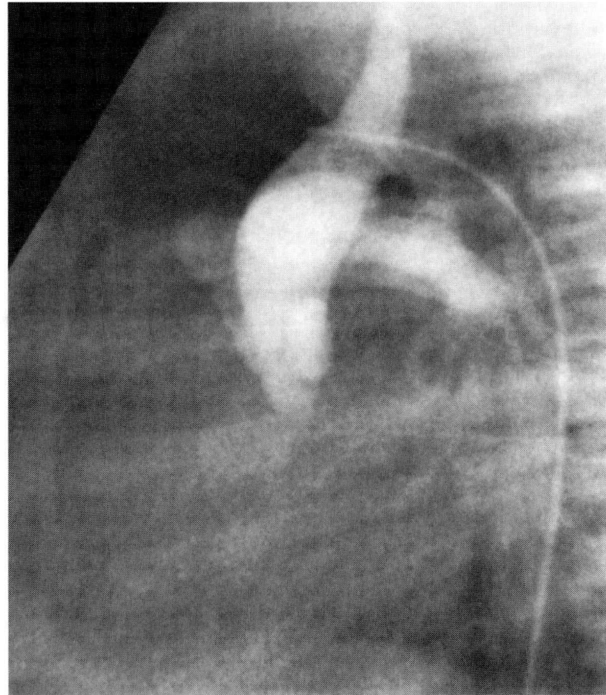

B

Figure 18-1. Frontal (A) and lateral (B) films of a retrograde aortic injection show contrast material entering the main pulmonary artery through an AP window before the arch is opacified. The lateral view shows retrograde flow in the pulmonary artery back to the level of the valve. The presence of two separate semi-lunar valves excludes truncus arteriosus.

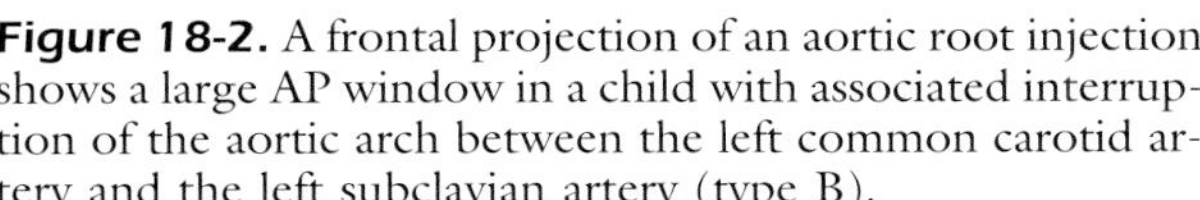

Figure 18-2. A frontal projection of an aortic root injection shows a large AP window in a child with associated interruption of the aortic arch between the left common carotid artery and the left subclavian artery (type B).

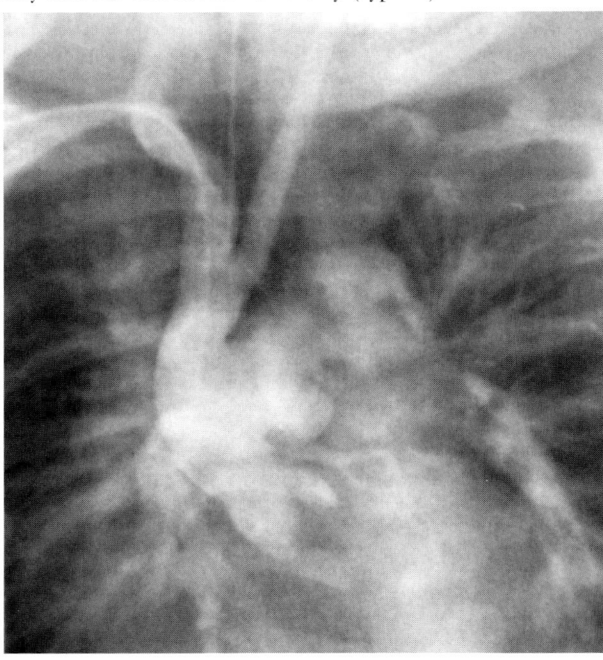

Figure 18-3. Angiogram in right anterior oblique projection, performed by passing a catheter from the pulmonary artery through a surgically created AP window into the ascending aorta. This connection was produced to bypass an area of subaortic stenosis in a child with a single ventricle.

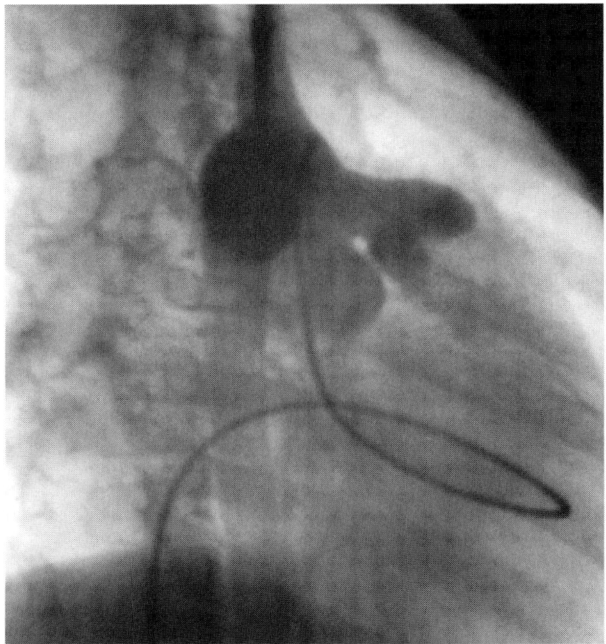

valve orifice between the ventricles and aorta is present, whereas in AP window the aortic valve is completely separated from the pulmonary valve. In lateral projection of the aortic injection contrast can be seen passing anterior to the aorta down to the level of the pulmonary valve (see Fig. 18-1).

Recently echocardiography combined with Doppler ultrasound has been described as useful in the diagnosis of AP window. Many of these reports describe single cases.[4,12,16–18] In a review of 15 cases, 6 of 7 AP windows were recognized on the initial examination when they were isolated lesions. In only 2 of 8 cases were they identified on the initial examination when they were associated with other cardiac lesions.[19]

Surgical therapy of AP window was first described using ligation. Most centers currently propose an open technique using cardiopulmonary bypass. The transaortic approach to the defect is the most popular, but transpulmonary, transdefect, and other variations have been described.[1,5,6,8,14,15,20,21] Early repair is recommended to prevent the development of pulmonary vascular disease.

Acknowledgments

I wish to thank Giuli Farquharson for secretarial assistance in the preparation of this manuscript.

References

1. Mori K, Ando M, Takao A, et al. Distal type of aortopulmonary window: report of 4 cases. Br Heart J 1978;40:681–689.
2. Ho SY, Gerlis LM, Anderson C, et al. Aortopulmonary window—morphology and associated lesions. Cardiol Young 1993;3(Suppl 1):141.
3. Kutsche LM, Van Mierop LHS. Anatomy and pathogenesis of aorticopulmonary septal defect. Am J Cardiol 1987;59:443–447.
4. Mendoza DA, Ueda T, Nishioka K, et al. Aortopulmonary window, aortic origin of the right pulmonary artery, and interrupted aortic arch: detection by two-dimensional and color Doppler echocardiography in an infant. Pediatr Cardiol 1986; 7:49–52.
5. van Son JAM, Puga FJ, Danielson GK, et al. Aortopulmonary window: factors associated with early and late success after surgical treatment. Mayo Clin Proc 1993;68:128–133.
6. Deverall PB, Aberdeen E, Bonham-Carter RE, et al. Aortopulmonary window. J Thorac Cardiovasc Surg 1969;57:479–486.
7. Neufeld HN, Lester RG, Adams P, et al. Aortopulmonary septal defect. Am J Cardiol 1962;9:12–25.
8. Prasad TR, Valiathan MS, Shyamakrishnan KG, et al. Surgical management of aortopulmonary septal defect. Ann Thorac Surg 1989;47:877–879.
9. Morrow AG, Greenfield LJ, Braunwald E. Congenital aortopulmonary septal defect: clinical and hemodynamic findings, surgical technic, and results of operative correction. Circulation 1962;25:463–476.
10. Krishnan P, Airan B, Sambamurthy S, et al. Complete transposition of the great arteries with aortopulmonary window: surgical treatment and embryologic significance. J Thorac Cardiovasc Surg 1991;101:749–751.
11. Ingram MT, Ott DA. Concomitant repair of aortopulmonary window and interrupted aortic arch. Ann Thorac Surg 1992; 53:909–911.
12. Carminati M, Borghi A, Valsecchi O, et al. Aortopulmonary window coexisting with tetralogy of Fallot: echocardiographic diagnosis. Pediatr Cardiol 1990;11:41–43.
13. Kothari SS, Rajani M, Shrivastava S. Tetralogy of Fallot with aortopulmonary window. Int J Cardiol 1988;18:105–108.
14. Ravikumar E, Whight CM, Hawker RE, et al. The surgical management of aortopulmonary window using the anterior sandwich patch closure technique. J Cardiovasc Surg (Torino) 1988;29:629–632.
15. Tiraboschi R, Salomone G, Crupi G, et al. Aortopulmonary window in the first year of life: report on 11 surgical cases. Ann Thorac Surg 1988;46:438–441.
16. Horimi H, Hasegawa T, Shiraishi H, et al. Detection of aortopulmonary window with ventricular septal defect by Doppler color flow imaging. Chest 1992;101:280–281.
17. Sreeram N, Walsh K. Aortopulmonary window with aortic origin of the right pulmonary artery. Int J Cardiol 1991;31:249–251.
18. Alboliras ET, Chin AJ, Barber G, et al. Detection of aortopulmonary window by pulsed and color Doppler echocardiography. Am Heart J 1988;115:900–902.
19. Balaji S, Burch M, Sullivan ID. Accuracy of cross-sectional echocardiography in diagnosis of aortopulmonary window. Am J Cardiol 1991;67:650–653.
20. Matsuki O, Yagihara T, Yamamoto F, et al. New surgical technique for total-defect aortopulmonary window. Ann Thorac Surg 1992;54:991–992.
21. Kitagawa T, Katoh I, Taki H, et al. New operative method for distal aortopulmonary septal defect. Ann Thorac Surg 1991; 51:680–682.

19

Aneurysms of the Thoracic Aorta

PATRICIA ANN RANDALL
ROBERT J. ASHENBURG

The normal aortic wall is composed of three layers: the intima, the media, and the adventitia. The intima, the innermost layer, is thin; it consists of a single thickness of endothelial cells and a supporting layer of connective tissue. The media, which is the middle layer, makes up the bulk (approximately 80 percent) of the aortic wall and is composed of lamellae of smooth muscle and elastic tissue, oriented in circular fashion around the aortic wall and held in place by areolar connective tissue. The adventitia, or the outermost layer, is also composed of areolar connective tissue with a fine fillwork of collagenous and elastic fibers. This portion of the aortic wall contains the vasa vasorum, which is the blood supply to the vessel wall.[1]

An aneurysm is defined as a localized, permanent dilatation of an artery due to disease affecting the vessel wall. Aneurysms can be classified as true or false. A true aneurysm results from a weakening of the vessel wall caused by atrophy and destruction of the elastic fibers in the media. The bulging wall of the true aneurysm still contains all three layers of the normal wall, albeit markedly thinned. A false aneurysm results from an actual disruption of the aortic wall and is contained only by the adventitia, perivascular connective tissues, and/or organized blood clot. Thus, the "wall" of a false aneurysm does not contain the usual three layers of the aortic wall.

Aneurysms can also be classified according to their appearance. The fusiform aneurysm is a diffuse, elongated widening of the caliber of the aorta and involves all walls. A saccular aneurysm projects outward from one side of the aortic wall and does not involve the complete circumference.

Both true and false aneurysms are found in the thoracic aorta. Table 19-1 lists the various types of aneurysms and their etiologies. Some overlap exists. True aneurysms are caused by sclerosis, syphilis, bacterial infection, and congenital abnormalities. False aneurysms are almost exclusively posttraumatic, with the exception of some mycotic aneurysms. Postoperative aneurysms are included under false aneurysms because they occur after surgical disruption of the aortic wall.

The incidence of aneurysms of the thoracic aorta ranges between 1 and 4 percent in various autopsy series.[2] True aneurysms were once dominated by the syphilitic variety, but improved diagnosis and treatment of that disease have made these relatively rare. With the extended life expectancy humans now enjoy, atherosclerotic aneurysms have increased in incidence and now represent the most common type of thoracic aortic aneurysm. The second most common types of aneurysms are posttraumatic false aneurysms, which have become more common secondary to rapid deceleration in this era of high-speed travel. Because thoracic aortic aneurysms are potentially life-threatening, it is important to recognize their presence and make a definitive diagnosis to facilitate prompt treatment. Technical advances achieved during the 1970s have greatly decreased the morbidity and mortality associated with surgical treatment. Medical treatment and support have also greatly changed, decreasing the morbidity and mortality of aortic aneurysms.

The signs and symptoms of thoracic aortic aneurysms usually reflect their location, area of involvement, and ability to affect contiguous structures. Aneurysms in the ascending aorta must grow very large before they produce their characteristic symptoms of chest pain, shoulder pain, or superior vena caval obstruction. However, they may be evident on plain chest film before symptoms occur. Aneurysms of the transverse arch are close to many vital structures in the narrow thoracic inlet. Early in their development, they can encroach on the trachea, esophagus, recurrent laryngeal nerve, and phrenic nerves, causing early symptoms. Aneurysms of the distal arch and descending thoracic aorta tend to produce symptoms such as pain, cough, and dyspnea or cause vertebral erosion at a late stage. Abnormalities of the descending aorta are usually evident on chest radiographs.

Death secondary to thoracic aortic aneurysms usu-

Table 19-1. Types of Aneurysms and Their Etiology

True Aneurysm	False Aneurysm
Atherosclerotic	Traumatic
Mycotic	Postoperative
Luetic	Some mycotic
Congenital	
Sinus of Valsalva	
Patent ductus arteriosus	

ally results from rupture, respiratory obstruction, infection, or cardiac failure. Rupture and massive hemorrhage are usually into the pericardial sac, pleural cavity, tracheobronchial tree, or esophagus.

Diagnosis

As stated previously, a definitive diagnosis is of critical importance whenever the possibility of aortic aneurysm exists. The means of diagnosis are discussed below in order of increasing invasiveness, as in other studies.[3]

Chest Radiography

Although thoracic aortic aneurysms are frequently visible on standard chest radiographs, their identification as aneurysms can often be difficult, and, unless they are considered in the differential diagnosis of a mediastinal mass, the diagnosis may be easily overlooked. As mediastinal masses, they present a smooth interface with adjacent lung and silhouette the aorta at their point of origin. Unfortunately, other mediastinal masses located adjacent to the aorta, or occasionally even parenchymal lesions invading the mediastinum, may have the same appearance and thus mimic each other.[4–6] Small polypoid aneurysms may present in an iceberg manner and thus appear to be separated from the aorta.[7] Curvilinear calcification increases the likelihood that the lesion is a vascular aneurysm, but other mediastinal masses, such as thymoma, thymic cyst, and bronchogenic cyst, may occasionally show similar calcifications.[8]

The plain chest radiograph can offer valuable information in the case of traumatic thoracic aneurysm, but the findings are nonspecific. Acutely, widening of the mediastinum and abnormalities of the aortic knob are most common. The aortic diameter may be increased; there may be a "double density" to the aortic shadow due to the enlarged posterior aorta superimposed over the normal anterior aorta; or the aortic contour may be irregular. Rightward deviation of the trachea and/or esophagus may be present. The left mainstem bronchus may be displaced downward. The descending aorta may be obscured, and a left pleural effusion usually suggests leakage of the aneurysm. Prominence of the left paraspinal stripe and capping of the left apex as well as deviation of a nasogastric (NG) tube are other secondary findings seen in acute transection and pseudoaneurysm formation. Chronically, the chest film shows the appearance of an aneurysm. Its location and correlation with the patient's history must make one suspicious that it is a traumatic aneurysm.

Findings on the chest radiographs secondary to nontraumatic aortic aneurysm are also often evident. Bronchial compression and obstruction may cause atelectasis or recurrent areas of pneumonia. Cardiac enlargement may be present due to systemic hypertension, aortic valve regurgitation, or coronary artery disease, all of which are frequently associated with aortic aneurysm. Aneurysms of the distal arch and descending thoracic aorta may cause erosion of adjacent vertebral bodies; the latter characteristically begins anteriorly, causing a concave defect and preserving the avascular intervertebral disks. Aneurysms of the ascending aorta may cause erosion of the posterior aspect of the sternum or clavicle if they become extensive.[9]

Fluoroscopy

Fluoroscopy may be helpful in localizing the lesion with more certainty, but it does not reliably differentiate vascular from nonvascular masses. Distinguishing between expansile and transmitted pulsation is virtually impossible. Usually only one margin of the mass is visible, and thrombus within an aneurysm may obliterate pulsations altogether. Therefore, this diagnostic test is seldom used. A barium swallow and conventional plain film tomography may show displacement of the esophagus and/or compression of the trachea. Although this may aid in confirming the presence of a lesion, it still does not make the diagnosis definitive.

Ultrasound

Traditional transthoracic ultrasonic evaluation of the aorta is possible if there is enough vessel dilatation to push the lung aside and move the aorta to the pleural surface. Preoperative demonstrations of sinus of Valsalva aneurysms have been made echocardiographically since 1974.[10] By using a substernal approach, the aortic arch can be measured and evaluated ultrasonically. The descending thoracic aorta and ascending aorta can be occasionally evaluated by scanning to the left of the spine posteriorly. Two-dimensional echo-

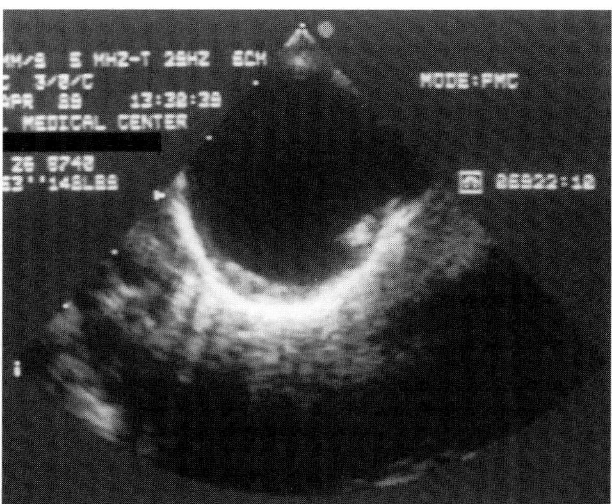

A

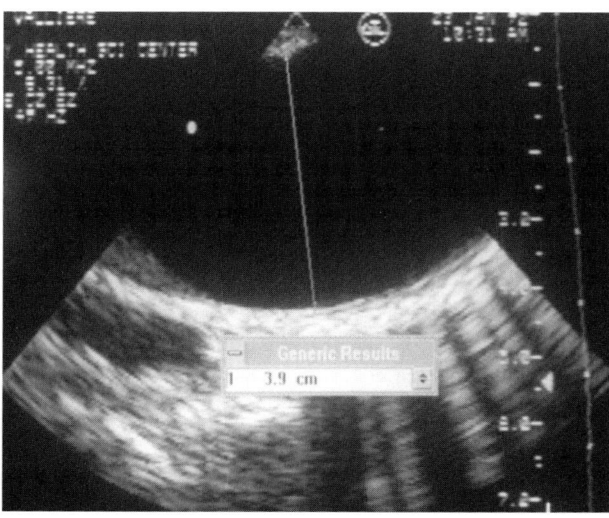

B

Figure 19-1. Transesophageal echocardiography (TEE). (A) Short axis view of a dilated ascending aorta. A plaque is noted in the 4 o'clock position with ulceration at 3 o'clock. (B) Short axis view of a descending aortic aneurysm. The aneurysm is adjacent to the esophagus and extends beyond the imaging plane both medially and laterally. The graphic accurately measures the diameter at this level. (Courtesy of Christopher Hare, RT, RDMS, and Raymond Carlson, M.D., SUNY Health Science Center, Division of Cardiology, Syracuse, N.Y.)

cardiography has definitively improved the accuracy of this noninvasive means for diagnosing thoracic aortic aneurysm.[11,12]

Transesophageal echocardiography (TEE) has further increased the accuracy of two-dimensional echocardiography in both the ascending and descending aorta. This is a more invasive technique in that the ultrasound probe must be passed down the esophagus. Since the esophagus courses adjacent to the descending aorta down to its distal attachment to the fundus of the stomach, transesophageal echocardiography can demonstrate the cross-sectional image of the descending aorta throughout its length. In cases of descending thoracic aortic aneurysm, the lateral borders often extend beyond the image area, and the transducer must be rotated to image the entire circumference of the aneurysm. The extent, shape, size, and wall thickness of an aneurysm are all well defined by this technique. The proximity of the TEE probe to these structures makes evaluation and characterization of the normal and abnormal aorta reliable (Fig. 19-1).[13]

Intravascular ultrasound of the aorta has been used and holds promise.[14]

Radionuclear Evaluation

Radionuclide angiography has been compared with contrast aortography for its usefulness in evaluating intrathoracic aneurysms.[15] This procedure does provide sufficient anatomic information for diagnosis while avoiding the risk of direct aortography. However, this technique has not gained great popularity because of its lack of resolution.

Leukocyte scintigraphy has been used successfully in the evaluation for mycotic aneurysms. Although this type of aneurysm is uncommon, its sequelae are frequently fatal. In the postoperative patient, this technique is sensitive to rule in or rule out infection at the site of the aneurysm or previous intervention.[16]

Computed Tomography

Conventional computed axial tomography (CT) has proven to be extremely valuable in differentiating aneurysms from other mediastinal masses.[17] Contrast enhancement can confirm the vascular nature of a lesion, and early diagnosis of some unusual types of thoracic aortic aneurysms has been achieved with this noninvasive technique.[18–20] CT has made a major impact on the workup and diagnosis of aneurysms since the 1980s. Thrombus within an atherosclerotic aneurysm will produce a peripheral rim or crescent that does not enhance. Calcifications can be more clearly demonstrated and precisely located. The presence of calcification in the wall of the aorta with layered intraluminal thrombus can be readily determined. This is a definitive means of differentiating atherosclerotic aneurysm with

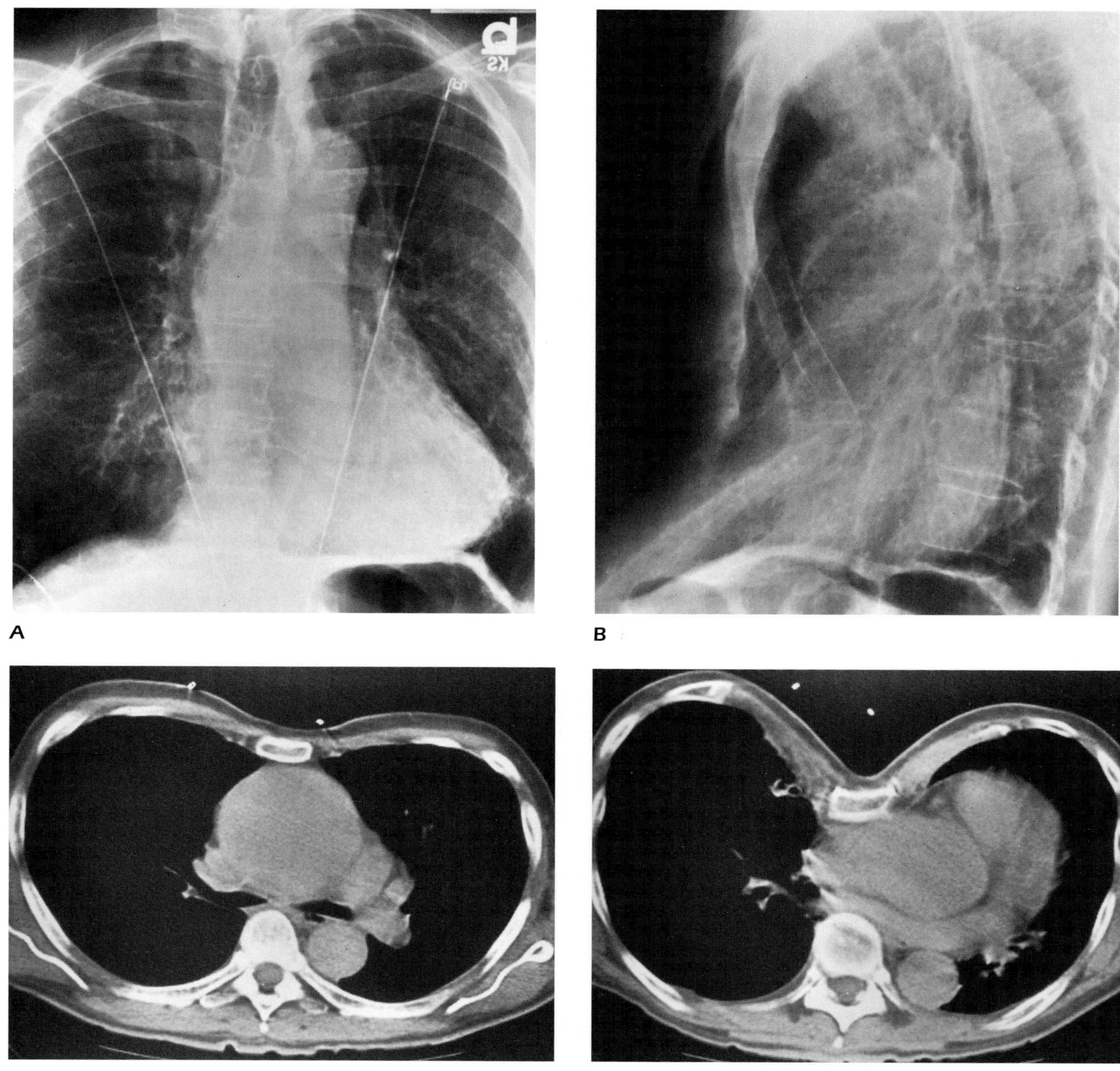

Figure 19-2. A tall, thin, 75-year-old man presented to the hospital with dyspnea and fatigue. His arterial blood gases revealed a PO_2 of 40. A ventilation-perfusion lung scan showed markedly decreased perfusion to the right lung. (A) PA chest radiograph shows marked cardiomegaly and prominence of the entire aorta. There is decreased pulmonary vasculature in the right lung as compared to the left. (B) Lateral film of the same patient demonstrates a marked pectus excavatum deformity. The marked cardiomegaly and enlarged ascending aorta are again visible. (C) Transaxial contrast-enhanced CT scan at the level of the carina. The large ascending aortic aneurysm is seen to be roughly twice the diameter of the descending aorta. (D) Transaxial contrast-enhanced CT scan at a slightly lower level shows the marked pectus deformity. The large ascending aortic aneurysm compresses the elongated right pulmonary artery, effectively obstructing flow to the right lung. (Courtesy of Department of Diagnostic Radiology, Mary Imogene Bassett Hospital and Clinics, Cooperstown, N.Y.)

thrombus from an aortic dissection with dilatation.[21] Penetrating atherosclerotic ulcers can be distinguished from aortic dissection.[22] The extent of an aneurysm as well as its relationship to contiguous structures can be demonstrated accurately. CT with contrast enhancement has also become a useful tool in following those patients in whom surgical intervention has been postponed. Dilated areas can be measured cross-sectionally to determine increased luminal dimensions and aneurysm growth.[23] Rupture of a thoracic aneurysm into the right chest is rare but has been demonstrated by CT preoperatively.[24] Compression of the right pulmonary artery by ascending aortic aneurysms has been demonstrated by CT.[25] A similar case is shown in Figure 19-2.

Until the 1990s, CT was not felt to be reliable or specific enough to play a role in the diagnosis of acute aortic transections and pseudoaneurysms. Recently, three separate groups have shown that dynamic CT in cases of thoracic aortic trauma is highly reliable as a screening test for aortic transection.[26–28] These authors state that unnecessary aortography was reduced significantly.

Ultrafast computed tomography (UFCT), by virtue of its excellent spatial resolution, rapid scan times, better vascular opacification, and decreased motion artifact, is ideally suited to imaging the thoracic aorta. The increasing use of UFCT is evident from the increased number of related articles in the literature.[29,30] Its accuracy and speed have made the technique a major step forward from conventional CT.

Spiral CT is another form of computed tomography that may yield additional benefits.[31] Its use with reduced volumes of contrast material will make it very competitive to UFCT and far better than conventional dynamic CT.[32]

Magnetic Resonance Imaging

Since the mid-1980s, magnetic resonance imaging (MRI) of the thoracic aorta has proven to be a reliable means of delineating the aorta from surrounding soft tissue structures without the administration of contrast material. Electrocardiogram (ECG) gated MRI examinations in the transverse, sagittal, and coronal as well as oblique planes have shown that high-quality examinations of the normal aorta and a variety of abnormalities are possible. MRI has a number of characteristics that are particularly well suited to the study of the aorta. These include excellent contrast between flowing blood and adjacent structures without the introduction of contrast media, images in any desired plane with high quality throughout a large field, and absence of any known biologic effect, which permits serial examinations to follow the patient without risk. The size and extent of aneurysm, presence of thrombus, relation to other arteries, and effect on adjacent structures are readily demonstrated by MRI. Because of these advantages, MRI has been considered by some to be the method of choice for the study of aortic pathology.[33,34] Cardiac MRI is able to provide useful noninvasive and pre- and postoperative information in perivalvular pseudoaneurysm due to endocarditis.[35] Two potential limitations to MRI are the difficulty in recognizing intimal calcification, which can be exquisitely identified by CT, and the difficulty in distinguishing intraluminal signal due to slow flow from true thrombus. This differentiation can usually be made by using other pulse sequences or fast scans using gradient recalled echoes.[36] MRI has proven to be very effective in evaluating Marfan syndrome, aortic dissection, aortic aneurysm, and some congenital aortic abnormalities such as coarctation (Fig. 19-3).[37,38] Use of gradient-echo sequences has enabled quantification of regurgitated cardiac lesions, and newer techniques permit MRI measurement of blood flow in the cardiovascular system.[39]

Both CT and MRI have acquired a definite role in the evaluation of aortic aneurysm and dissection. Both are relatively noninvasive and can be repeated for serial evaluation of disease progression or postoperative status.[40]

Aortography

Despite remarkable advances and refinements in cross-sectional and multiplanar imaging techniques, thoracic aortography remains the gold standard examination against which all other methods are compared. The diagnosis of thoracic aneurysmal disease may be suspected or confirmed with another modality, but surgical intervention is rarely undertaken without a thorough angiographic study. Specific advantages of angiography include (1) precise evaluation of the relationship of the aneurysm to branch vessels, (2) determination of the patency of branch vessels or possible associated branch vessel aneurysmal disease, and (3) evaluation of associated valvular dysfunction with ascending aortic disease.

The size of an aneurysm is best determined by cross-sectional imaging (i.e., CT or MRI) because angiography only depicts the luminal caliber and there is frequently extensive mural thrombus. However, one can overestimate the size of an aneurysm by CT if there is angulation of the aorta such that the true longitudinal axis is oriented in the axial plane. Correlation with angiography or MRI is then necessary.

Some aortic pathology (e.g., traumatic pseudoan-

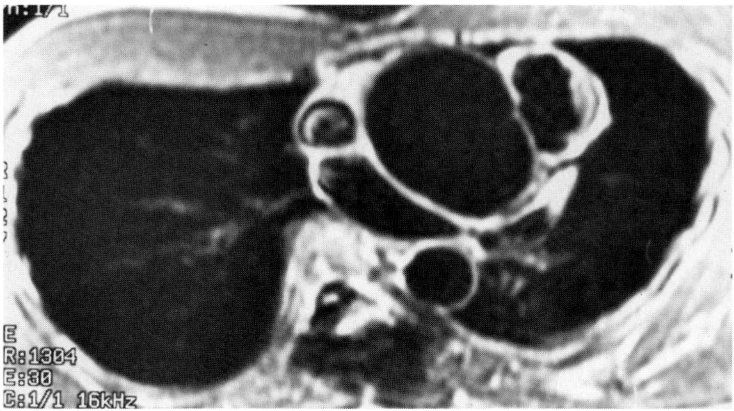

A

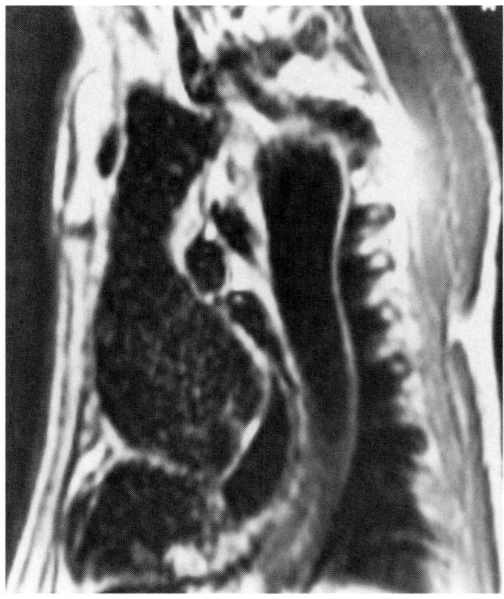

B

Figure 19-3. A 25-year-old asymptomatic man with known Marfan syndrome underwent an MRI to evaluate the size and extent of his ascending aortic aneurysm. (A) Transaxial T1-weighted MR image at the root of the thoracic aorta shows marked dilatation of the aortic root with compression of the left atrium against the thoracic spine in this patient with a narrow chest diameter. (B) Sagittal oblique T1-weighted MR image of the aorta demonstrates the "Erlenmeyer flask" dilatation of the sinuses of Valsalva and ascending aorta. This appearance is most commonly seen in Marfan syndrome. The entire aorta appears enlarged and tortuous. The arch portion is not imaged because it has deviated out of this plane. (Courtesy of Charles S. White, M.D., Department of Diagnostic Radiology, University of Maryland School of Medicine, Baltimore, MD.)

eurysm) is most conclusively imaged with angiography. Although somewhat controversial, thoracic aortography is generally considered the only examination sufficiently sensitive and specific to exclude a traumatic aortic rupture. One final and less compelling (although practical) argument for routine angiography is the fact that our surgical colleagues have been slow to embrace the newer modalities and remain comfortable with the proven technique of aortography.

Thoracic aortography is best performed using the standard Seldinger technique for aortic catheterization. The preferred access site is the femoral artery, although an axillary or brachial approach is sometimes necessary because of aortoiliac or femoral occlusive disease. Catheterization of the thoracic aorta is technically possible from a translumbar approach; however, this unusual method is rarely required.[41] Diagnostic images of the thoracic aorta can also be obtained with a right atrial injection and filming in the levo phase with digital subtraction technique. Images obtained with this "intravenous" digital technique are clearly suboptimal when compared with a direct arterial injection, and this method should be reserved as a secondary option.

Once access to the arterial system is obtained, the catheter, with leading guidewire, is advanced under fluoroscopic guidance into the ascending aorta within a few centimeters of the aortic valve. The catheter should be placed proximal enough so that the aortic root is opacified; yet it should not interfere with valvular function. An extremely tortuous thoracic or thoracoabdominal aneurysm often presents a formidable challenge when one is attempting to place a catheter into the ascending aorta from a femoral approach. The use of a floppy tipped guidewire or the use of torqueable catheters and/or guidewires may be helpful in this situation. Alternatively, catheterization from an axillary puncture can be performed to avoid the tortuous segment.

Improvements in catheter design over the past decade have focused on the miniaturization of catheter systems while allowing for adequate contrast delivery but at the same time reducing the arterial puncture defect. The numerous variations in catheter tip configurations are purported to deliver a more compact contrast bolus, thus improving vessel opacification. For thoracic aortography, with conventional cut-film technique, we prefer to use a 6 French pigtail catheter and generally inject 35 cc of contrast per second for 2 seconds. This relatively high rate of contrast delivery has been particularly helpful in trauma aortography, allowing excellent opacification of a long segment of the aorta in young individuals with good cardiac output. For older individuals with a diminished cardiac output and/or atherosclerotic aneurysm, the rate can be decreased and a 5 French catheter will suffice. For the average adult, a 90-cm catheter is of sufficient length; however, an extremely tortuous or unfolded aorta may call for a longer catheter. The catheter tip should have a pigtail configuration or slight modification to minimize aortic intimal injury or inadvertent selective catheterization of the coronary or innominate artery. If standard ionic contrast material is used, 76 percent medium is necessary. Low-osmolar contrast media should have a minimum of 350 mg of iodine per milliliter. These figures are for conventional angiography with a film changer. The contrast concentration as well as the rate and volume of contrast used would be lower for intraarterial digital technique.

The single best projection for evaluation of the thoracic aorta is the 45-degree left anterior oblique (LAO) or right posterior oblique (RPO) projection, which allows for unfolding of the arch and provides an excellent profile of the great vessel origins. For a thorough evaluation, a second view is mandatory, usually the contralateral oblique, although an anteroposterior (AP) image or true lateral projection is perfectly adequate. If simultaneous biplane imaging is possible, this is preferred to maximize information and minimize contrast. The field of view should be sufficient to visualize all aortic segments from the root to the distal descending aorta as well as the proximal segments of the great vessels. The rate of filming should be at least three images per second early in the run, especially in patients with a normal or increased cardiac output.

Although many angiographic laboratories continue to perform thoracic aortography with the cut-film technique, the pendulum is rapidly swinging toward the "filmless" catheterization laboratory using digital subtraction angiography (DSA). As outdated angiographic rooms become replaced, they are upgraded with high-quality digital imaging systems that are frequently devoid of film changers. Although intravenous digital imaging was hindered by poor visualization in patients with diminished cardiac output and never lived up to its high expectations, intraarterial DSA provides high-quality images with the advantages of lower contrast dose, shortened examination time, and reduced film costs. There has been some concern regarding the ability of DSA to identify subtle abnormalities. However, resolution is excellent with state-of-the-art equipment and 1024 × 1024 matrix size. Field coverage is not compromised because image intensifiers are available up to 16 inches in diameter. Intraarterial DSA for evaluation of the thoracic aorta is already the standard at many centers, and its prevalence will continue to increase over the next several years.

Arteriosclerotic Aneurysm

The most common etiology of thoracic aortic aneurysms at this time is arteriosclerosis. Such aneurysms are localized expressions of a diffuse disease process.[42] Joyce et al.[2] found that 73 percent of aneurysms in their series were arteriosclerotic in origin. A study by DeBakey et al.[43] reviewing their experience with 500 aneurysms of the descending aorta reported that 82 percent of these aneurysms were arteriosclerotic.

Pathogenesis

The pathogenesis of arteriosclerotic aneurysms was concisely described by Storer et al.[44] in 1967. Initially the intima thickens with age, and cholesterol is deposited subintimally. This deposition later ruptures into the lumen, resulting in an ulceration. Calcium is deposited at the ulcer site in an attempted healing process, and the typical calcified arteriosclerotic plaque is thus produced. The deeper portions of this lesion may disrupt the elastic fibers of the media, thereby weakening the vessel wall. The vessel slowly dilates and an aneurysm forms. Laminated clot may be deposited within the aneurysm, and adventitial fibrosis, if it occurs, may strengthen the abnormal aortic wall somewhat. However, if ischemic liquefaction necrosis should occur in the outermost layer of this laminated clot, further weakening of the aortic wall may lead to frank rupture. Arteriosclerotic aneurysms are usually fusiform, but occasionally they are saccular in morphology. They most commonly involve the distal aortic arch and descending aorta; only rarely is the ascending aorta affected. Arteriosclerotic aneurysms are found predominantly in males. However, the risk for rupture is higher for women than for men: in one study, 32 percent of women with arteriosclerotic aneurysms died after their rupture, compared to 23 percent of men (Fig. 19-4).[45] The mean age of these patients is generally 60 to 70 years. There is a high incidence of related cardiovascular disease: 50 percent of the patients have hypertension, coronary artery disease, or cerebrovascular disease, and many have associated abdominal aortic aneurysms.

Survival

The natural history of arteriosclerotic aneurysms was described by McNamara and Pressler in 1978.[46] In their 22 cases, the mean survival was 2.4 years with a 5-year survival of less than 20 percent. Fifty-six percent of the patients died from rupture of their aneurysm, and 32 percent died of unrelated cardiovascular dis-

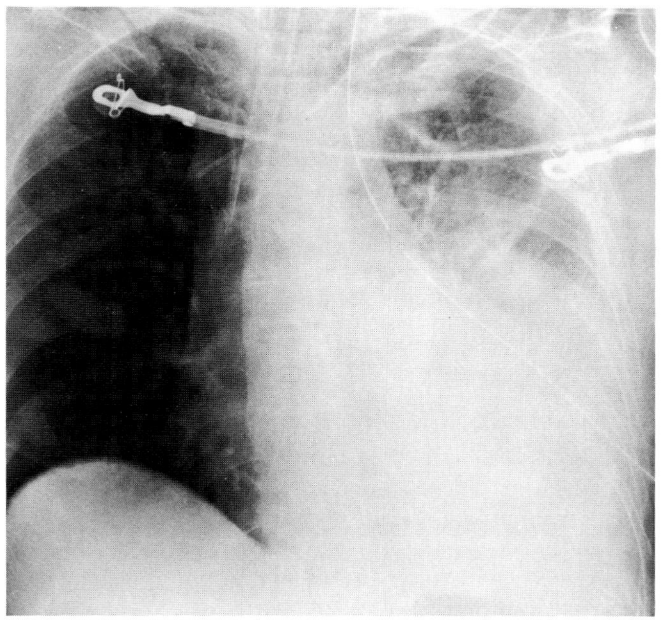

A

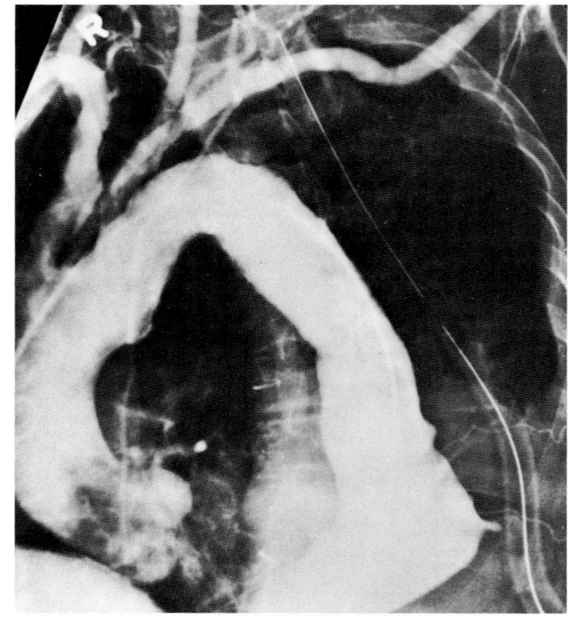

B

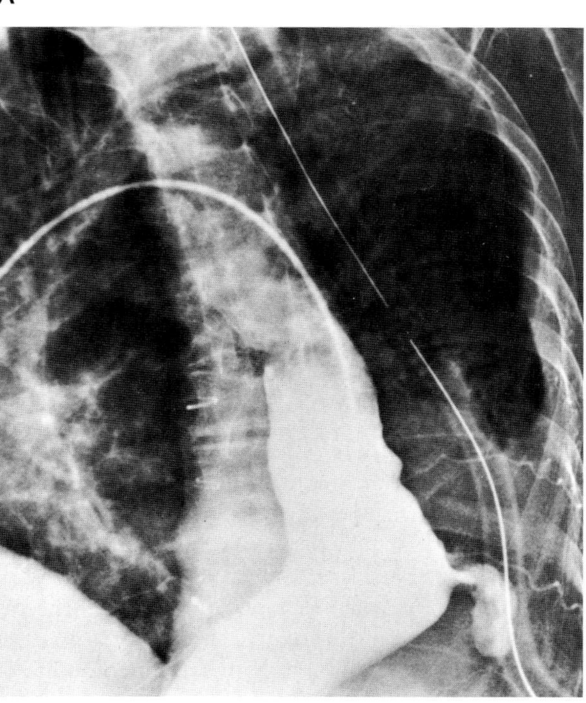

C

Figure 19-4. A 76-year-old woman with a recent complaint of increasingly severe back pain was admitted to the hospital. Previous chest film reportedly showed a saccular aneurysm of the descending thoracic aorta. (A) Initial portable supine AP chest radiograph shows cardiomegaly and a large pleural effusion on the left. The chest tube placed in the left thorax drained frank blood. An endotracheal tube is seen with the tip down into the right mainstem bronchus. The lower left cardiac border and descending thoracic aorta are totally obscured by the large left effusion. (B) Thoracic aortogram performed in the LAO position. The pigtail catheter is positioned in the ascending aorta, where the injection of contrast material demonstrates the ascending aorta to be fairly normal. Beyond the brachiocephalic branches, marked atherosclerotic changes are noted with ectasia and plaque throughout. There is an area of dilatation in the lower thoracic aorta with an outpouching of contrast material seen just above an intercostal artery. (C) A later film in the series more clearly shows the aneurysm in the descending thoracic aorta. More contrast material is noted extending from this outpouching into a pocket within the left pleural effusion. This is an excellent demonstration of a leaking atherosclerotic aneurysm. The patient was taken to surgery and these findings were confirmed.

ease. Pressler and McNamara[45] updated this series and noted that rupture accounted for 25 of 57 deaths (44 percent) in 76 patients with arteriosclerotic aneurysm not treated surgically. In the original series, all of the ruptures but one occurred in aneurysms greater than 10 cm in diameter, and a recent increase in size predicted the majority of these ruptures. Unlike the rupture of an abdominal aortic aneurysm, which can be contained by the retroperitoneal structures, rupture of a thoracic aortic aneurysm is not usually contained and rapidly becomes a fatal event.

Signs and Symptoms

The signs and symptoms of arteriosclerotic aneurysms are late clues to the diagnosis. Pain is the most common symptom and is related to compression or erosion of contiguous structures by the aneurysm. However, only 42 percent of patients with arteriosclerotic aneurysms have back or chest pain when first seen.[45] Occasionally, dyspnea and bronchospasm are seen because of compression of the bronchial tree.[47] These aneurysms can also compress the pulmonary artery and cause signs and symptoms suggestive of pulmonary emboli.[48,49] The literature has reported cases of rupture of a thoracic aortic aneurysm into a pulmonary artery.[50] Erosion of the vertebral bodies adjacent to these aneurysms has been described,[9] as has dysphasia and esophageal obstruction secondary to a tortuous thoracic aortic aneurysm.[51] These late signs relate to the large size of the aneurysm. Instances of upper GI bleeding and exsanguination from rupture of an arteriosclerotic aortic aneurysm into the esophagus have been reported.[25,52,53]

Frequently, saccular aneurysms are detected on routine chest radiographs and perceived as mediastinal masses.[54] It is important to distinguish these from neoplasms by various techniques, now most commonly CT and MRI. If a thoracic aneurysm ruptures, the patient most often has a left hemothorax, although right-sided effusions and hematomas can be seen when the tortuous and dilated aneurysm in the distal descending aorta extends into the right thorax.[55]

Multiple Aneurysms

Arteriosclerotic aneurysms may be multiple and extensive (Fig. 19-5). Because they frequently occur simultaneously in the abdominal and thoracic aorta, evaluation of both of these regions should be performed if this etiology is suspected. CT and MRI can be the first method of examination and aortography resorted to only when questions arise such as branch involvement. Occasionally aneurysms of the descending aorta are

Figure 19-5. A 69-year-old woman presented to an outside hospital with an abnormal chest radiograph. Multiple aneurysms of the descending aorta were noted. Her initial workup after routine PA and lateral chest radiographs included a contrast-enhanced CT scan. (A and B) PA and lateral chest radiograph demonstrates calcification within the walls of multiple aneurysms of the descending aorta. These are projected over one another on the frontal film but are actually in series throughout the elongated descending aorta beyond the brachiocephalic vessels. The overall heart size is upper limits of normal. There is no evidence of cardiac failure.

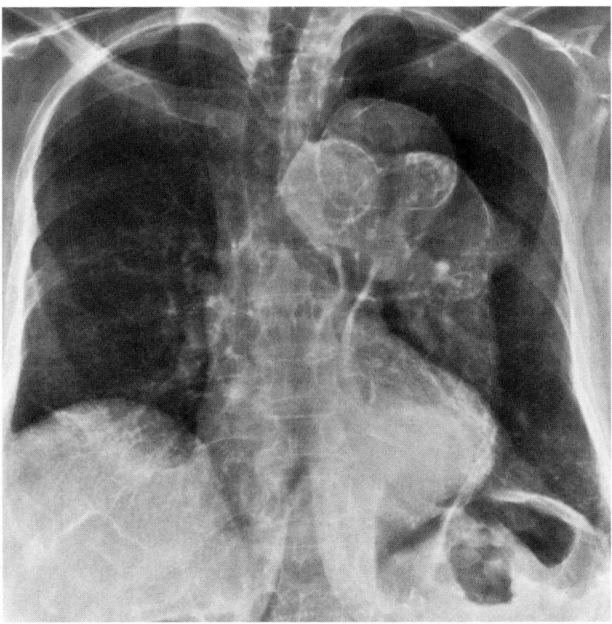

A

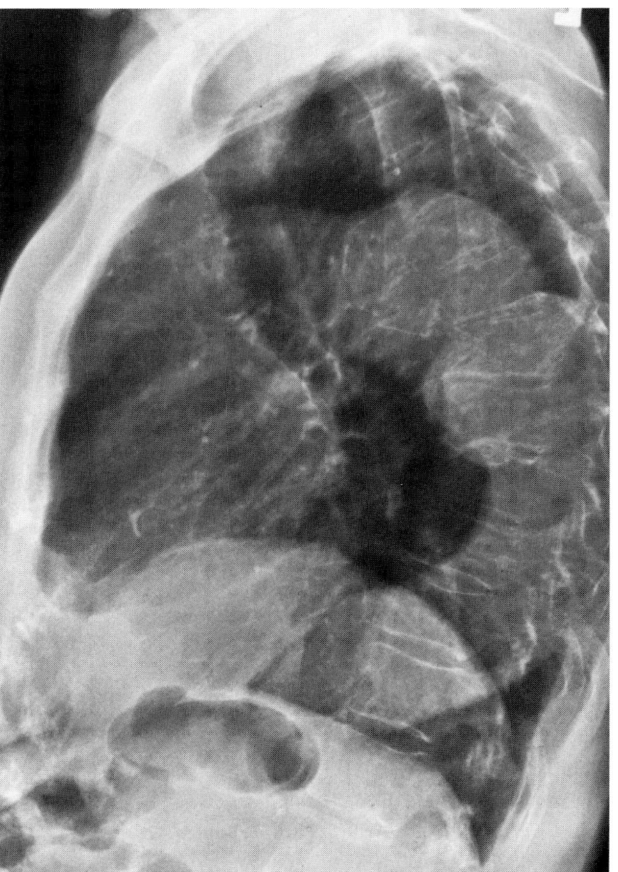

B

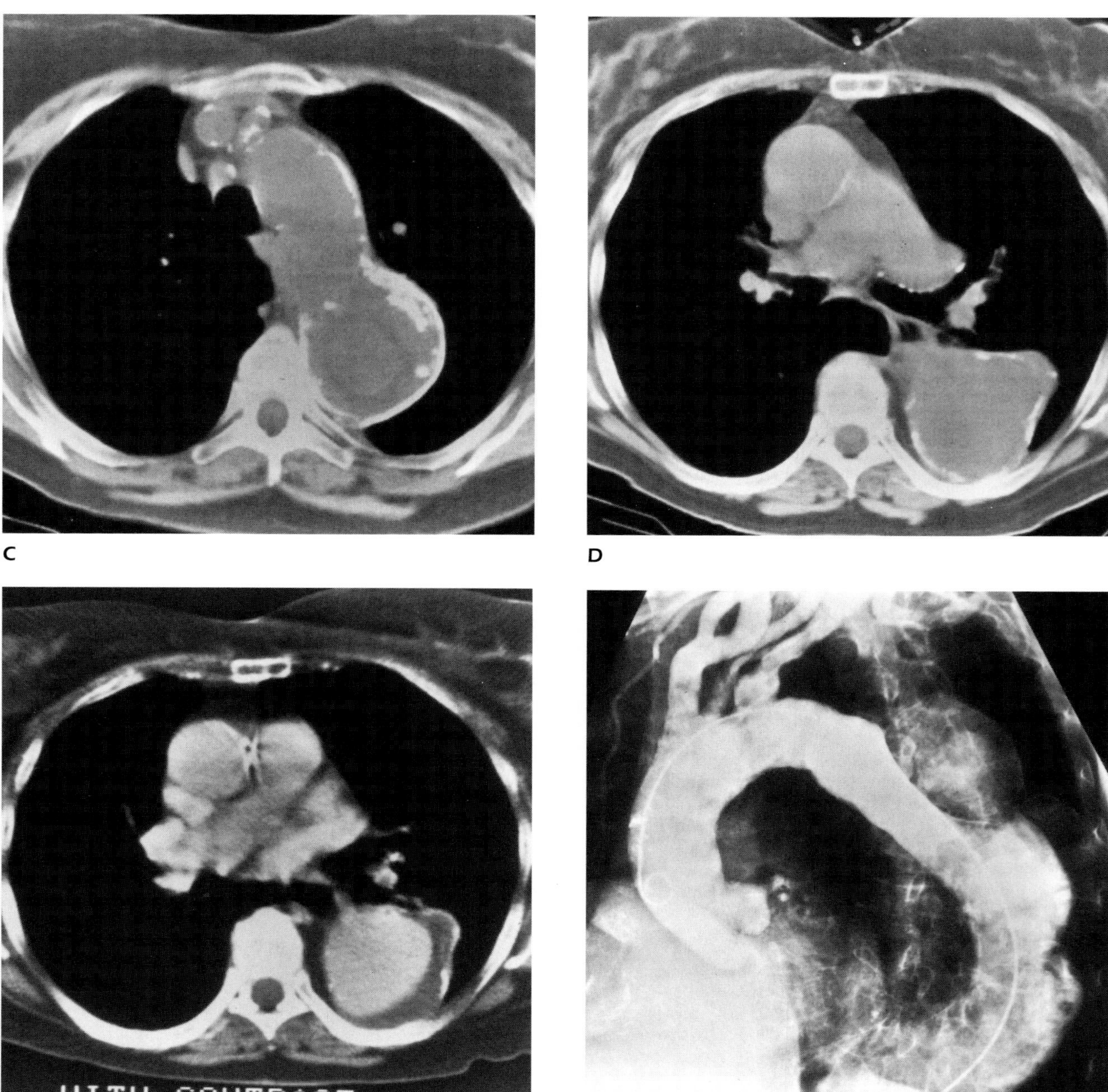

Figure 19-5 (continued). (C) Transaxial CT scan without contrast enhancement at the level of the aortic arch demonstrates the extensive intimal calcification of the aorta and brachiocephalic vessels. The presence of mural thrombus within the aneurysm of the proximal descending aorta is suspected because of the lucent circle within the distal portion of the arch. This may represent the interface between thrombus and flowing blood of the same density. (D) Transaxial CT scan without contrast enhancement at a lower level just below the carina. The normal size of the ascending aorta is compared to the aneurysmal enlargement of the descending aorta. Extensive peripherally located intimal calcification is noted. A lateral projection of the aorta may represent an other aneurysm. (E) Transaxial CT scan *with* contrast enhancement at approximately the same level as D. The lumen of the descending aorta is demonstrated, with extensive mural thrombus projecting into the aneurysm. (F) Thoracic aortogram in the same patient in the LAO projection demonstrates extensive atherosclerotic changes throughout the entire aorta and brachiocephalic vessels. The multiple aneurysmal dilatations with mural thrombus and ulceration are depicted just beyond the take-off of the left subclavian artery. Because of the extensiveness of the aneurysms and the relative asymptomatic status of the patient, no surgery was performed.

truly thoracoabdominal. These aneurysms are often associated with significant obstructive lesions in other major branches (coronaries, renals, brachiocephalics, iliacs, or peripheral vessels). Aortography may be needed before surgery for the complete evaluation of these suspected obstructions.

Arteria magna (a term used to describe multiple aneurysms in large-caliber, elongated, tortuous vessels with slow blood flow) was once considered a peculiar and unique form of arteriosclerosis. Reevaluation of this entity, which is seen predominantly in the elderly, reveals that the basic pathology appears to be a profound loss of elastic tissue in the media, with subsequent enlargement of both the vessel length and diameter. Patients with arteria magna frequently demonstrate thoracic aortic aneurysms, which are subject to fatal rupture just like regular arteriosclerotic aneurysms. This entity requires extensive diagnostic evaluation to delineate additional lesions and aneurysms.[56]

Surgical Intervention

Careful selection of patients for operative intervention is important. Surgical intervention is warranted in the presence of increasing symptoms and radiographic evidence of increasing aneurysm size. Resection of the aneurysm with graft replacement is a high-risk operation because of the patient's elderly age and concomitant related cardiovascular diseases. Ideally the goal is surgical intervention *just before* rupture. Once the presence of aneurysm has been established, serial follow-up studies to judge size, change in size, and relationship to symptoms must be performed. The operative mortality rate in ascending and descending aneurysms is approximately 5 to 10 percent. The mortality increases to approximately 15 percent for transverse arch and thoracoabdominal aneurysms.[43,46]

Traumatic Aortic Aneurysms

Traumatic aneurysms of the thoracic aorta are almost solely related to blunt, nonpenetrating trauma of the chest; they are also discussed in Chapter 21. They represent the prototype pseudoaneurysm, being contained only by adventitia or surrounding mediastinal tissues. Although they were originally described in the 16th century,[57] it was not until the autopsy study of Parmley in 1958 that a large series was published and statistics were generated documenting the significant mortality in the untreated patient.[58] These survival statistics are frequently quoted in the literature; however, it has been pointed out that they were accumulated when angiography was not widely available, and therefore an antemortem diagnosis was not possible. Because it is unknown how many patients with unsuspected aortic rupture are actually long-term survivors, the natural history in the untreated patient remains unknown.[59] Nevertheless, traumatic rupture of the aorta is a serious condition requiring expedient diagnosis and treatment.

The incidence of aortic rupture has increased steadily over the past several decades, now accounting for approximately 20 percent of all motor vehicle accident fatalities.[60–62] This is clearly related to our increasing use of and dependence on high-speed travel. The number of cases presenting to medical attention is also increasing, presumably as a result of improved emergency medical transport services and prehospital care. Although the majority of cases involve the young adult and adult population, there is a heightened awareness of the condition in the pediatric age group, and, in fact, it may be significantly underdiagnosed.[63] A high index of suspicion and appropriate imaging in the trauma patient will aid in diagnosis.

Mechanism of Injury

Aortic rupture occurs in the setting of an abrupt deceleration injury, most commonly motor vehicle accidents or falls from significant heights. Crush injuries and less significant falls have also been associated with this entity. The actual mechanism of injury is hypothesized to be related to shear stress on the aortic wall, occurring at sites where there is a transition from a relatively fixed segment of aorta to a more mobile segment. It is thought that differing rates of deceleration cause significant torsion and traction forces leading to circumferential tears and subsequent pseudoaneurysm development.[64,65] Other mechanisms have been suggested, including a transient rise in intraaortic pressure and inherent relative weakness of localized segments of the aortic wall, specifically the aortic isthmus.[66] These more traditional hypotheses have recently been challenged, and a new mechanism of injury has been proposed suggesting that the aorta is compressed by surrounding osseous structures. This hypothesis is supported by preliminary experimental findings.[67]

Location

Whatever the exact mechanism, it is certain that the isthmic portion of the aorta, just distal to the left subclavian artery, is the most susceptible to aortic rupture. In most published series of patients presenting alive at the hospital, this accounts for 95 percent of ruptures.

The proximal ascending aorta and the descending aorta at the diaphragm account for the remainder.[60,68,69] This is in great disparity to statistics derived from cases of rupture that do not survive to reach the hospital.[58] Approximately 20 percent of these tears are located in the ascending aorta. The disparity can be readily explained by the frequently associated cardiac injury in those with proximal aortic transection.[60,65,68,69] Multiple areas of rupture occur rarely, and are reported to be less than 5 percent (Fig. 19-6).[60,70]

Signs and Symptoms

The great difficulty and continuing problem with aortic rupture is determining which of the many patients who experience blunt chest trauma are actually likely to have an aortic transection. Historically, a significant deceleration injury or fall is nearly universally present. External signs of chest injury may be entirely absent in the presence of aortic injury. Physical signs and symptoms referable to aortic transection are nonspecific and have been reported in only approximately 40 percent of patients. They include chest or back pain, differential upper and lower extremity blood pressure, and the presence of a murmur.[59,60,71,72]

Diagnostic Imaging and Findings

Given the fact that the history and physical examination are of little help in selecting those patients at high risk for aortic transection, there is a great need for an easily obtainable, sensitive, and specific screening exam. None currently exists. The properly interpreted chest x-ray is highly sensitive (few false negatives) but has low specificity, and the study is all too frequently obtained in the supine patient, creating the false impression of a wide mediastinum. A great number of findings on the upright chest film have been described in association with aortic transection, including widening of the mediastinum, obscuration of the aortic knob

Figure 19-6. A 32-year-old man involved in a motor vehicle accident. Aortography was recommended because of superior mediastinal widening and an indistinct border of the aorta evident on supine chest film. (A) LAO projection from a thoracic aortogram shows characteristic saccular aneurysms in the proximal and mid-portion descending aorta (*arrows*). (B) Delayed contrast "washout" (*arrowheads*) is demonstrated on a later film from the same study. Multiple aortic tears frequently involve atypical locations, as demonstrated in this case with involvement of the mid-portion of the descending aorta.

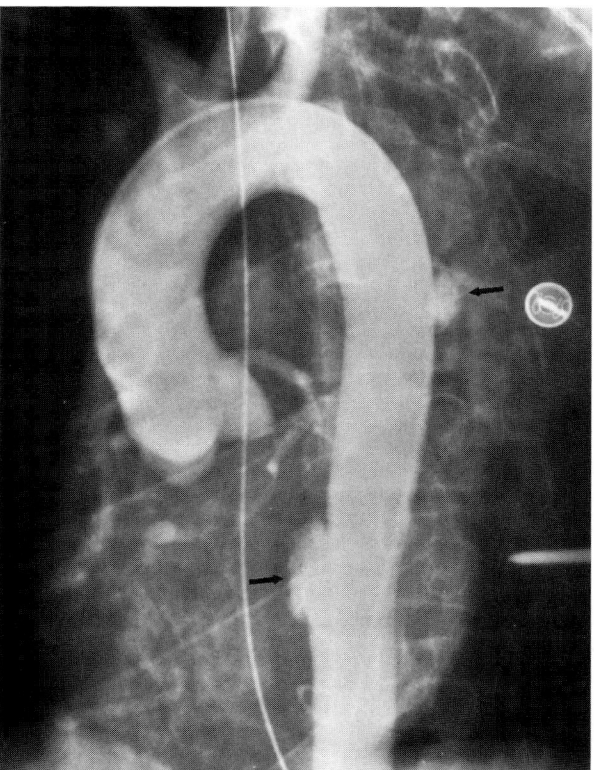

A

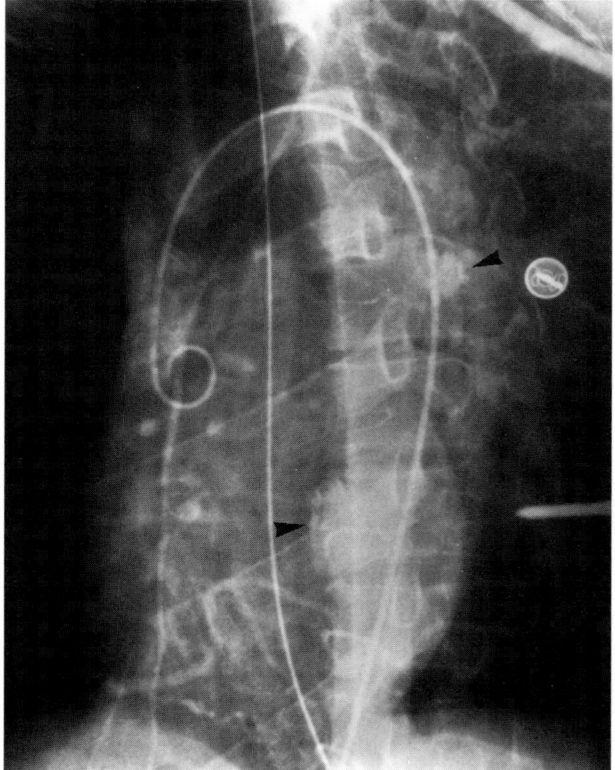

B

or descending aorta, deviation of the nasogastric tube or trachea, and depression of the left mainstem bronchus.[71,73,74] Although the presence of any of these signs should prompt further imaging evaluation (usually aortography), none is sufficiently sensitive or specific to accurately predict or exclude aortic injury.

Numerous studies have been reported regarding the use of CT in the setting of aortic trauma.[26-28,75-77] The role of CT continues to be controversial; however, a strong argument can be made for its selective use. From the available data certain conclusions can be drawn. There is no role for CT in attempting to identify the site of tear and then excluding the diagnosis when no morphologic abnormality is identified. Although identification of the torn segment has been reported in numerous studies, the axial plane of imaging is not optimal for detection.[61] The real utility of CT is in defining the absolutely normal mediastinum in low- and moderate-risk individuals in whom the screening chest x-ray is indeterminate or suboptimal.[74] Cases of aortic transection with a normal CT of the mediastinum have been reported,[27,77] but they are exceedingly unusual. Any abnormality on CT mandates further evaluation with aortography (Fig. 19-7). It should not be surprising that the majority of aortograms will still be normal, because the mediastinal bleeding detected by CT is almost never related to the aortic injury, but instead is due to bleeding from small mediastinal vessels. The presence of blood in the mediastinum only indicates the severity of trauma.

Certain other modalities deserve mention. MRI, with its excellent blood vessel visualization and multiplanar imaging capability, would seem an ideal choice as a noninvasive examination. In reality, the examination is difficult if not impossible to obtain in an expeditious manner with the uncooperative patient who has suffered multiple trauma. Life support equipment adds to the logistic problems.

Transesophageal echocardiography (TEE) provides an excellent image of the descending aorta and proximal ascending aorta and can be performed at the bedside. It has become well accepted in the diagnosis of aortic dissection and is undergoing evaluation at a number of centers in blunt trauma patients suspected of having aortic injury. Limitations at this time include the need for an available experienced operator, the limited visualization of the distal ascending aorta and proximal arch, and the inability to evaluate the great vessels.[13,78-83] Even if this modality becomes more universally available and acceptable, aortography will still be necessary for providing confirmation of the abnormality and more global imaging of the aorta and great vessels. This is similar to the way aortography is used for aortic dissection after the diagnosis is established with CT or TEE.

Angiography in the setting of trauma and possible aortic transection is a safe procedure with only rare complications. Nevertheless, careful attention to technique is required. A catheter should be advanced only under fluoroscopic guidance to avoid traumatizing the possibly transected segment. Resistance to catheter movement at the site of injury can also be better appreciated with visual as well as tactile input. In cases of possible transection, it is preferable to place a floppy guidewire into the ascending aorta before the catheter is actually placed. In most instances, the guidewire and catheter will pass easily through a disrupted segment into the ascending aorta, although resistance may be experienced. Formerly it was suggested that thoracic aortography did not increase the risk of rupture in those with a transected aorta. A recent report of two fatalities occurring during aortography has led to rethinking of this position. Those authors have suggested careful catheter and guidewire manipulations as well as alternative approaches if resistance to catheter advancement is met.[84] In the presence of extremely weak or absent femoral pulses (or if resistance is met), an axillary approach may be prudent (Fig. 19-8). Puncture of the right axillary artery is more likely to avoid the isthmus, that segment of the aorta most likely to be injured. If using an arm approach, one should also be aware of the potential for associated great vessel injury. A further alternative is a right atrial injection with digital imaging of the levo phase, completely avoiding possible sites of injury. As mentioned previously, for cut-film technique, a high-flow 6 French catheter is necessary for the preferred contrast injection of 35 cc per second. Many groups routinely use intraarterial DSA. They are able to achieve a high-quality examination with smaller catheter size (5 French) using less contrast material and completing the study in half the time.[85,86] Two views of the aorta should be obtained, the LAO being the most informative.[87]

Aortic transection usually presents an obvious angiographic abnormality. The typical appearance is that of a localized saccular outpouching occurring just distal to the left subclavian artery and frequently involving the entire circumference of the aortic wall (see Fig. 19-7). Other less common manifestations include narrowing of the aortic lumen at the site of transection or, rarely, complete occlusion or extravasation of contrast at the injured site (see Fig. 19-8). Subtle injuries at the isthmus are being discovered more frequently, and the great diagnostic difficulty is in distinguishing these more subtle tears from the ductus diverticulum

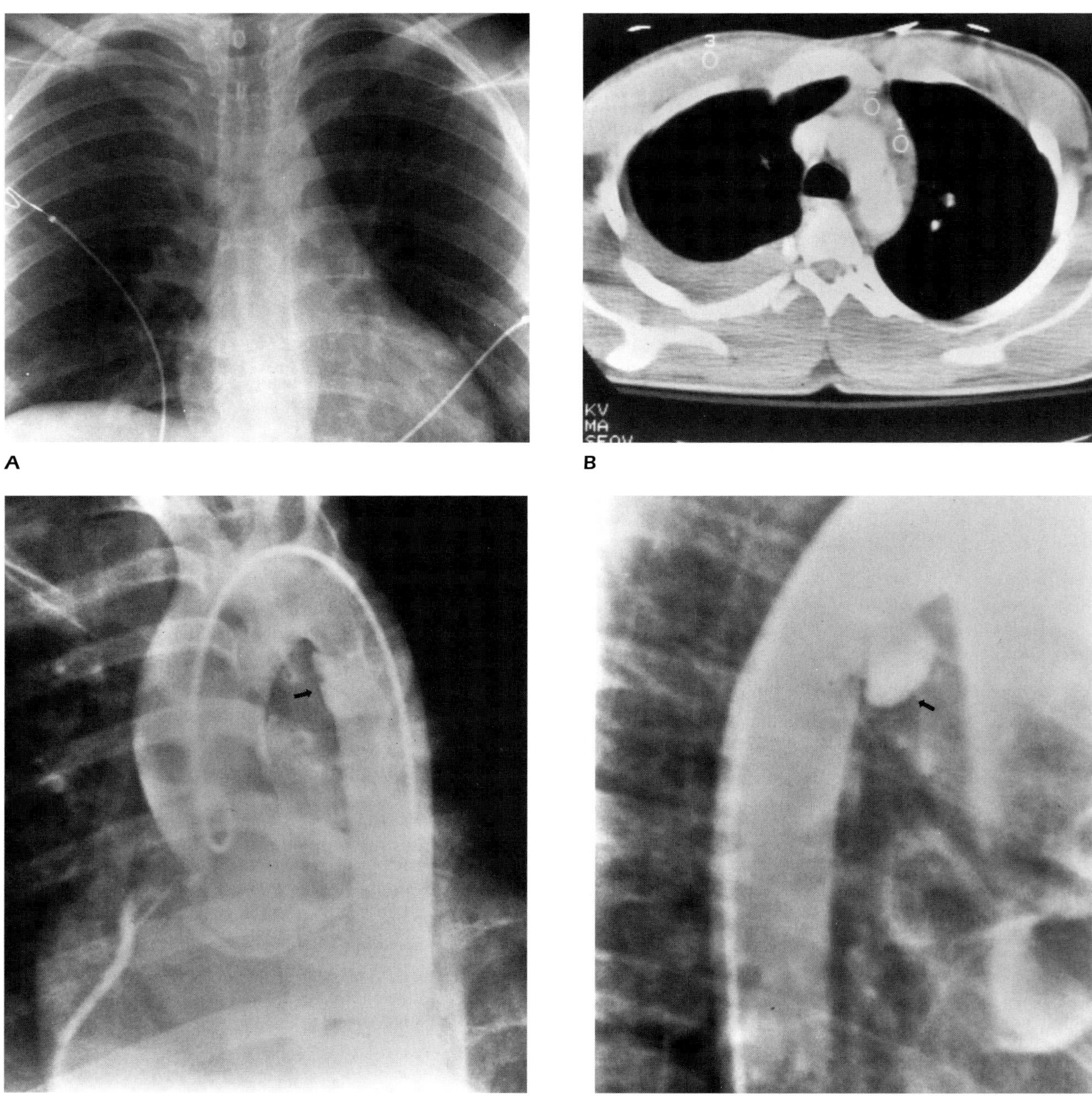

Figure 19-7. An 18-year-old man was involved in a high-speed motor vehicle accident and had clinical evidence of an acute abdomen, confirmed by blood in the peritoneal aspirate. A thoracic injury was not suspected clinically or with a screening chest film. (A) Even in retrospect, this frontal upright chest radiograph was interpreted as normal. (B) Although an aortic injury was not suspected, a limited CT of the chest was obtained as part of a trauma protocol. Transaxial image at the level of the aortic arch shows abnormal mediastinal blood, which necessitated further evaluation with thoracic aortography. LAO (C) and RAO (D) images from the aortogram demonstrate a traumatic pseudoaneurysm (*arrows*) in the typical location. (This case from Raptopoulos V, et al. Traumatic aortic tear: screening with chest CT. Radiology 1992;182:667–673.)

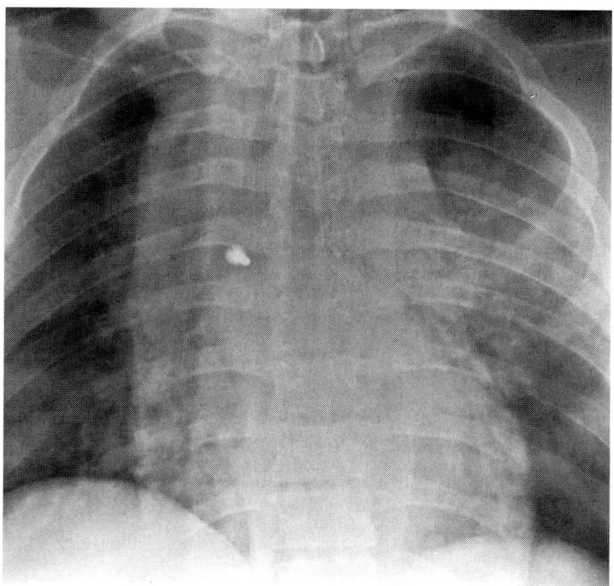

A

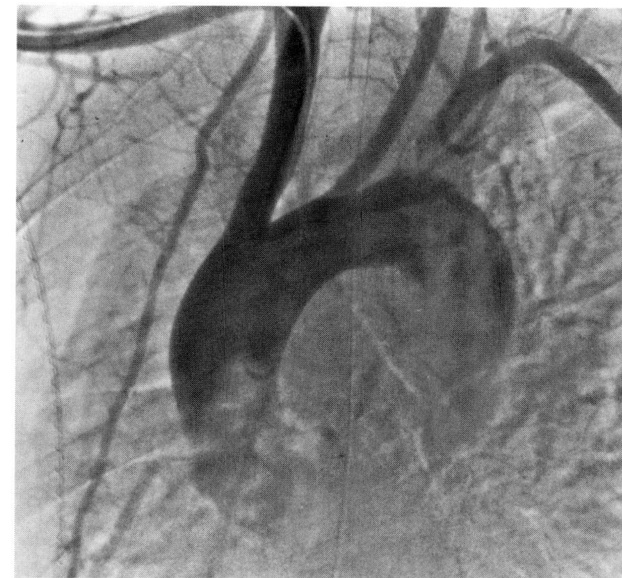

B

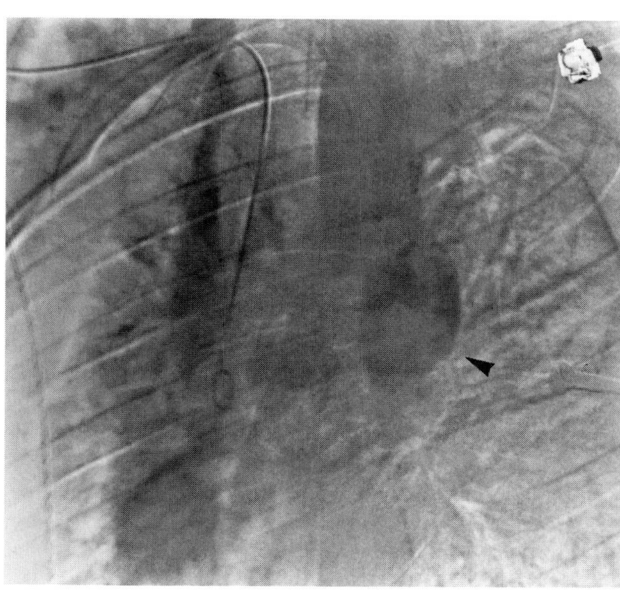

C

Figure 19-8. A 20-year-old male motorcycle accident victim was admitted to the hospital with severe lower extremity musculoskeletal injury and evidence of significant chest trauma. The patient was alert and conscious but had no palpable femoral pulses. This necessitated an axillary approach for catheterization. (A) Frontal chest radiograph demonstrates a wide "featureless" mediastinum with deviation of the trachea and nasogastric tube to the right at the level of the aortic arch. Early (B) and later (C) angiographic images from a thoracic aortogram obtained in the LAO projection. There is dilatation of the distal arch and proximal descending aorta with retention of contrast material in an extraluminal location (*arrowhead,* C). The distal aorta never opacified. Complete aortic transection was found at thoracotomy with distraction of the severed ends. Surgical repair was completed, but the patient expired in the operating room.

and ulcerated aortic plaques. The ductus diverticulum is located on the anteromedial surface of the proximal descending aorta and presents a smooth interface, with the remainder of the aortic wall usually forming obtuse angles (Fig. 19-9 A). Any deviation from these characteristics raises the likelihood of an aortic injury (Fig. 19-9). Ulcerated aortic plaques are a potential pitfall, and the aortogram should be scrutinized for other signs of atherosclerosis. The absence of other such signs or this appearance in a young individual favors a traumatic injury.[88,89] This may be an area where a completely normal CT is helpful in providing further confirmatory evidence. In certain cases a definitive opinion cannot be rendered, and exploratory thoracotomy has been recommended by some to avoid missing an occult tear.[88] Although unwarranted thoracotomy is not desirable, the aorta can be visually inspected and a tear can be confidently excluded or diagnosed. The aorta can be examined from its adventitial surface, and there should be no concern regarding spinal cord injury because aortic cross-clamping is unnecessary.

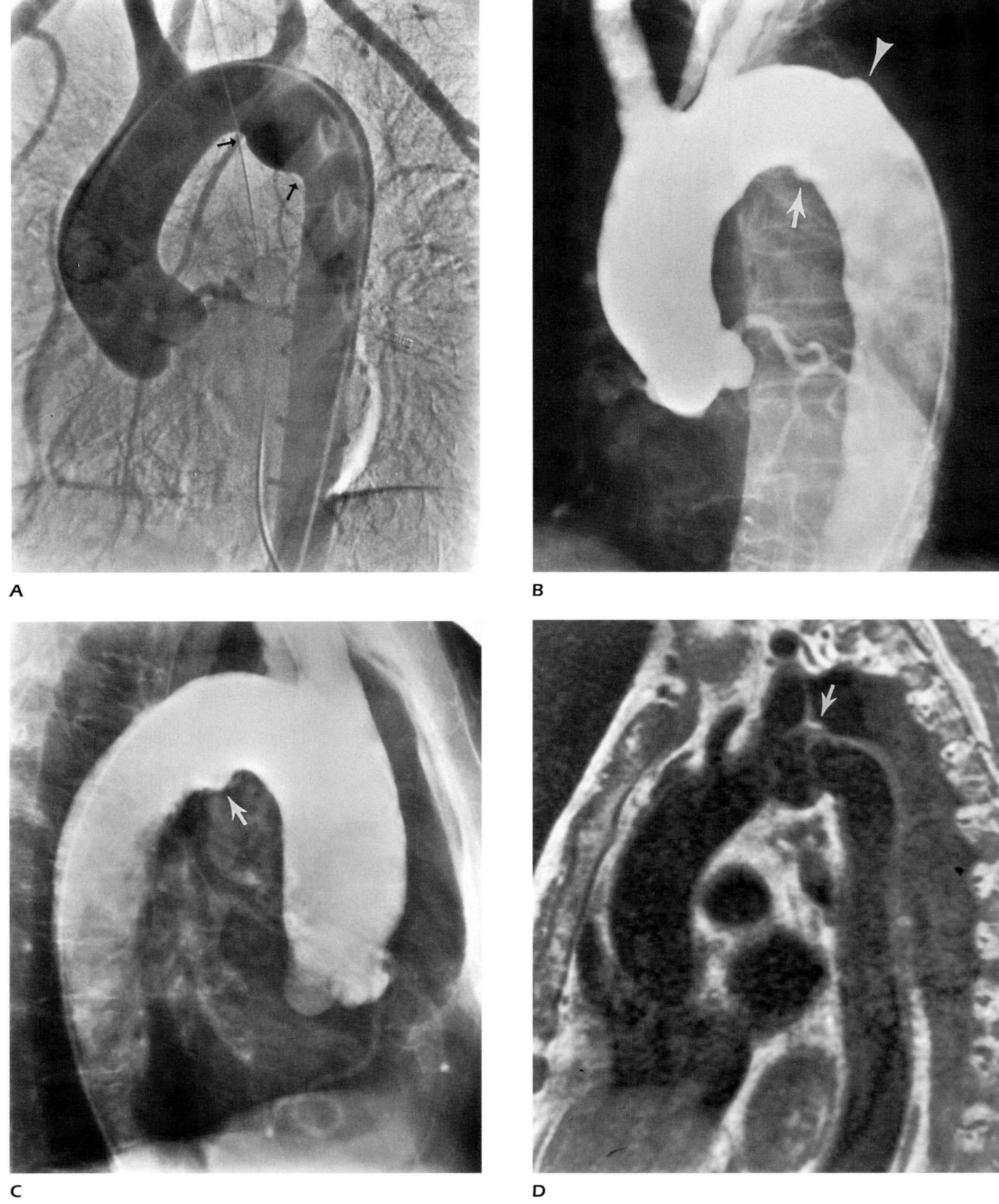

A B C D

Diagnostic Algorithm

With the prevalence of blunt chest trauma and the critical need for timely diagnosis of aortic injury, what diagnostic algorithm does one use? The chest radiograph, with all its limitations, remains the best screening examination, and every effort should be made to obtain an upright film. A completely normal chest film is extremely helpful, with a negative predictive value of 98 percent.[71,74] The definite presence of any abnormality associated with aortic transection, particularly mediastinal widening or obscuration of the aorta, requires that aortography be performed, though one must realize that a large number of *normal* angiograms will be obtained. More troublesome is the indeterminate chest film or questionably wide mediastinum in the low-risk patient. CT may provide assistance in the management of this group because a normal study should terminate the workup. As noted previously, any abnormality on the CT requires prompt aortography. A few patients in whom there is high suspicion of aortic injury and who are hemodynamically unstable may benefit from immediate thoracotomy without angiography.[90]

Surgical Treatment

If the patient is fortunate enough to arrive at the hospital alive and to undergo surgical repair, survival statistics are excellent, the associated mortality frequently being related to other injuries. The surgical technique, performed via left thoracotomy, involves either placement of an interposition graft or primary anastomosis. The most feared complication of surgery is paraplegia, occurring in up to 14 percent of patients regardless of specific technique (bypass versus clamp and sew).[91–94] Some injuries to the aorta have not been operated on immediately because of complicating associated injuries (Fig. 19-10).[95,96] Strict attention to maintenance of blood pressure is crucial until surgery can be performed on a more elective basis. Serial angiography may be helpful in assessing the stability of the injury.[70]

Chronic Traumatic Aneurysms

The preceding discussion has dealt primarily with the acute traumatic pseudoaneurysm. A small percentage of patients with aortic injury go undetected initially and present years later, having walled off the rupture with adventitia or surrounding mediastinal tissue. Their presentation is usually as an incidental finding on a chest film obtained for other reasons. The most commonly reported symptoms, if present, are cough, hoarseness, and chest pain. The appearance on the chest radiograph of a chronic pseudoaneurysm is entirely different from that of the acute pseudoaneurysm. There is usually a contour abnormality of the proximal descending aorta, often with associated calcification.[97] The diagnosis can be confirmed with CT or MRI, although angiography is usually obtained before surgery. A history of previous trauma can frequently be elicited from the patient. Although these chronic pseudoaneurysms have withstood the test of time and appear stable, the surgical dictum is for elective repair because there is a well-documented, definite occurrence of late rupture (see Fig. 19-10).[98,99]

Mycotic Aortic Aneurysms

Aneurysms arising from nonsyphilitic infections of an arterial wall were first referred to as *mycotic aneurysms* by Sir William Osler in 1885.[100] Although the term is an obvious misnomer because these aneurysms are almost exclusively of bacterial etiology,[101] it has been well established in the literature. *Infective aneurysms* would be a more correct term.

Pathogenesis

The normal arterial intima is extremely resistant to infection. It is generally felt that the development of a "mycotic" aneurysm requires both a source of infection and prior damage to the aortic wall. This damage is most frequently due to atherosclerosis,[102] but other

◀ **Figure 19-9.** The ductus diverticulum and diagnostic difficulties. (A) The typical ductus diverticulum is located on the anteromedial surface of the aorta just distal to the left subclavian artery. Note the smooth, obtuse angles formed with the aorta (*arrows*). The bulge may be less prominent than in this example and is then referred to as the *ductus bump*. (B and C) An elderly patient involved in a motor vehicle accident presented with poor definition of the descending aorta on a supine chest film (not shown). The bulge on the inferior and medial aspect of the aorta (*arrows*) is consistent with the ductus bump. However, the superior and lateral abnormality (*arrowhead*) is indicative of aortic injury. The patient expired from aortic transection while in transit to the operating room. (D) A 91-year-old man had a similar subtle abnormality detected by aortography at the time of injury. Conservative management was chosen because of the patient's advanced age. This sagittal MR image obtained 2 months later depicts the contour abnormality on the superior aspect of the aorta close to the subclavian artery (*arrow*).

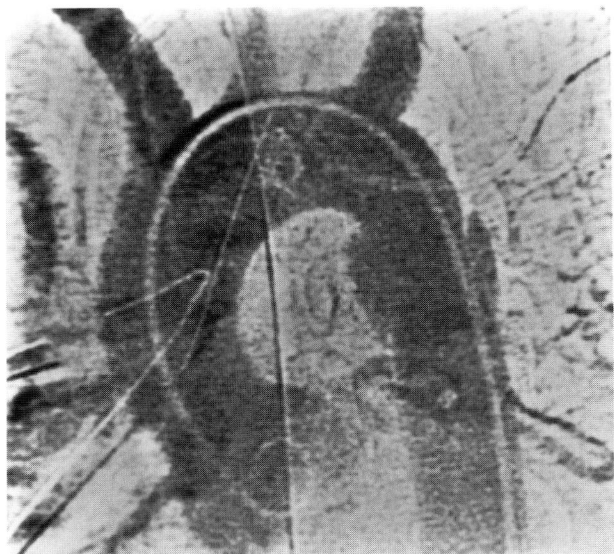

A

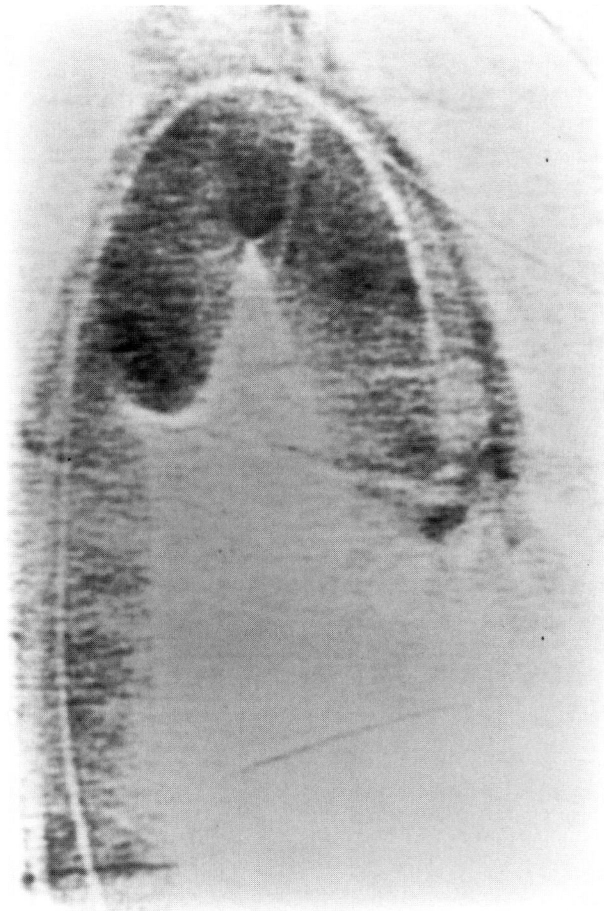

B

Figure 19-10. This 37-year-old man was severely injured in a helicopter crash. Surgical repair of the aortic injury could not be performed immediately because of multiple coexistent injuries. After a lengthy hospitalization, he was discharged and returned for elective surgical repair. (A and B) Intraarterial DSA images in the LAO and RAO projections obtained at the time of the acute injury show the typical appearance of aortic transection.

causes, such as cystic medial necrosis, trauma, congenital bicuspid aortic valve, or coarctation, have been described.[101,103] Infection of the aortic wall is thought to occur in one of four ways: (1) embolization of the infected material directly to the diseased intima or vaso vasorum; (2) direct extension from an intravascular source of infection such as bacterial endocarditis; (3) invasion of the aortic wall by an extravascular contiguous source of infection; or (4) lymphatic spread.[104] Colonization of a preexisting aneurysm by circulating bacteria does not constitute a "mycotic" aneurysm in the true sense and would best be entitled an *infected aneurysm.*

Classification

The classification of mycotic aneurysms was described by Crane in 1937[105] and was divided into primary and secondary types. Primary aneurysms are those produced by a distant or unknown source of infection. They are usually due to bacterial emboli that lodge in an already diseased intima or, less commonly, the vaso vasorum.[104] Secondary mycotic aneurysms are defined as arising from an intravascular source of infection such as bacterial endocarditis, or to extension from a contiguous extravascular inflammatory process, such as tuberculosis. In bacterial endocarditis, septic embolization to the vaso vasorum of adjacent but noncontiguous areas or direct extension to the sinuses of Valsalva is the probable mechanism of infection.[104] In the past, tuberculous "mycotic" aneurysms were usually the result of adjacent adenitis, osteitis, or pulmonary abscess.[106]

Before the mid-1940s, bacterial endocarditis was the most frequently reported cause of "mycotic" aneurysms in the thoracic aorta. With the development of antibiotics, however, the incidence of bacterial endocarditis and "mycotic" aneurysms caused by it has diminished significantly.[107] A definite source of infection is frequently unidentifiable in primary mycotic aneurysms, but when it is identified it is usually from a pneumonia, osteomyelitis, or cellulitis. Previous reports show that the incidence of "mycotic" aneurysms varied from 2 percent to approximately 3.5 percent of all thoracic aneurysms.[101,105] A series from Johns Hopkins published in 1978 reported five mycotic aneu-

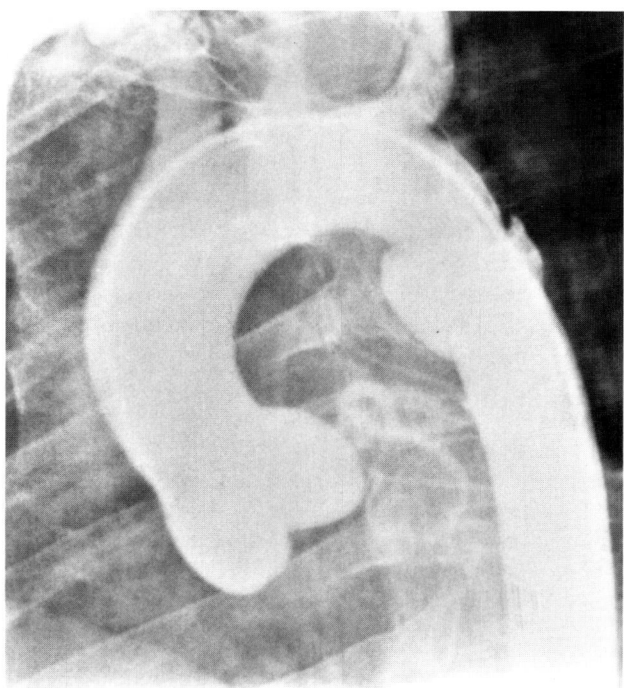

C

Figure 19-10 (continued). (C and D) Conventional aortography in the same projections 8 months later shows little change in the now chronic pseudoaneurysm. This was surgically repaired despite the apparent stability.

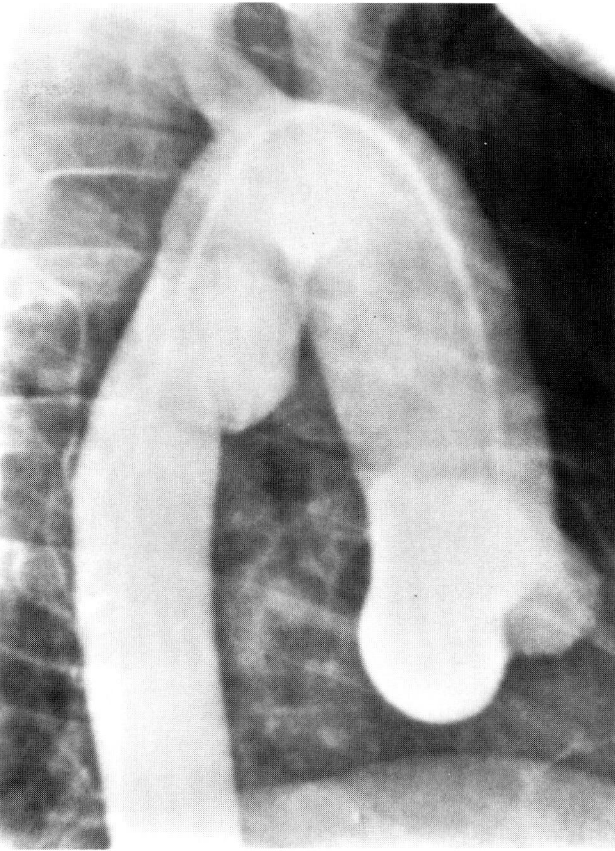

D

rysms involving the thoracic aorta; three were primary, only one was secondary, and the fifth was associated with coarctation.[107] "Mycotic" aneurysms are uncommon arterial lesions in infants,[108] but the increased use of umbilical artery catheters for monitoring has increased the incidence of septicemia and subsequent thoracic "mycotic" aneurysms at the previous location of the umbilical artery catheter tip.[109] Patients with prosthetic valves also have an increased incidence of subacute or acute bacterial endocarditis and subsequent "mycotic" aneurysm formation.[110]

Histologic Findings

Histologically, these aneurysms show loss of intima and destruction of the internal elastic lamina by an inflammatory process. The muscularis of the media and the adventitia will show varying degrees of destruction. Bacteria are often demonstrable histologically. Abnormalities of the adjacent aortic wall are also found.[101]

The infectious agents seen in secondary mycotic aneurysms are generally those responsible for the production of bacterial endocarditis (nonhemolytic streptococcus, pneumococcus, staphylococcus), although gonococcus and salmonella have also been reported.[103] When due to contiguous spread, the aneurysms are most commonly tuberculous.[106] Primary thoracic mycotic aneurysms show a high incidence of pneumococcus, but involvement with gonococcus, salmonella, staphylococcus, *Listeria,* and *Escherichia coli* also occurs.[101,104,107] *Staphylococcus aureus* has been found to be the most frequently identified organism in mycotic aneurysms occurring distal to the site of aortic coarctation.[111]

Signs and Symptoms

The clinical presentation of mycotic aneurysms varies widely, and these patients usually show a confusing variety of signs and symptoms. Nonspecific constitutional complaints such as weakness, malaise, low-grade fever, and chills may be present. The clinical picture of bacterial endocarditis, pneumonia, osteomyelitis, or some other primary process may also dominate. It is uncommon for mycotic aneurysms to reach the large size usually necessary to produce intrathoracic signs or symptoms. Chest pain may be present, and, although nonspecific, may indicate rapid enlargement or leaking.

Mycotic aneurysms not only represent a potential source of intravascular infection, but also have a great propensity for rupture, thus posing a significant threat to life.[112,113] Undiagnosed and untreated, they are almost uniformly fatal. With modern antibiotics and good surgical techniques, successful resection is usually possible.

Diagnostic Imaging and Findings

The radiographic findings in patients with mycotic aneurysms of the thoracic aorta are similar to those with other types of aneurysms, usually presenting as mediastinal widening or localized masses. They are almost always saccular in configuration but are rarely calcified. They are located most frequently in the ascending aorta, sinuses of Valsalva, or sites of previous surgery. Gas bubbles in the mediastinum have been reported in diabetics with mycotic aneurysm due to *E. coli*.[107] When rapid progression is seen on serial chest x-rays, it is suggestive of a mycotic etiology.

CT and MRI are the methods of choice for diagnosis.[35,38,114] Evaluation of contiguous structure, thinned areas of the wall, and possible leaking at a rupture site can be identified with contrast enhancement on CT or gradient-echo MRI studies. Ultrasound has a long history of utilization—especially for the evaluation of sinus of Valsalva aneurysms and their possible bacterial involvement.[115] Evaluation of the aortic root in these aneurysms may demonstrate sites of leakage back into cardiac chambers. Leukocyte scintigraphy has even been used recently in the diagnosis of mycotic aneurysm.[16] Thoracic aortography may be warranted to confirm findings or if questions remain unanswered.

Luetic Aneurysms

Syphilis in its late manifestations used to be the most common etiology of thoracic aortic aneurysms. A large autopsy series from the Boston City Hospital from 1902 to 1951 found 141 cases of syphilitic aneurysms of the thoracic aorta from a total of 338 aneurysms of the entire aorta.[101] With the continual improvement in detection and treatment of syphilis, however, the incidence has diminished dramatically. During the first 40 years of the Boston City Hospital series, syphilis was responsible for 52 to 70 percent of all aortic aneurysms. This incidence decreased to 25 percent for the last 10 years of that series. The discovery of penicillin some 40 years ago promised to eliminate syphilitic aortitis and subsequent aortic aneurysm formation despite the increase in the incidence of primary syphilis along with other sexually transmitted diseases in the last two decades.

Aortitis is said to occur in 10 percent of patients with untreated syphilis, usually presenting some 10 to 30 years after the primary infection. It does not appear to occur from congenital infections.[116] Aneurysm formation is a possible sequela of this treponemal infection of the aortic wall. The process begins when the organisms lodge in the vasa vasorum of the aorta during periods of spirochetemia. An obliterative endarteritis of the vasa vasorum occurs, producing necrosis and fragmentation of the elastic fibers of the media and frequently dystrophic calcification.[16,117] Severe focal destruction leads to aneurysm formation. The aortitis is asymptomatic and is diagnosable clinically only by its sequelae. Aortic regurgitation is two to three times more common than aortic aneurysm, whereas coronary ostial stenosis is much rarer.[116] The locations of luetic aneurysms in order of incidence are as follows[118]:

Ascending arch	36%
Transverse arch	34%
Descending arch	25%
Descending thoracic aorta	5%
Multiple sites	4%
Sinuses of Valsalva	1%

Signs and Symptoms

The clinical presentation varies with the site of involvement, although chest pain is the most common symptom. Ascending aortic aneurysms can grow large without being detected; compression of the superior vena cava, or anterior erosion of the chest wall or sternum may eventually occur. Aneurysms of the transverse arch are in close proximity to the structures passing through the narrow thoracic inlet; thus they may produce such symptoms as dysphasia, dyspnea, or hoarseness early in their course, while still small in size. Aneurysms of the descending arch and lower descending thoracic aorta produce symptoms late in their course, usually due to erosion of vertebrae or posterior ribs.[116,119] Undiagnosed and untreated, patients with luetic aneurysms have a very poor prognosis. Death frequently occurs within months of the onset of symptoms. In approximately 40 percent of cases, death is the result of aneurysm rupture, with cardiac or respiratory failure responsible for the remaining fatalities.

Diagnostic Imaging and Findings

Radiographic examination is extremely valuable, and its routine use is probably responsible for most diagnoses of luetic aneurysm.[116] Curvilinear calcification of the ascending aortic media is generally the earliest radiographic finding of luetic aortitis. Differentiation from atherosclerotic calcification is not always possible, although atherosclerosis tends to produce thicker, more regular plaques and to predominate in the distal arch and descending aorta.[117] Takayasu aortitis can show a similar appearance but is rarely seen in the ascending aorta.[118] When luetic aneurysms form, they present as thoracic masses, usually calcified[119] and predominantly in the ascending aorta and arch. They can frequently be quite large, although smaller ones in strategic locations may not be visualized even though symptomatic. Rarely, even the larger ones can be obscured by coexisting pleural effusion or pulmonary consolidation.[116]

CT, MRI, or echocardiography (especially TEE) can establish the presence of a luetic aneurysm with ease. Dilatation of the ascending aorta is usually demonstrated, and the aneurysm is most frequently saccular. Aortic regurgitation is often present. Quantitation of this can be done with Doppler or gradient-echo MRI. If aortography is needed to answer questions, a cine angiographic run with injection of contrast into the aortic root can also quantitate aortic regurgitation.

Congenital Aortic Aneurysms

Congenital aortic aneurysms most commonly involve the sinus of Valsalva. Since they were first reported in 1840, many cases of aneurysm of the sinus of Valsalva have been described in the literature. This type of aneurysm is considered rare, occurring in only 3.5 percent of series of congenital heart defects treated surgically.[120] Congenital and acquired types have been described, and some authors[121] have proposed a third division encompassing aneurysms associated with Marfan syndrome due to cystic medial necrosis. This subtype of "generalized dilatation of all three aortic sinuses" usually describes an aneurysm of the aortic root that extends through the annulus and involves the sinuses of Valsalva.[122]

Location

Congenital aneurysms tend to involve a single sinus,[120] although multiple sinus involvement has been reported.[121] Most aneurysms arise from the right sinus, with the noncoronary sinus being the second most common site.[123] Occasionally, these two sinuses are involved jointly.[124] If rupture into a cardiac chamber occurs from one of these aneurysms, it tends to be into the right ventricle or right atrium. Although aneurysms arising from the left sinus are rare, they have been reported.[124,125] Two theories have been proposed for the pathologic lesion in these aneurysms. According to the anatomic theory, there is a defect of the continuity between elastic tissue of the aortic media and the annulus fibrosa of the aortic valve ring, which creates a weakness of the wall.[124] According to the embryologic theory, there is incomplete fusion of the lamina spiralis with the bulbar septum.[126] Certain cardiovascular anomalies are frequently associated with sinus of Valsalva aneurysms.[127] These include ventricular septal defects, pulmonary insufficiency,[128] Turner syndrome,[129,130] and aortic lesions such as aortic stenosis, bicuspid aortic valve,[131,132] aortic regurgitation, patent ductus arteriosus, and coarctation. Acquired aneurysms of the sinus of Valsalva are less common. Before 1950, these were most commonly luetic in origin, but now they are almost exclusively due to bacterial endocarditis that occurs after such surgical procedures as coarctation repair or aortic valve replacement.[115,133–135] Aneurysms involving all three sinuses as well as the aortic root and ascending aorta are most commonly seen with idiopathic cystic medial necrosis. Fragmentation and rarefaction of the elastic fibers with mucoid degeneration in the aortic media are found histologically. This pattern is related to Marfan syndrome, the "forme fruste" of Marfan, Ehlers-Danlos syndrome, and other connective tissue disorders,[121] and osteogenesis imperfecta.[136] Aortic regurgitation is the most common finding associated with this type of aneurysm.[122]

Sinus of Valsalva aneurysms are usually asymptomatic before rupture unless their size encroaches on adjacent structures.[123,137] Aneurysms of the left sinus of Valsalva (congenital or acquired and rare) can produce obstruction of the left main coronary artery, causing anginal symptoms or myocardial infarction.[125] The more common right sinus of Valsalva aneurysm tends to project into and cause obstruction of the right ventricular outflow tract.[138] Patients may then manifest the symptoms of right ventricular pressure overload, such as dyspnea and chest pain. Rarely, a sinus of Valsalva aneurysm can protrude into the left ventricle. Here it may cause obstruction but most commonly causes conduction abnormalities with cardiac arrhythmias, left axis deviation, or right bundle branch block.[139]

Ruptured sinus of Valsalva aneurysms produce a spectrum of clinical findings depending on their route of rupture. There may be sudden onset of weakness, dyspnea, heart failure, atrioventricular block,[140] and a continuous, loud, to-and-fro murmur. Right sinus of Valsalva aneurysms tend to rupture into the outflow tract of the right ventricle, whereas noncoronary sinus of Valsalva aneurysms tend to rupture into the right atrium. Both of these produce large left-to-right shunts. Occasionally, there will be rupture into the left atrium or left ventricle; rarely, intrapericardial rupture occurs. Rupture into the left ventricle must be differentiated from aortic regurgitation caused by other etiologies.[141,142] Traumatic hemolysis has been reported with rupture of sinus of Valsalva aneurysms.[130]

Diagnostic Imaging and Findings

Diagnosis of an *unruptured* sinus of Valsalva aneurysm is difficult. The plain chest radiograph is usually normal, but occasionally the ascending aorta may be dilated. Sometimes this dilatation is marked, especially in cases of cystic medial necrosis, and rarely the ascending aorta may become so dilated that it is difficult to differentiate from an enlarged right atrium. Calcification rarely occurs in the congenital form of sinus of Valsalva aneurysms; when it does, it is usually secondary to bacterial endocarditis.

Ruptured sinus of Valsalva aneurysms produce radiographic findings that reflect their course of rupture and secondary results. If a large left-to-right shunt has been caused, the chest radiograph may show congestion, edema, increased pulmonary blood flow, and other signs. If the rupture causes a left-to-left shunt, the chest radiograph will look similar to an example of aortic regurgitation, with left ventricular dilatation and possible left heart failure due to overload. If the rupture is into the pericardium, signs of tamponade will be present.

Echocardiography has proven to be of value in the diagnosis of the sinus of Valsalva aneurysm. Ruptured sinus of Valsalva aneurysms have been diagnosed preoperatively by echocardiography[10] since 1974. It is important to know the echocardiographic features of the normal aortic root and valve to recognize the abnormal.[143] Two-dimensional echocardiography, either transthoracic or transesophageal, with Doppler has proven to be very helpful and accurate. The size and location of the aneurysm and the amount of aortic regurgitation can be determined and quantitated.

Contrast-enhanced CT and MRI (with and without gradient-echo imaging and in multiple planes) can likewise quantitate the size and location of the aneurysm, the course of rupture, and the degree of aortic regurgitation. Thoracic aortography may be performed in conjunction with coronary arteriography in those cases for planned surgery.[144] It may be needed for precise localization of the rupture site and fistulous tract before surgical intervention can be undertaken.[145] Other lesions may also be demonstrated that may need correction at the same time. A jet of contrast material passing from the aneurysm into the involved chamber can best be seen and appreciated with cine angiography in an oblique (LAO) projection.

Miscellaneous Thoracic Aortic Aneurysms

Congenital

A congenital aneurysm may be related to a patent ductus arteriosus (PDA). After PDA surgery, occasional patients may develop noninfected aneurysms in association with recanalized ligation of the ductus. These acquired aneurysms probably have a congenital predilection to form in this area. Falcone et al.[146] collected 60 cases of ductal aneurysms (i.e., aneurysms arising from the nonpatent ductus arteriosus). Congenital aneurysms located around the isthmus portion of the thoracic aorta are uncommon, but a series of nine cases was presented by Yuging et al.[147] On the basis of their series, they felt that the essential pathologic characteristics of the aneurysm were developmental dysplasia of the smooth muscle and elastic tissue as well as degeneration of the ground substance of the aortic wall.

Acquired

Rare thoracic aortic aneurysms are seen associated with other disease entities. Whether these are truly congenital or acquired is sometimes difficult to determine. Thoracic aneurysms have been demonstrated as part of the complex in tuberous sclerosis and neurofibromatosis.[148,149] The disease entity may cause an aortitis that results in aneurysm formation and subsequent complications. Multiple aortic aneurysms frequently occur in relapsing polychondritis; they are usually of the ascending aorta but may be multiple.[150] Involvement of the ascending aorta may result in aortic regurgitation and left ventricular failure.[151] Giant-cell aortitis has been described with aneurysmal dilatation of the ascending aorta and slight aortic regurgitation.

Aneurysms of the Intrathoracic Branches of the Aorta

Aneurysms of the major intrathoracic branches of the aorta have many of the same causes as have aneurysms that affect the aorta. The innominate and left subclavian arteries are most frequently involved, although the left common carotid, intercostal, and bronchial arteries can also be affected. The aorta may or may not be simultaneously involved. As in aneurysms of the aorta, arteriosclerosis and posttraumatic aneurysms predominate.[152]

Arteriosclerotic aneurysms usually occur in association with diffuse arteriosclerotic disease of the aorta, although they are occasionally isolated findings. Posttraumatic avulsion of one of the great vessels with subsequent false aneurysm formation is usually the result of blunt chest trauma and rapid deceleration. Violent anteroposterior compression of the chest wall can "squeeze" the superior arch and great vessels between the sternum and vertebral column; associated torsion and hyperflexion of the cervical spine may also be a factor.[153] The innominate artery is most frequently involved and, after the aorta, is the next most common thoracic vessel injured in patients surviving long enough to be evaluated. Injuries to the left subclavian artery and left common carotid arteries are much less common.

Mycotic aneurysms of the great vessels are usually related to contiguous infections of the soft tissues[107] or lung apex.[154]

Aneurysms of the great vessels are known to occur in association with congenital anomalies of the arch. The association of aneurysms of the intercostal arteries with coarctation is well known.[155]

Detection of these aneurysms is frequently an incidental radiographic finding, although visualization or palpation of a pulsatile mass may initiate the investigation. Severe trauma to the chest always warrants early radiographic evaluation. Aneurysms of the great vessels usually appear as superior mediastinal masses and, as such, must be differentiated from nonvascular lesions of the area. Aneurysms of the intercostal and bronchial arteries must be differentiated from pulmonary nodules. The presence of curvilinear calcification in these lesions may be helpful to rule in their vascular origin. In patients with acute trauma, superior mediastinal widening may be the only visualizable feature of the vascular injury that produced the false aneurysm. Marked ectasia of the innominate or left subclavian artery, which is more common than aneurysm, can simulate an aneurysm or even a pulmonary apical mass.[12,156] More specialized imaging methods can assist in differentiating ectasia and aneurysms. Suprasternal notch ultrasound may be helpful in evaluating the brachiocephalic vessels. Contrast-enhanced CT with narrow slices can be of particular value in differentiating tortuous vessels from adjacent structures. MRI can also be extremely helpful in differentiating tortuous vessels from aneurysms. Arteriography is needed less often and may be necessary only as part of surgical planning.

References

1. Williams PL, Warwick R, Dyson M, Bannister LH, eds. Gray's anatomy. 37th ed. New York: Churchill-Livingstone, 1989: 685–686.
2. Joyce JW, Fairbairn JF II, Kincaid OW, Jeurgens JL. Aneurysms of the thoracic aorta: a clinical study with special reference to prognosis. Circulation 1964;29:176–181.
3. Harder T, Nicholas V, Stendel A, Orrelano L. Radiological diagnosis of the thoracic aortic aneurysm. Thorac Cardiovasc Surg 1987;35:122–125.
4. Shahian DM, Javid H, Faver LP, Kittle CF, Matthew GR. Lesions of the thoracic aorta and its arch branches simulating neoplasm. J Thorac Cardiovasc Surg 1981;81:251–263.
5. Sos TA, Sniderman KW, Wixson DS. Pitfalls in plain film evaluation of the thoracic aorta: the mimicry of aneurysms and adjacent masses and the value of aortography. Part II. Descending thoracic aorta. Cardiovasc Radiol 1979;2:77.
6. Sprayregen S. Radiologic spectrum of arteriosclerotic aneurysms of aortic arch. N Y State J Med 1978;78:2198–2204.
7. Wixson D, Baltaxe HA, Sos TA. Pitfalls in plain film evaluation of the thoracic aorta: the mimicry of aneurysms and adjacent masses and the value of aortography. Part I. Transverse aortic arch. Cardiovasc Radiol 1979;2:69.
8. Heitzman ER. The mediastinum: radiologic correlations with anatomy and pathology. New York: Springer-Verlag, 1988: 294.
9. Kelley MA. Skeletal changes produced by aortic aneurysms. Am J Phys Anthropol 1979;51:35–38.
10. Cooperberg P, Mercer EN, Mulder DS, Winsberg F. Rupture of a sinus of Valsalva aneurysm: report of a case diagnosed preoperatively by echocardiography. Radiology 1974;113: 171.
11. Come PC, Sacks B, Vine H, McArdle C, Koretsky S, Weintraub R. Ultrasonic visualization of the posterior thoracic aorta in long axis: diagnosis of a saccular mycotic aneurysm. Chest 1981;79:470–472.
12. Mathew T, Nanda NC. Two-dimensional and Doppler echocardiographic evaluation of aortic aneurysm and dissection. Am J Cardiol 1984;54:379–385.
13. Shively BK. Transesophageal echocardiography in the assessment of aortic pathology. J Thorac Imaging 1990;5(4):40–47.
14. Williams DM, Simon HJ, Marx M, Starkey TD. Acute traumatic aortic rupture: intravascular ultrasound findings. Radiology 1992;182:247–249.
15. Bareotti A, Mariotti R, Bencivelli W, Mey M, Guzzardi R, Mariani M. Radionuclide angiography for intrathoracic aortic aneurysm evaluation: a comparison with contrast aortography. J Nucl Med Allied Sci 1980;24:233–238.
16. Ben-Haim S, Seabold JE, Hawes DR, Rooholamin SA. Leukocyte scintigraphy in the diagnosis of mycotic aneurysm. J Nucl Med 1992;33:1486–1493.
17. Smith TR, Khoury PT. Aneurysm of the proximal thoracic aorta simulating neoplasm: the role of CT and angiography. AJR 1985;144:909–910.

18. Posniak HV, Demos TC, Marsan RE. Computed tomography of the normal aortic and thoracic aneurysm. Semin Roentgenol 1989;24(1):7–21.
19. Godwin JD. Conventional CT of the aorta. J Thorac Imaging 1990;5(4):18–31.
20. Posniak HV, Olson MC, Demos TC, Benjoya RA, Marsan RE. CT of thoracic aortic aneurysm. Radiographics 1990;10: 839–855.
21. Heiberg E, Wolverson MR, Suridaram M, Shields JB. CT characteristics of aortic atherosclerotic aneurysm versus aortic dissection. J Comput Assist Tomogr 1985;9:78–83.
22. Kazerooni E, et al. Penetrating atherosclerotic ulcers of the descending thoracic aorta: evaluation with CT and distinction from aortic dissection. Radiology 1992;183:759–765.
23. Hirose Y, et al. Aortic aneurysms: growth rates measured with CT. Radiology 1992;185:249–257.
24. Kucich V, et al. Ruptured thoracic aneurysm: unusual manifestation and early diagnosis using CT. Radiology 1986;160: 87–89.
25. Cramer M, et al. Compression of the RPA by aortic aneurysm: CT demonstration. J Comput Assist Tomogr 1985;91(2): 310–314.
26. Madayag MA, et al. Thoracic aorta trauma: role of dynamic CT. Radiology 1991;179:853–855.
27. Morgan PW, et al. Evaluation of traumatic aortic injury: does dynamic contrast-enhanced CT play a role? Radiology 1992; 182:661–666.
28. Raptopoulos V, et al. Traumatic aortic tear: screening with chest CT. Radiology 1992;182:667–673.
29. Stanford W, et al. Ultra fast computed tomography in the diagnosis of aortic aneurysms and dissection. J Thorac Imaging 1990;5(4):32–39.
30. Stanford W, Rumberger JA, eds. Ultrafast CT in cardiac imaging: principles and practice. Mt. Kisco, NY: Futura, 1992: 287–310.
31. Costello P, et al. Assessment of the thoracic aneurysm by spiral CT. AJR 1992;158:1127–1130.
32. Costello P, et al. Spiral CT of the thorax with reduced volume of contrast material: a comparative study. Radiology 1992; 183:663–666.
33. Amparo EG, et al. Magnetic resonance imaging of aortic disease: preliminary results. AJR 1984;143:1203–1209.
34. Dinsmore RE, et al. Magnetic resonance imaging of the thoracic aortic aneurysms: comparison with other imaging methods. AJR 1986;146:309–314.
35. Akins EW, et al. Perivalvular pseudoaneurysm complicating bacterial endocarditis: MR detection in five cases. AJR 1991; 156:1155–1158.
36. Gefter WB, et al. Chest applications of magnetic resonance imaging: an update. Radiol Clin North Am 1998;26(3):577–579.
37. Webb WR, et al. MR imaging of thoracic disease: clinical uses. Radiology 1992;182:621–630.
38. Link KM, et al. The role of MR imaging in the evaluation of acquired diseases of the thoracic aorta. AJR 1992;158:1115–1125.
39. Mostbeck GH, et al. MR measurements of blood flow in the cardiovascular system. AJR 1992;159:453–461.
40. Rofsky NM, et al. Aortic aneurysm and dissection: normal MR imaging and CT findings after surgical repair with the continuous-suture graft-inclusion technique. Radiology 1993;186:195–201.
41. Bakal CW, Friedland RJ, Sprayregen S, et al. Translumbar arch aortography: a retrospective controlled study of usefulness, technique, and safety. Radiology 1991;178:225–228.
42. Ching CC, Hughes RK. Arteriosclerotic aneurysms of the thoracic aorta: late stage of a diffuse disease. Am J Surg 1967; 114:853.
43. DeBakey ME, et al. Surgical treatment of aneurysms of the descending thoracic aorta. J Cardiovasc Surg 1978;19:571–576.
44. Storer J, et al. Management of thoracic aneurysms. Int Surg 1967;47:344–355.
45. Pressler V, McNamara JJ. Thoracic aortic aneurysm: natural history and treatment. J Thorac Cardiovasc Surg 1980;79: 489–498.
46. McNamara JJ, Pressler VM. Natural history of arteriosclerotic thoracic aneurysms. Ann Thorac Surg 1978;26:468.
47. Gothe B, Harris L. Thoracic aortic aneurysm causing acute bronchospasm. Crit Care Med 1981;9:496–497.
48. Varkey B, Tristani FE. Compression of pulmonary artery and bronchus by descending thoracic aortic aneurysm: perfusion and ventilation changes after aneurysmectomy. Am J Cardiol 1974;34:610–614.
49. Zeit RM, Cope C, Lippman M. Compression of pulmonary artery by aortic aneurysm. JAMA 1981;246:1586–1587.
50. Guthaner D, Higgins CB, Wexler L. Angiographic demonstration of a thoracic aortic aneurysm with rupture into the pulmonary artery. J Can Assoc Radiol 1976;27:96–98.
51. Pezzella AT, Brown BE, Walls JT, Curtis JJ. Esophageal obstruction secondary to a tortuous thoracic aortic aneurysm: case report. Mo Med 1981;78:193–195.
52. Monro JL, Skidmore RD, Sbokos CG, Radcliffe T. Intraesophageal rupture of a thoracic aortic aneurysm. J Cardiovasc Surg 1975;16:302–307.
53. Sinar DR, Demaria A, Kataria YP, Thomas FB. Aortic aneurysm eroding the esophagus: case report and review. Am J Dig Dis 1977;22:252–254.
54. Higgins CB, Silverman NR, Harris RD, Albertson KW. Localized aneurysms of the descending thoracic aorta. Clin Radiol 1971;26:475–482.
55. Schechter LS, Held RT. Right-sided extrapleural hematoma: an unusual presentation of ruptured aortic aneurysm. Chest 1974;65:355.
56. Randall PA, Omar MM, Rohner R, Hedgcock M, Brenner RJ. Arteria magna revisited. Radiology 1979;132:295.
57. Sailer S. Dissecting aneurysm of the aorta. Arch Pathol Lab Med 1942:33:704–730.
58. Parmley LF, Mattingly TW, Manion WC, et al. Nonpenetrating traumatic injury of the aorta. Circulation 1958;17:1086–1101.
59. Pais SO. Assessment of vascular trauma. In: Mirvis SE, Young JW, eds. Imaging in trauma and critical care. Baltimore: Williams & Wilkins, 1992:485–496.
60. Stark P. Traumatic rupture of the thoracic aorta: a review. CRC Crit Rev Diagn Imaging 1984;21(3):229–255.
61. Sanders C. Current role of conventional and digital aortography in the diagnosis of aortic disease. J Thorac Imaging 1990; 5(4):48–59.
62. Sondenaa K, Tveit B, Kordt KF, et al. Traumatic rupture of the thoracic aorta. Acta Chir Scand 1990;156:137–143.
63. Spouge AR, Burrows PE, Armstrong D, et al. Traumatic aortic rupture in the pediatric population: role of plain film, CT, and angiography in the diagnosis. Pediatr Radiol 1991;21: 324–328.
64. Sevitt S. The mechanisms of traumatic rupture of the thoracic aorta. Br J Surg 1977;64:166–173.
65. Lundell CJ, Quinn MF, Finck EJ. Traumatic laceration of the ascending aorta: angiographic assessment. AJR 1985;145: 715–719.
66. Lundevall J. The mechanism of traumatic rupture of the aorta. Acta Pathol Microbiol Scand 1964;62:34–46.
67. Crass JR, Cohen AM, Motta AO, et al. A proposed new mechanism of traumatic aortic rupture: the osseous pinch. Radiology 1990;176:645–649.
68. Sanborn JC, Heitzman ER, Markarian B. Traumatic rupture of the thoracic aorta: roentgen-pathological correlations. Radiology 1970;95:293–298.
69. Daniels DL, Maddison FE. Ascending aortic injury: an angiographic diagnosis. AJR 1981;136:812–813.
70. Fleckenstein JL, Schultz SM, Miller RH. Serial aortography assesses stability of "atypical" aortic arch ruptures. Cardiovasc Intervent Radiol 1987;10:194–197.

71. Mirvis SE, Bidwell JK, Buddemeyer EU, et al. Imaging diagnosis of traumatic aortic rupture: a review and experience at a major trauma center. Invest Radiol 1987;22:187–196.
72. Groskin SA. Radiological, clinical and biomechanical aspects of chest trauma. Berlin: Springer-Verlag, 1991;110.
73. Mirvis SE, Bidwell JK, Buddemeyer EU. Value of chest radiography in excluding traumatic aortic rupture. Radiology 1987;163:487–493.
74. Mirvis SE, Rodriguez A. Diagnostic imaging of thoracic trauma. In: Mirvis SE, Young JW, eds. Imaging in trauma and critical care. Baltimore: Williams & Wilkins, 1992:93–106.
75. Egan TJ, Neiman NH, Herman RJ, et al. Computed tomography in the diagnosis of aortic aneurysm dissection or traumatic injury. Radiology 1980;136:141–146.
76. Mirvis SE, Kostrubink I, Whitley NO, et al. Role of CT in excluding major arterial injury after blunt thoracic trauma. AJR 1987;149:601–605.
77. Miller FB, Richardson JD, Thomas HA, et al. Role of CT in diagnosis of major arterial injury after blunt thoracic trauma. Surgery 1989;106:596–603.
78. Sparks MB, Burchard KW, Marrin CA, et al. Transesophageal echocardiography: preliminary results in patients with traumatic aortic rupture. Arch Surg 1991;126:711–714.
79. Brooks SW, Cmolik BL, Young JC, et al. Transesophageal echocardiographic examination of a patient with traumatic aortic transection from blunt chest trauma: a case report. J Trauma 1991;31(6):841–845.
80. Shapiro MJ, Yanofsky SD, Trapp JT, et al. Cardiovascular evaluation in blunt thoracic trauma using transesophageal echocardiography (TEE). J Trauma 1991;31(6):835–840.
81. Ellis JE, Bender EM. Intraoperative transesophageal echocardiography in blunt thoracic trauma. J Cardiothorac Vasc Anesth 1991;5(4):373–376.
82. Snow CC, Appelbe AF, Martin TD, et al. Diagnosis of aortic transection by transesophageal echocardiography. J Am Soc Echocardiogr 1992;5(1):100–102.
83. Brooks SW, Young JC, Cmolik B, et al. The use of transesophageal echocardiography in the evaluation of chest trauma. J Trauma 1992;32(6):761–766.
84. LaBerge JM, Jeffrey RB. Aortic lacerations: fatal complications of thoracic aortography. Radiology 1987;165:367–369.
85. Pozzato C, Fedriga E, Donatelli F, et al. Acute posttraumatic rupture of the thoracic aorta: the role of angiography in a 7-year review. Cardiovasc Intervent Radiol 1991;14:338–341.
86. Mirvis SE, Pais SO, Gens DR. Thoracic aortic rupture: advantages of intraarterial digital subtraction angiography. AJR 1986;146:987–991.
87. Parker LA, Delaney D, Friday JM. Oblique projections in aortography following blunt thoracic trauma. J Can Assoc Radiol 1989;40:172–173.
88. Morse SS, Glickman MG, Greenwood LH, et al. Traumatic aortic rupture: false-positive aortographic diagnosis due to atypical ductus diverticulum. AJR 1988;150:793–796.
89. Orron DE, Porter DH, Kim D, et al. False-positive aortography following blunt chest trauma: case report. Cardiovasc Intervent Radiol 1988;11:132–135.
90. Clark DE, Zeiger MA, Wallace KL, et al. Blunt aortic trauma: signs of high risk. J Trauma 1990;30(6):701–705.
91. Merrill WH, Lee RB, Hammon JW, et al. Surgical treatment of acute traumatic tear of the thoracic aorta. Ann Surg 1988; 207(6):699–706.
92. Turney SZ, Attar S, Ayella R, et al. Traumatic rupture of the aorta. J Thorac Cardiovasc Surg 1976;72(5):727–734.
93. Cowley RA, Turney SZ, Hankins JR, et al. Rupture of thoracic aorta caused by blunt trauma: a fifteen-year experience. J Thorac Cardiovasc Surg 1990;100:652–661.
94. Hilgenberg AD, Logan DL, Akins CW, et al. Blunt injuries of the thoracic aorta. Ann Thorac Surg 1992;53:233–239.
95. Pezzella AT, Todd EP, Dillon ML, et al. Early diagnosis and individualized treatment of blunt thoracic aortic trauma. Ann Surg 1978;44:699–703.
96. Fisher RG, Oria RA, Mattox KL, et al. Conservative management of aortic lacerations due to blunt trauma. J Trauma 1990;30(12):1562–1566.
97. Gundry SR, Burney RE, Mackenzie JR, et al. Traumatic pseudoaneurysms of the thoracic aorta: anatomic and radiologic correlations. Arch Surg 1984;119:1055–1060.
98. Finkelmeier BA, Mentzer RM, Kaiser DL, et al. Chronic traumatic thoracic aneurysm. Influence of operative treatment on natural history: an analysis of reported cases, 1950–1980. J Thorac Cardiovasc Surg 1982;84:257–266.
99. Heystraten FM, Rosenbusch G, Kingma LM, et al. Chronic posttraumatic aneurysm of the thoracic aorta: surgically correctable occult threat. AJR 1986;146:303–308.
100. Osler W. The Gulstonian lectures on malignant endocarditis. Brit Med J 1885;1:467–470.
101. Parkhurst GF, Decker JP. Bacterial aortitis and mycotic aneurysm of the aorta: a report of 12 cases. Am J Pathol 1955;31: 821–835.
102. Singh H, Parkhurst GF. Bacterial aortitis. N Y State J Med 1979;72:2779–2781.
103. Weintraub RA, Abrams HL. Mycotic aneurysms. Am J Roentgenol 1968;102:354–362.
104. Bennett DE. Primary mycotic aneurysms of the aorta. Arch Surg 1967;94:758–765.
105. Crane AR. Primary multilocular mycotic aneurysm of the aorta. Arch Pathol 1937;24:634–641.
106. Felson B, Akers PV, Hall GS, Schreiber JT, Greene RE, Pedrosa CS. Mycotic tuberculous aneurysm of the thoracic aorta. JAMA 1977;237:1104–1108.
107. Kaufman SL, White RI, Harrington DP, Barth KH, Siegelman SS. Protean manifestations of mycotic aneurysms. Am J Roentgenol 1978;131:1019–1025.
108. Wood BP, Young LW, Elbadawi NA. Primary mycotic aortic aneurysms in infancy and childhood. Am J Roentgenol 1973; 118:109–115.
109. Thompson TR, Tillei J, Johnson DE, et al. Umbilical artery catheterization complicated by mycotic aortic aneurysm in neonates. Adv Pediatr 1980;27:275–318.
110. Castaneda-Zuniga WR, Nath PH, Zollikofer C, Velasquez G, Valdez-Davila O, Edwards E. Mycotic aneurysm of the aorta. Cardiovasc Intervent Radiol 1980;3:144–149.
111. Bodner SJ, Zell AM, Killen DA. Ruptured mycotic aneurysm complicating coarctation of the aorta. Ann Thorac Surg 1973; 15:419–426.
112. Schneider JA, Rheuban KS, Crosby IK. Rupture of postcoarctation mycotic aneurysms of the aorta. Ann Thorac Surg 1979;27:185–190.
113. Estrera AS, Platt MR, Mills LJ, Nikaidoh H. Tuberculous aneurysms of the descending thoracic aorta: report of a case with fatal rupture. Chest 1979;75:386–388.
114. Vogelzang RL, Sohaey R. Infected aortic aneurysms: CT appearance. J Comput Assist Tomogr 1988;12(1):109–112.
115. Conde CA, Meller J, Donoso E, Dack S. Bacterial endocarditis with ruptured sinus of Valsalva and aorticocardia fistula. Am J Cardiol 1975;35:912–917.
116. Kampmeier RH. The late manifestations of syphilis. Med Clin North Am 1964;48:667–697.
117. Freundlich IM. Calcified luetic aneurysm of a sinus of Valsalva and ascending aorta. Ariz Med 1976;33:203–204.
118. Lande A, Berkmen YM. Aortitis: pathologic, clinical and arteriographic review. Radiol Clin North Am 1976;14:219–240.
119. Weisser RJ, Marshall RJ. Syphilitic aneurysms with bone erosion and rupture. West Va Med J 1976;72:1–4.
120. Sakakibara S, Konno S. Congenital aneurysms of the sinus of Valsalva: anatomy and classification. Am Heart J 1962;63: 708–719.
121. Ominsky SH, Kricun ME. Roentgenology of sinus of Valsalva aneurysms. Am J Roentgenol 1975;125:571–581.
122. Prian GW, Diethrich EB. Sinus of Valsalva abnormalities: a specific differentiation between aneurysms of and aneurysms involving the sinuses of Valsalva. Vasc Surg 1973;7: 155–164.
123. Mayer JH, Holder TM, Canent RV. Isolated, unruptured si-

nus of Valsalva aneurysms: serendipitous detection and correction. J Thorac Cardiovasc Surg 1975;69:429–432.
124. Boutefeu JM, Moret PR, Hahn C, Hauf E. Aneurysms of the sinus of Valsalva: report of seven cases and review of the literature. Am J Med 1978;65:18–24.
125. Garcia-Rinaldi R, VonKoch L, Howell JF. Aneurysm of the sinus of Valsalva producing obstruction of the left main coronary artery. J Thorac Cardiovasc Surg 1976;72:123–126.
126. Arey LB. Arey's developmental anatomy: a textbook of embryology. Rev. 7th ed. Philadelphia: Saunders, 1974:386.
127. Kakos GS, Kilman JW, Williams TE, Hosier DM. Diagnosis and management of sinus of Valsalva aneurysm in children. Ann Thorac Surg 1974;17:474–478.
128. Sanchez HE, Barnard CN, Barnard MS. Fistula of the sinus of Valsalva. J Thorac Cardiovasc Surg 1977;73:877–879.
129. Youker JE, Roe BB. Aneurysm of the aortic sinuses and ascending aorta in Turner's syndrome. Am J Roentgenol 1969; 23:89–93.
130. Ellman L, Know-Macauley H. Traumatic hemolysis with rupture of aneurysm of sinus of Valsalva. Arch Intern Med 1970; 126:1019–1021.
131. Howard RJ, Moller J, Castaneda AR, Varco RL, Nicoloff DM. Surgical correction of sinus of Valsalva aneurysm. J Thorac Cardiovasc Surg 1973;66:420–427.
132. Taguchi K, Sasaki N, Matsuura Y, Uemura R. Surgical correction of aneurysm of the sinus of Valsalva: a report of forty-five consecutive patients including eight with total replacement of the aortic valve. Am J Cardiol 1969;23:180–191.
133. Holmes EC, Bredenberg C, Brawley RK. Aneurysm of the sinus of Valsalva resulting from bacterial endocarditis. Ann Thorac Surg 1973;15:628–631.
134. Qizilbash AH. Mycotic aneurysm of the aortic sinus of Valsalva with rupture. Arch Pathol 1974;98:414–417.
135. DeSa-Neto A, Padnick MB, Desser KB, Steinhoff NG. Right sinus of Valsalva–right atrial fistula secondary to nonpenetrating chest trauma: a case report with description of noninvasive diagnostic features. Circulation 1979;60:205–209.
136. Heppner RL, Babbit HL, Bianchine JW. Aortic regurgitation and aneurysm of sinus of Valsalva associated with osteogenesis imperfecta. Am J Cardiol 1973;31:654–657.
137. Fishbein MC, Obma R, Roberts WC. Unruptured sinus of Valsalva aneurysm. Am J Cardiol 1975;35:918–922.
138. Kerber RE, Ridges JD, Kriss JP, Silverman JF, Anderson ET, Harrison DC. Unruptured aneurysm of the sinus of Valsalva producing right ventricular outflow obstruction. Am J Med 1972;53:775–783.
139. Heydorn WH, Nelson WP, Fitterer JD, Floyd GD, Strevey TE. Congenital aneurysm of the sinus of Valsalva protruding into the left ventricle: review of diagnosis and treatment of the unruptured aneurysm. J Thorac Cardiovasc Surg 1976; 71:839–845.
140. Anzai N, Okada T, Takanashi Y, Sano A, Yamada M. Ruptured aneurysm of aortic sinus of Valsalva into right atrium: associated atrioventricular block presumably caused by aneurysmal compression of His bundle. Chest 1976;70:309–311.
141. Spooner EW, Dunn JM, Behrendt DM. Aortico-left ventricular tunnel and sinus of Valsalva aneurysm: case report with operative repair. J Thorac Cardiovasc Surg 1978;75:232–236.
142. Yoshida S, Togashi M, Chida A, Miyahara M. Ruptured sinus of Valsalva aneurysm into the left ventricle. Jpn Heart J 1978; 19:954–960.
143. Rothbaum DA, Dillon JC, Chang S, Feigenbaum H. Echocardiographic manifestation of right sinus of Valsalva aneurysm. Circulation 1974;49:768–771.
144. DeBakey ME, Lawrie GM. Aneurysm of sinus of Valsalva with coronary atherosclerosis: successful surgical correction. Ann Surg 1979;189:303–308.
145. Meyer J, Wukasch DC, Hallman GL, Cooley DA. Aneurysm of fistula of the sinus of Valsalva: clinical considerations and surgical treatment in 45 patients. Ann Thorac Surg 1975;19: 170–179.
146. Falcone MW, Perloff JK, Roberts WC. Aneurysm of the nonpatent ductus arteriosus. Am J Cardiol 1972;29:422–426.
147. Yuging L, Xia W, Baolia J. Congenital aneurysm of thoracic aorta: radiologic-pathology study of 9 cases. Chin Med J 1981;94:213–220.
148. Dutton RV, Singleton EB. Tuberous sclerosis: a case report with aortic aneurysm and unusual rib changes. Pediatr Radiol 1975;3:184–186.
149. Petencost M, Stanley P, Takahashi M, Isaacs H Jr. Aneurysms of the aorta and subclavian and vertebral arteries in neurofibromatosis. Am J Dis Child 1981;475–477.
150. Cipriano PR, Alonso DR, Baltaxe HA, Gay WA Jr, Smith JP. Multiple aortic aneurysms in relapsing polychondritis. Am J Cardiol 1976;37:1097–1102.
151. Sohi GS, Desai AM, Ward WW, Flowers NC. Aortic cusp involvement causing severe aortic regurgitation in a case of relapsing polychondritis. Cathet Cardiovasc Diagn 1981;7: 79–86.
152. Thomas TV. Intrathoracic aneurysms of the innominate and subclavian arteries. J Thorac Cardiovasc Surg 1972;63:461–471.
153. Sethi GK, Scott SM, Bhayana J, Takaro T. Traumatic avulsion of the innominate artery: report of a case and review of literature. J Cardiovasc Surg (Torino) 1975;16:171–175.
154. Hara M, Bransford RM. Aneurysm of the subclavian artery associated with contiguous pulmonary tuberculosis. J Thorac Cardiovasc Surg 1963;46:256–264.
155. Stern WZ, Richardson JO Jr, Wolfe R. Multiple calcified aneurysms in coarctation of the aorta. Radiology 1970;96:331–334.
156. Christensen EE, Landay MJ, Dietz GW, Brinley G. Buckling of the innominate artery simulating a right apical lung mass. AJR 1978;131:119–123.

20

Dissecting Aortic Aneurysm

HERBERT L. ABRAMS
KRISHNA KANDARPA

Dissecting aneurysm is the condition produced by separation of the layers of the arterial wall by circulating blood. The intramural hematoma that develops is usually associated with widening of the diameter of the vessel. Although dissecting aneurysm was first established as a clinical entity in 1863, a review of the literature up to 1965 indicated that fewer than 1500 cases had been reported.[1] With the increasing proportion of aged individuals in the population and the high incidence of hypertension, dissection is being recognized today with increasing frequency. According to one author,[2] at least 2000 new cases occur each year in the United States; another source estimates that the annual incidence is 5 to 10 per million of population.[3]

Although dissection usually develops in people over 50 years of age, and more commonly in men,[4] it has been described in people from age 3 months to 100 years.[5] In the younger age group, it is likely to occur in association with Marfan syndrome, as a result of the faulty ground substance of the aortic wall. A high incidence has been noted during pregnancy. In a review of 49 cases of dissecting aneurysm in women below 40 years of age, 24 aneurysms were in pregnant women; an additional 12 such cases have been reported by Mandel.[6]

A dissecting aneurysm may result in death within a few hours to days in 80 to 90 percent of patients. According to one estimate, it is instantly fatal to 3 percent of patients, fatal within 15 minutes to 35 percent of patients, and fatal within 48 hours to 36 to 72 percent of patients.[7] However, 10 to 20 percent of patients may survive the initial attack for a variable period of time. About 50 percent of patients who survive the initial dissection die at a later date as the result of external aortic rupture into the pericardial, thoracic, or abdominal cavity.[8] Left untreated, 70 percent of patients die within 2 weeks and 90 percent die within 3 months of the initial episode.[7,9] In addition to Marfan syndrome and pregnancy, thoracic aortic dissection is also found in association with atherosclerosis, hypertension, bicuspid aortic valve, aortic stenosis, coarctation of the aorta, and trauma.[10] Iatrogenic cases have been reported following retrograde cardiac catheterization,[11] repair of aortic coarctation,[12] and cardiopulmonary bypass.[13] Chemicals that are toxic to the connective tissue play a known but uncertain role in its etiology; dissecting aneurysm has been caused in rats by the seeds of *Lathyrus odoratus* (sweet pea).[2] Aortic dissection has also been described following aortic valve replacement[14] and cannulation for perfusion.[15]

Pathology and Etiology

> The aorta was dilated and showed a transverse fissure an inch and a half long, through which some blood had lately passed under the external coat and formed an elevated ecchymosis.[16]

The above passage, which appeared in the 1761 postmortem report on George II of England, suggests the continued interest of pathologists in aortic dissection. The basic contributing factor in aortic dissection is thought to be a defective aortic media, either congenital or acquired. When it is congenital, as in Marfan syndrome, the mesodermal components of the media are easily disrupted. The defect is present at birth, but the resulting weakness of the media may not manifest itself until adult life. The incidence of aortic dissection in Marfan syndrome has caused considerable interest, particularly from a surgical point of view.[17] At one time, the nature of the disease was thought to suggest a poor prognosis for surgical repair, but fears as to delayed wound healing and disruption of sutures proved unwarranted in at least one instance.[17] Although in 1970 Voigt and Hansen[18] ascribed most dissecting aortic aneurysms in middle-aged men to heritable disorders, such as Marfan syndrome, other investigations[10,19] have ascribed only a small percentage of dissections (5 percent) to this syndrome.

The acquired type of aortic defect was long thought to be caused primarily by idiopathic cystic medial necrosis. This process, noted with extensive dissection, is characterized by degeneration of the aortic media and by deterioration of collagen and elastic tissue, and it is often accompanied by cystic change. It has been called the "pre-existing" but clinically inapparent aortic defect [which] is the sine qua non leading to dissecting aortic aneurysm."[20] In a later study by Wilson and Hutchins,[19] "cystic medionecrosis" was found in less than 10 percent of patients with dissection; these authors noted that the degenerative changes generally observed were not histologically specific to dissection. Other modern studies also suggest that the normal aging process of the aorta is involved; the changes found in normal medial degeneration, some authors maintain, are identical to those in dissection, *except in degree.*[3,21] Hypertension and collagen alterations may contribute to the process of injury and repair, ultimately leading to a *profoundly weakened support structure in the media*[21,22]—an apparent prerequisite for dissection regardless of etiology.[19] Subsequent constant exposure to cyclic hemodynamic stresses may result in intimal tears leading to intramural cleavage and spontaneous dissection.[19] Alternatively, rupture of the vasa vasorum may propagate a hematoma into the vessel wall, causing dissection in those cases in which an intimal tear does not appear to be involved. Less commonly, atherosclerosis of the intima and media is responsible, resulting in a more localized type of dissection.[5]

When atherosclerosis is responsible, its role is indirect in that it causes necrosis and structural weakening of the media and consequent aortic dilatation. Atherosclerotic intimal plaques may ulcerate and permit hemorrhage into the diseased media.

When dissection into the media occurs, it may split the aortic wall over a considerable distance. Transverse tears occur in the intima, allowing blood under systemic pressure to enter the dissection, further disrupting the aortic wall. In about 65 percent of patients the intimal tear is located at the aortic root, just above the level of the valve and the coronary arteries, in 10 percent it is in the transverse aortic arch, in 20 percent the tear occurs in the aortic arch just distal to the origin of the left subclavian artery, and in 5 percent it originates even more distally in the descending aorta.[23,24] Tears in the distal aortic arch may propagate in a retrograde direction into the ascending aortic region. The ascending aorta, which experiences considerable external motion and flexion with each cardiac systole, is especially prone to developing intimal tears; this tendency may be related to the hemodynamic stresses of episodic ejection of blood from the left ventricle under pressure.[3,25] Similarly, the relatively fixed region of the ligamentum arteriosum may provide a focus for high stresses, causing local intimal tears and distal dissections.

A significant but unexplained coincidence of pregnancy and aortic dissection exists. During pregnancy, a combination of hormonal imbalances, associated hypertension, and sclerosis and necrosis of both the medial layer and vasa vasorum is thought to play a contributory role.[6] First noted by Schnitker and Bayer in 1944,[26] the relationship has been well supported by statistical evidence. Some authors feel that as many as 50 percent of dissecting aneurysms in patients under 40 may occur in pregnant women.[3,6] A survey in London from 1968 to 1977 showed roughly half the deaths of women from aortic dissection to be associated with pregnancy in all stages of gestation.[25] Some authors have narrowed this incidence and maintain that it is highest during the third trimester.[2] Interest has focused on possible aortic changes during pregnancy. Cavanzo and Taylor[20] studied aortic sections in 43 women under the age of 40 who died of nonvascular disease during pregnancy; they compared these sections with a control group of 20 men and 20 nonpregnant women in the same age range and concluded that no difference existed between the aortas of pregnant women and those of the control group. The former showed no special attenuation of elastic and reticulin fibers, nor was there a pregnancy-related variation in the size and number of the smooth muscle fibers. Furthermore, animal experiments have shown aortic tensile strength to be the same in pregnant and nonpregnant rabbits.[20] Some authors, having ruled out intrinsic changes in pregnancy as being responsible for the high incidence of aortic dissection, suggest other possible factors: hypervolemia, frequent hypertension, and increased heart rate. Others insist that the aortic media in pregnant women shows degeneration of elastic fibers, which may lead to dissecting aneurysm.[27]

Classification and Course

Aortic dissection has been classified by different authors according to its site of origin, nature and duration of symptoms, and course. DeBakey's classification (Fig. 20-1) was previously widely used.[28] In that classification, type I aortic dissection initially involves the aortic root or ascending aorta and then extends to involve the transverse portion of the aortic arch and the descending aorta to a variable degree. Type II usually involves only the ascending aorta and is the classic variety found in association with Marfan syndrome. *The ascending aortic shadow is grossly enlarged, and the*

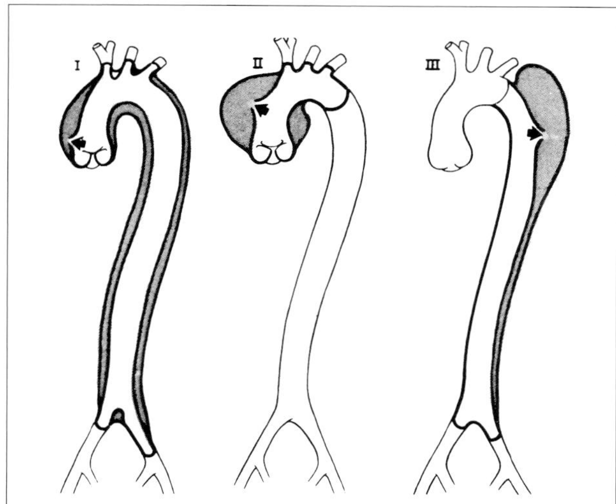

Figure 20-1. Diagram of types of dissection (from DeBakey[28]). Type I dissection, the commonest type, begins in the ascending aorta just above the aortic valve and extends along the arch of the aorta into the descending aorta to a varying extent. Type II, dissection typical of Marfan syndrome, involves only the ascending aorta and does not extend to the descending aorta. Type III dissection begins just beyond the origin of the left subclavian artery and usually extends caudally in the descending aorta to involve the abdominal aorta as well. At times retrograde dissection may occur to involve the arch and/or the ascending aorta.

transverse diameter is markedly increased in size. The wall is fragile and prone to rupture. Type III aortic dissection generally begins at or just beyond the origin of the left subclavian artery and most commonly extends caudally in the descending thoracic aorta toward the diaphragm (type IIIA), as well as into the abdominal aorta (type IIIB). An alternative classification proposed more recently categorizes all of the cases that involve the ascending aorta as type A, and all other cases as type B.[29] This (Stanford) classification, based on the differences in the prognosis and management of the two types, has recently become more established in practice.

Among 65 patients with aortic dissection analyzed at the Peter Bent Brigham Hospital (now The Brigham and Women's Hospital), 51 percent had type I, 7 percent type II, and 42 percent type III. This would correspond to 58 percent type A and 42 percent type B aortic dissections according to the newer Stanford classification. This contrasts with a series reported by Earnest et al.[30] in which 29 percent were type I, 21 percent type II, and 50 percent type III. However, in a more recent surgical series, Haverich et al.[24] reported a 71 percent incidence of type A (acute and chronic) and 19 percent incidence of type B dissections. In general, about two-thirds of all aortic dissections are said to involve the ascending aorta.[31]

To the above categories, Ambos et al.[31] add three groups:

Acute: survival less than 2 weeks
Subacute: survival 2 to 6 weeks
Chronic: survival more than 6 weeks

Others define chronic dissections as those in which survival exceeds 14 days[23,24]; after this period patients become more stable with improved early prognosis. Notably, 74 percent of deaths from complications of aortic dissection occur within the acute phase of 2 weeks. Haverich et al.[24] reported incidences of 29 percent type A and 17 percent type B chronic dissections in their series. Chronic dissections may be painless, well tolerated, and found only incidently during angiography, surgery, or autopsy. When chronic dissections reenter the true lumen, the patient may become asymptomatic. (Distal reentry points allow sufficient blood to lower extremities to equalize pulses.) In a series of 73 patients with aortic dissection who survived more than 6 weeks (i.e., those with chronic dissection), 90 percent were found to have reentry points.[32]

Depending on the length and position of the involved segment, the coronary, brachiocephalic, extremity, or visceral branches may be partially or completely obstructed, with consequent ischemia. As many as 70 percent of cases are said to terminate by rupture of the dissection externally into the pericardium.[33] Hemorrhage may occur into the pleural space, mediastinum, peritoneal cavity, or retroperitoneal tissues. In patients who survive the initial insult (approximately 10 percent), a second tear may develop in the intima, resulting in a reentry channel to the distal aorta. Under favorable conditions, the channel may become endothelialized.

Where external rupture occurs depends on the location of the primary tear: (1) if the primary tear is in the ascending aorta, 70 percent of ruptures are in the pericardium; (2) if the primary tear is in the aortic arch, 35 percent of ruptures are pericardial and 32 percent are left pleural; (3) if the primary tear is in the descending aorta, left pleural, mediastinal, and pericardial hemorrhage are most common; and (4) if the primary tear is in the abdominal aorta, external rupture occurs most commonly into the retroperitoneum.

With regard to involvement of branches of the aorta, if the primary tear is in the ascending aorta, the brachiocephalic, left common carotid artery, coronary artery, and renal arteries are involved, in descending order of frequency. If the tear begins in the descending aorta, it involves the iliac artery most commonly and the renal arteries second; renal artery involvement, when unilateral, is three times more common on the left side than on the right side.[34] This is explained by the fact that dissection is more common on the posterior left side, precisely where the left renal artery is located. The right renal artery originates in a somewhat more ventral position and therefore is not involved unless circumferential dissection of 270 degrees or more is present.

Clinical Findings

Sixty-five patients with aortic dissection were analyzed at the Peter Bent Brigham Hospital. They ranged in age from 27 to 78, mean age being 60. Sixty percent of the patients were men. No significant difference in age distribution was detected among the varying types of dissection. Slater and DeSanctis[35] found that patients with proximal dissections were younger and had a significantly higher incidence of Marfan syndrome.

In general, aortic dissections predominate in males with a male-female ratio of 3:1.[23,36,37] In people between the ages of 50 and 70 (approximately), dissecting aneurysm is more common by far in men, in a ratio of approximately 2:1.[2] However, in patients over 70, women with dissecting aortic aneurysms outnumber men, as shown in the following description of a "typical" case of dissecting aneurysm in a postmortem survey conducted at the University of Edinburgh: the patient was "an elderly hypertensive female, in whom dissection started in the ascending aorta and ruptured to produce hemopericardium: death occurred suddenly at home after a brief period of chest pain."[25] The peak incidence of aortic dissection is in the sixth and seventh decades.[2,38] Dissection is relatively rare in patients under 40, except for those with familial predisposition, such as Marfan syndrome, or congenital heart disease, such as coarctation of the aorta.[3] Aortic dissection is rare in young people; however, Voigt and Hansen[18] reported three cases of spontaneous rupture in patients under 30, and Kunita[37] reported aortic dissection in a 13-year-old boy. A 10-year study conducted by the office of the Tokyo Medical Examiner showed 102 autopsied cases of dissecting aneurysm between 1948 and 1958; only 5 of the subjects were younger than 40 years of age.[37]

As with other medical problems, a high index of clinical suspicion facilitates rapid diagnosis. The typical clinical history is one of severe, tearing chest pain, sudden in onset, with radiation to the arms or neck or posteriorly to the back—often reflecting the progressing path of the dissection.[23,36–38] The pain, which is present in 90 percent of patients,[38] is most severe at inception, unlike the crescendo pain associated with myocardial infarction.[2] In some patients, however, the symptoms may be less severe, and the chest pain may be mild. Syncope occurs in 10 to 15 percent of patients; syncope not due to stroke appears to be related to rupture into the pericardial space with cardiac tamponade.[38] In general, the symptom complex depends on the site of the initial dissection, the specific branches of the aorta involved in the dissection, and the location of the external rupture if present. The pain migrates from the point of origin to other sites, following the course of the dissecting tear as it extends throughout the aorta.[2,23,36–38] It may mimic coronary thrombosis but is more difficult to control with narcotics, and the typical electrocardiographic changes are usually absent unless the coronary arteries are compromised. Concomitant myocardial infarction occurs in about 1 to 2 percent of cases.[36] Hemiplegia may result from occlusion of the carotid artery; decreased pulsations in the arms or legs may result from involvement of the subclavian and iliac vessels; paraplegia may result from the interruption of the intercostal or lumbar arteries (Fig. 20-2). Pain is a clue to the site of aortic dissection. If it centers in the anterior thorax, it indicates proximal dissection; severe pain in the interscapular area is more common with a distal site of origin.[23,36–38] Absence of posterior back pain strongly suggests a nondistal dissection because more than 90 percent of patients with distal dissection report back pain.[2,38] Abdominal pain may be associated with occlusion of visceral arteries.

On physical examination, the heart is often enlarged and cardiac arrhythmias may be present. A significant percentage of patients are hypertensive or have a history of hypertension.[38] (Dalen et al. in 1974 documented a history of hypertension in 56 percent of patients.[39]) Slater and DeSanctis[35] confirmed the importance of hypertension and found that it was significantly more common in distal dissection, as was atherosclerosis. At the time of examination, the blood pressure may be normal or low, and there may be a significant difference in blood pressure between the two upper extremities.[17] If dissection involves the aortic ring, resulting in aortic insufficiency, the characteristic diastolic murmur will be heard.[36–38] Congestive heart failure may be found in patients with proximal dissection and free aortic regurgitation. Hematuria occurs in a small percentage of patients when the dissection involves the renal artery. Vasovagal symptoms (including drenching sweat, apprehension, and nausea)

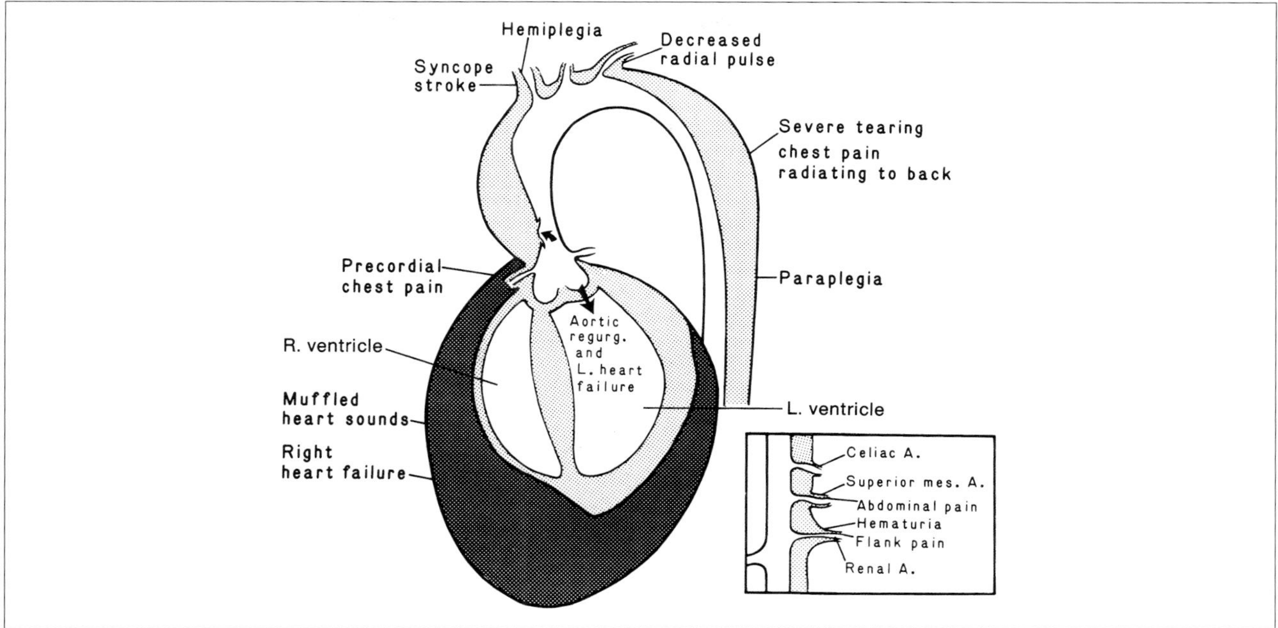

Figure 20-2. Diagrammatic representation of the effects of aortic dissection. Dissection may occur into the pericardium, with tamponade around the coronary arteries and the development of ischemia; into the aortic root, with impairment of valve closure and aortic regurgitation; into the neck vessels, with the development of cerebral symptoms or the loss of radial pulses; down the descending aorta, with obstruction of the intercostals and at times the bronchials, with severe back pain; into the celiac axis, with the symptoms of pancreatitis; into the superior mesenteric artery, with the symptoms of mesenteric ischemia; into the renal arteries, with the development of hypertension; and, in fact, into any branch of the abdominal aorta.

are common at the outset of aortic dissection.[2,36–38] Congestive heart failure may be the only symptom in patients with chronic aortic dissections; rapidly worsening failure should prompt the physician to order a diagnostic study (initially echocardiography or magnetic resonance imaging [MRI], and later angiography if necessary) by which an unsuspected aortic dissection may be picked up.[31] In a reported autopsy series of 30 aortic dissections, 10 percent of the patients presented with cardiac failure.[40]

Acute pericarditis has been reported as the presenting diagnosis in patients who were subsequently found to have suffered aortic dissection. Greenberg et al.[41] described two patients who presented with anterior pleuritic chest pain and clinical findings of acute pericarditis. At autopsy, both were found to have a dissecting aneurysm of the ascending aorta with extension into the pericardial space. In these patients, pericarditis was reactive, manifested by blood pigments and iron-containing macrophages in the pericardial sac, evidence of a slow leakage of blood at least several hours before death.[41]

Acute dissections (those in which survival is less than 2 weeks) usually show absent or unequal pulses, but chronic dissections often show normal pulses; the latter are usually DeBakey type III dissections that, because they begin after take-off of the brachiocephalic vessels, cause no decrease in blood flow to the head or arms.[31] In the subacute variety of this disease, the dissection may begin abruptly and progress rather gradually over a period of days or weeks.

Unusual symptoms have been reported, such as pleural effusion, decreased hearing, tinnitus, and ear and jaw pain.[42,43] The differential diagnosis includes coronary occlusion, pulmonary embolism, spontaneous pneumothorax, ruptured abdominal aneurysm, acute pancreatitis, mesenteric thrombosis, cerebrovascular accident, and transverse myelitis.

Radiographic Findings: Conventional Films

Although the plain film roentgen findings are not always pathognomonic, characteristic and rather persistent changes have been described.[1,8,33] One of the most valuable is a definite change in the diameter of the aorta shown on successive examinations, particularly

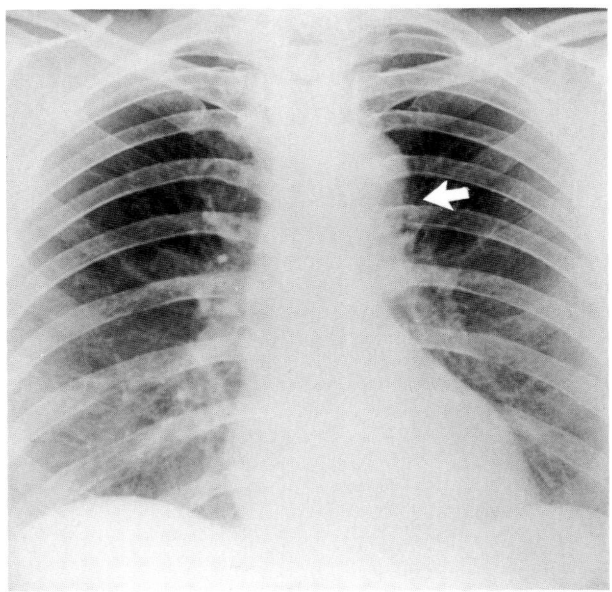

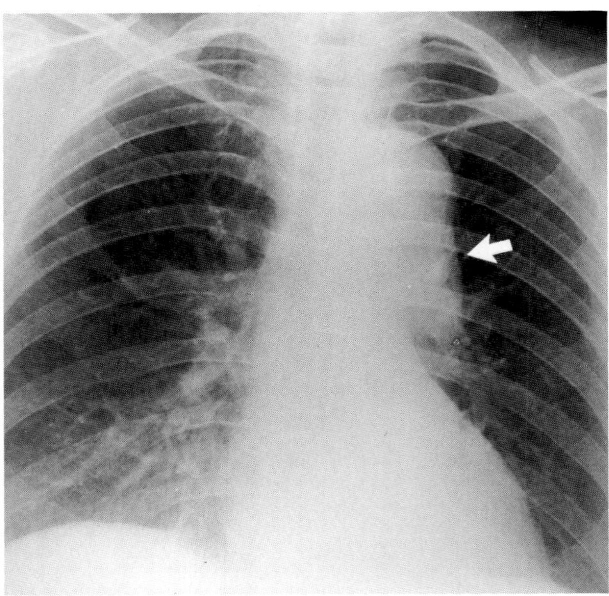

A

B

Figure 20-3. Chest film in aortic dissection showing the change in prominence of the aortic knob. The patient, a 60-year-old woman, entered the hospital complaining of back pain, at which time the initial film (A) was taken. The pain remitted, only to return 4 months later with more severity. At this time the patient was hospitalized, and the diagnosis of aortic dissection was made. The initial film (A) shows moderate prominence of the aortic knob, with poor definition of the descending aorta immediately below the knob (*arrow*). (B) Film 4 months later. A remarkable change in the configuration of the aorta has occurred, with a marked increase in prominence (*arrow*) of the descending aorta and the knob. As the descending aorta drops below the level of the carina, its margin becomes indistinct.

when these examinations are done over a short interval. (Unfortunately, prior films are not always available; nor are current films invariably adequate because the patient's condition frequently warrants bedside examination.) The changing aortic contour is usually best identified on the left side, at the level of the aortic knob, although the descending aorta may also show increased prominence (Fig. 20-3). A progressive increase in the prominence of the right aortic border may also be a valuable clue. Oblique and lateral films are helpful in evaluating aortic size. When diffuse prominence of the descending thoracic aorta is unaccompanied by apparent enlargement of the ascending aorta, dissection should be suspected (Fig. 20-4). Similarly, a disparity in the prominence of the ascending aorta may strongly suggest dissection that primarily involves the ascending portion (e.g., a type II dissection, typically encountered with Marfan syndrome) (Fig. 20-5). In general, aneurysms of luetic, atherosclerotic, or traumatic origin tend to produce a more localized area of dilatation. A loss of the usual sharpness of the aortic contour is also a useful diagnostic sign, particularly when serial changes are noted (Fig. 20-6). Various degrees of irregularity or knobbiness may occur along the outer diameter of the widened aorta (see Figs. 20-4 and 20-6). These may be related to extravasation of blood into the aortic wall and adjacent mediastinum or to a reactive, fibrinous, mediastinal pleurisy. Loss of the usual sharpness of the aortic contour may be further verified on overpenetrated views of the chest or with computed tomography or magnetic resonance imaging.

When the dissection involves the origins of the brachiocephalic vessels, there is usually widening of the superior mediastinal shadow on frontal films (Fig. 20-7) or a localized hump on the smooth superior contour of the aortic arch, best visualized in the lateral projection (Fig. 20-8B; see Fig. 20-4). Because the posterior portion of the aortic arch forms the aortic knob on the posteroanterior film, additional dilatation, particularly in the region of the left subclavian artery, will contribute to an increased size in the aortic knob, which may appear at a higher level than usually noted. The hump may also reflect the thickened aorta distal to the region of the subclavian artery produced by the dissection.

The demonstration of aortic wall thickening is also a valuable diagnostic aid (Fig. 20-9). The aortic wall

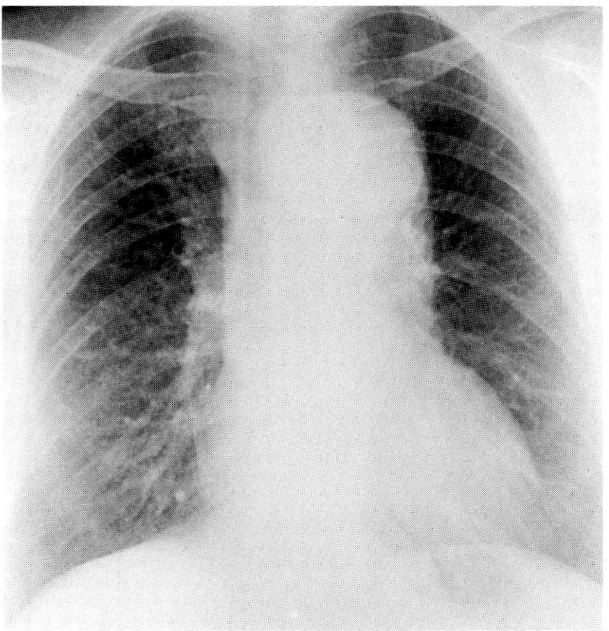

A

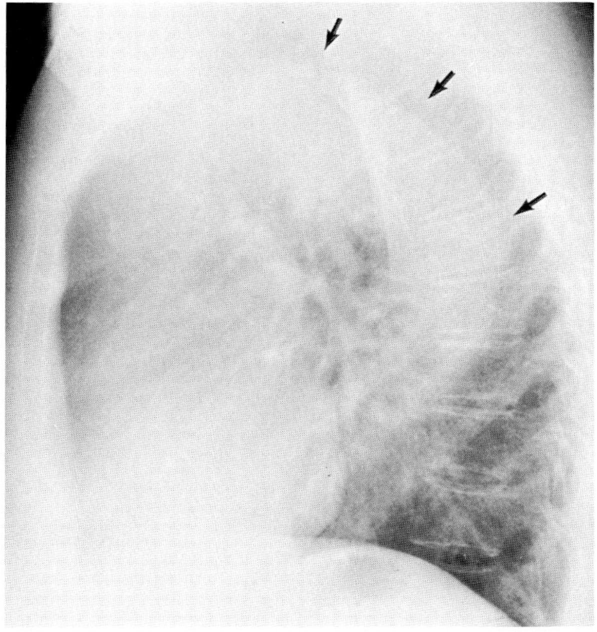

B

Figure 20-4. Chest film in aortic dissection showing the prominent descending aorta ("hump" sign) and the "disparity" sign. (A) Posteroanterior film. The region of the ascending aorta is normal. By contrast, the knob and the descending aorta demonstrate a marked increase in prominence, with displacement of the trachea to the right. Just before it merges with the heart shadow, the descending thoracic aortic shadow becomes ill defined. (B) Lateral film. The aortic shadow is both large and dense and presents as a zone of diffuse prominence in the distal arch and upper descending aorta (*arrows*). This represents the hump sign. The trachea is displaced and compressed in an anterior direction, the "tracheal push" sign. Note that the disparity, prominence, and size of the aortic knob and descending aorta as compared with the ascending aorta are strongly suggestive of aortic dissection.

is normally 2 to 3 mm thick,[10] and on occasion, with superimposition of a pericardial or pleural reflection, it may measure up to 5 mm. When this figure is surpassed, dissection should be suspected, particularly if there has been displacement of intimal calcification producing an unusually wide distance between the calcified intima and the outer aortic border. Eight of 46 patients in Eyler and Clark's series showed displacement of intimal calcification with the outer margin of the calcium 6 mm or more from the outer margin of the aortic wall.[1] Slater and DeSanctis[35] found this "calcium" sign to be more common in distal dissection. By contrast, atherosclerotic disease of the aorta does not cause central displacement of intimal calcification

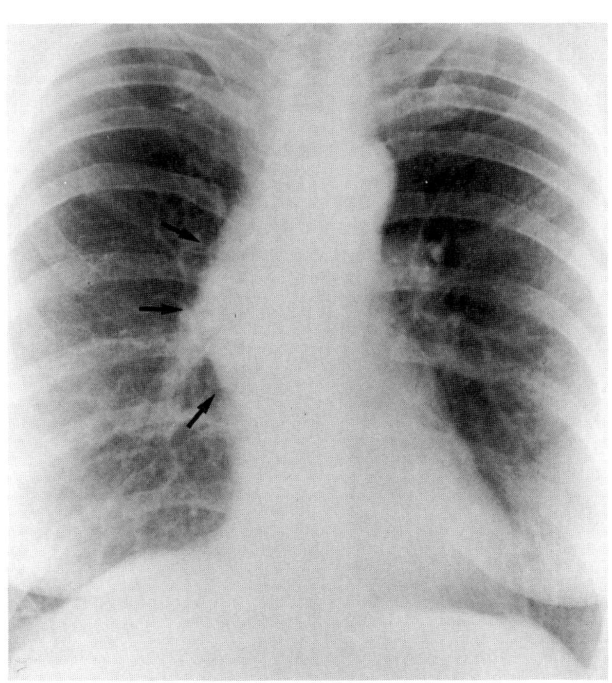

Figure 20-5. Chest film in aortic dissection showing the "disparity" sign. In the posteroanterior film, the ascending aorta (*arrows*) is markedly prominent as compared with the relatively normal aortic knob and descending aorta. This disparity suggests the possibility of type II dissection, as seen in Marfan syndrome, which is limited to the ascending aorta.

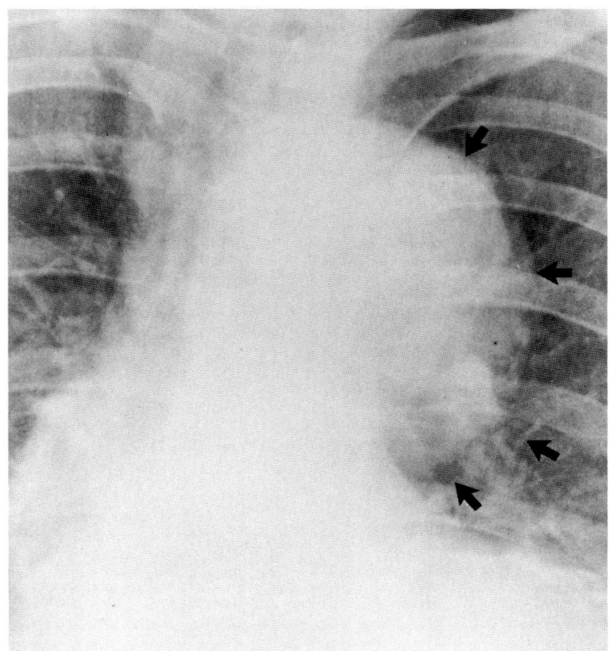

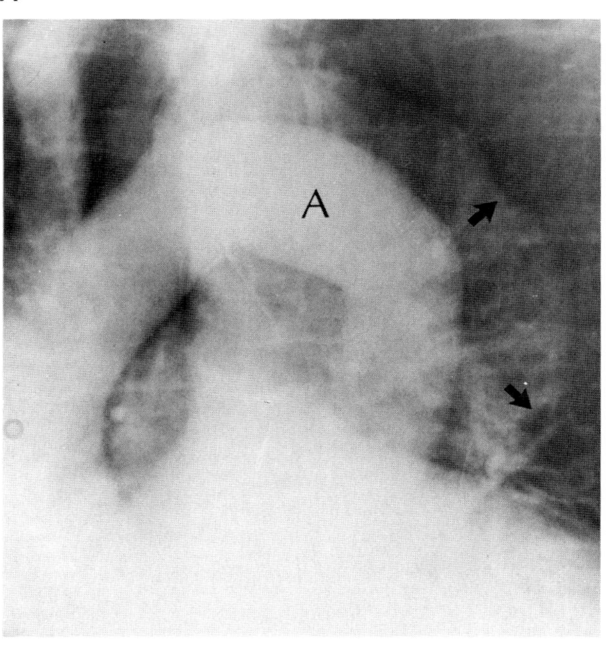

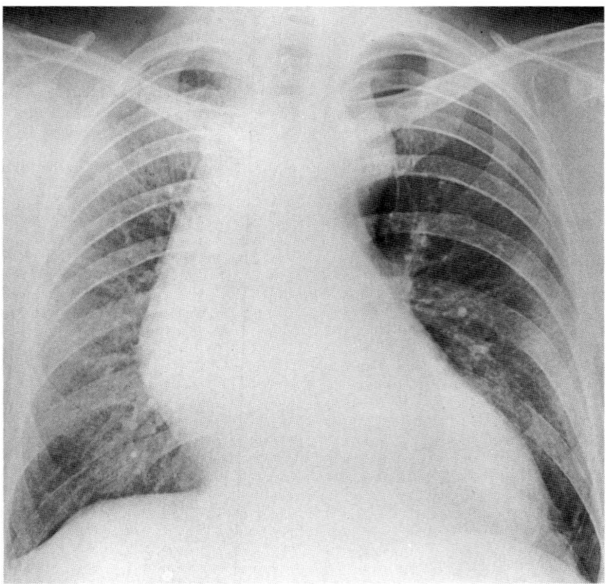

Figure 20-7. Chest film in aortic dissection showing a prominent mediastinal shadow. Posteroanterior chest examination demonstrates marked prominence of the ascending aorta and of the mediastinum. These findings strongly suggest the likelihood that the dissection has extended into the brachiocephalic vessels. Note also that there is cardiomegaly, caused by aortic insufficiency with dissection into the aortic root interfering with coaptation of the aortic cusps. (Courtesy of William Anderson, M.D.)

◂ **Figure 20-6.** Chest film in aortic dissection showing aortic marginal obscurity and irregularity. (A) In the posteroanterior chest film the aortic knob is grossly prominent (*upper arrows*), representing a "hump" sign. In addition, there is irregularity of the aortic margin below the knob and indistinctness as well (*lower arrows*). These signs are strongly suggestive of dissection. (B) Intravenous aortogram. The true lumen is well visualized (*A*), whereas the false lumen is completely thrombosed and therefore does not opacify. The aortic edge is irregular and ill defined (*arrows*).

Figure 20-9. Chest film in aortic dissection showing the "thickening wall" sign. (A) Posteroanterior film at the time of the patient's initial admission to the hospital with moderate back pain. The intima is defined by the calcific linear streak in the region of the aortic knob and is approximately 3 mm from the adventitial edge (*white arrow*). The aortic knob is moderately prominent (*black arrow*). (B) Posteroanterior film 5 months later. The patient experienced increasing chest pain and returned to the hospital, at which time a repeat chest examination was obtained. Increased prominence of the aortic knob is visible, and the calcified intimal plaque is now far more widely separated from the outer edge of the aorta (*arrows*) than on the previous film. This finding, present in only about 15 percent of patients, strongly suggests the likelihood of aortic dissection. ▸

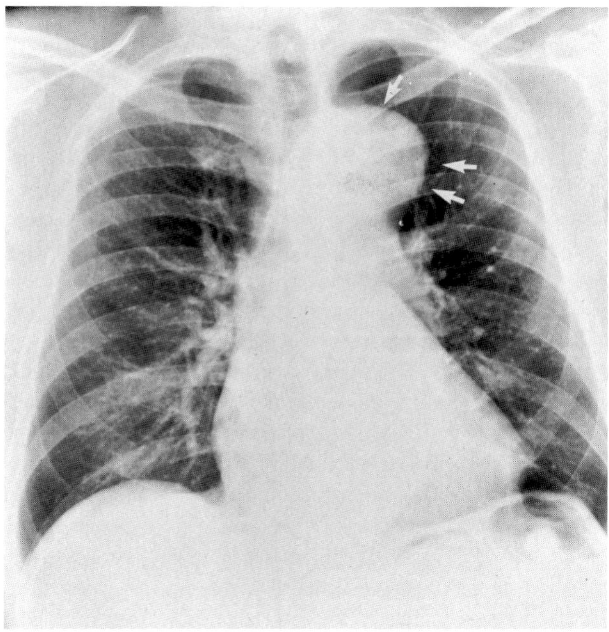

A

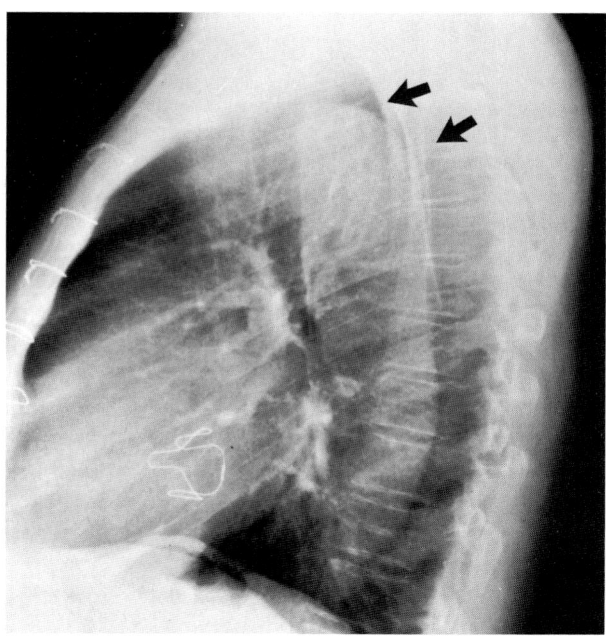

B

Figure 20-8. Chest film in aortic dissection showing the aortic "hump." (A) Posteroanterior film. The ascending aorta is normal, but there is a large hump in the region of the aortic knob (*arrows*). (B) Lateral film. Just as the transverse portion of the arch meets the descending portion, there is increased density and size of the aortic shadow (*arrows*). Note also the increased prominence of the descending thoracic aorta, indicating that the dissection has begun beyond the left subclavian artery and has extended into the abdomen.

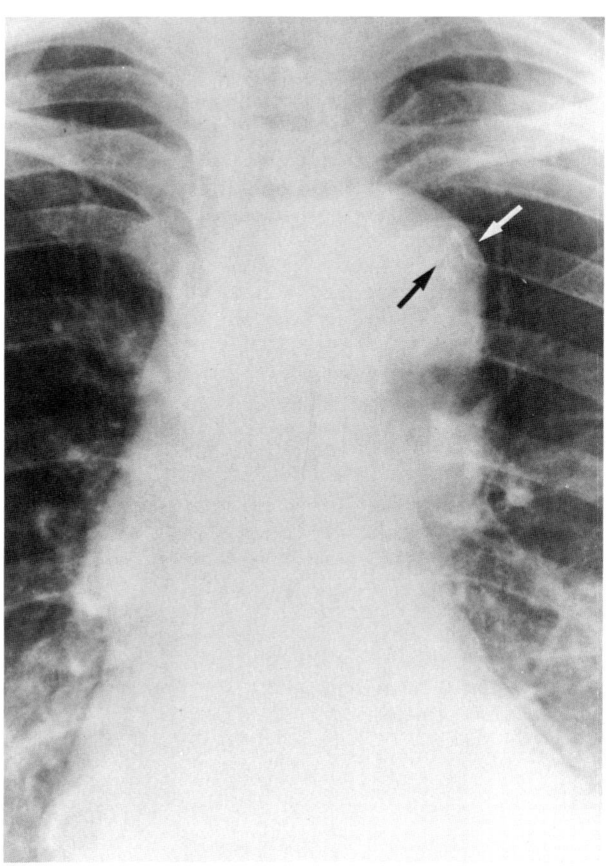

A

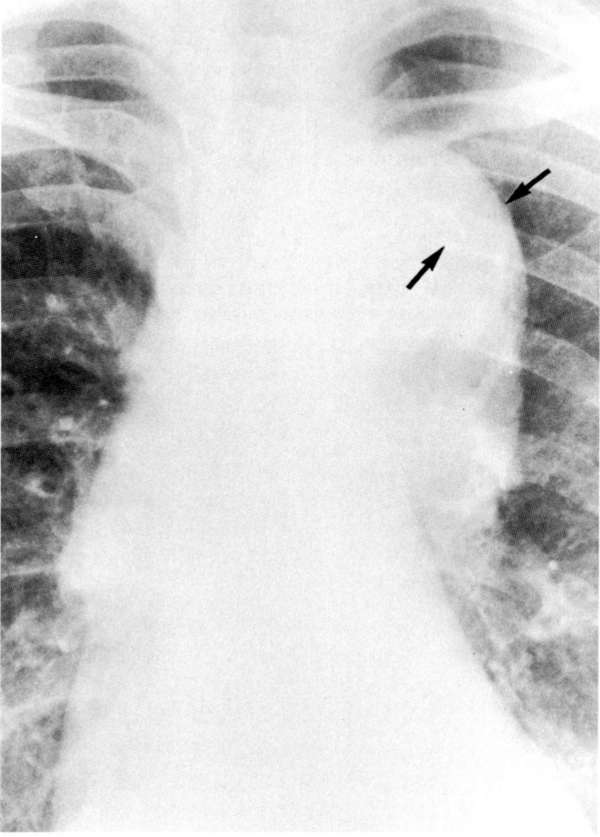

B

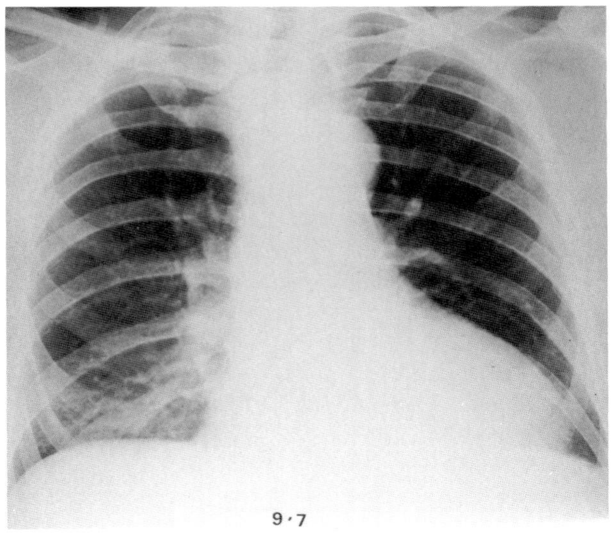

A

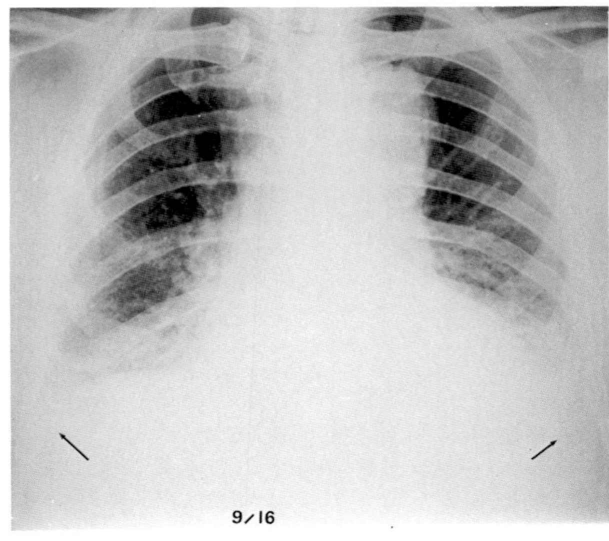

B

Figure 20-10. Chest film in aortic dissection showing rupture into the pleural cavity. The patient, a 65-year-old man, entered the hospital complaining of pain which radiated through to his back. The left radial pulse was diminished. (A) Posteroanterior chest film. Cardiomegaly is visible, and there is a slight prominence of the aortic knob. (B) Posteroanterior chest film made 9 days later. In the 1-week interval, the patient had stabilized and then developed sudden acute shortness of breath 3 hours before the second film was obtained. The film demonstrates bilateral pleural effusions (*arrows*), with elevation of the hemidiaphragm, cardiomegaly, and widening of the mediastinal shadow. The patient died shortly thereafter because of rupture of the dissection into the pleural space.

Figure 20-11. Chest film in aortic dissection showing mediastinal rupture. The patient, a 68-year-old man, entered the hospital with intractable chest pain. (A) Posteroanterior chest film on admission. The aortic knob is prominent, as is the descending aorta, which is also irregular in its lateral border. (B) Posteroanterior film 4 hours later. Three and one-half hours after admission, the patient suddenly became short of breath, and his blood pressure dropped. Portable chest film demonstrated gross widening of the mediastinum (*arrow*) and an apparent increase in heart size. Following the examination, the patient died. A gross dissection had communicated with the mediastinum, the site of massive bleeding.

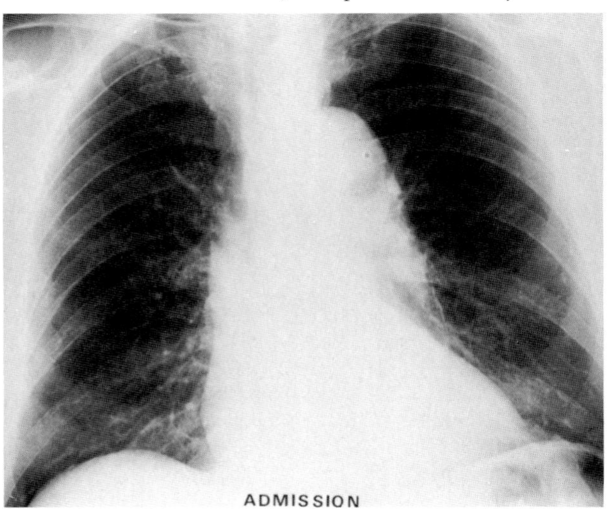

A

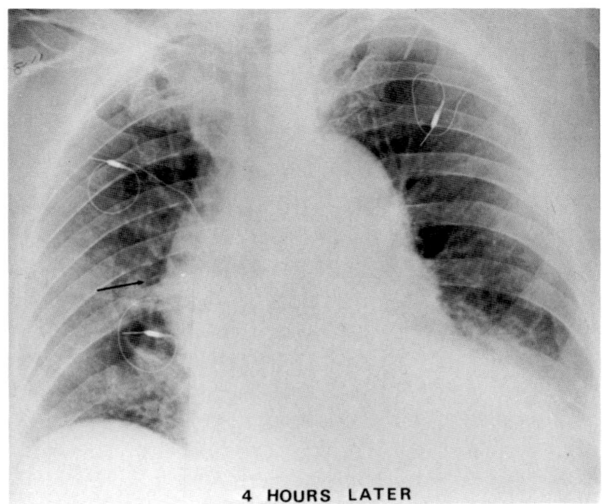

B

due to wall thickening. In some cases, the aortic diameter may decrease to a normal size and the contour may regain its usual degree of sharpness at or near the level of the diaphragm. This is a helpful diagnostic sign of reentry of the dissection into the main aortic channel.

If the dissection has involved the aortic ring, radiographs of the chest usually demonstrate evidence of cardiac enlargement due to the associated hypertension or aortic valve incompetence. Rupture into the pericardial cavity may also cause a gross increase in the size of the cardiac contour. Perforation into the pleural cavity, more commonly noted with distal dissection, results in hemothorax (Fig. 20-10). Mediastinal hematoma adds to the degree of mediastinal widening observed (Fig. 20-11). Compression atelectasis of chemical pneumonitis may be observed, particularly in the medial portions of the left lung.

The frequency of such plain film signs varies among different observers. In Table 20-1, our own findings are compared with composite data from the literature. In the Peter Bent Brigham Hospital series, serial changes in the aortic shadow were present in 80 percent of patients, a disparity in the prominence of the ascending and the descending aorta in 93 percent, an aortic hump in 75 percent, aortic edge irregularity and/or dullness in 68 percent, thickened aortic wall as judged by intimal calcification in 15 percent, mediastinal widening in 90 percent, tracheal displacement in 60 percent, cardiomegaly in 60 percent, and evidence of hemothorax in 15 percent. Although the plain film findings may be highly suggestive of the diagnosis, in some series up to 20 percent of the chest examinations have been normal.[30]

Table 20-1. Plain Film Findings in Aortic Dissection

Signs	Literature Incidence (%)	PBBH* Series Incidence (%)
Changes in the aortic shadow	90	80
Asymmetric enlargement of ascending or descending aorta	50	93
Aortic "hump"	?	75
Aortic edge irregularity and/or unsharpness	50	68
Displacement of calcified intima from edge	20	15
Mediastinal widening	30	90
Tracheal displacement	?	60
Cardiomegaly	80	60
Hemothorax	?	15

* PBBH = Peter Bent Brigham Hospital, Boston.

Aortography

Because advances in surgical technique have made correction of dissecting aneurysm possible in a significant number of patients, the diagnosis must be established rapidly with certainty and the site of dissection as well as its extent must be clearly defined. It is also essential to determine the degree of involvement of the brachiocephalic and other visceral vessels and to obtain information concerning the circulatory pattern, within both the true aortic lumen and the false channel. The presence and the exact location of sites of reentry into the main aortic channel are important. The surgical approach, and even the decision to attempt an operative repair, may depend in a large measure on the angiographic findings.

Intravenous aortography has been employed diagnostically in the past (see Fig. 20-6B), but frequently the anatomic detail has not been sufficient to offer optimal information. This is particularly true of patients with congestive heart failure and protracted circulation time; opacification of the vascular supply in the adventitia has led to misdiagnosis by simulating a small aortic dissection.[44]

Direct intraaortic injection (using a percutaneous retrograde transfemoral approach) of contrast material provides excellent delineation of anatomic features. Inadvertent cannulation of the false passage via both the transaxillary and the retrograde femoral approaches has been reported.[45] Injection of contrast material into the false passage carries a small potential risk, and careful monitoring of catheter position is required. Special catheters and techniques have made this a relatively safe procedure.[46,47]

In the technical approach to aortic dissection, it is essential to use the femoral artery with the best pulse. Once the guidewire has been replaced by the catheter, it should be advanced carefully, with contrast injections if necessary, and with pressure tracing as a control. The tip should ultimately reach the aortic valve to identify the true lumen and to inject contrast agent into it. If there is any suspicion that the catheter is in the false lumen, forcible injection should be avoided.

The right posterior oblique projection is usually most valuable in the evaluation of the entire aortic arch and the brachiocephalic vessels. Films should always be obtained in two projections if the anatomy is to be fully displayed and understood. On occasion it may be important to locate the reentry point; therefore, if the distal end of the lesion is not identified on the initial study, a second examination may be performed with proper centering of the film to include the lower thoracic and abdominal regions.

The purpose of aortography is to answer a number of important questions. The first question concerns the primary diagnosis: Is there a dissection? If so, what is the location of the proximal tear? What is the extent of the dissection? Is there vascular compromise of the coronary arteries, the brachiocephalic vessels, the renal or abdominal aortic branches, or the branches to the spine? Is aortic insufficiency or pericardial effusion present? What is the nature of the false lumen? All these questions are important not only in choosing an appropriate mode of therapy but also, if surgery is chosen, in defining the proper surgical approach.

The angiographic findings are variable and depend on the site, extent, and duration of the dissection. In a comprehensive review by Hirst et al.,[10] dissecting aneurysms involving the ascending aorta were far more common than those involving the descending aorta. A study of 65 patients at the Peter Bent Brigham Hospital shows a different breakdown by type from that reported by Earnest et al.[30] The explanation for the differences may well be that in autopsy series the ascending aortic dissections, which are far more hazardous, predominate, whereas the patients who survive for angiographic studies may well be those with dissection of the descending aorta, which has a much better prognosis. Other series of patients studied clinically[38] have shown a smaller percentage of dissections in the ascending aorta relative to the total than did the autopsy series of Hirst.[10]

One of the most common angiographic observations in aortic dissection is moderate to marked narrowing and distortion of the contrast column in the ascending aorta or in the region of or just distal to the left subclavian origin (Figs. 20-12 and 20-13). There is usually a large distance between the opaque stream and the soft tissue outline of the aorta because of the unopacified area of dissection impinging on the true lumen (see Figs. 20-6, 20-12, and 20-13). This may result in a tapered appearance of the contrast column near the left subclavian artery (Figs. 20-12 through 20-14). In some cases, the intimal flap may be delineated (Figs. 20-12 through 20-15) and the contrast column visualized as two separate lumens with a radiolucent wall between them (see Figs. 20-12, 20-13, and 20-15). This radiolucent line represents the intima and portions of the media that have been dissected from the aortic wall separating the true and false channels. The narrowed channel of the true aortic lumen may appear as a twisted piece of ribbon (see Fig. 20-12), presumably because of the spiraling nature of the dissection along the aortic media. The wall between the channels may be seen only in limited areas because of the relation of the projection to the spiraling course of dissection. In most cases, the false channel lies anteriorly and to the right in the ascending aorta, posteriorly and superiorly in the arch distal to the great vessels, and posterolateral to the left of the true channel in the lower thoracic aorta (see Fig. 20-12). If the dissection originates near the subclavian artery and dissects in retrograde fashion to the root of the aorta, initial injection of contrast material into the aortic root may demonstrate a nonopaque filling defect. As the contrast material fills the false channel near the subclavian artery, retrograde opacification of the false channel near the aortic root may be observed.

In our experience, the precise location of the intimal tear is defined in about 50 percent of patients; sometimes multiple tears are observed (Fig. 20-16). Earnest et al.[30] were able to identify the site of intimal tear in just 56 percent of the 52 patients in their series. When the brachiocephalic or other branch vessels are involved in the dissection, delayed and incomplete filling with contrast material and variable degrees of narrowing of the lumen may be identified (Figs. 20-12, 20-13, and 20-15 through 20-18). The angiographic studies may be nondiagnostic (1) if the intimal tear has sealed and the dissection is filled with clot or (2) if there is no intimal tear. The increased soft tissue density adjacent to and paralleling the contour of the contrast column is a helpful diagnostic sign (Fig. 20-19; see Fig. 20-6B).

Altered flow patterns may be observed, including stasis, reversal of flow within the false channel, and failure of major vessels such as the coronary, renal, or lumbars to fill, without evidence of a collateral circulation. At times, the intramural hematoma may be so large that the dissected aorta compresses adjacent venous structures (see Fig. 20-14). Aortic regurgitation is found in a small number of patients (see Fig. 20-13) and is an ominous sign.

The most common aortographic signs of dissection in our series were increased wall thickness (75 percent), lumen deformity (75 percent), and increased total aortic diameter (90 percent) (Table 20-2). Aortic regurgitation was observed in only 10 percent of patients, in contrast to the finding of Earnest et al.[30] that is was present in 33 percent of their patients.

Rarely, dissection may be present without symptoms, signs, or prior history suggestive of the event. The patient whose film is shown in Figure 20-20 entered the hospital because of hematuria. Urography revealed a mass lesion in the upper pole of the left

Text continues on page 509

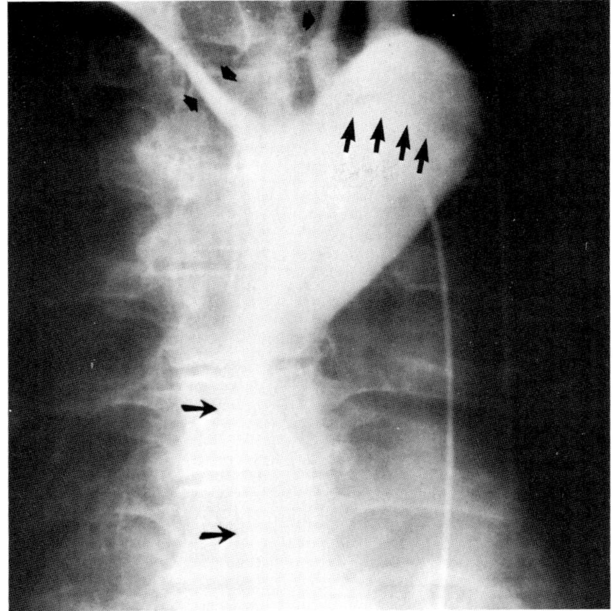

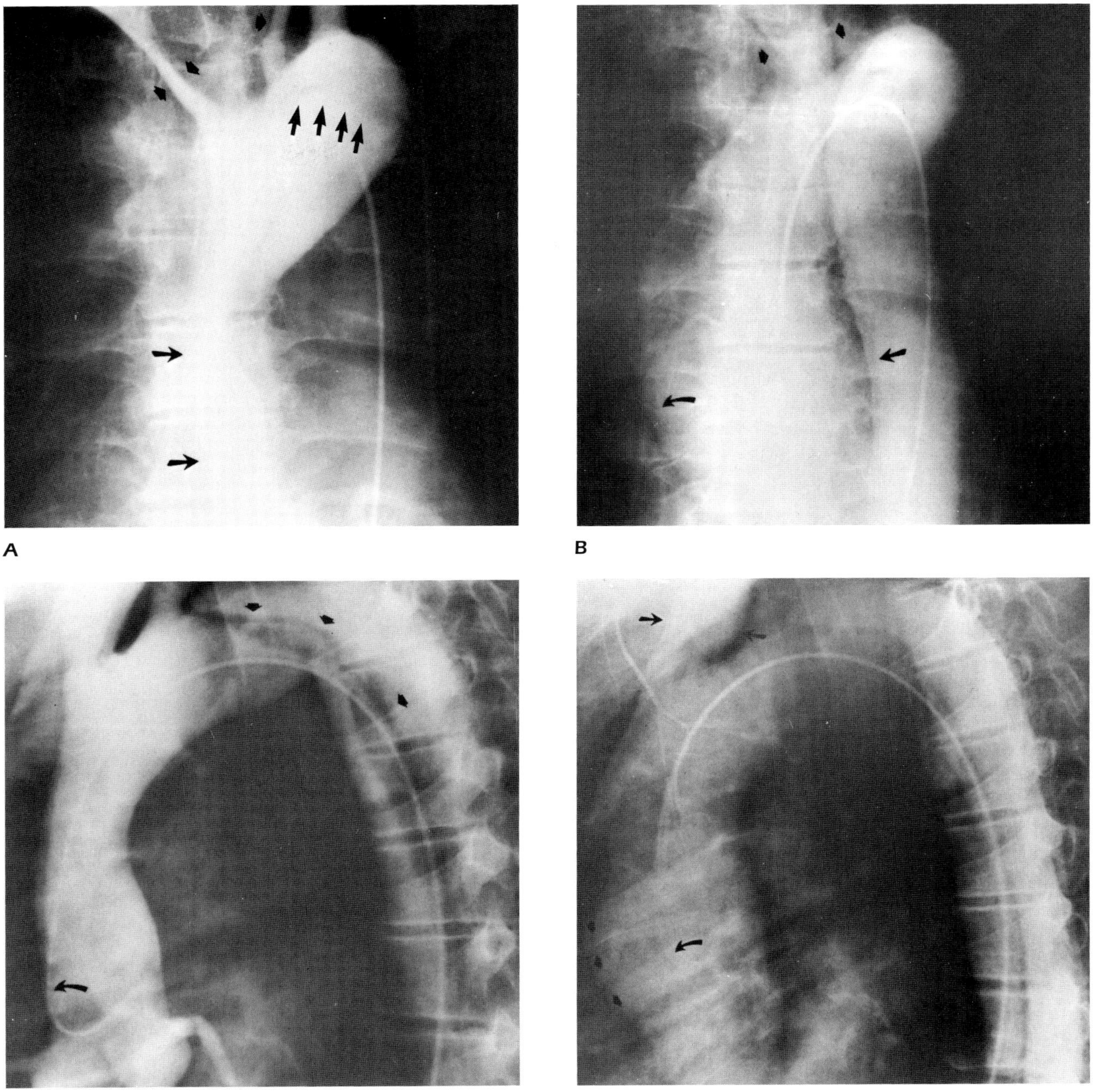

A

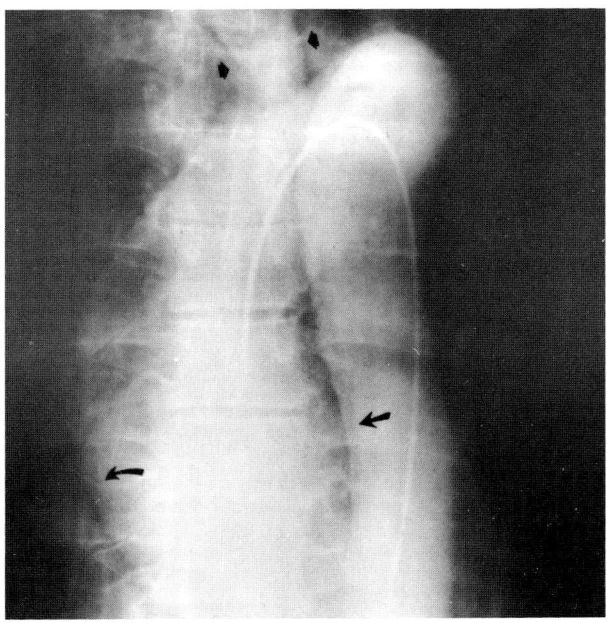

B

C

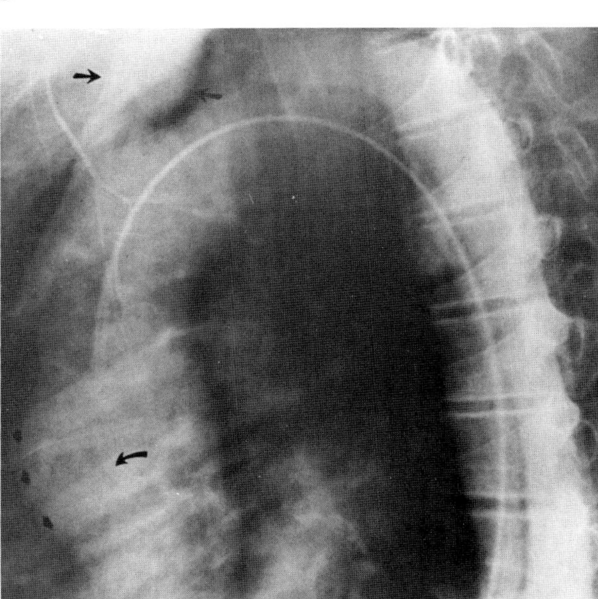

D

Figure 20-12. Angiography in dissection showing luminal deformity. (A) Anteroposterior view at 0.5 second. Contrast has been injected into the root of the aorta, producing visualization of a grossly deformed ascending aorta (*two lower arrows*). At its narrowest point the diameter of the true lumen has been reduced to 1.5 cm. The dissection extends well up into the innominate artery (*two arrowheads on right side*) and into the left common carotid artery as well (*upper arrowhead*). Through the shadow of the aortic knob, a faint radiolucency representing the intimal flap may be visualized (*four arrows*). (B) Anteroposterior film at 2 seconds. The false lumen has now become opacified (*lower arrow on right*), with extension of the opacification into the false lumen of the innominate artery (*arrowheads*). In the descending thoracic aorta, the edge of the intima is outlined against the medial wall of the aorta (*left lower arrow*). (C) Right posterior oblique film at 1 second. The J-shaped catheter may be seen in the aortic root with its anterior edge against the intimal lining (*lower arrow*). Moderate deformity of the ascending aorta is visible (*arrowheads*), but the extent is not possible to surmise from this single projection alone. Just beyond the subclavian artery the intimal flap is clearly delineated, with filling of both true and false lumen. (D) Right posterior oblique film at 2 seconds. With filling of the false lumen, its anterior edge is now visible (*three arrowheads*) and may be clearly defined separate from the intima, the site of which is indicated by the catheter position (*lower arrow*). Broadening of the shadow of the innominate artery (*upper arrows*) is attributable to the filling of the false lumen of the innominate. The false lumen in the region of the distal arch and descending aorta is now more opaque than the true lumen, in which the catheter may be seen extending cephalad from the diaphragm up to the level of the aortic arch.

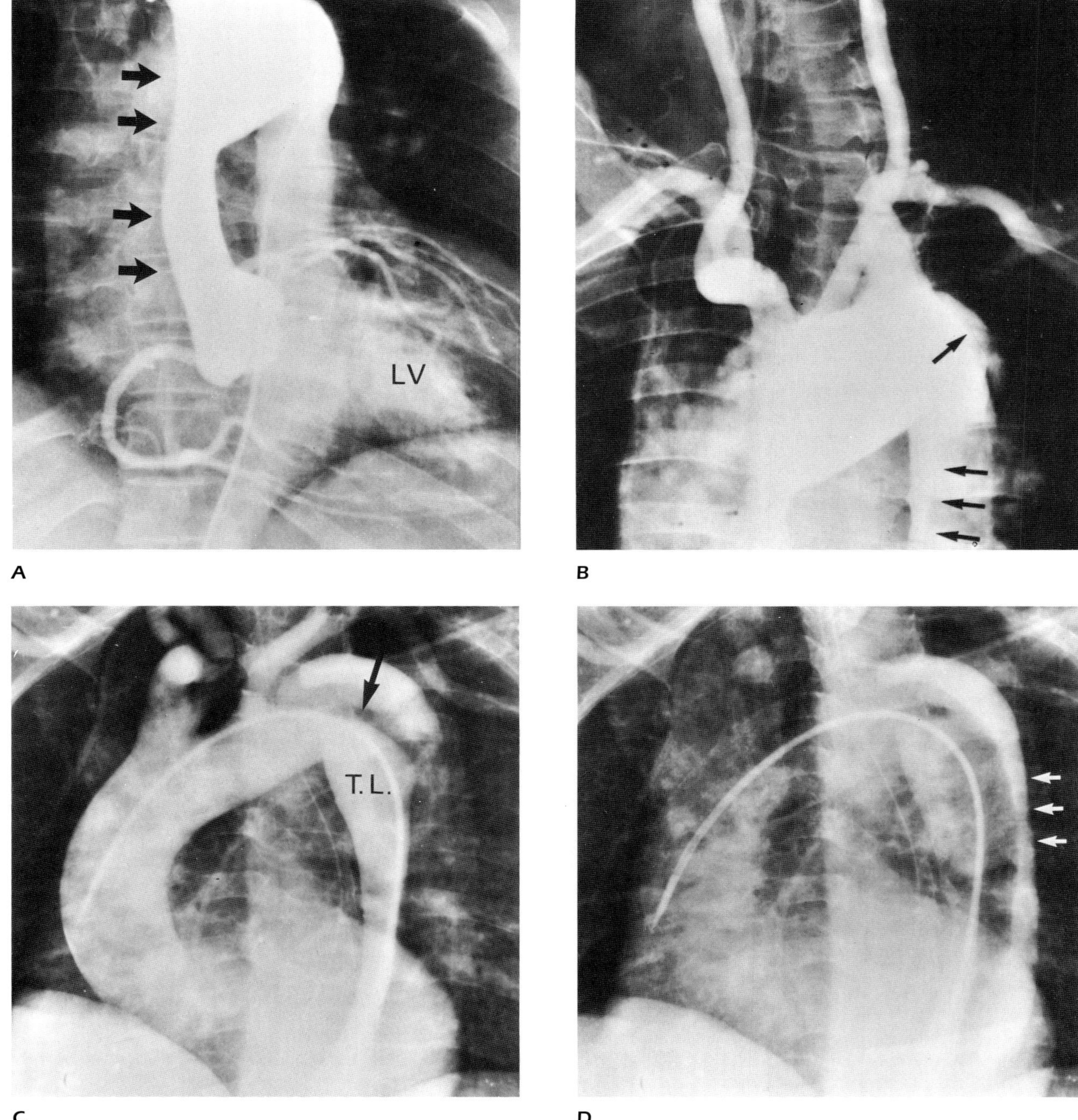

A

B

C

D

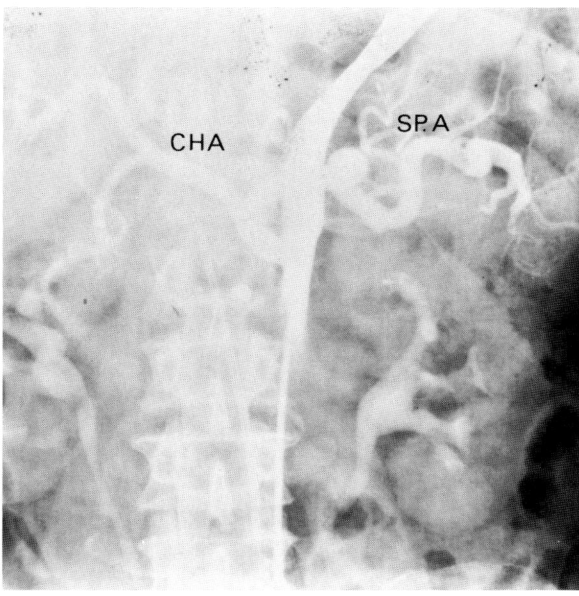

E

Figure 20-13. Angiography in dissection showing luminal deformity. The catheter is located in the ascending aorta just above the valve, at which site the injection has been made. (A) Anteroposterior projection. The ascending aorta is grossly deformed, in particular to the right and anterior (*arrows*). The deformity extends toward the neck, and the large size of the false lumen is depicted by the shadow to the right of the opacified aorta extending out to the border of the cardiomediastinal shadow. Note how well opacified the coronary arteries are, with no evidence of occlusion. Contrast has also refluxed into the left ventricle (*LV*). The border of the descending thoracic aorta is irregular and wavy because of the involvement of the dissection at this level. (B) Anteroposterior projection. Aortic arch and brachiocephalic vessels. The dissection extends cephalad to the site of origin of the innominate artery, which is moderately compressed. The intimal flap is seen at the site of the aortic arch on the left (*upper arrow*) with marked compression of the true lumen (*multiple arrows*) by the large intramural hematoma. (C) Right posterior oblique film at 1 second. The catheter tip is in the ascending aorta. The deformity of the ascending aorta is not as prominent in this projection. The intimal flap beyond the left subclavian artery is clearly seen (*arrow*) and separates the true lumen (*T.L.*) from the false lumen. Most of the false lumen is not opacified. (D) Right posterior oblique film at 3.5 seconds. The contrast agent has cleared from the ascending aorta and from the great vessels. The position of the true lumen is denoted by the position of the catheter. Note the dense opacification of the false lumen (*left lateral arrows*) with both delayed filling and delayed clearing of the contrast-filled area of dissection. (E) Anteroposterior film of abdominal aorta. The dissection extends well below the diaphragm, involving the abdominal aorta and its great branches. Although the celiac artery and its common hepatic (*CHA*) and splenic (*SP.A*) branches are patent and seemingly uncompromised by the dissection, compression of both renal arteries was present, and there was markedly delayed filling of the strikingly narrowed lumen of the abdominal aorta. The deformity of the abdominal aorta is pronounced, and its diameter has been reduced to less than one-third the normal size. (Courtesy of Laslo Szlavy, M.D.)

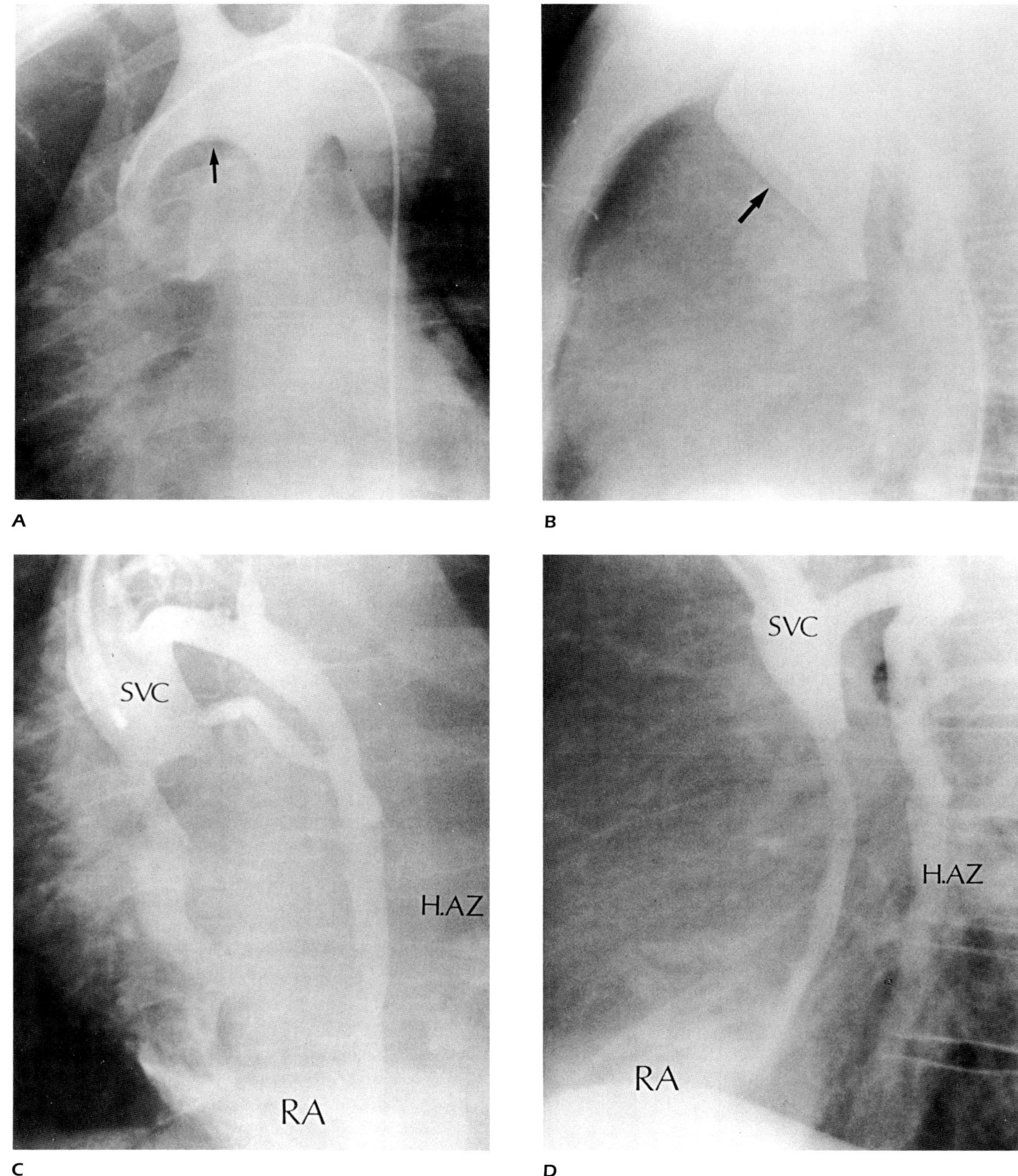
A
B
SVC
H.AZ
RA
C
SVC
H.AZ
RA
D

kidney. Abdominal aortography demonstrated an infiltrating renal cell carcinoma on the left, with multiple tumor vessels (see Fig. 20-20). An interesting additional finding was aortic dissection to the level of the renal arteries (see Fig. 20-20B, *arrow*), at which point the false lumen reentered the aorta.

Arterial compression, such as is visualized in Figure 20-18, is usually caused by a hematoma compressing the origin of the vessel. Alternatively, the dissection may extend into the branch of the aorta and compress the branch exactly as the aorta is compressed by the primary dissection. Finally, when compression of the origin by the primary dissection occurs, thrombosis may develop. At times, spontaneous relief of obstruction may occur if there is a rupture of the intramural segment of the artery, which then communicates freely with the false lumen. Spontaneous reentry of the dissection into the true aortic lumen also reduces the pressure of the intramural hematoma.

Problems in Establishing the Diagnosis of Aortic Dissection by Aortography

A number of difficulties may render the diagnosis of dissecting aortic aneurysm inexact.[44,48,49] Aortography appears to have about a 2 percent incidence of false-negative results in dissection.[50] Opacification of the false channel may be obscured at times, and multiple projections may be necessary for definitive evaluation. Improper location of the catheter relative to the intimal tear (entry site) may fail to opacify the false lumen. If equal and simultaneous opacification of true and false lumens occurs, it may appear simply as though the aorta is widened. Under these circumstances, the catheter position may be helpful, because, particularly during the injection, the catheter is propelled to the outer edge of the lumen and clearly reflects the position of the intima. In the past, mediastinal rupture of a thoracoabdominal aneurysm has been mistaken for dissection. In aortic regurgitation, there is prolonged opacification of the descending aorta in some patients, resembling the unusual flow patterns of dissection. Rarely, a very small dissection may be missed by aortography. In a number of instances, the width of the aortic wall had been misinterpreted as being excessive, at times leading to a mistaken diagnosis of dissection with thrombus or possible intramural hematoma. However, with the more widespread use of cross-sectional imaging (CT and MRI), early aortic dissection with intramural hemorrhage, but without intimal rupture, is being increasingly recognized.[51,52] Although 4 to 5 mm is generally considered the maximum thickness of the aortic wall, we have seen aortic wall thickness of as much as 10 mm in the presence of arteriosclerosis alone. Arteritis and aneurysm with laminated thrombus may also thicken the aortic wall. Adjacent neoplasm may give the appearance of a thickened aortic wall as it invades or compresses the aorta. Finally, mediastinal fat in some cases has been mistaken for the aortic edge, and the diagnosis of dissection has been made on that basis.[53,54] If there is any question about apparent wall thickening by fat, CT (decreased saturation of fat)[48,55] or MRI (increased signal intensity on spin-echo images) is useful for clarification of this finding.[48,55]

◀ **Figure 20-14.** Angiography in dissection showing the intimal flap. The catheter extends retrograde from the right femoral artery into the descending thoracic aorta, across the transverse portion of the arch, and into the ascending aorta. (A) Anteroposterior projection. There is total retrograde block to the flow of contrast agent because of the marked compression of the lumen by the intramural hematoma. The intimal flap (*arrow*) prevents movement of the catheter toward the aortic valve and also prevents the retrograde opacification of the true lumen of the ascending aorta. The dissection widens the mediastinum to a major degree and extends well up into the brachiocephalic arteries. The left subclavian artery is not visualized at this time because it is compressed, and clinically there is associated diminution of the left radial pulse. (B) Lateral film. The intimal flap (*arrow*) completely prevents the retrograde opacification of the proximal origin of the ascending aorta. A large soft tissue shadow fills the anterior mediastinum, representing the dilated dissecting aortic hematoma. (C) Superior vena cavogram, anteroposterior projection. There is marked compression of the superior vena cava (*SVC*) near its junction with the right atrium (*RA*). Most of the contrast agent flows into the azygos and hemiazygos (*H.AZ*) systems, reaching the right atrium from below through the inferior vena cava via communications between the azygos vein and the inferior vena cava. (D) Lateral projection. Marked compression of the superior vena cava is visible, with contrast spillover into the hemiazygos vein. It should be emphasized that the indication for the superior vena cavogram was the presence of clinical evidence of superior vena cava obstruction and the need to determine the site and cause of obstruction. The intimal flap in this patient has acted as a serious barrier to the retrograde flow of contrast agent. This is not always true, however, as is clear in Figures 20-12 and 20-13, in which the intimal flap is well defined but the hematoma in the wall of the aorta has failed to obstruct the retrograde passage of contrast and of the catheter. (Courtesy of William Anderson, M.D.)

Text continues on page 514

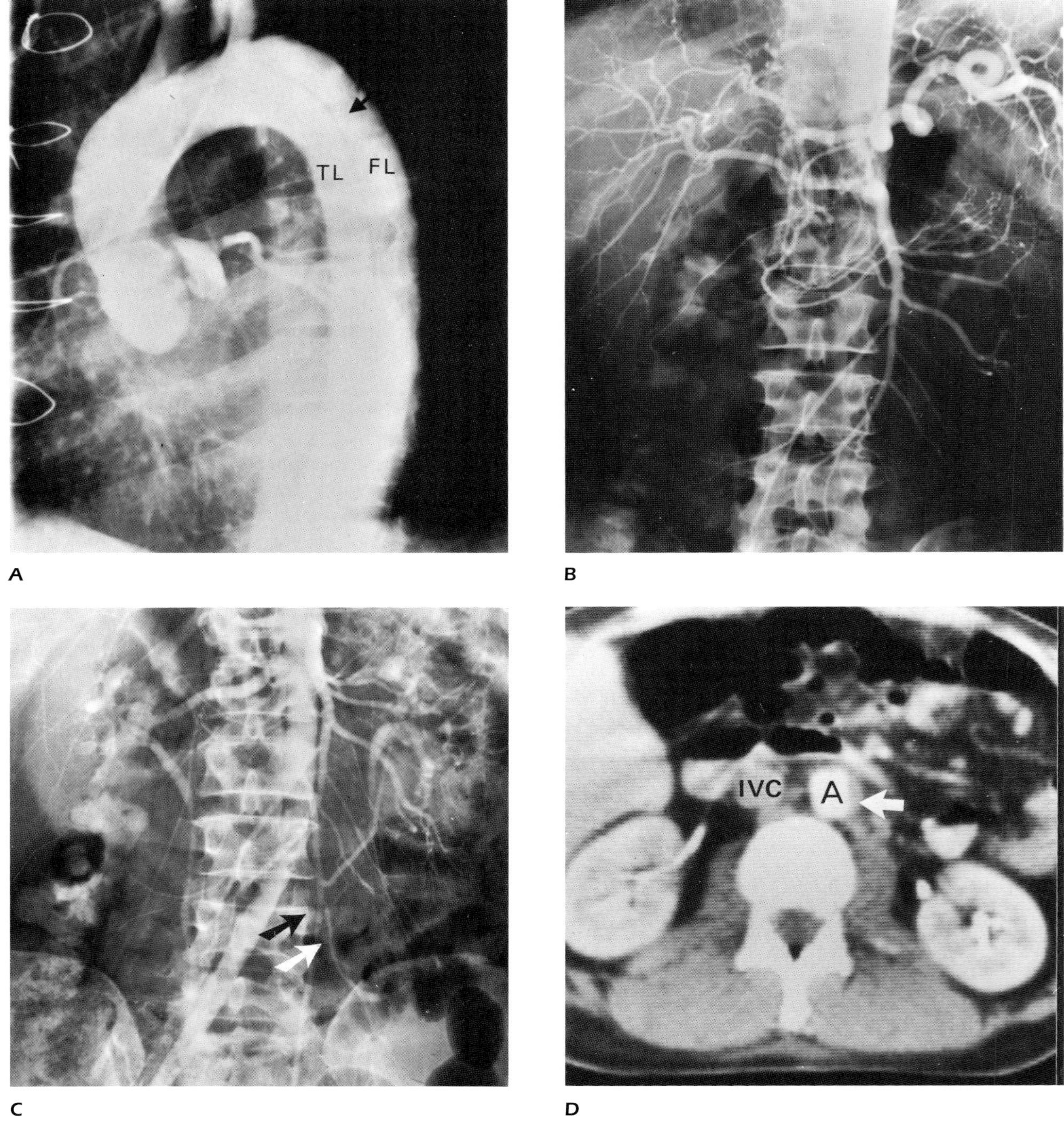
TL
FL
IVC
A
B
C
D

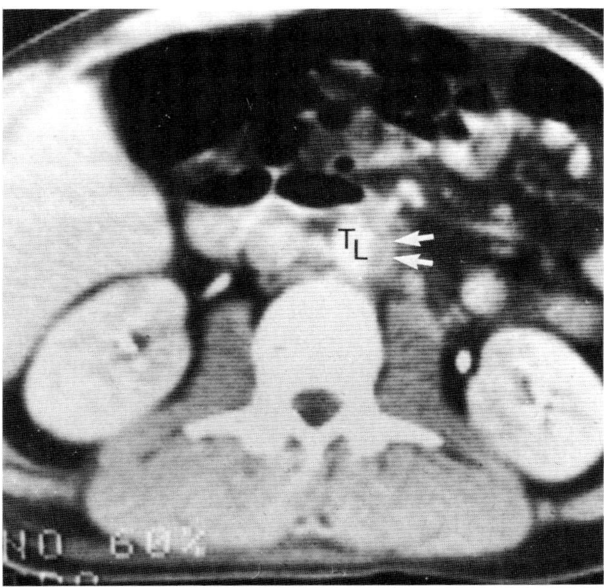

E

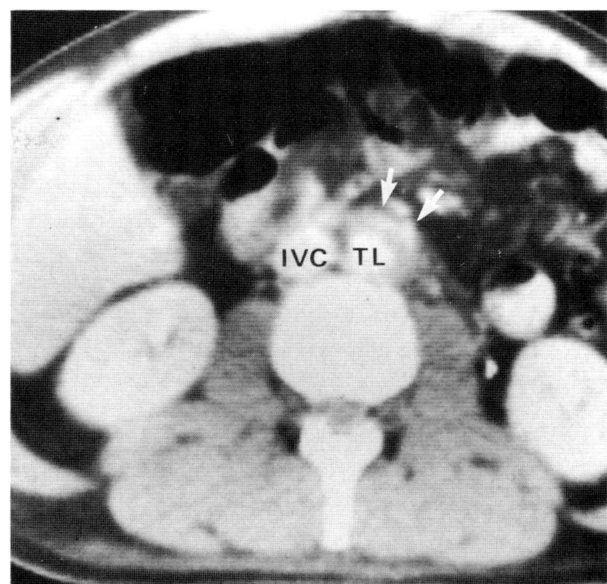

F

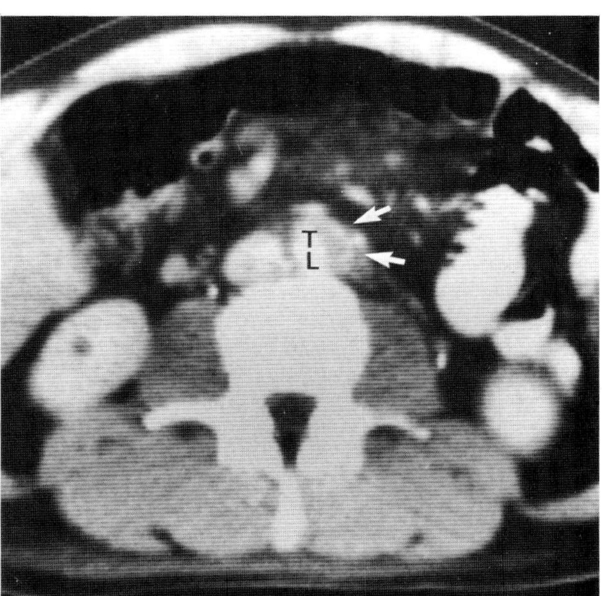

G

Figure 20-15. Angiography and CT in aortic dissection showing the intimal flap. The patient was a 60-year-old man with hypertension who was admitted to the hospital because of the sudden development of left leg discomfort on walking. Physical examination revealed the absence of a left femoral pulse. (A) Thoracic aortogram. Right posterior oblique projection. The classic appearance of a type III dissection begins just beyond the left subclavian artery, with a clearly defined intimal flap (*arrow*) separating true (*TL*) from false lumen (*FL*). (B) Abdominal aortogram with catheter entry via left axillary artery. There is filling of the celiac and superior mesenteric arteries, with compression of the mid and distal abdominal aorta by the intramural dissecting hematoma. (C) Abdominal aortogram at later phase. The narrowed mid and distal aorta is now visualized, with opacification of the right renal artery. The left renal artery is poorly visualized because its origin is compressed by the intramural hematoma. Contrast filling of the right common iliac artery is visible, but the left common iliac appears to be completely obstructed (*arrows*). (D) CT scan at the first lumbar vertebra. The aorta (*A*) is densely opacified, but its left lateral aspect is deformed by the intramural dissection (*arrow*). (E) CT scan at the level of L2. The aortic shadow is now more grossly altered, with the true lumen (*TL*) on the right side of the aorta, and the false lumen (*arrows*) visualized as a circumferential ridge of contrast. (F) CT scan at the level of the L2-L3 interspace. The false lumen (*arrows*) is now circumferential and surrounds the true lumen (*TL*), a band of diminished density visible between the two. (G) CT scan at the upper level of L3. The true lumen (*TL*) is now markedly compressed and displaced to the right. The false lumen is visualized as a thin band of increased density (*arrows*). The occlusion of the left common iliac artery is clearly explained by the size of the intramural hematoma on the left lateral aspect of the aorta just above the bifurcation.

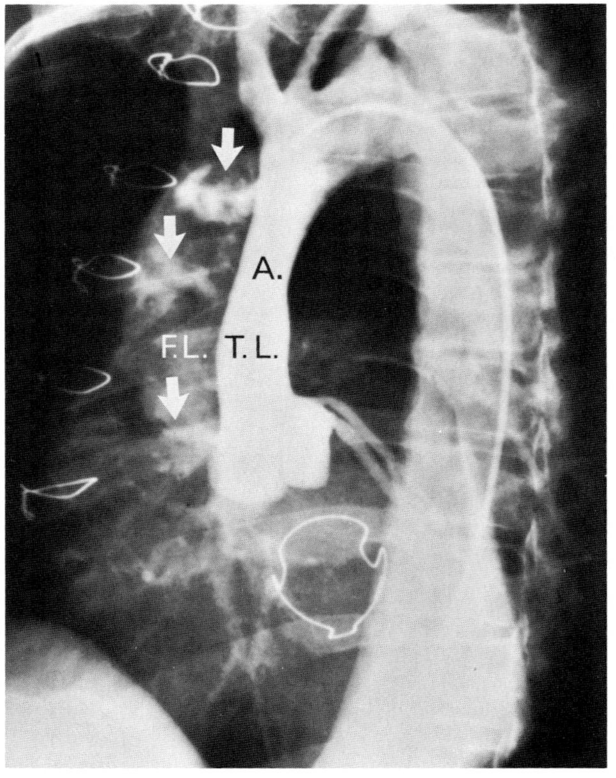

A

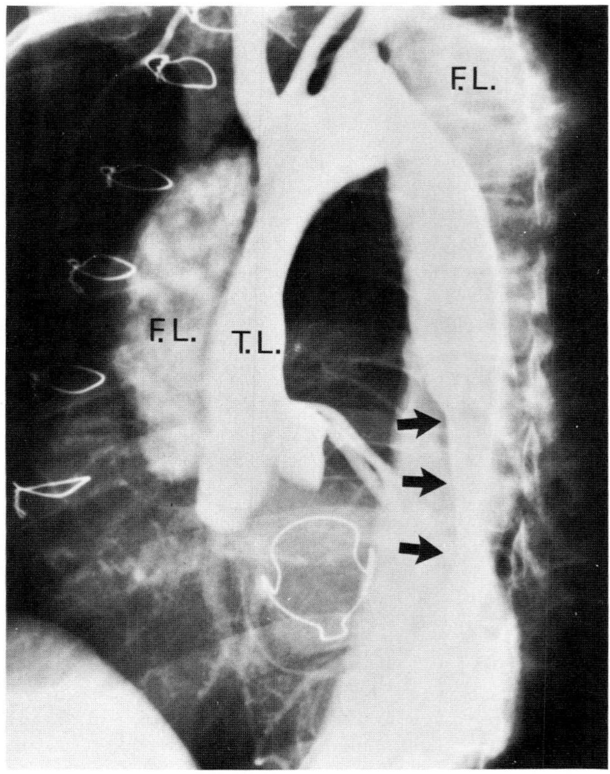

B

Figure 20-16. Angiography in dissection showing localization of the intimal tear. The patient, a 60-year-old man with mitral valve disease and mitral valve replacement, was admitted to the hospital complaining of chest pain. (A) Aortogram, right posterior oblique projection. Ascending aorta (*A.*) is markedly deformed from the level of the valve to the origin of the innominate artery. In addition, three discrete areas of communication between the true lumen (*T.L.*) and the false lumen (*F.L.*) may be visualized (*arrows*). Both the transverse portion of the arch and the descending aorta are markedly deformed. The left coronary artery is well visualized, but the right coronary artery appears obstructed. (B) The false lumen (*F.L.*) is now more densely opacified. This is true both in the region of the ascending aorta and just beyond the origin of the left subclavian artery. In addition, there is marked deformity of the descending aorta in its lower portion induced by circumferential dissection and hematoma surrounding the true lumen (*arrows*).

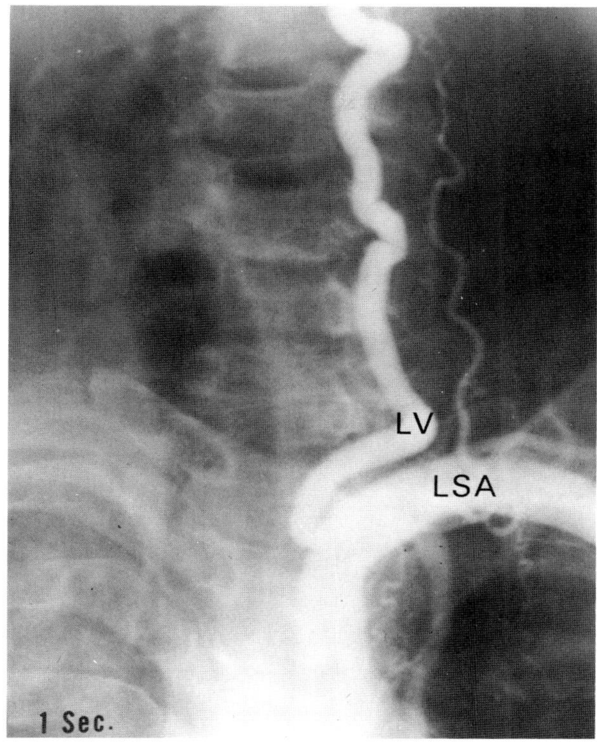

A

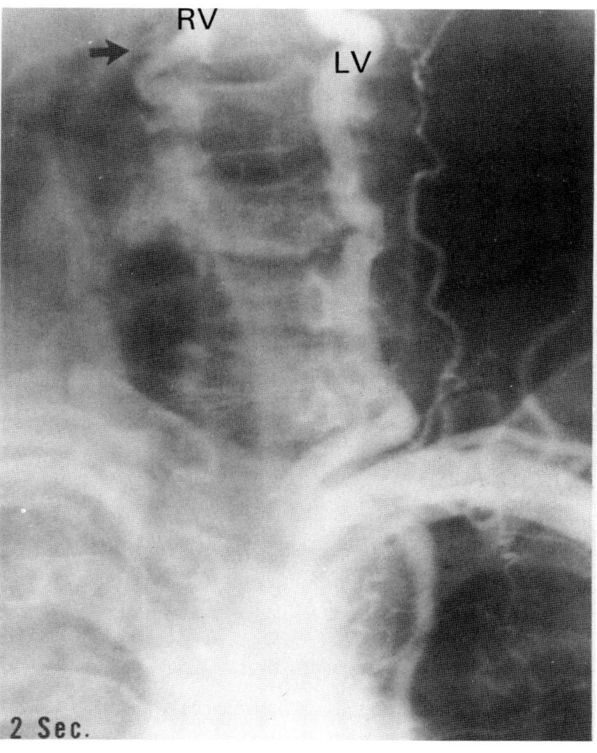

B

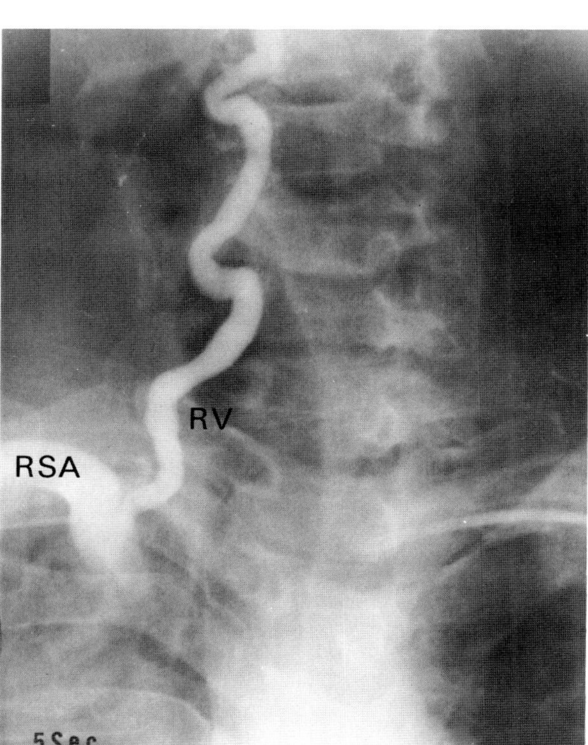

C

Figure 20-17. Angiography in aortic dissection showing branch artery compression. The patient has a type I dissection demonstrated on aortography. The innominate artery failed to opacify, and injection into the left subclavian artery was then performed. (A) Film at 1 second. The left subclavian artery (*LSA*) and the left vertebral (*LV*) artery are well visualized. (B) Film at 2 seconds. With the opacification of the left vertebral artery (*LV*), the right vertebral (*RV*) artery is now filling from the left vertebral artery via the basilar artery and is "stealing" blood from the posterior fossa (*arrow*). (C) Film at 5 seconds. There is now dense opacification of both the right vertebral (*RV*) artery and the right subclavian artery (*RSA*). The aortic dissection had completely occluded the origin of the innominate artery.

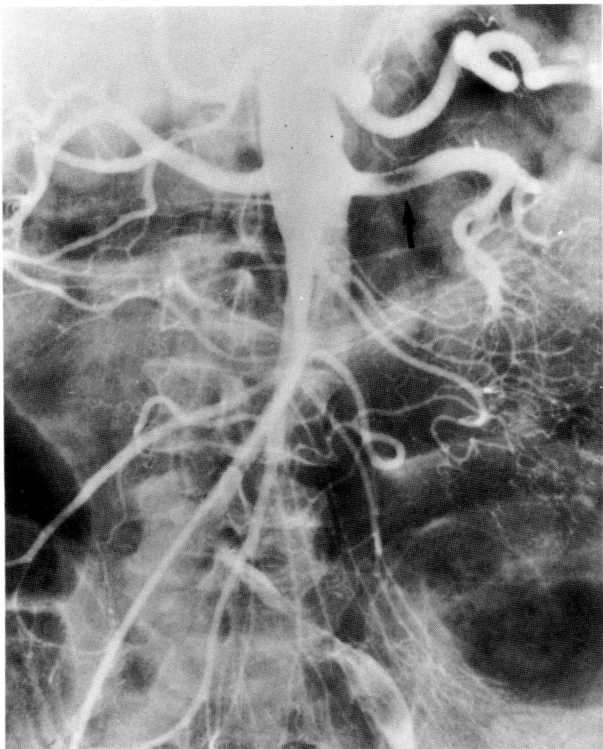

Figure 20-18. Angiography in aortic dissection showing branch artery compression. There is complete obstruction of the abdominal aorta, whereas the celiac, superior mesenteric, and renal arteries are patent and well filled. Note that the dissection has extended from the aorta into the left renal artery, with compression and diminished density of the renal artery 1 cm beyond its origin (*arrow*).

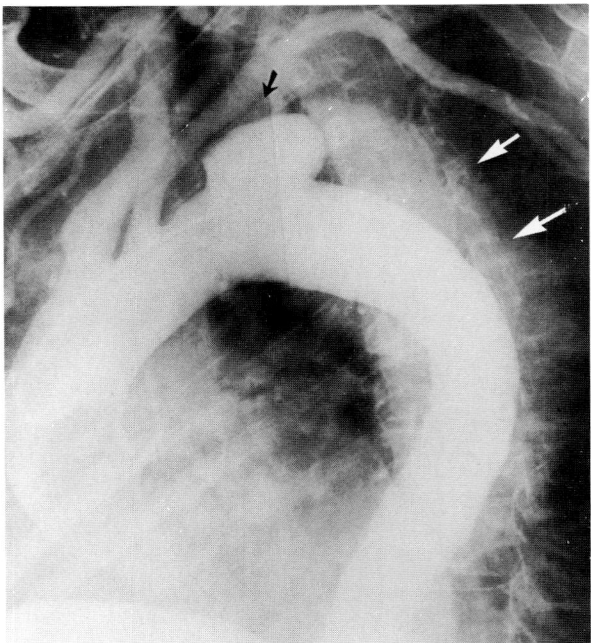

Figure 20-19. Angiography in aortic dissection showing chronic dissection with thrombus in the false lumen. Aortography demonstrates communication between the true lumen and the dissection (*top arrow*), but total lack of filling of the large area of intramural hematoma extending down the descending aorta (*lateral arrows*). The area of communication between the true lumen and the false lumen is relatively wide, but there is no flow through the false lumen.

Table 20-2. Aortographic Signs in Dissection

Signs	Incidence (%)
Increased wall thickness	75
Lumen deformity	75
Increased total aortic diameter	90
Definition of intimal tear	50
Double lumen	65
False lumen	65
Intimal flap	45
Aortic branch involvement	43
Altered flow pattern	50
Aortic regurgitation	10

Computed Tomography

Aortic dissection often occurs in elderly patients, some of whom have impaired renal and cardiovascular function and may not tolerate angiography well. For such patients, the noninvasive approach of computed tomography (CT) is useful as a diagnostic tool. It has proved helpful as an adjunct to angiography, being diagnostically corroborative in uncertain cases of aortic dissection with a subacute progression.[56] Recently, CT's acceptance among surgeons[23] has increased, and many are willing to operate based on CT findings alone, although it does not provide reliable information on branch vessels (especially the coronary arteries) or aortic valve function. CT has established itself as a noninvasive follow-up technique for patients who have had medical or surgical treatment for dissection. Whereas plain radiographs often do not detect the medial border of the aorta, CT can follow its widening well, and CT images, because they are cross-sectional, are not affected by slight changes in rotation of the patient.[57] Both CT and aortography detect the usual

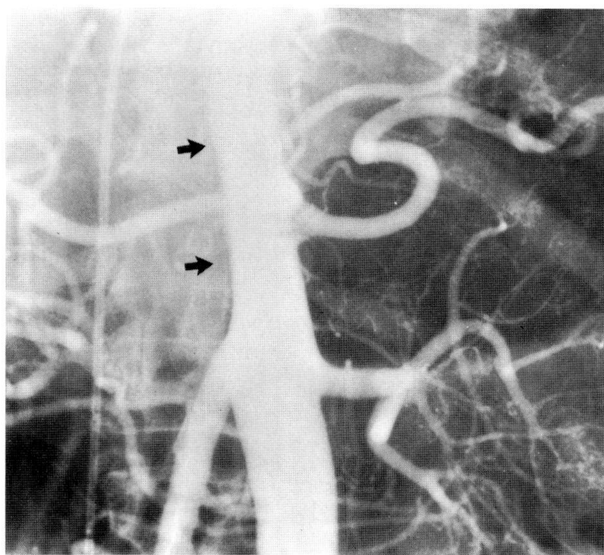

A

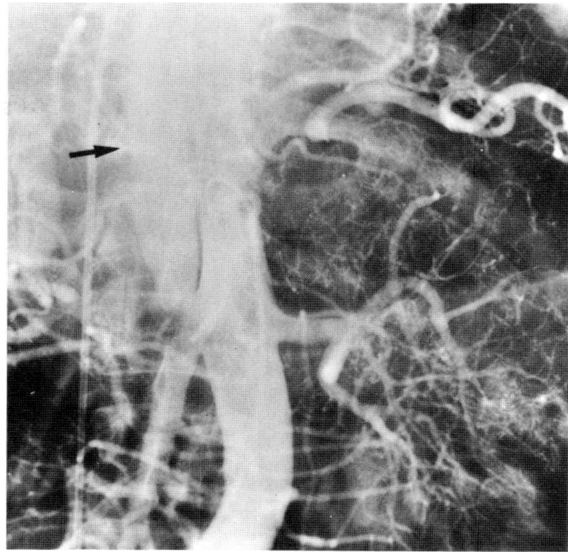

B

Figure 20-20. Angiography in aortic dissection showing asymptomatic dissection. The patient had abdominal aortography performed because of hematuria. (A) Abdominal aortography demonstrates compression of the abdominal aorta just above the origin of the right renal artery (*arrows*). In addition, there are some unusual vessels seen within the renal shadow on the left. (B) Anteroposterior film 1 second later. Filling of the false lumen of an aortic dissection is apparent (*arrow*). This was totally unsuspected in this patient. (C) Selective left renal arteriogram. Multiple abnormal tumor vessels are visible throughout the upper and mid portions of the left kidney, representing a renal cell carcinoma (*arrows*). It was the carcinoma that had caused the patient's bleeding, leading to the aortogram and the discovery of the dissection.

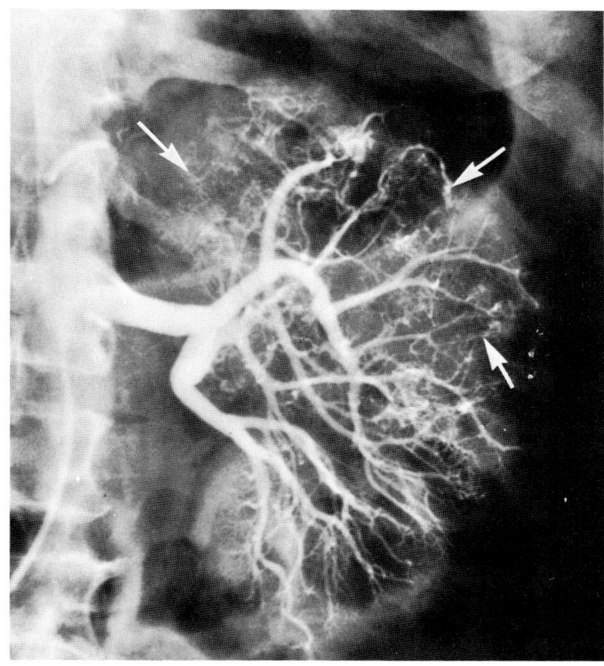

C

features of dissection: irregular lumen, disparate widening of the aorta, and stasis of contrast material in a channel. Early CT studies, which did not use contrast material, were unable to distinguish an aneurysm from a dissection or to identify intramural thrombus in an aneurysm.[57] Dynamic CT, with a bolus injection of contrast material, is generally capable of showing the relative rates of filling of the true and false channels in aortic dissection.[57,58] Bolus injection followed by a series of rapid injections and scans may define the intramural flap separating the false channel from the true one.[56]

In cases of possible dissection, CT has the following advantages over conventional radiography: (1) it detects calcification much more sensitively; (2) because of its cross-sectional images, it shows the precise relationship of calcification to the edge of the aortic wall; (3) it evaluates more adequately than aortography the apparent thickening of the aortic wall; and (4) because of its greater density resolution, it separates extraaortic fat and intraluminal (or intramural[51]) thrombus from other causes of widening.[57] Aortography, if not projected properly, may miss localized filling of a false channel; this problem does not occur in CT because projection is not a limitation.[57] One of the great strengths of CT is its ability to differentiate subtle variations in density.[59]

CT has its weaknesses as well.[58] It is unable to adequately define the status of aortic branch vessels or aortic insufficiency, if present. Because a CT section averages information over a finite thickness (usually 10 mm), it produces a composite image. A false appearance of displacement of intimal calcification may result and may suggest dissection rather than simple aneurysm. Correction is possible by rescanning the area and examining sections above and below.[57] Conventional CT is at times not reliable in demonstrating the intimal flap.

However, several recent advances,[58,60,61] including spiral (helical) computed tomography, which rotates the gantry about the patient as the table is advanced in the cranio-caudal direction, acquire continuous images rapidly and promise to improve the accuracy of CT in the diagnosis of aortic dissection.[60] In the future, spiral CT angiography may be able to better define branch vessel status. Thus CT fills a need for a reliable, noninvasive diagnostic technique in cases of suspected aortic dissection. It is often used alone and is a valuable adjunct to angiography. It is often able to rule out dissection and spare patients the rigors of angiography.

Newer Imaging Modalities

The newer noninvasive imaging modalities for the evaluation of dissecting aneurysms include transthoracic echocardiography,[59,62–64] transesophageal echocardiography,[65] and MRI,[48,59,62–64] in addition to CT[48,55,62,66–70] discussed above.

Transthoracic echocardiography has a sensitivity of 59 to 85 percent and a specificity of 63 to 96 percent for the diagnosis of aortic dissection.[59,62] Its sensitivity for dissections in the ascending aorta is somewhat higher, between 78 and 100 percent, but in the descending aorta it is much less, at about 55 percent[48,59]—limiting the modality's use in this region. With the addition of color Doppler[63] evaluation, the detection of flow in the false lumen, aortic insufficiency, and the site of intimal tear is simplified.

Transesophageal echocardiography has been increasingly employed in the diagnosis of aortic dissections, with a reported sensitivity of 97 percent and a specificity of 77[62] to 100 percent.[65] The sensitivity for the detection of the entry site appears to be around 77 to 87 percent.[59] Transesophageal echocardiography is also highly sensitive to aortic insufficiency (100 percent, specificity of 90 percent), and has a 100 percent negative predictive value for this finding; in addition, pericardial effusion is diagnosed with a sensitivity and a specificity of 100 percent. Furthermore, it appears to be more sensitive to proximal coronary artery involvement than the transthoracic method.[65] Despite its excellent performance, transesophageal echocardiography suffers from reverberation artifacts and limited views, perhaps accounting for the recently reported lower specificities of 68 to 77 percent.[59,62] Transesophageal echocardiography also carries a small risk of esophageal rupture, and rupture of the aorta following its use has been reported.[62] As with all ultrasound modalities, operator experience plays an important role in diagnosis with both the echocardiographic techniques discussed here.

Computed tomography has been extensively discussed in the previous section. In spite of the strengths and advantages outlined above, conventional CT is limited by the fact that it cannot adequately assess aortic branch vessels or aortic valve insufficiency. This has led some to argue that an approach using CT in combination with echocardiography (transthoracic) to detect valve involvement could provide all of the preoperative information needed.[64] The argument has been made that coronary artery involvement with aortic dissection, without accompanying symptoms or signs, is relatively rare and that perhaps routine evaluation of the coronary arteries (even with arteriography) may not be necessary.[71] Of course, transesophageal echocardiography may be better if this combined approach is taken. However, preferences of individual surgeons vary, and some are clearly willing to operate on CT findings alone,[23] when there is no clinical evidence of aortic insufficiency or coronary artery involvement. Future development of spiral CT angiography may render this modality even more attractive for the evaluation of the aorta and its branches.

Magnetic resonance imaging has advanced more rapidly since its introduction than perhaps any other new imaging modality introduced in the last 20 years. Routine MRI is done with spin-echo pulse sequences. These may be obtained in transverse, coronal, sagittal, or compound-angulated oblique projections, making MRI an extremely attractive modality for the evaluation of large vessels. With this imaging sequence, rapidly flowing blood appears black (no signal), and static blood or thrombus has an intermediate signal. Slowly flowing blood may be confused with mural thrombus; this may be clarified by obtaining images in other planes or using flow-sensitive imaging. With routine spin-echo images, aortic dissections are clearly demonstrated. The intimal tear is seen as a linear bright signal outlined by the dark true lumen and a false lumen of variable signal depending on the amount of flow within it. The other advantage of MRI is the ability to

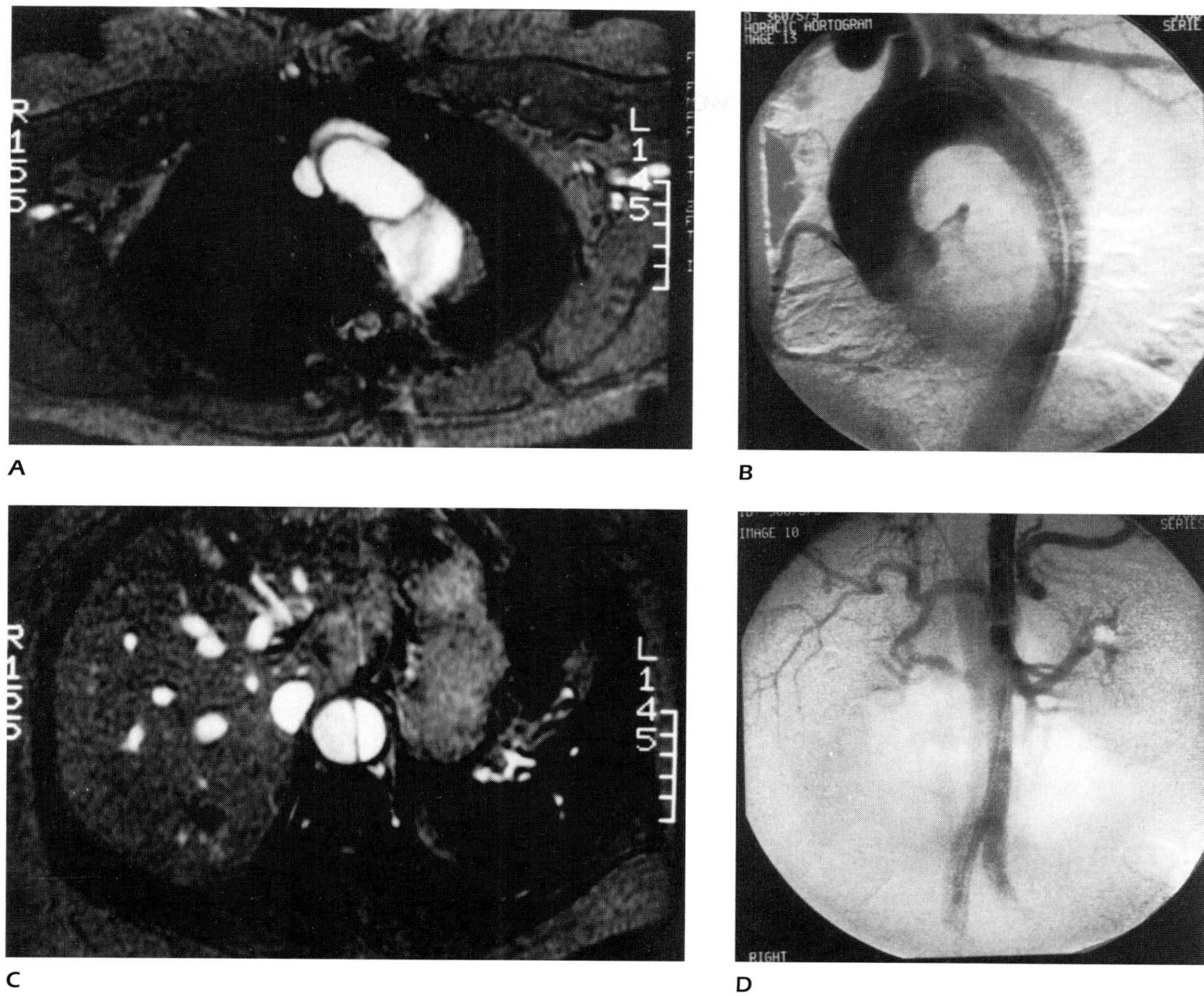

Figure 20-21. Magnetic resonance images (using gradient refocused echo pulse sequence, GRE-MRI) with corresponding intraarterial digital subtraction angiograms (IADSA) of a type B thoracic aortic dissection. (A) Axial GRE-MRI section at the level of the aortic arch. Bright white signal in the aorta medially is from fast-flowing blood in the true lumen. The less bright signal in the descending portion of the arch noted more laterally (to the left) and dorsally represents slower flow in the false lumen of the dissection. The section above showed the left subclavian artery to be arising from the true lumen. (B) The corresponding IADSA in left anterior oblique projection shows faint filling in the false lumen dorsolaterally, distal to the origin of the left subclavian artery. The brachiocephalic branches of the aorta are clearly seen arising from the true lumen of the aortic arch. The tip of the pigtail catheter is in the ascending aorta above the valve plane, and the shaft is noted in the true lumen in the descending aorta. (C) An axial GRE-MRI scan of the proximal abdominal aorta shows that the false lumen has spiraled to the right side of the abdomen (less intense signal) and that the true lumen (brighter white signal) is now on the left side of the abdomen. (D) Corresponding IADSA shows the false lumen to the right filling the renal artery on this side. The true lumen fills the celiac axis, the left renal artery, and the superior mesenteric artery. Note also that the false lumen extends into the right iliac artery. A right-sided false lumen as seen here occurs less frequently than a left-sided false lumen. All of the necessary information for the management of this patient was available from the magnetic resonance images.

obtain flow-sensitive gradient-refocused images that show fast-flowing blood as a bright (white) signal. Notably, flow in the true lumen is brighter than in the false lumen, making differentiation between them easy (Fig. 20-21). Velocity-mapping (velocity phase-encoding) techniques have also been used for distinguishing flow from intraluminal thrombus.[69] In addition, images may be obtained in cine mode, providing images resembling cine contrast angiography but without the same resolution.[68] These images are extremely useful for evaluating aortic insufficiency and moving intimal flaps.

Early reports suggested that MRI was highly sensitive (at a specificity level of 90 percent) for the diagnosis of aortic dissection, but that the sensitivity depended on the experience of the radiologist (83 to 100 percent, increasing with experience).[66] Advantages of MRI include its ability to detect aortic dissections without intimal tears[51,52] and the relatively rare entity of painless aortic dissection.[72] However, MRI has its pitfalls and artifacts[67] as well, and the diagnostic accuracy is improved when close attention is paid to avoiding them.

Finally, much has been written recently about the strengths and weaknesses of each of the imaging modalities used for evaluating aortic dissection.[37,48,55,62,70] A recent prospective study compared echocardiography (both transthoracic, TTE, and transesophageal, TEE), CT, and MRI (spin-echo, with cine MRI in selected patients); angiography results, operative findings, and autopsy findings were used as "gold standards." The sensitivities were as follows: MRI 98.3 percent, TEE 97.7 percent, and CT 93.8 percent; TTE, with 59.3 percent, was significantly lower. MRI and CT were highly specific at 97.8 percent and 87.1 percent, respectively; however, TTE and TEE did less well, with specificities of 83 percent and 77 percent, respectively. MRI, CT, and TEE were significantly more sensitive to detection of thrombus than TTE. MRI and TEE were highly accurate in detecting the entry site and aortic insufficiency, but CT was not. On the basis of these findings, they proposed an initial noninvasive diagnostic strategy whereby hemodynamically stable patients could be evaluated by MRI and unstable bed-bound patients could be evaluated by transesophageal echocardiography.

Ultimately, the diagnostic modality chosen will depend on the availability of each modality at a given institution and the preference of the local surgeon. Aortography will be chosen if the surgeon wants to have a complete vascular map and information on the patency of branch vessels and aortic insufficiency. On the other hand, if aortography is not readily available, and, depending on the clinical status of the patient (e.g., not a candidate for aortography, or no evidence for coronary or carotid artery, or aortic valve, involvement), the surgeon may operate on CT or MRI findings alone or in combination with transesophageal echocardiography. At times, TEE alone may provide all of the crucial information. Aortography continues to enjoy the status of a "gold standard." However, with the rapid technological advancements described above and with the new focus on "technology assessment" providing convincing studies that suggest better alternative imaging strategies, aortography's central role will be challenged in the future.

Management and Prognosis

Within the last decade, the management of dissecting aortic aneurysm has become more established.[23,24,36,37,71,73,74] Initially, upon presentation and regardless of the type of dissection, the objective is to stabilize the patient, and possibly prevent further dissection by decreasing the blood pressure and the velocity of left ventricular contraction in patients in whom dissection has been demonstrated. Patients qualifying for continued medical therapy are those with uncomplicated distal dissections (type B) whose lives or central function is not in immediate danger or those for whom surgery is contraindicated.

In contrast, immediate surgery is indicated in dissections involving the ascending aorta (type A), and when there is evidence of external rupture into the pericardium or pleural cavity, massive aortic regurgitation with heart failure, or occlusion of major branches to critical organs, such as the brain, heart, intestines, and kidneys. Thus contraindications to medical therapy at the time of admission include congestive heart failure, hemopericardium or evidence of rupture elsewhere, the new development of aortic regurgitation, and jeopardized carotid or coronary arteries.

The point has been made that when the false channel is visualized on aortography the mortality is far higher than when the false channel is not visualized.[74,75] On the other hand, if the cases from which these conclusions were drawn are arranged with regard to the location of the dissection, ascending aortic dissections have a mortality of 79 percent and descending aortic dissections have a mortality of 12 percent, simply reflecting the diminished hazard of dissections that begin in the descending aorta.[74,75]

In patients with ascending aortic dissection, early experience at the Peter Bent Brigham Hospital indicated that the survival of those treated surgically is three times as high as the survival rate of those treated medically (64 percent as opposed to 22 percent). In contrast, in patients with descending aortic dissection at the Peter Bent Brigham Hospital, earlier results indicated that medical therapy was successful in about 50 percent of patients, the remainder requiring surgery.

Because surgical correction is feasible and effective in aortic dissection, it is the treatment of choice, when performed promptly, for virtually all patients in whom the dissection is located in the ascending aorta. In contrast, patients with dissection of the descending aorta in the Brigham series had few urgent indications for surgical therapy. Medical therapy was therefore feasible and was instituted in all such patients. Experience indicates that it should be tried initially in patients with dissection of the descending aorta. Although surgical therapy is hazardous after medical therapy has failed, it should be undertaken nevertheless. Reported overall operative mortality ranges from 5 percent[23] to 22 percent,[24] being significantly higher in patients undergoing repair for acute (33 percent) versus chronic (9 percent) dissections.[24,73] Nearly 30 percent of all late deaths are due to subsequent aneurysm formation and rupture.[71] With proper postsurgical follow-up and treatment, the 10-year survival has been steadily improving and has recently been reported at 50 to 60 percent.[23,24] Other studies indicate that the overall 10-year survival of all patients treated for dissection is 40 percent, and for those leaving the hospital after initial treatment it is 60 percent.[23,24,37]

The foregoing data underline the urgent need to establish the diagnosis as soon as aortic dissection is suspected. Ascending aortic dissection may then be promptly approached surgically, whereas descending aortic dissection should be approached using a hypotensive regimen.[23,36,37,76,77] The aim of this treatment is to decrease blood pressure to the lowest level possible while maintaining adequate cerebral, cardiac, and renal perfusion.[23,36,37]

All of the modern assumptions about treatment, while based on solid data, are now undergoing reconsideration in the light of the established usefulness of stents in aortic dissection (see Chapter 23 in *Abrams' Angiography: Interventional Radiology*). As they become more widely used, they may replace medical and surgical therapy in many cases.

Until 20 years ago, the prognosis in aortic dissection was poor,[10] with one study reporting 80 percent of patients dying within 4 days of the onset and about 33 percent dying within the first 24 hours.[21] Modern medical, surgical, and interventional radiologic approaches are resulting in improved survival rates, and have placed in sharp focus the importance of both early suspicion of the diagnosis and definitive recognition and delineation of the anatomic abnormalities on an emergency basis.[29]

References

1. Eyler WR, Clark MD. Dissecting aneurysm of the aorta: roentgen manifestations including a comparison with other types of aneurysms. Radiology 1965;83:1047.
2. Braunwald E. Heart disease: a textbook of cardiovascular medicine. Philadelphia: Saunders, 1980.
3. Wheat MW Jr. Acute dissecting aneurysms of the aorta: diagnosis and treatment—1979. Am Heart J 1980;99:373.
4. Sutton D. Arteriography in the diagnosis of dissecting aneurysm. Clin Radiol 1960;11:85.
5. Holesh S. Dissecting aneurysm of the aorta. Br J Radiol 1960; 33:302.
6. Mandel W, Evans WE, Walsford RL. Dissecting aortic aneurysm during pregnancy. N Engl J Med 1954;251:1059.
7. Anagnostopoulos CE, Manakavalan JSP, Kittle CF. Aortic dissections and dissecting aneurysms. Am J Cardiol 1972;30:263.
8. Hemley S, Kanick V, Kittredge R, Finby N. Dissecting aneurysms of the thoracic aorta: their angiographic demonstration. AJR 1964;91:1263.
9. Pressler V, McNamara JJ. Thoracic aortic aneurysm: natural history and treatment. J Thorac Cardiovasc Surg 1980;79:489.
10. Hirst AE, Johns VJ Jr, Kime SW Jr. Dissecting aneurysm of the aorta: a review of 505 cases. Medicine (Baltimore) 1958;37: 217.
11. Wellons HA Jr, Singh R. Acute dissecting aortic aneurysm resulting from retrograde brachial arterial catheterization. Am J Cardiol 1974;33:562.
12. White CW, Zoller RP. Left aortic dissection following repair of coarctation of the aorta: the contribution of abnormal hemodynamics to medial degeneration. Chest 1973;63:573.
13. Benedict JS, Buhl TL, Henney RP. Acute aortic dissection during cardiopulmonary bypass: successful treatment of three patients. Arch Surg 1974;108:810.
14. Derkac W, Laks H, Cohn LW, Collins JJ. Dissecting aneurysm after aortic valve replacement. Arch Surg 1974;109:388.
15. Williams CD, Suwansirikul S, Engelman RM. Thoracic aortic dissection following cannulation for perfusion. Ann Thorac Surg 1974;18:300.
16. Nicholls F. Observations concerning the body of his late majesty. Philos Trans R Soc Lond (Biol) 1862;52:265.
17. Symbas PN, Baldwin BJ, Silverman ME, Galambos JT. Marfan's syndrome with aneurysm of ascending aorta and aortic regurgitation. Am J Cardiol 1970;25:483.
18. Voigt J, Hart Hansen JP. Spontaneous rupture of the aorta in young people: its relation to so-called medionecrosis cystica and Marfan's syndrome. Acta Pathol Microbiol Scand 1970; 212(Suppl):143.
19. Wilson SK, Hutchins GM. Aortic dissecting aneurysms: causative factors in 204 patients. Arch Pathol Lab Med 1982;106: 175.
20. Cavanzo FJ, Taylor HB. Effect of pregnancy on the human aorta and its relationship to dissecting aneurysms. Am J Obstet Gynecol 1969;105:567.
21. Schlatmann TJM, Becker AE. Pathogenesis of dissecting aneurysm of aorta: comparative histopathologic study of significance of medical changes. Am J Cardiol 1977;39:21.
22. Schlatmann TJM, Becker AE. Histologic changes in the normal aging aorta: implications for dissecting aortic aneurysm. Am J Cardiol 1977;39:13.
23. Crawford ES. The diagnosis and management of aortic dissection. JAMA 1990;264:2537.
24. Haverich A, Miller DC, Scott WC, Mitchell RS, Oyer PE, Stinson EB, Shumway NE. Acute and chronic dissections—determinants of long-term outcome for operative survivors. Circulation 1985;72 (Suppl 2):22.
25. Fothergill EF, Bowen DAL, Mason JK. Dissecting and atherosclerotic aneurysms: a survey of post-mortem examinations, 1968–1977. Med Sci Law 1979;19:253.
26. Schnitker MA, Bayer CA. Dissecting aneurysm of the aorta in young individuals, particularly in association with pregnancy, with report of a case. Ann Intern Med 1944;20:486.
27. Manalo-Estrella P, Barker AE. Histopathologic findings in human aortic media associated with pregnancy: a study of 16 cases. Arch Pathol 1967;83:336.
28. DeBakey ME, Cooley DA, Creech O Jr. Surgical considerations of dissecting aneurysm of the aorta. Am J Surg 1955;142:586.
29. Miller DC, Stinson EB, Oyer PE, Rossiter SJ, Reitz BA, Griepp RB, Shumway NE. Operative treatment of aortic dissections: experience with 125 patients over a sixteen-year period. J Thorac Cardiovasc Surg 1979;78:365.

30. Earnest FE IV, Muhm JR, Sheedy PF II. Roentgenographic findings in thoracic aortic dissection. Mayo Clin Proc 1979;54:43.
31. Ambos MA, Rothbert M, Lefleur R, Weiner S, McCauley D. Unsuspected aortic dissection: the chronic "healed" dissection. AJR 1979;132:221.
32. Prior JT, Buran RT, Perl T. Chronic (healed) dissecting aneurysms. J Thorac Surg 1957;33:213.
33. Wyman S. Dissecting aneurysm of the thoracic aorta: its roentgen recognition. AJR 1957;78:247.
34. Siegelman SS, Sprayregen S, Strasbert Z, Attai LA, Robinson G. Aortic dissection and the left renal artery. Radiology 1970;95:73.
35. Slater EE, DeSanctis RW. The clinical recognition of dissecting aortic aneurysm. Am J Med 1976;60:625.
36. Eagle KA, DeSanctis RW. Aortic dissection. Curr Probl Cardiol 1989;14:225.
37. Kunita Y. A pathological study of dissecting aneurysm in individuals under forty years of age including a case of a 13 year old boy. Acta Pathol Jpn 1978;28:253.
38. DeSanctis RW, Doroghazi RM, Austen WG, Buckley MJ. Aortic dissection. N Engl J Med 1987;317:1060.
39. Dalen JE, Alpert JS, Cohn LH, Black H, Collins JJ. Dissection of the thoracic aorta: medical or surgical therapy? Am J Cardiol 1974;34:803.
40. Erb BD, Tullis F. Dissecting aneurysms of the aorta: the clinical features of 30 autopsied cases. Circulation 1960;22:325.
41. Greenberg DI, Davia JE, McAllister HA, Cheitlin MD. Dissecting aortic aneurysm manifesting as acute pericarditis. Arch Intern Med 1979;139:108.
42. Nelson AR. Chronic hemothorax from contained aortic rupture. Ann Thorac Surg 1970;9:186.
43. Schechter GL, Brownson RJ. Aortic arch aneurysm and vertigo: a case report. Ann Otol 1970;79:185.
44. Kanick V, Hemby S, Kittredge R, Finby N. Some problems in the angiographic diagnosis of dissecting aneurysms of the thoracic aorta. AJR 1964;91:1283.
45. Hart WF, Berman EJ, LaCom RJ. Hazard of retrograde aortography in dissecting aneurysm. Circulation 1963;27:1140.
46. Baum S, Abrams HL. A J-shaped catheter for retrograde catheterization of tortuous vessels. Radiology 1964;83:436.
47. Caplan L, Furman S, Bosniak M, Robinson G. Right transaxillary thoracic aortography in the diagnosis of dissecting aneurysm. AJR 1965;95:696.
48. Petasnick JP. Radiologic evaluation of aortic dissection. Radiology 1991;180:297.
49. Shuford WH, Syber RG, Weens HS. Problems in the aortographic diagnosis of dissecting aneurysm of the aorta. N Engl J Med 1969;280:225.
50. Eagle KA, Quertermous T, Kritzer GA. Spectrum of conditions initially suggesting aortic dissection but with negative aortograms. Am J Cardiol 1986;57:322.
51. Yamada T, Tada S, Harada J. Aortic dissection without intimal rupture: diagnosis with MR imaging and CT. Radiology 1988;168:347.
52. Wolff KA, Herold CJ, Tempany CM, Parravano JG, Zerhouni EA. Aortic dissection: atypical patterns seen at MR imaging. Radiology 1991;181:489.
53. Price JE Jr, Gray RK, Grollman JH Jr. Aortic wall thickness as an unreliable sign in the diagnosis of dissecting aneurysm of the thoracic aorta. AJR 1971;13:710.
54. Shuford WH, Sybers RG, Weens HS, Lindsay J Jr, Hurst JW. Aortographic findings in dissecting aneurysm of the aorta. Am J Cardiol 1969;24:111.
55. Cigarroa JE, Isselbacher EM, DeSanctis RW, Eagle KA. Diagnostic imaging in the evaluation of suspected aortic dissection. N Engl J Med 1993;328:35.
56. Larde D, Belloir C, Vasile N, Frija J, Ferrano J. Computed tomography of aortic dissection. Radiology 1980;136:147.
57. Goodwin JD, Herfkens RL, Skioldebrand CG, Federie MP, Lipton MJ. Evaluation of dissections and aneurysms of the thoracic aorta by conventional and dynamic CT scanning. Radiology 1980;136:125.
58. Egan TJ, Nelman HL, Herman RJ, Malave SR, Sanders JH. Computed tomography in the diagnosis of aortic aneurysm dissection or traumatic injury. Radiology 1980;136:141.
59. Vasile N, Mathieu D, Keita K, Lellouche D, Bloch G, Cachera JP. Computed tomography of thoracic aortic dissection: accuracy and pitfalls. J Comput Assist Tomogr 1986;10:211.
60. Mast HL, Gordon DH, Kantor AM. Pitfalls in diagnosis of aortic dissection by angiography: algorithmic approach utilizing CT and MRI. Comput Med Imaging Graph 1991;15:431.
61. Costello P, Ecker CP, Tello R, Hartnell GG. Assessment of the thoracic aorta by spiral CT. AJR 1992;158:1127.
62. Nienaber CA, et al. The diagnosis of thoracic aortic dissection by noninvasive imaging procedures. N Engl J Med 1993;328:1.
63. Iliceto S, Nanda N, Rizzon P, Hsuing MC, Goyal RG, Amico A, Sorino M. Color Doppler evaluation of aortic dissection. Circulation 1987;75:748.
64. Tottle AJ, Wilde P, Hartnell GG, Wisheart JD. Diagnosis of acute thoracic aortic dissection using combined echocardiography and computed tomography. Clin Radiol 1992;45:104.
65. Ballal RS, et al. Usefulness of transesophageal echocardiography in assessment of aortic dissection. Circulation 1991;84:1903.
66. Kerstig-Sommerhoff BA, Higgins CB, White RD, Sommerhoff CP, Lipton MJ. Aortic dissection: sensitivity and specificity of MR imaging. Radiology 1988;166:651.
67. Solomon SL, Brown JJ, Glazer HS, Mirowitz SA, Lee JKT. Thoracic aortic dissection: pitfalls and artifacts in MR imaging. Radiology 1990;177:223.
68. Fruehwald FXJ, Fezoulidis J, Globits S, Mayr H, Wicke K, Glogar D. Cine-MR in dissection of the thoracic aorta. Eur J Radiol 1989;9:37.
69. Bogren HG, Underwood SR, Firmin DN, Mohiaddin RH, Klipstein RH, Ress RSO, Longmore DB. Magnetic resonance velocity mapping in aortic dissection. Br J Radiol 1988;61:456.
70. Barbant SD, Eisenberg MJ, Schiller NB. The diagnostic value of imaging techniques for aortic dissection. Am Heart J 1992;124:541.
71. Kern MJ, et al. Use of coronary arteriography in the preoperative management of patients undergoing urgent repair of the thoracic aorta. Am Heart J 1990;119:143.
72. Friese KK, Caputo GR, Higgins CB. Evaluation of painless aortic dissection with MR imaging. Am Heart J 1991;122:1169.
73. Dinsmore RE, Willerson JT, Buckley MJ. Dissecting aneurysm of the aorta: aortographic features affecting prognosis. Radiology 1972;105:567.
74. DeBakey ME, McCollum CH, Crawford ES. Dissection and dissecting aneurysms of the aorta: twenty-year follow-up of five hundred twenty-seven patients treated surgically. Surgery 1982;92:1118.
75. McFarland J, Willerson JT, Dinsmore RE, Austen WG, Buckley MJ, Sanders CA, DeSanctis RW. The medical treatment of dissecting aortic aneurysms. N Engl J Med 1972;286:115.
76. Jex RK, et al. Repair of ascending aortic dissection: influence of associated aortic valve insufficiency on early and late results. J Thorac Cardiovasc Surg 1987;93:375.
77. Wheat MW. Treatment of dissecting aneurysms of the ascending aorta: current status. Prog Cardiovasc Dis 1973;16:87.

21

Blunt Trauma to the Thoracic Aorta and Brachiocephalic Arteries

YORAM BEN-MENACHEM
RICHARD G. FISHER

In the United States, laceration of the thoracic aorta is sustained by approximately 8000 persons annually.[1] More than 80 percent of these victims die at the scene, en route to the hospital, or within an average of 24 minutes from arrival at the hospital, and almost half of those who live long enough to undergo thoracotomy for this injury do not survive.[2] In most events the cause of death is exsanguination from the transected aorta, although a significant minority of patients die of head injuries.[3] Although aortic laceration is primarily an adult injury, it occurs also in children below age 16.[4,5] Because in the pediatric age group this injury is rapidly fatal, it is rarely seen in children surviving road traffic accidents and, not being expected, is probably underinvestigated.[6]

The source of clinical material for this chapter is one author's teaching file, which includes 131 patients with 138 acute and 8 chronic aortic-brachiocephalic (ABC) injuries (Table 21-1), sustained in 132 accidents (Table 21-2).

Mechanisms of Injury

There is no consensus regarding the exact wounding mechanism responsible for rupture of the thoracic aorta and brachiocephalic arteries. Several theories have been proposed over the years; none offers complete and precise understanding of the event, but some—for lack of better explanation—have been repeatedly copied from one article or book to another, finally achieving the status of editorial dogma although never that of scientific conviction. Neither animal experiments nor work with human cadavers has been able to duplicate the event or to explain it. There is no doubt that ABC injuries are caused by a wide variety of mechanisms, and in very different accident environments (see Table 21-2), including such rare causes as equestrian accidents.[7] Sevitt[8] documented this fact and demonstrated that deceleration produces injuries of the aortic isthmus whereas direct impact causes trauma to the ascending aorta and the arch; because of the multiple sites of rupture, even at the isthmus—some injuries occur above the ligamentum arteriosum and some below it—Sevitt concludes that there are several different mechanisms.[9] For this reason, defining all blunt ABC injuries as "deceleration injuries" is a misleading oversimplification.

Some of the characteristics of the thoracic aorta, as documented in laboratory investigations, may help one to better understand the conditions under which it ruptures. Lundevall[10] has shown that the resistance of the isthmus to sudden tension and stretching is much less than that of the rest of the thoracic aorta. It has also been shown that vascular elements tolerate blunt forces very well because of their elastic fibers, but are extremely sensitive to shearing and twisting forces,[11] and that it is possible for the aorta to fail with a tear due to high pressure alone.[12] There is today enough evidence to show that rupture of the aortic isthmus in unrestrained frontal collisions (Fig. 21-1) is caused by a combination of sudden traction and a hydrostatic blowout, and that they can occur also with other mechanisms that create similar conditions. However, lacerations of the thoracic aorta are now seen with increasing frequency in victims of broadside impacts,[13] and other ABC injuries are produced by shearing and twisting forces, by crushing, or by contact wounding from fractures of the sternum.

Initial Assessment

For lack of a better method, triage of patients after violent blunt chest trauma begins with physical examination and the admission chest film. However, because

Table 21-1. Blunt Aortic-Brachiocephalic Trauma: Anatomic Sites of 146 Intrathoracic ABC Injuries in 131 Patients

Anatomic Site	Number	Percent
Aorta		
Ascending	6	
Arch	17	
Isthmus	89	
Descending	7	
Total	119[a]	81.5
Brachiocephalic Arteries		
Innominate		
Associated[b]	6	
Solitary	2	
	8[c]	
Subclavian		
Associated[b]	3	
Solitary	13[d]	
	16	
Carotid (all associated)	3	
Total	27	18.5

[a]Includes 8 chronic traumatic false aneurysms.
[b]Associated with laceration of the thoracic aorta or with another brachiocephalic artery.
[c]Includes 3 partial avulsions from the aortic arch by a fractured sternum.
[d]One patient injured both subclavian arteries.

Table 21-2. Blunt Aortic-Brachiocephalic Trauma: 132 Etiologies in 131 Patients*

Etiology		Number	Percent
In-vehicle, car			
Frontal, unrestrained	—driver	38	
	—driver ejected	4	
	—passenger	9	
Frontal, restrained	—driver	4	
	—passenger	2	
Broadside	—driver or passenger	13	
Exact mechanism unknown		16	
Total		86	65.1
Motorcycle		19	14.4
Pedestrians		9	6.8
Falls		5	3.8
Aircraft, frontal impact		1	0.8
Aircraft, broadside impact		1	0.8
Others and unknown		11	8.3

*One patient injured and reinjured the aortic isthmus in two separate accidents.

both are severely limited in their capacity to provide useful information, experienced physicians are directed by the mechanism of injury to suspect ABC trauma.

Clinical Presentation

An ABC laceration may be accompanied by any of 11 clinical signs, including (1) external evidence of trauma to the chest, (2) palpable sternal fracture, (3) expanding hematoma at the thoracic outlet, (4) interscapular murmur, (5) upper extremity hypertension, (6) diminished or absent pulses in the right upper limb, (7) diminished or absent femoral pulses (posttraumatic pseudocoarctation), (8) palpable fracture of the thoracic spine, (9) flail left chest, (10) elevated central venous pressure, and (11) hypotension.[14] These clinical signs often are obscured by those of other, more obvious injuries.[15]

Among those who die of a ruptured thoracic aorta at the scene of accident, at least 10 percent have no external signs of trauma to the body.[16] The same applies to survivors of road traffic accidents: up to 50 percent of patients with blunt ABC injuries have no external physical signs of thoracic injury.[14]

Accompanying Injuries

ABC injury is commonly associated with multiple other injuries, some of them potentially lethal. Although the highest percentage of a second fatal injury (41.2 percent) is found among those dead at the scene,[3] survivors sustain the same accompanying injuries as nonsurvivors—except for open cardiac injuries—although in smaller numbers: 2.6 associated injuries in survivors versus 4.0 in nonsurvivors of traumatic aortic rupture.[17]

Abdominal and posterior extraperitoneal injuries, commonly the cause of preventable death in patients with ABC trauma,[18] include lacerations and ruptures of the liver, spleen, stomach, colon, small intestine, kidneys, and diaphragm—even in seat belt users[19]—as well as of the abdominal aorta and its branches,[20] and major abdominal veins.[21] In frontal collisions and motorcycle accidents the distribution of abdominal injuries shows no predilection to site or side. In broadside impacts, on the other hand, the most severe if not the only abdominal injuries will be in the side of the abdomen that was on the receiving end of the impact;[22] the diagnosis of these injuries must be aggressively pursued, often irrespective of clinical symptoms. The recognition of the potential lethality of the thoracic aortic injury and of its accompanying abdominal injuries is a challenge that may call for extraordinary surgical judgment, because it is often difficult to assess the urgency of management of the various injuries. The tendency to take care of an obvious injury, such as a ruptured hemidiaphragm, may prove fatal (Fig. 21-2).[23]

Fractures of the upper thoracic spine often produce superior mediastinal hematomas identical to those accompanying ABC lacerations.[24] However, the presence of upper thoracic spinal fractures by no means excludes aortic injury in the "classic" site; indeed, recent evidence suggests the frequency of ABC injury is higher—and almost invariably fatal—in patients with

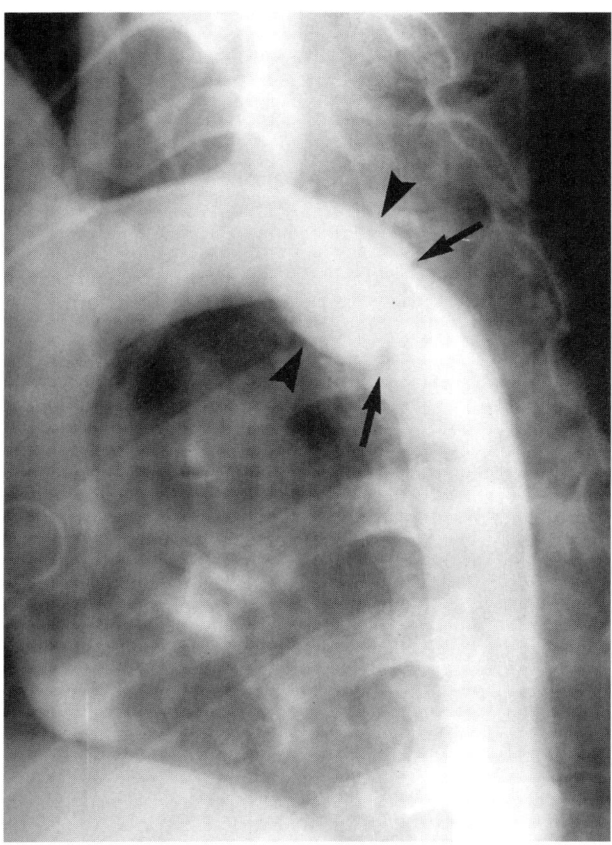

A

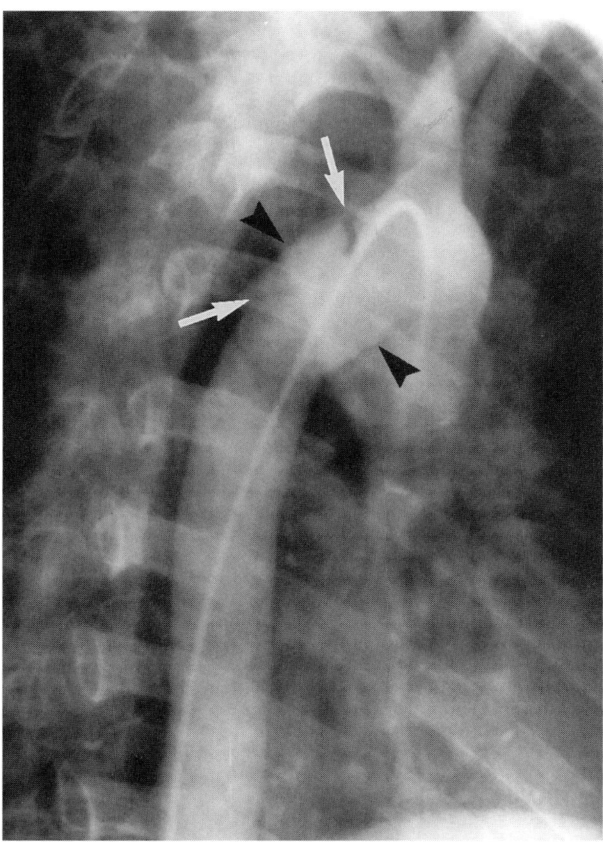

B

Figure 21-1. The isthmic transection, which accounts for 61 percent of all blunt ABC lacerations, is circumferential; therefore, both (A) right posterior oblique (RPO) and (B) left posterior oblique (LPO) projections show the tear lines in the intima and media (*arrows*) and the subadventitial collection of contrast medium (*between arrowheads*). The brachiocephalic arteries are intact. These are the correct projections, and centering, of thoracic aortography for blunt trauma.

vertebral fractures involving T1 to T8.[25] On the other hand, *fracture dislocations of the thoracolumbar spine* were found to be associated with transection of the lower thoracic aorta and the supraceliac abdominal aorta.[26]

Pelvic fractures and ABC injuries are closely associated. In a database of 63,763 patients with major trauma, the rate of occurrence of ruptured thoracic aorta in patients with pelvic fractures (1.6 percent) was

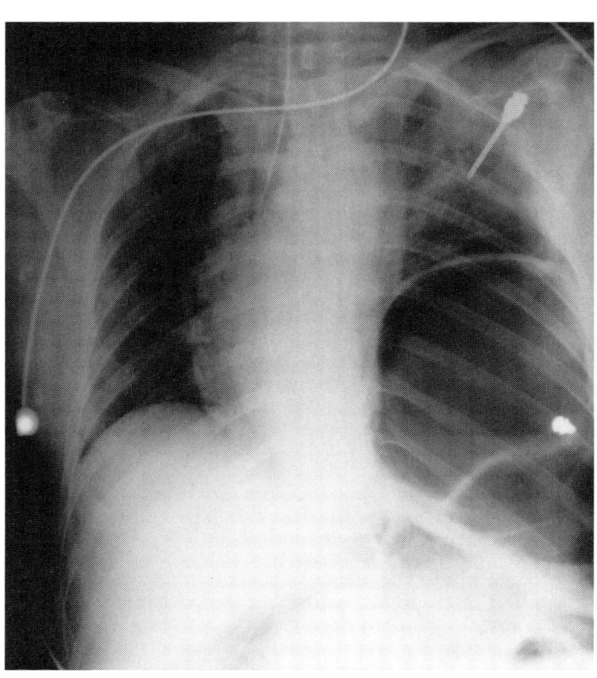

Figure 21-2. Admission chest film of a patient injured in an unrestrained frontal automobile collision. The superior mediastinal hematoma and the mechanism of injury should have directed the patient for emergency aortography, but were ignored in favor of the obvious evidence of a ruptured left hemidiaphragm. The patient bled to death from her transected thoracic aorta during laparotomy. (From Ben-Menachem Y. Imaging techniques in trauma. In: Maull KI, ed. Advances in trauma and critical care. Chicago: Mosby–Year Book, 1992;7:191–217. Used with permission.)

3.2 times that of the overall occurrence (0.5 percent), and 19.5 percent of patients with aortic injuries also had pelvic fractures—2.4 times the overall frequency of pelvic fractures (8.1 percent).[27] Furthermore, in patients whose pelvis was fractured by anteroposterior compression, the likelihood of rupture of the aorta is nine times greater than in the general trauma population.[28] Given that both injuries are potentially fatal, one would be well advised to possess a higher level of suspicion of ABC injury with respect to patients with pelvic ring disruptions.

Preliminary Radiography and Imaging

The admission chest film—cheap and noninvasive—is considered "easy reading" by most physicians. Unfortunately, not only is the chest film more difficult to read than most physicians admit, but it offers only a limited amount of gross information regarding the mediastinum and no information at all regarding vascular injuries.[29] This is especially evident in massive injuries, where a portable, supine chest film is the only one available.[30] Because none of the roentgen signs associated with mediastinal hematomas have statistically *predictive* significance in diagnosing a ruptured aorta,[15,31] they are not discussed here. For the purpose of emergency room reading of the chest film it suffices to remember that a hematoma blurs normal tissue planes[32] and displaces normal structures, but that its presence does not by any means guarantee the presence of a major arterial injury. Although patients with no mediastinal hematomas are unlikely to have sustained ABC injuries,[32,33] there still is ample evidence showing that even a patient with normal mediastinum may have an aortic tear.[34,35]

There is no correlation between *rib fractures* and ABC injuries.[36] Similarly, first and second rib fractures alone do not predict the presence of major intrathoracic vascular injuries.[37,38]

Given its limitations, the chest film cannot be expected to contain direct information of injury; what it does yield is, at best, circumstantial evidence. The need for rapid diagnosis of ABC injuries mandates further investigation, and the question then arises as to whether one must proceed with emergency aortography or continue with noninvasive studies in an attempt to avoid aortography.

At the time of writing of this chapter there is no substitute for aortography. The study one employs must provide direct evidence of all possible ABC injuries, and it must do so rapidly and reliably (i.e., with the least probability of false-positive or false-negative results). None of the available noninvasive modalities are capable of doing this.

Computed tomography (CT) carries a high rate of both false positives and false negatives.[39,40] Inserting CT into workup protocols of patients after severe trauma is frivolous and irresponsible: patients with ruptured aortas tend to die quickly, and every procedure or examination that postpones definite diagnosis may directly contribute to their demise.[23,41,42] Furthermore, because inclusion of CT in such protocols virtually guarantees that all patients with blunt chest trauma will undergo CT, one can expect a significant number of cases of "death by extrapolation."

Magnetic resonance imaging has too many technical and management obstacles and limitations to be regarded as a usable modality.

Transesophageal echocardiography offers a promise of rapid diagnosis on the triage table. However, although its preliminary results are encouraging,[43,44] this modality must be developed further to ensure complete diagnosis (including that of brachiocephalic artery trauma) and must be reliable enough to allow surgeons to make a decision to go to the operating theater without the need for angiography.

Angiography

Angiography is the only modality that can be relied on to document vascular injury or normalcy by direct evidence and with a negligible minimum of error.[15,32,45,46] It is also a safe procedure.[15] Therefore, whenever ABC injury is suspected, even from the slightest suspicion or evidence, aortography is mandatory and urgent.

Angiographic Technique

In setting up to perform thoracic aortography, the angiographer must plan thoracoabdominal aortography and also, if necessary, pelvic arteriography. This should be done as a matter of routine (except when the patient had a negative abdominopelvic CT scan immediately before angiography) in view of the frequent presence of associated injuries and pelvic fractures.[47,48] The abdominal aortogram should be done even if diagnostic peritoneal lavage was negative because the purpose of the angiogram is primarily to detect hemorrhage in the posterior and lateral abdominal extraperitoneum. Extension of the thoracic study to the abdomen and pelvis does not waste time—even when the thoracic aortogram is positive—because the extension requires only a few minutes and is usually completed long before the surgeon has alerted the thoracic surgeons and called to reserve an operating theater.

The preferred access is transfemoral, because it is safe to cross the injured aortic segment as long as the injury allows it.[49,50] If a femoral artery is not accessible, for any reason, a *right* axillary access should be used; because the majority of aortic injuries involve the isthmus, and some even extend proximally, a left axillary approach is hazardous and must be discouraged. The procedure should be performed via an introducer sheath (7 French, one-way flow). The introducer allows catheter exchange should there be a need for embolization; also, it can be left in the femoral artery at the end of the procedure to serve as an arterial line during the operation. Leaving the introducer in the access artery saves the 10 to 15 minutes that would be otherwise needed for puncture site hemostasis.

The preferred catheter for midstream aortography in trauma is a 7 French pigtail catheter (Royal Flush Plus by Cook), capable of administering 50 ml per second. The safest guidewire is a 0.038-inch, Teflon-coated, LLT, 2-mm J guidewire (Cook).

Figure 21-3. Improper performance of thoracic aortography for blunt trauma. The radiologist advanced the catheter—not a soft J-guidewire—into the proximal descending aorta and, when meeting resistance at the point of transection (*arrow*), forced the catheter against the resistance for over 5 cm (*arrowhead*), extending the subadventitial dissection to the origin of the left common carotid artery, and placing the patient at a high risk of a massive stroke. Moreover, the violent manipulation of the catheter could have brought on the completion of the transection, immediately killing the patient. See text and Figure 21-4 for comments and comparison.

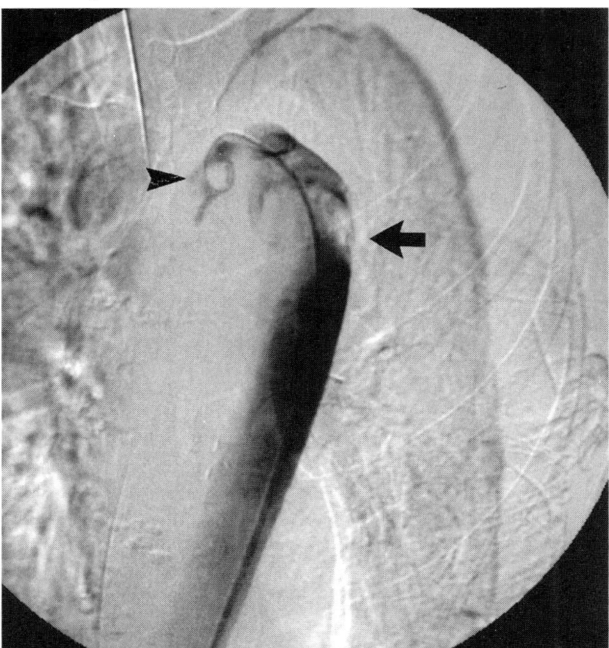

Working through the introducer, the guidewire must lead the way; the catheter tip should be at least 20 cm behind the guidewire's J. The guidewire must be advanced into and through the thoracic aorta slowly and under constant fluoroscopic view. If passage of the guidewire into the ascending aorta is smooth, the catheter can be advanced as well. Occasionally, the aortic injury interferes with passage of the guidewire. When this happens, one can both feel slight resistance to the guidewire's advance and see the guidewire buckle slightly at the site of injury (this is the reason for an LLT-J). *No attempt must ever be made to force the catheter through the resistance, nor should one inject contrast medium at the site of transection or below it:* not only will either of these aggravate the aortic injury, but they are likely to kill the patient (Fig. 21-3).[51] The transfemoral thoracic procedure must be abandoned and confined to the abdomen and pelvis. Instead, the thoracic aorta can be accessed via the axillary artery. However, because the diagnosis, in fact, has already been made, its documentation can be done by transvenous digital subtraction angiography (DSAV), provided the patient can stop breathing or be rendered apneic for image acquisition.[49] Access is via the femoral vein on the same side on which the artery was punctured (Fig. 21-4).

Figure 21-4. Transvenous DSA as substitute for transarterial aortography in a case of posttraumatic coarctation syndrome. When the leading guidewire met with resistance at the bottom of the lesion, it was removed and the transarterial study was aborted. The sterile right groin was reutilized to transvenously introduce an intraatrial catheter through which this study was performed. The transection is clearly seen (*between arrows*); this angiogram is probably sufficient to declare the rest of the thoracic aorta and the brachiocephalic arteries intact.

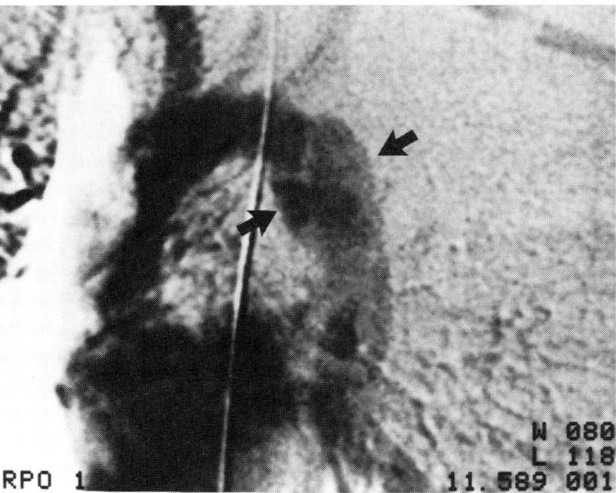

Contrast Medium Injection and Image Acquisition

The great majority of trauma patients exhibit high cardiac output and hyperdynamic circulation. The contrast medium injection rate and the filming or imaging program must accommodate these hemodynamics. The best studies of adult patients are achieved by injecting 50 ml of contrast medium at 50 ml per second, delivered at 1200 psi, for each thoracic aortogram. The abdominal aortogram for an adult trauma patient requires 60 ml at 35 to 40 ml per second.

Imaging can be on film or digital matrix (DSA) and must document the entire length of the thoracic aorta, as well as the intrathoracic and part of the extrathoracic courses of the brachiocephalic arteries. The thoracic aortogram must be done with two oblique views (the AP projection had been discarded as useless)[50–52]: 40 to 45 degrees RPO (right posterior oblique) and 45 to 50 degrees LPO (left posterior oblique). The film or screen image must show the entire thoracic aorta as well as the brachiocephalic arteries well beyond the thoracic outlet (see Fig. 21-1). If the RPO is positive, the LPO becomes unnecessary if it is not helpful to the surgeon. One must never rely on a negative, one-view aortogram. When a small laceration of the aorta involves the posteromedial wall alone, it can be seen only on the LPO projection. We have twice missed just such injuries by avoiding the LPO (Fig. 21-5), as have others.[53] The following are details on contrast medium and filming:

Imaging on film. Contrast medium: 370 mg iodine/ml, undiluted. Film program: 4 films per second for 2 seconds, 1 film per second for 4 seconds.

Digital imaging. Contrast medium: 370 mg iodine/ml, diluted with saline to 25 percent. Imaging sequence: 4 to 6 images per second until veins are seen.

The advantage of film over DSA is its finer image resolution and the reduced distortion by breathing and motion. However, today's state-of-the-art digital software produces excellent images with the distinct advantage of speed. The recommended modality is transarterial DSA (DSAA)[54] because of its sharp images, low volume of contrast medium, and immediate access to intervention by intraarterial catheter. DSAV is not recommended except when an arterial approach is impossible and the radiologist is highly skilled in reading the images. DSAV adds a risk of contrast overload and cardiac injury. Also, its images are noisy and of inferior quality, it is time-consuming, and it does not allow access to control of hemorrhage.[30,47] DSA's greatest disadvantage is its extreme susceptibility to motion. Unless the patient is most cooperative with breath holding—either willfully or by receiving a paralyzing agent and being disconnected from the respirator—image degradation precludes the use of DSA.

Figure 21-5. Missed aortic laceration due to incomplete examination. A 67-year-old man was injured in an unrestrained frontal automobile collision. (A) Aortography in RPO showed dissection due to atheromatous disease. The study was therefore altered from that for trauma (RPO/LPO) to that for dissection (RPO for thoracic aorta, anteroposterior (AP) for arch for neck, AP for thoracoabdominal aorta). (B) After the patient's death from the dissection, autopsy showed two traumatic lacerations in the posteromedial aspect of the aortic isthmus (*arrows*).

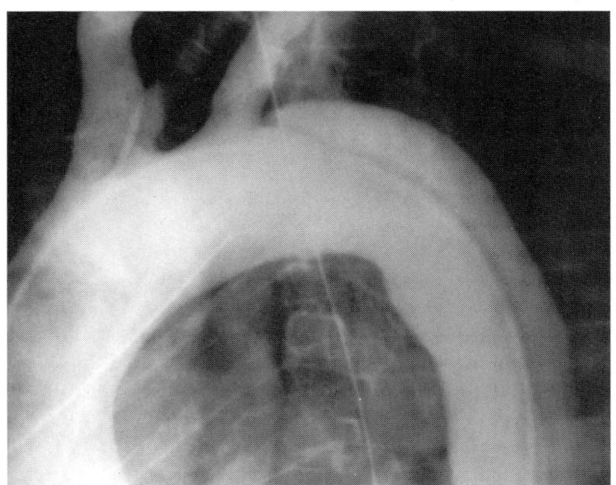

A

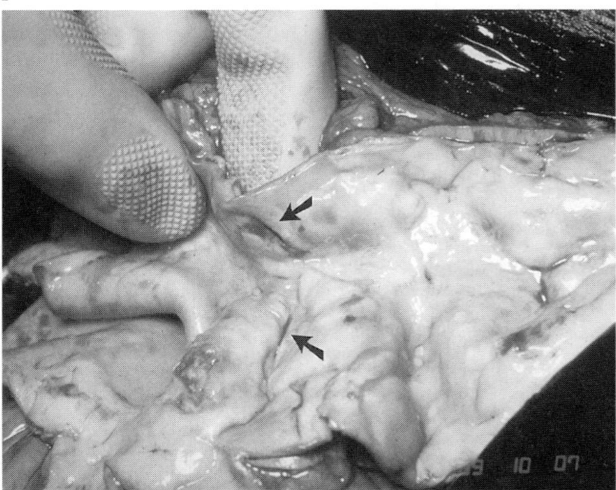

B

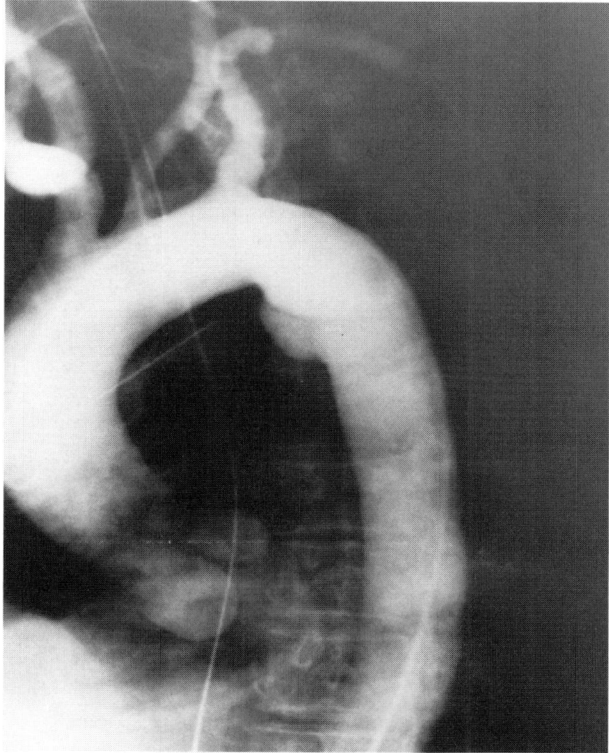

A

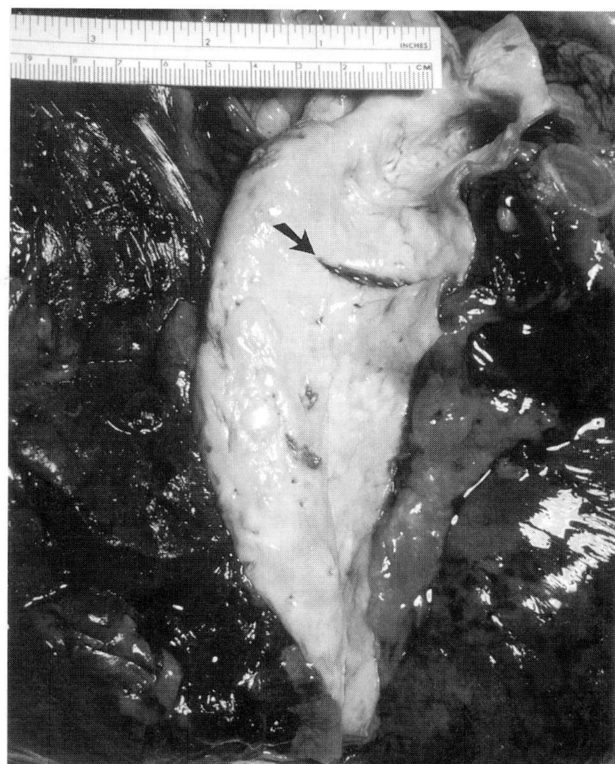

B

Figure 21-12. Typical broadside impact injury. (A) A small false aneurysm of the lesser curvature of the aorta is seen at the bottom of the arch. (B) The patient died of head injuries. Autopsy confirmed the site and size of the aortic laceration (*arrowhead*). (From Ben-Menachem Y. Rupture of the thoracic aorta by broadside impacts in road-traffic and other accidents: further angiographic observations and preliminary autopsy findings. J Trauma 1993;35:363–367. Used with permission.)

the injury is not rare—13 percent of patients in the author's files and 33 percent in Verdant's series.[69] Ten of the acute injuries in the author's experience have an almost identical angiographic presentation, namely, lacerations involving the lesser curvature of the aorta at the most distal segment of the arch, just above the isthmus. The laceration is usually transverse and incomplete and is accompanied by a relatively small false aneurysm, which might sometimes be confused with a normal "ductus bump" or a small ductus diverticulum.[49] It is important for the radiologist to recognize this specific injury and its cause because its relatively proximal location, at the bottom of the arch, leaves a shorter aortic segment with which to work; the radiologist should call the surgeon's attention to the fact.

The accompanying mediastinal hematoma varies in volume, and, as is the case with lacerations of the aorta by other mechanisms of injury, there is no association between the volume of the hematoma and the severity of the aortic laceration. The injury, as seen on the aortogram, is so distinct that in four of the author's patients assumption of a broadside impact was first made at the time of angiography based on the type and location of the aortic injury, and was later confirmed by the patient and/or by police.

Two of the 13 patients with acute injuries, whose angiographic findings differed from the rest of the group, included 1 with a transitory intramural hematoma of the proximal descending thoracic aorta and another who suffered reinjury of a chronic isthmic false aneurysm. One patient did not undergo angiography at all because a superior mediastinal hematoma on chest films was ignored and a positive chest CT was misread as negative.

Angiographic Findings

Most broadside impact lacerations are best, if not only, seen on the LPO projection. Their false aneurysms are smaller and are located higher than those of the torn isthmus. The anterolateral wall of the aorta is intact (Fig. 21-12). Rarely, a broadside collision may produce an aortic intramural hematoma, without

◀ **Figure 21-11.** Total (three-layer) transection of the isthmus. (A) The rugged outer border of the false aneurysm is an additional sign of impending fatal hemorrhage. (B) This opposite oblique projection was not necessary. This patient died in the operating theater of exsanguinating hemorrhage from both the aorta and the pulmonary artery.

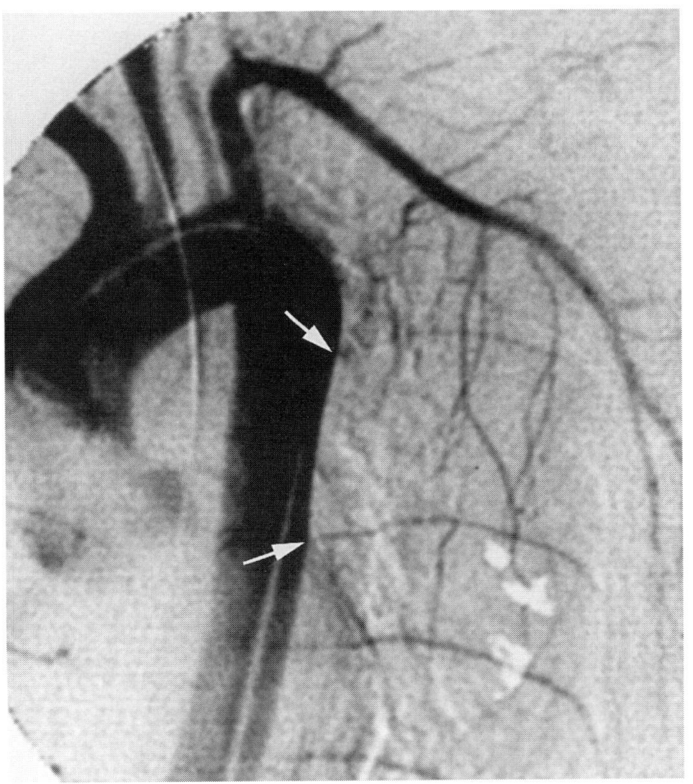

A

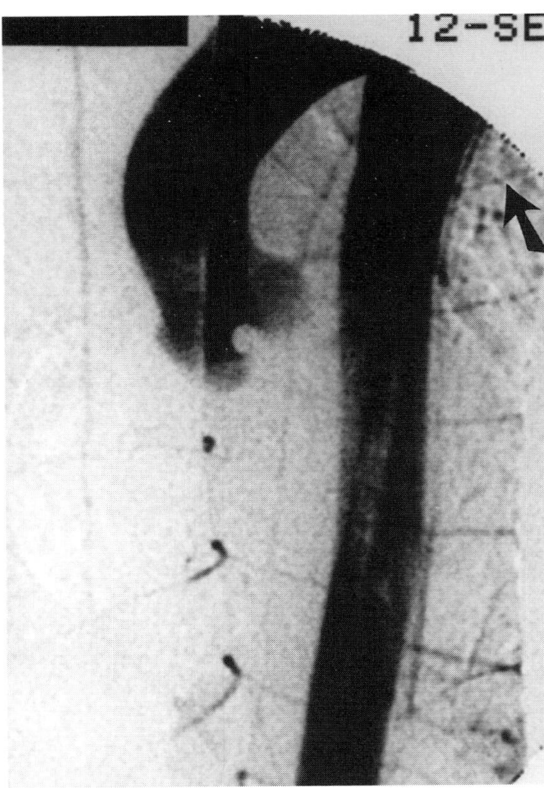

B

Figure 21-13. Minimal aortic injury in driver after left broadside impact. Thoracic aortogram on admission (A) shows slight concavity of a short segment of the proximal descending aorta (*between arrows*), representing a limited intramural hematoma; the sixth left posterior intercostal artery, which arises from this segment, is compressed at its origin by the intramural hematoma and remains unopacified. Follow-up aortogram 19 days later (B) shows normal aortic contour and reappearance of the sixth left posterior intercostal artery (*arrow*) after resorption of the hematoma. (From Ben-Menachem Y. Rupture of the thoracic aorta by broadside impacts in road-traffic and other accidents: further angiographic observations and preliminary autopsy findings. J Trauma 1993;35:363–367. Used with permission.)

laceration; this hematoma does not require surgical intervention and will be resorbed in a few weeks (Fig. 21-13).

Contact Wounding by a Fractured Sternum

To produce a cardiac or an aortic injury, the fractured sternum must buckle inward at the time of impact. Because there is usually outward buckling,[68] cardiovascular contact wounding is a rare and usually nonsurvivable event. Only three patients in the author's series suffered such a mechanism, and all had the same injury, namely, partial avulsion of the innominate artery from the aortic arch.[60] Innominate artery injuries can also be seen in crushing injuries to the chest (v.i.).

Angiographic Findings

The tear is evident at the point of origin of the innominate artery, involving either the proximal 1 cm of the artery or the aortic arch and innominate artery together. The artery may also sustain a second injury (Fig. 21-14).

ABC Injuries Associated with or Caused by Seat Belts

The defense offered by the automotive seat belt against severe injury is not absolute. When the force of impact is very high, a car occupant may sustain an aortic laceration despite the seat belt.[70,71] In addition, a restrained car occupant may be injured by the diagonal (i.e., shoulder) component of a seat belt. Usually, but

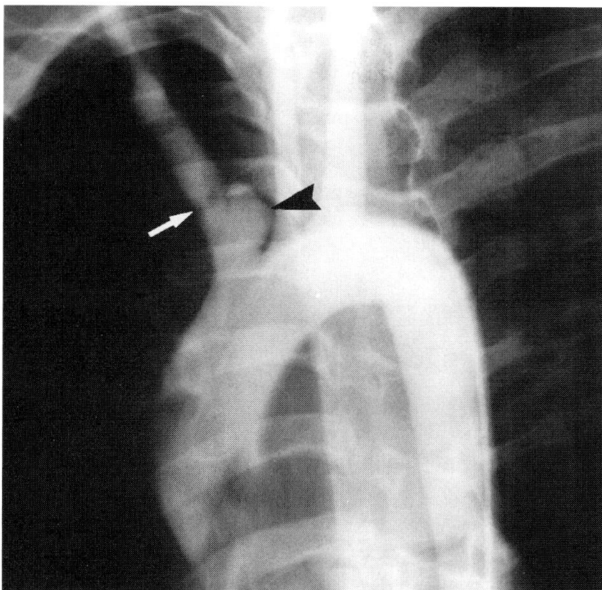

Figure 21-14. Contact wounding by a fractured sternum with partial avulsion of the innominate artery from the aorta. There is a false aneurysm at the site of injury (*arrowhead*). Disruption of the intima and media, of which only the distal boundary is seen on the aortogram (*arrow*), was shown at surgery to have begun at the aortoinnominate junction. (From Ben-Menachem Y. Avulsion of the innominate artery associated with fracture of the sternum. AJR 1988;150:621–622. Used with permission.)

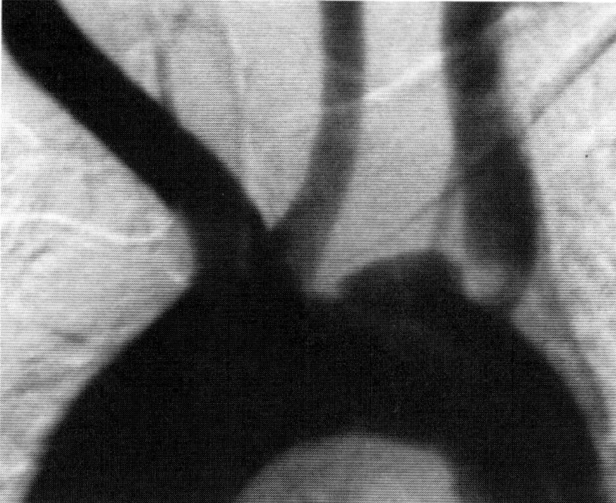

Figure 21-15. Seat belt injury, with partial avulsion of the left subclavian artery. The driver was seen in the emergency room with a prominent bruise on the left shoulder.

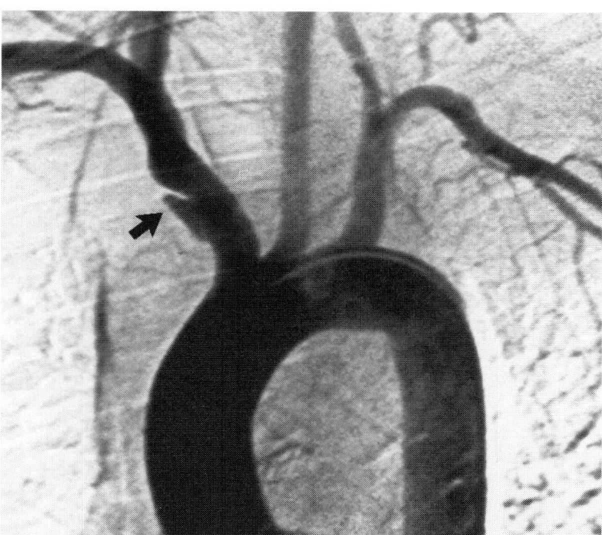

Figure 21-16. Seat belt injury, with incomplete transection of the innominate artery (*arrow*). This front seat passenger was seen in the emergency room with a prominent bruise on the right shoulder.

not necessarily (see Fig. 21-8), the injury involves the subclavian artery on the traumatized side (Fig. 21-15)[72] or the innominate artery in right-seat occupants (Fig. 21-16); however, a definite causal association is yet to be established because similar subclavian and innominate artery injuries may be sustained by car occupants not using seat belts.

Crushing ABC Injuries

The nature and severity of damage to intrathoracic structures depend on the width and center of the contact area, as well as on the intensity and direction of the crushing force. Vascular injuries seen in survivors of violent crushing trauma to the chest may involve mostly the brachiocephalic arteries and the top of the aortic arch, sometimes with partial avulsion of the innominate artery from the arch (Fig. 21-17).[73,74] In others, depending on the "epicenter" and direction of the crushing force, the descending aorta may be crushed (Fig. 21-18).

ABC Injuries by Other Mechanisms of Injury

As seen on Table 21-2, any violent blunt trauma to the chest may produce an ABC injury. Although the angiographic characteristics of many of these injuries are similar if not identical to those of ABC lacerations produced by the more "classic" wounding mechanisms, one cannot conclude that they share a common

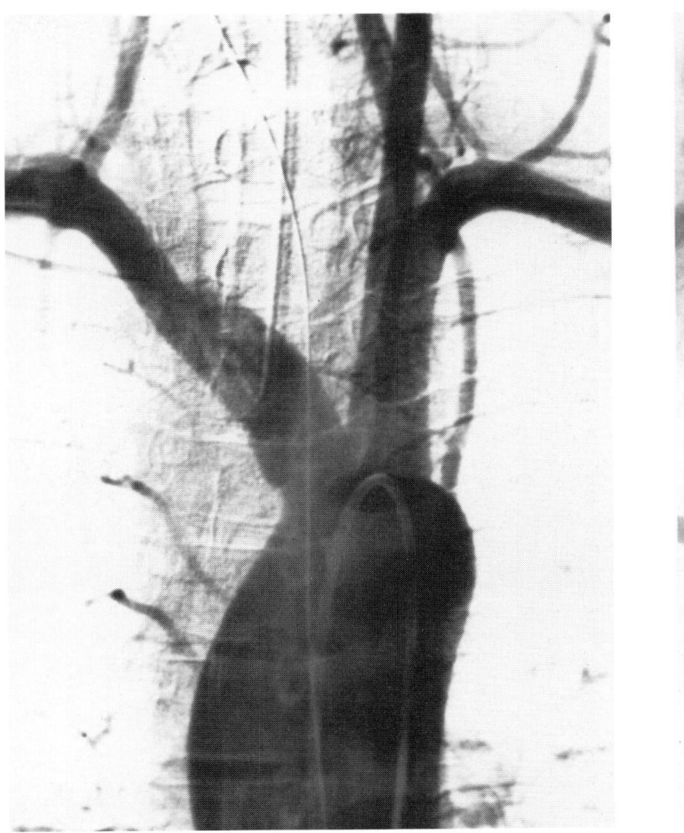

A

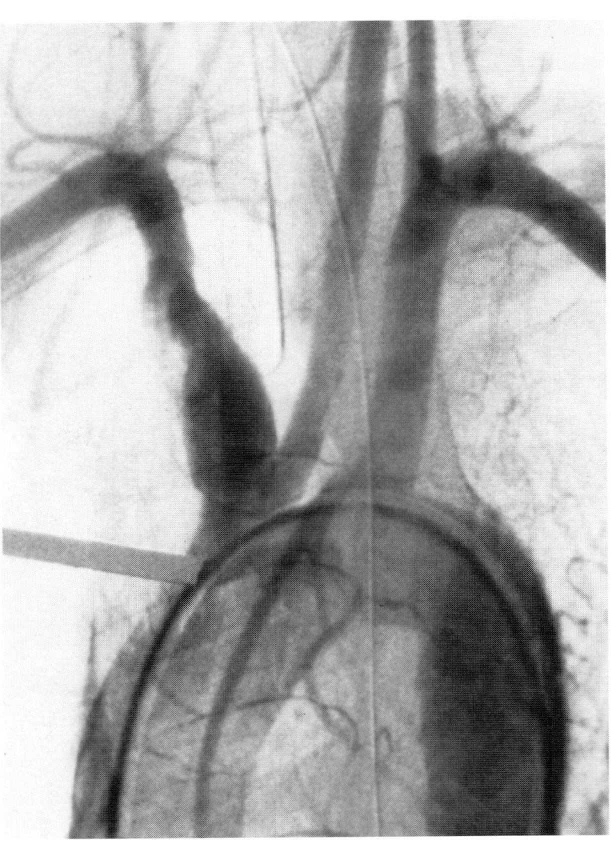

B

Figure 21-17. Crushing injury. The patient's chest was crushed under his own car. AP (A) and RPO (B) projections show subadventitial contrast medium throughout the artery's length.

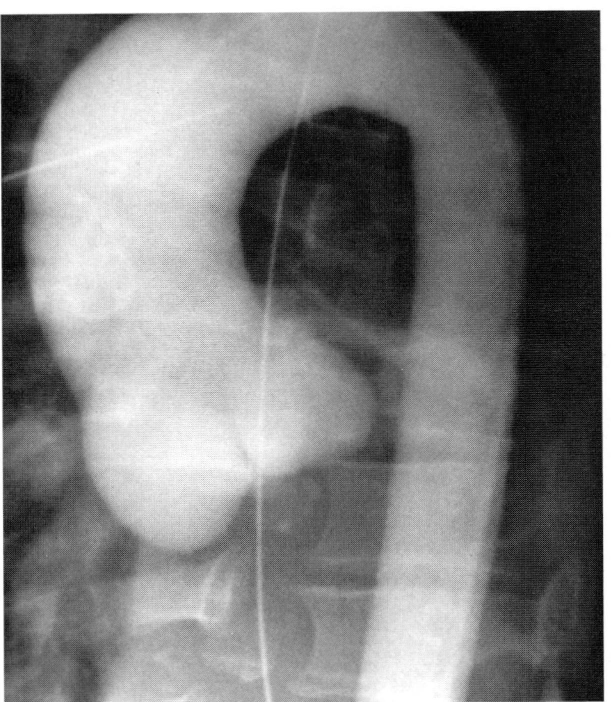

A

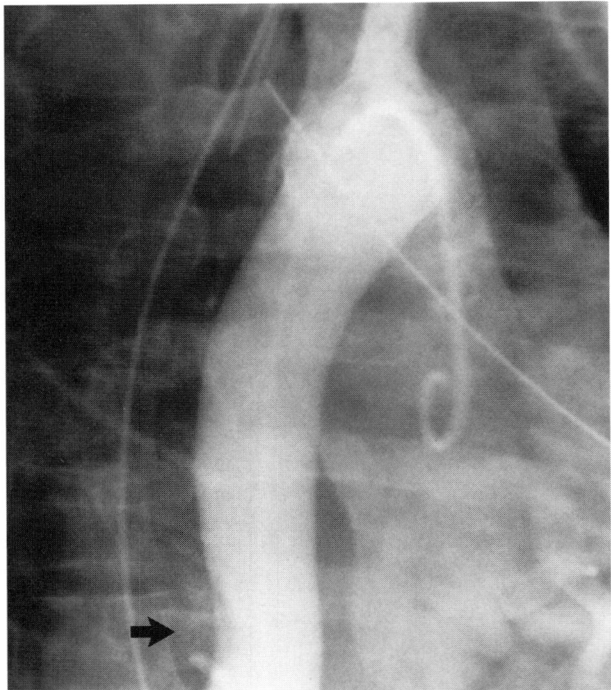

B

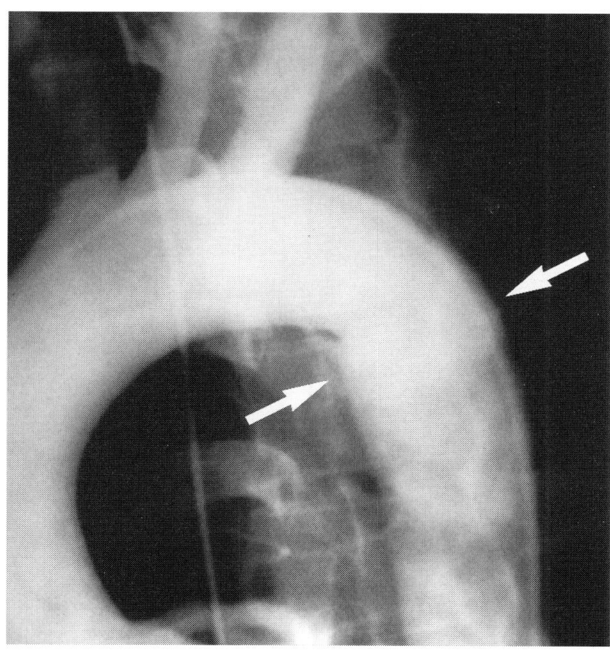

A

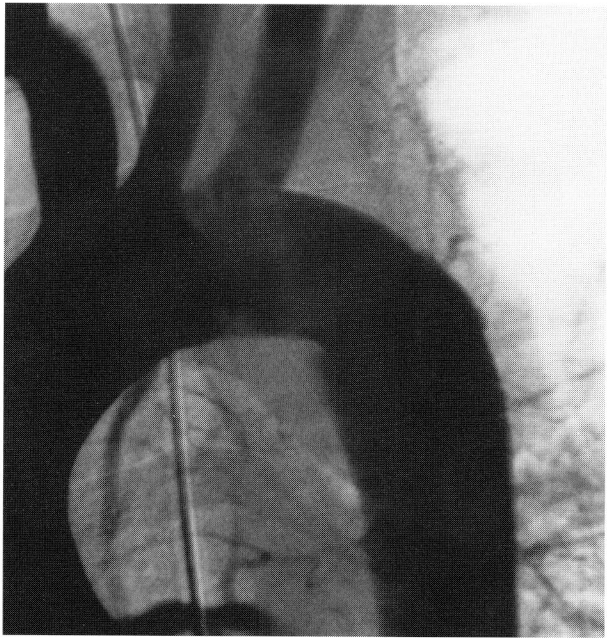

B

mechanism of injury. Very violent and complex mechanisms may still produce rather subtle injuries: the patient in Figure 21-19 was involved in a minor car accident on an elevated highway; he left his car to check on the other driver when a third vehicle collided with the car, which struck the patient, throwing him off the bridge, an approximately 60-foot drop.

Untreated ABC Injuries

Without treatment, up to 98 percent of patients with aortic laceration will die. In most of the 2 percent who survive, the false aneurysm remains; its periphery becomes fibrous and may eventually calcify (Fig. 21-20). A *chronic aortic false aneurysm is by no means harmless* and can complete its rupture unpredictably.[75] As a result, patients' long-range survival is less than 65 percent.[76] Survival after reinjury of a chronic traumatic false aneurysm is almost unheard of; to the best of the author's knowledge, the patient in Fig. 21-21 is the only known case. Surgical repair should be undertaken as soon as the diagnosis is made, even in asymptomatic patients. There is evidence to suggest that pregnancy may hasten the rupture of a chronic false aneurysm be-

C

Figure 21-19. Subtle injury. The patient was struck by a car and then fell 18 m off a bridge. A. Aortogram in RPO projection shows minimal findings (*between arrows*). B. Subtraction film of the same image shows the lesion better. C. Aortogram in LPO projection shows a small false aneurysm (*arrow*). At operation the transection involved most of the aortic circumference.

◀ **Figure 21-18.** Crushing injury of the aorta at T8 from a logging accident. The RPO view (A) is normal. An intramural hematoma is seen only on the LPO projection (*arrow*, B).

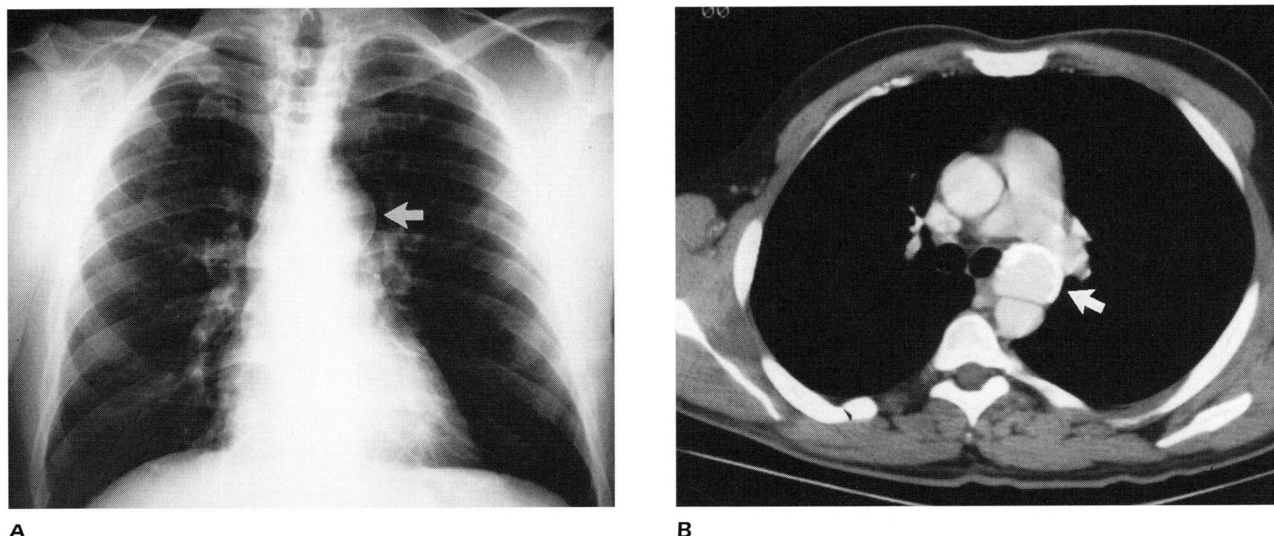

Figure 21-20. Chronic traumatic false aneurysm (12 years), an incidental finding in an asymptomatic patient. The calcified wall of the false aneurysm is seen on both chest film (*arrow,* A) and CT scan (*arrow,* B).

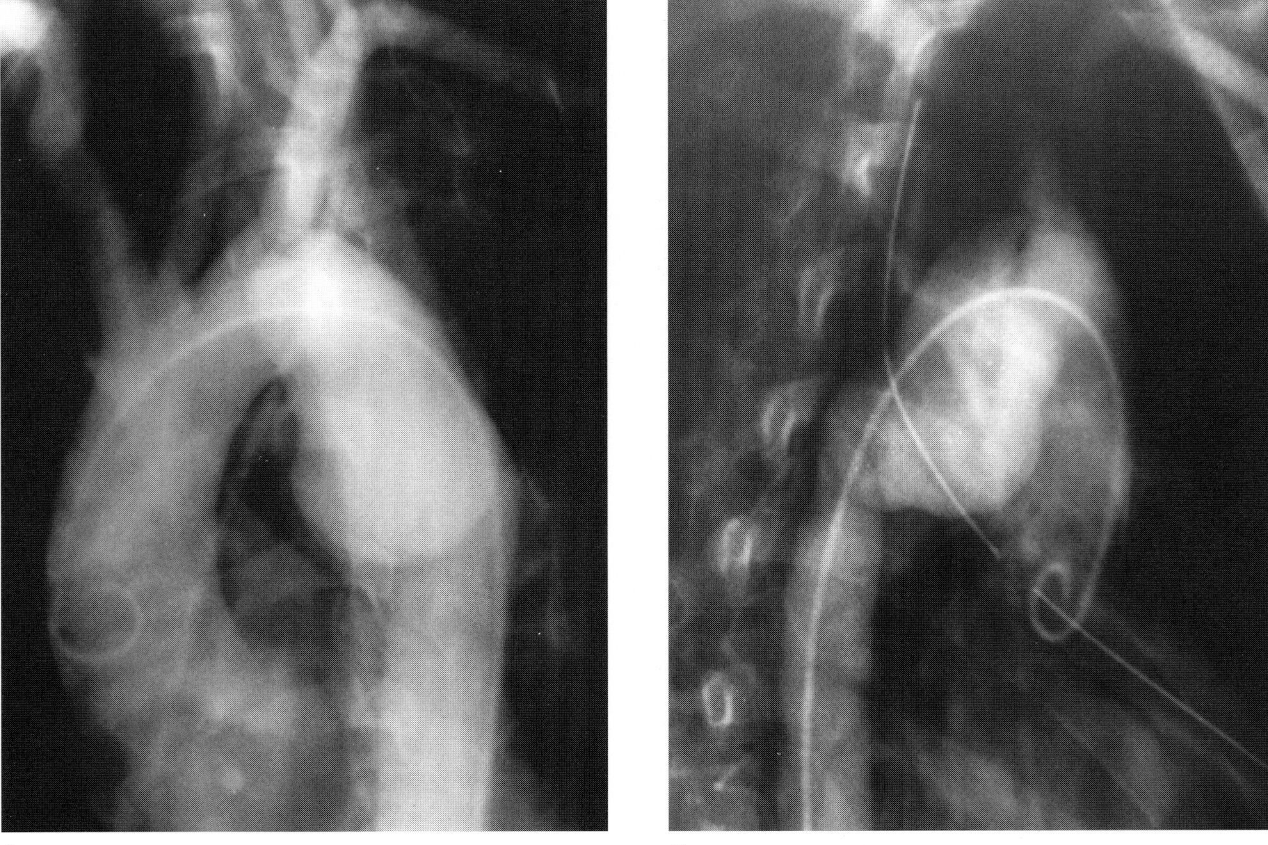

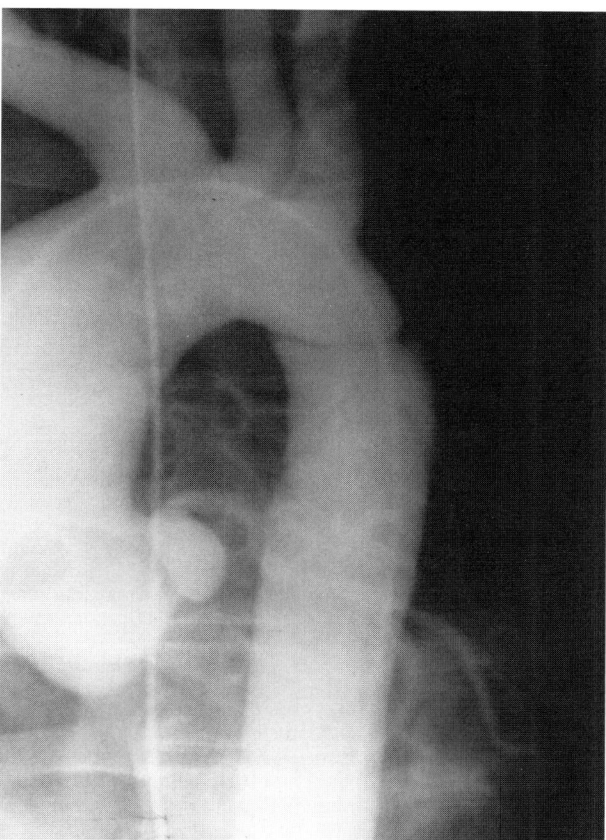

Figure 21-22. A matter of great urgency. This patient arrived in the emergency room less than 1 hour after an unrestrained frontal collision but did not undergo angiography for 6 hours and was not taken to the operating theater for another 4 hours; there, after the thoracic cavity was opened, the aorta burst and the patient expired. Physicians must appreciate that the injury seen here is a dynamic process: once the aorta begins its tearing, every pressure pulse produced by the normal heartbeat is an added traumatic event—100 times a minute, 60,000 times in 10 hours. This means that at any time the aorta will no longer be able to withstand the pressure.

cause of the generalized softening of all connective and fibrous tissues.[77]

Spontaneous healing of a lacerated aorta is an extremely rare event.[78,79] In all likelihood, healing can be expected only when the injury involves the intima alone. When the media is injured as well, a small false aneurysm should persist.[79]

Summary

The expected rapid and almost universal lethality of ABC injuries mandates early diagnosis and repair. The diagnosis must be suspected from the history of violent blunt trauma to the chest and from the presence of a superior mediastinal hematoma on the admission chest film, always bearing in mind that patients may not display external signs of recent trauma[16] and that the chest film is of limited value as a predictor of an ABC injury.[30,45,80] Moreover, because the chest film contains no reliable information to begin with, repeating it at regular intervals will not create more information and may actually hasten the patient's demise. To achieve a rapid diagnosis, one must not attend to obvious injuries (Fig. 21-22)[81,82]: these are superficial and therefore irrelevant injuries.[45,47]

The question is always asked, How does one establish the indication for aortography in blunt chest trauma? This is the wrong question, because this is not what the surgeon wants to know. *The only indication the surgeon seeks is to perform thoracotomy;* the aortogram is merely the means by which to establish that indication, and therefore the need for aortography is beyond question.[47]

References

1. Mattox KL. Decelerating aortic injury. In: Bergen JJ, Yao JST, eds. Vascular surgical emergencies. Orlando: Grune & Stratton, 1987:341–358.
2. Hartford JM, Fayer RL, Shaver TE, et al. Transection of the thoracic aorta: assessment of a trauma system. Am J Surg 1986; 151:224–229.
3. Sturm JT, McGee MB, Luxenberg MG. An analysis of risk factors for death at the scene following traumatic aortic rupture. J Trauma 1988;28:1578–1580.
4. Bergman K, Spence L, Wesson D, et al. Thoracic vascular injuries: a post mortem study. J Trauma 1990;30:604–606.
5. Eddy AC, Rusch VW, Fligner CL, et al. The epidemiology of traumatic rupture of the thoracic aorta in children: a 13-year review. J Trauma 1990;30:989–992.
6. Spouge AR, Burrows PE, Armstrong D, Daneman A. Traumatic aortic rupture in the pediatric population: role of plain film, CT and angiography in the diagnosis. Pediatr Radiol 1991;21:324–328.
7. Ingemarson H, Grevsten S, Thoren L. Lethal horse-riding injuries. J Trauma 1989;29:25–30.
8. Sevitt S. Traumatic ruptures of the aorta: a clinico-pathological study. Injury 1977;8:159–173.

◀ **Figure 21-21.** Reinjury of a chronic aortic false aneurysm. The driver, age 18, was in a left broadside collision. He was admitted with a left hemothorax, ruptured left hemidiaphragm, and fractured spleen, and was operated on immediately. Both views of a postoperative thoracic aortogram (A and B) show a large, smooth false aneurysm. The first injury was sustained 10 months earlier in a collision and ejection, high-speed motorcycle accident. At operation the fibrous sac of the chronic false aneurysm was found surrounded by a fresh hematoma from a reinjury.

9. Sevitt S. The mechanisms of traumatic rupture of the thoracic aorta. Br J Surg 1977;64:166–173.
10. Lundevall J. The mechanism of traumatic rupture of the aorta. Acta Pathol Microbiol Scand 1964;62:34–46.
11. Mays ET. Wounding forces. In: Mays ET, ed. Clinical evaluation of the critically injured. Springfield, IL: Charles C Thomas, 1975:14–45.
12. Mohan D, Melvin JW. Failure properties of passive human aortic tissue: II. Biaxial tension tests. J Biomech 1983;16:31–44.
13. Feczko JD, Lynch L, Clark MA, et al. An autopsy case review of 142 nonpenetrating (blunt) injuries of the aorta. J Trauma 1992;33:846–849.
14. Mattox KL. Injury to the thoracic great vessels. In: Moore EE, Mattox KL, Feliciano DV, eds. Trauma. 2nd ed. E. Norwalk: Appleton & Lange, 1991:393–408.
15. Fisher RG, Hadlock F, Ben-Menachem Y. Laceration of the thoracic aorta and brachiocephalic arteries by blunt trauma: report of 54 cases and review of the literature. Radiol Clin North Am 1981;19:91–110.
16. Greendyke RM. Traumatic rupture of the aorta: special reference to automobile accidents. JAMA 1966;195:119–122.
17. Eddy AC, Rusch VW, Marchioro T, et al. Treatment of traumatic rupture of the thoracic aorta: a 15-year experience. Arch Surg 1990;125:1351–1356.
18. Townsend RN, Colella JJ, Diamond DL. Traumatic rupture of the aorta—critical decisions for trauma surgeons. J Trauma 1990;30:1169–1174.
19. Arajarvi E, Santavirta S, Tolonen J. Abdominal injuries sustained in severe traffic accidents by seatbelt wearers. J Trauma 1987;27:393–397.
20. Ben-Menachem Y. Blunt thoracoabdominal trauma. In: Ben-Menachem Y. Angiography in trauma: a work atlas. Philadelphia: Saunders, 1981:124–131.
21. Ben-Menachem Y, Fisher RG, Ward RE. Are "occult" intraabdominal and extraperitoneal injuries really occult? Radiol Clin North Am 1981;19:125–140.
22. Blackbourne BD. Injury-vehicle correlations in the investigation of motor vehicle accidents. In: Wecht CH, ed. Legal medicine 1980. Philadelphia: Saunders, 1980:1–19.
23. Ben-Menachem Y. Imaging techniques in trauma. In: Maull KI, ed. Advances in trauma and critical care. Chicago: Mosby–Year Book, 1992;7:191–217.
24. Rogers LF. Common oversights in the evaluation of the patient with multiple injuries. Skeletal Radiol 1984;12:103–111.
25. Sturm JT, Hines JT, Perry JF Jr. Thoracic spinal fractures and aortic rupture: a significant and fatal association. Ann Thorac Surg 1990;50:931–933.
26. Stambough JL, Frree BA, Fowl RJ. Aortic injuries in thoracolumbar spine fracture-dislocations: report of three cases. J Orthop Trauma 1989;3:245–249.
27. Ochsner MG, Champion HR, Chambers RJ, Harviel JD. Pelvic fracture as an indicator of increased risk of thoracic aortic rupture. J Trauma 1989;29:1376–1379.
28. Ochsner MG, Hoffman AP, DiPasquale D, et al. Associated aortic rupture—pelvic fracture: an alert for orthopedic and general surgeons. J Trauma 1992;33:429–434.
29. Dontigny L. Comments to the 42nd Annual Session of the American Association for the Surgery of Trauma, 1982. J Trauma 1983;23:298–299.
30. Ben-Menachem Y. Chest trauma. In: Sperber M, ed. Radiologic diagnosis of chest disease. New York: Springer-Verlag, 1990:501–523.
31. Gundry SR, Burney RE, Mackenzie JR, et al. Assessment of mediastinal widening associated with traumatic rupture of the aorta. J Trauma 1983;23:293–299.
32. Stark P, Cook M, Vincent A, Smith DC. Traumatic rupture of the thoracic aorta: a review of 49 cases. Radiologue 1987;27: 402–406.
33. Mirvis SE, Bidwell JK, Buddemeyer EU, et al. Value of chest radiography in excluding traumatic aortic rupture. Radiology 1987;163:487–493.
34. Woodring JH, King JG. The potential effects of radiographic criteria to exclude aortography in patients with blunt chest trauma. J Thorac Cardiovasc Surg 1989;97:456–460.
35. Cohen AM, Crass JR. Traumatic lacerations of the aorta and great vessels with a normal mediastinum at radiography. J Vasc Intervent Radiol 1992;3:541–544.
36. Shackford SR, Virgilio RW, Smith DE, et al. The significance of chest wall injury in the diagnosis of traumatic aneurysms of the thoracic aorta. J Trauma 1978;18:493–497.
37. Fisher RG, Ward RE, Ben-Menachem Y, et al. Angiography and the fractured first rib: too much for too little? AJR 1982; 138:1059–1062.
38. Woodring JH, Fried AM, Hatfield DR, et al. Fractures of first and second ribs: predictive value for arterial and bronchial injury. AJR 1982;138:211–215.
39. Hilgenberg AD, Logan DL, Akins CW, et al. Blunt injuries of the thoracic aorta. Ann Thorac Surg 1992;53:233–239.
40. Pozzato C, Fedriga E, Donatelli F, Gattoni F. Acute posttraumatic rupture of the thoracic aorta: the role of angiography in a 7-year review. Cardiovasc Intervent Radiol 1992;14:338–341.
41. Wills JS, Lally JF. Use of CT for evaluation of possible traumatic aortic injury. AJR 1991;157:1123–1124.
42. McLean TR, Olinger GN, Thorsen MK. Computed tomography in the evaluation of the aorta in patients sustaining blunt chest trauma. J Trauma 1991;31:254–256.
43. Brooks SW, Young JC, Cmolik B, et al. The use of transesophageal echocardiography in the evaluation of chest trauma. J Trauma 1992;32:761–768.
44. Sparks MB, Burchard KW, Marrin CAS, et al. Transesophageal echocardiography: preliminary results in patients with traumatic aortic rupture. Arch Surg 1991;126:711–714.
45. Ben-Menachem Y. Radiology. In: Moore EE, ed. Early care of the injured patient. Philadelphia: BC Decker, 1990:84–90.
46. Sturm JT, Hankins DG, Young G. Thoracic aortography following blunt chest trauma. Am J Emerg Med 1990;8:92–96.
47. Ben-Menachem Y, Fisher RG. Radiology. In: Feliciano DV, Moore EE, Mattox KL, eds. Trauma. 3rd ed. Norwalk, CT: Appleton & Lange, 1995:203–234.
48. Ward RE, Miller P, Clark DG, et al. Angiography and peritoneal lavage in blunt abdominal trauma. J Trauma 1981;21: 848–853.
49. Ben-Menachem Y. Angiography in diagnosis of vascular trauma. In: Taveras JM, Ferrucci JT, eds. Radiology: diagnosis–imaging–intervention. Philadelphia: Lippincott, 1988;2:1–14.
50. Ben-Menachem Y. Blunt chest trauma. In: Ben-Menachem Y. Angiography in trauma: a work atlas. Philadelphia: Saunders, 1981:110–123.
51. LaBerge JM, Jeffrey RB. Aortic lacerations: fatal complications of thoracic aortography. Radiology 1987;165:367–369.
52. Parker LA Jr, Delany D, Friday JM. Oblique projections in aortography following blunt thoracic trauma. J Can Assoc Radiol 1989;40:172–173.
53. Williams DM, Simon HJ, Marx MV, Starkey TD. Acute traumatic aortic rupture: intravascular US findings. Radiology 1992;182:247–249.
54. Mirvis SE, Pais SO, Gens DR. Thoracic aortic rupture: advantages of intraarterial digital subtraction angiography. AJR 1986;146:987–991.
55. Morse SS, Glickman MG, Greenwood LH, et al. Traumatic aortic rupture: false-positive aortographic diagnosis due to atypical ductus diverticulum. AJR 1988;150:793–796.
56. Devineni R, McKeenzie FN. Avulsion of a normal aortic valve cusp due to blunt chest injury. J Trauma 1984;24:910–912.
57. Weaver FA, Suda RW, Stiles GM, Yellin AE. Injuries to the ascending aorta, aortic arch and great vessels. Surg Gynec Obstet 1989;169:27–31.
58. Ben-Menachem Y. Rupture of the thoracic aorta by broadside impacts in road-traffic and other accidents: further angiographic observations and preliminary autopsy findings. J Trauma 1993;35:363–367.

59. Graham JM, Feliciano DV, Mattox KL, Beall AC Jr. Innominate vascular injury. J Trauma 1982;22:647–655.
60. Ben-Menachem Y. Avulsion of the innominate artery associated with fracture of the sternum. AJR 1988;150:621–622.
61. Asfaw I, Ramadan H, Talbert JG, Arbulu A. Double traumatic rupture of the thoracic aorta. J Trauma 1985;25:1102–1104.
62. Stothert JC Jr, McBride L, Tidik S, et al. Multiple aortic tears treated by primary suture repair. J Trauma 1987;27:955–956.
63. Parmley LF, Mattingly TW, Manion WC, et al. Nonpenetrating traumatic injury of the aorta. Circulation 1958;17: 1086–1101.
64. Gotzen L, Flory PJ, Otte D. Biomechanics of aortic rupture at classical location in traffic accidents. Thorac Cardiovasc Surg 1980;28:64–68.
65. Crass JR, Cohen AM, Motta AO, et al. A proposed new mechanism of traumatic aortic rupture: the osseous pinch. Radiology 1990;176:645–649.
66. Cohen AM, Crass JR, Thomas HA, et al. CT evidence for the "osseous pinch" mechanism of traumatic aortic injury. AJR 1992;159:271–274.
67. Ben-Menachem Y. The mechanism of injury. In: Ben-Menachem Y. Angiography in trauma: a work atlas. Philadelphia: Saunders, 1981:25–46.
68. Sevitt S. Fatal road accidents: injuries, complications, and causes of death in 250 subjects. Br J Surg 1968;55:481–505.
69. Verdant A. Major mediastinal vessel injury: an underestimated lesion. Can J Surg 1987;30:402–404.
70. Arajarvi E, Santavirta S. Chest injuries sustained in severe traffic accidents by seatbelt wearers. J Trauma 1989;29:37–41.
71. Hayes CW, Conway WF, Walsh JW, et al. Seat belt injuries: radiologic findings and clinical correlation. Radiographics 1991;11:23–36.
72. Ruskey J, Lieberman ME, Shaikh KA, et al. Unusual subclavian artery lacerations resulting from lap-shoulder seatbelt trauma: case reports. J Trauma 1989;29:1598–1600.
73. Thieman KC, Grooters RK. Double disruption of an innominate artery secondary to blunt trauma. Ann Thorac Surg 1982; 33:285–289.
74. Gardner MAH, Bidstrup BP. Intrathoracic great vessel injury resulting from blunt chest trauma associated with posterior dislocation of the sternoclavicular joint. Aust N Z J Surg 1983; 53:427–430.
75. Heystraten FM, Rosenbusch G, Kingma LM, Lacquet LK. Chronic posttraumatic aneurysm of the thoracic aorta: surgically correctable occult threat. AJR 1986;146:303–308.
76. Pratt A, Warembourg H Jr, Watel A, et al. Chronic traumatic aneurysms of the descending thoracic aorta (19 cases). J Cardiovasc Surg 1986;27:268–272.
77. Townsend JN, Davies MK, Jones EL. Fatal rupture of an unsuspected post-traumatic aneurysm of the thoracic aorta during pregnancy. Br Heart J 1991;66:248–249.
78. Wigle RL, Moran JM. Spontaneous healing of a traumatic thoracic aortic tear: case report. J Trauma 1991;31:280–283.
79. Fisher RG, Oria RA, Mattox KL, et al. Conservative management of aortic lacerations due to blunt trauma. J Trauma 1990; 30:1562–1566.
80. Ben-Menachem Y. Overview of the role of the radiologist in emergency department care. In: Campbell RE, Harle TS, eds. A categorical course in emergency department care. Oak Brook: RSNA Publications, 1990:9–13.
81. Dove DB, Stahl WM, DelGuerico LRM. A five-year review of deaths following urban trauma. J Trauma 1980;20:760–766.
82. Blair E, Topuzlu C, Davis JH. Delayed or missed diagnosis in blunt chest trauma. J Trauma 1971;11:129–145.

22

Additional Applications of Thoracic Aortography

HERBERT L. ABRAMS

Aortic Stenosis

Aortic stenosis may be valvular, subvalvular (subaortic), or supravalvular in location. In most cases the valvular form is acquired, probably on the basis of rheumatic infection.[1,2] Campbell and Kauntze, however, contend that many cases are congenital but do not cause symptoms until late in life.[3] Under any circumstances, pathologically there is thickening, fusion, and often calcification of the valve cusps.[4] In subaortic stenosis the lesion usually consists of a firm, fibrous band or ring of tissue 2 to 4 mm in thickness that extends from 1 to 10 mm into the ventricular cavity and is located 1 to 20 mm below the aortic valve.[5,6] It has been considered analogous to infundibular stenosis of the right ventricle and is possibly related to an arrested involution of the bulbus cordis during fetal life. Idiopathic hypertrophic subaortic stenosis differs from the congenital lesion in that it is functional in character and is associated with marked hypertrophy of the entire ventricular wall.

Congenital aortic stenosis is important to document because it is a cause of sudden death in the young. In general, the effect on the heart depends on the extent to which left ventricular work is increased by the obstructing lesion. If it is slight, there may be only minimal left ventricular hypertrophy; if severe, marked hypertrophy and dilatation of the left ventricle may develop.

On physical examination a harsh systolic murmur, frequently accompanied by a thrill, is heard at the base of the heart. The pulse pressure is usually small, and the aortic second sound is of normal or diminished intensity. The electrocardiogram shows evidence of left ventricular hypertrophy. Conventional roentgenologic studies reveal varying degrees of left ventricular enlargement and prominence of the ascending aorta. At fluoroscopy calcification of the valve may be visible; and the amplitude of pulsation of the proximal ascending aorta, particularly in the left anterior oblique view, may be accentuated, whereas that of the aortic knob is usually diminished.

The comparative dimensions of the ascending aorta can be significant indicators of disease etiology. This notion is based on the ratio between two widths: that of the mid–ascending aorta and that of the aortic root. Supravalvular aortic dilatation is consistently greater in patients with congenital stenosis than in those with stenosis of rheumatic origin.[7] Aortic measurement can also be a clue to the site of suspected valve defects. The normal width of the mid–ascending aorta ranges between 2.5 and 3.0 cm in patients studied by aortography. In patients with aortic regurgitation, however, the aortic width is greatly enlarged, and it is larger than normal in patients with valvular aortic stenosis. The mean values of the width of the aortic arch are approximately equal in two disease states: aortic regurgitation alone and aortic regurgitation combined with mitral insufficiency. Only when aortic regurgitation is associated with stenosis does it not produce striking enlargement of the aortic arch—probably because the stenosis reduces the volume of blood that is ejected into the aorta.[8]

Aortic stenosis has been studied both by angiocardiography and by aortography. Grishman et al., using intravenous angiocardiography, reported dilatation and hypertrophy of the left ventricle as well as dilatation of the thoracic aorta.[9] Kjellberg et al. noted thickened, fused aortic valves in one patient.[10] Lehman et al. used direct needle ventriculography as a means of showing the aortic valve and demonstrated thickening and deformity of the valve cusps.[11] The aortographic studies of the congenital aortic stenosis by Downing demonstrated mainly dilatation of the ascending aorta.[12] Ödman and Philipson have also reported studies of the valvular apparatus by thoracic aortography.[13] They have emphasized the necessity for biplane studies with a rapid exposure rate and coordinated electrocardiographic and exposure registration. The essential findings in their series were thickening and restricted

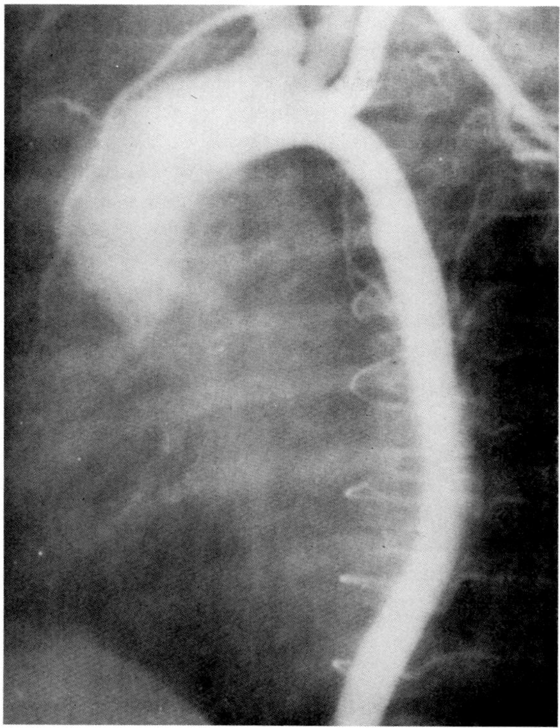

A

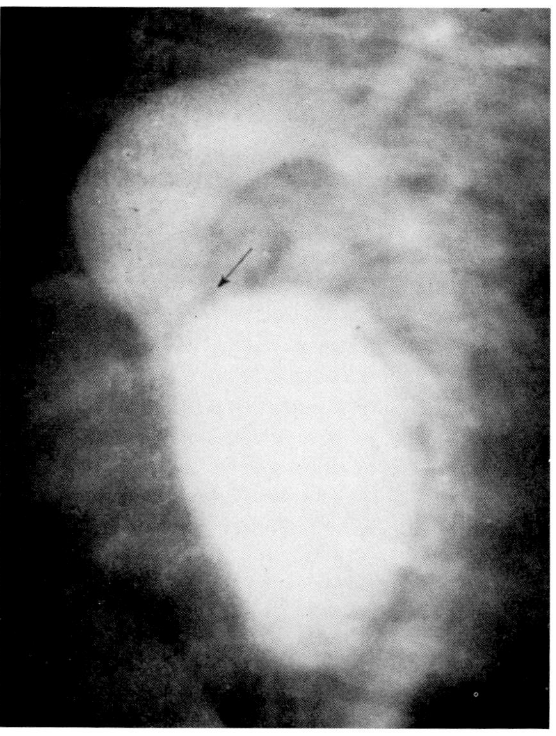

B

Figure 22-1. Congenital aortic stenosis. This infant entered the hospital in congestive heart failure. Initially, no murmurs were heard. Conventional chest roentgenograms demonstrated gross cardiac enlargement. The pulses were generally weak, but there was no disparity between upper and lower extremity blood pressures. After diagnostic studies demonstrated the presence of congenital aortic stenosis, thoracotomy was performed. When the aorta was opened, fusion of the aortic valve cusps was visible with the kind of pinhole opening more commonly seen in the presence of pulmonic stenosis. It was possible to obtain a satisfactory cleavage plane, and before surgical closure the cusps appeared to appose well without significant aortic insufficiency. About 4 hours after surgery, the infant suddenly died. Autopsy demonstrated repair of the aortic stenosis and endocardial fibroelastosis involving mainly the left ventricle. (A) Retrograde brachial aortogram. The opaque medium has been injected through the right brachial artery and demonstrates the entire aortic arch. There is gross dilatation of the ascending aorta and a rather peculiar funnel-shaped deformity of its base. (B) Angiocardiogram. Film obtained 5 seconds after injection. A large, thick-walled left ventricle is visible. Narrowing of the valve area (*arrow*) is noted with gross poststenotic dilatation similar to that seen in retrograde brachial aortogram.

mobility of the aortic valves, a narrowed jet that reflected the size of the aortic orifice, and irregular filling of the dilated ascending aorta.

It is apparent that contrast studies have a definite place in the analysis of aortic stenosis. Figure 22-1 demonstrates a case of congenital aortic stenosis studied both by retrograde aortography and by angiocardiography. The deformity of the valve is apparent in both studies, and there is striking poststenotic dilatation. At surgery the valves were fused and had a pinhead opening similar to that commonly seen in congenital pulmonic stenosis.

The diagnosis of aortic valve stenosis using aortography is partially inferential. The size of the valve orifice is estimated mainly from the negative jet of nonopacified blood coming from the left ventricle. Obviously, it would be desirable to demonstrate the actual size of the orifice by opacified blood. To accomplish opacification, a high concentration of the opaque medium in the left ventricle must be attained. This is best achieved by transseptal left heart catheterization or by retrograde transaortic valve catheterization of the left ventricle. Filling of the left ventricle with contrast agent in aortic stenosis demonstrates impeded mobility of the valve cusps, thickening, "doming," and a jet of contrast expelled into the aorta during ventricular systole. All these findings are demonstrated on large films and on cine, but the jet, the impeded valve movement, and the valve calcification are best visualized with motion picture studies.

Supravalvular Aortic Stenosis

Supravalvular aortic stenosis may occur as an isolated entity, but its frequent association with peripheral pulmonary artery stenosis, physical and mental retardation, and a characteristic abnormal facies with maldeveloped dentition has been emphasized.[14] These findings constitute one or more new and fascinating syndromes. In addition, some studies[15,16] indicate that hypercalcemia in infancy may be another facet of the syndrome and may actually be responsible for the various developmental abnormalities. As a cause of obstruction to left ventricular outflow, which is clearly operable, its recognition and differentiation from valvular or subvalvular stenosis are important before surgery.

All of the previously reported cases of supravalvular aortic stenosis may be classified according to the system developed by Taybi and his coworkers[17]:

Type I. Hypoplastic ascending aorta
- A. Tubular narrowing of the entire ascending aorta
- B. Narrowing more marked in the proximal region

Type II. Normal or dilated ascending aorta with stenosis immediately above the aortic valve leaflets due to an internally protruding circumferential ridge and/or an externally detectable narrowing of the aorta above the sinuses of Valsalva

Type III. A thin, membranous diaphragm

Most cases fall in Taybi's type I or II with a definite localized area of narrowing just above the aortic valve and/or hypoplasia of the entire ascending aorta. Rarely, type III, consisting of a true diaphragm, may be clinically significant.[18]

The pathology of this lesion has been well described by Perou.[19] He has pointed out that "microscopically, aortic coarctation and supravalvular aortic stenosis are very similar. The basic microscopic lesion of true supravalvular aortic stenosis seems to be an angulation and exaggerated infolding with thickening and focal disorganization of the media capped by a zone of intimal thickening or hypertrophy showing various degenerative changes."

Abnormality of the aortic valves is frequently associated with the supravalvular lesion: in 25 percent of cases, according to Edwards.[4] The valve may be bicuspid, and various degrees of thickening and fibrosis of the leaflets can be present. The free edge of all or part of one or more cusps may form adhesions to the aorta at the site of stenosis and result in aortic insufficiency or in partial to complete obstruction of the involved coronary artery. The coronary arteries are usually markedly dilated and tortuous because they arise proximal to the stenosis and are perfused at a high pressure head. Valvular calcification is not seen, and poststenotic dilatation of the ascending aorta is uncommon in supravalvular stenosis. Therefore, if an adult patient with physical signs of aortic stenosis does not have valvular calcification or a dilated ascending aorta, supravalvular aortic stenosis should be considered.[20]

The resemblance of the patients to one another and the dissimilarity to their own family members are striking. The facial resemblance seems derived largely from soft tissue similarity because no common abnormalities were found in roentgenograms of the skull reviewed by Williams et al.[21] The face is usually full with a broad forehead, widely set eyes, heavy cheeks, wide mouth, pouting lips, pointed chin, and prominent ears. The dental defects include generalized hypoplasia of the teeth, particularly the upper and middle incisors; malformations of the deciduous molars; partial anodontia; and late mineralization.[14]

On physical examination a systolic ejection murmur and systolic thrill are frequently louder in the neck and suprasternal notch than in the right first or second intercostal space, although not invariably. The aortic second sound is usually normal. Discrepancy in the pulses and blood pressures in the arms due to associated obstructive lesions in the greater vessels may be noted.

Generally, a left ventricular or combined hypertrophy pattern is identified on the electrocardiogram, depending on the presence or absence of pulmonic branch stenoses.

Radiologically, the absence of poststenotic dilatation serves as a useful, although by no means infallible, differentiating point from valvular aortic stenosis. An analysis of 121 cases, in 70 of which x-ray films were reproduced or descriptions included, indicated absence of a prominent ascending aorta and presence of a small aortic knob in over 90 percent of cases.[22] Sixty percent had slight to moderate cardiac enlargement, and the remainder were normal. Discrete left ventricular enlargement or prominence was thought to be present in 57 percent of cases. In 10 percent, left atrial enlargement was also noted. Coincident right ventricular enlargement was apparent in 14 percent of cases, usually those with associated multiple branch stenoses. The irregular, sausagelike appearance of the central branches of the pulmonary arteries described in the presence of multiple branch stenoses was rarely recorded.

Cardiac Catheterization

The physiologic findings in valvular, subvalvular, and supravalvular stenosis have been well described by Hancock.[23] It is important that the catheter side holes be as far distal in the catheter as possible when the stenotic segment is short. If the constriction is well beyond the valve, three distinct pressure zones exist: (1) high ventricular systolic pressure, (2) similarly high proximal aortic systolic pressure, and (3) distal to the stenosis, an abrupt fall in systolic pressure with relatively little change in diastolic pressure.

Angiography

Contrast study of the thoracic aorta is by far the best method of determining the presence, location, and degree of supravalvular aortic stenosis. Motion picture techniques are admirable for demonstrating the flow through the distended coronary bed, and they afford better delineation of aortic valve motion. Associated lesions such as fusion of valve leaflets can be identified readily. At the time of thoracic aortography, pressures are obtained at the ventricular, supravalvular, and suprastenotic area.

Preoperative study is essential to determine the presence or absence of hypoplasia of the aorta above the site of stenosis, to allow the surgeon to plan the approach, and to obtain some estimate of the operative risk. In all of our cases the supravalvular narrowing was localized to the site just above the sinuses of Valsalva (Fig. 22-2). In two instances diffuse hypoplasia of the ascending aorta accompanied the stenosis. The sinuses of Valsalva were large, and gross dilatation of the coronary arteries was a prominent feature.

Angiocardiographic studies were performed in 69 cases recorded in the literature.[22] In two-thirds the injection was made into the left ventricle, and in the remaining one-third a supravalvular injection was performed. A few patients were studied after injection into the right cardiac chambers. Cine recording was employed in one-quarter of the cases and large-film recording in three-quarters.

Left ventricular enlargement was noted in about 25 percent of cases, whereas hypertrophy was rarely described although obviously present in some cases. Abnormal limitation of movement of the aortic valve leaflets was apparent in 10 percent of cases. The appearance of the aorta was very similar in most cases, with a localized segment of narrowing immediately above the sinuses of Valsalva or within 1 to 2 cm beyond. Above the localized segment the aorta was of normal size in 60 percent of cases, hypoplastic in 30 percent, and dilated in 10 percent. In three cases there was hypoplasia of the entire aorta. The stenosis was mild in 21 percent, moderate in 56 percent, and severe in 17 percent. The length of the narrowed segment varied between 0.5 and 3.0 cm. Among 35 cases in which pulmonic stenosis coexisted with supervalvular aortic stenosis, it involved branches on both sides in 57 percent, on one side in 20 percent, the main pulmonary artery in 9 percent, and the pulmonic valve in 14 percent.

Brachiocephalic Branch Stenosis

Occasional cases have been reported in which stenotic lesions have been observed in the brachiocephalic vessels. Often suspicion of such a finding is first evident when a pulse or blood pressure differential is noted during the physical examination. This was true of two of our own cases in which stenosis was evident. The fact that three of our four cases demonstrated some degree of narrowing of one or more of the branch vessels of the aortic arch strongly indicates that the incidence of this associated anomaly is higher than has been reported. A review of 121 published cases described a relatively small number of localized brachiocephalic lesions, but careful analysis of the roentgenographic illustrations indicated that some lesions were not discussed.[22] Also, in many of the cases previously recorded in the literature, bilateral upper extremity blood pressures were not reported and may well have failed to reflect the stenosis that was present.

Aortic Insufficiency

Rheumatic valvulitis is the commonest cause of an incompetent aortic valve.[24] With a rheumatic lesion, insufficiency produces more marked cardiac enlargement than stenosis, and with severe degrees of regurgitation the so-called cor bovinum develops.

Aortic insufficiency is an important lesion to detect and quantitate. The present state of valve replacement requires precise preoperative assessment of lesions potentially correctable by surgery. In association with mitral stenosis, the degree of aortic insufficiency may be masked, and corrective mitral valve surgery may render an apparently mild lesion more severe. Aortic insufficiency unsuspected before surgery may complicate open heart repair of mitral valve disease.

When insufficiency is gross and the clinical signs are unequivocal, there is no problem. In more subtle cases its presence and degree may be difficult to detect. The murmur may be absent when significant degrees of aortic insufficiency are found. Thus increasing reliance has been placed on thoracic aortography as a means

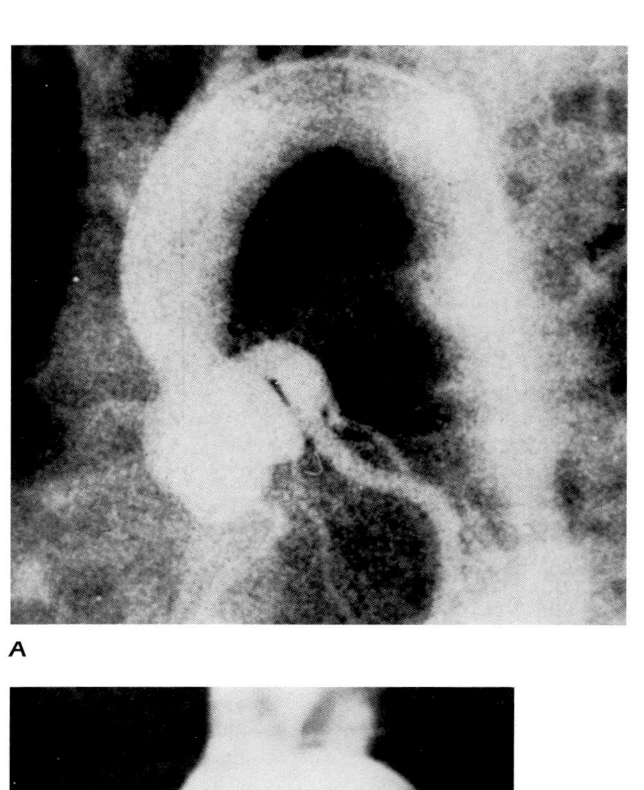
A

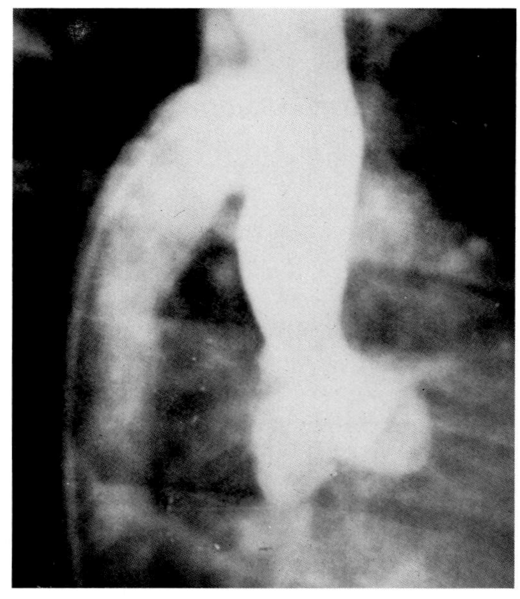
B

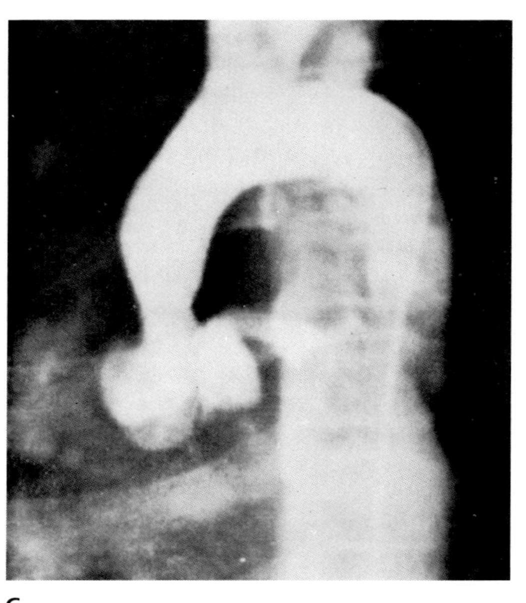
C

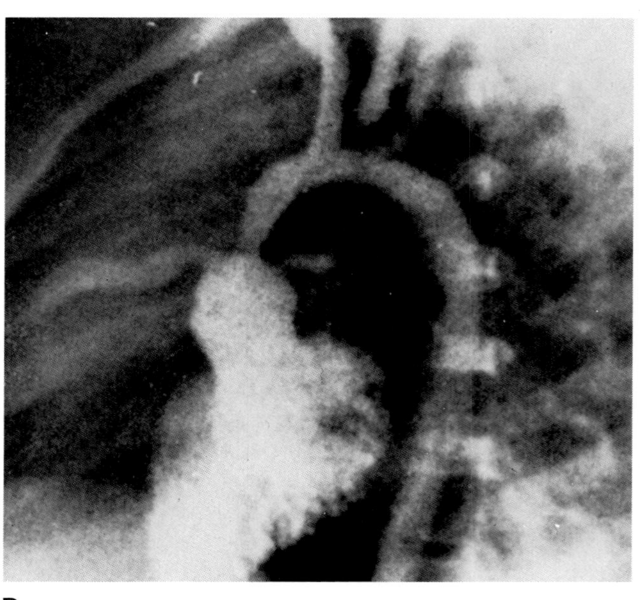
D

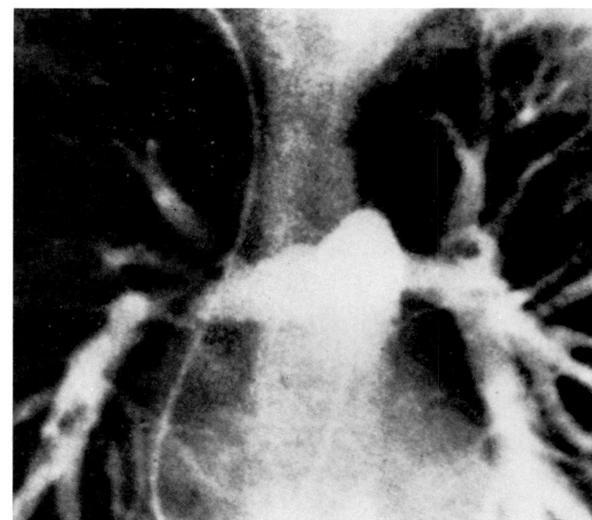
E

of determining the presence and severity of aortic insufficiency.[25-29]

When contrast material is noted in the ventricular cavity after a supravalvular injection, it represents unequivocal evidence of reflux through the aortic valve. But the pathologic significance of reflux must be carefully assessed. The pertinent question is whether it always implies malfunction of the aortic valve. The evidence is conflicting.

Experimental studies of aortic insufficiency in 1956 led to the conclusion that "the normal aortic valve does not permit reflux into the left ventricle."[30] This statement was based on an analysis of 10 injections of contrast material into the ascending aorta in normal dogs using a no. 7 Lehman aortic catheter.[31] Single-spot roentgenograms rather than serialographic methods were used for roentgen recording. By contrast, Nelson et al. in 1958, concerned with quantitating aortic insufficiency in humans, performed experiments on 14 dogs which indicated that "injection of contrast material through open-end catheters near the aortic valve would produce evidence of 'aortic regurgitation' in animals proved at autopsy to have normal valves. The regurgitating consistently occurred during systole when the valves were open. . . ."[32] The open-end catheter was abandoned and replaced by a side-opening closed-end catheter. When the tip was placed 2 to 3 cm cephalad to the valves, this technique precluded "obtaining false radiographic evidence of aortic insufficiency."[32]

Sloman and Jefferson, in agreement with Nelson et al., found that the jet from a single-end-hole catheter often forced contrast material through the open aortic valve during ventricular systole.[33] With side holes and an open-end hole, less reflux into the left ventricle was observed. With a closed-end catheter, no reflux was visualized in 14 dogs.

Two years after their original paper, Nelson et al. in 1960 reiterated their endorsement of closed-end catheters after 350 injections in 50 dogs.[34] They emphasized the competence of the aortic valve under these conditions, although some of their illustrations suggested that regurgitation might have occurred.

Kjellberg et al. in 1961 also indicated that the open-end catheter was a source of error that could be eliminated by using a nonrecoiling catheter with a closed tip.[35] Runco et al. stated that they specifically looked for and found no instance of false-positive aortic regurgitation in over 70 patients with competent aortic valves studied by coronary arteriography.[36]

Mouquin et al., in reporting a cinematographic study of the aortic valve, stated that the valves were tightly closed in diastole with no leakage observable, not even minimal and transient leakage.[37] In 1962 Figley et al., in a study of coronary arteriography in dogs, found that doses of 1 ml per kilogram of body weight occasionally resulted in aortic incompetence and that doses of 0.5 ml per kilogram produced no reflux unless the blood pressure was temporarily reduced. "Aortic incompetence was not dependent upon catheter position in one of the sinuses of Valsalva, nor did injection here regularly produce incompetence."[38] Figley described an instance of reflux in both systole and diastole. Lehman et al. in 1962 stated, on the basis of their experience with 273 examinations, that "the competent aortic valve will not allow a significant reflux of contrast material into the left ventricle under the conditions of catheter thoracic aortography as we employ it. We have observed, on rare occasions, with a transient bradycardia or asystole, a slight 'puff' of opaque medium issuing through a competent valve and entering the left ventricle."[26]

Amplatz in 1962 noted "excellent correlation between the surgical findings and the angiographic ap-

◀ **Figure 22-2.** The appearance of supravalvular aortic stenosis. (A) Moderate. Thoracic cineaortogram, enlargement of a 35-mm frame. Just above the origin of the coronary arteries there is a localized zone of stenosis that demonstrated a systolic pressure gradient of 58 mmHg. The coronary arteries are strikingly dilated. There is also mild narrowing of the left common carotid artery and the left subclavian artery. (B and C) Moderate. Left anterior and right anterior oblique projections. A polyethylene catheter has been passed from the right femoral artery into the ascending aorta. With the injection of the contrast agent, a discrete zone of supravalvular stenosis is demonstrated. In contrast to valvular stenosis, poststenotic dilatation is not evident. The left coronary artery is dilated and arises just proximal to the zone of stenosis. A withdrawal pressure trace from the left ventricle was obtained and demonstrated a gradient in the supravalvular area of 46 mmHg. Surgical correction of the supravalvular aortic stenosis was successfully undertaken. (D) Marked. Thoracic cineaortogram, enlargement of a 35-mm frame. The injection is performed with the catheter in the left ventricle. The study demonstrates an enlarged left ventricle, which is also somewhat trabeculated. About 2 cm above the valve there is an area of marked narrowing of the aorta, which is hypoplastic above the site of stenosis. The mean systolic pressure gradient was 87 mmHg. The coronary arteries are huge. Stenosis of the origin of the left common carotid as well as minimal narrowing of the proximal portion of the innominate artery are also visible. The descending thoracic aorta is normal in caliber. (E) Pulmonary cinearteriogram, same case as (D), enlargement of a 35-mm frame. Profound stenosis is visible at the origin of a number of branch pulmonary arteries, particularly on the right but on the left as well.

pearance of the regurgitating jet. In a large group of patients, aortic insufficiency was demonstrated by this technique and confirmed on surgical intervention, although the lesion was not suspected clinically."[25] In 1963 Abrams reported briefly on the presence of reflux occurring "predominantly during the period of protodiastole" in a small series of dogs studied by thoracic aortography. There was absence of systolic reflux and increased diastolic reflux when the intrathoracic pressure was elevated.[39]

Rowe et al. in 1964 observed that contrast material rarely showed aortic incompetence when sampling of an indicator in the left ventricle after supravalvular injection failed to reveal it. They stated: "Indeed aortic insufficiency may be simulated by the rapid injection of contrast substance through a normal aortic valve during systole, particularly when open-end catheters are used."[40]

Segal et al., in 1964, in discussing "silent" rheumatic aortic valve regurgitation, indicated that severe reflux could be demonstrated by cineaortography in the absence of the characteristic diastolic murmur. They emphasized that the injection should be made at least 1 inch above the valve to avoid spurious regurgitation.[27] Massumi in 1964 reported a case in which factitious regurgitation occurred because the catheter in the aortic sinus actually impeded valve movement. Regurgitation occurred both in systole and in diastole. He suggested that thoracic aortography for aortic insufficiency should be performed with the catheter tip 5 cm above the valve.[41] Herbert in 1965 also emphasized the possibility of radiologic errors in the diagnosis of aortic insufficiency. He pointed out that in coronary arteriography simulated aortic insufficiency might occur when a long catheter slips through the valve because of recoil, with the contrast hiding the catheter tip. At the end of the injection the tip might return to its supravalvular position. Even if the injection into the left ventricle failed to occur directly, the catheter might interfere with the cusp motion. He suggested that turbulence alone might prevent complete closure of the valve and simulate aortic insufficiency.[42]

Thus many agree that aortography is the most sensitive means of diagnosing aortic valvular incompetence, and several remark that it often shows regurgitation when none was suspected clinically.[25,26,28] Most observers feel that the normal aortic valve does not permit any regurgitation except when the injection is made through an end-hole catheter, in which case the jet may go through the open valve during systole. Massumi states that factitious regurgitation is probably not rare,[41] whereas others disregard this possibility entirely.[25,37,43,44]

The literature, then (in its infinite variety), appears to support the following statements:

1. The normal aortic valve permits no reflux under normal circumstances.[26,30,43,45]
2. Factitious reflux through a normal aortic valve may occur with the end-hole catheter but only with the end-hold catheter.[26,33–35]
3. Factitious reflux may occur during systole with a rapid injection—especially, but not exclusively, with an end-hole catheter.[40]
4. Factitious reflux may occur if the catheter tip interferes with the valve action.[27,32,41,42]
5. Factitious reflux may result from a high injection volume.[38]
6. Factitious reflux may occur secondary to transient, unobserved slipping of the catheter tip through the valve.[42]
7. The use of a closed-end catheter prevents factitious reflux.[32,33,35]
8. Reflux may occur normally through the aortic valve with moderate volumes of contrast agent and moderate injection pressures.[39]

Our own experimental studies have led us to believe that reflux can occur through normal aortic valves and may indeed be physiologic.[45] The difficulty is to define what significant reflux is. A quantitative approach is helpful. A trace or a 1+ reflux is certainly not significant. Systolic reflux, if it occurs in humans, is not significant. The higher the catheter in the ascending aorta in humans, the more significant reflux becomes. Meaningful regurgitation should occur throughout diastole up to the point of ventricular systole. It should be at least 2+ on a scale of 4 (Fig. 22-3), should opacify not merely a small segment of the outflow tract but some of the apical portion of the ventricle as well, and should occur consistently in repeated heart cycles. The ventricular cavity should contain contrast material after the termination of injection. Although the presence of regurgitation is accurately displayed by aortography, angiographic grading may vary significantly from measured regurgitant volume, especially if the left ventricle is enlarged.[46]

On rare occasions artifactual aortic insufficiency or normal aortic insufficiency made more prominent by increased intrathoracic pressure may fulfill these criteria. It may then be necessary to repeat the examination with the catheter somewhat higher and the intrathoracic pressure normal. A similar volume of contrast agent, slower injection rate, and cine recording will augment the accuracy of the procedure.

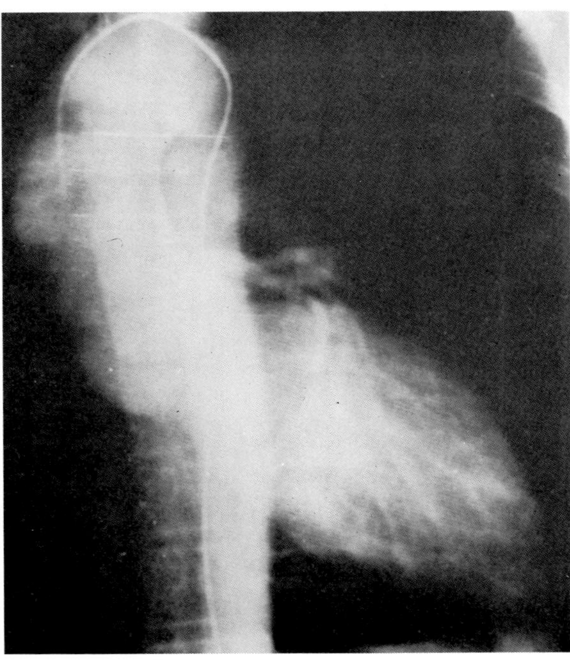

A

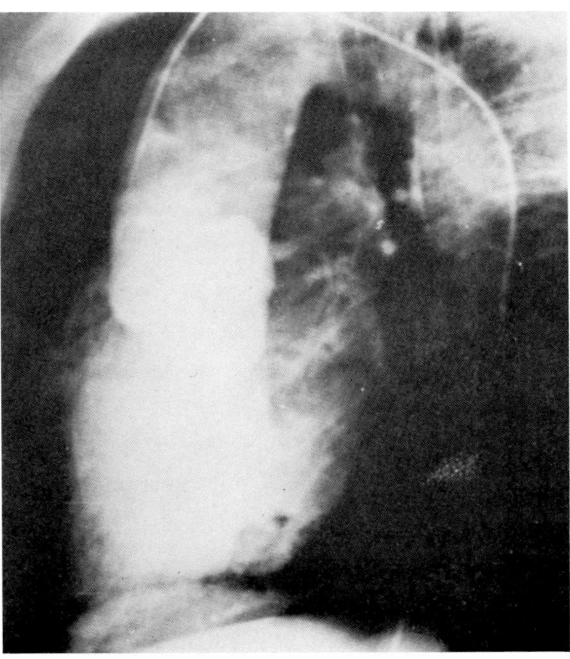

B

Figure 22-3. Aortic insufficiency. (A) Frontal projection. (B) Lateral projection. The catheter has been placed in the ascending aorta, which is grossly dilated. With the injection of 50 ml of 76 percent Renografin, gross reflux into a large left ventricle is visible. The contrast agent remained in the ventricular cavity throughout sequential heart cycles. The reflux is significant, grade 3, and indicates gross valvular disease.

Anomalies of the Aortic Arch

Developmental anomalies of the aortic arch vessels are due to the persistence of embryonic aortic arches or to the involution of vascular channels that normally persist.[47] Those that warrant attention are a persistent right aortic arch; double aortic arch; other vascular rings; and aberrant subclavian, common carotid, and innominate arteries. Clinically these conditions are often asymptomatic because they do not disturb circulatory dynamics significantly. When symptoms do occur, they are referable to pressure on the trachea and esophagus and may include dysphagia, dyspnea, wheezing, and even cyanosis (rarely). Careful fluoroscopic and radiographic study of the superior mediastinum, with particular attention to the relationship of the aortic arch and its major branches to the trachea and barium-filled esophagus, usually permits a general and frequently a specific identification of the nature of the anomaly.[48–51] Instillation of Lipiodol into the trachea may be desirable to determine both the presence and the degree of compression.

In most instances aortography is unnecessary. Rarely, it may not be possible to provide definitive information about the aortic arch without recourse to special studies. Retrograde aortography may demonstrate clearly the anatomy of the root of the aorta and its great branches, and at times angiocardiography may be equally helpful.

The order of filling and washout is of utmost importance in studying these anomalies; careful attention must be paid to both, because the differential diagnosis is based on the sequence of opacification. In adults, the percutaneous femoral approach is optimal. For infants with a suspected vascular ring, catheter or retrograde brachial aortography offers good detail and a high degree of opacification. Serial biplane films or cine technique should be used, the latter being best for showing the rapid blood flow to infants.[52] Although digital subtraction angiography may be employed effectively, it may occasionally be misleading.[53]

In frontal projection the appearance of the opacified right-sided aortic arch is distinctive.[54] The ascending aorta rises more obliquely to the right than usual, and the arch is seen on the right of the trachea rather than on the left. The course of the descending aorta on either the right or the left of the spine is delineated by the opaque material. Rarely, a right aortic

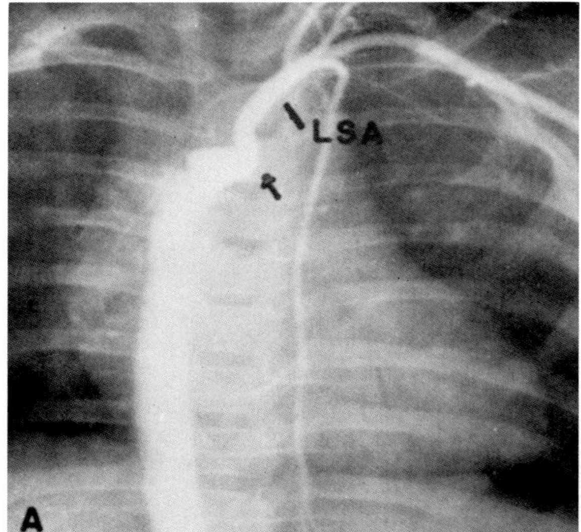

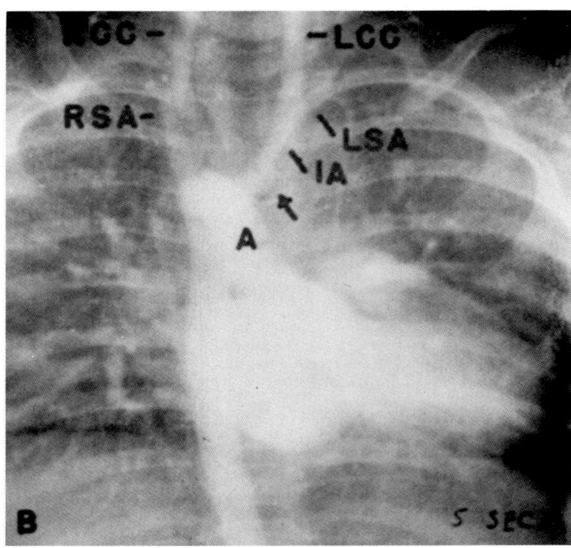

Figure 22-4. Right aortic arch with retroesophageal aortic diverticulum in a 13-month-old girl. (A) Retrograde aortogram at 1 second demonstrates the left subclavian artery (*LSA*) entering a small round pouch (*arrow*) to the left of the right descending aorta. This pouch is the "aortic diverticulum." (B) Angiocardiogram at 5 seconds shows the aorta ascending on the right in continuity with the right descending aorta. The right subclavian (*RSA*) and common carotid (*RCC*) arteries arise as individual trunks from the aorta instead of from a right innominate artery. The aortic diverticulum (*arrow*) gives rise to the left innominate artery (*IA*), from which the left common carotid (*LCC*) and the left subclavian (*LSA*) arteries spring. On conventional roentgenologic studies the barium-filled esophagus demonstrated a large, semicircular indentation in its posterior margin at the level of the aortic diverticulum.

arch with a retroesophageal aortic diverticulum may be demonstrated (Fig. 22-4), generally indicating the absence of any severe intracardiac anomalies. Mirror-image branching of the brachiocephalic vessels, when found, is usually associated with an intracardiac defect.[55] Unusual anomalies, such as left aortic arch with right descending aortic or cervical aortic arches, are readily diagnosed by aortography, although magnetic resonance imaging (MRI) achieves this noninvasively.[56] In the presence of a double aortic arch, the patency and relative size of both arches may be established and thus permit positive preoperative differentiation from ligamentous vascular rings. The position of the descending aorta and the origin, course, and relationships of the major arterial branches of the arch are also classified. An isolated innominate artery has been demonstrated by ventriculography in association with a right-sided arch. Late films showed contrast flow down the left carotid and left vertebral arteries to outline an isolated innominate trunk that communicated through a left ductus arteriosus with the pulmonary artery.[57] In the study of other types of vascular rings, the contrast agent demonstrates that part of the constricting ring is not patent. It also permits reasonably accurate determination of the location, length, and topographic relationships of the ligamentous portion of the ring when correlated with the conventional roentgen studies. Aberrant vessels are usually easily identified and rarely require aortography.

Rare anomalies have been disclosed on occasion by arteriography—a persistent trigeminal artery, for example, which was revealed during common carotid studies with filling of the apex of the basilar artery, the posterior cerebral arteries, and the superior cerebellar artery. Trigeminal arteries are extremely uncommon, with an incidence of only 0.08 to 0.6 percent in arteriographic series. Constant structures in the early human embryo, they serve as major branches of the internal carotid artery that initially constitute the primary blood supply to the bilateral longitudinal neural arteries. With the appearance of the posterior communicating arteries, the trigeminals cease to be major pathways to the human hindbrain. At this point, they normally begin to involute and are no longer evident after the vertebral arteries appear.[47] Often they do not cause any clinical neurologic syndrome. Transient ischemic attacks have been reported in patients with persistent trigeminal arteries, with symptoms resolving after endarterectomy. Such reports emphasize the importance of ruling out the anterior circulation as a source of microemboli.[47]

Sequestration of the Lung

There has been increasing recognition that intralobar pulmonary sequestration is by no means a rare anomaly.[58] In this condition a portion of the lower lobe is partially or completely separated from the normal bronchial tree. In frequent association with this separated lung, one or more anomalous systemic arteries may be encountered entering the pulmonary tissue.[59] The anomaly may be discovered at any age and is usually associated with recurrent pulmonary infection. Radiographically, the lesion is seen more commonly on the left than on the right. There may be pulmonary consolidation, multiple thin-walled cysts, or an apparent paravertebral mass. At bronchography no contrast medium enters the involved portion of lung. One or more systemic vessels feed the sequestrated lung and usually arise from the thoracic aorta.[60]

A number of cases of sequestrated lung have proved troublesome at surgery when there has been no prior knowledge of the presence of anomalous arteries (particularly if the arteries arise from the subdiaphragmatic aorta). These vessels have been demonstrated in the past with contrast medium in the aorta.[61] Figure 22-5 illustrates a case in which the sequestrated lung was fed by three large vessels arising from the aorta. The venous return from this sequestrated segment of lung was systemic: The opaque medium entered the hemiazygos vein and reached the superior vena cava through the azygos vein. Hence, these vessels did not communicate or anastomose with the pulmonary vessels.

Evaluation of Aortic Grafts

A late common complication of valve replacement with aortic grafts is hemorrhage at the anastomotic site. Radiology is important in managing the patients.[62] Arterial graft thrombosis can be influenced by the thrombosing tendency of blood flowing through the graft, and by turbulence or stagnation of blood flow in the graft. Anastomotic constriction at the suture lines is obviously related to the latter. Studies of canine aortas correlated the observed patency of aortic grafts with arteriographic evidence of constriction at the suture lines. Arteriographic evidence of suture-line narrowing proved to be an acceptable indicator of subsequent patency.[63] Although visual observation of grafts at surgery may show them to have a pulsatile flow of blood, aortograms can demonstrate a significant (and unrecognized) anastomotic constriction. Sometimes only careful selective cineangiography will disclose a small leak beneath an anastomosis. Because leakage occurs only in systole, it is usually not demonstrated on cut-film aortography. Rapid intracoronary and pericoronary injections during cine recording are required. With this technique, it is important to inject the contrast medium rapidly, to produce reflux from the coronary ostium.[62]

Truncus Arteriosus

A truncus arteriosus is a single great arterial vessel which, arising from the heart, gives rise to the coronary arteries, the pulmonary arteries (or, in their absence, collateral lung vessels), and the systemic arteries.[64,65] The pulmonary artery may arise as a single vessel from the trunk and then branch, whereas the main hilar branches may arise individually from the ascending portion of the trunk. In the absence of pulmonary arteries, bronchial arteries or other collateral vessels supply the lungs and there is then decreased pulmonary blood flow. At times the pulmonary arteries receive blood through a patent ductus arteriosus; most of these cases, however, probably represent examples of pulmonary atresia.[66] Angiocardiography is the preferred method of studying truncus arteriosus and analyzing both the intracardiac and the extracardiac elements in the anomaly (Fig. 22-6).[67] Selective injection of contrast medium into the common trunk shows simultaneous filling of the ascending aorta and the pulmonary artery.[68] However, evidence of pulmonary arteries arising directly from the trunk may also be demonstrated with aortography.[58,69,70] This, of course, constitutes an important piece of information, because a lesion of this kind is inoperable. With filling of the aorta, the opaque material passes immediately into the pulmonary arteries and is demonstrated in the lung fields, filling the branch vessels.

The Status of Subclavian Pulmonary Artery Anastomoses

In the care of patients with tetralogy of Fallot who have undergone the Blalock-Taussig procedure, it is sometimes difficult to be certain whether the anastomotic site actually remains patent. This is particularly important when it is planned to subject these patients to open heart surgery and total repair, because patency of this anastomotic site in the absence of a continuous murmur may occur and may cause difficulty at surgery. Thoracic aortography clarifies the problem.[71] With the catheter in the ascending aorta or in the transverse por-

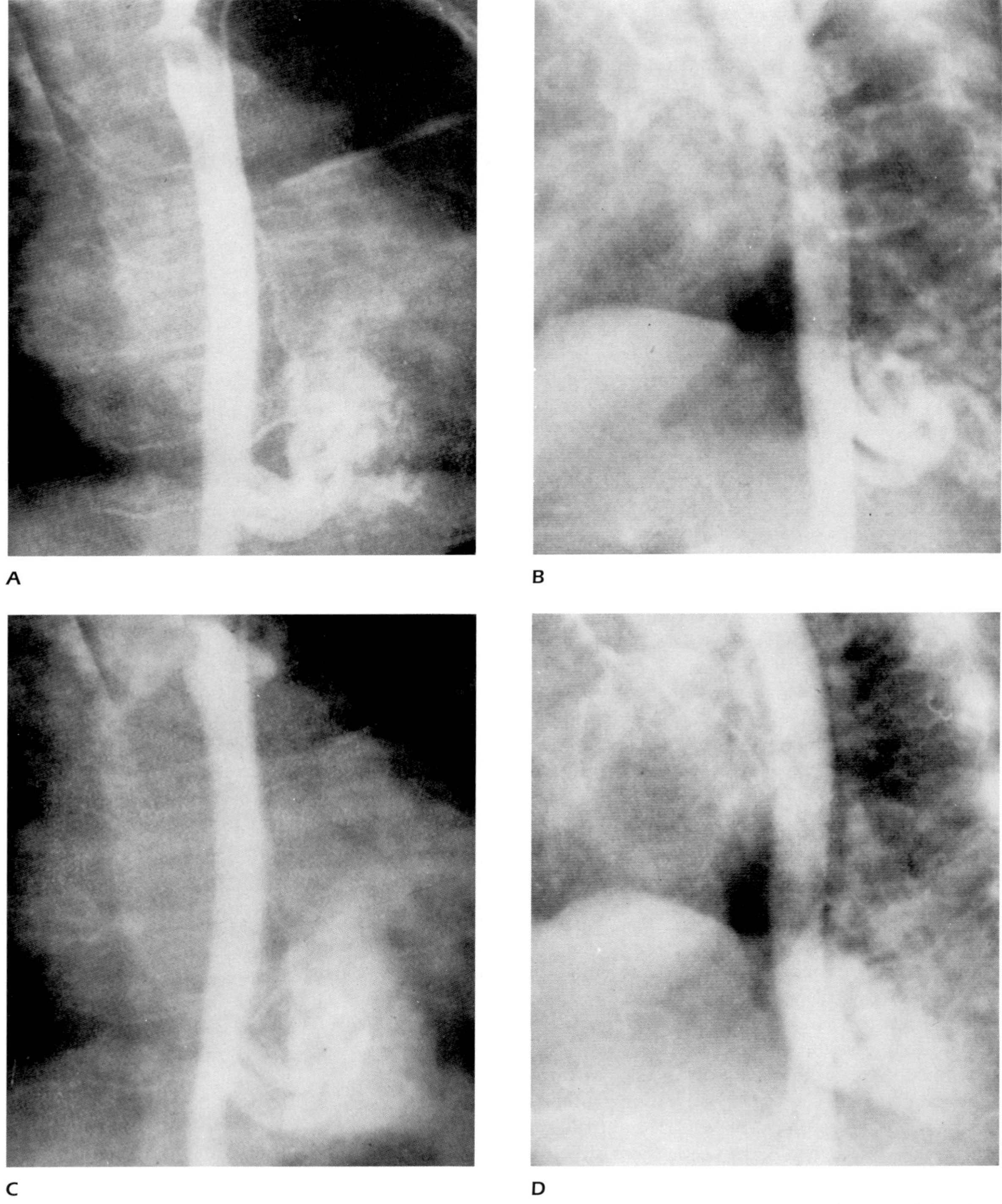

Figure 22-5. Sequestration of the lung associated with anomalous arteries from the aorta in a 1-year-old girl. Conventional chest films demonstrated a patchy density in the left lower lobe adjacent to the spine. A retrograde brachial aortogram demonstrated three large vessels entering the area of consolidation. (A) Posteroanterior projection, ½ second. The descending thoracic aorta is densely opaque, and three large vessels may be seen entering the consolidated portion of the left lower lobe. (B) Lateral projection, ½ second. The posterior origin of the vessels is clearly seen. (C) Anteroposterior projection, 2 seconds. The opaque medium is now in the capillary bed and fills the consolidated area densely. (D) Lateral projection, 2 seconds, showing similar findings to those in the frontal projection.

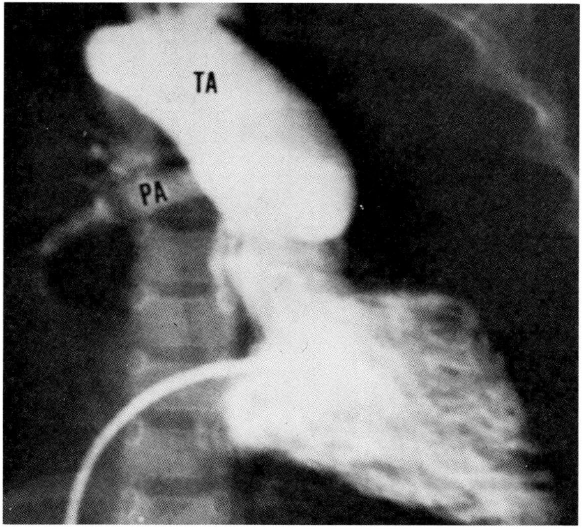

A

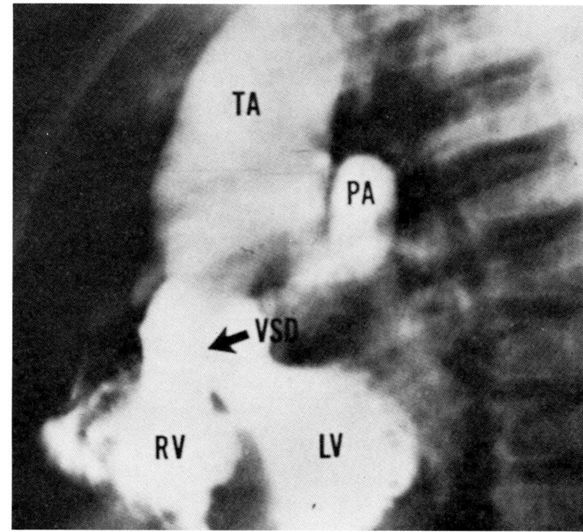

B

Figure 22-6. Truncus arteriosus. (A) Posteroanterior projection. (B) Lateral projection. The catheter has been passed from the inferior vena cava to its intraventricular position. With contrast injection a single large trunk is visible overriding the ventricular septum with the pulmonary artery arising posteriorly from the trunk. A ventricular septal defect (*VSD*), which is always present in a true truncus arteriosus, is visible. Although angiocardiography is usually more useful than thoracic aortography in the study of truncus arteriosus, the exact definition of the origin of the pulmonary arteries in the trunk is frequently better accomplished by aortography. *TA,* truncus arteriosus; *PA,* pulmonary artery; *RV,* right ventricle; *LV,* left ventricle.

tion of the arch, it is possible to opacify the great vessels of the arch and to demonstrate whether there is passage of the opaque medium through the anastomotic site into the pulmonary vessels. In Figure 22-7, for example, the opaque medium is clearly seen entering the left lung through a subclavian artery that is only partially occluded by laminated clot.

Buckling of the Great Vessels

Buckling of the innominate[72] and the common carotid[73] arteries is usually seen in patients over the age of 50 with a pulsatile mass at the base of the neck on the right side. Frequently the chest roentgenogram is the first indication of the mass, and on physical examination the pulsation may be felt. The appearance of the mass may be sufficiently suggestive to cause exploratory thoracotomy to be performed.[72]

Buckling can be demonstrated simply by aortography or angiocardiography.[74] Whenever there is a suspicion of this lesion and/or whenever the possibility of thoracotomy is entertained for a supposed mediastinal mass in the region of the buckled vessels, contrast studies are indicated.[74]

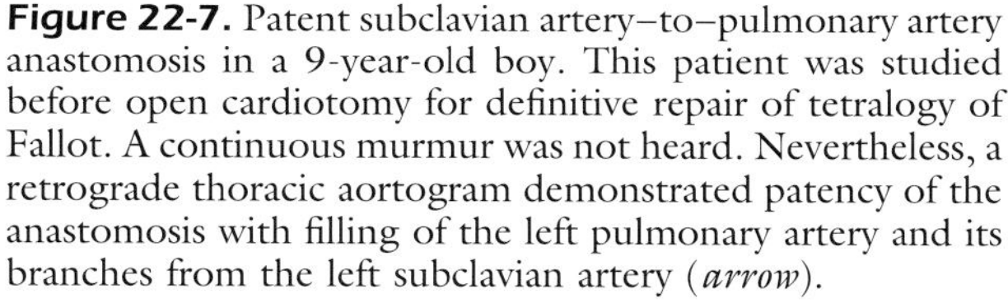

Figure 22-7. Patent subclavian artery–to–pulmonary artery anastomosis in a 9-year-old boy. This patient was studied before open cardiotomy for definitive repair of tetralogy of Fallot. A continuous murmur was not heard. Nevertheless, a retrograde thoracic aortogram demonstrated patency of the anastomosis with filling of the left pulmonary artery and its branches from the left subclavian artery (*arrow*).

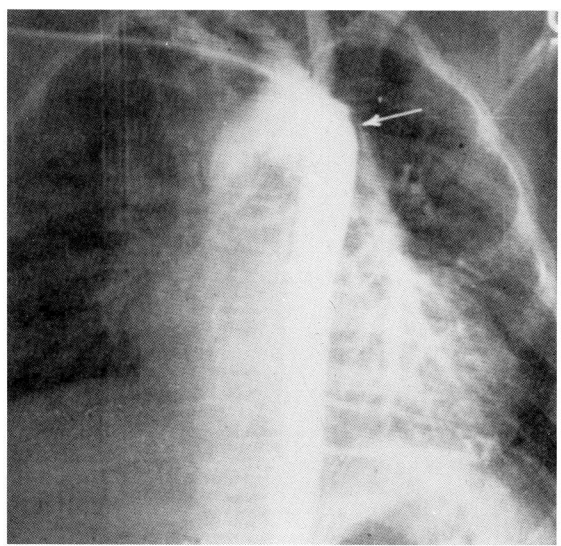

Figure 22-8. Vertebral flow reversal syndrome. (A) One second. An aortic arch injection has been made with the patient in the right posterior oblique projection. The stump of the left subclavian artery is seen with no contrast passing beyond it. Atheromatous changes are visible in the innominate and right subclavian arteries. (B) At 6 seconds, the left vertebral artery (*LVA*) is visualized filling from above. (C) At 8 seconds, contrast filling of the left subclavian artery (*LSA*) is observed in continuity with the retrograde left vertebral filling.

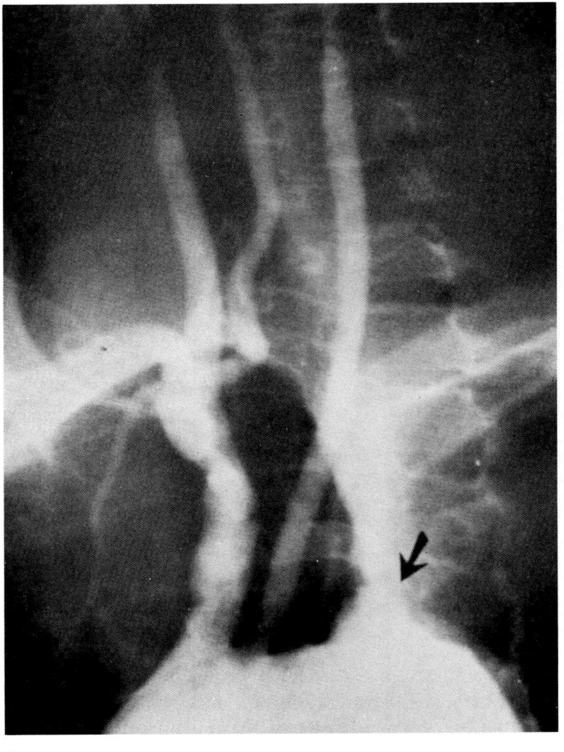

A

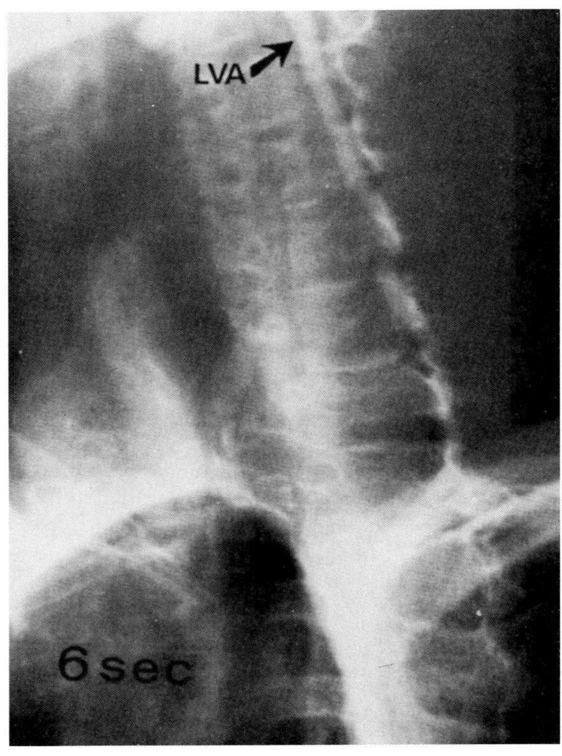

B

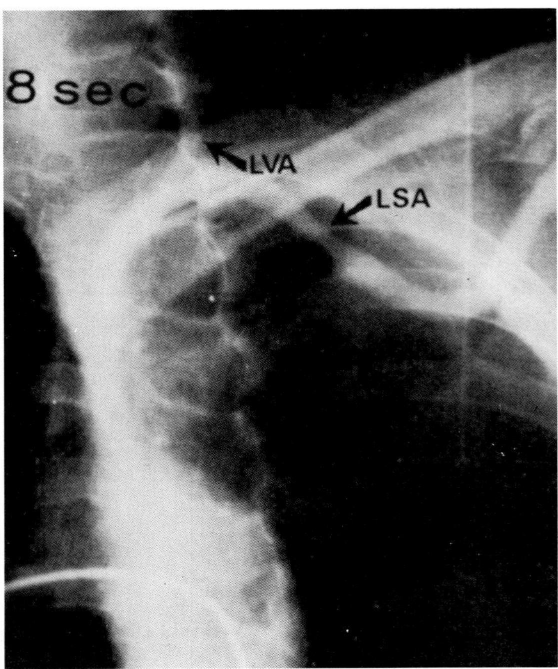

C

Pseudocoarctation

Pseudocoarctation, an anomaly that is congenital rather than acquired, is also called *kinking of the aorta*. Several suggestions have been made as to its cause, among them the failure to atrophy of the distal right arch and its subsequent incorporation into the distal left arch.[75] It usually comes to the attention of the radiologist on a conventional posteroanterior chest film.[76] Because it may simulate a tumor, defining its exact nature is of great importance. The radiologic appearance is similar to that of coarctation, but there is generally no diminution in pressure or pulse in the lower extremities, and the area of apparent narrowing of the aorta on conventional films has no dynamic effect. The presence of pressure gradients in some cases of pseudocoarctation and their occasional absence in classic coarctation have led some investigators to believe that the distinction between the two entities may be artificial. Pressure gradients across the kinked area of pseudocoarctation have been well documented. The relationship, however, remains conjectural.[75] Both angiocardiography[61,77] and aortography[78] have been employed in the study of kinking of the aorta. Contrast studies enable clear delineation of the aorta in this region, the exclusion of a nonvascular mass, and the demonstration of the aortic deformity.

Study of the Brachiocephalic Vessels

The so-called aortic arch syndrome has been receiving increased attention. As originally described, it was characterized by arteritis and thrombosis of the great vessels arising from the arch and occurred mainly in young women in association with cerebral and ocular symptoms as well as symptoms referable to the upper extremities.[79] Takayasu disease is one variant of this syndrome. It is characterized by occlusion of the brachiocephalic trunks and their orifice; a flame-shaped termination is characteristic. In extreme forms—the classic arteriographic appearance of a bold aortic arch—all or most of the trunks are occluded, and the entire circulation of the brain is accomplished by collateral vessels.[80] One of the rarer anomalies of the brachiocephalic vessels is absence of the common carotid artery, with separate origins of the internal and external carotid arteries. In about half of such cases, absence of a common carotid artery is associated with additional vascular anomalies: double aortic arch, right aortic arch, and aberrant right subclavian artery.[81] The study of the origin of the great vessels to the brain, head, and neck has proved increasingly important as concepts of cerebral insufficiency have developed and as the possibility of removing stenosing lesions of the carotid arteries has been realized.[82] Thus thoracic aortography with flooding of the aortic arch has been widely used as a means of showing all of the great vessels arising from the arch simultaneously and of demonstrating the extracranial course and character of the carotid vessels. Study of these vessels in the presence of arteriosclerotic disease has brought to light the so-called vertebral flow reversal syndrome,[83] in which complete occlusion of the left subclavian artery may be accompanied by retrograde filling of the left vertebral artery from the basilar artery with distal filling of the left subclavian artery from the vertebral artery (Fig. 22-8).

Acknowledgments

Some of the work described in this chapter was supported in part by grants HE11668 and HE05832 from the United States Public Health Service, National Institutes of Health.

References

1. Mitchell AM, Sackett EH, Hunzicker WJ, et al. The clinical features of aortic stenosis. Am Heart J 1954;48:684.
2. Taussig H. Congenital malformations of the heart. New York: Commonwealth Fund, 1947.
3. Campbell M, Kauntze R. Congenital aortic valvular stenosis. Br Heart J 1953;15:179.
4. Edwards JE. Pathology of left ventricular outflow tract obstruction. Circulation 1965;31:586.
5. Gruenwald P. Subaortic stenosis of the left ventricle: report of six cases. J Tech Meth 1947;27:187.
6. Young D. Congenital subaortic stenosis. Am Heart J 1944;28:440.
7. Gishen P, Lakier JB. The ascending aorta in aortic stenosis. Cardiovasc Radiol 1979;2:85.
8. Harris VJ. The size and configuration of the aorta in acquired heart disease: correlation with physiologic data. J Am Wom Assoc 1979;34:303.
9. Grishman A, Steinberg MF, Sussman ML. Congenital aortic and subaortic stenosis with associated anomalies of the aorta. Med Clin North Am 1947;31:543.
10. Kjellberg SR, Mannheimer E, Rudhe U, et al. Diagnosis of congenital heart disease. Chicago: Year Book, 1955.
11. Lehman JS, Musser BG, Lykens HD. Cardiac ventriculography. AJR 1957;77:267.
12. Downing DF. Congenital aortic stenosis: clinical aspects of surgical treatment. Circulation 1956;16:188.
13. Ödman P, Philipson J. Aortic valvular diseases studied by percutaneous thoracic aortography. Acta Radiol (Stockh) 1958; 182(Suppl):1.
14. Beuren AJ, Schulze C, Eberle P, et al. The syndrome of supravalvular aortic stenosis, peripheral pulmonary stenosis, mental retardation and similar facial appearance. Am J Cardiol 1964; 13:471.
15. Black JA, Bonham Carter RE. Association between aortic stenosis and facies of severe infantile hypercalcemia. Lancet 1963; 2:745.

16. Garcia RE, Friedman WF, Kaback MM, et al. Idiopathic hypercalcemia and supravalvular aortic stenosis: documentation of a new syndrome. N Engl J Med 1964;271:117.
17. Taybi H, Petry E, Merritt A, et al. Congenital supravalvular aortic stenosis and associated pulmonary vascular anomalies. Scientific Exhibit, 49th Annual Meeting of the Radiological Society of North America, Chicago, November, 1963.
18. Cheu S, Fiese MJ, Hatayoma E. Supra aortic stenosis. Am J Clin Pathol 1957;28:293.
19. Perou ML. Congenital supravalvular aortic stenosis. Arch Pathol Lab Med 1961;71:453.
20. Klatte EC, Yune H, Bryan B. Radiographic manifestations of aortic stenosis and aortic valvular insufficiency. Semin Roentgenol 1979;14:122.
21. Williams JCP, Barratt-Boyes BG, Lowe JB. Supravalvular aortic stenosis. Circulation 1961;24:1311.
22. Kupic EA, Abrams HL. Radiological aspects of operative heart disease: VIII. Supravalvular aortic stenosis. AJR 1966;98:822.
23. Hancock EW. Differentiation of valvar, subvalvar, and supravalvar aortic stenosis. Guy's Hosp Rep 1961;110:1.
24. Segal J, Harvey WP, Hufnagel C. A clinical study of 100 cases of severe aortic insufficiency. Am J Med 1956;21:200.
25. Amplatz K. The roentgenographic diagnosis of mitral and aortic valvular disease. Am Heart J 1962;64:556.
26. Lehman JS, Boyle JJ Jr, Debbas JN. Quantitation of aortic valvular insufficiency by catheter thoracic aortography. Radiology 1962;79:361.
27. Segal BL, Likoff W, Kaspar AJ. "Silent" rheumatic aortic regurgitation. Am J Cardiol 1964;14:628.
28. Taubman JO, Goodman DJ, Steiner RE. The value of contrast studies in the investigation of aortic valve disease. Clin Radiol 1966;17:23.
29. Castellanos A, Garcia O. The diagnosis of aortic insufficiency in the living subject and the cadaver by means of retrograde aortography. Rev Cubana Pediatr 1953;25:455.
30. Wilder RJ, Moscovitz HL, Ravitch MM. Transventricular and aortic angiocardiography and physiologic studies in dogs with experimental mitral and aortic insufficiency. Surgery 1956;40:86.
31. Wilder RJ, Moscovitz HL, Ravitch MM. Roentgen contrast diagnosis of experimental mitral and aortic insufficiency in dogs by transventricular injection and retrograde catheterization. J Thorac Cardiovasc Surg 1957;33:147.
32. Nelson SW, Molnar W, Kiabsen KP, et al. Aortic valvulography and ascending aortography. Radiology 1958;70:697.
33. Sloman G, Jefferson K. Cine-angiography of the coronary circulation in living dogs. Br Heart J 1960;22:54.
34. Nelson SW, Molnar W, Christoforidis A, et al. Coronary arteriography: development of a method in animals with particular attention to physiologic effects. Radiology 1960;75:34.
35. Kjellberg SR, Nordenström B, Rudhe U, et al. Cardioangiographic studies of the mitral and aortic valves. Acta Radiol (Stockh) 1961;204(Suppl):1.
36. Runco V, Molnar W, Meckstroth CV, et al. The Graham Steell murmur versus aortic regurgitation in rheumatic heart disease. Am J Med 1961;31:71.
37. Mouquin M, Brun P, Geschwind H, et al. Étude cinetique des valves aortiques: premiers éléments tiers de la cine angiocardiographieu. Arch Mal Coeur Vaiss 1962;55:1.
38. Figley M, Haight C, Sloan H, et al. Coronary arteriography—some physiologic observations during development of a controlled experimental study. Univ Mich Med Bull 1962;28:237.
39. Abrams HL. Present status of biplane cineangiocardiography. JAMA 1963;184:747.
40. Rowe G, Castillo C, Alfonso S, et al. Diagnostic cine angiocardiography. Vasc Dis 1964;1:45.
41. Massumi RA. Factitious aortic regurgitation: report of a case. Dis Chest 1964;46:734.
42. Herbert WW. Radiographic errors in the diagnosis of aortic insufficiency. Vasc Dis 1965;2:87.
43. Colapinto RS, Thorfinnson PC, Holmes RB. Aortic insufficiency—a cine-radiologic assessment. J Can Assoc Radiol 1962;13:112.
44. Hansen PF, Davidsen HG. Thoracic aortography in aortic valvular disease and subaortic stenosis. Dan Med Bull 1964;11:8.
45. Fabian CE, Abrams HL. Reflux through normal aortic valves. Invest Radiol 1968;3:178.
46. Croft CH, Lipscomb MD, Mathis K, et al. Limitations of qualitative angiographic grading in aortic or mitral regurgitation. Am J Cardiol 1984;11:1593.
47. Moore TS, Morris JL. Aortic arch vessel anomalies associated with persistent trigeminal artery. AJR 1979;133:309.
48. Abrams HL. Left ascending aorta with right arch and right descending aorta. Radiology 1951;57:58.
49. Lubert M, Epstein HC, Mendelsohn H, et al. An unusual variant of double aortic arch. AJR 1952;67:763.
50. Neuhauser EBD. The roentgen diagnosis of double aortic arch and other anomalies of the great vessels. AJR 1946;56:1.
51. Paul RN. Left aortic arch with right descending aorta. J Pediatr 1948;32:19.
52. Garti IJ, Aygen MM, Levy MJ. Double aortic arch anomalies: diagnosis by counter-current right brachial arteriography. AJR 1979;133:251.
53. Trigaux JP, Schoevaerdts JC, van Beers B, et al. Pitfalls of digital angiography in the diagnosis of right aortic arch. Eur J Radiol 1987;7:216.
54. Castellanos A, Pereiras R, Lopez AG. Arco aortico a la derecha en el nino: Estudio general. Valor de la angiocardiografia. Arch Inst Cardiol Mex 1945;15:301.
55. Van der Horst RL, Fisher EA, DuBrow IW, et al. Right aortic arch, right patent ductus arteriosus, and mirror-image branching of the brachiocephalic vessels. Cardiovasc Radiol 1978;1:147.
56. Jaffe RB. Radiographic manifestations of congenital anomalies of the aortic arch. Radiol Clin North Am 1991;29:319.
57. Martin EC, Mesko ZG, Griepp RB, et al. Isolation of the left innominate artery, a right arch, and a left patent ductus arteriosus. AJR 1979;132:833.
58. Pryce DM. Lower accessory pulmonary artery with intralobar sequestration of lung: a report of 7 cases. J Pathol 1946;58:457.
59. Wall CA, Lucido JL. Intralobar bronchopulmonary sequestration. Surg Gynecol Obstet 1956;103:701.
60. Bruwer AJ, Clagett OT, McDonald JR. Intralobar bronchopulmonary sequestration. AJR 1954;71:751.
61. Kenney LJ, Eyler WR. Preoperative diagnosis of sequestration of the lung by aortography. JAMA 1956;160:1464.
62. Nath PH, Zollikofer C, Castaneda-Zuniga WR, et al. Radiological evaluation of composite aortic grafts. Radiology 1979;131:43.
63. Mortensen JD. Importance of immediate postoperative arteriography in evaluation of arterial graft patency rates. Trans Am Soc Artif Intern Organs 1978;24:692.
64. Anderson RC, Obata W, Lillehei CS. Truncus arteriosus. Circulation 1957;16:586.
65. Humphreys EM. Truncus arteriosus communis persistens: criteria for identification of common arterial trunk with report of case with 4 semilunar cusps. Arch Pathol Lab Med 1932;14:671.
66. Collett RW, Edwards JE. Persistent truncus arteriosus: a classification according to anatomic types. Surg Clin North Am 1949;29:1245.
67. Abrams HL, Kaplan HS. Angiocardiographic interpretation in congenital heart disease. Springfield, IL: Charles C Thomas, 1956.
68. Zamora C, Jain SC, Munoz-Castellanos L, et al. Truncus arteriosus communis, an unusual anatomical variant of type I. Cathet Cardiovasc Diagn 1980;6:81.
69. Contro S, Miller RA, White HA, et al. Syndrome of truncus arteriosus communis with large pulmonary flow: resemblance to patent ductus arteriosus. Circulation 1956;14:921.
70. Singleton EB, McNamara DG, Cooley DA. Retrograde aortog-

raphy in the diagnosis of congenital heart disease in infants. J Pediatr 1955;47:720.
71. Castellanos A, Garcia O, Pereiras R. On the value of retrograde aortography in the study of the congenital cardiac lesions operated. Rev Cubana Pediatr 1953;25:413.
72. Honig EI, Dubilier W Jr, Steinberg I. Significance of the buckled innominate artery. Ann Intern Med 1953;39:74.
73. Deterling RA Jr. Tortuous right common carotid artery simulating aneurysm. Angiology 1952;3:483.
74. Hsu I, Kistin AB. Buckling of the great vessels: a clinical and angiographic study. Arch Intern Med 1956;98:712.
75. Winer HE, Kronzon I, Glassman E, et al. Pseudocoarctation and mid-arch aortic coarctation. Chest 1977;72:519.
76. Bruwer AJ, Burchell HB. Kinking of aortic arch (pseudocoarctation, subclinical coarctation). JAMA 1956;162:1445.
77. Steinberg I. Aneurysm of aortic sinuses with pseudocoarctation of the aorta. Br Heart J 1956;18:85.
78. DiGuglielmo L, Guttadauro M. Kinking of aorta: report of 2 cases. Acta Radiol (Stockh) 1955;44:121.
79. Koszewski BJ, Hubbard DF. "Pulseless disease" due to brachial arteritis. Circulation 1957;16:406.
80. Landé A, Bard R, Bole P, et al. Aortic arch syndrome (Takayasu's arteritis): arteriographic and surgical considerations. J Cardiovasc Surg (Torino) 1978;19:507.
81. Bryan RN, Drewyer RG, Gee E. Separate origins of the left, internal and external carotid arteries from the aorta. AJR 1978; 130:362.
82. DeBakey MD, Morris TC Jr, Jordan GL, et al. Segmental thrombo-obliterative disease of branches of aortic arch. JAMA 1958;166:998.
83. Reivich N, Holling EH, Roberts B, et al. Reversal of blood flow through the vertebral artery and its effect on cerebral circulation. N Engl J Med 1961;265:878.

23

Technique of Coronary Arteriography

DAVID C. LEVIN

The modern era of coronary arteriography began with the development by Sones and Shirey[1] of a safe technique for selectively catheterizing the coronary arteries. This landmark in the diagnosis of acquired heart disease occurred over 3 decades ago. Although considerable improvement in equipment and techniques has taken place since then, the Sones method is still widely used.

The Sones method of performing coronary arteriography entails surgical exposure of the brachial artery. In the early and mid-1960s, percutaneous transfemoral selective coronary arteriography was introduced by several groups of radiologists—notably Ricketts and Abrams,[2] Judkins,[3] and Amplatz et al.[4] Both Judkins and Amplatz et al. developed preformed catheters that are available from several manufacturing companies. The Judkins technique, because of its ease, speed, reliability, and a somewhat lower complication rate, has become the most widely used approach for coronary arteriography in the United States.[5] This chapter is principally devoted to a discussion of the Judkins technique and also discusses other techniques.

Guidewires and Catheters

In performing percutaneous transfemoral arteriography of all types, most angiographers routinely use a 0.035-inch guidewire with a 3-mm J tip. The guidewire should be at least 145 cm in length. The use of the J tip promotes easy passage of the guidewire through tortuous iliac arteries and, compared with straight-tipped guidewires, lessens the likelihood of dissection of an atherosclerotic plaque. In patients with severe atherosclerosis or marked tortuosity of vessels, it may not be possible to pass even this standard J wire satisfactorily. In that case, we switch to tapered-core J wires, movable-core J wires, or multicurved J wires, all of which provide more tip flexibility. It is advisable that the catheterization-angiographic laboratory keep a variety of different guidewires on hand to facilitate wire passage in difficult cases.

The Judkins and Amplatz catheters are shown in Figure 23-1. These catheters are available in both polyurethane and polyethylene. A metal braid is incorporated into the wall of the shaft of the catheter to allow for better "torque" control. The Judkins left coronary catheter is available in three sizes, commonly referred to as JL4, JL5, and JL6. The numbers 4, 5, and 6 refer to the length in centimeters of the secondary arm (the portion of the catheter that remains outside the coronary ostium in the ascending aorta). For average-sized patients with average-sized thoracic aortas, the JL4 catheter is appropriate. If patients are tall or have somewhat elongated or tortuous thoracic aortas, a JL5 catheter should be used. For patients with very elongated thoracic aortas or marked poststenotic dilatation, a JL6 may be necessary. The Judkins right coronary catheters are available in sizes JR4, JR5, and JR6. Again, the numerical designation refers to the length of the secondary arm of the catheter. Selecting the proper-sized catheter is not quite as critical in catheterizing the right coronary artery as it is on the left side. The catheters come in a standard 100-cm length, although they can be specially ordered in a greater length. In most adult patients, either 7 or 8 French catheters are used; in either case, the tip tapers down to a size 5 French.

It is useful to have the capability of altering these catheters in the laboratory if the patient's anatomy requires it. For example, in a short patient with an unusually small ascending aorta, a JL4 catheter might

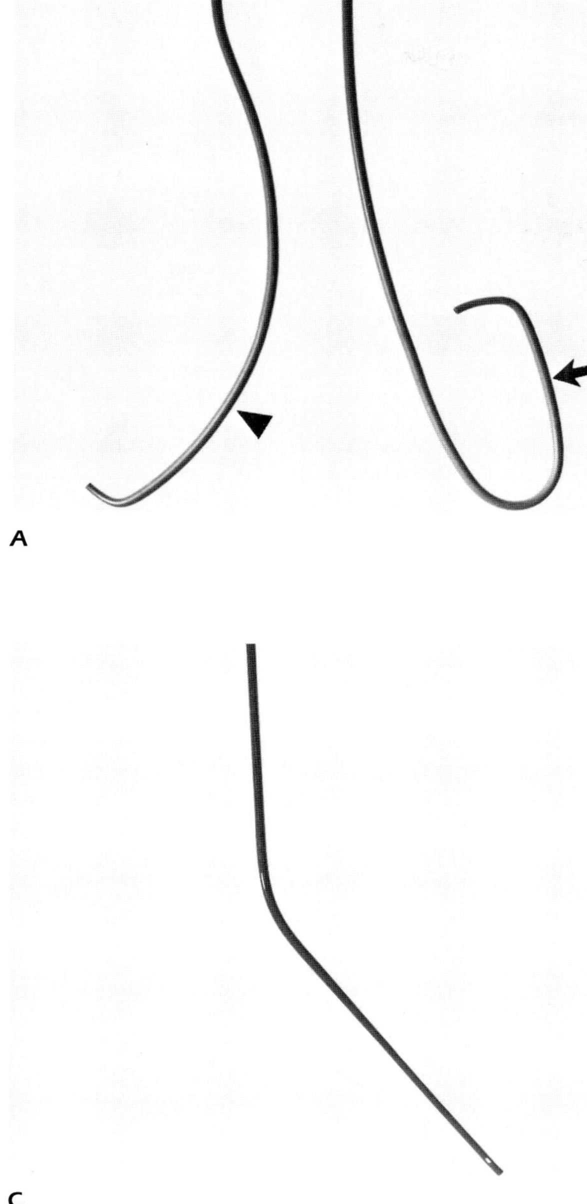

A

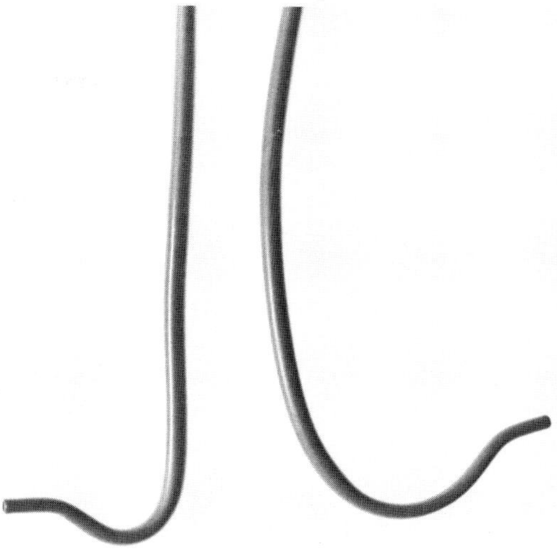

B

C

Figure 23-1. The most commonly used catheters for coronary arteriography. (A) Right and left Judkins catheters. The *arrowhead* points to the secondary arm of the Judkins right coronary catheter; the *arrow* points to the secondary arm of the Judkins left coronary catheter. (B) Amplatz right and left coronary catheters. (C) Sones coronary catheter.

have too long a secondary arm to enter the left coronary ostium properly. It may instead tend to become positioned in the left sinus of Valsalva below the left coronary ostium, rather than in the coronary artery. When this occurs, the steam jet emanating from a tea kettle can be used to alter the shape of the catheter. In this particular case, one would first straighten out the secondary curve of the catheter and then rebend the catheter to make an even shorter secondary arm. Curves can be easily removed and rebent by passing a polyethylene catheter briefly through the steam jet while holding it in a desired configuration. Subsequent immersion of the newly shaped segment of catheter in cold water will fix the new configuration, and the catheter will retain this new shape quite effectively. This procedure can only be satisfactorily carried out with polyethylene catheters. Polyurethane catheters cannot be reshaped this easily; this is one of the disadvantages of that particular material.

Another catheter alteration that may facilitate coronary arteriography is simply cutting the primary catheter tip with a sterile blade to shorten it, if for some reason the tip proves to be too long. In doing this, the angiographer should make certain that the cut is clean and smooth, so that no ragged edges are left on the catheter tip to promote thrombus formation.

The Amplatz catheters come in the same length, French sizes, and materials, although as Figure 23-1 shows, the tip configuration is markedly different from that of the Judkins catheters. The Amplatz left coronary catheters are sized AL1 to AL4. The Amplatz right coronary catheters are sized AR1 and AR2. These numerical designations refer to the overall size of the curved portion of the catheter. In most patients in whom Amplatz catheters are employed, the AL1 or AL2 catheter can be used for the left coronary artery and the AR1 catheter for the right coronary artery. The larger shapes are used in patients with more dilated aortic roots. There are some patients whose anatomy is such that the Judkins catheter simply will not enter one or the other of the coronary arteries. In this situation, the corresponding Amplatz catheter should be used. The configurations of the Judkins and Amplatz catheters are sufficiently different so that, if the Judkins catheter cannot be selectively placed in the left or right coronary artery, the corresponding Amplatz catheter almost always can. Any laboratory that primarily uses the Judkins percutaneous femoral approach to coronary arteriography should always keep a supply of Amplatz catheters in stock to use when needed.

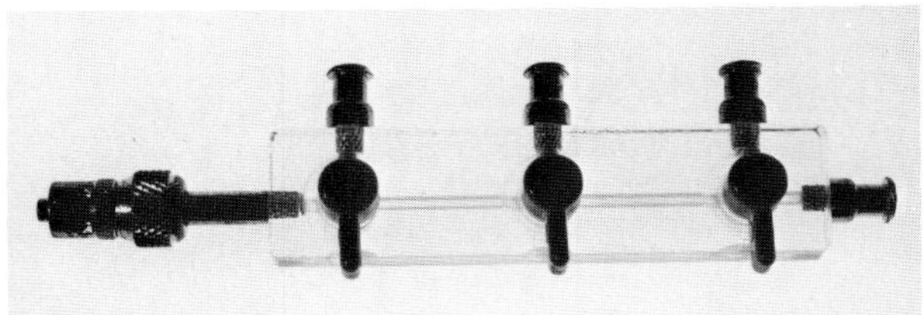

Figure 23-2. The three-stopcock manifold used for coronary arteriography. On the *far left* is the rotating adapter, which is connected directly to the coronary artery catheter. On the *far right* is a female Luer-Lok fitting, which is attached to a 10-ml syringe. The three female Luer-Lok fittings at the top are connected, respectively *from left to right,* to lines leading to the pressure transducer, saline flushing solution, and contrast material for arteriography. By manipulating the three keys on the manifold, the angiographer has the option of monitoring catheter tip pressure, filling the syringe with flushing solution and then injecting it through the catheter, or filling the syringe with contrast material and then injecting it through the catheter. Catheter tip pressure should be constantly monitored except when the catheter is being flushed with saline or contrast material is being injected for arteriography.

Manifold and Arterial Sheath

Two important additional pieces of equipment in coronary arteriography are the manifold and the arterial sheath.

The three-stopcock manifold, which is used in most laboratories employing the Judkins technique, is shown in Figure 23-2. This device allows easy manipulation of the catheter and rapid switching over from pressure monitoring to contrast injections or flushing of the catheter with saline, all in a closed system that allows maintenance of sterile technique. One end of the manifold has a rotating adapter that is attached to the coronary catheter. The other end of the manifold has a Luer-Lok fitting to which a 10-ml syringe is attached. The three side ports receive lines that lead to the pressure transducer, heparinized saline, and contrast material, respectively.

The arterial sheath is shown in Figure 23-3. This device allows the angiographer to monitor catheter tip pressure and femoral artery pressure simultaneously, using only the single femoral arterial puncture. The sheath is inserted into the femoral artery at the beginning of the procedure and is somewhat larger than the outer diameter of the catheter, thus allowing arterial blood to fill the shaft of the sheath surrounding the catheter. The pressure of this arterial blood is monitored through a side-arm extension tube, which is attached to a separate transducer. A small rubber valve at the distal end of the sheath maintains hemostasis and serves as a portal of entry for the catheter. The ability to monitor catheter tip pressure through the manifold and femoral artery pressure through the sheath side arm simultaneously allows immediate detection of damping of catheter tip pressure that may signify occlusion of a stenotic coronary ostium by the catheter. Even relatively minor amounts of damping can be rapidly detected with this technique. It is also helpful in measuring pressure gradients across a stenotic aortic valve. Additional advantages of the sheath are that it allows quick changes of catheters without the necessity of groin compression and lessens the discomfort caused by catheter manipulation. The major disadvantage is that a larger hole is created in the artery because of the extra size of the sheath. For example, if a 7.3 French coronary catheter is used, an 8 French sheath must be used to allow sufficient space around the outer border of the catheter for satisfactory pressure transmission. The wall thickness of an 8 French sheath is such that the outer diameter is 9 French. Thus the insertion hole in the artery is almost two French sizes larger than it ordinarily would be. In a review of our experience with this sheath in 562 patients undergoing coronary arteriography, we found no significant increase in local arterial complications.[6]

Arterial Puncture and Catheterization of the Left Ventricle

The point of maximal impulse of the femoral artery is palpated, usually at about the level of the inguinal crease. One should plan on entering the artery at this level, so the small skin puncture in turn should be sev-

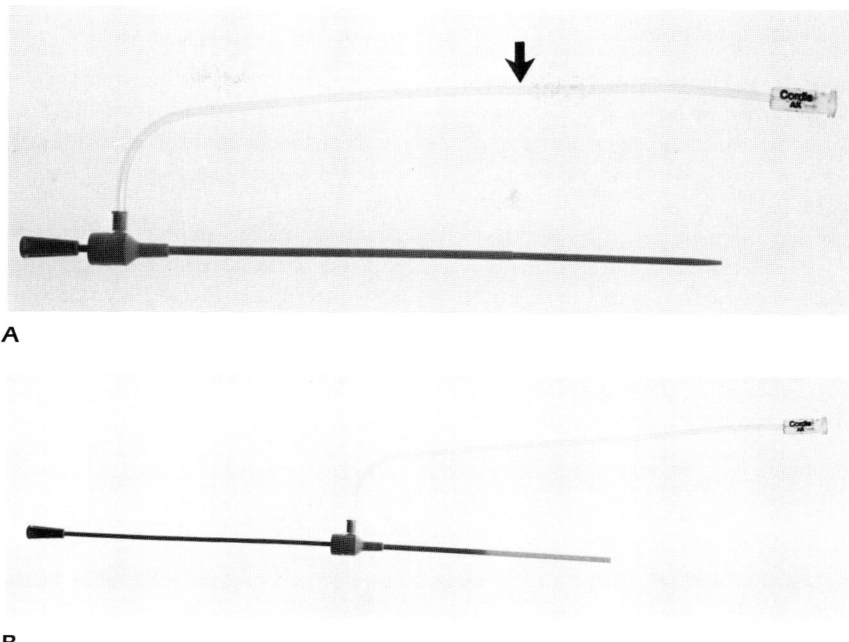

Figure 23-3. Arterial sheath used in coronary arteriography. (A) The sheath with the introducer fully inserted. (B) The sheath with the introducer partially withdrawn. After the entire device is inserted over the guidewire at the beginning of the procedure, the introducing catheter is withdrawn, leaving only the sheath and the side-arm extension tube (*arrow*, A), which leads to a pressure transducer.

eral centimeters distal to this point. The inguinal crease is located at different levels, depending on the obesity of the patient, but in any event the angiographer should always check to make sure it is well below the inguinal ligament (which stretches from the superior pubic ramus to the anterior superior iliac spine). If the arterial needle enters the femoral artery above the inguinal ligament, uncontrollable pelvic hemorrhage may result. The skin puncture should be placed slightly lateral to where the arterial pulse can be palpated, so the needle tip has to be directed very slightly medially to enter the artery. Because the femoral artery takes a turn toward the midline at this level, having the needle tip pointing medially helps ensure that the guidewire will be directed along the long axis of the artery, rather than impinging on the lateral wall of the artery, as would probably occur if the needle tip entered the vessel from the medial side.

Infiltration of the skin and subcutaneous tissues with Xylocaine should be carried out slowly and carefully. This can be one of the more painful parts of the procedure if it is not done carefully. It is of great importance in coronary arteriography to have the patient as relaxed as possible throughout the entire procedure; meticulous and effective local anesthesia can help greatly in achieving relaxation. Exploring the subcutaneous tissues gently with the anesthetic needle, one can often feel the femoral sheath. If possible, this should be anesthetized because it contains numerous nerve endings. The femoral nerve just lateral to the artery should also be anesthetized. We generally use approximately 8 ml of 1 percent Xylocaine; the use of much larger amounts of anesthetic may make it difficult subsequently to palpate the femoral pulse.

After local anesthesia has been induced, the point of maximal impulse of the femoral artery is once again palpated and, with this as a landmark, the arterial needle is inserted with a rapid and firm motion, the angle between the needle and the skin surface being kept at approximately 30 degrees. The advancement of the needle is generally continued until it reaches bone or until it has passed all the way in as far as its hub. We do not attempt to make a "one wall" puncture because this is time-consuming and usually unsuccessful. The advancement of the needle can be another painful part of the procedure, and in the interests of maintaining good rapport it is wise to forewarn the patient. Once the needle has been introduced, it is slowly withdrawn with two hands until a pulsatile flow of blood is obtained. At this point, the needle is fixed in position and the guidewire is introduced through it.

As previously indicated, the guidewire initially used

in femoral artery puncture should always have a J tip because the angiographer has virtually no way of knowing whether the patient has tortuous or atherosclerotic iliac arteries. In either or both of these situations, the use of a straight guidewire could result in dissection of the vessel or restriction of wire passage by a plaque.

Once the guidewire has been passed into the midabdominal aorta, the artery above the puncture site is compressed, the needle is removed, and a 5 French Teflon dilator is introduced for the purpose of spreading apart the subcutaneous soft tissues and the wall of the femoral artery. The dilator is then removed and the previously described arterial sheath is inserted over its introducer. When inserting this sheath, the angiographer will often feel some resistance at the point where the sheath meets the wall of the femoral artery. The most effective way of overcoming this resistance is to grasp the sheath tightly at a point 1 to 2 cm above the skin surface and then advance it with a short, sharp motion. This generally enables the sheath to pass smoothly through the wall of the femoral artery. Once the sheath has been passed in to its hilt, both the introducer and the guidewire can be removed. The small rubber hemostasis valve prevents back-bleeding. The side arm is flushed and connected to the transducer, which then allows continuous monitoring of femoral artery pressure. Once the sheath has been secured and a satisfactory pressure tracing is obtained, the angiographer is ready to catheterize the left ventricle with the pigtail catheter.

The pigtail catheter is partially straightened by having a guidewire passed through it so that 1 to 2 mm of the guidewire protrudes beyond the end of the pigtail catheter. This very short guidewire "leader" is used to get the tip of the pigtail catheter through the small rubber valve of the arterial sheath. Once the catheter tip is through the valve, the guidewire is again advanced into the lower abdominal aorta, and at that point the catheter is allowed to follow it. When the guidewire and catheter are in the lower thoracic aorta, the guidewire is removed and the catheter is carefully flushed with saline and attached to the manifold. The angiographer should now check both pressures—one from the catheter tip, which is monitored through the manifold, and the other from the femoral artery, which is monitored through the side arm of the arterial sheath.

If the pressure tracings are satisfactory, the catheter is advanced around the aortic arch, through the aortic valve, and into the left ventricle. There is virtually always resistance to passage of the pigtail catheter at the aortic valve. In the nonstenotic valve, this can generally be overcome by gentle to-and-fro movement of the catheter tip. Rotation of the pigtail into a different plane often helps. Whenever the catheter tip is rotated with the left hand, a corresponding turn of the rotating adapter on the manifold should always be made with the right hand. In this way, "torque" is satisfactorily transmitted along the shaft of the catheter to the tip. Another maneuver that is frequently helpful in crossing the aortic valve is the formation of a small loop at the level of the valve. Once the loop is formed, gradual withdrawal of the catheter frequently will result in prolapse of the pigtail tip across the aortic valve into the left ventricle. If all else fails, a J guidewire or tapered-tip straight guidewire can be passed through the catheter and used to probe the aortic valve. One or the other of these maneuvers virtually always will enable the angiographer to enter the left ventricle successfully.

When the catheter enters the left ventricle, it frequently irritates the ventricle and produces a number of premature ventricular contractions. These are detected on the electrocardiogram and the pressure tracings. It is important to change the depth and angle of the catheter tip within the left ventricle to seek a position in which ectopic activity is absent. Ideally, the tip of the catheter should be either in the midportion of the ventricle or near the apex. If the catheter tip is too close to the aortic valve, much of the contrast injected during left ventriculography will pass immediately out the aortic valve without satisfactorily opacifying the ventricular cavity.

When a stable catheter position has been achieved, left ventricular pressure is recorded. The angiographer should pay careful attention to ensure that an accurate left ventricular end-diastolic pressure is clearly noted on the pressure tracing. Left ventriculography can then be performed.

Left Ventriculography

In our laboratory, left ventriculography is generally performed by injecting 40 to 45 ml of Renografin-76 at a flow rate of 13 to 15 ml per second. If the patient is severely ill or in congestive heart failure, a smaller total volume of contrast is used. If the patient has a very large left ventricle, a larger total volume may be used. An injection rate of over 15 ml per second is rarely needed, even in patients with a large left ventricle. During the approximately 3 seconds of elapsed time required for the contrast to be injected, the angiographer should be ready to terminate the injection instantly if one or more of the contrast jets from a side hole of the catheter is dissecting through the endocardium. This complication is not uncommon, especially if great care is not exercised in properly positioning the catheter before left ventriculography is performed. When it occurs, it is rarely serious, but obviously it should be avoided if at all possible. The maximum injection rate of 15 ml per second can be used with either 7 or 8 French pigtail catheters. The entire sequence is filmed on 35-mm cine film at a rate of 30 to 60 frames per second.

If the cineangiographic laboratory being used has only single-plane cineangiographic capability and the patient is being studied for suspected coronary disease, the best projection for left ventriculography is the 30-degree right anterior oblique (RAO) projection. This projection visualizes the left ventricle perpendicular to its long axis, so that the ventricular contour is seen in profile. The principal areas of importance (anterior wall, apex, inferior wall, and mitral valve) are all seen well in this projection. The septum and true posterior wall are not seen in the RAO projection, but these are generally considered to be of somewhat lesser importance. If biplane cine equipment is available, a corresponding 60-degree left anterior oblique (LAO) view should be simultaneously obtained. This view does visualize the interventricular septum and true posterior wall of the left ventricle. If the mounting unit for the second cine plane is capable of obtaining cranial angulation views, we feel the optimal LAO view of the left ventriculogram is that obtained with approximately 25 to 30 degrees of cranial angulation, in addition to the 60-degree LAO angulation. This avoids the foreshortening that ordinarily occurs in the standard 60-degree LAO projection and gives a more complete view of both the interventricular septum and true posterior wall of the left ventricle and another look at the mitral valve as well. It is especially valuable for detecting abnormalities of the outflow portion of the ventricle.

If the laboratory is equipped with dual-mode image intensifiers (generally a 6-inch–9-inch combination is used), the left ventriculogram should be obtained with the larger mode so that the entire ventricle is imaged in the radiographic field. Evaluation of regional wall motion and determination of ventricular volumes are more accurate if the necessity of panning can be avoided.

In evaluating a cine left ventriculogram, the angiographer initially assesses regional wall motion qualitatively. The ventricle should show uniform inward motion of all regions during systole. Regional wall motion abnormalities are designated as hypokinesia, akinesia, or dyskinesia. A hypokinetic segment is one that exhibits reduced inward motion during systole. An akinetic segment is one that shows no inward motion whatsoever during systole. A dyskinetic segment is one that bulges paradoxically during systole. In most cases, regional akinesia or dyskinesia indicates severe scarring of that portion of the myocardium, although such a finding occasionally occurs in the presence of structurally normal, viable myocardium that is severely ischemic. It is important to know whether an akinetic or dyskinetic segment of left ventricle myocardium is irreversibly damaged or only ischemic, and for this purpose augmented or interventional left ventriculography can be repeated. This can be accomplished in one of three ways: administration of epinephrine, administration of nitroglycerin, or introduction of an extrasystole, which is followed by a compensatory pause and then a potentiated contraction. Whether the method uses an unloading effect (nitroglycerin) or an inotropic effect (epinephrine or postextrasystolic potentiation),[7–9] it may unmask areas that still retain some contractile reserve. This improvement in regional contractility on potentiated left ventriculography suggests that the involved area is merely ischemic, rather than irreversibly scarred.

In addition to assessment of regional wall motion, global left ventricular function is assessed from the left ventriculogram by determining the ejection fraction. This, in turn, entails calculation of left ventricular volume at end-systole and end-diastole. The calculations are generally based upon the area-length method originally described by Dodge et al.[10] and subsequently expanded by a number of other groups.[11,12] According to this method, the left ventricle is assumed to be represented by an ellipsoid, the volume (V) of which is determined by the formula $V = 4\pi/3 \cdot L/2 \cdot D_1/2 \cdot D_2/2$ as determined from simultaneous frontal and lateral left ventriculograms. L = the longest measured axis from the two views, D_1 = the minor axis from one projection, and D_2 = the minor axis from the other projection. L is measured directly from the projected image of the cineangiogram, but D_1 and D_2 are calculated by means of a second formula for the area of an ellipse: $A = \pi DL/4$, where A = the area of the left ventricle (measured by planimetry), D = the minor axis, and L = the long axis. After determination of the area of the left ventricle by planimetry, the formula is solved for D_1 and D_2, respectively, and these values are then used in the original formula for left ventricular volume. Corrections for magnification and pincushion distortion of the image intensifier must be made, and a regression equation should be used to correct inherent errors in the system and also to correct for the fact that most laboratories use RAO and LAO left ventriculography, rather than frontal and lateral ventriculography. The formula can also be applied in computing left ventricle volumes from single-plane left ventriculograms. For details regarding these calculations, the reader is referred to textbooks on cardiac catheterization.[13] Ejection fraction is the stroke volume (end-diastolic minus end-systolic volume) divided by end-diastolic volume.

Ejection fraction is probably the most widely used index of global left ventricular function in patients with coronary artery disease. The lower limit of normal in most laboratories is 55 percent. Patients with ejection fractions below 40 percent are considered to have significantly impaired left ventricular function, and below 30 percent, function is considered severely impaired. The ejection fraction is an important consideration in making the decision regarding medical versus surgical therapy and is also a major factor in determining prognosis.

Catheterizing the Coronary Arteries

After left ventriculography has been performed, left ventricular pressure should again be measured. It will generally be found that the contrast injection has produced a significant elevation of left ventricular end-diastolic pressure (LVEDP).[14] This is likely to be well tolerated as long as the LVEDP remains below 30 mmHg, above which point pulmonary edema may occur. If the post–left ventriculography LVEDP is noted to have reached this level, consideration should be given to administrating a diuretic or possibly even to terminating the procedure and postponing coronary arteriography until the next day, particularly if the patient shows symptoms of congestive heart failure.

If the LVEDP following ventriculography remains within acceptable limits, the pigtail catheter is withdrawn from the left ventricle under constant pressure recording to ascertain whether there is a pressure gradient across the aortic valve. Once the catheter is in the descending thoracic aorta, the guidewire is inserted and the pigtail catheter is exchanged for a Judkins left coronary catheter.

For catheterizing either coronary artery, the patient or the image intensifier should be positioned so that the angiographer views the patient in the LAO projection. In this projection, the right coronary artery will originate from the right side of the arota and the left coronary artery will originate from the left side of the aorta.

To catheterize the left coronary artery, the left coronary catheter is advanced slowly around the aortic arch, as shown in Figure 23-4. It is very important that it be advanced *slowly* and that it be rotated so the two curves of this catheter can be seen clearly in profile at all times. If the catheter is advanced too rapidly, it may snap suddenly into the left coronary artery, causing dissection of the wall of the vessel. If the catheter is allowed to rotate so that it no longer retains its profile position, as shown in Figure 23-4B and C, the catheter tip may coil up, making it impossible to catheterize the left coronary artery without uncoiling it with a guidewire in the abdominal aorta. To ensure that the catheter maintains a proper profile, the operator should rotate the catheter with the left hand near the groin puncture site while the right hand correspondingly turns the rotating adapter of the manifold to which the catheter is attached.

If the angiographer advances the catheter slowly, maintaining the profile position, the catheter tip will slowly pass down the left posterolateral aspect of the ascending aorta and enter the left coronary ostium. Passage of the left coronary catheter into the ostium can generally be recognized as an abrupt leftward motion of the catheter tip. When this motion is seen, the angiographer should immediately look at the catheter tip pressure as displayed on the pressure recorder. If the catheter tip pressure is unchanged and is roughly equivalent (both in systole and in diastole) to the femoral artery pressure, which is being concurrently monitored through the side arm of the sheath, it is safe to assume that the catheter tip is free within the luminal portion of the main left coronary artery. This status can be verified by a small test injection of contrast. If, however, there is significant damping of the catheter tip pressure or "ventricularization" (normal systolic pressure but a very low diastolic pressure), this may suggest a significant stenosis of the main left coronary artery and indicate that the catheter tip has passed through it and created a total or near-total obstruction. Dangerous ischemia can result, and when such pressure changes are seen, the catheter should be immediately withdrawn from the left coronary ostium. It is also conceivable, though less likely, that damping or ventricularization of the pressure tracing can be caused simply by abutment of the catheter tip on the side of a nonstenotic left main coronary artery. One must err on the conservative side in such a situation and assume that a left main coronary stenosis is present until proved otherwise. The catheter should be reinserted very carefully into the main left coronary artery. If the same pressure abnormality is noted, the catheter should once again be withdrawn and a nonselective injection of contrast performed with the catheter tip just outside the left coronary ostium. This will enable the angiographer to detect a main left coronary stenosis if one is present. If, on the other hand, the catheter tip pressure is normal and a small test injection of contrast verifies that the catheter is within a nonstenotic

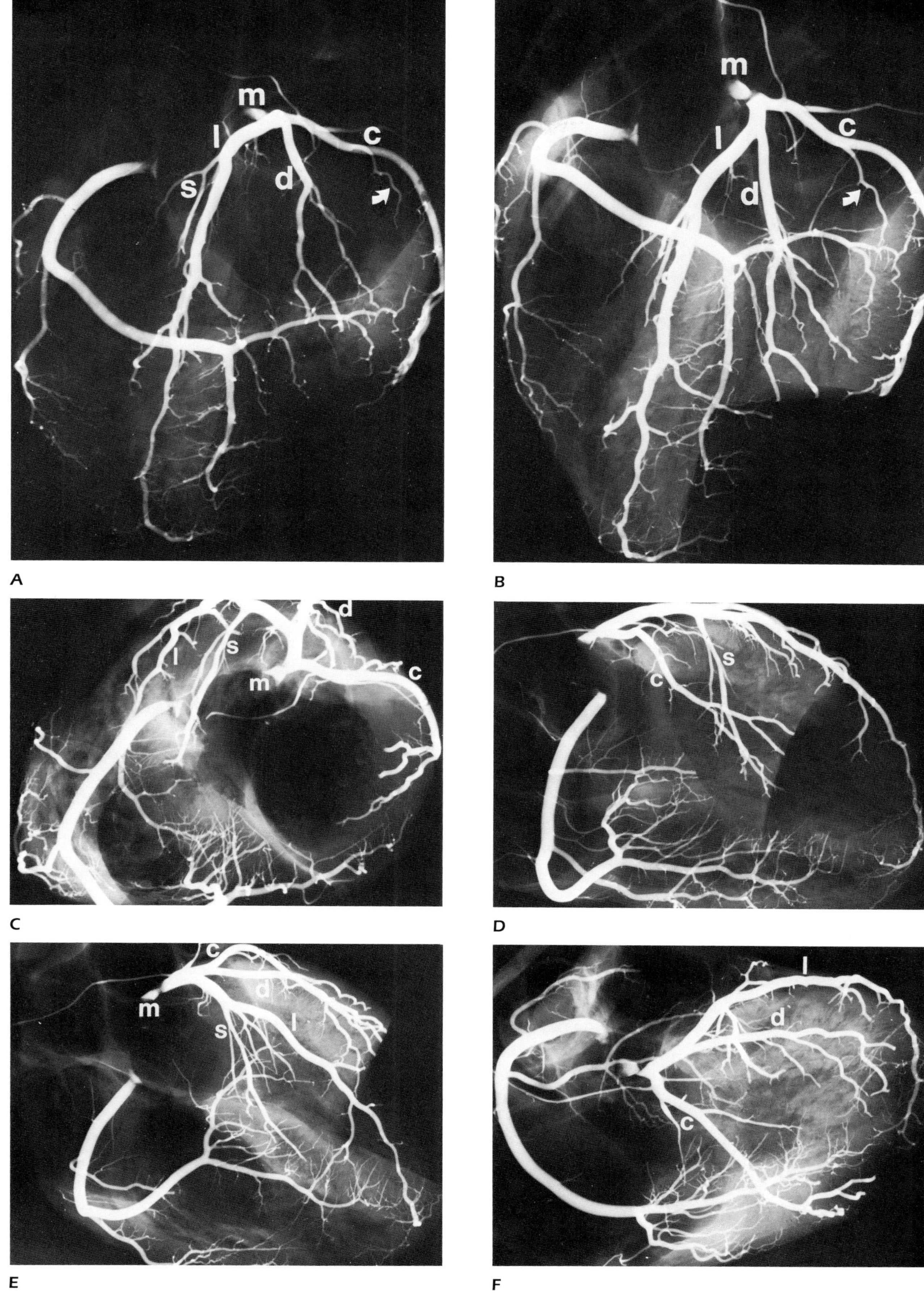

m
l
c
s
d
A
m
l
c
d
B
d
l
s
m
c
C
s
c
D
c
m
d
s
l
E
l
d
c
F

multiangulation rotational mounting units that are available from several equipment manufacturers. Sagittal angulation of the x-ray beam to at least some degree is now routinely incorporated into virtually all LAO and RAO projections.

Electrocardiographic and Hemodynamic Changes Associated with Coronary Arteriography

Injection of Renografin-76 into the coronary arteries produces rather striking electrocardiographic (ECG) and hemodynamic changes in many patients. Selective injection of contrast into the right coronary artery generally produces T-wave inversion in leads II, III, and aVF. Sinus bradycardia and systemic hypotension lasting from 10 to 30 seconds are also common. Less important changes during right coronary arteriography include decreased Q-wave amplitude and prolongation of the Q–T interval. Injection of contrast into the left coronary artery usually produces peaking of the T wave in leads II, III, and aVF. Sinus bradycardia and transient systemic hypotension also occur, although they tend to be less pronounced during left coronary injection than during right coronary injection in many patients. Other less important changes during left coronary arteriography include a decrease in P-wave amplitude, a decrease in the height of the R wave, and prolongation of the Q–T interval. If the right coronary artery is totally occluded, a biphasic response may be noted with left coronary injection if the distal right coronary artery is supplied by collaterals from the left side. That is, the left coronary injection will initially produce T-wave elevation, but within a few seconds, as the contrast passes through collaterals to the distal right coronary tree, the characteristic T-wave inversion generally associated with right coronary arteriography will develop.

In some individuals, selective coronary arteriography may produce profound sinus bradycardia and hypotension and even sinus arrest. If severe bradycardia occurs, it should be treated by intravenous injection of 1 mg atropine. Instructing the patient to give several vigorous coughs is also helpful; this markedly raises arterial pressure and forces oxygenated blood through the coronary arteries to replace the injected contrast material. If sinus arrest occurs and does not respond to coughing, the angiographer should deliver a vigorous blow to the patient's chest with his or her fist. This will almost always successfully restore normal sinus rhythm.

The cause of the adverse effects of contrast injection upon cardiac rhythm and contractility is not entirely clear. They appear to be due to a combination of hyperosmolarity, cation content, and direct anion toxicity of the myocardium.[19–21] The sodium content of contrast material used for coronary arteriography is particularly important. Renografin-76, an aqueous solution of 66 percent *N*-methylglucamine diatrizoate and 10 percent sodium diatrizoate, contains 0.19 mEq per cubic centimeter. Although the lowest possible sodium content has been felt to be desirable in other circulations, it has been found that in the performance of coronary arteriography, if the sodium content of the contrast agent is substantially below this level, an increased incidence of ventricular fibrillation occurs.[22,23] Even if Renografin-76 is used, potentially lethal arrhythmias, such as ventricular fibrillation or ventricular tachycardia, may occasionally occur. These should be treated immediately with D.C. countershock.

Drugs Used During Coronary Arteriography

Premedication

A rapid, efficient, and uncomplicated angiographic procedure is facilitated by having a cooperative and relaxed patient. Adequate premedication is very helpful in this regard. Different angiographers prefer different combinations of drugs, and numerous regimens are equally effective. The dosage depends on the size and anxiety level of the patient. In some laboratories, Valium, 5 to 10 mg, and Benadryl, 25 to 50 mg, are administered intramuscularly immediately before the patient is sent for coronary angiography. Others prefer to use stronger premedication, such as a combination of Demerol, 50 to 75 mg, and Nembutal, 50 to 75 mg, intramuscularly.

Heparin

We strongly recommend heparinization of all patients during coronary arteriography. The heparin is administered through the pigtail catheter at the start of the procedure, after this catheter has been passed into the lower thoracic aorta. An average-sized adult patient receives 4000 to 5000 units. The author's experience suggests that heparinization of patients decreases the mortality and morbidity of coronary arteriography, although published data in some studies suggest that heparin does not have a significant beneficial effect.[5] At the end of the procedure, the anticoagulant effect of heparin is reversed by intravenous administration of protamine sulfate. This drug is given at a dosage schedule of 10 mg for each 1000 units of heparin that had been administered earlier. Protamine should be given by slow intravenous injection over approximately a 5-minute period.

Nitroglycerin

Nitroglycerin has a number of effects on the cardiovascular system, not all of which are completely understood. From the point of view of the coronary angiographer, its principal effect is to decrease vasomotor tone in the large (epicardial) coronary arteries. It is given prophylactically to offset the possibility of catheter-induced spasm and should be administered sublingually at a dosage of 0.3 mg shortly before the coronary arteriogram is to be obtained. Nitroglycerin has a short duration of action (20–30 minutes), and catheter-induced spasm can occur even with the administration of 0.3 mg. Therefore, additional doses may be necessary during the procedure if spasm is suggested for any reason.

In some patients, particularly those with suspected Prinzmetal variant angina, spontaneous spasm may, in fact, be the principal cause of the patient symptoms. If spontaneous spasm is suspected as an important factor in the clinical pattern, nitroglycerin should not be used because this would obviously mask the very phenomenon the angiographer is attempting to demonstrate. In patients in whom spasm is not suspected clinically, we favor routine use of sublingual nitroglycerin just before coronary arteriography.

Atropine

Atropine has certain potentially beneficial effects in patients undergoing coronary arteriography. It lessens the likelihood of a vasovagal reaction and also diminishes the sinus bradycardia that frequently occurs after selective injection of contrast material into the coronary arteries. However, it almost invariably increases heart rate, an effect that is somewhat undesirable because this not only increases myocardial oxygen demand but makes adequate opacification of the coronary arteries more difficult to achieve. In our laboratory, atropine, 0.6 mg, is given intravenously just before coronary arteriography if the patient has a slow heart rate. If the patient has sinus tachycardia, the drug is withheld. However, it may be given during the procedure (at a dosage of 1 mg intravenously) if, after the initial contrast injections, a profound sinus bradycardia or sinus arrest occurs.

Ergonovine Maleate

Prinzmetal angina is described later in Chapter 28. Briefly, it is characterized by chest pain, which, as opposed to typical angina pectoris, is unrelated to exercise or other inciting factors and is often cyclic in nature in that it tends to occur at the same time every day. The chest pain is accompanied by S–T segment elevation on the ECG, often simulating acute myocardial infarction. However, both the chest pain and ECG changes are transient and revert either spontaneously or in response to sublingual nitroglycerin. In their original description of this syndrome, Prinzmetal et al.[24] postulated that these findings were due in part to coronary artery spasm. The suggestion has been verified subsequently by numerous investigators. Spasm can occur at sites within the coronary arteries that are narrowed by atherosclerotic disease but can also occur at sites that are angiographically entirely normal. When a patient is suspected of having Prinzmetal angina and does not happen to have a spontaneous attack during coronary arteriography, the arteriographer may wish to provoke spasm to demonstrate its existence. This can be done by the intravenous administration of ergonovine maleate. This drug has been found to produce spasm in the vast majority of patients who have Prinzmetal angina but in very few patients who do not.

Ergonovine maleate can be given according to several different dosage schedules.[25-27] In most laboratories, progressively increasing intravenous boluses of the drug are given, starting at a dosage of 0.05 to 0.1 mg and going as high as 0.4 mg. After each bolus is administered, the patient is carefully observed for the development of chest pain or of S–T segment elevation on the ECG. If either develops, coronary arteriography is immediately repeated. If neither develops, arteriography is performed after 5 to 10 minutes and the next higher dose is then administered. Once spasm has been documented, nitroglycerin should be given immediately by the sublingual route. If this does not reverse the spasm at once, intravenous nitroglycerin should be administered. If the attack is severe and refractory to intravenous nitroglycerin, this drug can be injected directly into the involved coronary artery. Intravenous or intracoronary nitroglycerin should be administered in bolus doses of 100 to 300 μg. A report in 1980[28] documented three deaths resulting from ergonovine-induced coronary vasospasm. Although the ergonovine test has been widely used in many laboratories with complete safety, this report emphasizes that it is not a totally innocuous test and should be performed only with extreme caution.[29,30] Because Prinzmetal angina can be reliably diagnosed clinically, many laboratories have abandoned the use of ergonovine.

Other Techniques of Coronary Arteriography

Sones Technique

Although the Judkins technique is now the most widely used approach to coronary arteriography, the Sones technique was the first approach ever taken in common practice and is still used in a number of laboratories. This technique requires a surgical cutdown of the brachial artery, usually performed on the right side, although some angiographers prefer to use the left arm instead. The details of the Sones approach have been previously published,[1,31,32] and the reader is referred to the sources mentioned for specifics. Briefly, the Sones catheter is available in either woven Dacron or polyurethane construction. The catheter is shown in Figure 23-1. It has an end hole and four small side holes very close to the catheter tip. It is available in sizes 7 and 8 French, with a tip that tapers to 5 French. After performance of the brachial artery cutdown, the catheter is advanced through the subclavian artery (generally without the use of a guidewire, although a wire can be helpful where there is tortuosity of or atherosclerotic plaque formation in the subclavian artery). Once the catheter has traversed the subclavian and innominate arteries and has reached the ascending aorta, it is connected to the manifold, which was described earlier in this chapter. Pressure monitoring, filming technique, and safety precautions are virtually the same for the Sones technique as they are for the Judkins technique.

In the Sones approach, the same catheter is used for entering both the right and left coronary arteries. To catheterize the left coronary artery, the catheter is advanced to the aortic valve while the heart is being viewed in the LAO projection. There are several different methods of achieving entry into the left coronary ostium, but the most common is to form a loop on the right aortic cusp so that the shaft of the catheter and the tip form approximately a 45-degree angle with the tip pointed toward the left. Alternating advancement and withdrawal of the catheter will then generally allow engagement of the left coronary ostium. When the ostium has been entered, stable seating of the catheter tip can be accomplished in some patients by advancing the catheter, whereas in others it requires slight retraction to shorten the loop. One of the relative disadvantages of the Sones technique in comparison with the Judkins technique is that the catheter position tends to be somewhat less stable.

To enter the right coronary artery, a slightly smaller loop is formed. The catheter is slowly withdrawn while being rotated in a clockwise direction. Here also, several different types of maneuvers may be required to engage the right coronary ostium. When the catheter tip does enter the right coronary artery, it may pass quite far down the vessel, necessitating slow withdrawal to avoid spasm or failure to opacify the proximal portion of the artery.

If the brachial artery approach is used and the Sones catheter cannot be introduced into one or both coronary arteries, the Amplatz catheters may be useful in achieving successful entry.

Amplatz Technique

The Amplatz catheters were originally designed for use with the percutaneous femoral artery approach. These catheters are seen in Figure 23-1. For catheterizing the left coronary artery, the broad secondary curve of the left Amplatz catheter is allowed to rest on the right aortic cusp. Choosing the proper-sized catheter is crucial; the left Amplatz catheters come in four different sizes (AL1–AL4). Once the proper-sized catheter is chosen and the secondary curve is resting on the right aortic cusp with the tip pointing to the left, gentle alternating advancement and retraction of the catheter will allow the catheter tip to engage the left coronary artery. After entry has been achieved, it is generally desirable to stabilize the position of the catheter tip by slightly retracting the catheter.

Catheterization of the right coronary artery with the Amplatz catheter (the right coronary catheter comes in sizes AR1 and AR2) is accomplished by manipulating the catheter in much the same fashion as the right Judkins catheter was handled. That is, the catheter tip generally points initially to the left; the catheter is slowly withdrawn and rotated clockwise so that the tip points toward the right and can engage the right coronary ostium.

As indicated above, the Amplatz catheters are useful in both the femoral and brachial approaches if the Judkins or Sones catheters cannot be maneuvered into the desired vessel. We have also found the right Amplatz catheter (AR1) to be valuable in postcoronary bypass angiography. With this single catheter, it is generally possible to catheterize selectively saphenous vein grafts extending from the aorta to the right coronary, LAD, or circumflex arteries.

Bourassa Technique

Several years after the Judkins and Amplatz techniques were developed, Bourassa et al. at the Montreal Heart Institute[33] developed a new set of catheters. Their technique also employs the percutaneous femoral approach. The catheters are somewhat similar in shape to the Judkins catheters. The technique is not widely used in this country, and we have no experience with it.

Schoonmaker-King Technique

In 1974, Schoonmaker and King[34] described a single catheter that could be inserted percutaneously via the femoral artery approach and used to catheterize both coronary arteries. It obviates the need for catheter exchange and offers the theoretical advantage of being able to catheterize the right and left coronary arteries more quickly. This technique too has never achieved wide popularity. Although we have no experience with it, others have found that the catheter tip often cannot be selectively seated in the left coronary ostium, so that a nonselective cusp injection must be relied on.[35] Therefore, El Gamal et al.[35] modified the catheter shape somewhat, but even with the modification, they were able to catheterize both coronary arteries successfully in only 86 percent of their procedures.

References

1. Sones FM, Shirey EK. Cine coronary arteriography. Mod Concepts Cardiovasc Dis 1962;31:735.
2. Ricketts HJ, Abrams HL. Percutaneous selective coronary cine arteriography. JAMA 1962;181:620.
3. Judkins MP. Selective coronary arteriography: I. A percutaneous transfemoral technique. Radiology 1967;89:815.
4. Amplatz K, Formanek G, Stanger P, Wilson W. Mechanics of selective coronary artery catheterization via femoral approach. Radiology 1967;89:1040.
5. Davis K, Kennedy JW, Kemp HG Jr, Judkins MP, Gosselin AJ, Killip T. Complications of coronary arteriography. Circulation 1979;59:1105.
6. Barry WH, Levin DC, Green LH, Bettmann MA, Mudge GH Jr, Phillips D. Left heart catheterization and angiography via the percutaneous femoral approach using an arterial sheath. Cathet Cardiovasc Diagn 1979;5:401.
7. Horn HR, Teichholz LE, Cohn PF, Herman MV, Gorlin R. Augmentation of left ventricular contraction pattern in coronary artery disease by an inotropic catecholamine: epinephrine ventriculogram. Circulation 1974;49:1063.
8. Hefant RH, Pine R, Meister SG, Feldman MS, Trout RG, Banka VS. Nitroglycerin to unmask reversible asynergy: correlation with post coronary bypass ventriculography. Circulation 1974;50:694.
9. Dyke SH, Cohn PF, Gorlin R, Sonnenblick EH. Detection of residual myocardial function in coronary artery disease using postextrasystolic potentiation. Circulation 1974;50:306.
10. Dodge HT, Sandler H, Ballew DW, Lord JD Jr. Use of biplane angiocardiography for the measurement of left ventricular volume in man. Am Heart J 1960;60:762.
11. Rackley CE. Quantitative evaluation of left ventricular function by radiographic techniques. Circulation 1976;54:862.
12. Wynne J, Green LH, Mann T, Levin DC, Grossman W. Estimation of left ventricular volumes in man from biplane cine angiograms filmed in oblique projections. Am J Cardiol 1978; 41:726.
13. Rackley CE, Hood WP Jr, Grossman W. Measurements of ventricular volume, mass and ejection fraction. In: Grossman W, ed. Cardiac catheterization and angiography. Philadelphia: Lea & Febiger, 1980:232–244.
14. Levin DC, Baltaxe HA. Effect of radiopaque contrast material upon left ventricular end diastolic pressure. NY State J Med 1972;72:2619.
15. Sos TA, Lee JG, Levin DC, Baltaxe HA. New lordotic projection for improved visualization of the left coronary artery and its branches. AJR 1974;121:575.
16. Lesperance J, Saltiel J, Petitclerc R, Bourassa MG. Angulated views in the sagittal plane for improved accuracy of cinecoronary angiography. AJR 1974;121:565.
17. Aldridge HE, McLoughlin MJ, Taylor KW. Improved diagnosis in coronary cinearteriography with routine use of 110° oblique views and cranial and caudal angulations: comparison with standard oblique views in 100 patients. Am J Cardiol 1975;36:568.
18. Arani DT, Bunnell IL, Greene DG. Lordotic right posterior oblique projection of the left coronary artery: a special view for special anatomy. Circulation 1975;52:504.
19. Ovitt T, Rizk G, Frech RS, Cramer R, Amplatz K. Electrocardiographic changes in selective coronary arteriography: the importance of ions. Radiology 1972;104:705.
20. Trägårdh B, Bove AA, Lynch PR. Mechanism of production of cardiac conduction abnormalities due to coronary arteriography in dogs. Invest Radiol 1976;11:563.
21. Higgins CB. Effects of contrast media on the conducting system of the heart: mechanism of action and identification of toxic component. Radiology 1977;124:599.
22. Paulin S, Adams DF. Increased ventricular fibrillation during coronary arteriography with a new contrast medium preparation. Radiology 1971;101:45.
23. Snyder CF, Formanek A, Frech RS, Amplatz K. The role of sodium in promoting ventricular arrhythmia during coronary arteriography. AJR 1971;113:567.
24. Prinzmetal M, Kennamer R, Merliss R, Wada T, Bor N. Angina pectoris: 1. A variant form of angina pectoris. Preliminary report. Am J Med 1959;27:375.
25. Heupler FA Jr, Proudfit WL, Razavi M, Shirey EK, Greenstreet R, Sheldon WC. Ergonovine maleate provocative test for coronary artery spasm. Am J Cardiol 1978;41:631.
26. Curry RC Jr, Pepine CJ, Sabom MB, Feldman RL, Christie LG, Conti R. Effects of ergonovine in patients with and without coronary artery disease. Circulation 1977;56:803.
27. Cipriano PR, Guthaner DF, Orlick AE, Ricci DR, Wexler L, Silverman JF. Effects of ergonovine maleate on coronary arterial size. Circulation 1979;59:82.
28. Buxton A, et al. Refractory ergonovine-induced coronary vasospasm: importance of intracoronary nitroglycerin. Am J Cardiol 1980;46:329.
29. Watanabe K, et al. Electrophysiologic study and ergonovine provocation of coronary spasm in unexplained syncope. Jpn Heart J 1993;34(2):171–182.
30. Harding MB, et al. Ergonovine maleate testing during cardiac catheterization: a 10-year perspective in 3,447 patients without significant coronary artery disease or Prinzmetal's variant angina. J Am Coll Cardiol 1992;20(1):107–111.
31. Conti CR, Levin DC, Grossman W. Coronary angiography. In: Grossman W, ed. Cardiac catheterization and angiography. Philadelphia: Lea & Febiger, 1980:147–169.
32. Gensini GG. Coronary arteriography. Mt. Kisco, NY: Futura, 1979:79–130.
33. Bourassa MG, Lesperance J, Campeau L. Selective coronary arteriography by percutaneous femoral artery approach. AJR 1969;107:377.
34. Schoonmaker FW, King SB. Coronary arteriography by the single catheter percutaneous femoral technique. Circulation 1974; 50:735.
35. El Gamal M, Siegers L, Bonnier H, Borsje P, Relik T, van Gelder L, de Vries D. Selective coronary arteriography with a preformed single catheter: percutaneous femoral technique. AJR 1980;135:630.

24

Complications of Coronary Arteriography

JOHN E. ARUNY

The angiographic determination of coronary artery anatomy, hemodynamics, and ventricular function has an important position in the algorithm for the diagnosis and management of atherosclerotic heart disease. The relative importance of this information in the decision analysis has supported the increasing numbers of coronary angiograms being performed. It is interesting to note that coronary angiography and interventional procedures are now being performed with increasing frequency in community hospitals away from university medical centers. Every et al. report that the proportion of hospitals with on-site cardiac catheterization facilities in the metropolitan Seattle area has increased from 31 to 69 percent, resulting in nearly identical services in several neighboring hospitals.[1] Therefore, the complications of these procedures are being recognized more frequently and at a number of smaller institutions.

Mortality

Several large studies have been published dealing with the mortality of coronary arteriography.[2–14] A summary of the larger and more recent studies is given in Table 24-1.

Two early surveys conducted by Adams and Abrams in which the responders were guaranteed anonymity were compared. It was revealed that between the surveys of 1970–1971[7] and those of 1973–1974[6] the overall mortality rate had decreased from 0.45 to 0.14 percent. This drop reflected a marked decrease in the mortality with the femoral approach developed by Ricketts and Abrams[15] and modified by Judkins,[16] from 0.78 to 0.16 percent.[13] These results were confirmed by Davis et al. in the Coronary Artery Surgery Study (CASS), a study of 13 institutions (7553 patients) that showed a mortality rate of 0.20 percent.[3] This was 3.6 times lower than the mortality rate using the brachial technique ($p < 0.05$) and established the femoral approach as a safe and time-efficient procedure.

In the previous edition of this textbook Abrams summarized the mortality data on 191,165 cases published between 1964 and 1979. The overall mortality rate was 0.24 percent. The mortality rate from 135,525 cases published from 1975 to 1979 was significantly decreased to 0.17 percent.[13]

The first of the cooperative, multicenter studies that defined the risks of cardiac catheterization was sponsored by the National Heart Institute.[2] The mortality rate for patients from 2 to 59 years of age was 0.14 percent. Wyman et al. reported data from 2883 procedures, of which 1609 were diagnostic procedures and 933 were percutaneous transluminal coronary angioplasty (PTCA). Their mortality rate for diagnostic procedures was 0.12 percent, and for PTCA it was 0.3 percent.[12]

The Society for Cardiac Angiography and Interventions (SCA&I) in its 1982 Registry reported complications data for 53,581 procedures. The overall mortality rate was 0.14 percent.[4] When stratified according to age, the mortality rate in the age group of 1 to 60 years was 0.07 percent and in the over-60 years was 0.25 percent. Following their initial report in 1982, the SCA&I reported an additional 222,553 patients in 1989 from its Registry.[5] These patients underwent selective coronary arteriography between July 1, 1984, and December 31, 1987. The overall mortality rate was 0.10 percent. Mortality rates were similar regardless of technique, with the femoral approach used in 68 percent and the brachial approach in 32 percent.

When the two Registry reports are compared, it is found that in the first report 33 percent of the patients were older than 60 years of age compared with 50 percent in the second Registry report. Also, 48 percent were class III or class IV compared with 58 percent of the patients in the second report. The rates of major complications were very similar for the two reports: 1.77 percent (1982) and 1.74 percent (1989). However, it must be emphasized that the mortality rate fell, despite the facts that the patients were characterized as being older and more seriously ill.

In 1990 the SCA&I computerized its reporting system and reported a survey of 63 facilities for a total of

Table 24-1. Mortality and Major Morbidity of Coronary Arteriography

	Adams and Abrams[7]	Takaro et al.[8]	Bourassa and Noble[9]	Adams and Abrams[6]	Hansing[10]	Davis et al.[3]	*Abrams[13]	Kennedy[4]	Morton and Beanlands[11]	Wyman et al.[12]	Johnson et al.[5]	Noto et al.[14]
Years of survey	1970–71	1968–72	1970–74	1973–74	1972–77	1975–76	1964–79	1979–81	1977–82	1986–87	1984–87	1990
Number of patients	46,904	3050	5250	89,079	14,050	7553	191,165	51,974	7552	1609	222,553	71,916
Mortality	0.45%	1.7%	0.23%	0.14%	0.19%	0.20%	0.24%	0.11%	0.09%	0.12%	0.10%	0.11%
MI	0.6%	—	0.09%	0.18%	0.13%	0.25%	0.33%	0.07%	0.11%	—	0.06%	0.05%
Stroke	0.43%	—	0.13%	0.09%	0.06%	0.03%	—	0.07%	0.12%	0.1%	0.07%	0.07%
Major vascular	0.12%	—	—	0.12%	—	0.74%	—	—	—	1.6%	0.46%	0.43%

*Summary of 30 studies cited in the previous edition of this book.

Table 24-2. Mortality Rates Based on the Extent of Angiographically Demonstrated Coronary Artery Disease

Coronary Angiography	Mortality Rate (%)
Normal coronary arteries	0.02
< 50% stenosis	0.01
One-vessel critical disease	0.05
Two-vessel critical disease	0.07
Three-vessel critical disease	0.12
Left main critical disease	0.55

Data from Johnson LW, et al. Coronary arteriography 1984–1987: a report of the Registry of the Society for Cardiac Angiography and Interventions: I. Results and complications. Cathet Cardiovasc Diagn 1989;17:5–10.

71,916 patients from January 1 through December 31, 1990. The mortality for diagnostic procedures was 0.11 percent, remaining remarkably constant from prior registry reports.[14]

Risk Factors

Severe Coronary Artery Disease

Several studies have confirmed that the risk of death following diagnostic coronary arteriography increases with the severity of the angiographically demonstrated coronary artery disease.

The 1973–74 survey of Adams and Abrams[7] reported that 47 percent of deaths occurred in patients with three-vessel disease, 15 percent of reported deaths occurred with two-vessel disease, and only 2 percent of deaths occurred with one-vessel disease. In the CASS study, 12 of 15 patients who died within 48 hours after arteriography had severe three-vessel disease. Eleven of the 12 had greater than 70 percent stenosis of all the major arteries.[3] The SCA&I reported in 1989 for the period from 1984 to 1987 that death was less likely but not unreported in patients with less severe disease.[5] The mortality rates for patients with increasing grades of coronary artery disease are listed in Table 24-2.

Left Main Coronary Artery (LMCA) Disease

In the CASS study, 38 percent of patients who died had stenoses of the LMCA and 0.76 percent (5 of 657 cases) with LMCA disease died, whereas only 0.12 percent (8 of 6884 cases) without LMCA disease died. The adjusted ratio of these two proportions is 6.8, which is an estimate of the relative risk of death attributable to LMCA disease.[3] The 1973–1974 survey by Adams and Abrams reported that 46 percent of all deaths occurred in patients with a significant LMCA lesion.[7] Some earlier works failed to demonstrate an increased risk with LMCA disease.[17–19] However, the SCA&I reported in 1989 that death occurred in 0.55 percent of patients with LMCA disease and other major complications occurred in 3.8 percent of all patients with angiographically demonstrated LMCA disease.[5]

The patient with LMCA disease is at increased risk for death and other major complications during diagnostic coronary arteriography. Clinical findings that suggest LMCA disease include severe, long-standing angina with the recent development of a crescendo pattern unresponsive to medication or ischemic changes on the resting ECG, angina associated with dyspnea, or greater than 2-mm S–T segment depression on the exercise electrocardiogram.[20,21] Nuclear myocardial stress-rest scintigraphy with ^{201}Tl or ^{99m}Tc-isonitril agents performed before coronary angiography can be helpful to assess the extent of disease. Scans that show multiple transient perfusion defects in the septal, anterior, and lateral segments that reperfuse at rest may indicate LMCA disease. Alternatively, the entire myocardium may show uniform depression of uptake of the radiopharmaceutical during exercise. This uniform depression of uptake may be difficult to detect without the application of quantitative techniques. A "normal" scintigraphic appearance of the myocardium with significant ECG changes during exercise should suggest LMCA disease.

Because LMCA disease is a powerful risk factor for diagnostic coronary angiography, these patients should be given special attention. Special care should be exercised when engaging the ostium. If damping of the pressure tracing is encountered, the catheter should be removed without injecting contrast. The number of selective injections is limited to the few necessary to define the anatomy, and the procedure time is kept to a minimum.

Unfortunately, not all of these patients are identified before angiography. Some investigators begin by imaging the LMCA to best advantage to quickly establish if there is LMCA disease. Meyerovitz et al. described the use of the 16-degree to 25-degree caudally angulated posteroanterior (PA) view to best image the LMCA.[22] This angulated view allows better visualization of the LMCA bifurcation, which would have been obscured by the superimposition of the left circumflex (LCX) coronary artery and left anterior descending (LAD) coronary artery origins. This angulated view also has the advantage of markedly improving visualization of the LCX in 78 to 89 percent of subjects.

Depressed Left Ventricular Ejection Fraction

In the CASS study, 5682 patients and 11 of 13 patients who died had their ejection fractions (EF) calculated angiographically. The mean EF for the group was 0.60 ± 0.15, and for those who died 0.40 ± 0.17.[3]

Table 24-3. Mortality Rates Stratified by the Left Ventricular Ejection

	Ejection Fraction		
	> 0.50	0.30–0.49	< 0.30
CASS Study mortality[3]	0.07% (3/4286)	0.46% (5/1091)	1.2% (3/251)
SCA&I Study mortality[5]	0.03% (40/128,074)	0.12% (41/34,083)	0.30% (20/6726)

The relative risk of death with an EF of less than 0.30 compared with a normal EF is 9.0 (95 percent confidence limit: 2.6–31.4). Table 24-3 compares the mortality rates stratified as to ejection fraction from the CASS and SCA&I study groups and demonstrates a close relationship between EF and risk of death.

Functional Class

The risk of death increases with the increase in grade of the functional class. The SCA&I study stratified patients according to the New York Heart Association's functional classes (Table 24-4).[5] The mortality rates were as follows: class I: 0.02 percent (5/25,662), class II: 0.02 percent (13/53,924), class III: 0.05 percent (32/65,754), and class IV: 0.29 percent (131/45,290).

Other Factors

Other factors associated with death and their relative risks and 95 percent confidence interval obtained from the CASS study[3] were as follows:

Multiple premature ventricular contractions	6.8 (1.7–26.9)
Hypertension	4.2 (1.4–13)
Congestive heart failure	5.3 (1.8–15)

Heparin Use

The use of heparin was monitored in the CASS study. The mortality with heparin was 0.16 percent and without the use of heparin was 0.18 percent. The difference was not significant ($p > 0.75$).[3]

Morbidity

Nonfatal Acute Myocardial Infarction (AMI)

The occurrence of an AMI is confirmed by the appearance of positive ECG changes or elevated cardiac enzymes recorded within 24 hours of the procedure. However, in the CASS study, the protocol called for recording of AMIs at 24 hours and from 24 to 48 hours following the procedure, which contributed to a higher reported incidence of AMI.

Table 24-4. New York Heart Association's Criteria for Functional Capacity

Class I: No limitation of physical activity. Ordinary physical activity does not cause undue fatigue, palpitation, dyspnea, or anginal pain.

Class II: Slight limitation of physical activity. Comfortable at rest, but ordinary physical activity results in fatigue, palpitation, dyspnea, or anginal pain.

Class III: Marked limitation of physical activity. Comfortable at rest, but less than ordinary activity causes fatigue, palpitation, dyspnea, or anginal pain.

Class IV: Unable to carry on any physical activity without discomfort. Symptoms of cardiac insufficiency, or of the anginal syndrome, may be present even at rest. If any physical activity is undertaken, discomfort is increased.

Adapted from Sokolow M, McIlroy MB. Clinical cardiology, 2nd ed. Los Altos, CA: Lange, 1979.

Catheter-related AMI during coronary angiography may be related to prolonged wedging of the catheter in the coronary ostium, severely restricting coronary blood flow. Alternatively, introduction of the catheter deep into the coronary ostium with irritation of the intima may induce a myogenic reflex resulting in prolonged vasospasm. The incidence of spasm varies from 0.26 to 2.9 percent.[23,24]

Subintimal coronary artery dissection has a reported incidence of 0.05 percent in diagnostic angiograms.[25–29] It would appear to be more common in the right coronary artery. However, left coronary dissections result in myocardial infarction in the majority of cases, whereas only 50 percent of right coronary artery dissections lead to infarction.[26] Dissections occur from the mechanical force of the catheter tip impacting on diseased vessel intima. Forceful contrast injection then initiates or extends the dissection process through the media of the vessel. Careful attention to the pressure tracing and a gentle test injection with the catheter tip in a nonwedge position to confirm free flow around the catheter tip should help minimize the risk of subintimal dissection. The experienced operator will avoid torquing the catheter once it is engaged in the coronary ostium and can often recognize if the catheter is engaged too deeply from its appearance on fluoroscopy.

Thrombotic occlusion of a coronary artery from platelets embolizing from the catheter tip has been thoroughly investigated. Platelets invariably adhere to the catheter and guidewire surfaces, as has been demonstrated on both electron microscopic and angiographic bases.[30,31] Takaro et al. proposed a mechanism whereby thrombotic material on the outer surface of a catheter is picked up by the guidewire and transferred to the tip of a second catheter during the exchange process.[32] When the guidewire is removed in the ascending aorta, this material can migrate from the catheter tip into a coronary artery or the cerebral circulation. Silverman and Wexler modified their technique so that catheters were exchanged in the descending thoracic aorta and vigorous flushes with heparinized saline were performed.[33] This significantly reduced their incidence of myocardial infarctions.

Overall, the reported incidence of AMI associated with diagnostic coronary angiography ranges from 0.05 to 0.6 percent (see Table 24-1). When only the more recent studies recorded after 1979 are considered, the rate of AMI averages 0.061 percent.

Stroke

Neurovascular complications are embolic in nature, with a similar etiology as in AMI. Catheter exchanges in the distal thoracic aorta significantly reduce the rate of cerebral embolic complications.[33] The overall incidence of stroke ranges from 0.03 to 0.43 percent (see Table 24-1). Studies recorded after 1979 average a stroke rate of 0.07 percent.

Contrast Media–Related Morbidity

Intravascular contrast media are derivatives of triiodinated benzoic acids. They are divided into ionic agents, or those that dissociate into charged particles in solution, and nonionic agents, or those that do not. Table 24-5 lists the most commonly used contrast media for coronary angiography and compares their physical properties to those of blood plasma. The majority of ionic media are sodium and methylglucamine salts with very high osmolalities in relation to blood.

The high-osmolality contrast agents (HOCAs) can be subdivided on the basis of their calcium-binding properties. Renografin-76 contains sodium EDTA and citrate to sequester trace quantities of heavy metals and to act as buffering agents. These additives also chelate calcium. The localized binding of calcium in the coronary arteries can have significant hemodynamic and electrophysiologic consequences.[34] The binding of calcium causes a decline in myocardial contractile force, which correlates with decreased concentration of calcium in coronary venous blood following injection. Ventricular fibrillation may be precipitated by delayed repolarization, which is decreased when calcium is added to contrast agents that contain calcium-binding properties. Hypaque-76 and Angiovist do not contain citrate and therefore have less calcium-binding activity. They use calcium-enriched sodium EDTA as a sequestering agent.

The nonionic media produce only half the number of osmotically active particles in solution than the ionic agents. One exception is an ionic agent, sodium methylglucamine ioxaglate (Hexabrix, Mallinckrodt Diagnostics). This agent has six iodine atoms bonded to a double ring structure and, although ionic, has an osmolality that is only about twice that of blood.

Many of the adverse effects attributed to contrast media in coronary angiography appear to be related to their high osmolalities and ionic content. Several trials have confirmed a decreased incidence of adverse effects with low-osmolality contrast agents (LOCAs).[35–38] However, the incremental cost of these agents is significant.

A recent randomized trial reported that treatment for adverse events during diagnostic coronary angiography was required in 213 of 737 patients who received HOCAs (29 percent) but in only 69 of 753

Table 24-5. Commonly Used Contrast Media for Coronary Angiography and Their Physical Properties Compared to Plasma

	Mg iodine/ml	Osmolality (mOsm/kg)	Viscosity (37°C)	Na Conc. (mEq/ml)	Calcium Binding	Additives
Plasma	0	285	—	145–155	—	—
Ionic—high osmolar (HOCA)						
Angiovist	370	2076	8.4	160	No	.01% NaCaEDTA
Hypaque-76	370	2016	8.32	160	No	.01% NaCaEDTA
Renografin-76	370	1940	8.4	190	Yes	.32% NaCitrate .04% NaEDTA
Ionic—low osmolar						
Ioxaglate	320	600	7.5	150	No	.01% NaCaEDTA
Nonionic—low osmolar (LOCA)						
Iopamidol	370	796	9.4	minimal	No	.05% NaCaEDTA
Iohexol	350	844	10.4	minimal	No	.01% NaCaEDTA
Ioversol	320	720	5.8	minimal	No	.02% NaCaEDTA

patients who received nonionic agents (9 percent) (95 percent confidence interval for the percent difference). If all patients in their trial had been given nonionic contrast material, the incremental cost per procedure would have been $89.[36] A second randomized double-blind trial evaluated 505 patients undergoing coronary angiography with a nonionic LOCA (iohexol) and an HOCA that does not avidly bind calcium (Hypaque-76). The 253 patients who received an HOCA were three times more likely to have a moderate adverse reaction but no more likely to have a severe reaction. The incremental cost per moderate reaction avoided by giving an LOCA to all patients would be $5842.[35]

Because cost restrictions may prevent the general use of these agents that are 15 to 25 times more expensive than HOCAs, selective use on a risk-related basis may be more cost-effective. Factors that appear to place patients at increased risk for contrast-related adverse events include unstable angina, severe coronary disease, and age greater than 60 years. The definitive resolution of this issue has not yet been generally agreed upon and remains hotly debated.

Dose-related adverse effects following intracoronary artery injection of iodinated contrast are usually transient but, if persistent, may require treatment, as described in the following paragraphs.

Arrhythmias

Bradycardia. Slowing of the sinus node rate is frequently observed following intracoronary injection of contrast. It is observed within 2 to 10 seconds after either left or right intracoronary injection and spontaneously resolves by 40 to 60 seconds. The average decrease is 3 to 5 beats per minute with an LOCA injection and 9 to 12 beats per minute if an HOCA is used.[34] Persistent bradycardia requires treatment because this will delay washout of contrast from the coronary artery, possibly initiating ventricular arrhythmias in response to myocardial hypoxia. The predominant cause of sinus slowing is a vagus nerve–related reflex response.[39] The trigger appears to be the hypertonicity of the contrast rather than its ionic composition.[40] This same vagal response may produce transient second-degree atrioventricular (AV) nodal block, particularly in patients who have been taking calcium channel blockers.[41] Atropine has been useful in reducing the vagal response to contrast injection.[42]

Ventricular Fibrillation. Intracoronary contrast injection and ventriculography will reduce the fibrillation threshold in a dose-related fashion with the effect lasting for approximately 1 minute.[43] The incidence of ventricular fibrillation during coronary angiography varies between 0.1 and 1.2 percent of patients being studied. A Mayo Clinic study of 7915 patients undergoing diagnostic coronary angiography had a 0.5 percent rate of ventricular fibrillation. A profile of a patient who develops fibrillation includes normal ventricular function (79 percent), fibrillation following injection of the right coronary artery (62 percent), and onset within 10 seconds after injection completed (95 percent).[44]

Animal studies indicate that the newer nonionic, low-osmolality agents lower the fibrillation threshold to a lesser degree.[45] Large studies in humans have not been reported. A significant difference in the incidence of fibrillation occurs between contrast agents that bind calcium (Renografin-76) and those that do not (Hypaque-76, Angiovist, and LOCA).[34] One study showed a decrease in the incidence of ventricular fibrillation from 0.6 to 0.1 percent when the investigators switched to a contrast agent that did not bind calcium.[46] Other investigators have confirmed the importance of injecting contrast that does not reduce the local concentration of intracoronary calcium.[47,48]

Myocardial Effects

Selective injection of the coronary arteries with standard ionic media depresses myocardial function transiently.[49] There may be a rebound in ventricular performance above baseline 20 to 30 seconds following injection and cardiac output increases secondary to reduced peripheral vascular resistance. Sodium-containing ionic contrast media depress contractile performance by causing an imbalance in the ratio of extracellular sodium to calcium ions. Thus the concentration of calcium is reduced by the preservatives in the contrast and the sodium concentration is increased by the sodium ions in the contrast media. Nonsodium nonionic contrast agents produce no myocardial depressant effects.[50]

Complications Related to the Vascular Access Site

Several recent, large studies have shown the incidence of peripheral vascular injury to be between 0.4 and 1.0 percent.[51–55] Regardless of the type of injury, there is a direct association between early recognition of the injury and successful repair with minimal complications. Babu et al. reviewed 16,350 patients: 10,500 patients underwent brachial artery access and 5850 patients underwent femoral access. Surgical intervention was necessary in 0.57 percent of the brachial arterial injuries and in 0.23 percent of the femoral artery injuries. Only 1.7 percent of the 56 patients who had early repair had a complication. Twenty-eight percent with delayed intervention suffered significant complications.[52]

A recent report studied 503 consecutive patients who underwent a cardiac catheterization or interventional procedure. The factors that contributed to femoral artery complications were restarting heparin after sheath removal, the number of procedures done during one hospitalization, noncompliance of the patient with bedrest after the procedure, the number of arterial punctures to initiate the procedure, and preprocedure treatment with corticosteroids.[56]

Thrombosis and Embolism

These are the most important and frequent complications at the site of vascular access. The mechanism of injury is that thrombus that has formed on the wall of the catheter or introducer sheath is stripped off. This thrombus may adhere to the vessel wall at the puncture site or travel distally to occlude a smaller peripheral branch. Subintimal dissection may also occur with passage of the guidewire or catheter into a false channel. Subsequently, an intimal flap occurs and becomes separated from the media. The flap then extends into the lumen of the vessel and occludes flow, often resulting in further thrombus formation as platelets aggregate on the newly exposed media.

Factors that increase the risk of thrombotic vascular complications include preexisting vascular disease with atherosclerotic plaque that narrows the lumen and may be a site for subintimal passage of a guidewire or catheter. Patients with valvular heart disease have been reported to have a higher incidence of vascular complications.[57] Other factors include small femoral arteries, the length of the procedure, puncture of the superficial femoral or profunda femoral artery, and an underlying hypercoagulable state.

Arteriovenous Fistulas

Arteriovenous fistulas occur from simultaneous injury to the adjacent artery and vein. A review of 23,291 cardiac catheterizations in five hospitals showed an incidence of 0.017 percent.[58] Congestive heart failure and limb ischemia were the most frequent presenting symptoms. These symptoms developed from 2 to 10 months after catheterization.

Retroperitoneal Hematoma

This is an unusual but a potentially serious complication. A retrospective review of 9585 femoral artery catheterizations revealed an overall prevalence of 0.5 percent, with the highest frequency being after coronary artery stenting (3 percent).[59] Signs and symptoms included suprainguinal tenderness and fullness in 100 percent, severe back and lower quadrant pain in 64 percent, and femoral neuropathy in 36 percent. Only 16 percent of these patients required operations. Most were treated with transfusion alone.

Neuropathy

This rare but potentially debilitating complication of cardiac catheterization, whose pathophysiologic condition is not well understood, is probably related to nerve compression or traction from an adjacent hematoma. In a recent review of 9585 cardiac catheterizations, the incidence of this complication was 0.21 percent.[60] Two groups of patients can be identified. One group had a retroperitoneal hematoma as the dominant finding. These patients had a lumbar plexopathy involving the femoral, obturator, or lateral femoral cutaneous nerve. These patients had undergone excessive anticoagulation, and the neuropathy more frequently occurred after procedures that required larger sheaths. The pain was severe and was sometimes delayed until the second postprocedure day. Motor neuropathy developed in 13 of 16 patients with this presentation, and 6 patients required intensive inpatient rehabilitation.

The second presentation of these patients was with a groin hematoma or false aneurysm, which resulted in paresthesias involving the medial and intermediate cutaneous branches of the femoral nerve. This pain was relatively mild and resolved in all patients.

Pseudoaneurysm

These false aneurysms are rare, occurring in 0.04 percent of patients in the 1979 report of Adams and Abrams.[6] These aneurysms are reported to have a higher incidence in patients with aortic insufficiency and hypertension.[61] They had generally been considered an indication for surgery, but recently they have been successfully treated with local compression using an ultrasound transducer.[62,63] Careful attention to the placement of the puncture site is essential because it has been reported that low femoral puncture sites below the femoral head have a high incidence of pseudoaneurysm formation.[64]

Other Complications

Dissection of the ascending aorta has rarely been reported, with surgical repair necessary if an intimal flap develops.[65] Other, sporadically occurring complications include congestive heart failure, acute pulmonary edema, splenic infarction, prolonged hypotension, intramyocardial and intrapericardial injection of contrast agents, pyrogenic reactions, pulmonary embolism, mesenteric thrombosis, and infection.[66,67] Contrast nephropathy and acute anaphylactic reactions are known complications of peripheral and cardiac angiography.

Complications in the Pediatric and Neonatal Age Group

Risk stratification in the neonate undergoing catheterization has been proposed by Stanger and coworkers and is based on assessment of the potential for deterioration during the procedure[67]:

Low risk: nondistressed nonacidotic neonate with (a) $PaO_2 > 25$ mmHg and (b) controlled congestive heart failure

Medium risk: (a) $PaO_2 < 25$ mmHg and (b) neonates with severe congestive heart failure, poorly controlled with digitalis and diuretics

High risk: (a) ventilatory assistance, (b) profound hypoxemia with acidosis, and (c) poor perfusion resulting in shock or severe acidosis ($pH < 7.1$)

Mortality

Mortality rates in the pediatric population fluctuate depending on how mortality is defined. Death within 24 hours of the procedure from any cause places the mortality rates in the 5 to 15 percent range. Deaths during the procedure are approximately 1 percent. The results of two large studies that reported their mortalities stratified according to age are listed in Table 24-6. It can be seen that the mortality risk declines significantly after the newborn period.

Vascular Complications

The complication rate for vascular damage is directly related to the small size of the femoral artery in relation to the arterial sheath or catheter. The highest rates occur in infants weighing less than 10 kg.[69] Besides having a small stature, children with cyanotic heart disease are frequently found to be polycythemic, a condition that increases blood viscosity, decreases flow rates, and predisposes these patients to vascular thrombosis. Arterial spasm is much more a problem in children than in adults. The loss of smooth muscle cells at the puncture site has been related to a decreased ability of the smooth muscle to relax after arterial spasm.[70]

Overall, the incidence of acute complications at the vascular access site varies between 3 and 40 percent.[71,72]

The late complications of femoral artery catheterization in children are well known. They include limb growth retardation, claudication, and chronic ischemia. A recent study followed 58 children who underwent femoral artery catheterization before 5 years of age and who were restudied with angiography from 5 to 14 years after the original study.[73] The patients had bone length radiographs and duplex arterial sonography as well. Arterial occlusion was present in 33 percent of patients and 37 percent of limbs. Leg growth retardation was present in 8 percent (4 of 51 children). The mean ankle-brachial index in the catheterized limbs was 0.79. There was a significant inverse relationship between the ankle-brachial index and leg growth retardation. Only one patient had claudication. Thus, although femoral artery occlusion is common after catheterization, arterial repair in the absence of symptoms is probably not indicated.

Arrhythmias

Bradycardia is a more serious event in the infant undergoing cardiac catheterization than in the adult. The infant is more dependent on heart rate to maintain cardiac output and has less of an ability to increase stroke volume. The potential for severe hemodynamic consequences is increased in the face of bradycardia even for a short period. The infant's heart is more easily disturbed by catheter manipulation, and various degrees

Table 24-6. Mortality Rates for Cardiac Catheterization in the Pediatric Population

		Death Within 24 hr		Death due to Study	
Age Group	**Number of Patients**	**Number**	**Percent**	**Number**	**Percent**
New England Regional Infant Cardiac Program[68]					
0–30 days	155	10	6.4	1	0.6
31–60 days	52	1	1.8	0	—
2–12 months	105	1	0.95	0	—
American Heart Association Cooperative Study[61]					
0–30 days	325	20	6.2	17	5.2
31–60 days	155	9	5.8	7	4.5
2–12 months	681	8	1.2	4	1.1
1–14 years	2889	3	0.1	3	0.1

of AV block are produced that are usually transient but that may be sustained and require therapy.

Supraventricular tachycardia (SVT) occurs in approximately 4 percent of cases, with the frequency highest in the newborn.[61–67,68] SVT has the potential for being poorly tolerated in patients with poor ventricular function or subpulmonic outflow obstruction.[74]

The importance of arrhythmia monitoring and treatment can be seen in that 9 of the 55 deaths in the Cooperative Study[61] were the results of severe bradycardia, heart block, or tachycardia.

Continuous Quality Improvement (CQI) and Total Quality Management (TQM)

This system of continuous monitoring of the activities of the catheterization laboratory has been shown to be effective in maintaining adequate standards of performance to advance the quality of care. Heupler and the members of the Laboratory Performance Standards Committee of the SCA&I recently published a paper outlining the methodology to establish a program of CQI/TQM.[75]

CQI/TQM differs from standard quality assurance methods in the following ways:

1. It emphasizes analysis of the processes of care rather than individual physician performance.
2. Its goal is to continuously improve performance, not merely to meet guidelines.
3. It involves not just physicians in the quality improvement process, but all members of a department, as well as appropriate members of related departments.
4. It involves many functions in the department, not just those selected for inspection.[76]

Modern CQI programs consist of five steps:

1. Identification of quality indicators, which should be precise, reliable, and valid
2. Systematic collection of data regarding these quality indicators
3. Analysis of these data to identify deficiencies
4. Development and implementation of an action plan to address probable causes of these deficiencies
5. Systematic repeat collection of data to analyze the impact produced by the intervention

The effective implementation of this type of program will require cooperation from all members of the team involved in the catheterization laboratory. Once in place, it will continue to monitor the activities of the catheterization service, including the complication rates, and ensure the preservation of quality in the face of ever-expanding regulation.

References

1. Every NR, Larson EB, Litwin PE, Maynard C, Fihn SD, Eisenberg MS, et al. The association between on-site cardiac catheterization facilities and the use of coronary angiography after acute myocardial infarction. N Engl J Med 1993;329:546–551.
2. Braunwald E, Gorlin R. Cooperative study on cardiac catheterization: total population studied, procedures employed, and incidence of complications. Circulation 1968;37(Suppl III): 8–16.
3. Davis K, Kennedy JW, Kemp HG, Judkins MP, Gosselin AS, Killip T. Complications of coronary arteriography from the collaborative study of Coronary Artery Surgery (CASS). Circulation 1979;5:1105–1111.
4. Kennedy JW. Complications associated with cardiac catheterization and angiography. Cathet Cardiovasc Diagn 1982;8: 5–11.
5. Johnson LW, Lozner EC, Johnson S, Krone R, Pichard AD, Vetrovec GW, Noto TJ, and the Registry Committee of the Society for Cardiac Angiography and Interventions. Coronary arteriography 1984–1987: a report of the Registry of the Society for Cardiac Angiography and Interventions: I. Results and complications. Cathet Cardiovasc Diagn 1989;17:5–10.
6. Adams DF, Abrams HL. Complications of coronary arteriography: a follow-up report. Cardiovasc Radiol 1979;2:89.
7. Adams DF, Abrams HL. The complications of coronary arteriography. Circulation 1973;48:609.
8. Takaro T, Hultgren HN, Littmann D, et al. An analysis of deaths occurring in association with coronary arteriography. Am Heart J 1973;86:587.
9. Bourassa MG, Noble J. Complication rate of coronary arteriography: a review of 5250 cases studied by a percutaneous femoral technique. Circulation 1976;53:106.
10. Hansing CE. The risk and cost of coronary angiography: II. The risk of coronary angiography in Washington state. J Am Med Assoc 1979;242:735.
11. Morton BC, Beanlands DS. Complications of cardiac catheterization: one centre's experience. Can Med Assoc J 1984;131: 889.
12. Wyman RM, Safian RD, Portway V, Skillman JJ, McKay RG, Baim DS. Current complications of diagnostic and therapeutic cardiac catheterization. J Am Coll Cardiol 1988;12:1400–1406.
13. Abrams HL. Complications of coronary arteriography. In: Abrams HL, ed. Abram's angiography: vascular and interventional radiology. 3rd ed. Boston: Little, Brown, 1983:504.
14. Noto TJ, Johnson LW, Krone R, Weaver WF, Clark DA, Kramer JR, Vetrovec GW, and the Registry Committee of the Society for Cardiac Angiography and Interventions. Cardiac Catheterization 1990: a report of the registry of the society for cardiac angiography and interventions (SCA&I). Cathet Cardiovasc Diagn 1991;24:75–83.
15. Ricketts HJ, Abrams HL. Percutaneous selective coronary cinearteriography. JAMA 1962;181:620.
16. Judkins MP. Percutaneous transfemoral selective coronary arteriography. Radiol Clin North Am 1968;6:492.
17. DeMots H, Bonchek LI, Rosch J, Anderson RP, Starr A,

Rahimtoola SH. Left main coronary artery disease: risks of angiography, importance of coexisting disease of other coronary arteries and effects of revascularization. Am J Cardiol 1975;36:136.
18. Mehta J, Hamby RI, Voletti C, Wisoff BG, Hartstein ML. Main left coronary artery disease: risk of coronary angiography and bypass surgery. N Y State J Med 1975;75:2193.
19. Khaja FU, Sharma SD, Easley RM, Heinle RA, Goldstein S. Left main coronary artery lesions: risks of catheterization; exercise testing and surgery. Circulation 1974;50(Suppl II):136.
20. Cohen MV, Cohn PF, Herman MV, Gorlin R. Diagnosis and prognosis of main left coronary artery obstruction. Circulation 1972;45(Suppl I):57.
21. Lavine P, Kimbiris D, Segal BL, Linhart JW. Left main coronary artery disease: clinical arteriographic and hemodynamic appraisal. Am J Cardiol 1972;30:791.
22. Meyerovitz MF, Reagan K, Friedman PL. Caudal-posteroanterior view in coronary arteriography. Radiology 1989;171:866–868.
23. Lavine P, Kimbiris D, Linhart JW. Coronary artery spasm during selective coronary arteriography: a review of 8 years experience. (Abs) Circulation 1973;48(Suppl IV):89.
24. Chahine RA, Raizner AE, Ishimori T, et al. The incidence and clinical implications of coronary artery spasm. Circulation 1975;52:972.
25. Takaro T, Hultgren HN, Littmann D, et al. An analysis of deaths occurring in association with coronary arteriography. Am Heart J 1973;86:587.
26. Morise AP, Harding NJ, Bovill EG, et al. Coronary artery dissection secondary to coronary arteriography: presentation of three cases and review of the literature. Cathet Cardiovasc Diagn 1981;7:283.
27. Feit A, Kahn R, Chowdry I, et al. Coronary artery dissection secondary to coronary arteriography: case report and review. Cathet Cardiovasc Diagn 1984;10:177.
28. Weiner RD, Boston BA, Mintz GS, et al. Catheter induced coronary artery dissection. Circulation 1981;64(Suppl IV):108.
29. Haas JM, Peterson CR, Jones RC. Subintimal dissection of the coronary arteries: a complication of selective coronary arteriography and the transfemoral percutaneous approach. Circulation 1968;38:678.
30. Talano JV, Tonaki H, Meadows WR, et al. Platelet aggregates in preformed polyurethane catheters following coronary arteriography: an electron microscopy study. Circulation 1972; 45,46(Suppl II):32.
31. Wilner GD, Casarella WJ, Baier R, et al. Thrombogenicity of angiographic catheters. Circ Res 1978;43:424.
32. Takaro T, Pifarre R, Wuerflein RD, et al. Acute coronary occlusion following coronary arteriography: mechanisms and surgical relief. Surgery 1972;72:1018.
33. Silverman JF, Wexler L. Complications of percutaneous transfemoral coronary arteriography. Clin Radiol 1976;27:317.
34. Matthai WH Jr, Hirshfeld JW Jr. Choice of contrast agents for cardiac angiography: review and recommendations based on clinically important distinctions. Cathet Cardiovasc Diagn 1991;22:278–289.
35. Steinberg EP, Moore RD, Powe NR, et al. Safety and cost effectiveness of high-osmolality as compared with low-osmolality contrast material in patients undergoing cardiac angiography. N Engl J Med 1992;326:425–430.
36. Barrett BJ, Parfrey PS, Vavasour HM, et al. A comparison of nonionic, low-osmolality radiocontrast agents with ionic, high-osmolality agents during cardiac catheterization. N Engl J Med 1992;326:431–436.
37. Hill JA, Winniford M, Cohen MB, et al. Multicenter trial of ionic versus nonionic contrast media for cardiac angiography. Am J Cardiol 1993;72:770–775.
38. Regan K, Bettman MA, Finkelstein J, et al. Double-blind study of a new nonionic contrast agent for cardiac angiography. Radiology 1988;167:409–413.
39. Eckberg DL, White CW, Kioschos MJ, et al. Mechanisms mediating bradycardia during coronary arteriography. J Clin Invest 1974;54:1455.
40. Higgins CB. Effects of contrast media on the conducting system of the heart. Radiology 1977;124:529.
41. Higgins CB, Kuber M, Slutsky RA. Interaction between verapamil and contrast media in coronary arteriography: comparison of standard ionic and new nonionic media. Circulation 1983;68:628.
42. Shah A, Ghog J, Fisher VJ. Complications of selective coronary arteriography by the Judkins technique and their prevention. Am Heart J 1975;90:353.
43. Wolf GL, Kraft L, Kilzer K. Contrast agents lower ventricular fibrillation threshold. Radiology 1978;129:215.
44. Nishimura RA, Holmes DR, McFarland TM, et al. Ventricular arrhythmias during coronary angiography in patients with angina pectoris or chest pain syndromes. Am J Cardiol 1984;53:1496.
45. Wolf GL, Mulry CS, Kilzer K, et al. New angiographic agents with less fibrillatory propensity. Invest Radiol 1981;16:320.
46. Murdock DK, Johnson SA, Loeb HS, Scanlon PJ. Ventricular fibrillation during coronary angiography: reduced incidence in man with contrast media lacking calcium binding additives. Cathet Cardiovasc Diagn 1985;11:153–159.
47. Bayshore TM, Davidson CJ, Mark DB, et al. Iopamidol use in the cardiac catheterization laboratory: a retrospective analysis of 3313 patients. Cardiology 1988;5:6–9.
48. Missri J, Jeresaty RM. Ventricular fibrillation during coronary angiography: reduced incidence with nonionic contrast media. Cathet Cardiovasc Diagn 1990;19:4–7.
49. Yamazaki H, Banka VS, Bodenheimer MM, et al. Differential effects of Renografin-76 on the ischemic and non-ischemic myocardium. Am J Cardiol 1981;47:597–602.
50. Baltaxe HA, Sos TA, McGrath MB. Effects of the intracoronary and intraventricular injections of a commonly available vs a newly available contrast medium. Invest Radiol 1976;11:172–181.
51. Oweida SW, Roubin GS, Smith RB, Salam AA. Postcatheterization vascular complications associated with percutaneous transluminal coronary angioplasty. J Vasc Surg 1990;12:310–315.
52. Babu SD, Piccorelli GO, Shah PM, Stein JH, Clauss RH. Incidence and results of arterial complications among 16,350 patients undergoing coronary catheterization. J Vasc Surg 1989; 10:113–116.
53. Kaufman J, Moglia R, Lacy C, Dinerstein C, et al. Peripheral vascular complications from percutaneous transluminal coronary angioplasty: a comparison with transfemoral cardiac catheterization. Am J Med Sci 1989;297:22–25.
54. Lilly MP, Reichman W, Sarazen AA Jr, et al. Anatomic and clinical factors associated with complications of transfemoral arteriography. Ann Vasc Surg 1990;4:264–269.
55. McCann RL, Schwartz LB, Pieper KS. Vascular complications of cardiac catheterization. J Vasc Surg 1991;14:375–381.
56. Bogart DB, Bogart MA, Miller JT, et al. Femoral artery catheterization complications: a study of 503 consecutive patients. Cathet Cardiovasc Diagn 1995;34:8–13.
57. Barnes RW, Petersen JL, Krugmire RB, et al. Complications of percutaneous femoral arterial catheterization. Am J Cardiol 1974;33:259.
58. Glaser RL, McKellar D, Scher KS. Arteriovenous fistulas after cardiac catheterization. Arch Surg 1989;124:1313–1315.
59. Kent KC, Moscucci M, Mansour KA, et al. Retroperitoneal hematoma after cardiac catheterization: prevalence, risk factors and optimal management. J Vasc Surg 1994;20:905–913.
60. Kent KC, Moscucci M, Gallagher SG, et al. Neuropathy after cardiac catheterization: incidence, clinical patterns, and long-term outcome. J Vasc Surg 1994;19:1008–1014.
61. Braunwald E, Swan HJC, eds. Cooperative study on cardiac catheterization. Circulation 1968;3(Suppl).
62. Sorrell KA, Feinberg RL, Wheeler JR, et al. Color-flow duplex-directed manual occlusion of femoral false aneurysms. J Vasc Surg 1993;17:571–577.

63. Fellmeth BD, Roberts AC, Bookstein JJ, et al. Postangiographic femoral artery injuries: non-surgical repair with US-guided compression. Radiology 1991;178:671–675.
64. Altin RS, Flicker S, Naidech HJ. Pseudoaneurysm and arteriovenous fistula after femoral artery catheterization: association with low femoral punctures. AJR 1989;152:629–631.
65. Carter AJ, Brinker JA. Dissection of the ascending aorta associated with coronary angiography. Am J Cardiol 1994;73:922–923.
66. Adams DF, Fraser D, Abrams HL. Hazards of coronary arteriography. Semin Roentgenol 1972;4:357.
67. Stanger P, Heymann MA, Tarnoff H, et al. Complications of cardiac catheterization of neonates, infants, and children. Circulation 1974;50:595.
68. Cohn HE, Freed MD, Hellerbrand WF, et al: Complications and mortality associated with cardiac catheterization in infants under one year: a prospective study. Pediatr Cardiol 1985;6:123.
69. Wessel DL, Keane JF, Fellows KE, et al. Fibrinolytic therapy for femoral arterial thrombosis after cardiac catheterization in infants and children. Am J Cardiol 1986;56:347.
70. Franken EA, Girod D, Sequeira FW. Femoral artery spasm in children: catheter size is the principal cause. Am J Radiol 1982;138:295.
71. Kirkpatrick SE, Takahashi M, Petry EL, et al. Percutaneous heart catheterization in infants and children. Circulation 1970;42:1049.
72. Freed MD, Rosenthal AR, Fyler D. Attempts to reduce arterial thrombosis after cardiac catheterization: use of percutaneous technique and aspirin. Am Heart J 1974;87:283.
73. Taylor LM, Troutman R, Feliciano P, et al. Late complications after femoral artery catheterization in children less than five years of age. J Vasc Surg 1990;11:297–306.
74. King SB, Franch RH. Production of increased right to left shunting by rapid heart rates in patients with tetralogy of Fallot. Circulation 1971;44:265.
75. Heupler FA, Al-Hani AJ, Dear WE, et al. Guidelines for continuous quality improvement in the cardiac catheterization laboratory. Cathet Cardiovasc Diagn 1993;30:191–200.
76. Berwick DM. Peer review and quality management: are they compatible? Quality Rev Bull 1990;17:246–251.

25

Normal Coronary Anatomy

SVEN PAULIN

Understanding abnormal processes within the coronary circulation requires a precise knowledge of the coronary anatomy and its variations. As in other fields of medicine, much insight in cardiac anatomy derives from extensive studies in cadavers.

Postmortem Studies

Postmortem techniques for anatomic delineation of the heart and coronary arteries include manual dissection, dye techniques, and dye and corrosion techniques.

Manual Dissection

Manual dissection of the coronary vessels from their origin in the aortic root to their apparent distal termination—where they attenuate to such a degree that they cannot be followed farther by visual inspection—was the customary procedure for the classical anatomist. Fundamental traits in the anatomy of the coronary arteries as they are perceived today were known as early as the sixteenth century.[1–3] The manual dissection method, which is the most commonly practiced, is a time-consuming and painstaking procedure when optimally performed, requiring the devoted attention of a highly skilled and knowledgeable pathologist. In 1904, the Italian anatomist Banchi[4] presented a detailed description of the anatomy of the coronary artery and originated a still widely used classification system of arterial preponderance. Banchi's work is a typical example of the potential of this simple approach when expertly performed.

However, this technique may lead to misinterpretations, particularly if performed more casually and by less experienced observers. As was pointed out by Jenner[5] and convincingly illustrated by James,[6] anatomic details and important pathologic lesions may be overlooked because of the rich epicardial fat accumulation that can conceal arterial structures. Today's time-pressed pathologist rarely has the time and interest to reproduce the accuracy and exactitude that were apparently characteristic of the work of the classic anatomist.

More recently, McAlpine[7] has presented postmortem specimens of unusual clarity and detail (Fig. 25-1) using perfusion fixation of the heart, that is, distention of cardiac chambers and arteries. By using high-flow pumps delivering the fixation solutions, he reproduced the spatial relationship of chambers, as well as of the coronary arteries and veins as they are seen by the cardiac surgeon. In combining meticulous dissection and sequential photography—at times enhanced by specifically directed light sources to highlight anatomic and topographic detail—this elaborate technique presents illustrations of convincing clarity. In coronary artery studies, the technique appears to be particularly powerful for demonstrating variations in the position and direction of coronary artery orifices, the larger primary and secondary coronary branches, and their relationship to gross cardiac anatomy.

Dye Techniques

Injection of dyes into the coronary arteries before dissection is an adjunctive method that greatly facilitates the procedure and improves its accuracy. Replacing the dyes with radiopaque fluids creates the possibility of postmortem angiography, which allows for careful study of the vessels without disturbing their anatomic integrity. Hildebrand introduced such a technique to general postmortem studies in 1900,[8] and Fryett later applied it to the coronary circulation in 1905,[9] as did Jamin and Merkel in 1907.[10] The last two authors performed a detailed study based on a series of 37 human postmortem coronary angiograms applying stereoscopic techniques.

Gross established a standardized approach and published a classic monograph entitled *The Blood Supply to the Heart*.[11] He used pressure-controlled injection of barium mixture followed by stereoscopic roentgen-

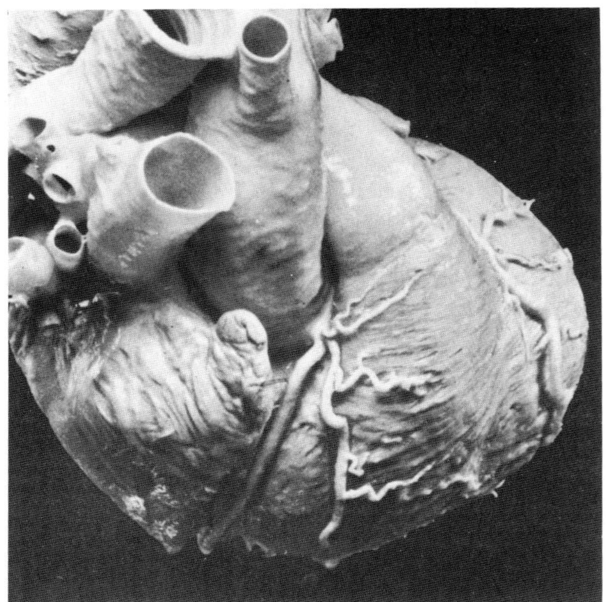

Figure 25-1. Anterior cranial view of postmortem heart specimen prepared according to McAlpine's technique. Note the detailed illustration of coronary artery branches and their topographic relationship to the great vessels and myocardial wall. (From McAlpine WA. Heart and coronary arteries: an anatomical atlas for clinical diagnosis, radiological investigation and surgical treatment. New York: Springer-Verlag, 1975. Used with permission.)

ographic exposures and dissection. Among his followers, Campbell in 1929[12] and Fulton in 1960[13] made outstanding contributions and deserve special mention because of their exquisite technique and their contributions to the present understanding of anatomic detail.

Schlesinger,[14] apparently unconvinced by the stereoscopic technique's ability to unravel overlapping coronary vessels and to differentiate such occurrences from anastomotic channels, modified Gross's technique by injecting lead phosphate agar, which, because of its different consistency, permitted "unrolling" of the unfixed heart onto a single-plane surface. Schaper[15] used this technique particularly when comparing distal coronary artery extensions and anastomoses of the human coronary circulation with those of other species (Fig. 25-2).

A slightly different injection technique not using radiography but exposing the interior vascular anatomy of the heart was described by Spalteholz in 1907.[16] His technique dehydrates and clears the surrounding tissue with benzene and copper sulfate, revealing the chrome-yellow, gelatin-filled arteries to visual inspection. Shortcomings, such as the difficulty of producing with consistency these at times very beautiful and instructive preparations, were probably the reason for their limited popularity.

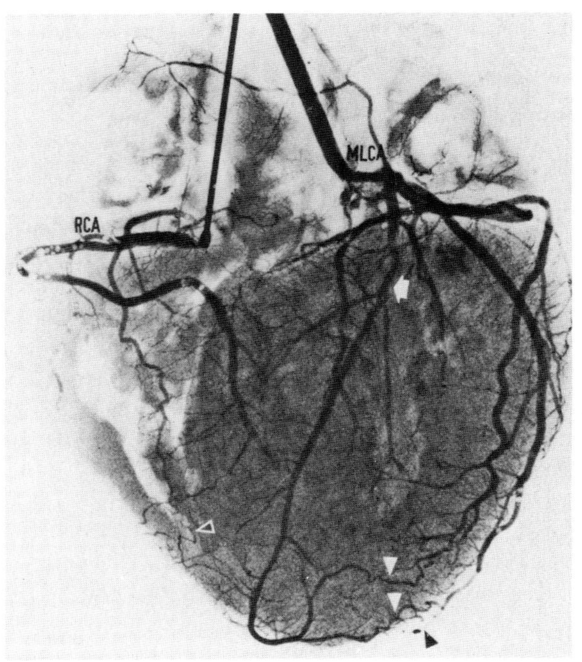

A

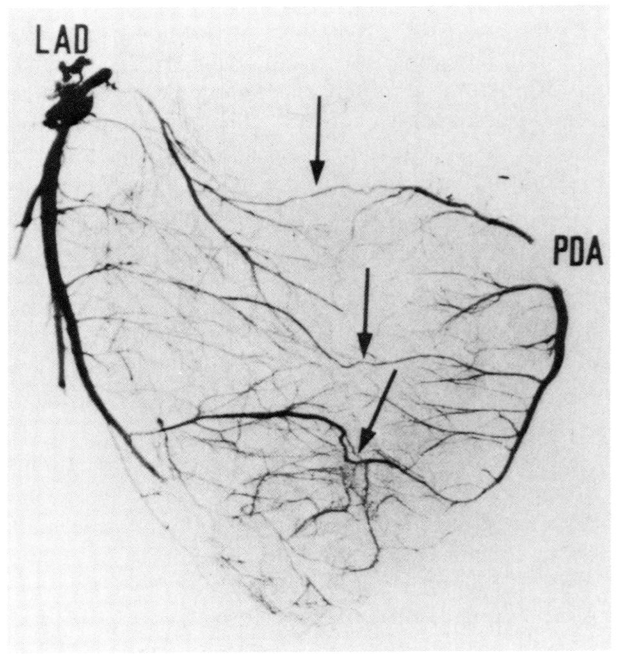

B

Dye and Corrosion Techniques

The injection-corrosion technique, which involves filling the vasculature with a mass that hardens and then corrodes the organ, is the most selective technique for studies of vascular detail. It overcomes the shortcomings of the radiographic injection technique, which projects the three-dimensional vascular tree onto a single plane image, because the resulting vascular cast can be inspected from an unlimited number of directions and can also be submitted to mechanical isolation. Hyrtl in 1873[17] and Nussbaum in 1912[18] originally performed this method using metal alloys with a low melting point. Advances in the field of plastics have greatly improved and refined it.[19–21]

This method is particularly suitable for studying the anatomy of the arterial vessels. When performed in combination with casts of the heart chambers, it provides excellent topographic information. Using coloring agents as a code for different coronary arteries and cardiac chambers, James[6] prepared a series of 95 perfect casts from patients who had died of noncardiac causes and in whom there was no gross evidence of coronary heart disease. His classic book, *Anatomy of the Coronary Arteries,* which was based on this material and was published in 1961, not only excelled in its esthetically attractive illustrations (Fig. 25-3) and lucid descriptions, but also became an important source of information for the first generation of coronary angiographers.

All these postmortem methods have also been used successfully for studies that correlate vascular findings with clinical symptoms and signs of coronary artery disease. The extensive studies by Schlesinger[22,23] and his Boston colleagues[24] during the 1940s and 1950s immensely furthered knowledge of the pathologic involvement of the coronary arteries and their relation to localized myocardial disease and clinical symptomatology. However, their results and those of others[25] were sometimes conflicting. Quite clearly, the postmortem angiogram, obtained "post facto," is limited in its ability to assess the natural history or the prognosis of coronary artery disease. Nevertheless, postmortem examination can be the ultimate method of information when the in vivo angiographic examination raises questions concerning anatomy and topography.

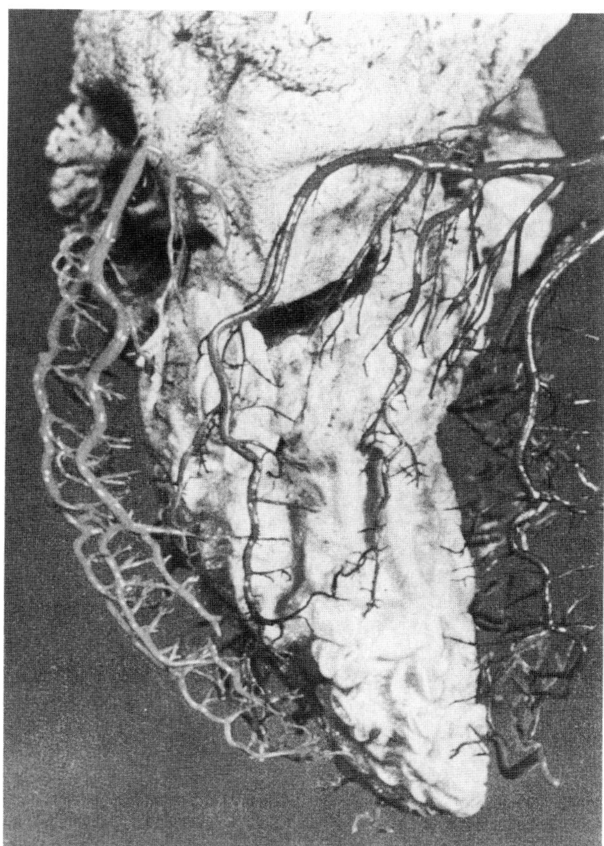

Figure 25-3. Injection-corrosion preparation of normal coronary arteries using coloring agents to code extension of right versus left coronary artery. In this black and white reproduction, the red left coronary (*left side* of picture) appears in lighter tone than the blue right coronary artery. Also observe the topographic relationship to the case of the left ventricular cavity. (From James TN. Anatomy of the coronary arteries. New York: Hoeber Medical Division, Harper & Row, 1961. Used with permission.)

◀ **Figure 25-2.** Postmortem arteriogram of human heart. (A) Demonstration of distal coronary artery extensions and anastomoses (*arrowheads*). The *arrow* points to the left anterior descending coronary arteries. *RCA,* right coronary artery; *MLCA,* main left coronary artery. (B) A barium sulfate mixture was injected selectively into the coronary arteries of a pig under controlled pressure for subsequent direct-contact radiography of the isolated interventricular septum. This radiograph convincingly demonstrates collateral anastomoses (*arrows*) from the posterior descending artery (*PDA*) to the experimentally stenosed left anterior descending (*LAD*) artery. (From Schaper W. The collateral circulation of the heart. Clinical Studies Series. New York: Elsevier, 1971; 1. Used with permission.)

General Description of Coronary Circulation and Cardiac Topography

Any person who performs clinical coronary arteriography must be familiar with cardiac anatomy and physiology, particularly the coronary circulation, the detail of which exceeds the information usually presented in standard textbooks. The interested reader can find a vast literature of excellent articles and texts dealing with all facets of this subject.[4,6,7,13,16,26–35] For practical reasons, the following sections focus on details that are considered important both for the technical performance of the examination and for adequate interpretation of in vivo coronary arteriography. Thus the description of the coronary orifices is relatively extensive because of the implication for their successful catheterization and their potential involvement by pathologic changes; the less frequently demonstrated and rarely involved cardiac veins are dealt with in more general terms.

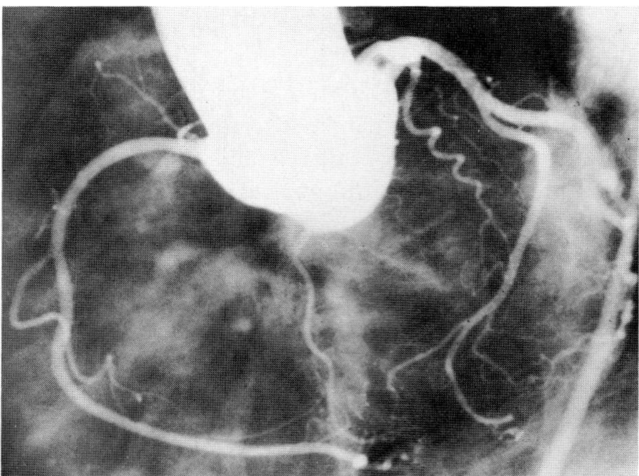

Figure 25-4. Nonselective in vivo coronary arteriogram in LAO projection illustrating the almost complete vascular ring formed by the right and left circumflex coronary arteries in their position in the atrioventricular ring.

The Coronary Arteries

The arterial components of the coronary circulation can be divided into two compartments: (1) the larger and mostly subepicardially located extramural coronary arteries, and (2) the great number of much smaller, intramurally located coronary branches that distribute blood flow into the capillary bed. Whereas the former are accessible to direct angiographic demonstration in the living patient, the latter, in most instances, are not visible because of their small calibers.

The human coronary circulation has two major arterial vessels, the right and the left coronary arteries, which arise from the corresponding sinuses of the aortic valve apparatus. The third sinus is the noncoronary cusp. Both arteries have a tendency to occupy the atrioventricular sulcus on either side, thus forming an almost complete ring around the atrioventricular plane. From this plane, numerous branches arise at rather acute angles in the direction of the cardiac apex to supply the myocardial walls (Fig. 25-4). The classical anatomist recognized this general pattern of arterial supply and compared it to the appearance of a crown; hence their Latin name, *arteriae coronariae.*

The *right coronary artery* departs from the aorta via its mostly anteriorly directed orifice and runs in the right atrioventricular sulcus (Fig. 25-5). It lies below the epicardium and is surrounded by the right atrial appendage. It then travels on the surface of the heart, occasionally covered by small myocardial bridges. Its course, which begins between the aortic root and the main trunk of the pulmonary artery, subsequently extends downward along the right side of the heart to the diaphragmatic surface and forms a semicircle. This portion is therefore also known as the *right circumflex artery* in analogy to the corresponding coronary artery on the left side.

In the majority of human hearts, the right coronary artery reaches the crux of the heart, the latter representing the intersection of the atrioventricular sulcus with the posterior interventricular groove, which indicates the border between the walls of the right and left ventricle. With regard to the interior topography, the atrioventricular sulci correspond to the fibrous ring—the skeleton of the heart—to which the four cardiac valves are related. The posterior interventricular groove and the more shallow posterior interatrial groove indicate the posterior attachment of the interventricular and interatrial septum, respectively. At the crux, the right coronary artery divides its arterial distribution in two directions. One branch continues to the left in the area of the posterior atrioventricular sulcus; the other turns toward the apex to supply the area of the posterior interventricular groove.

From the aortic orifice to its division at the crux, the right coronary artery gives off branches in the anterior direction toward the right ventricular wall and in the posterior direction toward the right atrium. Its first branch is usually directed anteriorly and passes around the anterior aspect of the outflow tract of the right ventricle close to the level of the pulmonic valve. This *pulmonary conus branch* is relatively constant in its distribution but frequently has its own orifice closely adjacent but clearly separate from the main right coro-

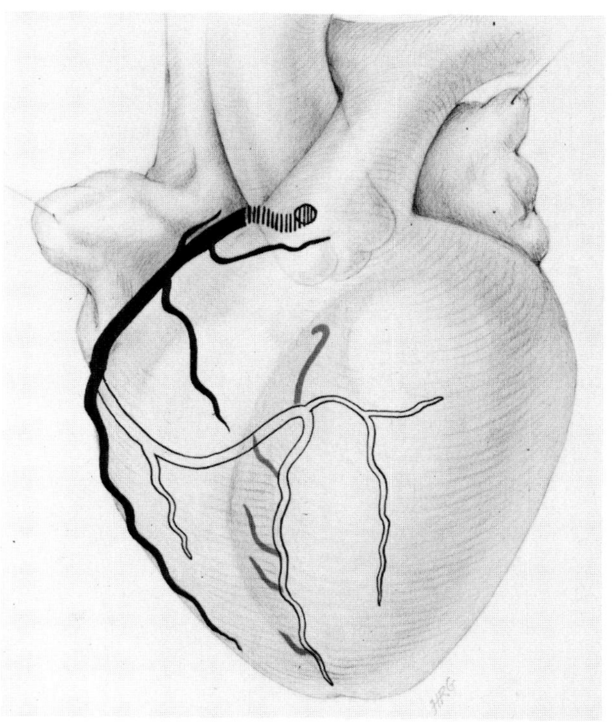

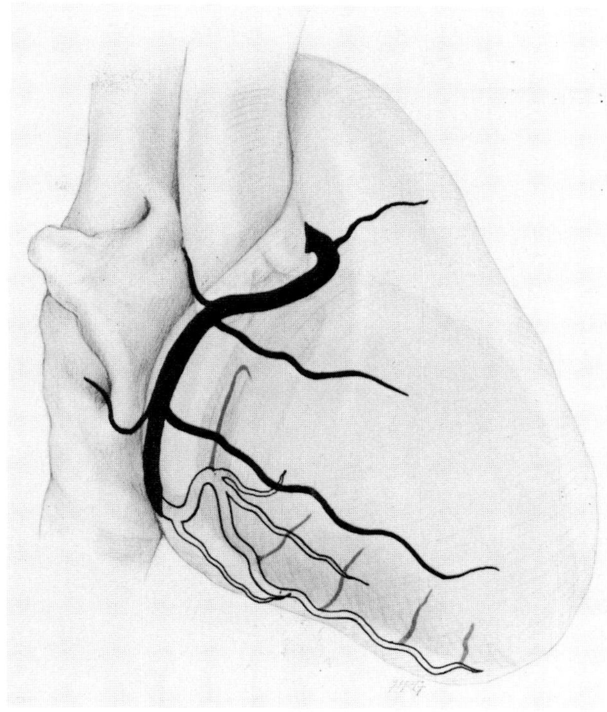

A B

Figure 25-5. Drawing of right coronary artery in LAO (A) and RAO (B) views. Vessels on near side are black; those on far side are outlined. Vessels in interventricular septal levels are shaded. See text for anatomic detail.

nary artery ostium in the right coronary sinus. Because of this rather frequent appearance (almost 50 percent), this usually small branch has been denoted as the *third coronary artery.* The subsequently arising anteriorly directed branches vary greatly in number and size. One of these is usually the largest and extends toward the apical region of the heart. Because it is close to the acute margin of the right ventricle, its designation is the *acute marginal branch.* Branches to the diaphragmatically oriented portion of the right ventricle are fewer and smaller than the relatively large *posterior descending coronary artery.* This artery, characterized by its origin near the crux from the right coronary artery, distributes preferentially in the posterior interventricular sulcus and adjacent areas.

A varying number of branches may supply the posterior aspect of the left ventricle, depending on the degree to which the right coronary artery extends to the left of the crux. Very small septal branches usually arise from the posterior descending coronary artery to distribute in the posterior third of the interventricular septum. These *posterior septal branches* are consistently much smaller than the anterior septal branches that arise from the left anterior descending coronary artery.

Branches of the right coronary artery directed posteriorly toward the right atrium are small. A relatively constant one is the *anterior atrial branch,* which ramifies over the anterior atrial wall and parts of the atrial appendage. It usually arises as the second branch, the first being the pulmonary conus branch. In hearts in which it extends to the ostium of the superior vena cava to supply the sinus node, the anterior atrial artery is clearly the widest of the atrial branches. Its designation as the *ramus ostii venae cavae superioris* or *sinus node artery* is self-explanatory. Small, rather inconstant atrial branches originate from the right circumflex artery at the acute margin and at the diaphragmatic surface to supply the lateral and posterior walls of the atrium, respectively. They have been described as the *intermediate* and *posterior atrial branches.*

After arising from the left sinus of Valsalva, the *left coronary artery* runs in the groove between the left atrial appendage and the main trunk of the pulmonary artery (Fig. 25-6). Initially it courses backward to the left, but then turns in the ventral direction before bifurcating into the *left circumflex artery* and the *anterior descending artery.* The latter vessel is a direct continuation of the main trunk of the left coronary artery,

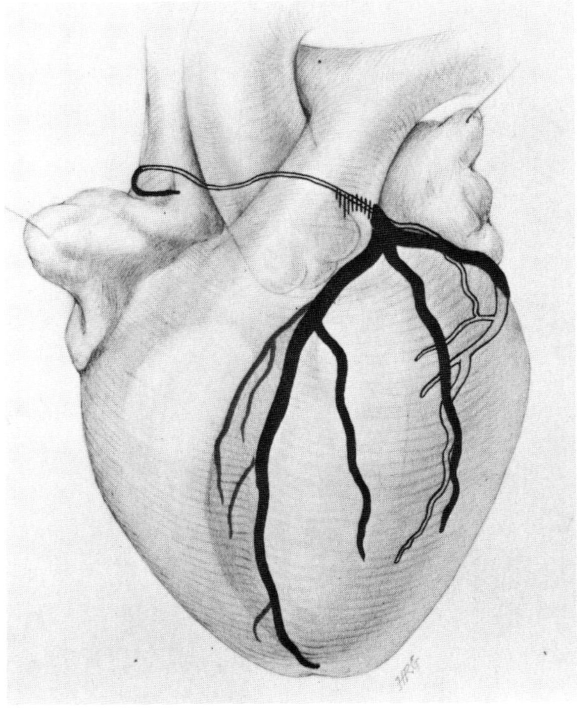

A

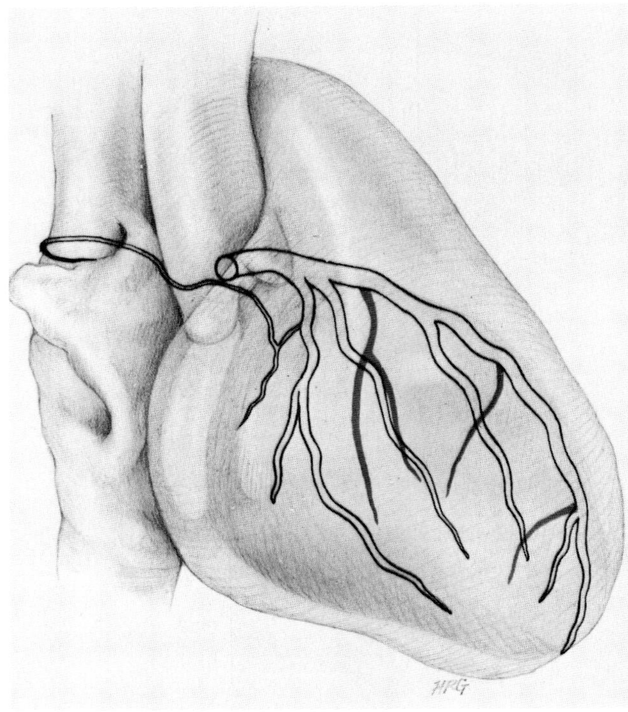

B

Figure 25-6. Drawing of left coronary artery in LAO (A) and RAO (B) views. Vessels on near side are black; those on far side are outlined. Vessels in interventricular septal levels are shaded. See text for anatomic detail.

whose length between the ostium and the bifurcation varies from a few millimeters to a few centimeters. Only extremely small, inconstant branches depart from the main trunk.

The anterior descending artery, after its origin from the left main bifurcation of the main stem, curves around the left margin of the pulmonary conus and enters the anterior interventricular groove forming the border between the left and right ventricles on the anterior wall of the heart. It runs under the left atrial appendage for the first few centimeters of its course, but it subsequently lies on the cardiac surface directly below the visceral layer of the pericardium. Sometimes buried in the myocardium for a short or longer portion, it invariably returns to the surface before reaching the apical region, where it generally curves around to the diaphragmatic wall to supply various-sized areas with its terminal branches.

The anterior descending artery supplies subepicardially located branches to the anterior walls of both the right and left ventricles, as well as branches directed centrally to the interventricular septum. A small branch, running toward the conus branch from the right coronary artery, is rather consistent. Otherwise, *branches to the right ventricle are small and few,* particularly when compared to the diagonal branches, which are significantly wider and larger and which are given off in the direction of the anterolateral wall of the left ventricle.

A varying number of branches arising from the anterior descending artery in the apical and diaphragmatic direction supply the anterior two-thirds of the interventricular septum. The first, and usually the largest, of these *anterior septal branches* arises from the proximal portion of the anterior descending artery close to the bifurcation of the main trunk. It frequently divides into two or more secondary septal branches.

The *left circumflex artery,* in contrast to the anterior descending artery, rises almost perpendicularly from the main trunk and follows a course in the left atrioventricular sulcus. Its length in this location varies, as do the number and size of its branches to the adjacent areas of the left and posterior walls of the left ventricle. These variations in size and extension are related in a reciprocating fashion to those occurring in the most distal distribution of the right coronary artery. Among the anteriorly directed side branches from the left circumflex artery, a relatively large branch is usually visible and located approximately halfway between the anterior and posterior free walls of the left ventricle. Its path corresponds to the area of the obtuse margin; thus the term *left circumflex obtuse marginal branch* identifies this vessel. In some hearts, an artery running toward the midportion of the lateral wall of the left ventricle arises from the angle between the division of the anterior descending and the circumflex arteries. This creates the appearance of a trifurcation of the left main trunk. This branch is sometimes so large that it may even reach the apical region. Appropriate terms for this vessel are *left intermediate artery, ramus medianus,* or *arteria intermedia.*

The *anterior atrial artery* departs from the left circumflex artery in a dorsal direction toward the left atrium and extends over the cranial wall of the atrium and its appendage. A more constant small artery, the *intermediate left atrial artery,* may arise at the level of the obtuse margin. Parallel to the circumflex artery, there is often a branch coursing around the lateral wall of the left atrium, known as the *left atrial circumflex artery.* Both these left-sided atrial arteries may traverse the midline of the heart either at the cranial or posterior aspect of the atria and extend to the junction between the superior vena cava and the right atrium. Either may supply the sinus node, in which case it is the strongest of all atrial branches and is identified as a left-sided *sinus node artery.*

Reciprocity exists between the right and left coronary arteries of the human heart; a large distribution of one takes place at the cost of the other. Variations of this nature have the greatest implication with regard to the blood supply of the crux and the posterior interventricular sulcus. In roughly 90 percent of the cases, the right coronary artery reaches and supplies this area; otherwise, the left circumflex artery provides the supply. Consequently, the supply of the posterior third of the interventricular septum and the atrioventricular node by the *posterior septal branches* depends on the integrity of the coronary artery that serves this area. The concept of right or left coronary preponderance is based on these variations in contribution. When right and left coronary artery branches share rather equally in the supply of the crux, the term *balanced* or *codominant coronary distribution* has been applied.

Reciprocal variations in distribution between the right and left coronary arteries also exist regarding the termination of the left anterior descending artery and the right posterior descending artery. The concept of coronary artery preponderance of the human heart, however, does not include them.

The Intramural Circulation

In contrast to the epicardially located large coronary arteries and their branches, the intramural or intramyocardial portion of the coronary arterial supply consists of numerous small branches that perpendicularly enter the wall. According to Baroldi and Scomazzoni,[26] the intramural branches penetrate its entire thickness. They give rise to smaller branches at different levels, which ramify in multiple planes parallel to the wall's internal surface. James[6] observed that the intramural arteries of the right ventricular myocardium are at a more acute angle from the extramural circulation and therefore follow a more oblique course while penetrating the myocardium.

Further ramifications into the capillary network occur in all directions and at all levels from these secondary intramural branches. A distinction can be made between two types of intramural branches: (1) those that after a short distance immediately subdivide into a meshlike pattern, preferentially supplying the outer layers, and (2) those that are longer and penetrate deeper to supply the more endocardially located layers, including the subendocardial zone. The latter variety's longer course through the contracting myocardium exposes them to a phasically occurring compression, which accounts for the systolic reduction of coronary blood flow and probably explains the increased vulnerability of the subendocardial layers of the myocardium to partial ischemia.

Numerous vascular connections exist in the intramural circulation (Fig. 25-7). Thus, anastomoses are known to occur among intramural arteries, between intramural arteries and intramural veins, and among intramural veins. In addition, each of these vascular compartments may communicate with the left ventricular cavity via three directions: (1) the so-called arterial sinusoidal vessels, (2) the slightly larger and more direct connecting arterioluminal vessels on the precapillary arterial side, and (3) the thebesian vessels on the venous side. The return of the coronary blood flow occurs predominately through the intramural venous compartment, which is topographically similar to the corresponding arteries. The lower pressure in the intramural veins makes them more compressible during myocardial contraction, a mechanism that is believed to account for acceleration of coronary venous flow during systole.

Pathologic conditions of the intramural coronary arteries and of the extramural circulation differ considerably. There are no reports of arteriosclerotic disease in the intramural arteries without involvement of the epicardial vessels.[26] Certain forms of cardiomyopathy,

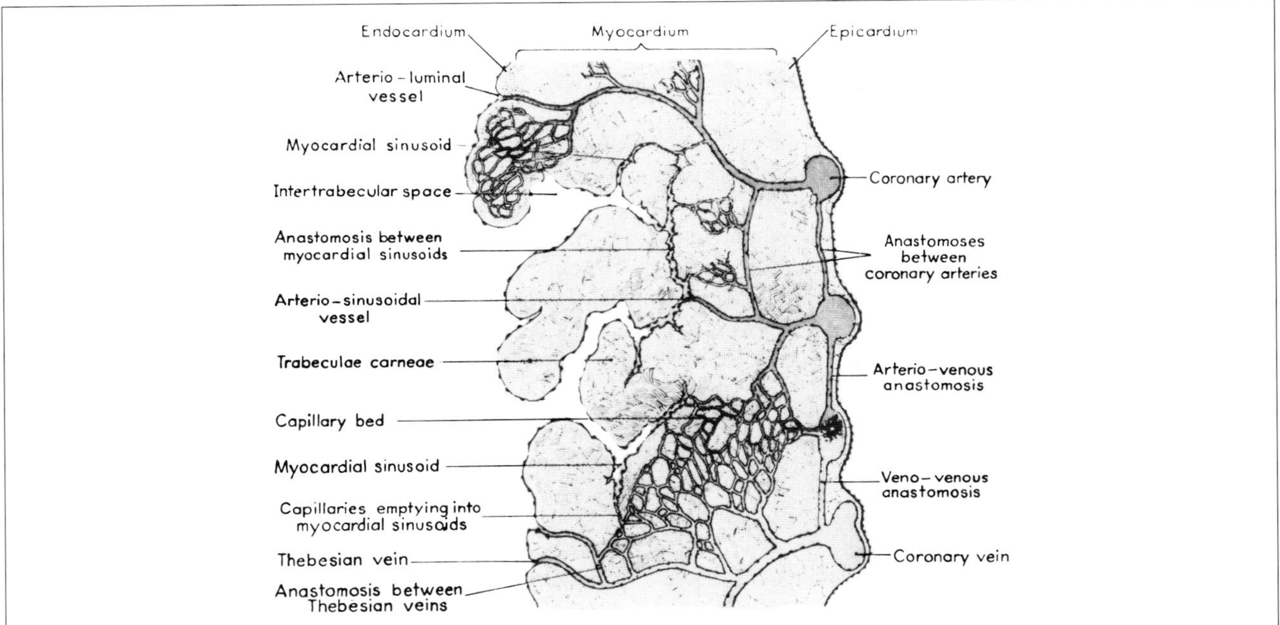

Figure 25-7. Schematic illustration of intramural coronary circulation. (From Gould SE, ed. Pathology of the heart. Springfield, IL: Charles C Thomas, 1953. Used with permission.)

however, characteristically involve these intramural vessels exclusively.[36–38]

The Coronary Veins

The extramural portion of the coronary venous system has two components: the larger and more important connects the major portion of coronary veins with the large venous coronary sinus; the smaller anterior cardiac venous system is characterized by independent drainage into the right atrium.

The *coronary sinus* is located in the left atrioventricular sulcus and opens into the right atrium at its posterior lower margin; its orifice is guarded by an incomplete valve (*thebesian valve*). The most distant vein draining into the coronary sinus system is usually the *anterior interventricular vein,* which forms at the anterior surface of the heart and drains the area supplied by the anterior descending artery. The vein is often duplicated until it curves at a rather sharp angle to follow the left atrioventricular sulcus. From this point on, it is also known as the *great cardiac vein* (Fig. 25-8), continuing directly into the large venous coronary sinus. The point of demarcation between the latter two portions of this capacious venous channel is determined by the entrance of the oblique vein of Marshall, the adult residual of the fetal left superior cardinal vein that sometimes persists as the left marginal vein connecting at the level of the obtuse margin of the heart. In the event of a persisting left superior vena cava, the vein of Marshall will accomplish a conduit for systemic venous blood into the right atrium via the coronary venous sinus, a finding well remembered by any angiographer who has encountered catheter passage through this route. The *middle vein,* which runs from the apex toward the base in the area of the posterior interventricular sulcus, and the *left posterior vein,* which extends over the dorsal and lateral aspect of the left ventricle, are major, usually well-defined vessels, all draining either into the great cardiac vein or the venous coronary sinus.

The *anterior cardiac venous system* has numerous variations. A relatively constant vein follows the acute margin of the heart and is called the *right marginal vein.* The topographic division into the two cardiac venous systems does not reflect a functional separation; indeed, the two systems anastomose freely, particularly near the anterior interventricular sulcus, the cardiac apex, and the conus pulmonalis.

Angiographic Anatomy

As is obvious from the preceding general description, the epicardially located coronary arterial tree surrounds the globe-shaped heart, resulting in great variations of the spatial orientation of its individual branches. Angiographic demonstration, which images

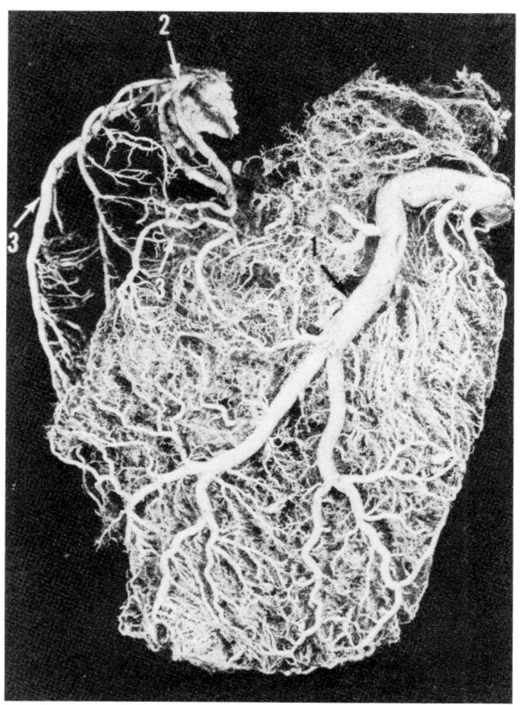

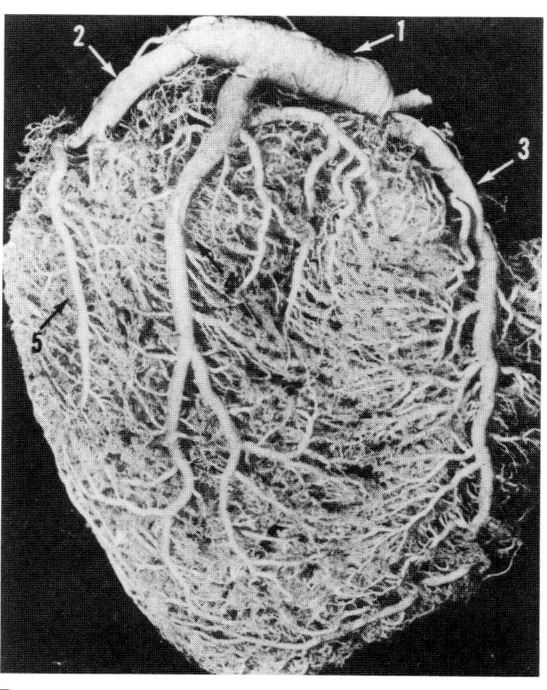

Figure 25-8. Cast of coronary veins demonstrating the great cardiac vein on the anterior aspect (A) and its continuation into the coronary sinus on the posterior aspect (B) of the heart. (A) *2* and *3*, small anterior veins draining separately into right atrium. (B) *1*, coronary sinus; *2*, great cardiac vein; *3*, middle vein. (From Baroldi G, Scomazzoni G. Coronary circulation in the normal and pathologic heart. Washington, DC: Office of the Surgeon General, Department of the Army, 1967. Used with permission.)

three-dimensional structures on a single plane, meets special challenges when applied to the visualization of the coronary arteries.

The methods of choice for selective coronary arteriography are radiographic image-intensification techniques combined with cinematography, which became popular in the early 1960s. They are more flexible than large, direct serial angiography, which requires bulky film changers. The initial introduction of patient-supporting rotatable cradles permitted the operator to perform several selective injections in a number of different obliquities. Presently available technical arrangements preserve the patient's supine position and make use of modern support stands for the radiographic equipment that facilitates the use of angulations of the central x-ray beam in all directions, including the patient's long body axis, an important feature for the proper depiction of certain critical anatomic sites of the coronary arterial tree. Image-storing devices for immediate replay enhance recognition of subtle changes and variations and allow one to perform the additional projections that are deemed to be optimal. The operator must therefore be thoroughly familiar with equipment design and function (Fig. 25-9), for its optimal use in the individual case.[39] In addition, profound and detailed familiarity with coronary artery anatomy and topography is one of the most important requirements for success.

The Aortic Root and the Coronary Ostia

Independent of technique, the topography of the ascending aorta and the aortic bulb and the size and position of the coronary artery orifices may influence the successful performance of a coronary arteriogram. A detailed description of the common anatomy and the most common variations of the structures therefore appears to be in order. Deformations attributable to congenital and acquired pathology are not included in this presentation. The same is true for ectopic coronary arteries arising from the pulmonary artery, which result in a typical clinical entity (Bland-White-Garland syndrome),[40] as well as other aberrations that are known to be of pathologic significance.[41]

The *aortic bulb* constitutes a mild dilatation of the ascending aorta in direct connection with the aortic valve (Fig. 25-10). It comprises the *three sinuses of Valsalva* and is caudally bordered by the three thin, about

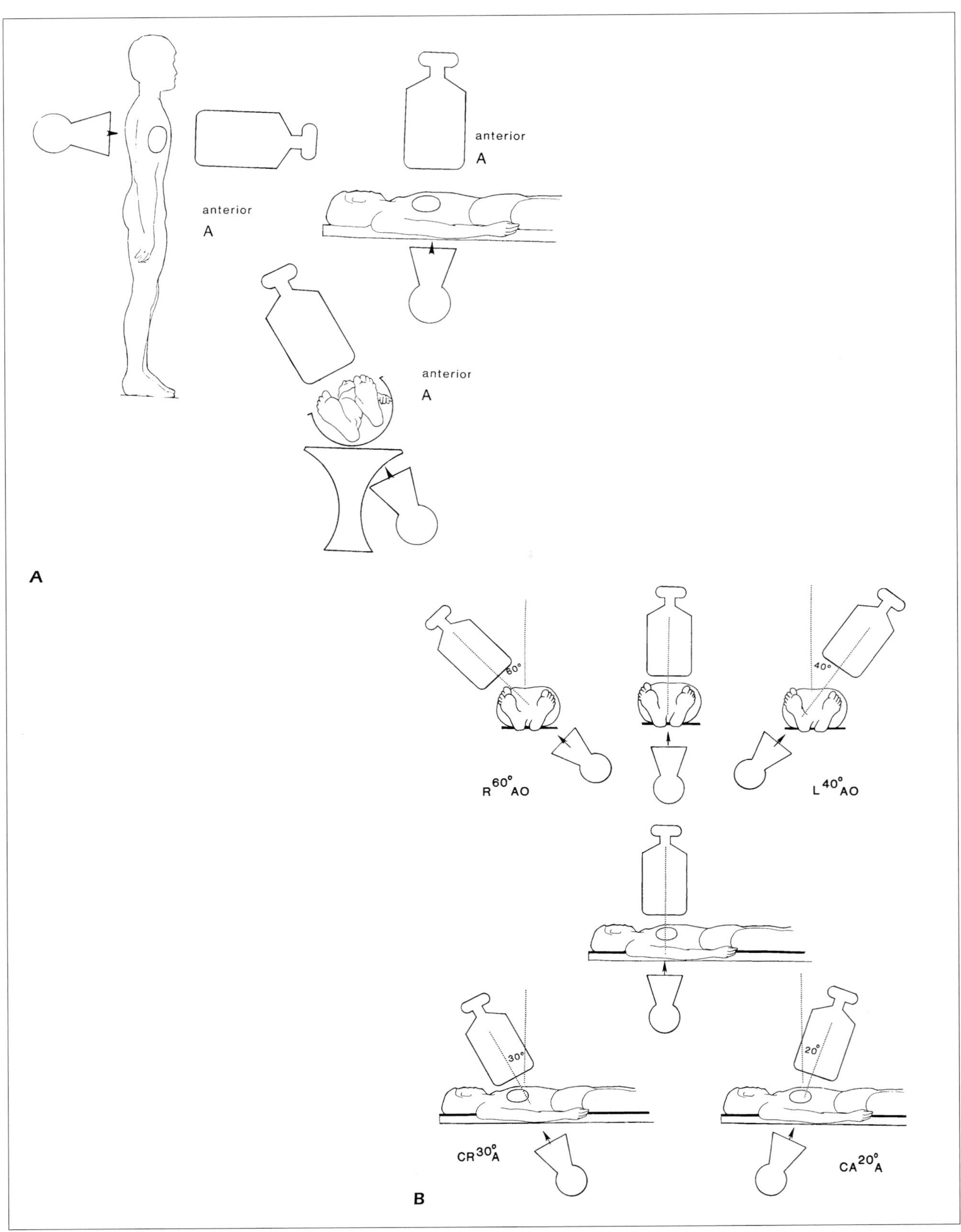
anterior
A
anterior
A
anterior
A
A
60°
40°
R 60° AO
L 40° AO
30°
20°
CR 30° A
CA 20° A
B

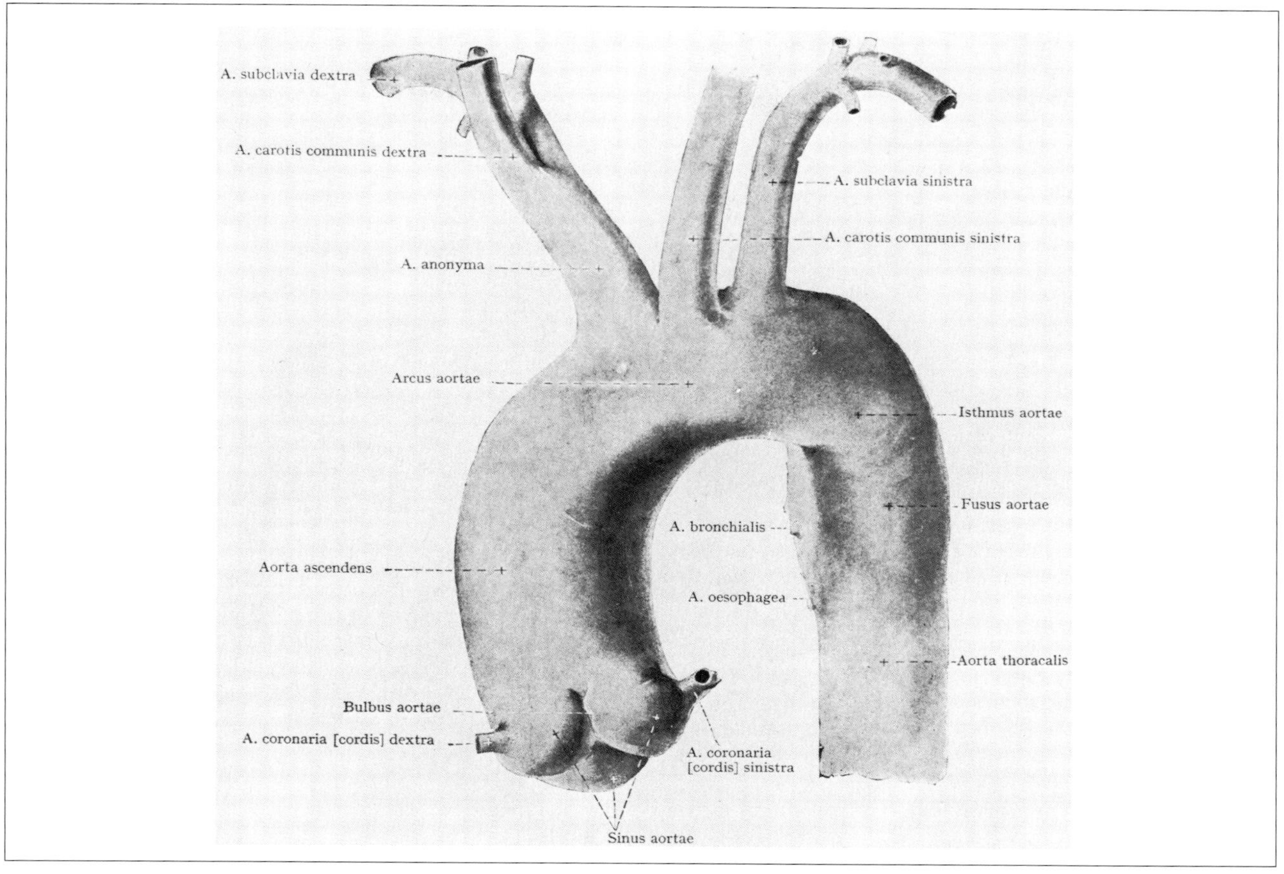

Figure 25-10. The aortic bulb and thoracic aorta in LAO position according to Spalteholz. (From Paulin S. Coronary angiography: a technical, anatomic and clinical study. Acta Radiol (Stockh) 1964;233 (Suppl). Used with permission.

equally sized, semilunar valve leaflets. The parts of the sinuses facing the periphery form semicircular bulges. As a rule, the border between the aortic bulb and the ascending aorta is discernible as a slight indentation in the tangential contour of an aortogram, also denoted as the *supravalvular ring.*

According to current terminology, the designations of the three semilunar valves are *right coronary cusp, left coronary cusp,* and *noncoronary cusp.* It is not advisable to apply old anatomic nomenclature, using *anterior, posterior,* and *lateral cusps,* because these relate to the orientation of the isolated heart on the dissection table and have little to do with the topography as seen on the in vivo angiographic examination. Considering the standard radiologic oblique projections, the left anterior oblique (LAO) and the right anterior oblique (RAO), and their relation to the long axis of the body, the left coronary cusp orients to the left but slightly posteriorly and cranially, the right coronary cusp is anterior but slightly to the right and more caudal, and the noncoronary cusp is posterior and slightly to the right but most caudal in relation to the others (Fig. 25-11). Obviously, a perfect tangential angiographic depiction of the aortic valve plane would require a certain degree of craniocaudal tilt of the central x-ray beam.

◄ **Figure 25-9.** Terminology for radiographic projections. (A) The image intensifier sees the patient in the anterior projection (*A*), whether standing, supine, or rotated. (*B*) The supine patient is seen from the foot end in RAO and LAO projection on either side of the straight anterior view (*upper row*). Cranial (*CR*) and caudal (*CA*) projections are demonstrated from the side (*lower row*). The degree of angulation is indicated in elevated numbers. (From Paulin S. Terminology for radiographic projections in cardiac angiography. Cathet Cardiovasc Diagn, 1981;7:351. Used with permission.)

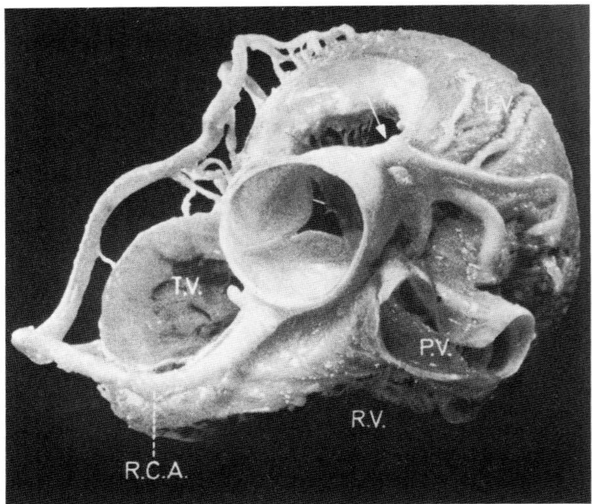

Figure 25-11. Postmortem specimen of the heart as seen from above. Observe the topographic relationship between the aortic valve cusp, the wall of ascending aorta, and the coronary arteries. *T. V.,* tricuspid valve; *P. V.,* pulmonary vein; *R. V.,* right ventricle; *R.C.A.,* right coronary artery. *Arrow* points at the main left coronary trunk. (From McAlpine WA. Heart and coronary arteries: an anatomical atlas for clinical diagnosis, radiological investigation and surgical treatment. New York: Springer-Verlag, 1975. Used with permission.)

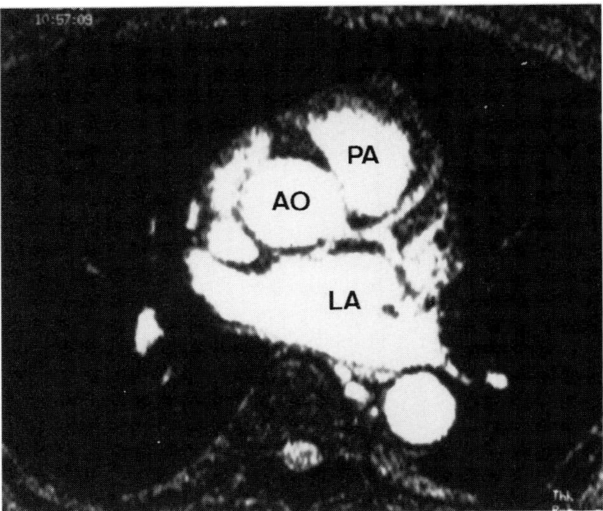

Figure 25-12. Magnetic resonance image of horizontal plane section through heart at level of the aortic root, demonstrating take-off of left main coronary artery and bifurcation into left anterior descending and circumflex arteries. This view is not accessible with conventional angiography. *AO,* aorta; *PA,* pulmonary artery; *LA,* left atrium. (Courtesy of Robert R. Edelman, M.D., Beth Israel Hospital and Harvard Medical School, Boston.

Delineation of the aortic root and proximal coronary arteries in a horizontal plane, as can be illustrated in a postmortem specimen and in schematic drawings (see Figs. 25-11, 25-13, 25-19, 25-21, and 25-28), is not practical using contrast radiography, but has become possible with other imaging techniques such as ultrafast CT, transesophageal echocardiography, and MRI. In the future, these techniques[42,43] may identify abnormalities in the anatomy of the coronary artery in relation to their take-off from the aorta, with alleged potential clinical consequences (Fig. 25-12). Such observations made on postmortem studies[44] have so far defied recognition by in vivo coronary arteriography.

Figure 25-13. Most common position of the coronary ostia as given by May.[45] (From Paulin S. Coronary angiography: a technical, anatomic and clinical study. Acta Radiol (Stockh) 1964;233(Suppl):48. Used with permission.)

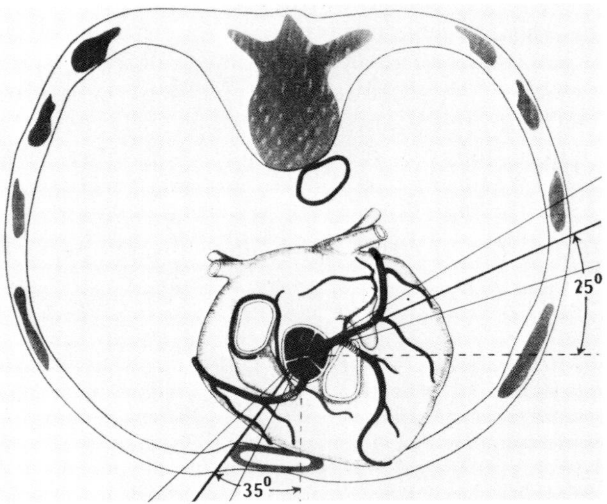

The two large coronary arteries do not arise diametrically opposite each other. According to May,[45] who described the surgical anatomy of the coronary arteries, the left coronary artery leaves the aortic bulb in a sinistrodorsal direction approximately 25 degrees from the frontal plane (Fig. 25-13). In exceptional cases, however, he observed the coronary ostium displaced so far forward that it lay parallel to the frontal plane or even ventral to it. The right coronary artery arose anteriorly to the right, forming an angle of about 35 degrees (variation of 10 degrees) with the sagittal plane. McAlpine[7] recorded similar results on 50 specimens specifically so examined.

These anatomic features require moderate rotation of the patient from the sagittal plane into an LAO projection for tangential radiographic depiction of the left coronary ostium. An additional 30-degree rotation to a steeper LAO projection is optimal for depiction of the right coronary ostium (Fig. 25-14).

Failure to delineate the proximal left coronary ar-

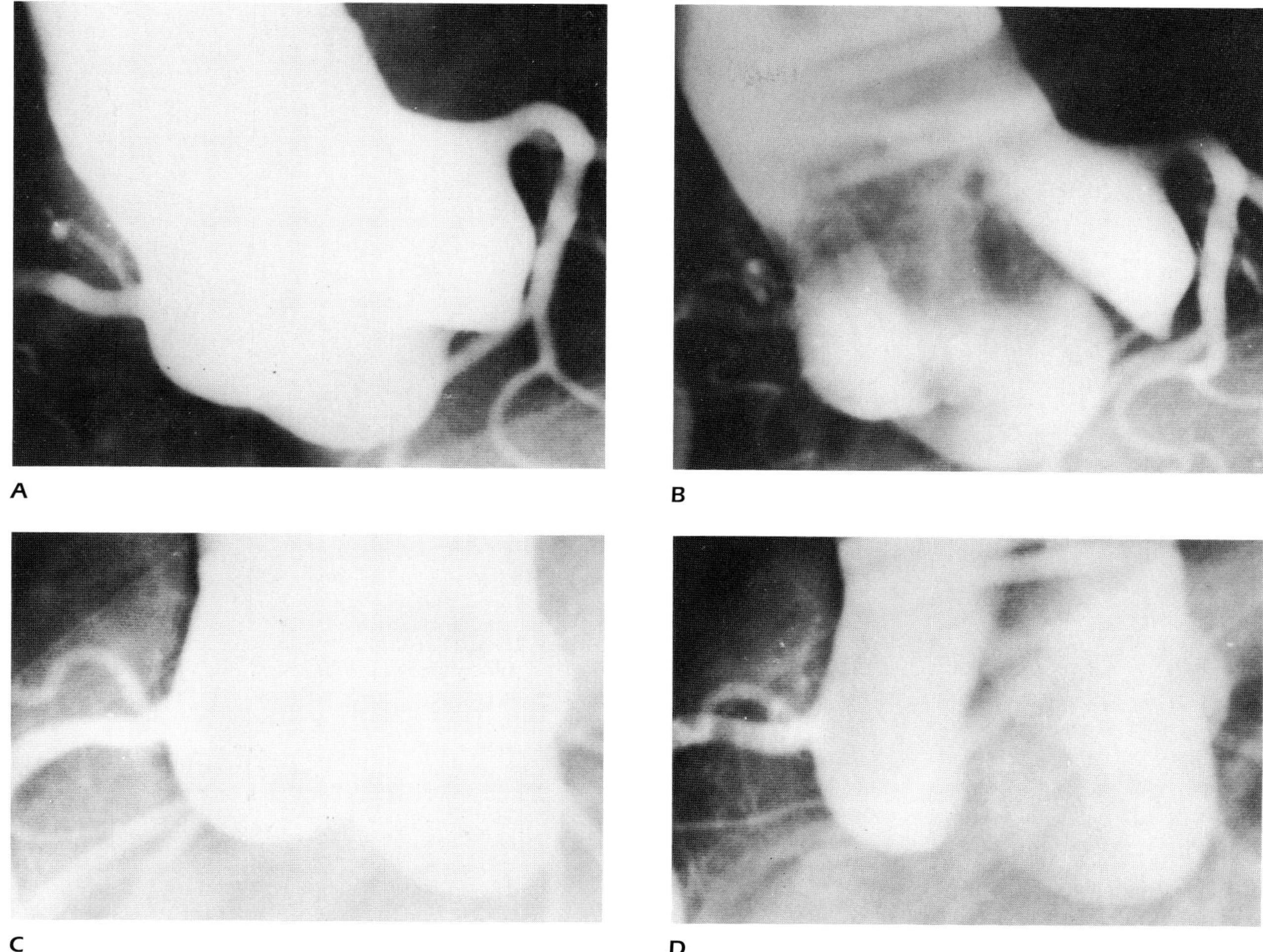

Figure 25-14. Example of tangentially depicted coronary ostia. Left coronary ostium in LAO view (A and B), permitting free communication between the aortic lumen and the coronary orifices (C and D).

tery in the usual rotation results from the rare instances in which the left coronary artery turns directly to the left. An additional selective injection in the posteroanterior projection usually renders the desired tangential demonstration, provided that increased radiographic penetration compensates for the unavoidable superimposition with the spine in this projection. Steeper rotation into the LAO projection, similar to that required for the right ostium, compensates for unusual posterior placement of the orifice. Occasionally, and particularly in horizontal hearts, superimposition with the proximal portions of the left anterior descending (LAD) artery may create problems. Cranial tilts, obtained either with special devices or by elevating the patient in a semierect position, are likely to yield optimal results. Unsuccessful tangential exposure of the right coronary artery ostium is often the result of insufficient rotation into the LAO projection. It is important to remember that a steep LAO and close to lateral projection is essential for this purpose, even if such performance might be somewhat inconvenient to obtain with presently available equipment.

Slight variations in the position of the coronary ostia, such as displacement close to a commissure, are common (Fig. 25-15)[46,47] but probably less important for selective catheterization. These minor degree variations also seem to be unrelated to the length of the left main coronary artery,[7] to the type of coronary artery dominance,[48] or to both.[49] This is probably also the case for small positional variations in cranial displacements that Vladover and colleagues[47] observed in a high percentage of unselected adult hearts.

More important in this respect is greater cranial displacement, that is, when dislocation of the ostium is a few centimeters or more higher up so that it arises from the wall of the ascending aorta itself (Fig. 25-16).

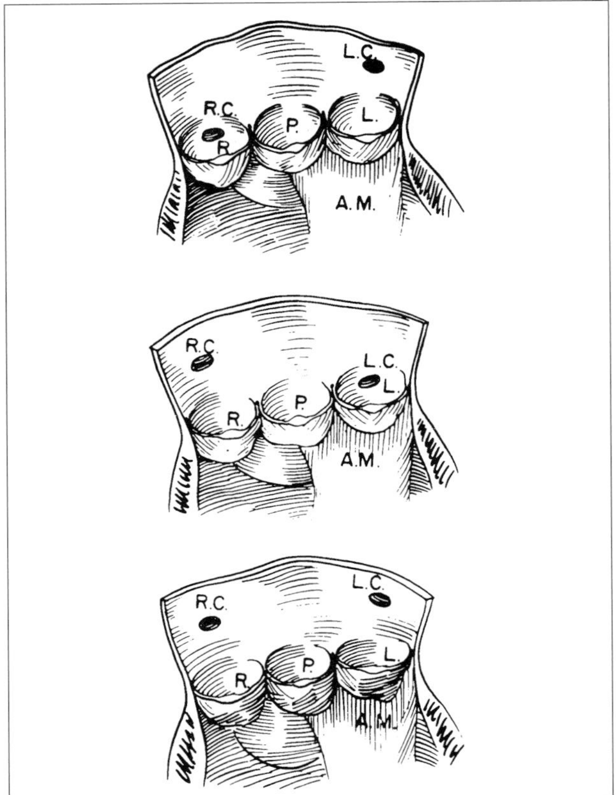

Figure 25-15. Illustration of common minor positional variations of coronary ostia. *L.C.,* left coronary artery ostium; *R.C.,* right coronary artery ostium; *R.,* right aortic sinus; *P.,* posterior (noncoronary) aortic sinus; *L.,* left aortic sinus; *A.M.,* anterior leaflet of the mitral valve. (From Vladover RZ, Neufeld HN, Edwards JE. Pathology of coronary disease. Semin Roentgenol 1972;1:376–394. Used with permission.)

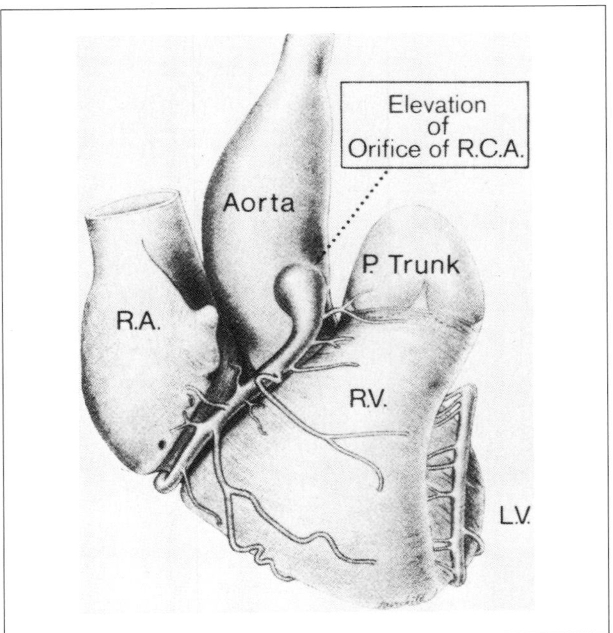

Figure 25-16. Elevation of right coronary orifice with additional displacement to the left. *P. Trunk,* pulmonary trunk; *R.A.,* right atrium; *R.V.,* right ventricle; *L.V.,* left ventricle; *R.C.A.,* right coronary artery. (From McAlpine WA. Heart and coronary arteries: an anatomical atlas for clinical diagnosis, radiological investigation and surgical treatment. New York: Springer-Verlag, 1975. Used with permission.)

Such cranial displacement occurs frequently in Marfan's syndrome, in which it is secondary to dilatation and elongation of the ascending aorta, but it has also been seen in autopsies of apparently normal hearts.[7,46,47] It is readily demonstrable in a nonselective coronary arteriogram,[50] in which such significant displacement was found on the right side in 4 and on the left side in 1 out of 208 cases (Figs. 25-17 and 25-18).[48] With selective technique such variation may remain unnoticed, but, as pointed out by Amplatz et al.,[51] cranial displacement usually creates more technical difficulties for selective catheterization, since it often requires more extensive catheter manipulations or the use of catheters of special design. At times, unsuccessful cannulation attempts may call for an additional nonselective bolus injection for guidance. Extreme ectopia with a coronary artery arising from a branch of the aorta (e.g., the internal mammary artery) seems to be rare and predominantly occurs in patients with other cardiovascular anomalies.[52,53]

The origin of the coronary arteries varies with respect not only to position but also to number. Less than two coronary ostia are presented by the so-called monostic coronary circulation, or *single coronary artery.* This anomaly is more commonly associated with other cardiac malformations, but may occur as an isolated condition. In the latter situation it is useful to classify these arterial variants as either aplasia-type or joining abnormalities.

Aplasia of one coronary artery is found when one coronary artery is distributed so extensively over the whole heart that no trace of the other artery remains (Fig. 25-19). Such a variant corresponds to the true type of single coronary artery first described in Hyrtl.[17] This rare anomaly has been observed at autopsies,[46,47,54] and one rather convincing in vivo radiographic demonstration has been reported (Fig. 25-20).[55] Obviously angiographic exclusion of the presence of an extremely small right coronary may be less conclusive than what can be accomplished by careful postmortem examination, the method by which Ogden[56] was able to differentiate between a true *single left coronary artery* and a very marked left preponderant circulation.

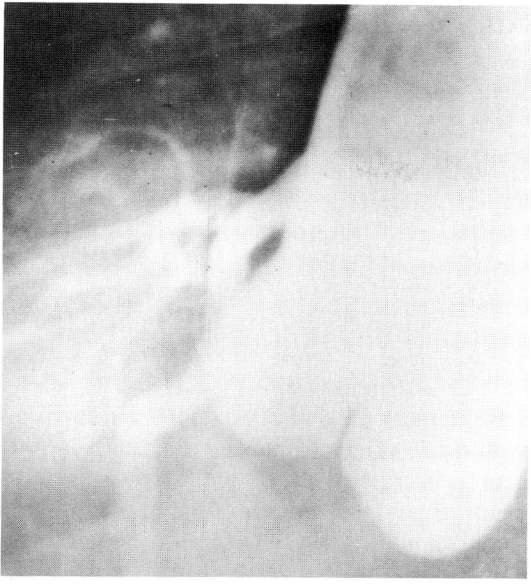

A

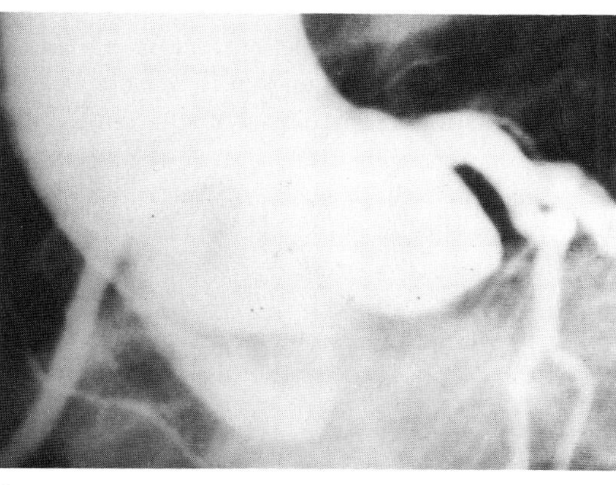

B

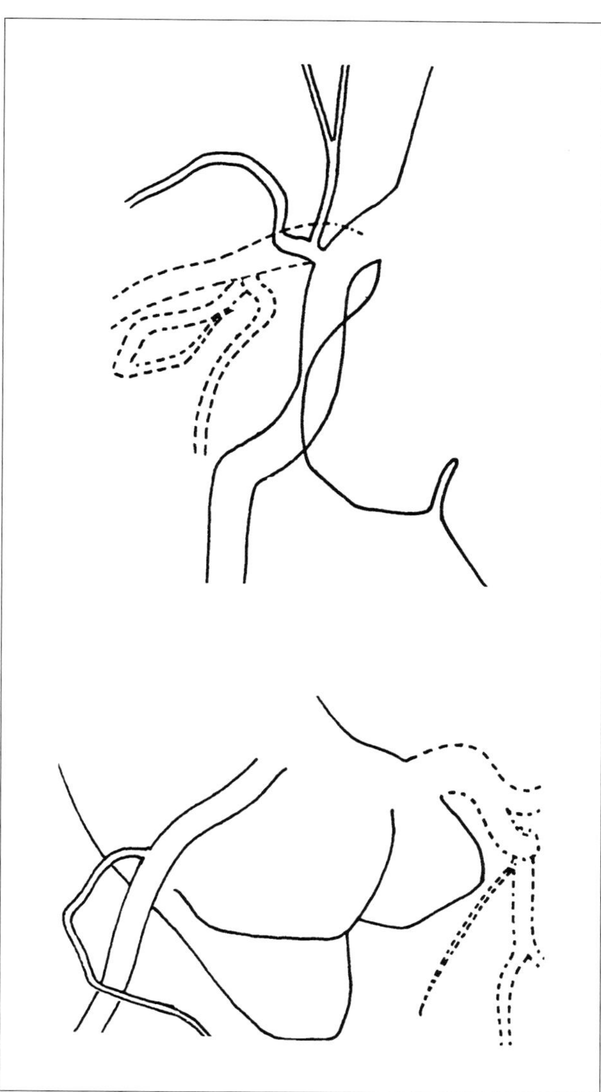

Figure 25-17. Nonselective in vivo coronary arteriography demonstrating unusually high position of right coronary ostium above the right coronary cusp in the lower part of the ascending aorta. In lateral view (A) and LAO view (B) the coronary artery orifice is identified in a similar location as illustrated in Figure 25-16. Line drawings on the *right* highlight findings on corresponding radiographs on *left*.

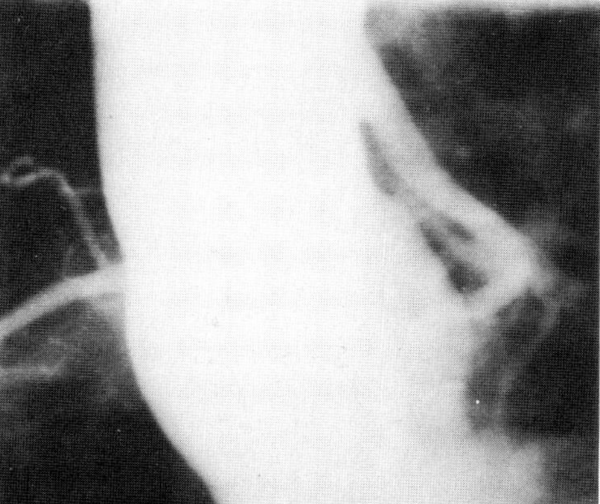

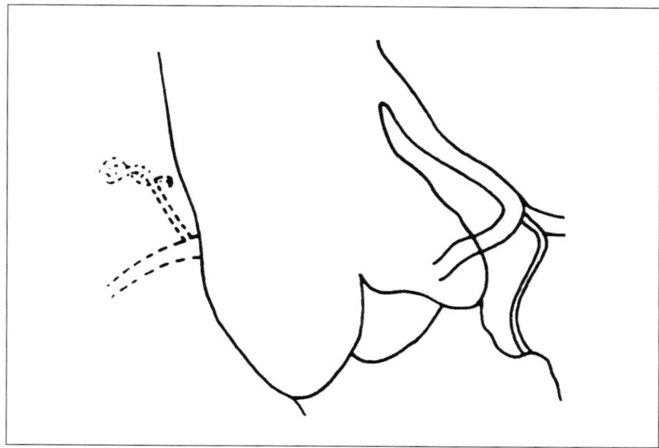

Figure 25-18. *Left:* Variant of left coronary main orifice position arising from the ascending aorta well above the coronary sinus in LAO position. *Right:* line drawing of radiograph. (From S. Coronary angiography: a technical, anatomic and clinical study. Acta Radiol (Stockh) 1964; 233(Suppl):55. Used with permission.)

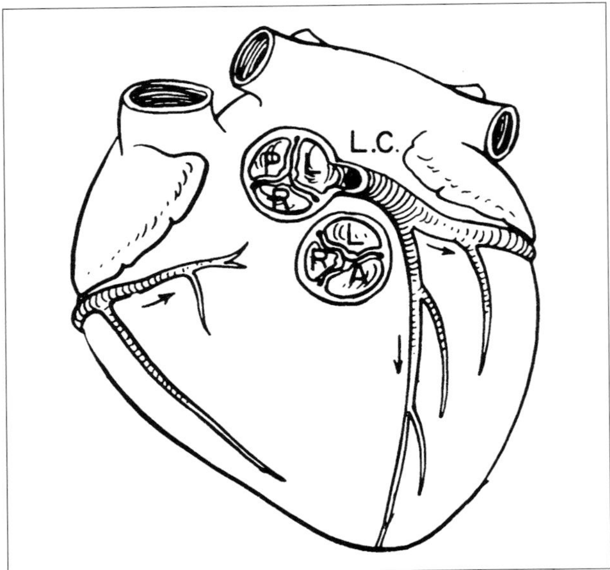

Figure 25-19. Aplasia of right coronary artery. The single left coronary artery (*L.C.*) distributes over the whole heart. *P*, posterior (noncoronary) sinus; *L*, left aortic sinus, *R*, right aortic sinus. Also shown are the left (*L*), right (*R*), and anterior (*A*) pulmonary valves. (From Vladover RZ, Neufeld HN, Edwards JE. Pathology of coronary disease. Semin Roentgenol 1972;1:376–394. Used with permission.)

A true *single right coronary artery,* which appears to be even more infrequent, presents a "hyperdominant" right coronary artery occupying the entire circumference of the left atrioventricular groove and terminating as a normally located anterior descending artery.

A joining abnormality can be characterized as a single coronary artery to which parts of the opposite artery are abnormally connected. The distal distribution shows the trait of the anatomy of two normal coronary arteries (Fig. 25-21). Again, joining abnormalities resulting in a monostic circulation are rare; of 600 autopsy cases studied by White and Edwards,[57] they found only one joining abnormality with a single ostium in the right sinus of Valsalva delivering a normal right coronary artery from which an early departing large branch coursed like a left coronary artery. As more information from autopsy and angiographic studies accumulated, there were more reports of similar abnormalities involving either the right or the left coronary artery.[46,58–64] A classification system for these coronary arteries has been proposed by Lipton et al. (Fig. 25-22).[55]

An important feature appears to be the location of the abnormally joining arterial segment. The anomalous courses may be anterior, that is, traversing the anterior interventricular border in front of the pulmonary artery or the pulmonary conus, or may be found posterior to the main pulmonary artery and just in front of the ascending aorta. A third location for such connecting segment exists posteriorly to the aorta in the depth of the transverse pericardial sinus. Finally, there may be connections passing through the interventricular septum. The single right coronary artery

Figure 25-20. Selective in vivo coronary angiogram demonstrating single left coronary artery of similar appearance to that in Figure 25-19. (A) LAO projection; (B) RAO projection. (From Lipton MJ, et al. Isolated single coronary artery: diagnosis, angiographic classification and clinical significance. Radiology 1979;130:39. Used with permission.)

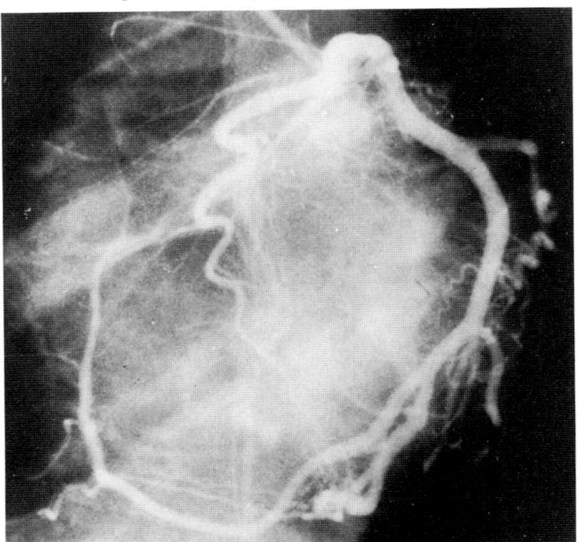

A

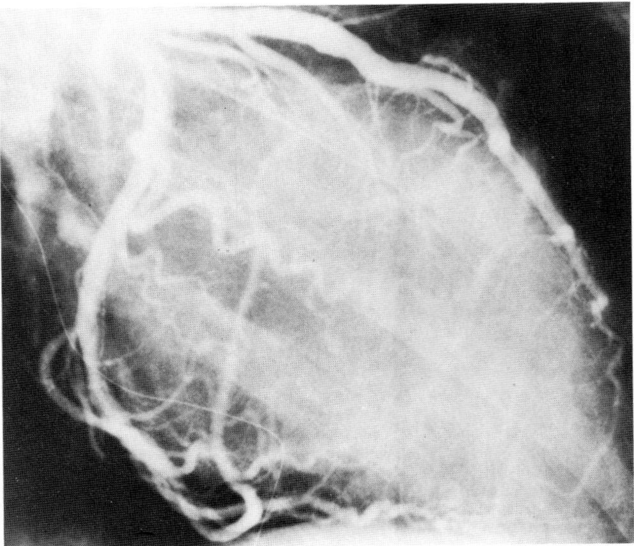

B

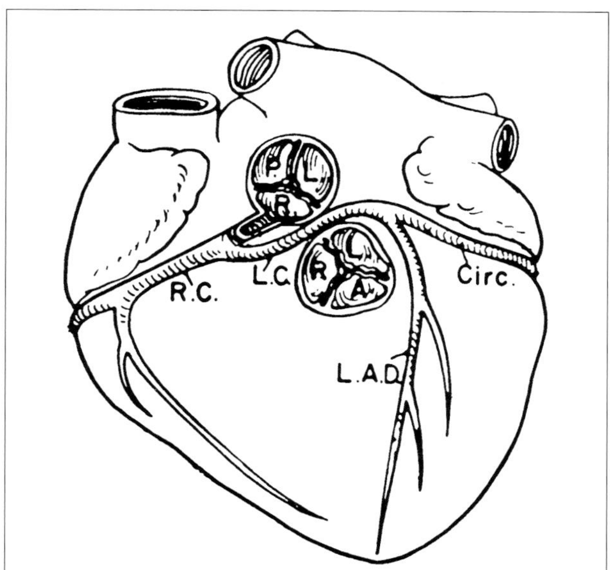

Figure 25-21. Drawing of abnormally joining left coronary artery (*L.C.*), which arises from the proximal right coronary artery (*R.C.*). Coronary orifice in left sinus of Valsalva is absent. *Circ.*, circumflex coronary artery; *L.A.D.*, left anterior descending coronary artery; *P.*, posterior (noncoronary) sinus; *L*, left aortic sinus; *R*, right aortic sinus. Also shown are the left (*L*), right (*R*), and anterior (*A*) pulmonary valves. (From Vladover RZ, Neufeld HN, Edwards JE. Pathology of coronary disease. Semin Roentgenol 1972;1:376–394. Used with permission.)

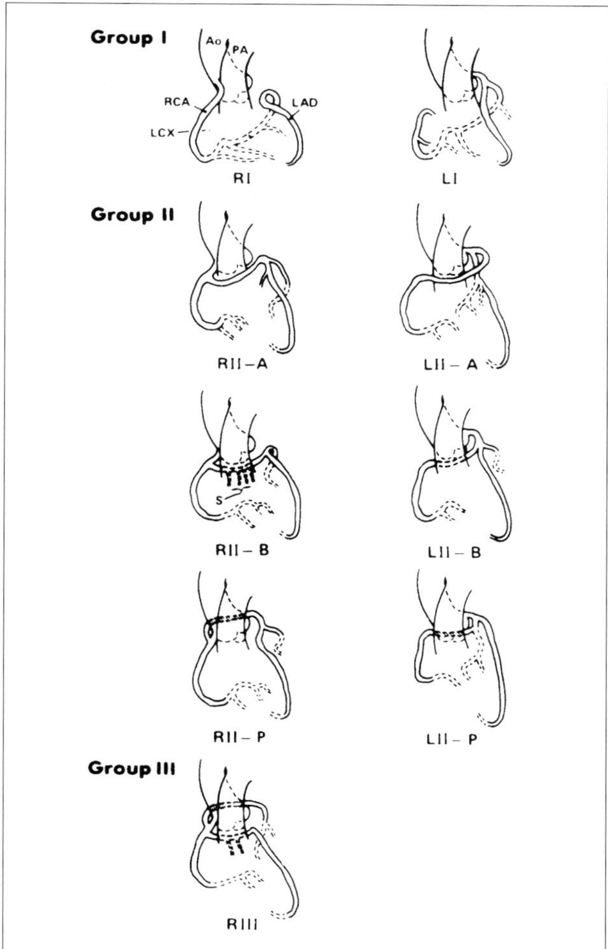

Figure 25-22. Schematic illustration of types of single coronary artery distribution (*R*, right; *L*, left; *A*, anterior; *B*, between; *P*, posterior to the great vessels). *RCA*, right coronary artery; *LAD*, left anterior descending coronary artery; *LCX*, left circumflex coronary artery; *AO*, aorta; *PA*, main pulmonary artery. Shading of the transverse trunk indicates that this artery courses posterior to the aorta. (From Lipton MJ, et al. Isolated single coronary artery: diagnosis, angiographic classification and clinical significance. Radiology 1979;130:39. Used with permission.)

ostium appears to have a wider variety of these joining anomalies than does the left.[7] The latter type of single coronary ostium on the left side with the right coronary artery joining abnormally occurred most frequently in autopsy material as reported by Kragel and Roberts.[65] In either situation, it is most important to attain proper angiographic identification of a retropulmonary position of an arterial segment, since mechanical compression of such a vessel between the aorta and the pulmonary artery has been alleged to be the potential cause of regional ischemia.[41,66] For in vivo examination, the RAO projection appears to be the most suitable to make this distinction. Insertion of a right-sided cardiac catheter into the main pulmonary artery at the time of examination may provide a useful landmark for exactly determining the vessel segment's position.

A condition that can be identified as a subform of a joining abnormality is the anomalous origin of the left coronary artery from the right anterior aortic sinus. Although similar to the single coronary arteries described above, there still exist two coronary artery orifices, albeit arising from the same cusp in close vicinity to each other. An excellent description and classification has been rendered by Ishikawa and Brandt,[67] which distinguishes between the different positions of the proximal portion of an ectopic LAD: epicardially in front, deeply embedded in the interventricular septum, or posteriorly to the pulmonary artery but in front of the aorta (Figs. 25-23 and 25-24). The authors concluded that the septal intramyocardial variant is the most common and did in their experience not show any relationship to sudden death or myocardial ischemia.

Supernumerary coronary arteries arising separately from the aorta are more frequent and are discernible as separate coronary artery branches (Fig. 25-25).

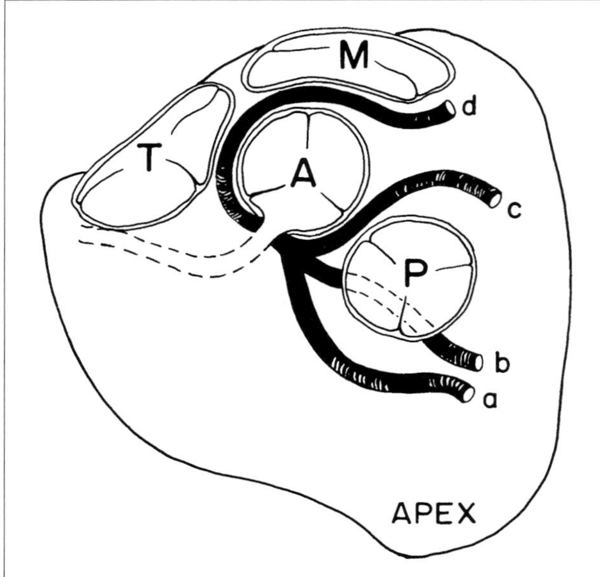

Figure 25-23. The three possible courses of an anomalous left main coronary artery arising from the right anterior aortic sinus of Valsalva: *a,* epicardially in front; *b,* deeply embedded in the interventricular septum; *c,* posteriorly to the main pulmonary artery, but in front of the aorta. In *d* the common left circumflex artery, arising abnormally from the right side, is illustrated for completeness. (See also Fig. 25-28.) M, mitral valve; T, tricuspid valve; A, aorta; P, pulmonary artery. (From Ishikawa T, Brandt P. Anomalous origin of the left main coronary artery from the right anterior aortic sinus: angiographic definition of anomalous course. Am J Cardiol 1985;55:770–776. Used with permission.)

Banchi[4] observed the separate orifice of a small pulmonary conus branch from the right coronary sinus in 33 percent of cases, and he named this occurrence *arteria accessoria*. Schlesinger et al.[68] focused specifically on this finding in a postmortem injection study and re-

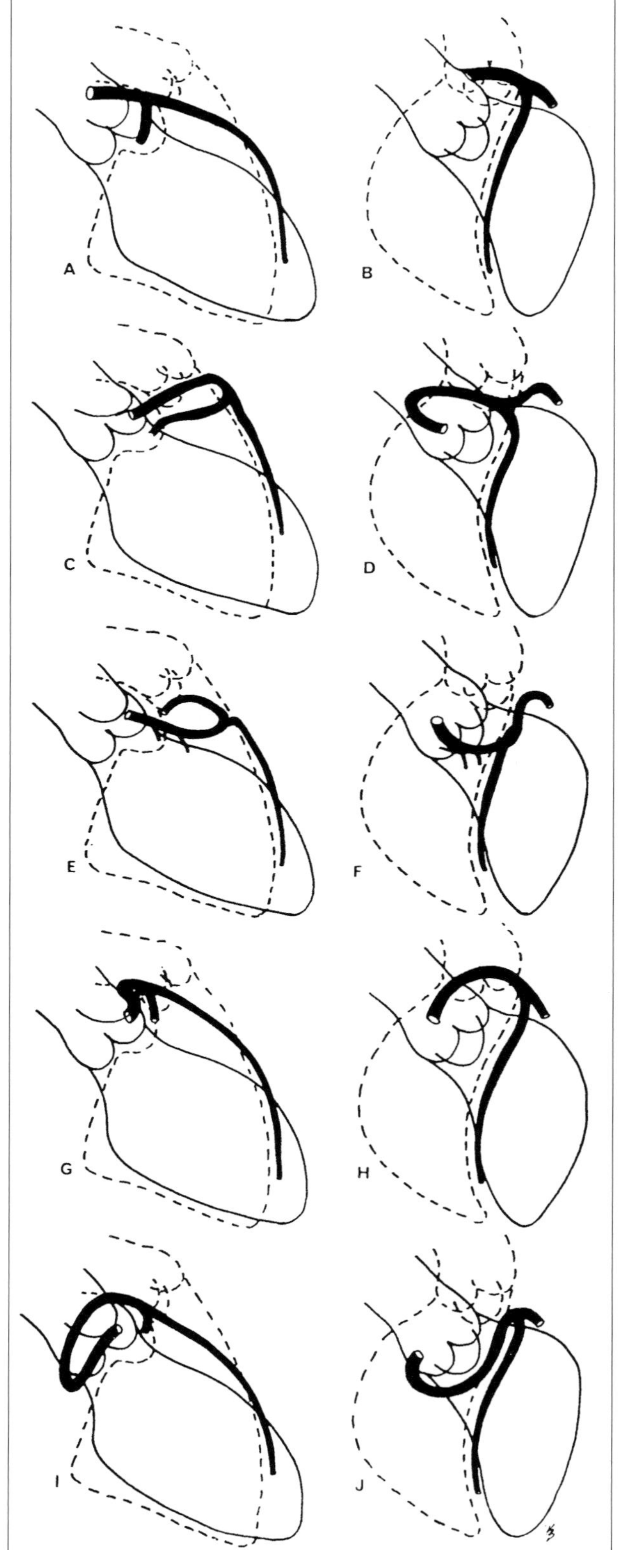

Figure 25-24. Angiographic appearances in right anterior oblique (A,C,E,G,I) and left anterior oblique (B,D,F,H,J) projections of the left main coronary artery, most of its anterior descending branch, and the proximal part of its left circumflex branch. Compare normal origin and course (A and B) with anomalous origin from the anterior aortic sinus, with anterior free wall course showing a cranial anterior loop (C and D), septal course with a caudal anterior loop (E and F), interarterial course with a cranial posterior loop (G and H), and retroaortic course with a caudal posterior loop (I,J). The left ventricle and aortic valve are shown by the *continuous line* and the right ventricle and pulmonary valve by *the interrupted line*. Septal branches of the left main coronary artery are indicated in (E and F). (From Ishikawa T, Brandt P. Anomalous origin of the left main coronary artery from the right anterior aortic sinus: angiographic definition of anomalous course. Am J Cardiol 1985;55:770–776. Used with permission.)

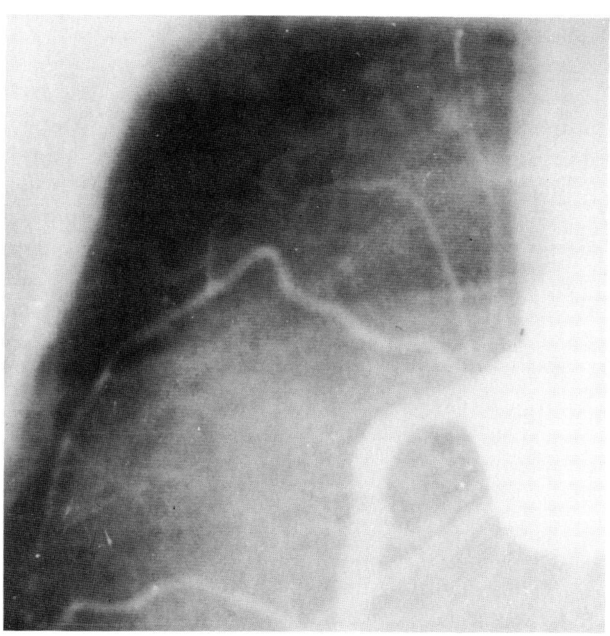

A

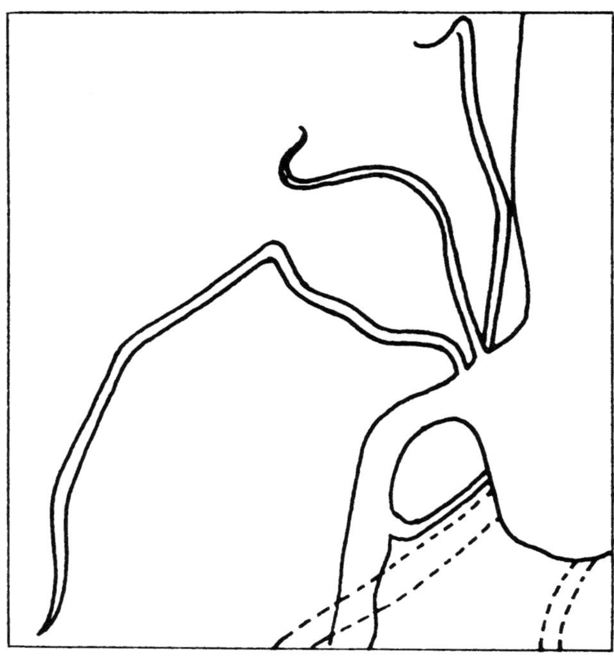

B

Figure 25-25. (*A*) Radiographic detail of nonselective coronary arteriogram demonstrating two supernumerary branches arising in the right coronary cusp adjacent to but separate from the right coronary artery orifice. The most cranial branch running parallel and close to the wall of the ascending aorta is likely to supply periaortic adipose tissue. The second branch distributes over the anterior surface of the pulmonary conus. Note the proximal position of the next branch to the right ventricular wall. (*B*) Line tracing highlighting features on radiographic.

ported a 51 percent incidence. They pointed out that the caliber of the conus artery at the ostium may be 2.0 mm or more but that its commonest diameter is 0.4 to 1.0 mm.

Since the third coronary artery is generally small, it is not surprising that in vivo angiography records a lower incidence of its presence. Semiselective technique demonstrated this third coronary artery in only 38 percent of cases. In a few cases, however, even two small supernumerary branches were observed. Detailed postmortem anatomic studies[4,7] support the assumption that the smaller and more cranially directed vessel represents a so-called adventitial branch distributing along the wall of the large vessels within the pericardial reflection. These studies also indicate that on rare occasions the supernumerary orifices may involve a right superior septal branch, a slightly larger preventricular branch to the anterior free wall of the right ventricle, or the right sinus node artery (Fig. 25-26).

Selective coronary arteriography must, by necessity, leave these arteries undetected unless specific efforts for their cannulation are made. The majority of cases hardly warrant such an approach, except when the absence of detectable vessels in a larger territory suggests that the missed supernumerary branch has an unusually large distribution. In addition, obstructive coro-

Figure 25-26. Schematic illustration of potential anatomic variations encountered in areas adjacent to right coronary artery orifice. (From McAlpine WA. Heart and coronary arteries: an anatomical atlas for clinical diagnosis, radiological investigation and surgical treatment. New York: Springer-Verlag, 1975. Used with permission.)

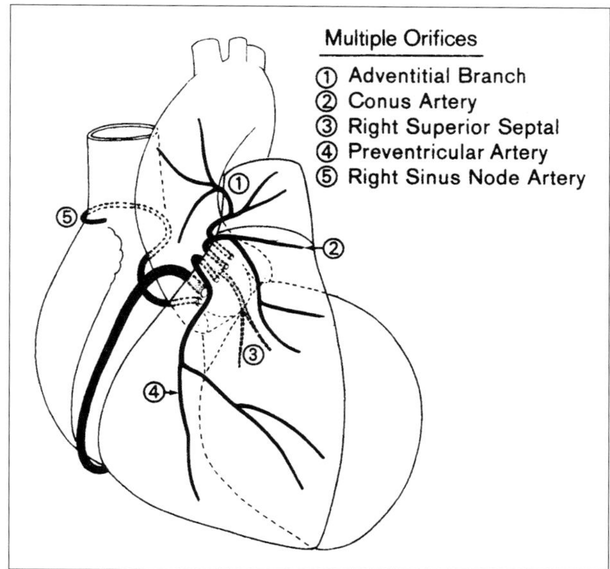

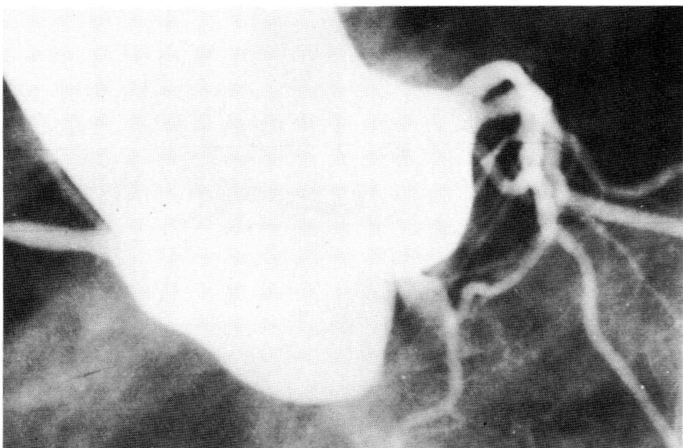

Figure 25-27. Separate orifices for left anterior descending and left circumflex arteries arising from the left coronary sinus adjacent to each other. (From Paulin S. Coronary angiography: a technical, anatomic and clinical study. Acta Radiol (Stockh) 1964;233(Suppl):55. Used with permission.)

nary artery changes may increase the importance of a separately arising conus or right septal branch because their communication with the corresponding left-sided branches may create major pathways for collateral flow.[6,48,69,70]

Supernumerary coronary ostia on the left side appear to be very rare. When they occur, they most frequently represent separately arising orifices of the left anterior descending and the left circumflex arteries, which implies that the left coronary main stem does not exist (Fig. 25-27). Autopsy cases report such an occurrence in 0.2 to 1.0 percent of cases.[6,46,68,71] Angiographically such a dual left ostium was depicted only once out of 208 cases (see Fig. 25-27).[48] A subform of this variant, more often noted in selective studies, is a common ostium for both of these arterial branches, implying an extremely short main trunk for the left coronary artery. In this situation, the tip of a selectively introduced catheter may enter too deeply into one branch without adequately filling the other. Awareness of this will guide the angiographer to withdraw the catheter correspondingly or to cannulate each vessel separately for adequate and complete examination. Optimal separation of the most proximal arterial portions in the presence of a common ostium is usually accomplished in LAO projection to which a steep caudal tilt has been added.

A relatively prevalent distribution abnormality that sometimes includes a supernumerary orifice is an abnormal origin of the left circumflex artery from the right side. In such an anomaly the left anterior descending artery still originates from the site of the normal left coronary artery ostium, whereas the left circumflex arises from the most proximal portion of the right coronary artery or has a separate orifice in the right coronary cusp (Fig. 25-28). An experienced examiner will be alerted to this anomaly by the appearance of an unusual long left coronary artery before it bifurcates with either a first septal or a first diagonal branch. In different series of autopsy studies this abnormality was revealed with an incidence of between 0.3 and 2.0 percent.[6,46,57,68] Invariably the proximal portion of this aberrant left circumflex artery curves dorsally to the aorta in close vicinity to the valve plane to reach the area of its normal distribution. This explains why one can recognize its presence readily on an RAO left ventriculogram as an end-on-seen vessel coursing posteriorly to the contrast filled aortic root, if such examination precedes the selective coronary arteriogram. It is not hard to recognize on in vivo angiograms, and was reported in 3 of 208 cases examined by nonselective coronary angiography[48] and in 19 of 4350 cases examined by selective technique.[72] It is also interesting that this relatively common variant was recently observed in a familial cluster of one parent and two offspring.[73]

Similar distribution abnormalities may involve the anterior descending artery, which then connects to the proximal right coronary artery. This variant appears to be extremely rare in normal hearts but occurs quite frequently in congenital abnormalities of the heart involving the outflow tract of the right ventricle, particularly in tetralogy of Fallot.[33,56,74]

The author has not found an account in the literature of a supernumerary coronary artery arising from the noncoronary cusp unless it was associated with other severe congenital cardiac malformations.[56,75] Ectopic origin of one of the coronary arteries from the noncoronary cusp has been reported as rather common in cases with complete transposition of the large vessels by Vladover et al.,[47] but this may also be explained by difficulties in identifying the individual cusps appropriately. In the presence of normal gross cardiac anatomy, a coronary artery arising from the posterior noncoronary cusp is extremely rare. The few cases described so far in the English literature[56,62,76,77] showed such abnormal take-off location as an isolated abnormality in the presence of an otherwise normal left coronary artery anatomy.

Although it has been suggested in the literature that variations and distribution abnormalities of the coronary ostia and the large coronary arteries may be a cause of sudden death in adolescents and adults[78,79] or could relate to the etiology of ischemic heart disease,[80–84] these concepts have never been substantiated. Certainly in an individual with a single coronary artery the presence of an obstructive lesion in proximal location is more dangerous because of the larger myocar-

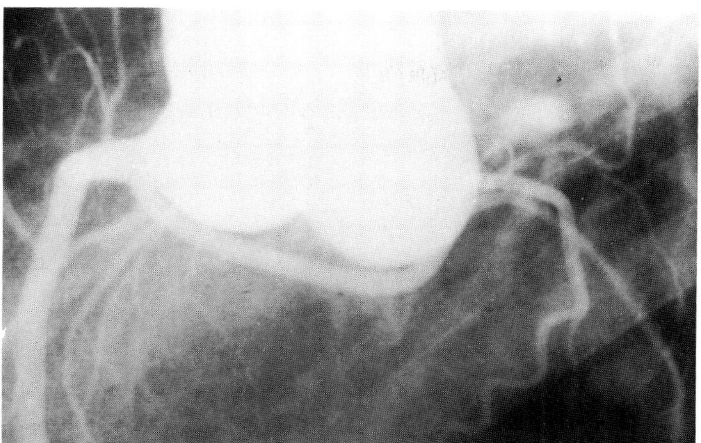

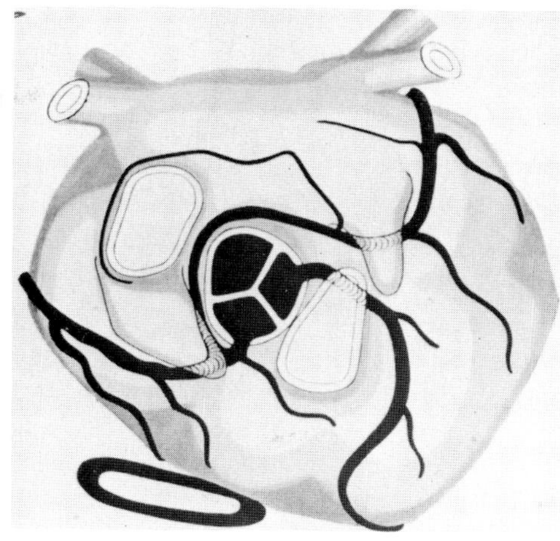

Figure 25-28. Abnormal origin of left circumflex artery from the proximal part of the right coronary artery. Only the anterior descending artery arises from the left ostium. Radiograph in left lateral view demonstrates the left circumflex artery running behind the aorta on the level of the valvular plane until it reaches the left atrioventricular sulcus. In the schematic drawing, this type of distribution is illustrated as seen from above. (From Paulin S. Coronary angiography: a technical, anatomic and clinical study. Acta Radiol (Stockh) 1964;233(Suppl):56. Used with permission.)

dial territory at risk and the reduced availability of intercoronary anastomoses for development of collateral circulation. On the other hand, the rather common variant in which the left circumflex artery arises from the right side has a similar distribution among patients with normal and abnormal coronary arteriograms and is therefore unlikely to be a risk factor for coronary artery disease. Distribution abnormalities of this kind may place the patient at greater risk in the event of cardiac surgical interventions. Obviously, during aortic valve replacement the surgeon would like to be alerted that a sizable coronary artery is located in the immediate posterior vicinity of the valve, and a similar situation exists during surgical correction of tetralogy of Fallot in which a high incidence of LAD arising from the right side has been reported,[74] its presence posing the danger of unintentional transection. Still, it must be emphasized that all the distributional coronary anomalies and variations just described can occur singly, without additional cardiac abnormalities, and can exist without evidence that they cause symptoms or alter the patient's prognosis.

The Right Coronary Artery

The right coronary artery, which runs in the right atrioventricular sulcus and, in most cases, reaches the crux and adjacent areas of the posterior wall of the left ventricle, is angiographically well demonstrated in the standard left and right oblique projections (LAO and RAO). In both projections superposition with the dense structures of the spine is avoided and the distribution of the artery and its branches, including their relation to the gross topography of the heart, can be assessed.

In the LAO projection the right coronary artery forms a wide semicircle with its convexity directed to the right side of the patient (Fig. 25-29). The side

Figure 25-29. Selective coronary angiogram of right coronary artery in LAO position. This represents the most common type of right coronary artery distribution, which reaches the crux and supplies a few minor branches to the adjacent area of the posterior wall of the left ventricle.

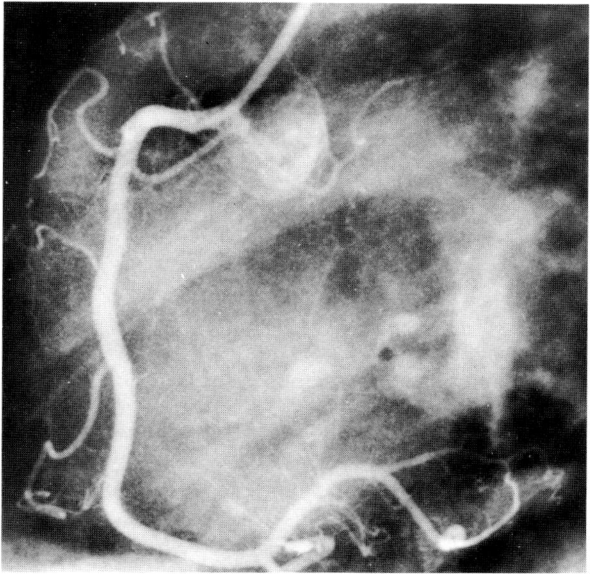

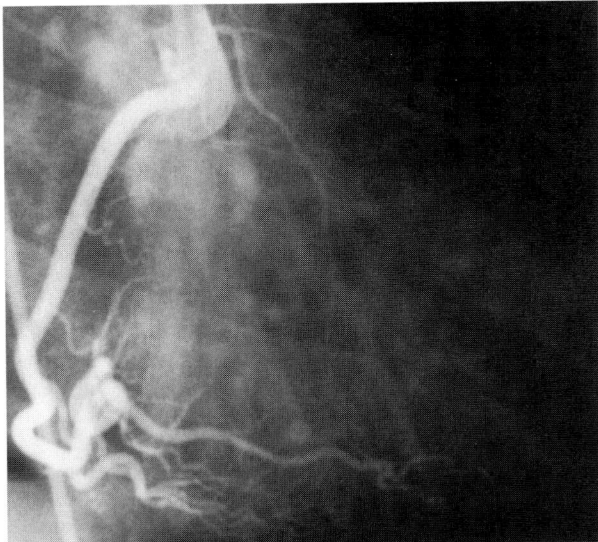

Figure 25-30. Distal portion of right coronary artery in RAO projection. Note the superimposition of multiple arterial branches at the posterior aspect of the heart.

branches arising from it course in either the anterior or the posterior direction. This implies that they are markedly foreshortened in this view. The RAO projection, which tangentially depicts the atrioventricular plane, shows the right circumflex artery as a fairly straight, downward-directed vessel from which side branches arise either in a posterior direction to the right atrium or anteriorly to the right ventricular wall (Fig. 25-30). Branches at the posterior aspect of the right and left ventricular walls are often superimposed in this view, but identification of their origin from the right circumflex artery can be helpful in assessing their location. The inverted U turn of the right coronary artery at the crux is a landmark indicating the border between the tricuspid and the mitral valves at the fibrous ring. It is also the origin of the centrally running atrioventricular node artery. Identification of the right coronary artery U turn is usually easier in the LAO projection.

The number and size of coronary branches supplying the right ventricular wall vary greatly. Between two and seven (average four) individual side branches may originate separately from the right coronary artery between its ostium and the crux (Table 25-1). It is usually possible to identify one of these branches as the largest; it extends the farthest anteriorly and at times reaches the apical region of the heart. Contrary to the general concept that the take-off of this marginal branch strictly determines the acute margin, it has been observed to arise frequently from the more proximal part of the right coronary artery. Occasionally it is an exceptionally large conus branch extending far down to the anterior aspect of the right ventricular wall (Fig. 25-31). This variant is identical to the *pre-infundibular artery*[71] or *preventricular artery*.[7] In roughly 15 percent of cases, a number of almost equal-sized branches arising from the coronary artery share the supply of the right ventricular wall (Fig. 25-32).

Table 25-1. Number and Type of Branches to the Right Ventricle from the Circumflex Artery: 135 Cases in Which This Artery Reaches the Crux

		Largest Branch with Orifice			
Number of Branches	Number of Cases	Close to Ostium	In Proximal Third	In Middle Part	Equalized Branches
2	12	1	10	1	0
3	39	0	17	18	4
4	59	1	17	28	13
5	20	0	5	10	5
6–7	5	0	4	1	0
Total	135	2	53	58	22

Figure 25-31. Detail from coronary arteriogram in LAO projection demonstrating a large branch to the acute margin of the right ventricle arising extremely proximally from the right circumflex artery. (From Paulin S. Coronary angiography: a technical, anatomic and clinical study. Acta Radiol (Stockh) 1964;233(Suppl):71. Used with permission.)

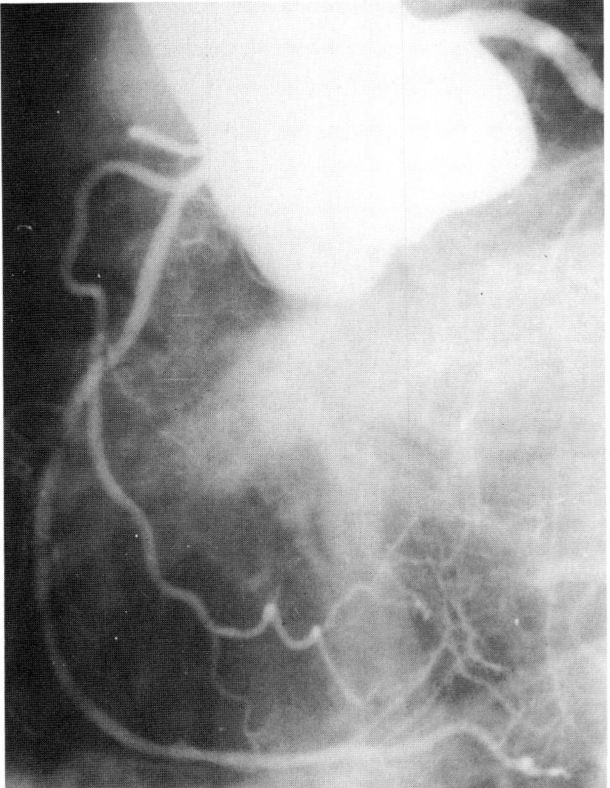

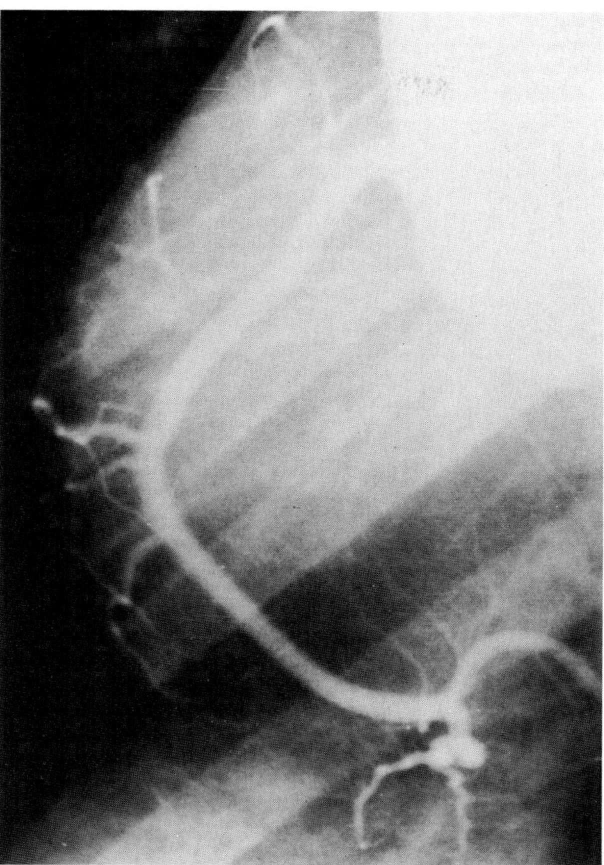

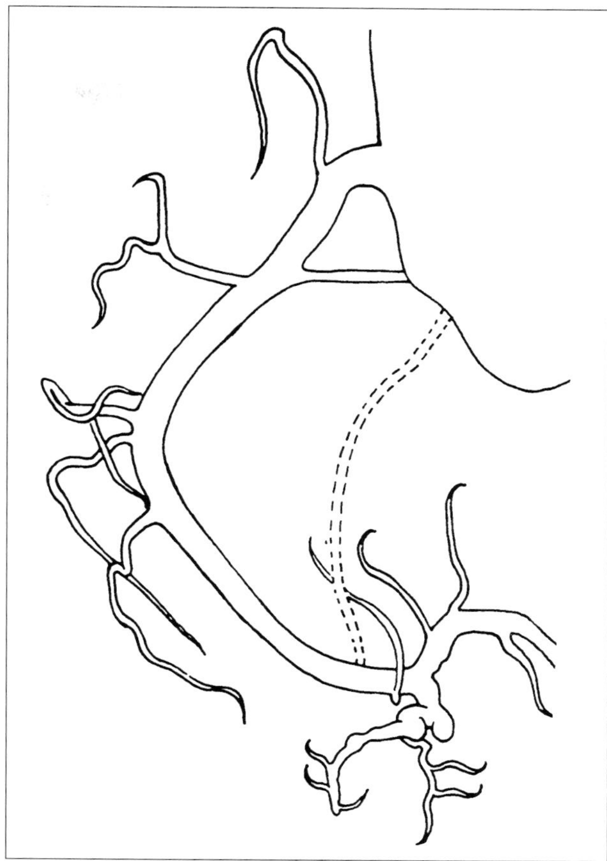

A B

Figure 25-32. (A) Multiple branches of approximately the same size running from the right circumflex artery to the right ventricle, demonstrated in LAO projection. (B) Line tracing of (A). (From Paulin S. Coronary angiography: a technical, anatomic and clinical study. Acta Radiol (Stockh) 1964;233(Suppl): 72. Used with permission.)

More important than the demonstration of these common pattern variations is recognizing those arterial branches that extend beyond the limit of the right ventricle, a finding that indicates their participation in the supply of the left ventricular wall or interventricular septum.[48] Levin and Baltaxe[85] emphasized that such extension occurs frequently in the distribution of the posterior right ventricular and acute marginal branches as they course medially and reach the posterior interventricular sulcus in the apical half (Fig. 25-33).

Adding a cranial tilt to the LAO projection significantly improves the delineation of vascular branches and their topographic relationship to the atrioventricular and the interventricular grooves. The cranial tilt corrects for the horizontal component of the heart's long axis, which otherwise is the cause for considerable foreshortening of the distal branches running from the base of the heart in an apical direction (Fig. 25-34).

Visualization of the right coronary artery by selective injection permits the identification of the basal part of the posterior interventricular septum, determined by the typical U turn of the right coronary artery at the crux. Precise identification of the cardiac apex, however, is usually not achieved because right coronary branches rarely reach this region. Simultaneous filling of both coronary arteries, as accomplished in nonselective coronary arteriography, provides the simultaneous demonstration of the rather constant sharp turn of the distal LAD artery slightly to the right of the cardiac apex (Fig. 25-35). A line drawn between the U turn of the crux and the apical position of the LAD artery fairly accurately defines the position of the posterior interventricular groove.

Analysis of vascular distribution in relation to the posterior interventricular border thus defined demonstrates that in the majority of cases this area is supplied by two or more branches running from behind on the right obliquely to the left. The implication is that acute

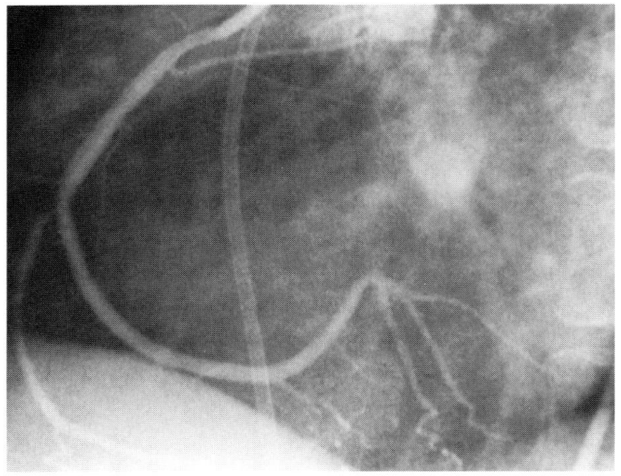

A

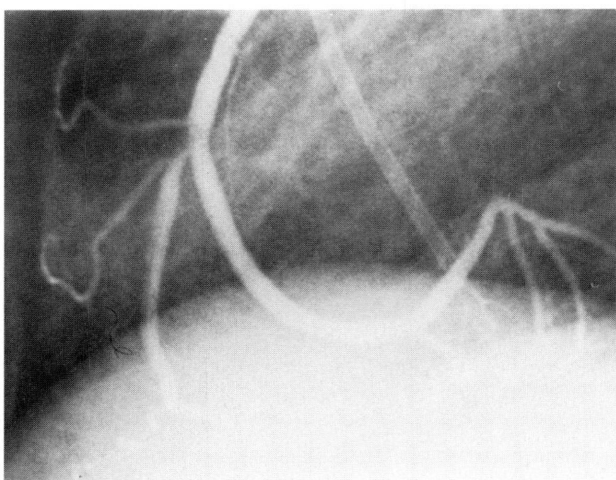

B

Figure 25-33. Selectively injected right coronary artery in LAO (A) and lateral (B) projection. Note the proximal division of the right coronary artery into two major branches, one of which supplies the crux and the posterior aspect of the left ventricle; the other transverses diagonally over the posterior aspect of the right ventricle to reach the area of the posterior interventricular sulcus close to the apex.

marginal as well as posterior right ventricular branches may not only contribute to the supply of the interventricular septum but may also deliver blood flow to various parts of the posterior wall of the left ventricle.

Another helpful angiographic sign is that these branches are usually wider in caliber than those that are limited to the right ventricular wall, reflecting the larger flow requirements of the left ventricular myocardium. On the basis of all such angiographic findings, it becomes apparent that the so-called typical distribution of the distal right coronary artery, that is, one single posterior descending artery precisely identifying the border between right and left posterior ventricular walls, represents a minority, since it is found in less than 10 percent of the cases.[48] The implications of such variations in relation to the location of significant lesions and their importance for the performance of bypass surgery or angioplasty are obvious.[85]

Precise superimposition of coronary and cardiac anatomy may be more problematic on a selective coronary cineangiogram, where only one coronary artery and its branches are visible at a time. For a selective injection of the right coronary artery, the LAO projection to which a cranial tilt has been added helps un-

Figure 25-34. Shallow LAO view of distal right coronary artery (A) with 25-degree cranial tilt added (B). Whereas the posterior descending and distal posterior left ventricular branches appear crowded in (A), they are well separated in (B).

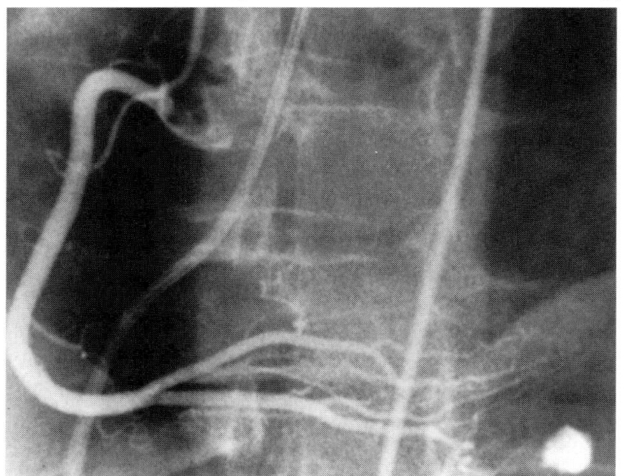

A

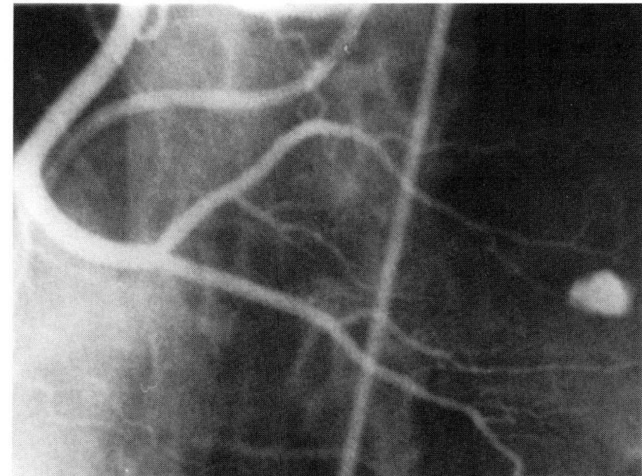

B

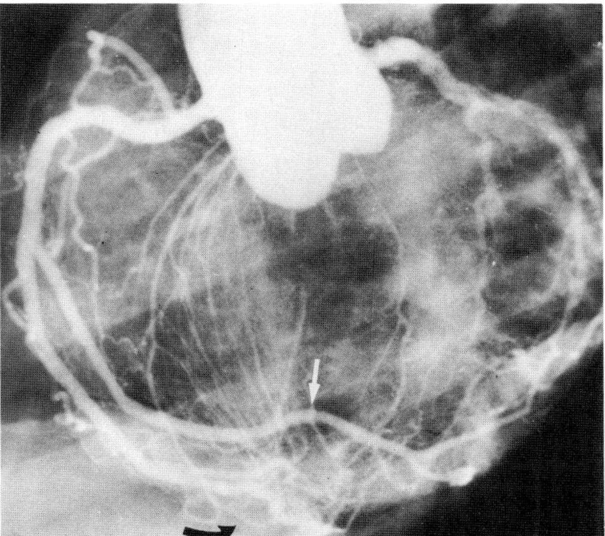

Figure 25-35. Semiselective coronary arteriogram in LAO view. *Arrows* indicate the U-turn of the right coronary artery at the crux and the distal left anterior descending artery at the apex of the heart. An imaginary line drawn between these two points is traversed by at least three arterial branches from the right to the left. See text for details. (From Paulin S, Coronary angiography: a technical, anatomic and clinical study. Acta Radiol (Stockh) 1964;233(Suppl):81. Used with permission.)

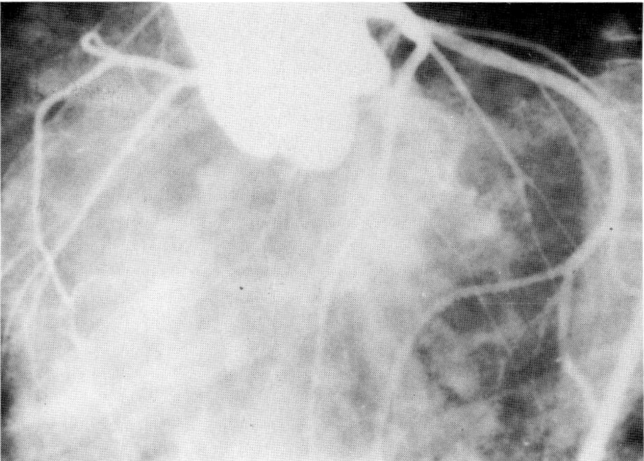

Figure 25-36. Nonselective angiogram in LAO projection showing the small distribution of the right coronary artery in a left-predominant system. Proximal bifurcation of the right coronary artery into two branches of almost equal size is common in such a situation.

ravel the multiple distal branches much better than the conventional LAO view (see Fig. 25-34). For practical interpretation purposes, one will denote as the posterior descending artery (PDA) a sizable branch that is located in the middle of the posterior cardiac wall, irrespective of whether it arises from the coronary artery more proximally at the acute margin or from the U turn at the crux. Additional, more distally arising branches of the right coronary artery must consequently supply the posterior left ventricular wall. More proximally arising branches can still reach and traverse the posterior interventricular groove; however, this is more likely in the apical area.

Left coronary artery preponderance confines the distribution of the right coronary artery to the right side of the heart. The reduced blood supply demand of the right ventricular myocardium explains the small caliber and slender appearance of the right coronary artery and its branches in these cases (Fig. 25-36).[48] This finding should not lead to the erroneous diagnosis of right coronary artery hypoplasia.[81,86,87] Somewhat characteristic for all patients with left coronary preponderance and a small right coronary artery distribution is that the latter artery divides its major branches at a rather acute angle. As a result, the right ventricular acute marginal branches run downward more obliquely toward the posterior interventricular sulcus, rather than the apex.[6] The angiographic appreciation of such a pattern on a selective right coronary angiogram immediately indicates the presence of a left preponderant coronary artery system.

The Left Coronary Artery

The main trunk of the left coronary artery usually has two main divisions: the *left anterior descending (LAD) artery* and the *left circumflex (LCX) artery.* If one looks at the isolated heart from above (e.g., Figs. 25-11 and 25-19), one observes that the left main coronary artery after its slightly posteriorly oriented exit from the aorta curves anteriorly into the direction corresponding to that of the LAD artery. This curve extends practically over 90 degrees or more in the majority of cases where the main stem is at least 1 to 2 cm long. It implies that, although the left coronary ostium may be optimally depicted in LAO projection, its distal portion, which is the site of predilection for atherosclerotic lesions in the main stem, is poorly shown. Obviously a RAO projection is much better suited. However, and because of the marked foreshortened presentation of the proximal LCX artery in conventional RAO view, an added caudal view is preferred, since it is likely to optimally show the main stem bifurcation. Certain laboratories use such caudal tilt RAO projection routinely as the initial view of choice when studying unstable patients.[88]

The LAD artery is the most constant coronary arterial structure with regard to its topographic location in the anterior interventricular sulcus. In the conven-

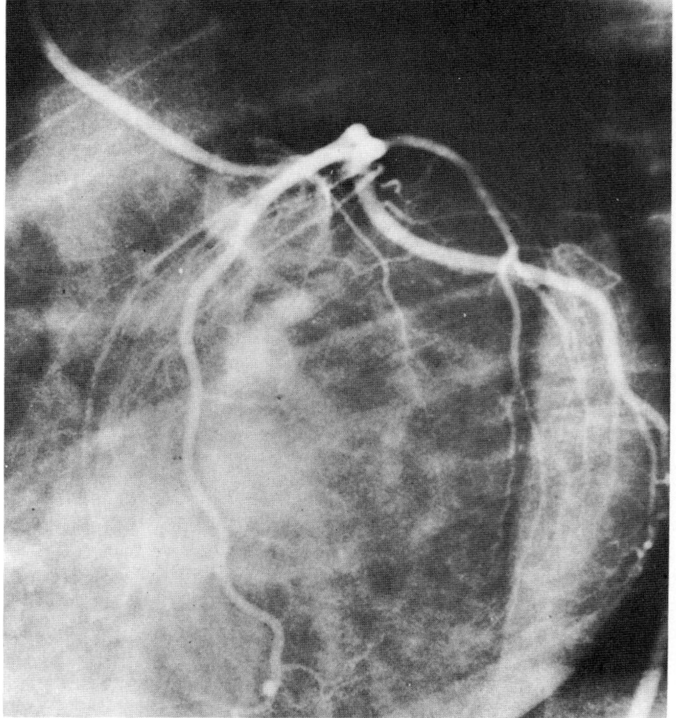

A

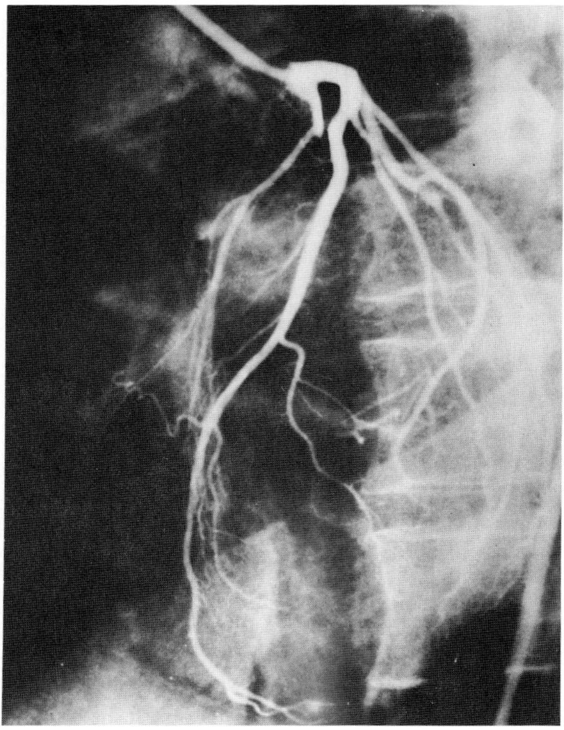

B

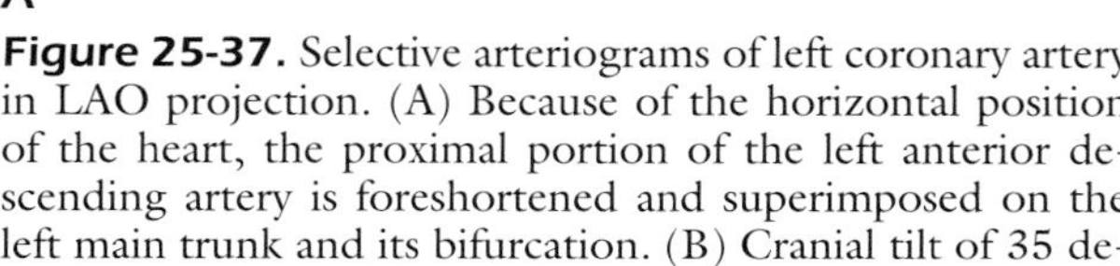

Figure 25-37. Selective arteriograms of left coronary artery in LAO projection. (A) Because of the horizontal position of the heart, the proximal portion of the left anterior descending artery is foreshortened and superimposed on the left main trunk and its bifurcation. (B) Cranial tilt of 35 degrees improved the demonstration of the proximal left anterior descending artery separated from the left main trunk and the septal branches. Note the reverse S configuration of the LAD that reaches the apex of the heart.

tional LAO view its proximal portion may be very much foreshortened, particularly in horizontally positioned hearts, where it may even overlap with the left coronary artery main trunk (Fig. 25-37). Exposures in cranially tilted views correct for this shortcoming and improve the demonstration of the left coronary artery bifurcation. The position of the distal LAD artery in the apical region is relatively constant and corresponds to the slight indentation on the epicardial surface between the right and left ventricles a few millimeters to the right of the true cardiac apex. Its location at this point creates a useful angiographic landmark of its topographic relationship to the cardiac chambers.

The RAO projection best displays the LAD artery in its entire extension because it runs perpendicular to

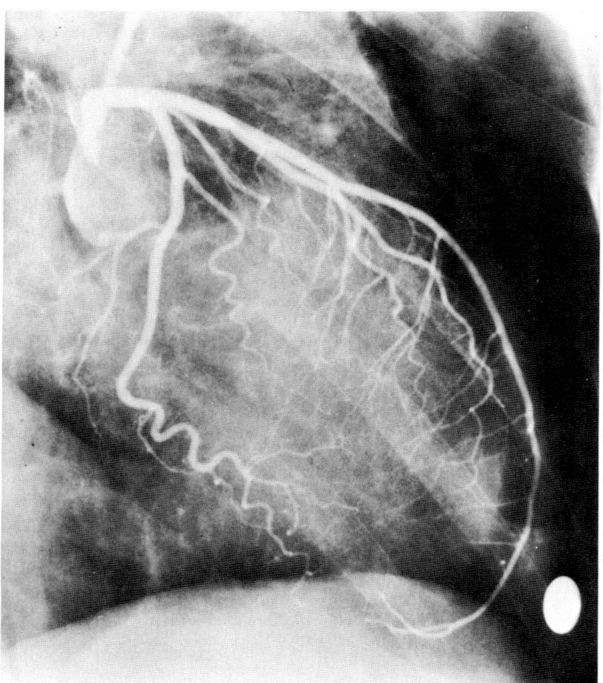

Figure 25-38. Selective left coronary arteriogram in RAO projection. The left anterior descending artery runs along the anterior epicardial surface of the heart and reaches and surrounds the apex of the heart to supply a small area of the posterior wall of the left ventricle as well. The left circumflex artery, after running in the left atrioventricular sulcus, sends a large myocardial branch to the posterolateral aspect of the left ventricular wall. See text for details.

the x-ray beam along the anterior epicardial surface of the heart (Fig. 25-38). In most cases, the LAD artery extends its distal distribution, after having curved around the apex, to the diaphragmatic aspect of the heart, where it may supply an area of various sizes. In some instances it has substituted completely for the PDA,[26] but this is rare. Short anterior descending arteries do occur in a small percentage of cases, and in these situations the PDA or other adjacent secondary coronary branches correspondingly extend farther to the apex. A number of postmortem and in vivo series (Table 25-2) have analyzed the termination point of the LAD artery and have found that it reaches the apex in more than 90 percent of the cases.

A variation of considerable practical importance is the occurrence of a relatively large side branch running close and parallel to this artery, giving the impression of a twin trunk (Fig. 25-39).[6] Obviously, there exists the possibility of a false angiographic diagnosis when complete and flush occlusion occurs at the take-off in one or the other of these arteries. A not uncommon similar variant of the LAD artery was reported by Spindola-Franco et al.[89] to occur in approximately 1 percent of cases and was described as a dual LAD. The definition of this variant is that the artery divides proximally into two vessels, the shorter of which occupies the proximal portion of the interventricular groove, and the longer division leaves this sulcus only to return to it so as to terminate in the apical region. The midportion of this long and deviating vessel may run to the left (type 1), to the right (type 2), or be posteriorly embedded in the interventricular septum (type 3) in relation to the epicardially located groove. A fourth type of dual LAD represents an ectopic origin of the longer division from the right coronary arterial sinus, resembling the anatomy described by Ishikawa and Brandt and others.[67,90–93] The authors appropriately emphasized the importance of these variations for the practical planning of surgical therapy (Fig. 25-40).

Table 25-2. Termination Point of the Anterior Descending Artery According to Different Authors

Author	% Before Apex	% at Apex	% Distal to Apex	Number of Cases
Banchi (1904)[4]	6	78	16	100
Gross (1921)[11]	2	38	60	100
Crainicianu (1922)[71]	2	23	75	200
James (1961)[6]	17	23	60	106
Paulin (1964)[48]	6	12	82	112

There are three types of side branches to the LAD artery: branches to the right ventricular wall, branches to the left ventricular wall, and septal branches.

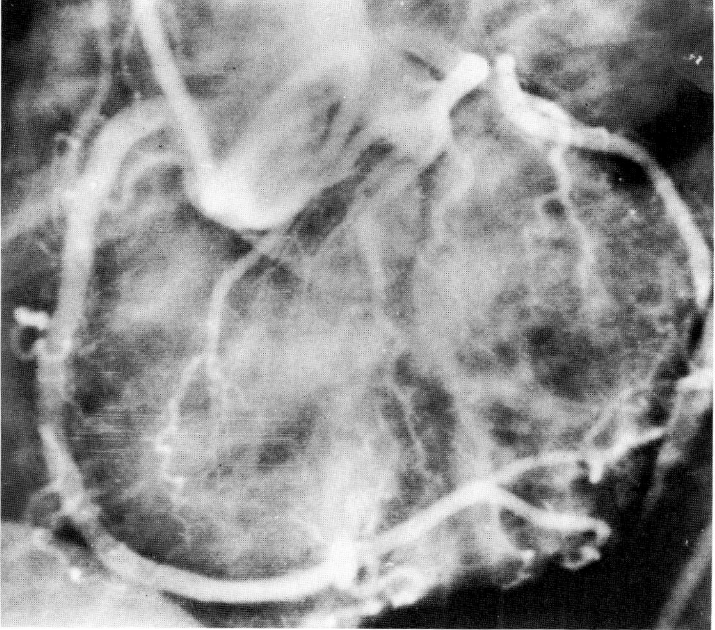

A

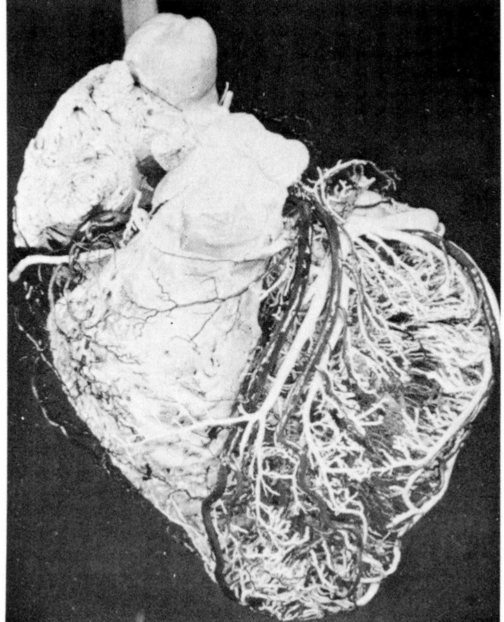

B

Figure 25-39. Nonselective coronary arteriogram in LAO projection demonstrates the presence of a large first diagonal branch to the left anterior descending artery resulting in a "twin trunk" formation. A similar anatomic variant is illustrated at the *right* in a postmortem injection-corrosion preparation. (From James TN. Anatomy of the coronary arteries. New York: Hoeber Medical Division, Harper & Row, 1961. Used with permission.)

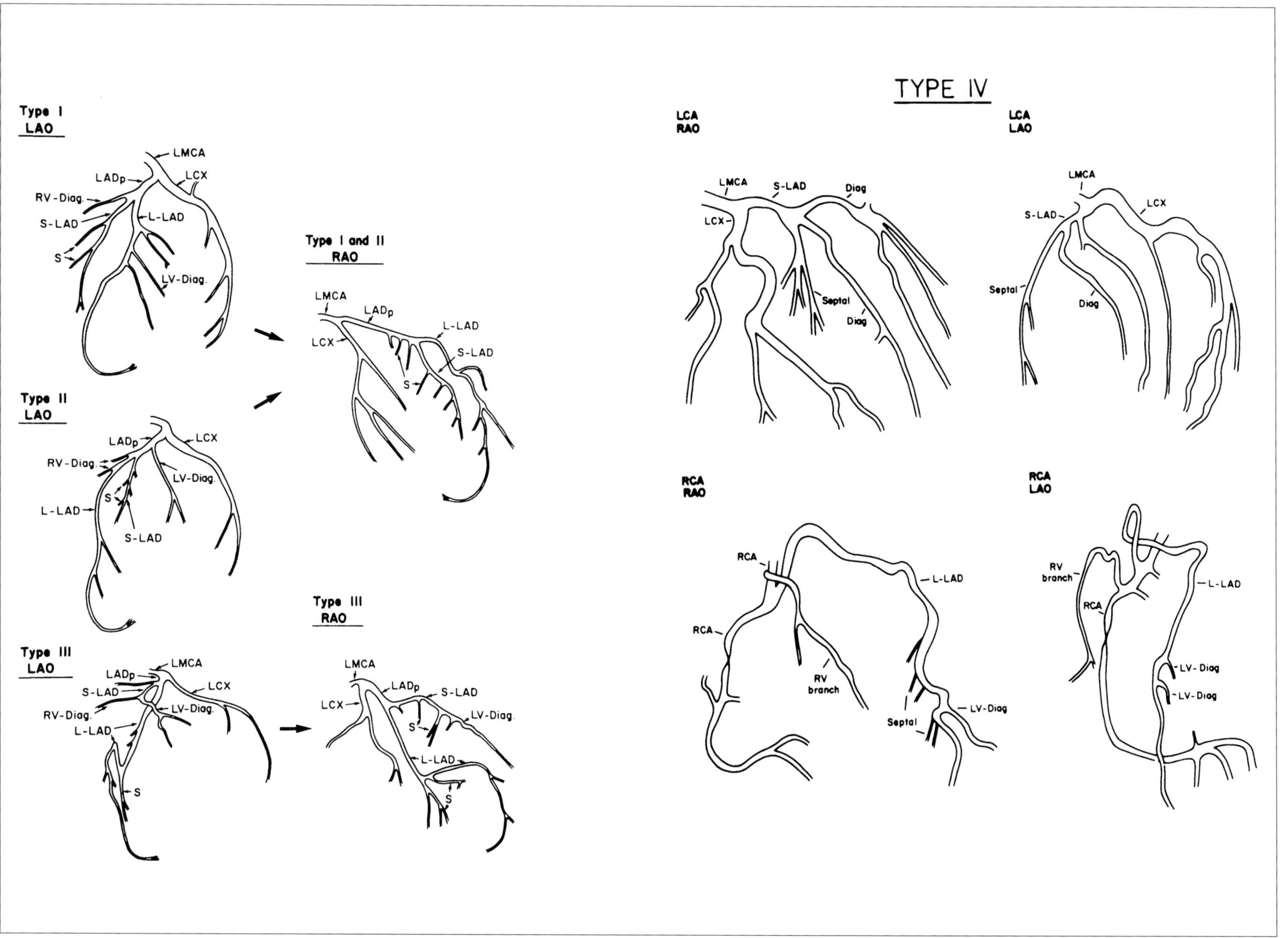

Type I LAO
LMCA
LADp
LCX
RV-Diag.
S-LAD
L-LAD
S
LV-Diag.
Type II LAO
LADp
LCX
RV-Diag.
LV-Diag.
S
L-LAD
S-LAD
Type III LAO
LMCA
LADp
S-LAD
LCX
RV-Diag.
LV-Diag.
L-LAD
S
Type I and II RAO
LMCA
LADp
L-LAD
LCX
S-LAD
S
Type III RAO
LMCA
LADp
S-LAD
LCX
LV-Diag.
S
L-LAD
S
TYPE IV
LCA RAO
LMCA
S-LAD
Diag
LCX
Septal
Diag
LCA LAO
LMCA
S-LAD
LCX
Septal
Diag
RCA RAO
RCA
L-LAD
RCA
RV branch
LV-Diag
Septal
RCA LAO
RV branch
L-LAD
RCA
LV-Diag
LV-Diag

Right ventricular branches are few, small, and inconsistent. They are not relevant to the supply of the more important myocardium of the left ventricle. In the LAO projection there is possible confusion with septal branches, but the RAO projection allows effortless appreciation and differentiation.

Branches to the left ventricle are considerably larger and longer. They invariably arise from the LAD artery at an acute angle and run in the apical direction to supply the anterolateral aspect of the left ventricle. In the generally prevailing terminology of in vivo angiography, these left-sided lateral branches of the LAD artery are called *diagonal branches.* Consistent use of this terminology avoids confusion with the *intermediate branch* (an additional branch arising directly at the site of the left coronary artery bifurcation) and the *marginal branches,* a term reserved for those left ventricular branches that arise from the LCX artery. The number of diagonal branches varies from one to six, sometimes including an *intermediate branch* (Table 25-3).

The *anterior septal branches* deriving from the LAD artery are discernible in the RAO projection as originating at an acute angle and directing their course diaphragmatically. In the LAO projection they have a tendency to overlap with each other and with the LAD artery. The number of detectable septal branches varies, but individual identification of one to six is possible. Obviously, angiography does not always demonstrate the smallest ones, which explains why *postmortem* studies may detect a larger number of septal branches. The largest septal branch is usually the most proximal one, also known as the *first septal perforator,* which frequently splits into two or more secondary branches. One of these at times is observable as advancing farther to the right in its extension into the moderator band of the right ventricle. It is identical to the limbic artery described by Gross.[11] Otherwise, the septal branches terminate angiographically in the posterior half of the septum short of communicating with the corresponding smaller posterior coronary arterial supply.

Another variant of septal supply involves the presence of a very large first or second septal perforator branch running in the anterior portion of the septum somewhat parallel to the LAD artery (Fig. 25-41). Similarity to the dual LAD exists, and differentiation on in vivo angiography may be impossible because of the inability to outline precisely the subepicardial location of the interventricular groove.

Table 25-3. Number and Type of Branches to the Left Ventricle from the Anterior Descending Artery: 112 Cases Without Stenosis of This Artery

Number of Branches	Intermediate Branch Present	Intermediate Branch Absent	Total
1	3	11	14
2	12	28	40
3	14	24	38
4	5	8	13
5	5	1	6
6	0	1	1
Total	39	73	112

A normal in vivo coronary arteriogram does not demonstrate direct communications between anterior and posterior septal branches, but cases with significant obstructive lesions often show them. They illustrate the importance of the septal route as an intercoronary anastomotic pathway. A septal artery arising from the main trunk of the left coronary artery is rare; if present, it is usually small (Fig. 25-42A).[48] Bream[94] described several cases in which the first septal perforator had its origin from the proximal portion of the first diagonal, intermediate, or circumflex branch, establishing differently directed collateral pathways in the presence of obstructions. More constant and demonstrable by angiography in about 10 percent of patients[48] is a *right septal branch* arising from the proximal right coronary artery to run via the *crista supraventricularis* of the right ventricle before it reaches the midpoint of the anterior septum (see Fig. 25-42B). It usually arises as the second branch of the right coronary artery and, on rare occasions, has its own supernumerary ostium in the right coronary sinus[12,75] (see Fig. 25-26).

In the LAO projection the left circumflex artery curves first laterally away from the left main trunk before it continues to surround the left circumference of the atrioventricular border. The RAO view makes it difficult to observe the sometimes marked angle in the origin of the LCX artery at the bifurcation of the left main coronary trunk because of radiographic foreshortening. Proper angiographic delineation of this area and that of the main bifurcation constitutes a challenge, as mentioned above, and may require additional projections preferentially including caudal tilt (Fig. 25-43). In its further run, the LCX artery is di-

◄ **Figure 25-40.** Line drawings of cases illustrating different types of the "dual LAD." See text for details. (From Greenberg M, Spindola-Franco H. Dual left anterior, descending coronary artery (Dual LAD). Cathet Cardiovasc Diagn 1994;31:250. Used with permission.)

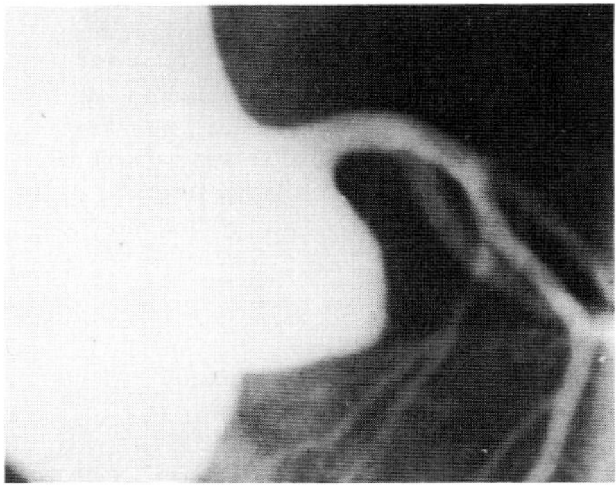

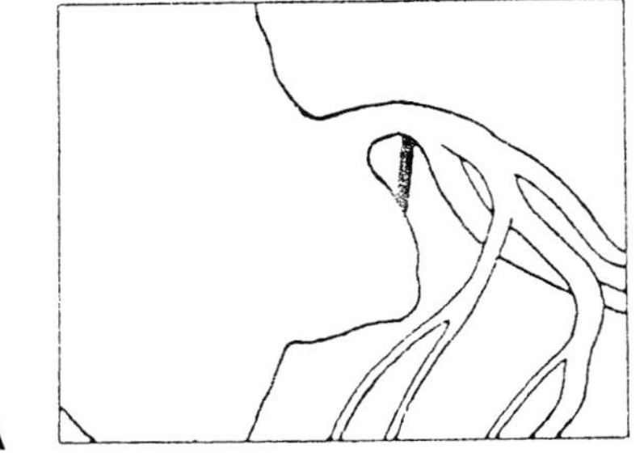

A

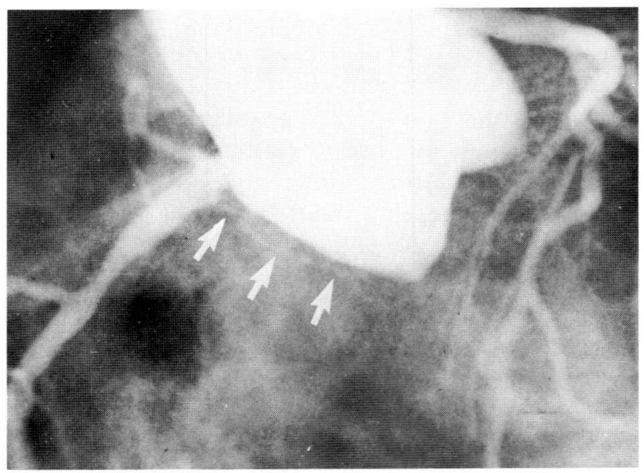

B

Figure 25-41. Examples of variations occurring in the supply of the proximal interventricular septum. (A) First septal perforator is seen to arise from the left coronary artery main trunk. (B) So-called right-sided first septal perforator (*arrows*).

rected fairly straight downward in the atrioventricular groove. The atrioventricular groove is frequently detectable on high-quality fluoroscopy or cinematography because of the accumulation of fatty tissue, which results in a typical band of increased translucency. In addition, the identification of the contrast-filled venous coronary sinus during the late phases of the cineangiogram can confirm the position of the left-sided atrioventricular groove. Again, these findings present important landmarks for the proper identification of arterial distribution. They also help avoid confusing the LCX artery with parallel branches located adjacent to it at the atrial or ventricular level.

In the LAO projection, the two circumflex arteries (from the right and left side) form an almost complete ring at the periphery of the atrioventricular plane of the heart. If both coronary arteries fill at the same time, the magnitude of each with regard to caliber and extent reflects the degree of preponderance. Consequently, because the incidence of right coronary artery preponderance in human hearts is high, the LCX artery is likely to be smaller. In particular, the most distal extension of the LCX artery beyond the origin of the last obtuse marginal branch to the myocardial wall projects as a very narrow artery embedded in the atrioventricular sulcus.

The size and number of side branches to the posterolateral aspect of the left ventricular wall vary and relate somewhat to the length of the LCX artery (Table 25-4, Fig. 25-44). As is noted also on the right

Figure 25-42. Cine coronary angiogram of LAD and unusually large first septal perforator branch with multiple secondary branches: LAO (A) and RAO (B) projection with added cranial tilt. See text for details.

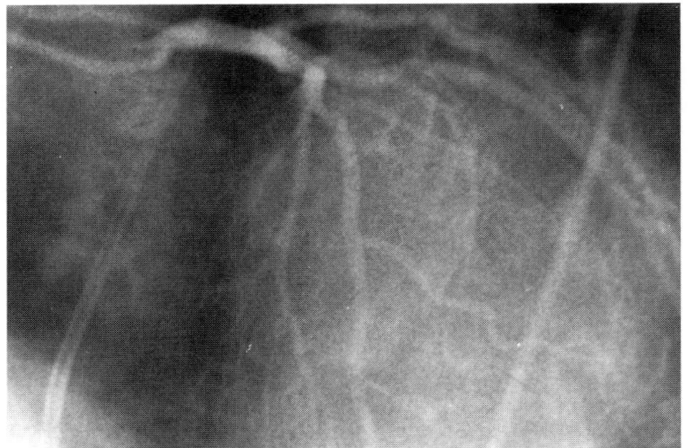

A

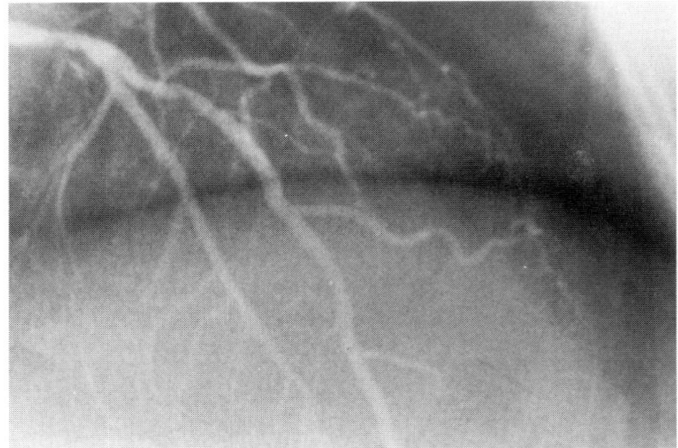

B

side, the secondary branches generally arise from the circumflex artery at an acute angle and course in the ventral-caudal direction. Like other vessels running from the base of the heart to the apex, these secondary branches on the surface of the contracting myocardial wall exhibit a certain tortuosity that accentuates during systole. This observation may facilitate their differenti-

Figure 25-43. Selective left coronary arteriograms of two patients in RAO projection with a 20-degree caudal tilt. This compensates for the lateral angle in the proximal left circumflex artery and appropriately visualizes the bifurcation of the main coronary artery. *Arrows* point at the proximal left circumflex artery.

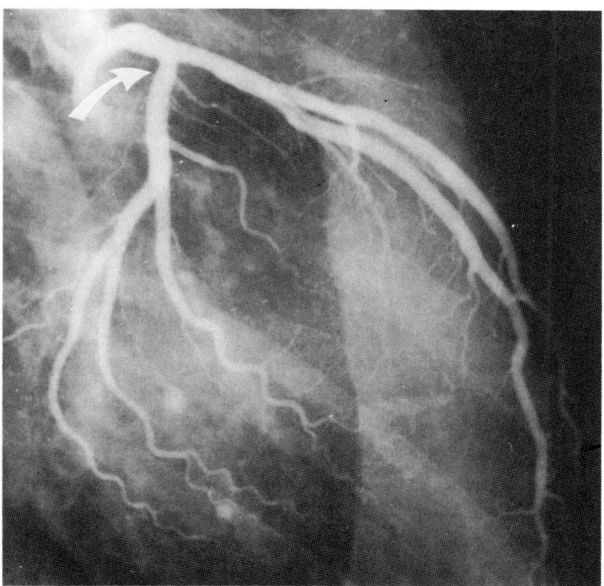

A

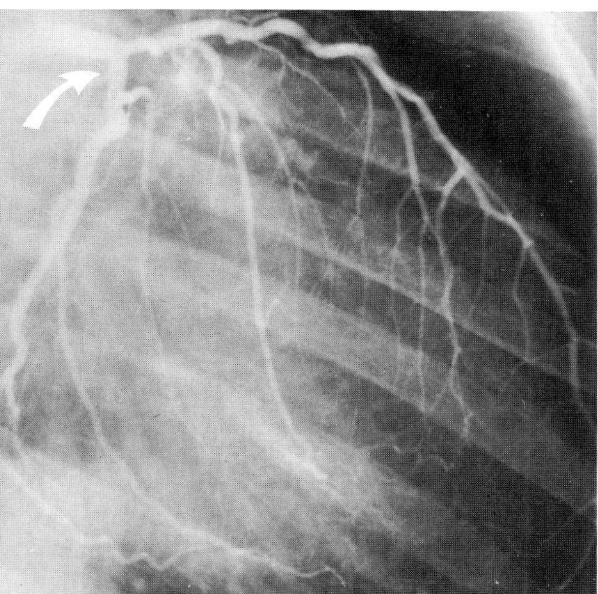

B

Table 25-4. Number of Branches to the Left Ventricle from the Left Circumflex Artery in Relation to Area of Distribution of This Artery: 167 Cases Without Obstruction of This Artery

Number of Branches	Area of Distribution			Total
	Small	Medium	Large	
1	28	2	0	30
2	42	31	4	77
3	3	29	6	38
4–6	0	12	10	22
Total	73	74	20	167

Figure 25-44. Drawings of small (A) and large (B) variety of the left circumflex artery (*shaded*) in lateral view. Note the variations in caliber, particularly of the distal extension of the left circumflex artery. *Broken lines* denote the position of the right coronary artery.

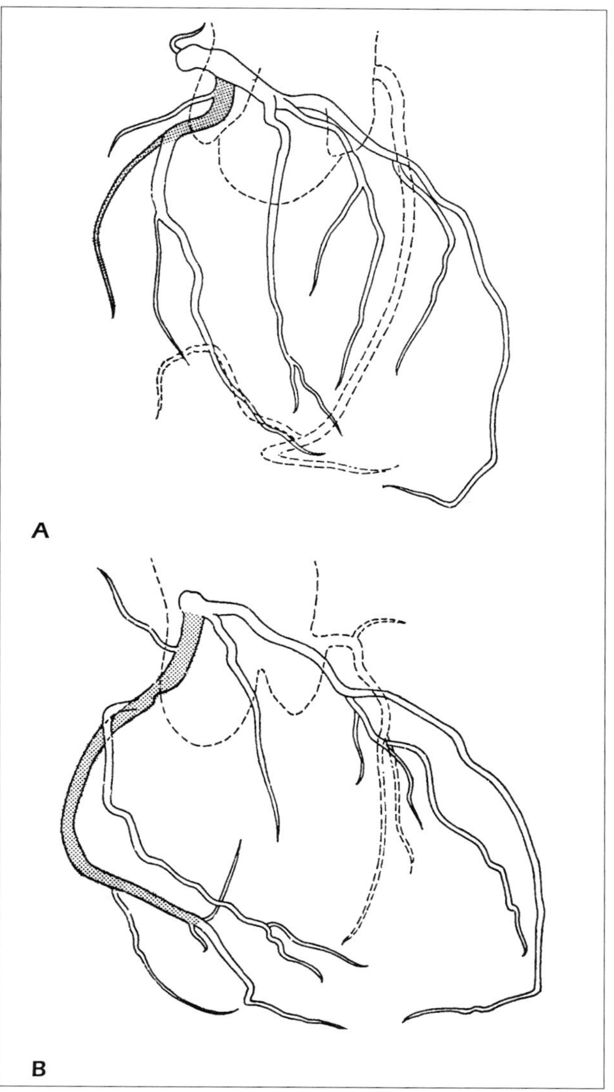

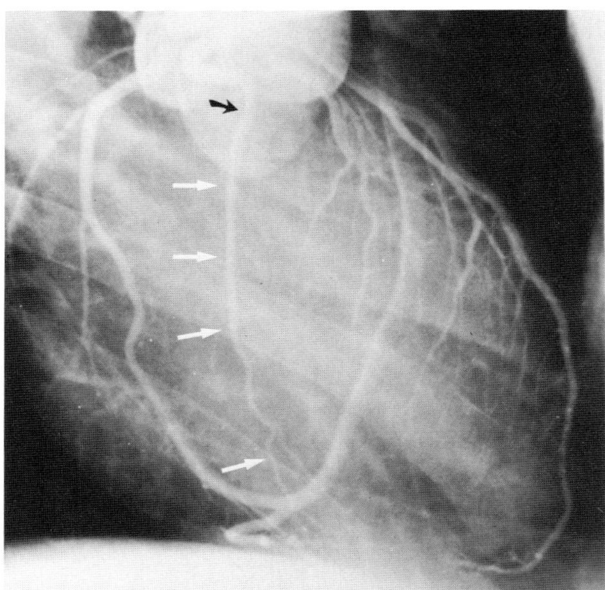

Figure 25-45. Nonselective coronary arteriogram in lateral view illustrating the presence of a large diagonal branch (*arrows*).

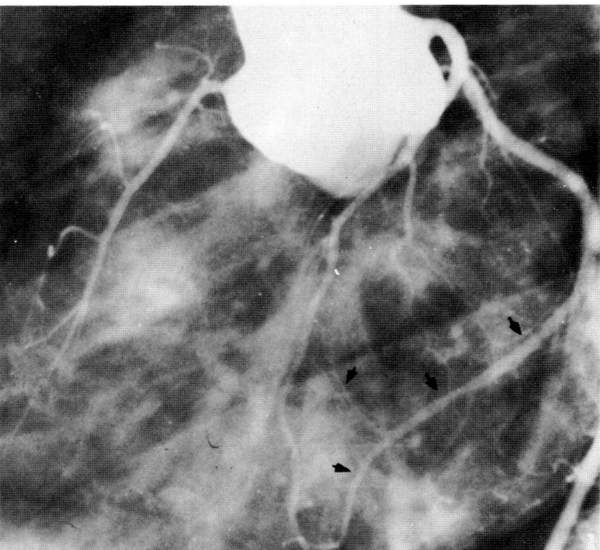

Figure 25-46. Nonselective coronary angiogram in LAO position illustrating marked left coronary artery preponderance. *Arrows* indicate the large left circumflex artery terminating in the posterior interventricular descending branch. The origin of the atrioventricular node artery can be observed *between the second and third arrows.* Note the shallow inverted U turn frequently seen in this type of distribution.

ation because vessels traveling in the atrioventricular groove and at the atrial wall lack this change in tortuosity.

In the same way as on the right side, one of the side branches of the LCX artery may be found dominant in size and usually courses along the lateral wall of the left ventricle to form a boundary between the anterolateral and diaphragmatic surfaces of the left ventricular wall. Its position corresponds to the obtuse margin of the heart, and it is consequently known as the *left circumflex obtuse marginal branch.* If such a large branch has an early origin very near the left main stem bifurcation, it may resemble a *trifurcation.* If this coincides with the early origin of a diagonal and/or an *intermediate branch,* the division of the left coronary main trunk gives the impression of a division into multiple radiating branches of relatively equal size, a pattern described by James as octopuslike.[6]

The rich variations occurring in the arterial supply have produced a confusing terminology, as is apparent in the existing anatomic and angiographic literature. When performing angiographic interpretations it is recommended to reserve the term *intermediate branch* or *ramus intermedius* for a vessel that arises purely as a third branch in midposition within the division of the left coronary main trunk and is traveling an oblique course over the middle of the left ventricle to extend at least half the distance to the apex. Such a large vessel in intermediate position exists in about one-third of normal cases.[48] Applying this concept strictly, other arterial branches supplying this area should be identified as side branches of the LAD artery (the diagonal branches) (Fig. 25-45) or of the LCX artery (the marginal branches). Parenthetically, the incidence of a large intermediate branch in European hearts[48] did not differ from the results obtained in hearts of South African Bantu,[95] in which the presence of a similarly defined intermediate artery was alleged to explain the lower incidence of ischemic heart disease in this population. Thus, there is no evidence to support the idea that variations of arterial supply of this nature present a specific coronary risk factor.

In cases with left preponderance, the LCX artery reaches the crux and supplies the myocardial areas adjacent to it. Consequently, the caliber of the LCX artery is much larger throughout its course in the left-sided atrioventricular sulcus (Fig. 25-46). Variations in its proximal distribution do not differ from those described earlier, and only one to two *posterior left ventricular branches* as well as a posterior interventricular branch, that is a *left posterior descending artery (PDA),* are added. Orientation of the side branches to the LCX artery in a direction more nearly parallel to the atrioventricular sulcus (similar to what has been described for the right side) does occur but is less frequent. The U turn at the crux, so characteristic when supplied by the right coronary artery, has a tendency to be more shallow and therefore is less distinct in angiographic examination of cases with left preponderance.

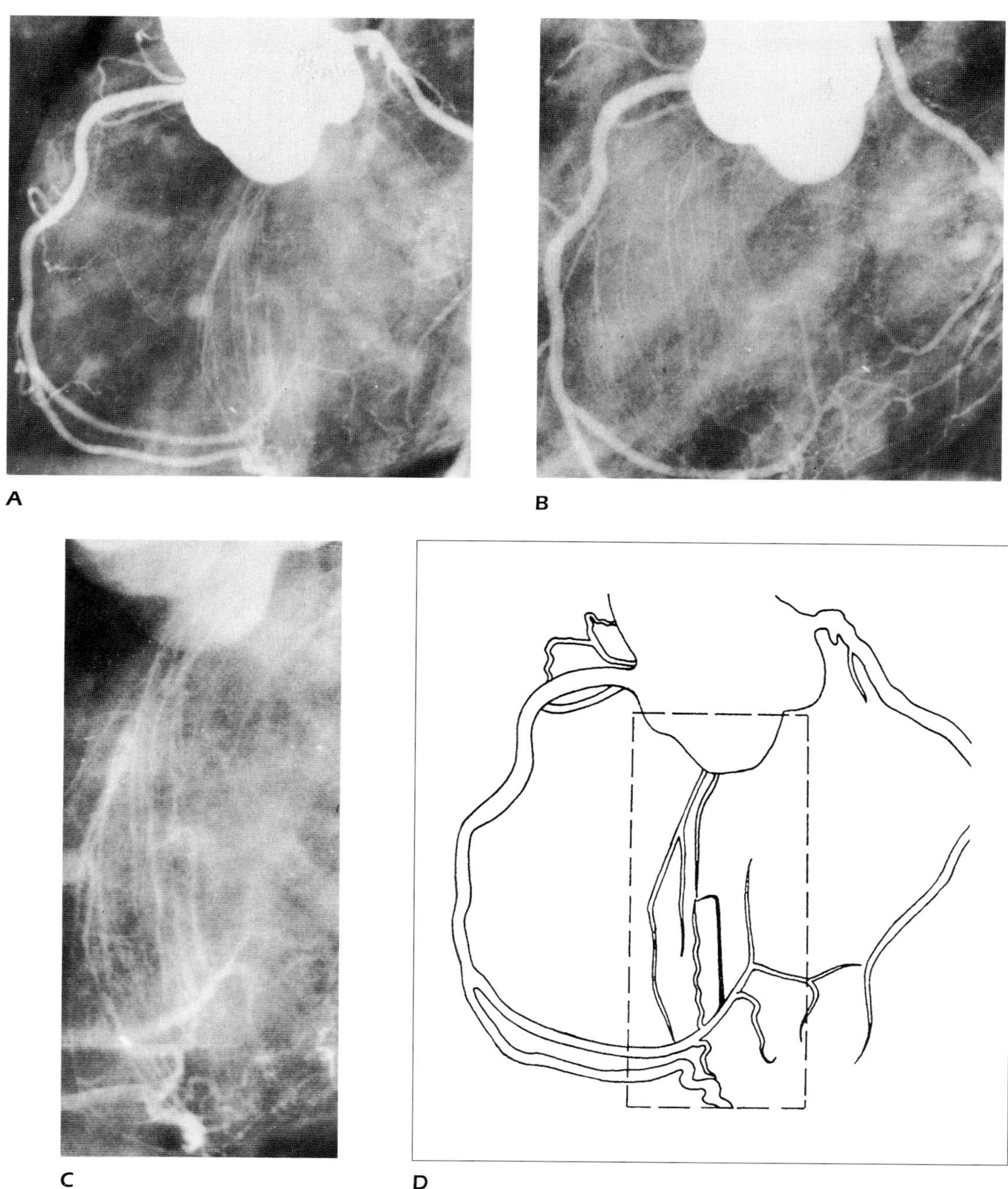

Figure 25-55. Atrioventricular node artery arising from the U turn of the right coronary artery at the crux. In left anterior oblique (A) and left lateral (B) views, it runs toward the non-coronary sinus. The small bend in the distal part of the vessel (detail in C) presumably represents its ramification to the bundle of His. Line tracing (D) in the LAO projection highlights topographic features. Broken-line square corresponds to detail radiograph in (C). (From Paulin S. Coronary angiography: a technical, anatomic and clinical study. Acta Radiol (Stockh) 1964;233(Suppl):118. Used wtih permission.)

localized and prolonged contrast staining of the intramural structures. Angiographers should avoid this occurrence because of the increased risk for contrast-induced side effects.

Nordenström et al. suggested that myocardiography could be a useful tool for detecting myocardial abnormalities.[107] Such an assumption appeared to be valid in light of postmortem angiographic studies that found diminished intramural circulation in areas of old myocardial infarction.[26] Densitometric quantita-

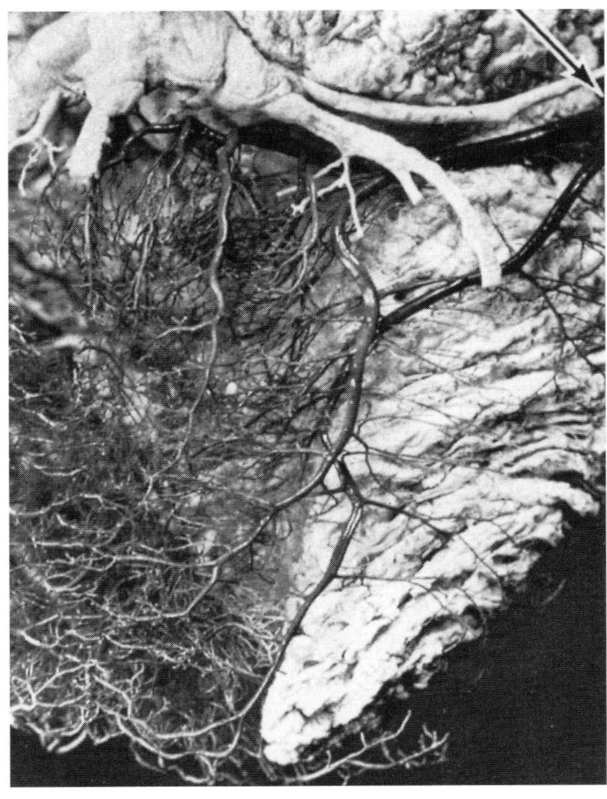

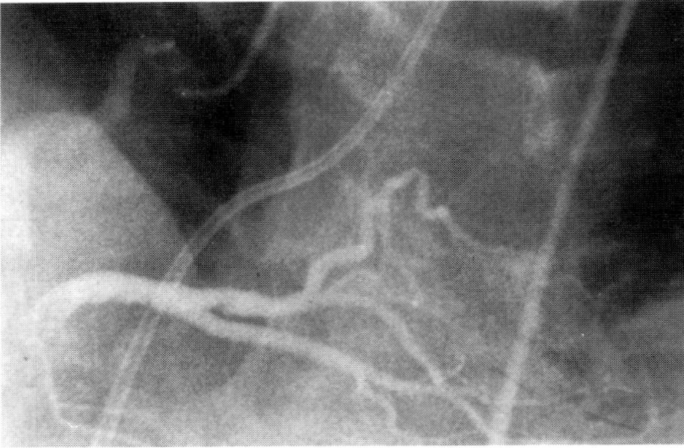

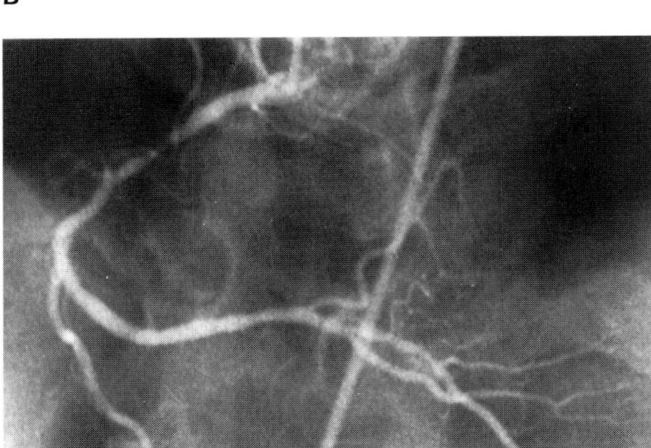

Figure 25-56. (A) Detail of posterior view of coronary cast demonstrating two competing posterior descending arteries arising from the right coronary artery, which bifurcates at the acute margin of the heart (*arrow*). The two branches cross over each other in the posterior interventricular groove. Cine coronary arteriogram demonstrates conclusively in shallow LAO projection (B) and with added cranial tilt (C) a similar crossover phenomenon in the distal right coronary artery. (Part A from James TN. Anatomy of the coronary arteries. New York: Hoeber Medical Division, Harper & Row, 1961. Used with permission.)

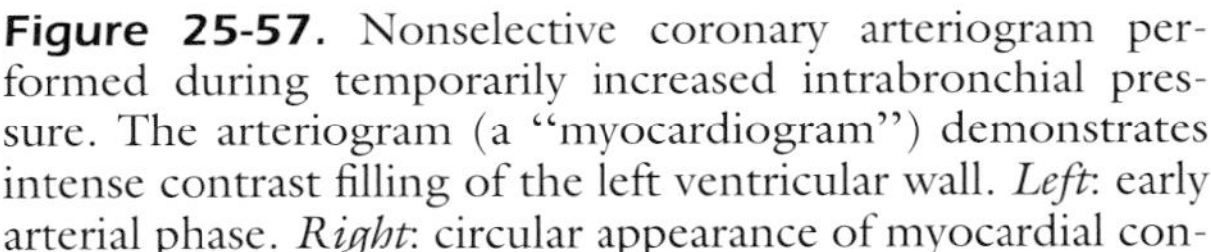

Figure 25-57. Nonselective coronary arteriogram performed during temporarily increased intrabronchial pressure. The arteriogram (a "myocardiogram") demonstrates intense contrast filling of the left ventricular wall. *Left*: early arterial phase. *Right*: circular appearance of myocardial contrast accumulation in septal and lateral wall of left ventricle. (From Nordenström B, Ovenfors CO, Törnell G. Myocardiography and demonstration of the cardiac veins in coronary angiography. Acta Radiol (Stockh) 1962;57:11. Used with permission.)

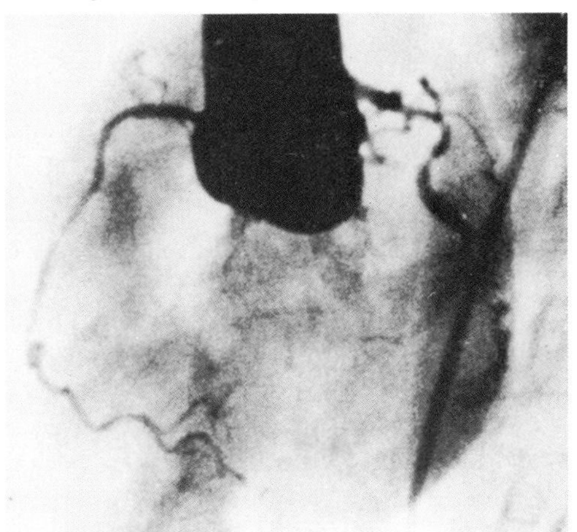

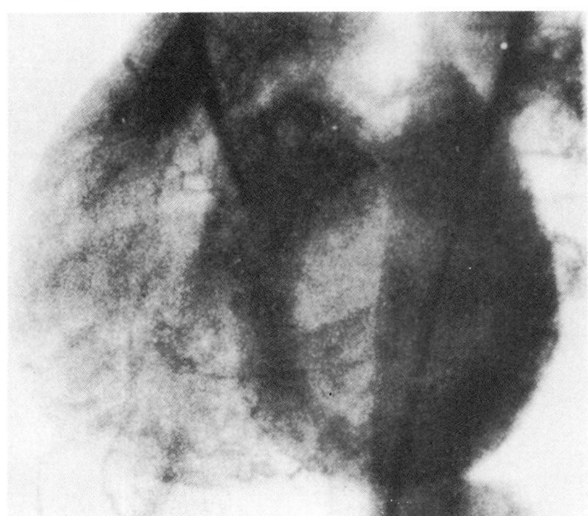

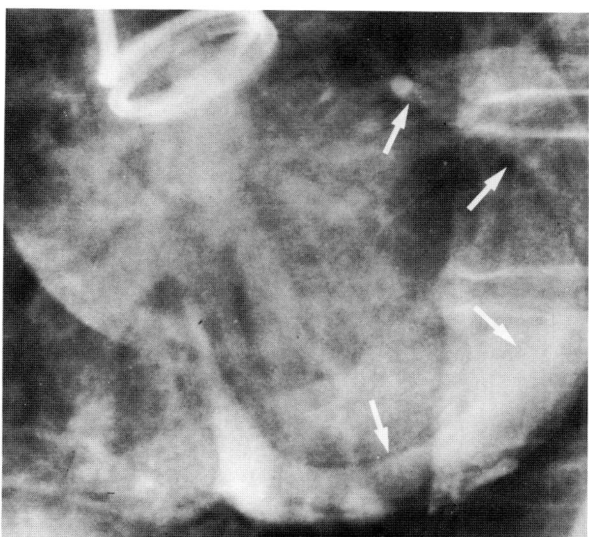

Figure 25-58. Late phase of nonselective coronary angiogram in LAO projection. The contrast medium outlines the coronary sinus and veins (*arrows*).

tions of this phenomenon from cine films[108] and with the video imaging technique[109] have been tried, and it was suggested that such techniques may have potential use for the identification of myocardial injuries. These techniques have been superseded by other more potent and less invasive imaging techniques, such as radionuclide scanning of the myocardium.

The large coronary veins, most of which converge in the venous coronary sinus, are visualized rather constantly a few seconds after a successful selective injection into the coronary artery, albeit at much lower contrast concentration (Fig. 25-58). Cinematography gives a higher yield than large-film serial radiography and readily illustrates the phasic propagation of the contrast medium into the right atrium during systole. As previously mentioned, localization of the great cardiac vein and the coronary sinus may help as a landmark for proper identification of the left-sided atrioventricular sulcus in which these venous structures run. Their intimate topographic relationship to the arterial U turn at the crux should also be recognized. Peripheral venous branches parallel the arterial supply to a certain extent, and examiners should not confuse their filling with delayed appearance of arterial branches. Early and abundant vein filling is characteristic of congenital abnormalities such as arteriovenous fistulas. Otherwise the demonstration of the coronary veins does not seem to have practical diagnostic importance.

Quantitation of Coronary Artery Distribution

The coronary arteriogram aims primarily at the topographic and anatomic delineation of arterial abnormalities, which in the majority of clinical cases are represented by obstructive lesions. The difficulties in quantifying these changes and their translation into functional terms, that is, in determining their significance with regard to flow reduction,[110-112] are not dealt with here.

On the other hand, it is logical to assume that the clinical importance and the potential hazard of a given lesion or other local vascular abnormality will have some relation to its location within the arterial tree. The seriousness of a left main stem stenosis is widely recognized and must increase by necessity if it happens to occur in the presence of a left-dominant circulation. An occlusion of an ordinary right coronary artery is usually better tolerated and may be practically inconsequential when the artery is nondominant, that is, when it is very small and confines its distribution solely to the right ventricular myocardium.

Similar considerations suggest that, in the presence of myocardial hypertrophy of one or the other chamber, the related increased flow demand will cause widening of the relevant artery and branches, but should not have such effect on the others. The same holds for a coronary artery or branch that may carry additional collateral flow. For these and similar reasons, the effort to classify the interrelationship between right and left coronary arteries with regard to variations in distribution and relative caliber dimensions is not merely an academic exercise but a matter of practical importance.

It is unlikely that distributional variations have any influence on the total blood supply of normal hearts, nor has it been possible to verify the hypothesis that certain types of distribution predispose to coronary artery disease.[113,114] The predominance of one vessel over the other in an organ that is supplied by a dual artery system can be determined by the magnitude of flow that occurs in each. Such selective flow determinations are now possible in the living patient using intravascular ultrasonic flow probes and applying pulsed Doppler velocimetry.[115] The technique is promising and correlates positively with simultaneously performed coronary venous sinus thermodilution flow determinations. At the present time, however, sufficient validation is lacking, and there are no data available on comparisons between flow values in relation to anatomically defined distribution patterns. Blood flow measurements that can be carried out less invasively use diffusible radiolabeled tracers[116,117] and express the existing flow in terms of milliliter per unit myocardial mass, thus not permitting a comparison of flow in absolute values.

Selective flow determinations have been obtained, however, in postmortem examination of human hearts in which fluid perfusions of separate arteries were used to measure their individual flow capacity. Although one can question the validity of such studies in relation to what may exist in a living organism because of the obviously altered peripheral resistance in the specimen, it is interesting to note that their results indicate a dominance of the left coronary artery in the majority of cases. Crainicianu[71] found in a series of 100 specimens of apparently normal hearts that 72 had a larger flow in the left coronary artery, 12 had equal flow, and only 16 had a flow that was greater in the right coronary artery. Schoenmackers,[118,119] when performing a quantitative morphologic study of the coronary arteries, also found a preponderance of the left coronary artery in a great majority of cases. Similarly, Fischer,[120] in postmortem perfusion experiments, found that the right coronary artery definitely exceeded 50 percent of the total perfusion capacity in only 1 of 10 normal hearts.

James[6] quantitated the contribution of the right versus the left coronary artery to the supply of the cardiac structures using his coronary cast specimens. "If one considers," he stated,

> how much greater the mass of the LV myocardium is than that of the right, and the fact that by far most of the LV free wall, by far most of the interventricular septum, and a considerable portion of the atria and free wall of the right ventricle are regularly supplied by the left coronary artery, it is clear that the left coronary artery is preponderant in virtually all normal human hearts and in some is overwhelmingly so. (pp. 79–80)

In a more recent study in which postmortem planimetry of multiple sequential coronary slices was performed, Kalbfleisch and Horst[121] substantiated James's findings when comparing arterial dominance in relation to myocardial mass subserved. For the total material of 171 cases the left coronary arteries supplied roughly two-thirds of the total myocardial mass. When only the supply of the left ventricular wall and that of the septum was considered, the same value rose to 79 percent. Even in cases with marked right coronary preponderant distribution, the left coronary artery still supplied more than 50 percent of the total. In only two cases (1 percent) an extremely extensive right coronary distribution was accountable for a more than 50 percent supply by that artery.

A dominance of the left over the right coronary artery has also been brought out in studies determining the relative caliber of these arteries at their take-off from the aorta. Such a study was first performed by Halbertsma[122] as early as in 1863 describing that a larger ostium of the left coronary artery was present in 16 out of 20 autopsy specimens. In 1 heart the calibers of both ostia were equal, and in the remaining 3 the right was slightly wider. Halbertsma's investigation must have been of decisive importance because it contradicted the prevailing notion that the right coronary was generally the larger of the two.[123–125]

Crainicianu[71] also measured the arterial calibers of the 100 specimens that he had used for flow capacity determinations; 72 had a larger caliber on the left, and 16 were larger on the right. In 12 hearts both arteries had the same width.

Baroldi and Scomazzoni,[26] measuring the inner coronary diameters of postmortem casts, found variations of from 1.5 to 5.5 mm. The mean value for the left coronary artery was 4.0 mm versus 3.2 mm on the right. Similarly, McAlpine[7] found a larger mean value for the left coronary artery when measuring the size of the coronary orifices as seen from the inner side of the aorta. Interestingly, he emphasized that these were most often elliptic in appearance, in contrast to the more circular shape of the more distal arterial lumen.

The first study that addressed arterial caliber comparisons in in vivo coronary arteriograms[48] also found that a distinct majority of left coronary arteries were wider (67 percent), whereas the right coronary was wider in only 5 percent of cases as measured on large-sized radiographs of apparently normal coronary angiograms. Similar relationships between left and right coronary arteries were found in a sizable cineangiographic study.[126]

All these findings indicate that the left coronary artery is most often the larger, and they contradict the generally prevailing notion that a right coronary artery preponderance exists in most human hearts. The explanation for this apparent paradox is that the conventional classification systems for coronary artery distribution attend to certain topographic peculiarities rather than defining the mass of cardiac tissue supplied by either one. In 1904, Banchi[4] introduced the term *coronary artery prevalence,* focusing on the distribution of coronary artery extension at the posterior aspect of the heart, that is, the area of the crux and the adjacent parts of the ventricles (Fig. 25-59). Since in 80 percent of his cases the right coronary artery supplied that area, Banchi called this appearance the "normal" distribution pattern. He spoke of a right prevalence in those roughly 10 percent in which this artery extended significantly further to the left to supply also varying areas of the left ventricular posterior and lateral wall. In the remaining 10 percent the left circumflex

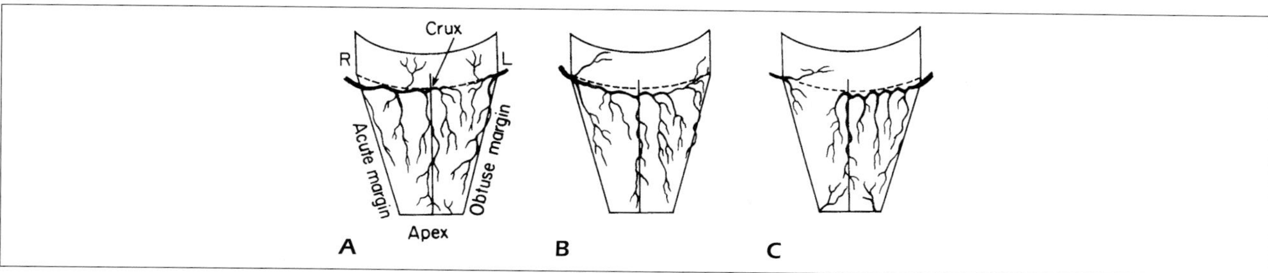

Figure 25-59. Drawing illustrating arterial supply of the posterior wall of the heart. Vertical midline identifies interatrial and interventricular sulcus; diagonal line to the left identifies the acute margin and that to the right the obtuse margin of the heart. The three examples illustrate the vascular supply of this region and its variations according to Banchi.[4] (A) The most common and normal distribution pattern of the human heart. (B) Dominance of the right coronary artery. (C) Dominance of the left coronary artery. See text for details.

artery reached the crux and supplied the posterior interventricular sulcus and adjacent areas and hence were identified as left prevalence. Schlesinger[23] also paid attention to variations of coronary artery distribution in the posterior wall of the heart and modified the terminology of the system by assigning the term *right coronary artery preponderance* to 48% of his cases. He apparently applied this term to many cases that Banchi would have called "normal." Schlesinger also introduced the term *balanced distribution,* which was characterized by a left circumflex artery supplying the posterior aspect of the left ventricular wall totally, but the posterior descending artery still deriving from the right side. He denoted all cases in which the posterior descending artery connected to the left circumflex artery as "left preponderance." Schlesinger's widely popularized terminology can be held responsible for the controversy and misunderstanding that permeate the relevant literature. Since in vivo angiography more easily identifies the posterior descending artery than the true position of the crux, the term *right preponderance* tends to be used for cases that represent Schlesinger's "balanced supply." Hamby[29] recommended that angiographers use the term *balanced coronary distribution* only when both coronary arteries give rise to separate descending arteries in parallel positions, or when the right and left coronary arteries join at the crux with one posterior descending artery arising from both. Such situations, however, are extremely rare.

Anatomists and angiographers who have devoted extensive work to this subject are uniform in their criticism that classification systems that denote the human coronary circulatory system as right preponderance in a majority of cases are unfortunate,[12,22,34,84,127,128] because this leads to the belief that the right coronary artery is preponderant in the blood supply of the heart as well.[26,27,29,48,59,70] It should also be recognized that most systems pay attention to only one topographic area of coronary arterial interplay, the crux. They do not address variations in distribution between the right and left coronary arteries as they frequently may occur at the free walls of the ventricles and the apical region. Baroldi and Scomazzoni[26] have tried to overcome these shortcomings by adding subgroups, but they have also recognized that such detailed grouping of the large number of variations may become impractical.

Recognizing the multitude of variations in the human coronary circulation, it is fair to say that all people carry their own individual "vascular fingerprint." The development of a system that determines the distribution of one artery and its branches in their relationship to the total wall area of the left ventricle may be considered a useful approach for quantitating a particular vessel's relative contribution.[70,129] Guided by postmortem angiograms followed by segmentation of the left ventricles and the septum's myocardium into equal segments, such a system was developed (Fig. 25-60). Important radiologic landmarks, detectable in most high-quality coronary angiograms, are (1) the atrioventricular ring, which is apparent as a translucent line of fat between the atria and ventricles; (2) the location of the aortic root; (3) the typical inverted U turn of the coronary artery that reaches the site of the crux; and (4) the characteristic, almost 180-degree curve, of the distal LAD artery near the apex. Superimposition of the existing arterial tree over this scheme can be surprisingly accurate and reproducible.[130]

Not only is such a system practically independent of all the frequently occurring arterial variations, but it also avoids nomenclature controversies that can make communications difficult.[131] Furthermore, the system helps to detect avascular zones that otherwise can be easily overlooked, particularly when a minor branch may be completely amputated at its origin. Obviously, this system also allows for quantification of the myo-

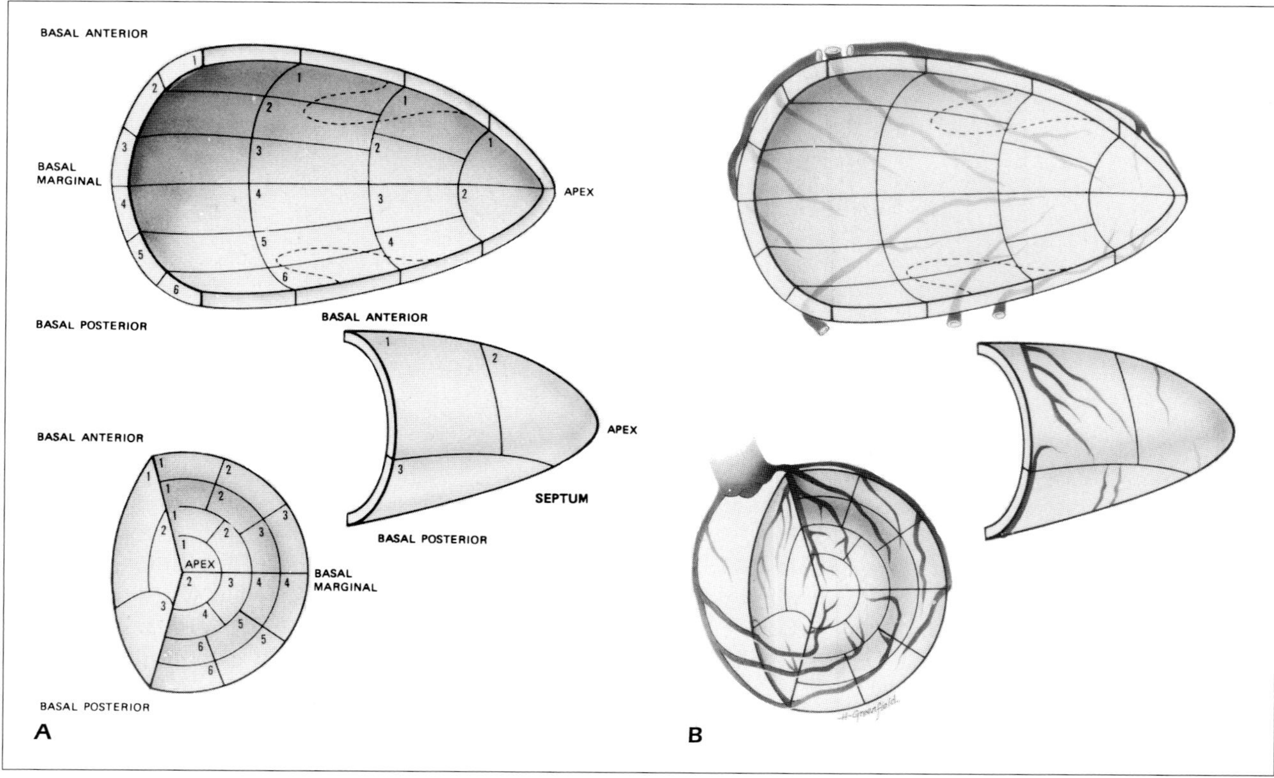

Figure 25-60. (A) Schematic division of the left ventricular wall, including the interventricular septum, into 21 approximately equal segments. (B) Radiographically identifiable landmarks such as the position of the aortic root, the inverted U turn at the crux, the typical bend of the distal left anterior descending artery at the apex, and the position of the coronary arteries in the atrioventricular ring permit consistent and reproducible superimposition of the coronary arterial tree over the scheme in (A). This approach permits quantification of the myocardial area in relation to the supply deriving from the right or the left coronary artery. See text for details.

cardial area in jeopardy by expressing the number of segments dependent on a proximally located stenosis or occlusion.

The Diagnostic Value of a Normal Coronary Angiogram

The diagnostic and prognostic consequences of normal results from coronary angiography are as important as the angiographic demonstration of pathologic lesions. Angiographically, the exclusion of abnormalities may pose a greater challenge to the performer than the demonstration of advanced pathology. This also justifies the preceding detailed discussion of the normal angiographic anatomy and its variations. The author's personal experience and that of others has often helped to identify and solve situations that may cause diagnostic uncertainties. It is hoped that the following account will be useful to the reader, particularly if she or he is likely to embark actively in the performance and the interpretation of angiographic examinations of the coronary circulation.

Roentgenographic contrast media are heavier than blood and also differ with regard to their physical properties.[130] Consequently, there is a possibility of incomplete mixing and layering in the depending part of an artery (Fig. 25-61), especially when the injection is made slowly.

Cine coronary angiograms are most frequently performed with a vertical x-ray beam, resulting in poor appreciation of this layering phenomenon, which in the presence of a tortuous arterial configuration may simulate a stenosis. The author also has frequently observed that an initial careful and slow selective injection into the main left stem will adequately fill the left circumflex artery system without filling the anterior descending artery. A subsequent faster injection usually results in complete contrast filling of the entire left system, clearly indicating that the layering mechanism was operative and prevented the heavy contrast medium from filling the upwardly directed LAD during the slower injection.

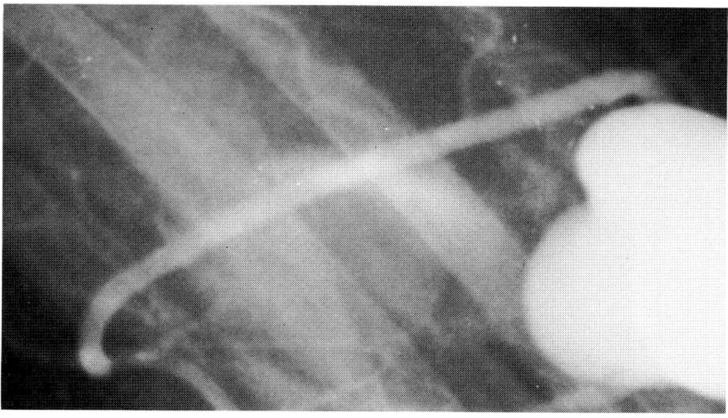

A

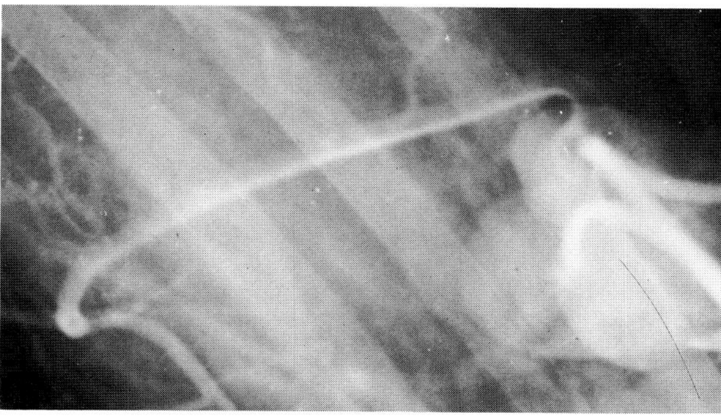

B

Figure 25-61. Radiographic detail of right coronary artery obtained with horizontal x-ray beam. (A) Complete contrast filling of the right coronary artery is demonstrated. (B) After the contrast injection into the aortic root is terminated, there is layering of the contrast medium in the dependent part of the right coronary artery because its specific weight is greater than that of blood.

Layering of contrast medium in conjunction with test injections in the ascending aorta and aortic bulb during the search for the coronary ostia may also create interpretive difficulties. For example, the left coronary artery may not fill at all following a manual injection into the left coronary cusp of a patient in LAO position supported by a rotating cradle. A similar manual injection in unchanged catheter position will show the vessel very adequately after the patient has been rotated into the RAO position, now with the coronary artery ostium in a dependent location.

Failure to demonstrate either coronary artery, in spite of catheter placement had similar nonselective injection in the corresponding coronary sinus, does not always indicate pathology. As described before, positional variations of the coronary ostia are common. Systematic catheter palpation of the wall of the aortic root is likely to be successful in many cases. If not, a large contrast bolus, delivered with the power injector, is mandatory to adequately fill the entire ascending aorta.

Occasionally, catheters for selective coronary artery catheterization advance more deeply into the coronary artery than is desired. The result may be insufficient opacification of the most proximal parts of the arteries. It is advisable in these situations to continue the injection during a gentle pullback maneuver, which usually solves the problem.

Vascular spasm at the site of the catheter tip may also pose diagnostic difficulties and is more frequently observed in the right coronary artery.[132,133] Repeat examination after nitroglycerin administration is likely to diminish, if not abolish, this phenomenon.

Some angiographers propose that using specific coronary artery dilators such as nitroglycerin, dipyridamole, and Isordil routinely could improve the diagnostic yield of coronary arteriography.[134,135] In the absence of arterial pathology, mild to moderate dilatation of the large epicardial coronary arteries and their branches can usually be accomplished. This does not permit any conclusion about flow augmentation, however, because simultaneous changes in heart rate and perfusion pressure occur in most instances (Fig. 25-62). Having a particular vessel respond to these stimuli may be helpful in excluding the possibility of diffuse and evenly distributed arteriosclerotic changes, which may be visible as narrow but apparently unobstructed vessels.[136]

The size of the individual coronary arteries and their branches relates strongly to the territorial size of their distribution. The smaller blood flow requirement of the right ventricular myocardium explains why the arterial branches supplying the wall of the right ventricle have a more attenuated appearance than those of the left ventricle. The small size of the right coronary artery is particularly striking when its distribution is confined to the right ventricular wall. In such a situation, when the right coronary artery diameter may be less than 2.0 mm, it is inappropriate to diagnose arterial hypoplasia, a poorly defined entity that is difficult to document even on postmortem examination.

Not only is a small coronary artery technically more difficult to cannulate, but its presence also poses an increased risk that the tip of the catheter may significantly obstruct the arterial lumen. If complete occlusion results from a wedged catheter in the arterial orifice, the subsequent injection of contrast medium will exert excessive pressures within that vascular system of limited flow capacity. If the initial contrast test injection does not run off into the periphery, this could indicate such a potentially dangerous situation. In these cases, it is strongly recommended to withdraw

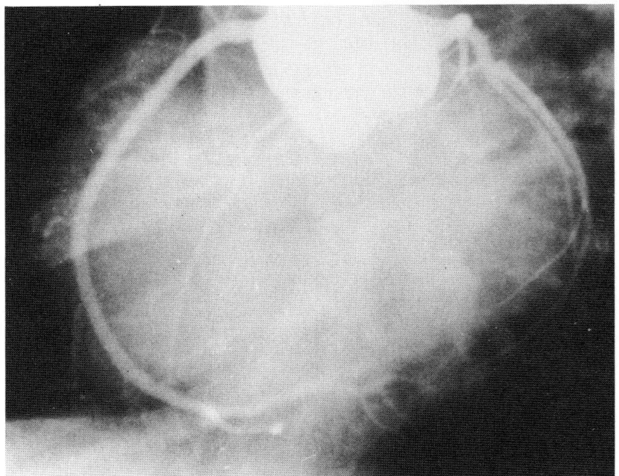

A

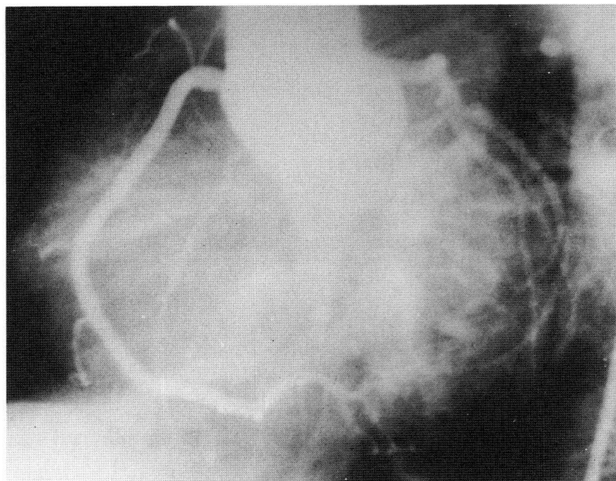

B

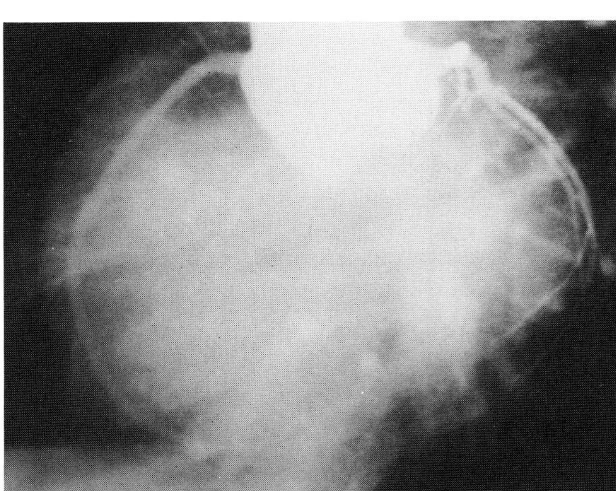

C

Figure 25-62. Comparable nonselective angiograms of a patient with undemonstrable pathologic changes in the coronary artery. (A) Under basal conditions. (B) Under the influence of Arfonad. (C) Under the influence of Aramine. In (B) the coronary arteries are generally slightly wider and in (C) slightly narrower than in (A). Mean arterial blood pressure and heart rate were simultaneously recorded. With Arfonad, the blood pressure was lower and the heart rate was increased, whereas with Aramine the blood pressure as well as the heart rate was increased when compared to basal conditions. (From Paulin S. Coronary angiography: a technical, anatomic and clinical study. Acta Radiol (Stockh) 1964; 233(Suppl):171. Used with permission.)

the catheter immediately, even if the pressure recorded via the catheter does not show any significant change from the original pattern. Apart from causing a higher incidence of arrhythmias and long-lasting electrocardiographic changes that usually coincide with a temporary myocardial contrast stain, such an injection can lead to an early and profound contrast passage to the corresponding veins. This in turn can lead to the erroneous diagnosis of a coronary arteriovenous fistula.[137] In another personally encountered instance in which the proximal part of the right coronary artery tightly encircled the catheter tip, the manual injection of the contrast medium resulted in the filling of a large anastomotic channel leading into the left circumflex coronary artery. Contrast filling continued and eventually demonstrated the entire left coronary artery, including the main stem, from which contrast regurgitated into the left coronary arterial sinus. Such extensive and easy transit of contrast media from one coronary arterial bed to the other is highly suggestive of intercoronary collateralization, which, however, in this case was not caused by an angiographically demonstrable unilateral obstruction. It is conceivable that the performance of the wedged catheter arteriogram may have coincided with the existence of an unusual intercoronary anastomosis similar in type to that described by Hines and colleagues[138] and others.[139]

The definition of a normal coronary arteriogram appears to have undergone some changes during the last decade, a time period characterized by the rapid proliferation of nonsurgical interventions in the coronary arteries. This has led to a tendency among cardiac interventionalists to declare a coronary artery or branch as normal whenever local lesions do not exceed a certain threshold of luminal narrowing believed to be hemodynamically significant, and therefore lacks a valid indication for the performance of intravascular angioplasty. It should be clear that such criteria are in conflict with those established by pathologists.[140] Although in vivo coronary arteriography does not match the postmortem examination's ability to assess the pathologic processes occurring in the arterial wall, irregularities of the arterial lumen and adjacently located calcium deposits are—isolated or combined—indirect but compelling evidence of arterial atherosclerosis, albeit in its preclinical state. It would be inappropriate to curtail the angiogram's sensitivity in this respect, particularly because these early findings are likely to contain important prognostic information.

Since one can postulate that there are technical limitations to detecting minute, discrete changes in the luminal contour of vessels, the question has been raised whether a general compromise of the coronary arterial system, that is, diffuse and general reduction of the coronary artery dimensions, could identify pathology.[48,121,126] Angiographic measurements made on large-size radiograph coronary arteriograms of apparently normal patients with normal-sized hearts under resting conditions have shown that the diameter of the proximal right coronary artery may range from 1.5 to 5.0 mm, and that of the left main coronary trunk from 3.0 to 6.0 mm (Table 25-5). A more recent study addressed measurements of practically all major primary and secondary branches of the epicardially located coronary arterial tree.[141] In a carefully selected material of clinically and angiographically normal cases (83 cases out of 9160 cineangiograms), the average values were 4.6 mm for the left main stem, 4.0 mm for the right, 3.4 mm for the left circumflex artery, and 3.8 mm for the left anterior descending artery. Again, the values varied when applied to subgroups that represented the most common distribution patterns. The calibers of secondary and tertiary branches measured roughly between 1.0 and 2.0 mm in diameter and showed a positive relationship to the angiographically determined length of the branch. Comparison with the available coronary arteriograms of 10 normal female patients again confirmed that women have smaller coronary arteries than men, even after normalization for body surface area.

The author's effort, using computer-aided technology to establish detailed nomograms for normal dimensions for all coronary arteries and branches, was confronted with the same problems as have been encountered previously, namely, obtaining a large enough patient material that fulfilled the criteria for coronary normalcy in combination with certain less frequently occurring types of distribution.[48] If one adds to this the difficult task of eliminating the potentially disturbing influences on constant vessel dimensions, such as medications, different vascular tone, and other physiologic and technical factors that are poorly controlled during the examination, the practical value of these detailed vessel measurements for diagnostic purposes in the individual case can be seriously questioned.

Table 25-5. Caliber of Right and Left Coronary Arteries: 39 Selected Cases

Caliber (mm)	Right Coronary Artery (Number of Cases)	Left Coronary Artery (Number of Cases)
1.5	1	0
2.0	1	0
2.5	3	0
3.0	5	2
3.5	8	4
4.0	17	15
4.5	2	6
5.0	2	8
5.5	0	3
6.0	0	1
Total	39	39

Perhaps the most difficult situation for correct angiographic interpretation is the complete amputation of a coronary branch exactly at the site of its origin and the absence of any collateral filling of its distal extension. Such missing branches, when occurring in the terminal distribution of the right or left circumflex artery, may result in unexplained vascular gaps between their territories. The angiographer should not accept this as normal without carefully assessing possible pathology. Similar interpretive difficulties may be encountered regarding the left anterior descending artery if a large septal perforator or diagonal branch simulates normal anatomy. The examiner should not accept an artery that does not show the typical curve at the apex of the heart as being the LAD artery unless visualization of the correspondingly increased extension of the posterior descending branch or a variation such as a so-called dual LAD explains the short variant.

Phasic segmental narrowing during systole indicates the intramyocardial position of a large coronary artery. This may occur in any location and can be single or multiple. This narrowing has a statistically significantly higher incidence in the left anterior descending artery.[103,104] Rapid serial films or cinematography will usually permit its differentiation from pathologic stenosis.[142] Although autopsy studies find myocardial bridges around the epicardial coronary arteries of practically all normal hearts, it is possible that the less frequently observed systolic stenoses on coronary arteriograms may have some functional or clinical importance, particularly when they are very marked, extensive in length, or multiple (Fig. 25-63).[6,143,144]

Considerations concerning the spatial orientation of the epicardially located coronary arteries (as treated in detail in the foregoing), which practically surround

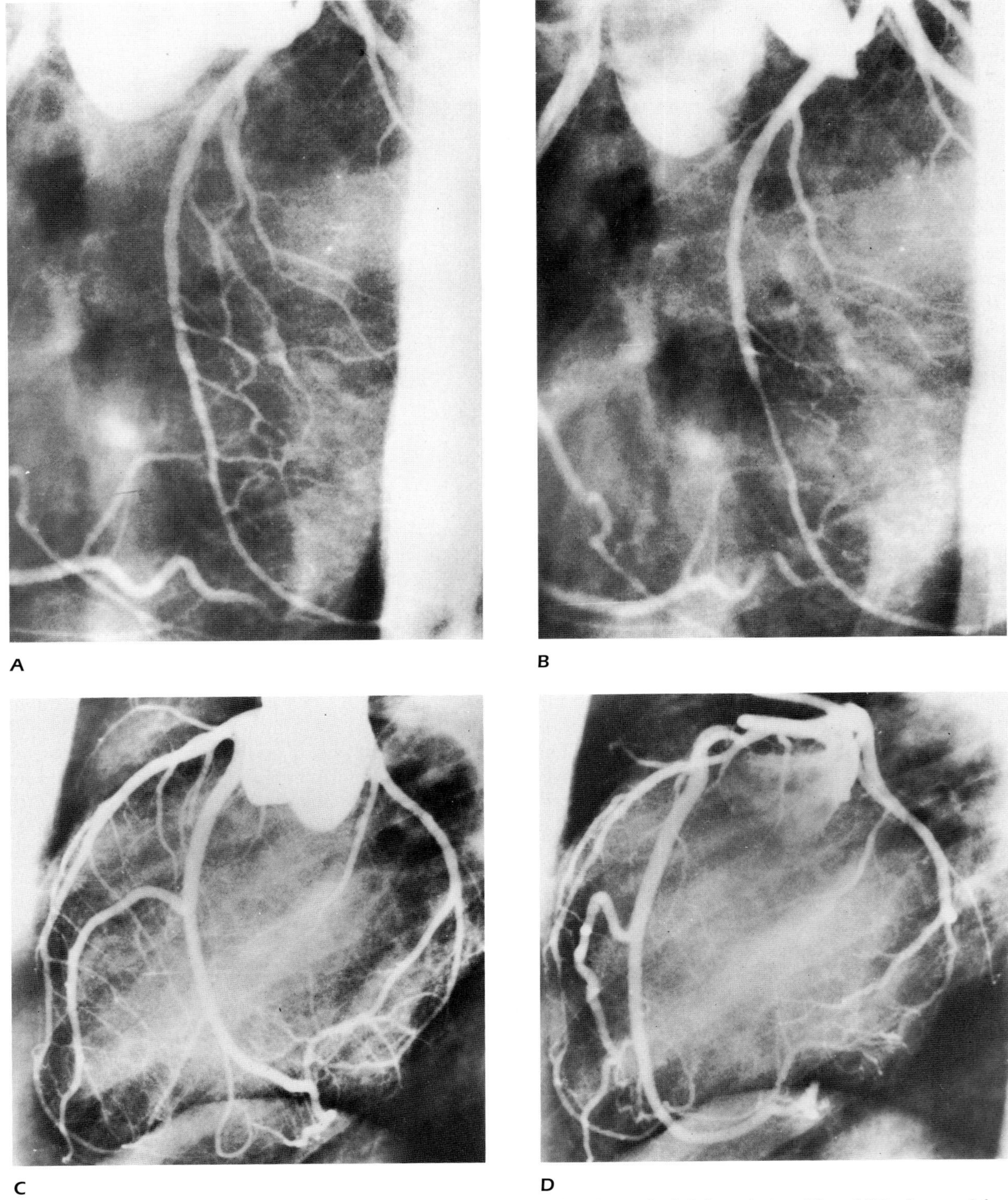

Figure 25-63. Nonselective coronary arteriogram demonstrating an intramural segment of the distal left anterior descending artery. In LAO projection, the inconspicuous caliber of the artery during diastole (A) is changed to a significant narrowing approximately 2 cm long during systole (B). In the left lateral view (C and D), the arterial segment of phasic systolic narrowing is clearly displaced inward and below the epicardial surface of the heart. This 24-year-old woman suffered from anginal pain coinciding with electrocardiographic evidence of ischemia.

the roughly globe-shaped heart, dictate that the conventional two-directional projections, as used in the past, do not suffice for proper demonstration of all relevant vascular structures. This warning is especially relevant to the area of the left coronary artery bifurcation and its adjacent segments, but may apply to any other area of the coronary arterial tree where vessels may be depicted as foreshortened or convoluted in a particular projection. The introduction of cranial- and/or caudal-tilt devices has overcome this problem to a large extent. The angiographer can now perform an optimal examination that more confidently excludes the presence of obstructive lesions and more accurately demonstrates the anatomic integrity of the coronary arteries.

Provided that it is complete and obtained according to technically high standards, a coronary arteriogram demonstrating smoothly delineated arterial contours with regularly occurring divisions and evenly distributed branches represents normal nonobstructed coronary arteries. It cannot exclude temporary causes of regional ischemia, such as intraluminal thrombus formation followed by spontaneous or therapeutic lysis, or spontaneously occurring spasm, which has been identified unequivocally to be the potential cause of typical angina pectoris, electrocardiographic abnormalities, and even myocardial infarction.[145] Consequently, cardiac challenge to the point of anginal symptoms, by using intravenous injections of ergonovine maleate, has been advocated in these puzzling cases to unveil their tendency to develop local arterial spasm during the performance of the angiogram.[146–149]

References

1. Fallopius G. Medici mutinensis observationes. Venice, 1562. Cited by Gross.[11]
2. Riolanus J. Anthropographia, lutetiae Parisiorum. Paris, 1649.
3. Vieussens R. Nouvelles découvertes sur le coeur. Paris, 1796. Cited by James.[6]
4. Banchi A. Mortfologia della arteriae coronariae cordis. Arch Ital Anat Embriol 1904;3:87.
5. Baron J. The life of Edward Jenner. London: Colburn H, 1838;1.
6. James TN. Anatomy of the coronary arteries. New York: Hoeber Medical Division, Harper & Row, 1961.
7. McAlpine WA. Heart and coronary arteries: an anatomical atlas for clinical diagnosis, radiological investigation and surgical treatment. New York: Springer-Verlag, 1975.
8. Hildebrand. Über die Methode durch Einbringen von schattengebenden Flüssigkeiten Hohlorgane des Körpers im Röentgenogramm sichtbar zu machen. ROEFO 1907;11:96.
9. Fryett AG. Arch Roentg Ray. London, 1905;51:112. Cited by Gross.[11]
10. Jamin F, Merkel H. Die Koronararterien des menschlichen Herzens unter normalen und pathologischen Verhältnissen. Dargestellt in stereoskopischen Röntgenbildern. Jena: Fischer, 1907.
11. Gross L, ed. The blood supply to the heart in its anatomical and clinical aspects. New York: Hoeber Medical Division, Harper & Row, 1921.
12. Campbell JS. Stereoscopic radiography of the coronary system. Q J Med 1929;22:247.
13. Fulton WFM. Observation on the coronary arteries. MD thesis, Glasgow, 1960.
14. Schlesinger MJ. An injection plus dissection study of the coronary artery occlusions and anastomoses. Am Heart J 1938;15:528.
15. Schaper W. The collateral circulation of the heart. Clinical studies series. New York: American Elsevier, 1971;1.
16. Spalteholz W. Uber die Arterien der Herzwand. Verhande d deutsch path gesellsch. Leipzig, 1909.
17. Hyrtl J. Die Corrosion-Anatomie und ihre Ergebnisse Wien. 1873. Cited by Gross.[11]
18. Nussbaum A. Über das Gefässystem des Herzens. Arch Mikrobiol Anat 1912;80:450.
19. Batson OV. Latex emulsion in human vascular preparations. Science 1939;90:518.
20. Stern H, Razenhofer ER, Liebow AA. Preparation of vinylite casts of the coronary vessels and cardiac chambers. Lab Invest 1954;3:337.
21. Wagner A, Poindexter CA. Demonstration of the coronary arteries with nylon. Am Heart J 1949;37:258.
22. Schlesinger MJ. Relation of anatomic pattern to pathologic conditions of the coronary arteries. Arch Pathol Lab Med 1940;30:403.
23. Zoll PM, Wessler S, Schlesinger MJ. Interarterial coronary anastomosis in the human heart, with particular reference to anemia and relative cardiac anoxia. Circulation 1951;4:797.
24. Blumgart HL, Zoll PM, Wessler S. Angina pectoris: clinical pathologic study of 177 cases. Trans Assoc Am Physicians 1960;63:262.
25. Allison RB, Rodriguez FL, Higgins EA, et al. Clinicopathologic correlations in coronary atherosclerosis: four-hundred thirty patients studied with postmortem coronary angiography. Circulation 1963;27:170.
26. Baroldi G, Scomazzoni G. Coronary circulation in the normal and pathologic heart. Washington, DC: Office of the Surgeon General, Department of the Army, 1967.
27. Gensini GG. Coronary arteriography. Mt. Kisco, NY: Futura, 1975.
28. Gould SE, ed. Pathology of the heart. Springfield, IL: Charles C Thomas, 1953.
29. Hamby RI. Clinical anatomical correlates in coronary artery disease. Mt. Kisco, NY: Futura, 1971.
30. Hood JH. Anatomy of coronary arteries. Semin Roentgenol 1973;8:3.
31. James TN. Anatomy of the coronary arteries in health and disease. Circulation 1965;32:1020.
32. James TN, Burch GE. The atrial coronary arteries in man. Circulation 1958;17:90.
33. James TN, Burch GE. The blood supply of the human interventricular septum. Circulation 1958;17:391.
34. Smith GT. The anatomy of the coronary circulation. Am J Cardiol 1962;9:327.
35. Soto B, Russell RO Jr, Moraski RE. Radiographic anatomy of the coronary arteries: an atlas. Mt. Kisco, NY: Futura, 1976.
36. James TN. Pathology of small coronary arteries. Am J Cardiol 1967;20:691.
37. Thorén C. Cardiomyopathy in Friedreich's ataxia: with studies of cardiovascular and respiratory function. Acta Paediatr Scand 1964(Suppl 153).
38. Varnauskas E, Ivemark B, Paulin S, et al. Obscure cardiomyopathies with coronary artery changes. Am J Cardiol 1967;19:531.
39. Paulin S. Terminology for radiographic projections in cardiac angiography. Cathet Cardiovasc Diagn 1981;7:351.

40. Keith JD. The anomalous origin of the left coronary artery from the pulmonary artery. Br Heart J 1959;21:149.
41. Liberthson RR, Dinsmore RE, Bharati S, et al. Aberrant coronary artery origin from the aorta: diagnosis and clinical significance. Circulation 1974;50:774.
42. Paulin S, vonSchulthess GK, Fossel ET, et al. MR imaging of the aortic root and proximal coronary arteries. AJR 1987; 148:665–670.
43. Manning WJ, Li W, Edelman RR. A preliminary report comparing magnetic resonance coronary angiography with conventional angiography. N Engl J Med 1993;328:828–832.
44. Virmani R, Chun PK, Goldstein RE, et al. Acute take-off of the coronary arteries along the aortic wall and congenital coronary ostial valve-like ridges: association with sudden death. J Am Coll Cardiol 1984;3:766–771.
45. May AM. Surgical anatomy of the coronary arteries. Dis Chest 1960;38:645.
46. Hackensellner HA. Koronaranomalien unter 1000 auslesefrei untersuchten Herzen. Anat Anz 1955;100:123.
47. Vladover RZ, Neufeld HN, Edwards JE. Pathology of coronary disease. Semin Roentgenol 1972;1:376–394.
48. Paulin S. Coronary angiography: a technical, anatomic and clinical study. Acta Radiol (Stockh) 1964;233.
49. Virmani R, Chun PK, Rabinowitz M, et al. Length of the left main coronary: lack of correlation to coronary dominance and bicuspid aortic valve—an autopsy study of 54 cases. Arch Pathol Lab Med 1984;108:638–641.
50. DiGuglielmo L, Guttadauro M. Anatomic variations in the coronary arteries: an arteriographic study in living subjects. Acta Radiol (Stockh) 1954;41:393.
51. Amplatz K, Formanek G, Stranger P, et al. Mechanics of selective coronary artery catheterization via femoral approach. Radiology 1967;89:1040.
52. Alexander RW, Griffith GC. Anomalies of the coronary arteries and their clinical significance. Circulation 1956;14:800.
53. Evans W. Congenital stenosis (coarctation) atresia and interruption of the aortic arch (a study of 28 cases). Q J Med 1933; 26:1.
54. Krumbhaar EB, Erlich WE. Varieties of single coronary artery in man occurring as isolated cardiac anomalies. Am J Med Sci 1938;196:407.
55. Lipton MJ, Barry WH, Obrez L, et al. Isolated single coronary artery: diagnosis, angiographic classification and clinical significance. Radiology 1979;130:39.
56. Ogden JA. Congenital abnormalities of the coronary arteries. Am J Cardiol 1970; 25:474.
57. White NK, Edwards JE. Anomalies of the coronary arteries: report of four cases. Arch Pathol 1948;45:766.
58. Hillestad L, Eie H. Single coronary artery: a report of three cases. Acta Med Scand 1971;189:409.
59. Allen GL, Snider TH. Myocardial infarction with a single coronary artery. Arch Intern Med 1966;117:261.
60. Longnecker CG, Reemtsma K, Creech O Jr. Surgical implications of single coronary artery: a review and two case reports. Am Heart J 1961;61:382.
61. Murphy M. Single coronary artery. Am Heart J 1967;74:557.
62. Click R, Holmes DR, Vliestra RE, et al. Anomalous coronary arteries: location, degree of atherosclerosis and effect on survival—a report from CASS. J Am Coll Cardiol 1989;13:531–537.
63. Roberts WC, DiCicco BS, Waller BF, et al. Origin of the left main- from the right coronary artery or from the right aortic sinus with intramyocardial tunneling to the left side of the heart via the ventricular septum: the case against clinical significance of myocardial bridges or coronary tunnel. Am Heart J 1982;104:303–305.
64. Roberts WC. Major anomalies of coronary arterial origin seen in adulthood. Am Heart J 1986;111:942–962.
65. Kragel AH, Roberts WC. Anomalous origin of either the right or left main from the aorta with subsequent coursing between the aorta and pulmonary trunk: analysis of 32 necropsy cases. Am J Cardiol 1988;62:771–777.
66. Cheitlin MD, DeCastro CM, McAllister HA. Sudden death as a complication of anomalous left coronary origin from the anterior sinus of Valsalva. Circulation 1975;50:780.
67. Ishikawa T, Brandt P. Anomalous origin of the left main coronary artery from the right anterior aortic sinus: angiographic definition of anomalous course. Am J Cardiol 1985;55:770–776.
68. Schlesinger MJ, Zoll PM, Wessler S. The conus artery: a third coronary artery. Am Heart J 1949;38:823.
69. Bream PR, Souza AS Jr, Elliott LP, et al. Right superior septal perforator artery: its angiographic description and clinical significance. AJR 1979;133:67.
70. Vieweg WVR, Smith DC, Hagan AD. A clinically useful coding system for normal coronary artery anatomy. Cathet Cardiovasc Diagn 1975;1:171.
71. Crainicianu A. Anatomische Studien über die Coronararterien und experimentelle Untersuchungen über ihre Durchgängigkeit. Virchows Arch Pathol Anat 1922:238:1.
72. Engel HJ, Torres C, Page HL. Major variations in anatomical origin of the coronary arteries: angiographic observations in 4,250 patients without associated congenital heart disease. Cathet Cardiovasc Diagn 1975;1:157.
73. Rowe L, Carmody T, Askenazi J. Anomalous origin of the left circumflex coronary artery from the right aortic sinus: a familial clustering. Cathet Cardiovasc Diagn 1993;29:277–278.
74. Meng CCL, Eckneer FA, Lev M. Coronary artery distribution in tetralogy of Fallot. Arch Surg 1965;90:363.
75. Elliot LP, Neufeld HN, Anderson RC, et al. Complete transposition of the great vessels: I. An anatomic study of sixty cases. Circulation 1963;27:1105.
76. Cohen DJ, Kim D, Baim DS. Selective injection of a left coronary artery arising anomalously from the "non-coronary" sinus of Valsalva. Cathet Cardiovasc Diagn 1991;22:190–192.
77. Lawson MA, Daily SM, Soto B. Selective injection of a left coronary artery arising anomalously from the posterior aortic sinus. Cathet Cardiovasc Diagn 1993;30:300–302.
78. Benson PA. Anomalous aortic origin of coronary artery with sudden death: case report and review. Am Heart J 1970;79: 254.
79. Cohen LS, Shaw LD. Fatal myocardial infarction in an 11-year-old boy associated with a unique coronary artery anomaly. Am J Cardiol 1967;19:420.
80. Dadswell JV. Congenital anomaly of the left circumflex coronary artery. J Pathol 1960;79:204.
81. Grossman LA, Burko H. Diminutive coronary arteries and congenital coronary anomalies. J Tenn Med Assoc 1968;61: 687.
82. Laurie W, Woods JD. Single coronary artery: a report of two cases. Am Heart J 1964;67:95.
83. Manninen V, Rissanen VT, Halonen PL. Coronary ostium outside the aortic sinus: a factor in the etiology of ischemic heart disease? Adv Cardiol 1970;4:94.
84. Ravin A, Geever EF. Coronary arteriosclerosis, coronary anastomoses and myocardial infarction: a clinicopathological study based on an injection method. Arch Intern Med 1946; 78:125.
85. Levin DC, Baltaxe HA. Angiographic demonstration of important anatomic variations of the posterior descending coronary artery. AJR 1972;116:41.
86. Greenberg M, Spindola-Franco H. Dual left anterior descending coronary artery (Dual LAD). Cathet Cardiovasc Diagn 1994;31:250.
87. Berkheiser SWL. Significance of coronary artery hypoplasia and congenital variations associated with coronary heart disease. Aerospace Med 1969;40:188.
88. Baim DS, Grossman W. Coronary angiography. *In:* Baim DS, Grossman W, eds. Cardiac catheterization angiography and intervention. 4th ed. Philadelphia: Lea & Febiger, 1991; chap. 13.
89. Spindola-Franco H, Grose R, Salomon N. Dual left anterior coronary artery: angiographic description of important varia-

tions and surgical implication. Am Heart J 1983;105(3):445–455.
90. Bittner V, Nath HP, Cohen M, et al. Dual connection of the left anterior descending coronary artery to the left and right coronary arteries. Cathet Cardiovasc Diagn 1989;16:168–172.
91. Ilia R, Gilutz H, Gueron M. Mid left anterior descending coronary artery originating from the right coronary artery. Int J Cardiol 1991;33:162–165.
92. Voudris V, Salachas A, Saounotsou M, et al. Double left anterior descending artery originating from the left and right coronary artery: a rare coronary artery anomaly. Cathet Cardiovasc Diagn 1993;30:45–47.
93. Selig MB, Jafari N. Anomalous origin of the left main coronary artery from the right coronary artery ostium—interarterial subtype: angiographic definition and surgical treatment. Cathet Cardiovasc Diagn 1994;31:41–47.
94. Bream PR. The anomalous first septal perforator artery: its origin from the first diagonal, first left marginal, and circumflex arteries. Circulation 1979;60:631.
95. Pepler WJ, Meyer BJ. Interarterial coronary anastomoses and coronary arterial pattern: a comparative study of South African Bantu and European hearts. Circulation 1960;22:14.
96. Keith A, Flack M. The form and nature of the muscular contractions between the primary divisions of the vertebrate heart. J Anat 1907;41:172.
97. James TN. The connecting pathways between the sinus node and the A-V node and between the right and left atrium in the human heart. Am Heart J 1963;66:498.
98. Bachmann G. The interauricular time interval. Am J Physiol 1916;41:309.
99. Koch W. Üeber die Blutversorgung des Sinusknotens und etwaige Beziehungen des Letzteren zum Atrioventrikularknoten. München Med Wochenschr 1909;56:2362.
100. Dragneff S. Recherches anatomiques sur des Artères coronaires du coeur chez l'homme. Thesis No. 26, Nancy, 1897. Cited in Spalteholz.[16]
101. Haas G. Über die Gefässversorgung des Reizleitungssystems des Herzens. Anat Hefte 1911;43:629. Cited in Spalteholz.[16]
102. Keith A. The auriculo-ventricular Bundle of His. Lancet 1906;1:623.
103. Geiringer E. The mural coronary. Am Heart J 1951;41:359.
104. Polacek P. Relation of myocardial bridges and loops on the coronary arteries to coronary occlusions. Am Heart J 1961; 61:44.
105. Bilazarian SD, Jacobs AK, Fonge R, et al. Case report of a coronary anomaly: crossing of two obtuse marginal arteries. Cathet Cardiovasc Diagn 1991;23:130–132.
106. Nordenström B. The Thebesian circulation in coronary angiography. Angiology 1965;16:616.
107. Nordenström B, Ovenfors CO, Törnell G. Myocardiography and demonstration of the cardiac veins in coronary angiography. Acta Radiol (Stockh) 1962;57:11.
108. Sandor T, Paulin S, Shridar B. Densitometric evaluation of myocardial contrast accumulation. 1977; Boston, MA: S.P.I.E. Application in Optical Instrumentation in Medicine, VI. 1977;127:349.
109. Ritman EL, Robb RA, Johnson SA, et al. Quantitative imaging of the structure and function of the heart, lung and circulation. Mayo Clin Proc 1978;53:3.
110. Hood JH. Cine-angiocardiography, rendition of movement and information content. Br J Radiol 1970;43:423.
111. Paulin S. Grading and measuring coronary artery stenosis. Cathet Cardiovasc Diagn 1979;5:214.
112. Smith HC, Frye RL, Donald DE, et al. Roentgen videodensitometric measure of coronary blood flow: determination from simultaneous indicator-dilution curves at selected sites in the coronary circulation and in coronary-saphenous vein grafts. Mayo Clin Proc 1971;46:800.
113. Pitt B, Zoll PM, Blumgart HL. Anatomy of coronary arterial occlusions. Abstracts of the 35th Scientific Sessions of the American Heart Association. Circulation 1962;26:773.
114. Truex RC. The distribution of the human coronary arteries. Cited in Eikoff W, Moyer JH, eds. Coronary heart disease. New York: Grune & Stratton, 1963.
115. Eichhorn EJ, Alvarez LG, Jessen ME, et al. Measurement of coronary and peripheral artery flow by intravascular ultrasound and pulsed Doppler velocimetry. Am J Cardiol 1992; 70(4):542–545.
116. Asokan SK, Fraser RC, Kolbeck RC, et al. Variations in right and left coronary blood flow in man with and without occlusive coronary disease. Br Heart J 1975;37:604.
117. Wisenberg G, Schelbert HR, Hoffman EJ, et al. In vivo quantitation of regional myocardial blood flow by positron emission computed tomography. Circulation 1981;63:1248.
118. Schoenmackers J. Zur quantitativen Morphologie der Herzkranzschlagadern. Z Kreislaufforsch 1945;37:617.
119. Schoenmackers J. Die Herzkranzschlagadern bei der anteriokardialen Hypertrophie. Z Kreislaufforsch 1949;38:321.
120. Fischer S. Pathology of coronary occlusion with special reference to anticoagulant medication. Copenhagen: Store Nordiske Videnskabsboghandel, 1963.
121. Kalbfeisch H, Horst W. Quantitative study on the size of coronary artery supplying areas postmortem. Am Heart J 1977; 94:183.
122. Halbertsma HJ. Ontleedkundige aanteekeningen. Nederl T Geneesk 1863;7:693.
123. Albrecht E. Der Herzmuskel und seine Bedeutung fur Physiologie Pathologie und Klinik des Herzens. Berlin 1903. Cited in Tandler J. Anatomie des Herzens. Jena: Fischer, 1913.
124. Cruveilhier J. Traité anatomie descriptive. Paris, 1834. Cited in Spalteholz.[16]
125. Henle J. Handbuch der Gefässlehre des Menschen. Braunschweig: Vieweg & Sohn, 1868;87.
126. MacAlpin RN, Abbasi AS, Grollman JH, et al. Human coronary artery size during life: a cinearteriographic study. Radiology 1973;108:567–576.
127. Fulton WFM. The coronary arteries: arteriography, microanatomy and pathogenesis of obliterative coronary artery disease. Springfield, IL: Charles C Thomas, 1965.
128. Kuwabara M. Studies on coronary sclerosis: I. Incidence and distribution of coronary sclerosis. Acta Gerontol Jpn 1959; 31:1.
129. Brandt PWT, Partridge JB, Wartie WJ. Coronary arteriography: method of presentation of the arteriogram report and a scoring system. Clin Radiol 1977;28:361.
130. Paulin S. A new classification for evaluation of vascular changes in the coronary arteriogram. Presented at the Annual Meeting of the Association of University Radiologists, Vancouver, B.C., 1973.
131. O'Reilly RJ. Coronary angiographic nomenclature: current status and a plea for standardization. Radiology 1975;115: 229.
132. Paulin S, Schlossman D. Coronary angiography: technique and normal anatomy. Clin Radiol Nucl Med 1973;4:333.
133. O'Reilly RJ, Spellberg RD, King TW. Recognition of proximal right coronary artery spasm during coronary arteriography. Radiology 1970;95:305.
134. Gensini GG, Kelly AE, DaCosta CB, et al. Quantitative angiography: the measurement of coronary vasomobility in the intact animal and man. Chest 1971;60:6.
135. van Tassel R, Moore R, Amplatz K. Determination of the true size of the coronary artery in coronary arteriography. AJR 1972;116:62.
136. Likoff W, Kasparian H, Lehman JS, et al. Evaluation of "coronary vasodilators" by coronary arteriography. Am J Cardiol 1964;13:7.
137. Spindola-Franco H, Eldh P, Adams DF, et al. Coronary vascular patterns during occlusion arteriography. Radiology 1975;114:59.
138. Hines BA, Brandt PW, Agnew TH. Unusual intercoronary communication: a case report. Cardiovasc Intervent Radiol 1981;4(4):259–263.
139. Phillips DA, Berman J. A variation in the origin of the poste-

rior descending coronary artery. Cardiovasc Intervent Radiol 1984;7(2):75–77.
140. Glagov S, Weisenberg RK, Stancunavicius R, et al. Compensatory enlargement of human atherosclerotic coronary arteries. N Engl J Med 1987;316:1371–1375.
141. Dodge JT Jr, Brown BG, Bolsen EL, et al. Lumen diameter of normal coronary arteries: influence of age, sex and anatomic variation in left ventricular hypertrophy or dilation. Circulation 1992;86:232–246.
142. Portsmann W, Iwig J. Die intramurale Koronarie im Angiogramm. ROEFO 1960;92:129.
143. Paulin S. Nonselective coronary arteriography. Semin Roentgenol 1972;7:369.
144. Greenspan M, Iskandrian AS, Catherwood E, et al. Myocardial bridging of the left anterior descending artery: evaluation using exercise thallium-201 myocardial scintigraphy. Cathet Cardiovasc Diagn 1980;6:173.
145. Oliva PB, Potts DE, Pluss RG. Coronary arterial spasm in Prinzmetal angina: documentation by coronary arteriography. N Engl J Med 1973;288:745.
146. Eliot RS, Bratt GT. The paradox of myocardial ischemia and necrosis in young women with normal coronary arteriograms: relationship to anomalous hemoglobin-oxygen dissociation. Am J Cardiol 1968;21:98.
147. Kemp HG, Elliott WC, Gorlin R. The anginal syndrome with normal coronary arteriography. Trans Assoc Am Physicians 1967;80:59.
148. Likoff W, Segal BL, Kasparian H. Paradox of normal selective coronary arteriograms in patients considered to have unmistakable heart disease. N Engl J Med 1967;276:1063.
149. Neil WA, Kassebaum DG, Judkins MP. Myocardial hypoxia as the basis for angina pectoris in a patient with normal coronary arteriograms. N Engl J Med 1968;279:789.

26

Angiography in Coronary Disease

HERBERT L. ABRAMS
KRISHNA KANDARPA
JOHN E. ARUNY

Until a decade ago, the number of deaths from coronary artery disease had increased strikingly in association with a marked prolongation of the average life span. Since Herrick's original description in 1912 of the clinical features of acute coronary occlusion,[1] there had been relatively little progress toward better understanding or more rational management. Fortunately, in recent years there has been a decline in the incidence of coronary artery disease,[2,3] in part because of the recognition[4] and correction of risk factors predisposing to atherosclerosis. New preventive[5,6] and therapeutic interventions[7–15] promise further reductions in the morbidity and mortality associated with this disease, which remains the leading cause of death in the United States.[16]

Surgeons as far back as 1935[17] attempted to augment myocardial blood supply. A variety of procedures was proposed before Bailey et al. performed the first coronary endarterectomy in 1957.[18] In the ensuing years, internal mammary implantation into the myocardium was employed, discarded, and immediately replaced by the modern method of saphenous vein bypass.[7,8,19,20] Meanwhile, it had become evident that, without a detailed radiologic map of the coronary circulation in vivo, no rational therapeutic approach could evolve, prosper, and be evaluated.

Coronary arteriography began with the elegant anticipatory studies of Rousthoi[21] and Reboul and Racine.[22] In 1948 Radner[23] described the technique of radial artery catheterization and thus made possible the development of an effective diagnostic method. Jonsson et al.[24] applied Radner's technique, and Di-Guglielmo and Guttadauro[25] analyzed Jonsson's data. In the late 1950s many workers, including Dotter and Frische,[26] Lehman et al.,[27] and Bellman et al.,[28] approached this problem. These workers used a bolus injection in the root of the aorta, an approach still in use today when attempts at selective catheterization fail.[29] In 1962 Sones and Shirey reported success with the method of selective brachial arteriography that Sones had employed first in 1959,[30] and in the same year Ricketts and Abrams described percutaneous transfemoral selective coronary arteriography with preshaped catheters.[31] Modifications of this technique have been developed by others,[32–34] and Judkins's modification is now more widely used for coronary arteriography than any other method.[32] Over the past decade, the number of cardiac catheterizations and surgical bypass procedures has more than doubled, and the use of coronary balloon angioplasty has risen exponentially.[16] In recent years all three of these procedures have had a doubling time of 5 years, despite the decline in the incidence of coronary artery disease.

Abbreviations

The following abbreviations are used in illustrations throughout this chapter. The reader should refer to this list whenever required.

Coronary Arteries and Branches

A	Atrial artery
AM	Acute marginal branch
AV	Atrioventricular node branch
C	Conus branch
D	Diagonal branch
DRC	Distal right coronary artery
EC	Epicardial branch
LACX	Left atrial circumflex artery
LAD	Left anterior descending coronary artery
LCA	Left coronary artery
LCiA	Left circumflex artery
LCX	Left circumflex artery
LM	Left main coronary artery
OM	Obtuse marginal branch
PD	Posterior descending artery
RC	Right coronary artery (distal segment)
RCA	Right coronary artery
RM	Ramus medianus

S	Septal branch
SA	Sinus node branch
SN	Sinus node branch

Radiographic Projections

AP	Anteroposterior projection
RAO	Right anterior oblique or left posterior oblique projection
LAO	Left anterior oblique or right posterior oblique projection

Indications for Coronary Arteriography

The pathology of the coronary arteries as visualized in vivo by coronary arteriography is inextricably intertwined with the criteria by which a patient is selected for this technique. It is essential, therefore, that the indications for coronary arteriography be defined and that the patient population be placed clearly in perspective as the types of pathoanatomic change uncovered are reviewed.

The indications may conveniently be divided into therapeutic and diagnostic (Table 26-1), with the understanding that a clear separation of the two is impossible because the arteriogram is always a diagnostic tool.[35] In this chapter, the term *coronary arteriography* will be assumed to include contrast left ventriculography and pressure measurements; without them, no coronary arteriogram is complete.

Table 26-1. Indications for Coronary Arteriography

Therapeutic Indications	Diagnostic Indications
Incapacitating angina pectoris	Angina with normal ECG at rest and in exercise
Unstable angina pectoris	Mild angina, young adults or those with poor family history
Stable angina, recent increase in severity	Prinzmetal variant angina
Recent angina, progressive increase in severity	Atypical chest pain
Angina at rest: "coronary insufficiency"	Asymptomatic patients, abnormal ECG
Angina: mild, but probably 3-vessel or left main disease	Asymptomatic, high-risk factors
Strongly + exercise test	Unexplained heart failure
Resting S–T segment depression	
Dyspnea with angina	
Multiple infarcts, short time in the young	
Complications of coronary disease	
Aneurysm	
Mitral regurgitation	
Septal perforation	
Intractable heart failure	
Valvular disease with angina	
Postprocedural evaluation of coronary arteries	
Correctable congenital lesions	
Evaluation of medical therapy	
Intractable ventricular arrhythmias	

Therapeutic Indications

Incapacitating Angina Pectoris

The single most important indication for coronary arteriography is incapacitating angina pectoris. Without a preoperative anatomic map of the extent and distribution of the coronary disease, the potential usefulness of revascularization cannot be determined. Furthermore, neither the type of procedure nor the site of profitable intervention(s) can be rationally defined. With the widespread use of coronary artery revascularization, the cardiologist and the cardiac surgeon are confronted with the need for high-quality radiologic studies that define the morphology of the lesions and that indicate their hemodynamic significance, the nature of the vascular bed beyond the stenosis, and the condition of the ventricular myocardium. Following surgery, improvement in angina pectoris may be anticipated in 75 to 85 percent of patients.

Unstable Angina Pectoris

This category of patients includes three groups: those with stable angina and a recent increase in severity, those with recent angina with a progressive increase in severity, and those with angina at rest or "acute coronary insufficiency." The mortality of such patients is almost twice as high when they are treated medically as when they are treated surgically.[36] These patients should be studied by coronary arteriography, ventriculography, and cardiac catheterization, after aggressive medical management in an effort to stabilize their condition. Before surgery, an arteriographic map and knowledge of ventricular function must be attained.

Angina Pectoris: Mild but with Likelihood of Three-Vessel Disease or Left Main Disease

This group of patients consists of those in whom the objective is the prolongation of life, rather than the amelioration of symptoms alone. There seems little question that in left main coronary disease surgical mortality is less than medical mortality.[37] Furthermore, in three-vessel disease surgery may provide a better prognosis than medical therapy or angioplasty. The important problem is how to identify patients with mild angina who fit into this category on the basis of clinical and laboratory parameters. Major clues to the existence of left main disease and three-vessel disease include a strongly positive exercise test, resting S–T segment depression, and dyspnea with angina or an anginal equivalent. Patients with such symptoms or signs deserve coronary arteriography.

Coronary Heart Disease with Multiple Infarcts in a Short Time

In patients with multiple infarcts, especially young patients, it may be essential to determine the status of the coronary circulation with a view to surgical revascularization of the circulatory bed beyond the stenoses or occlusions. Nevertheless, revascularization has not been proved to affect the incidence of recurrent infarcts. Furthermore, there is inadequate evidence that life is prolonged in such patients.

Complications of Coronary Disease: Possible Surgical Candidates

Ventricular Aneurysm. The presence of a ventricular aneurysm may contribute significantly to inefficient performance by the left ventricle, with consequent left heart failure. Under these circumstances, removal of the aneurysm may be a prerequisite to attaining some element of hemodynamic stability. The coronary arteriogram is an essential aspect of the diagnostic workup of ventricular aneurysm to determine the feasibility of combined revascularization surgery.

Mitral Insufficiency. Papillary muscle infarction may produce mitral insufficiency of profound degree, at times sufficiently severe that it may be an emergency indication for surgery. Whereas the ventriculogram establishes the diagnosis of mitral regurgitation, the coronary arteriogram permits the surgeon to plan simultaneous revascularization to augment myocardial blood flow at the time of prosthetic valve replacement.

Septal Perforation. Infarction involving the ventricular septum may produce a perforation and a consequent left-to-right shunt. When this shunt is associated with the compromise of the arterial bed that produced the infarct initially, it may represent an insuperable volume load and contribute significantly to heart failure. Although the diagnosis of septal perforation can be made by left ventriculography, the coronary arteries should also be visualized with the objective of simultaneous revascularization if required.

Coronary Disease with Intractable Heart Failure. Although many patients in this category are not candidates for surgery because of the poor condition of the myocardium, occasionally either a reparable mechanical element or sufficient viable muscle with good distal coronary arteries may warrant surgery. It is important to choose carefully those patients for whom surgery offers a reasonable possibility of improvement, rather than subjecting all such patients to catheterization and angiography.

Valvular Heart Disease with Angina Pectoris

In this group of patients, particularly in those with aortic stenosis, it is impossible to be certain whether the myocardial ischemia is due to the fixed cardiac output and a tight valve orifice or to coronary disease per se. Decreased coronary flow reserve (compromised vasodilator response) in a hypertrophied left ventricle has been proposed as a mechanism for angina in patients with aortic stenosis and normal coronary arteries.[38] The prognosis of patients with severe aortic stenosis and severe coronary disease is worse than that of individuals with valve disease alone but is improved when aortocoronary bypass surgery is performed at the time valve replacement or valve surgery is undertaken.

In planning aortic valve replacement, knowledge of coronary anatomy is essential to ensure adequate myocardial perfusion and particularly adequate flow distal to severe stenosis, as well as to avoid superselective catheterization and perfusion.

Postprocedural Evaluation of Coronary Arteries

It is essential to evaluate the degree to which myocardial revascularization procedures have improved the delivery of blood to the myocardium. Although the coronary arteriogram affords a relatively gross anatomic view, at least it can indicate that a saphenous vein bypass is patent, that its size seems adequate, and that contrast agent appears to be flowing to those areas of the myocardium that would otherwise be ischemic. Isotopic studies with myocardial scans add significant information. Coronary arteriography is particularly important in patients who either have had no symptomatic relief or have had recurrence of symptoms, to determine whether the revascularized artery is patent or closed, whether the number of grafts was adequate, whether disease in the native circulation has progressed, and whether additional procedures are required.

Correctable Congenital Lesions

Coronary arteriography should be undertaken in any suspected case of a congenital lesion of the coronary circulation that may be operable. The precise diagnosis can be made in no other way. In the presence of coronary arteriovenous fistula or anomalous origin of the left coronary artery, it is essential to define the anatomy preoperatively. Frequently the arteriogram is obtained simply because the diagnosis is uncertain. In other congenital cardiac anomalies with a known high incidence of coronary vessel abnormalities, such as transposition of the great vessels, it is also important to define with precision the exact course and status of the coronary vessels.

Evaluation of Medical Therapy

There is no uniformity of opinion that the institution of medical therapy must be accompanied by a coronary arteriogram, although in some centers this is considered essential. It seems clear, however, that, without confirmation of the diagnosis and delineation of the extent of coronary disease before the institution of drug therapy, effects of the drugs on the disease process will be impossible to assess. Long-term anticoagulants, long-term vasodilators, beta blocking agents, lipid-lowering agents, and fibrinolytic agents are all being employed in the medical treatment of coronary disease. If these forms of therapy are evaluated solely on the basis of relief, objective data on arterial lesions per se will be difficult to attain in large series. Obviously, both hemodynamic and coronary angiographic data would be invaluable in the assessment of the effect of such drugs or of any new ones that are developed. Nevertheless, this is an unusual indication for coronary arteriography in most centers today.

Intractable Ventricular Arrhythmias

Coronary arteriography is indicated in patients in whom arrhythmias cannot readily be controlled by antiarrhythmic drugs. On rare occasions, such an arrhythmia may be the major indication of the presence of occult coronary disease and myocardial ischemia. Because individual patients with such conditions have responded to coronary bypass surgery, it must be considered a potential indication under appropriate circumstances.[39,40]

Diagnostic Indications

Angina Pectoris in the Presence of Normal Resting and Exercise Electrocardiograms

The absence of typical electrocardiographic supporting evidence of myocardial ischemia warrants careful study of the coronary arterial bed as a means of assessing the accuracy of diagnosis, translating the exercise test into morphologic terms, and determining whether true angina can exist without major disease in the coronary arteries.[41] The data acquired may furnish important evidence that the locus of the ischemia is in the small coronary vessels beyond the capacities of roentgenographic resolution.[42]

Mild Angina Pectoris in Young Adults or Those with a Poor Family History

In this group of patients it is essential to know the degree of coronary artery involvement from both prognostic and therapeutic points of view. Proudfit et al.[43] failed to find any correlation between coronary arteriography and the duration or distribution of chest pain or its precipitating factors. Baltaxe et al.[44] were unable to document the expected correlation between the levels of hypercholesterolemia and the severity of coronary disease defined by the coronary arteriogram. Precise anatomic and hemodynamic evaluation in these patients is of great importance.

Prinzmetal Variant Angina

This group of patients with angina pectoris at rest and S–T elevation includes individuals with organic disease of the coronary arteries and associated spasm, as well as some without any definite organic disease. Coronary arteriography is indicated to confirm the diagnosis of Prinzmetal angina by demonstrating the presence of spasm. In the absence of spasm on the arteriogram, pharmacologic maneuvers such as the administration of ergonovine may demonstrate the presence of spasm. Furthermore, because some of the patients have moderately severe to severe organic coronary disease, it is important to assess this feature early in the course, and to consider the possibility of surgical therapy if the disease worsens. Whereas aortocoronary bypass may be essential for individuals with fixed stenosing lesions, those with normal vessels are treated with long-term vasodilator therapy.[45]

Atypical Chest Pain with or Without Normal Resting and Exercise Electrocardiograms

It is important to determine whether atypical chest pain is related to coronary disease, particularly in patients placed on a rigid dietary and exercise regimen and informed of the presence of coronary disease without adequate supporting evidence. The risk of cardiac neurosis, despondency, and fear of death in a patient with normal coronary circulation requires consideration. The major contribution of arteriography for such a patient is the demonstration of a normal coronary vascular bed. The decision to perform arteriography in this group can be made only on an individual basis. Other patients exhibit chest pain suggestive of angina or prior myocardial infarction, or show electrocardiographic abnormalities suggesting healed myocardial infarction. Here it is important to determine whether the risk of the procedure is less than that of remaining ignorant about the status of the coronary vascular bed.

Asymptomatic Patients with Abnormal Electrocardiograms

In some cases nonspecific changes in the S–T segments or in the T waves have been considered prima facie evidence of coronary disease. On this basis, patients have been disqualified for life insurance. Pilots, subjected to an annual physical examination in which a minor alteration of the electrocardiogram has been apparent, have been permanently grounded. Yet it is well known that changes in the resting electrocardiogram may occur under a variety of circumstances without myocardial ischemia. A positive exercise test may also be observed in patients without coronary disease—as in the hyperventilation syndrome. Under these circumstances, the coronary arteriogram furnishes unequivocal evidence of the presence or absence of disease in the major arterial branches. Begg et al.,[46] for example, have used selective coronary arteriography to define the lack of statistical correlation between coronary atherosclerosis and heart block.

Asymptomatic Patients with High-Risk Factors

As coronary arteriography has become more widely applied, questions have been raised as to the importance of evaluating the status of the coronary bed in patients with diabetes, hypertension, hyperlipidemia, and other factors augmenting the incidence and severity of coronary disease. These risk factors are by no means widely accepted indications, nor is there any uniformity of opinion that in the asymptomatic patient the presence of high-risk factors justifies the procedure.

Unexplained Heart Failure

The precise cause of heart failure cannot always be determined by clinical and conventional laboratory means. In some patients, the cause may well be coronary disease, whereas in others it may be myocarditis, cardiomyopathy, pericardial disease, or even occult valvular disease. In such individuals, because of the possibility of appropriate therapeutic interventions once the nature of the underlying disease has been demonstrated, catheterization and coronary arteriography may be indicated. Thus careful patient selection is required.

Ventriculography: Indications and Role

Coronary arteriography and left ventricular catheterization with ventriculography are complementary studies in the investigation of ischemic heart disease. The former delineates the arterial lesions, whereas the latter demonstrates their effect on ventricular function and gross morphology. The indication for ventriculography may be simply stated: *It should be performed in all patients undergoing coronary arteriography unless there is a specific contraindication.*

The depressant effect of intracoronary and intraventricular contrast medium on the myocardium[47–49] has largely determined the optimal sequence of investigation: left ventricular pressure recordings before and after ventriculography, followed by coronary arteriography.

Calculation of ventricular volume and ejection fraction from the ventriculogram is essential to the assessment of the hemodynamic effects of coronary artery disease. Left ventricular wall thickness and mass can be estimated from the ventriculogram,[50] and good autopsy correlations have been obtained.[51] Systolic wall thickening (normally 70–106 percent) is markedly reduced in dyskinetic areas.[52] The ejection fraction is the most useful quantitative parameter in assessing left ventricular function in the patient with coronary artery disease.

The Normal Ventriculogram

The normal pattern of ventricular contraction (synergy) has been described by Herman et al.[53] as a uniform, almost concentric, inward motion of all points along the inner ventricular surface during systolic ejection. McDonald[54] has pointed out that systolic increase in wall thickness, approximation of trabeculae, papillary muscle-filling defects, and mitral valve movements make ventricular cavity contraction less symmetric than that of the epicardial surface. The transverse diameter of the ventricle narrows in isovolumetric systole. Karliner's group[55] stated that the long axis remained constant during systole, but McDonald[54] described descent of the base in the preejection phase.

An outward bulge of the high posterior left ventricular wall in early systole was described in some normal patients examined fluoroscopically.[56] We have seen this occasionally in the LAO projection of normal ventriculograms.

Ventricular relaxation also occurs symmetrically but in a somewhat stepwise fashion because of the effect of aortic valve closure, mitral valve opening, and atrial systole.

Left Ventricular Asynergy

In 1935, Tennant and Wiggers[57] described abnormality of left ventricular contraction after experimental coronary occlusion in dogs. The following three decades saw numerous reports of fluoroscopic and kymographic recognition of this in patients with coronary artery disease.[58–60] In 1965, Harrison[61] introduced the term *asynergy* to describe the poor teamwork of the musculature of the ventricle in such patients, and in 1967 the concept of asynergy was amplified.[53,62,63]

Herman et al.[53] classified asynergy on the basis of cineventriculographic appearances and described four distinct types: *akinesis,* a total lack of motion of a portion of the left ventricular wall; *asyneresis,* diminished or inadequate motion of part of the wall; *dyskinesis,* paradoxical systolic expansion; and *asynchrony,* a disturbed temporal sequence of contraction. *Hypokinesis* was reserved for a generalized reduction in left ventricular contraction but has now become interchangeable with *asyneresis* when the local area is specified (e.g., anterior wall hypokinesis). Recognition of these contraction abnormalities is not usually difficult, although a premature ventricular beat can mimic all forms of asynergy.[64]

Asynergy may be quantitated by plotting against time the percentage change from end-diastolic length of multiple axes and hemiaxes drawn on frame-by-frame silhouettes of the projected cineventriculogram.[65] Superimposition of end-systolic on end-diastolic silhouettes is less tedious but will not reveal asynchrony.

Although common, the exact incidence of asynergy in ischemic heart disease is unknown. The patients who undergo ventriculography are preselected, and, because an area of asynergy may be histologically normal, pathologic changes are misleading. The following figures are a rough guide: in angina pectoris with no electrocardiographic evidence of myocardial infarction but arteriographically documented coronary artery disease, Bjork et al.[66] found 11 of 21 patients (52 percent) with ventricular dysfunction (asynergy). Asynergy was seen, by radarkymography, in 44 of 56 patients (79 percent) with acute myocardial infarction and in 36 of 54 patients (67 percent) with previous myocardial infarction.[67] Seventy-six percent of post-myocardial infarction patients studied by biplane ventriculography have asynergy.[68]

The sites of asynergy can be consistently related to significant disease in the appropriate coronary artery.[62,69,70] Its prevalence increases with the number of vessels involved.[71] Areas of asynergy may be single or multiple and on pathologic examination may show normal myocardium, fibrous replacement of muscle, and complete, incomplete, or acute infarction.[53] Even a ventriculographic aneurysm may show only scattered fibrosis in predominantly viable muscle.[62]

There seems no doubt, therefore, that asynergy occurs not only in areas of postinfarction scar but also in areas of acute or chronic myocardial ischemia. Thus it may be due to replacement of myocardium by fibrosis or to more subtle derangement in the contractile process.[72] Catecholamines also appear to have some role in asynergy; infusion of epinephrine may in some cases improve contraction in asynergic areas,[69] and beta-adrenergic blockade can induce or exaggerate asynergy.[73]

After Harrison suggested that ventricular asynergy might be important in the genesis of cardiac failure in coronary disease,[61] convincing supporting evidence was produced by subsequent workers.[69] An asynergistic area of sufficient size may give rise to ventricular failure despite normal myocardium in the remainder of the ventricle. The therapeutic implication is that asynergistic areas may be surgically resectable or may be improved by successful aortocoronary saphenous vein bypass.

A detailed discussion of ventricular aneurysm, mitral regurgitation, and postinfarction ventricular septal defects is beyond the scope of this chapter. In all these conditions, ventriculography is essential.

Finally, it must be clear that the ventriculogram is a required element in all patients in whom the coronary circulation is examined by arteriography. It is not enough to depict the degree and location of disease in the coronary arteries; its impact on the left ventricle must also be clarified.

The Roentgen Pathology of Coronary Disease

An understanding of the pathologic anatomy of coronary arteriosclerosis assists in translating roentgen findings into their pathologic counterparts. The progress of arteriosclerotic disease appears to be related to repeated thrombosis on the surface of the initial plaque. The deposited thrombus becomes organized, and from the edges the endothelium spreads over its free surface.

Arteriography depicts the gross pathology of arteriosclerotic disease and provides an excellent road map of its distribution. However, serious discrepancies may occur when attempting to assess the physiologic compromise caused by individual lesions, as will be noted later.

A number of particular changes are visible in many patients with coronary disease. Many of these are related to the caliber of the arteries.

Vessel Caliber

The vessel may be normal, narrow, or dilated. Vessels may remain normal in caliber even when there is extensive involvement of their walls with atherosclerosis. Unless the lumen is compromised, atherosclerosis need not present a clinical problem. Atheroma, thrombus, and underlying hemorrhage provoke luminal narrowing. Stenosis, as noted shortly, may be concentric or eccentric. The changes occur predominantly in the central portions of the large coronary arteries rather than in the small peripheral branches but may involve all segments of a particular vessel. Finally, the dilated artery is associated with alteration and destruction of the muscular and internal elastic layers of the blood vessel wall as a manifestation of atherosclerosis. When the vessels become rigid, tortuosity may develop. Dilated coronary arteries are also noted in the absence of intimal thickening with Mönckeberg sclerosis, which is found far less commonly in the coronary arteries than in peripheral arteries.

In evaluating alterations in lumen caliber, normal variations must be kept in mind. Females show consistently smaller arteries than males; with increasing age, arterial size as measured at autopsy increases; and patients with clinical hypertension have increased coronary artery dimensions.[74]

The Arterial Orifice

The orifice of the coronary vessels may be ring-shaped, with the origin of equivalent size to the maximum diameter of the vessel (see Figs. 26-1D and 26-5E). It may also be funnel-shaped, with gradual diminution in size of the lumen as it extends from its origin in the aorta (see Figs. 26-1E and 26-2F). Orificial narrowing occurs with or without involvement of the distal part of the vessel, although the most common cause, arteriosclerosis, is usually associated with disease in other areas of the coronary vascular bed. Particularly in luetic aortitis, the vessel beyond the stenosed origin may be entirely normal. Other causes of orificial narrowing and occlusion include dissecting aortic aneurysm, embolism, and arteritis.

Marginal Irregularity

Minor irregularities of the wall are an early manifestation of arteriosclerosis (Fig. 26-1). They are invariably due to intimal plaques and can almost always be seen in patients over the age of 45 if definition is adequate. The proliferation of the intima that begins at birth is not considered abnormal until the intimal thickness is greater than the media.[75] The thickened intima is composed predominantly of collagen and elastic fibers but also contains smooth muscle cells that may be lipid-filled. The plaques occur irregularly along the length of the vessels, but frequently in the more pronounced form proximally.

Filling Defects

With increase of the plaque size or with accretions by fresh or organized thrombus, larger filling defects extending from the wall into the lumen may be visualized (Fig. 26-2). At times these may be due to hemorrhage beneath the plaque. Filling defects are usually eccentric, may produce stenosis, and ultimately, with increasing thrombus formation, can lead to complete obstruction.

Stenosis

Stenosis involves vessel narrowing and is distinguishable from filling defects only in a quantitative sense. It implies luminal narrowing of greater or lesser degree (Fig. 26-3). Stenosis may be eccentric or concentric, and it reflects increased deposition of atherosclerotic material in the intimal layer, thrombus, or hemorrhage in a subatheromatous location. Obstructive lesions secondary to trauma are rare but have been observed. The amount of disease in the wall of the coronary vessel does not necessarily reflect the degree of luminal compromise.[76] A reduction in transverse diameter of 50 percent may be translated into a 75 percent decrease in cross-sectional area—a level of luminal compromise considered hemodynamically significant (see Fig. 26-11). The angiographic estimation of stenosis severity correlates poorly with its actual physiologic importance as determined by a loss in coronary reactive hyperemic response.[77] This is discussed in more detail in the section on appraisal of significant disease.

Diffuse Narrowing

At times, intimal and wall thickening may occur in remarkably uniform fashion and result in narrowed vessels with a relatively smooth lumen or slight marginal irregularity (Fig. 26-4). The distinction of these vessels from vessels that are normally hypoplastic may be difficult. The evaluation must take into account whether there is a right- or left-dominant coronary artery system. More often, diffuse narrowing is associated with segments of irregularity and stenosis. In some patients the diffusely narrowed vessel may be the site of moderate or marked arteriosclerosis alone, whereas in others

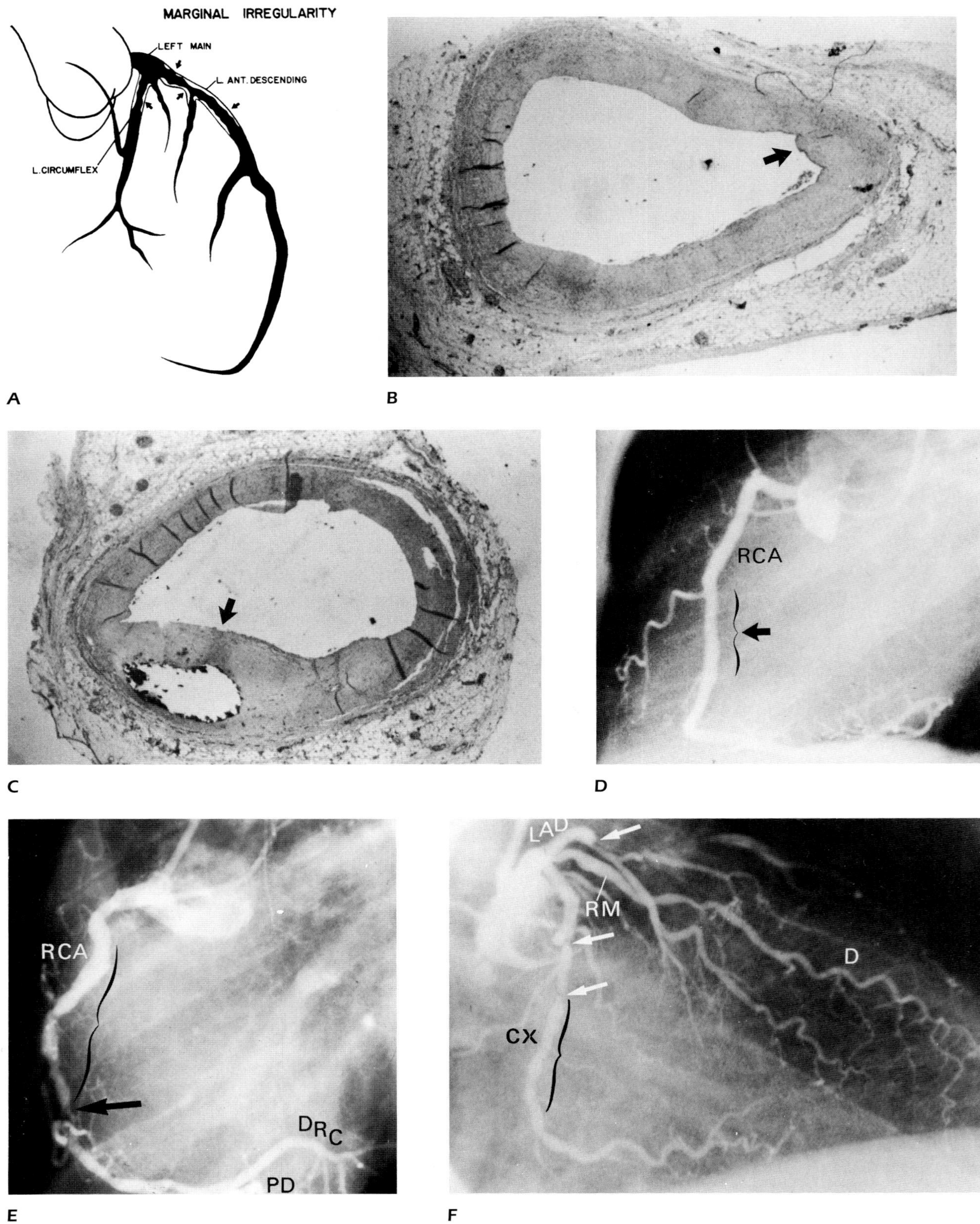
MARGINAL IRREGULARITY
LEFT MAIN
L. ANT. DESCENDING
L. CIRCUMFLEX
A
B
C
RCA
D
RCA
D$_{RC}$
PD
E
LAD
RM
D
CX
F

organized thrombus may be superimposed on atheroma (see Fig. 26-4B).

Occlusion

With increasing obstruction and slowing of blood flow, the tendency toward thrombus formation increases and complete thrombosis of the vessel ultimately occurs (Fig. 26-5). On arteriography, this is seen as a cutoff of the opaque column. In a single projection, when multiple branches are side by side or overlap, complete stenosis may be difficult to define; thus it is essential that the vessels be viewed from a number of different angles. The duration of occlusion is reflected in part by the size and number of the collateral vessels supplying the region distal to it. With abrupt complete occlusion, however, there may be immediate filling and visualization of the small collateral pathways normally available in the majority of individuals[78] or almost complete absence of collateral vessels. Furthermore, intraluminal thrombus usually produces abrupt change in the caliber of the vessel, whereas chronic arteriosclerotic occlusion is generally more gradual and tapered in appearance. Although arteriographically the distinction between thrombotic and arteriosclerotic occlusion is sometimes difficult, abrupt termination of the contrast column in the absence of developed collateral vessels, or only minimal collateral filling, strongly suggests acute thrombosis (see Fig. 26-5G).

Embolus

Unusually, embolic occlusion may be defined in the coronary vessels (Fig. 26-6). Like its counterpart in the large peripheral arteries, embolus generally differs from thrombosis or chronic arteriosclerotic occlusion in appearance, with the contrast column defining a discrete edge based on the concave tip of the embolus. Pathologically, the embolus is separate from the arterial intima and frequently has a "tail" (see Fig. 26-6B). It projects into the contrast-filled lumen with a distinctively rounded edge (see Fig. 26-6C).

Although coronary emboli used to be considered a rarity, it is now apparent that there are many causes and that embolus is not infrequent at autopsy.[79] The commonest causes include infective and noninfective endocarditis, intracardiac mural thrombus (as in coronary disease, ventricular aneurysm, or mitral stenosis), and intracavitary neoplasm, particularly myxoma. Iatrogenic factors include cardiac catheterization, selective angiography, and the adjuncts of cardiac surgery—especially prosthetic valves, cardioversion, and external cardiac massage.

Coronary embolus may well explain many cases of myocardial infarction with apparently normal coronary arteries on arteriography.[80] In such patients, lysis or fragmentation of the embolus has presumably occurred following the infarct.

Dilatation and Tortuosity

Dilatation of the vessel wall, localized or diffused, may be the predominant manifestation of the arteriosclerotic process (Fig. 26-7). At times, this is associated with classic Mönckeberg sclerosis, whereas in most patients it is due to fragmentation and breakdown of the muscular and the internal elastic layers of the vessel wall. Intimal change and luminal compromise may be absent or insignificant in some patients, whereas in others they may alternate with segments of dilated artery. Elongation and tortuosity of the vessel occur as a result of circumferential as well as longitudinal dilatation. Tortuosity may also be found in vessels that are otherwise small; under these circumstances, it may be a variant or it may reflect an increased resistance to flow. Particularly when a vessel participates as a collateral channel, it is likely to enlarge longitudinally as well as circumferentially and then appear sinuous and tortuous.

◀ **Figure 26-1.** Marginal irregularity. (A) Diagrammatic representation of selective left coronary arteriogram, RAO projection. Instead of the smooth borders of a normal artery, the edge shows many serrated indentations (*arrows*). (B) Low-power photomicrograph. The *arrow* points to a small plaque, representing early atherosclerosis. (C) A larger plaque and thrombus are visible (*arrow*), with recanalization of thrombus. (D) Selective right coronary arteriogram, LAO projection. There is no evidence of stenosis or occlusion, but the margin is irregular (*brace*). Such vessel irregularity is almost invariably due to intimal plaques when the irregularity is relatively slight. Note the normal ring shape of the vessel as it arises from the aorta, the origin being equal in diameter to the remainder of the proximal portion of the vessel. (E) Selective right coronary arteriogram, LAO projection. The right coronary artery is irregular throughout its course, showing a combination of minimal atherosclerosis, seen as marginal irregularity, and some larger filling defects (*arrow*) and stenosis (*brace*). The orifice is funnel-shaped, a normal appearance. (F) Selective left coronary arteriogram, RAO projection. Marginal irregularity is visible in the distal circumflex (*brace*). Multiple stenoses are also present in the circumflex artery (*arrows*), and a large filling defect is visible near the origin of the ramus medianus. Complete obstruction of the left anterior descending coronary artery is visible 2 cm beyond its origin (*upper arrow*).

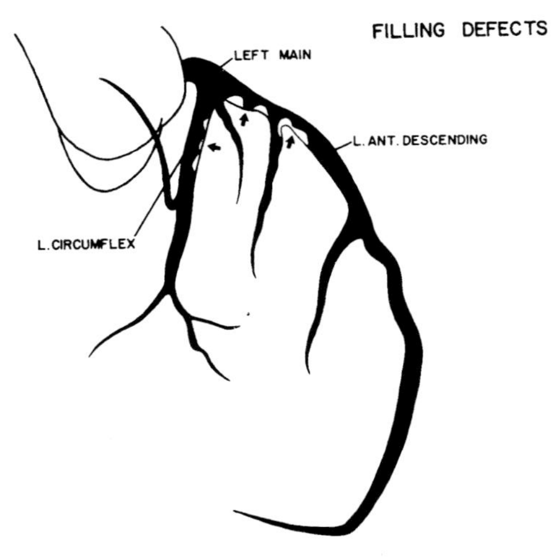
FILLING DEFECTS
LEFT MAIN
L. ANT. DESCENDING
L. CIRCUMFLEX

A

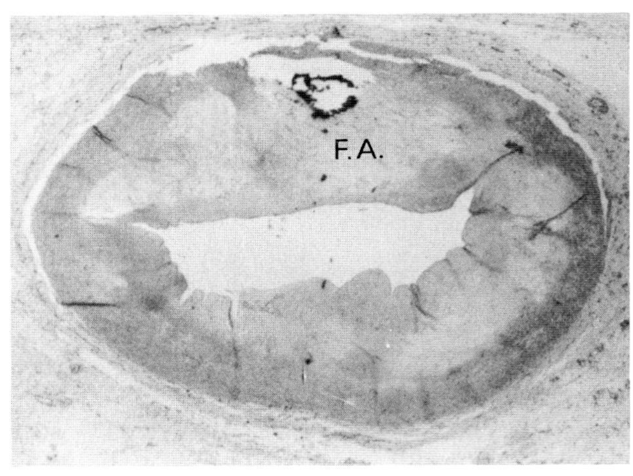
F.A.

B

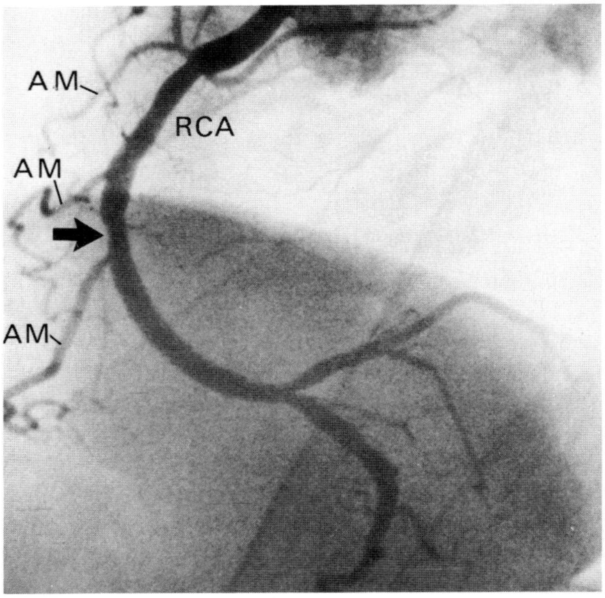

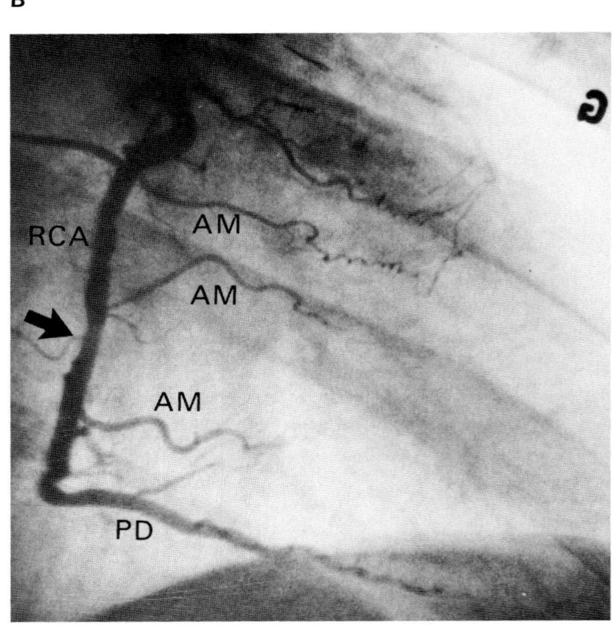
RCA
AM
AM
AM
PD

D

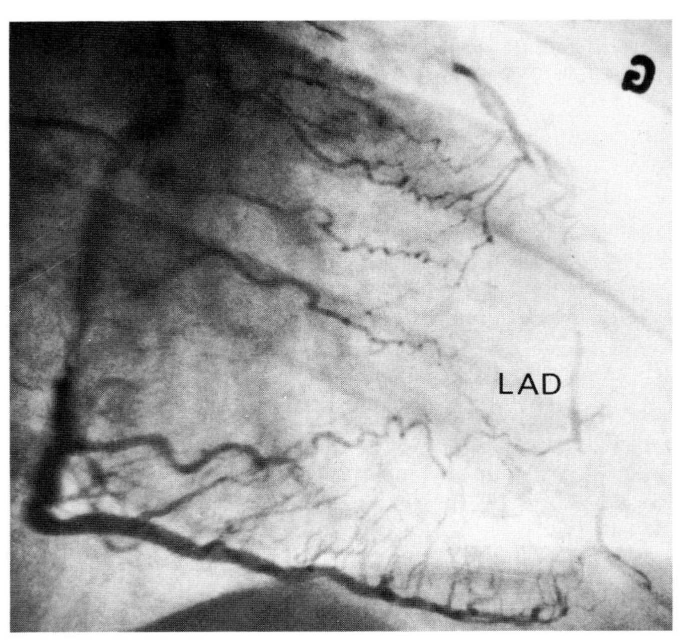
LAD

E

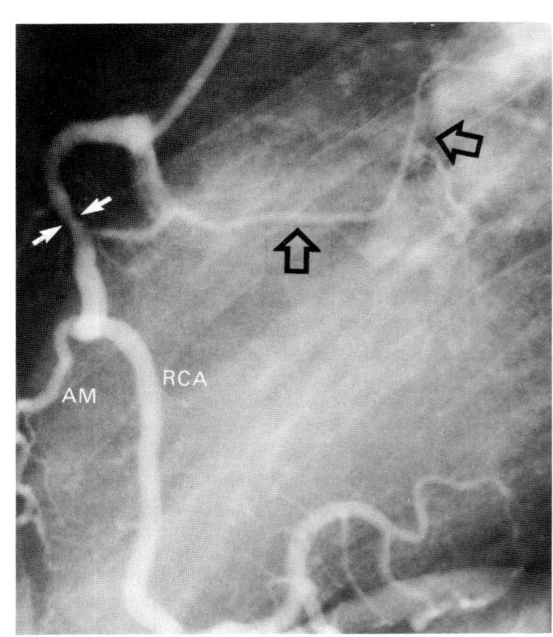
AM
RCA

F

Aneurysm

Local dilatation of the wall between two segments of vessel that may be normal in caliber is generally related to thinning and weakening of the media. The aneurysm (Fig. 26-8) may contain laminated thrombus. Localized aneurysm of coronary arteries is unusual, but Daoud et al. found it in 1.4 percent of 694 autopsies performed in patients over the age of 16 years.[81] It was located most commonly in the right coronary artery, followed by left main, LAD, and circumflex. Coronary aneurysms are often multiple[82] and appear to have an association with abdominal aortic aneurysm. Although usually asymptomatic, they apparently predispose to myocardial infarction. Rupture of a coronary artery may result in cardiac tamponade and death. Coronary artery aneurysm is most often arteriosclerotic,[83] with congenital origin next in frequency.[84,85] Coronary arterial aneurysms may also be due to mucocutaneous lymph node syndrome (Kawasaki disease)[86,87] and periarteritis nodosa,[88,89] or they may be mycotic,[90,91] dissecting,[92–94] or luetic.[95]

Kalke and Edwards[96] classified coronary aneurysms as follows:

I. Localized
   A. Congenital
   B. Acquired
      1. Atherosclerosis
      2. Inflammation
      3. Trauma
      4. Neoplasm
      5. Arteriovenous fistula
II. Dissecting
   A. Primary
   B. Secondary to aortic dissecting aneurysm
III. Diffuse arteriovenous fistula

Rarely, visualization of an annular calcification may suggest the diagnosis,[97] but a conclusive diagnosis during life can be made only by coronary artery imaging. Dissection is a rare complication.[92] Aneurysm of a coronary artery in patients with syphilis has also been reported.[95,98] Surgical treatment of coronary artery aneurysm is feasible.[84]

Ulceration

With undermining of the atheromatous plaque, a subatheromatous ulcer may form. This may have the appearance of a localized area of aneurysm formation because the contrast medium may project outside the expected lumen of the vessel. The process is best detected when the ulcer is filled with contrast agent and when undermined edges are visible (Fig. 26-9).

Calcification

A frequent accompaniment of atheroma formation, thrombus, and subatheromatous hemorrhage, calcification (Fig. 26-10) is usually visible during fluoroscopy before the coronary arteriogram. It is most extensive in the proximal segments of the vessels.[75]

When looked for fluoroscopically, it is recognized in 15 to 20 percent of patients over the age of 40.[99–101] At autopsy, it is found in as many as 70 percent of unselected subjects.[102,103]

The presence of calcification in the coronary arteries is associated with hemodynamically significant disease of at least one vessel in 50 to 75 percent of patients examined by arteriography.[104,105] This finding does not necessarily imply that the narrowing is located at precisely the site of the calcification. In the rare cases in which the calcification is medial, as in Mönckeberg sclerosis, the lumen may be normal or even dilated. Although patients with coronary calcification have a high incidence of significant disease,[104,105] they do not have an increased mortality as compared with those coronary disease patients in whom calcification is not visible.[99]

Text continues on page 650

◂ **Figure 26-2.** Filling defects. (A) Diagrammatic representation of selective left coronary arteriogram, RAO projection. (B) Low-power photomicrograph. Fatty atheroma (*F.A.*) is visible, resulting in marked thickening of the intima. There are multiple foam-filled, lipid-containing cells. (C) Selective right coronary arteriogram, LAO projection. A localized indentation (*arrow*) is visible in the right coronary artery proximal to the origin of the third acute marginal branch. (D) Same patient as in (C). Selective right coronary arteriogram, RAO projection. The region of the plaque covers a larger area (*arrow*) than is visible in (C). (E) Same patient as in (C) and (D). Multiple epicardial branches have extended over the surface to communicate with segments of the LAD, which is occluded 3 cm beyond its origin. Septal branches from the right posterior descending coronary artery also act as collateral vessels. (F) Selective right coronary arteriogram, LAO projection. The *small arrows* point to filling defects in the proximal right coronary artery. The *large open arrows* identify the sinoatrial node branch. Filling defects such as those seen in (C), (D), and (F) are due to large intimal plaques, fresh or organized thrombus overlying the plaques, hemorrhage beneath the plaques, or a combination of these factors. The orifice of the right coronary artery has a larger diameter than the proximal artery, a normal "funnel" shape.

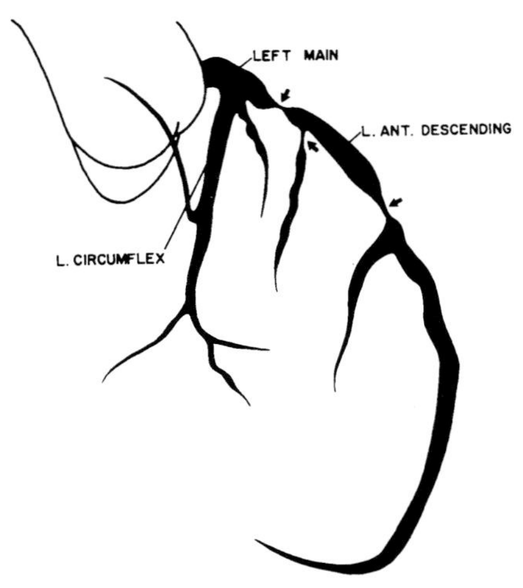

A

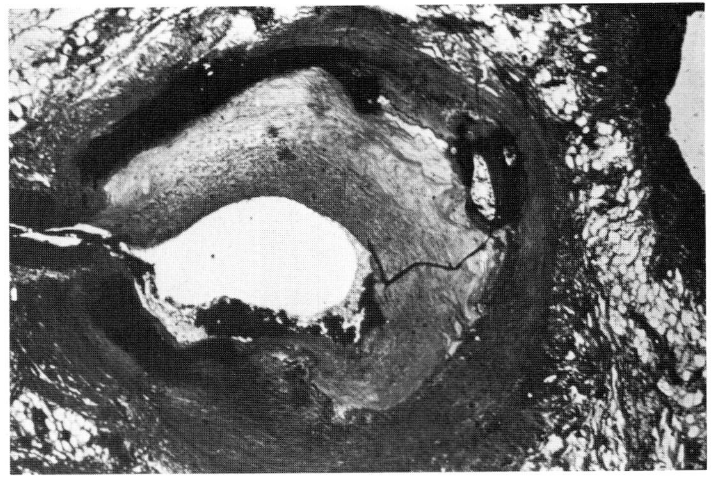

B

CONFIGURATION	APPEARANCE	RATIO OF SMALLEST TO GREATEST DIAMETER	ORDER OF FREQUENCY
ROUND		0.9–1.0	4
OVAL		0.6–0.8	1
BEAN		0.4–0.6	2
CRESCENT		0.3–0.5	3
ELONGATED		0.2–0.3	5
SLIT-LIKE		0.1–0.2	—
ECCENTRIC	—	—	59%
CONCENTRIC	—	—	41%

C

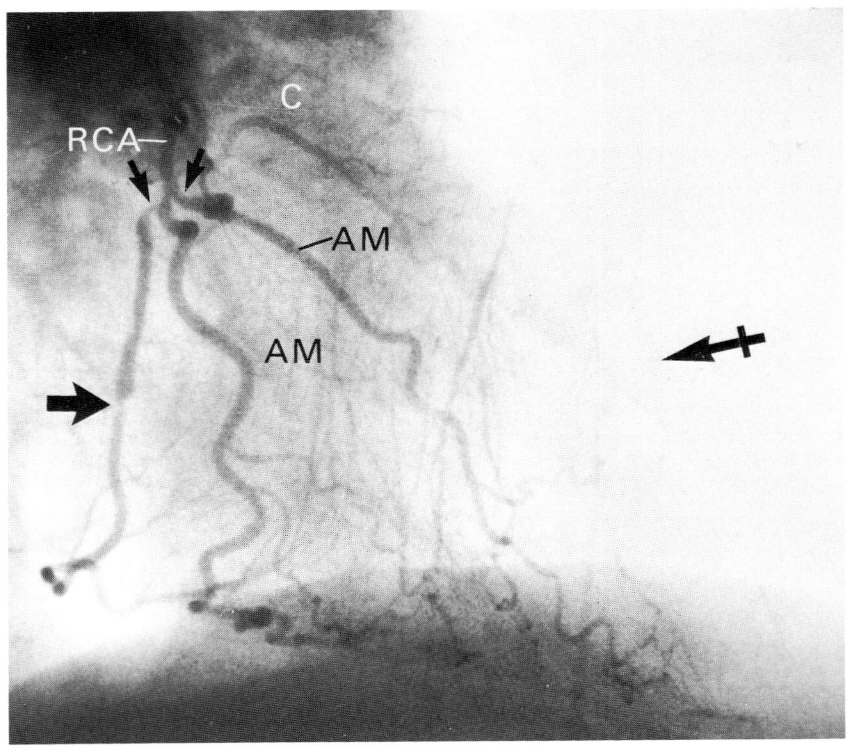

D

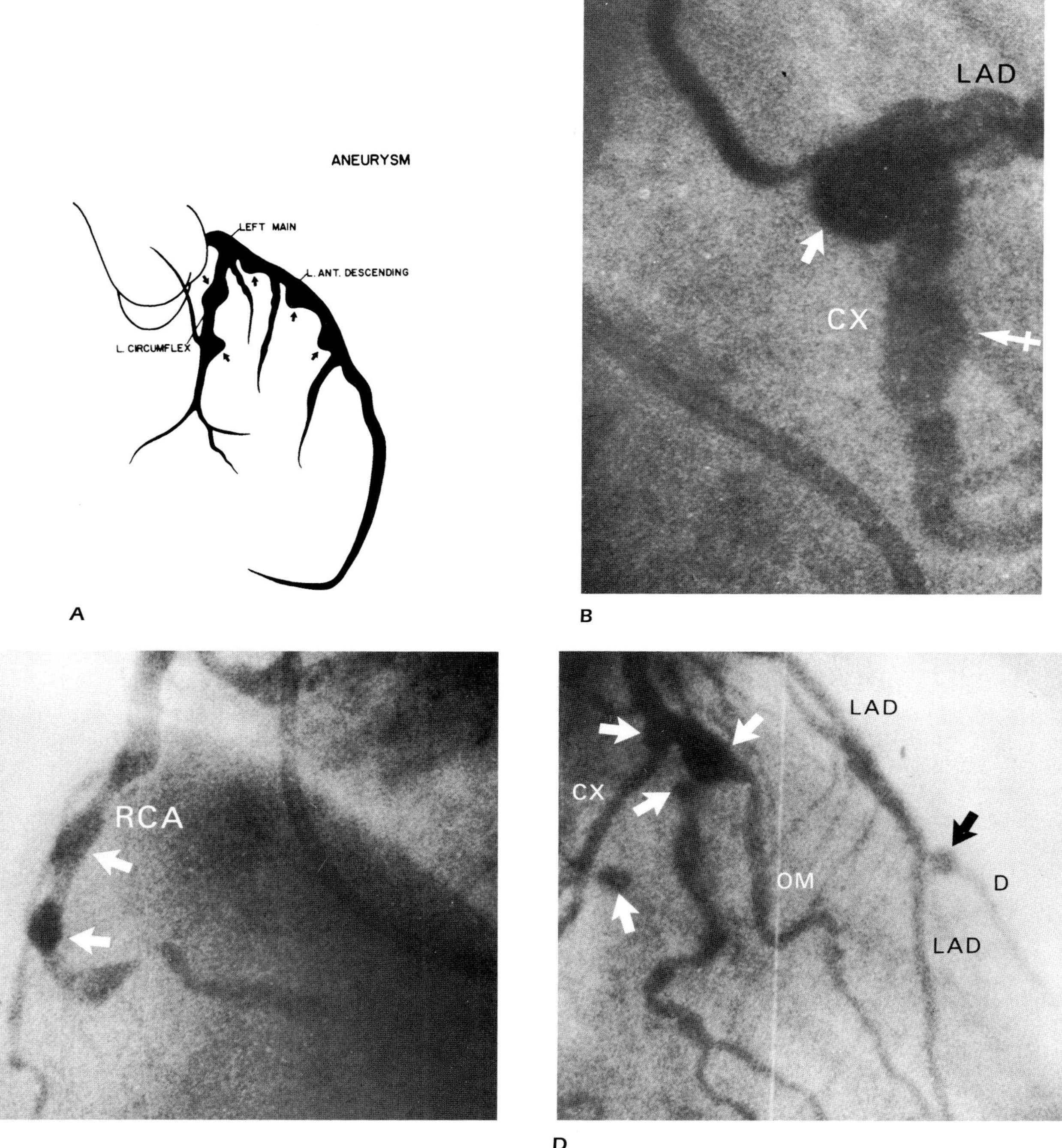

Figure 26-8. Aneurysm. (A) Diagrammatic representation of selective left coronary arteriogram, RAO projection. *Arrows* point to multiple bulges indicating the presence of multiple aneurysms. (B) Selective left coronary arteriogram, cine frame, RAO projection. A large aneurysm (*arrow*) of the left main coronary artery is defined, together with a more fusiform aneurysm (*barred arrow*) of the circumflex artery. (C) Selective right coronary arteriogram, cine frame, LAO projection. Multiple aneurysms are visible (*arrows*) in a dilated right coronary artery. These focal dilatations of the vessel wall are related to thinning and weakening of the media, just as is dilatation. (D) Selective left coronary arteriogram, cine frame, RAO projection. Multiple aneurysms (*arrows*) are visible in the LAD, circumflex, and obtuse marginal branches.

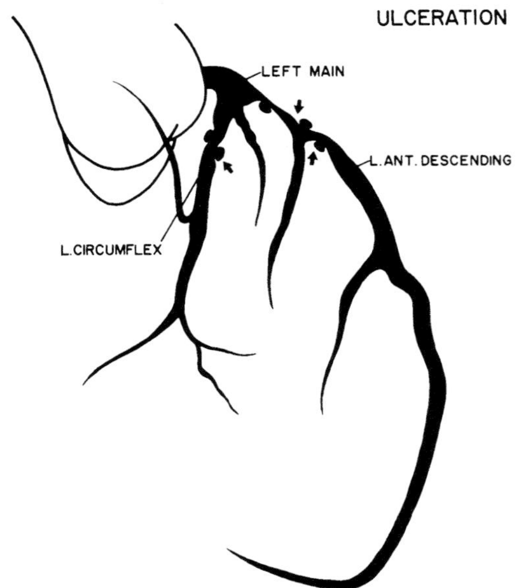

A

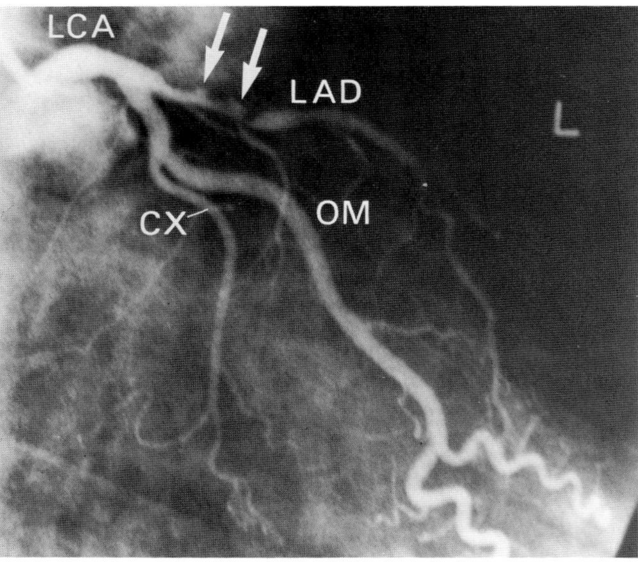

B

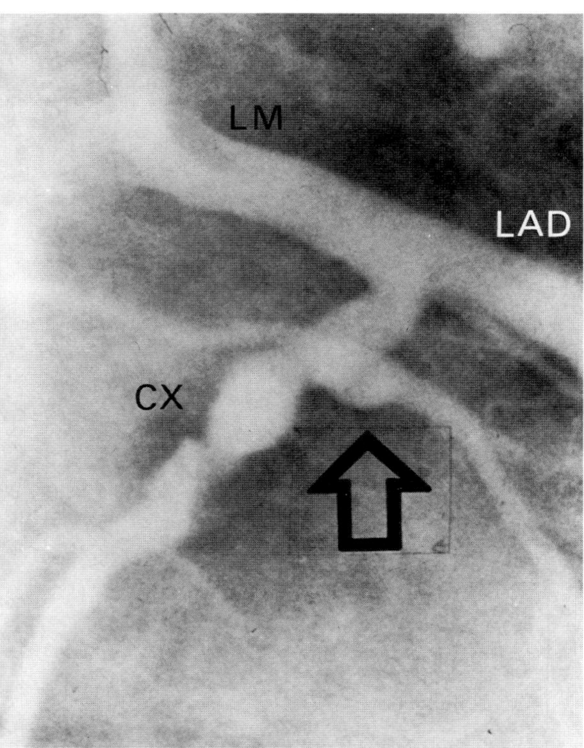

C

Figure 26-9. Ulceration. (A) Diagrammatic representation of selective left coronary arteriogram, RAO projection. *Arrows* point to multiple areas in which there has been undermining of plaques, with localized "ulceration." (B) Selective left coronary arteriogram, RAO projection. Just beyond the bifurcation of the left coronary artery into the LAD and circumflex branches, a long area of atheromatous involvement and narrowing is visible, with two subatheromatous ulcers (*arrows*) readily defined. (C) Selective left coronary arteriogram, RAO projection. Coronary artery ulceration. The left main coronary artery is normal, as is the visualized area of the left anterior descending artery. The circumflex vessel is involved with coronary atherosclerosis, and at the origin of the obtuse marginal branch from the circumflex artery (*arrow*) an undermined plaque is visible, with opacification by contrast agent representing a subatheromatous ulceration.

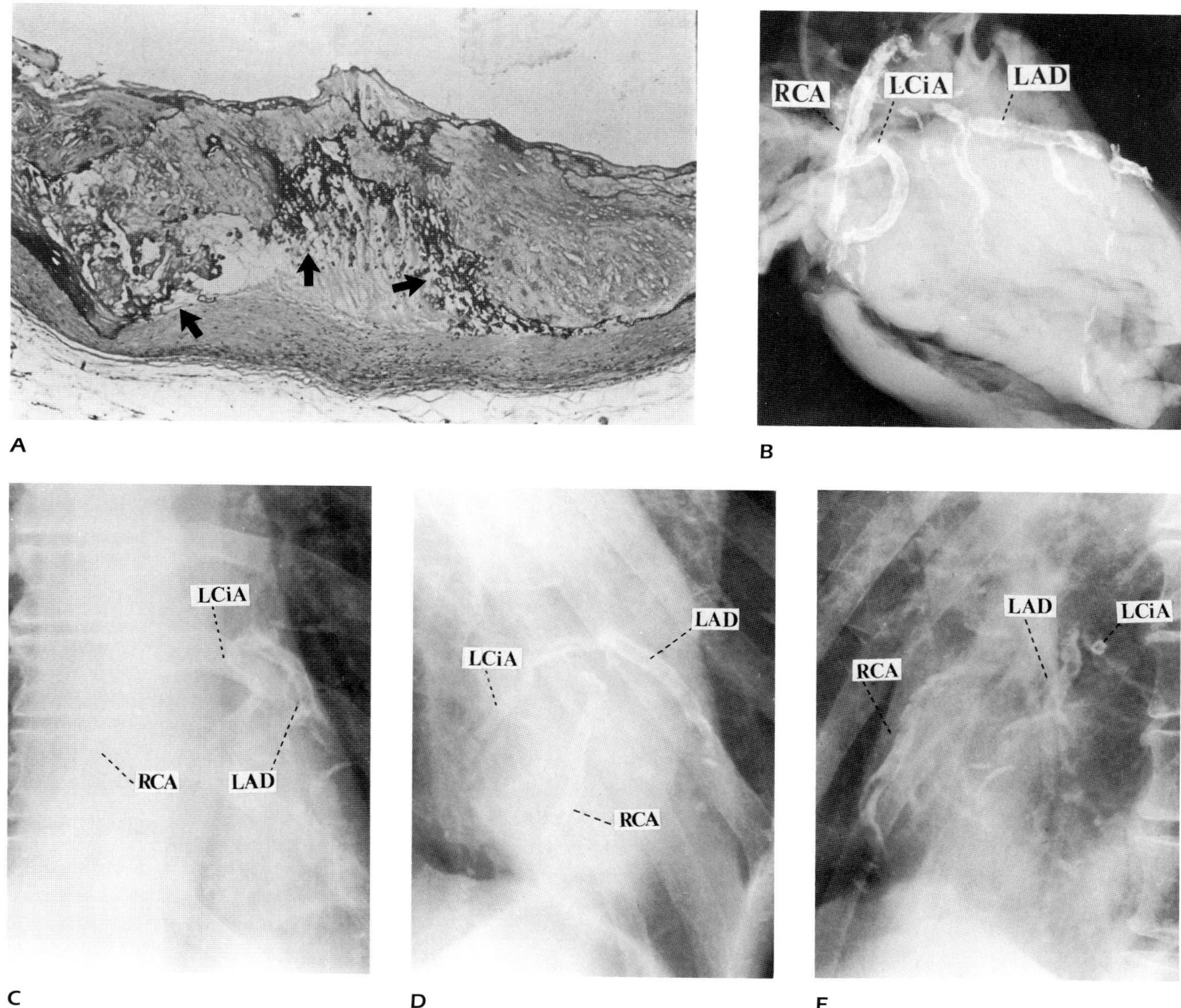

Figure 26-10. Calcification. (A) Photomicrograph of section of left anterior descending coronary artery showing marked atheromatous thickening of the intima. Calcification of the wall (*arrows*) is prominent, and is found microscopically at autopsy in the coronary arteries of a majority of patients over 60. (B) X-ray film of postmortem heart. Dense calcification is visible in virtually all branches of the coronary arteries, including the left anterior descending, the left circumflex and the right coronary arteries. Note that the lumen in the presence of calcification may be adequate, but that in this patient severe atherosclerosis has occluded the distal left anterior descending coronary artery and narrowed multiple branches. (C, D, and E) AP, RAO, and LAO chest films of a 73-year-old man who entered the hospital with pneumonia. Extensive calcification is visible in the major coronary arteries, including the left anterior descending, the left circumflex, and the right coronary artery branches. The calcification extends through the proximal portion of the arteries into the midportion of the left anterior descending and circumflex vessels, and more distally in the right coronary artery. It outlines a lumen that appears to be adequate in all branches.

Eusterman and colleagues[110] demonstrated marked discrepancies between postmortem angiographic and pathologic estimates of stenosis. These were particularly striking in focal lesions, in which underestimation was the rule rather than the exception. In 60 percent of nonfocal disease there was agreement between the two methods. Hale and Jefferson, in a correlative clinical pathologic study, found that arteriography underestimated disease and concluded that "the worst possible assessment is probably the most accurate."[111] In a similar study, Kemp et al. found a 16 percent error rate, mainly underestimation.[112]

Other investigations have not dispelled the concept that arteriography underestimates the severity of disease. Vlodaver et al. found this to be the case in one-third of coronary artery segments in which angiographic and pathologic findings were compared.[113] In yet another study, among 23 patients who died following coronary surgery, 9 (40 percent) had discrepancies between angiographic and postmortem findings.[114] Schwartz et al. noted 20 percent disagreement between cineangiographic and pathologic estimates of the degree of stenosis, three-quarters of them underestimates.[115]

In a study by Arnett et al.[116] in which angiographic findings were verified histologically, the degree of narrowing was also found to have been frequently underestimated angiographically. In all patients, a significant narrowing of at least one coronary artery was underestimated by one of three experienced angiographers who reviewed the antemortem angiograms. There were no overestimations. In the coronary arteries and their subdivisions narrowed histologically by 50 percent or less, there was a good correlation between the angiographic and histologic studies. In those narrowed 51 to 75 percent, underestimation occurred in 87.5 percent, and in those narrowed 76 to 100 percent, underestimation occurred in 40.5 percent. The authors suggested that the underestimation may arise because of the diffuse nature of the disease—the "normal" areas used as a baseline in the patients may themselves be diseased and so lead to underestimations of the degree of stenosis.

Murphy et al., comparing postmortem studies with angiography during life in patients who died within months after the arteriogram was obtained, found an unusually high accuracy of 86 percent.[117] False positives were most frequently seen in the right, left main, and circumflex marginal arteries on single or combined views. The LAD had few false positives. False negatives were most often seen in the posterior descending, proximal LAD, first diagonal, proximal and distal circumflex, and obtuse marginal arteries.[117]

A study by Staiger et al.[118] of 203 arteries at postmortem showed angiographic underestimation of severity in 47 percent, overestimation in 9 percent, and agreement in 44 percent. This study was of particular importance in that *70 percent of the vessels with "critical" (60–90 percent) stenosis were underestimated angiographically.* The authors suggested that in doubtful cases the indications for surgery should be broadened.

The importance of discrepancies in angiographic-pathologic correlation has been emphasized by Grondin et al.[114] In four of nine patients in whom there were important disagreements, death was thought to be related to the inexactness of the appraisal of coronary disease by angiography.

In summary, some observers have found good correlation between angiography and autopsy findings.[106,107,111,112,117,119] The majority of careful studies, however, have shown serious discrepancies and have raised important questions about the precision of the method in severe disease.

Explanation for Angiographic-Pathologic Discrepancies

It can be argued that the pathologist is by no means the court of last resort; the coronary arteries at postmortem are remote from the vascular bed of the functioning heart in vivo, perfused with relatively large volumes of fluid at high pressure. This line of reasoning would suggest that the pathologist overestimates rather than that the radiologist underestimates. It would hardly explain the discrepancies between postmortem arteriograms and pathologic studies obtained following coronary artery injection under pressure, with fixation of the injection mass.[109,110,118]

Some of the difficulties in correlating antemortem angiograms and postmortem pathologic studies are related to the progressive character of arteriosclerosis as a disease, and the fact that the postmortem studies have been performed months to years after the angiographic studies. This does *not* explain the poor correlation between *postmortem* arteriograms and pathologic examinations.

One problem that must be dealt with is the method of assessing stenosis of a coronary artery on arteriography. For the most part, this is based on a decrease in luminal diameter as compared to what is assumed to be the normal caliber. Because atherosclerosis is a diffuse disease, however, what appears to be normal may actually be a narrowed segment.[116] Furthermore, the pathologist is analyzing a blood vessel in cross section, whereas the arteriogram provides a two-dimensional view of altered diameter (Fig. 26-11).[80]

There are many other sources of error in the assessment of stenosis. Underestimation may be based on

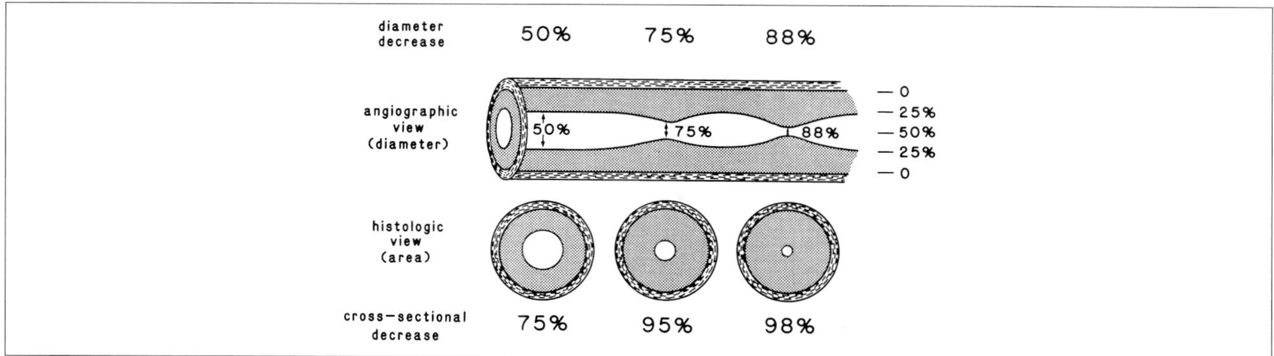

Figure 26-11. Diagrammatic representation of angiographic versus postmortem view and analysis of coronary artery stenosis. (From Arnett EN, Roberts WC. Acute myocardial infarction and angiographically normal coronary arteries: an unproven combination. Circulation 1976;53: 395. Used with permission.)

foreshortening, vessel overlap, eccentric lesions, severe proximal lesions, long segments with uniform involvement, and recanalization. Recanalization is of particular interest in that it is well documented arteriographically and may occur following total obstruction.[120] Recanalization is only rarely visualized because most patients are studied only once.

Overestimation may be based on spasm, myocardial bridging, anomalous origins, failure of some vessels to fill because of superselectivity, left coronary artery dominance, and layering of the contrast agent. Technical errors, such as obturation arteriography, slow contrast injection, poor filling, poor processing, and failure to recognize anatomic variants, may also make a significant contribution to lack of precision (see Chapter 28).

Limitations of Visual Interpretation of Angiograms

An equally important aspect has to do with the visual interpretation of the *degree* of coronary stenosis. Several studies have shown significant interobserver and intraobserver variability in the assessment of the degree of stenosis.[121,122] This disparity was as true of cineangiography as of 70-mm film and was observed with both subjective assessment of the degree of stenosis and objective measurement with calipers. In the study by Zir et al.,[122] only 65 percent of the time did all four readers agree that there was a significant stenosis in the proximal and/or mid–left anterior descending coronary artery. In one interesting analysis by Myers et al.[123] comparing 35-mm cine and 70-mm spot films, three experienced observers' variability was lowest on the cine, suggesting that the number of films per second may be more important than their resolution. Detre et al.[124] found that interobserver disagreement was largest when intraobserver inconsistency between two different readings was greater. Intraobserver agreement, on the other hand, correlated with the amount of experience in interpreting coronary arteriograms. DeRouen et al. found disagreement about the number of vessels with 70 percent stenosis in 31 percent of interpretations by 11 readers.[125] Most disagreements were observed in assessments of distal arterial segments, nonopacified segments, and films taken in severe disease or those that were technically inadequate. Fisher et al.[126] evaluated the reproducibility of interpretation of 870 coronary arteriograms in the Coronary Artery Surgery Study (CASS) by readers at two different centers. They found that the interpretation of proximal segment lesions was least reproducible ($p < 0.02$) in the left main coronary artery. The number of vessels with a 70 percent or greater stenosis was equal for all readers in approximately two-thirds of the films, but differed by one vessel in one-fifth of them. Reproducibility of interpretation was better among the studies judged to be of higher quality—emphasizing the importance of proper technique in the acquisition of angiograms.

Another source of potential error is represented by the physical limitations of the method. In a study using plastic tubes 1.5 to 5.0 mm in diameter as models, Bjork and O'Keefe found a progressive increase in deviation from the true diameter: 0.6 percent of the 5-mm tube, 4.8 percent of the 4-mm tube, 6.2 percent of the 3-mm tube, and 16 percent of the 1.5-mm tube.[121]

The visual estimation of *percent diameter stenosis,* which was once considered the "gold standard" for assessing the severity of disease, is now recognized for correlating poorly with more accurate measures of the "true" physiologic (or hemodynamic) significance of a stenosis.[77,127] However, the latter methods (e.g., translesional pressure gradient, intracoronary Doppler velocity measurements to assess coronary flow reserve, etc.) are not readily available in many catheterization suites and have some limitations of their own. Thus there remains a need for rapid and accurate estimation of stenosis severity in individual vessels, for example, when deciding about proceeding with angioplasty while the patient is on the table. In such cases, recent studies[128] suggest using simple quantitative coronary arteriography (e.g., computerized automatic edge detection, now more widely available on digital angiography units) or the *mean visual value* of the data from a (preferably large) panel of angiographers. The benefit of this proposed strategy is the improved accuracy and consistency in the estimation of the arteriographic severity of a stenosis, but not its true physiologic severity.

Grading of the Coronary Arteriogram

In many of the studies designed to relate the coronary arteriograms to the clinical and laboratory abnormalities of coronary disease, the arteriogram has been described as "abnormal," or a lesion as "potentially significant." Frequently, the abnormalities have been described or reproduced without any attempt to quantitate the observed changes.[129–131] In an effort to qualitatively describe the degree of disease on coronary arteriography, several grading systems have been suggested.[132–135] No standardized approach, widely applicable to all laboratories in which coronary arteriography is being performed, has evolved.

Proudfit et al.[135] used the following arteriographic classification of coronary disease: (1) none: normal vessels; (2) slight: minimal lesions (up to 30 percent narrowing); (3) moderate: 30 to 50 percent narrowing; (4) severe: 50 to 90 percent narrowing; (5) subtotal: 90 percent or more narrowing; and (6) total: complete obstruction. This classification was then redivided into none, minimal (less than 30 percent narrowing), and significant (30–100 percent). "Significant" was distinguished from "severe," which included severe, subtotal, and total.

Hultgren et al.[136] employed a grading system that took into account the severity of disease in all the major coronary arteries. Although only of historical interest now, such a classification embodies a broad statement as to the overall extent of major vessel disease.

Later, Brandt et al.[137] used a system in which the estimate of the severity of stenosis is expressed as a percentage of cross-sectional area lost. They also introduced a scoring system to evaluate the amount of myocardium jeopardized, by taking into account the number of vessels involved and the degree of stenoses within them.

No classification currently in use has been entirely satisfactory. The following classification provides a potentially common basis for understanding degrees of "abnormality" or "significance" in a broader framework than a single laboratory.

Normal vessels
- Grade 0

Abnormal vessels
- Grade I. Insignificant disease (mild)
  - A. Vessel irregularity
  - B. Stenosis (reduction in vessel diameter) of less than 50 percent, no slowing of flow, no collateral channels
- Grade II. Significant disease
  - A. Stenosis of less than 50 percent with segments longer than 1 cm involved with slowed flow or collateral channels (moderate)
  - B. Stenosis of 50 to 80 percent (moderate)
  - C. Stenosis greater than 80 percent (severe)
  - D. Occlusion (severe)

The number of major vessels involved is indicated parenthetically as 1, 2, 3, or 4. The specific major vessel is indicated by initial as follows: l = left main coronary, a = left anterior descending, r = right coronary, and c = left circumflex. A patient with occlusion of the right, left anterior descending, and circumflex arteries would be classified as grade II (D3, arc) (see Fig. 26-45). A patient with occlusion of the right and left anterior descending coronaries would be classified as grade II (D2, ar) (see Fig. 26-40). A patient with greater than 80 percent stenosis of the LAD artery and normal circumflex and right coronary arteries would be classified as grade II (Cl, a). In practice, to render this a useful classification that rapidly indicates the extent of disease, the following classes are employed:

Class 0. All individuals with normal arteries or a maximum grade I disease in up to four arteries
Class 1. Significant disease in one artery
Class 2. Significant disease in two arteries
Class 3. Significant disease in three arteries
Class 4. Significant disease in four arteries

Thus a class 4 would necessarily be a grade II (D4, larc). The above classification permits a relatively simple description in a form useful for analysis and comparison.

The interested reader is referred to a recent report from the Society for Cardiac Angiography & Interventions (SCA&I) on a totally computerized cardiac catheterization laboratory reporting system that is useful for data collection and analysis, clinical reporting, monitoring, and quality assurance purposes.[138]

Quantitative Coronary Arteriography

As alluded to earlier, the notion that the visual estimation of the degree of stenosis on arteriography reflects its actual physiologic significance has been discredited recently by several workers.[77,139,140] In addition, the relationship between the true hemodynamic compromise caused by a stenosis and the degree of narrowing demonstrated angiographically is poor, even if the more reproducible methods such as manual calipers, hand tracing, or expensive computerized edge detection techniques are used for quantification.[77,141] Common reasons for the limitations of these methods include the inability to identify a normal adjacent segment for comparison when diffuse disease is present, eccentricity of lesions resulting in inadequate demonstration on the acquired projections, and occasionally superimposed unrecognized spasm.

Earlier, Gould et al.[142] elegantly demonstrated the relationship between *coronary flow reserve* (the ratio of flow rate at maximum metabolic demand to flow rate at rest, normally 4:5) to percent diameter stenosis of isolated experimental lesions in carefully conducted studies in dogs with otherwise normal coronary arteries and hearts. They showed that, at rest, the point of critical ischemia (abrupt drop in blood flow) occurred at 90 percent diameter stenosis. With induced hyperemia, the point of critical ischemia occurred at about 50 percent, and the ability of the vessel to mount a hyperemic response was completely abolished at 90 percent stenosis. They concluded that the coronary flow reserve, a measure of the distal myocardial vasculature's ability to mount a vasodilator response to an increase in metabolic demand, progressively decreased with increasing severity of the stenosis and showed associated regional ^{99m}Tc-MAA-perfusion abnormalities.

Based on the above concepts, many workers have tried to quantitate coronary artery functional capacity in humans by studying the relationships between stenosis severity, or estimated translesional pressure gradients (or stenosis resistance) using fluid dynamic computations based on stenosis dimensions, and coronary flow reserve.[127,143–145] Unfortunately, with the exception of animal studies[127,146,147] and certain studies involving highly selected groups of patients with clearly defined coronary artery disease (e.g., isolated stenosis in a single vessel without collaterals and with limited symptoms) in which general relationships between coronary flow reserve and stenosis geometry are noted,[148–152] these concepts are otherwise difficult to apply in daily practice to individual patients. In fact, visual estimation of percent diameter is still widely used in most clinical catheterization laboratories even today.[153] However, rapid improvements in digital angiography may result in more widespread use of the more accurate and reproducible computer edge detection estimates of stenosis severity, and perhaps even coronary flow reserve using videodensitometric techniques and digital subtraction angiography.[146] Presently, *qualitative* descriptors of lesions (see section on angiographic morphology) are being recognized for their greater importance in determining a lesion's stability and its relation to clinical ischemic syndromes.[154] Nonetheless, the methods of *quantitative* coronary arteriography *must* be used for any clinical research on the natural history of coronary artery disease or its modulation with treatment.[139]

Appraisal of Significant Disease

Degree of Narrowing or Obstruction

When the coronary arteriogram shows normal vessels or only marginal irregularity or small filling defects, there is little likelihood of a hemodynamically significant lesion. When the artery is completely obstructed, or presents only a pinhole opening, there is equal certainty that perfusion beyond the arteriosclerotic lesion must be affected by the disease process.[155] Between these two extremes a large range of appearances and various degrees of stenosis must be evaluated. The most important single determinant of the hemodynamic effect of stenosis is the cross-sectional area of the vessel at the site of narrowing. The number of stenoses and their length, although less important,[156] nevertheless may also seriously affect distal perfusion.

Arterial stenosis may be divided into three major categories. The first group includes lesions with less than 50 percent narrowing of the luminal diameter. These lesions are usually not hemodynamically significant.[134–136] The second group consists of lesions with 50 to 70 percent decrease in diameter, and they are usually hemodynamically significant. The third group includes those with a decrease in diameter of two-thirds or more, which are invariably hemodynamically significant.

In experimental studies, a 75 percent reduction in the lumen of a large artery is required to decrease flow. In practice, a reduction of the diameter of the coronary artery by 50 percent or more is generally considered significant, representing as it does a 75 percent reduction in cross-sectional area. A two-thirds decrease in diameter represents a 90 percent decrease in cross-sectional area, and a 75 percent decrease in diameter implies a 95 percent reduction in cross-sectional area (see Fig. 26-11).[75,137] Long segments or multiple short segments of narrowing may cause significant ischemia before they are as severe as stenosis involving only a short segment. Thus fixed narrowings of 40 to 60 percent over 15 mm may produce decreases in coronary blood flow similar to those caused by short segments of luminal narrowing of 90 percent.[157]

Collateral Circulation

The presence of a developed collateral circulation always denotes a hemodynamically significant lesion. Evidence indicates that there are communications between the right and left coronary arteries larger than 40 μ in 33 to 78 percent of all cases, regardless of age.[158] Collaterals progressively involute during the first decade of life and reappear during the second decade. In the normal adult heart substantial collaterals are demonstrable. They are markedly increased in patients who have anemia. Reiner et al.'s data[158] are in contrast to those of Zoll, Wessler, and Schlesinger,[159] which showed collaterals in only about 9 percent of normal hearts. The latter emphasized that collaterals form only when the narrowing of the coronary arteries exceeds 75 percent of their diameter. With complete occlusion, their figures showed a frequency of approximately 80 percent, and with complete chronic occlusion, the incidence increased to 100 percent. Reiner et al.'s data suggest that collaterals are always present but become used significantly when occlusive coronary disease develops.

Major collateral pathways by which the myocardium receives its blood supply after arterial occlusion can be clearly delineated by arteriography (see Chapter 27). In the postmortem heart of the patient with coronary disease, extracoronary collaterals can be demonstrated in 77 percent of subjects[160]; during life the percentage shown is significantly less. It is likely that the severity of clinical manifestations is related not only to the degree of demonstrated stenosis in the major coronary branches but, to a major extent, to the presence and size of anastomotic channels.

Arteriographic Velocity of Flow

The velocity of flow in the coronary artery may be evaluated visually by cineangiography, but digital arteriography with videodensitometric analysis is more accurate and reproducible. Visual arteriographic appraisal frequently depends on comparing the filling rate in one vessel with that in another. Such comparisons may be invalidated by the presence of two- and three-vessel disease. Slow flow through and beyond an area of stenosis is often detectable both as delayed filling and as delayed washout. Its presence implies a significant lesion. Absolute velocity of flow may be quantified in humans by use of an intracoronary Doppler catheter,[77,150,161–163] which can also be used to determine in vivo coronary vasodilator reserve (see section on quantitative coronary arteriography in text preceding).

Ventriculography

As noted elsewhere in this chapter, ventriculography is an important indicator of the hemodynamic significance of coronary artery lesions. The ventriculogram most closely reflects myocardial damage after infarction, and, although it may be abnormal in ischemia, in many patients with single-vessel disease and no prior infarction, both the ventriculogram and ventricular hemodynamics may be normal.[164]

The Role of Radionuclide Studies

Just as contrast radiography is invaluable in reflecting ventricular contractility and function, so radionuclide cineangiography of the left ventricle[165] is useful in the evaluation of left ventricular function. Myocardial perfusion scanning with isotopes reflects the dynamic effects of arterial lesions on flow beyond the diseased portion of the vessel to the myocardial zone subserved by the vessel.[166] By and large, the sensitivity of such methods as thallium myocardial perfusion scintigraphy to the presence of coronary disease proved by ateriography is about 75 to 90 percent, and its specificity is even higher.[167] Quantitative thallium stress testing for the detection of coronary artery disease in patients with unstable angina has a sensitivity and a specificity of about 85 to 90 percent. Gould et al.[168] have reported that positron emission tomography (^{82}rubidium PET), using intravenous dipyridamole and hand grip exercise, has a sensitivity of 95 percent and a specificity of 100 percent for detecting stenotic disease causing a decrease in coronary flow reserve to below 3 (as determined by quantitative coronary arteriography). More importantly, it appears that PET is better able to identify viable myocardium and to differentiate it from scar tissue than planar thallium scanning alone[169] and thallium SPECT (single proton emission computed tomography) scanning.[170] Because radionuclide studies are noninvasive in character, they are a valuable adjunct to coronary arteriography and frequently strengthen the appraisal of the hemodynamic significance of the arterial lesion.

The Relationship of the Angiographic Morphology of Coronary Artery Lesions to Clinical Syndromes

Autopsy studies indicate that, early in the disease process, atherosclerotic human coronary arteries undergo a compensatory enlargement in lumen area in response to plaque development, and that a hemodynamically significant stenosis occurs later, only after the lesion occupies at least 40 percent of the area within the internal elastic lamina.[171] This may explain why patients with "chest pain" and insignificantly narrowed coronary arteries have a good long-term prognosis, with subsequent cardiac events most likely related to disease progression.[172] However, early symptoms may be related to a defective endothelial vasodilator response or other biochemical abnormalities in atherosclerotic arteries.[173]

Levin and Fallon[174] compared postmortem coronary arteriographic morphology to histologic examination of subtotal stenoses. Classifying lesion borders into angiographically smooth (hourglass-shaped lesions without intraluminal lucencies) and angiographically irregular (with intraluminal lucencies) types, they showed that a large majority of the latter lesions, but only a small minority of the former, had complex pathologic morphology consisting of plaque rupture, hemorrhage, and superimposed thrombus. Such intracoronary thrombosis occurs more frequently in the early hours of acute myocardial infarction,[175] and is also noted in victims of sudden death.

Early clinical studies demonstrated a relationship between unstable angina and progression in the extent and severity of coronary artery disease on angiograms.[176] Subsequently, an increased frequency of intracoronary filling defects, presumably thrombi, on angiograms of patients with unstable angina (37 percent, versus 0 percent for those with stable angina) was reported.[177] Ambrose et al.,[178] extending the work of Levin and Fallon,[174] demonstrated clinically that eccentric asymmetric stenoses with narrow necks and/or irregular borders (type II eccentric) were significantly more frequently seen on the angiograms of patients with unstable angina, whereas eccentric stenoses with broad necks and/or smooth borders (type I eccentric) were more frequently seen with stable angina. They speculated that the type II lesions probably represented acutely ruptured atherosclerotic plaques and/or partially occlusive thrombi that were actively causing symptoms through transient reduction in perfusion due to local alterations in vasomotor tone, and proposed that this type of lesion was an "angiographic marker" for unstable angina pectoris. These findings have been corroborated by others.[179–181] The degree of ulceration of a plaque has also been reported to be a marker for a "high-risk" lesion related to unstable angina and subsequent myocardial infarction.[163,182,183]

Further evidence supporting the theory that acute symptoms are related to abrupt rupture of preexisting plaque causing acute coronary occlusion was provided by Little et al.,[184] who found that stenosis severity on an initial angiogram does not accurately predict the site or time of a subsequent infarct-related occlusion. Moreover, a significant number of subsequent occlusions occurred at sites that were previously noted to have nonsevere plaques.[182] Ambrose et al.[185] reported similar findings, but found in addition that non–Q-wave infarctions were more likely to occur because of more severe preexisting stenoses than Q-wave infarctions, presumably because the myocardium was protected in the former case by the development of collateral vessels.[186] Ellis et al.[187] evaluated the angiographic morphology of left anterior descending artery lesions of 118 patients treated medically (from the Coronary Artery Surgery Study [CASS]) who had anterior myocardial infarctions (AMI) in the subsequent 3 years and compared them to 141 patients who did not have subsequent AMI. They found that lesion roughness was highly correlated to the risk of future myocardial infarction, being second in importance only to stenosis severity. Lesion roughness presumably predisposes to increased local thrombus formation.

Sansa et al.[188] reported that patients with intracoronary thrombi and eccentric or multiple lesions on their angiograms were less likely to respond to medical therapy than patients with concentric stenoses or even total occlusions. Emergency bypass surgery was more commonly needed for the former group. Similarly, complex stenosis morphology and intracoronary thrombus have been reported to be associated with a higher incidence of in-hospital cardiac complications such as infarction, bypass surgery, and death.[189] Subsequently, intracoronary thrombus was noted to be the best angiographic predictor of cardiac events, but the frequency of its detection was related to the time between symptoms (angina at rest) and the performance of the angiogram.[190] Thus the presence of intraluminal thrombus serves as an angiographic marker and suggests a common mechanism for the acute ischemic syndromes of unstable angina, prolonged rest angina, and myocardial infarction.[191,192]

Plaque rupture and thrombus formation appear to be the central event in the continuum of acute coronary syndromes from unstable angina and myocardial infarction[186] to sudden cardiac arrest and death.[193–196] In light of these recognized clinical implications, all diagnostic interpretations of coronary arteriograms must include an appropriate qualitative description of lesion morphology.

Angina and Myocardial Infarction with Angiographically Normal Coronary Arteries

Patients exhibiting angina with normal coronary arteries, as compared to those with coronary artery disease, are younger as a group,[197] are more commonly women,[198] are less frequently relieved by nitroglycerin,[197] and have a life expectancy similar to that of the general population.[199] Although the "normal" coronary arteries in some of these patients have been attributed to poor angiographic technique,[200] there are many well-documented cases in which excellent studies have been performed.[201] Among the numerous explanations, spasm,[202] small-vessel disease (as in collagen disorders or amyloidosis,[200] myocardial bridges, mitral valve prolapse, altered oxyhemoglobin dissociation,[198] cardiomyopathy,[203] arterial thrombi,[204] and platelet thrombi have all been suggested as potential sources of the myocardial ischemia in these patients.

Many of the same factors have been considered responsible for myocardial infarction in patients with normal coronary arteries. The combination of spasm and platelet aggregates has been viewed as a possible mechanism in documented cases of infarction examined by arteriography within 12 hours of the onset of symptoms.[205]

Papanicolaou et al.[172] studied the prognosis of 1977 symptomatic patients with angiographically normal and insignificantly narrowed major epicardial coronary arteries. With the exception of mitral valve prolapse, patients with the other explanations listed above for ischemic symptoms, and specifically those with spasm, were excluded. Patients from both groups had a 98 percent survival rate at 10 years. The myocardial infarction–free survival rate was higher for patients with normal coronary arteries than for those with initially insignificant disease (98 percent versus 90 percent at 10 years). However, both groups continued to have chest pain, which resulted in the use of medication, hospitalization, and job disability.

Nordenstrom[206] has described a number of patients with angina pectoris who have wide or normal central coronary arteries without evidence of arteriosclerosis but with a marked lack of small branches from these arteries. Although such evidence suggests peripheral small-vessel obstruction as a cause of angina in these patients, the conclusion has not been adequately corroborated by pathologic study. The matter of small-vessel disease continues to be a subject of debate,[207–210] but one thing is clear: there are syndromes in which small-vessel disease occurs that is beyond the resolution of the best coronary arteriography.[211] Arnett and Roberts believe, however, that "the most reasonable explanation appears to be acute coronary embolism with subsequent clot lysis, retraction, or recanalization."[80] Patients with ventricular aneurysm and normal coronary arteries represent an equally mystifying and poorly explained group.[212] Resolution and fragmentation of thrombus, spasm, and hemorrhage into a plaque with regression or absorption of hemorrhage have been suggested as factors underlying initial coronary obstruction, infarction, and aneurysm formation with subsequent disappearance of obstruction.[212]

The Arteriogram in Coronary Arteriosclerosis

The Left Coronary Artery

The left coronary artery represents the major source of blood supply to the left ventricle, and consequently disease in the main vessel or any of its branches may have a critical effect on the muscle. The left coronary artery supplies the free wall of the left ventricle, the apex, the anterior area of the interventricular septum, and, to a lesser and variable extent, the posterior left ventricular myocardium. Disease in any one of the branches subserving these areas may produce ischemia and/or infarction, with consequent alteration of the contractile capacity of the involved area.

Arteriosclerotic disease may affect the left coronary artery at any point along its distribution. Because the left ventricle is the major pumping chamber of the heart, disease in this vascular bed critically influences viability of the myocardium and ultimate prognosis.

Left Main Coronary Artery

The left main coronary artery extends from the orifice to the bifurcation into the left anterior descending and the circumflex arteries. Alternatively there may be a trifurcation into the left anterior descending, ramus medianus, and left circumflex arteries. Under these circumstances, the ramus medianus or intermediate branch covers much of the anterolateral portion of the ventricle, in precisely the areas where the diagonal arteries are generally distributed.

Hemodynamically significant stenosis of the left main coronary artery is particularly important because it jeopardizes the portions of muscle subserved by both the left anterior descending and the circumflex arteries, and therefore the major portion of the left ventricular myocardium. Furthermore, in patients with disease of the left main coronary artery, arteriography, surgery, and medical therapy all carry a higher risk than in patients with any other individual branch disease.

The mortality of coronary arteriography in patients with left main disease has averaged 2.3 percent of all cases reported in the literature in the past, with a range of 1 to 16 percent.[213] Despite the fact that mortality in many laboratories today is much lower than these figures, the suspicion of left main disease necessitates special precautions. A sinus injection should be performed initially. If left main disease is present, the study should be somewhat limited. In particular, positioning of the catheter tip should be undertaken cautiously. The catheter tip should be withdrawn immediately if there is any damping of the pressure trace. On completion of the contrast injection, immediate catheter withdrawal from the artery is indicated. Repeat injection should be avoided whenever possible. Nitroglycerin should be used when angina develops.

When a left main coronary lesion is present and selective right coronary arteriography is performed, depending on catheter position and injection rate there may be temporary ischemia of the left ventricular myocardium, and arrhythmias may result. Similarly, when the catheter enters the left main coronary artery in the presence of unsuspected left main coronary disease, occlusion may occur as the catheter reaches the stenosed area, and the blood supply to the left ventricle then must come through collateral pathways.

The length of the left main coronary artery is variable,[214] and in conventional coronary arteriograms, lesions within the left main may be obscured either by foreshortening or by overlap. As a consequence, it is essential to obtain cranial and caudal angled views of the left main, as of the left anterior descending coronary artery, in any cases in which disease is suspected.[215–217]

Figures 26-12 and 26-13 illustrate the classic appearance of left main coronary disease. The bolus study in Figure 26-12A shows complete occlusion less than 1 cm beyond the orifice, whereas Figure 26-12B shows stenosis at and beyond the orifice. In Figure 26-12C, the left main trunk is short, and a severe stenotic lesion is located just proximal to the bifurcation. The coexistence of severe LAD and circumflex lesions with a tight distal left main stenosis is demonstrated in Figure 26-12D to F. In Figure 26-12F, the angled view indicates the presence of virtual occlusion of the left main coronary artery. Figure 26-13 emphasizes the importance of angled views in revealing the full extent of left main disease.[216,217]

The arteriographic definition of the degree of left main stenosis is an important predictor of survival with medical therapy. Although the 3-year survival rate with 70 percent stenosis or greater is only 49 percent, with stenosis less than 70 percent a 3-year survival rate of 66 percent has been found.[218] The operative mortality in left main coronary disease in the past has averaged 12 percent[213,219–224] but is presently approximately 2.5 percent, increasing to 4 percent when there is abnormal left ventricular function.[225] Despite the relatively high operative mortality, the Veterans Administration Cooperative Study appears to have shown conclusively that the prognosis of patients treated surgically is better than it is for those treated medically.[222]

The identification of this group of patients, therefore, has been a matter of overriding interest to physicians. "Crescendo" angina has been considered one of the presenting syndromes associated with ischemia of left main coronary disease; although it may well alert the physician to the possible presence of left main disease, it is per se an unreliable predictor of left main disease.[226]

The electrocardiogram, in left main disease, frequently shows at least 2 mm of S–T segment depression on exercise, although it may be normal at rest. The absence of chest pain or of electrocardiographic changes during exercise renders the possibility of a left main lesion somewhat unlikely.[226]

Left main disease frequently coexists with lesions in the left anterior descending, circumflex, and right coronary arteries (see Fig. 26-12). In isolated form it is relatively rare. Nevertheless, approximately 7 percent of all patients who are studied by coronary arteriography, usually because of angina pectoris, demonstrate left main coronary artery disease.[138] When such patients are found in whom crescendo angina is an important aspect of the clinical presentation, an aggressive approach to surgical therapy is usually warranted.

Lesions affecting the left main coronary artery may be precisely at or near the orifice (see Fig. 26-12A and B) and, if so, may be caused by luetic aortitis as well as by arteriosclerosis. When ostial stenosis is severe, the angiographic catheter may obstruct the vessel completely, with an abrupt onset of acute myocardial ischemia.[227] Bypass surgery in orificial stenosis can be successfully performed, with relief of symptoms. When orificial stenosis is arteriosclerotic in origin, it is usually associated with arteriosclerosis of the sinus of Valsalva from which the coronary artery arises.[227] Disease may be present throughout any portion of the left main coronary artery (see Fig. 26-12C to F), which is variable in length and tends to be shorter in the presence of aortic stenosis. Some left main lesions occur almost at the bifurcation (see Fig. 26-12C) and may then in-

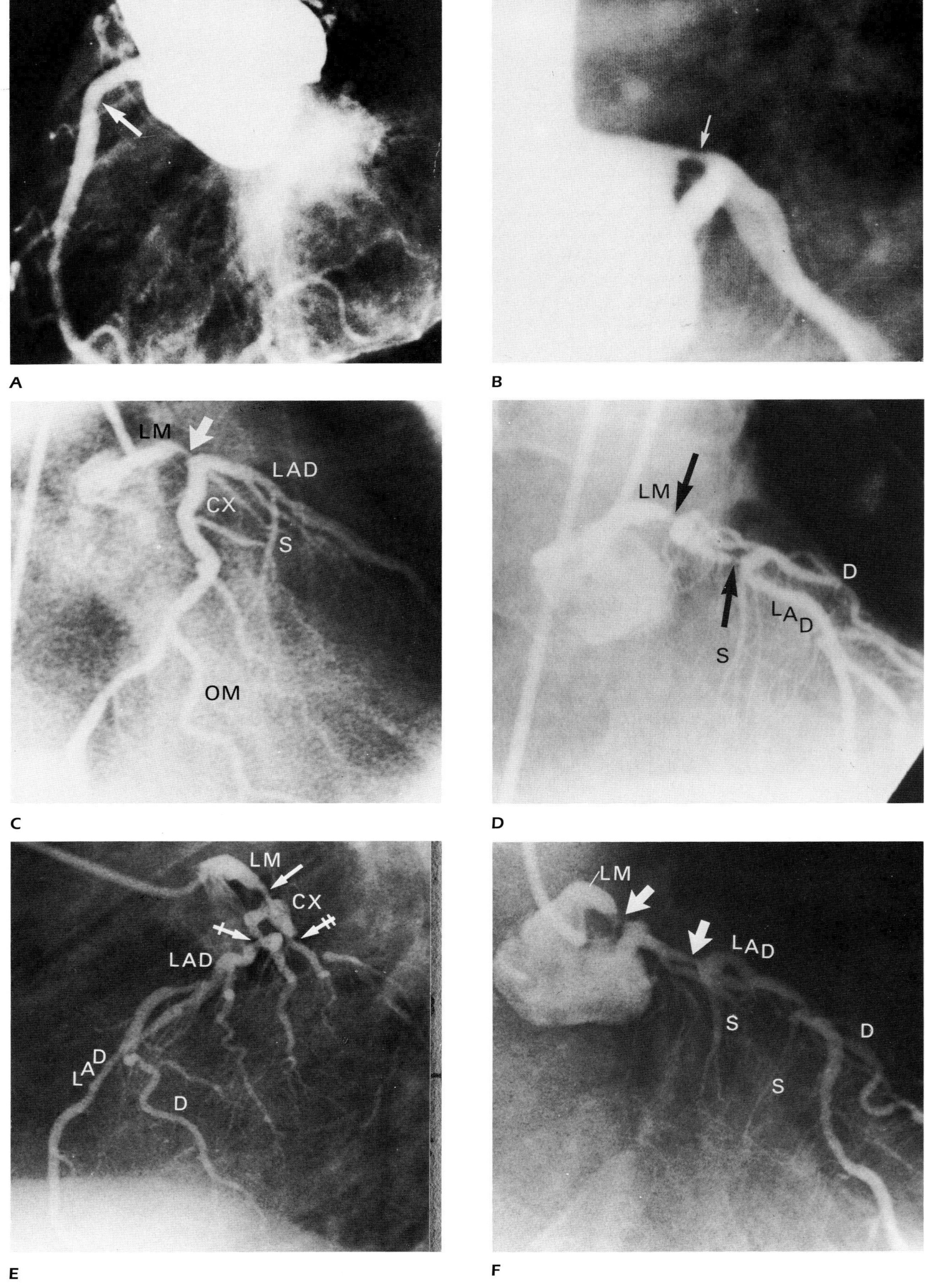
A
B
LM
LAD
CX
S
OM
C
LM
D
LAD
S
D
LM
CX
LAD
LAD
D
E
LM
LAD
S
D
S
F

volve the left anterior descending and/or the circumflex artery.

Left Anterior Descending Branch

The left anterior descending coronary artery has been called the artery of sudden death. Because it supplies the anterolateral wall and the apex of the ventricle, sudden occlusion in the absence of collateral vessels may produce massive infarction and necrosis of a large portion of the left ventricular myocardium. In women under the age of 50 studied for chest pain, the LAD is the vessel most frequently involved.[228] In all patients, if only single-vessel disease is present, it is most commonly in the LAD.[229]

The LAD arises at the bifurcation of the left main coronary artery and passes anteriorly and to the left in the anterior interventricular groove. Its length is variable. In most instances, it bends over the apex of the heart to supply the apical segment in its entirety. A long LAD may extend over the apex and into the inferodiaphragmatic area, supplying myocardium that usually receives its blood supply from the posterior descending artery. Occlusion of such a long vessel may produce a larger area of infarction than occlusion of a short LAD. With a short LAD, the apex receives some of its blood supply from other branches, which will continue to supply apical muscle even after LAD obstruction.

It is well known that single-vessel coronary disease has a better survival rate at 5 and 10 years than double- or triple-vessel disease.[230,231] Although the annual mortality of patients with single-vessel disease is less than 3 percent,[232] if the single vessel involved is the LAD the mortality is nearly double, at 5 percent.[233] The site of stenosis of the LAD is an important determinant of prognosis.[234] If infarction is associated with isolated LAD stenosis, the prognosis is worse than with inferior myocardial infarction.[230] From a hemodynamic point of view, ejection fraction is unaffected by isolated stenosis of the LAD unless myocardial infarction is present.[164] Nevertheless, subtle contraction abnormalities are visible in LAD stenosis even in the absence of myocardial infarction. The interpretation of LAD disease requires a careful documentation in a number of different projections of the presence, the location, and the degree of the disease. For example, it is essential that its relationship to the first septal artery be identified, because there are data indicating that left ventricular performance and prognosis in the presence of stenosis or occlusion of the LAD proximal to the first septal artery are worse than with patients in whom the first septal artery remains as an important collateral pathway for distal left coronary artery perfusion.[164,235] Lesions may be eccentric or concentric and may occur at the origin of the LAD or at any point in its course. Approximately three-quarters of all lesions occur within the first 3 or 4 cm of the branch, and the most severe narrowing usually develops in the first 2 cm.[75] It is important to be fully conversant with the distribution of diagonal branches from the LAD, because the absence of a diagonal branch could represent either a congenital abnormality or complete occlusion. The distinction between the two may generally be accomplished by observing the distribution pattern of diagonal branches over the ventricular myocardium. A significant gap frequently means that occlusion of a branch has occurred.

In the LAO projection, complete occlusion of the LAD may be overlooked because of a large septal branch that appears to run in the area of the LAD. Similarly, a large diagonal branch may be mistaken for the LAD. Under these circumstances, the RAO projection is often helpful, but at times the frontal and

◀ **Figure 26-12.** Left main coronary artery disease. (A) Bolus aortogram, LAO projection, showing occlusion adjacent to the orifice. There is complete occlusion of the left main coronary artery 1 cm beyond its origin. The left anterior descending coronary artery filled via collateral branches from the right coronary artery. Note the discrete plaque in the right coronary artery just beyond the origin (*arrow*). (B) Stenosis adjacent to the orifice; bolus aortogram, LAO projection. There is marked stenosis of the LCA near its origin (*arrow*). Narrowing is present at the orifice and extends into the vessel for about 6 mm. The vessels beyond the narrowing appear to be relatively smooth and free of disease. (Courtesy of Sven Paulin, M.D.) (C) Stenosis, distal left main coronary artery. Selective left coronary arteriogram, RAO projection. Marked stenosis is visible (*arrow*), involving the distal one-third of a short left main coronary artery. There is minimal arteriosclerosis in the LAD but no other apparent major areas of disease in the left system. (D, E, and F) Severe left main coronary disease. RAO projection (D) shows marked stenosis of the left main coronary artery and the LAD (*arrows*). Lateral projection (E) better defines the length of the stenotic segment in the left main coronary artery (*arrow*). The left anterior descending coronary artery stenosis is apparent (*barred arrow*), as is severe disease in the left circumflex artery (*double-barred arrow*). Note also stenosis of the origin of the diagonal branch. RAO projection with caudal angulation (F) clearly shows virtual occlusion of the left main coronary artery (*proximal arrow*) and severe stenosis of the LAD (*distal arrow*). The distal LAD is remarkably normal in caliber. The absence of filling in the circumflex artery reflects the presence of occlusion. Note also that the LAD lesion is proximal to the first septal branch, precluding its use as an effective collateral in the event of more distal disease.

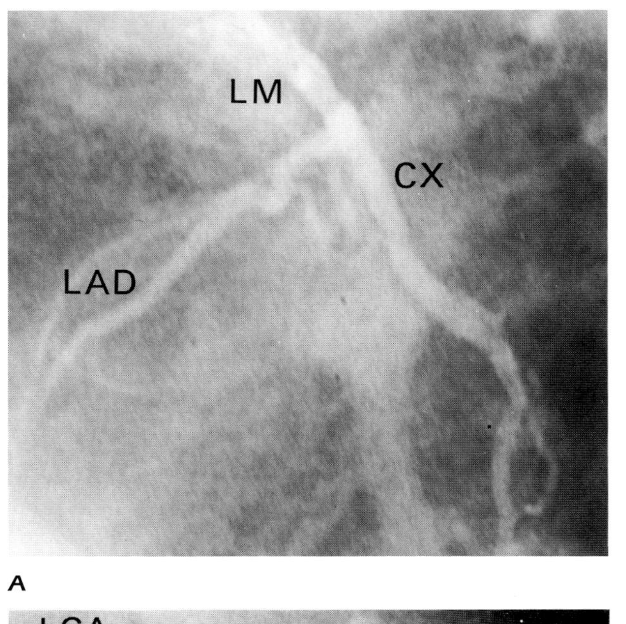

A

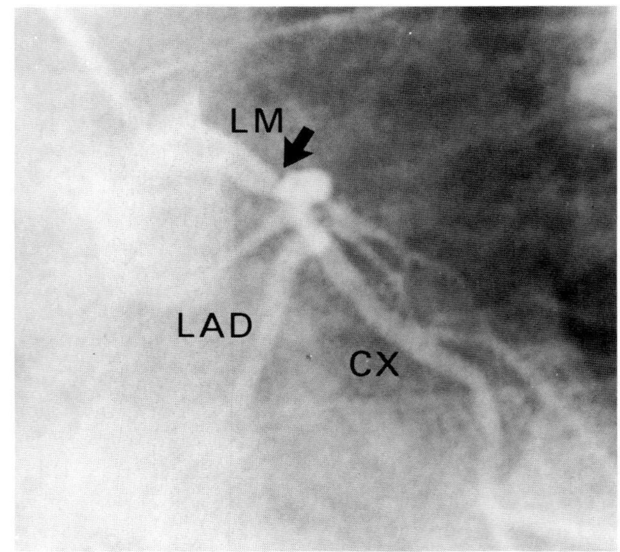

B

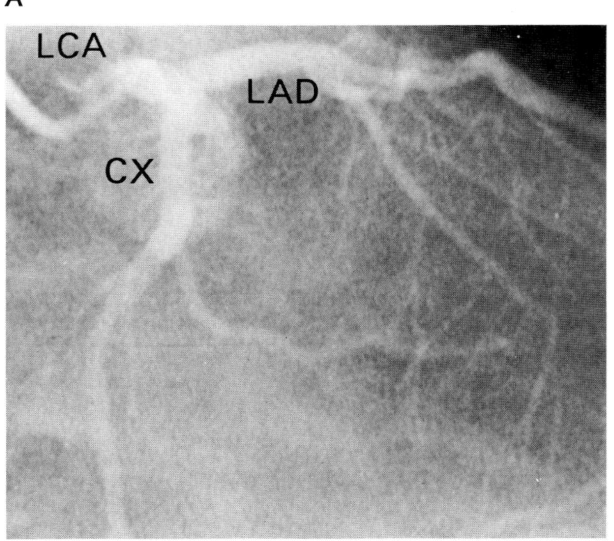

C

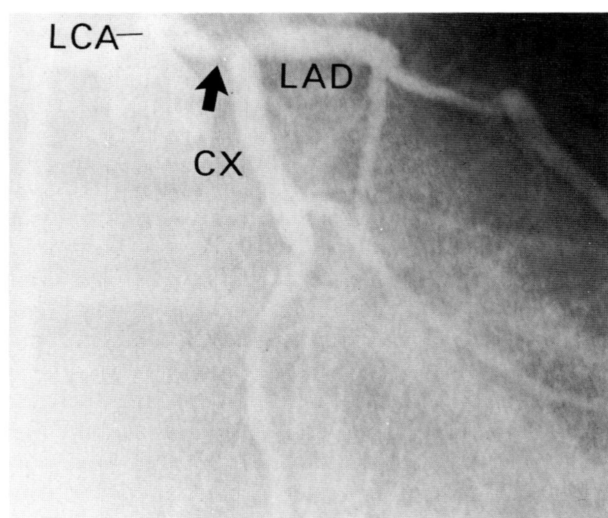

D

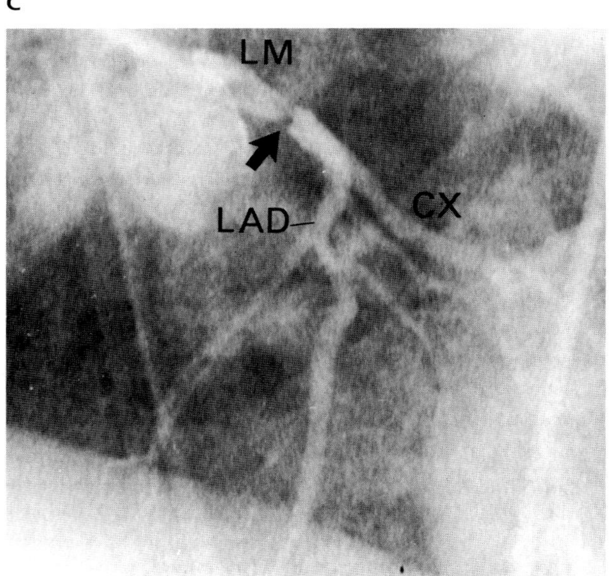

E

Figure 26-13. Left main coronary artery stenosis. Selective left coronary arteriogram, selected cine frames. (A) Lateral projection. No definite stenosis in the LAD, left main, or circumflex arteries is visible. (B) LAO projection. A suggestion of stenosis in the left main artery (*arrow*) is now seen, but the degree of narrowing cannot be assessed. (C) RAO projection. No evidence of narrowing of the major coronary arteries is seen. (D) RAO projection with caudal angulation. It is now apparent that there is significant stenosis of the left main coronary artery (*arrow*) just proximal to the bifurcation into the circumflex and left anterior descending arteries. Stenosis of the LAD is also present. (E) LAO projection with cranial angulation. Profound stenosis of the left main coronary artery is visible (*arrow*), best assessed in this projection. The LAD stenosis is less obvious than in (D).

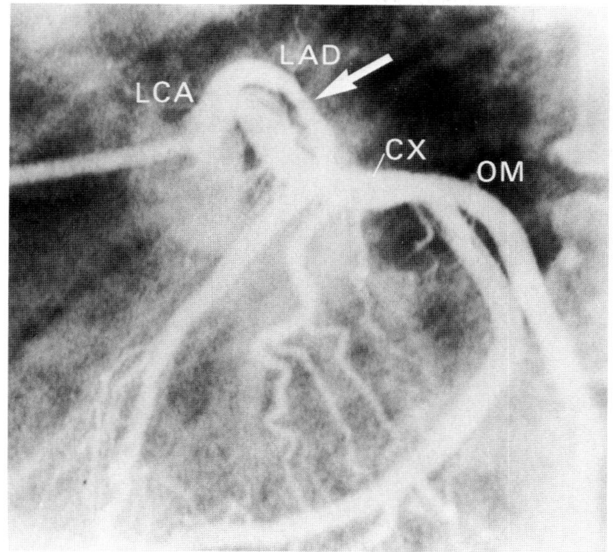

A

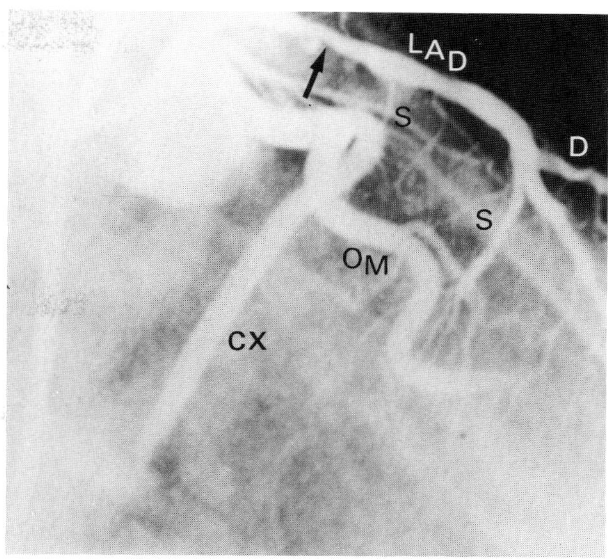

B

C

D

Figure 26-14. LAD stenosis, single vessel, mild. Selected frames from selective left cineangiogram. (A) LAO projection. There is a tubular segment of narrowing in the left anterior descending coronary artery (*arrow*). Note the large size of the obtuse marginal and circumflex branches. (B) RAO projection. The *arrow* indicates the location of the left anterior descending stenosis. (C and D) Selective right coronary arteriogram, LAO and RAO projections. The right coronary artery is a relatively small vessel, which fails to extend beyond the crux and does not give rise to a posterior descending branch. This appearance is characteristic of left coronary artery dominance, with the large left coronary artery branches supplying the posterior aspects of both the left and the right ventricles.

lateral projections may also be necessary to confirm the precise anatomy of the stenosed or obstructed LAD.

The hemodynamic significance of LAD stenosis is not always easy to assess. In Figure 26-14, for example, there is mild single-vessel disease extending over an area of approximately 1 cm. It is proximal to the origin of the first septal branch, so that its location is unfavorable, but it is at the borderline of hemodynamic significance.

This case also illustrates left coronary dominance with branches uniformly large except at the site of disease, whereas the right coronary artery appears hypoplastic but actually represents a nondominant vessel. In Figure 26-15, a moderate degree of stenosis is apparent in the proximal LAD, involving a relatively long segment, as compared with the severe localized stenosis visible in Figure 26-16. The severe type of single-vessel disease apparent in Figure 26-17 is located just

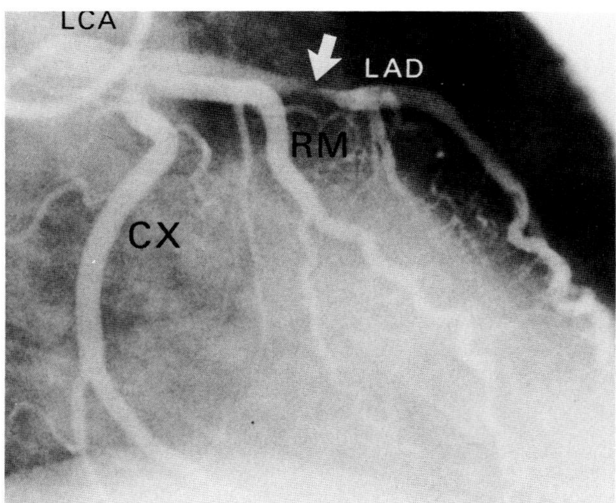

Figure 26-15. LAD stenosis, single vessel, moderate. Selective left coronary arteriogram, RAO projection. A relatively long segment of the LAD is more or less symmetrically involved by arteriosclerosis (*arrow*). Note the large ramus medianus.

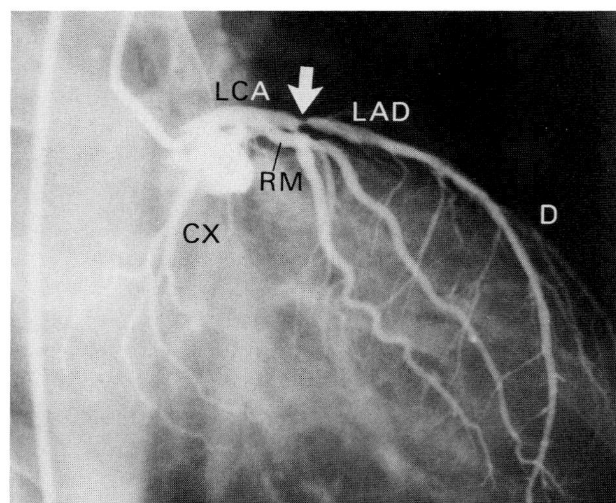

Figure 26-16. LAD stenosis, single vessel, severe. Selective left coronary arteriogram, RAO projection. A localized short segmental area of involvement (*arrow*) is apparent. The other branches appear normal. This patient demonstrates the anatomy that might well be amenable to balloon angioplasty.

beyond the origin of the first septal branch and is therefore more favorable from a prognostic point of view.

The patient illustrated in Figure 26-18 had a long segment of disease involving only the LAD, with all other branches widely patent. Figure 26-19 demonstrates almost complete obstruction of the proximal LAD, with a distal vessel that is satisfactorily patent

Figure 26-17. LAD stenosis, single vessel, severe, eccentric. Selective left coronary arteriogram, RAO projection. Note that the location of the stenosis (*arrow*) is just distal to the first septal branch, permitting it to play a role as a collateral vessel to fill the distal LAD. The prognosis of LAD disease is better when the stenosis is distal to rather than proximal to the septal branch.

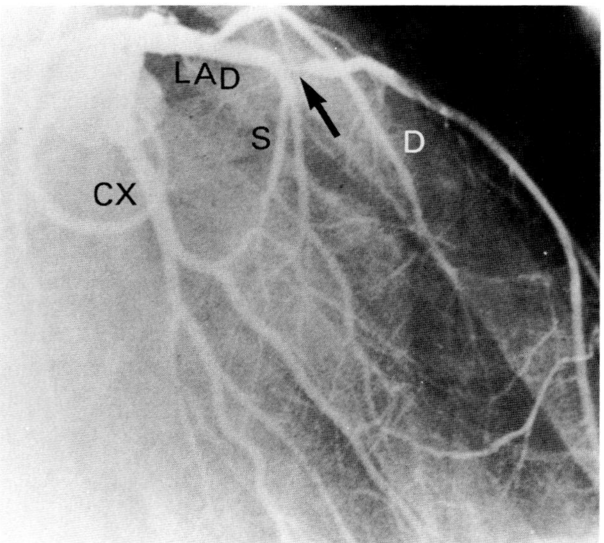

Figure 26-18. LAD stenosis, single vessel, severe. Selective left coronary arteriogram, lateral projection. A long segment of marked narrowing is present (*arrow*). All other branches of the left coronary artery are widely patent and show no evidence of coronary disease. (Courtesy of Melvin Judkins, M.D.)

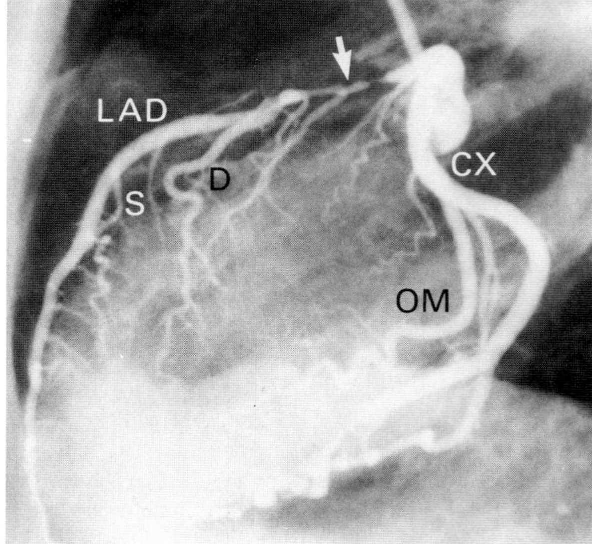

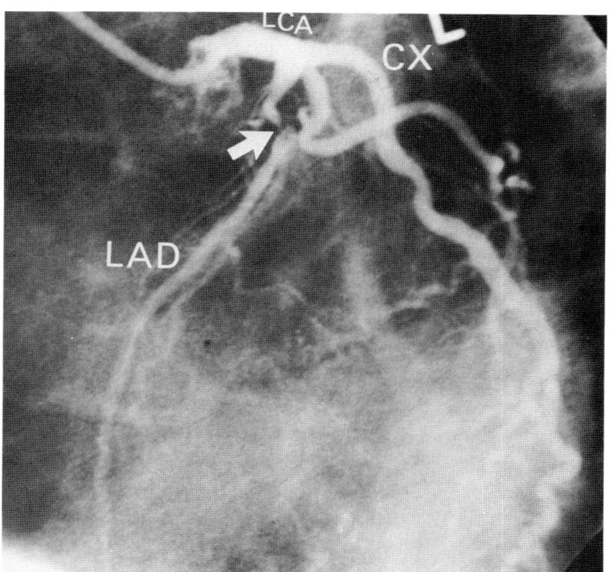

Figure 26-19. LAD disease, severe. Selective left coronary arteriogram, LAO projection. The left anterior descending coronary artery demonstrates the most severe degree of stenosis (*arrow*), with only a pinpoint lumen remaining.

throughout its course. In Figure 26-20, the disease is obscured in the LAO projection, whereas the RAO projection reveals a long segment of profound stenosis in the LAD. Coronary bypass surgery in the presence of such a lesion has not been shown to extend life and therefore must be justified on the basis of symptom remission.

LAD obstruction is not always apparent in a single projection. In Figure 26-21, for example, the RAO projection demonstrates the LAD in apparent continuity with a distal vessel that is shown to be the diagonal branch in the LAO projection. Complete obstruction of the LAD is present. Similarly, in Figure 26-22, the LAO projection shows a vessel in continuity with a proximal LAD that proved to be a septal branch, clearly revealed in the RAO projection (see Fig. 26-22B). In the RAO projection, total obstruction of the LAD (*arrows*) is demonstrated, with obstruction as well of the left circumflex artery, just after the origin of the large obtuse marginal (*large single arrow*). Despite the presence of complete obstruction, the distal LAD is patent and well visualized after right coronary arteriography, since it fills from multiple septal branches as well as the conus and epicardial branches

Figure 26-20. LAD stenosis, severe. Selective left coronary arteriogram of a 57-year-old man with intractable angina pectoris. (A) LAO projection. The catheter is in the orifice of the left coronary artery. Mild stenosis of the left circumflex branch is visible with atheromatous change distally. The anterior descending artery appears slender and somewhat irregular, but no definite stenosis is apparent. The bifurcation of the left main coronary artery into its respective branches is the site of overlapping vessels (*upper arrow*). Note also that a portion of the left anterior descending artery is obscured by reflux into the left aortic sinus (*lower arrow*). (B) RAO projection. The catheter is in the left main coronary artery. Profound stenosis in the anterior descending artery, obscured by foreshortening of the artery in the LAO projection, is now visible, and recanalization has almost certainly occurred. The middle segment of the LAD is also involved. On the basis of the single LAO projection, it would have been impossible to properly assess the degree of disease.

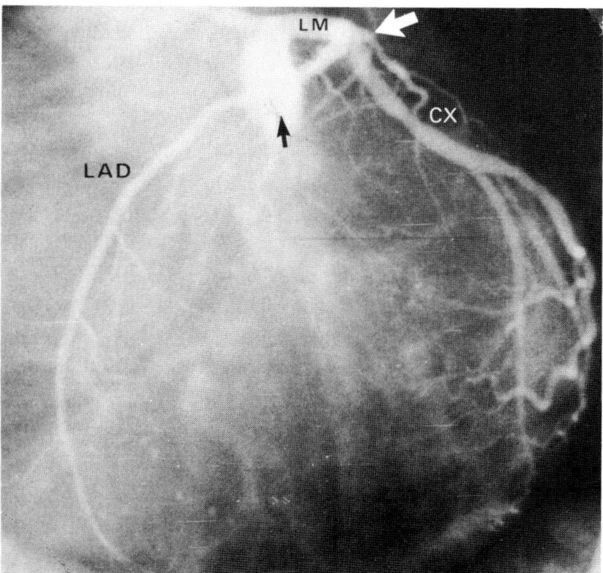

A

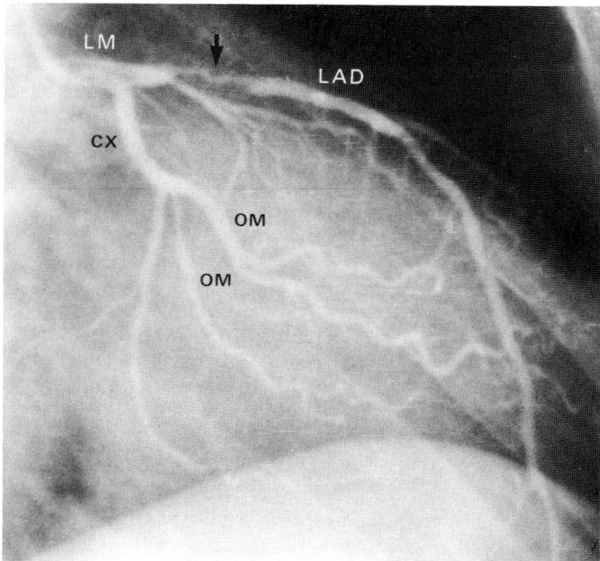

B

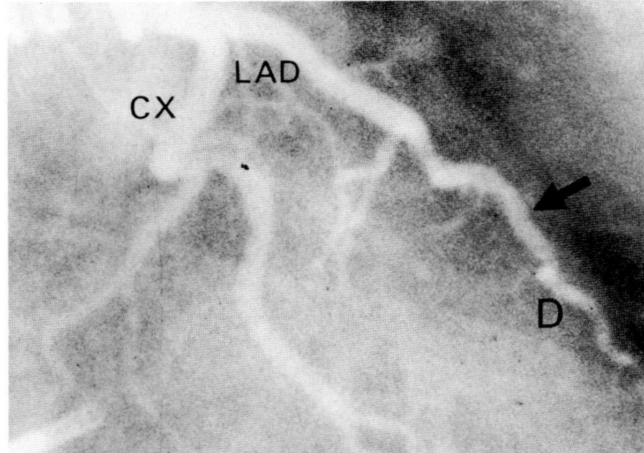

A

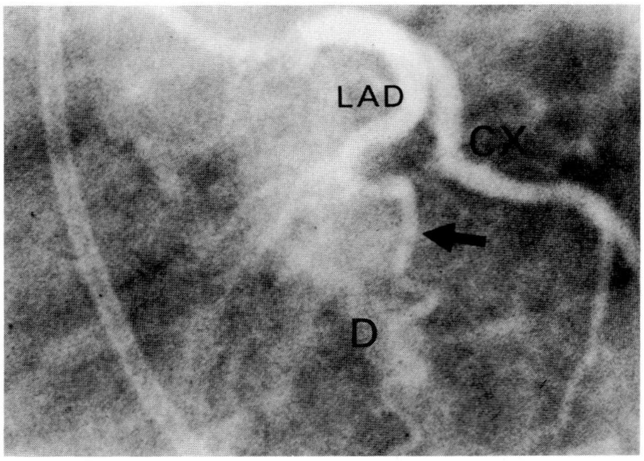

B

Figure 26-21. LAD obstruction. Selective left cine coronary arteriogram. (A) RAO projection. The proximal LAD appears to be normal and extends into a distal vessel that, in this projection, might readily be assumed to be the LAD but is actually the diagonal branch. The LAD is occluded at the origin of the large diagonal branch (*arrow*). (B) LAO projection. Complete occlusion of the LAD has occurred; no vessel filling is visible in its normal location. Instead, the vessel that appears to be the distal LAD in the RAO projection is now clearly defined as a diagonal branch (*arrow*). Such anatomic arrangements explain the need for multiple projections.

from the right coronary artery (see Fig. 26-22C and D).

The anatomy shown in Figure 26-23 is of great interest because the LAD is totally obstructed, with stenosis of the diagonal branch as well. Involvement of this branch, which assumes increasing importance in the presence of LAD disease, now places a good deal of the free wall of the ventricle in jeopardy.

Defining the presence of proximal occlusion or stenosis of the LAD is not an adequate outcome of a coronary arteriogram. The quality of the distal vessel must be established for surgical considerations to be appropriately evaluated. Because the distal coronary artery may fill either by bridging collaterals or perhaps by a series of collateral pathways from the right coronary artery, it is essential that every effort be made to show as fully as possible the total area of the LAD that is patent beyond an occlusion. It is equally important to show more distal stenosis in the presence of an occluded artery, because this may dictate to the surgeon that the bypass should be placed beyond the stenotic lesion.

Diagonal Arteries

The diagonal branches of the LAD are almost as important as the LAD itself, except for the fact that they do not supply the apex. Originating from the LAD, they pass caudally, ventrally, and to the left to supply the free wall of the left ventricle (Figs. 26-23 through 26-26). Sometimes they are very large trunks that supply a major portion of the lateral wall. Occlusion of such branches may be responsible for a large area of ischemia. The ramus medianus, or intermediate branch, arises from the left coronary artery as a separate trunk at a trifurcation of that vessel into the LAD, the circumflex, and the ramus. When present, it usually supplants and replaces the diagonal arteries and almost invariably bifurcates into vessels of relatively equal size.

Figure 26-22. LAD obstruction. (A) LAO projection, selective left coronary arteriogram. The proximal LAD is filled and extends into a branch in the area usually occupied by the LAD but actually representing the septal branch. Marked stenosis of the circumflex artery, not visible on the subsequent RAO projection, is best seen in this LAO projection (*arrow*). (B) RAO projection. The LAD is totally obstructed (*small arrows*). A large diagonal branch originates proximal to the site of occlusion, and there is also filling of the first septal branch. The proximal circumflex stenosis visible in (A) is obscured in this projection because of superimposition. This view reveals the presence of a rudimentary circumflex artery (*large arrow*) beyond the origin of a large obtuse marginal branch. (C) LAO projection, selective right coronary arteriogram. The catheter is in the mouth of the right coronary artery. The vessel fills well, without evidence of significant obstruction. Retrograde filling of the totally obstructed LAD via collateral vessels is apparent. The most important collateral route appears to be via septal branches. (D) RAO projection, selective right coronary arteriogram. The posterior descending coronary artery, extending along the posterior interventricular groove, gives rise to multiple septal branches that fill the LAD (*arrows*). ►

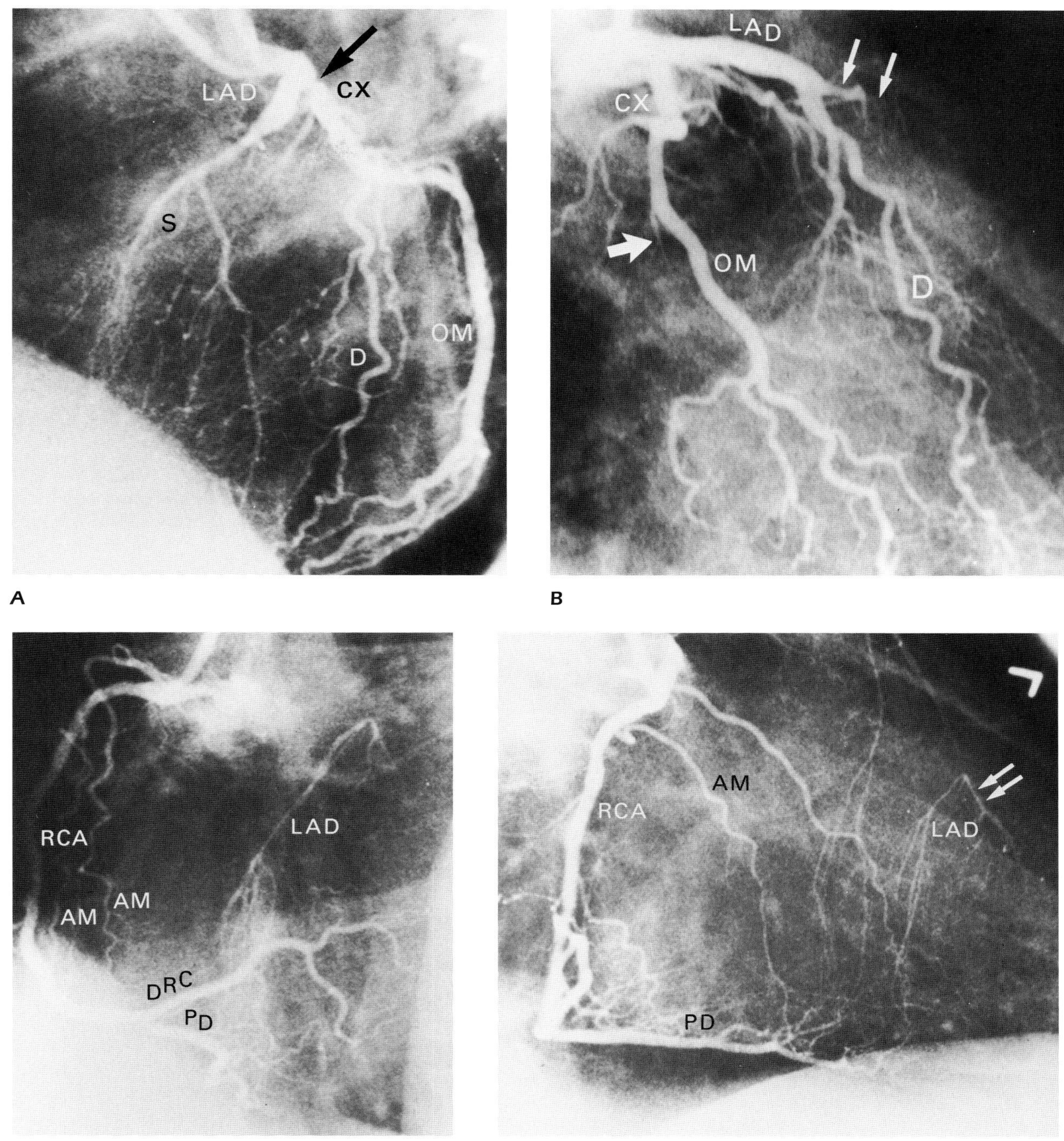
LAD
CX
S
D
OM
A
LAD
CX
OM
D
B
RCA
LAD
AM
AM
DRC
PD
C
AM
RCA
LAD
PD
D

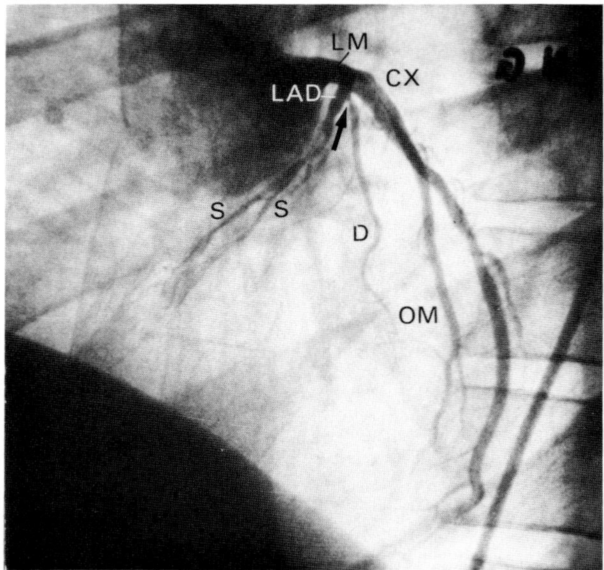

Figure 26-23. LAD obstruction and diagonal branch stenosis. Selective left coronary arteriogram, LAO projection. Complete occlusion of the LAD has occurred, with filling of a few septal branches visible in the area usually filled by the LAD in this projection. The diagonal branch, which assumes increasing importance in the presence of LAD disease, is stenosed at its origin (*arrow*).

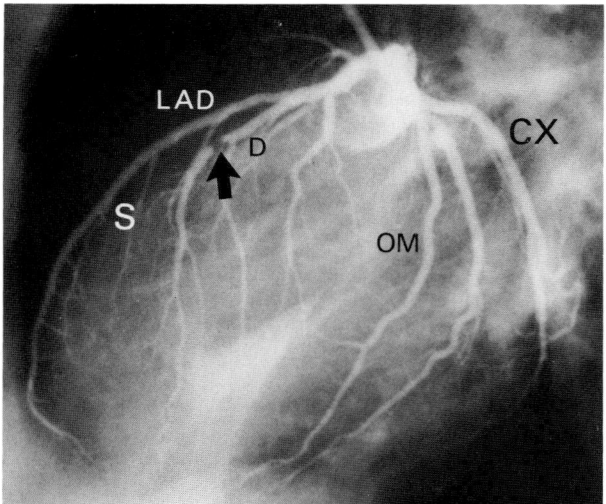

Figure 26-24. Diagonal branch stenosis, single-vessel disease. Selective left coronary arteriogram, lateral projection. Profound stenosis with subtotal occlusion of the vessel is visible in the diagonal branch (*arrow*) of the LAD. All other branches are normal in caliber.

The right one is generally distributed more toward the interventricular groove, and the left more toward the free margin of the left ventricle.

Diagonal branch stenosis may occur at the origin of the branch from the LAD (see Fig. 26-23) or at any point along its course. It may be slight in degree, moderate (see Fig. 26-23), or marked. It may occur as single-vessel disease (see Fig. 26-24) but more com-

Figure 26-25. Diagonal branch stenosis, with multibranch disease (LAD, CX, OM). Selective left coronary arteriogram, RAO projection. (A) Early phase. Marked stenosis of the diagonal branch (*arrow*) representing virtual occlusion, with possible recanalization, is visible. In addition, stenosis of the LAD immediately beyond the origin of the diagonal is noted. A mild degree of narrowing of the origin of the first septal branch is also present. (B) Later phase. Besides the lesions visible in (A), there is also stenosis of the circumflex artery (*arrow*) and the obtuse marginal branch (*barred arrow*).

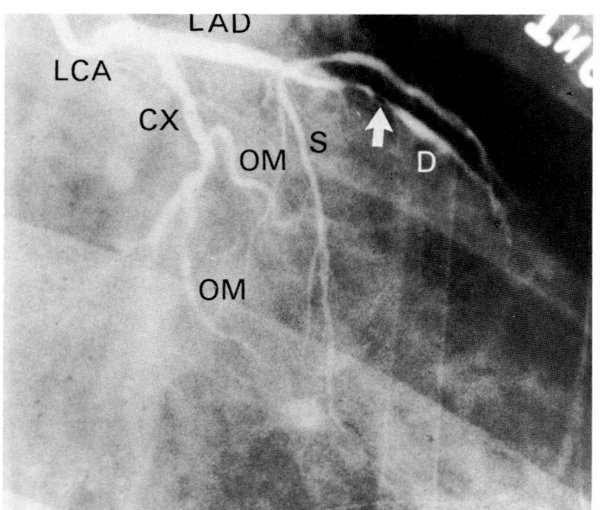

A

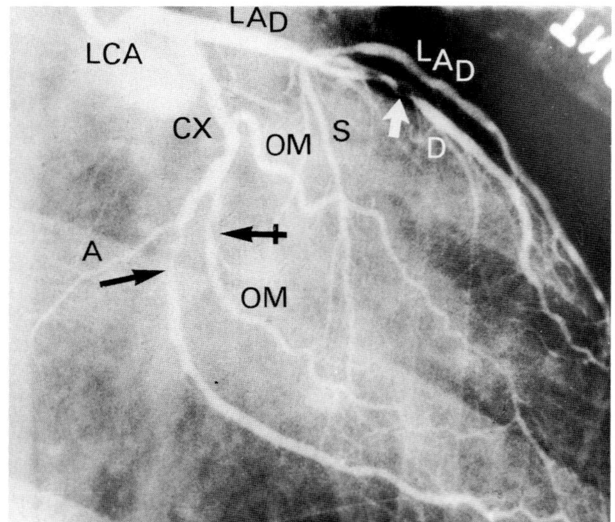

B

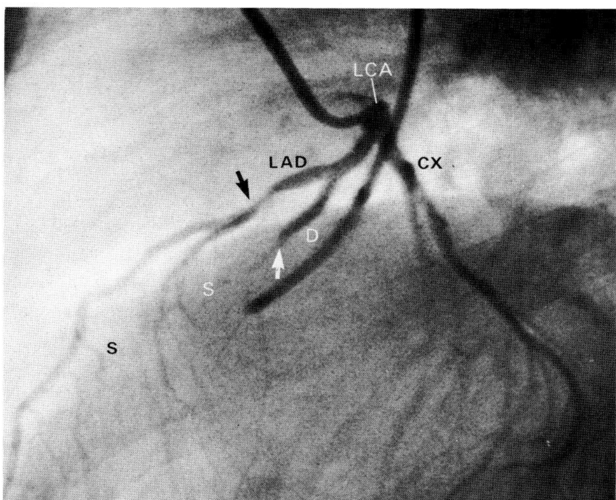

Figure 26-26. Diagonal branch occlusion. Selective left coronary arteriogram, lateral projection. The diagonal branch is occluded proximally (*white arrow*), with no filling beyond this area. In addition, severe LAD stenosis proximal to the first septal branch is apparent (*black arrow*).

monly accompanies disease in other arteries. Multiple stenoses of varying severity may be observed within the same diagonal artery (see Fig. 26-30).

The importance of diagonal branch involvement is indicated by the diminished left ventricular performance when LAD stenosis occurs proximal to the origin of the first diagonal branch.[164] When LAD stenosis or occlusion occurs beyond the first diagonal branch, the diagonal may participate in supplying the anterolateral wall of the left ventricle and the apex of the heart. When stenosis occurs proximally, the diagonal branch is not available to collateralize the region normally supplied by the LAD.

Septal Branches

The septal arteries are of major importance as collateral pathways between the right and left coronary arteries. Stenosis, which is unusual, at times involves both the LAD near the septal orifice and the septal branch itself. In Figure 26-12D, stenosis is visible just proximal to the first septal artery. The mortality of LAD narrowing proximal to the first septal branch has been found to be as much as three times as long as that of disease beyond the first septal branch.[235]

There is tremendous variation in the size of the septal branches, and there is some variation in the number visualized. Not infrequently they can be seen throughout much of the course of the LAD (see Fig. 26-16). In some patients, they may be mistaken for the LAD when that artery is occluded and when the arteriogram is obtained in the LAO projection (see Fig. 26-22A). With retrograde filling of the obstructed LAD from the right coronary artery, the septals may be visualized (see Fig. 26-22C). Figure 26-25A illustrates a case in which the first septal branch is narrowed at its origin in association with a large plaque in the LAD. Severe stenosis of the second septal artery is visible in the arteriograms shown in Figure 26-28, the adjacent LAD being widely patent but with a plaque present. In the patient whose arteriogram is shown in Figure 26-45B, with severe proximal LAD stenosis, a few septal branches are visualized, but they appear relatively narrow.

In the coronary arteriographic study it is essential that such vessels as the septal branches be visualized in as fine detail as possible, and that their number and the presence of disease be fully delineated.

Left Circumflex Branch

The left circumflex artery extends as a continuation of the left main vessel in a dorsal direction, circling posteriorly in the left atrioventricular groove. At a variable distance beyond its origin, it gives off one or more obtuse marginal branches. The circumflex artery then continues in the atrioventricular groove, reaching the crux (defined as the intersection between the atrioventricular groove and the posterior interventricular groove) of the heart frequently as a relatively small vessel.

The degree to which the circumflex artery supplies the posterior portion of the left ventricle is a reflection of the presence or absence of left coronary dominance. In general, the distal right coronary artery extends as the posterior interventricular artery to supply the posterior aspect of both left and right ventricles. In about 10 to 15 percent of patients, the left coronary artery, via the circumflex, may supply a considerable portion of the vascular bed to this area.

Depending on whether the circulation is left-dominant, balanced, or right-dominant, the circumflex artery, on reaching the crux, bifurcates into a posterolateral left ventricular branch and the posterior descending artery. The posterior descending branch may replace the normal branch of the right coronary, may be diminutive, or may be nonexistent.

Circumflex disease is less commonly seen than LAD disease but may be present at any site throughout the length of the vessel. It is rarely found as single-vessel involvement (Fig. 26-27); frequently LAD or RCA disease is also present (Figs. 26-28 and 26-29). When present, it may be associated with either free wall ischemia or infarction or posterior wall ischemia or infarction, depending on the site of the stenosis or occlusion of the circumflex artery. Particularly if it occurs proximal to the origin of obtuse marginal vessels, the

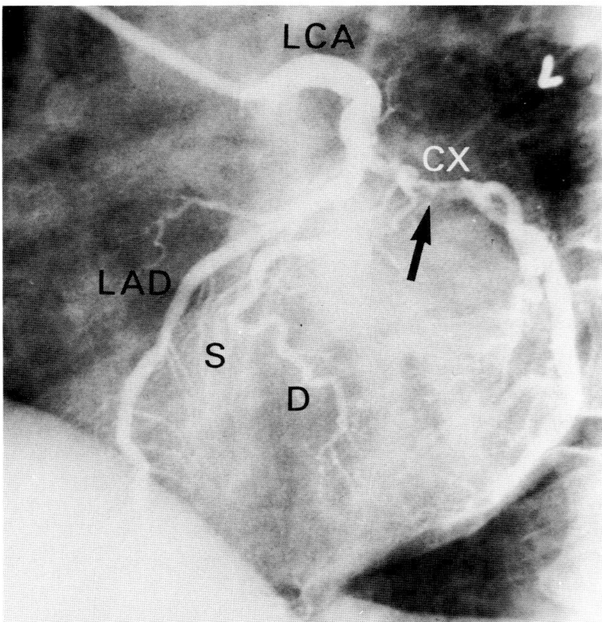

Figure 26-27. Left circumflex artery stenosis, single-vessel disease. Selective left coronary arteriogram, LAO projection. Stenosis of the proximal portion of the circumflex coronary artery is present (*arrow*), with severe irregular narrowing of the vessel. The LAD is widely patent, with minimal stenosis in the midportion.

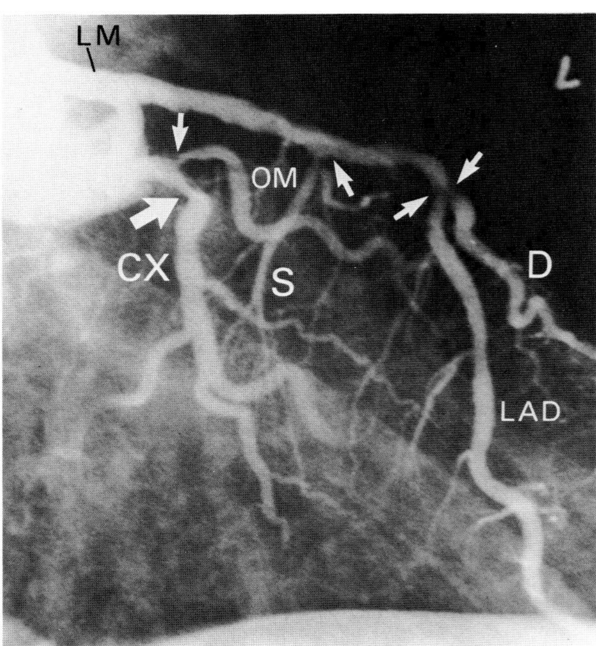

Figure 26-28. Left circumflex stenosis, proximal, associated with multibranch stenoses. Selective left coronary arteriogram, RAO projection. The *large arrow* indicates the site of severe circumflex disease. *Small arrows* demonstrate narrowing of the origin of the obtuse marginal, septal, LAD, and diagonal branches. Note also that there is marginal irregularity in virtually all of the LAD, indicating the presence of varying degrees of coronary disease.

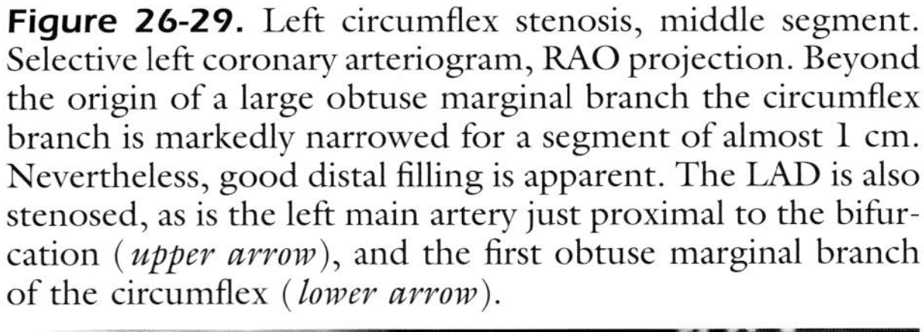
Figure 26-29. Left circumflex stenosis, middle segment. Selective left coronary arteriogram, RAO projection. Beyond the origin of a large obtuse marginal branch the circumflex branch is markedly narrowed for a segment of almost 1 cm. Nevertheless, good distal filling is apparent. The LAD is also stenosed, as is the left main artery just proximal to the bifurcation (*upper arrow*), and the first obtuse marginal branch of the circumflex (*lower arrow*).

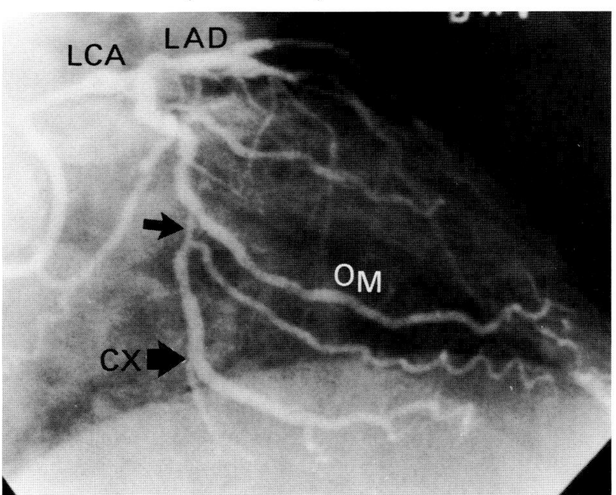

Figure 26-30. Selective left coronary arteriogram, lateral projection. The left circumflex artery is the site of two severe areas of stenosis (*black arrows*), with little distal filling beyond the second stenosis. Whereas the LAD is the site of only minimal disease, its diagonal branch demonstrates two areas of stenosis (*white arrows*).

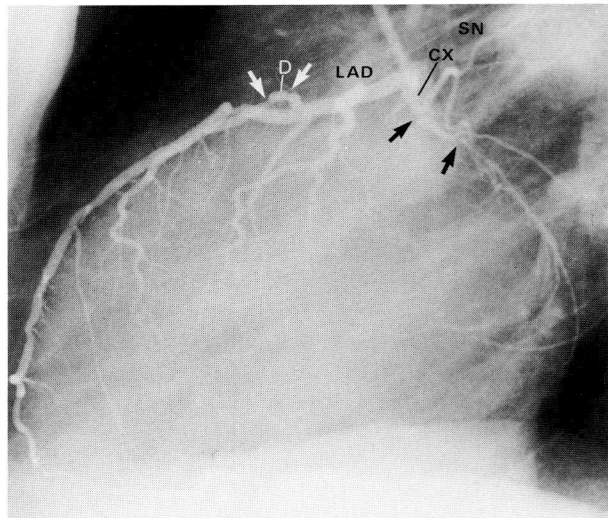

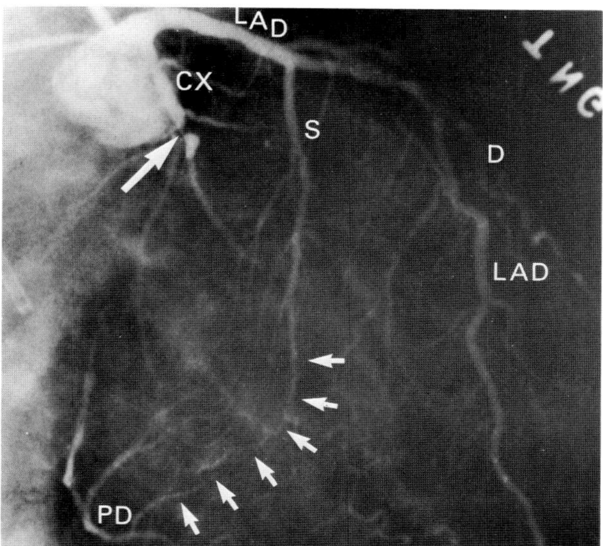

Figure 26-31. Left circumflex stenosis, severe, with virtual occlusion. Selective left coronary arteriogram, RAO projection. A pinhole opening is visible (*large arrow*) in the left circumflex artery in association with severe narrowing of the obtuse marginal artery. The patient also had right coronary artery obstruction, and the large first septal branch gives rise to multiple branches that fill the posterior descending coronary artery (*small arrows*).

posterior free wall of the left ventricle may be grossly involved or in jeopardy.

At times, a long segment of proximal disease is present (see Figs. 26-25B and 26-27). The anatomy in Figure 26-25B is more favorable from a prognostic point of view in that the stenosis is distal to the origin of two obtuse marginal arteries; in Figure 26-27 it is proximal to the origin of the obtuse marginal, and there is severe, irregular narrowing with intraluminal thrombus. The common association of circumflex disease with other branch involvement is illustrated in Figure 26-28 and 26-32. In Figure 26-28 the circumflex stenosis is distal to the origin of the first obtuse marginal artery, but intrinsic stenosis of the obtuse marginal, LAD, diagonal, and septal branches is apparent. In Figure 26-29, a longer area of stenosis just beyond the origin of the obtuse marginal branch is accompanied by severe LAD disease. Two segments of almost complete obstruction of the circumflex artery are delineated in Figure 26-30, with marked impairment of the distal circulation of the posterior free wall of the left ventricle. The LAD in Figure 26-30 is patent and long, extending over the apex in the interventricular groove, but the diagonal branch is stenosed in two separate areas.

The circumflex branch may be so severely diseased

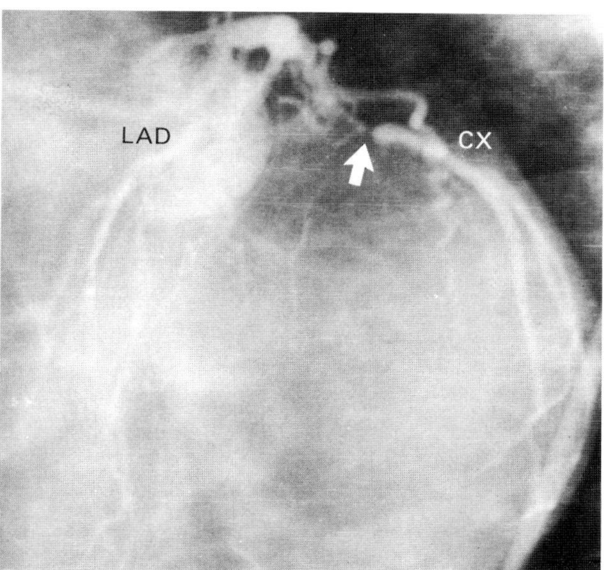

A

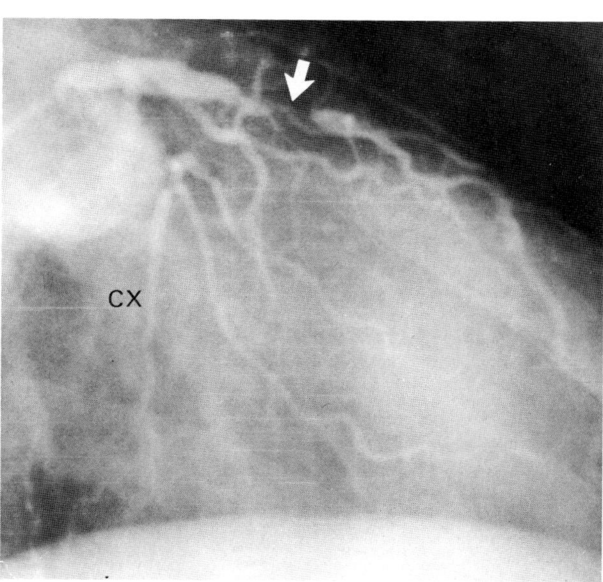

B

Figure 26-32. Left circumflex disease, severe, with virtual occlusion. Selective left coronary arteriogram. (A) LAO projection. Severe narrowing of the circumflex artery (*arrow*) is apparent. The LAD is poorly defined. (B) RAO projection. Marked narrowing of the circumflex artery is again visible, although there is filling of distal branches. This projection also demonstrates that marked stenosis of the LAD (*arrow*) is present. Thus this is at the very minimum two-vessel disease, but the patient also had occlusion of the right coronary artery and so actually had three-vessel disease.

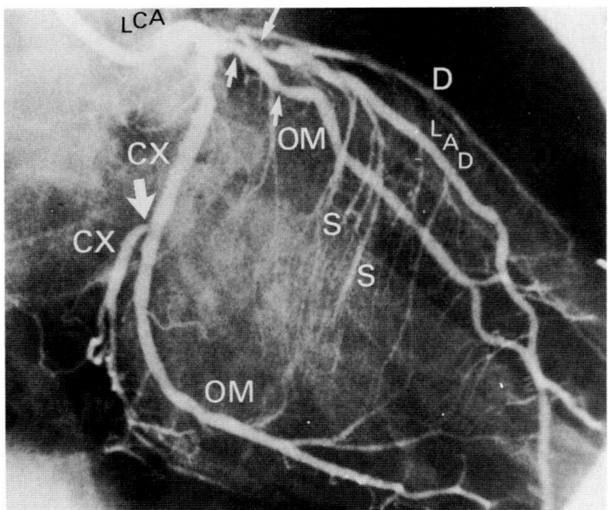

Figure 26-33. Obtuse marginal stenosis in association with circumflex and LAD stenosis. Selective left coronary arteriogram, RAO projection. Two localized segments of stenosis are visible in the first obtuse marginal branch, the proximal less severe than the more distal (*arrows*). In addition, severe stenosis of the LAD (*upper arrow*) is visible. The circumflex artery is somewhat irregular but widely patent until the point of origin of the second large obtuse marginal branch, at which point circumflex stenosis is visible (*large arrow*). Multiple septal branches are filled and provide collateral flow to the posterior descending right coronary artery in association with right coronary artery obstruction.

that it cannot furnish collaterals to the distal right coronary artery, even with RCA obstruction. In Figure 26-31, for example, both the circumflex and the obtuse marginal branches are almost completely obstructed, and the first septal branch is the major avenue of collateral flow to the obstructed right coronary artery, with retrograde filling of the posterior descending artery and RCA. When circumflex obstruction exists as a part of three-vessel disease (Fig. 26-32), the location is of great importance; if proximal, it precludes utilization of obtuse marginal branches for collateral flow to the posterior myocardium. Circumflex stenosis, like all other types of arteriosclerotic disease, often occurs at bifurcations (Figs. 26-33 and 26-34). At times it is difficult to distinguish complete occlusion of the circumflex artery (see Fig. 26-34) from a diminutive branch in the presence of two obtuse marginal arteries, or from the anatomic variation in which the circumflex branch leaves the atrioventricular sulcus and is continuous with a posteroventricular branch. Although there is usually a distal circumflex artery, its size is strikingly variable.

Obtuse Marginal Arteries

The obtuse marginal artery is frequently larger than the circumflex artery beyond the origin of the obtuse marginal branch. When circumflex stenosis occurs

Figure 26-34. Obtuse marginal stenosis with circumflex obstruction. Selective left coronary arteriogram. (A) RAO projection. The proximal LAD is patent, although diseased in its distal segment. The circumflex artery is stenotic proximally (*arrow*) but occluded beyond the origin of the large obtuse marginal. Notice as well the severe degree of stenosis precisely at the origin of the obtuse marginal branch (*arrow*). (B) Lateral projection. No evidence of localized stenosis of the obtuse marginal or circumflex arteries is visible in this projection. Instead, there appears to be an area of narrowing that is relatively elongated (*arrow*) in the obtuse marginal branch. (Courtesy of Melvin Judkins, M.D.)

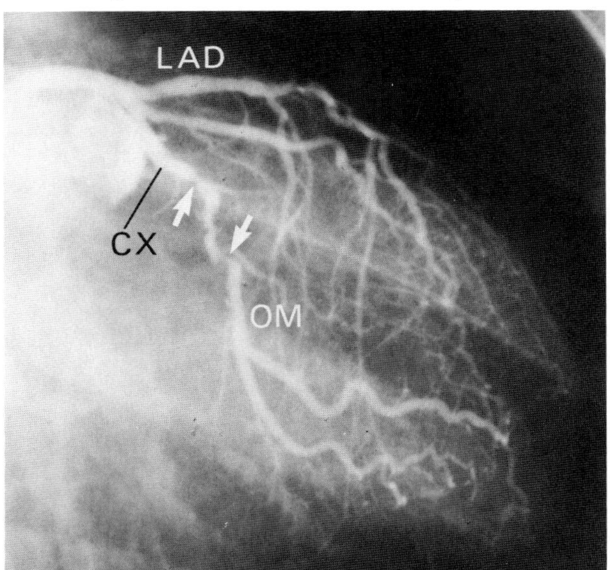

A

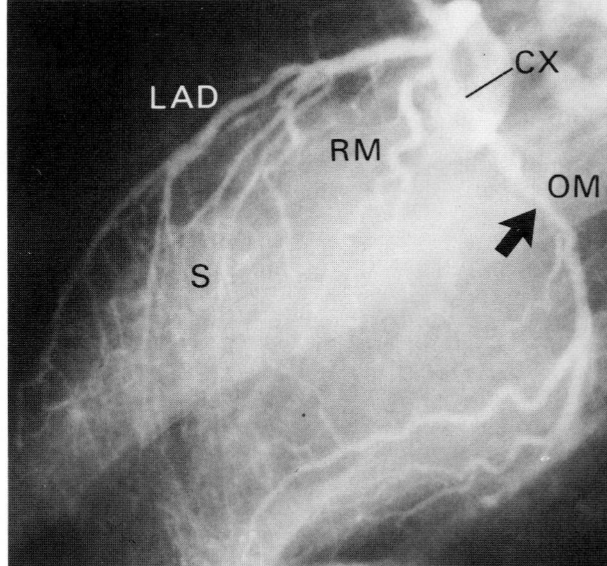

B

proximal to the origin of the obtuse marginal arteries, it diminishes the capacity of these branches, even if not diseased, to perfuse the posterior portion of the free margin of the left ventricle (see Fig. 26-27). Equally often, when intrinsic disease of the circumflex artery is present, the obtuse marginal branches are also involved (see Figs. 26-28, 26-30, and 26-31). Stenosis of the obtuse marginal artery is most likely to be located in its proximal portion, immediately beyond its origin (see Figs. 26-28, 26-31, 26-33, and 26-34). Multiple stenoses are commonly present (see Figs. 26-33 and 26-35). Although the disease tends to be proximal in location more often than distal, at times stenoses of the distal artery are present (Fig. 26-35). When multiple large obtuse marginal branches are present (see Figs. 26-25 and 26-33), the site of origin from the circumflex artery is variable; some may be proximal (see Fig. 26-33), whereas others arise more distally. With either proximal circumflex disease or with obtuse marginal disease that is severe and obstructing, the obtuse marginal artery can no longer serve as a collateral channel to an obstructed right coronary artery (by communicating with its left posterolateral branch) or to an obstructed LAD (through the diagonal and other branches). As in designating the degree and location of stenosis in all other branches, it is essential to indicate the exact site of stenosis, because this may impinge on both the surgical and the prognostic implications of the diseased coronary vascular bed. Conversely, a patent obtuse marginal artery may be a massive trunk collateralizing both the apex and the lateral wall of the left ventricle as well as the posterior descending coronary artery (see Fig. 26-44).

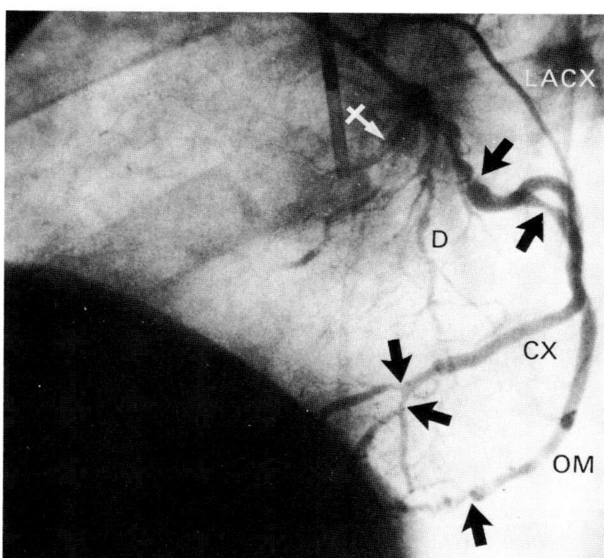

Figure 26-35. Obtuse marginal stenosis with multiple vessel involvement. Selective left coronary arteriogram, LAO projection. The *barred white arrow* points to the site of obstruction of the LAD, but there are also multiple areas of stenosis in the diagonal branch. The proximal circumflex artery is severely involved (*black arrow*), as is the obtuse marginal branch shortly after its origin (*black arrow*). Moreover, severe disease in the distal obtuse marginal as well as in the circumflex artery and its branches is apparent (*black arrows*). This patient illustrates the fact that when there is severe disease of the obtuse marginal artery in a number of different areas it is usually accompanied by extensive involvement of other coronary branches.

The Right Coronary Artery

Because the left ventricle is the systemic pumping chamber and hence is responsible for visceral blood flow, disease of the left coronary system has always been considered the most important element in arteriosclerotic heart disease. Right ventricular infarction is far less common than left, and from a hemodynamic point of view disease of the right coronary artery, even with myocardial infarction, has a much less important effect on systemic circulatory function than does disease of the left ventricle. Thus stenosis involving only the right coronary artery has a favorable prognosis whether treated medically or surgically.[230,231,233] Furthermore, resting hemodynamics in patients so afflicted may be similar to the hemodynamics in patients with normal coronary arteries.[229] With marked stenosis or complete occlusion, myocardial infarction may occur, and subsequently asynergy has been observed.[236]

Nevertheless, right coronary artery disease is closely linked to survival data when other coronary arteries are involved. Thus two-vessel disease involving the right coronary artery and left anterior descending coronary artery has an annual mortality similar to that of two-vessel disease involving the left anterior descending and left circumflex branches. One possible explanation is the role that the right coronary artery may play as a collateral pathway in the presence of left coronary disease. Obstructive disease of the right coronary artery clearly limits its capacity to perfuse such collateral branches as the conus artery, the acute marginal vessels, the posterior descending coronary artery, and septal branches. As a consequence, it is essential to define precisely the location, extent, and degree of disease involving the right coronary artery, both for prognosis and for planning surgical therapy.

The right coronary artery arises in the right anterior sinus of Valsalva, extending caudally and to the right in the right atrioventricular groove down to the crux of the heart. The first and highest branch of the right coronary artery is the conus artery, which represents an important collateral pathway to the left anterior descending artery. The conus artery arises anteriorly, and at the level of its point of origin the sinus node artery may be visible, arising in a dorsal direction and also representing an important collateral pathway. Beyond the origin of the conus artery, one or more acute marginal branches subserving the anterior epicardium of the right ventricle arise at variable points along the course of the right coronary artery. At the crux of the heart, the right coronary artery makes a sharp bend, gives rise to the artery to the atrioventricular node, and then travels in a ventral direction along the posterior interventricular groove as the posterior descending coronary artery. In 85 to 90 percent of patients this vessel is responsible for supplying blood to a major portion of both the right and left ventricles. After giving rise to the posterior descending artery, the right coronary artery continues as one or more posterolateral branches.

Because the conus branch frequently arises as an independent artery, failure to opacify it with a main right coronary artery injection does not imply either its absence or the presence of disease. It is an important branch to opacify, because it often serves as a collateral route to the left anterior descending coronary artery when the latter is diseased. Occlusion of the right coronary artery at the orifice may occur in the presence of luetic aortitis, aortic dissection, arteritis, ankylosing spondylitis, embolus, or arteriosclerosis. Occlusion at the orifice of the vessel can be readily demonstrated by bolus aortography, and orificial stenosis may also require a bolus study (Fig. 26-36). In selective studies, the catheter tip may pass beyond the stenotic zone and fail to reveal the area of narrowing.

Major coronary disease in the right coronary artery is usually found within the proximal one-third (Fig. 26-37), to a lesser degree in the middle one-third (Fig. 26-38), and least commonly in the distal one-third of the right coronary artery (Fig. 26-39).

Stenosis in the proximal right coronary artery is most frequently sharply localized, covering no more than 1 or 2 mm in length (see Fig. 26-38). When stenosis is severe and thrombosis and complete obstruction occur, the segment involved is usually 1 to 2 cm or more in length because of thrombosis distal and proximal to the obstructed segments (Figs. 26-40 through 26-42). With stenosis or occlusions, bridging collaterals may well be present and may afford adequate filling of the distal vessel (see Fig. 26-41). At times, an acute marginal branch in continuity with the RCA may obscure the presence of occlusion in the LAO projection (see Fig. 26-42A); the RAO may then reveal total absence of RCA filling beyond the origin of the marginal branch (see Fig. 26-42B).

With complete obstruction, particularly if it extends into the midportion of the right coronary artery, col-

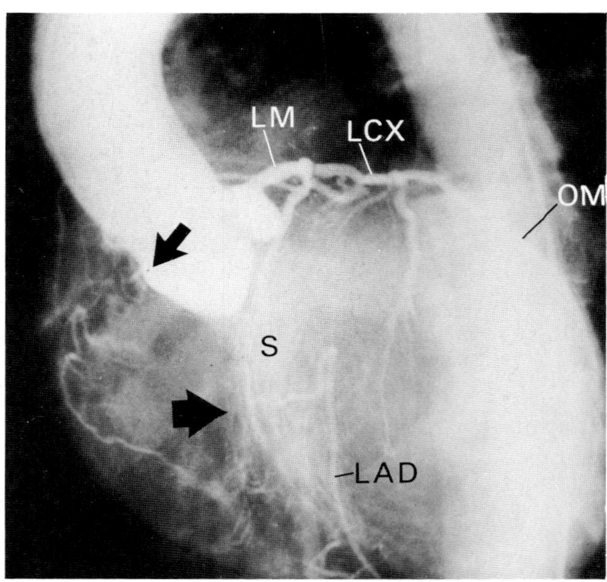

A

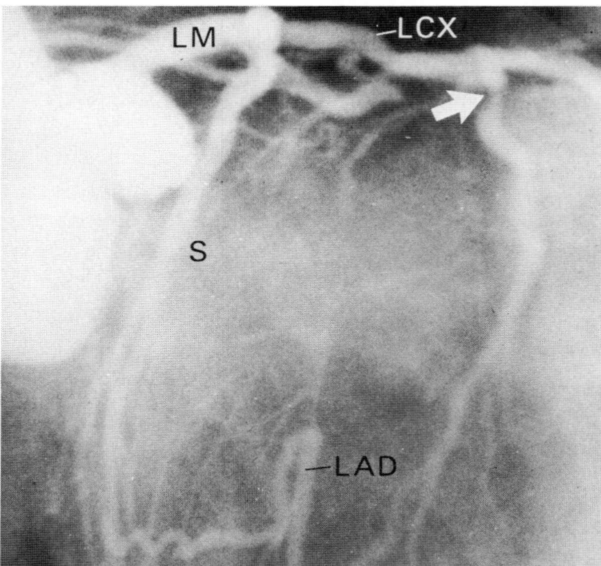

B

Figure 26-36. Right coronary artery obstruction at the origin. Bolus aortogram. (A) LAO projection. There is complete occlusion of the right coronary artery at its origin from the aorta (*upper arrow*). A few epicardial branches in the region of the right coronary artery fill via collateral channels. Notice also that the LAD is obstructed and fills via collaterals from a proximal septal branch (*lower arrow*). (B) Enlargement of (A) demonstrating nicely the communication between the septal branch, which fills proximally, and the obstructed left anterior descending coronary artery, which fills in its distal two-thirds. Note the disease in the circumflex branch as well (*arrow*).

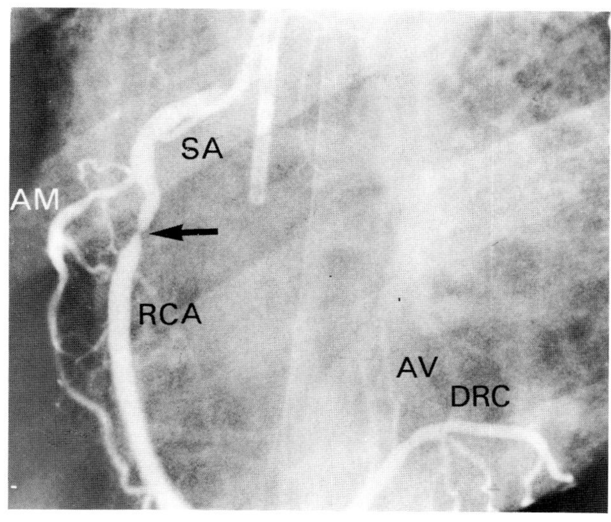

A

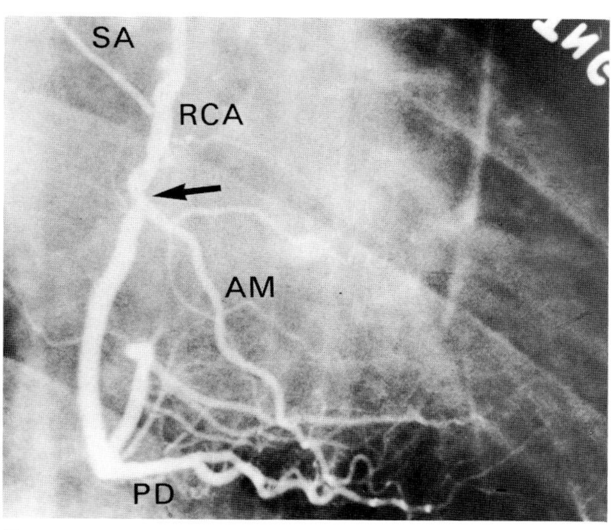

B

Figure 26-37. Right coronary artery stenosis, severe, proximal. Selective right coronary arteriogram. (A) LAO projection. Localized, relatively severe concentric stenosis is visible in the proximal right coronary artery (*arrow*). The distal branch fills well. (B) RAO projection. The site of stenosis is largely obscured by the acute marginal branch originating proximal to the stenosis and superimposed on it (*arrow*).

Figure 26-38. Right coronary artery stenosis, severe, middle segment. Selective right coronary arteriogram. (A) LAO projection. A long area of stenosis is visible in the midportion of the right coronary artery (*arrow*). (B) RAO projection. The stenosis is relatively symmetric in character and has produced striking narrowing throughout a segment of approximately 1 cm of the vessel (*arrow*).

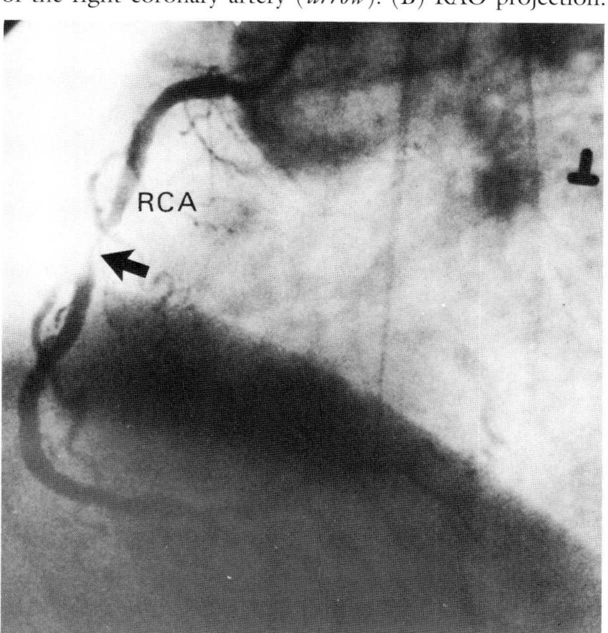

A

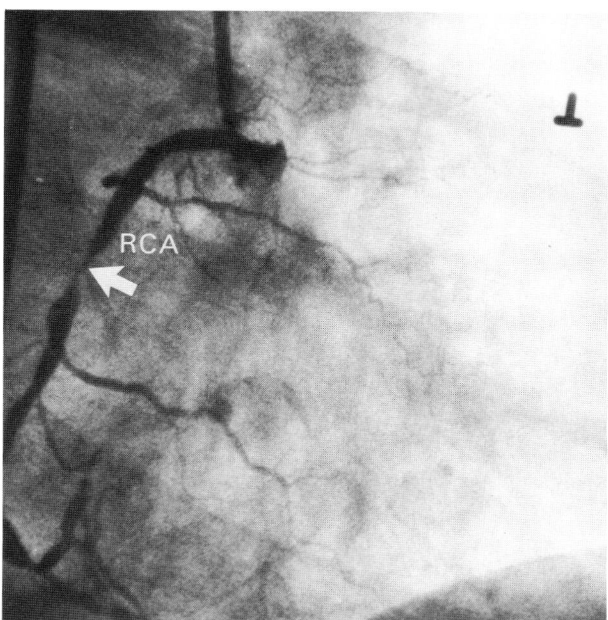

B

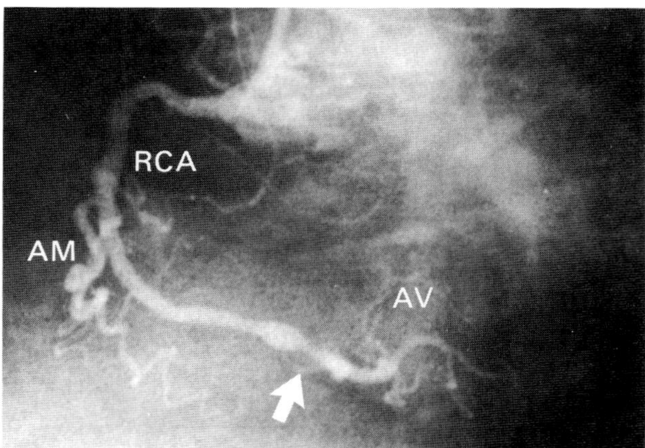

Figure 26-39. Right coronary artery stenosis, moderate, distal. Selective right coronary arteriogram, LAO projection. Marginal irregularity is present in the proximal right coronary artery and the midportion, without severe stenosis. In the distal right coronary artery, just proximal to the origin of the atrioventricular node branch, an area of moderate stenosis (*arrow*) is apparent.

lateral flow from the left system via septal, epicardial, obtuse marginal, circumflex, or anterior descending communications may permit perfusion of the distal right coronary artery that is adequate to preserve the viability of the right ventricular myocardium (Figs. 26-43 and 26-44).

Multivessel Disease

In the presence of angina pectoris, approximately 30 percent of patients have three-vessel, 30 percent have two-vessel, and 30 percent have one-vessel disease; about 10 percent of patients have normal coronary arteries. Mortality is directly related to the number of major vessels involved.[231] Furthermore, the fact that coronary disease is inherently a diffuse disorder suggests that although single-vessel disease may be diagnosed by arteriography, many of the patients may have multivessel disease. As has already been noted, it is essential that all vessels are carefully explored and that a complete description of the degree and location of all lesions is furnished.

With one-, two-, or three-vessel disease, left ventricular function may be significantly compromised after myocardial infarction. In the absence of myocardial infarction, the left ventricular ejection fraction is diminished with three-vessel disease.

Figure 26-43 demonstrates severe two-vessel disease involving the LAD and the right coronary artery, which is completely occluded. The obtuse marginal branch acts as a collateral pathway to fill the posterior descending coronary artery. In Figure 26-44, complete obstruction of the LAD is indicated by the *large arrow*, and severe stenosis by the *small arrow*. The right coronary artery is totally obstructed, and the

Figure 26-40. Right coronary artery obstruction. Selective right cineangiogram, LAO projection. (A) Early filling. Complete obstruction of the right coronary artery is apparent (*arrow*). The conus branch fills and extends toward the LAD. In addition, a large epicardial collateral is visible. (B) Later phase. Both the epicardial collateral and the conus branch have contributed to the filling of the left anterior descending coronary artery, which is totally obstructed proximally. Although the opacified LAD appears narrow, it is probably of entirely adequate caliber for bypass grafting.

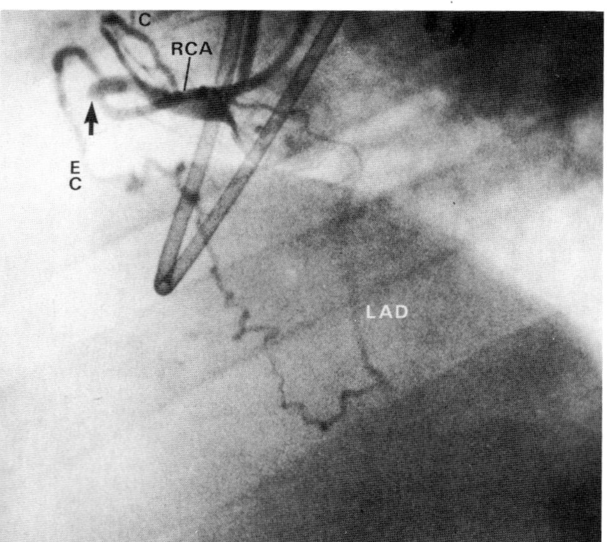

A

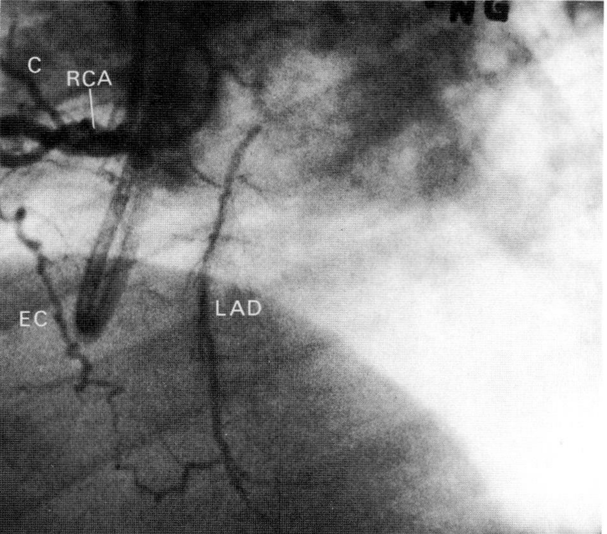

B

huge obtuse marginal artery supplies branches both to the apex and to the posterior descending artery. The patient whose arteriogram is shown in Figure 26-45 had complete occlusion of the proximal LAD, stenosis of the diagonal branch at its origin, subtotal occlusion of the circumflex artery, and total occlusion of the right coronary artery. Nevertheless, the LAD filled via collaterals from the right coronary artery and demonstrated an excellent distal vessel, entirely suitable for coronary bypass surgery.

Therapeutic Alternatives in Coronary Artery Disease

The coronary arteriogram, the ventriculogram, and the hemodynamic data obtained during catheterization provide key information for making decisions about further therapy. The arteriogram is a road map

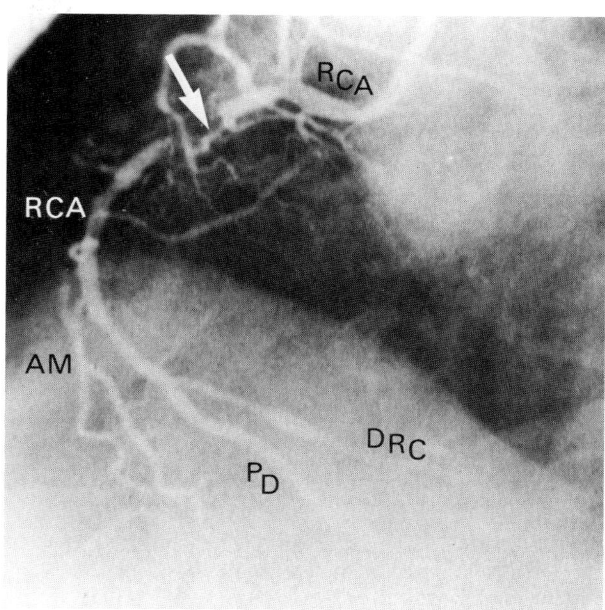

Figure 26-41. Right coronary artery obstruction, proximal, with bridging collaterals. Selective right coronary arteriogram, LAO projection. There is a 1-cm segment of total occlusion of the right coronary artery (*arrow*), with bridging vessels demonstrating the patency of the distal right coronary artery and the posterior descending branch.

Figure 26-42. Right coronary artery obstruction, middle segment. Selective right cine coronary arteriogram. (A) LAO projection. The acute marginal branch (*arrow*) appears to be continuous with the right coronary artery and of course originates from it. With this projection alone, it might be difficult to be certain that right coronary artery obstruction was present. (B) RAO projection. The main right coronary artery fills to the level of the origin of the distal acute marginal branch, at which point it is completely obstructed (*arrow*).

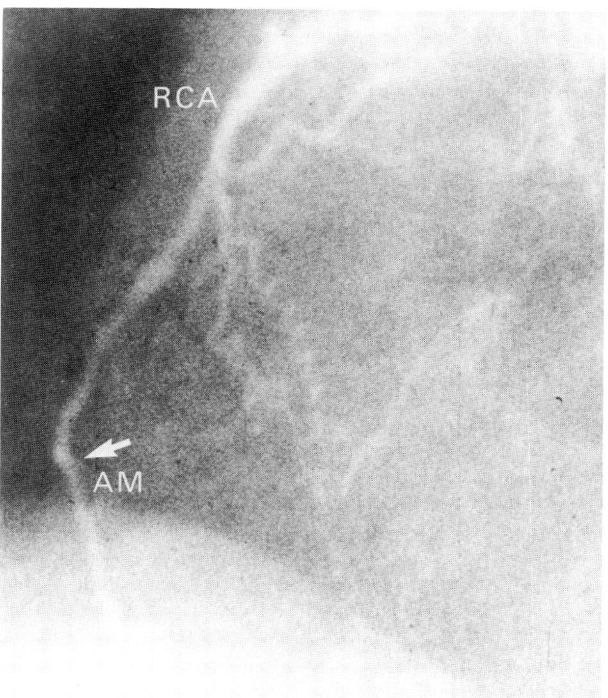

A

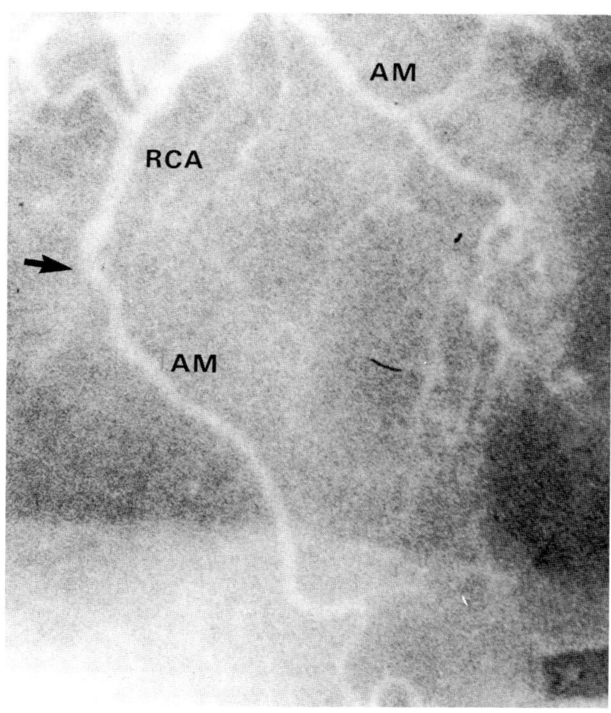

B

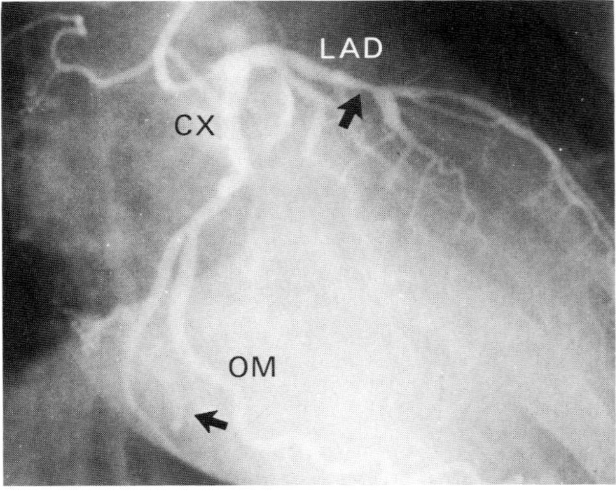

A

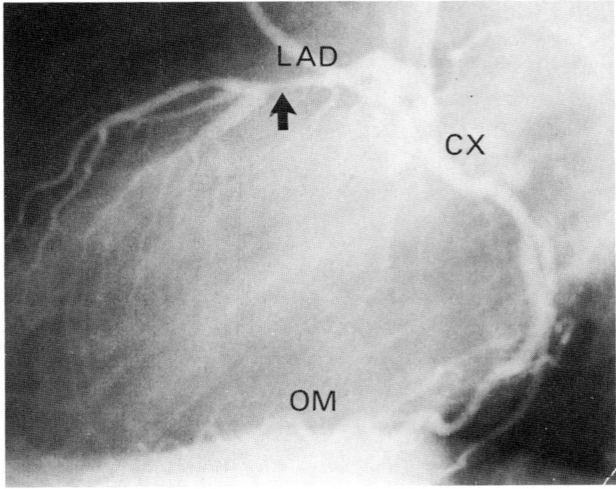

B

Figure 26-43. Multivessel disease, LAD and RCA. This 48-year-old man had severe angina of 6 months' duration. Same patient as in Figure 26-5D, showing right coronary artery obstruction. (A) RAO projection. There is severe narrowing (*upper arrow*) and occlusion of the LAD with filling of septal and diagonal branches. In addition, there is filling of the right coronary artery (*lower arrow*), which was completely obstructed on the right coronary arteriogram (see Fig. 26-5D). (B) Lateral projection. Severe stenosis of the proximal LAD (*arrow*) is associated with occlusion and absence of filling of the distal LAD.

of the coronary arteries and gives information on the anatomy, the number of vessels involved, the number of lesions, and the presence of diffuse disease. The ventriculogram, and complementary radionuclide studies (generally stress thalium studies) or echocardiographic and MRI studies, provide functional information that must be interpreted in the context of the patient's presentation—unstable angina or myocardial infarction, severity of symptoms, ability to tolerate physical effort—and his or her willingness to undergo invasive procedures such as percutaneous transluminal angio-

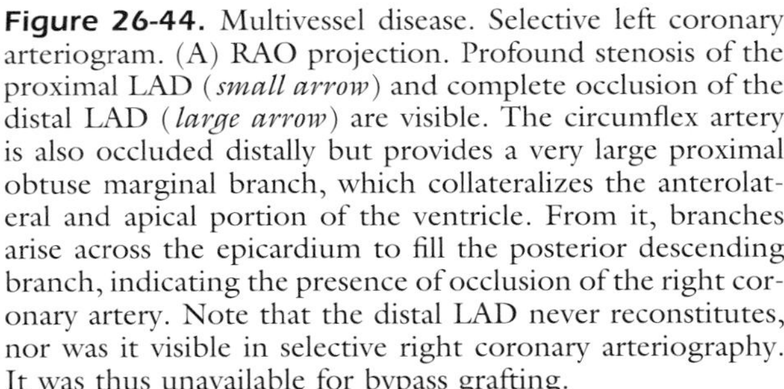

Figure 26-44. Multivessel disease. Selective left coronary arteriogram. (A) RAO projection. Profound stenosis of the proximal LAD (*small arrow*) and complete occlusion of the distal LAD (*large arrow*) are visible. The circumflex artery is also occluded distally but provides a very large proximal obtuse marginal branch, which collateralizes the anterolateral and apical portion of the ventricle. From it, branches arise across the epicardium to fill the posterior descending branch, indicating the presence of occlusion of the right coronary artery. Note that the distal LAD never reconstitutes, nor was it visible in selective right coronary arteriography. It was thus unavailable for bypass grafting.

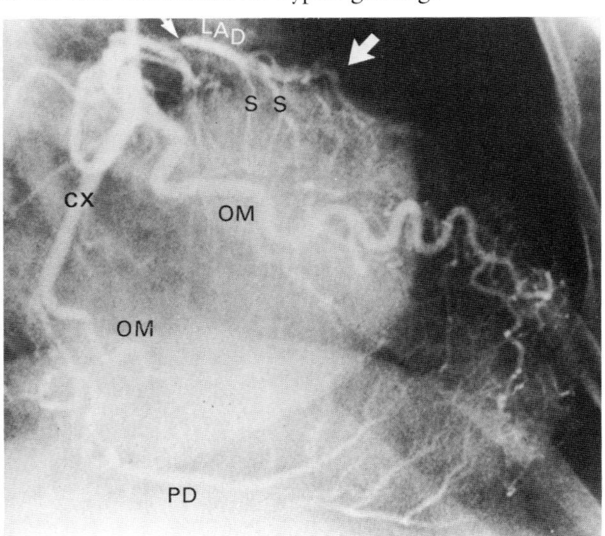

Figure 26-45. Multivessel disease. (A) Selective left coronary arteriogram, LAO projection. There is complete occlusion of the LAD (*arrow*). (B) Selective left coronary arteriogram, RAO projection. In addition to the stenosis (*upper arrow*) and occlusion (beyond) of the LAD, there is stenosis of the diagonal branch at its origin and virtually complete occlusion of the circumflex branch (*lower arrow*). (C and D) Selective right coronary arteriogram, LAO projection, early and late films. The right coronary artery (RCA) is completely obstructed (*arrow*), and the large conus branch fills epicardial collaterals that communicate with the LAD and fill a septal branch as well. (E and F) Selective right coronary arteriogram, RAO projection, early and late films. In the early phase, complete occlusion of the RCA is visible, with a large conus branch that extends across the right ventricle to the very apex of the heart and fills the LAD. Branches extend as well from this conus branch to the proximal LAD, with septal filling, and to the posterior descending artery. In the later phase (F), virtually all of the LAD is opacified, and multiple septal branches are visible. ▶

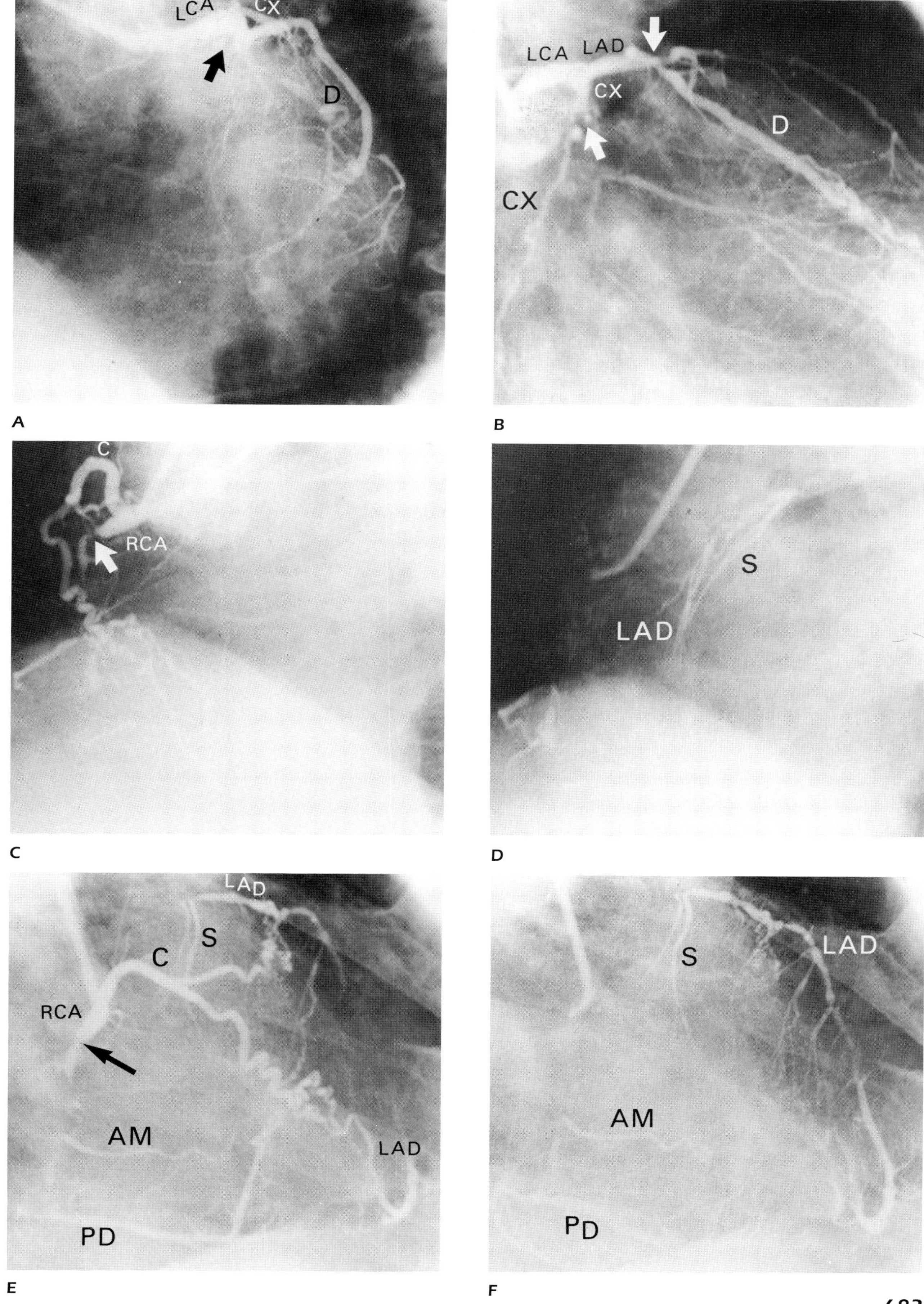
LCA
CX
D
A
LCA
LAD
CX
D
CX
B
C
RCA
C
S
LAD
D
LAD
S
C
RCA
AM
LAD
PD
E
S
LAD
AM
PD
F

plasty or bypass surgery, should they be the appropriate therapeutic choices.

Patients with stable angina who have no complicating factors related to their coronary artery disease generally can be treated medically with nitrates, beta blockers, and calcium channel blockers. Patients with unstable angina may also be treated similarly, but they must be hospitalized and evaluated to rule out infarction and other complications. This evaluation should include a coronary arteriogram after the patient is stabilized. Variant angina is treated with nitrates and calcium channel blockers, but beta blockers are avoided because of the possibility of unopposed alpha-adrenergic vasoconstriction. Should medication fail in the treatment of severe stable angina or unstable angina, then revascularization by either angioplasty or bypass grafting should be considered. Patients with variant angina are generally not candidates for revascularization unless significant fixed stenoses are also present.

Patients presenting with acute myocardial infarction should have supportive treatment and prompt thrombolytic therapy, followed by elective angioplasty or bypass surgery of the culprit vessel. These patients may be candidates for earlier attempts for revascularization if medication fails and there is evidence that the infarction may be extending. Complications such as rupture of the papillary muscle, ventricular septum, or a large symptom-producing ventricular aneurysm (congestive heart failure, recurrent emboli, or refractory arrhythmias) should be treated surgically.

The choice between percutaneous transluminal coronary angioplasty (PTCA) and coronary artery bypass surgery (CABG) must be based on the immediate and long-term risks and benefits of each procedure. Angioplasty is less invasive and more immediately available than surgery, but should only be performed if surgical backup is available for immediate intervention in case of a complication such as extensive occluding dissection. Emergency bypass surgery is needed in about 2 percent of PTCA patients.[15] A minimal degree of non-occlusive intimal dissection is usually seen after angioplasty, and its absence may actually predispose to early restenosis.[237]

Operative mortality for bypass surgery is under 1 percent with normal left ventricular function, and under 2 percent when abnormal. For PTCA, in-hospital death rates are 0.2 percent, 0.9 percent, and 2.8 percent with one-, two-, and three-vessel disease, respectively. Perioperative myocardial infarction occurs in 5 to 10 percent of CABG patients, versus 3.5 to 5.1 percent in patients undergoing PTCA.

Angioplasty is technically successful about 90 percent of the time and is best when performed on an isolated proximal lesion in a patient with good ventricular function. However, it is increasingly being attempted[15] on patients with multiple lesions and poorer ventricular function despite the increased difficulty. Surgery relieves or reduces chest pain in about 90 percent of patients, with recurrent angina noted in 2 to 4 percent of patients per year. This compares with an overall clinical success rate of about 80 percent with PTCA and a 30 percent restenosis rate within 6 months. About 50 percent of surgical grafts occlude in 10 years; however, internal mammary artery grafts have a greater than 90 percent patency rate at 10 years. The long-term benefits of bypass surgery are well established. Survival after surgery is about 80 percent at 8 years, with 50 percent of patients being symptom-free at 5 years. In patients who have had a successful angioplasty, most with single-vessel disease, 70 percent have been reported to be pain-free at 4 years.[15,238] Eighty-three percent of patients with multivessel disease undergoing angioplasty were free from cardiac events at 3 years.[239]

Surgery improves the symptoms and the survival of patients with significant ($\geq$ 50 percent) left main coronary artery stenosis,[240] and remains the procedure of choice in this setting. Because of this, and the fact that a complicating occlusion can jeopardize a large portion of the left ventricular myocardium, angioplasty has no role in the treatment of a left main stenosis unless it is protected distally by a graft. Surgery also improves survival in patients with three-vessel disease with normal left ventricular function who have severe symptoms or positive exercise tolerance test (ETT).[241,242] Thus PTCA should not be attempted in patients with multiple-vessel disease with severe diffuse atherosclerosis. More complete clinical and morphologic criteria for performing coronary angioplasty are provided by the ACC/AHA Task Force Report.[237]

Special Problems in Coronary Arteriography

Coronary Artery Spasm

Spasm of the coronary arteries represents an extremely important aspect of coronary disease for the cardiovascular radiologist for two reasons. First, it may well be mistaken for organic disease of the coronary arteries, and second, its presence may explain symptoms and signs in patients with or without demonstrably abnormal coronary arteries.

Some evidence of coronary artery spasm has been reported in 0.2 to 3.4 percent of all patients under-

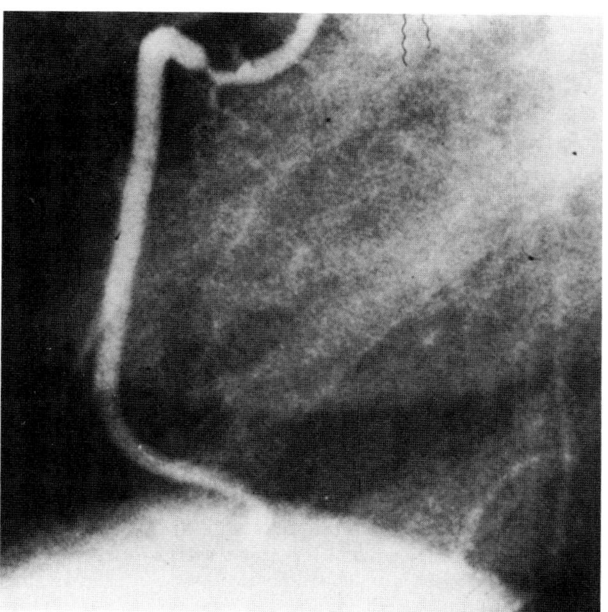

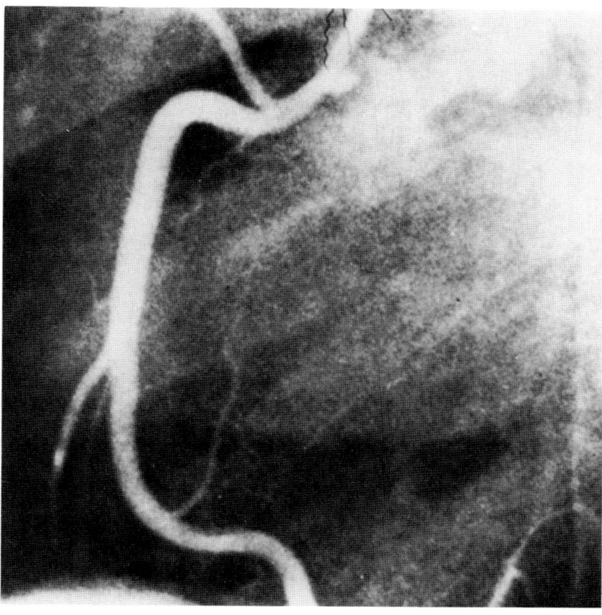

Figure 26-46. Coronary artery spasm, catheter-induced. Right coronary arteriogram, RAO projection. (A) Initial injection. Localized narrowing just at the catheter tip is visible. (B) After the removal of the catheter and the introduction of nitroglycerin, the narrowing is no longer visible. (Courtesy of Hugo Spindola Franco, M.D.)

going selective coronary arteriography.[224,243,244] In patients who do not receive vasodilators before coronary arteriography, spasm is seen in about 1 to 3 percent.[245–248] For the most part, this relatively high incidence of spasm is caused by mechanical stimulation of the arteries by the catheter tip and does not produce myocardial ischemia.

Catheter-Induced Spasm

Iatrogenic spasm of the coronary arteries in humans is produced by the introduction of a selective catheter into the coronary artery, with manipulation of the catheter and presumably local irritation of the vascular wall. It is distinguished by its location usually close to the tip of the catheter. Almost invariably it occurs in the right coronary artery. Its appearance is that of a short, concentric, usually rather smooth area of narrowing (Fig. 26-46A), with the length of the narrow segment generally but not invariably less than 0.5 mm. Symptoms are relatively unusual in the presence of catheter-induced spasm.

Perhaps the most important aspect of catheter-induced spasm is its prompt response to removal of the catheter or to the administration of nitroglycerin (see Fig. 26-46B).[249] On rare occasions, catheter-induced spasm may fail to respond promptly to nitroglycerin administration.

Spontaneously Occurring Spasm (Prinzmetal Variant Angina)

In 1959, Prinzmetal et al. described a type of variant angina in which the pain was typical but occurred spontaneously at rest, without relationship to exercise or emotion, and was associated with elevated S–T segments in the electrocardiogram.[250,251] With the disappearance of pain, the elevated S–T segments returned to normal. As Prinzmetal variant angina was explored more thoroughly, it became clear that it was associated primarily with coronary artery spasm—a concept that has been called a "proved hypothesis."[249,252,253] The endothelium, medial smooth muscle cells, autonomic nerves, and mural and sympathetic nerve chemoreceptors appear to be involved in a complex feedback system that may result in vasospasm.[254,255]

The broader implications of spontaneously occurring spasm of the coronary arteries have been effectively explored by Maseri and his associates,[256] as well as by many other investigators.[202] Spasm severe enough to obstruct the coronary branches has been documented in angina at rest.[257] It has also been shown convincingly that angina at rest followed by myocardial infarction may be accompanied by severe spasm in specific cases.[256,258] Maseri has suggested and believes he has verified that spasm causes acute myocardial infarction in some patients in whom infarction follows

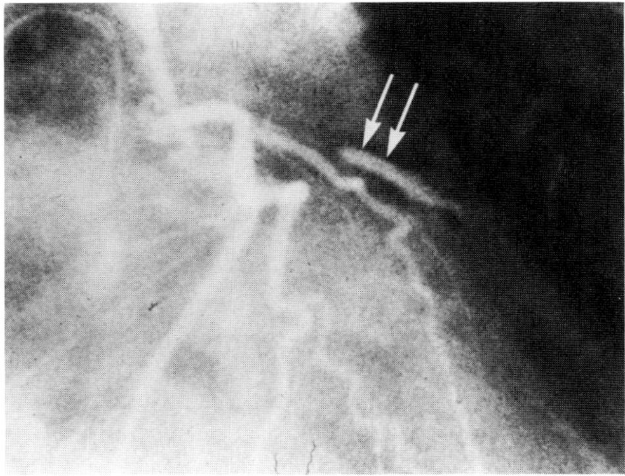

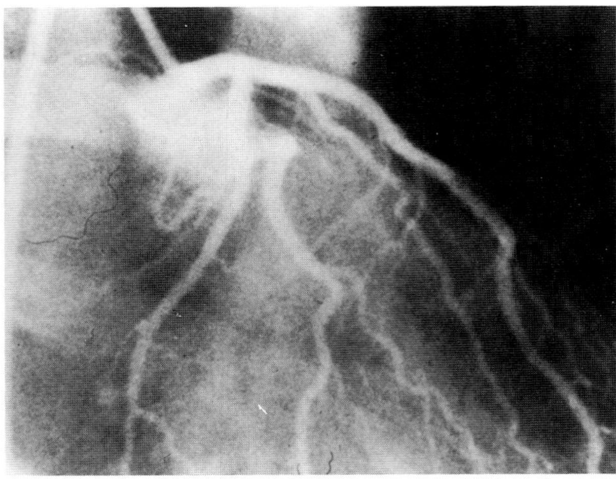

A B

Figure 26-47. Coronary artery spasm, spontaneous. Selective left coronary arteriogram, RAO projection, of a 31-year-old man with Prinzmetal variant angina. (A) Initial examination. Profound narrowing of the proximal and distal segments of the LAD is visible (*arrows*). The midsegment of the LAD is opacified through epicardial collateral flow. Note the absence of arteriosclerotic change in the other visualized branches. (B) Angiogram after the administration of 1/150 of a grain of sublingual nitroglycerin. The LAD coronary artery now appears entirely normal. (Courtesy of Hugo Spindola Franco, M.D.)

acute ischemic attacks. Radioisotope studies have shown decreased perfusion, just as angiography has shown severe vasospasm.[257,259,260] In many patients, spasm has been observed in vessels that are the site of atherosclerotic lesions,[257,259–262] but clearly atherosclerotic disease is not a prerequisite for the development of vasospasm.[249,257,263]

Coronary arteriography may play an important role in confirming the diagnosis of Prinzmetal variant angina by demonstrating the presence of spasm during an ischemic attack. Angiographically, the spasm observed in Prinzmetal angina is frequently irregular and eccentric, and it involves a longer segment of the artery than does catheter-induced spasm. Rarely it is smooth, and it may change in location with different injections. It may be located many centimeters from the tip of the catheter and extend over a length of 0.5 to 2.5 cm or more in many patients.[249] Although the spasm usually responds to nitroglycerin (Fig. 26-47), the response is not uniform.

Prinzmetal angina may occur with normal arteries or with coronary atherosclerosis. Normal vessels have been found angiographically in only 18 percent of patients in whom spasm during angina has been documented by angiography. Both in patients with normal coronary arteries and in those with organic coronary disease, the spasm occurs most commonly in a single vessel. When the spasm coexists with organic coronary disease, it is found in the vessel with an organic lesion in 90 percent of patients, and in only 10 percent does it occur in an apparently normal portion of the vessel.[261]

Induced Coronary Spasm in Patients with Prinzmetal Angina

Provocative pharmacologic testing for coronary spasm has been widely used as a means of confirming the origin of ischemic pain.[264] Progressive doses of 0.1 to 0.3 mg of ergonovine maleate are administered (Fig. 26-48), with the production of sometimes remarkable spasm in coronary arteries that may otherwise appear normal. Ergonovine should not be administered without full preparation for immediate nitroglycerin administration if arrhythmias, coronary artery occlusion, or severe ischemic pain develops. As a potentially hazardous intervention, it should be employed with great care and discretion in the choice of patients.

Myocardial Bridging

Flow in the left coronary artery differs distinctly from that in the right coronary artery. Left coronary flow drops profoundly during isovolumetric contraction, and systolic flow in general is less than diastolic. In midsystole, however, there is a slight increase in coronary flow during maximum ejection and further reduc-

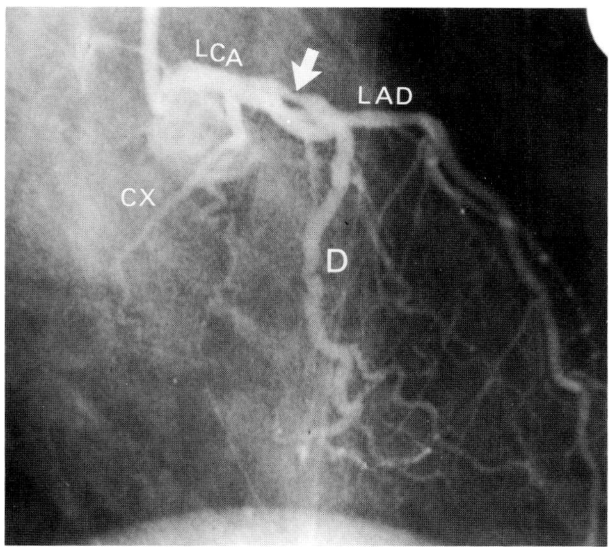

A

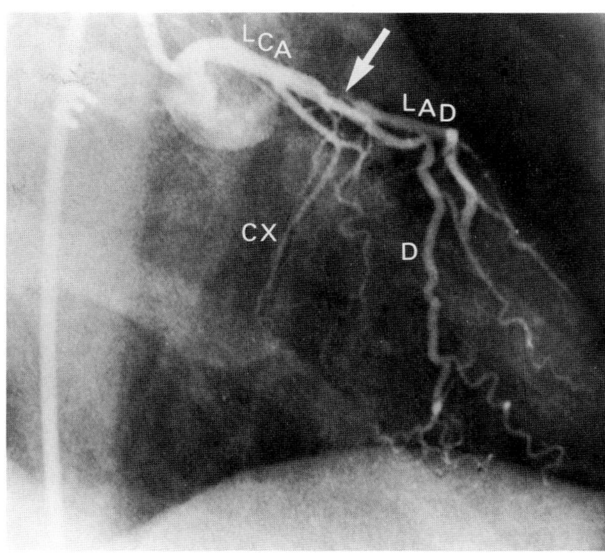

B

Figure 26-48. Coronary artery spasm, pharmacologically induced. Selective left coronary arteriogram, RAO projection, of a 46-year-old man who had episodes of severe chest pain at rest, associated with elevation of the S–T segment in the electrocardiogram. (A) Initial angiogram. Moderate stenosis of the LAD is visible (*arrow*). Minimal irregularity is present in other vessels. (B) Angiogram after ergonovine administration. Striking narrowing of all branches of the left coronary artery has developed. The organic lesion in the proximal LAD (*arrow*) appears more severe, whereas the distal LAD is totally obstructed. This response to 0.1 mg of ergonovine is typical of the hyperreactivity demonstrated in patients with Prinzmetal angina.

tion during reduced ejection. With protodiastole and isovolumetric relaxation, coronary arterial flow increases significantly and remains at a relatively high level throughout diastole. The opening of the aortic valve is synchronous with a moderate systolic increase in coronary flow, and the closure of the aortic valve at the end of systole is accompanied by a sharp rise in coronary flow associated with decreased intracavitary and intramyocardial pressure. This flow pattern contrasts with that in other viscera during systole; when the velocity of flow through most viscera increases, in the left coronary artery it decreases.

Myocardial contraction may affect flow patterns strikingly under special circumstances. With marked ventricular hypertrophy, as in aortic stenosis, the heightened intramyocardial pressure during systole sometimes produces cessation of coronary blood flow or even reversal of flow.

This phenomenon may also be observed during ventricular systole in septal branches markedly compressed by septal contraction (Fig. 26-49).

A similar compression effect on epicardial branches may be observed when the vessel is deep to the epicardium within the myocardium or bridged by muscular bands.[265–268] Myocardial bridging may be diagnosed with certainty when the artery is normal or near normal during diastole but narrowed during ventricular contraction (Fig. 26-50). This finding occurs in about 5 percent of human hearts and is most frequently seen in the left anterior descending artery. Until recently, it was thought to be an innocuous phenomenon, an angiographic curiosity without major clinical relevance. Because coronary blood flow is predominantly diastolic (see above), systolic compression should not affect myocardial perfusion significantly. A number of observers have concluded that bridging of the left anterior descending coronary artery may produce myocardial ischemia.[266–268] Others have suggested that bridging may affect the development of arteriosclerosis in the involved vessel.[269] In some symptomatic patients, periarterial muscle resection has been accompanied by relief of chest pain symptoms.[270] Nevertheless, the evidence is conflicting, and some data indicate that neither the exercise electrocardiogram nor exercise ^{201}thallium myocardial scintigraphy reflects ischemia in the presence of well-documented myocardial bridging.[271]

Aside from its direct clinical relevance, clear recognition of myocardial bridging is essential to permit adequate differentiation from organic coronary disease.

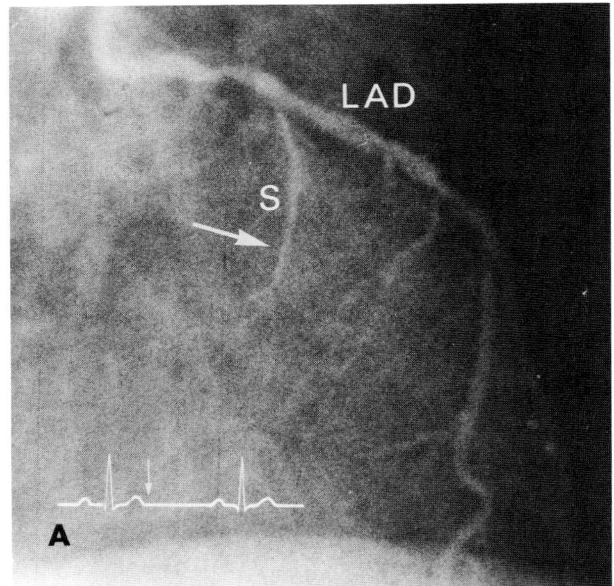

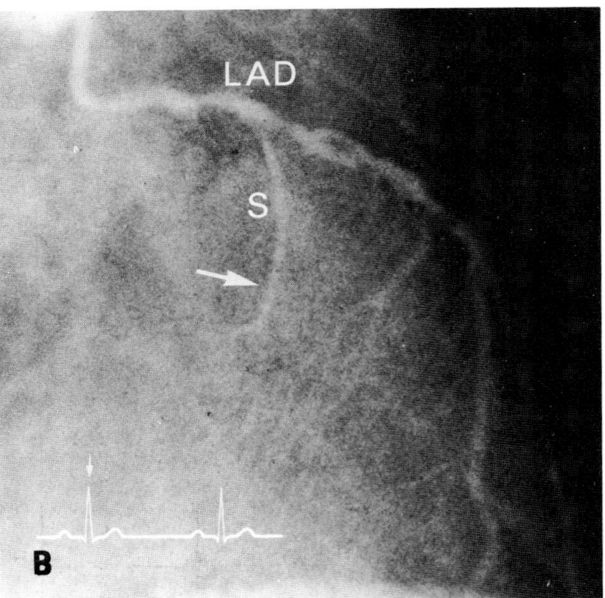

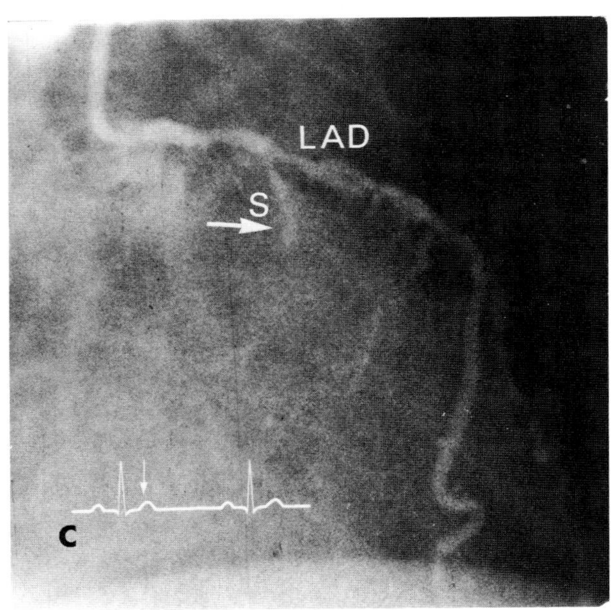

Figure 26-49. Compression of septal branches during ventricular systole. Cine frames of selective left coronary arteriogram, RAO projection, of a 66-year-old man with angina pectoris who demonstrated two-vessel disease on angiography. The first septal artery (*arrow*) is visualized beyond an ostial stenosis. There was antegrade flow in protodiastole, in diastole (A), and throughout atrial systole and ventricular isometric contraction (B). Reversal of flow occurred at the onset of the ejection period (C), with contraction of the ventricular septum.

Determinants of Operability

Presence of Hemodynamically Significant Stenosis or Occlusion

The application of PTCA or revascularization surgery depends on the arteriographic demonstration of hemodynamically significant stenosis. The criteria of "significance" have already been discussed above.

The Vessel Beyond the Lesion

The coronary arteriogram is not always capable of demonstrating precisely the degree of arteriosclerotic involvement beyond a significant stenosis. A reduced lumen caliber in the distal vessel may become much larger when the perfusion pressure is increased at surgery or after a recanalization procedure. Conversely, a narrowed vessel may reflect extensive involvement by atherosclerosis, making the bypass procedure technically difficult. Finally, it should be emphasized that failure to demonstrate a distal vessel need not imply its absence. The surgeon may find an acceptable distal vessel or may widen an existing channel to an acceptable degree by endarterectomy.

The "runoff" to the distal perfusable myocardial capillary bed is highly significant. In some instances, the vessel beyond the stenosis may be adequate in size but may perfuse only a small amount of myocardium. A surgical bypass or recanalization procedure will then be accompanied by low flow, which is associated with a high incidence of procedural failure. Very slow emptying of the vasculature beyond a stenotic lesion may

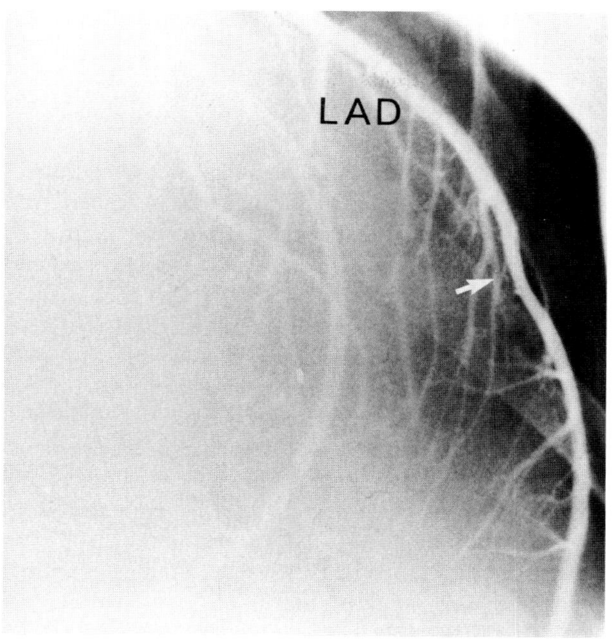

A

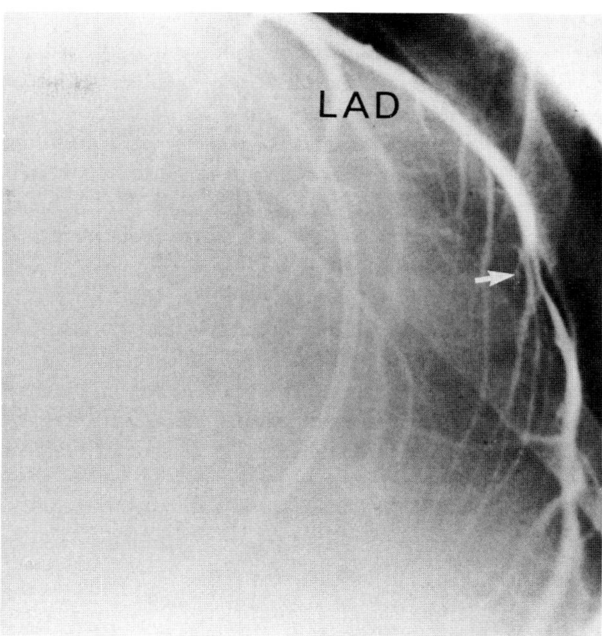

B

Figure 26-50. Myocardial bridging. Selective left coronary arteriogram, RAO projection, of a 55-year-old man who complained of chest pain on exercise. The resting and exercise electrocardiograms were normal. (A) Ventricular diastole. The LAD appears normal (*arrow*). (B) Ventricular systole. The LAD is strikingly but symmetrically narrowed (*arrow*), the typical appearance of a myocardial bridge.

reflect either the severity of the stenosis or a limited amount of perfusable myocardium.

The Ventricular Myocardium

A ventriculogram is probably the most useful parameter in evaluating the operability of the patient once the presence and location of a coronary stenotic lesion have been established. Asynergy in the ventriculogram is useful in determining the physiologic significance of stenoses that are difficult to assess purely by arteriography. Unfortunately, the converse is not true. The function of the ventricular myocardium is assessed by the left ventriculogram. The ventriculogram may show frank ventricular aneurysm, requiring removal at the time of coronary artery bypass, or may indicate that the only area served by the obstructed vessel is a thin-walled, noncontractile segment that would not benefit from repairing the obstructed artery. Ventriculography is particularly useful in detecting patients who will tolerate the surgical procedure poorly because of inadequate myocardial contractility in the entire ventricle. When the ejection fraction is less than 20 to 30 percent, the risk of the surgical procedure is considerably elevated. Biplane assessment of the ventricle under these circumstances is helpful because the ejection fraction calculated from the biplane assessment may differ from that calculated by single-plane ventriculography alone.[272]

The Arteriogram in Angina Pectoris

In classic angina pectoris, occlusive disease of the major coronary arteries is usually demonstrable. The left anterior descending branch is involved in most patients with angina, and angina is more likely in the presence of disease involving at least two coronary arteries.[135] Although data have been presented indicating that angina pectoris may occur with only a single mild arterial lesion,[172,273] other investigators have found severe coronary disease in virtually all such patients.[131,134,136,274]

Proudfit, Shirey, and Sones[275] noted that 94 percent of patients with clinical angina pectoris had evidence of moderate or severe obstruction of one or more major vessels. In 95 percent of patients thought to be free of coronary artery disease, the arteriograms showed no significant abnormalities. In patients with myocardial infarction, arterial narrowing was demonstrated almost uniformly, and virtually all patients had severe obstructive disease (usually associated with total or almost total occlusion).

Campeau and colleagues[276] also studied the correlation between the arteriogram and angina pectoris. Of their patients presumed not to have coronary insufficiency, 96 percent had no arteriographic evidence of obstructive coronary disease. Only 80 percent of their patients with typical angina, however, had significant stenosis of one or more major coronary arteries. Ninety percent of those with myocardial infarction had significant obstructive coronary disease documented by coronary arteriography.

In our experience, angina pectoris is accompanied by one-vessel disease in 30 percent of patients, by two-vessel in 30 percent, by three-vessel in 30 percent, and by normal coronaries in about 10 percent. Patients with angina and a normal resting electrocardiogram have an incidence of lesions similar to that of patients with abnormal electrocardiograms but of lessened severity.[274] No definite correlation could be found between the severity of the arteriographic abnormalities and the duration of clinical symptoms.[274] By the time symptoms occur, diffuse involvement of the coronary arteries is frequently present. A group of patients with atypical chest pain warrants additional comment. Characteristically, they have a history of painful episodes suggesting acute myocardial ischemia but no electrocardiographic changes during pain and negative exercise tests. The arteriograms have usually been abnormal.[136]

The Positive Exercise Test

It is possible to relate the exercise test to morphologic change in the coronary arteries during life, and thus to "define" it arteriographically. In general, there has been a high correlation of the positive exercise test with demonstrated arteriosclerotic disease of the major coronary arteries.[277] In our own series, all cases with a positive test in the absence of valvular disease or digitalis administration were associated with an abnormal arteriogram.[136] Davis[130] reported that exercise tests in his series were positive only in patients with abnormal studies. In Paulin's extensive report, positive exercise tests were rare in patients with normal arteriograms.[134] Most patients with positive exercise tests had severe obstructive changes as demonstrated by arteriography. Kemp and Elliott[278] reported a somewhat higher incidence (20 percent) of positive double Master tests in the presence of angina and a normal coronary arteriogram. A negative exercise electrocardiogram does not exclude positive arteriographic findings: arteriography reveals significant coronary artery stenosis in 25 percent of the patients. Boelling et al.[279] found good correlation of the "roentgenographic exercise test" with coronary arteriography. This test, now of historical interest only, consisted in evaluating heart size on standard chest roentgenography before and after a 100-yard walk at a swift pace.

Surgical Aspects

Surgical and percutaneous recanalization procedures require knowledge of the localization of lesions, the status of the distal vascular bed, and the degree to which patency persists after repair. Preoperative and postoperative coronary arteriography fills these needs. Aside from determining the presence of lesions that would render a revascularization feasible, the arteriogram demonstrates patency and perfusion of the coronary bed after a successful procedure.[280] This is the most definitive method of study available at present. The degree of augmented blood flow to ischemic myocardium, a critical factor, may be evaluated with isotopic studies.

Coronary arteriography demonstrates luminal changes from intimal hyperplasia and medial fibrosis associated with the rejection phenomenon[281] after cardiac transplantation.

Prognostic Implications of Arteriography

The radiographic assessment of coronary pathology is closely related to the overall prognosis of coronary disease and represents an important predictor of survival potential (Table 26-2). For example, the presence of only single-vessel disease judged to be hemodynamically significant is associated with an annual mortality rate that varies from 1.6 to 3.0 percent.[104,282] With two-vessel disease, the mortality rate more than doubles,

Table 26-2. Prognostic Implications of Coronary Arteriography*

Radiographic Assessment of Pathology (Arteriography)	Annual Mortality (%)	Survivors at 5 Years (%)
One-vessel disease	1.6–3.0	85–92
Left main	6.0–7.8	37–51
LAD	4.2	
RCA	2.0	
LCA	2.6	
Two-vessel disease	3–7	62–85
Three-vessel disease	6–11	47–64
Asynergy	Doubles mortality	
Low ejection fraction	Doubles mortality	
Congestive heart failure	Triples mortality	

*Involvement of one, two, or three vessels connotes at least one hemodynamically significant lesion in each vessel.

reaching 3 to 7 percent per year. With three-vessel disease, it triples, reaching 6 to 11 percent.[283–285] The presence of asynergy doubles the mortality rate, and an increase in the heart volume raises the mortality rate considerably.[284] Furthermore, if the chest film reveals evidence of congestive heart failure with redistribution and pulmonary venous hypertension, the overall mortality of one-, two-, and three-vessel disease goes up by a factor of 5.[284]

In assessing one-vessel disease, one must be aware that the average mortality rate does not describe the life expectancy for particular vessel involvement. For example, with LAD stenosis, the mortality is twice as high as it is with right coronary or left circumflex stenosis. Left main coronary artery stenosis involves a mortality almost double that of LAD stenosis and well over twice as high as the average of one-vessel disease.

In summary, beyond its specifically diagnostic and therapeutic implications, the coronary arteriogram furnishes important information as to the likelihood of survival in medically treated individuals simply on the basis of the number of vessels involved with hemodynamically significant disease and the evidence of altered heart volume and performance. The ejection fraction as determined from the ventriculogram is of great importance in the prognosis of patients treated both medically and surgically.[286,287] When the ejection fraction is greater than 50 percent, the probability of 4-year survival is high. When the ejection fraction is less than 25 percent, the probability of 2-year survival is low in patients treated either medically or surgically.[287] Similarly, in unstable angina, the presence of a low ejection fraction and an increased ventricular volume as assessed angiographically is associated with a doubling of the mortality rate at the end of 1 year.[288]

When analysis of the arteriogram is used to predict successful bypass surgery, the most important factor is the size of the vessel to which the bypass is anastomosed. If the vessel is 1.5 mm or less in diameter, if it perfuses a limited area of cardiac muscle, or if there is moderate to severe distal atherosclerosis, a very high incidence of bypass occlusion may be anticipated.[258]

Other Causes of Coronary Artery Disease

Numerous diseases besides arteriosclerosis may cause occlusive disease of the coronary arteries (Table 26-3). Some of these are so unusual as to be pathologic curiosities. Others warrant specific mention.

Dissecting Aortic Aneurysm with Coronary Involvement

Dissecting aneurysm involving the ascending aorta may obstruct a coronary orifice or may extend along an artery.[289,290] Compression by extravasated blood or by hemopericardium is an alternative mechanism of involvement.[291] In a review of 505 cases of dissecting aneurysms proved by autopsy or operation, one or both coronary arteries were involved in 39 cases.[292] It is worth emphasizing that thoracic aortography in a patient with dissecting aneurysm often does not show the coronary ostia adequately. Primary dissecting aneurysm of the coronary arteries[92] is far less common than involvement secondary to aortic dissection.

Table 26-3. Occlusive Abnormalities Other Than Arteriosclerosis

Inflammatory and autoimmune
- Syphilis
- Granulomatous arteritis
- Sclerosing aortitis
- Nonspecific infections
- Lupus erythematosus
- Scleroderma
- Periarteritis nodosa
- Rheumatoid arthritis
- Ankylosing spondylitis
- Degos syndrome

Traumatic
- Closed chest trauma
- Laceration
- Traumatic injury
- Iatrogenic injury
- Radiation injury

Metabolic
- Diabetes
- Mucopolysaccharidosis
- Homocystinuria
- Fabry disease
- Amyloidosis
- Juvenile intimal sclerosis
- Progeria
- Pseudoxanthoma elasticum
- Oral contraceptives and postpartum

Functional—spasm
- Prinzmetal angina
- Iatrogenic (catheter)
- Nitrate withdrawal

Embolic
- Infective endocarditis
- Prosthetic valve embolus
- Myxoma
- Atrial or ventricular thrombus
- Iatrogenic

Miscellaneous
- Aortic dissection
  - Cystic medial necrosis
  - Relapsing polychondritis
  - Arteriosclerosis
  - Syphilis

Acquired aneurysms

Modified from Morettin LB, Radiol Clin North Am 1976;14:189. Used with permission.

Syphilis

Tertiary syphilis is no longer a frequent cause of coronary artery disease, but occasional cases are observed.

Ostial stenosis or occlusion is a typical manifestation and may be a result of medial disease of the aortic wall. Particularly when this involves the left coronary orifice, the patient is at high risk. Furthermore, if surgery for aortic aneurysm is contemplated, difficulty in cannulating the ostium may well occur.

Trauma

Thrombosis of coronary arteries may follow nonpenetrating wounds of the chest. To make this diagnosis, the history of recent trauma must be present, without evidence of recent occlusive disease or of lesions in other vessels.[78,293,294]

Lacerations of the coronary artery are extremely rare and are generally due to penetrating stab wounds. Because these have a very high mortality,[295] prompt diagnosis is essential, and the patients should be approached with an aggressive view toward defining the presence of coronary arterial bleeding. With selective coronary arteriography, the injured coronary artery can be demonstrated, and operative intervention may then be planned.[295]

Autoimmune and Metabolic Diseases

Lupus erythematosus, rheumatoid arthritis, and periarteritis nodosa may all involve the coronary arteries with occlusive disease.[296,297]

A number of metabolic diseases can affect the coronary arteries, including diabetes, Hurler disease, and progeria. Coronary artery disease may also follow the use of oral steroids for contraception.[298]

Intimal or Medial Fibroplasia

Fibroplasia occurs most commonly in the renal arteries. It has been described but rarely verified in the coronary arteries. "Membranous" stenosis has been observed arteriographically but has generally been produced by atypical plaque formation (Fig. 26-51), although congenital membranes may occur in rare patients coming to clinical attention.

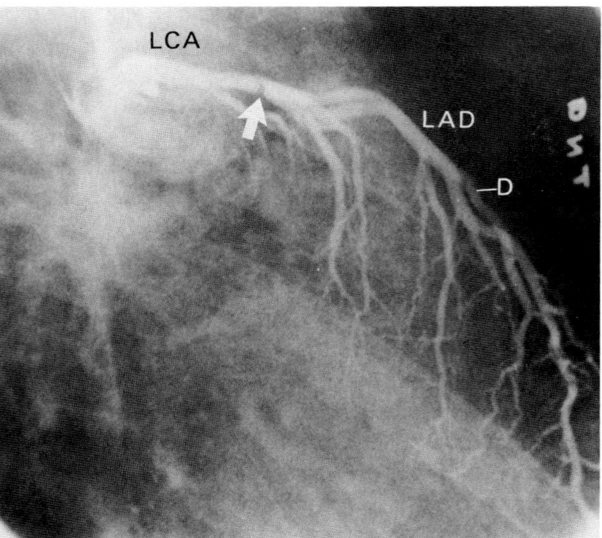

Figure 26-51. Membranous stenosis of the coronary artery. A localized membranous stenosis of the LAD (*arrow*) is visible. This intrudes on the lumen very much as a congenital membrane does but almost invariably turns out to be an unusual atherosclerotic plaque. Although cases of dysplastic disease of the coronary arteries have been described, their presence as an important element in coronary disease in humans is disputed by most observers.

Emerging Methods for Evaluating Coronary Artery Disease

Several new methods for anatomical, and potentially functional, imaging of the coronary arteries and ventricles have been introduced. Although these techniques are unproven for routine clinical use, they hold future promise as powerful imaging modalities. Transthoracic echocardiography and transesophageal echocardiography have proven their clinical usefulness in evaluating the chambers of the heart and proximal aorta, but are limited in their ability to evaluate the coronary arteries. Spiral (dynamic) computed tomography has been applied successfully in the evaluation of coronary artery bypass graft patency, demonstrating an 87 percent sensitivity and 100 percent specificity compared to conventional angiography.[299] However, the experience is limited and, like standard computed tomographic evaluation of the cardiac chambers,[300,301] is not widely available. The most promising of the newer modalities is magnetic resonance imaging. It has already demonstrated its ability to provide both static and cine images of the cardiac chambers[302] and is proving to be useful in evaluating the ventricular manifestations of ischemic heart disease.[301,303–306] MR angiography (MRA) as well is being applied to the evaluation of the coronary arteries. Recently, Manning et al.[307] demonstrated an overall sensitivity of 90 percent and a specificity of 92 percent for MRA, compared to conventional angiography, in the detection of stenoses greater than or equal to 50 percent by diameter. The sensitivity and specificity were 100 percent for detecting lesions in the left main coronary artery, 87 percent and 92 percent for the LAD, 71 percent and 90 percent for the LCX, and 100 percent and 78 percent for the RCA, respectively. They concluded that MRA may be useful for excluding clinically important stenoses in patients referred for conventional contrast arteriography. In the future, it appears that MRI, with its ability to demonstrate anatomic lesions and to quantify blood flow and ventricular wall motion, could potentially serve as a screening modality for patients with suspected coronary artery disease. However, it still suffers from significant motion artifacts, poor image resolution, and the inability to accommodate severely ill patients.

References

1. Herrick JB. Clinical features of sudden obstruction of the coronary arteries. JAMA 1912;59:2015.
2. Levy RI, Moskowitz J. Cardiovascular research: decades of progress, a decade of promise. Science 1982;217:121–129.
3. Kuller LH, Traven ND, Rutan GH, Perper JA, Ives DG. Marked decline of coronary artery disease mortality in 35–44 year old white men in Allegheny County, Pennsylvania. Circulation 1989;80:261–266.
4. Kagan A, Kannel WB, Dawber TR, Revotski N. The coronary profile. Ann NY Acad Sci 1963;97:883.
5. Brown G, Alber JJ, Fisher LD, et al. Regression of coronary artery disease as a result of intensive lipid-lowering therapy in men with high levels of apolipoprotein B. N Engl J Med 1990;323:1289–1298.
6. Ornish D, Brown S, Scherwitz LW, et al. Can lifestyle changes reverse coronary artery disease? Lancet 1990;336:129–133.
7. Favaloro RG, Effler DB, Groves LK, Sones FM, Fergussen DJG. Myocardial revascularization by internal mammary artery implant procedures. J Thorac Cardiovasc Surg 1967;54:359.
8. Proudfit WL, Sones FM, Shirey EK, Fergussen DJG, Sheldon WC. Revascularization of the myocardium. Dis Chest 1969;55:315.
9. Seaman AJ, Griswold HE, Reume RB, Fitzmann L. Long-term anticoagulant prophylaxis after myocardial infarction. N Engl J Med 1969;281:115.
10. ISIS Steering Committee. Intravenous streptokinase given within 0–4 hours of onset of myocardial infarction reduced mortality in ISIS-2. Lancet 1987;28:502.
11. Serruys PW, Simoons ML, Suryapranata H, et al. Preservation of global and regional left ventricular function after early thrombolysis in acute myocardial infarction. J Am Coll Cardiol 1986;7:729–742.
12. TIMI Study Group. The thrombolysis in myocardial infarction (TIMI) trial. N Engl J Med 1985;312:932–936.
13. Peduzzi P, Hultgren H, Miller C, et al. Veterans Administration Cooperative Study of medical versus surgical treatment of stable angina—progress report: V. The five-year effect of coronary bypass surgery on the relief of angina. Prog Cardiovasc Dis 1986;28:267–272.
14. Hultgren H, Peduzzi P, Shapiro W, et al. Veterans Administration Cooperative Study of medical versus surgical treatment of stable angina—progress report: VII. Effect of medical versus surgical treatment on exercise performance at five years. Prog Cardiovasc Dis 1986;28:279–284.
15. NHLBI PTCA Registry: principal investigators and their associates. Percutaneous transluminal coronary angioplasty in 1985–1986 and 1977–1981. N Engl J Med 1988;318:265–270.
16. American Heart Association. 1992 heart and stroke facts. Dallas: American Heart Association, 1992.
17. Beck CS. Development of a new blood supply to the heart by operation. Ann Surg 1935;102:801.
18. Bailey CP, May A, Lemmon WM. Survival after coronary endarterectomy in man. JAMA 1957;164:641.
19. Effler DB, Groves LK, Sones FM. Myocardial revascularization by internal mammary implantation. Vasc Dis 1966;3:42.
20. Sheldon WC, Rincon G, Pichard AD, Razani M, Cheanvechai C, Loop FD. Surgical treatment of 741 patients followed 3–7 years. Prog Cardiovasc Dis 1975;18:237.
21. Rousthoi P. Uber Angiokardiographie: Vorufige Mitteilung. Acta Radiol (Stockh) 1933;14:419.
22. Reboul H, Racine M. La ventriculographie cardiac experimentale. Presse Med 1933;1:763.
23. Radner S. Thoracic aortography by catheterization from the radial artery. Acta Radiol (Stockh) 1948;29:178.
24. Jonsson G, Broden B, Karnell J. Thoracic aortography. Acta Radiol (Stockh) 1951;89(Suppl):1.
25. DiGuglielmo L, Guttadauro MA. A roentgenologic study of the coronary arteries in the living. Acta Radiol (Stockh) 1952; 97(Suppl):1.
26. Dotter CT, Frische LJ. Visualization of the coronary circulation by occlusion aortography: a practical method. Radiology 1958;71:502.
27. Lehman JS, Boyer RA, Winter FS. Coronary arteriography. AJR 1959;81:749.
28. Bellman S, Frank HA, Lambert PB, Littman D, Williams JA. Coronary arteriography: 1. Differential opacification of the aortic stem by catheters of special design—experimental development. N Engl J Med 1960;262:325.
29. Paulin S. Coronary angiography: a technical, anatomic, and clinical study. Acta Radiol (Stockh) 1964;233(Suppl):1.
30. Sones F, Shirey EK. Cine coronary arteriography. Mod Concepts Cardiovasc Dis 1962;31:735.
31. Ricketts HJ, Abrams HL. Percutaneous selective coronary cinearteriography. JAMA 1962;181:620.
32. Judkins MP. Selective coronary arteriography: 1. A percutaneous transfemoral technic. Radiology 1967;89:815.
33. Judkins MP. Percutaneous transfemoral selective coronary arteriography. Radiol Clin North Am 1968;6:467.
34. Lee GB, Amplatz K. Coronary arteriography: selective vs. non-selective methods. Minn Med 1968;51:343.
35. Adams DF, Abrams HL, Ruttley M. The roentgen pathology of coronary artery disease. Semin Roentgenol 1972;7:319.
36. Hultgren HN. Medical versus surgical management of unstable angina. Am J Cardiol 1976;38:479.
37. Takaro T, Hultgren HN, Detre KM. VA cooperative study of coronary arterial surgery: left main disease. Circulation 1975; 52(Suppl):11–143.
38. Marcus ML, Doty DB, Hiratzka LF, Wright CB, Eastham CL. Decreased coronary reserve: a mechanism of angina pectoris in patients with aortic stenosis and normal coronary arteries. N Engl J Med 1982;307:1362–1366.
39. Bryson AL, Parisi AF, Schecter E, et al. Life threatening ventricular arrhythmias induced by exercise: cessation after bypass surgery. Am J Cardiol 1973;32:995.
40. Graham AF, Miller DC, Stinson EB, et al. Surgical treatment of refractory life threatening ventricular tachycardia. Am J Cardiol 1973;32:909.
41. Kemp HG, Elliott WC. The anginal syndrome with normal coronary arteriography. Trans Assoc Am Physicians 1967;80:59.
42. James T. Pathology of small coronary arteries. Am J Cardiol 1967;20:679.
43. Proudfit WL, Shirey EK, Sheldon WC, Sones FM. Certain clinical characteristics correlated with extent of obstructive lesions demonstrated by selective cine-coronary arteriography. Circulation 1968;38:947.
44. Baltaxe HA, Amplatz K, Varco RL, Buchwald H. Coronary arteriography in hypercholesterolemic patients. AJR 1969; 105:784.
45. Maseri A, Severi S, deNes M, et al. "Variant" angina: one aspect of a continuous spectrum of vasospastic myocardial ischemia. Am J Cardiol 1978;42:1019.
46. Begg FR, Magovers GJ, Cushing WJ, Kent EM, Fisher DL. Selective cine coronary arteriography in patients with complete heart block. J Thorac Cardiovasc Surg 1969;57:9.
47. Bouchard RJ, Karliner JS, Gault JH. Effect of contrast medium on left ventricular performance in man. Circulation 1970;41–42(Suppl):138.

48. Kong Y, Morris JJ Jr, McIntosh HD. Assessment of regional myocardial performance from biplane coronary cineangiograms. Am J Cardiol 1970;25:374.
49. Rahimtoola SH, Gau GT, Raphael MJ. Cardiac performance after diagnostic coronary arteriography. Circulation 1970;41:537.
50. Rackley CE, Dodge HT, Coble YD Jr, Hay RE. A method of determining left ventricular mass in man. Circulation 1964;29:666.
51. Kennedy JW, Reichenbach DD, Baxley WA, Dodge HT. Left ventricular mass: a comparison of angiocardiographic measurements with autopsy weight. Am J Cardiol 1967;19:221.
52. Eber LM, Greenspan HM, Cooke JM, Gorlin R. Dynamic changes in left ventricular free wall thickness in the human heart. Circulation 1969;39:455.
53. Herman MV, Heinle RA, Klein MD, Gorlin R. Localized disorders in myocardial contraction: asynergy and its role in congestive heart failure. N Engl J Med 1967;277:222.
54. McDonald G. The shape and movements of the human left ventricle during systole: a study of cineangiography and by cineradiography of epicardial markers. Am J Cardiol 1970;26:221.
55. Karliner JS, Bouchard RJ, Gault JH. Dimensional changes of the human left ventricle prior to aortic valve opening: a cineangiographic study in patients with and without left heart disease. Circulation 1971;44:312.
56. Keats TE, Martt JM. False paradoxic movement of the posterior wall of the left ventricle simulating myocardial aneurysm. Radiology 1962;78:381.
57. Tennant R, Wiggers CJ. Effect of coronary occlusion on myocardial contraction. Am J Physiol 1935;112:351.
58. Kurtzman RS, Lofstrom JE. Detection and evaluation of myocardial infarction by image amplification and cinefluorography. Radiology 1963;81:57.
59. Master AM, Gubner R, Dack S, Jaffe HL. The diagnosis of coronary occlusion and myocardial infarction by fluoroscopic examination. Am Heart J 1940;20:475.
60. Sussman ML, Dack S, Master AM. Roentgenkymogram in myocardial infarction: abnormalities in left ventricular contraction. Am Heart J 1940;19:453.
61. Harrison TR. Some unanswered questions concerning enlargement and failure of the heart. Am Heart J 1965;69:100.
62. Gorlin R, Klein MD, Sullivan JM. Prospective correlative study of ventricular aneurysm: mechanism concept and clinical recognition. Am J Med 1967;42:512.
63. Mein MD, Herman MV, Gorlin R. A hemodynamic study of left ventricular aneurysm. Circulation 1967;35:614.
64. Eber LM, Cooke JM, Gorlin R. The dynamic characterization of ventricular premature beats in man. J Clin Invest 1968;47:27a.
65. Herman MV, Elliott WC, Gorlin R. An electrocardiographic, anatomic, and metabolic study of zonal myocardial ischemia in coronary heart disease. Circulation 1967;35:834.
66. Bjork L, Cullhed I, Hallon A. Cineangiographic studies of the left ventricle in patients with angina pectoris. Circulation 1967;36:868.
67. Kazamias TM, Gander MP, Ross J Jr, Braunwald E. Detection of left-ventricular-wall motion disorders in coronary-artery disease by radarkymography. N Engl J Med 1971;285:63.
68. Baxley WA, Reeves TJ. Abnormal regional myocardial performance in coronary artery disease. Prog Cardiovasc Dis 1971;13:405.
69. Herman MV, Gorlin R. Implications of left ventricular asynergy. Am J Cardiol 1969;23:538. Semin Roentgenol 1969;4:346.
70. McConahay DR, McCallister BD, Hallermann FJ, Smith RE. Comparative quantitative analysis of the electrocardiogram and vectorcardiogram: correlation with the coronary arteriogram. Circulation 1970;42:245.
71. Helfant RH, Kemp HG, Gorlin R. Coronary atherosclerosis, coronary collaterals, and their relation to cardiac function. Ann Intern Med 1970;73:189.
72. Katz AM, Hecht HH. The early "pump" failure of the ischemic heart. Am J Med 1969;47:497.
73. Helfant RH, Herman MV, Gorlin R. Abnormalities of left ventricular contraction induced by beta adrenergic blockade. Circulation 1971;43:641.
74. Restrepo C, Eggen DA, Guzman MA, Tejada C. Postmortem dimensions of the coronary arteries in different geographic locations. Lab Invest 1973;28:244.
75. Roberts WC. Coronary heart disease: a review of abnormalities observed in the coronary arteries. Cardiovasc Med 1977;2:29.
76. Abramson DI. Blood vessels and lymphatics. New York: Academic, 1980:812.
77. White CW, Wright CB, Doty DB, Hiratzka LF, Eastham CL, Harrison DG, Marcus ML. Does visual interpretation of the coronary arteriogram predict the physiologic importance of coronary stenosis? N Engl J Med 1984;310:819–824.
78. Benray J, Price EC, Massin FK, Bowers JC, Cooley DA. Coronary occlusion secondary to nonpenetrating chest trauma. Tex Med 1975;71:60.
79. Roberts WC. Coronary embolism: a review of causes, consequences, and diagnostic considerations. Cardiovasc Med 1978;3:699.
80. Arnett EN, Roberts WC. Acute myocardial infarction and angiographically normal coronary arteries: an unproven combination. Circulation 1976;53:395.
81. Daoud AS, Pankin D, Tulgan H, Florentin RA. Aneurysms of the coronary artery: report of ten cases and review of the literature. Am J Cardiol 1963;11:228.
82. Sayegh S, Adad W, Macleod CA. Multiple aneurysms of the coronary arteries. Am Heart J 1968;76:266.
83. Eshchar Y, Yahini JH, Deutsch V, Neufeld HN. Arteriosclerotic aneurysm of the coronary artery. Chest 1977;72:374.
84. Dawson JE Jr, Ellison RG. Isolated aneurysm of the anterior descending coronary artery—surgical treatment. Am J Cardiol 1972;29:868.
85. McMartin DE, Stone AJ, Franch RH. Multiple coronary-artery aneurysms in a child with angina pectoris. N Engl J Med 1974;290:669.
86. Onuchi Z, Simazu S, Kiyosawa N, Takamatsu T, Hamaoka K. Aneurysms of the coronary arteries in Kawasaki disease: an angiographic study of 30 cases. Circulation 1982;66:1–6.
87. Sasaguri Y, Kato H. Regression of aneurysms in Kawasaki disease: a pathological study. J Pediatr 1982;2:225–231.
88. Bertelsen S, Lindahl A. Aneurysms of the coronary arteries: report of two cases. Acta Med Scand 1964;175:589.
89. Chamberlain JL III, Perry LW. Infantile periarteritis nodosa with coronary and brachial aneurysms: a case diagnosed during life. J Pediatr 1971;78:1039.
90. Crook BRM, Raftery EB, Oram S. Case report—mycotic aneurysms of coronary arteries. Br Heart J 1973;35:107.
91. Konecke LL, Spitzer S, Mason D, Kasparian H, James PM Jr. Traumatic aneurysm of the left coronary artery. Am J Cardiol 1971;27:221.
92. Claudon DG, Claudon DB, Edwards JE. Primary dissecting aneurysm of coronary artery: a cause of acute myocardial ischemia. Circulation 1972;45:259.
93. Roy JJ, Klein HZ. Dissecting aneurysm of the coronary artery. JAMA 1971;218:1047.
94. Whitehead R, Dunnill MS. Primary dissecting aneurysms of coronary arteries. J Pathol 1969;99:33.
95. Denham SW. Syphilitic aneurysm of the left coronary artery. Arch Pathol 1951;51:661.
96. Kalke B, Edwards JE. Localized aneurysms of the coronary arteries. Angiology 1968;19:460.
97. Ellis R, Kurth RJ. Calcified coronary artery aneurysms. JAMA 1968;203:51.
98. Scott DH. Aneurysm of the coronary arteries. Am Heart J 1948;36:403.
99. Hudson NM, Walker JK. The prognostic significance of coronary artery calcification seen on fluoroscopy. Clin Radiol 1976;27:545.

100. McGuire J, Schneider HJ, Chou TC. Clinical significance of coronary artery calcification seen fluoroscopically with the image intensifier. Circulation 1968;37:82.
101. Tarnpas JP, Soule AB. Coronary artery calcification: its incidence and significance in patients over 40 years of age. AJR 1966;97:369.
102. Frink RJ, Achor RWP, Brown AL, Kincaid OW, Brandenburg RO. Significance of calcification of the coronary arteries. Am J Cardiol 1970;26:241.
103. McCarthy DR, Palmer FJ. Incidence and significance of coronary artery calcification. Br Heart J 1974;36:499.
104. Bartel AG, Chen JT, Peter RH, Behar VS, Kong Y, Lester RG. The significance of coronary calcification detected by fluoroscopy. Circulation 1974;49:1247.
105. Hamby RI, Tabrah R, Wisoff BG, Hartstein ML. Coronary artery calcification: clinical implications and angiographic correlates. Am Heart J 1974;87:565.
106. Schlesinger MJ, Zoll PM. Incidence and localization of coronary artery occlusions. Arch Pathol 1941;32:178.
107. Littman D, Dean D, Crowley F, Gelson I, Williams J. Clinical coronary angiography. Am J Cardiol 1961;7:570.
108. Sloman G, Hare WSC. Clinical application of coronary angiography. Med J Aust 1960;47:611.
109. Gray CR, Hoffman HA, Hammond WS, Miller KM, Oseasohn RO. Correlation of arteriographic and pathologic findings in coronary arteries in man. Circulation 1962;26:494.
110. Eusterman JH, Achor RWP, Kincaid OW, Brown AL Jr. Atherosclerotic disease of the coronary arteries: a pathologic-radiologic correlative study. Circulation 1962;26:288.
111. Hale G, Jefferson K. Technique and interpretation of selective coronary arteriography in man. Br Heart J 1963;25:644.
112. Kemp HG, Evans H, Elhott WC, Gorlin R. Diagnostic accuracy of selective coronary cinearteriography. Circulation 1967;36:526.
113. Vlodaver Z, Frech R, Van Tassel RA, Edwards JE. Correlation of the antemortem coronary arteriograms and the postmortem specimen. Circulation 1973;47:162.
114. Grondin CM, Dyrda J, Pasternac A, Campeau L, Bourassa M, Lespérance J. Discrepancies between cineangiographic and postmortem findings in patients with coronary artery disease and recent myocardial revascularization. Circulation 1974;49:703.
115. Schwartz JN, Kong Y, Hackel DB, Bartel AG. Comparison of angiographic and postmortem findings in patients with coronary artery disease. Am J Cardiol 1975;36:174.
116. Arnett EN, Isner JM, Redwood DR, Kent KM, Baker WP, Ackerstein H, Roberts WC. Coronary artery narrowing in coronary heart disease: comparison of cineangiographic and necropsy findings. Ann Intern Med 1979;91:198.
117. Murphy ML, Galbraith JE, de Soyza N. The reliability of coronary angiogram interpretation: an angiographic-pathologic correlation with a comparison of radiographic views. Am Heart J 1979;97:578.
118. Staiger J, Dieckmann H, Adler CP, Barmeyer J, Sandritter W. Postmortem angiographic and pathologic-anatomic findings in coronary heart disease: a comparative study using planimetry. Cardiovasc Intervent Radiol 1980;3:1.
119. Forsberg SA, Alestig D, Bjure J, Haggendahl E, Paulin S, Varnauskas E, Werkö L. Post mortem, coronary arteriographic, clinical, and electrocardiographic findings in 80 patients investigated with coronary arteriography. Acta Med Scand 1971;189:463.
120. Zollikofer CL, Vlodaver Z, Nath HP, Castaneda-Zuniga W, Valdez-Davila O, Amplatz K, Edwards JE. Angiographic findings in recanalization of coronary arterial thrombi. Radiology 1980;134:303.
121. Bjork L, O'Keefe A. Estimation of coronary artery stenosis. Acta Radiol (Stockh) 1976;17:777.
122. Zir LM, Miller SW, Dinsmore RE, Gilbert JP, Harthorne JW. Interobserver variability in coronary angiography. Circulation 1976;53:4.
123. Myers MG, Shulman HS, Saibil EA, Naqui SZ. Variation in measurement of coronary lesions on 35 and 70 mm angiograms. AJR 1978;130:913.
124. Detre KM, Wright E, Murphy ML, Takaro T. Observer agreement in evaluating coronary angiograms. Circulation 1975;52:979–986.
125. DeRouen TA, Murray JA, Owen W. Variability in the analysis of coronary arteriograms. Circulation 1977;55:324.
126. Fisher LD, Judkins MP, Lespérance J, et al. Reproducibility of coronary arteriographic readings in the Coronary Artery Surgery Study (CASS). Cathet Cardiovasc Diagn 1982;8:565–575.
127. Kirkeeide RL, Gould KL, Parsel L. Assessment of coronary artery stenoses by myocardial perfusion imaging during pharmacologic coronary vasodilation: VII. Validation of coronary flow reserve as a single integrated functional measure of stenosis severity reflecting all its geometric dimensions. J Am Coll Cardiol 1986;7:103–113.
128. Beauman GJ, Vogel RA. Accuracy of individual and panel visual interpretations of coronary arteriograms: implications for clinical decisions. J Am Coll Cardiol 1990;16:108–113.
129. Collier RE, Matson JL, Tomme JW, Hyland JW. Correlation of myocardial photoscanning and coronary angiography in angina pectoris. Radiology 1968;91:310.
130. Davis FW Jr. Objective evaluation of ischemic heart disease. Am Heart J 1962;63:136.
131. Kattus AA, MacAlpin R, Longmire WP, O'Loughlin BJ, Biship H. Coronary angiograms and the exercise electrocardiogram in the study of angina pectoris. Am J Med 1963;34:19.
132. Gensini GG, Buonanno C. Coronary arteriography: a study of 100 cases with angiographically proved coronary artery disease. Dis Chest 1968;54:90.
133. Likoff W, Kasparian H, Segal BL, Novack P, Lehman JS. Clinical correlation of coronary arteriography. Am J Cardiol 1965;16:159.
134. Paulin S. Coronary angiography: a technical, anatomic, and clinical study. Acta Radiol (Stockh) 1964;233(Suppl):1.
135. Proudfit WL, Shirey EK, Sheldon WC, Sones FM. Certain clinical characteristics correlated with extent of obstructive lesions demonstrated by selective cini-coronary arteriography. Circulation 1968;38:947.
136. Hultgren H, Calciano A, Platt F, Abrams H. A clinical evaluation of coronary arteriography. Am J Med 1967;42:228.
137. Brandt PWT, Partridge JB, Wattie WJ. Coronary arteriography: method of presentation of the arteriogram report and a scoring system. Clin Radiol 1977;28:361.
138. Noto TJ, Johnson LW, Krone R, et al. Cardiac Catheterization 1990: A report of the Registry of the Society for Cardiac Angiography and Interventions (SCA&I). Cathet Cardiovasc Diagn 1991;24:75–83.
139. Marcus ML, Skorton DJ, Johnson MR, Collins SM, Harrison DG, Kerber RE. Visual estimates of percent diameter coronary stenosis: "a battered gold standard." J Am Coll Cardiol 1988;11:882–885.
140. Gould KL. Percent coronary stenosis: battered gold standard, pernicious relic or clinical practicality? J Am Coll Cardiol 1988;11:886–888.
141. Harrison DG, White CW, Hiratzka LF, et al. The value of lesion cross-sectional area determined by quantitative coronary angiography in assessing the physiologic significance of proximal left anterior descending coronary arterial stenoses. Circulation 1984;69:1111–1119.
142. Gould KL, Lipscomb K, Hamilton GW. Physiologic basis for assessing critical coronary stenosis: instantaneous flow response and regional distribution during hyperemia as measures of coronary flow reserve. Am J Cardiol 1974;33:87–94.
143. Marcus ML, White CW, Kirchner PT. Is it time to evaluate the utility of noninvasive approaches for the diagnosis of coronary artery disease? J Am Coll Cardiol 1986;8:1033–1034.
144. Herold EM, Borer JS. Efforts toward quantification of coronary artery functional capacity. J Am Coll Cardiol 1986;7:114–115.

145. Marcus ML, Hiratzka LF, Doty DB, Wright CB, Harrison DG, White CW. Coronary obstructive lesions: assessing their physiological significance in humans. Ann Thorac Surg 1987; 42(Suppl S):5–8.
146. Cusma JT, Toggart EJ, Folts JD, et al. Digital subtraction angiographic imaging of coronary flow reserve. Circulation 1987;75:461–472.
147. Gould KL, Kirkeeide RL, Buchi M. Coronary flow reserve as a physiologic measure of stenosis severity. J Am Coll Cardiol 1990;15:459–474.
148. McMahon MM, Brown BG, Cukingnan R, et al. Quantitative coronary angiography: measurement of the "critical" stenosis in patients with unstable angina and single-vessel disease without collaterals. Circulation 1979;60:106–113.
149. Wijns W, Serruys PW, Reiber JHC, et al. Quantitative angiography of the left anterior descending coronary artery: correlations with pressure gradient and results of exercise thallium scintigraphy. Circulation 1985;71:273–279.
150. Wilson RF, Laughlin DE, Ackell PH, et al. Transluminal, subselective measurement of coronary artery blood flow velocity and vasodilator reserve in man. Circulation 1985;72:82–92.
151. Wilson RF, Marcus ML, White CW. Prediction of the physiologic significance of coronary arterial lesions by quantitative lesion geometry in patients with limited coronary artery disease. Circulation 1987;75:723–732.
152. Zijlstra F, Ommeren JV, Reiber JHC, Serruys PW. Does the quantitative assessment of coronary artery dimensions predict the physiologic significance of coronary stenosis? Circulation 1987;75:1154–1161.
153. Hermiller JB, Cusma JT, Spero LA, Fortin DF, Harding MB, Bashore TM. Quantitative and qualitative coronary angiographic analysis: review of methods, utility, and limitations. Cathet Cardiovasc Diagn 1992;25:110–131.
154. Fuster V, Badimon L, Badimon JJ, Cheseboro JH. The pathogenesis of coronary artery disease and the acute coronary syndromes. N Engl J Med 1992;326:242–250.
155. May AG, Van de Berg L, DeWeese JA, Rob CG. Critical arterial stenosis. Surgery 1963;54:250.
156. Brice JG, Dowsett DJ, Lowe RD. Haemodynamic effects of carotid artery stenosis. Br Med J 1964;2:1363.
157. Feldman RL, Nichols WW, Pepine CJ, Conti CR. Hemodynamic significance of the length of a coronary arterial narrowing. Am J Cardiol 1978;41:865.
158. Reiner L, Molnar J, Jiminez FA, Freudenthal RR. Interarterial coronary anastomoses in neonates. Arch Pathol 1961;71:103.
159. Zoll PM, Wessler S, Schlesinger MJ. Interarterial coronary anastomosis in the human heart with particular reference to anemia and relative cardiac anoxia. Circulation 1951;4:797.
160. Petelenz T. Radiological picture of extracoronary arteries of myocardium in man. Cardiologia (Basel) 1965;46:65.
161. Marcus ML, Wright CB, Doty DB, et al. Measurements of coronary velocity and reactive hyperemia in the coronary circulation of humans. Circ Res 1981;49:877–891.
162. Sibley DH, Millar HD, Hartley CJ, Whitlow PL. Subselective measurements of coronary blood flow velocity using a steerable Doppler catheter. J Am Coll Cardiol 1986;8:1332–1340.
163. Wilson RF, Holida MD, White CW. Quantitative angiographic morphology of coronary stenoses leading to myocardial infarction or unstable angina. Circulation 1986;73:286–293.
164. Kumpuris AG, Quinones MA, Kanon D, Miller RR. Isolated stenosis of left anterior descending or right coronary artery: relation between site of stenosis and ventricular dysfunction and therapeutic implications. Am J Cardiol 1980;46:13–20.
165. Borer JS, Bacharach SL, Green MV, Kent KM, Epstein SE, Johnston GS, Mack B. Real-time radionuclide cineangiography in the non-invasive evaluation of global and regional left ventricular function at rest and during exercise in patients with coronary artery disease. N Engl J Med 1977;296:839.
166. Zaret BL, Strauss HW, Martin ND, Wells HP Jr, Flamm MD Jr. Noninvasive regional myocardial perfusion with radioactive potassium. Study of patients at rest, with exercise, and during angina pectoris. N Engl J Med 1973;288:809.
167. Lenaers A. Thallium-201 myocardial perfusion scintigraphy during rest and exercise. Cardiovasc Radiol 1979;2:195.
168. Gould LK, Goldstein RA, Mullani NA, et al. Noninvasive assessment of coronary stenoses by myocardial perfusion imaging during pharmacologic coronary vasodilation: VIII. Clinical feasibility of positron cardiac imaging without a cyclotron using generator-produced rubidium-82. J Am Coll Cardiol 1986;7:775–789.
169. Brunken R, Schwaiger M, Grover-McKay M, Phelps M, Tillisch J, Schelbert H. Positron emission tomography detects tissue metabolic activity in myocardial segments with persistent thallium perfusion defects. J Am Coll Cardiol 1987;10: 557–567.
170. Tamaki N, et al. Value and limitation of stress T1-201 tomography: comparison with perfusion and metabolic imaging with positron tomography. Circulation 1987;76(Suppl IV):4.
171. Glagov S, Weisenberg E, Zarins CK, Stankunavicius R, Kolettis GJ. Compensatory enlargement of human atherosclerotic coronary arteries. N Engl J Med 1987;316:1371–1375.
172. Papanicolaou MN, Califf RM, Hlatky MA, et al. Prognostic implications of angiographically normal and insignificantly narrowed coronary arteries. Am J Cardiol 1986;58:1181–1187.
173. Ludmer PL, Selwyn AP, Shook TL, et al. Paradoxical vasoconstriction induced by acetylcholine in atherosclerotic coronary arteries. N Engl J Med 1986;315:1046–1051.
174. Levin DC, Fallon JT. Significance of the angiographic morphology of localized coronary stenoses: histopathologic correlations. Circulation 1982;66:316–320.
175. Dewood MA, Spores L, Notkske R, et al. Prevalence of total coronary occlusion during the early hours of transmural infarction. N Engl J Med 1980;303:897–902.
176. Moise A, Theroux P, Taeymans Y, et al. Unstable angina and progression of coronary atherosclerosis. N Engl J Med 1983; 309:685–689.
177. Capone G, Wolf NM, Meyer B, Meister SG. Frequency of intracoronary filling defects by angiography in angina pectoris at rest. Am J Cardiol 1985;56:403–406.
178. Ambrose JA, Winters SL, Stern A, et al. Angiographic morphology and the pathogenesis of unstable angina pectoris. J Am Coll Cardiol 1985;5:609–616.
179. Haft JI, Goldstein JE, Niemeira ML. Coronary arteriographic lesion of unstable angina. Chest 1987;92:609–612.
180. Kranjec I, Delaye B, Didier B, Delahaye F, Grand A. Angiographic morphology and intraluminal coronary artery thrombus in patients with angina pectoris: clinical correlations. Eur Heart J 1987;8:106–115.
181. Cowley MJ, DiSciascio G, Rehr RB, Vetrovec GW. Angiographic observations and clinical relevance of coronary thrombus in unstable angina pectoris. Am J Cardiol 1989;63:108E–113E.
182. Brown BG, Gallery CA, Badger RS, et al. Incomplete lysis of thrombus in the moderate underlying atherosclerotic lesion during intracoronary infusion of streptokinase for acute myocardial infarction: quantitative angiographic observations. Circulation 1986;73:653–661.
183. Nagakawa S, Hanada Y, Koiwaya Y, Tanaka K. Angiographic features in the infarct-related artery after intracoronary urokinase followed by prolonged anticoagulation. Circulation 1988;78:1335–1344.
184. Little WC, Constantinescu M, Applegate RJ, et al. Can coronary angiography predict the site of a subsequent myocardial infarction in patients with mild-to-moderate coronary artery disease? Circulation 1988;78:1157–1166.
185. Ambrose JA, Tannenbaum MA, Alexopoulos D, et al. Angiographic progression of coronary artery disease and the development of myocardial infarction. J Am Coll Cardiol 1988;12: 56–62.
186. Ambrose JA, Hjemdahl-Monsen CE, Borrico S, Gorlin R, Fuster V. Angiographic demonstration of a common link be-

tween unstable angina pectoris and non–Q-wave acute myocardial infarction. Am J Cardiol 1988;61:244–247.

187. Ellis S, Alderman EL, Cain K, Wright A, Bourassa M, Fisher L. Morphology of left anterior descending coronary artery territory lesions as a predictor of anterior myocardial infarction: a CASS registry study. J Am Coll Cardiol 1989;13: 1481–1491.
188. Sansa M, Cernigliaro C, Bolognese L, Bongo SA, Rossi L, Rossi P. Angiographic morphology and response to therapy in unstable angina. Clin Cardiol 1988;11:121–126.
189. Williams AE, Freeman MR, Chisholm RJ, Patt NL, Armstrong PW. Angiographic morphology in unstable angina pectoris. Am J Cardiol 1988;62:1024–1027.
190. Freeman MR, Williams AE, Chisholm RJ, Armstrong PW. Intracoronary thrombus and complex morphology in unstable angina: relation to timing of angiography and in-hospital cardiac events. Circulation 1984;80:17–23.
191. Cowley MJ, DiSciascio G, Rehr RB, Vetrovec GW. Angiographic observations and clinical relevance of coronary thrombus in unstable angina pectoris. Am J Cardiol 1989;63:108E–113E.
192. Rehr R, DiSciascio G, Vetrovec G, Cowley M. Angiographic morphology of coronary artery stenoses in prolonged rest angina: evidence of intracoronary thrombosis. J Am Coll Cardiol 1989;14:1429–1437.
193. Lo YA, Cutler JE, Blake K, Wright AM, Kron J. Swerdlow CD. Angiographic coronary morphology in survivors of cardiac arrest. Am Heart J 1988;115:781–785.
194. Gorlin R, Fuster V, Ambrose JA. Anatomic-physiologic links between acute coronary syndromes. Circulation 1986;74: 6–9.
195. Ambrose JA. Coronary arteriographic analysis and angiographic morphology. J Am Coll Cardiol 1989;13:1492–1494.
196. Fuster V, Badimon L, Cohen M, Ambrose JA, Badimon JJ, Cheseboro J. Insights into the pathogenesis of acute ischemic syndromes. Circulation 1988;77:1213–1220.
197. Kemp HG Jr, Vokonas PS, Cohn PF, Gorlin R. The anginal syndrome associated with normal coronary arteriograms. Am J Med 1973;54:735.
198. Eliot RS, Bratt GT. Paradox of myocardial ischemia and women with normal coronary arteriograms: relationship to anomalous hemoglobin-oxygen association. Am J Cardiol 969;23:633.
199. Friesinger GC, Page EE, Ross RS. Prognostic significance of coronary arteriography. Trans Assoc Am Physicians 1969;83: 78.
200. James T. Pathology of small coronary arteries. Am J Cardiol 1967;20:679.
201. Selzer A. Cardiac ischemic pain in patients with normal coronary arteriograms. Am J Med 1977;63:661.
202. Oliva PB, Potts DE, Pluss RG. Coronary arterial spasm in Prinzmetal angina. N Engl J Med 1973;288:745.
203. Richardson PJ, Livesay B, Oram S. Angina pectoris with normal coronary arteriogram: transvenous myocardial biopsy in diagnosis. Lancet 1974;2:677.
204. Gault JH, Gentzier RD II. The anginal syndrome without evidence of coronary artery disease. Adv Intern Med 1976; 21:335.
205. Oliva PB, Breckinridge JC. Acute myocardial infarction with normal and near normal coronary arteries: documentation with coronary arteriography within 12½ hours of onset of symptoms in two cases (three episodes). Am J Cardiol 1977; 40:1000.
206. Nordenstrom B. A peripheral type of vascular change in the coronary arteries. Vasc Dis 1965;2:293.
207. Campeau L, et al. Clinical significance of selective coronary cinearteriography. Can Med Assoc J 1968;99:1063.
208. Likoff W, Segal BL, Kasparian H. Paradox of normal selective coronary arteriograms in patients considered to have unmistakeable heart disease. N Engl J Med 1967;267:1063.
209. Mason JW, Strefling A. Small vessel disease of the heart resulting in myocardial necrosis and death despite angiographically normal coronary arteries. Am J Cardiol 1979;44:171.
210. Neil WA, Kassebaum DG, Judkins MP. Myocardial hypoxia as the basis for angina pectoris in a patient with normal coronary arteriograms. N Engl J Med 1968;279:789.
211. Hultgren HN. Medical versus surgical management of unstable angina. Am J Cardiol 1976;38:479.
212. Esente P, Gensini GG, Huntington PP, Kelly AE, Black A. Left ventricular aneurysm without coronary arterial obstruction or occlusion. Am J Cardiol 1974;34:152.
213. Cohen MV, Gorlin R. Main left coronary artery disease, clinical experience from 1964–1974. Circulation 1975;52:275.
214. Abedin Z, Goldberg J. Origin and length of left main coronary artery: its relation to height, weight, sex, age, pattern of coronary distribution, and presence or absence of coronary artery disease. Cathet Cardiovasc Diagn 1978;4:335.
215. Aldridge HE. Better visualization of the asymmetric lesion in coronary arteriography utilizing cranial and caudal angulated projections. Chest 1977;71:502.
216. Sos TA, Baltaxe HA. Cranial and caudal angulation for coronary angiography revisited. Circulation 1977;56:119.
217. Sos TA, Lee JG, Levin DC, Baltaxe HA. New lordotic projections for improved visualization of the left coronary artery and its branches. AJR 1974;121:575.
218. Conley MJ, Ely RL, Kisslo J, Lee KL, McNeer F, Rosati RA. The prognostic spectrum of left main stenosis. Circulation 1978;57:947.
219. Cohen MV, Cohn PF, Herman MV et al. Diagnosis and prognosis of main left coronary artery obstruction. Circulation 1972;45,46(Suppl):1–57.
220. Iskandrian A, Segal BL, Mundth ED. Appraisal of treatment for left main coronary artery disease. Am J Cardiol 1977;40: 291.
221. Sung RJ, Mallon SM, Richter SE, et al. Left main coronary artery obstruction. Circulation 1975;51,52(Suppl):1–112.
222. Takaro T, Hultgren HN, Lipton MJ, et al. The VA cooperative randomized study of surgery for coronary arterial occlusive disease: II. Subgroup with significant left main lesions. Circulation 1976;54(Suppl III):107.
223. Talano JV, Scanlon PJ, Meadows WR, et al. Influence of surgery on survival in 145 patients with left main coronary artery disease. Circulation 1975;51,52(Suppl):1–105.
224. Zeft HJ, Manley JC, Huston JH, Tector AJ, Auer JE, Johnson, WD. Left main coronary artery stenosis: results of coronary bypass surgery. *Circulation* 1974;49:68.
225. CASS principal investigators and their associates. Coronary Artery Surgery Study (CASS): a randomized trial of coronary artery bypass surgery. Survival data. Circulation 1983;68: 939–950.
226. Lavine PG, Kimbiris D, Linhart SW. Coronary artery spasm during selective coronary arteriography: a review of 8 years' experience. Circulation 1973;48(Suppl IV):89.
227. Pritchard CL, Kudo JG, Barner AB. Coronary osteal stenosis. Circulation 1975;52:46.
228. Welch CC, Proudfit WL, Sheldon WC. Coronary arteriographic findings in 1,100 women under age 50. Am J Cardiol 1975;35:211.
229. Hamby RI, Gupta MP, Young MW. Clinical and hemodynamic aspects of single vessel coronary artery disease. Am Heart J 1973;85:458.
230. Bruschke AVG, Proudfit WL, Sones FM Jr. Progress study of 590 consecutive non-surgical cases of coronary disease followed 5–9 years. Circulation 1973;47:1147.
231. Burggraf GW, Parker JO. Prognosis in coronary artery disease: angiographic, hemodynamic, and clinical factors. Circulation 1975;51:146.
232. Webster JS, Moberg C, Rincon G. Natural history of severe proximal coronary disease as documented by cineangiogram. Am J Cardiol 1974;33:195.
233. Sheldon WC, Rincon G, Pichard AD, Razani M, Cheanvechai C, Loop FD. Surgical treatment of 741 patients followed 3–7 years. Prog Cardiovasc Diagn 1975;18:237.

234. Kouchoukos NT, Oberman A, Russell RO, Jones WB. Surgical versus medical treatment of occlusive disease confined to the left anterior descending coronary artery. Am J Cardiol 1975;35:836.
235. Platia E, Griffith L, Humphries JO. Location and severity of coronary artery narrowing as predictors of survival. Circulation 1975;51,52(Suppl):II–91.
236. Bakst A, Lewis BS, Mitha AS, Gotsman MS. Isolated obstruction of the right coronary artery. Chest 1974;65:18.
237. ACC/AHA Task Force Report: guidelines for percutaneous transluminal coronary angioplasty. J Am Coll Cardiol 1988; 12:529–545.
238. Kent KM, Cowley MJ, Kelsey CF, et al. Long term follow-up of the NHLBI-PTCA Registry. Circulation 1986;74 (Suppl II):280.
239. Roubin G, Weintraub WS, Sutor C, et al. Event free survival after successful angioplasty in multivessel coronary artery disease. J Am Coll Cardiol 1987;9:15A.
240. Takaro T, Hultgren HN, Lipton MJ, et al. The VA cooperative study of surgery for coronary arterial occlusive disease: II. Subgroup with significant left main lesions. Circulation 1976;54(Suppl III):107–117.
241. Kaiser GC, Davis KB, Fisher LD, et al. Survival following coronary artery bypass grafting in patients with severe angina pectoris (CASS). J Thorac Cardiovasc Surg 1985;89:513–524.
242. Ryan TJ, Weiner DA, McCabe CH, et al. Exercise testing in the Coronary Artery Surgery Study randomized population. Circulation 1985;72(Suppl V):31–38.
243. Chahine RA, Raizner AE, Ishimori T, Luchi RJ, McIntosh HD. The incidence and clinical implications of coronary artery spasm. Circulation 1975;52:972.
244. Gensini GG. Incidence of documented myocardial ischemia, angina and infarction in patients with normal coronary angiograms. In: Maseri A, Klassen GA, Lesch M, eds. Primary and secondary angina pectoris. New York: Grune & Stratton, 1978:129–143.
245. Buda AJ, Levene DL, Myers MG, Chisholm AW, Shane SJ. Coronary artery spasm and mitral valve prolapse. Am Heart J 1978;95:457.
246. Cheng TO, Bashour T, Kelser GA Jr, Weiss L, Bacos J. Variant angina of Prinzmetal and normal coronary arteriograms: a variant of the variant. Circulation 1973;47:476.
247. Demany MA, Tambe A, Zimmerman HA. Coronary arterial spasm. Dis Chest 1968;53:714.
248. Linhart JW. Prinzmetal variant of angina pectoris. JAMA 1974;228:342.
249. Friedman AC, Spindola-Franco H, Nivatpumin T. Coronary spasm: Prinzmetal's variant angina vs. catheter-induced spasm; refractory spasm vs. fixed stenosis. AJR 1979;132:897.
250. Prinzmetal M, Ekmekci A, Kennamer R, et al. Variant form of angina pectoris: previously undelineated syndrome. JAMA 1960;174:1794.
251. Prinzmetal M, Kennamer R, Merliss R, et al. A variant form of angina pectoris: preliminary report. Am J Med 1959;27: 375.
252. Meller J, Pichard A, Dack S. Coronary arterial spasm in Prinzmetal's angina: a proved hypothesis. Am J Cardiol 1976;37: 938.
253. Yasue H, Tony M, Shimam H, Tanakas AF. The role of the autonomic nervous system in the pathogenesis of Prinzmetal's variant form of angina. Circulation 1974;50:534.
254. Wilerson JT, et al. Conversion from chronic to acute coronary artery disease: speculation regarding mechanisms. Am J Cardiol 1984;54:1349–1354.
255. Feldman RL. Coronary thrombosis, coronary spasm and coronary atherosclerosis, and speculation on the link between unstable angina and acute myocardial infarction. Am J Cardiol 1987;59:1887–1190.
256. Maseri A, et al. Coronary vasospasm as a possible cause of myocardial infarction: a conclusion derived from the study of "preinfarction" angina. N Engl J Med 1978;299:1271.
257. Maseri A, Severi S, Denes M, et al. "Variant" angina: one aspect of a continuous spectrum of vasospastic myocardial ischemia. Am J Cardiol 1978;42:1019.
258. Lespérance J, Bourassa MG, Biron P. Aorta to coronary artery saphenous vein grafts: preoperative angiographic criteria for successful surgery. Am J Cardiol 1972;30:459.
259. Dhurandhar RW, Watt DJ, Silver MD, Tremble AS, Adelman AG. Prinzmetal's variant form of angina with arteriographic evidence of coronary arterial spasm. Am J Cardiol 1972;30: 902.
260. Gianelly R, Mugler F, Harrison DC. Prinzmetal's variant of angina pectoris with only slight coronary atherosclerosis. Calif Med 1968;108:129.
261. MacAlpin RN. Relation of coronary arterial spasm to sites of organic stenosis. Am J Cardiol 1980;46:143.
262. Ludmer PL, Selwyn AP, Shook TL, et al. Paradoxical vasoconstriction induced by acetylcholine in atherosclerotic coronary arteries. N Engl J Med 1986;315:1046–1051.
263. Whiting RB, Klein MD, Vander Veer J, et al. Variant angina pectoris. N Engl J Med 1970;282:709.
264. Heupler FA, Proudfit WL, Razavi M, Shirey EK, Greenstreet R, Sheldon WC. Ergonovine maleate: provocative test for coronary arterial spasm. Am J Cardiol 1978;41:631.
265. Amplatz K, Varco RL, Buchwald H. Coronary arteriography in hypercholesterolemic patients. AJR 1969;105:784.
266. Faruqui AM, Maloy WC, Felner JM, Schlant RC, Logan WD, Symbas P. Symptomatic myocardial bridging of coronary artery. Am J Cardiol 1978;41:1305.
267. Ishimori T, Raizner AE, Verani MS, Miller RR, Chahine RA. Documentation of ischemic manifestations in patients with myocardial bridges. Clin Res 1979;27:176A.
268. Noble J, Bourassa MG, Petitclerc R, Dyrda I. Myocardial bridging and milking effects of the left anterior descending coronary artery: normal variant or obstruction? Am J Cardiol 1976;37:993.
269. Polacek P. Relation of myocardial bridges and loops on the coronary arteries to coronary occlusion. Am Heart J 1951;41: 359.
270. Noble J, Grodin P, Bourassa MG. Successful periarterial muscle resection for myocardial bridging and milking effect of the left anterior descending artery. Am J Cardiol 1977;39:267.
271. Greenspan M, Iskandrian AS, Catherwood E, Kimbiris D, Bemis CE, Segal BL. Myocardial bridging of the left anterior descending artery: evaluation using exercise thallium-201 myocardial scintigraphy. Cathet Cardiovasc Diagn 1980;6: 173.
272. Cohn P, Gorlin R, Adams DF, Chahine R, Vokonas P, Herman M. Biplane versus single plane ventriculography in coronary artery disease. Am J Cardiol 1974;31:1.
273. Cohen LS, Elliott WC, Mein MD, Gorlin R. Coronary heart disease: clinical, cinearteriographic and metabolic consideration. Am J Cardiol 1966;17:153.
274. Parker JO, DiGiorgi S, West RO. Selective coronary arteriography. Can Med Assoc J 1966;95:291.
275. Proudfit WL, Shirey EK, Sones FM Jr. Selective cine coronary arteriography: correlation with clinical findings in 1,000 patients. Circulation 1966;33:901.
276. Campeau L, Lespérance J, Bourassa MG, Ashekian PB. Myocardial infarction without obstructive disease at coronary arteriography. Can Med Assoc J 1968;99:837.
277. Astrand I, Lundman T. The exercise electrocardiogram in coronary heart disease. Scand J Clin Lab Invest 1968;22:301.
278. Kemp HG, Elliott WC. The anginal syndrome with normal coronary arteriography. Trans Assoc Am Physicians 1967;80: 59.
279. Boelling GM, Phillips WJ, Frerking HW, Paine R. Roentgenographic exercise test: a new test of myocardial state. JAMA 1967;202:275.
280. Grondin CM, et al. Atherosclerotic changes in coronary vein grafts six years after operation: angiographic aspect in 110 patients. J Thorac Cardiovasc Surg 1979;77:24.
281. Lower RR, Kontos HA, Kosek JC, Sewell DH, Graham WH.

Experiences in heart transplantation. Am J Cardiol 1968;22: 766.

282. Effler DB, Groves LK, Sones FM. Myocardial revascularization by internal mammary implantation. Vasc Dis 1966;3:42.
283. Lichtlen PR. Natural history of coronary artery disease based on coronary angiography: a critical review. Cleve Clin J Med 1978;45:153.
284. Oberman A, Jones WB, Riley CP. Natural history of coronary artery disease. Bull NY Acad Med 1972;48:1109.
285. Reeves TJ, Oberman A, Jones WB, Sheffield LT. Natural history of angina pectoris. Am J Cardiol 1974;33:423.
286. Cohn PF, Gorlin R, Cohn LH, et al. Left ventricular ejection fraction as a prognostic guide in the surgical treatment of coronary and valvular heart disease. Am J Cardiol 1974;34:136.
287. Vlietstra RD, et al. Survival predictors in coronary artery disease: medical and surgical comparisons. Mayo Clin Proc 1977;52:85.
288. Plotnick GD, Conti CR. Unstable angina: angiography, short- and long-term morbidity, mortality and symptomatic status of medically treated patients. Am J Cardiol 1977;63: 870.
289. Khan R, Amaram S, Gomes JA, Kelen GJ, Lynfield J, El-Sherif N. Myocardial infarction following acute aortic dissection. Cathet Cardiovasc Diagn 1980;6:181.
290. Lantos G, Sos TA, Sniderman KW, Saddekni S, Hilton S. Dissecting hematoma of the thoracic aorta extending into a coronary artery: angiographic demonstration. Radiology 1980; 135:329.
291. Oram S, Holt MC. Coronary involvement in dissecting aneurysm of the aorta. Br Heart J 1950;12:10.
292. Hirst AE Jr, Johns VJ Jr, Kime SW Jr. Dissecting aneurysm of the aorta: a review of 505 cases. Medicine (Baltimore) 1958;37:217.
293. Jenkins JL, Nishimura A. Coronary artery obstruction and myocardial infarction resulting from nonpenetrating chest trauma. Tex Med 1975;71:78.
294. Parmley LF, Manion WC, Mattingly TW. Nonpenetrating traumatic injury of the heart. Circulation 1958;18:371.
295. Pepine CJ, Beasley DW, Schang SJ, Bemiller CR. Angiographic diagnosis of coronary artery lacerations. J Thorac Cardiovasc Surg 1992;63:183.
296. Morettin LB. Coronary arteriography: uncommon observations. Radiol Clin North Am 1976;14:189.
297. Tsakrakiides VG, Blieden LC, Edwards JE. Coronary atherosclerosis and myocardial infarction in association with lupus erythematosus. Am Heart J 1974;87:637.
298. Ivey NS, Norris HJ. Intimal vascular lesions associated with female reproductive steroids. Arch Pathol 1973;96:227.
299. Tello R, Costello P, Ecker C, Hartnell G. Spiral CT evaluation of coronary artery bypass graft patency. J Comput Assist Tomogr 1993;17:253–259.
300. Foster CJ, Sekiya T, Brownlee WC, Griffin JF, Isherwood I. Computed tomographic assessment of left ventricular aneurysms. Br Heart J 1984;52:332–338.
301. Sechtem U, Sommerhoff BA, Markiewicz W, White RD, Cheitlin MD, Higgins CB. Regional left ventricular wall thickening by magnetic resonance imaging: evaluation in normal persons and patients with global and regional dysfunction. Am J Cardiol 1987;59:145–151.
302. Ehman RL, Julsrud PR. Magnetic resonance imaging of the heart: current status. Mayo Clin Proc 1989;64:1134–1146.
303. Just H, Holubarsch C, Friedburg H. Estimation of left ventricular volume and mass by magnetic resonance imaging: comparison with quantitative biplane angiocardiography. Cardiovasc Intervent Radiol 1987;10:1–4.
304. Akins EW, Hill JA, Sievers KW, Conti CR. Assessment of left ventricular wall thickness in healed myocardial infarction by magnetic resonance imaging. Am J Cardiol 1987;59:24–28.
305. Katz J, Milliken MC, Stray-Gundersen J, et al. Estimation of human myocardial mass with MR imaging. Radiology 1988; 169:495–498.
306. Axel L, Dougherty L. MR imaging of motion with spatial modulation of magnetization. Radiology 1989;171:841–845.
307. Manning WJ, Li W, Edelman RR. A preliminary report comparing magnetic resonance coronary angiography with conventional angiography. N Engl J Med 1993;328:828–832.

27

Coronary Collateral Circulation

SVEN PAULIN

Visualization of coronary collaterals in coronary arteriography performed in vivo constitutes an important finding and, particularly in the presence of coronary artery disease, allows for observations related to the hemodynamic consequences of the disease process. Undoubtedly, the presence of collateral flow indicates that a compensatory mechanism has developed to ameliorate the detrimental effect of blood flow cessation caused by the obstruction of the arterial pathways. It also appears logical to assume that the incidence of demonstrable collaterals in coronary arteriography ought to correlate positively with the severity and extension of obstructive arterial lesions. However, the mere morphologic demonstration of abnormal collateral connections in an angiogram does not, in itself, reveal the magnitude of collateral flow that occurs or that these pathways may be able to carry. Thus it would be inappropriate to interpret such a finding categorically as either an indication of severe regional ischemia or a sign of effective biologic compensation.[1]

Historically, the first report on coronary collaterals was rendered in 1669 by Richard Lower,[2] who observed that fluid injected into one coronary artery of a specimen emerged from the other. Lower seems to have concluded not only that the two coronary arteries communicated with each other in their periphery via anastomoses but that these also guarded against deficiencies of "heat and nourishment." Similar observations were also made by Vieussens[3] and were subsequently accepted generally.[4,5] Hyrtl,[6] who had developed an injection-corrosion technique, raised severe doubts about the existence of peripheral anastomoses, and Henle,[7] in his extensive text on human blood vessels, specifically supported these concerns by stating that the assumption of a communication between the coronary arteries was most likely erroneous. He suggested that the distal bent of the right coronary artery in the posterior aspect of the atrioventricular sulcus at the crux was missed and the distal left circumflex artery was wrongly identified as its continuation. If this explanation did not exclude the possibility of other more hidden or smaller communications, the publication of the experimental examinations by Cohnheim and von Schulthess-Rechberg were more decisive in this regard.[8] They had difficulties in demonstrating arterial connections following infusion experiments and noted that clamping of either coronary artery in a dog resulted in cessation of effective cardiac contractions within less than 2 minutes. They concluded that coronary interarterial anastomoses must be absent or at least functionally insignificant and consequently declared the coronaries to be true end-arteries, a concept that perplexed the profession for almost half a century and that, as we know now, was erroneous. Schaper[9] attributed this fundamental mistake largely to the authors' examination technique, in which plaster of Paris was injected selectively into the coronary arteries, and its rapid hardening prevented demonstration of the more delicate structures of the vascular periphery. This interesting historical note emphasized the importance of the statement by James[10] that any discussion of anastomoses and collaterals should be preceded by a definition of the method employed for the study, particularly its limitations.

Technically more advanced methods using pressure injections of fluids of the correct viscosity and containing appropriately small particles have successfully clarified specific questions with regard to vascular communications in the coronary circulation. Thus many workers have shown conclusively that multiple communicating prearteriolar channels are present in practically all normal human hearts and exist with approximately equal frequency between branches of the same artery and between the right and left coronary arteries, denoted as intracoronary and intercoronary anastomoses, respectively.[11–14] These normally occurring connections are characterized by their rather straight appearance and small caliber. They differ from the usually very tortuous and much wider collaterals frequently found in obstructive disease.

The initial assumption by Blumgart et al.[15] that normal coronary arterial anastomoses are smaller than 40 μ in diameter must be considered too conservative in light of the results of later experiments. Prinzmetal et al.[16] demonstrated that glass spheres of up to 170 μ in diameter injected in suspension in one coronary artery of a normal specimen could be identified in the arterial territory of the opposite side. Vastesaeger et al.[17] determined from postmortem angiograms that the ordinarily small normal channels could at times have a wider diameter of close to 1.0 mm and made such a finding in 7.5 percent of apparently normal hearts. Baroldi and Scomazzoni[18] analyzed a large collection of postmortem injection-corrosion specimens that had been produced with uniform technique and found that in all cases anastomotic communications existed in large numbers and in varying sizes. In specimens that represented normal hearts, the caliber of the individual anastomoses varied between 150 and 350 μ, with an average value of 200 μ. After quantifying these channels—expressing their number and size in a so-called anastomotic index—the same authors found that these smaller types of communicating channels were increased in specimens free from coronary artery disease but representing myocardial hypertrophy or chronic hypoxia. Whether these variations were more the expression of individual constitutional differences or the result of increased intensities and duration of repeat stimuli capable of augmenting collateral circulation, or a mixture of both, remained unclear. Nevertheless, the findings indicate that varying numbers of preformed anastomotic channels may be present independent of the development of atherosclerotic obliterative processes in the coronary arteries.

In the presence of moderate coronary artery disease—that is, of a degree believed to be clinically insignificant—the same coronary vascular casts also demonstrated a higher anastomotic index, and increasingly so when combined with myocardial hypertrophy. In hearts with severe stenoses, other types of connecting channels were recognized with increasing frequency. These channels, most often located at or close to the epicardial surface of the myocardial wall, were less numerous but rather wide, up to 1.0 mm or more in caliber. Baroldi and Scomazzoni found in each instance of true occlusion just such an enlarged and tortuous collateral conduit coming either from the proximal portion of the same occluded vessel or from other patent vessels to connect with the distal portion of the artery. They coined the term *satellite anastomotic circulation* to define these channels (Fig. 27-1). They are identical in appearance, size, and location to the collaterals demonstrable in postmortem angiographic studies of the type performed by Schlesinger and colleagues.[15,19]

Since it is reasonable to assume that these wide, elongated, and tortuous satellite anastomoses represent preexisting dormant channels that have changed under the stress of a major unidirectional pulsatile flow demand caused by a unilateral obstruction, one may

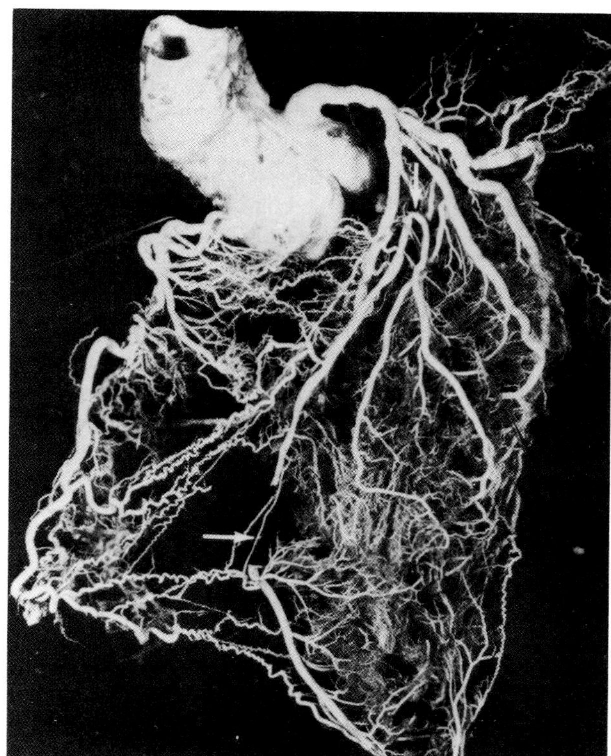

Figure 27-1. Plastic cast of injection-corrosion specimen illustrating several tortuous "satellite" anastomotic channels connecting with arterial segments located distal to occlusions (*arrows*) of the left anterior descending artery. (From Baroldi G, Scomazzoni G. Coronary circulation in the normal and pathologic heart. Washington, DC: Office of the Surgeon General, Department of the Army, 1967. Used with permission.)

deduce that their gross morphologic features may represent a reliable, albeit crude, indicator that they have functional importance. James[10] found that these larger connections could be found in almost all areas of the heart, but that, if visible on the surface of the free walls, they were commonly located near the interventricular sulci, the apex cordis, the crux, and the free walls of the atria. The connections were more concealed when they occurred in both the interventricular and interatrial septa. Although they were more frequently encountered in the few samples of advanced coronary artery disease in his collection of casts, there was undeniable evidence of subepicardially located anastomoses with calibers as large as 300 μ or more in numerous normal cases. James pointed out that with his casting technique using Vinylite solution of much higher viscosity than blood, he could not precisely assess their true incidence, but he felt strongly that his findings supported previous observations made by others[17,20,21] that large, epicardially located, interarterial connections can be present in hearts from patients without signs of having suffered from myocardial hypoxemia.

In a coronary angiogram of a living patient, the situation differs considerably. The numerous intramural individual anastomoses are so small that their depiction is unlikely because of the limited resolution power of the available radiographic imaging systems. Furthermore, even in the less frequent instances in which preformed larger epicardial anastomoses may exist, the lack of a significant pressure gradient between entrances to the communicating channel prevents their filling with contrast medium. The consistent absence of demonstrable coronary collaterals in nonselective coronary arteriograms of patients with normal or only slightly stenotic coronary arteries supports the opinion that these structures are functionally dormant.[22] This also holds for selective coronary arteriography, provided that the only temporary and small pressure elevations generated by the manual injection into the unobstructed coronary artery are not strong enough to fill them. If, however, the catheter tip occludes the mouth of the artery—because of the unusual small size of the artery or catheter-induced spasm—transmission of the injection pressure may force the contrast medium through collateral pathways into the noninjected but apparently unobstructed artery or branches of the opposite side. Filling of collaterals following an appropriate selective injection in a nonwedged artery position strongly suggests the presence of hemodynamically significant obstruction somewhere in the coronary circulation.

Hemodynamic and circulatory considerations indicate that coronary arterial obstructions must reach a narrowing of at least 50 percent in diameter (equivalent to 75 percent transectional area reduction) before a significant reduction in perfusion pressure and flow can be expected. Bookstein and Kahn[23] performed experimental studies in calves to elucidate the relationship between arterial narrowing and the occurrence of detectable coronary collaterals using cineangiographic technique. Experimentally induced stenoses of less than 50 percent diameter reduction never resulted in a significant pressure gradient, and they observed no collaterals. They found that stenoses of higher degree induced the appearance of collateral flow only when these were effective enough to create an angiographically disturbed progression of the contrast medium in the relevant stenosed artery. The authors concluded that morphologic quantitation of a narrowed vessel alone is of only limited value in determining the hemodynamic significance of a stenosis, whereas the filling of collaterals into the area of its supply reveals the hemodynamic impact to a more reliable degree.

The results of these experiments agree well with the numerous reported observations in clinical coronary angiography, namely, that coronary collaterals are detectable only when the arterial obstructions are well advanced.[24,25] The level of luminal arterial encroachment at which collaterals begin to be angiographically detectable depends on the type of scoring system. In general, a diameter narrowing of 70 percent or more should be present. The author's own results have consistently shown that when an arterial stenosis is so advanced that it results in delayed contrast filling, the likelihood of detectable coexisting collaterals is very high. Thus, in a group of patients with advanced stenoses and occlusions but not including cases with a history of recent-onset angina or infarctions, evidence of lesion-related collaterals in nonselectively performed large-sized serial radiographs was as high as 98 percent. Levin[26] found demonstrable collaterals in approximately 70 percent of angiograms showing at least 90 percent stenosis or occlusion. Weintraub et al.[27] also found a good correlation between high-grade lesions and collaterals in patients with unstable ischemia requiring intraaortic balloon support. When collaterals were absent the culprit lesion resulted in delayed contrast filling on the cineangiogram and identified the area of acute ischemia. Thus one can conclude that differences in the reported incidence of collaterals may be influenced not only by the lack in preciseness with which an angiogram can determine the degree of arterial luminal narrowing, but also by clinical difficulties in obtaining accurate timing of the onset of the myocardial ischemia.

The large epicardial coronary anastomoses are most likely to occur in sites where the distal distributions of both coronary arteries meet (Fig. 27-2). Thus, not surprisingly and in accordance with postmortem findings, the most common site of these large collateral pathways detectable by angiography is the interventricular septum, where numerous communications between left anterior and right posterior septal branches exist. (Eighty percent of human hearts have posterior septal branches arising from the distal *right* coronary artery and anterior septal branches arising from the *left* anterior descending artery.) Other sites are the apex, where the terminal ramifications of the anterior and posterior descending arteries are located, the joining point between the left and right circumflex arteries near the atrioventricular sulcus, the epicardial surface of the free walls of the right and left ventricles, and communications between left and right atrial arteries.

In contrast to these intercoronary collaterals, less frequently encountered connections exist between two branches of the same coronary artery, called intracoronary collaterals. The term *extracoronary collaterals* is restricted to those anastomoses that connect the cor-

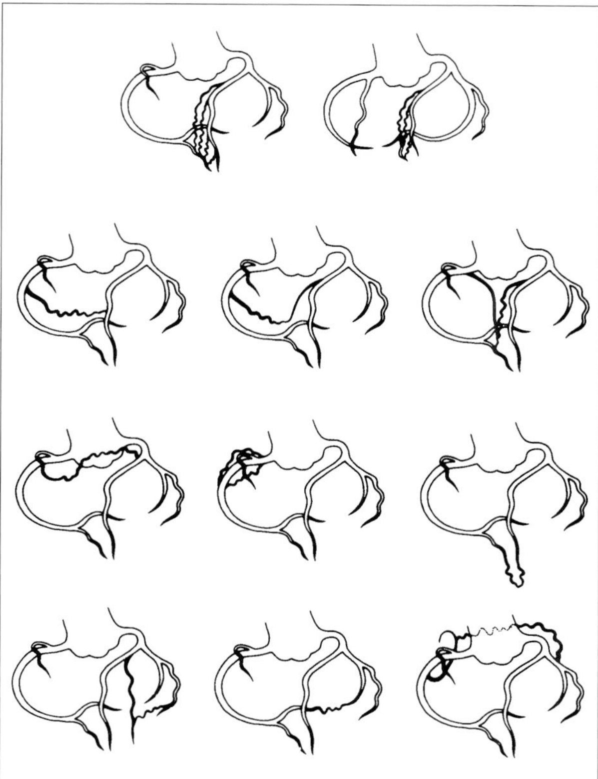

Figure 27-2. Schematic presentation of interarterial connections frequently encountered in coronary arteriography. (A) Septal collaterals. (A′) Same collaterals as in (A) with large distribution of left circumflex artery. (B) Epicardial collateral of right ventricular wall. (C) Collateral in moderator band. (D) Collateral in crista supraventricularis. (E) Epicardial collateral at pulmonary conus. (F) Direct bypassing collateral. (G) Epicardial collateral at apex. (H) Collateral in left ventricular wall. (I) Collateral in atrioventricular sulcus. (J) Collateral in atrial wall. (From Paulin S. Interarterial coronary anastomoses in relation to arterial obstruction demonstrated in coronary arteriography. Invest Radiol 1967; 2:147. Used with permission.)

onary arteries with other arterial systems, usually the bronchial arterial circulation. Angiography in vivo most likely underestimates the true incidence of their occurrence because rarely is a selective bronchial arteriogram performed, a prerequisite for their angiographic demonstration.

In the following paragraphs the most frequent and characteristic collaterals are listed and described.

Intercoronary Collaterals

Collaterals of the interventricular septum ordinarily present as multiple connections between the numerous, relatively large anterior septal branches of the left anterior descending artery and the smaller posterior septal branches deriving from the posterior interventricular artery (Fig. 27-3). Their individual size is usually less than 1.0 mm and they are characterized by a moderate tortuosity. These findings point to the fact that they are embedded in the septal myocardium and are not in a true epicardial location. At times, septal collateral flow may be dominated by a relatively large first septal perforator branch that arborizes into multiple distal minor branches in the posterior basal aspect of the septum. The direction of contrast flow in these collaterals is entirely dependent on the site of the most significant arterial obstruction and is thus either posteroanterior or anteroposterior (Fig. 27-4).

Whereas the exact location of an occlusion in the right coronary artery has little influence on the extent of septal collaterals, more peripherally located obstructions in the left anterior descending artery will exclude some of the more proximally located anastomoses. In the presence of a left-preponderant circulation, the septal collaterals are practically identical, but since they connect to posterior septal branches deriving from the left circumflex artery, they represent, by definition, *intracoronary* collateral pathways (Fig. 27-5).

Epicardial collaterals of the right ventricular wall comprise one or two rather large and tortuous communications between the largest branch of the right coronary artery near the right ventricular wall and the anterior descending artery (Fig. 27-6). They are typically wider and more tortuous than individual septal collateral connections and frequently enter the left anterior descending artery at a sharp angle at about the junction of its middle and distal third. They are rarely seen alone but are encountered in approximately a third of the cases in hearts that have collaterals in the interventricular septum as well.

Collaterals in the moderator band are, with a few exceptions, solitary, rather straight vessels. They join the large first septal perforator of the anterior descending artery with the distal branches of the acute marginal branch of the right coronary artery. These collaterals are identical in location and distribution to the ramus limbi described by Gross,[28] which forms the distal extension of the first septal branch and runs in the moderator band to the anterior wall of the right ventricle. Although various in size, these anastomoses are usually small in caliber and never reach the large size seen in most of the epicardial collaterals with which they frequently coexist.

Pulmonary conus collaterals are mostly solitary tortuous anastomoses that are usually rather wide (Fig. 27-7). They are identical to the arterial ring of Vieussens[3] around the root of the pulmonary artery, which is the communication of the pulmonary conus branch of the right coronary artery with the corresponding,

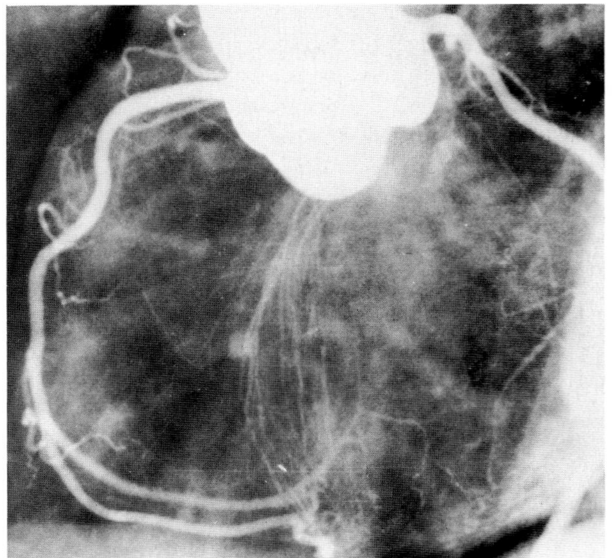

A

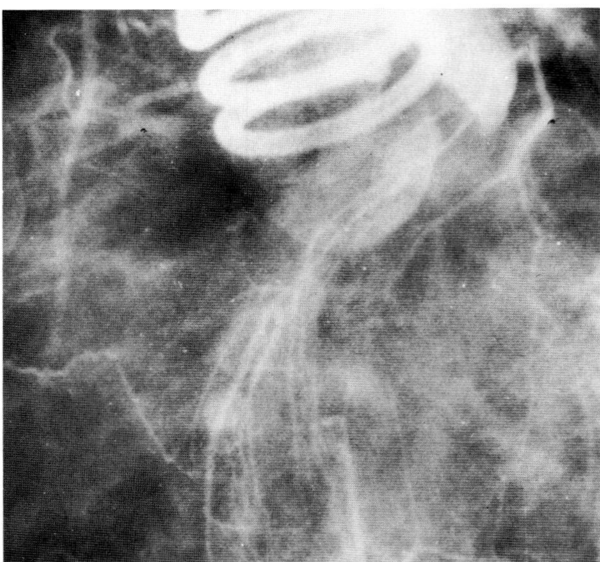

B

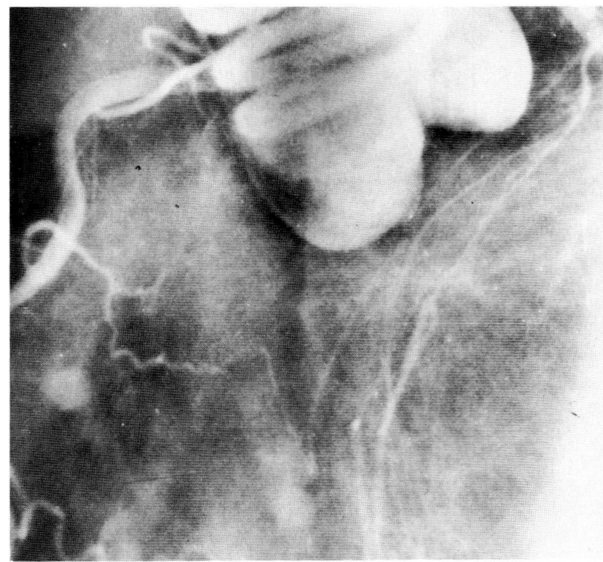

C

Figure 27-3. Coronary arteriogram in LAO projection. (A) Numerous tortuous collaterals with irregular walls arising from distal extension of the right coronary artery and supplying the occluded anterior descending artery. (B and C) Stereoscopic detail images of additional interarterial collateral connection between the acute marginal branch from the right coronary artery and the artery in the moderator band connecting with the first septal branch of the occluded left anterior descending (LAD) artery. (From Paulin S. Interarterial coronary anastomoses in relation to arterial obstruction demonstrated in coronary arteriography. Invest Radiol 1967;2:147. Used with permission.)

usually smaller, branch deriving from the proximal left anterior descending artery. Although this anastomosis represents the potentially shortest collateral circuit, it is not encountered frequently because it requires a most proximally located obstruction of the right coronary artery or the left anterior descending artery. In approximately one-third of the cases, semiselective coronary angiography has identified the right conus branch as having a separate orifice from the aorta and therefore as representing a communication between the aorta and the proximally occluded anterior descending artery. The potential undetected presence of this important collateral in selective coronary arteriography should be noted.

Epicardial collaterals at the apex represent communications between the most distal extension of the LAD and the posterior descending artery (Fig. 27-8). Various in size, they are similar in appearance to other epicardially located tortuous channels. They occur less frequently than septal collaterals.

Connections in the atrioventricular sulcus link the distal extension of the right coronary artery with that of the left circumflex artery (Fig. 27-9). In accordance with the most common distribution pattern, they are most often seen in the region between the obtuse margin and the crux. Their existence is determined by obstructive lesions in the right coronary artery and the left circumflex artery and thus has no relationship to obstructions within the territory of the left anterior descending artery. In the presence of isolated right coronary artery obstruction, they occur less frequently than

Text continues on page 708

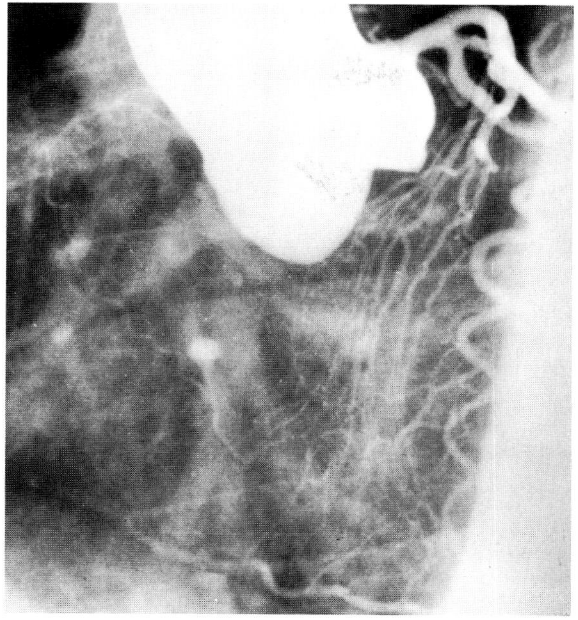

A

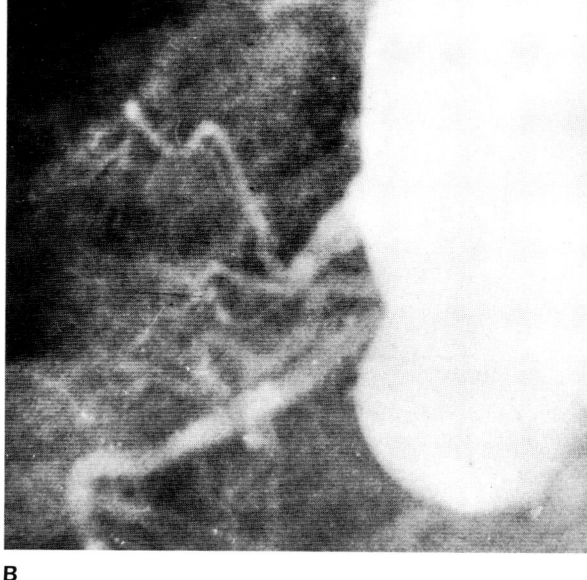

B

C

Figure 27-4. Nonselective coronary arteriogram with proximal occlusion of right coronary artery. (A) LAO projection demonstrating numerous interventricular septal anastomoses. (B) Detail of angiogram in lateral projection identifying the short remaining stump of the occluded proximal right coronary artery, from which high-positioned collateral side branches are recognizable. (C) Lateral view showing numerous collateral anastomoses along the entire surface of the right ventricle during the late arterial filling phase. (From Paulin S. Coronary angiography: a technical, anatomic and clinical study. Acta Radiol 1964;233(Suppl):156. Used with permission.)

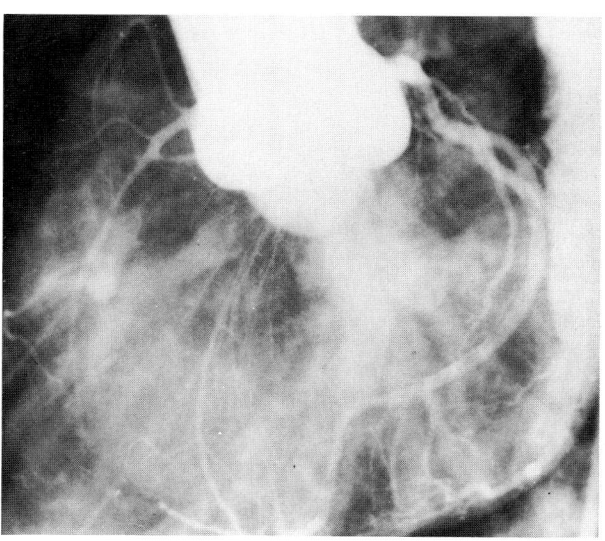

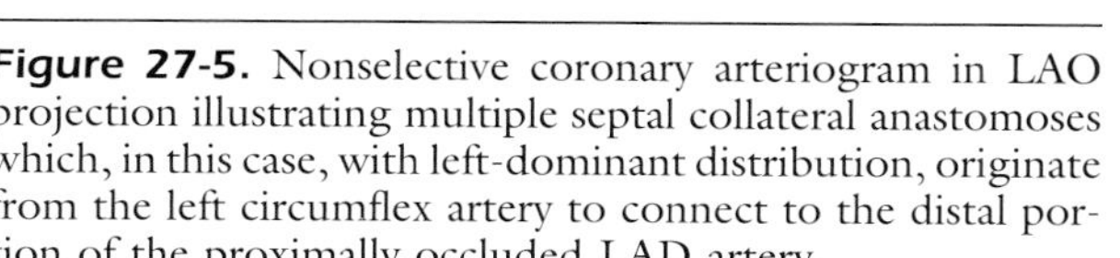

Figure 27-5. Nonselective coronary arteriogram in LAO projection illustrating multiple septal collateral anastomoses which, in this case, with left-dominant distribution, originate from the left circumflex artery to connect to the distal portion of the proximally occluded LAD artery.

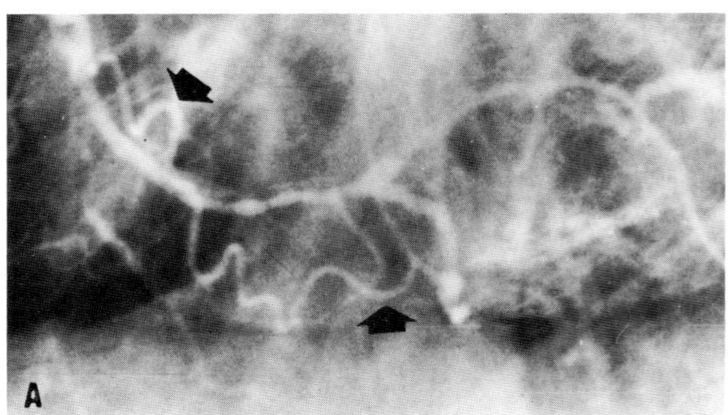

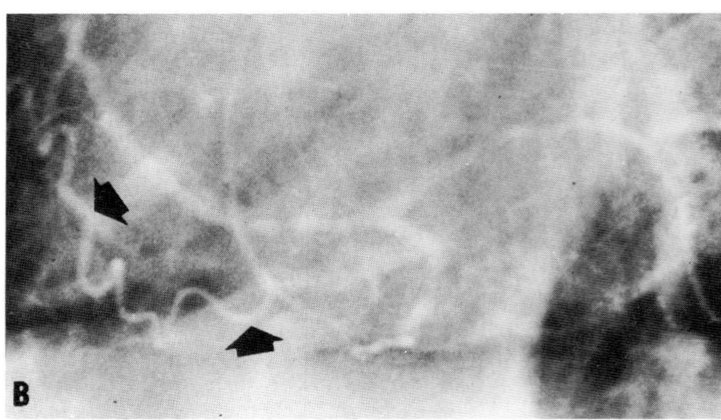

Figure 27-6. (A and B) Stereoscopic pair of films in LAO projection demonstrating tortuous epicardial anastomoses (*arrows*) between acute marginal branch of right coronary artery and descending anterior artery. There was a complete occlusion of the anterior descending artery. (From Paulin S. Coronary angiography: a technical, anatomic and clinical study. Acta Radiol 1964;233(Suppl):160. Used with permission.)

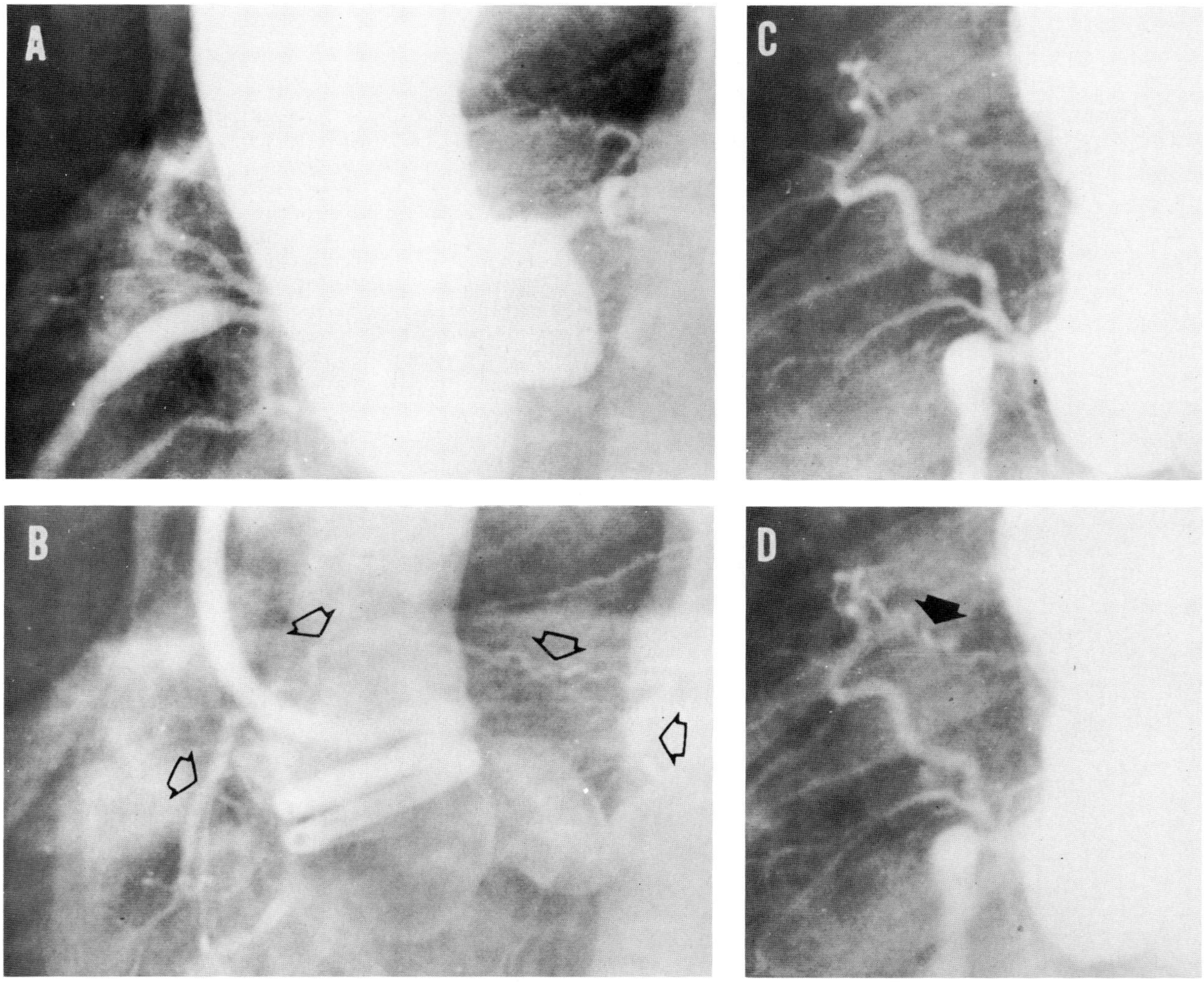

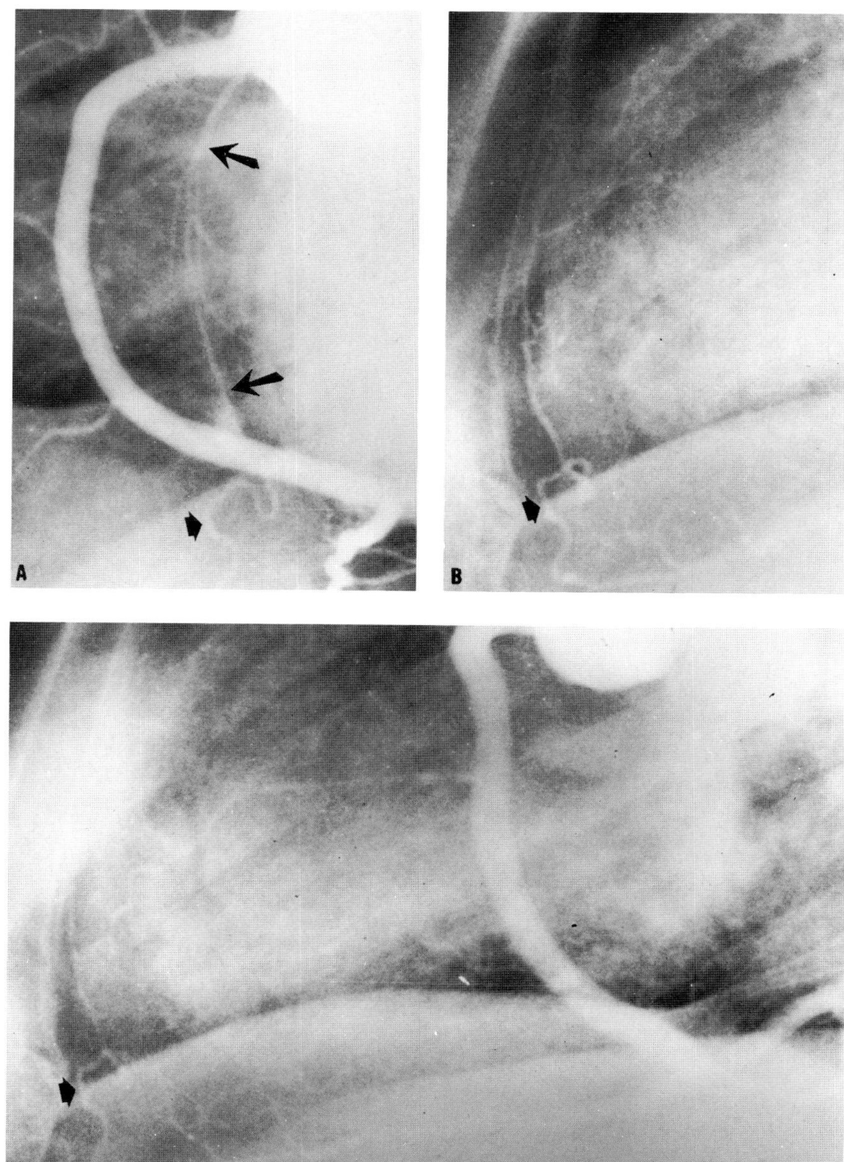

Figure 27-8. Coronary arteriogram of patient with marked narrowing of a long segment of the anterior descending artery (*long arrows*). (A) LAO projection. (B and C) Stereoscopic pair of films in left lateral view. *Short arrow* points to a rather wide and tortuous anastomosis between the posterior descending and the anterior descending artery at the apex of the heart. Note the wide caliber of the apparently normal right circumflex coronary artery. (From Paulin S. Interarterial coronary anastomoses in relation to arterial obstruction demonstrated in coronary arteriography. Invest Radiol 1967;2:147. Used with permission.)

◄ **Figure 27-7.** Stenosis of both main coronary arteries near their orifices and occlusion of proximal part of LAD artery. (A and B) LAO projection. (C and D) Left lateral views. *Arrows* identify a wide and tortuous anastomosis between a separately arising pulmonary conus branch and the occluded anterior descending artery. This anastomosis, which is located in front of the ascending aorta, is identical with the so-called Vieussens coronary arterial ring. (From Paulin S. Interarterial coronary anastomoses in relation to arterial obstruction demonstrated in coronary arteriography. Invest Radiol 1967;2:147. Used with permission.)

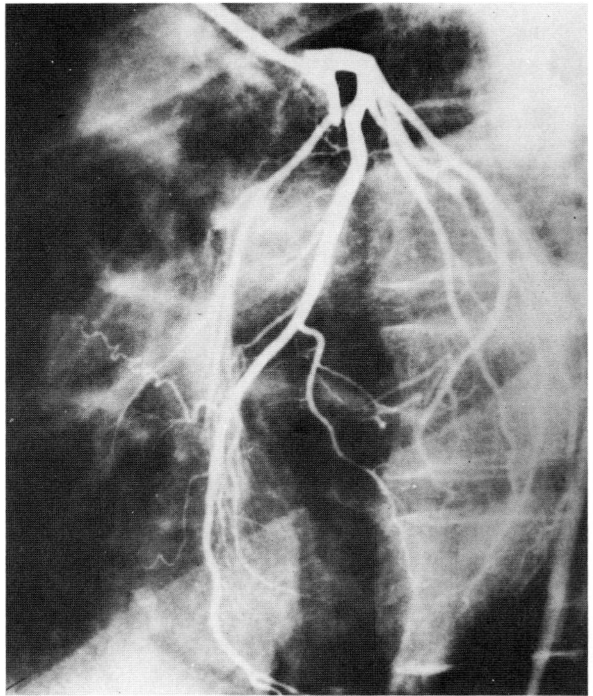

A

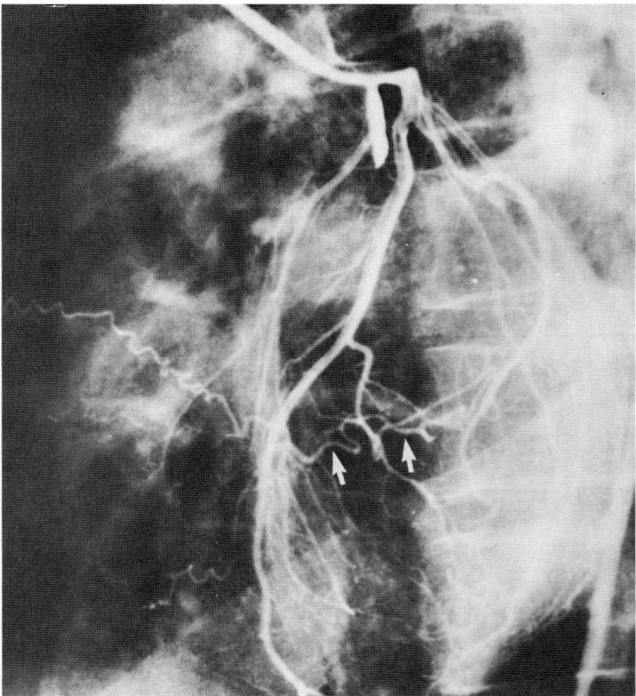

B

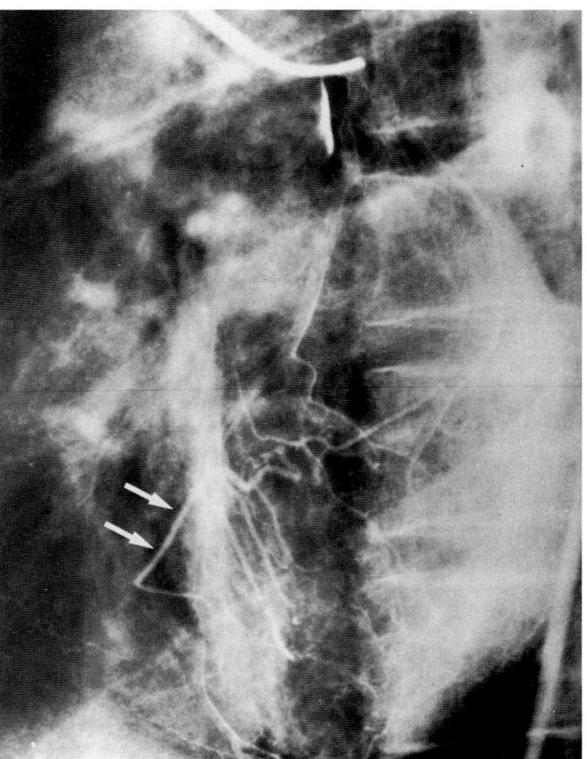

C

Figure 27-9. Left-sided selective coronary arteriogram in LAO projection demonstrating a wide and tortuous anastomosis (*arrows,* B) extending from the left circumflex artery and adjoining the distal right coronary artery at the site of the crux (*arrows,* C). Note also the tortuous vessel, approximately 1.0 mm wide, arising from the LAD midportion toward the left upper portion of the image. This is an epicardial collateral to a large, acute marginal branch. The selective right coronary arteriogram, not shown here, did indeed disclose a proximal total occlusion. Time interval between (A), (B), and (C) approximately 2 seconds.

septal collaterals or other collaterals connecting branches of the right with the left anterior descending artery. However, the relative incidence of connections in the atrioventricular sulcus seems to increase in two-vessel disease, affecting both the right and left anterior descending coronary arteries. Differentiation between this anastomosis and one running at the atrial level, usually involving the so-called left atrial circumflex artery, may be difficult if not impossible to establish. The former, however, tends to become larger.

Collaterals at the free posterior ventricular wall form connections between branches of the obtuse marginal artery from the left circumflex artery to the posterior descending artery of the right coronary artery. The incidence of these collaterals and their relationship to obstructive lesions are similar to those of collaterals

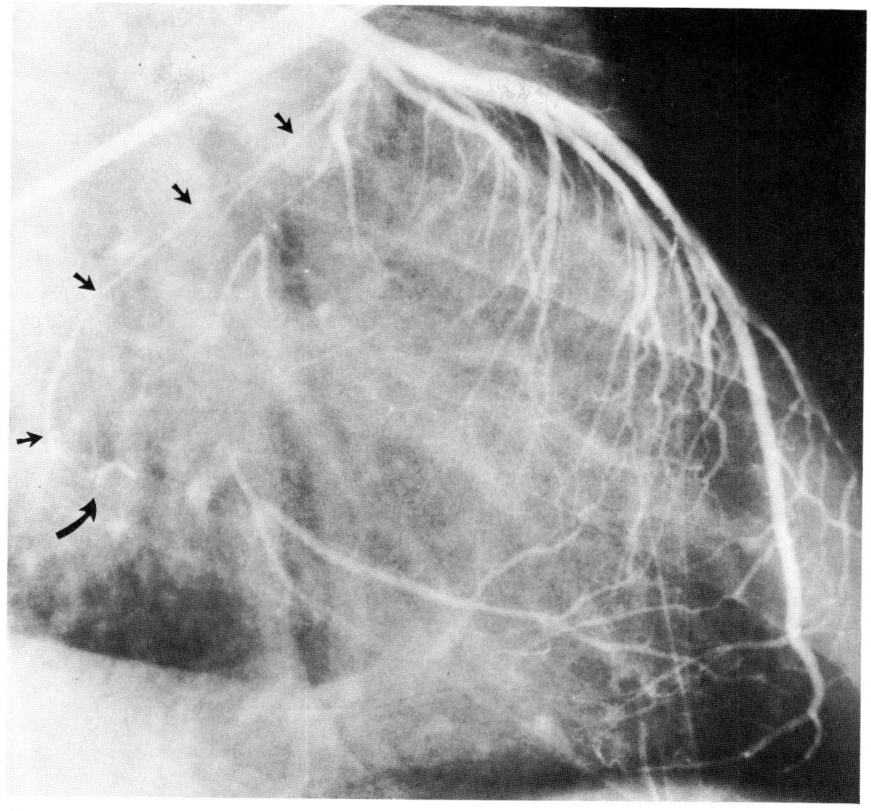

A

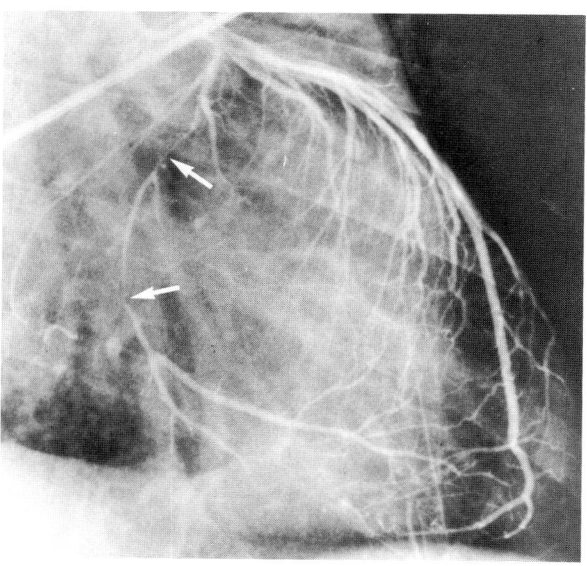

B

Figure 27-10. Left-sided selective coronary arteriogram in RAO projection illustrating two high-grade stenoses in the left circumflex artery (*arrows,* B). Progression of contrast through these stenoses was very much delayed (time interval from (A) to (B) 3 seconds). Dorsally (*small arrows,* A), a parallel running artery filled faster and reached segments of the distal right coronary artery (*curved arrow,* A), which was proximally occluded. The "left atrial circumflex artery," thus presented, served in this instance as an anastomosing channel.

occurring in the left atrioventricular sulcus, but their topographic localization differs.

Atrial collaterals—interarterial coronary collaterals at the atrial level—are characterized by their location posterior to the atrioventricular sulcus. Anatomically they present the shortest collateral pathways from the most proximal arterial segments of both coronary arteries to the distal coronary arterial distribution at the posterior aspect of the heart.[10] Often the largest of the atrial collateral anastomoses includes the sinus node artery or the atrioventricular node artery arising from either side and continuing in a tortuous fashion to the contralateral side of the circulation. Another relatively well defined atrial artery participating in these collaterals is the so-called left atrial circumflex artery that runs parallel and slightly posterior to the left circumflex artery in the atrioventricular sulcus (Fig. 27-10).

Although these channels may vary considerably in their locations, typical examples of intercoronary collaterals at the atrial level are a right-sided sinus node artery, with branches extending over the lateral and posterior free wall of the left atrium to connect with the left circumflex artery, and a left atrial circumflex artery that has established an anastomosis with the atrioventricular node artery arising from the distal right circumflex coronary artery.

Atrial collaterals may also occur within the atrial septum, which is the site of Kugel's artery,[29,30] or *arteria anastomotica auricularis magna* (Fig. 27-11). As this name implies, it creates an arterial connection between the proximal and anteriorly located portions of the coronary arteries and the distal portion of the artery supplying the dorsal area of the heart—the crux. Unlikely to be seen on an angiogram of a normal heart because of the small size and flow, filling of these vessels may be observed in the event of atrial collateral circulation development.[31–33] Its take-off may occur from the proximal portion of either the left or right coronary artery, not infrequently incorporating the proximal portions of other atrial branches, such as the sinus node artery, the left atrial circumflex artery, or the right-sided septal branch in the crista supraventricular

Figure 27-11. Diagrams of transverse sections of the heart at the level of the atrioventricular sulcus. (A), (B), and (C) are the three variations of the arteria anastomotica auricularis magna described by Kugel.[29] (D) Shows the right-sided variant as outlined by James.[10] Also see text on atrial collaterals. (From Cohen MV. Coronary collaterals: clinical and experimental observation. Mt. Kisco, NY: Futura, 1985. Used with permission.)

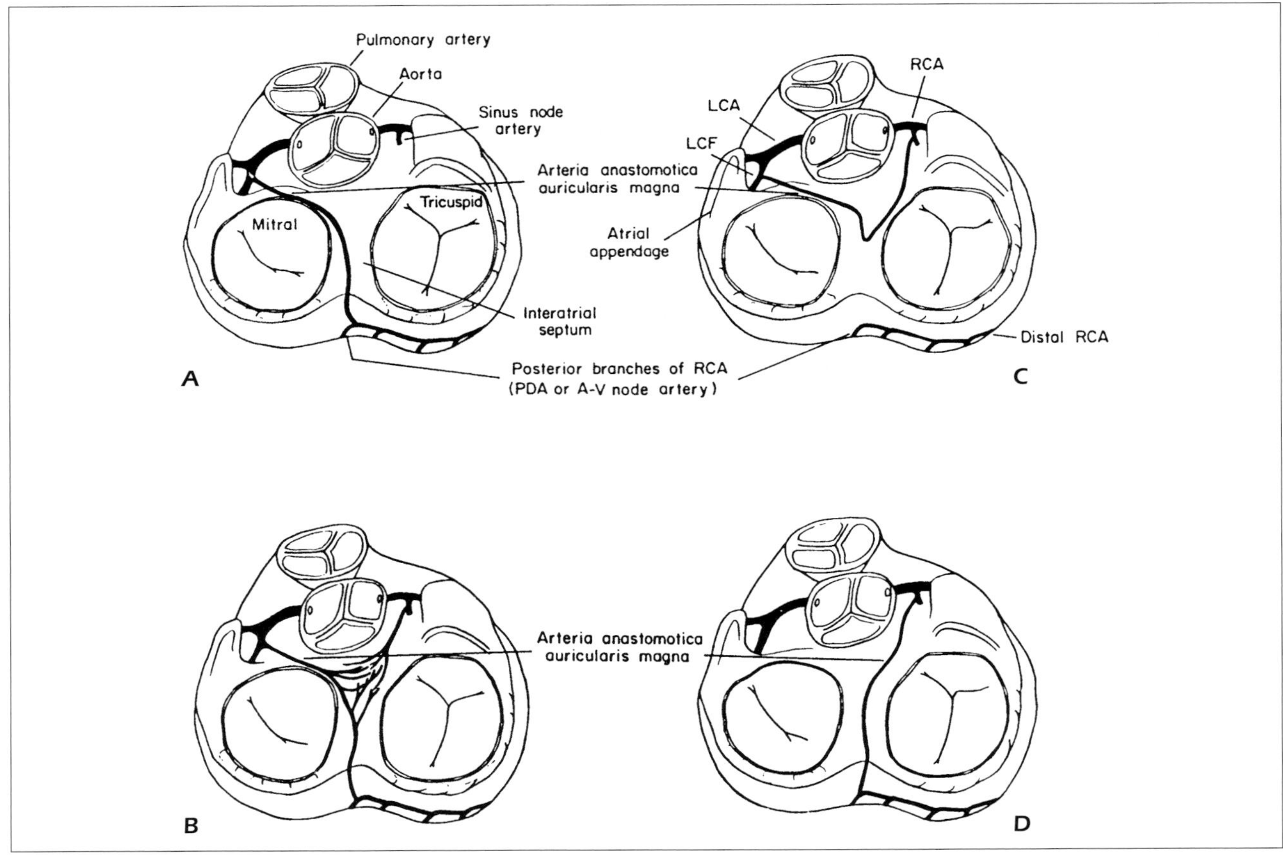

ularis. It then courses in the most anterior portion of the atrial septum close to the atrioventricular valve rings, to communicate with the distal branches of the coronary artery that supply the crux. In this distal portion of the collateral pathway the atrioventricular (AV) node artery may be included. By definition, collaterals along Kugel's artery are intercoronary only in those instances in which they connect the proximal left with the distal right coronary artery and vice versa. If a collateral connects the same artery, as has been reported by Grollman and Heger,[34] it is an intracoronary collateral.

The term "artery" for the vascular structures described by Kugel[29] constitutes a misnomer, inasmuch as it does not represent a single vessel with constant take-off, course and termination. When elucidating the shortest pathways connecting the left and right coronary arteries on injected specimens of 50 apparently normal human hearts, Kugel identified as the most common variant (66%) a small atrial artery arising from the proximal left circumflex artery running via the interatrial septum toward the crux where it communicated with the distal branches of the right coronary artery. The second most common type (26%) had a similar origin, but rather than to connect posteriorly, it made a sharp turn and reversed its run in the septum toward the right side where it finally connected with the proximal right coronary artery. The third variant (8%) was described as a network of small vessels in the anterior area of the atrial septum connecting with both coronary arteries proximally as well as distally with the artery supplying the crux. James[10] agreed generally with Kugel's concept of the anastomosing atrial vessel and declared it to be one of the most strategically placed arteries in the entire heart, but pointed out that it also may arise from the proximal right coronary artery. One of his illustrated casts shows this connection to occur in the crista supraventricularis of the right ventricle. James also pointed out that the vessel in its course at the anterior margin of the atrial septum and close vicinity to the junction with the ventricular septum has free connections to practically all other atrial branches, including the sinus node and AV node arteries, thus providing a potential route of collateral circulation to the ventricular myocardium of the posterior portions of the heart. Baroldi and Scomazzoni[18] apparently were less impressed by Kugel's description, for they were unable to identify on their more than 500 coronary casts a clearly defined single arterial pathway among the numerous anastomotic channels connecting all atrial branches in the form of a net of vessels all about the same small caliber. Their extensive description of larger so-called satellite collaterals bypassing severe stenoses, or occlusions, included descriptions of several connections at the atrial level, interestingly located at the free walls rather than the septum.

Atrial collaterals have no direct relationship to obstructions in the left anterior descending artery. It is conceivable, however, that simultaneously existing occlusions of this artery and of either the right or the left circumflex artery may increase the incidence of atrial collaterals. The relatively low incidence of atrial collaterals described in clinically performed coronary arteriography[22,25,26,35] is surprising in light of the findings on postmortem casts by James,[10] who describes these anastomoses as a frequent and major route of collateral circulation. A possible explanation lies in the fact that atrial arteries connect with extracardiac anastomoses through which unopacified blood may enter and prevent their filling.

Intracoronary Collaterals

By definition, intracoronary collaterals are connections between branches of the same coronary artery. In general, in a coronary arteriogram obtained in vivo their incidence is lower than that of intercoronary collaterals. With regard to the right coronary artery, the potential routes are as follows.

At the free wall of the right ventricle, collaterals connect proximal branches with more distally located branches. An example of this category is a conus branch communicating with an acute marginal branch of the most proximally occluded right coronary artery.

Collaterals in the crista supraventricularis are identical with the ramus cristae supraventricularis or the right septal perforator branch, arising as the second or third branch of the right coronary artery and running toward the superior and posterior part of the interventricular septum to communicate with the distal right coronary artery via coexisting septal collaterals or the atrioventricular node artery. Because it is very difficult to identify angiographically the precise location of the margin between the interatrial and interventricular septa, some of these anastomoses may be identical with interatrial anastomoses as described by Kugel.[29]

Direct bypass collaterals at the site of occlusion are defined as multiple, small, tortuous vessels in the direct vicinity of a most proximal occlusion, connecting the proximal artery with the distal obstructed part of the same vessel. James[36] feels that these do not represent arterial anastomoses but rather are enlarged vasa vasorum or adventitial arteries that form a multichannel cuff around the obstructed segment. This observation may explain their less frequent angiographic depiction in coronary arteriography, as well as the fact that they

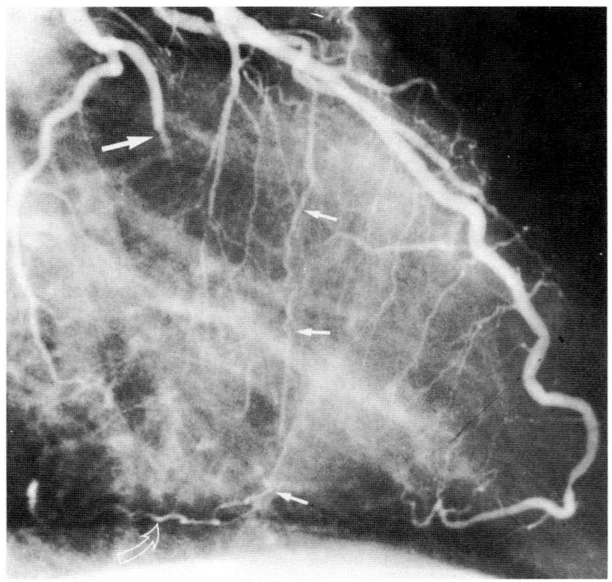

A

B

Figure 27-12. Selective left coronary arteriogram in RAO projection identifying occlusion in midportion of obtuse marginal branch (*large straight arrow,* A). Several tortuous septal anastomoses (*small arrows,* A) are seen to fill from the unobstructed proximal LAD, filling some portions of the posterior descending branch of the occluded right coronary artery. (Selective injection of right coronary artery, not illustrated here, showed proximal occlusion.) In (B), 3 seconds later, filling of the distal obtuse marginal artery (*curved arrows*) has been accomplished by anastomosis deriving from the distal right coronary artery (*small white arrows*) and the distal LAD (*small black arrows*), creating channels at the surface of the posterior lateral wall of the left ventricle.

are relatively more often seen in multivessel occlusions.[22]

Intracoronary collaterals are more frequent in the distribution of the left coronary artery than of the right. The reason probably lies in the anatomy of the left coronary artery, separating, as it does, into two major branches the left anterior descending and the left circumflex artery, each of which may be the site of a high-grade proximal stenosis or occlusion. Indeed, in most cases, these collaterals serve as connections between branches deriving from these two major territories. The potential locations of the collaterals are as follows:

1. At the lateral aspect of the free left ventricular wall, epicardially located coronary collaterals connect branches of the obtuse marginal artery from the left circumflex artery with diagonal branches deriving from the left anterior descending artery. If an intermediate ramus exists, it might substitute as a donor or recipient (Fig. 27-12).
2. Collaterals confined to the left anterior descending artery distribution can be found between the left anterior descending artery and one or more of its diagonal branches, or they may be found in the interventricular septum, connecting proximal to distal septal branches and thus bypassing a correspondingly located short occlusion in the left anterior descending artery.
3. Collateral channels confined to the territory of the left circumflex artery may be found at the latero-posterior wall of the left ventricle connecting a high obtuse marginal with a second, lower-positioned, obtuse marginal artery. Similarly located occlusions in the left circumflex artery may also be collateralized by the left atrial circumflex artery.
4. Direct bypass collaterals at the site of occlusion are similar to those described for the right coronary artery above.

Extracoronary Collaterals

Potential routes for extracoronary collaterals exist between the pericardial reflections along the pulmonary veins and the posterior aspect of the left atrial wall, where small posterior mediastinal arterial structures—mostly deriving from the bronchial circulation—may communicate with atrial arteries.[37] Collateral flow toward the heart in these pathways is unlikely to be detected in selective coronary arteriography because the recipient coronary arteries—ordinarily the right coronary artery and the left circumflex artery—receive an additional, peripheral inflow of unopacified blood. Björk[38] was able to present some angiographic evidence of such bronchial-coronary communications in nonselective coronary arteriography, a technique that also, to some extent, delivers contrast medium to the bronchial circulation. The yield of such a finding might be considerably higher when selective bronchial artery angiography is performed, as was demonstrated by Johnsson in a few cases.[39]

Coronary-to-bronchial anastomoses, indicating a centrifugal collateralization away from the coronary arteries, have been reported by Smith et al.[40] They do not indicate coronary artery disease, but are probably related to abnormal processes in the bronchial circulation, for they may occur in pulmonary conditions such as obstructive airway disease.[41]

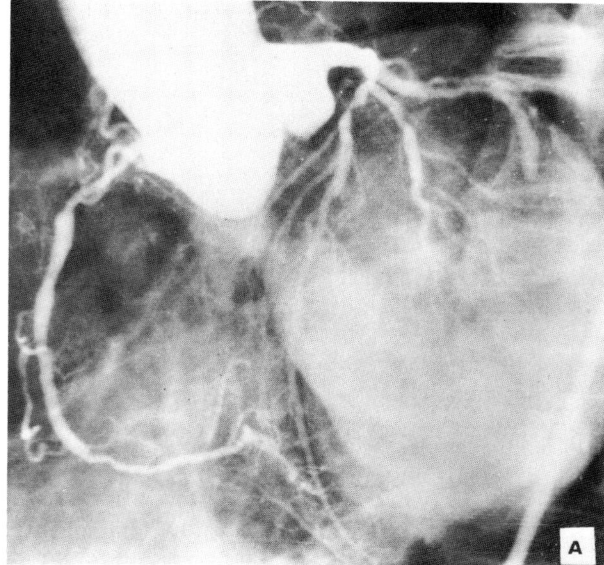

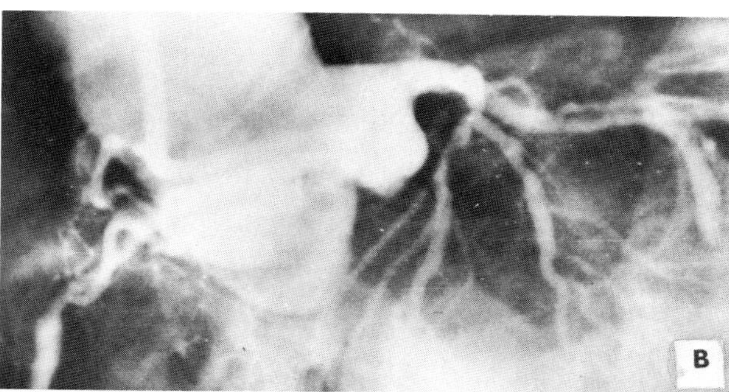

Figure 27-13. Nonselective arteriogram in LAO projection. Multiple stenoses are seen in the right and left anterior descending arteries, and the left circumflex artery is occluded in its midportion. A tortuous arterial connection emerges from the proximal left circumflex artery and traverses to the right, behind the aorta, to connect with a wide and tortuous sinus node artery. The direction of contrast flow in this anastomosis indicated that the proximal narrowing of the right coronary artery is of hemodynamic significance. Multiple septal collaterals and an easily identifiable artery in the crista supraventricularis represent additional collateral pathways. (From Paulin S. Coronary angiography: a technical, anatomic and clinical study. Acta Radiol 1964;233(Suppl):157. Used with permission.)

Variability in Collaterals

The types of coronary collaterals just described may be found isolated or in combination with each other, their overall incidence increasing with the number of arteries and major branches that contain significant obliterations (Fig. 27-13 through Fig. 27-21). In multivessel disease, collateral pathways may be found to exist in sequence. For example, collaterals deriving from an obtuse marginal artery may supply a proximally occluded left anterior descending artery from which septal collaterals feed secondarily the distal portion of an occluded right coronary artery. The listing of all different topographic sites in which collaterals have been described does not include a quantitation of their true size or an estimate of the amount of flow that may occur through them. Such quantitation is difficult in the analysis of coronary angiograms and probably susceptible to considerable subjectivity.

Significant variability in individual cases, however, is indisputable. The variations may be explained in part by technical factors, such as the resolution power of different radiographic equipment, the degree of dilution of contrast medium in the coronary arteries, and the hemodynamic conditions that exist at the time of the examination.[42] Nevertheless, these factors do not explain why certain collateral communications are easily demonstrable in some cases but absent in others with essentially the same obstructive lesions. Differences in collateral pathways may be due to earlier differences in the collateral demand of evolving obstructive lesions occurring over different time spans but resulting in identical final vessel obstruction at the time of the examination. Another explanation is the normal anatomic variability in potentially collateral routes present before the start of the disease.

Text continues on page 721

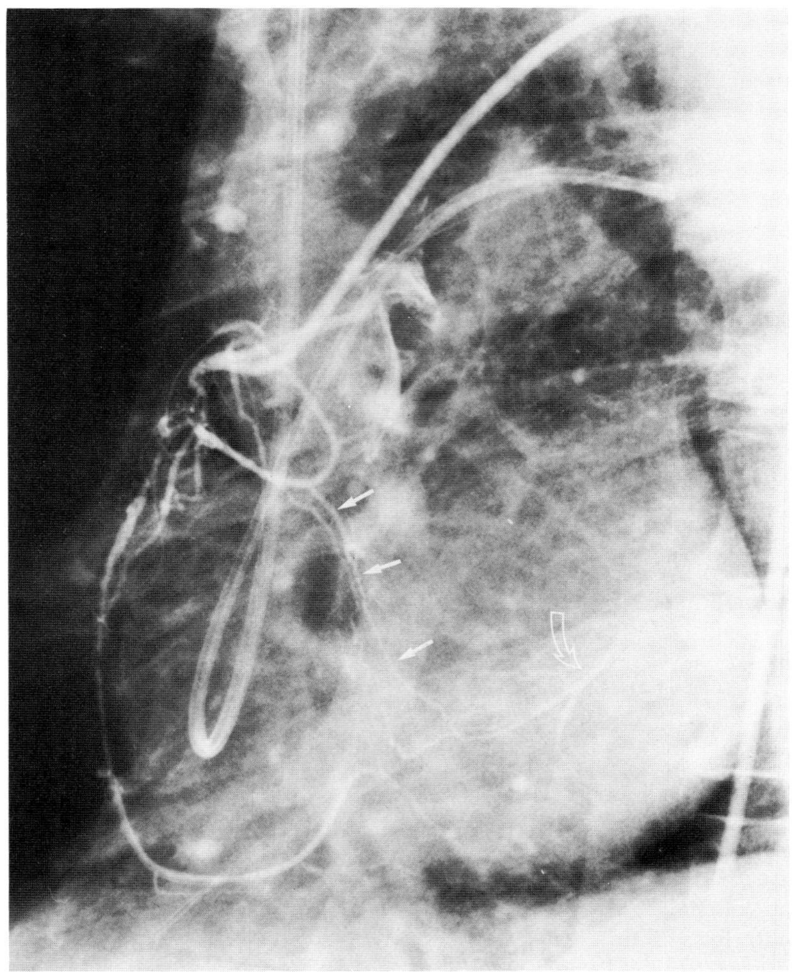

A

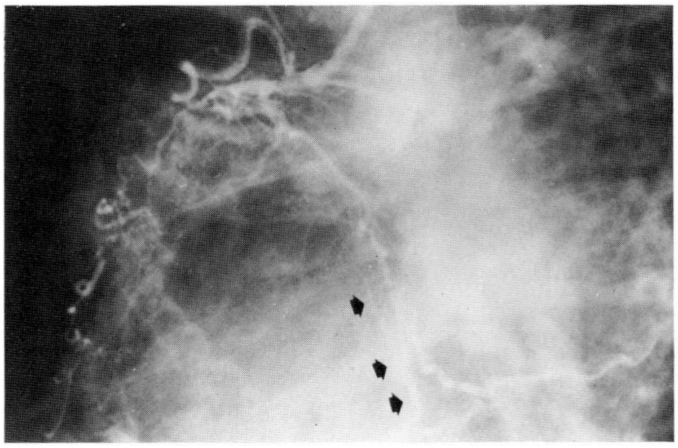

B

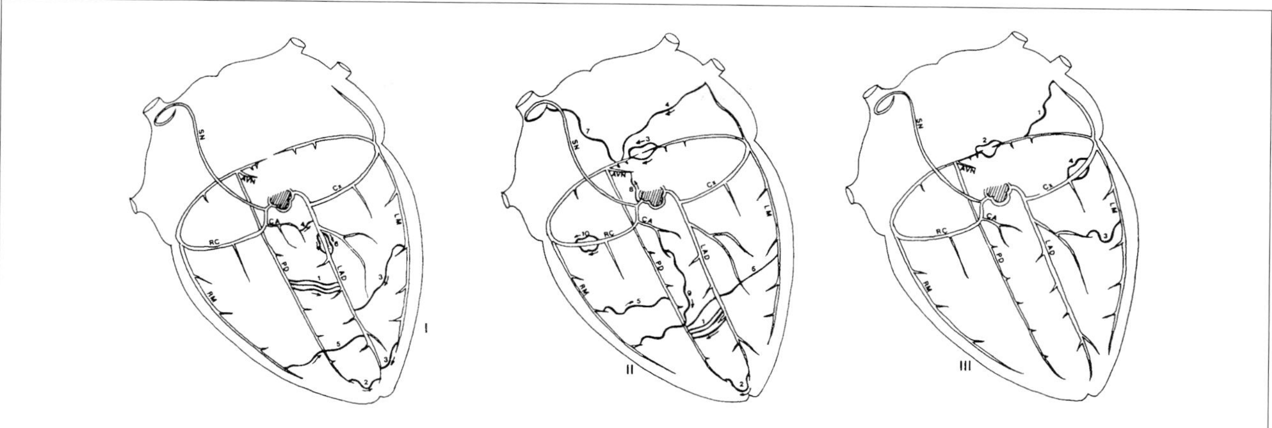

Figure 27-15. Schematic illustration of intercoronary and intracoronary collaterals. Severe stenosis or occlusion located in (I) left anterior descending artery, (II) right coronary artery, and (III) left circumflex artery. (I) *1,* septal anastomoses; *2,* anastomosis over the apex; *3,* left marginal anastomosis to the LAD; *4,* Vieussens circle; *5,* right marginal anastomosis to the LAD; *6,* intracoronary anastomoses across occlusion. (II) *1,* septal anastomoses; *2,* apical anastomosis; *3,* left circumflex anastomoses with distal RC; *4,* atrial circumflex anastomosis with distal RC; *5,* right marginal anastomosis with posterior descending; *6,* left marginal anastomosis with posterior descending; *7,* sinus node artery anastomosis with distal RC; *8,* Kugel's artery; *9,* conus artery anastomosis of the right marginal branches; *10,* intercoronary anastomoses across occlusion. (III) *1,* anastomosis from the left atrial circumflex to the circumflex; *2,* anastomoses from the right coronary artery to the left circumflex; *3,* diagonal over the left marginal to the left circumflex; *4,* intercoronary anastomoses bridging the occlusions. *CX,* left circumflex artery; *RC,* right coronary artery; *AVN,* atrioventricular node artery; *LAD,* left anterior descending artery; *PD,* posterior descending artery; *LM,* left marginal artery of the obtuse angle; *RM,* right marginal artery of the acute angle; *SN,* sinus node artery; *CA,* conus artery. (From Jochem W, et al. Radiographic anatomy of the coronary circulation. AJR 1972;116:50. Used with permission.)

◂ **Figure 27-14.** Selective right coronary arteriograms in LAO projection in two patients with advanced occlusive disease. The right coronary arteries are totally occluded approximately 2 cm distal to their orifices, and a network of multiple tortuous coronary collaterals is seen in the expected location of their continuation. (A) A wide sinus node artery is seen in typical loop shape. From its midportion a branch takes off to the left and downward. It continues in a tortuous anastomosis (*straight arrows*), eventually connecting to the distal left circumflex artery (*curved arrow*), which it fills in retrograde fashion. (B) In another patient a wide crista supraventricularis branch originates from the proximal right coronary artery and connects via a very wide and tortuous anastomosis with the left circumflex artery. Observe also an additional anastomosis to the right of the atrioventricular node artery (*arrows*), the latter running approximately parallel to the tortuous anastomosis. This represents an in vivo demonstration of Kugel's anastomosis in the interatrial septum, the shortest collateral pathway to the posterior surface of the heart.

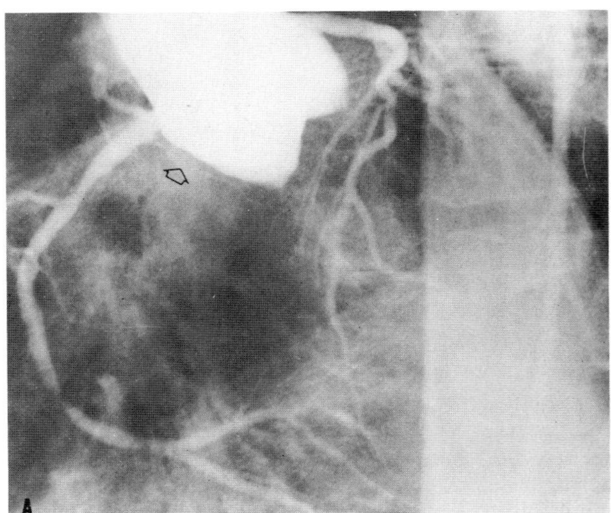

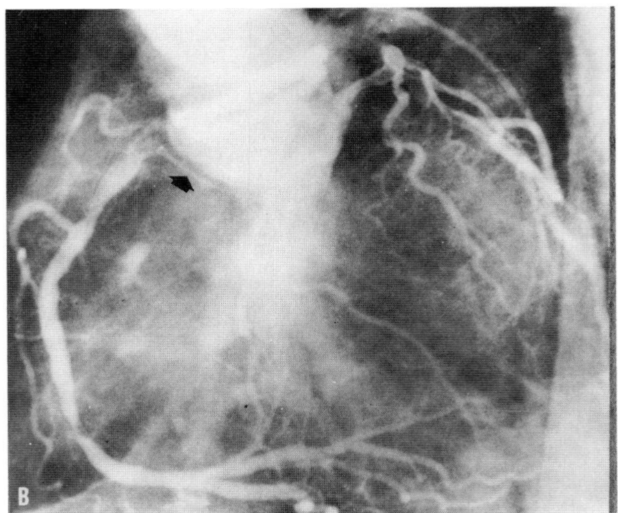

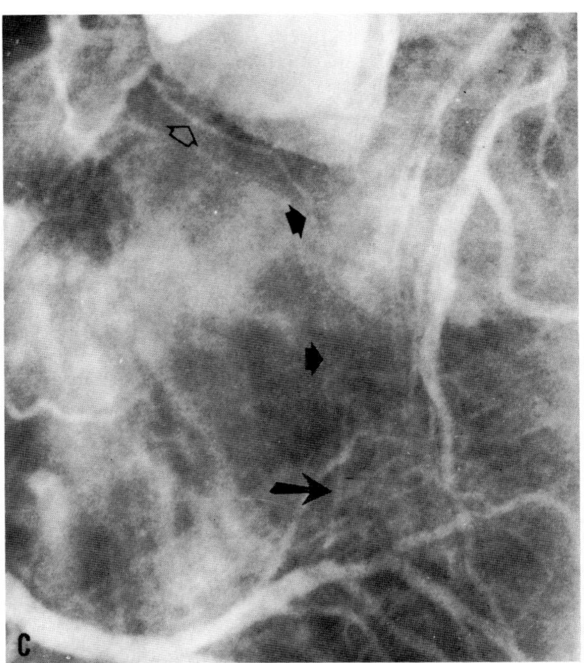

Figure 27-16. Nonselective coronary arteriogram in LAO projection. (A and B) Paired films in stereoscopic projection. Narrow stenosis in the distal right circumflex coronary artery results in retarded filling of the distal part of the right coronary artery. *Arrows* point at an unusual right branch of the right coronary artery at the site of the crista supraventricularis. (C) Detail film illustrating extension of this branch (*short arrows*) into the posterior part of the interventricular septum and the vicinity of atrioventricular node artery (*long arrow*). (From Paulin S. Interarterial coronary anastomoses in relation to arterial obstruction demonstrated in coronary arteriography. Invest Radiol 1967;2:147. Used with permission.)

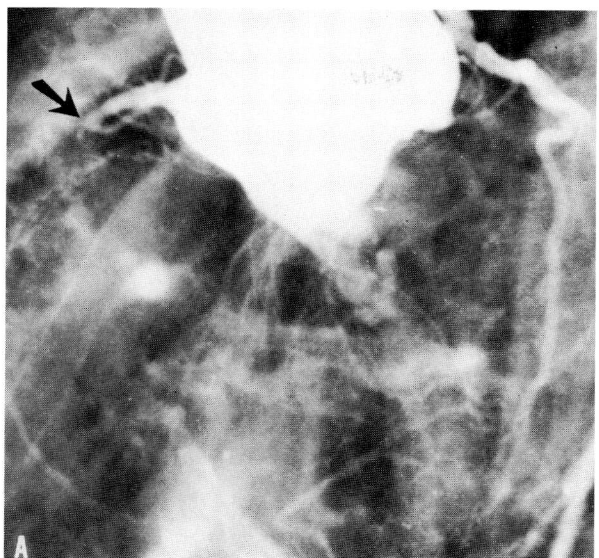

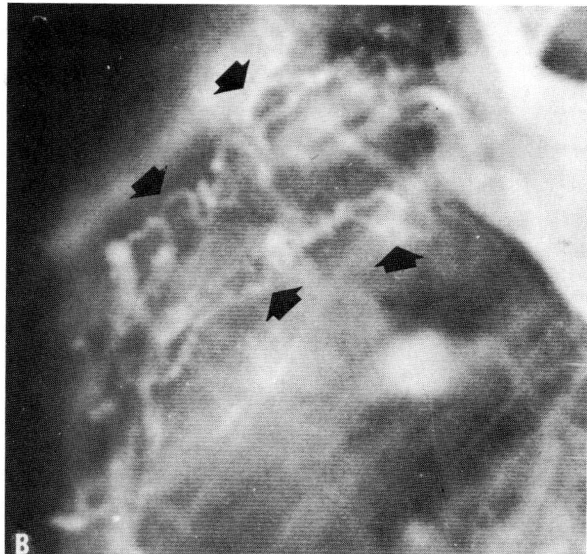

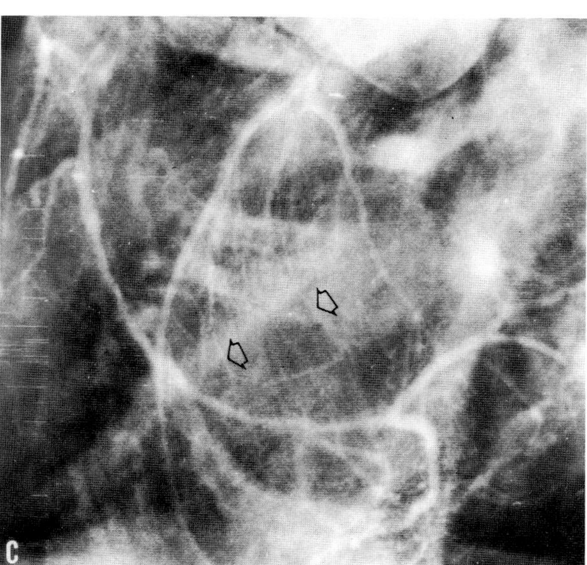

Figure 27-17. Occlusion of proximal part of right coronary artery (*arrow*, A) with tortuous bypass collaterals in the vicinity of obstruction. All films in LAO projection. (A) Early phase of filling. (B) Detail showing collateral (*arrows*) close to occlusion. (C) Approximately 2 seconds after start of injection there is filling of the distal part of the right coronary artery and the numerous collaterals in the interventricular septum (*arrows*), and eventual filling of the distal anterior descending artery, which was occluded proximally. (From Paulin S. Interarterial coronary anastomoses in relation to arterial obstruction demonstrated in coronary arteriography. Invest Radiol 1967;2:147. Used with permission.)

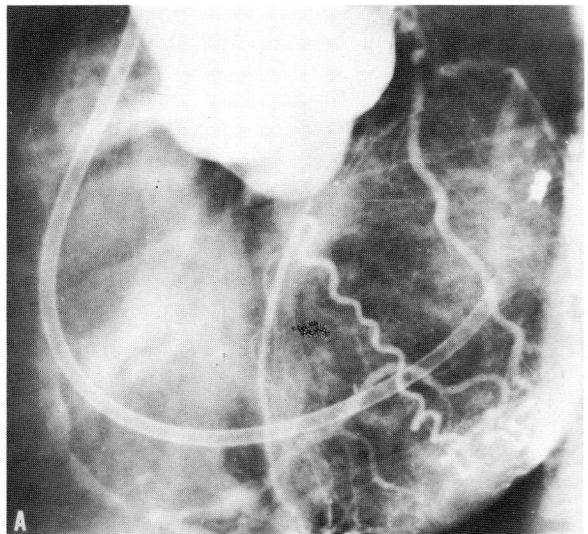

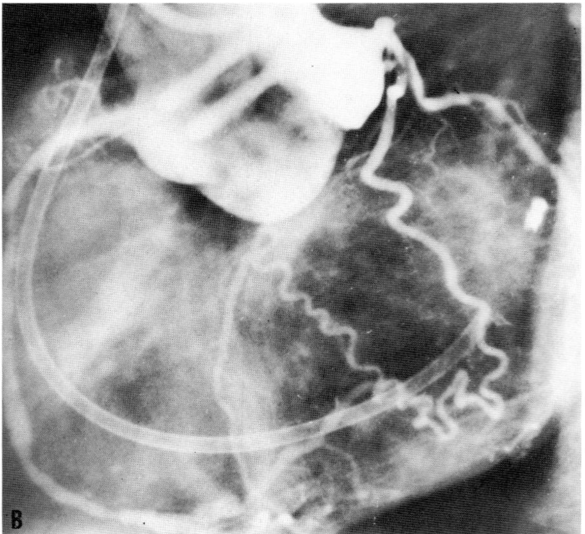

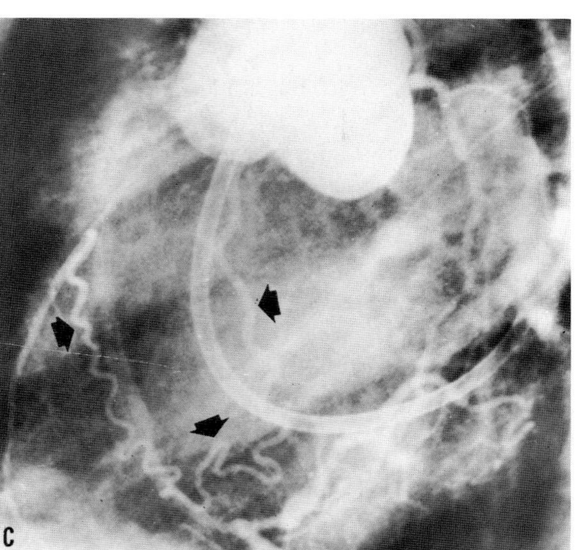

Figure 27-18. Coronary arteriogram of patient with obliteration of proximal third of anterior descending artery. Diffuse wall irregularities in the right coronary artery coincide with virtual absence of any filling of side branches to the right ventricle. (A and B) Stereoscopic pairs in LAO projection demonstrating wide tortuous intraarterial anastomoses at the surface of the left ventricular anterior wall. (C) Lateral view showing the same anastomosis (*arrows*) between the intermediate branch and the large diagonal branch of the anterior descending artery. Catheter in coronary sinus was used with simultaneous coronary flow determinations. (From Paulin S. Interarterial coronary anastomoses in relation to arterial obstruction demonstrated in coronary arteriography. Invest Radiol 1967;2:147. Used with permission.)

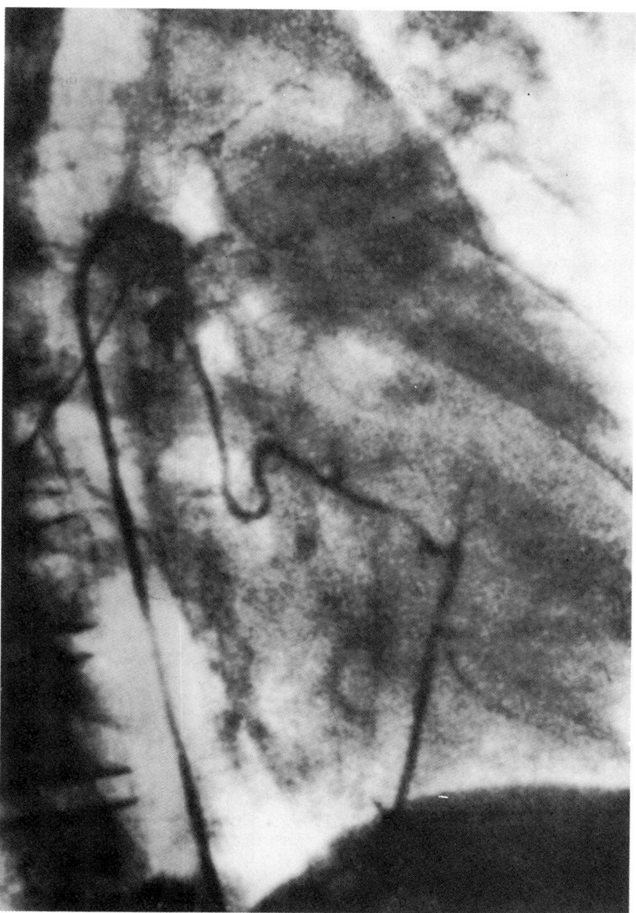

Figure 27-19. Selective bronchial arteriogram in RAO projection identifying anastomoses between the bronchial circulation and the right coronary artery via the sinus node branch. The proximal right coronary artery was occluded in this patient. (From Johnsson KA. Collateral circulation between bronchial and coronary arteries. Acta Radiol (Stockh) 1969;8:393. Used with permission.)

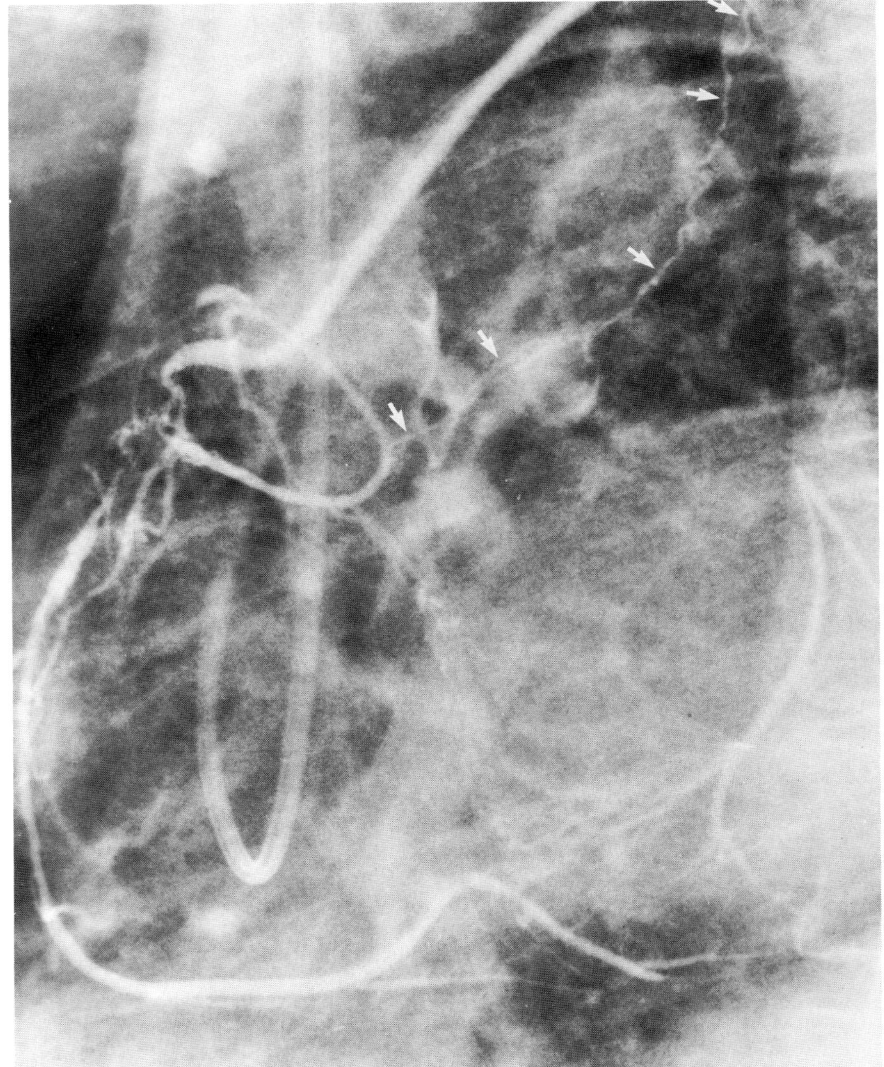

Figure 27-20. Selective right coronary arteriogram in LAO projection. The proximal right coronary artery is occluded in a short segment, and its distal filling is accomplished by direct bypassing collaterals. A large sinus node artery is identified by its typical counterclockwise turn around the ostium of the superior vena cava. At about the midportion of the sinus node artery a narrow, but readily identifiable, collateral is seen to run in a left upward direction and to reach high up in the superior mediastinum (*arrows*). Although not specifically elaborated in this patient, such anastomotic channels may herald abnormalities in the bronchial circulation secondary to obstructive airway disease or pulmonary vascular abnormalities. (Distal filling of an occluded left circumflex artery can be identified to the right of the picture and was accomplished via anastomoses in the interatrial and interventricular septa.)

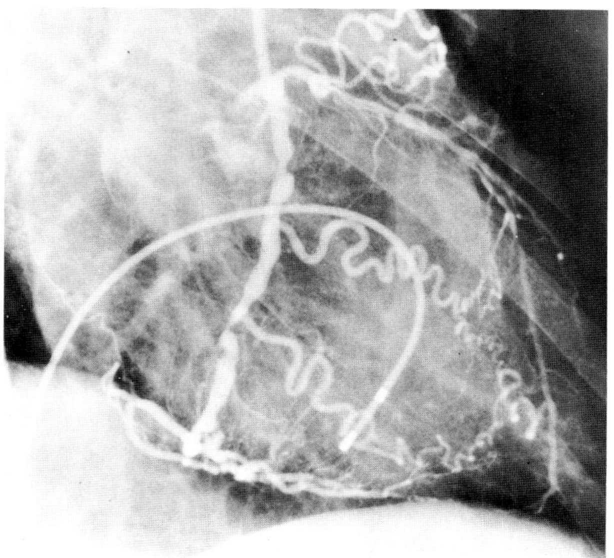

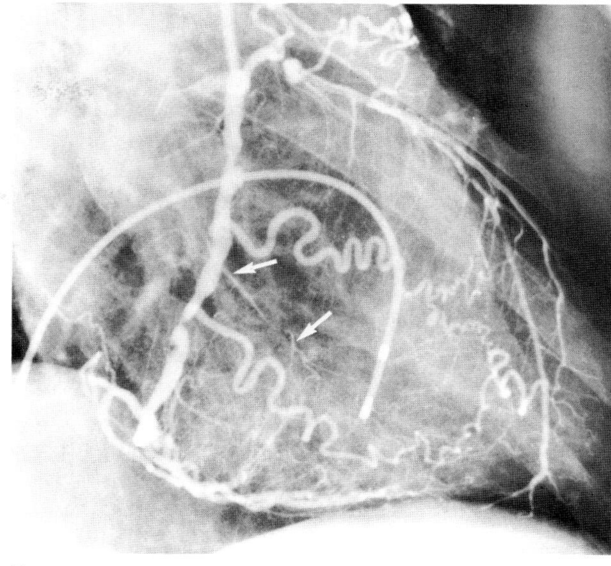

Figure 27-21. Selective right coronary arteriogram in RAO projection in the presence of left main coronary artery occlusion. Multiple, very wide, and tortuous collaterals are seen to anastomose with the left anterior descending artery. Rapid and good filling of the proximally occluded left anterior descending artery, including multiple septal and large diagonal branches (time interval between [A] and [B] is 1.5 seconds), contrasts with the rather faint filling of a narrow segment of the left circumflex artery (*arrows,* B). The selective biplane left ventricular angiogram (not illustrated here) disclosed the most marked wall motion abnormality in the left lateral wall. Note the pacing catheters placed in the right ventricle, a precaution during the angiographic examination of this very symptomatic patient.

Angiographic Assessment of Collateral Function

The general concept that coronary collaterals should present at least a partial compensation for regional flow deficits as in other organ systems[43] was challenged by Helfant, Kemp, and Gorlin.[44] These authors compared ventricular contractility in patients with single or multiple stenosis greater than 75 percent with or without collateral circulation. They found that depression of left ventricular function was slightly more prevalent in the group with collaterals and concluded that their presence did not protect the myocardium. Similarly, Miller et al.[45] reported a higher incidence of left ventricular wall motion abnormalities in patients with collateral vessels. McConahay et al.[46] found that collateral vessels did not reduce the incidence of asynergy, and Björk[47] reported no difference in maximal work capacity, left ventricular systolic and diastolic size, or regional wall motion impairment in patients with and without collaterals. Smith et al.[48] found no increase in myocardial blood flow in patients with coronary collaterals as measured by xenon-133 washout at the time of coronary artery bypass surgery. Bartel et al.[49] and Harris et al.[50] were unable to find a difference in graded exercise performance between patients with and without angiographically documented collaterals.

These findings, which were uniformly interpreted as presenting evidence against any significant functional importance of coronary collaterals, raised considerable controversy. They were certainly incompatible with reported cases in which total occlusion of the left main coronary artery was demonstrated in living patients.[51–54]

Proponents of a different view[26,55] sugested several reasons why the above-mentioned results appeared to underestimate the importance of coronary collateral circulation. First, the mere presence of detectable collaterals does not indicate their importance in transporting flow. Although it is likely that large and multiple collaterals have greater functional potentials, the crucial angiographic observation is to assess their ability to accomplish adequate and rapid phasic filling with the injected contrast material in the periphery of the occluded coronary artery, including its good distal runoff. None of the studies just cited had paid specific attention to such findings. Second, the analyzed obstructive lesions did not represent high-grade subtotal and total occlusions only, but included stenosis of approximately 75 percent of the transectional area, an angiographic finding that does not constitute a homogeneous population.[56] In this category of stenosis the cases with collaterals may represent patients who have more advanced coronary artery disease and thus logically may be expected to have a higher incidence of left ventricular myocardial damage. Third, determination of left ventricular function in terms of cardiac output at rest and/or at exercise is not specific enough to correlate collateral circulation with regional wall motion impairment. Such a determination would require a specific study of the area of potential myocardial injury that is subserved by the angiographically demonstrated collateral anastomoses. Indeed, Levin et al.[57] found, in a series of complete arterial obstructions, a positive correlation between the quality of collateral flow (as determined by the degree of visualization and filling of the distal segments of an occluded artery) and regional ventricular wall motion. In particular, the assessment of adequate distal arterial runoff of the contrast material identified cases with strikingly better myocardial contractility in the relevant area, whereas akinesis was a dominant finding when the collateral contrast flow was clearly retarded. Hecht et al.[55] concluded from their study, in which collaterals were quantitated with regard to their effectiveness, that the coronary collateral circulation plays a role in the preservation of left ventricular function.

An interesting finding encountered frequently in selective coronary arteriography when adequate collateral peripheral filling is present is the so-called reciprocating pattern, indicating competitive flow between opacified and unopacified pathways.[58] The reciprocating pattern should also indicate preserved myocardial contractility resulting in systolic and diastolic phasic changes in peripheral resistance.

As mentioned earlier, the intensity and direction of collateral flow may be subject to alterations in conjunction with changes in hemodynamics and cardiac stress. Frick and colleagues[59] performed a comparative analysis of coronary collaterals in ischemic heart disease by carrying out angiography at rest and during ischemia induced by pacing. Regional myocardial perfusion responses, as determined by xenon-133 washout curves, yielded suggestive evidence that the angiographically demonstrated collaterals were intimately involved in the enhancement of flow. However, the data showed that in some patients the collateral circulation reacted to regional ischemia by enhancement, whereas in others it was decreased, raising the possibility of "collateral steal" under certain circumstances. Although not demonstrated conclusively in this clinical experimental study, evidence of a "myocardial steal syndrome" following the administration of lidoflazine, a long-acting coronary vasodilator, was shown in animal experimental models of chronic coronary artery occlusion by Schaper and colleagues.[60] Thus it is appropriate to emphasize that angiographic evidence of collaterals can only mirror collateral flow as it occurs at the time of the examination.[61] Appreciation of this fact would probably eliminate much of the remaining controversy on this subject.[62]

Clinical studies on coronary collaterals comparing them with well-defined end points are in strong support of their functional importance. Numerous reports have accumulated describing patients with complete occlusion of the left main coronary artery with collateralization from either a normal or abnormal right coronary artery,[61,63,64] and remarkable cases have been encountered in which both proximal and right and left main coronary arteries were totally occluded and the supply depended on an ectopically arising conus artery providing collateralization.[65,66] Since most of these reports make mention of relatively well preserved left ventricular function, the postulate that these angiographically detectable collaterals have no functional importance appears absurd. There exists, of course, postmortem evidence of left main coronary artery occlusions, many of which might have had evidence of poor collaterals. Such ominous combinations may be encountered during the angiographic examinations of terminal patients unlikely to recover unless immediate recanalization attempts, such as angioplasty or emergent bypass surgery, are performed successfully (unpublished data).

Other data that were strongly supportive, albeit less conclusive, derived from Fuster et al.'s large study[67] in which a subgroup of patients with a total occlusion somewhere in the large proximal coronary arteries on 1-year follow-up examination only demonstrated evidence of subendocardial injury. The authors suggested that the well-detectable epicardially located collaterals in all these cases were probably responsible for limiting the infarction to the inner wall. The same authors also separated a group of 58 patients with transmural myocardial infarction related to a coronary occlusion; 32 reported postinfarction angina whereas the remaining 26 were free of symptoms. Whereas the former subgroup had a high incidence of collateral filling to the distal portion of the artery, the latter asymptomatic subgroup showed collaterals only in about one-third. Considering the limitations in the spatial resolution power of myocardial scanning techniques, these results are open to speculation in either direction. Thus the presence of collaterals could suggest that some islands of surviving myocardium were still present resulting in angina, whereas the true and definitive transmural infarction explains its absence.

Supportive evidence for a functional role of angiographically demonstrable collaterals is also present in the accumulating data from follow-up angiograms after bypass surgery, and from the experience that has been gained with the performance of angioplasty and thrombolytic therapy.[68,69] It is generally agreed that when a bypass graft is patent and effective, the relevant preoperatively shown collaterals disappear, or may even seem to be filled in reverse direction toward the less affected but nonrevascularized stenosed coronary artery.[70] If a graft occludes, the collateral circulation returns to the preoperative level, provided that the complicating event did not result in a major myocardial injury. Similarly, collaterals usually disappear following successful thrombolysis or balloon angioplasty.

Angiographic evidence of collaterals, particularly of a type that supplies prompt and high-concentration contrast filling of the distal vessel according to previously established criteria,[26,55] have rendered valuable information. Thus patients with angiographically visible collateral flow of good quality at the time of thrombolytic therapy initiation have a significant advantage.[68] As a group they have better values of left ventricular ejection fraction on follow-up examination, with the benefit seen not only in those patients who had successful thrombolysis but also in those in which the vessel occlusion remained. Rentrop et al.[71] performed a clinical evaluation of symptom onset and time interval in patients receiving thrombolytic treatment during acute myocardial infarction. Their results suggested that the presence of coronary collaterals extends the time window for the beneficial effect of this therapy. Hirai et al.[72] have found a link between the presence of collaterals and protection from left ventricular aneurysm formation following myocardial infarction. Thus the angiographic depiction of coronary collaterals and the analysis of their mode of filling[26,55,61] have gained greater attention recently.

Although there should be little remaining doubt that this angiographic finding identifies an important alternate source of arterial blood flow in the presence of obstructive coronary artery disease, the observations made so far strongly support the assumption that even the most efficient collaterals do not reach the capacity of the original normal arteries or that of an efficient bypass graft.

Angiographic Pitfalls

In the event of a narrow and hemodynamically effective stenosis or occlusion of the coronary artery, it is most likely that the collateral flow uses the path of least resistance. Anastomoses, therefore, should be detectable most often in areas where these relatively wide, preformed interarterial connections are present. The more proximally a given obstruction is located, the greater the number of potential collateral pathways participating in this compensatory flow. If a given obstruction is not accompanied by filling of collaterals, that fact may be explained by the following circumstances:

1. The hemodynamic importance of a stenosis at the time of the examination is less than was suggested angiographically, and the pressure drop is not sufficient to induce collaterals.
2. The stenosis is hemodynamically important and reduces flow, but the event is recent and collateralization has not yet developed.
3. The collateral flow occurs from an artery that has not been injected properly, such as a supernumerary coronary arterial branch or a bronchial artery–coronary artery anastomosis.
4. An occlusion has resulted in a complete avascular scar.
5. A stenosis or occlusion is compensated for by multiple small vascular anastomoses with an individual caliber below the threshold for angiographic demonstration. Filling of the distal tree may be seen in spite of "absent collaterals."

References

1. Gorlin R. Coronary collaterals. Cited in Gorlin R, ed. Coronary artery disease. Philadelphia: Saunders, 1976:59.
2. Lower R. Tractatus de Corde. Item de motu & colore sanguinis et chyli in eum transitu. Amstelodami, 1669. Cited in Spalteholz W. Die Arterien der Herzwand. Leipzig: Hirzel, 1924.
3. Vieussens R. Nouvelles decouvertes sur le coeur. Paris, 1706. Cited in James.[10]
4. Hunter J. Essays and observations; 1861. In: Owen R, ed. The pathophysiology of myocardial perfusion. London: van Voorst 1861;1:126.
5. Ruysch F. Opera Omnia Anatomico-Medico-Chirurgica. Amstelodami, 1737. Cited in Schaper W. The collateral circulation. In: Schaper W, ed. The pathophysiology of myocardial perfusion. New York: Elsevier North–Holland, 1979:415.
6. Hyrtl J. Die Corrosion Anatomie und ihre Ergebnisse. Wien: Wilhelm Braumüller, 1873.
7. Henle J. Handbuch der Gefässlehre des Menschen. Braunschweig: Vieweg & Sohn, 1868.
8. Cohnheim J, von Schulthess-Rechberg A. Über die Folgen der Kranzarterienverschliessung auf das Herz. Virchows Arch Pathol Anat 1881;85:503.
9. Schaper W. The collateral circulation. In: Schaper W, ed. The pathophysiology of myocardial perfusion. New York: Elsevier North–Holland, 1979.
10. James TN. Anatomy of the coronary arteries. New York: Hoeber Medical Division, Harper & Row, 1961.
11. Spalteholz W. Die Coronararterien des Herzens. Verh Anat Ges 1907;21:141–153.
12. Crainicianu A. Anatomische Studien über die Coronararterien und experimentelle Untersuchungen über ihre Durchgangigkeit. Virchows Arch A Pathol Anat Histopathol 1922;238: 1–75.
13. Campbell JS. Stereoscopic radiography of the coronary system. Q J Med 1929:22:247–267.

14. Gross L, Kugel MA. The arterial blood vascular distribution to the left and right ventricles of the human heart. Am Heart J 1933;9:165–177.
15. Blumgart HL, Schlesinger MJ, Davis D. Studies on the relation of the clinical manifestations of angina pectoris, coronary thrombosis, and myocardial infarction to the pathologic findings. Am Heart J 1940;19:1.
16. Prinzmetal M, Simkin B, Bergman HC, et al. Studies on the coronary circulation: II. The collateral circulation of the normal human heart by coronary perfusion with radioactive erythrocyte and glass spheres. Am Heart J 1974;33:420.
17. Vastesaeger MM, van der Straeten PP, Friart J, et al. Les anastomoses intercoronariennes telles qu'elles apparaissent à la coronarographie post mortem. Acta Cardiol (Brux) 1957;12:365.
18. Baroldi G, Scomazzoni G. Coronary circulation in the normal and pathologic heart. Washington, DC: Office of the Surgeon General, Department of the Army, 1967.
19. Schlesinger MJ. An injection plus dissection study of the coronary artery occlusions and anastomoses. Am Heart J 1938;15: 528.
20. Baroldi G, Mantero O, Scomazzoni G. The collaterals of the coronary arteries in normal and pathologic hearts. Circ Res 1956;4:223.
21. Bellman S, Frank HA. Intercoronary collaterals in normal hearts. J Thorac Surg 1958;36:584.
22. Paulin S. Interarterial coronary anastomoses in relation to arterial obstruction demonstrated in coronary arteriography. Invest Radiol 1967;2:147.
23. Bookstein JJ, Kahn DR. Appraisal of coronary arteriography in evaluating the hemodynamic significance of experimental coronary artery stenosis. Radiology 1967;88:672.
24. Conti CR, Pepine CJ, Feldman RL, et al. The angiographic definition of critical coronary stenosis. Acta Med Scand 1978; 615(Suppl):9.
25. Gensini GG, DaCosta BCB. The coronary collateral circulation in living man. Am J Cardiol 1969;24:393.
26. Levin DC. Pathways and functional significance of the coronary collateral circulation. Circulation 1974;50:69.
27. Weintraub RM, Aroesty JM, Paulin S, et al. Medically refractory unstable angina pectoris: I. Long-term follow-up of patients undergoing intraaortic balloon counter pulsation and operation. Am J Cardiol 1979;43:877.
28. Gross L. The blood supply of the heart. New York: Hoeber Medical Division, Harper & Row, 1921.
29. Kugel MA. Anatomical studies on the coronary arteries and their branches: I. Arteria anastomotica auricularis magna. Am Heart J 1927/28;3:260.
30. Cohen MV. Coronary collaterals: clinical and experimental observation. Mt. Kisco, NY: Futura, 1985.
31. Levin DC, Kauff M, Baltaxe HA. Coronary collateral circulation. Am J Roentgenol 1974;119:463–473.
32. Smith C, Amplatz K. Angiographic demonstration of the Kugel's artery (arteria anastomotica auricularis magna). Radiology 1973;106:113–118.
33. Soto B, Jochem W, Karp RB, et al. Angiographic anatomy of the Kugel's artery: arteria anastomotica auricularis magna. Am J Roentgenol 1973;119:503–507.
34. Grollman J, Heger L. Angiographic anatomy of the left Kugel's artery. Cathet Cardiovasc Diagn 1978;4:127–133.
35. Jochem W, Soto B, Karp RB, et al. Radiographic anatomy of the coronary circulation. AJR 1972;116:50.
36. James TN. The delivery and distribution of coronary collateral circulation. Chest 1970;58:183.
37. Moberg A. Anastomoses between extracardiac vessels and coronary arteries. Acta Med Scand 1968;485(Suppl).
38. Björk L. Anastomoses between the coronary and bronchial arteries. Acta Radiol (Stockh) 1966;4:93.
39. Johnsson KA. Collateral circulation between bronchial and coronary arteries. Acta Radiol (Stockh) 1969;8:393.
40. Smith S, Adams D, Herman M, et al. Coronary to bronchial anastomoses: an in vivo demonstration by selective coronary arteriography. Radiology 1972;104:289.
41. Spindola-Franco H, Weisel A, Delman AJ. Pulmonary steal syndrome: an unusual case of coronary-bronchial pulmonary artery communication. Radiology 1980;126:25.
42. Tuna N, Amplatz K, Johnson E. The significance of coronary collateral circulation, coronary angiogram and electrovectorcardiographic correlations. In: Proceeding of the Satellite Symposium of the 25th International Congress of Physiological Sciences. Brussels, Belgium: Presses Academiques Europeennes, 1972.
43. Hollenberg NK. Collateral arterial growth and reactivity: lessons from the limb and renal blood supply. In: Schaper W, Schaper J, eds. Collateral circulation, heart, brain, kidney, limbs. Dordrecht: Kluwer Academic Publishers, 1993.
44. Helfant RH, Kemp HG, Gorlin R. Coronary atherosclerosis, coronary collaterals and their relation to cardiac function. Ann Intern Med 1970;73:189.
45. Miller RR, Mason DT, Salel A, et al. Determinants and functional significance of the coronary collateral circulation in patients with coronary artery disease. Am J Cardiol 1972;29:281.
46. McConahay DR, McCallister BD, Hallermann FJ, et al. Comparative quantitative analysis of the electrocardiogram and the vectorcardiogram. Circulation 1970;42:245.
47. Björk L. Angiographic demonstration of collaterals of the coronary arteries in patients with angina pectoris. Acta Radiol (Stockh) 1969;8:305.
48. Smith SC, Gorlin R, Herman MV, et al. Myocardial blood flow in man: effect of coronary collateral circulation and coronary bypass surgery. J Clin Invest 1972;51:2556.
49. Bartel AG, Behar VS, Peter RH, et al. Graded exercise stress tests in angiographically documented coronary artery disease. Circulation 1974;49:348.
50. Harris CN, Kaplan MA, Parker DP, et al. Anatomic and functional correlates in intercoronary collateral vessels. Am J Cardiol 1972;30:611.
51. Goldberg S, Grossman W, Markis JE, et al. Total occlusion of the left main coronary artery: a clinical hemodynamic and angiographic profile. Am J Med 1978;64:3–8.
52. Goldberger AL, Costello DL, Moores WY. Normal left ventricular function with total occlusion of right and left main coronary arteries. Cathet Cardiovasc Diagn 1980;6:185.
53. Greenspan M, Iskandrian AS, Segal BL, et al. Complete occlusion of the left main coronary. Am Heart J 1979;98:83.
54. Valle M, Virtanen K, Hekali P, et al. Survival with total occlusion of the left main coronary artery: significance of the collateral circulation. Cathet Cardiovasc Diagn 1979;5:269–275.
55. Hecht H, Aroesty J, Morkin E, et al. The role of the coronary collateral circulation in the preservation of left ventricular function. Radiology 1975;114:305–313.
56. Paulin S. Grading and measuring coronary artery stenosis. Cathet Cardiovasc Diagn 1979;5:213.
57. Levin DC, Sos TA, Lee JG, et al. Coronary collateral circulation and distal coronary runoff: the key factors in preserving myocardial contractility in patients with coronary artery disease. AJR 1973;119:474.
58. Spindola-Franco H, Adams DF, Herman MV, et al. Reciprocating flow in the coronary circulation. Radiology 1973;107:497.
59. Frick MH, Valle M, Korhola O, et al. Analysis of coronary collaterals in ischemic heart disease by angiography during pacing induced ischemia. Br Heart J 1976;38:186.
60. Schaper W, Lewi P, Flameng W, et al. Myocardial steal produced by coronary vasodilation in chronic artery occlusion. Basic Res Cardiol 1973;68:3.
61. Paulin S. Functional alterations in the coronary circulation as mirrored in the angiogram. Cardiovasc Intervent Radiol 1983; 5:177–185.
62. Carroll RJ, Verani MS, Falsetti HL. The effect of collateral circulation on segmental left ventricular contraction. Circulation 1974;50:709.
63. Goldberger AL, Costello DL, Moores WY. Normal left ventricular function with total occlusion of right and left main coronary arteries. Cathet Cardiovasc Diagn 1980;6:185–190.
64. Frye RL, Gura GM, Chesebro JH, et al. Complete occlusion

of the left main coronary artery and the importance of coronary collaterals. Mayo Clin Proc 1977;52:742–745.
65. Rathor AL, Gooch AS, Maranhao V. Survival through conus artery collateralization in severe coronary heart disease. Chest 1973;63:840–843.
66. Paulin S. Coronary angiography: a technical, anatomic and clinical study. Acta Radiol 1964;233(Suppl):1–215.
67. Fuster V, Frey RL, Kennedy MA, et al. The role of collateral circulation in the various coronary syndromes. Circulation 1979;59:1137–1144.
68. Topol EJ, Ellis SG. Coronary collaterals revisited: accessory pathway to myocardial preservation during infarction. Circulation 1991;83(3):1084–1086.
69. Habib GB, Heibig MD, Forman SA, et al. Influence of coronary collateral vessels on myocardial infarct size in humans: results of Phase I thrombolysis in myocardial infarction (TIMI) trial. Circulation 1991;83(3):739–746.
70. Valle M. Postoperative coronary angiography. Acta Radiol (Stockh) 1973;333(Suppl):51.
71. Rentrop KP, Feit F, Sherman W, et al. Late thrombolytic therapy preserved left ventricular function in patients with collateralized total coronary occlusion: primary end point findings of the second Mount Sinai-New York University Reperfusion Trial. J Am Coll Cardiol 1989;14:58–64.
72. Hirai T, Fujita M, Nakajima H, et al. Importance of collateral circulation for prevention of left ventricular aneurysm formation in acute myocardial infarction. Circulation 1989;79:791–796.

28

Pitfalls in Coronary Arteriography

DAVID C. LEVIN

In virtually every cardiac catheterization-angiographic laboratory, the incidence of normal coronary arteriograms in patients with clinically suspected coronary artery disease is somewhere between 15 and 25 percent. These patients with strong clinical symptoms but normal coronary arteriograms represent one end of a broad spectrum. At the other end are patients with relatively minor symptoms (or no symptoms at all, with a positive stress electrocardiogram) who prove to have severe and diffuse coronary artery disease at coronary arteriography. The frequent discrepancy between clinical pattern and arteriographic findings is one of the most intriguing aspects of coronary artery disease. However, it raises the possibility that the arteriogram in some cases may not present a true picture of the pathologic anatomy of the coronary arterial tree. Several studies comparing in vivo or postmortem coronary arteriograms with serial sections of the coronary arteries at autopsy have emphasized the possible inaccuracy of the coronary arteriogram.[1-3]

This chapter discusses various pitfalls in coronary arteriography that could result in inaccuracies in the studies. These pitfalls should be carefully kept in mind by the angiographer in an effort to avoid mistakes. They include absence or early bifurcation of the left main coronary artery, left main coronary stenosis, separate origin of the conus artery from the right sinus of Valsalva, eccentric atherosclerotic lesions that cannot be visualized in all projections, coronary artery spasm, failure to visualize certain segments of the coronary arteries because of superimposed branches, myocardial bridging, recanalization of coronary artery occlusions, small-vessel obstruction, angiographic artifacts related to flow and pressure changes induced by contrast injections, and anomalous origins or anatomic variations of the coronary arteries. (Anomalies and anatomic variations are discussed in Chapter 29.)

Absence or Early Bifurcation of the Main Left Coronary Artery

In approximately 2 percent of human hearts, the main left coronary artery either is absent or extends for no more than 1 to 2 mm before bifurcating into left anterior descending (LAD) and circumflex branches.[4-7] In those instances in which the main left coronary artery is completely absent, the LAD and circumflex branches arise from the left sinus of Valsalva via separate ostia that are immediately adjacent to each other. In either instance, an attempt at catheterizing the left coronary artery will result in entry of the catheter tip into one or the other of these two branches. The resulting arteriogram will therefore visualize only that branch, possibly leading the angiographer to assume erroneously that the other branch is totally occluded at its origin. This mistake may sometimes, but not always, be avoided if there is sufficient reflux of contrast material back into the sinus of Valsalva to opacify the other vessel, at least partially. If the left ventriculogram fails to demonstrate contraction abnormalities in the distribution of a vessel presumed to be occluded without collateral circulation, the possibility of nonvisualization of a separate branch should be considered.

Figure 28-1 is an example of this anatomic pattern. In a patient with angina pectoris but without a previous history of myocardial infarction, a selective left coronary arteriogram demonstrated only a left circumflex artery. Even with reflux of contrast material into the left sinus of Valsalva, there was no visualization of the LAD branch. No collateral circulation to the LAD was seen during right coronary arteriography either. Complete proximal obstruction of the LAD without any collateral circulation is almost invariably accompanied by severe contraction abnormalities of the ante-

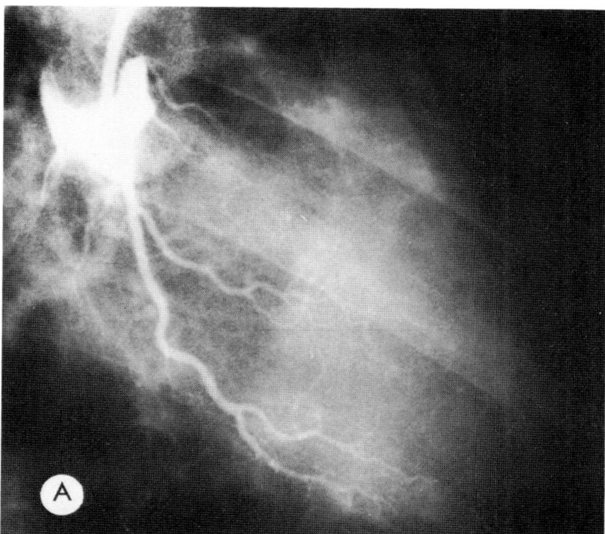

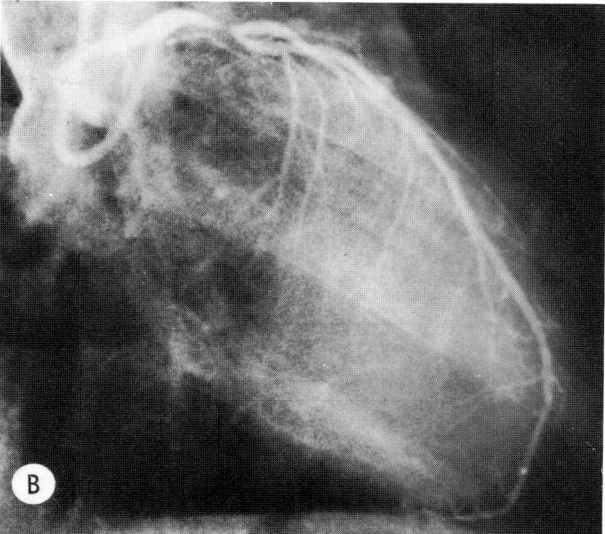

Figure 28-1. Separate origin of the LAD and circumflex branches from the left sinus of Valsalva in a patient who has no main left coronary artery. (A) Selective left circumflex arteriogram, RAO projection. A left Judkins catheter had been used and had been selectively positioned in what was initially thought to be the left coronary artery. However, the vessel proved to be only a circumflex branch. Even though there is considerable spillover of contrast into the left sinus of Valsalva, no LAD was visualized, thereby raising the possibility of total LAD occlusion. (B) Selective LAD injection subsequently performed with a left Amplatz catheter, RAO projection. The LAD arose separately from, but very close to, the origin of the left circumflex artery. A severe stenosis of the proximal segment of the vessel is seen. (From Levin DC, Baltaxe HA, Lee JG, Sos TA. Potential sources of error in coronary arteriography: I. In performance of the study. AJR 1975;124:378. Used with permission.)

rior wall of the left ventricle. In this case, the left ventriculogram was entirely normal, suggesting the possibility that a separate LAD was present and had simply not been visualized on the initial "left coronary arteriogram." After an exchange of catheters and a careful probing of the left sinus of Valsalva, the separate LAD ostium was selectively entered and a satisfactory arteriogram obtained, demonstrating a proximal LAD stenosis. This discrepancy between the ventriculographic and the coronary arteriographic findings should suggest the possibility of separate origin whenever left coronary arteriography fails to demonstrate one or the other of the two major left coronary branches. It may also be, of course, that the vessel actually is occluded. However, in this event there will generally be some degree of contraction abnormality. Finally, the nonvisualized vessel could arise from an ectopic origin, as described in Chapter 29.

When a separate origin of the LAD and circumflex arteries is suspected because of nonvisualization of one or the other vessel, it may be helpful to withdraw the catheter so it is nonselectively positioned in the left sinus of Valsalva and to perform a forceful injection of contrast medium. This may result in at least partial visualization of the second vessel.

Stenosis of the Main Left Coronary Artery

Stenosis of the main left coronary artery is the most serious of all possible coronary artery lesions. Its presence is an indication for emergency bypass surgery. It also significantly increases the risk of the angiographic procedure, because the catheter tip may cause dissection of the atherosclerotic plaque as it enters the main left coronary artery. The presence of main left coronary stenosis is frequently associated with S–T segment depression of greater than 2 mm on a stress electrocardiogram. When such a finding is noted during preoperative evaluation of the patient, subsequent left coronary arteriography should be performed with even more than the usual precautions.

Even if the arteriogram is safely obtained, it is conceivable that the lesion may not be satisfactorily detected on the study. First of all, the left main coronary artery may be inadequately visualized because of superimposition of the LAD and circumflex branches on the standard oblique projections. The left main coronary artery is best visualized on a straight anteroposterior view, or in the angulated views described in

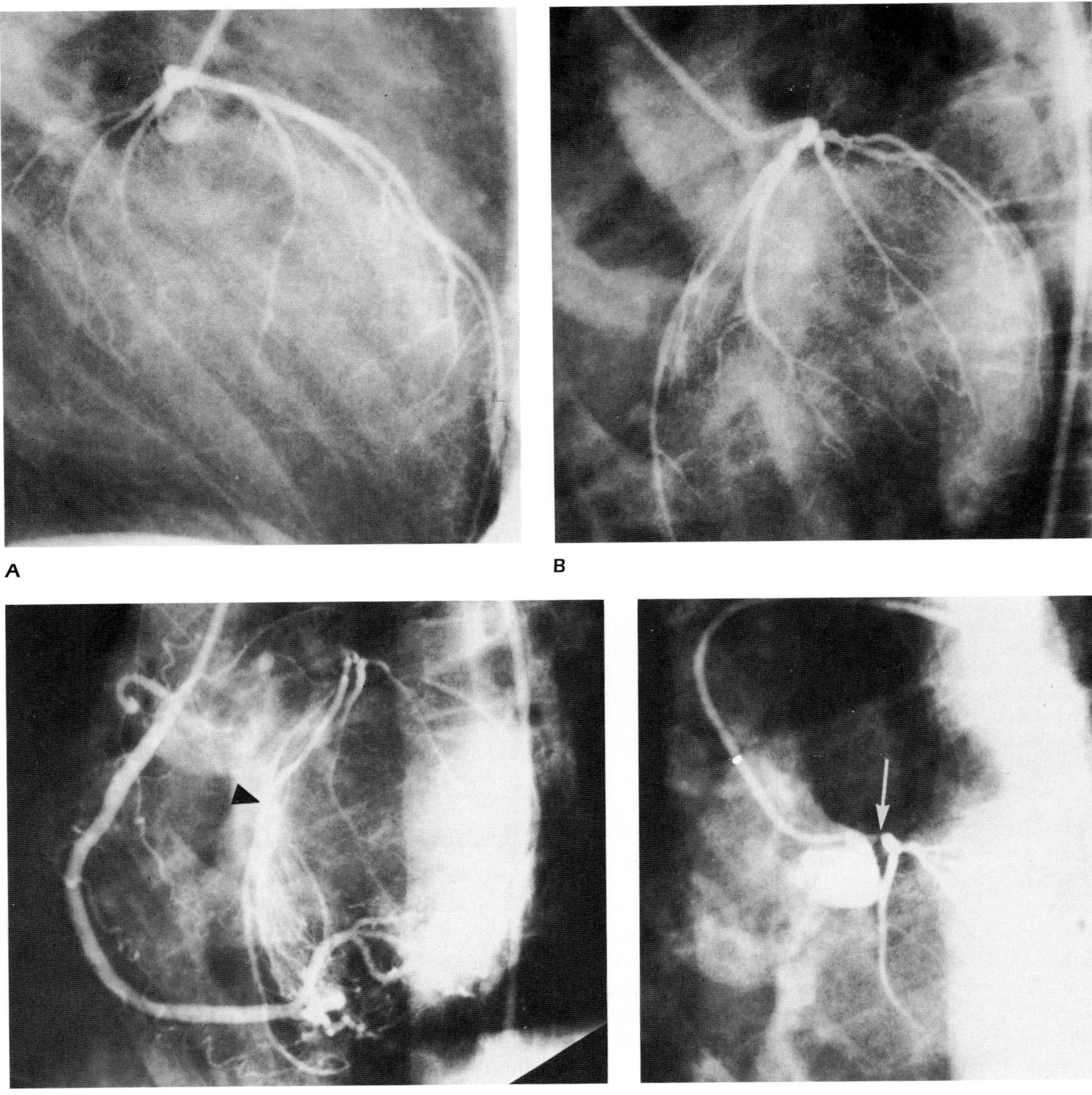

Figure 28-2. Severe stenosis of the main left coronary artery, which was not appreciated initially because the catheter tip had traversed the lesion and the contrast injection did not opacify the proximal segment of the left main coronary artery. (A and B) Initial RAO and LAO views of the left coronary arteriogram. No significant lesions of the LAD or circumflex arteries are noted. However, the main left coronary artery is not opacified and there is no reflux of contrast back through the left coronary ostium into the left sinus of Valsalva. In patients with patent left main coronary arteries, a selective left coronary arteriogram generally provides adequate visualization of this vessel by reflux of contrast material back through the left coronary ostium. (C) Right coronary arteriogram, LAO projection. There is extensive collateral circulation from the right coronary artery with retrograde filling of both the LAD (*arrowhead*) and circumflex arteries. The demonstration of this collateral circulation provides unequivocal evidence of a hemodynamically significant lesion of the left coronary system. Since both the LAD and circumflex arteries fill via collateral circulation, a left main coronary lesion would be suspected. (D) Repeat left coronary arteriogram, LAO projection. In this instance, the catheter was purposely positioned nonselectively in the left sinus of Valsalva just outside the left coronary ostium. Note that the left main coronary artery is severely stenotic (*arrow*). This lesion was not demonstrated on the initial left coronary arteriogram because the catheter tip had passed beyond it and was almost totally occluding the vessel so that contrast reflux did not occur. (From Levin DC, Baltaxe HA, Lee JG, Sos TA. Potential sources of error in coronary arteriography: I. In performance of the study. AJR 1975;124:378. Used with permission.)

Chapter 23. These views should always be obtained as a standard part of the angiographic procedure.

Second, failure to detect a left main coronary artery stenosis can also occur if the catheter tip, upon entering the left coronary ostium, traverses the stenosis so that the contrast medium subsequently injected passes entirely in the antegrade direction and never opacifies the stenotic proximal portion of the left main coronary artery. In a case of this kind (Fig. 28-2), initial catheterization of the left coronary artery resulted in what appeared to be normal left coronary arteriograms. The right coronary arteriogram obtained immediately thereafter revealed, surprisingly, extensive collateral circulation from the right coronary to the LAD and circumflex arteries. This indicated that a left main coronary stenosis was probably present, a finding that was confirmed by performance of a nonselective contrast injection into the left sinus of Valsalva just outside the left coronary ostium. In this case, selective catheterization of the left coronary artery had resulted in passage of the catheter tip through the stenotic lesion, and the subsequent antegrade flow of contrast material failed to opacify the stenotic segment.

In most cases, during selective left coronary arteriography with a forceful hand injection of contrast material, there is reflux of at least some of the contrast back through the left coronary ostium into the left sinus of Valsalva. This results in satisfactory visualization of the proximal portion of the left main coronary artery. If this does not occur, a stenotic lesion at the origin of the vessel should be suspected. Another clue to the presence of such a lesion can be obtained from the constant monitoring of catheter tip pressure. If the catheter passes through a left main coronary stenosis, a total or near-total occlusion may be produced. The pressure in the left coronary system will then drop below the aortic pressure. This decline can be detected either as a significant damping of the pressure tracing or as "ventricularization" (a drop in the diastolic pressure only, so that the pressure contour resembles that obtained in the left ventricle).

When lack of visualization of the left coronary ostium or a pressure drop occurs, left main coronary stenosis should be strongly suspected. It can be confirmed, as shown in Figure 28-2, by withdrawing the catheter so it is positioned nonselectively in the left sinus of Valsalva just outside the left coronary ostium and performing a forceful contrast injection.

Separate Origin of the Conus Artery

One of the many anatomic variations of the coronary arteries is in the origin of the conus branch. This vessel is traditionally considered the first branch of the right coronary artery. It passes anteriorly over the right ventricular infundibulum and ends by ramifying near the anterior interventricular groove. Its principal importance in human coronary artery disease is to serve as a major source of collateral circulation to the LAD when that vessel is obstructed. An example of this collateral pathway is seen in Figure 28-3A.

In actuality, the conus artery originates from the proximal right coronary artery in only about 50 percent of human hearts.[4,8] In the other 50 percent, the conus artery arises in the right sinus of Valsalva from a small separate ostium that lies very close to the right coronary ostium. In these cases, a selective right coronary arteriogram may fail to opacify the conus artery unless there is enough reflux of contrast material into the right sinus of Valsalva to fill the small separate conus ostium satisfactorily. A study of a large series of adult coronary arteriograms indicated that in 20 percent of cases the conus artery was not opacified satisfactorily during the procedure.[9] Presumably, most or all of the patients in whom the conus artery is not satisfactorily opacified come from the group having a separate conus origin.

In patients with LAD obstruction whose conus artery is not satisfactorily opacified during right coronary arteriography, an important source of collateral circulation to the LAD may be missed. This is a matter of some concern, because the decision to undertake bypass surgery is influenced by the degree to which the distal segment of an obstructed artery fills via collateral circulation. It has been shown that the chances of successful bypass are considerably enhanced if the distal segment of the obstructed artery is well filled by angiographically visible collaterals.[10–12]

Figure 28-3B is a typical example of conus artery anatomy in which this vessel is well opacified during right coronary arteriography, even though the conus artery appears to have a separate origin immediately adjacent to that of the right coronary artery itself. On the other hand, Figure 28-3C is an example of a case in which selective right coronary arteriography failed to visualize a conus artery at all. The angiographer interpreting coronary angiograms should always carefully note whether the conus artery is opacified in patients who have LAD obstruction. If it is not, the angiographer should recognize that the study may be incomplete in this respect—that is, that he or she may have failed to demonstrate a significant source of collateral circulation to the LAD. If failure to visualize the conus artery is recognized during the course of the angiographic procedure, the catheter tip may be partially withdrawn from the right coronary ostium so that nonselective opacification of the right sinus of

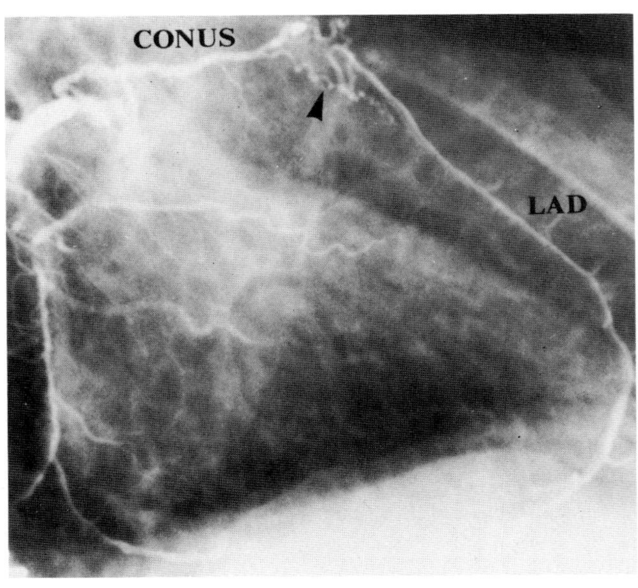

A

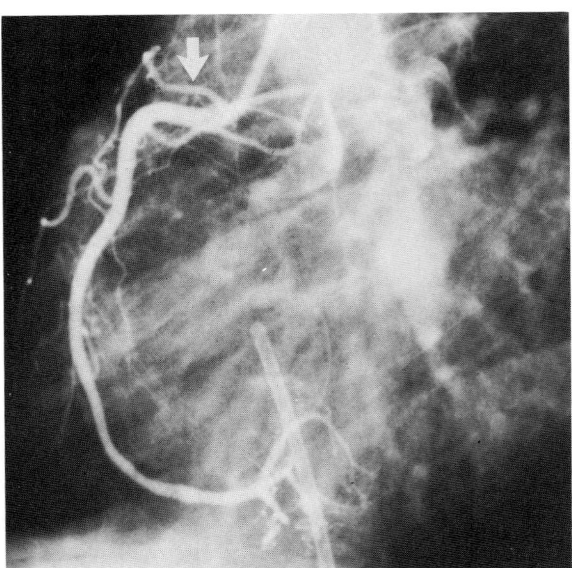

B

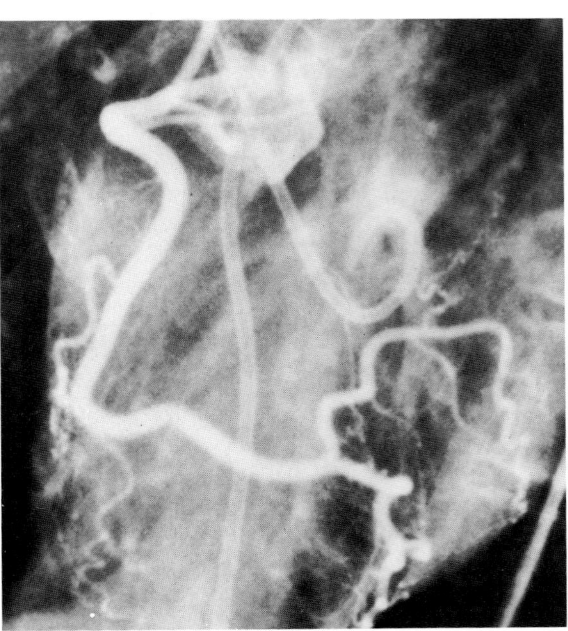

C

Figure 28-3. Right coronary arteriograms in three patients demonstrating different aspects of the conus artery anatomy. (A) Right coronary arteriogram, RAO projection, in a patient with total obstructions of both the LAD and right coronary arteries. The distal LAD is filled via collateral circulation (*arrowhead*) emanating from the conus branch of the right coronary artery. (B) Right coronary arteriogram, LAO projection. The conus artery (*arrow*) is well opacified, even though it appears to have a separate origin in the right sinus of Valsalva immediately adjacent to the right coronary ostium. (C) Right coronary arteriogram, LAO projection. The conus artery is not visualized, probably because of a separate origin. (A, from Levin D, Kauff M, Baltaxe HA. Coronary collateral circulation. AJR 1973;119:463. Used with permission.)

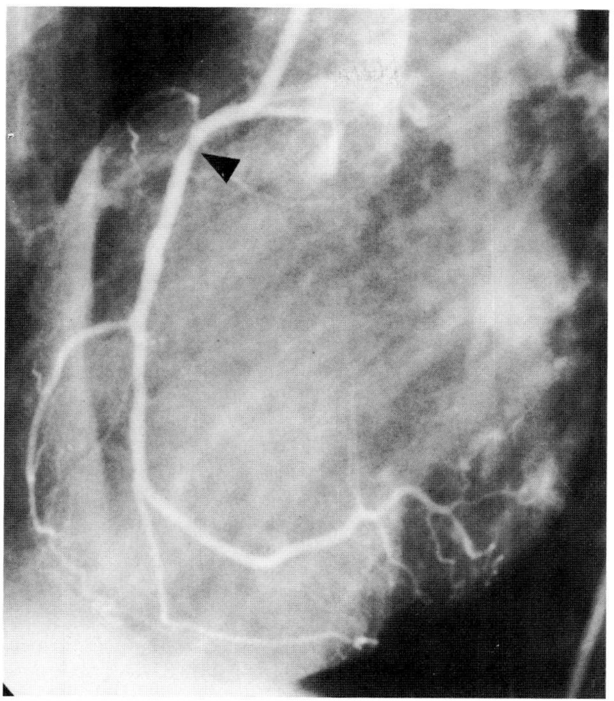

A

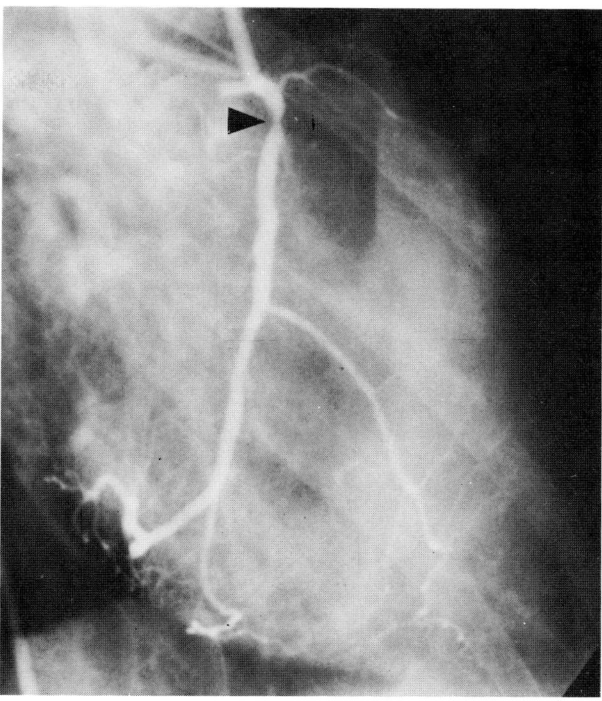

B

Figure 28-4. Eccentric stenosis of the proximal right coronary artery that is well seen in the RAO projection but is not appreciated in the LAO projection. (A) The right coronary arteriogram in the LAO projection shows diffuse atherosclerotic plaque formation. The lesion in the proximal right coronary artery (*arrowhead*) does not appear to be significant in this projection. (B) The right coronary arteriogram in the RAO projection shows that the lesion (*arrowhead*) is considerably more significant than one might have suspected merely by viewing the LAO projection. This finding is due to the eccentricity that characterizes many coronary stenoses. (From Levin DC, Baltaxe HA, Lee JG, Sos TA. Potential sources of error in coronary arteriography: I. In performance of the study. AJR 1975;124:378. Used with permission.)

Valsalva can be obtained. Contrast material may then enter the separate conus ostium, resulting in satisfactory conus artery visualization.

Eccentric Stenoses

Atherosclerotic narrowings of the coronary arteries are often eccentric or slitlike. If the x-ray beam happens to pass through such a lesion perpendicular to the long axis of the lumen, the vessel may appear to be of relatively normal caliber. However, if the x-ray beam passes parallel to the long axis of the lesion, the narrowing will be apparent. Figure 28-4 shows a stenosis of the proximal right coronary artery that appears to be of only very mild degree in the left anterior oblique (LAO) view, whereas it is seen to be much more severe in the right anterior oblique (RAO) projection. No coronary artery lesion can be properly evaluated angiographically by visualizing it in only a single projection. At least two projections 90 degrees apart are required.

Coronary Artery Spasm

Spasm within the major epicardial coronary arteries can be a major problem for the angiographer and can have important clinical implications. There are two types of spasm: catheter-induced spasm occurring during angiography and spontaneous spasm.

For reasons that are not entirely clear, catheter-induced spasm is much more common in the right coronary artery than in the left coronary artery. Whenever a selective right coronary arteriogram demonstrates a proximal narrowing of the right coronary artery near the tip of the catheter, the possibility of catheter-induced spasm must be considered. If this possibility is raised, a repeat arteriogram should be obtained after the administration of sublingual nitroglycerin. This drug reduces vasomotor tone in large coronary arteries[13,14] and should be given prophylactically in most patients before catheterizing the coronary arteries to prevent spasm from occurring. However, the duration of

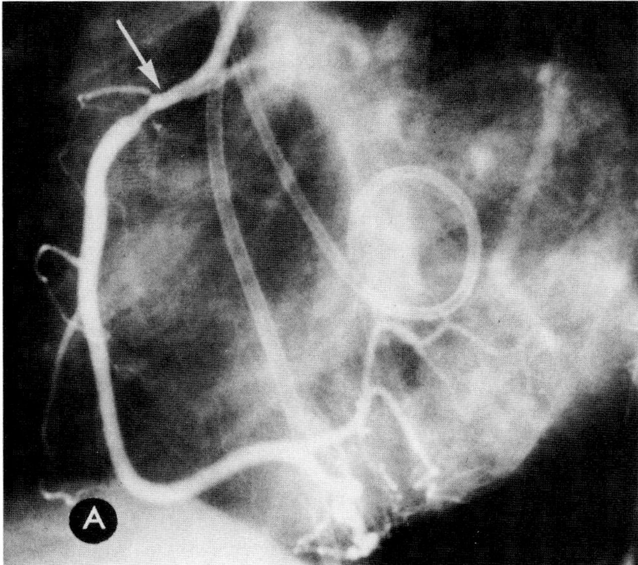

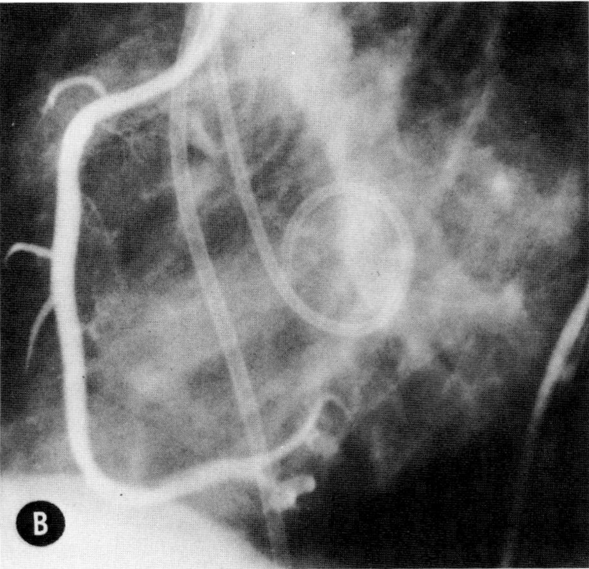

Figure 28-5. Catheter-induced spasm of the proximal right coronary artery. (A) Right coronary arteriogram, LAO projection, prior to administration of sublingual nitroglycerin. Note the irregular narrowing (*arrow*) of the proximal portion of the right coronary artery. (B) Repeat right coronary arteriogram several minutes after administration of sublingual nitroglycerin. The catheter-induced spasm has disappeared. (From Levin DC, Baltaxe HA, Lee JG, Sos TA. Potential sources of error in coronary arteriography: I. In performance of the study. AJR 1975;124:378. Used with permission.)

action of sublingual nitroglycerin is relatively short (20–30 minutes). Thus, if the drug was given some time before angiography was performed, its effect might have worn off and a repeat dose would have to be administered when proximal right coronary artery narrowing is seen.

Figure 28-5 shows the catheter-induced spasm of the right coronary artery. Figure 28-5A is the initial selective right coronary arteriogram in the LAO projection. A significant narrowing of the proximal right coronary artery is seen. Figure 28-5B shows a repeat right coronary arteriogram obtained 10 minutes later after the administration of sublingual nitroglycerin. The vessel is now seen to be entirely normal.

Catheter-induced spasm of the right coronary artery rarely causes pain, but it obviously can result in misinterpretation of the arteriogram if repeat studies are not obtained after the administration of nitroglycerin. The rarity of catheter-induced spasm of the left coronary artery means that if a narrowing of the left main coronary artery is seen at angiography, such a narrowing is much more likely to be of organic than of functional origin.

An even larger problem is that of spontaneous coronary artery spasm. This entity was first recognized by Prinzmetal et al. in 1959.[15] They and numerous subsequent authors described an unusual form of angina in which the onset of chest pain was not provoked by the usual factors, such as exercise, emotional upset, cold, or ingestion of a meal. Variant angina, sometimes referred to as *Prinzmetal angina,* generally commences at rest without any known provoking factor. The pain may be cyclic in nature, tending to occur at the same time each day. In addition to this unusual pain pattern, the electrocardiographic (ECG) changes are unusual. The patients exhibit transient S–T segment elevation, a finding that is ordinarily associated with myocardial injury and acute myocardial infarction. As opposed to true myocardial infarction, however, this S–T segment elevation rapidly reverts to normal when the pain disappears spontaneously or is aborted by the administration of nitroglycerin.[15,16] Although Prinzmetal et al. correctly postulated that variant angina was related to transient coronary artery spasm, this was not angiographically demonstrated until the early 1970s.[17–19] It soon became apparent that, in most patients with clinical manifestations of Prinzmetal angina, spasm was superimposed on an area of significant stenosis, resulting in transient complete occlusion. However, in approximately one-fourth of patients with this syndrome, the spasm was noted to occur in areas of the coronary arteries that were entirely normal organically.[20]

It is of course not always possible or convenient to

perform coronary arteriography at the exact time a patient is experiencing an episode of chest pain. Thus the documentation of spasm as a cause of chest pain might prove difficult to achieve in many cases. Intravenous ergonovine maleate has been used to provoke spasm in patients clinically suspected of having Prinzmetal angina.[21–24] After initial coronary arteriograms have been obtained in such cases, intravenous ergonovine is administered in increasingly large boluses until the patient reports the occurrence of chest pain or the ECG demonstrates S–T segment elevation. At this point, repeat arteriography of either the right or left coronary artery is quickly performed, depending on the location of the ECG changes. It has been found that the vast majority of patients with Prinzmetal angina will develop angiographically demonstrable spasm in response to the administration of ergonovine.[21–24] Once spasm has been demonstrated, nitroglycerin should be administered quickly to abort the episode. If symptoms and ECG changes persist after the administration of sublingual nitroglycerin, the drug should be given intravenously or even by direct injection into the coronary artery. Because of risks associated with this test, many laboratories have given it up. Although ergonovine almost invariably produces spasm in patients with Prinzmetal angina (those with both angiographically normal and organically diseased coronary arteries), it rarely provokes spasm in patients with truly normal coronary arteries.

Evidence has come to light suggesting that, in addition to Prinzmetal angina, spasm may be implicated in other, more common manifestations of coronary artery disease. Maseri et al.[25] have proposed that spasm may be a cause of unstable or preinfarction angina. The same group, as well as Oliva and Breckinridge,[26] have evidence suggesting that spasm also plays a major role in acute myocardial infarction. Rothman et al.[27] present the idea that spasm may be the cause of symptoms in a significant proportion of the puzzling group of patients with angina and normal coronary arteriograms.

Thus, although the original concept of human coronary artery disease was that fixed organic obstruction produced a deficit in blood flow and led to the clinical signs and symptoms, it has become increasingly plain that spasm plays an important role in various forms of myocardial ischemia and can occur both in diseased and in organically normal coronary arteries. It can produce Prinzmetal angina, unstable or preinfarction angina, and acute myocardial infarction, and it may ultimately prove to be associated with some cases of typical and atypical angina as well. Of the many unanswered questions about spasm, not the least concerns the mechanism by which it occurs. Obviously, the angiographer must realize that a coronary artery that appears normal arteriographically may actually be causing major manifestations of coronary artery disease if it develops spontaneous spasm. Furthermore, localized lesions that seem to be of mild or moderate degree can become severe or totally obstructing with the superimposition of spasm. Finally, a lesion seen on the arteriogram may itself represent spasm, rather than a fixed atherosclerotic stenosis. Whenever a lesion seen on the arteriogram is suspected of being partially or entirely due to spasm, a repeat arteriogram should be obtained after the administration of nitroglycerin.

The inability to predict precisely when spasm is or is not present represents one of the major pitfalls of coronary arteriography.

Failure to Detect Obstructions due to Superimposition of Other Branches

Occlusions of the major coronary arteries tend to occur at branch points. If a vessel becomes occluded at its origin and there are other coronary artery branches overlying it in the various projections, the obstruction might go undetected. This can be a problem in any branch but is of particular concern in patients with LAD obstructions. The LAD generally has one or more large diagonal branches supplying the anterolateral aspect of the left ventricle and sometimes closely paralleling the course of the LAD. The branches are highly variable in number, site of origin, and distribution. It may be difficult to differentiate diagonal branches from the LAD in all projections. Figure 28-6 shows a large diagonal branch of the LAD. The diagonal branch is approximately the same size as the LAD and occupies the same general area in both LAO and RAO projections. If the LAD were to become occluded immediately beyond the origin of the diagonal branch, the obstruction could be missed because the diagonal branch could be mistaken for the LAD. If no collateral circulation to the distal LAD were present, the obstruction might not be detected. The LAD has certain anatomic characteristics that usually, but not invariably, enable the angiographer to identify it. First, the LAD usually passes all the way around the cardiac apex and terminates along the diaphragmatic surface of the cardiac apex, whereas the diagonal branches usually do not reach the diaphragmatic surface of the heart. Second, the LAD always gives off small septal perforating branches that pass vertically down in the interventricular septum, whereas diagonal branches generally do not give off these septal perforating arteries.

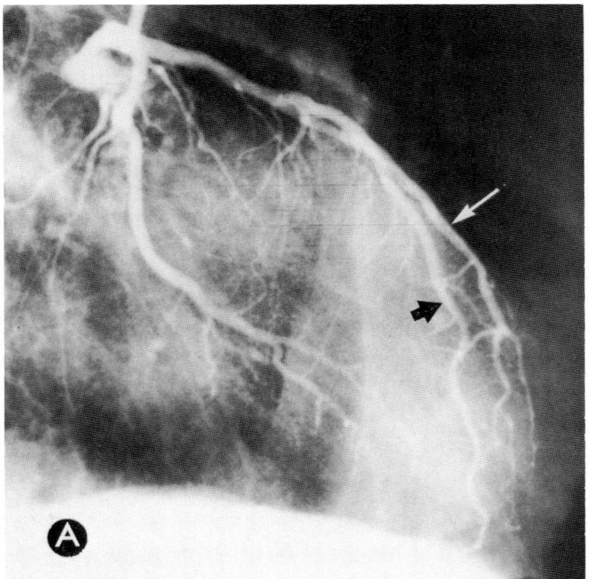

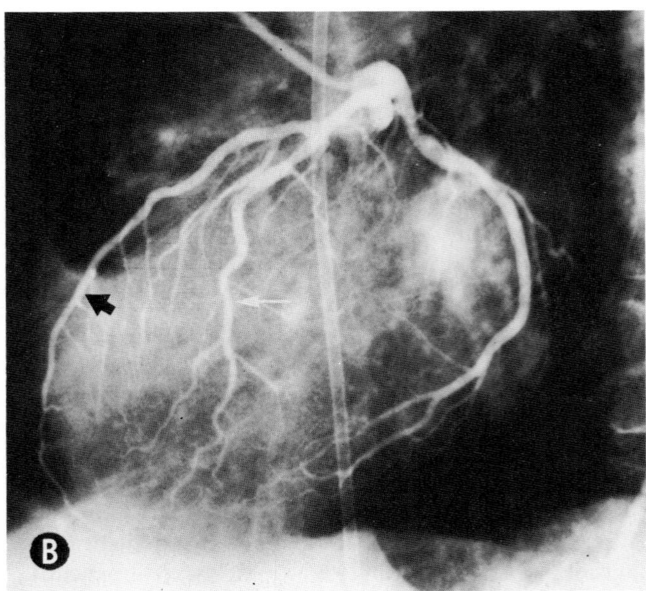

Figure 28-6. Left coronary arteriogram in a patient with a single large diagonal branch of the LAD. (A) RAO projection. (B) LAO projection. The *black arrows* point to the LAD, the *white arrows* to the large diagonal branch. Note that the diagonal branch has a course quite similar to that of the LAD in both projections. However, the LAD gives rise to a number of septal branches and also passes around the cardiac apex. These two characteristics generally allow the angiographer to differentiate the LAD from its diagonal branches. (From Levin D, Baltaxe HA, Sos TA. Potential sources of error in coronary arteriography: II. In interpretation of the study. AJR 1975;124:386. Used with permission.)

Another branch that can be mistaken for the LAD is the first septal perforator. When the LAD becomes occluded beyond the origin of the first septal perforator, the latter vessel often undergoes marked enlargement in an attempt to supply collateral circulation through connections in the interventricular septum to the more distal septal branches. The first septal branch may actually become as large as the LAD. In the LAO projection, the large first septal branch is often superimposed directly upon the LAD, and because of this relationship an LAD obstruction can be obscured. The problem is usually recognizable in the RAO projection, although sometimes the first septal branch pursues a course similar to that of the LAD in this view also. Figure 28-7 reveals obstruction of the LAD immediately beyond the origin of the first septal perforator. The septal branch has undergone marked enlargement in an attempt to supply collateral circulation and is the same size as one would expect the LAD to be. In the LAO projection, it is difficult to ascertain that the LAD is occluded because the large first septal branch overlies it and takes the same course it does. In the RAO projection, the first septal branch also takes a course somewhat similar to that of the LAD, but an experienced angiographer should be able to recognize that this branch lies within the septum, rather than on the epicardial surface of the anterior interventricular groove.

The angiographer must always keep in mind these potential difficulties in identifying LAD obstructions. Particular attention should be paid to the late phase of the left coronary cineangiograms, in which late filling of the distal segment of an obstructed LAD might provide the best clue to obstruction of this vessel.

Stenoses (rather than total occlusions) of major coronary arteries may also go undetected because of superimposition of overlying branches on the standard oblique projections. This problem can be most effectively resolved with the use of angulation of the x-ray beam in both cranial and caudal directions during coronary arteriography in the LAO or RAO projections. The addition of cranial or caudal angulation to the more commonly used oblique projections frequently alleviates superimposition problems by shifting branches away from the parent vessels. The technique and angiographic anatomy of the cranial or caudal angulation views are discussed in more detail in Chapter 23.

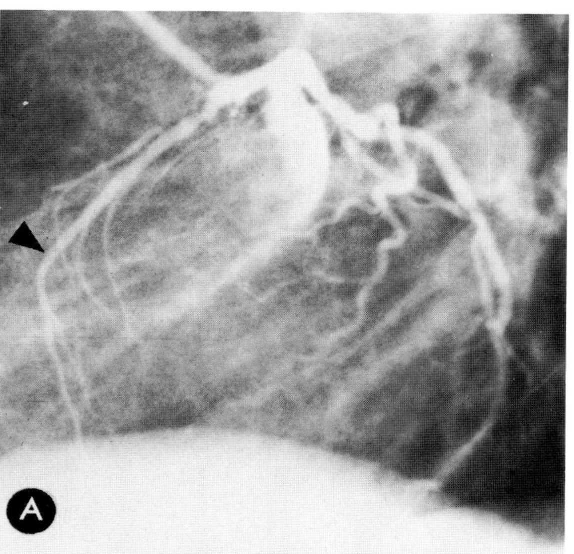

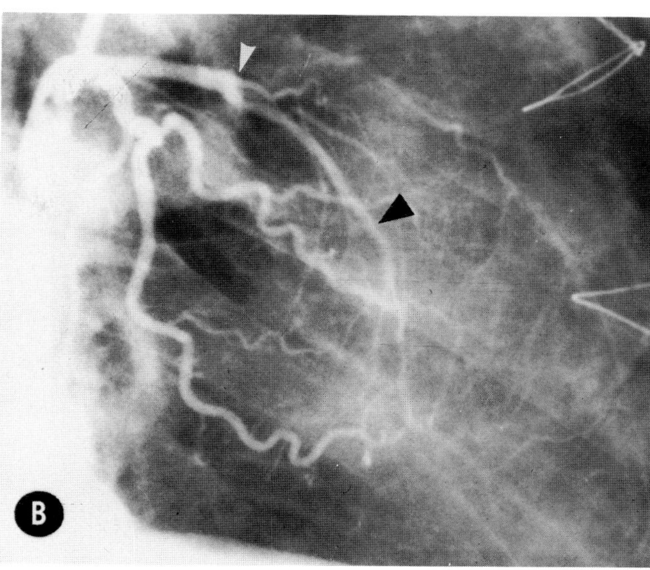

Figure 28-7. Left coronary arteriogram in a patient with total LAD occlusion. (A) LAO projection. The total LAD occlusion cannot be appreciated because of marked compensatory enlargement of the first septal branch (*arrowhead*). In the LAO projection, the first septal branch is often superimposed directly upon the course of the LAD. (B) RAO projection. The *white arrowhead* indicates the point of total LAD obstruction. The *black arrowhead* points to the enlarged first septal branch. In this projection, the first septal branch runs parallel to the LAD but is within the interventricular septum and posterior to the normal epicardial position of the LAD. (From Levin D, Baltaxe HA, Sos TA. Potential sources of error in coronary arteriography: II. In interpretation of the study. AJR 1975;124:386. Used with permission.)

Myocardial Bridging

The major coronary arteries pass along the epicardial surface of the heart. On occasion, however, short segments of vessels, particularly the LAD, pass down into the myocardium. In this event, systolic contraction of the overlying or bridging myocardial fibers can narrow the involved segment of the coronary artery on cineangiography. The vessel will appear narrowed during systole but will return to a normal or nearly normal caliber during diastole. Edwards et al.[28] noted myocardial bridging in 5.4 percent of human hearts, an incidence that approximately matches the author's own experience.

Figure 28-8 shows myocardial bridging of the LAD. The angiographic detection of a myocardial bridge in a vessel other than the LAD is rare.

Although most cases of myocardial bridging are not thought to be clinically or hemodynamically significant, in some reported cases there was strong clinical evidence that the myocardial bridge was severe enough to produce ischemia.[29–32] It would seem that if a bridge is very long or very severe and is present in a patient with no other lesions to explain ischemic symptoms, the bridge should be strongly considered a possible etiologic factor. Regardless of whether the bridge is producing symptoms, the angiographer should recognize that coronary artery narrowings (particularly of the LAD) that occur during systole and disappear during diastole are caused by contraction of overlying myocardial fibers rather than by atherosclerotic stenoses.

Recanalization of Occluding Thrombi

The angiographer visualizing a localized subtotal narrowing of a coronary artery generally terms it a *stenosis,* thereby implying that it represents an atherosclerotic lesion that has not yet occluded the lumen. In actual fact, a significant number of such lesions may be previously occluding thrombi that have gone on to recanalize. Previous pathologic studies have shown that more than one-third of totally occluded coronary arteries undergo recanalization.[33,34] The angiographic appearance of a recanalized segment of a coronary artery may be indistinguishable from that of a preocclusive atherosclerotic stenosis (Fig. 28-9). Sometimes, however, the recanalization appears angiographically as an irregular, serpiginous channel traversing the obstructed segment. Although the latter cases are relatively char-

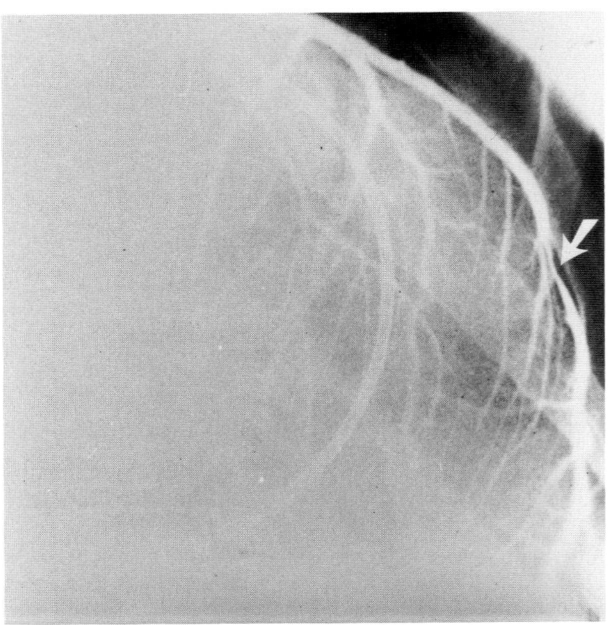

A

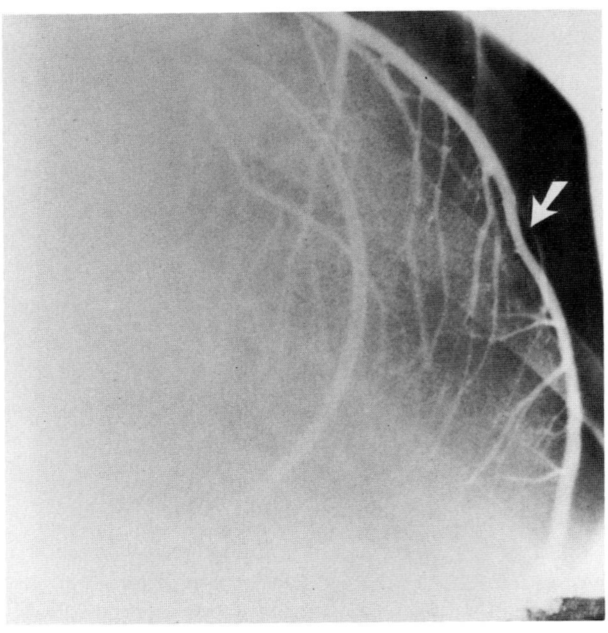

B

Figure 28-8. Myocardial bridging of the LAD seen in RAO projections of the left coronary arteriogram. (A) During systole, the bridged segment (*arrow*) appears extremely narrowed. (B) During diastole, the same segment reverts to nearly normal caliber.

Figure 28-9. Right coronary arteriogram, LAO projection. An apparent stenosis of a long segment of the midportion of the vessel is seen (*arrow*). The patient died a week later, and at autopsy this segment was found to be a recanalized old thrombus. This lesion would be quite difficult to differentiate angiographically from an atherosclerotic plaque that had not yet totally occluded the artery.

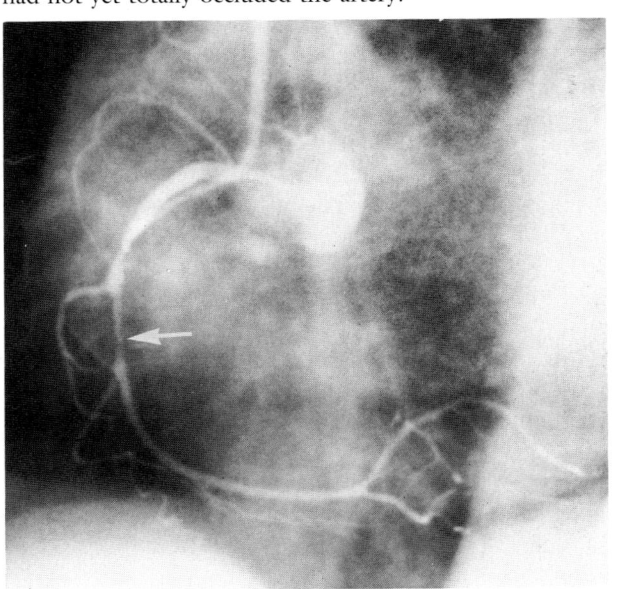

acteristic, the angiographer must bear in mind that he or she is not always able to differentiate preocclusive stenosis from postocclusive recanalization. It has been suggested[35] that recanalized lesions are somewhat more dangerous than stenoses in that they are prone to undergo complete occlusion due to intramural hemorrhage or thrombosis.

Obstructive Disease of Small Coronary Artery Branches

Small branches of the coronary arteries may be variable in origin and distribution. Complete occlusion of such a branch may therefore be difficult to detect. Detection may depend on visualization of a small stump at the origin of a branch or late opacification of the distal segment via collateral circulation. The angiographer should always carefully scrutinize the late phase of the angiogram, which may provide the only demonstration of small-vessel reconstitution. If the anatomic field incorporated on the cine frame is very small, because of excessive overframing or the use of a small image intensifier mode, it may be necessary during the angiographic filming sequence to pan rapidly from one portion of the heart to another. The result could be failure to visualize a late-filling distal segment lying outside the radiographic field. In our laboratory, the 6-inch mode of the image intensifier is used for coronary cineangiography; this allows for sufficient magnification with relatively little requirement for panning and therefore can be expected to include most of the important coronary vessels during all phases of the contrast injection.

The clinical significance of small-vessel occlusion is not yet entirely clear. There is a well-known group of patients who have clinical symptoms suggestive of coronary artery disease but who prove at angiography to have normal coronary arteries. The possibility has been raised by some authors that this discrepancy could be explained by small-vessel disease that cannot be appreciated angiographically. In an era of constantly improving x-ray technology leading to improved resolution capability, failure to detect small-vessel occlusions should become a relatively insignificant problem as long as an adequately sized field is visualized on the cineangiogram.

Angiographic Artifacts Related to Flow and Pressure Changes Induced by Contrast Injections

For many years, flow patterns seen on angiographic studies were thought to be accurate representations of the patient's native circulatory dynamics. It was assumed that, because the caliber of a catheter tip selectively positioned in the origin of a major artery was considerably smaller than the caliber of the artery, the force of the contrast injection would be instantaneously dissipated out into the aorta and that consequently the injection would not alter flow and pressure in the catheterized artery. However, experimental and clinical studies have shown that this is not the case.[36,37] In actuality, selective injection of contrast or any other fluid into a major artery through a standard, nonoccluding catheter will significantly raise both flow and pressure in that artery for the duration of the injection.

Figure 28-10. Right coronary arteriogram in a patient with total obstruction of the LAD and right coronary arteries. (A) The initial right coronary arteriogram, LAO projection, demonstrates minimal filling of the distal segment of the LAD (*arrow*) via collateral circulation. (B) The RAO projection of the right coronary arteriogram, several minutes later, demonstrates much more extensive filling of the distal LAD (*straight arrow*) via collateral circulation from the conus branch (*curved arrow*) of the right coronary artery. This occurred because during repositioning of the patient the catheter tip inadvertently slipped superselectively into the conus branch. The contrast injection then considerably increased flow and pressure in the conus branch, resulting in greater filling of the distal segment of the LAD.

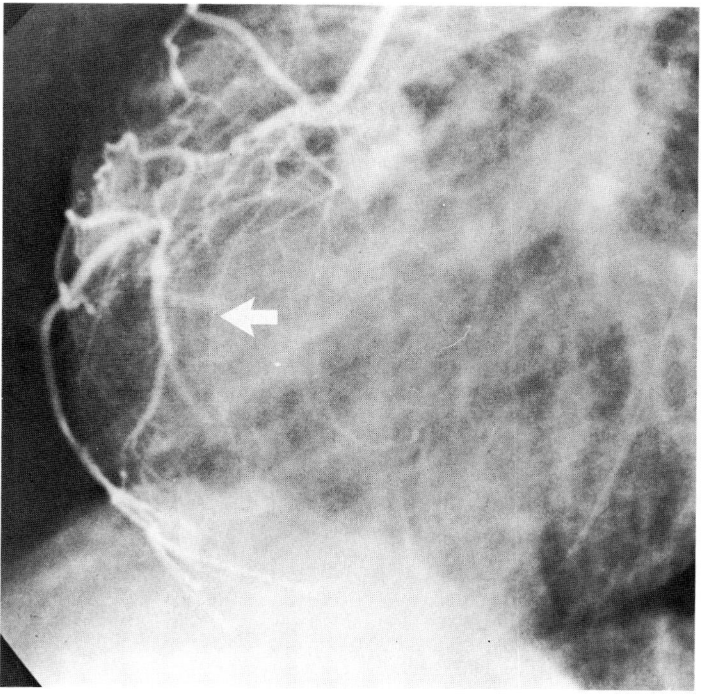

A

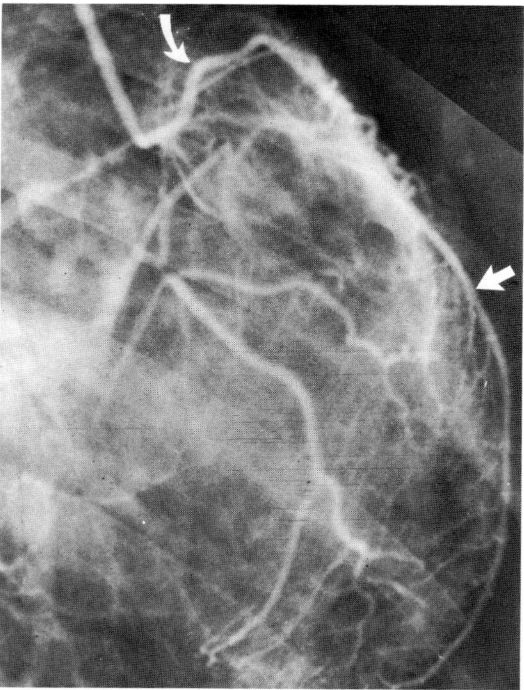

B

During angiographic studies, the result will be the artifactual forcing of additional contrast through the arterial tree and a tendency to accentuate filling of branch vessels and also of collateral circulation. The degree to which this artifactual accentuation occurs is a function both of the force of the injection and of the relative sizes of the catheter tip and the artery into which it has been inserted. The smaller the size of the artery relative to the size of the catheter tip, the greater the expected rise in flow and pressure resulting from the contrast injection. In the performance of coronary arteriography, these factors are not predictable or reproducible from one case to another or even from one injection to another in the same patient. The angiographer must bear in mind that the speed of flow seen on the arteriogram, the degree of opacification of distal branches, and the degree of opacification of collaterals and distal segments of obstructed vessels to a great extent depend on the transient increase in flow and pressure that occurs during selective injection.

An example of this type of artifact is provided in Figure 28-10. The patient had obstruction of both the right coronary and LAD. The initial right coronary arteriogram in the LAO projection demonstrated minimal filling of the distal segment of the LAD through conus-LAD collaterals. The patient was then rotated into the RAO position, and during this change in position the catheter tip inadvertently slipped superselectively into the origin of the conus branch. The catheter did not occlude the origin of the conus branch, because there was no detectable drop in monitored catheter tip pressure. However, the resulting angiogram showed a marked increase in the degree of collateral circulation from the conus branch to the LAD and much more prominent opacification of the distal LAD than had been noted on the previous LAO projection. The striking discrepancy in the filling of the distal LAD on the two injections is a dramatic example of how collateral circulation and opacification of distal segments of obstructed coronary arteries can vary with angiographic technique, catheter position, and so forth. The possibility of artifacts of this type must be taken into account in any attempt to evaluate and quantify collateral filling and flow velocity.

Anomalous Origins or Anatomic Variations of the Coronary Arteries

This topic is discussed in detail in Chapter 29. It is mentioned here only for the sake of completeness in a discussion of pitfalls of coronary arteriography. When a coronary artery does not originate from the aorta in the usual position, it may be difficult or impossible to catheterize it selectively. Anomalous origins are rare but, when present, may prove a significant technical challenge to the angiographer. Anatomic variations of the branches are generally apparent if the parent vessel can be selectively catheterized, but here too the angiographer must recognize the variant distribution patterns and must take particular care to call their presence to the attention of the surgeons.

References

1. Gray CR II, Hoffman HA, Hammond WS, Miller KL, Oseasohn RO. Correlation of arteriographic and pathologic findings in the coronary arteries in man. Circulation 1962;26:494.
2. Eusterman JH, Achor RWP, Kincaid OW, Brown AL Jr. Atherosclerotic disease of the coronary arteries: pathologic radiologic correlative study. Circulation 1962;26:1288.
3. Vlodaver Z, Frech R, Van Tassel RA, Edwards JE. Correlation of antemortem coronary arteriogram and postmortem specimen. Circulation 1973;47:162.
4. James TN. Anatomy of the coronary arteries. New York: Hoeber Medical Division, Harper & Row, 1961.
5. Vlodaver Z, Neufeld HN, Edwards JE. Pathology of coronary disease. Semin Roentgenol 1972;7:376.
6. Levin DC, Baltaxe HA, Lee JG, Sos TA. Potential sources of error in coronary arteriography: I. In performance of the study. AJR 1975;124:378.
7. Hermiller JB, et al. Unrecognized left main coronary artery disease in patients undergoing interventional procedures. Am J Cardiol 1993;71(2):173–176.
8. Schlesinger MJ, Zoll PM, Wessler S. The conus artery: a third coronary artery. Am Heart J 1949;38:823.
9. Levin DC, Beckmann CF, Garnic JD, Carey P, Bettmann MA. Frequency and clinical significance of failure to visualize the conus artery during coronary arteriography. Circulation 1981; 63:833.
10. Lespérance J, Bourassa MG, Biron P, Campeau L, Saltiel J. Aorta to coronary artery saphenous vein grafts: preoperative angiographic criteria for successful surgery. Am J Cardiol 1972; 30:459.
11. Levin DC, Carlson RG, Baltaxe HA. Angiographic determination of operability in candidates for aorto-coronary bypass. AJR 1972;116:66.
12. Rösch J, Dotter CT, Antonovic R, Bonchek L, Starr A. Angiographic appraisal of distal vessel suitability for aortocoronary bypass surgery. Circulation 1973;48:202.
13. Likoff W, Kasparian H, Lehman JS, Segal BL. Evaluation of "coronary vasodilators" by coronary arteriography. Am J Cardiol 1964;13:7.
14. Winburg MM, Howe BB, Hefner MA. Effect of nitrates and other coronary vasodilators on large and small coronary vessels: an hypothesis for the mechanism of action of nitrates. J Pharmacol Exp Ther 1969;168:70.
15. Prinzmetal M, Kennamer R, Merliss R, Wada T, Bor N. Angina pectoris: I. Variant form of angina pectoris. Am J Med 1959; 27:375.
16. MacAlpin RN, Kattus AA, Alvaro AB. Angina pectoris at rest with preservation of exercise capacity: Prinzmetal's variant angina. Circulation 1973;47:946.
17. Dhurandhar RW, Watt DL, Silver MD, Trimble AS, Adelman AG. Prinzmetal's variant form of angina with arteriographic evidence of coronary arterial spasm. Am J Cardiol 1972;30:902.
18. Cheng TO, Bashour T, Kelser GA, Weiss L, Bacos J. Variant angina of Prinzmetal with normal coronary arteriogram: variant of the variant. Circulation 1973;47:476.

19. Oliva PB, Potts DE, Pluss RG. Coronary arterial spasm in Prinzmetal angina: documentation by coronary arteriography. N Engl J Med 1973;288:745.
20. Levin DC, Wolk M, Summers DN. Prinzmetal's variant angina pectoris. AJR 1974;122:812.
21. Schroeder JS, Bolen JL, Quint RA, Clark DA, Hayden WG, Higgins CB, Wexler L. Provocation of coronary spasm with ergonovine maleate: new test with results in 57 patients undergoing coronary arteriography. Am J Cardiol 1977;40:487.
22. Curry RC Jr, Pepine CJ, Varnell JH, Sabom MB, Conti CR. Clinical usefulness and safety of the ergonovine test in patients with chest pain. Am J Cardiol 1978;41:369.
23. Heupler FA Jr, Proudfit WL, Razavi M, Shirey EK, Greenstreet R, Sheldon WC. Ergonovine maleate provocative test for coronary arterial spasm. Am J Cardiol 1978;41:631.
24. Cipriano PR, Guthaner DF, Orlick AE, Ricci DR, Wexler L, Silverman JF. The effects of ergonovine maleate on coronary arterial size. Circulation 1979;59:82.
25. Maseri A, et al. Coronary vasospasm as a possible cause of myocardial infarction: a conclusion derived from the study of "preinfarction" angina. N Engl J Med 1978;299:1271.
26. Oliva PB, Breckinridge JC. Arteriographic evidence of coronary arterial spasm in acute myocardial infarction. Circulation 1977; 56:366.
27. Rothman M, Bergman G, Atkinson L, Jewett D. The value and limitations of ergometrine in predicting vasospastic angina. Circulation 1978;57(Suppl II):180.
28. Edwards JC, Burnsides C, Swarm RL, Lansing AI. Arteriosclerosis in intramural and extramural portions of coronary arteries in the human heart. Circulation 1956;13:235.
29. Noble J, Bourassa MG, Petitclerc R, Dyrda I. Myocardial bridging and milking effect of the left anterior descending coronary artery: normal variant or obstruction? Am J Cardiol 1976; 37:993.
30. Faruqui AMA, Maloy WC, Felner JM, Schlant RC, Logan WD, Symbas P. Symptomatic myocardial bridging of coronary artery. Am J Cardiol 1978;41:1305.
31. Bestetti RB, Costa RS, Kazava DK, Oliveira JS. Can isolated myocardial bridging of the left anterior descending coronary artery be associated with sudden death during exercise? Acta Cardiol 1991;46(1):27–30.
32. Parashara DK, Ledley GS, Kotler MN, Yazdanfar S. The combined presence of myocardial bridging and fixed coronary artery stenosis. Am Heart J 1993;125(4):1170–1172.
33. Snow PJD, Jones AM, Daber KS. Coronary disease: a pathological study. Br Heart J 1955;17:503.
34. Friedman M. The coronary canalized thrombus: provenance, structure, function and relationship to death due to coronary artery disease. Br J Exp Pathol 1967;48:556.
35. Friedman M. Pathogenesis of coronary plaques, thromboses and hemorrhage: an evaluation review. Circulation 1975; 51,52(Suppl III):34.
36. Levin DC, Phillips DA, Lee-Son S, Maroko PR. Hemodynamic changes distal to selective arterial injection. Invest Radiol 1977; 12:116.
37. Levin DC. Augmented arterial flow and pressure resulting from selective injections through catheters: clinical implications. Radiology 1978;127:103.

29

Anomalies and Anatomic Variations of the Coronary Arteries

DAVID C. LEVIN

This chapter deals with three different categories of abnormal or unusual coronary anatomy. The first includes those coronary artery anomalies that alter myocardial perfusion. Because of the alteration in perfusion, clinical symptoms usually develop. The four principal anomalies in this category are (1) coronary artery fistulas, (2) anomalous origin of the left coronary artery from the pulmonary artery, (3) congenital stenosis or atresia of the coronary arteries, and (4) origin of the left coronary artery from the right sinus of Valsalva with subsequent passage of the vessel between the aorta and the right ventricular infundibulum.

The second category includes coronary artery anomalies that do *not* alter myocardial perfusion. These are positional anomalies only, in which the major coronary arteries have aberrant origins from the aorta but are still perfused at normal aortic pressure by normally oxygenated blood. In and of themselves they are not associated with clinical symptoms. Included in this category are (1) origin of the circumflex artery from the right coronary artery or right sinus of Valsalva, (2) origin of the left anterior descending (LAD) artery from the right sinus of Valsalva or right coronary artery, (3) single coronary artery, (4) origin of all three coronary arteries from either the right or the left sinus of Valsalva via two or three separate ostia, and (5) high origin of the coronary arteries.

The third category deals with simple anatomic variations of the coronary artery branches in patients whose coronary anatomy is otherwise considered normal.

Coronary Anomalies That Alter Myocardial Perfusion

Coronary Artery Fistulas

The author reviewed 342 previously reported cases of this lesion and 21 cases of his own.[1] The lesions are congenital precapillary connections between a major coronary artery and a cardiac chamber, the coronary sinus, superior vena cava, or pulmonary artery. They represent the most prevalent form of hemodynamically significant coronary artery anomalies. These fistulas may vary in size from very small to massive. When the fistula drains into a right-sided cardiac chamber, the coronary sinus, superior vena cava, or pulmonary artery, a left-to-right shunt is created. Approximately half of all patients with coronary fistulas develop symptoms of congestive heart failure because of a large shunt, subacute bacterial endocarditis, myocardial ischemia or infarction resulting from a coronary steal, or rupture of an aneurysmal fistula. The other half may remain asymptomatic but are frequently subjected to cardiac catheterization and angiography because of a loud continuous precordial murmur.

Among the 363 cases that the author and colleagues either studied or reviewed,[1] 50 percent of the fistulas arose from the right coronary artery or its branches, 42 percent from the LAD or circumflex arteries or their branches, and 5 percent from multiple vessels. In 3 percent, the vessel of origin was not indicated. The most common drainage area was the right ventricle (41 percent of cases), followed by the right atrium (26 percent), pulmonary artery (17 percent), coronary sinus (7 percent), left atrium (5 percent), left ventricle (3 percent), and superior vena cava (1 percent). It can be seen from these data that the potential for a left-to-right shunt exists in over 90 percent of these lesions.

Angiography provides the most definitive means of diagnosing the lesions because it is the only method of precisely localizing the point of origin and point of drainage. Selective coronary arteriography usually demonstrates that the donor vessel is enlarged, although the degree will vary directly with the size of the shunt. The enlargement extends only to the point of origin of the fistula; the distal portion of the involved coronary artery beyond the fistula is usually of normal caliber. The actual site of communication between the involved coronary artery and the recipient

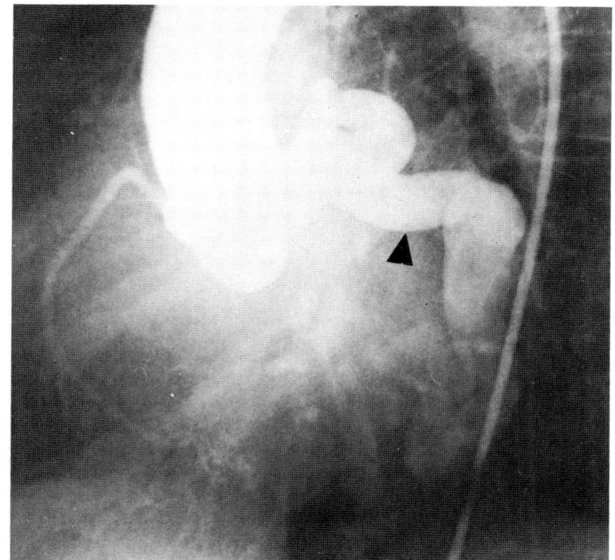

A

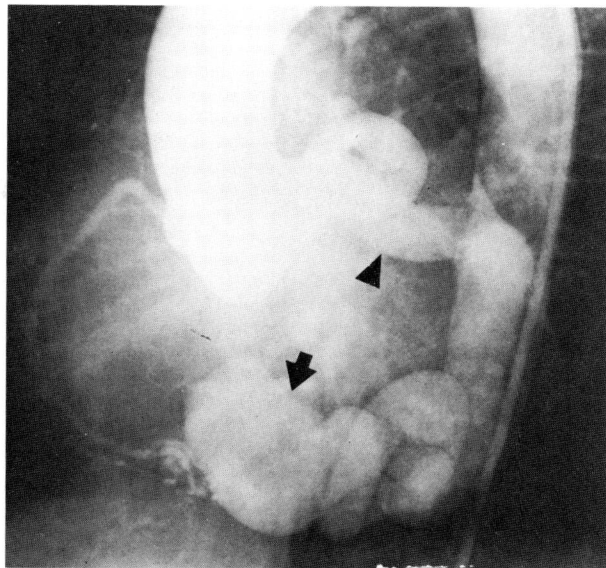

B

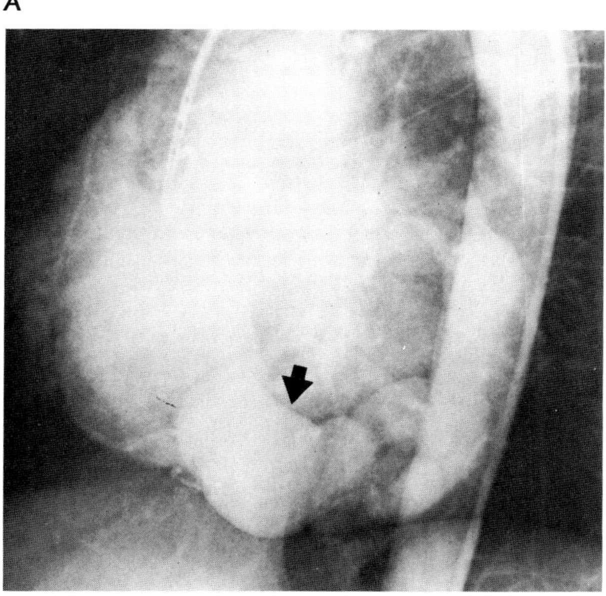

C

Figure 29-1. Congenital fistula from the left circumflex artery to the coronary sinus. (A) Ascending aortogram, early phase, shows early filling of a massively dilated left circumflex artery (*arrowhead*). (B) Slightly later during the injection, the coronary sinus (*arrow*) is opacified. (C) During the late phase of the injection, the reopacified right atrium is seen, indicating a large left-to-right shunt. (From Levin DC, Fellows KE, Abrams HL. Hemodynamically significant primary anomalies of the coronary arteries: angiographic aspects. Circulation 1978;58:25. Used with permission.)

chamber or vessel is usually clearly identified angiographically. If the shunt is very large, it may be visualized on a supravalvular aortogram. However, if the shunt is somewhat smaller, selective arteriography may be necessary to localize the communication precisely. Precise localization of shunts is important because they may be multiple and because effective surgical therapy requires that all communications be obliterated.

Figure 29-1 demonstrates a left circumflex artery–coronary sinus fistula. The communication is very large and is clearly visualized on supravalvular aortography. Figure 29-2 shows a much smaller communication between the distal right coronary artery and the right ventricle. This lesion could be visualized only on selective coronary arteriography. In this case, the donor right coronary artery is just somewhat enlarged.

Fistulas between the LAD and the pulmonary artery are relatively common, tend to be small, and are often composed of multiple serpiginous channels. Surgical ligation may not be necessary because of the small size of the shunt.[2]

Coronary artery fistulas are usually isolated anomalies. In approximately 3 percent of cases, however, the contralateral coronary artery is absent.[3] Among the author's 21 cases, there was one instance of coronary artery fistula associated with congenital absence of the contralateral coronary artery.

Origin of the Left Coronary Artery from the Pulmonary Artery

Origin of a coronary artery from the main pulmonary artery instead of from the aorta is the second most common hemodynamically significant anomaly of the coronary system. In the vast majority of cases, the left

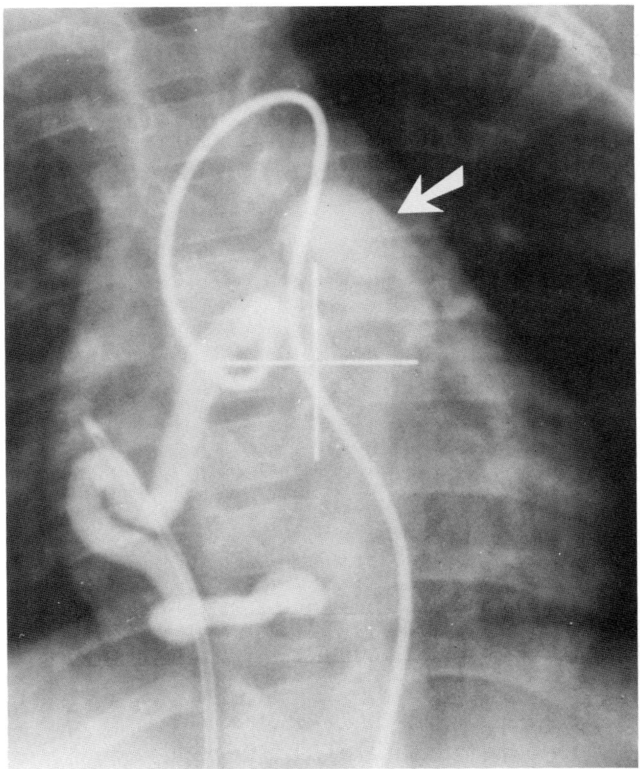

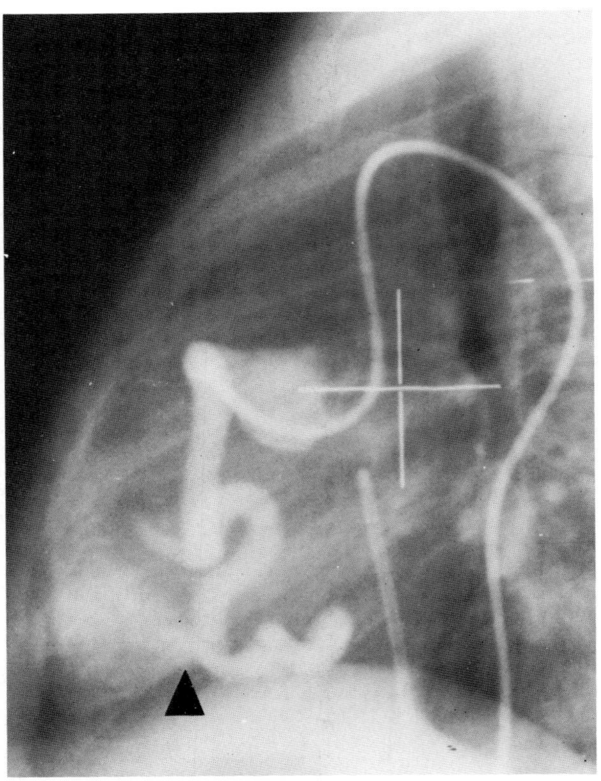

A B

Figure 29-2. Nonsimultaneous frontal and lateral views of a selective right coronary arteriogram in a patient with a congenital right coronary to right ventricular fistula. (A) The frontal view demonstrates opacification of the main pulmonary artery (*arrow*) as a result of the left-to-right shunt. (B) The fistula itself (*arrowhead*) is best seen on the lateral projection. Contrast is seen passing directly from the distal right coronary artery into the right ventricle. (From Levin DC, Fellows KE, Abrams HL. Hemodynamically significant primary anomalies of the coronary arteries: angiographic aspects. Circulation 1978;58:25. Used with permission.)

coronary artery originates from the pulmonary artery, but small numbers of cases of right coronary origin from the pulmonary artery, LAD origin from the pulmonary artery, and origin of both coronary arteries from the pulmonary artery have been reported. This discussion deals only with origin of the left coronary from the pulmonary artery.

The majority of patients with this anomaly develop symptoms and signs of myocardial ischemia early in infancy, and many die within the first 2 years of life. Chest radiographs in such patients demonstrate cardiomegaly. Approximately 25 percent of patients with the anomaly survive infancy but may develop mitral regurgitation, angina, or a continuous murmur later in life.[4,5]

The typical angiographic findings in this disease are reflected in Figure 29-3. Selective coronary arteriography is generally not required in making the diagnosis; supravalvular aortography will suffice. A high-volume injection of contrast with the catheter positioned a short distance above the aortic valve demonstrates absence of an aortic origin of the left coronary artery. The right coronary artery is large, and as the film sequence progresses, collateral circulation can be seen

Figure 29-3. Anomalous origin of the left coronary artery from the pulmonary artery. (A) Simultaneous frontal and lateral views of an ascending aortogram, early phase, show an enlarged right coronary artery (*arrowheads*), but the left coronary artery does not fill directly from the ascending aorta. The left anterior descending (*curved arrow*) and circumflex arteries are seen to opacify as a result of collateral flow from the right coronary artery. (B) Slightly later during the same contrast injection, the left anterior descending (*curved arrow*) and circumflex arteries are fully opacified, and there is retrograde flow back through the left coronary ostium into the main pulmonary artery (*black arrow*). (From Levin DC, Fellows KE, Abrams HL. Hemodynamically significant primary anomalies of the coronary arteries: angiographic aspects. Circulation 1978;58:25. Used with permission.) ▶

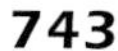

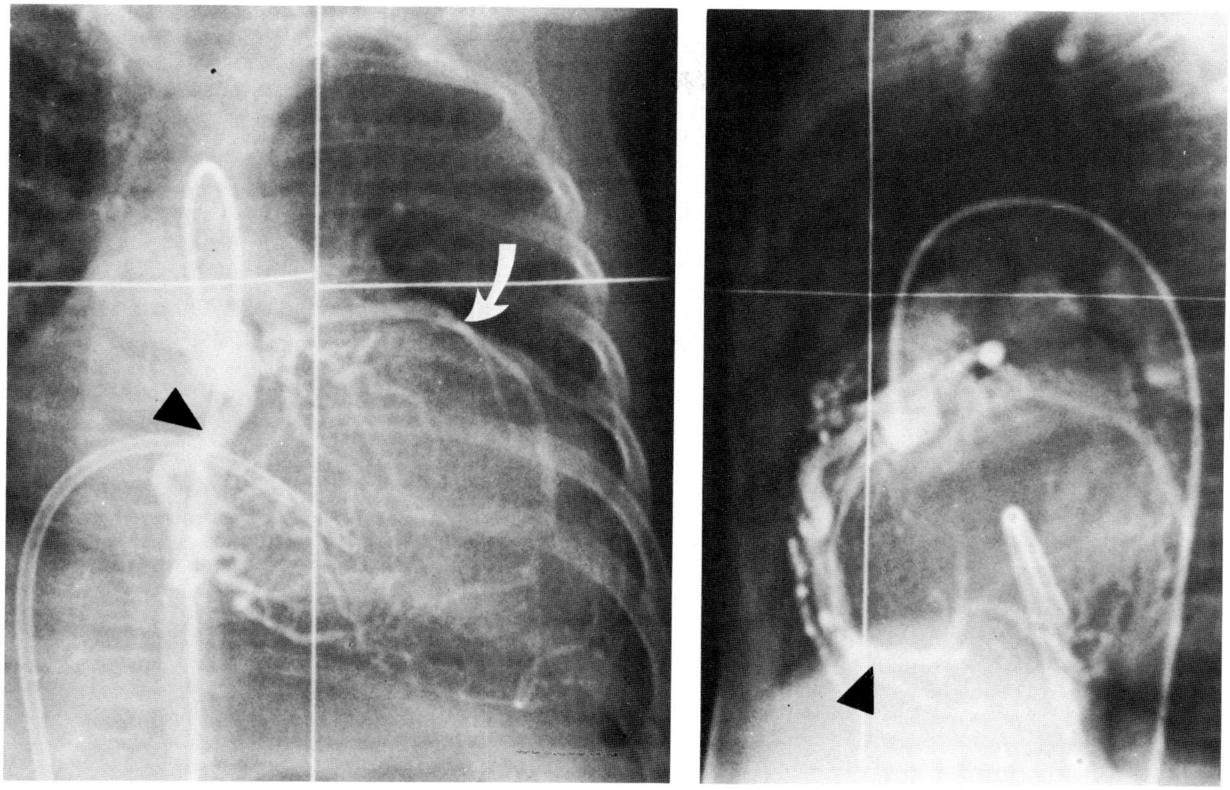

A

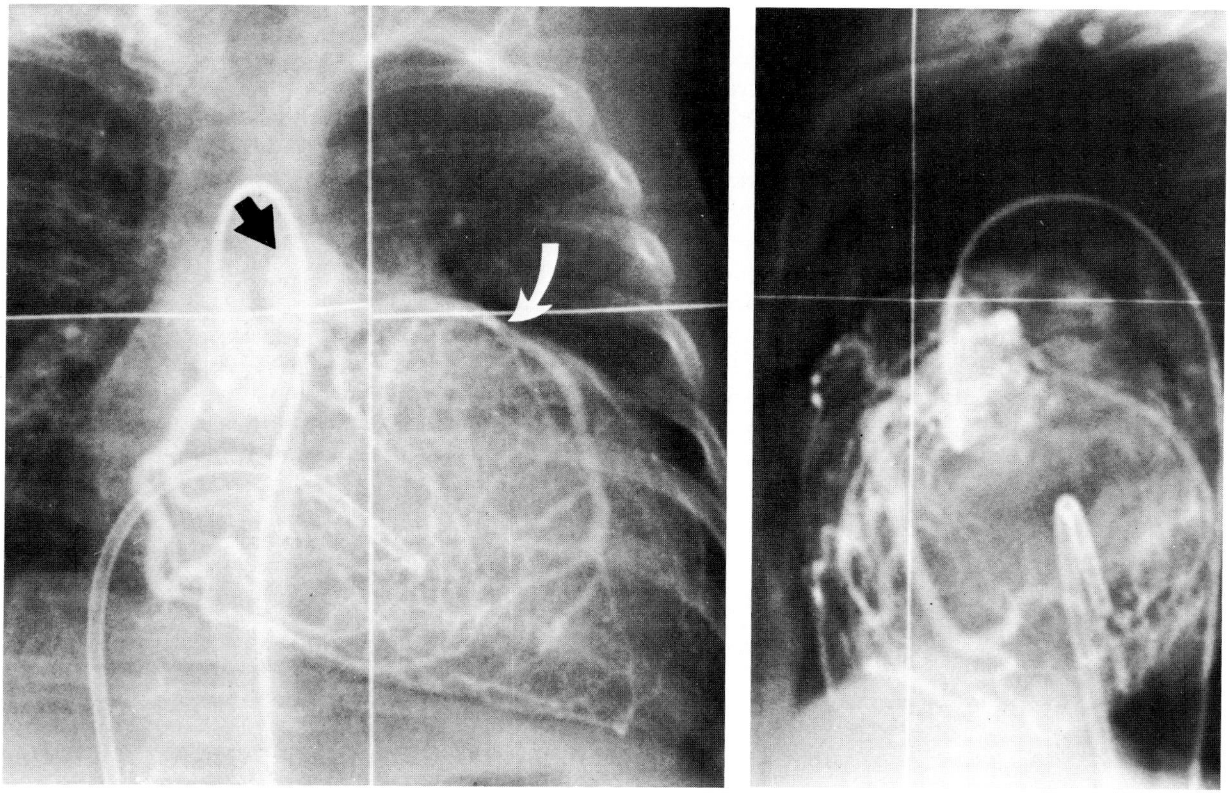

B

extending from the right coronary artery to the LAD and circumflex branches of the left coronary artery. The contrast will then usually be noted to flow in a retrograde fashion back to the point of origin of the left coronary artery from the pulmonary artery, with subsequent opacification of the pulmonary artery. The degree of collateralization, visualization of the left coronary branches, and visualization of the pulmonary artery are variable from patient to patient. In general, it can be stated that the clinical course of the patient will be more favorable if the collateral circulation (and resultant left-to-right shunting) is well developed than if it is poorly developed.[6]

Profound left ventricular myocardial ischemia develops in these patients because the left coronary artery is initially perfused by blood of low oxygen content and at low pressure. The usual benefits of collateral circulation are not fully realized because blood reaching the left coronary branches through the developing collaterals to a large extent fails to perfuse myocardium, draining off instead into the low-pressure pulmonary arterial tree. A left-to-right shunt and coronary "steal" are thereby created.

Congenital Coronary Stenosis or Atresia

Congenital coronary artery occlusion is a rare anomaly. It may occur as an isolated lesion or in association with other congenital diseases such as calcific coronary sclerosis, supravalvular aortic stenosis, homocystinuria, Friedreich's ataxia, Hurler syndrome, progeria, and rubella syndrome.[1] An angiographic example of congenital atresia of the left coronary artery in a patient with supravalvular aortic stenosis is shown in Figure 29-4. The findings are somewhat similar to those in anomalous origin of the left coronary artery from the pulmonary artery, in that the left coronary branches fill via collateral circulation from the right coronary. However, the blind ending of the proximal left coronary artery is clearly seen, and there is of course no drainage back into the pulmonary artery in this case. The patient was a 17-year-old boy with no signs or symptoms of myocardial ischemia.

Origin of the Left Coronary Artery from the Right Sinus of Valsalva

This is likewise a rare congenital lesion in which the left coronary artery arises from the proximal right coronary artery or directly from the right coronary ostium in the right sinus of Valsalva. The left coronary artery then takes a sharp leftward turn and passes between the right ventricular infundibulum and the aorta. After emerging from behind the main pulmonary artery, the vessel bifurcates in the usual manner into LAD and circumflex branches. A diagram of the anatomy of the lesion is shown in Figure 29-5. This lesion represents only one of the numerous forms of single coronary artery, discussed in greater detail later in the chapter. It is the only form of single coronary artery that is clearly associated with an alteration in myocardial perfusion. Cheitlin et al.[7] reviewed 33 cases and found that sudden unexplained death occurred in 9 (27 percent). These deaths tended to occur at a young age and frequently following vigorous exercise. The authors felt that death probably resulted from acute occlusion of the left coronary artery, which could take place at either of two sites, as shown in the diagram. One potential site is the abrupt leftward turn immediately beyond the origin of the aberrant left coronary artery; the other is the narrow passageway between the right ventricular infundibulum and the aorta. Narrowing at either or both of these sites could be produced or accentuated by the increased flow through the two great vessels that accompanies vigorous exercise. Regardless of the exact mechanism, there seems to be little question that this is a highly dangerous lesion and should be treated by bypass surgery.

There have also been isolated reports of cases in which myocardial ischemia may have developed in patients whose right coronary artery originated from the left sinus of Valsalva and then passed between the right ventricular infundibulum and the aorta,[8] or in which the left coronary artery originated from the right sinus of Valsalva but passed either anterior to the pulmonary artery or posterior to the aorta.[9] Because of the rarity of these cases, their hemodynamic significance is not entirely clear.

Figure 29-4. Congenital atresia of the origin of the left coronary artery in a patient with supravalvular aortic stenosis. (A) Left ventriculogram in frontal and lateral projections. Marked left ventricular hypertrophy and narrowing of the aorta (*thick arrow*) just above the sinus portion are noted. A large right coronary artery is seen (*thin arrow*), but there is no evidence of a left coronary artery arising from the aorta. (B) Selective right coronary arteriogram in frontal and lateral projections. The right coronary artery is large, and there is extensive collateral circulation with retrograde filling of the left anterior descending (*arrow*) and circumflex arteries. The retrograde contrast flow opacifies the blind proximal pouch of the atretic left coronary artery (*arrowhead*) near the left sinus of Valsalva. ▶

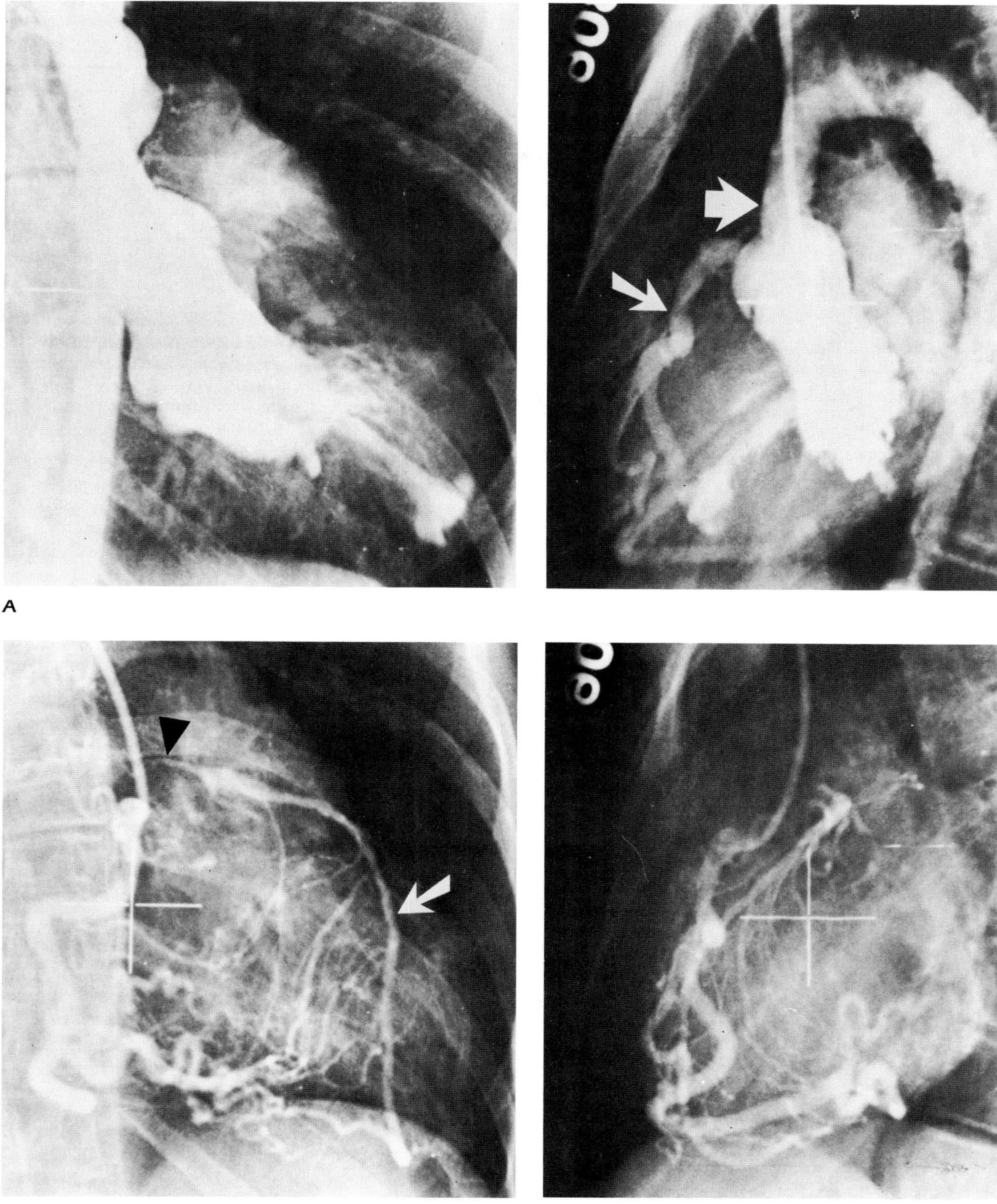

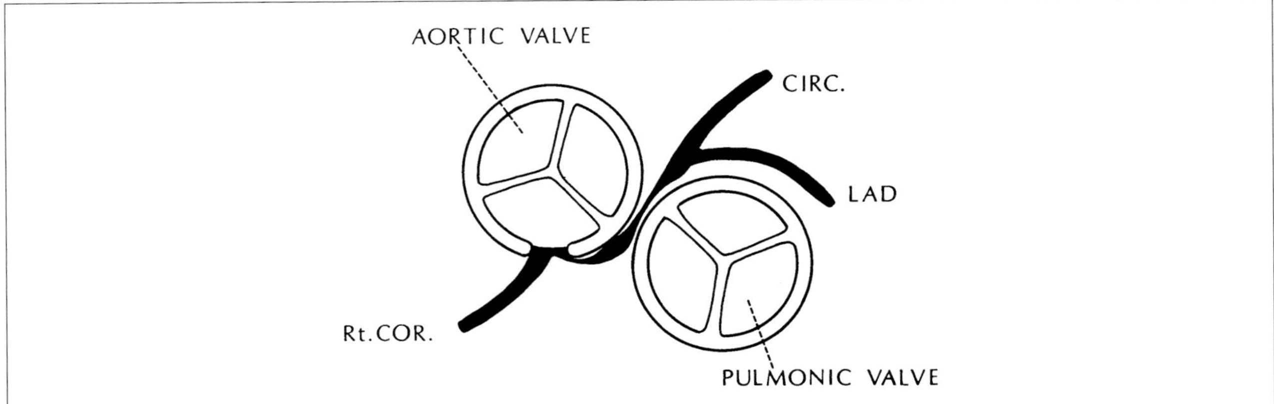

Figure 29-5. Anomalous origin of the left coronary artery from the right sinus of Valsalva with subsequent passage of the vessel between the aorta and the right ventricular infundibulum, viewed from above with the anterior chest wall facing the bottom of the page. There are two potential sites of narrowing: the first immediately beyond the origin of the left coronary artery where it takes a sharp turn to the left, the second as it passes between the aorta and the right ventricular infundibulum. (From Levin DC, Fellows KE, Abrams HL. Hemodynamically significant primary anomalies of the coronary arteries: angiographic aspects. Circulation 1978;58:25. Used with permission.)

Coronary Anomalies That Do Not Alter Myocardial Perfusion

The anomalies discussed in the previous section all result, in one way or another, in alteration of perfusion of myocardium supplied by the affected coronary artery. This section deals with anomalies that have no inherent effect on myocardial perfusion. They are positional anomalies only; the affected coronary arteries originate from the aorta but in an unusual location. Because of the aortic origin of these vessels, the blood supply of the myocardium is entirely normal. The anomalies may prove troublesome for the angiographer because the coronary ostium cannot be found in the usual or expected position. As a group, these anomalies occur in 0.6 to 1.0 percent of all adult patients undergoing coronary arteriography.[9–12]

Origin of the Circumflex Artery from the Right Sinus of Valsalva

Among the five major categories of anomalous aortic origins of the coronary arteries, by far the most common is anomalous origin of the circumflex artery from the right sinus of Valsalva. It represents between one-half and two-thirds of all anomalous coronary artery origins from the aorta.[9–12] In these cases, the circumflex artery originates from the right sinus of Valsalva either through its own separate ostium or from a common ostium with the right coronary artery. The circumflex artery then passes around the posterior aspect of the aortic root toward the left atrioventricular groove. Once it reaches this groove, it resumes the normal course of a circumflex artery. An example of the anomaly is shown in Figure 29-6. A left coronary ostium is present but it gives rise only to the LAD. The diagnosis is easily made if the circumflex artery has a common origin with the right coronary artery. The selective right coronary arteriogram will then opacify both the right coronary and the circumflex arteries simultaneously. However, if the circumflex artery has a separate origin in the right sinus of Valsalva, a selective right coronary arteriogram may fail to opacify it satisfactorily, even if there is reflux of contrast into the right sinus during the selective right coronary arteriography. Whenever both selective right and left coronary arteriograms fail to demonstrate any portion of the left circumflex artery, one possibility to be considered is anomalous origin of the circumflex artery from a separate ostium in the right sinus of Valsalva. Further probing in the right sinus with the catheter tip should then be carried out to try to locate an aberrant ostium. Other possibilities include absence of a left main coronary artery with separate origins of the LAD and circumflex branches in the left sinus of Valsalva, and total occlusion of the left circumflex artery immediately at its origin.

Origin of the LAD from the Right Sinus of Valsalva

In Ogden's experience,[13] origin of the LAD from the right sinus of Valsalva is almost as common as origin of the circumflex artery from the right sinus of Valsalva.

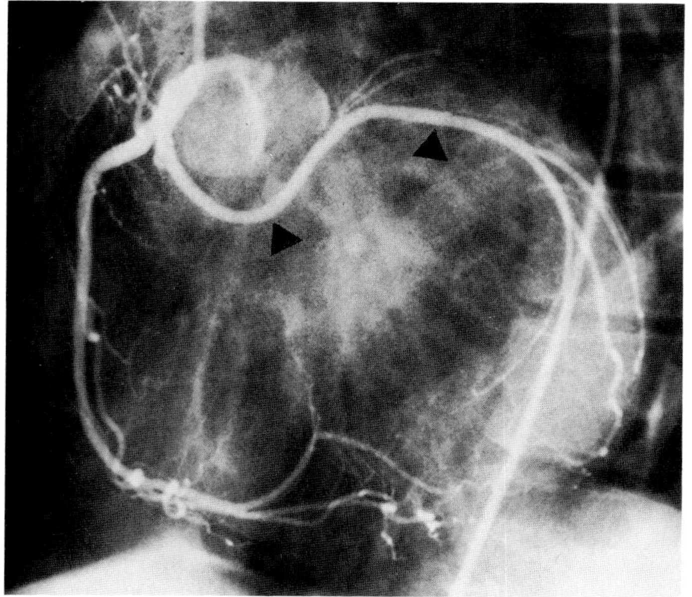

A

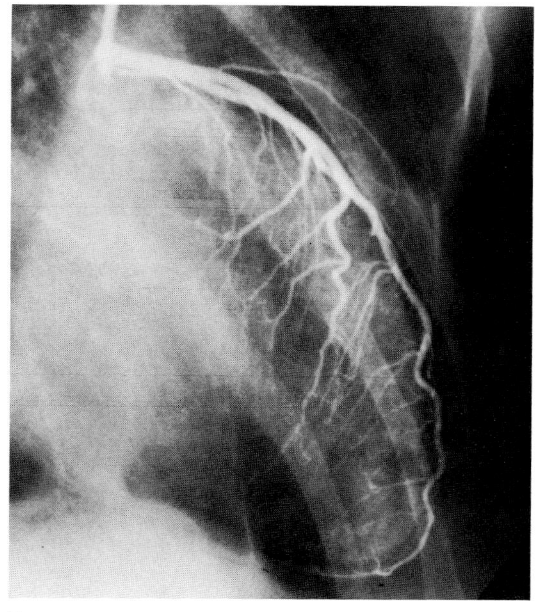

B

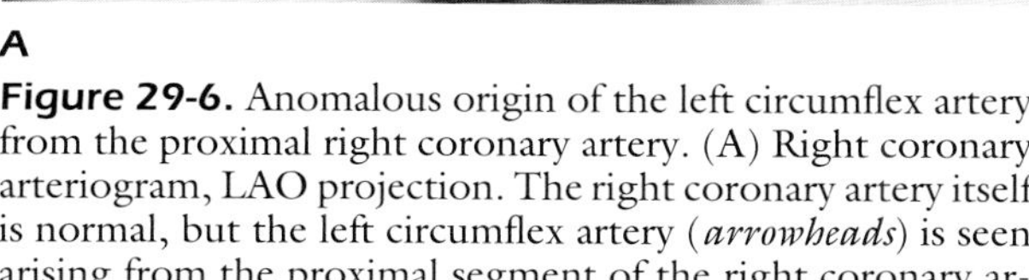

Figure 29-6. Anomalous origin of the left circumflex artery from the proximal right coronary artery. (A) Right coronary arteriogram, LAO projection. The right coronary artery itself is normal, but the left circumflex artery (*arrowheads*) is seen arising from the proximal segment of the right coronary artery, then passing behind the aortic root, and then resuming its normal position in the left atrioventricular groove. (B) Left coronary arteriogram, RAO projection. Only a left anterior descending artery is seen.

However, in the author's own experience and that of previously published reports,[9–12] this is a rare anomaly. When it is present, the right coronary artery has a normal origin and distribution. The LAD originates in the right sinus of Valsalva or from a common trunk with the right coronary artery, then passes anteriorly over the right ventricular infundibulum toward the anterior interventricular groove.[10,13] When it reaches this groove, it turns forward and subsequently pursues the course of a normal LAD. Angiographically, this anomaly is somewhat similar to anomalous origin of the circumflex artery from the right sinus. Selective left coronary arteriography reveals only a circumflex artery. Selective right coronary arteriography will opacify the anomalous LAD if it arises as a common trunk; otherwise it may only be satisfactorily seen by spillover of contrast material or probing in the right sinus of Valsalva for the separate LAD ostium. When a selective left coronary arteriogram demonstrates the presence only of a circumflex artery, the possibilities to be considered include absence of a left main coronary artery with separately originating LAD and circumflex branches in the left sinus of Valsalva, complete occlusion of the LAD immediately at its origin, and anomalous origin of the LAD from the right sinus of Valsalva. Again, it is wise to bear in mind that the latter is probably a rare anomaly.

Single Coronary Artery

Next to origin of the circumflex artery from the right sinus of Valsalva, single coronary artery is probably the most prevalent of the anomalies in this group. There are numerous varieties of this anomaly, and perhaps the best classification system is that of Lipton et al.[14] According to their system, the pattern is first designated as an R or L pattern, depending on whether it is a single right or single left coronary artery. It is then designated as group I, II, or III, depending on the course of the anomalous artery. Finally, group II is subdivided as indicated below. The exact classification system is as follows:

Group R I

There is a single right coronary artery. This vessel and its posterior descending and posterior left ventricular branches are normal. Instead of terminating along the diaphragmatic surface of the left ventricle, however, the right coronary artery continues all the way around the left atrioventricular groove. As it passes up the left atrioventricular groove, it gives off obtuse marginal branches and finally reaches the anterior interventricular groove along the upper anterior aspect of the heart. At this point it gives off the LAD as its terminal branch.

Group L I

This is the converse of R I. There is a single left coronary artery. The LAD and circumflex arteries and their branches are normal. However, the circumflex continues beyond the crux of the heart and passes up the right atrioventricular groove in the territory normally supplied by the right coronary artery. It gives off acute marginal branches and finally terminates along the upper portion of the right atrioventricular groove.

Group R IIA

There is a single right coronary artery. The right coronary and its posterior descending and posterior left ventricular branches are normal. The left coronary artery originates from the proximal right coronary artery, passes anterior to the right ventricular infundibulum, and gives off the LAD as it crosses the anterior interventricular groove. It then continues down the left atrioventricular groove as the circumflex artery. The *A* in this designation refers to the fact that the aberrant left coronary artery passes anterior to the aorta.

Group L IIA

This is the converse of R IIA. There is a single left coronary artery. The right coronary artery originates from the area of the left coronary bifurcation or the LAD, passes anterior to the right ventricular infundibulum, then reaches the right atrioventricular groove where it continues as a normal right coronary artery.

Group R IIB

There is a single right coronary artery. The left coronary artery originates from the proximal right coronary artery, but instead of passing anterior to the right ventricular infundibulum, it passes between the infundibulum and the aorta. After emerging from between the two, it bifurcates as usual into LAD and circumflex branches. The *B* designation refers to the passage of the aberrant left coronary artery between the right ventricular infundibulum and the aorta.

Group L IIB

This is similar to group L IIA except that the anomalous right coronary artery here also passes between the right ventricular infundibulum and the aorta.

Group R IIP

Again there is a single right coronary artery. The left coronary artery originates from the proximal right coronary but passes posterior to the aortic root (hence the *P* designation) on its way toward the left atrioventricular groove. After emerging from behind the aorta, it bifurcates into LAD and circumflex branches.

Group L IIP

There is a single left coronary artery. The right coronary artery arises from the left coronary bifurcation or from the proximal circumflex and passes posterior to the aortic root on its way toward the right atrioventricular groove. Once it reaches the right atrioventricular groove, it resumes a normal course of a right coronary artery.

Group R III

In this group there is a single right coronary artery. The LAD originates from the proximal right coronary artery, then passes between the right ventricular infundibulum and the aorta on its way toward the anterior interventricular groove. The left circumflex artery also originates from the proximal right coronary but passes behind the root of the aorta on its way toward the left atrioventricular groove.

Group R IIB represents the only form of single coronary artery that has proved to be of some danger from the clinical viewpoint. As discussed earlier, it is felt to be due to the potential for acute occlusion of the left coronary artery before or in the tunnel between the right ventricular infundibulum and the aorta.

Origin of All Three Coronary Arteries from Either Right or Left Sinus of Valsalva via Two or Three Separate Ostia

This anomaly is similar to single coronary artery, in that there is complete absence of coronary ostia in either the left or right sinus of Valsalva. The "missing" coronary arteries arise in the opposite sinus of Valsalva and may have distribution patterns resembling those just described for single coronary artery. However, instead of arising as a single trunk with the contralateral coronary artery, they arise via additional but separate ostia in the contralateral sinus. Figure 29-7 shows the origin of all three coronary arteries from the right sinus of Valsalva via three separate ostia.

High Origin of the Coronary Arteries

In the vast majority of human hearts, the left and right coronary arteries originate in the sinuses of Valsalva. Rarely, one or both coronary arteries may originate higher up the ascending aorta, above the sinuses of Valsalva and the ridge marking the junction of the sinus and tubular portions of the aorta. Cases of this type have been reported by Ogden[13] and Alexander and Griffith.[15]

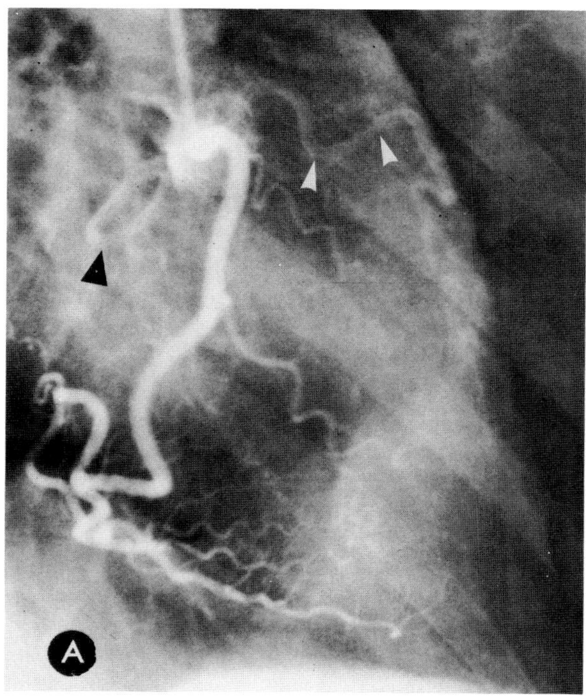

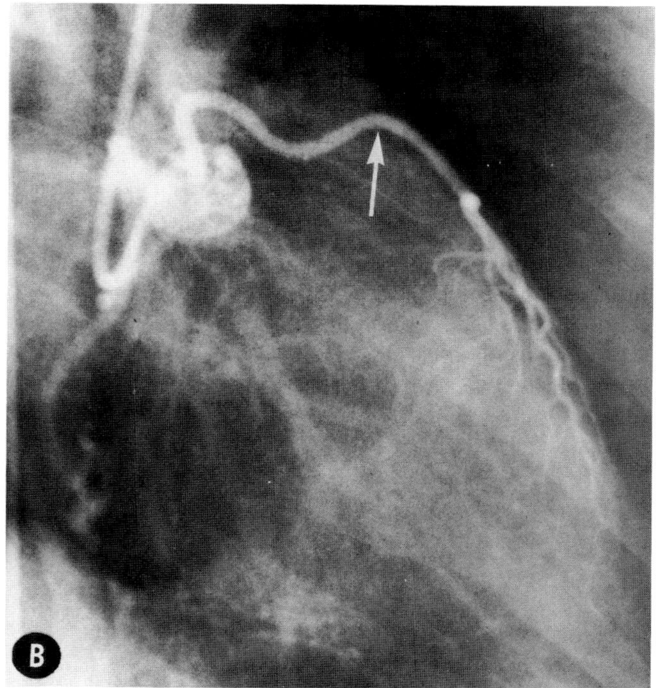

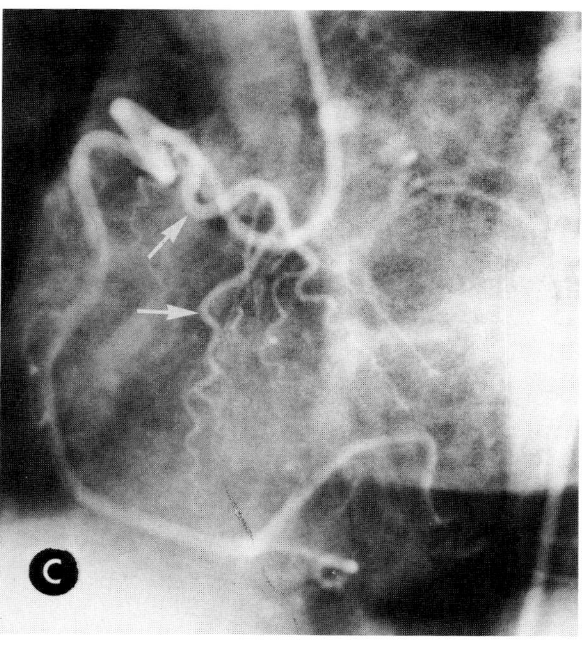

Figure 29-7. Origin of all three coronary arteries from the right sinus of Valsalva via three separate ostia. (A) Right coronary arteriogram, RAO projection. The right coronary artery is normal. As a result of reflux of contrast from the right coronary back into the right sinus of Valsalva, there is faint opacification of anomalously originating left anterior descending (*white arrowheads*) and circumflex (*black arrowhead*) arteries. (B and C) RAO and LAO views of a selective injection into the anomalously originating left anterior descending artery. The catheter tip can be seen pointing into the right sinus of Valsalva during this injection. The *arrows* point to the anomalous left anterior descending artery, which originates from the right sinus, then appears to pass behind the right ventricular infundibulum, and finally emerges in the anterior interventricular groove. Beyond this point it pursues a normal course along the anterior interventricular groove.

Anatomic Variations of the Coronary Arteries

The question of when an anomaly becomes a normal anatomic variant is often a matter of semantics. This discussion assumes that anything occurring in more than 1 percent of human hearts represents an anatomic variation rather than a true anomaly. As in most other organs of the human body, there are numerous anatomic variations in the origin and distribution of the major coronary artery branches. The most important of these are the following.

Coronary Artery Dominance

The term *dominance* is somewhat misleading but has been widely used in the medical literature to indicate which of the two major arteries supplies blood to the diaphragmatic aspects of the interventricular septum and left ventricle. The blood supply of the diaphragmatic surface of the interventricular septum is via the posterior descending artery, whereas the blood supply of the diaphragmatic aspect of the remainder of the left ventricle is via one or more posterior left ventricular (sometimes also referred to as *left posterolateral*) branches. In approximately 85 percent of human hearts, the right coronary artery is dominant. In such cases, the right coronary artery passes all the way around the right atrioventricular groove to the crux (the junction along the diaphragmatic surface of the heart of the right and left atrioventricular grooves with the posterior interventricular groove). At or near the crux, the dominant right coronary artery gives off the posterior descending branch. It then continues toward the diaphragmatic surface of the left ventricle, where it terminates by giving off one or more posterior left ventricular branches. In 7 to 8 percent of human hearts, the left circumflex artery is dominant. With this anatomic arrangement, the right coronary artery is small and never reaches the crux. The left circumflex artery is large and supplies not only the usual obtuse marginal branches but also the posterior left ventricular and posterior descending branches. In the final 7 to 8 percent of human hearts, there is codominance or a "balanced" circulation. In these hearts, the right coronary artery reaches the crux, where it gives off the posterior descending artery as its terminal branch. The posterior left ventricular branches arise from the left circumflex artery as the terminal branches of that vessel.

The clinical importance of a given coronary artery is directly related to the amount of left ventricular myocardium it supplies. In patients with dominant left coronary arteries, the right coronary artery supplies little or no left ventricular myocardium. The latter vessel is therefore not generally a clinically significant vessel in these patients. At the present time, there is felt to be no indication for bypass of a stenotic or occluded nondominant right coronary artery.

Origin of the Conus Artery

The conus artery is generally considered to be the first branch of the right coronary artery. In approximately 50 percent of hearts, however, the conus branch does not originate from the right coronary artery but from a small separate ostium in the right sinus of Valsalva near the right coronary ostium.[16,17] In patients with a separate conus ostium, selective right coronary arteriography may fail to opacify the conus branch unless there is sufficient reflux of contrast from the right coronary artery into the right sinus of Valsalva to fill the small separate ostium. In a large series of adult patients undergoing coronary arteriography, it was found[18] that in 20 percent of cases the conus artery was not satisfactorily visualized on right coronary arteriography. The conus artery is not a very important vessel, but in patients with LAD obstruction it becomes a major source of collateral blood supply.

Origin of the Sinoatrial Node Artery

This vessel arises from the proximal right coronary artery in slightly more than half of human hearts and from the left circumflex artery in slightly less than half of human hearts.[19] It is the principal source of blood supply to both atria. Regardless of whether it arises from the right coronary or left circumflex artery, it is usually associated with a smaller atrial branch arising on the contralateral side; the smaller atrial branch is often referred to as a *left* (or *right*) *atrial circumflex branch*. After originating from the proximal right or proximal circumflex artery, the sinoatrial node artery passes posteriorly in the atrial septum toward the sinus node and ends by giving off branches to the node and also to the free walls of both atria.

Atrioventricular Node Artery

The atrioventricular node artery generally originates at the crux of the heart from whichever vessel is dominant (either the right coronary or left circumflex artery). It can be identified as a small twig that passes vertically upward in the lower portion of the atrial septum toward its termination in the region of the atrioventricular node. On occasion there will be two small branches present instead of one single branch, and sometimes there are branches to the atrioventricular node from both the right coronary and left circumflex arteries, particularly in the presence of a balanced circulation.

Anatomic Variations of the Posterior Descending Artery

In most patients with a dominant right coronary artery, the posterior descending branch originates at or near the crux (Fig. 29-8) and then passes forward along the posterior interventricular groove to supply the diaphragmatic aspect of the interventricular septum. In an analysis of a large series of coronary arteriograms,[20] there were found to be significant anatomic variations in the origin of the posterior descending artery in 23 percent of patients with dominant right coronary systems. These variations include partial supply of the posterior descending territory by either posterior right ventricular or acute marginal branches, double posterior descending artery, and early origin of the posterior descending artery proxi-

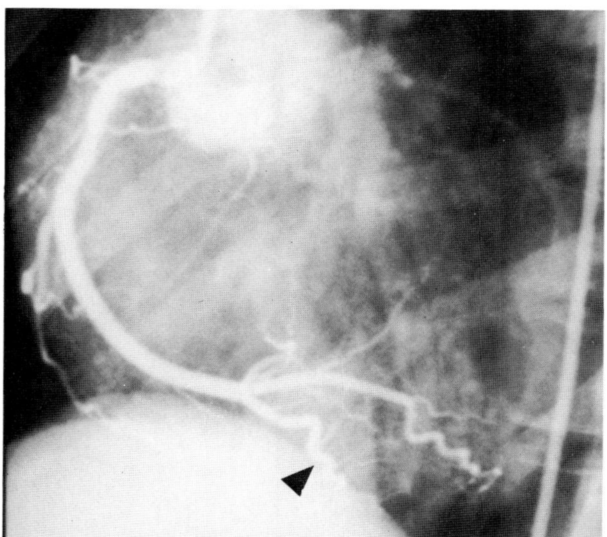

Figure 29-8. Single posterior descending artery arising at the crux of the heart in a patient with right coronary dominance. Right coronary arteriogram, LAO projection. The *arrowhead* points to the posterior descending branch.

mal to the crux. These variations are shown diagrammatically in Figure 29-9. Figure 29-10 is an example of a coronary angiogram showing early origin of the posterior descending branch well before the crux. In Figure 29-11 a portion of the normal posterior descending artery distribution is seen to be supplied by an acute marginal branch of the right coronary artery. Figure 29-12 shows a double posterior descending artery. This case also demonstrates the surgical significance of these variations. In addition to a lesion of the distal right coronary, there is a separate lesion at the origin of one of the two large posterior descending branches. Because of the large size of the latter and the separate lesion at its origin, two separate bypasses would have to be placed to revascularize this right coronary system adequately.

Absence or Early Bifurcation of the Left Main Coronary Artery

In the author's experience and that of James,[17] approximately 2 percent of human hearts have either absence or very early bifurcation of the left main coronary artery. If the left main coronary artery is totally absent,

Figure 29-9. Anatomic variations in the course and distribution of the posterior descending artery in 23 percent of patients with dominant right coronary systems. (A) Early origin of the posterior descending artery proximal to the crux. (B) Partial supply of the posterior descending artery by an acute marginal artery. (C) Double posterior descending artery. (D) Partial supply of the posterior descending distribution by a posterior right ventricular branch. *PD*, posterior descending artery; *PLV*, posterior left ventricular branches; *AM*, acute marginal branch; *PR V*, posterior right ventricular branch.

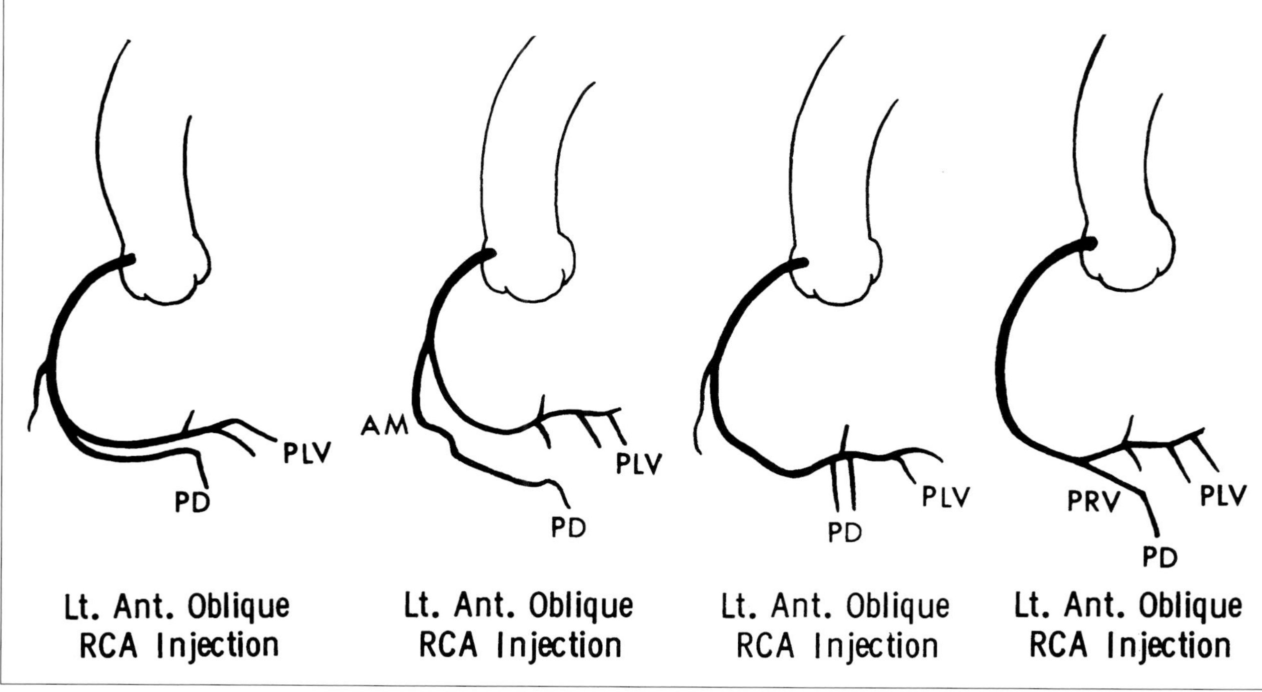

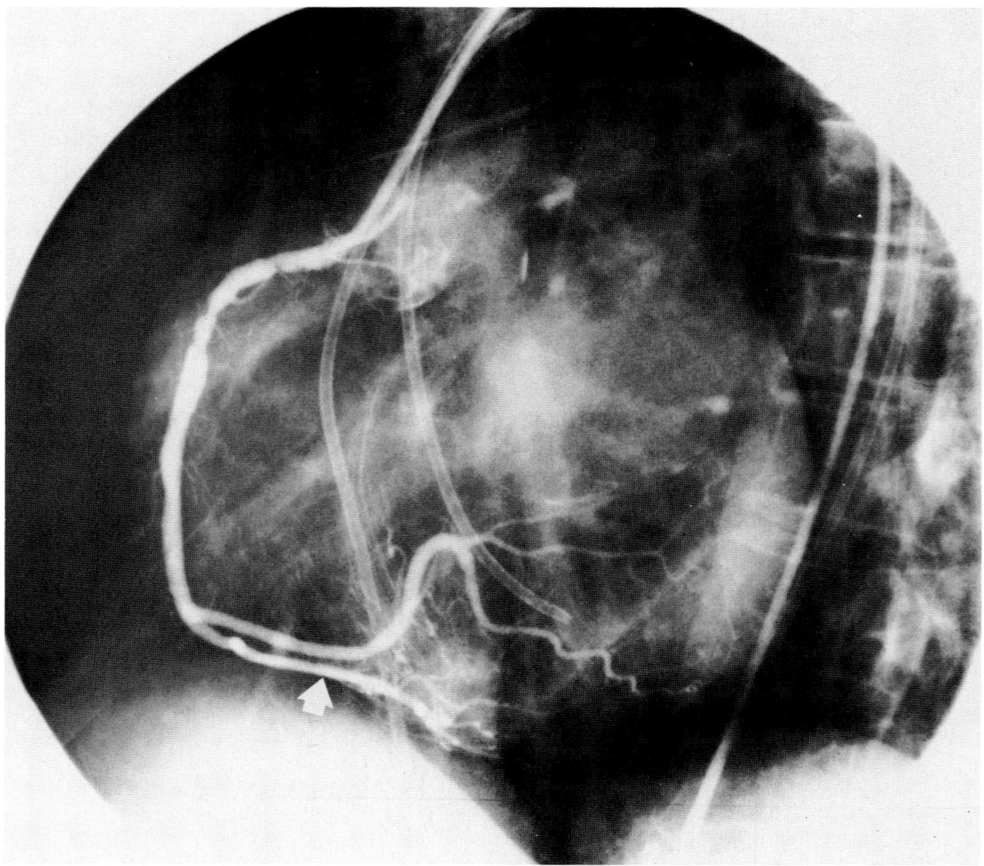

Figure 29-10. Right coronary arteriogram, LAO projection, in a patient whose posterior descending artery (*arrow*) originates from the right coronary artery well before the crux.

there are two separate ostia, one for the LAD and one for the circumflex artery, located side by side in normal position in the left sinus of Valsalva. Alternatively, a single left coronary ostium may be present with immediate branching into LAD and circumflex arteries so that, in effect, there is again absence of the left main coronary artery. Finally, a very short left main coronary may be present, extending for only 1 to 2 mm, after which there is the expected bifurcation into LAD and circumflex branches. Whenever these anatomic patterns are present, they can prove troublesome to the angiographer because an attempt at selective catheterization of the left main coronary artery will result in superselective entry of the catheter tip into the LAD or the circumflex branch. The resulting arteriogram may show only that branch and thus lead to the erroneous diagnosis of total occlusion of the other branch at its origin. The other branch may be visualized in some cases as a result of reflux of contrast material back into the left sinus of Valsalva, but this does not occur in every case. Whenever the LAD or circumflex artery is not visualized at all during left coronary arteriography, the possibility of separate origin of that branch should be strongly considered. A nonselective injection of contrast into the left sinus of Valsalva should be made to try to visualize the origin of that branch. The latter can then be selectively catheterized in most instances with additional catheter manipulation or the use of a catheter of a different shape.

Ramus Medianus

The term *ramus medianus* has been used to designate a large branch arising at the left main coronary division and passing between the LAD and circumflex branches to supply a portion of the free wall of the left ventricle. In such a case, there is a left coronary trifurcation, rather than a bifurcation. A recent angiographic study has shown that a ramus medianus is present in 37 percent of human hearts.[21] The ramus medianus is often as large as the LAD and larger than the circumflex artery and must therefore be carefully studied for signs

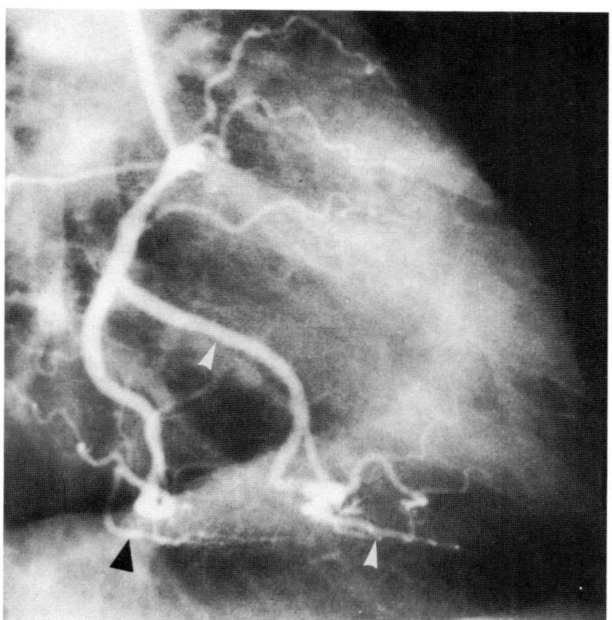

Figure 29-11. Right coronary arteriogram, RAO projection, in a patient whose posterior descending distribution is supplied largely by an acute marginal branch of the right coronary artery. The *white arrowheads* indicate the acute marginal branch. Note that the distal segment of this vessel occupies the posterior interventricular groove, which is the area normally occupied by the distal posterior descending artery. The *black arrowhead* points to a small posterior descending branch that occupies its normal position but does not extend all the way to the cardiac apex.

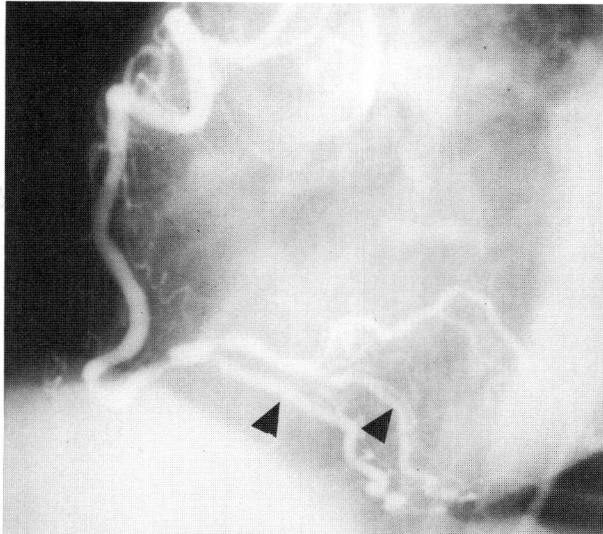

Figure 29-12. Selective right coronary arteriogram, LAO projection, in a patient with two posterior descending branches (*arrowheads*) that lie very close to each other and follow a parallel course.

of disease, even though angiographers tend to devote most of their attention to the LAD and circumflex branches. Because the ramus medianus may be superimposed on portions of the left main coronary or the LAD or circumflex branches in the standard oblique projections, cranial or caudal angulation of the x-ray beam may be necessary to visualize the entire length of this vessel properly.

Diagonal Branches of the LAD

The LAD gives rise to a variable number of diagonal branches that supply the anterolateral aspect of the free wall of the left ventricle. These vessels are similar in size and distribution to the ramus medianus when the latter is present. Seventy-three percent of adult patients undergoing coronary arteriography have either one or two diagonal branches,[21] but as many as five may be present in some cases. Complete absence of diagonal branches is rare. If no diagonal branches are seen, or if there is a paucity of such branches supplying the free wall of the left ventricle, the possibility of occlusion at the origin of a diagonal branch should be considered. Visualization of the distal segments of such branches via collateral circulation should be carefully sought on the arteriogram. Because of the great variability from patient to patient in the number of diagonal branches, it is impossible to predict how many should be present in any given case. An angiographic example of the anatomy of the ramus medianus and diagonal branches is seen in Figure 29-13.

Length of the LAD

The LAD generally passes all the way around the cardiac apex and terminates along the diaphragmatic surface of the heart. However, one angiographic study[22] showed that in 22 percent of patients the LAD failed to reach the diaphragmatic surface but instead terminated at or even before the cardiac apex. In these cases, the posterior descending branch of the right coronary artery was longer than usual and supplied some or all of the cardiac apex. An example of this anatomic arrangement is shown in Figure 29-14. The less apical myocardium the LAD supplies, the smaller and shorter this vessel will appear. Thus a short LAD with a narrow distal caliber is not necessarily a diseased vessel if some or all of the cardiac apex is supplied by the posterior descending artery. In patients with a short LAD, proximal lesions of this vessel assume less significance and bypass may be more difficult because of its relatively narrow distal caliber. Lesions of the midportion of

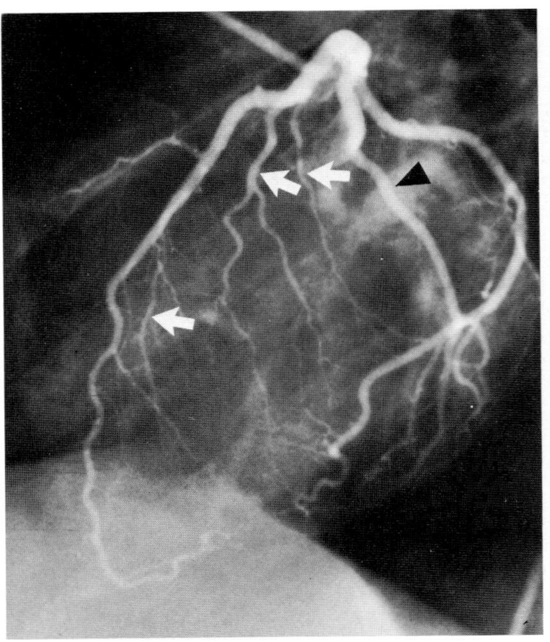

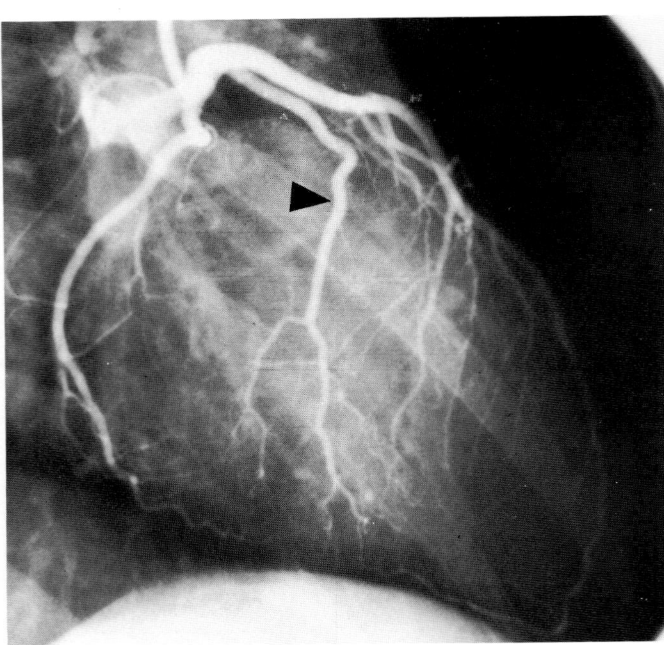

A B

Figure 29-13. Left coronary arteriogram in a patient with a ramus medianus and three small diagonal branches. (A) LAO projection. A large ramus medianus (*arrowhead*) is seen arising at the division of the left main coronary artery. Three smaller diagonal branches (*arrows*) are seen arising farther distally from the left anterior descending artery. (B) RAO projection. *Arrowhead* shows ramus medianus.

Figure 29-14. Short left anterior descending artery. (A) Left coronary arteriogram, RAO projection. The left anterior descending artery (*arrow*) is relatively small and short and terminates before reaching the cardiac apex. (B) Right coronary arteriogram, RAO projection. The posterior descending branch (*arrow*) is unusually long and supplies the cardiac apex.

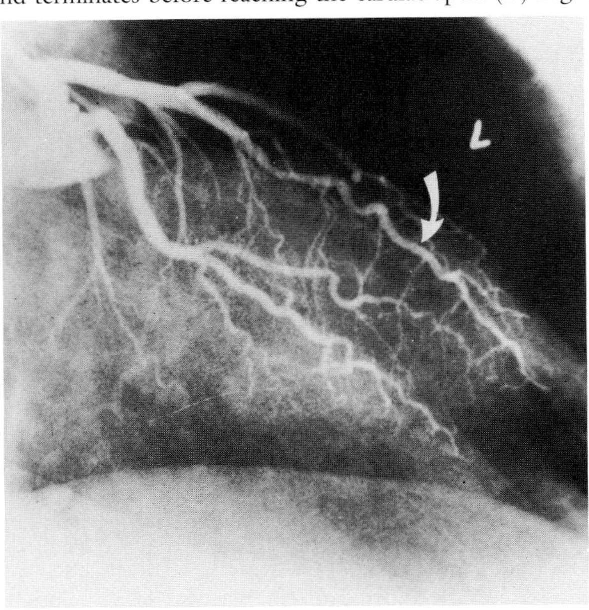

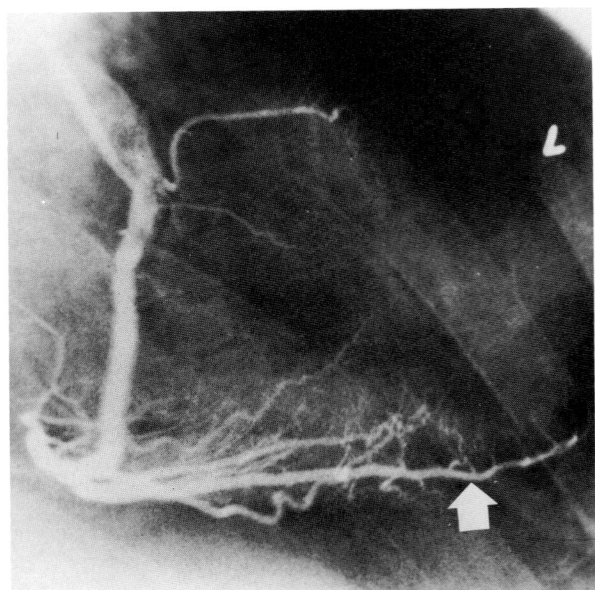

A B

such arteries may be of almost no clinical significance and may not require bypass.

Length and Size of the Circumflex Artery

In the 15 percent of human hearts in which there is a balanced circulation or left circumflex dominance, the circumflex artery is invariably quite large. However, in the 85 percent of patients with dominant right coronary systems, the left circumflex artery may vary substantially in size and length, depending on the degree of right coronary dominance. In patients with very strong right coronary dominance, the distal right coronary artery may ascend the left atrioventricular groove for a considerable distance and supply branches to the diaphragmatic and lateral aspects of the left ventricle. In such cases, the circumflex artery will tend to be small and short and may terminate after giving off only one obtuse marginal branch. Where right coronary dominance is relatively weak, the right coronary artery will terminate shortly beyond the crux by giving rise to only one or two branches to the diaphragmatic aspect of the left ventricle. In these cases, the circumflex artery can be expected to be larger and to supply some branches to the lateral and diaphragmatic aspects of the left ventricle.

Myocardial Bridging

The major coronary arteries pass, for most of their length, along the epicardial surface of the heart. Occasionally, however, short segments of these arteries dip down into the myocardium, so that the overlying myocardial fibers form a bridge over the involved segment of the vessel. Myocardial bridging occurs in approximately 5 percent of human hearts[23] and is most frequent in the LAD. It can be identified angiographically as transient narrowing of a segment of a coronary artery that occurs during systole but reverts to a more normal caliber during diastole. The systolic narrowing of the artery is caused by contraction of the overlying myocardial fibers. An illustration of myocardial bridging is shown in Figure 28-8.

References

1. Levin DC, Fellows KE, Abrams HL. Hemodynamically significant primary anomalies of the coronary arteries: angiographic aspects. Circulation 1978;58:25.
2. Björk VO, Björk L. Coronary artery fistula. J Thorac Cardiovasc Surg 1965;49:921.
3. Oldham HN Jr, Ebert PA, Young WG, Sabiston DC Jr. Surgical management of congenital coronary artery fistula. Ann Thorac Surg 1971;12:503.
4. Wesselhoeft H, Fawcett JS, Johnson AL. Anomalous origin of the left coronary artery from the pulmonary trunk: its clinical spectrum, pathology and pathophysiology based on a review of 140 cases with seven further cases. Circulation 1968;38:403.
5. Wilson CL, Dlabal PW, Holeyfield RW, Akins CW, Knauf DG. Anomalous origin of left coronary artery from pulmonary artery: case reports and review of literature concerning teenagers and adults. J Thorac Cardiovasc Surg 1977;73:887.
6. Perry LW, Scott LP. Anomalous left coronary artery from pulmonary artery. Report of 11 cases; review of indications for and results of surgery. Circulation 1970;41:1043.
7. Cheitlin MD, DeCastro CM, McAllister HA. Sudden death as a complication of anomalous left coronary origin from the anterior sinus of Valsalva: a not-so-minor congenital anomaly. Circulation 1974;50:780.
8. Thompson SI, Vieweg WVR, Alpert JS, Hagan AD. Anomalous origin of the right coronary artery from the left sinus of Valsalva with associated chest pain: reports of two cases. Cathet Cardiovasc Diagn 1976;2:397.
9. Liberthson RR, et al. Aberrant coronary artery origin from the aorta. Diagnosis and clinical significance. Circulation 1974;50:774.
10. Engel HJ, Torres C, Page HL Jr. Major variations in anatomical origin of the coronary arteries: angiographic observations in 4,250 patients without associated congenital heart disease. Cathet Cardiovasc Diagn 1975;1:157.
11. Chaitman BR, Lesperance J, Saltiel J, Bourassa MG. Clinical, angiographic, and hemodynamic findings in patients with anomalous origin of the coronary arteries. Circulation 1976;53:122.
12. Kimbiris D, Iskandrian AS, Segal BL, Bemis CE. Anomalous aortic origin of coronary arteries. Circulation 1978;58:606.
13. Ogden JA. Congenital anomalies of the coronary arteries. Am J Cardiol 1970;25:474.
14. Lipton MJ, Barry WH, Obrez I, Silverman JF, Wexler L. Isolated single coronary artery: diagnosis, angiographic classification, and clinical significance. Radiology 1979;130:39.
15. Alexander RW, Griffith GC. Anomalies of the coronary arteries and their clinical significance. Circulation 1956;14:800.
16. Schlesinger MJ, Zoll PM, Wessler S. The conus artery: a third coronary artery. Am Heart J 1949;38:823.
17. James TN. Anatomy of the coronary arteries. New York: Hoeber Medical Division, Harper & Row, 1961:38–41.
18. Levin DC, Beckmann CF, Garnic JD, Carey P, Bettmann MA. Frequency and clinical significance of failure to visualize the conus artery during coronary arteriography. Circulation 1981;63:833.
19. James TN. Small arteries of the heart. Circulation 1977;56:2.
20. Levin DC, Baltaxe HA. Angiographic demonstration of important anatomic variations of the posterior descending coronary artery. AJR 1972;116:41.
21. Levin DC, Harrington DP, Bettmann MA, Garnic JD, Davidoff A, Lois J. Anatomic variations of the coronary arteries supplying the anterolateral aspect of the left ventricle. Invest Radiol 1982;17:458.
22. Levin DC. Unpublished data.
23. Edwards JC, Burnsides C, Swarm RL, Lansing AI. Arteriosclerosis in intramural and extramural portions of coronary arteries in the human heart. Circulation 1956;13:235.

30

Coronary Arteriography Following Bypass Surgery

DIANA F. GUTHANER
MICHAEL R. REES
LEWIS WEXLER

Techniques of Bypass Surgery

The aim of bypass surgery is to augment myocardial perfusion by providing alternative vascular pathways for blood to bypass diseased coronary segments. The technique of aortocoronary bypass grafting using autologous saphenous veins to the right coronary artery was first performed at the Cleveland Clinic by Favaloro in May 1967.[1] This was then extended to all major coronary vessels in 1969 by Johnson and colleagues.[2] These techniques have proved to be a major advance in the treatment of coronary artery disease, with significant improvements in survival and relief of symptoms for 5 years after surgery;[3] however, over 10 years the survival for saphenous vein grafting is the same as for medical treatment. The survival for surgical patients has been improved with the introduction of internal thoracic artery grafts. At 20 years, the survival for patients with one or two internal thoracic artery grafts is 50.0 to 63.5 percent, compared to a survival for saphenous vein grafting of 38 percent.[4] Other conduits that have been used include the radial artery, which has been abandoned because of poor results,[5] the gastroepiploic artery,[6] the inferior epigastric artery,[7] and bovine and synthetic grafts.[8]

Sites of Origin from Aorta

Coronary artery bypass grafts (CABG) are attached to the anterolateral surface of the ascending aorta a few centimeters above the coronary sinuses. The site of anastomosis in the aorta is usually made via a vertical knife cut or a triangular scissors cut, but may be made via a circular punch. This latter technique can make the origin of the graft appear widened or saccular and in rare cases can lead to an aneurysm forming at the site of the punched-out area in the aorta. Left ventricular lateral wall grafts to the diagonal and marginal arteries are usually anastomosed cephalad to the left anterior descending graft origin, and left coronary grafts are attached higher than the right grafts (Fig. 30-1). Occasionally, sequential grafts to the posterolateral branches and/or the left circumflex artery arise on the right side of the aorta just in front of the superior vena cava.

In some institutions graft origins are marked by metallic clips placed superiorly, inferiorly, or encircling the ostium, or by metallic rings facilitating subsequent selective catheterization. However, these markers often migrate in relation to the graft and consequently may be misleading to the angiographer.

Course of Grafts

Anterior to Pulmonary Artery

Grafts to the left coronary circulation arise from the aortic root anteriorly and course cephalad to the left, looping over the main pulmonary artery (Fig. 30-2). The grafts then pursue an oblique course caudad to reach the lateral aspect of the left ventricle and interventricular septum (see Fig. 30-1). The lateral wall grafts course in a more horizontal direction. Grafts that pass between the sternum and a very anteriorly positioned pulmonary artery may be subject to tethering due to fibrosis, presumably secondary to trauma of the graft (Fig. 30-3).

Posterior to Pulmonary Artery

Occasionally grafts to the posterior and posterolateral ventricular surface, distal circumflex branches, or obtuse marginal arteries course between the superior vena cava and the aorta, posterior to the pulmonary artery in the transverse sinus above the left atrium, to reach the posterolateral cardiac surface (Fig. 30-4).

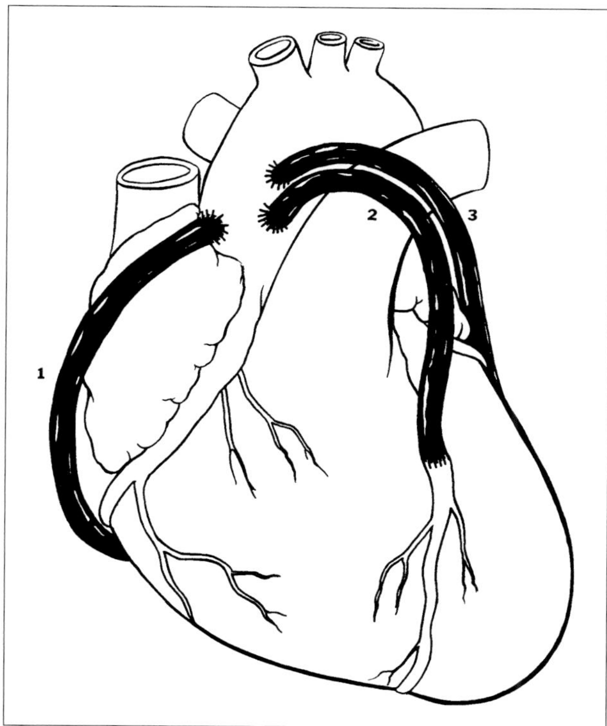

Figure 30-1. Diagrammatic representation of the origin and course of saphenous vein aortocoronary bypass grafts to the right coronary artery (*1*), left anterior descending coronary artery (LAD) (*2*), and left ventricular lateral wall (*3*).

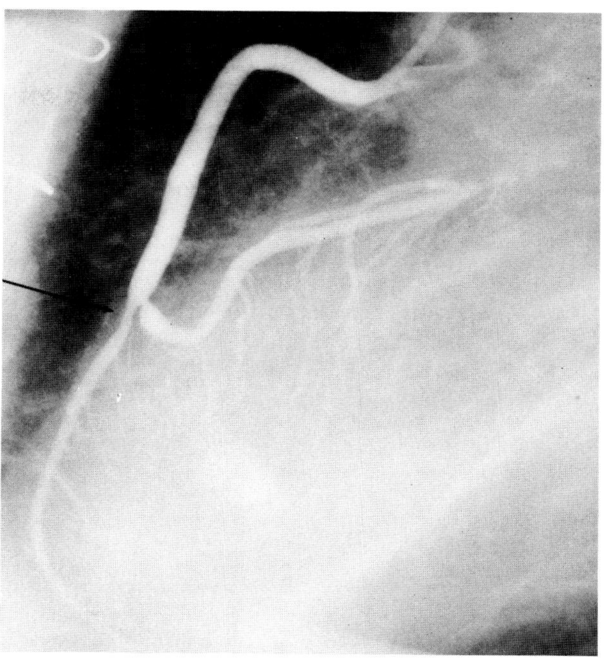

Figure 30-2. Selective LAD graft injection, lateral projection, demonstrating a widely patent graft, antegrade filling of the distal LAD, and retrograde filling of the proximal LAD. Tenting of the native coronary artery has occurred at the distal graft anastomosis (*arrow*).

Figure 30-3. (A) Selective LAD graft angiogram, lateral projection, shows filling of a patent graft containing a proximal stenosis and native LAD. The proximal portion of the graft courses anteriorly as it arches over the pulmonary artery (*arrow*). (B) Selective right graft injection, lateral projection, demonstrates an unusual anterior course of this graft, which is tethered retrosternally (*arrow*). Good distal and proximal filling of the native right coronary artery is seen.

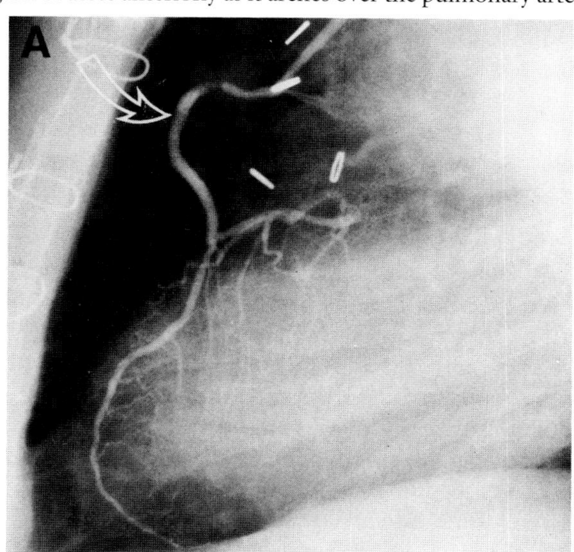

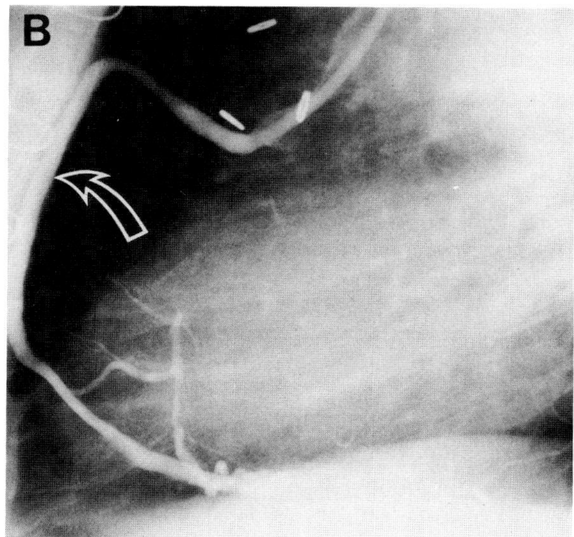

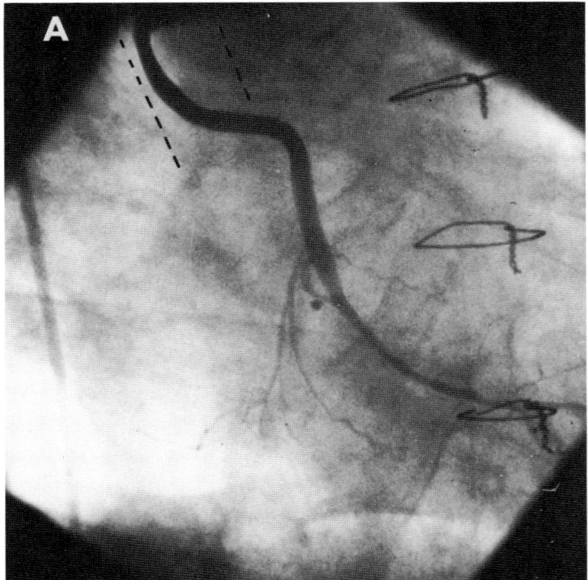

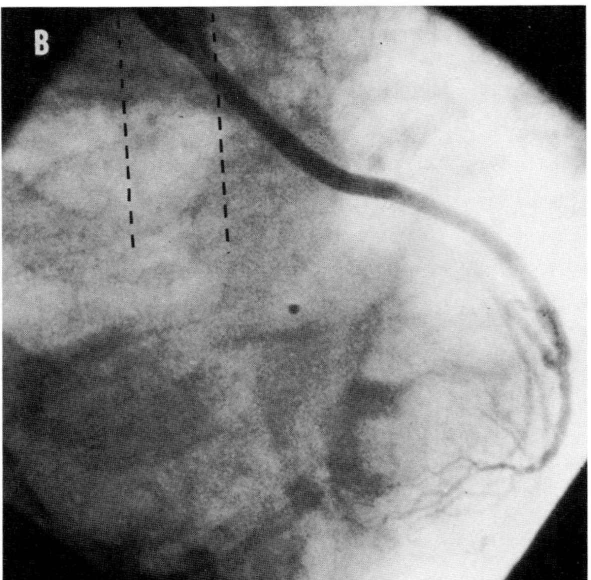

Figure 30-4. Selective obtuse marginal graft injections, RAO (A) and LAO (B) projections, demonstrate the artery's posterior aortic origin and posterior course above the left atrium to reach the lateral wall of the left ventricle. The *broken lines* indicate the approximate position of the aortic walls.

Anatomic Considerations

Saphenous vein coronary grafts use reversed veins and when opacified demonstrate linear radiolucent filling defects of venous valves. Occasionally tied-off side branches from the vein graft are seen as outpouchings.

In contrast to the grafts to the left coronary circulation, which course in varying obliquities anterior to the pulmonary artery, grafts to the right coronary artery course vertically in an inferior direction from their aortic origin parallel to the atrioventricular groove to reach the distal right coronary artery (Fig. 30-5; see Fig. 30-1).

Y Grafts

A graft that takes origin from another graft having two distal end-to-side anastomoses to native coronary arteries—the Y graft—is no longer performed. Graft patency was found inferior because of the propensity of branch thrombosis and subsequent propagation of thrombus to involve the main limb.

Types of Insertion

End-to-Side

The standard distal anastomosis of the vein graft is an end-to-side anastomosis into the distal coronary artery. The distal vein is cut obliquely to ensure adequate lumen at the anastomosis. To facilitate this anastomosis, the left anterior descending coronary artery is mobilized and lifted up. If the vein graft is short, further retraction produces tenting or kinking of the left anterior descending artery at the anastomosis (see Fig. 30-2).

Side-to-Side (Jump Graft)

"Snake" or jump grafts have become popular as a method for achieving grafts to several branches using one saphenous vein. Sequential side-to-side anastomoses are performed between the vein graft and several coronary arteries with a terminal end-to-side anastomosis (Fig. 30-6). Although there have been no systematic follow-up studies of these grafts to the best of our knowledge, patency rates appear clinically favorable.

Internal Mammary Artery Graft

Over the last 15 years, bypass grafting using the internal mammary artery has become the operation of choice for patients under the age of 65 requiring surgery to the left anterior descending coronary artery. This is because this artery remains virtually free of atheroma and retains the property of relaxation and flow regulation that is lost with venous conduits.[9] The patency rate for internal mammary artery grafts to the left anterior descending artery at 10 years is 90 percent.[10,11] There is some evidence that internal mammary grafts to other vessels do not have such a high patency rate,[12]

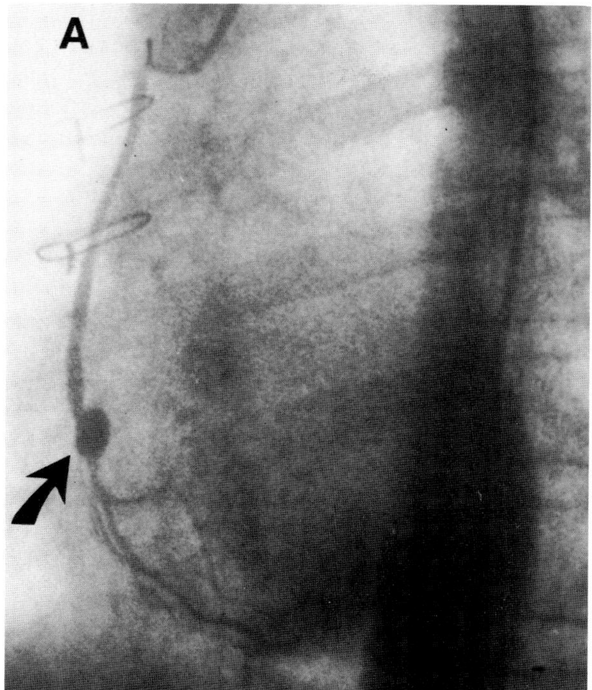

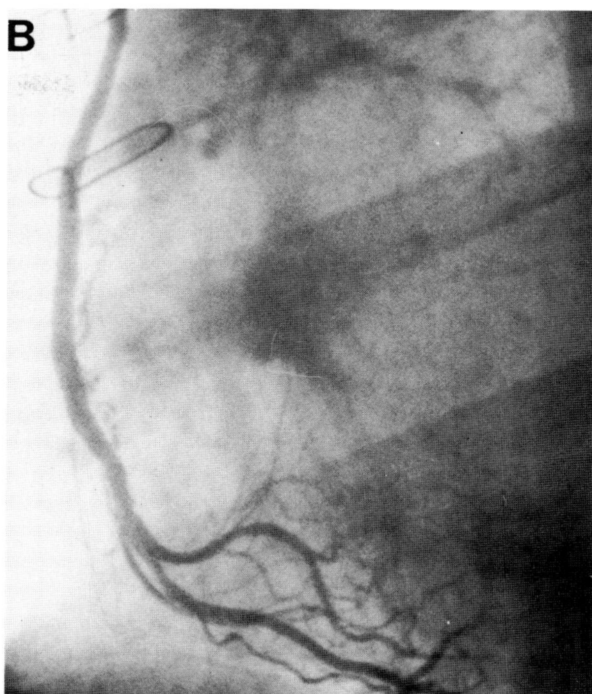

Figure 30-5. (A) Selective right graft injection at early study after surgery. A pseudoaneurysm is seen at the distal anastomotic site (*arrow*), which at follow-up 8 years after surgery (B) is no longer opacified.

although separate mammary grafts to the left anterior descending and circumflex arteries in left main stem disease can provide adequate blood flow to the entire left coronary system.[13] Patients with bilateral internal mammary grafts have the same survival rates as patients with single internal mammary grafts,[14] but there seems to be a higher morbidity from devascularization of the sternum than with venous grafting.[15]

Figure 30-6. Selective "jump" graft injections in RAO (A) and LAO (B) projections showing the first anastomosis (side-to-side) into a diagonal branch (*black arrows*) and a final anastomosis (end-to-side) into the LAD distally (*open arrows*).

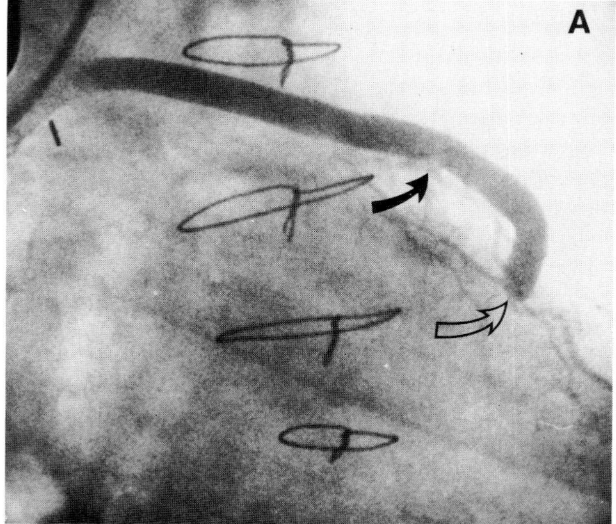

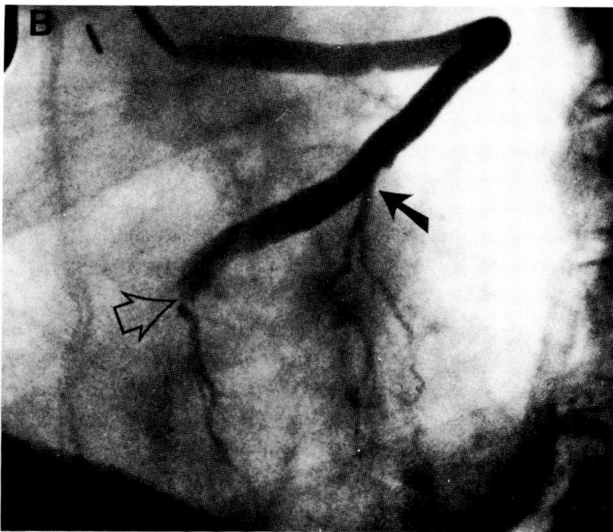

Angiography

Objectives of Angiographic Study

Although routine postoperative angiography is performed in some centers, the indication for performing graft angiography is usually a persistence or recrudescence of symptoms. Left ventricular function and segmental wall motion, graft patency and flow, and status of the native coronary circulation are all indicators of the adequacy of myocardial perfusion and the success of myocardial revascularization.

Angiographic evaluation, therefore, includes left ventriculography, measurement of aortic and left ventricular pressures, selective bypass angiography, and arteriography of the native coronary arteries to assess progression of atheroocclusive disease.[16]

Left Ventriculography

Left ventriculography provides a method of evaluating left ventricular wall motion.[17] Preoperative assessment is enhanced by interventional techniques using nitroglycerin or postextrasystolic potentiation.[18] These techniques allow one to predict potential reversibility of left ventricular contraction abnormalities. Myocardium that is ischemic but viable will presumably improve with revascularization compared with areas of previous myocardial infarction and myocardial fibrosis with irreversible contraction disorder. A normally contracting left ventricular wall segment must receive adequate blood supply, at least at rest, and be subserved by a patent graft, adequate collateral, or nonocclusive disease in the native coronary arteries. The functional status of the left ventricle as assessed by angiography remains an excellent determinant of operative risk and long-term survival after surgery.

Coronary Circulation

Graft Angiography

Catheter Selection and Use. Selective graft angiography is a modification of the techniques of coronary arteriography.[19] For a percutaneous approach to the grafts, an Amplatz right coronary catheter with a 2-cm primary curve and horizontal catheter tip[20,21] or a specifically designed Judkins graft catheter similar to a right coronary catheter but modified so that the tip has a smooth, downward-pointing terminal curve (3 cm) may be used (Fig. 30-7). But any catheter may be modified to accommodate the aortic width in a given patient and reach anteriorly to the graft orifices. The Judkins graft catheter is useful to engage the posterior grafts and may be employed like a Sones catheter by shaping its curve on the aortic valve. The same catheter can often be used for selective native right coronary injection, eliminating an additional catheter exchange. A final catheter exchange is made for a Judkins left coronary catheter to visualize the native left circulation.

Although the authors use the percutaneous transfemoral approach[22] or, in the presence of iliofemoral obstructive disease, the transaxillary route, the brachial approach of Sones is also feasible. The standard Sones catheters are then used to engage the graft orifices.[23] Selective graft and coronary injections are performed in multiple obliquities with axial angulation when indicated.

Selective catheterization of the internal mammary artery is usually performed with a preshaped catheter that has a hook-shaped distal end. Alternatively, a Judkins right coronary catheter modified with a more acutely angled tip can be used. The subclavian artery is engaged either by manipulation of the catheter or more often by the combination of a catheter and guidewire. The internal mammary catheter is then positioned in the subclavian artery usually distally to the internal mammary artery and slowly withdrawn until the internal mammary artery is engaged. Care should be taken because the internal mammary artery is small and the catheter can occlude this vessel more easily than a saphenous graft, with subsequent ischemia and precipitation of ventricular fibrillation.

Functional Considerations of Graft Injection. In most cases there is complete and prompt washout of contrast medium from the vein graft when the graft functions normally.[24] When the vein graft is disproportionately larger than the native coronary artery, however, slow flow in the graft and slow washout may be seen.

When a segment of the coronary artery receives blood flow from both the native circulation and a patent well-functioning graft, injection of either the graft or the native artery will demonstrate the segment. Often a bidirectional flow pattern[25] will be seen on graft injection, with alternate filling and emptying of the segment due to competitive flow of nonopaque blood from the unopacified circulation.

If the flow from the native circulation is minimal because of stenosis or occlusion, there will be no competitive flow when the graft is injected. Usually antegrade flow takes place from the graft into the coronary vessel distal to the anastomosis. There is often retrograde flow as well, with back-filling of significant branches of the native coronary artery. With a stenotic or poorly functioning vein graft, decreased antegrade filling of the distal coronary artery occurs.

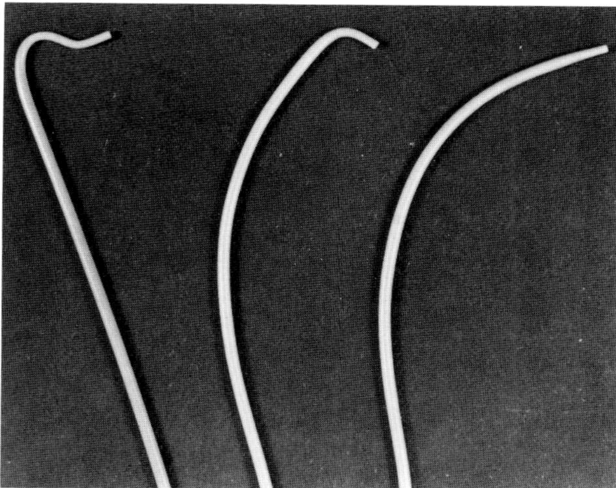

Figure 30-7. Catheters used for selective catheterization of coronary bypass grafts. *Left,* Amplatz right coronary catheter; *right,* modified right coronary catheter (graft catheter); *center,* standard Judkins right coronary catheter for comparison.

Status of Native Circulation

Functional Considerations of Native Coronary Injection. In the presence of a patent graft, selective injections into a native coronary artery may produce no opacification distally as nonopacified blood from the graft fills the distal vessel. The appearance of occlusion of the native coronary artery when, in reality, it is patent is called *pseudoocclusion* (Fig. 30-8). Injection of the graft may produce retrograde flow past the stenosis and prove the pseudoocclusion.[26,27] In the presence of a stenotic or occluded graft, only minimal or no washout of contrast by nonopacified blood flow is seen on selective coronary arteriography. Occasionally, native coronary injection may produce retrograde filling of a portion of a poorly functioning graft as a result of the lower pressure in the distal vein graft. Therefore, it is important to observe the flow patterns in the coronary vessels, since they give clues to the patency of grafts when their orifice is not readily engaged for contrast injection.

Collateral Circulation. If an obstructive lesion is successfully bypassed, intercoronary collateral circulation regresses. A good correlation has been demonstrated

Figure 30-8. (A) Selective LAD injection fails to fill the distal LAD (pseudoocclusion). (B) Selective LAD graft injection fills the distal and proximal LAD in both an antegrade and a retrograde fashion. (From Guthaner D, Wexler L. The radiologic evaluation of patients with coronary bypass. In: Moseley RD Jr, et al, eds. Current problems in diagnostic radiology. Chicago: Year Book, 1976. Used with permission.)

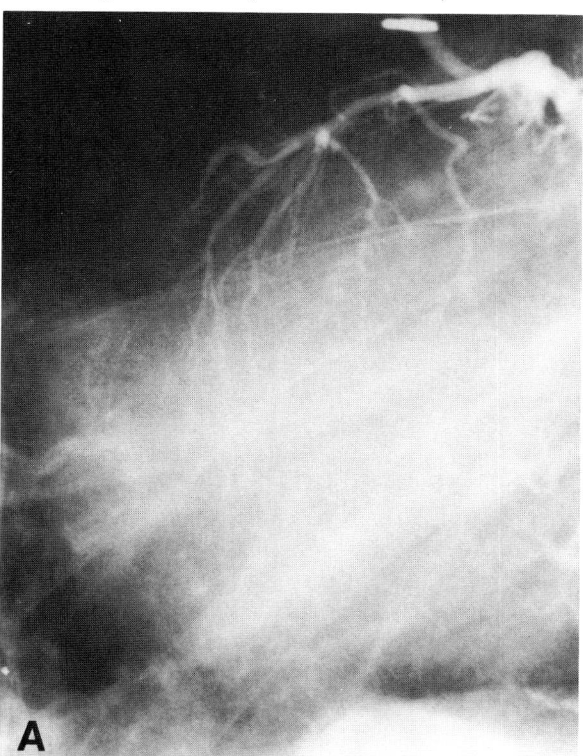

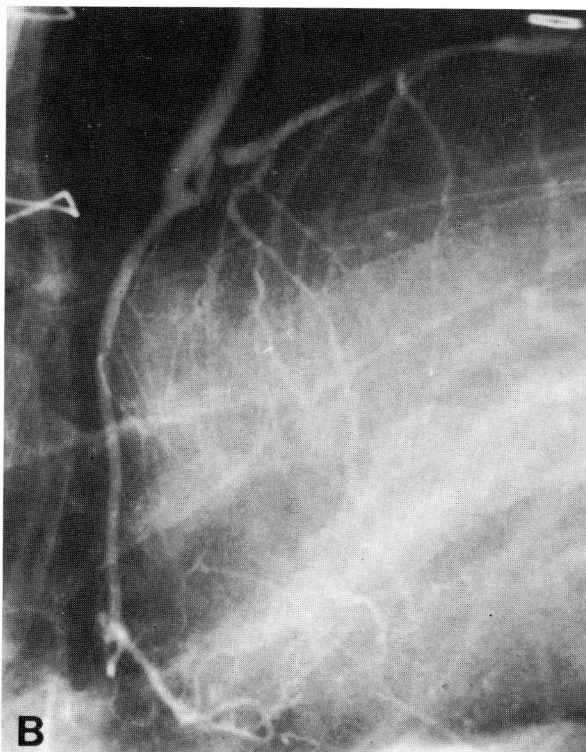

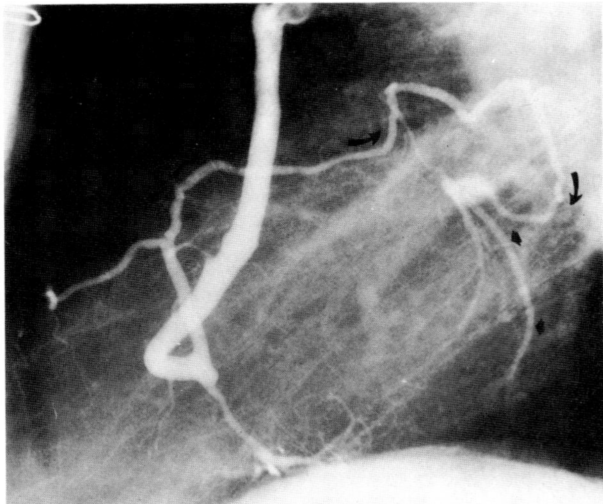

Figure 30-9. Right coronary graft injection fills the distal right coronary artery and an extensive collateral network (*long arrows*) from the sinoatrial branch of the right coronary artery that courses around the left atrium to the distal circumflex marginal system (*short arrows*). The occluded circumflex artery is dependent on the patent right graft.

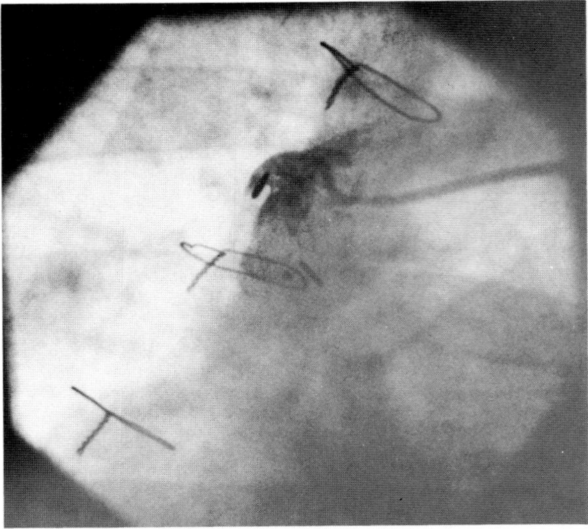

Figure 30-10. Attempted selective graft injection in an axial LAO projection demonstrating an outpouching beyond the aortic wall due to proximal occlusion of the graft. Metallic clips mark the aortic ostia of the grafts.

between graft patency and angiographic disappearance of preexistent collaterals.[28] Collateral flow patterns may therefore be another useful indicator of graft patency. In the presence of an occluded or stenotic graft, collaterals supplying the grafted artery will persist.[29,30] Reversal of collateral flow may occur when a patent graft to a previously occluded vessel now provides flow to another nonbypassed coronary artery or to a bypassed vessel whose graft is occluded or contains a significant stenosis (Fig. 30-9).

Angiographic Findings

Proximal Anastomosis

At the proximal anastomosis the proximal segment of the bypass graft is funnel-shaped and tends to arise from the aorta perpendicularly or at an acute angle. Ostial and proximal stenoses are optimally visualized in profile, requiring orthogonal projections for evaluation of the degree of stenosis. Most proximal stenoses are eccentric in nature, but occasionally concentric narrowing is seen as a result of periaortic fibrosis secondary to surgery, or sometimes to radiation therapy to the mediastinum. Intimal hyperplasia with accelerated atherosclerosis may also occur in the proximal graft segment.

In a small series of patients[31] followed for 5 to 7 years after surgery, proximal graft stenoses were found in 20 percent of patients, but it was impossible to predict long-term graft patency on the basis of early angiographic appearances. In another series,[32] graft occlusion was reported in 21.6 percent of stenotic grafts, whereas there were no late occlusions in normal-appearing grafts.

Graft occlusion may be confirmed by probing in the region of the aortic ostium to visualize the outpouching or small stump of the graft. The catheter tip may become engaged at the site of an occluded graft and is best seen at selective angiography (Fig. 30-10) in the appropriate obliquity that places the catheter tip projecting beyond the aortic wall. Supravalvular aortography may also be used to demonstrate grafts. Those arising from the right anterolateral aspect of the aorta to the right coronary artery are best seen in a steep left anterior oblique projection, and grafts to the left coronary system in a shallow right anterior oblique projection. However, aortography is not an infallible approach to visualizing occluded grafts. Contrast layering posteriorly may not fill the anteriorly located grafts, or the obliquity may not be optimum for visualizing the ostium of an occluded graft in profile. Nonfilling of a graft on supravalvular aortography is a considerably less reliable indicator of graft occlusion than visualization of the stump in profile, or selective catheterization and angiography of the stump.

Body of Graft

Irrespective of the original size of the vein used for grafting, its caliber gradually approaches the size of the native coronary artery during the first year.[33,34] The diffuse diameter reduction is produced by the development of intimal hyperplasia throughout the graft length and is related to arterialization of the vein graft.[35] Intimal hyperplasia may occur diffusely over a long segment or focally, often originating at the site of a venous valve. Pathologically, intimal fibrous proliferation is associated with circumferential fibrous myointimal thickening, proliferation of smooth muscle cells, and subsequent medial fibrosis. Although obliterative intimal hyperplasia is demonstrated in the first year after surgery, further significant reduction in caliber and late occlusion are not common.[36] In one series, although focal stenoses developed at a yearly rate of 15 percent, there was no change in the diffusely narrowed graft segments at late follow-up.[32] It would therefore appear that intimal hyperplasia may progress but is not a significant factor in long-term graft occlusion.[32,37–41]

Angiographically, intimal hyperplasia may be seen as diffuse, smooth narrowing or a shagginess involving a long or short segment of the entire length of the graft (Fig. 30-11). There may be associated accelerated atherosclerosis with eccentric, irregular lesions, platelet deposition, and thrombus formation.

Occasionally, an anteriorly positioned venous graft or a mobilized internal mammary artery may become adherent to the sternum as a result of postoperative scarring and fibrosis (see Fig. 30-3B).

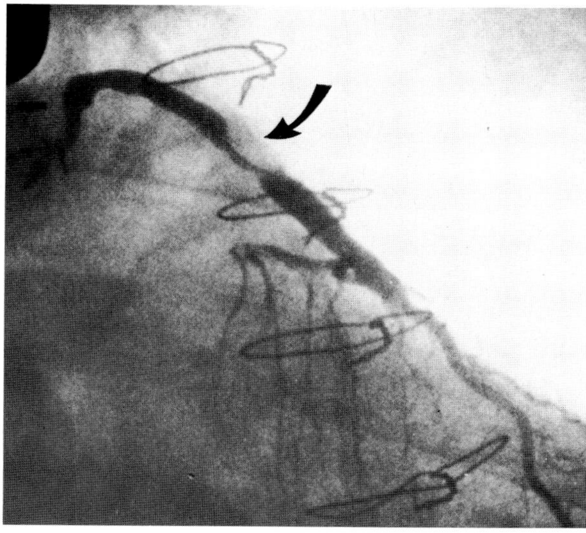

Figure 30-11. Selective LAD graft angiogram 5 years postoperatively demonstrates a focal stenosis in the midportion of the body of the vein graft (*arrow*) due to intimal hyperplasia. The graft remains patent, filling both the distal and proximal LAD.

Distal Anastomosis

The distal anastomoses are performed either end-to-side or side-to-side (in jump grafts). Often a left anterior descending artery graft is short, and retraction of the coronary artery at the distal anastomotic site occurs (see Fig. 30-2). Narrowing of the native coronary artery in this situation is unlikely to progress to significance.

Stenoses may occur in (1) the distal graft or (2) the native coronary artery at the distal anastomotic site. Predictive factors for long-term graft patency are not apparent angiographically in the presence of a distal anastomotic stenosis.[31,42]

False aneurysms or pseudoaneurysms occur rarely at the anastomotic site (see Fig. 30-5). They probably result from leakage at the suture line. Some heal themselves by thrombosis (see Fig. 30-5), some remain, and in some the thrombus extends to partially compromise the lumen of the graft.

Progression of Disease in Native Vessels

Nonbypassed Vessels

Progression of coronary atheroocclusive disease continues in an unpredictable fashion. Several series have shown that late symptomatic deterioration is related to the continued march of the atherosclerotic disease process (Fig. 30-12).[42]

Bypassed Vessels

Progression of coronary artery occlusive disease proximal to the graft anastomosis is accelerated,[36,43] probably because decreased blood flow through the stenotic segment predisposes to thrombosis. This progression may involve branches such as diagonals arising proximal to the graft anastomosis. Accelerated progression of occlusive disease distal to the graft anastomosis is a controversial question. Several groups reported increased progression,[26,44] supposedly due to increased turbulence of blood flow downstream. The authors have not confirmed these reports and have found no significant difference in disease progression in grafted vessels distal to the anastomosis compared to nongrafted vessels in the same patient.[31,32,45]

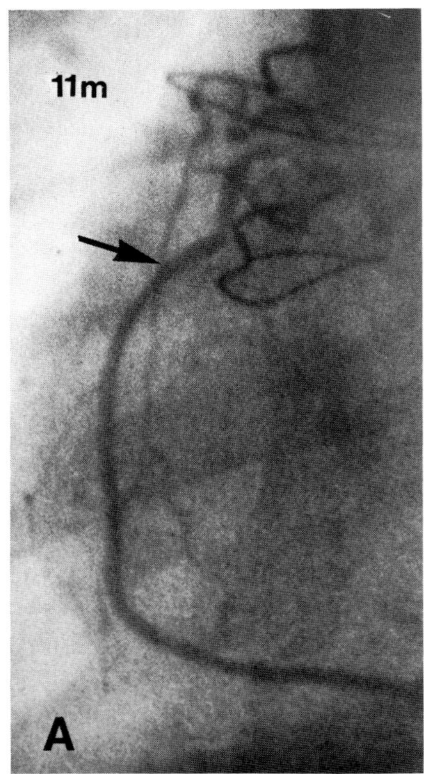

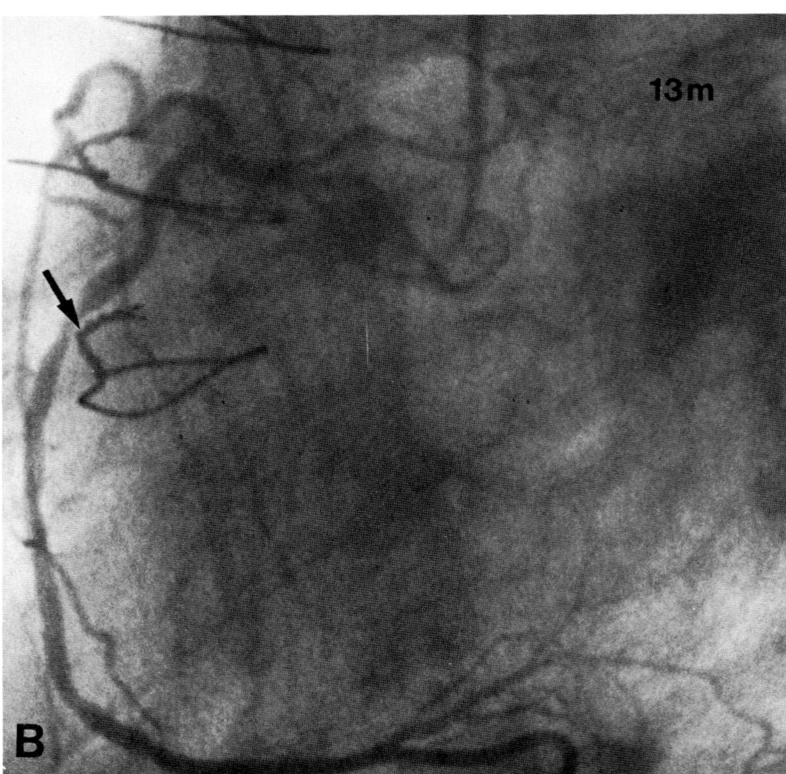

Figure 30-12. (A) Selective right coronary arteriogram, 11 months after bypass surgery to another vessel (*arrow*). (B) At 13 months following surgery, a tight stenosis is seen in the nonbypassed right coronary artery in a segment free from angiographic evidence of disease on the previous study (*arrow*).

Internal Mammary Graft Disease

The internal mammary artery shows greater long-term patency than saphenous grafts. Autopsy studies have shown that atherosclerosis occurs in only 4 percent of routine autopsies in patients with internal mammary grafts.[46] Early disease in this vessel at 1 to 6 months tends to occur at the site of anastomosis with the native coronary artery or occasionally at the origin of the vessel. Such lesions are usually treatable by coronary angioplasty.[47] Disease of the subclavian artery can also affect the flow in the internal mammary artery.

Clinical Significance

Although the final place of myocardial revascularization by direct coronary artery bypass grafting in the therapeutic approaches to coronary artery disease has not yet been established, the procedure enjoys continued popularity. The relief of angina and survival after coronary bypass surgery are related to the completeness of revascularization and graft patency. Studies

Figure 30-13. Computed tomographic scan after coronary artery bypass surgery to the LAD. After administration of a bolus of contrast medium, the ascending (*Ao*) and descending (*DAo*) aorta is opacified. The graft (*arrow*) is seen arising from the aorta anteriorly, passing anterior to the pulmonary artery (*PA*), toward the interventricular groove. (From Guthaner DF, Brody WR, Ricci M, Oyer PE, Wexler L. The use of computed tomography in the diagnosis of coronary artery bypass graft patency. Cardiovasc Intervent Radiol 1980;3:3. Used with permission.)

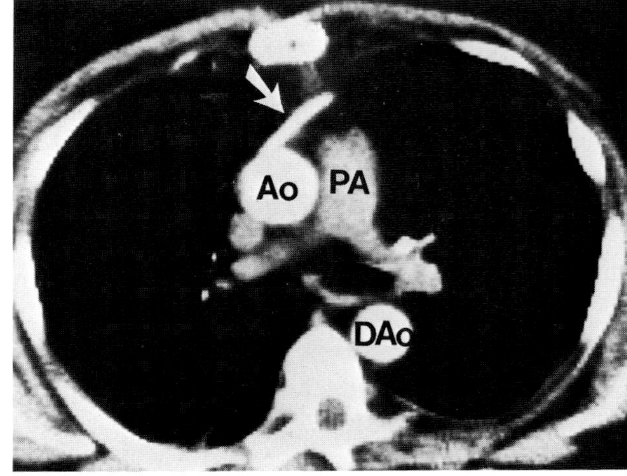

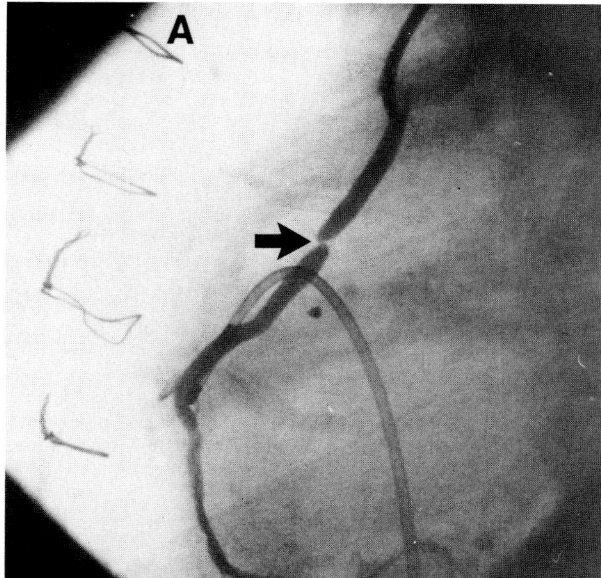

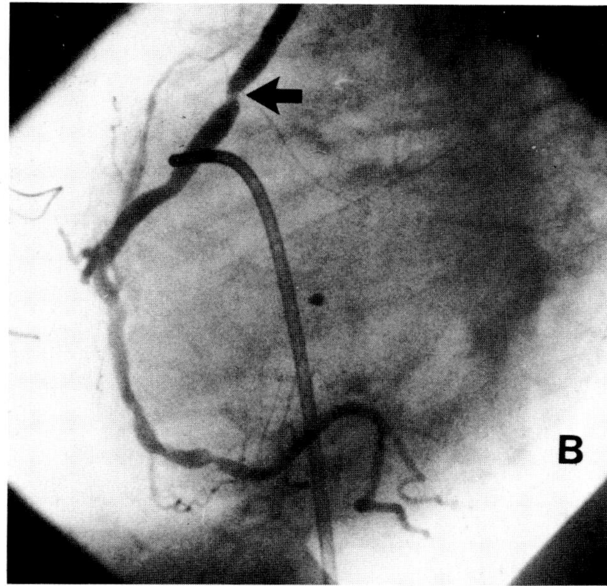

Figure 30-14. (A) Selective right graft angiogram demonstrating a tight stenosis in its midportion (*arrow*). (B) Following balloon inflation and graft dilatation, selective graft injection shows increased graft caliber (*arrow*).

have shown that bypass surgery offers excellent symptomatic relief for patients with atheroocclusive coronary artery disease. Graft patency correlates well with symptomatic relief.[48,49] However, long-term studies suggest that relief of angina may be only short-term, with recrudescence of angina or symptomatic deterioration from atherosclerotic disease.[42,50–53] But whether there is also increased longevity can be resolved only as results of long-term follow-up studies become more widely available. Several retrospective studies suggest improved prognosis with surgery in patients with "critical" lesions, two- and three-vessel disease, and left main coronary artery disease.[52–54]

Graft patency is related to multiple factors, such as the surgical technique, the quality of the autologous vein used, the site of coronary anastomosis, abnormalities of lipids and platelets, left ventricular wall motion, and the area of left ventricular wall supplied. The most significant factor is the condition of the recipient coronary artery and the size of the distal runoff. This can be estimated at the time of surgery by measuring blood flow in the graft after anastomoses are completed. Patency is better in high-flow grafts (greater than 45 ml/min) and poor in low-flow grafts (less than 20 ml/min).[55] Graft occlusion tends to occur in the first few months postoperatively (10–30 percent),[48,52,56] and if the graft is patent at 1 year, the long-term prognosis is excellent,[32,45] with an average annual attrition rate approaching 2 percent.

The use of computed tomography and magnetic resonance imaging continues to be only of some interest for determining graft patency.[57] This technique would facilitate screening of patients after surgery (Fig. 30-13).

With the development of angioplasty techniques for peripheral vessel dilatation, there has been successful application of the technique to coronary artery occlusive disease[58] (Fig. 30-14) and to venous grafts. This technique has become a helpful adjunct to surgery, particularly when used to dilate stenotic vein grafts without a second operation.

References

1. Favaloro RG. Saphenous vein graft in the surgical treatment of coronary artery disease: operative technique. J Thorac Cardiovasc Surg 1969;58:178.
2. Johnson WD, Flemma RJ, Lepley D Jr, Ellison EH. Extended treatment of severe coronary artery disease: a total surgical approach. Ann Surg 1969;170:460–470.
3. Proudfit WL, Kramer JR, Goormastic M, Loop FD: Ten year survival of patients with mild angina or myocardial infarction without angina: a comparison of medical and surgical treatment. Am Heart J 1990;119:942–948.
4. Cameron A, Brogno DA, Green GE. Internal thoracic artery grafts, twenty years clinical follow up. Circulation 1991; 84(Suppl II):463.
5. Carpentier A, Guermonprez JL, Deloche A, Frechette C, DuBost C. The aorta-to-coronary radial artery by-pass graft. Ann Thorac Surg 1973;16:111–121.

6. Pym J, Brown PM, Charrette EJP, Parker JO, West RO. Gastroepiploic-coronary anastomosis: a viable alternative bypass graft. J Thorac Cardiovasc Surg 1990;99:251–255.
7. Puig LB, Ciongolli W, Cividanes GVL, Dontos A, Kopel L, Bittencort D, et al. Inferior epigastric artery as a free graft for myocardial revascularisation. J Thorac Cardiovasc Surg 1990; 99:251–255.
8. Foster ED, Kranc MA. Alternative conduits for aortocoronary bypass grafting. Circulation 1989;79(Suppl I):34.
9. Luscher TJ, et al. Differences between endothelium dependent relaxation in arterial and venous coronary bypass grafts. N Engl J Med 1988;319:462.
10. Ivert T, Huttunen K, Landou C, Bjork VO. Angiographic studies of internal mammary artery grafts 11 years after coronary artery bypass grafting. J Thorac Cardiovasc Surg 1988;96:1.
11. Acinapura AJ, et al. Internal mammary artery bypass grafting: influence on recurrent angina and survival in 2,100 patients. Ann Thorac Surg 1989;48:186.
12. Huddleston CB, et al. Internal mammary grafts: technical factors influencing patency. Ann Thorac Surg 1986;42:583.
13. Barner HB, Naunheim KS, Willman VL, Fiore AC. Revascularization with bilateral internal thoracic artery grafts in patients with left main coronary stenosis. Eur J Cardiothorac Surg 1992;6:66.
14. Galbut DL, et al. Seventeen year experience with bilateral internal mammary artery grafts. Ann Thorac Surg 1990;49:195.
15. Seyfer AE, Shriver CD, Miller TR, Graeber GM. Sternal blood flow after median sternotomy and mobilization of the internal mammary arteries. Surgery 1988;104:899.
16. Guthaner DF, Wexler L. The radiologic evaluation of patients with coronary bypass. Curr Probl Diagn Radiol 1976;6:19.
17. Martin EC, Wixson D, Baltaxe HA. Regional ejection fractions in patients with patent and thrombosed grafts after coronary artery vein bypass surgery. Invest Radiol 1977;12:205.
18. Banka VS, Bodenheimer MM, Shah R, Helfant RH. Intervention ventriculography: comparative value of nitroglycerin, post-extrasystolic potentiation and nitroglycerin plus postextrasystolic potentiation. Circulation 1976;53:632.
19. Judkins MP. Selective coronary arteriography: I. A percutaneous transfemoral technic. Radiology 1967;89:815.
20. Amplatz K, Formanek G, Stanger P, Wilson W. Mechanics of selective coronary artery catheterization via femoral approach. Radiology 1967;89:1040.
21. Baltaxe HA, Amplatz K, Levin DC. Coronary angiography. Springfield, IL: Charles C Thomas, 1973.
22. Ricketts HJ, Abrams HL. Percutaneous selective coronary cine arteriography. JAMA 1962;181:620.
23. Sones MF Jr, Shirey EK. Cine coronary arteriography. Mod Concepts Cardiovasc Dis 1962;31:735.
24. Baltaxe HA, Carlson RG, Lillehei CW. Roentgenographic appearance of aortocoronary artery bypass using a reversed saphenous vein. Circulation 1970;110:734.
25. Levin DC, Baltaxe HA, Carlson RG. Angiographic demonstration of bidirectional coronary artery blood flow following aortocoronary bypass vein grafts. AJR 1971;113:554.
26. Griffith LSC, Achuff SC, Conti CR, Humphries JO, Brawley RK, Gott VL, Ross RS. Changes in intrinsic coronary circulation and segmental ventricular motion after saphenous-vein coronary bypass graft surgery. N Engl J Med 1973;288:589.
27. Ross AM, Hammond GL, Cohen LS, Wolfson S. Angiographic evaluation of saphenous vein bypass grafts: artifactual "occlusion" caused by dual sources of flow. Am J Cardiol 1977;39: 384.
28. Glassman E, Spencer FC, Krauss KR, Weisinger B, Isom OW. Changes in underlying coronary circulation secondary to bypass grafting: circulation secondary to bypass grafting. Circulation 1974;49,50(Suppl II):80.
29. Levin DC, Sos T, Beckmann C, Sniderman K. Effect of coronary bypass surgery on collateral circulation. Circulation 1979; 59,60(Suppl II):162.
30. McLaughlin PR, et al. Saphenous vein bypass grafting: changes in native circulation and collaterals. Circulation 1975;52(Suppl I):1.
31. Guthaner DF, Robert EW, Alderman EL, Wexler L. Long-term serial angiographic studies after coronary artery bypass surgery. Circulation 1979;60:250.
32. Campeau L, Lesperance J, Corbara F, Hermann J, Grondin CM, Bourassa MG. Aortocoronary saphenous vein bypass graft changes 5 to 7 years after surgery. Circulation 1978;58(Suppl I):170.
33. Spray TL, Roberts WC. Changes in saphenous veins used as aortocoronary bypass grafts. Am Heart J 1977;94:500.
34. Vlodaver Z, Edwards JE. Pathologic changes in aortic coronary arterial saphenous vein grafts. Circulation 1971;44:719.
35. Brody WR, Angell WW, Kosek JC. Histologic fate of the venous coronary artery bypass in dogs. Am J Pathol 1972;66:111.
36. Bourassa MG, Lesperance J, Corbara F, Saltiel J, Campeau L. Progression of obstructive coronary artery disease 5 to 7 years after aortocoronary bypass surgery. Circulation 1978;58:100.
37. Grondin CM, Lepage G, Castonguay YR, Meere C, Grondin P. Aortocoronary bypass graft: initial blood flow through the graft and early postoperative patency. Circulation 1971;44: 815.
38. Grondin CM, Lesperance J, Bourassa MG, Pasternac A, Campeau L, Grondin P. Serial angiographic evaluation in 60 consecutive patients with aortocoronary artery vein grafts 2 weeks, 1 year and 3 years after operation. J Thorac Cardiovasc Surg 1974;67:1.
39. Lawrie GM, Lie JT, Morris GC, Beazley HL. Vein graft patency and intimal proliferation after aortocoronary bypass: early and long-term angiopathologic correlations. Am J Cardiol 1976; 38:856.
40. Lawrie GM, Morris GC, Chapman DW, Winters WL, Lie JT. Patterns of patency of 596 vein grafts up to seven years after aortocoronary bypass. J Thorac Cardiovasc Surg 1977;73:443.
41. Lesperance J, Bourassa MG, Saltiel J, Grondin CM. Late changes in aortocoronary vein grafts: angiographic features. AJR 1972;116:74.
42. Robert EW, Guthaner DF, Wexler L, Alderman EL. Six-year clinical and angiographic follow-up of patients with previously documented complete revascularization. Circulation 1978; 58(Suppl I):194.
43. Aldridge HE, Trimble AS. Progression of proximal coronary artery lesions to total occlusion after aortocoronary saphenous vein bypass grafting. J Thorac Cardiovasc Surg 1971;62:7.
44. Maurer BJ, Oberman A, Holt JH Jr, Kouchoukos NT, Jones WB, Russell RO, Reeves TJ. Changes in grafted and nongrafted coronary arteries following saphenous vein bypass grafting. Circulation 1974;50:293.
45. Lesperance J, Bourassa MG, Saltiel J, Campeau L, Grondin CM. Angiographic changes in aortocoronary vein grafts: lack of progression beyond the first year. Circulation 1973;48:633.
46. Kay HR, Korns ME, Flemma RJ, Tector AJ, Lepley D. Atherosclerosis of the internal mammary artery. Ann Thorac Surg 1976;21:504–507.
47. Shimshak TM, Giorgi LV, Johnson WL, Mcconahay DR, Rutherford BD, Ligon R, Hartzler GO. Application of percutaneous coronary angioplasty to the internal mammary artery graft. J Am Coll Cardiol 1988;12:1205–1214.
48. Alderman EL, Matloff HJ, Wexler L, Shumway NE, Harrison DC. Results of direct coronary artery surgery for the treatment of angina pectoris. N Engl J Med 1973;288:535.
49. Matloff HJ, Alderman EL, Wexler L, Shumway NE, Harrison DC. What is the relationship between the response of angina to coronary surgery and anatomical success? Circulation 1973; 47, 48(Suppl III):168.
50. Cameron A, Kemp HG Jr, Shimomura S, Santilli E, Green GE, Hutchinson JE, Mekhjian HA. Aortocoronary bypass surgery: a 7-year follow-up. Circulation 1979;60:1.
51. Campeau L, Lesperance J, Hermann J, Corbara F, Grondin CM, Bourassa MG. Loss of the improvement of angina between 1 and 7 years after aortocoronary bypass surgery: correla-

tions with changes in vein grafts and in coronary arteries. Circulation 1979;60(Suppl I):1.
52. Sheldon WC, Rincon G, Effler DB, Proudfit WL, Sones FM Jr. Vein graft surgery for coronary artery disease: survival and angiographic results in 1000 patients. Circulation 1973;47, 48(Suppl III):184.
53. Tecklenberg PL, Alderman EL, Miller DC, Shumway NE, Harrison DC. Changes in survival and symptom relief in a longitudinal study of patients after bypass surgery. Circulation 1975; 51, 52(Suppl I):98.
54. Takaro T, Hultgren HN, Detre KM. VA cooperative study of coronary arterial surgery: II. Left main disease. Circulation 1975;52:143.
55. Walker JA, Freidberg HD, Flemma RJ, Johnson WD. Determinants of angiographic patency of aortocoronary vein bypass grafts. Circulation 1972;45(Suppl I):86.
56. Lesperance J, Bourassa MG, Biron P, Campeau L, Saltiel J. Aorta to coronary artery saphenous vein grafts: preoperative angiographic criteria for successful surgery. Am J Cardiol 1972; 30:459.
57. Guthaner DF, Brody WR, Ricci M, Oyer PE, Wexler L. The use of computed tomography in the diagnosis of coronary artery bypass graft patency. Cardiovasc Intervent Radiol 1980; 3:3.
58. Grüntzig AR, Senning A, Siegenthaler WE. Nonoperative dilatation of coronary artery stenosis: percutaneous transluminal coronary angioplasty (PTCA). N Engl J Med 1979;301:61.

31

Pulmonary Arteriography: Indications, Technique, Normal Findings, and Complications

ROBERT E. BARTON
PAUL C. LAKIN
JOSEF RÖSCH

Historical Overview

In its early stages pulmonary arteriography was a part of cardiac visualization, or angiocardiography. Two techniques were used: a needle technique and a catheter technique. With the needle technique contrast medium was injected through one or two needles introduced into an antecubital vein or veins. The needle technique was perfected by Robb and Steinberg[1] in the 1930s and was used extensively by Dotter.[2] With the catheter technique, which was pioneered by Forssmann in the early 1930s,[3,4] a catheter was introduced by a cubital vein cutdown and contrast medium was injected directly into the heart or into the superior vena cava (SVC). Both of these techniques were still in use when pulmonary arteriography came into clinical use more than 3 decades later. In 1963 Williams and associates,[5] using the technique of Robb and Steinberg, reported the first large series in which pulmonary embolism was diagnosed angiographically.

With development of the Seldinger technique of percutaneous catheter introduction,[6] the needle technique was completely abandoned and catheter pulmonary arteriography began its rapid development. Sasahara and colleagues[7] in 1964 first reported using selective pulmonary arteriography to detect pulmonary emboli, and selective arteriography soon became the standard for visualizing the pulmonary circulation.[8-11] Dotter[2] described it as "a technically sophisticated means of obtaining highly detailed studies of local, gross pulmonary vascular anatomy in normal and diseased states." Studies were usually performed through an antecubital vein cutdown, but other routes such as jugular,[12] axillary,[13] and subclavian[14] veins were also used. General purpose straight or slightly bent catheters were initially employed, but these permitted only limited selective catheterization and their use entailed some risks.[8,15] Selective pulmonary arteriography usually involved injecting contrast into the main pulmonary artery. Improved catheters followed, however, that permitted more selective catheterization and visualization of individual pulmonary arteries. Segmental arteriography capable of demonstrating emboli in very small branches was described by Bookstein[16] in 1969. Cut-film serialography, which yields high-quality images of the entire lung, emerged as the preferred means of recording the studies.

Two final developments in the late 1960s brought pulmonary arteriography to its present status as a simple and safe procedure yielding optimal visualization of the entire pulmonary circulation or its parts. In 1969 Ranniger[15] demonstrated that selective pulmonary arteriography could be performed safely from the femoral approach using the Seldinger technique. This approach proved much simpler and faster than the traditional antecubital cutdown, and made pulmonary arteriography more practical in emergency situations. It was Grollman and colleagues,[17] however, who in 1970 described the method that would become the standard technique of performing pulmonary arteriography. They reported using a new "pulmonary artery–seeking" pigtail catheter that was introduced through the femoral approach to perform bilateral selective pulmonary artery injections. This method greatly simplified pulmonary arteriography and resulted in far fewer catheter-related complications. Bilateral selective injections provided much better image quality than the main pulmonary artery injections that were commonly used at that time. The Grollman technique remains in widespread use today.

Subsequent developments such as digital subtraction arteriography,[18,19] balloon occlusion pulmonary arteriography,[20,21] and pulmonary cineangiography[22] have served to complement rather than replace conventional cut-film pulmonary arteriography. Recent advances in imaging modalities such as CT and MRI are promising and may permit noninvasive evaluation of the pulmonary circulation in certain situations, but to date none of the newer imaging modalities rivals selective arteriography. Pulmonary arteriography as it is performed today is simple, safe, and reliable. It remains the best way to visualize the pulmonary vasculature.

General Anatomic and Functional Considerations

The pulmonary vascular bed differs substantially from the systemic vascular bed in anatomic structure, dynamics, and function.

Anatomically, there are three types of pulmonary arteries.[23] (1) *Elastic pulmonary arteries* include the main pulmonary artery and its branches down to the extralobular branches that are 1 mm in diameter. These contain primarily layers of elastic fibers with a minimal number of muscle cells. (2) *Muscular pulmonary arteries* are 100 to 1000 μm in diameter and accompany pulmonary branchioles within the lobules. These have a distinct muscular layer interspersed between the internal and external elastic laminae. (3) *Pulmonary arterioles* supply alveolar ducts and alveoli and are less than 100 μm in diameter. They contain progressively fewer muscle cells and are primarily endothelial tubes with minimal elastic support.

Hemodynamically, the pulmonary circulation is a low-resistance, low-pressure, highly distensible system. The absence of terminal muscular arterioles and the voluminous thin-walled pulmonary capillaries contribute to the low resistance and high distensibility of the pulmonary circulation. The pulmonary vascular resistance is about one-sixth of the systemic circulation, with the pulmonary arterial pressure averaging about 22/8 mmHg (mean 13 mmHg). The degree of distensibility of the normal pulmonary vascular bed allows the pulmonary blood flow to triple without a significant increase in pulmonary artery pressure. The work of the right ventricle is thus much less than that of the left, and consequently the right ventricle has considerably less muscle than the left. Although there is little vasomotor control, the pulmonary circulation is responsive to neurohumoral stimuli and to pharmacologic agents. Pulmonary arterial muscular tone responds to abnormal alveolar O_2 or CO_2 and abnormal arterial blood pH or low PO_2.[24,25] Serotonin, histamine, prostaglandin F_{2a} (PGF_{2a}), thromboxane A_2, leukotrienes, and platelet-activating factor are among the naturally occurring compounds that can increase pulmonary vascular resistance.[26]

The principal *function* of the pulmonary circulation is the exchange of oxygen and carbon dioxide between alveolar air and blood in the pulmonary capillaries. Because of its position, the pulmonary vascular bed also functions as a filter for foreign particles, thrombi, and other embolic debris circulating in the systemic venous blood. By virtue of its separate blood supply via systemic bronchial arteries, the pulmonary vascular tree can filter out even major emboli without self-destruction. Bronchial arteries dilate to supply necessary oxygenated blood to portions of the lung where pulmonary arterial flow is reduced or arrested.

Indications

The most common indication for pulmonary arteriography is suspected pulmonary embolism. Selective arteriography is the most reliable means of establishing or excluding the diagnosis of acute pulmonary embolism; however, its precise role has been controversial. The invasive nature of angiography and its perceived risks have led many to turn to other modalities, predominately lung ventilation-perfusion scanning, to diagnose this entity. In 1977 Robin[27] asserted that overreliance on perfusion scanning had led to pulmonary embolism being overdiagnosed and overtreated. This, together with the realization that heparinization, the preferred treatment for pulmonary embolism, was a major cause of drug-related mortality and morbidity,[28–30] prompted critical reevaluation of the roles of the various diagnostic modalities. The limitations of lung scanning have since become clear, and the safety[31–34] and reliability[35,36] of pulmonary arteriography have been firmly established.

Several reports in the past 15 years have helped to clarify the relative roles of pulmonary arteriography and ventilation-perfusion scanning in the evaluation of suspected pulmonary embolism.[34,36–40] Foremost among these is the prospective investigation of pulmonary embolism diagnosis (PIOPED) study. In view of the controversy that has existed regarding the diagnosis of pulmonary embolism, several points from this study are worth noting.

First, a normal ventilation-perfusion scan virtually excludes the possibility that pulmonary embolism has occurred. In the PIOPED study[36] only 4 percent of patients with a normal scan were subsequently shown to have pulmonary emboli. Others have shown even lower false-negative rates.[41]

A low-probability scan is somewhat less useful. Patients with such a scan are generally felt to have about a 10 percent chance of having had a pulmonary embolus.[42] In the PIOPED study[36] the actual probability was at least 12 percent. The value of a low-probability scan in excluding embolism is enhanced when clinical assessment of the patient is taken into consideration. In the PIOPED study[36] the incidence of documented pulmonary embolism in patients with a low-probability scan who were considered clinically unlikely to have pulmonary embolism was only 4 percent. On the other hand, pulmonary emboli were demonstrated angiographically in 16 percent and 40 percent, respectively, of those with intermediate and high clinical probability. Therefore, the low-probability ventilation-perfusion scan appears highly reliable only when it agrees with the clinical impression.

An intermediate-probability scan is generally agreed to be of no value in either establishing or excluding the diagnosis of pulmonary embolism. Patients in this group have about a 30 percent probability of having had a pulmonary embolus[29,36,41,42] and should undergo pulmonary arteriography. In the PIOPED study[36] 40 percent of the patients fell into this group.

A high-probability ventilation-perfusion scan is fairly specific in diagnosing pulmonary embolism, but occurs in only about 40 percent of patients with emboli.[36] High-probability scans have a positive predictive value of about 90 percent.[36,41] When scan results agree with the clinical assessment and there is no history of prior emboli, the reliability increases to 98 percent.[36] However, in patients who have had pulmonary emboli in the past, a new high-probability scan has a positive predictive value of only 74 percent.[36]

These findings indicate that ventilation-perfusion scanning is most useful at the extremes. The lung scan alone is usually sufficient when normal, or when a high- or low-probability study agrees with the clinical assessment. Unfortunately, many patients with suspected pulmonary embolism do not fall into one of these categories. According to the investigators in the PIOPED study,[36] "the scan combined with clinical assessment permitted a noninvasive diagnosis or exclusion of acute pulmonary embolism for a minority of patients." This is not to say that ventilation-perfusion scanning is of no value. Scintigraphy yields a highly reliable diagnosis in more than one-third of cases. In the remainder it may direct the angiographer to those areas of the lung where emboli are most likely to be found.

Based on these data, the indications for pulmonary arteriography in the diagnosis of acute pulmonary embolism at our institution are similar to those listed by Kramer et al.[43]:

1. An intermediate or indeterminate lung scan
2. A high-probability lung scan in someone with a relative contraindication to anticoagulation or a history of prior pulmonary embolism
3. A low-probability lung scan in someone in whom there is a moderate to high clinical suspicion of pulmonary embolism
4. Before insertion of an inferior vena cava (IVC) filter
5. Before anticipated surgical or catheter embolectomy

These indications are not absolute, however. As with any procedure, the risks of the procedure must be weighed against the benefits of establishing an accurate diagnosis.

Acute pulmonary embolism is not the only indication for pulmonary arteriography. It is also important for diagnosis and interventional treatment of pulmonary arteriovenous fistulas, for evaluation of vascular extension of lung tumors, and for evaluation of pulmonary hypertension. Pulmonary arteriography should also be done in patients with recurrent hemoptysis not explained by bronchial arteriography. Lesions such as Rasmussen aneurysms or pulmonary vascular involvement from necrotic parenchymal infections can account for hemoptysis in approximately 5 percent of cases.

Procedure of Selective Pulmonary Arteriography

Preparation

As in any angiographic study, the clinical problem is reviewed and the patient is visited by the angiographer, who personally obtains informed consent. Laboratory studies such as for serum creatine and potassium levels are checked and a history of allergic reaction to prior contrast injections is sought. Chest radiographs are reviewed for pulmonary pathology and heart size, particularly the size of the right atrium. The latter is important for selection of a proper catheter. When pulmonary embolism is suspected, ventilation-perfusion scans may be helpful by directing the angiographer to appropriate areas of the lungs. Venous ultrasound examinations or contrast venograms should also be reviewed because they might reveal thrombosis of the preferred entry site, necessitating selection of an alternative approach. Finally, the ECG must be examined for evidence of a left bundle branch block, which, if present, could be converted to complete heart block during passage of a catheter through the right ventricle.[44]

Premedication may include mild sedatives for apprehensive patients. Narcotic drugs are not needed because the procedure is not painful. Patients with or subject to bradycardia and vasovagal reflex should be given intravenous atropine (0.4–1.0 mg). Atropine as well as Xylocaine should be immediately available for emergencies.

Monitoring

Pressure and electrocardiographic monitoring are essential parts of selective pulmonary arteriography, both for the patient's safety and to facilitate a comprehensive and functional study. A defibrillator and an emergency cart as used for any heart catheterization must be available in the angiographic suite. A transvenous pacemaker should also be immediately available when performing pulmonary arteriography in a patient with left bundle branch block.[44]

Approach Routes

Regardless of the chosen (or imposed) approach route, percutaneous entry into a peripheral access vein is practically always possible by the standard Seldinger technique using one of the several approaches discussed below.

Transfemoral Route

The transfemoral route is the most commonly used approach. Access is easily achieved, even repeatedly, and it favors the easy and safe catheter manipulation required for selective pulmonary artery catheterization. The venous entry is performed under local anesthesia, 1 to 2 cm medial to the femoral artery and 2 to 3 cm lower than the usual site of corresponding arterial puncture. The right femoral vein entrance is preferred because of the decreased angle of the right iliac vein with the IVC. This is particularly important when additional interventional procedures such as placement of IVC filters or occlusion of abnormal pulmonary vessels are considered. The left common iliac vein is oriented almost perpendicularly to the right iliac vein and IVC.[45] This angle makes interventional procedures done from the left femoral venous approach more difficult.

Despite its advantages, however, the transfemoral approach is best avoided in patients with either documented or suspected thrombosis of the ipsilateral femoral and iliac veins or the IVC. In questionable cases contrast medium should be injected through the needle or a small catheter placed in the common femoral vein to confirm patency of the iliac veins and the IVC.

Although other routes are preferred, the femoral approach may be used safely even when an IVC filter is present.[46] Within several weeks of introduction, caval filters become incorporated into the wall of the cava, making dislodgment during catheter manipulation extremely unlikely. Before a catheter is passed through a filter, however, a cavagram should be performed to look for thrombus. Pigtail catheters should also be straightened with a guidewire as they are both advanced and withdrawn through the filter. We have used the femoral approach in patients with all filter types currently available in the United States except the Bird's Nest (Cook, Inc.) with no problems.

Transjugular Route

The right internal jugular vein offers the next best alternative to the femoral venous approach. The left internal jugular vein or large external jugular veins are also suitable options. The internal jugular vein is easily entered, although experience is required for safety. To avoid pneumothoraces we use an anterior approach, high on the neck, about 4 to 5 cm below the angle of the mandible. The puncture is done between the carotid artery, which is pushed medially, and the sternocleidomastoid muscle. Placing the patient in a slight Trendelenburg position or elevating the legs before the puncture facilitates entry into the jugular vein.

Transbrachial Route

The transbrachial approach is rarely needed. It is best performed by percutaneous entry into the median basilic vein, the largest of the antecubital veins. The median basilic vein is less likely to offer resistance to catheter passage toward the axillary vein. The cephalic vein is less desirable for catheterization because the sharp bend it makes at the shoulder limits catheter manipulation. Catheterization of the pulmonary artery from the left brachial approach is somewhat easier than from the right because the catheter course from the left side is more of a circle and thus requires less manipulation.[45]

Other entry sites of access for pulmonary arteriography from "above," such as the axillary[13] or subclavian[14] vein, have been used only rarely. However, angiographers and interventionalists are becoming increasingly familiar with these approaches through the insertion of long-term central venous lines, making them possible options in difficult cases. Ultrasound guidance facilitates entry into the axillary and subclavian veins and makes it very safe.

Catheters for Selective Pulmonary Arteriography

The types and configurations of catheters used for selective pulmonary arteriography have varied with the experience and preference of individual angiographers. We will discuss those catheters and their shapes that we consider most efficient for performing selective pulmonary examinations.

Preshaped Pigtail Catheter

A pigtail catheter with a 90-degree bend 3 to 6 cm from the pigtail that has both an end hole and side holes is the most efficient and safe catheter for selective pulmonary arteriography. Grollman et al.[17] pioneered this catheter in 1970 under the name of *pulmonary artery–seeking pigtail catheter*. Their original catheter also had a secondary curve along the shaft, which was subsequently removed.[47] Today this is the most commonly used catheter for selective pulmonary arteriography from either the femoral or transjugular approach. It is available commercially (Cook, Inc.), but some angiographers prefer to make it by shaping a conventional (straight) pigtail catheter.

An 8 French catheter is preferable to the 6 or 7 French catheter because it has better torque control and stability. The length of the distal curve should correspond to the width of the right atrium and should optimally be long enough to reach the tricuspid valve. Evaluation of heart size on chest film is useful in selecting or shaping the catheter to correspond to the patient's anatomy. The length of the curve can also be extended by using a deflector wire (Cook, Inc.).[17]

The pigtail end should be tight (slightly less than 1 cm) and can be oriented in the superior direction toward the outflow tract or in the inferior direction toward the ventricular apex.[45] The orientation of the pigtail makes little difference to an experienced angiographer using an 8 French catheter, which can usually be easily rotated and advanced through the right ventricular outflow tract. In less experienced hands, the superior orientation of the pigtail is preferable because it facilitates pulmonary artery catheterization with the use of a guidewire, minimizing the need for catheter rotation.[48] With the pigtail turned upward, however, the catheter has a tendency to pass preferentially into upper lobe pulmonary artery branches. The pigtail, therefore, must be positioned beyond their origin for good opacification of the entire pulmonary vasculature with contrast injection.

A variety of modifications to the basic Grollman design have been described, including short or long distal curves, double curves, and inferiorly oriented pigtails.[45] All of these designs can be used safely and successfully in performing high-quality pulmonary arteriograms.

Curved Catheter Without Pigtail

The same curves as described above but without the pigtail are sometimes needed for superselective catheterization of peripheral pulmonary artery branches for more detailed diagnosis and for interventional procedures. Depending on the situation, a catheter with an end hole and side holes or only an end hole and with a bend 2 to 4 cm from its tip is used. Angiographers should adjust the shape in steam or hot water, depending on the anatomy of the vessel to be catheterized. A gentle curve is used for catheterization of upper lobe branches and a sharper curve for lower lobe branches. A Headhunter H1 catheter is also a good option. It must be emphasized that advancement of these nonpigtail catheters through the heart should only be performed with a soft J guidewire leading the way.

Balloon Catheter

Occlusion balloon catheters or Swan-Ganz balloon catheters are used in special situations for occlusion pulmonary arteriography. Balloon occlusion pulmonary arteriography allows detailed evaluation of the pulmonary architecture with the use of less contrast material.[20,21] When flow-directed catheters are used, steerable guidewires may be required to direct the catheter into the pulmonary arterial branches of interest.

Guidewires

Guidewires play an important role in selective pulmonary artery catheterization. J-tipped wires are the only type that should be used for manipulation in the heart. Because of their round tips, they readily bounce off the heart wall, thus avoiding cardiac perforation. We prefer a long-tapered guidewire with a 3-mm radius J tip. A deflector guidewire (Cook, Inc.) can be useful for extending the length of the catheter curve in the right atrium and also for selective catheterization of the right pulmonary artery.

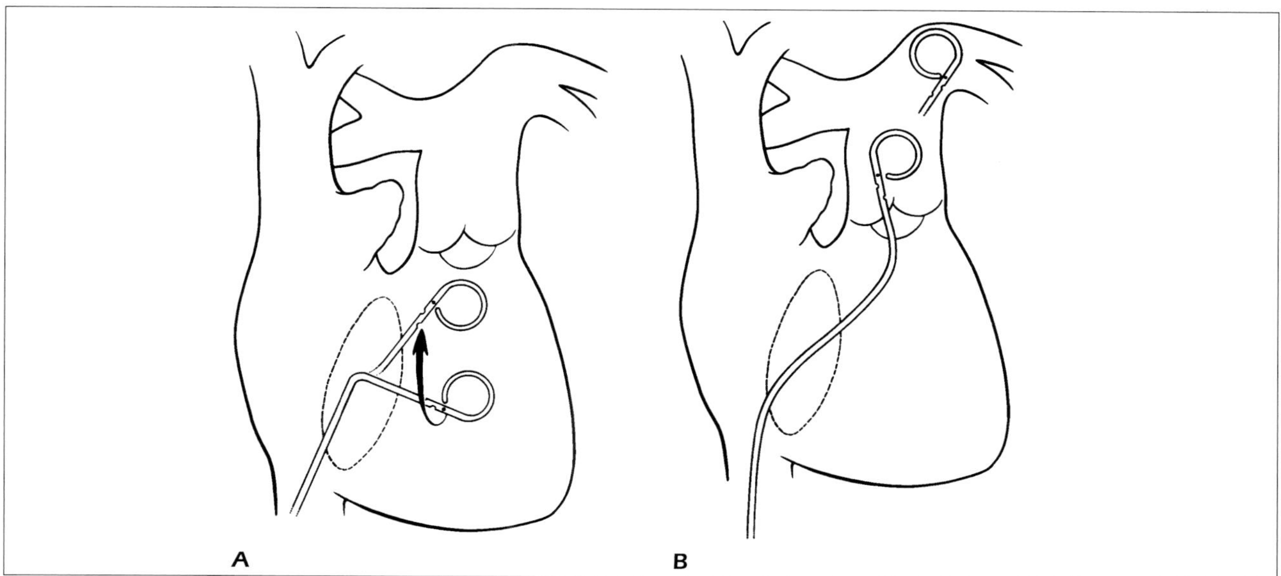

Figure 31-1. Catheterization with the Grollman catheter. (A) After the catheter has been advanced into the right ventricle, counterclockwise rotation will bring the tip into the pulmonary outflow tract. (B) Continued rotation and advancement will cause the catheter to pass into the left pulmonary artery.

Catheterization

The catheter insertion site should be on the extremity not involved or suspected of being involved with deep venous thrombosis. If there is an undue resistance to J-guidewire passage, a test injection should be made in the vein entered to exclude the presence of thrombus. As Dotter warned in an earlier edition,[2] "dislodging a thrombus from an iliac vein would make a diagnosis but might break the patient." If thrombosis of the inferior or superior vena cava is suspected, a conventional venogram should be done before the pulmonary artery catheter is advanced.

Transfemoral Catheterization

The preshaped pigtail catheter is advanced over a guidewire into the right atrium. After the guidewire is withdrawn, the catheter is rotated to the left so the pigtail tip lies at the tricuspid valve. The catheter is then advanced slightly so the tip enters the right ventricle. Ventricular pressure can now be measured. If the distal limb of the catheter is too short so that the tricuspid valve cannot be crossed, the curve can be lengthened using tip-deflecting wire (Cook, Inc.).[17] With the catheter tip just in the right ventricle, counterclockwise rotation and advancement of the catheter will often bring it into the ventricular outflow tract and left pulmonary artery without the use of a guidewire (Fig. 31-1). If the catheter tends to advance preferentially toward the ventricular apex, it can be straightened by carefully advancing the stiff end of a guidewire just beyond the curve in the catheter. The straightened catheter can then be rotated easily toward the ventricular outflow tract and into the pulmonary artery.[49] When using the stiff end of a guidewire, one must always be careful to keep the end of the wire inside the catheter.

In difficult cases the pulmonary artery can be catheterized using a long-tapered J wire introduced through a Grollman catheter with the pigtail oriented upward.[48,50] After the Grollman catheter has been advanced into the right ventricle, the guidewire is advanced out the end of the catheter (Fig. 31-2). The taper of the guidewire mandril causes the pigtail to open gradually, directing the wire superiorly into the pulmonary artery. The catheter is then advanced into the pulmonary artery over the wire.

An alternative approach is to perform the procedure with a straight pigtail catheter.[51] Once the catheter is in the right atrium, it is curved using a tip-deflecting wire (Cook, Inc.) or the bent stiff end of a guidewire and rotated toward the tricuspid valve (Fig. 31-3). The guidewire or deflector wire is then fixed in place and the catheter is advanced off the wire, entering the right ventricle. Once the catheter tip has crossed the tricuspid valve, tension on the deflector wire is released, allowing the catheter to straighten. The straight catheter can then usually be advanced directly into the left

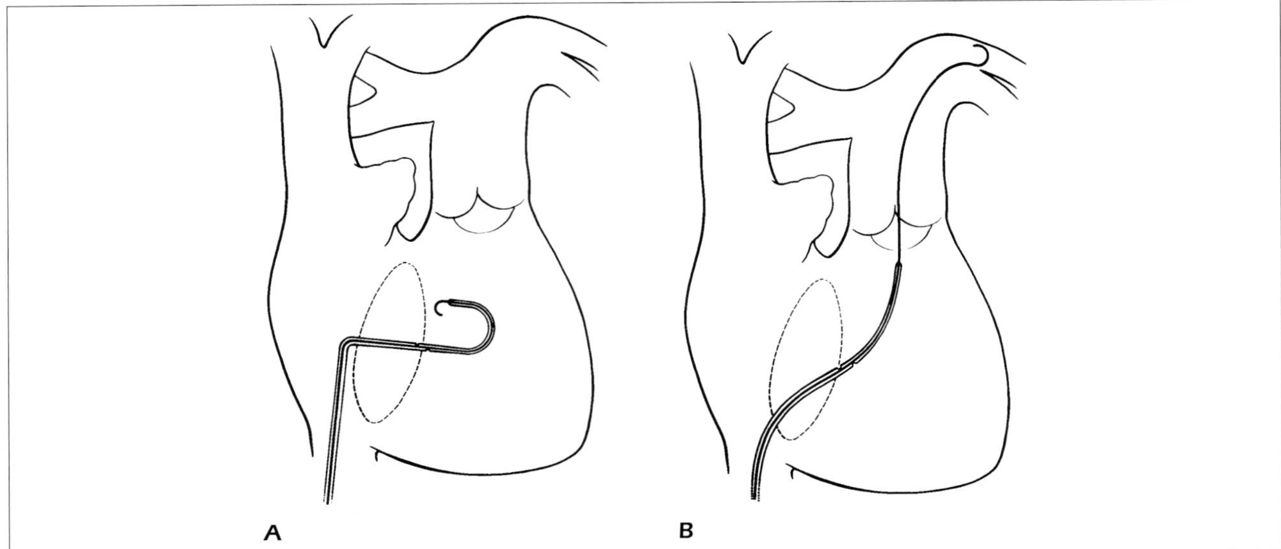

Figure 31-2. Catheterization with a guidewire. (A) After the Grollman catheter has been advanced into the right ventricle, a long, tapered, J-tipped guidewire is advanced out the end of the catheter, causing the pigtail to open gradually. (B) Advancing the guidewire will cause it to pass directly into the left pulmonary artery. The wire is then held in place and the catheter is advanced over it.

pulmonary artery. The deflector wire is used to curve the catheter again when it is placed into the right pulmonary artery.

Selective catheterization of the left pulmonary artery is typically easy because it originates in a cephalad direction. Catheterization of the right pulmonary artery, which branches horizontally from the main pulmonary artery at a right angle, requires more manipulation. From the left pulmonary artery, the curved catheter is withdrawn into the main pulmonary artery and is rotated clockwise to the right. Occasionally the catheter can then be advanced easily into the right pulmonary artery, but often a J-tipped guidewire must be used. When the right pulmonary artery originates in a downward angle, use of a Cook deflector wire will adjust the catheter curve and facilitate catheterization.

The catheter position is tested with hand injections of contrast and saline. All branches supplying the catheterized lung, including early branches to the upper lobe, should fill on the test injection. With a hard saline test injection the catheter should be stable and not recoil from its position. Before removal of the catheter from the pulmonary artery, the pigtail tip should be straightened with a guidewire to prevent damage to the heart valves as the catheter is withdrawn.

Transjugular Approach

With the transjugular approach or other approaches from "above," a catheter with a downturned pigtail tip and a 45-degree to 90-degree curve is again positioned in the right ventricle just beyond the tricuspid valve. If the catheter will not advance on its own into the pulmonary artery, a tapered tip J guidewire is then inserted and the cranially oriented pigtail directs it into the outflow track of the right ventricle and the pulmonary artery. The catheter is then easily advanced over the guidewire. Either the right or the left pulmonary artery can then be catheterized with appropriate rotations.

Pressures

Monitoring of right heart pressures is an important part of pulmonary arteriography. Ideally, pressures should be recorded in the right atrium, right ventricle, and pulmonary arteries. At the least, pressures from the pulmonary arteries should be obtained before and after contrast injection. If the mean pulmonary artery pressure is greater than about 40 mmHg, right ventricular pressures must be obtained because an end-diastolic pressure above 20 mmHg has been associated with an increased risk of death following contrast injection.[31] Mild, transient elevation of pulmonary arterial pressure immediately after contrast medium injection is common,[52,53] but a severe rise in pressure should be viewed as a warning sign that should prompt the angiographer to carefully consider if further injections are warranted. No maximum pulmonary artery or right ventricular pressure above which pulmonary arteriography is absolutely contraindicated has ever been

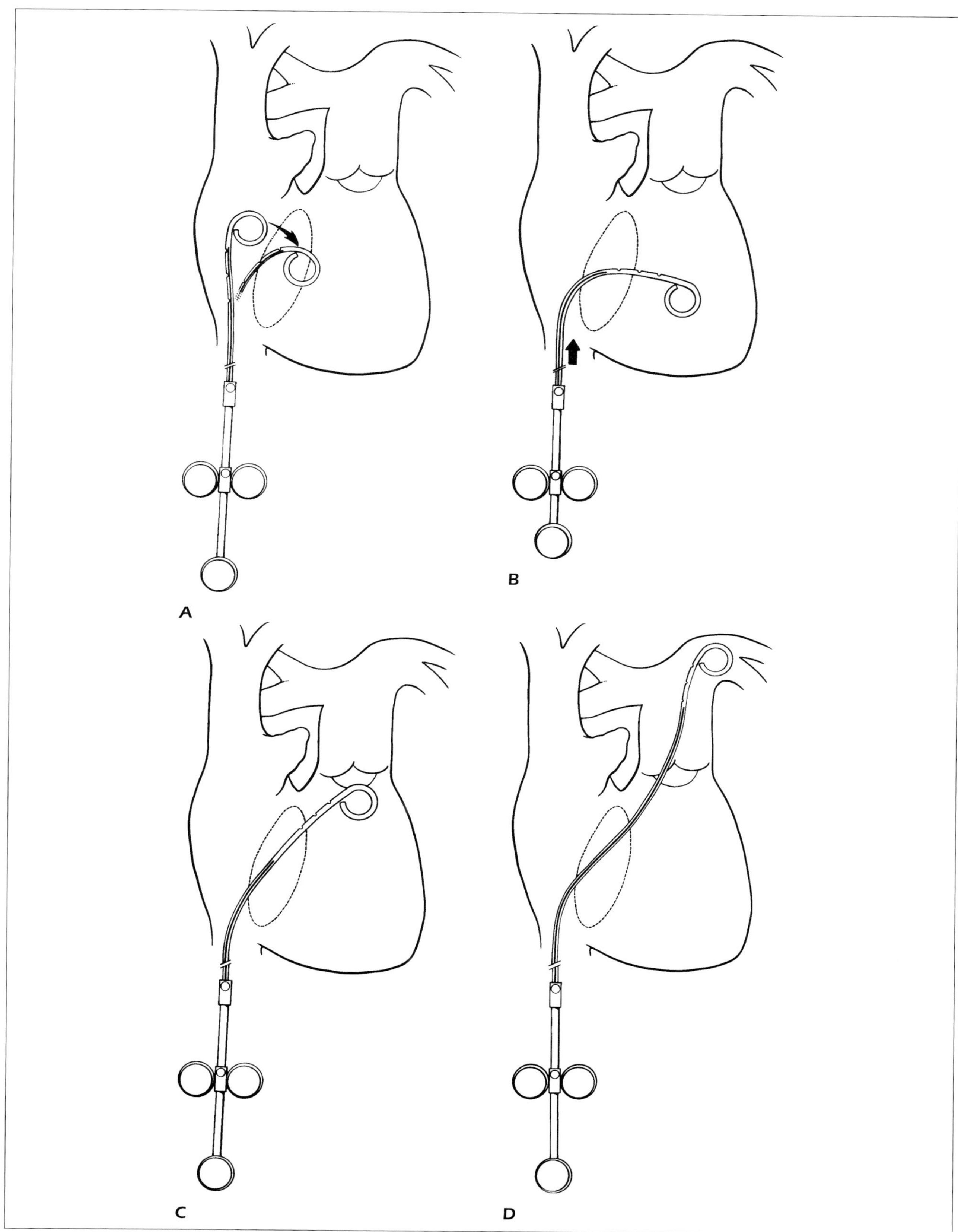

Figure 31-3. Catheterization using deflector wire. (A) A straight pigtail catheter is placed in the right atrium, curved by a tip-deflecting wire, and rotated toward the tricuspid valve. (B) The catheter is then advanced off the wire and into the right ventricle. (C) Once the tricuspid valve has been crossed, tension on the deflector wire is released, allowing the catheter to straighten. (D) The catheter is then advanced directly into the pulmonary artery.

established. As with any procedure, the risks must be weighed against the necessity of establishing an accurate diagnosis. In high-risk patients, a limited study directed by a ventilation-perfusion scan might be more appropriate than conventional angiography.

Contrast Medium Injections

Selective pulmonary arteriography has been performed safely for many years using high-osmolar, ionic contrast agents such as Renografin-76 (meglumine diatrizoate, Squibb, Inc.). In fact, in all of the major studies demonstrating the safety of pulmonary arteriography, virtually all of the angiograms were performed using high-osmolar contrast media.[31,32] Since the introduction of low-osmolar, nonionic contrast agents in the late 1980s, however, there has been a progressive shift to their use. Today, the nonionic agents are more widely used than the ionic contrast agents for pulmonary arteriography.[54] Some use them almost exclusively, but we prefer to use nonionic contrast media on a selective basis. Because they have less adverse hemodynamic effects than their ionic counterparts,[52,53] nonionic contrast media are used in all high-risk patients with pulmonary hypertension in our practice. The nonionic contrast media also produce less patient discomfort and coughing, which leads to improved image quality.[55,56]

For main pulmonary artery injections, which are performed only rarely, an injection of contrast at a rate 30 to 35 ml per second for 2 seconds is needed. Injection into the right pulmonary artery calls for 25 to 30 ml per second for 2 seconds, and injection into the left pulmonary artery requires 22 to 26 ml per second for 2 seconds. Injections into lobar and segmental pulmonary arteries require much less contrast medium; often amounts from 5 to 15 ml per second for 2 seconds are satisfactory. Injections should always be adjusted to the flow in the pulmonary arteries as assessed by a test injection.

Imaging

Conventional Large-Film Serial Arteriography

Large cut-film serial arteriography remains the gold standard for the evaluation of the pulmonary vascular tree and is appropriate for most patients. Images are obtained of the lung as contrast is injected selectively into either the right or left pulmonary artery. Filming of both lungs while contrast is injected into the main pulmonary artery is no longer performed. Advantages of cut-film arteriography include a large field of view, very high resolution, and the ability to obtain diagnostic examinations even in a relatively uncooperative patient. Serial large-film pulmonary arteriography is best done in angiographic systems with high-quality fluoroscopy and a 14 by 14 inch large film changer capable of filming at least three films per second. High-speed film screen combinations are optimal because they permit the use of shorter x-ray exposure times. Appropriate placement of aluminum wedge filters improves image quality by ensuring more even exposures over the entire film.

Filming is usually first done in anteroposterior projection during deep inspiration. Additional films in oblique and lateral projections are obtained as needed. The right posterior oblique projection is very useful for evaluation of the central left pulmonary artery branches. Lower lobe branches of both lungs are best seen on ipsilateral posterior oblique views.[57] Magnification can add to the quality of the selective studies of the lobar and segmental branches. Exposure rates are ordinarily three to four films per second for 3 seconds, followed by one exposure per second for the next 3 seconds. A test injection of contrast material before selection of the film sequence helps in choosing the proper rate of filming, particularly in patients with heart disease and slow circulation.

Alternatives to Serial Large-Film Arteriography

Digital subtraction pulmonary arteriography (DSA) is a potential alternative to serial large-film arteriography in selected cases.[18,19,21] Recent improvements in digital imaging systems, particularly the introduction of 14- to 16-inch image intensifiers with high-resolution video systems, have made DSA very attractive. Larger pulmonary arteries can be well evaluated by intravenous DSA. Images are obtained as contrast is injected into the SVC, IVC, or right atrium at a rate of 15 to 20 ml per second for 2 seconds during suspended respiration. Using this technique, emboli can be demonstrated in up to third-order pulmonary artery branches. For more detailed evaluation of peripheral branches, selective pulmonary arteriography must be performed.

The principal drawback to DSA is its susceptibility to motion artifacts. Suspended respiration is essential for good image acquisition, and patients who cannot suspend respiration for 10 to 15 seconds are not candidates for DSA pulmonary arteriography. Cardiac motion may hinder evaluation of areas of the lungs near the heart borders even in cooperative patients. DSA is sometimes advocated to allow an examination to be completed using a minimum of contrast material. If additional views are required because the DSA images are nondiagnostic, however, the potential savings in contrast are lost. The primary use of intravenous DSA may lie in permitting pulmonary arteriography to be safely performed in patients with particularly irritable ventricles in whom selective catheterization is contraindicated because of the risk of serious arrhythmias.

Nonsubtracted digital arteriography is another attractive technique for pulmonary arteriography. Examinations are performed in a manner identical to cut-film arteriography except that digital images are acquired. Because subtraction is not employed, patient motion is usually not a problem. Images acquired appear similar to cut-film images. The primary advantage of this technique is decreased examination time. Scout films are not required, and images are immediately available for viewing. However, image quality remains inferior to that of large serial cut films.

Balloon occlusion arteriography[20,21] can be used to supplement the conventional study for detailed evaluation of selected areas of the lung. A Swan-Ganz catheter with the balloon inflated is advanced into the pulmonary artery using flow direction. Steerable guidewires are then used to facilitate catheterization of the lobar or segmental arteries to be studied. After the balloon is inflated to occlude the artery to be studied, 5 to 15 ml of contrast medium is injected and images are obtained. Cut film can be used with magnification technique, or digital or cine filming may be employed. Balloon occlusion angiography is useful in evaluating areas of the pulmonary vasculature that appear suspicious on the initial angiogram. It can also be used instead of conventional arteriography in high-risk patients to evaluate areas shown to be abnormal by lung ventilation-perfusion scanning.

Cineradiography[22,45] may be helpful in patients with severe tachypnea and tachycardia, because the very short exposure times minimize adverse effects of motion. Some newer imaging systems can produce digital cine images at rates up to 30 frames per second. Digital systems have the advantage of permitting high-quality images to be viewed immediately, something not possible with conventional cinefluorography. We have found this technique very useful in quickly assessing areas of the pulmonary vasculature that are poorly demonstrated on the initial cut-film arteriogram.

Normal Findings

The interpretation of pulmonary arteriograms requires that certain facts be borne in mind. The volume, wall thickness, and relative position of cardiovascular structures vary during the cardiac cycle. Variations in the respiratory phase also significantly change the apparent form, position, and degree of filling of the opacified structures. The pulmonary vessels of youth differ from those of old age.

Technical factors, especially the site of injection and the amount of injected contrast agent, significantly influence pulmonary arteriograms. Injection into the pulmonary artery can provide reasonably good visualization of large and medium-sized arteries but often results in poor visualization of the peripheral branches (Figs. 31-4 and 31-5). Selective injections will provide excellent visualization of all grossly discernible branches of the vascular system supplied by the catheterized artery (Figs. 31-6 and 31-7). The visualization of small peripheral branches is favored by superselective injections and magnification filming techniques. When insufficient contrast medium is injected, anteriorly oriented branches may be underfilled because of gravitational layering of contrast agent or systolic washout of contrast. These factors must be considered in differentiating between normal and pathologic findings. The crossing of arteries or of an artery and a bronchus can simulate intraluminal filling defects. Supplementary studies in oblique or lateral projections will ordinarily resolve such problems.

The arterial phase of the pulmonary arteriogram is followed in 2 to 3 seconds by a capillary phase. Pulmonary veins immediately then fill with no cephalocaudal differential in flow patterns in the supine position. In the midlung fields, the pulmonary veins lie below their corresponding arteries and converge to enter the left atrium. In the upper lobes, the veins lie lateral to their corresponding arteries. Normally, the left atrium fills well in 4 to 6 seconds, following which there is sequential filling of the left ventricle and the thoracic aorta.

Main Pulmonary Artery

The main pulmonary artery is a short, broad vessel arising from the pulmonary conus of the right ventricle at the pulmonary semilunar valves. It runs upward and slightly medially and posteriorly to its bifurcation into the left and right pulmonary arteries. The bifurcation of the main pulmonary artery varies in appearance, its angle ranging between 100 and 180 degrees (Fig. 31-8). The diameter of the right pulmonary artery measures between 17 and 30 mm (mean 23.4 mm). The caliber of the main pulmonary artery varies between 20 and 30 mm (mean 26.4 mm).[58] The sum of the diameter of the left and right main branches is greater than the diameter of the main pulmonary artery. The size of the main pulmonary artery and its branches also varies with systole and diastole.[59,60] Dotter[58] demonstrated that a slight increase of the caliber of the pulmonary artery occurs with advancing age.

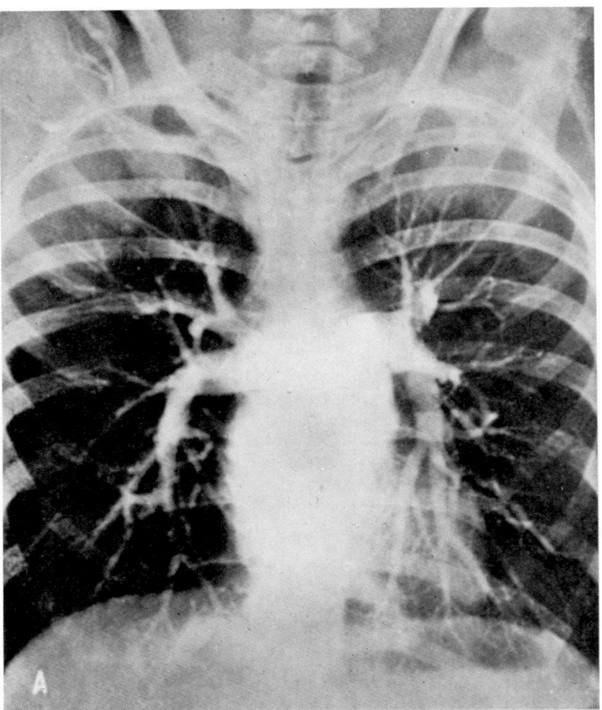

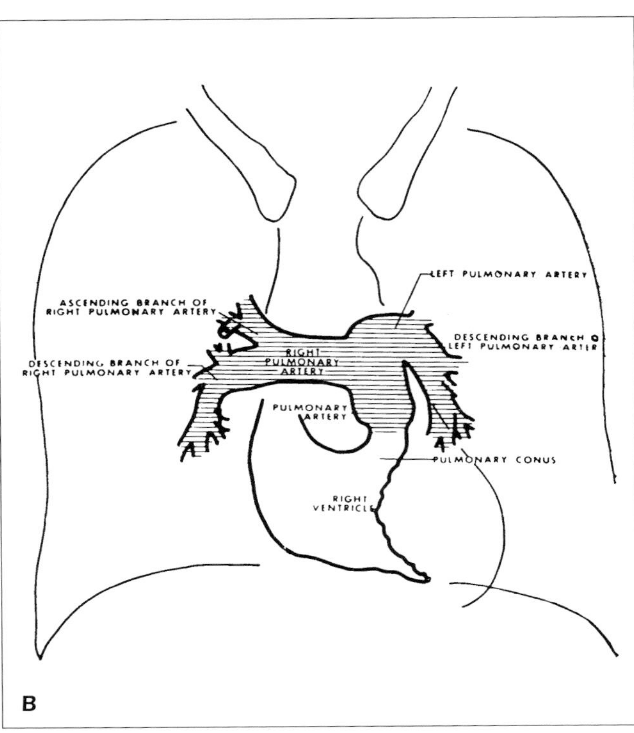

Figure 31-4. Normal pulmonary arteries, posteroanterior angiocardiogram, in a 17-year-old man. (A) The left pulmonary artery rises convexly about 1 cm above the level of the horizontally coursing right pulmonary artery. (B) Tracing of (A); the pulmonary artery and both main branches are accentuated. Angiocardiography fails to provide good definition of the peripheral branches.

Figure 31-5. Normal pulmonary arteries, left lateral projection at 2.5 seconds, in a 49-year-old man. (A) The right pulmonary artery is seen from the end, and the left branch is viewed from the side. (B) Tracing of (A); the pulmonary artery and both main branches are accentuated.

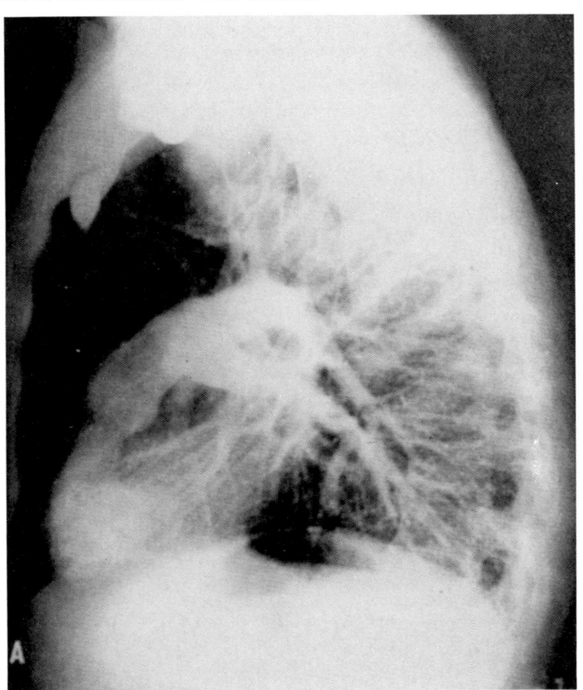

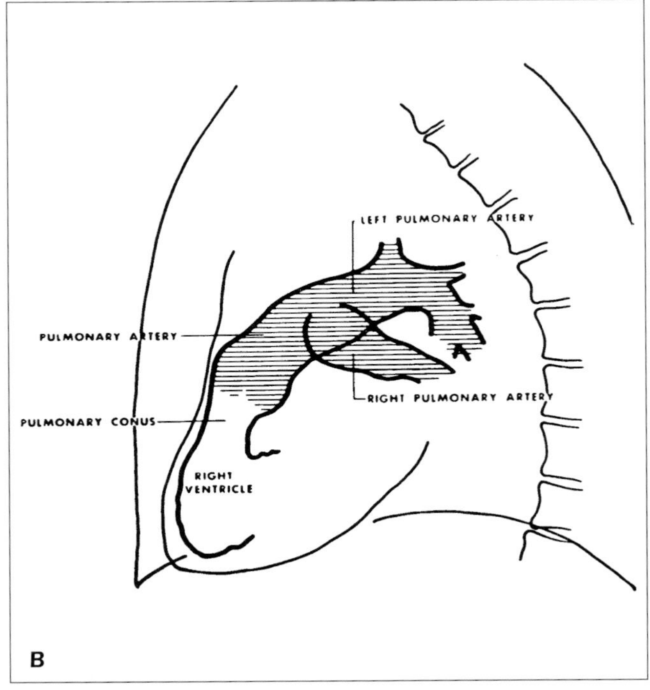

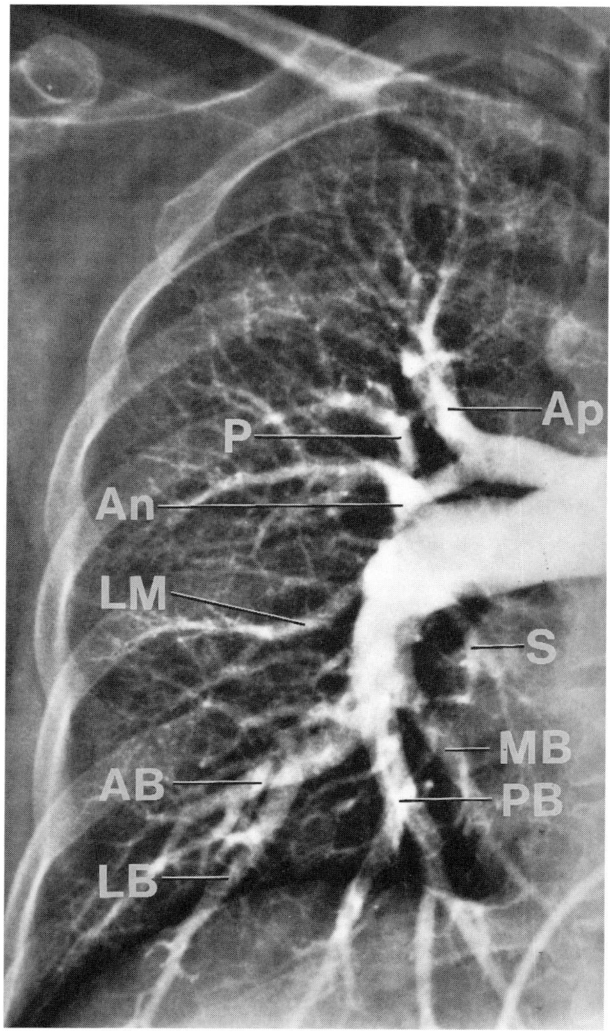

A

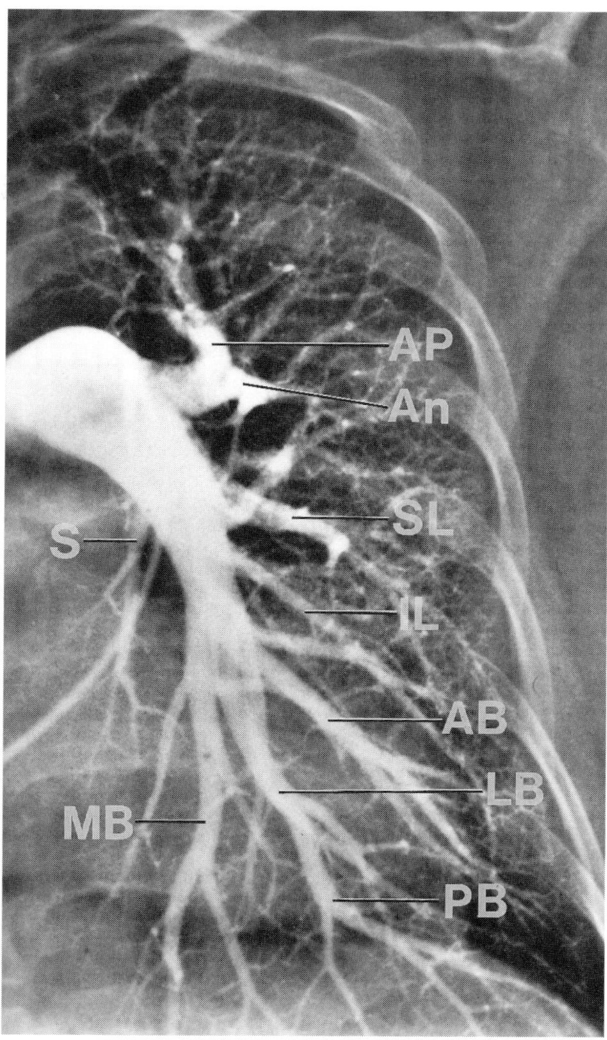

B

Figure 31-6. Normal right and left selective pulmonary arteriograms, separately injected in a 58-year-old man in the anteroposterior projection. *An,* anterior segmental, upper lobe; *Ap,* apical segmental, RUL; *P,* posterior segmental, RUL; *AP,* apical-posterior segmental, LUL; *SL,* superior segmental, lingula, LUL; *IL,* inferior segmental, lingula, LUL; *LM,* lateral segmental, RML; *S,* superior segmental, RML; *AB,* anterior basal segmental, lower lobe; *LB,* lateral basal segmental, lower lobe; *PB,* posterior basal segmental, lower lobe; *MB,* medial basal segmental, lower lobe.

Right Pulmonary Artery

The right pulmonary artery is slightly smaller in caliber than the main artery and runs a horizontal, sometimes slightly downward, course across the heart to the hilus of the right lung, where it divides into ascending and descending branches. It lies behind the ascending aorta, the SVC, and the right upper lobar pulmonary vein and in front of the tracheal bifurcation and esophagus.[61–63]

Left Pulmonary Artery

The left pulmonary artery is a continuation of the main pulmonary artery, running superiorly, posteriorly, and to the left, where it turns sharply to the left and downward in the hilus of the left lung. It lies in front of the descending aorta and beneath the curve of the aortic arch, to which it is connected by the ligamentum arteriosum. In the frontal angiogram, the proximal left pulmonary artery is foreshortened and its projected

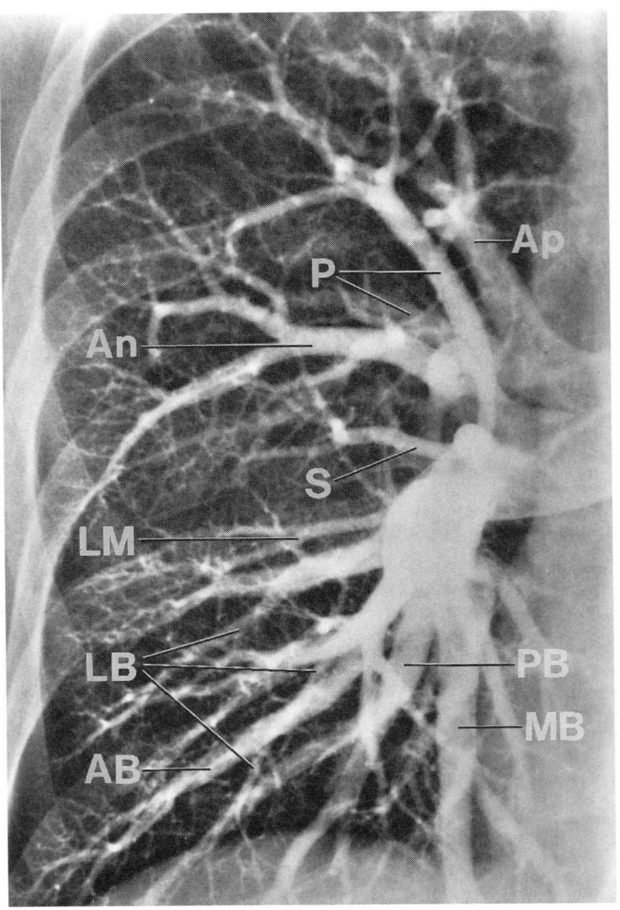

A

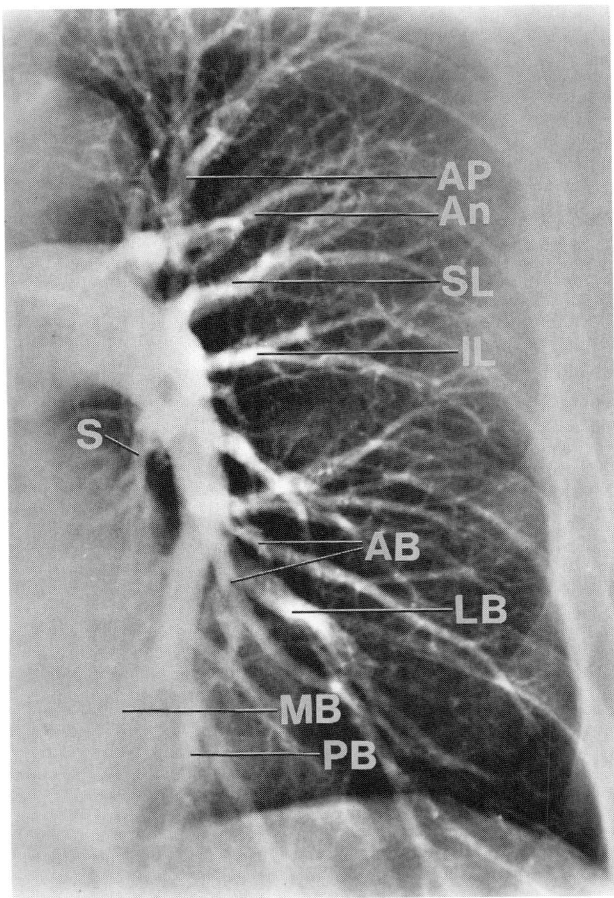

B

Figure 31-7. Normal selective pulmonary arteriogram. (A) The right pulmonary arteriogram in the anteroposterior projection demonstrates an anatomic variant with the posterior ramus of the posterior segmental artery (RUL) and the anterior segmental artery (RUL) both arising from the descending branch of the right pulmonary artery. (B) Left pulmonary arteriogram, anteroposterior projection.

image can be compared to looking at a vertical candy cane in such a way that the short curved part appears almost as a straight line. Either the lateral or the right posterior oblique projection is necessary for its detailed evaluation (see Fig. 31-7).

Pulmonary Artery Branches

The pulmonary artery segmental branches in both lungs usually follow the segmental bronchi, although there are frequent variations. There may not be separate segmental branches for each segment, or there may be two branches in relation to a single lobar or segmental bronchus. Variations are most often seen in the upper lobes. Beyond their origins, the segmental arteries remain in close relation to the bronchi, although the peripheral pulmonary arterial branches are more numerous than those of the bronchial tree.

The segmental arteries and their branches gradually taper toward the periphery, exhibiting two types of arterial branching. In *bifurcational* branching, the parent artery divides into two branches of similar size at an angle of 10 to 60 degrees. In *collateral* branching, the trunk divides into two branches of dissimilar size, the larger of which continues in the direction of the parent trunk. The other, smaller, branch comes off at an angle of from 30 to 80 degrees. In both types, the sum of the branch diameters exceeds that of the trunk.

Right Lung

The right pulmonary artery divides at the right hilus into two main branches: the ascending branch, which supplies the right upper lobe, and the descending branch, which supplies the right middle and lower lobes.

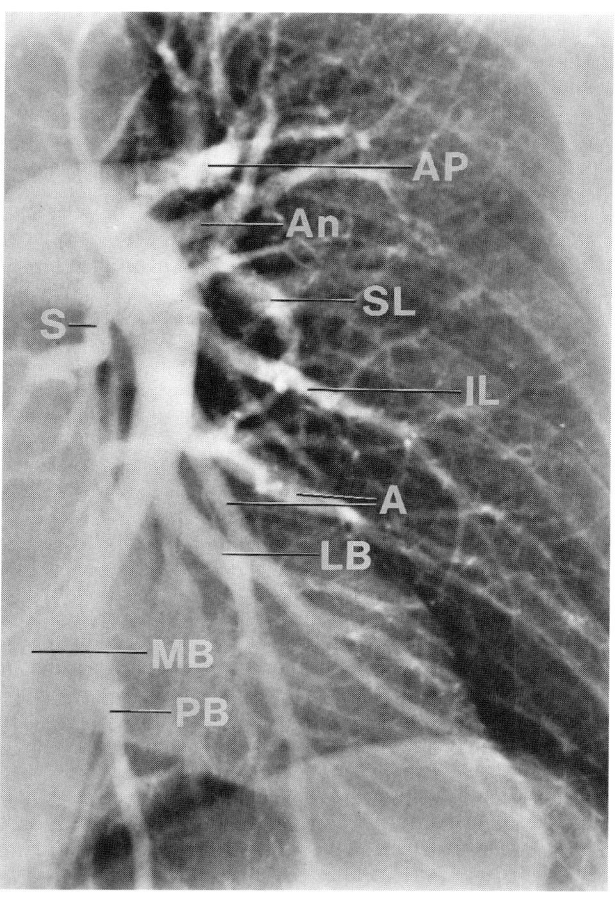

C

Figure 31-7 (continued). (C) Right posterior oblique projection of the left pulmonary demonstrating improved visualization of the origins of the segmental arteries in the lingular segments (LUL) and the basal segments (LLL). (Legend same as Fig. 31-6.)

The *ascending branch of the right pulmonary artery* supplies the *right upper lobe* (RUL). It first courses upward a short distance and trifurcates into three segmental arteries: the apical, the posterior, and the anterior segmental arteries.

The apical segmental artery is the largest of the segmental arteries to the RUL and courses superiorly and slightly laterally in the frontal view.[64] It promptly divides into two easily identified major rami, the apical and the posterior rami, which supply the apical and posterior portions of the apical bronchopulmonary segment of the RUL.

The posterior segmental artery of the RUL arises from the trifurcation of the ascending branch of the right pulmonary artery and proceeds posteriorly to supply the posterior bronchopulmonary segment of the RUL. In the frontal arteriogram, it runs obliquely and laterally, lying between the apical and anterior segmental arteries. The posterior segmental artery gives rise to two major rami, a posterior ramus and a lateral ramus. In a variation of this anatomy, the posterior segmental artery may arise as a branch of the anterior segmental artery, in which case it usually originates from the descending rather than the ascending branch of the right pulmonary artery (see Fig. 31-7).

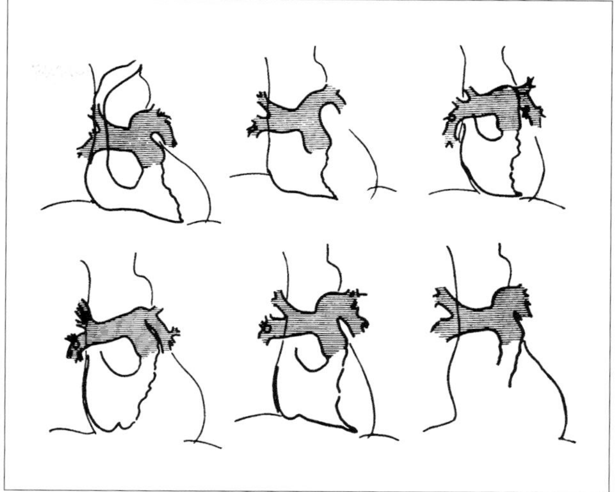

Figure 31-8. Variations in the angiocardiographic appearance of the normal pulmonary artery and main branches, posteroanterior projection (traced from angiocardiograms).

The anterior segmental artery of the RUL supplies the bronchopulmonary segment of the same name and is the most inferior artery of the trifurcation of the ascending branch of the right pulmonary artery. After a short course, it divides into an anterior ramus and a lateral ramus. The anterior ramus courses inferiorly and paramediastinally (in the frontal view) and anteriorly (in the lateral view), and the lateral ramus courses horizontally toward the periphery.

The *descending branch of the right pulmonary artery* supplies the right middle and lower lobes. It proceeds directly downward from the right hilus and the first branches to come off are the middle lobe artery of the right middle lobe (RML) and the superior segmental artery of the right lower lobe (RLL), followed by the medial basal segmental artery and the anterior basal segmental artery. The parent vessel then splits to form the posterior basal segmental artery and the lateral basal segmental artery. These branches are quite constant, with each supplying the correspondingly bronchopulmonary segment of the RLL.

The middle lobe artery arises from the descending branch of the right pulmonary artery opposite the origin of the superior segmental artery (RLL). It proceeds anteriorly and inferiorly, soon bifurcating into lateral and medial segmental arteries, which supply the respective bronchopulmonary segments of the *right middle lobe*. In the frontal view, the medial segmental artery of the RML courses inferiorly, parallel to the heart border. It is difficult to identify this vessel in the frontal projection because it is often superimposed on the descending branch of the right pulmonary artery. The lateral segmental artery (RML) is seen in the frontal projection to run laterally and slightly downward, parallel to and below the horizontal fissure and above the anterior and lateral basal segmental arteries to the lower lobe.

The superior segmental artery of the *right lower lobe* courses posteriorly upward and laterally to supply the uppermost part of the RLL.

The medial basal segmental artery of the RLL arises as the third major branch of the descending branch of the right pulmonary artery and comes off distal to the origin of the superior segmental artery (RLL). In the frontal projection, the vessel pursues a course downward and medially and overlapping the right atrial border.

The anterior basal segmental artery of the RLL arises from the anterolateral aspect of the descending branch of the right pulmonary artery inferior to the origin of the medial basal segmental artery, and courses laterally and anteriorly, supplying the bronchopulmonary segment of the same name. In the frontal projection, it is the most lateral basal segmental artery and extends into the right costophrenic sulcus.

The lateral basal segmental artery of the RLL arises with the posterior basal segmental artery as a bifurcation of the descending branch of the right pulmonary artery and proceeds inferiorly and laterally to supply the bronchopulmonary segment of the same name. It is seen in the frontal projection to run between the anterior and posterior basal segmental arteries.

The posterior basal segmental artery of the RLL, the largest of the segmental arteries of the right lung, arises with the lateral basal segmental artery as a bifurcation of the descending branch of the right pulmonary artery and proceeds inferiorly and posteriorly, its branches reaching to the most posterior and dependent portion of the right lung. In the frontal projection, it is seen to lie between the medial basal segmental artery and the lateral basal segmental artery.

Left Lung

The *left pulmonary artery* bifurcates in the left hilus into the ascending branch, which supplies the upper two segments of the left upper lobe (LUL), and the descending branch, which supplies the lingula and the left lower lobe (LLL).

The *ascending branch of the left pulmonary artery* arises 2 to 4 cm from the origin of the parent vessel. It runs superiorly and bifurcates immediately into the apical-posterior segmental artery and the smaller anterior segmental artery.

The apical-posterior segmental artery of the *left upper lobe* originates superiorly at the bifurcation of the ascending branch of the left pulmonary artery and runs a short course superiorly and posteriorly. In the frontal projection, the apical-posterior segmental artery is seen as a short trunk projecting superiorly and dividing into two major rami, apical and posterior, which supply the correspondingly named portions of the apical-posterior bronchopulmonary segment of the left upper lobe. The apical ramus may be identified as the medial and usually larger of the two and is seen to course superiorly toward the apex of the left lung. The posterior ramus follows an oblique course superiorly and laterally.

The anterior segmental artery of the LUL arises inferiorly at the bifurcation of the ascending branch of the left pulmonary artery and courses anteriorly, giving rise to anterior and lateral rami, which supply the correspondingly named portions of the anterior segment of the left upper lobe. In the frontal projection, the anterior segmental artery is seen as a foreshortened trunk seeming to take origin from the inferior margin of the ascending branch of the left pulmonary artery and paralleling the descending branch of the left pulmonary artery for a short distance before its division into anterior and lateral rami. The anterior ramus runs inferiorly, whereas the lateral ramus runs horizontally toward the periphery of the lung.

The *descending branch of the left pulmonary artery* courses downward into the left lung in a smooth continuation of the arc of the left pulmonary artery. It gives origin to the lingular artery, the superior segmental artery (LLL), and the arteries supplying the basal bronchopulmonary segments of the LLL.

The lingular artery arises from the left descending pulmonary artery approximately 2 cm inferior to the bifurcation of the left pulmonary artery. It comprises a short vascular trunk (appearing to arise from the lateral aspect of the descending pulmonary artery) and almost immediately divides into its two segmental components. The superior segmental artery of the lingula is the superiorly placed division coursing horizontally and slightly downward to the periphery and is usually located at the level of the left fourth anterior interspace. The inferior segmental artery of the lingula runs an oblique downward course from its point of origin toward (but not reaching) the left costophrenic sulcus. It runs above and, in general, parallel to the anterior basal segmental artery of LLL.

The segmental arteries to the *left lower lobe* are comparable to those of the right lower lobe. Until 1989, the anterior and medial basal segments were combined

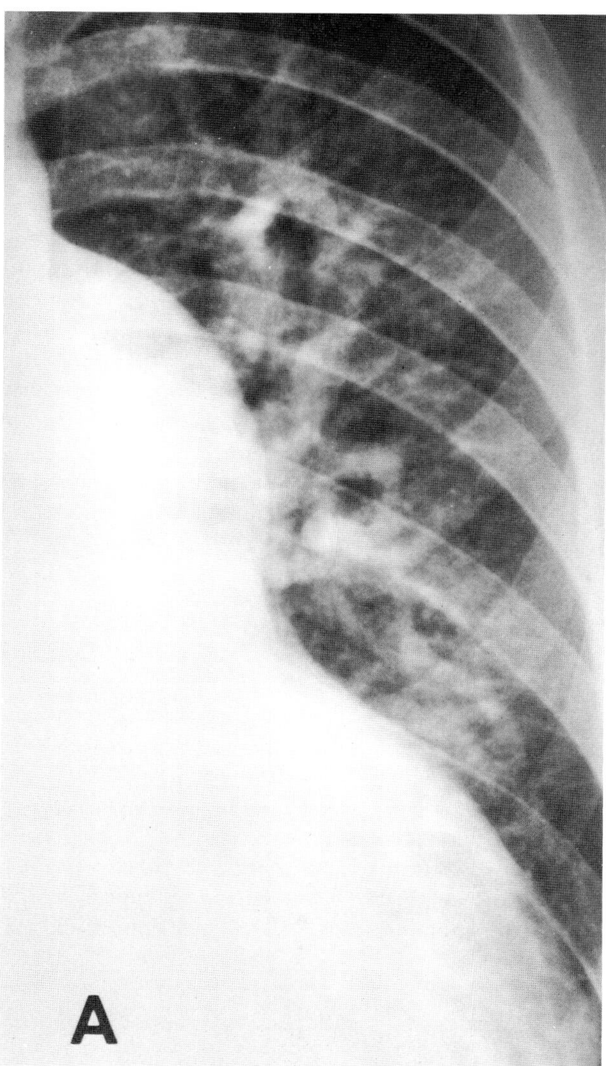

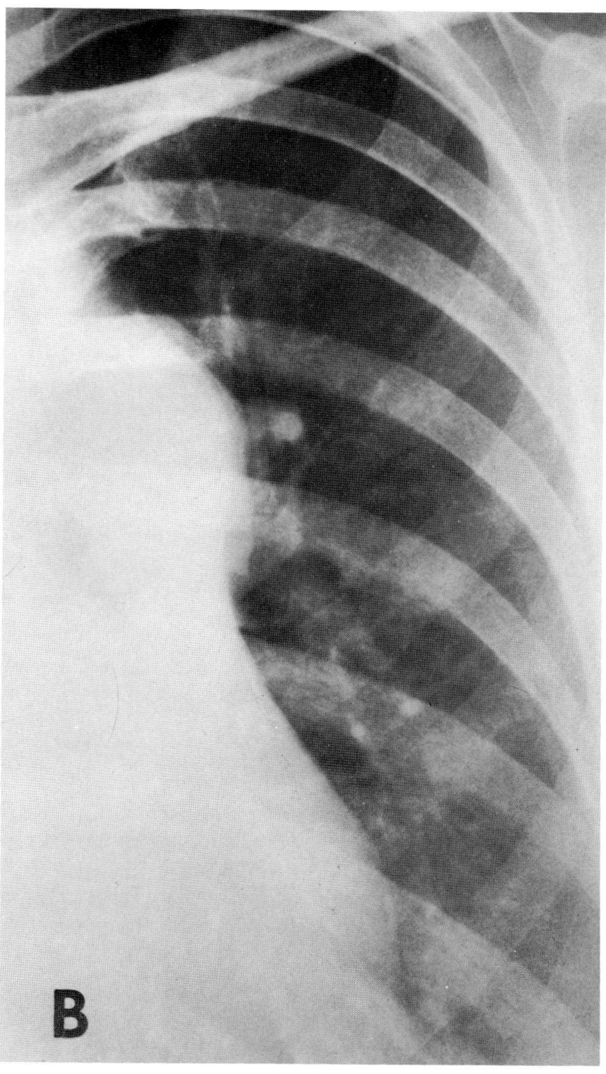

Figure 32-1. Hemodynamically induced pulmonary vascular changes. (A) Diffuse pulmonary artery enlargement reflects increased flow and pressure due to left-to-right shunting in an interventricular septal defect. (B) Peripheral pulmonary hypovascularity reflects decreased flow and pressure in pulmonary valvular stenosis. Arteriography is not needed to assess such changes.

pearance in association with defects of the ventricular septum. Interventricular defects large enough to be physiologically significant are often accompanied by gradually rising pulmonary pressures over a period of years. When cyanosis appears with interventricular defects, it reflects the elevation to systemic levels of right ventricular *systolic* pressure, whereas in interatrial septal defects it reflects the elevated ventricular *diastolic* pressure of decompensation. Another important difference between the two conditions is related to the chronicity of the hypertension. In interventricular defects, long-standing pulmonary hypertension often exists in the absence of greatly increased pulmonary flow; adjustments can therefore be made gradually. In interatrial septal defects, the added load of pulmonary hypertension on the right ventricle (already taxed to provide the high pulmonary flow required to achieve a useful systemic cardiac output) constitutes a "last-straw" situation.

No attempt will be made here to categorize the various changes associated with all of the different congenital cardiac lesions. The abnormalities identified depend not only on the underlying lesion but also where in the "life cycle" of the pathology we are examining the patient. In tetralogy of Fallot one may see relatively normal appearing pulmonary vessels, al-

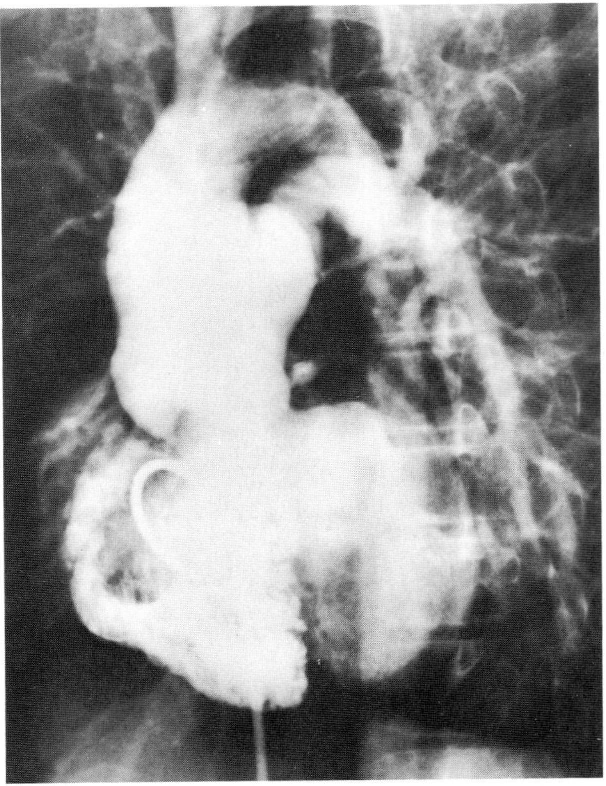

Figure 32-2. Common truncus arteriosus, type 1. Selective right ventricular injection. Left and partly hidden right pulmonary arteries arise from the ascending aorta. There is a large defect in the upper part of the interventricular septum.

though diminution of the size of the entire pulmonary vascular bed is more common. Successful corrective surgery results in near-normal pulmonary vascularity.

In cyanotic patients, generous-sized pulmonary arteries suggest common truncus arteriosus (Fig. 32-2). Similarly, transposition is likely if the main pulmonary artery takes origin behind rather than to the left of the aortic root. Irregular, mottled, hilar vascular shadows that fill poorly during pulmonary arteriography indicate the presence of systemic-to-pulmonary collateral pathways in pseudotruncus arteriosus, pulmonary atresia, and other functionally similar malformations. Thoracic aortography will demonstrate both aortic and pulmonary arterial opacification. Selective injection of bronchial, intercostal, or other aortopulmonary collateral vessels provides detailed information although not necessarily a complete anatomic diagnosis (Figs. 32-3 through 32-6).

Pulmonary Stenosis and Poststenotic Dilatation

Isolated pulmonary valvular stenosis can cause diagnostically useful changes in the conventional and angiographic appearance of the pulmonary vessels.[3] Poststenotic dilatation may affect the pulmonary artery centrally, as in valvular stenosis (Fig. 32-7), or peripherally, as in multiple pulmonary artery stenoses (Fig. 32-8). The subject of poststenotic dilatation has received considerable study.[4–6] Dotter proposed the fol-

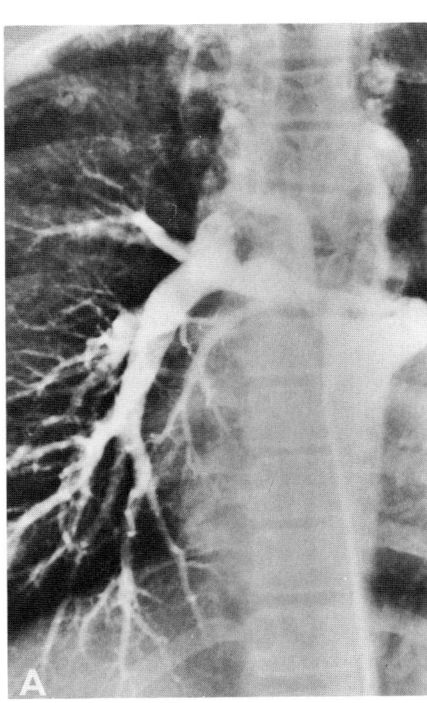

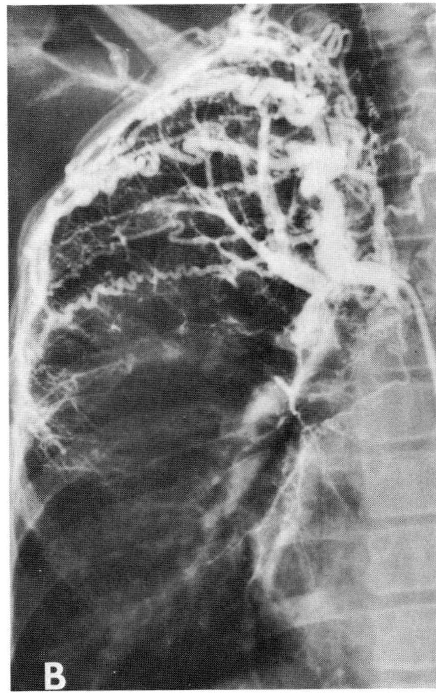

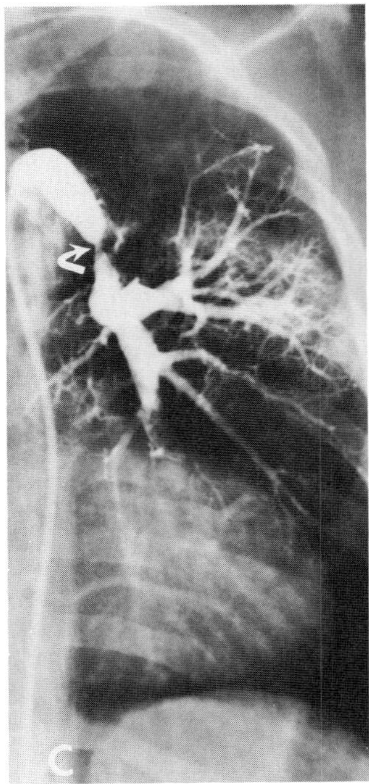

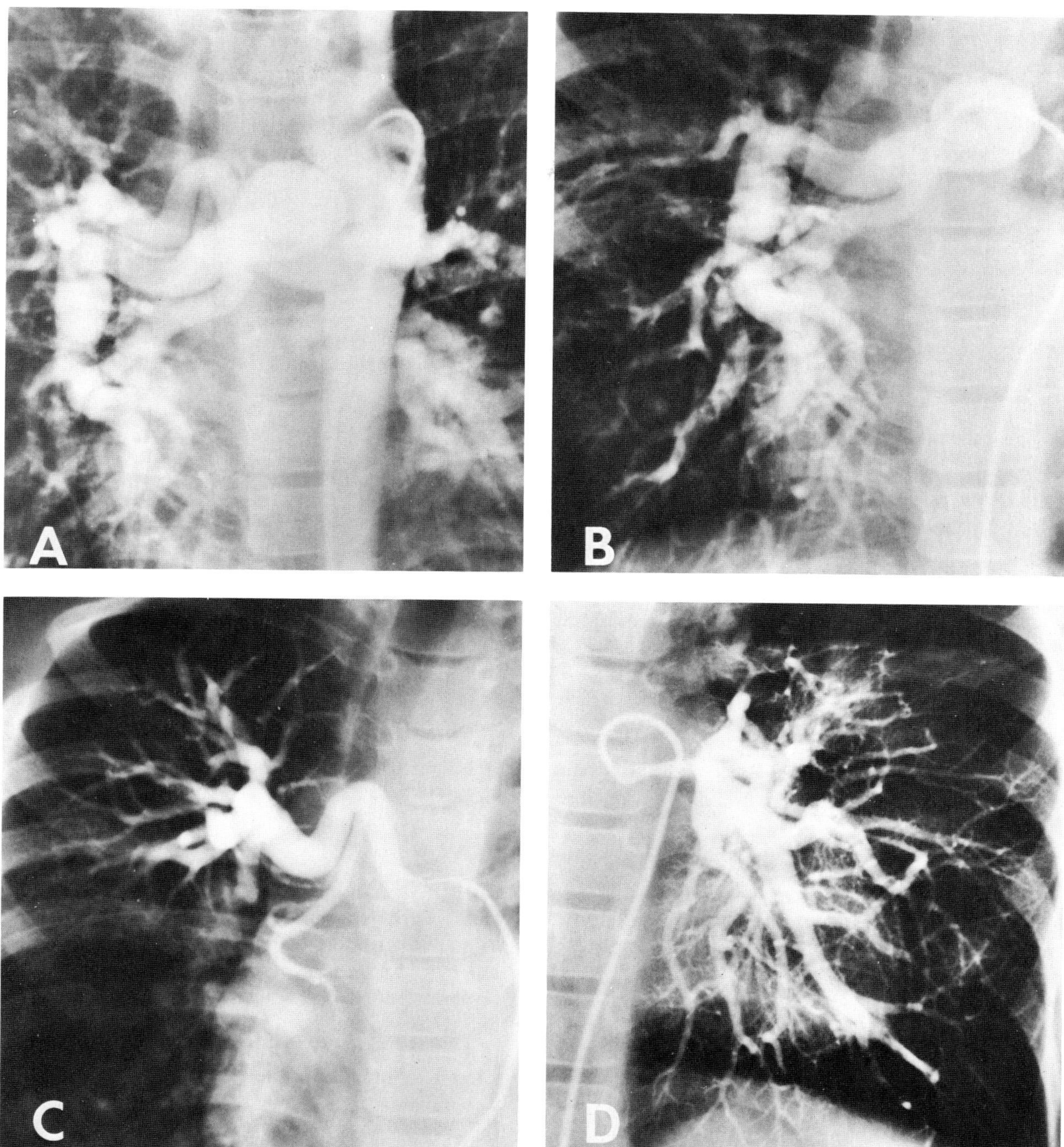

Figure 32-4. Aortopulmonary collateral vessels in pseudotruncus arteriosus (pulmonary atresia, ventricular septal defect). (A) An aortic injection shows filling of dilated hilar pulmonary arteries via a patent ductus and aortopulmonary collateral vessels. (B to D) Selectively injected bronchial collateral vessels fill the pulmonary arteries, which do not communicate directly with the heart.

◀ **Figure 32-3.** Aortopulmonary collateral vessels in pseudotruncus arteriosus. (A) A selective injection of an aortopulmonary collateral vessel fills the arteries to the lower right lung. (B) A selective bronchial injection with filling of the right upper lobe arteries and tortuous, enlarged intercostal collateral vessels. (C) A selective injection of a large collateral vessel shows a stenosis (*arrow*) impairing the filling of the pulmonary artery that partially supplies the left lung.

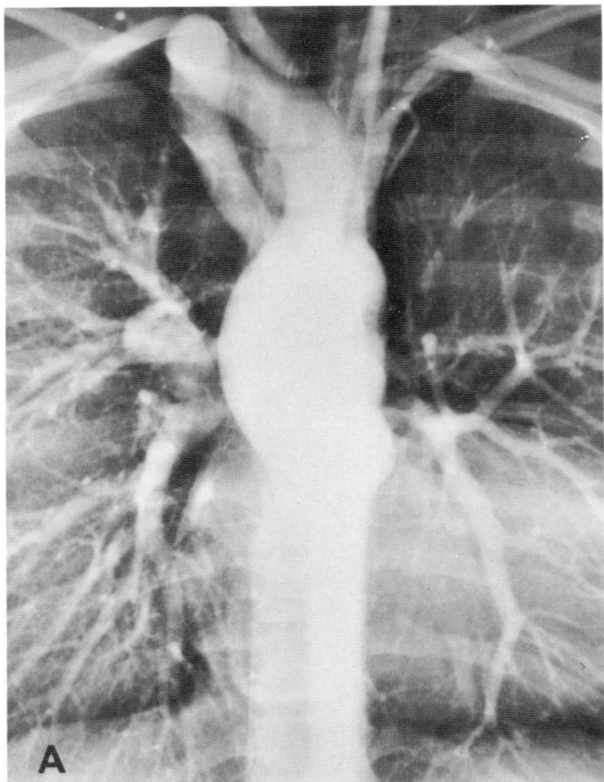

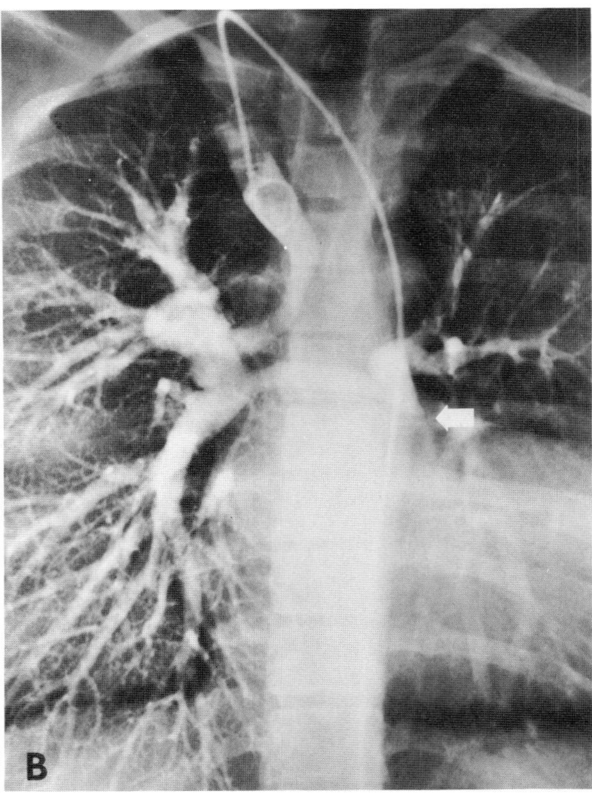

Figure 32-5. Pulmonary artery atresia, pulmonary blood flow via right subclavian and bronchial artery collateral vessels. (A) An aortic injection shows bilateral filling of the pulmonary arteries mostly via a huge descending branch of the right subclavian artery. (B) A selective injection of the right subclavian artery shows the route of blood flow into the malformed central pulmonary arteries. The site of the atresia of the main pulmonary artery is evident (*arrow*). The left lower lobe fills via the bronchial artery (not selectively injected). A large ventricular septal defect was present.

lowing explanation of the mechanism of its formation.[7] Blood velocity varies at different sites within the cardiovascular system, at different times in the cardiac cycle, and at different levels of cardiac output. In general, the closer to the heart, the higher the peak and the mean velocity attained by the blood. The restrictions to blood flow in the tetralogy of Fallot and coarctation of the aorta are partially compensated for by collateral pathways, but in pure valvular stenosis the entire output must be forced through an extremely small orifice during the same time as normally would be required for its passage through an area considerably larger. The resulting high-velocity jet impinges on the wall of the pulmonary artery and tends to push it out, causing local, asymmetric elongation and dilatation of the main and left pulmonary arteries along the principal axis of the jet stream. This elongation accounts for the high position of the left pulmonary artery in adults with mild to moderate congenital pulmonary valvular stenosis.

A second factor in the mechanism producing poststenotic dilatation is lateral wall force due to turbulence. Turbulent flow occurs normally and pathologically at many sites within the cardiovascular system, but never more dramatically than in association with severe pulmonary or aortic valve stenosis, either congenital or acquired.[8] The presence and character of turbulence are determined by (1) geometric factors, namely, luminal and mural anatomy; (2) fluid (blood) viscosity; and (3) velocity of flow. In valvular stenosis, the abrupt transition in vascular caliber from the small stenotic orifice to the large, comparatively stagnant, poststenotic pulmonary artery and the high velocity of the jet cause a turbulent vortex, which in diagrammatic cross section could be represented as two oppositely directed circular flow paths centrally related to each other on opposite sides of the jet stream. Actually, in the three-dimensional patient, this pattern traced by moving blood is more like a lopsided doughnut.

This pattern of flow was demonstrated radiographically by Dotter, who used a simple model (Fig. 32-9). This demonstrated the abnormal pattern of post-

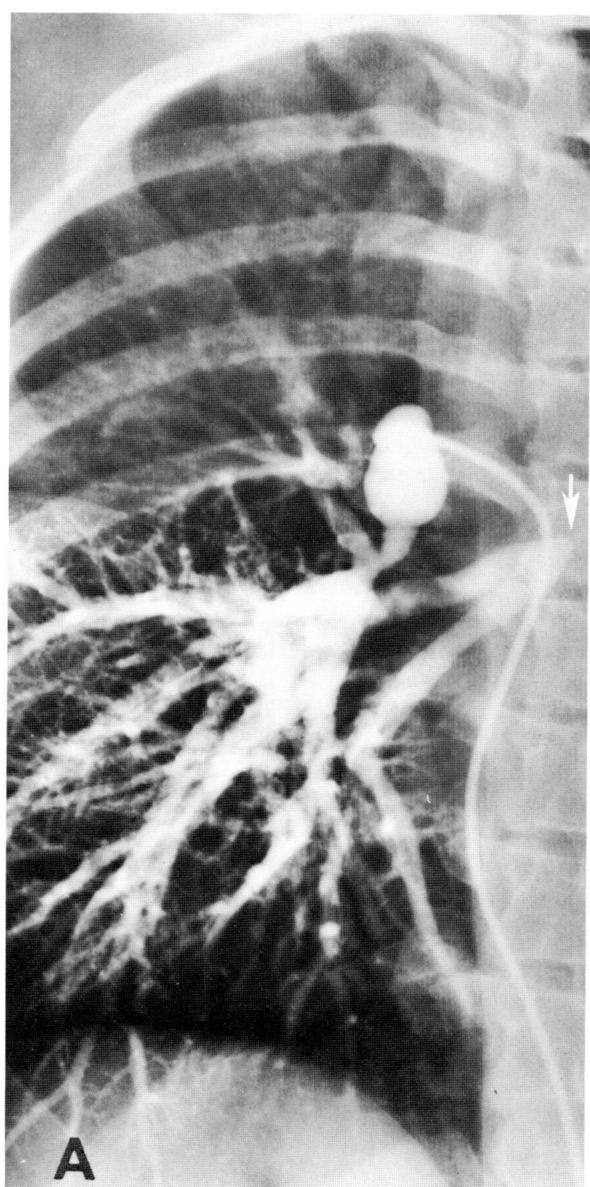

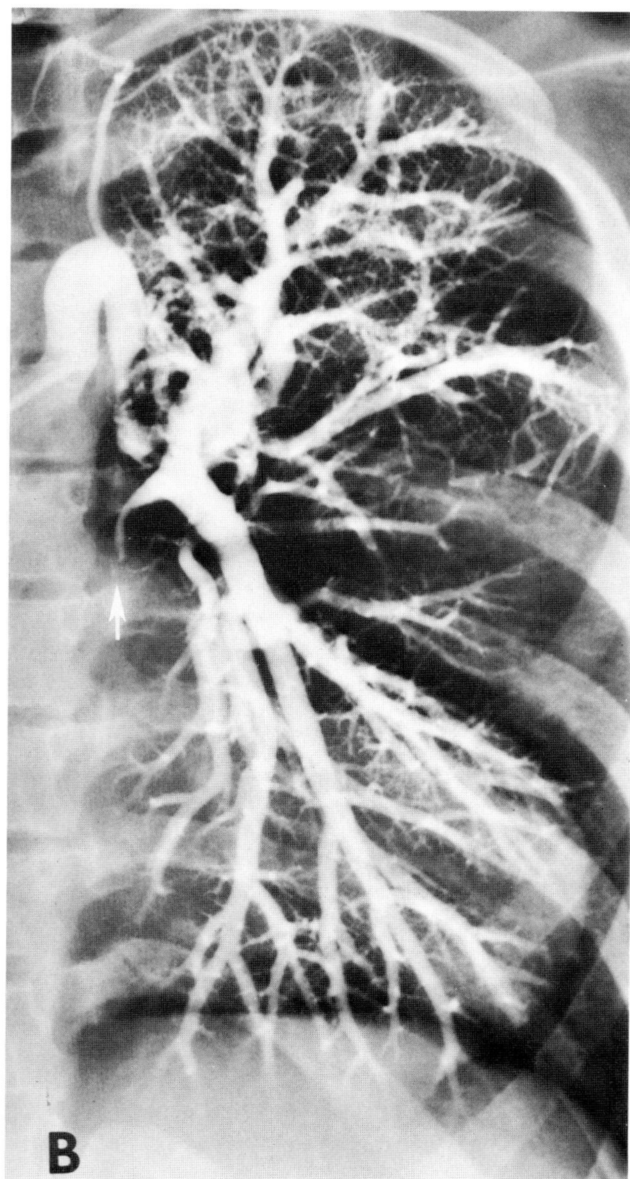

Figure 32-6. Pulmonary atresia, bronchial aortopulmonary collateral vessels. (A) A selective right bronchial injection fills centrally atretic (*arrow*) pulmonary arteries to the right middle lobe and the right lower lobe. (B) A selective left bronchial injection fills the centrally atretic (*arrow*) left pulmonary arteries through an apparently stenotic point of communication. The right upper lobe arteries fill via uninjected collateral vessel(s).

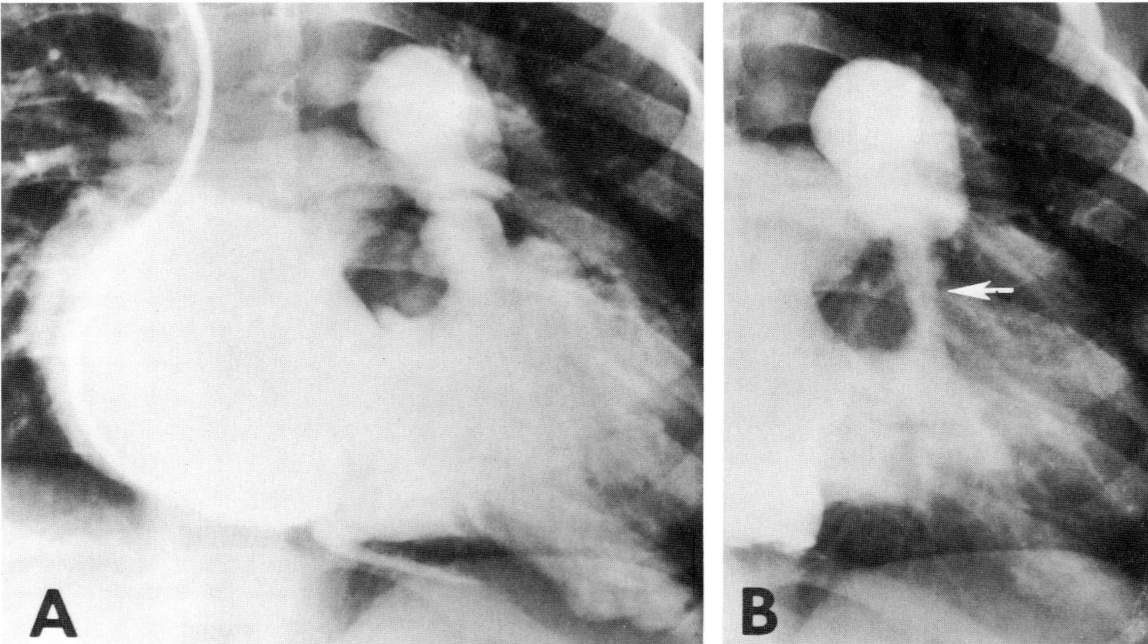

Figure 32-7. Isolated congenital pulmonary valve stenosis. A right atrial injection shows a dilated right atrium and an enlarged thick-walled right ventricle. (A) The early systolic phase shows a domelike unsegmented pulmonary valve. (B) The late systolic phase shows an apparent narrowing of the right ventricular infundibulum (*arrow*), reflecting marked right ventricular hypertrophy caused by the primary valvular stenosis.

Figure 32-8. Multiple congenital pulmonary artery branch stenoses. A selective pulmonary arteriogram shows numerous, bilateral perihilar stenoses with corresponding poststenotic dilatations.

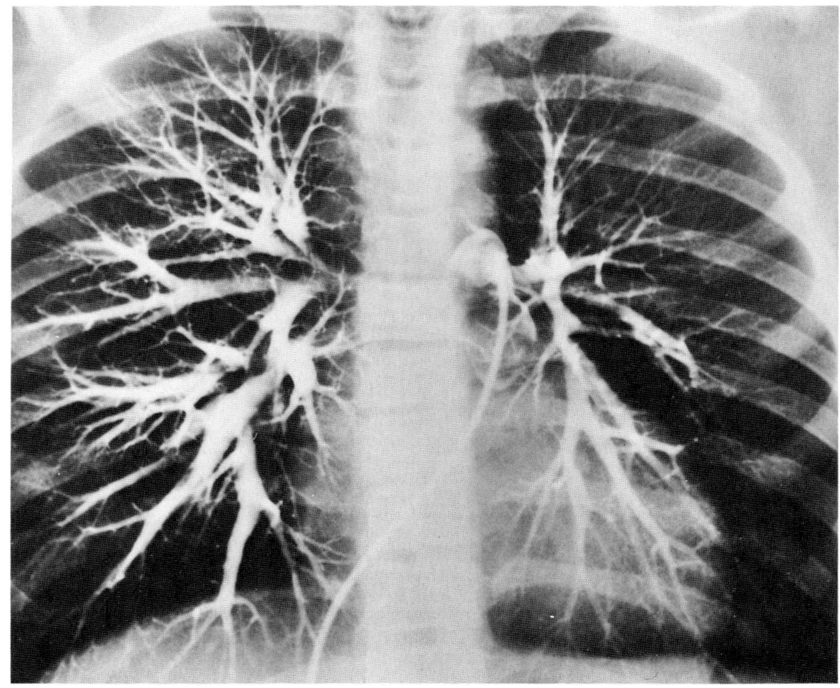

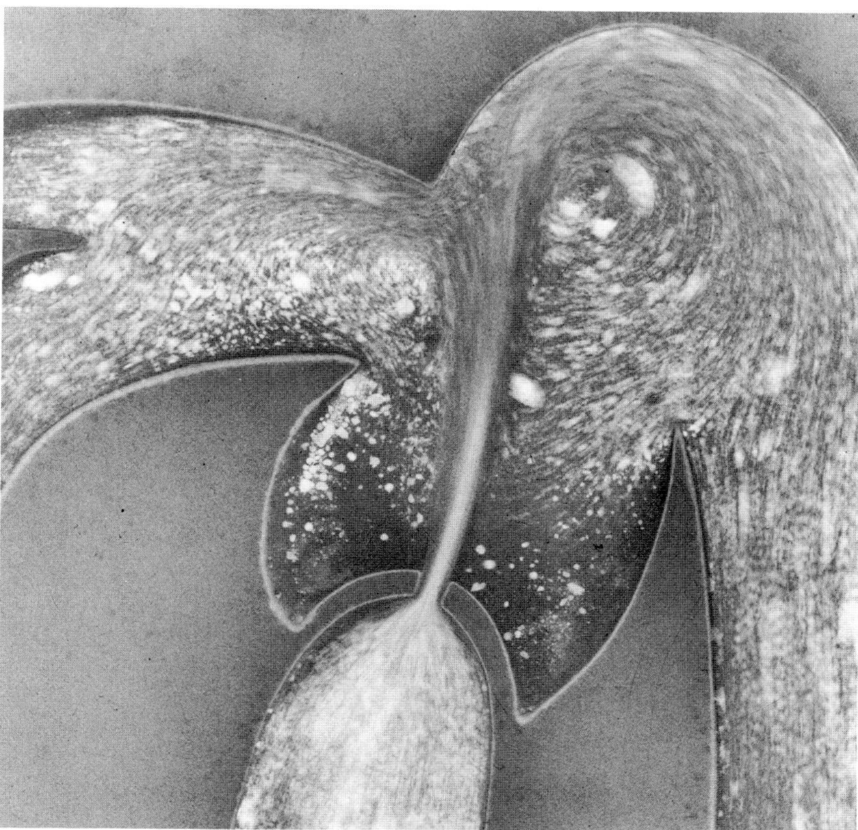

Figure 32-9. Radiographic study of turbulence in plastic model simulating pulmonary valve stenosis. Particles of barium carbonate suspended in motor oil were forced through the cavity with a syringe and interconnecting rubber tubing. The pattern of particle motion is clearly shown in this 1/10 second (12-impulse) summed-image exposure. A stethoscope clearly demonstrated a "systolic murmur" that varied in pitch and intensity with the velocity of the injection.

stenotic flow and also offered a simple, logical explanation of poststenotic dilatation at any site in the cardiovascular system. Blood has mass and, of necessity, exhibits all the physical properties of mass, including inertia. Masses traveling in circular paths exert centrifugal force. In traversing the circular pathways evident in Figure 32-9, blood exerts centrifugal force along the entire vortical periphery. In the center of the vessel, where circular vortical flow paths are adjacent, opposing force vectors are canceled. The net effect is that while poststenotic blood pressures as measured through a catheter are lower than prestenotic pressures, lateral pressure against the walls of the vessel causes poststenotic dilatation. In addition, focal pressure due to the jet impact probably plays a further role in misshaping blood vessels.

In severe pulmonary stenosis with an overriding aorta or interventricular septal defect, the low volume of transstenotic pulmonary flow usually provides insufficient energy to cause poststenotic dilatation. In pure pulmonary stenosis with a comparable severe valve area reduction, life may be literally too short for the development of poststenotic dilatation.

Multiple Pulmonary Artery Stenoses

Multiple sites of peripheral pulmonary stenosis cause poststenotic dilatation.[9–12] This is recognizable on conventional chest radiographs and strikingly apparent on pulmonary arteriograms, resulting in a bizarre appearance (see Fig. 32-8). Transstenotic catheter pressure measurements show pressure gradients that vary from one stenosis to another. Although it might be assumed that multiple pulmonary stenoses would be necessarily associated with distal pulmonary hypotension, that is not always so.

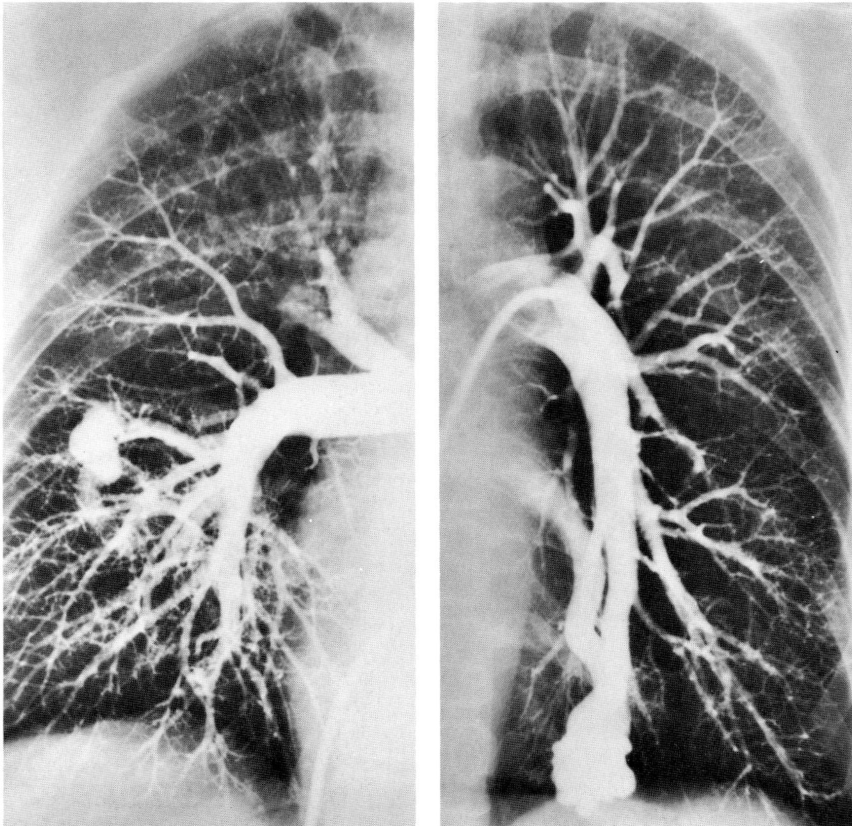

Figure 32-10. Multiple pulmonary arteriovenous fistulas. Right and left selective pulmonary arteriograms show typical lesions in each lung.

Pulmonary Artery Sling

Although pulmonary artery sling is uncommon, it carries a 50 percent mortality rate. This anomaly of the aortic arch system results in the left pulmonary artery (or rarely the left lower lobar artery only) arising from the right pulmonary artery. The artery then passes posterior to the trachea and anterior to the esophagus as it courses to the left lung. On the plain film, a soft tissue mass will be seen between the trachea and esophagus.[13] Pulmonary angiography will confirm the diagnosis. However, MRI may now be the preferred modality according to some authors.[14]

Pulmonary Arteriovenous Fistula

Pulmonary arteriovenous fistula is a relatively frequent congenital anomaly. It is often hereditary,[15,16] and, because it can be treated by transcatheter techniques, is of considerable interest to interventional radiologists. In about a third of the patients with pulmonary arteriovenous fistula, multiple telangiectases of skin and mucous membranes are present with the pulmonary lesions as components of the Osler-Weber-Rendu disease. Classically, pulmonary arteriovenous fistulas are direct communications between branches of pulmonary arteries and veins, usually with considerable dilatation of the affected vessels, which are detectable on conventional chest radiographs. Multiple sites of involvement are common (Figs. 32-10 and 32-11). Except for the recognition of telangiectatic lesions, discernible bruits, and occasionally detectable cyanosis, physical examination is not very helpful. Marked pulmonary artery enlargement occurs in approximately 2 percent of cases of pulmonary arteriovenous fistula, usually in patients who also have mitral stenosis (Fig. 32-12). Hemodynamic studies have shown total pulmonary vascular resistance to be normal in the face of large arteriovenous communications, perhaps because of a compensatory increase in the resistance of the unaffected portions of the pulmonary vascular bed.[17]

The complications of pulmonary arteriovenous fistula include pulmonary hemorrhage (with anemia, if severe), brain abscess, coronary and cerebral embo-

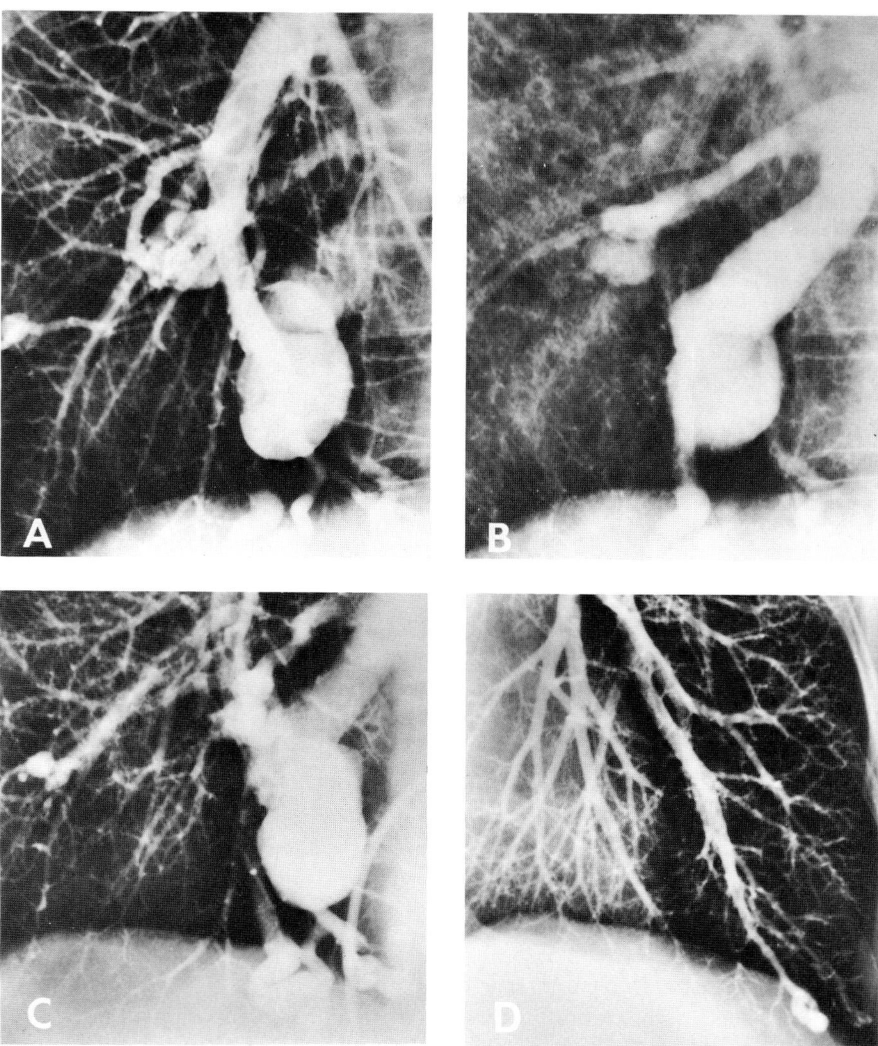

Figure 32-11. Multiple pulmonary arteriovenous fistulas. One large and four smaller fistulas in a right lung shown in the frontal view during (A) arterial and (B) venous filling. (C) A slightly oblique view of same. (D) A small lesion arising from the left lateral basal artery. Percutaneous transluminal obliteration of the large lesion at the right base would require measures to prevent undesired systemic embolization of an occlusive device or a secondary thrombus.

lism, cyanosis, and polycythemia.[18] Heart failure is not ordinarily caused by pulmonary arteriovenous fistulas because, unlike peripheral vascular fistulas, these lesions rarely cause significant alterations in ventricular hemodynamics. Because the presence of the lesion carries significant potential complications, its suspected presence is a strong indication for pulmonary angiography. The disproportionate vascular resistances offered by the fistula and the unaffected portions of the pulmonary bed result in an increase in blood flow through the lesion at the expense of the remaining lung, resulting in excellent visualization of the lesion. This self-selectivity favors the angiographic detection of previously unsuspected small communications occurring at other sites in the pulmonary vascular bed (see Fig. 32-10). Because there are multiple lesions in many of the patients affected, it is important that no part of the lung fields be excluded from examination. Selective studies in multiple projections (see Fig. 32-11) are necessary for treatment planning, whether by surgical resection or by transcatheter occlusion (Fig. 32-13).[19–22]

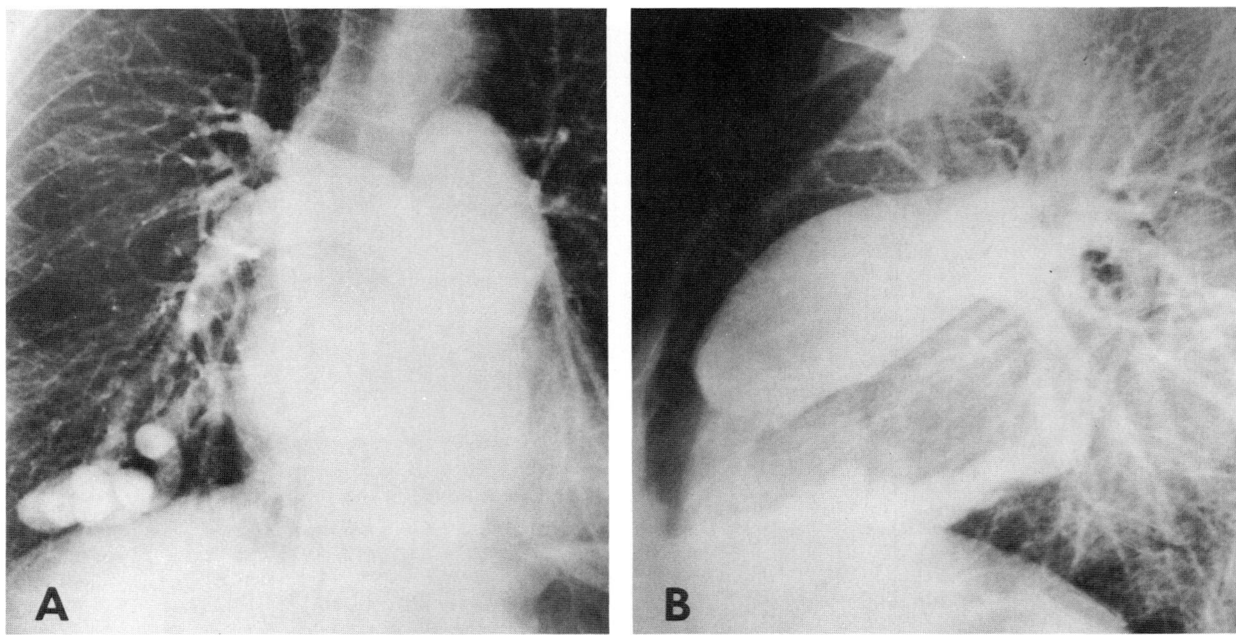

Figure 32-12. Pulmonary arteriovenous fistula complicated by mitral stenosis. (A) A frontal angiocardiogram. (B) A lateral angiogram. Marked central pulmonary arterial enlargement reflects the mitral stenosis, not the fistula.

Patent Ductus Arteriosus and Aorticopulmonary Window

In both these lesions, left-to-right shunting occurs from the aorta into the pulmonary arteries.[2] One of the earliest known retrograde aortograms (done in the 1940s by Pereiras et al.)[23] demonstrated a patent ductus clearly enough to be used as an illustration in this chapter (Fig. 32-14) a half century later. Figure 32-15 demonstrates the tortuous, dilated pulmonary arteries evident secondary to the combined dilating effects of increased flow and pressure present 4 weeks after the successful surgical closure of a congenital aorticopulmonary window.

In patent ductus arteriosus, the development of pulmonary hypertension sometimes results in the shunting of unoxygenated blood from the pulmonary artery through the ductus and into the distal aortic arch.[24] In this situation, right heart or main pulmonary artery injection of contrast agent will opacify not only the pulmonary arteries but also the descending aorta.

Miscellaneous Congenital Pulmonary Vascular Abnormalities

The contributions of pulmonary arteriography to the study of other congenital defects affecting the pulmonary vascular bed are generally straightforward and do not require detailed discussion.

Idiopathic pulmonary artery dilatation[25] is a diagnosis made by exclusion. Contrast visualization alone does not provide this exclusion, although good-quality studies aid by showing normal valvular function. Catheter pressure measurements across the pulmonary valve are needed to rule out a pressure gradient.

Isolated *pulmonary artery atresia* and *coarctation* are uncommon congenital abnormalities. Congenital absence or hypoplasia of a branch pulmonary artery[26–31] can readily be studied by means of pulmonary arteriography with selective injections (Fig. 32-16). Coarctation of the central pulmonary artery appears to occur in association with patent ductus arteriosus,[32] whereas interruption of a right or left pulmonary artery is more common in conjunction with tetralogy of Fallot.[33] Angiographically, the unaffected pulmonary artery will be larger than normal whereas the pulmonary vasculature on the affected side will be bizarre, frequently filling from bronchial collaterals or occasionally from intercostal or phrenic arteries. Associated rib notching may be present. In all such cases, studies should include aortography or selective arteriography of the involved systemic arteries in order to visualize the vessels supplying the area of lung in which pulmonary arteries are deficient (see discussion of pulmonary sequestration below).

Hypoplasia of the right or left pulmonary artery may not be congenital in origin. Because autopsy stud-

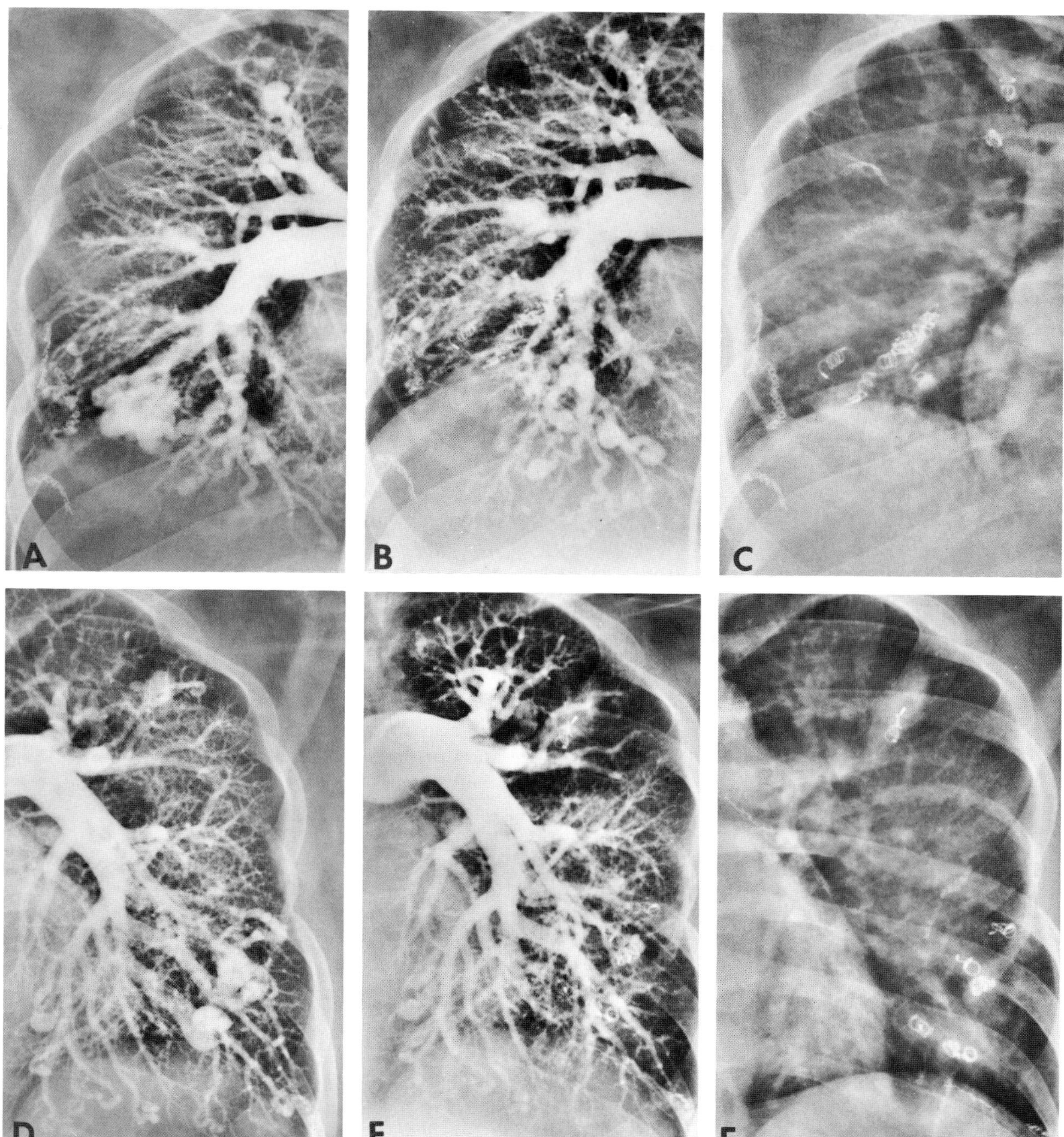

Figure 32-13. Multiple bilateral pulmonary arteriovenous fistulas treated by catheter occlusion. A 32-year-old woman after bilateral lobectomies with persistent cyanosis and recurrent cerebral abscesses. (A) Preocclusion right pulmonary angiogram. (B) Right pulmonary angiogram after the occlusion of eight fistulas with Gianturco coil springs. (C) Conventional radiograph showing sites of occlusion. (D) Preocclusion, left pulmonary angiogram. (E) After the occlusion of eight fistulas with coil springs. (F) Conventional radiograph. Though other smaller fistulas remain, transcatheter occlusion led to an immediate reduction of the right-to-left shunt from 27 to 8 percent of the cardiac output and to the disappearance of cyanosis.

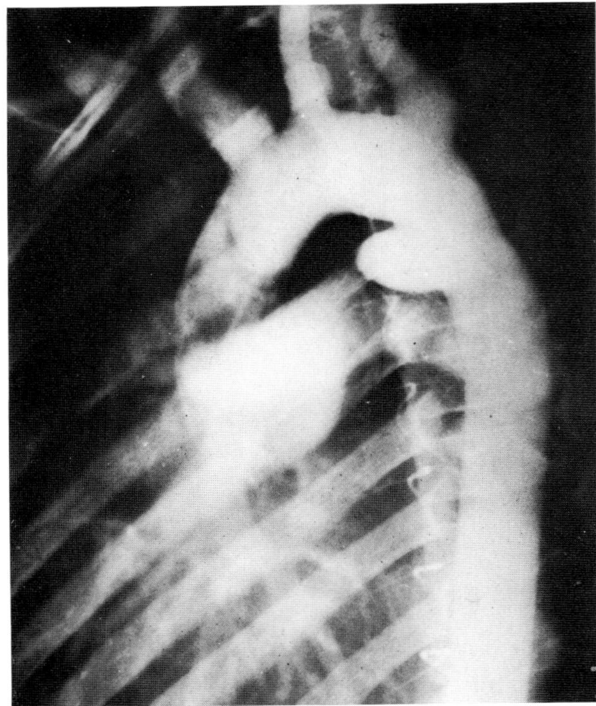

Figure 32-14. Patent ductus arteriosus; a retrograde aortogram made approximately a half century ago. The conical ductus shunts blood from the aorta into the pulmonary artery. (From Pereiras R, et al. Aortografia retrograda superior desde la arteria carotida primitiva en el niño y en el adulto. Rev Cubana Cardiol 1950;11:65. Used with permission.)

ies of thousands of newborn infants have failed to reveal the condition and because unilateral destructive pulmonary disease can produce identical changes (including the development of large, collateral bronchial arteries), it is probable that here the term *congenital* may be a misnomer.[34] The size of a pulmonary artery tends to reflect its functional usefulness, as is evidenced by the prompt diminution in flow and vessel size after ligation of the corresponding bronchus.

Pulmonary sequestration is a mass of nonfunctioning pulmonary parenchyma that fails to communicate with the tracheobronchial tree and has an anomalous systemic arterial supply. In *intralobar sequestration,* the segment is enclosed in the pulmonary visceral pleura and occurs on the left side in two-thirds of the patients, most commonly in the basilar segments. In most patients, the venous drainage is to the left atrium, although it is occasionally to the right atrium. It usually presents in older children or adults, typically with recurrent pulmonary infections.[35] In *extralobar sequestration,* the segment is enclosed in its own visceral pleura but again occurs most commonly in the left base, usually between the left lower lobe and the left hemidiaphragm. However, extralobar sequestrations have been reported in intrapericardial, subdiaphragmatic, retroperitoneal, and anterior mediastinal locations.[36–38] Again, a systemic artery, usually from the thoracic aorta but occasionally from the abdominal aorta or one of its branches, supplies the segment. In contrast, the drainage is into a systemic vein, usually

Figure 32-15. Pulmonary vascular dilatation due to a congenital aortopulmonary window. Marked changes shown by angiocardiography done a month following successful surgical correction.

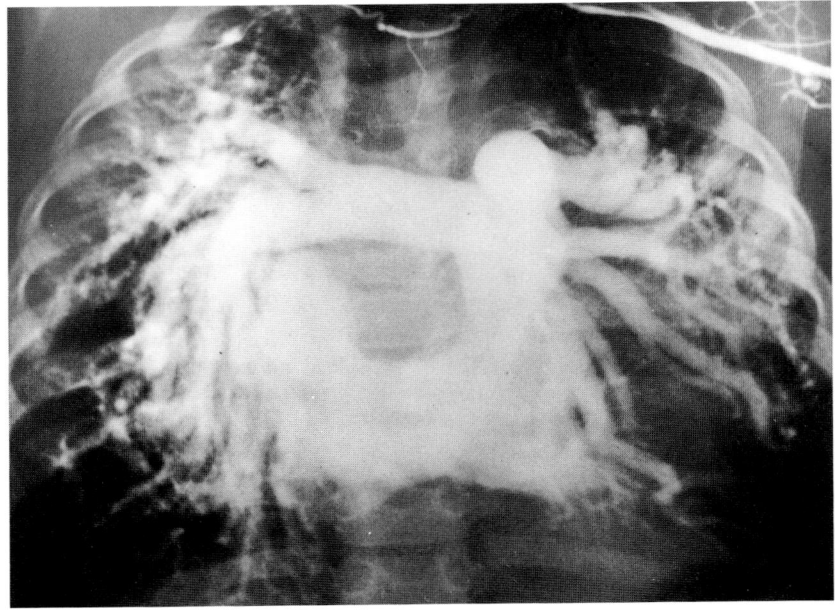

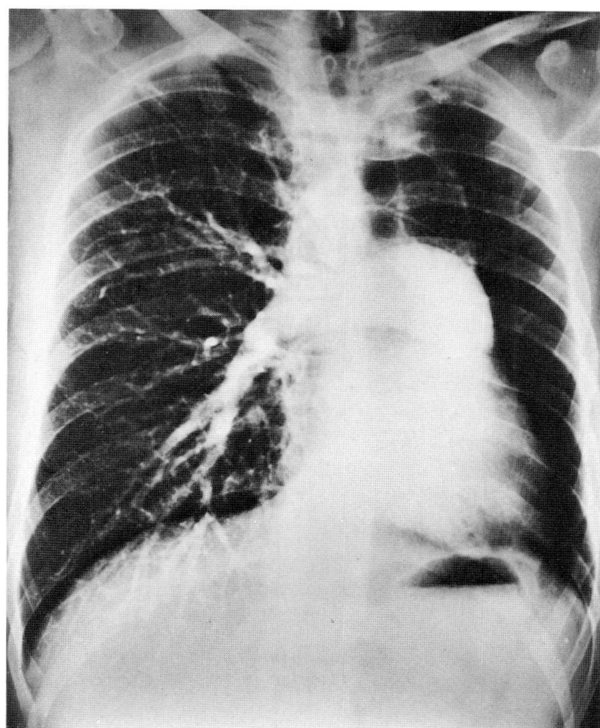

Figure 32-16. Hypoplasia or aplasia, left pulmonary artery. Intravenous frontal angiogram. The heart is rotated, and the right lung is herniated into the left chest. The right pulmonary vessels are dilated. There are no discernible left pulmonary arteries.

the inferior vena cava (IVC) or the azygos or hemiazygos system. The patients usually present early in life because of symptoms that include cyanosis, dyspnea, or feeding difficulty. In all instances, pulmonary arteriography will demonstrate the nonperfused segment, and thoracic or abdominal aortography with appropriate selective systemic arteriography will demonstrate the anomalous arterial supply to the sequestered segment.

Congenital lobar emphysema (controversy exists as to the etiology of this entity) produces marked displacement of the pulmonary arteries, well shown arteriographically (Fig. 32-17).

The definitive anatomic diagnosis of *anomalous origin of a coronary artery from the pulmonary artery* and *coronary artery–pulmonary artery fistula*[39,40] is made by selective arteriography from the aortic or pulmonary side, depending on the nature of the lesion and the direction of flow (Fig. 32-18). These anomalies may result in myocardial ischemia, particularly in later life if an associated coronary artery stenosis occurs. Reversibility of the associated myocardial ischemia may be demonstrated with stress thallium tomography.[41]

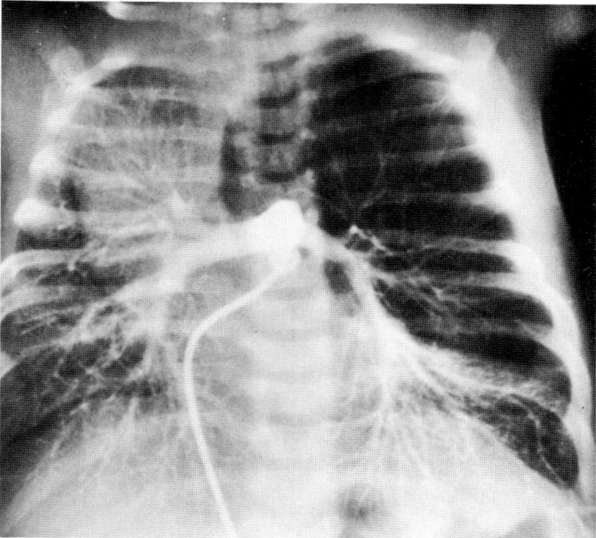

Figure 32-17. Congenital lobar emphysema, a selective pulmonary arteriogram. A large emphysematous area occupies most of the left hemithorax with vascular and mediastinal displacement and crowding of pulmonary arterial branches to the compressed left lower lobe. There is severe functional impairment. The etiology is uncertain.

Minor developmental variations in pulmonary segmental arteries occur frequently but are rarely a matter of clinical concern. If planned segmental pulmonary resection is preceded by arteriographic examination, these minor alterations will be recognized in advance. Studies should include visualization of the pulmonary veins as well as the arteries, because the intersegmental location of the veins may be helpful in planning surgery.

Acquired Abnormalities

Angiography demonstrates changes in the pulmonary vessels caused by a wide variety of conditions. Functional alterations are important, but a classification based solely on them would be no more useful than a lengthy, etiologic breakdown. Therefore, the role and findings of pulmonary angiography will be considered under groupings justified by clinical usage rather than under a detailed enumeration of specific conditions.

Pulmonary Heart Disease

By common usage, the terms *pulmonary heart disease* and *cor pulmonale* refer to instances in which a significant abnormal load is imposed on the right ventricle because of pulmonary disease.[42] In the absence of

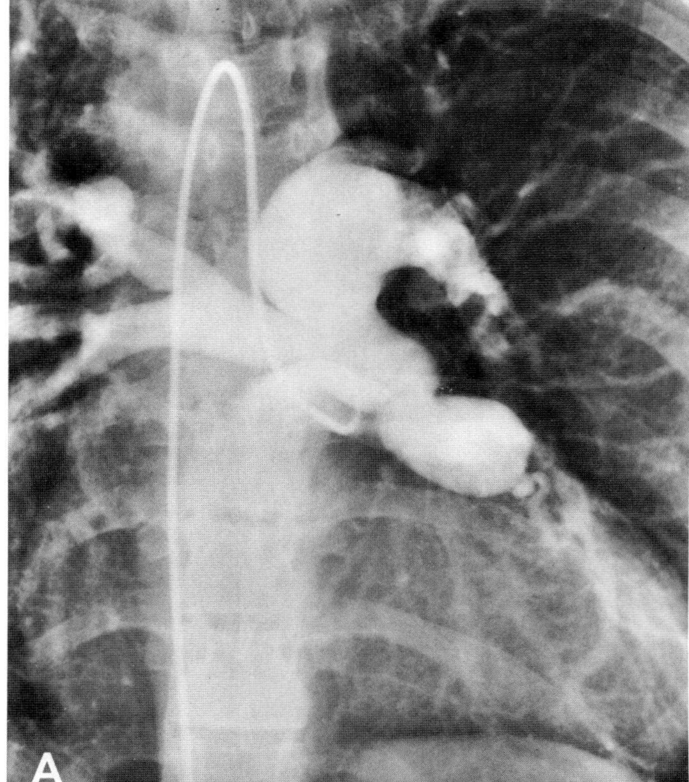

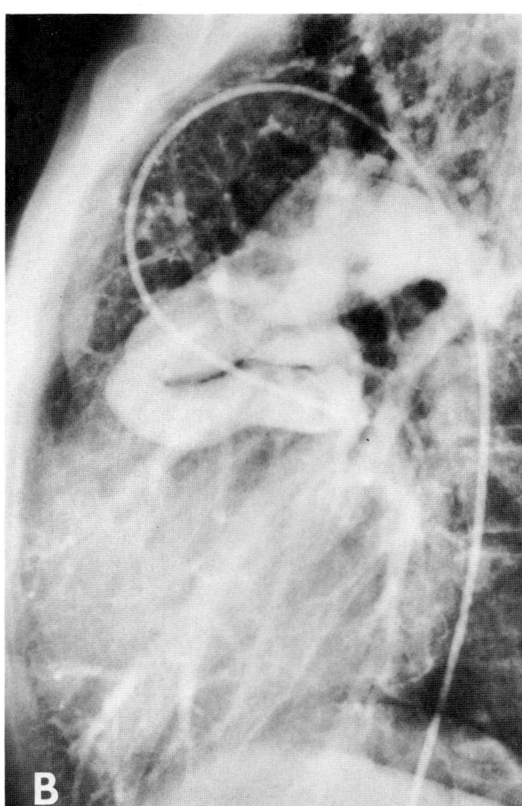

Figure 32-18. Anomalous left coronary artery–pulmonary artery fistula in tetralogy of Fallot. Frontal and lateral selective injections into the aortic end (*right-sided arch*) of the tortuous communication disclose that major pulmonary arterial filling occurs by this unusual route. Pulmonary atresia prevents pulmonary blood flow by the normal route.

chamber dilatation, right ventricular enlargement cannot be identified by conventional roentgenologic means.[43–45]

The earliest anatomic response of the right ventricle to increased pulmonary vascular resistance is hypertrophy. Hypothetically, unless chamber dilatation is also present, doubling of the right ventricular muscle mass adds only about a centimeter to the transverse diameter of the heart (assuming a doubling of the right ventricle's maximum normal wall thickness). This minor widening falls within the limits of normal systolic-diastolic variation. This is illustrated by Figure 32-19,

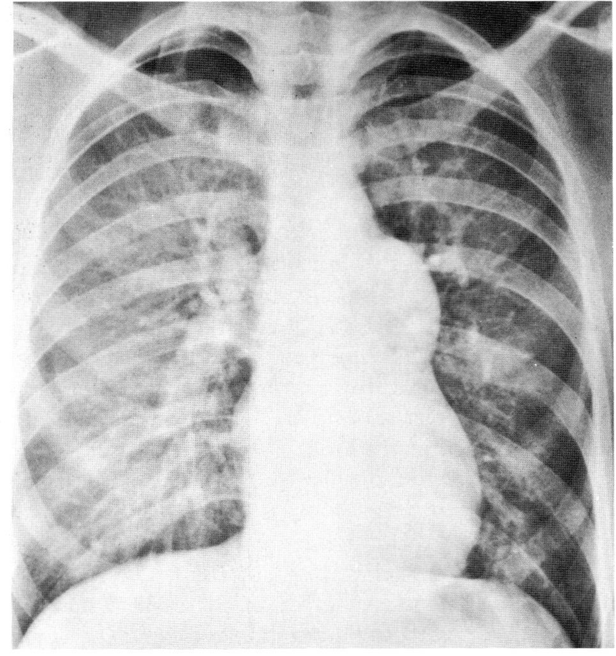

Figure 32-19. Protracted severe pulmonary hypertension without demonstrable right ventricular enlargement. Chest film of a 23-year-old man who was cyanotic for the last 9 years because of a high interventricular septal defect and pulmonary artery pressures approaching systemic levels. Despite this, there was no radiologically recognizable enlargement of the heart. The pulmonary arteries are grossly dilated because of increased pressure and flow. An electrocardiogram showed right ventricular hypertrophy.

the chest film of a 23-year-old man with an interventricular septal defect and pulmonary hypertension. Clinically, his right ventricle had been operating for 9 years at near-systemic pressure levels without perceptible cardiac enlargement on his chest radiograph. The electrocardiogram revealed right ventricular hypertrophy, and the chest film disclosed central pulmonary arterial dilatation as the only evident morphologic abnormality.

Occasionally, a normal right ventricle may appear to be enlarged when, as the result of a congenital anomaly, the left ventricle has undergone reciprocal underdevelopment. The small, characteristically boot-shaped heart seen in tetralogy of Fallot is illustrative. In many cases of pulmonary heart disease, pulmonary vascular enlargement is accompanied by ventricular dilatation and therefore perceptible x-ray enlargement of the right ventricle.

The principal contributions of radiology to the study of pulmonary heart disease lie in the study of the lungs and the pulmonary vascular bed.[46] The echocardiogram is a superior means of recognizing right ventricular hypertrophy, whereas pulmonary function studies and cardiac catheterization offer more reliable hemodynamic appraisals. The foregoing defines rather than discredits the contribution of radiology. The following discussion of pulmonary arteriography will emphasize its value.

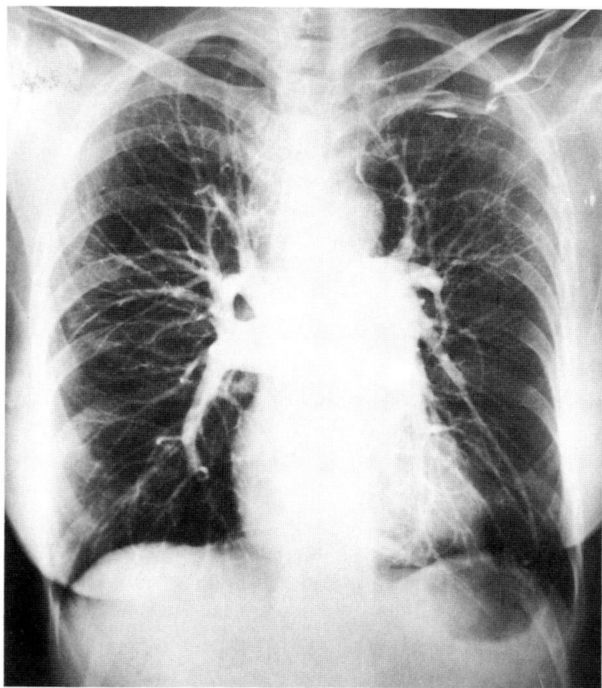

Figure 32-20. Generalized pulmonary emphysema. Emphysema and moderate pulmonary hypertension (43/21 mmHg) in a 52-year-old woman. Angiocardiogram shows central pulmonary arterial enlargement due to the hypertension. The peripheral pulmonary arterial branches are widely separated and thinned. The right ventricle is not demonstrably enlarged.

Pulmonary Emphysema and Pulmonary Hypertension

In mild, diffuse pulmonary emphysema, radiographic changes are usually absent. When the disease is sufficiently advanced to produce the classic alterations on conventional roentgenograms, pulmonary arteriography can be expected to show central pulmonary arterial dilatation due to secondary pulmonary hypertension and peripheral distributive changes, including wider spacing between adjacent pulmonary arterial branches and an increase in the take-off or subdivision angle (Fig. 32-20). With pulmonary hypertension of greater severity and longer duration, greater degrees of central pulmonary arterial dilatation appear, and, in addition to the architectural changes already mentioned, there is narrowing of the widely spaced peripheral branches of the pulmonary artery. With severe emphysema, particularly in highly localized forms, the arteriographic findings are striking.[47] As shown in Figure 32-21, in bullous emphysema, pulmonary arteriography provides clinically important information by delineating with accuracy air-containing cysts or bullae and by demonstrating the displacement and crowding of adjacent vessels. Poorly perfused, locally overdistended parts of the lung compress otherwise normal adjacent lung tissue. The resulting combination of faulty ventilation and perfusion usually adds up to gross respiratory insufficiency. The effects of essentially local changes are hidden in the average values obtained by ordinary pulmonary function tests, including nonsegmental bronchospirometry. In bullous emphysema, pulmonary arteriography provides a means of planning resectional surgery. Figure 32-22 illustrates the appearance of the lungs in a patient with bullous emphysema in whom resection of a markedly emphysematous, cystic left upper lobe was followed by reexpansion of the compressed lower lobe and an end to 3 years of respiratory invalidism.

Obliterative Pulmonary Diseases

The spectrum of diseases causing lung destruction or scarification includes many that result in anatomic or functional obliteration of the pulmonary arterial bed.[48] Broadly speaking, the disappearance of pulmonary arteries in chronic upper lobe tuberculosis may be indis-

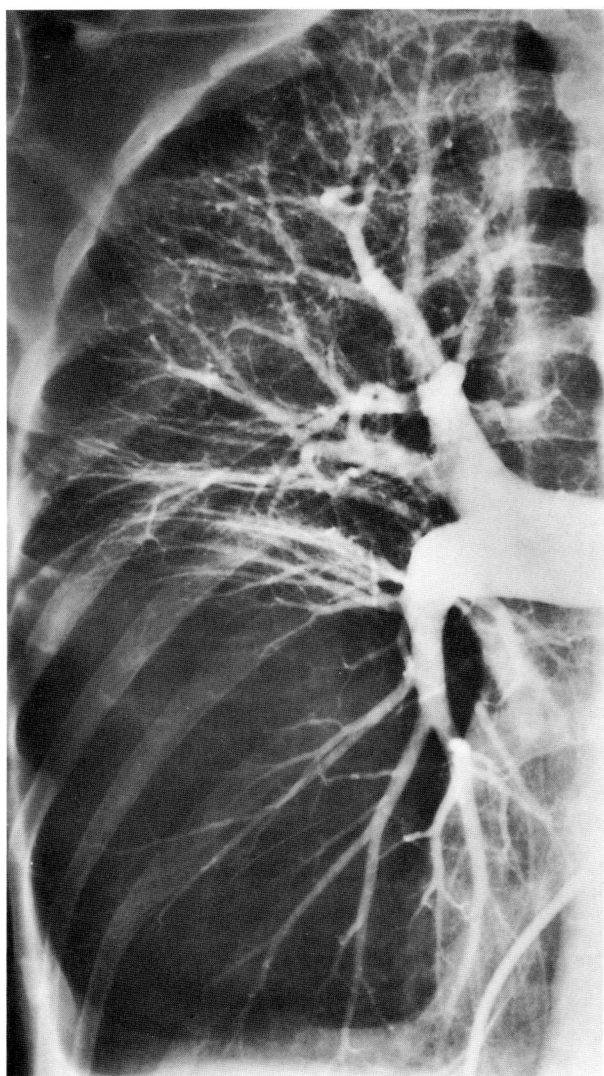

Figure 32-21. Localized bullous emphysema in a 65-year-old man. Right selective pulmonary arteriogram shows a large, lucent, poorly perfused anterior right lower lobe bulla elevating and jamming together the right middle lobe vessels. There is impaired ventilation of the bulla, as well as adjacent, compressed, but otherwise normal lung. A bullectomy led to marked functional improvement.

tinguishable from similarly local obliterative changes associated with other infections, certain tumors, post-irradiation fibrosis, and so on.

Acute primary pulmonary tuberculosis can lead to a general reduction in blood flow to the entire affected lung (Fig. 32-23). Active, upper lobe reinfection-type tuberculosis can, through caseous necrosis, destroy the integrity of blood vessels with arteriographically demonstrable (and, incidentally, catheter-controllable) intrapulmonary or intracavitary hemorrhage from pulmonary vessels. Long-standing chronic pulmonary tuberculosis nearly always results in thrombofibrotic destruction of affected pulmonary artery branches.[49] As in other chronic infections, such as bronchiectasis, this often leads to the development of systemic-to-pulmonary collateral vessels taking origin in bronchial, pleural, and chest wall arteries.[50,51] In such instances, severe hemoptysis can result, and transpleural collateral vessels can turn an attempted lobectomy into a bloody mess. The risk can easily be identified by selective catheterization of the systemic collateral source arteries (Fig. 32-24) and also reduced by transcatheter vaso-occlusion.

Despite these considerations, it is often difficult in local or diffuse pulmonary arterial obliteration to distinguish among numerous possible causes. Figure 32-25 shows grossly obvious but anatomically similar changes resulting from destructive pulmonary sarcoidosis in one patient and, in another patient, the diffuse fibrosis associated with scleroderma. Both patients died of cor pulmonale. Figure 32-26 shows peripheral arterial changes attributed to vasculitis in a patient with chronic disseminated lupus erythematosus and mild pulmonary hypertension. Although it is clear that useful arteriographic distinctions can be made, it is equally clear that numerous etiologically different, chronic, sclerosing diseases eventually produce an arteriographically anonymous hypovascularity.

It has been suggested that acute pulmonary infections cause reactive pulmonary arterial hypervascularity similar to that surrounding peripheral abscesses. This may apply to bronchial arterial responses, but pulmonary arterial flow does not appear to respond similarly to acute local infections. Usually the opposite occurs—that is, a decrease in regional pulmonary blood flow. In pneumonia, for example, an apparent hypervascularity can be simulated by associated atelectasis, edema, consolidation, and exudation in the lung and adjacent pleura (Fig. 32-27). Acute lung abscesses, unlike those in the liver or the peripheral soft tissues, are likely to cause a local reduction, not an increase, in pulmonary arterial flow. Both animal studies and isotopic scanning show that bronchial ligation and alveolar flooding characteristically cause decreased local pulmonary arterial blood flow. The clinical equivalent can be shown by selective pulmonary arteriography in acute lobar pneumonia. Digital subtraction studies should help distinguish between density allegedly due to hypervascularity and that due to superimposed nonvascular abnormalities.

Despite the shortcomings of pulmonary arteriography in the precise differentiation of various pulmonary

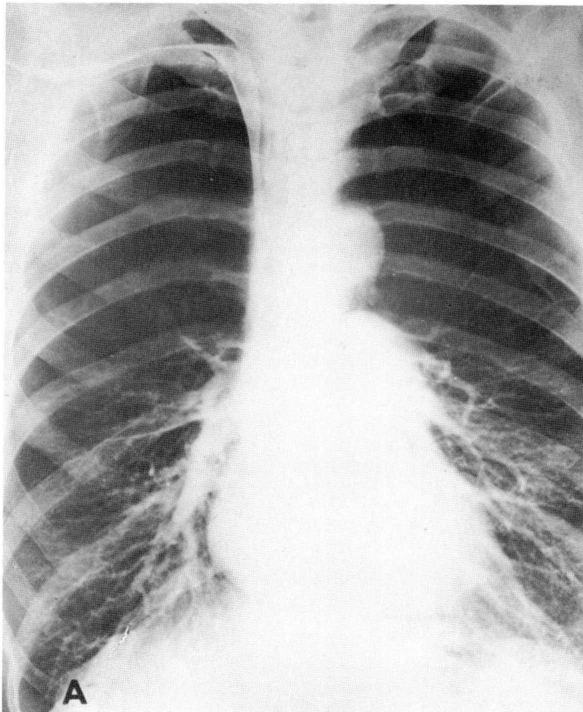

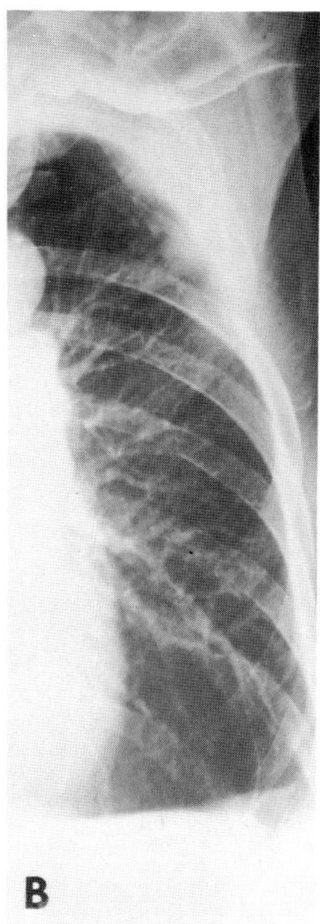

Figure 32-22. Bullous emphysema with postsurgical improvement. (A) Nonselective pulmonary angiogram shows depression and crowding of the pulmonary arteries due to a bilateral upper lobe bullous emphysema in a 40-year-old man disabled by dyspnea. After resection of the left upper lobe, he returned to work for the first time in 3 years. (B) Follow-up arteriogram shows normal-appearing pulmonary arteries to the reexpanded left lower lobe.

destructive processes, there may be light around the corner. Arteriographic studies incorporating macroradiography, bronchial arteriography, and digital subtraction, as well as computed tomography and MRI, may lead to improved differential diagnosis. Unfortunately, except where pulmonary embolization is suspected, few patients with lung disease are referred for pulmonary arteriography, and its broader diagnostic potential in lung disorders remains unexploited. Also overlooked is its ability to delineate the extent and severity of diseases and their secondary changes, a capability that can facilitate therapeutic decision, such as whether and how best to do pulmonary resection.

Among the many pulmonary diseases causing diminished and/or nonfilling of pulmonary arteries are the following: chronic tuberculosis, pneumoconiosis, pulmonary fibrosis (idiopathic, postinflammatory, postirradiation), sarcoidosis, scleroderma, actinomycosis, bronchiectasis, lung tumors, and pulmonary embolism with or without infarction. Suspected pulmonary embolism, the most common clinical indication for pulmonary arteriography, warrants particular consideration here.

Figure 32-23. Reduced pulmonary blood flow in primary tuberculosis in a 12-year-old girl. An angiogram $2\frac{1}{2}$ seconds after an arm vein injection shows reduced pulmonary blood flow through the affected left lung, where an exudative process of several months' duration was beginning to regress. There is no evidence of arterial compression.

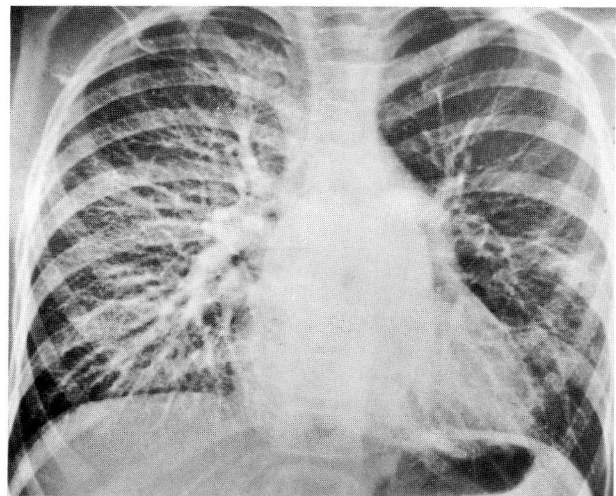

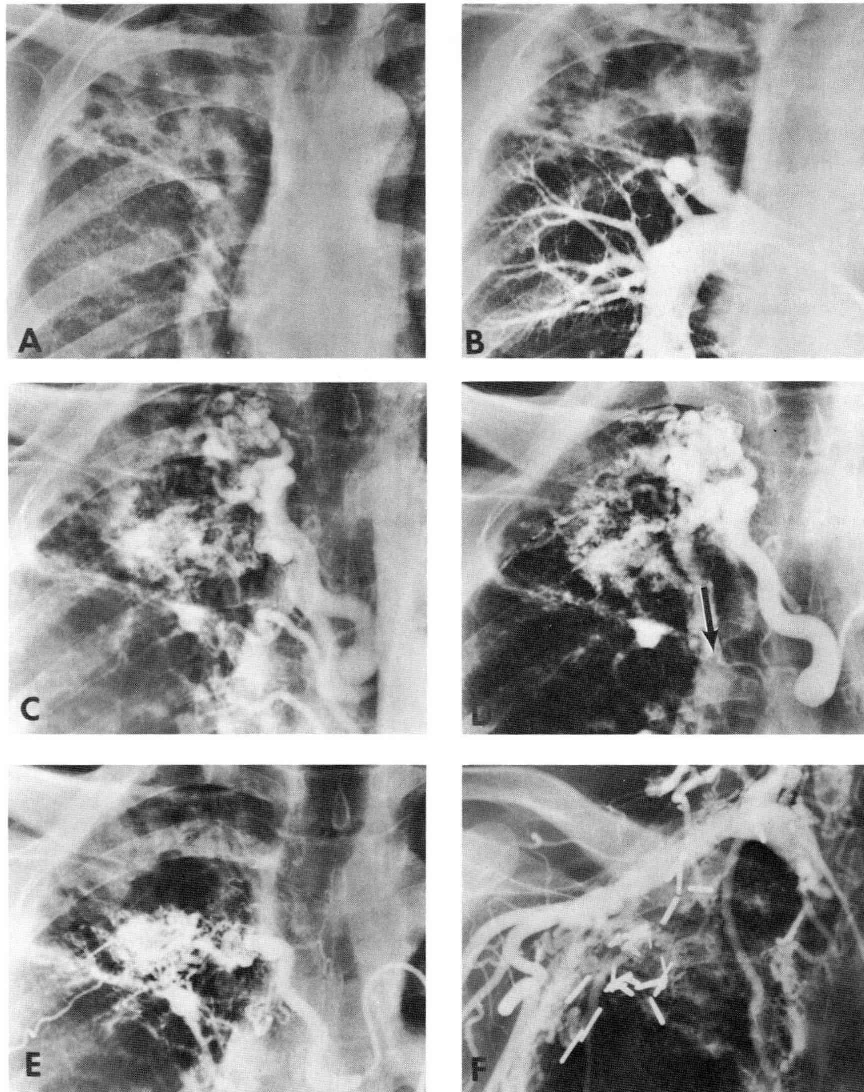

Figure 32-24. Systemic-pulmonary collateral flow in chronic tuberculosis of the right upper lobe with hemoptysis. Chronic, active, reinfection-type tuberculosis with recurrent hemoptysis in a 37-year-old man. A hemorrhage ended an attempted resection. (A) Conventional x-ray. (B) Pulmonary arteriogram shows nonfilling of the right upper lobe branches. (C) Aortic injection shows filling of the large bronchial arteries to the diseased area. (D and E) Selective bronchial arteriography shows retrograde flow into the right upper lobe pulmonary arteries (*arrow*). (F) Selective subclavian study shows large transpleural collateral vessels. Bleeding from them forced the termination of an attempted resection. A subsequent selective catheter occlusion of systemic collateral vessels ended the recurrent hemoptysis.

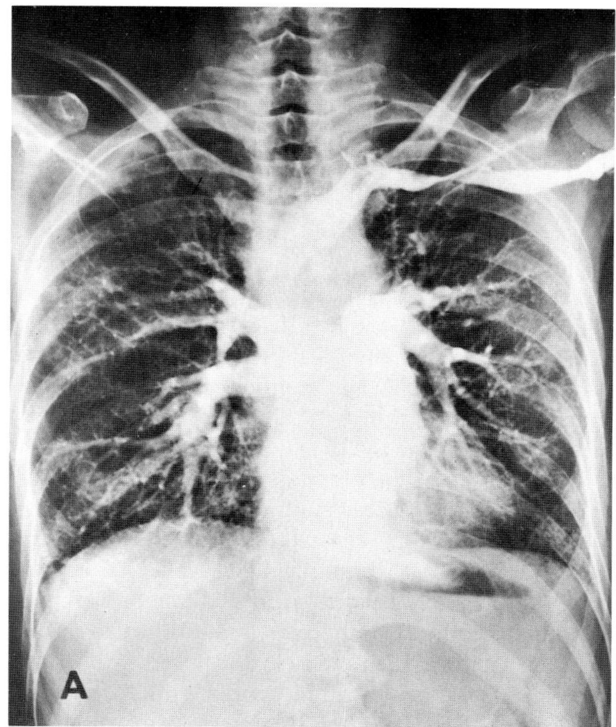

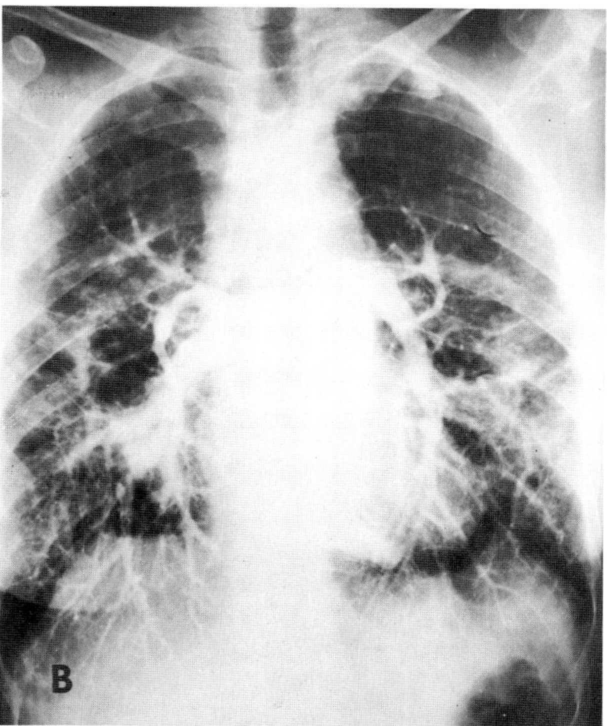

Figure 32-25. Scleroderma and pulmonary sarcoidosis. (A) Scleroderma in a 44-year-old woman. Diffuse nodular pulmonary fibrosis had been shown on a conventional chest roentgenogram. A nonselective pulmonary arteriogram shows central dilatation, peripheral branch distortion, and obliteration. (B) Biopsy-proved sarcoidosis in a 45-year-old woman. Infiltrations and bullae had been shown on a conventional chest film. A pulmonary angiogram shows irregular distortion of segmental arteries. The pulmonary artery pressure was 75/23 mmHg.

Pulmonary Embolism

Although pulmonary embolism is a common condition, the diagnosis may be difficult. Estimates of the incidence of symptomatic episodes are as high as 630,000 annually in the United States.[52] The estimated annual death rate due to pulmonary embolism varies from 50,000 to 200,000.[52,53] The indications for pulmonary angiography as well as its validity and complications have been described in multiple reports over the past 20 years. The largest series and most credible study is the prospective investigation of pulmonary embolism diagnosis (PIOPED) study.[54,55] Pulmonary angiography has been demonstrated to be a safe and

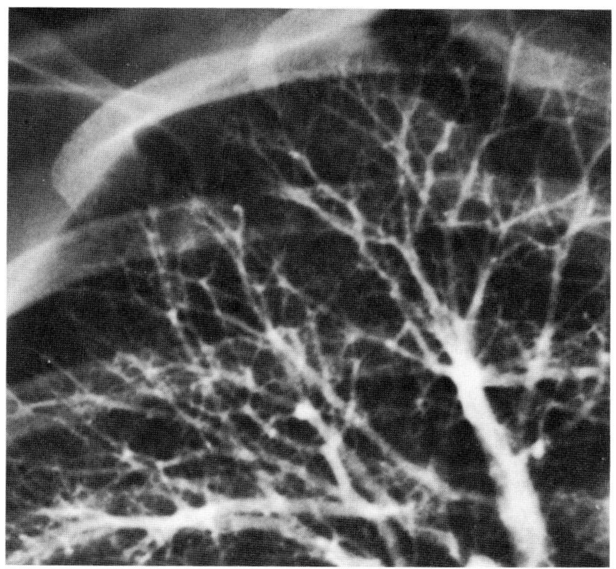

Figure 32-26. Chronic systemic lupus erythematosus with obstructive pulmonary vasculitis in a 28-year-old woman. Dyspnea, congestive heart failure, and right ventricular and central pulmonary arterial enlargement. The pulmonary artery pressure was 75/30 mmHg. An arteriogram shows generalized, peripheral, small artery tapering without an emphysematous branching pattern and chronic small and medium vessel vasculitis.

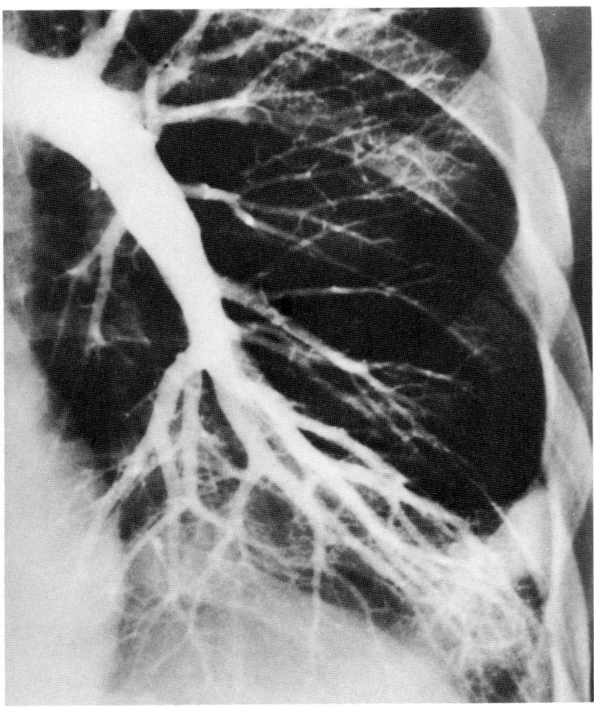

Figure 32-27. Acute pneumococcal pneumonia with atelectasis and adjacent pleural reaction in a 22-year-old man. There was an acute onset of pleuritic pain, fever, dyspnea, and hemoptysis. A selective pulmonary arteriogram did not show suspected pulmonary embolism, but, instead, atelectatic crowding of arteries at and adjacent to the site of infiltration and local pleural thickening or effusion. The pneumonia responded promptly to penicillin.

cost-effective modality in the diagnosis of pulmonary embolism when used in conjunction with perfusion-ventilation lung scans and ultrasonography of the legs as a part of a diagnostic management strategy.[56,57]

Although the terms *pulmonary infarction* and *pulmonary embolism* may be frequently used interchangeably clinically, they are certainly not synonymous. True infarction—the obstruction of a pulmonary artery with the subsequent necrosis of pulmonary tissue—occurs in a small minority of patients with pulmonary embolism.[58–61] Occasionally, fleeting areas of consolidation occur after an episode of pulmonary embolism, but these appear to represent areas of hemorrhage and/or edema and not necrotic tissue. These will be seen to resolve on serial chest films.[62]

Selective pulmonary arteriography is the best way to demonstrate pulmonary emboli. The resolution rate for pulmonary emboli varies considerably and may vary from a day to months. Although it is preferable to do the angiogram promptly following the onset of symptoms, a short delay of the study does not preclude the firm diagnosis of pulmonary embolism. A delay of several days will result in a less accurate examination.

Major central and segmental emboli are readily visualized as sharply bordered, rounded intraluminal filling defects by selective pulmonary arteriography (Figs. 32-28 through 32-36). If the embolus appears to cause complete occlusion of an artery, then one must see contrast surround the offending thrombus and outline the trailing edge of the clot. Although one may see parenchymal hypovascularity or slowing of pulmonary arterial or venous flow, these are only secondary signs of pulmonary embolism, and therefore one must not make the diagnosis of pulmonary embolism without visualization of the clot. Other secondary signs are recanalization of an occluded vessel, pruning or attenuation of branches, and demonstration of tortuous arterial collaterals. Small, peripheral clots may require segmental injections and magnification filming (Fig. 32-37).[63–66] These techniques may be useful but are usually not essential for distinguishing embolism from various nonembolic pulmonary vascular obliterations (neoplastic, postinflammatory, and other types of fibrotic obliterations). Large central emboli, such as saddle emboli to the right pulmonary artery, ordinarily make themselves known, and they are easily demonstrated. Multiple small peripheral emboli can persist and can cause pulmonary hypertension with right ventricular failure. These, when organized, are likely to exhibit a lacy network rather than sharply bordered defects. Unlike acute pulmonary emboli, they are often associated with bronchial artery dilatation and pleural collateral flow,[59] especially if infarction has occurred. If a patient with a normal pulmonary angiogram has recurrent symptoms, repeat pulmonary angiography should be considered because the patient may have a subsequent pulmonary embolus or the initial embolus may have been missed.[67]

Recurrent pulmonary microemboli may cause pulmonary hypertension and cor pulmonale and, although difficult to document, should be considered in cases of cor pulmonale that develop over a period of several months or even years. Sometimes the emboli may be demonstrated by using magnification techniques or balloon occlusion angiography.[63,68–71] In addition, pulmonary tumor microemboli that resulted in cor pulmonale have been described in autopsy specimens to both the alveolar and septal arteries but have not been demonstrated angiographically.[72,73] However, secondary signs of pulmonary hypertension may indeed be identified, including multiple subsegmental perfusion abnormalities, dilatation of the central pulmonary arteries, and tortuous pruned peripheral arteries.[74–76] Finally, acute cor pulmonale has been described secondary to pulmonary microemboli of

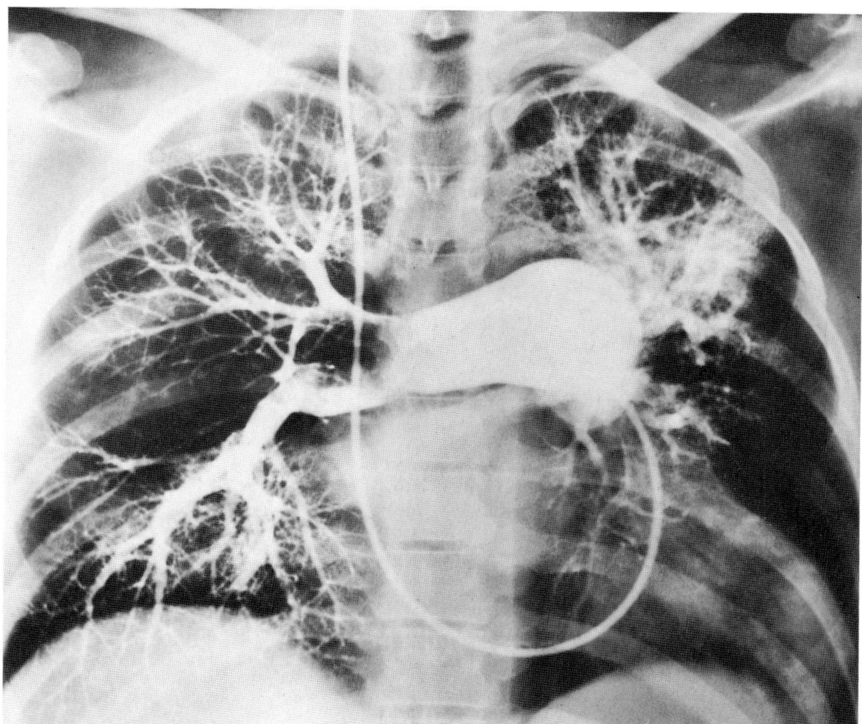

Figure 32-28. Repeated acute, massive, pulmonary embolism in a 23-year-old woman. The initial embolism (10 days earlier) had been treated by ligation of the inferior vena cava. A main pulmonary arteriogram shows a large embolus blocking flow to the lingula and the left lower lobe, compensatory hyperflow in the left upper lobe causing early left atrial filling, and dilated central pulmonary arteries. The mean pulmonary artery pressure was 36 mmHg. The patient eventually recovered on heparin therapy.

Figure 32-29. Acute massive right pulmonary embolus, smaller left pulmonary embolus. Sudden hypotensive collapse. A hyperlucent right lung had been shown on a chest film. An arteriogram shows a sharply bordered defect of a large right saddle embolus with nearly complete obstruction of flow and smaller perfusion and filling defects in the left upper (*arrow*) and lower lobes. Heparin did not prevent autopsy confirmation. The hyperlucency of the right lung was due to a lack of blood in the vessels.

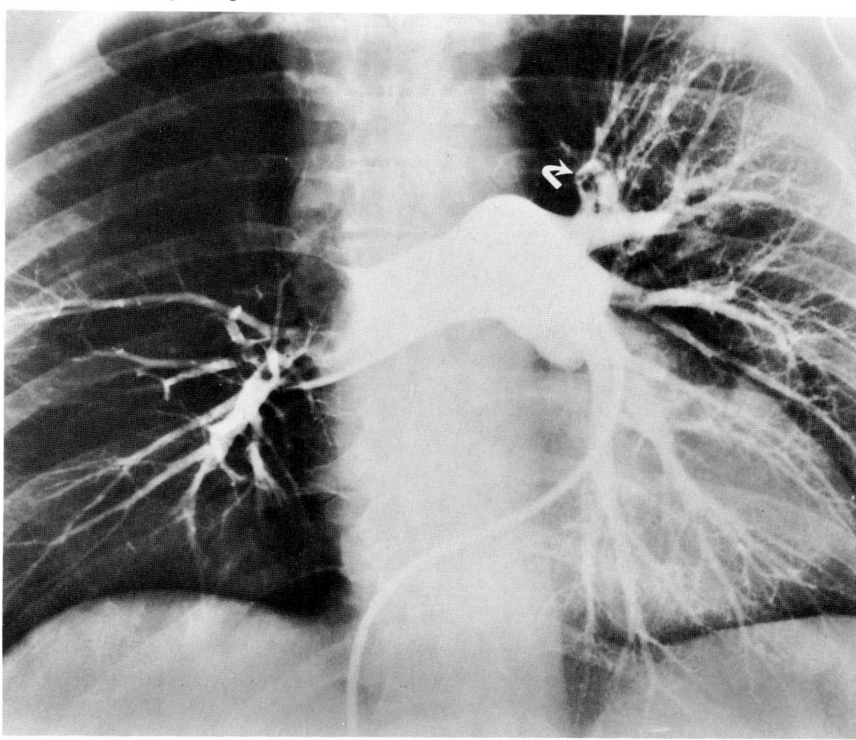

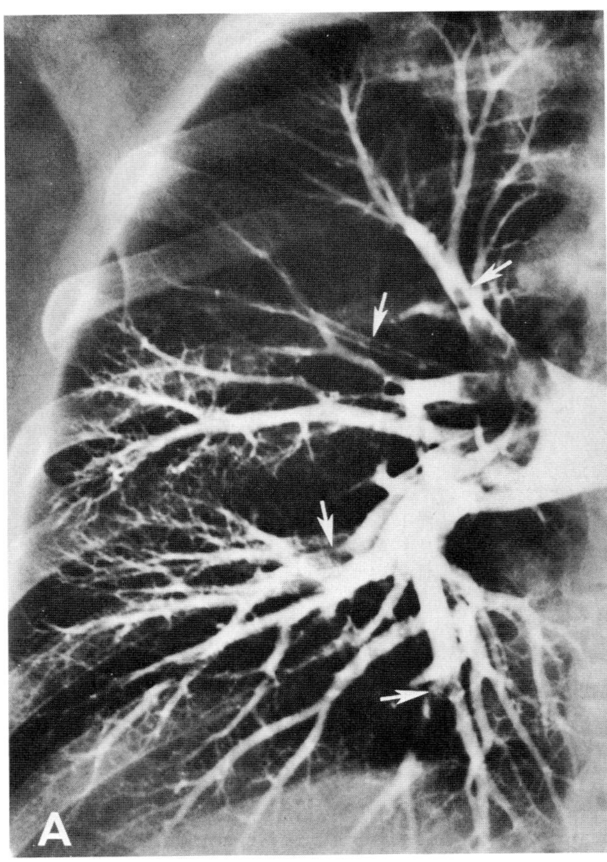

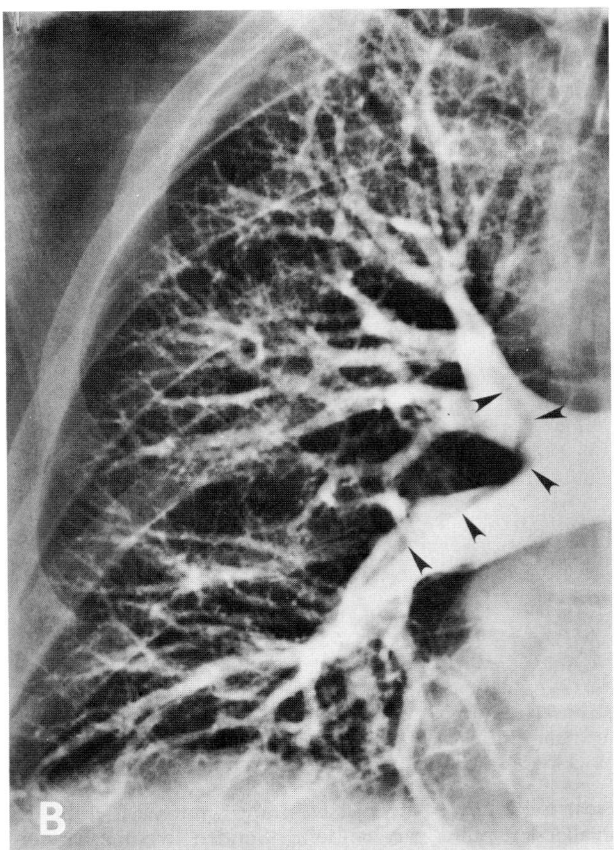

Figure 32-30. Two different acute right saddle emboli. (A) A large, rounded, central, partially obstructing saddle embolus with multiple peripheral filling defects (*arrows*). (B) A similarly situated, small, stringlike, virtually nonobstructive embolus (*arrowheads*) in another patient whose thrombosed vein was obviously much smaller and whose clot was gone within 72 hours, during which time streptokinase was given intravenously. Both patients recovered.

necrotic tissue from a retroperitoneal hematoma with associated muscle necrosis.[77]

Arteriography done immediately and at serial intervals following standardized, acute, pulmonary embolization in dogs[78] has strengthened the belief that death due to pulmonary embolism is caused by mechanical blockage of the pulmonary circulation and not to reflex spasms.[79] Postmortem studies, including arteriography before sectioning, have indicated that when a relatively small pulmonary embolus causes sudden death, it usually constitutes a terminal insult to a vascular system already severely restricted by prior embolization or some other cause.[80]

Conventional and more recently spiral volumetric CT has been used in the diagnosis of pulmonary embolism.[81–84] In 42 patients, Remy-Jardin et al. reported no false positives, but nine intersegmental lymph nodes were misinterpreted as filling defects.[83] Figure 32-38 demonstrates both the filling defects and the decreased pulmonary arterial flow secondary to pulmonary emboli. MR pulmonary angiography using time-of-flight technique has also been compared with conventional pulmonary angiography. In 20 patients with suspected pulmonary embolism, a sensitivity of 92 to 100 percent and a specificity of 62 percent were reported for the detection of pulmonary emboli.[85]

Figure 32-32. Postpartum pulmonary emboli. (A) Control right pulmonary angiogram shows clots at the bifurcation and in several branches (*arrows*). The mean pulmonary artery pressure was 50 mmHg. (B) Following a 4-day streptokinase infusion, the clots are smaller, and the peripheral flow is improved. The mean pulmonary artery pressure was 15 mmHg. ▶ (C) A week later, the lysis has been completed by the patient's own fibrinolytic mechanism. A similar involvement and course were shown on the left pulmonary angiogram.

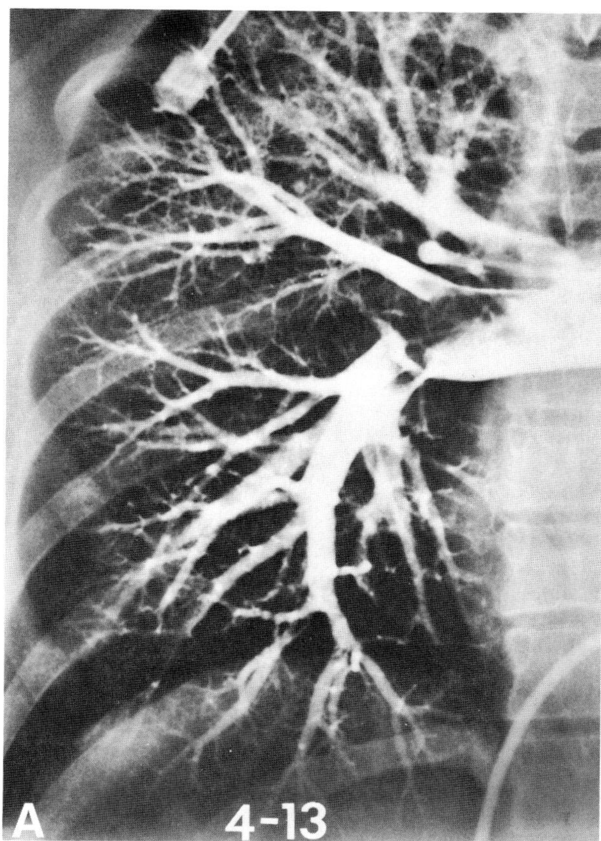

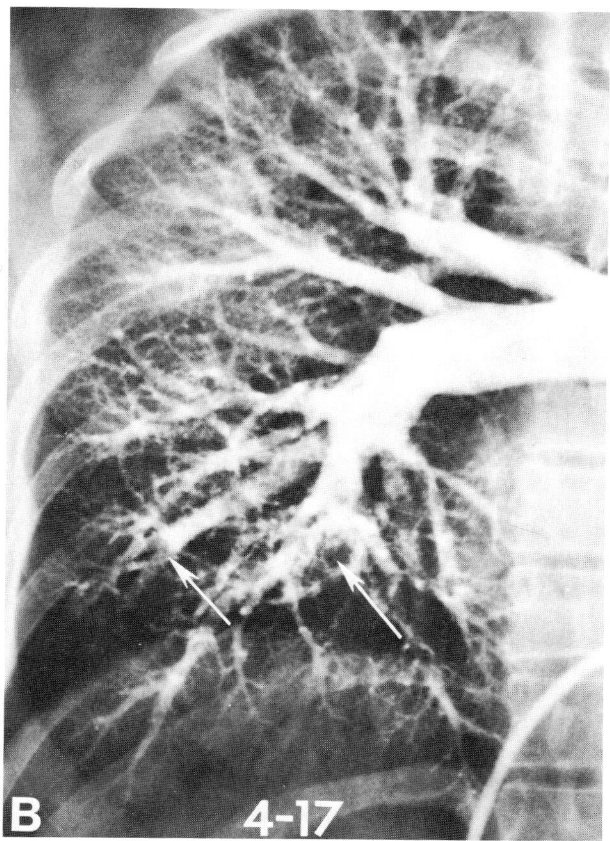

Figure 32-31. Streptokinase-accelerated lysis in pulmonary embolism in an 18-year-old girl. The patient, while taking birth control pills, developed left leg thrombophlebitis and sudden bilateral central pulmonary embolism, with dyspnea, cyanosis, and elevated right heart pressures. (A) Control right pulmonary arteriogram prior to starting the intravenous streptokinase infusion. (B) The large clot was gone in only 4 days. The peripheral migration of partially lysed fragments (*arrows*) may have aided in the dramatic clinical improvement, which occurred within 48 hours. Streptokinase was continued for 72 hours to speed the lysis of the remaining emboli as well as the persisting deep vein thrombi. The patient made a prompt, complete recovery without postthrombotic syndrome.

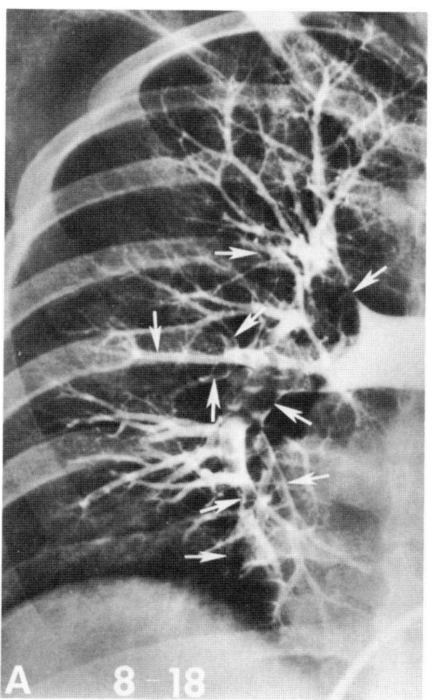

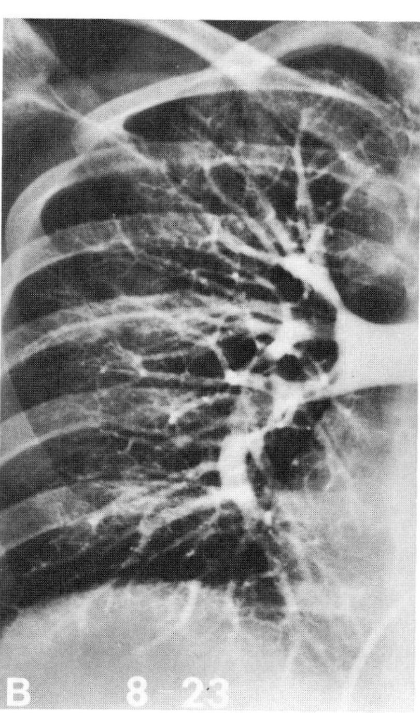

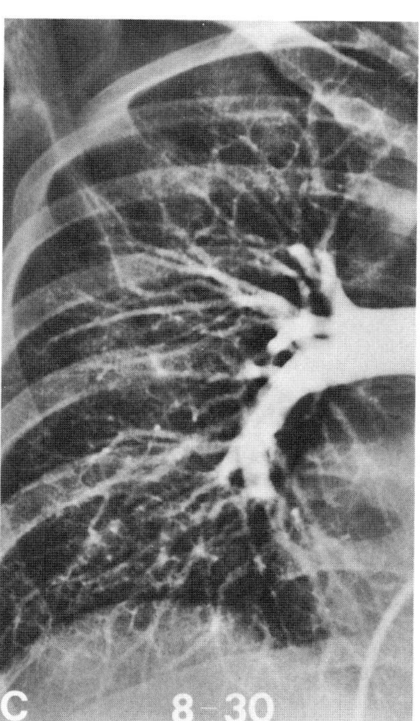

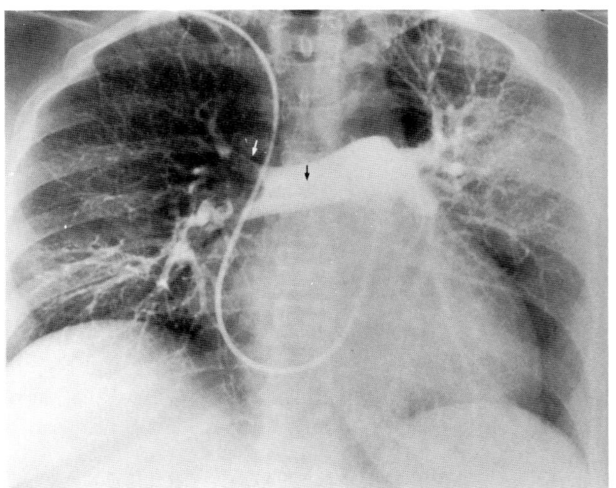

A

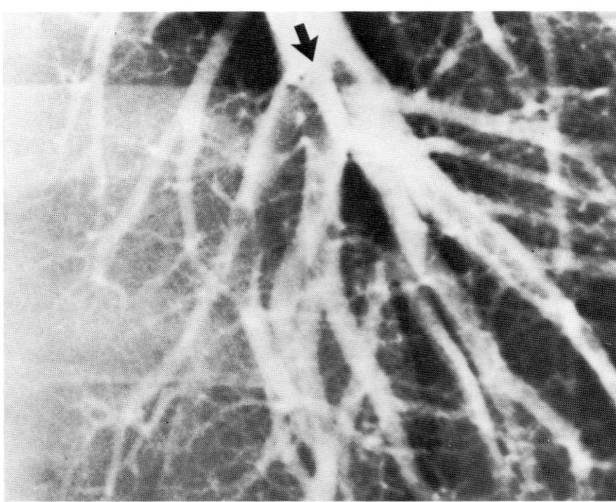

B

Figure 32-33. (A) A large saddle embolus in the right pulmonary artery. The embolus extends back from the bifurcation of the right pulmonary artery (*white arrow*) toward the main pulmonary artery (*black arrow*). (B) Lobar and segmental emboli in the left lower lobe artery (*arrow*). Many smaller emboli are seen outlined by the contrast material in the segmental branches. (Courtesy of Richard H. Greenspan, M.D.)

Pulmonary arterial catheterization can play an even more active role if used not just to diagnose but also to relieve hemodynamically intolerable pulmonary embolization. At far less risk than thoracotomy, catheters can favorably tip the hemodynamic balance by removing[86] or displacing large, centrally lodged emboli.[87] Dotter reported a patient in whom catheter dislodgment allowed peripheral migration of a saddle embolus from the bifurcation of the right pulmonary artery, which appeared to result in immediate clinical improvement by opening up blocked proximal branches.[88] If given sufficient time, the patient's own thrombolytic capabilities will result in the dissolution of fresh clots. Obviously, partial peripheral obstruction is less hazardous to the patient's health than is massive central obstruction. Transluminal therapy offers the advantage of not imposing the physiologic burden of thoracotomy on an already dangerously overloaded circulation.

Figure 32-34. A large perfusion defect involving the right middle and lower lobes, unrelated to pulmonary emboli. Neither the trailing edge of an embolus nor an intraluminal defect is visualized. The patient had unilateral emphysema (Swyer-James or Macleod's syndrome). (Courtesy of Richard H. Greenspan, M.D.)

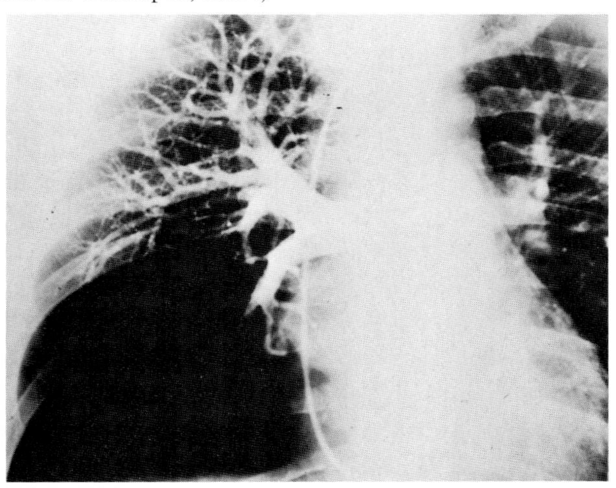

Pulmonary arteriography is also a safe and valuable adjunct to case selection and the assessment of progress in the fibrinolytic treatment of life-threatening pulmonary embolism. The results of a national cooperative study of streptokinase and urokinase[89] are consistent with our earlier clinical experience with streptokinase[90] and subsequent randomized, heparin-controlled study of its sometimes striking value in major pulmonary embolus (see Figs. 32-31 and 32-32).

Lung Cancer and Other Intrathoracic Tumors

The analysis of pulmonary angiograms in 100 consecutive, microscopically proven cases of bronchogenic carcinoma has shown that significant information can be gained in affected patients.[91,92] Positive findings associated with pulmonary and mediastinal tumors[93] include vascular obstruction, encasement, dislocation,

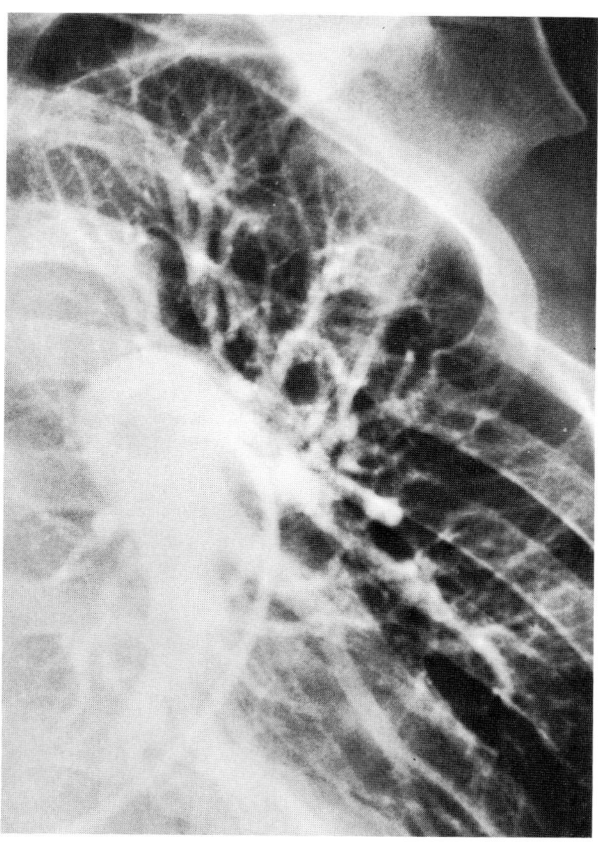

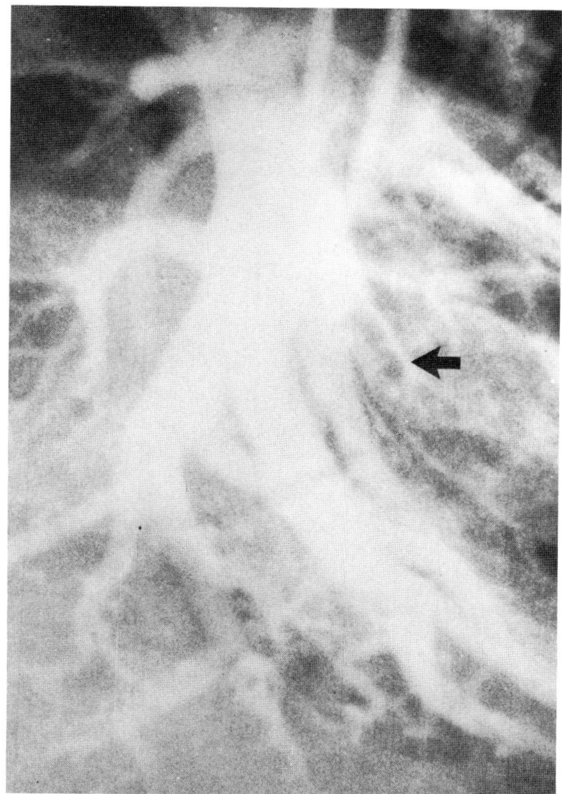

Figure 32-35. (A) An angiogram done from the left pulmonary artery in a very slight left posterior oblique projection in a patient with left lower lobe volume loss having symptoms of pulmonary embolism. A perfusion scan defect was present at the left base. The vessels are crowded and appear abnormal, but a definite diagnosis of embolus cannot be made. (B) A more peripheral selective examination using a 30-degree oblique position demonstrates an intraluminal filling defect (*arrow*) diagnostic of pulmonary embolism. (Courtesy of Richard H. Greenspan, M.D.)

and intraluminal invasion (Fig. 32-39).[94–96] High-resolution computed tomography may also demonstrate the compression or encasement of pulmonary vessels as well as venous and bronchial compression or invasion.[97]

Pulmonary arteriograms are of little value in revealing the blood supply to pulmonary and other intrathoracic tumors, because the blood supply comes principally via systemic arteries. Selective bronchial arteriography is more pertinent in this connection.[98,99]

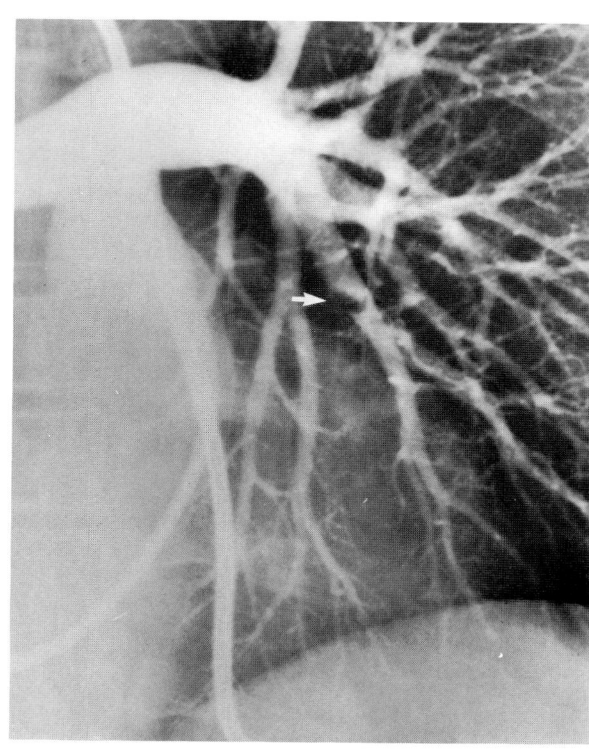

Figure 32-36. A single embolus (*arrow*) that projects into a branch of the left lower lobe artery is clearly delineated. Contrast material is seen faintly outlining the embolus in the segmental vessel. (Courtesy of Richard H. Greenspan, M.D.)

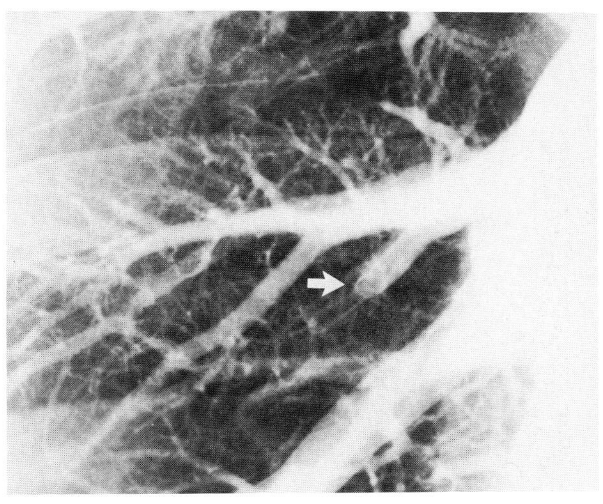

A

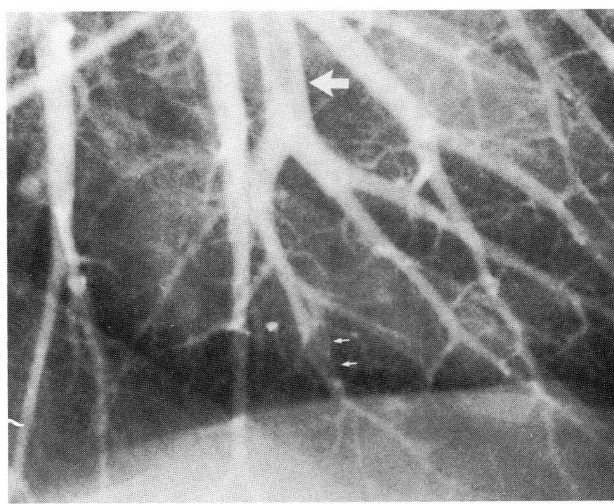

B

Figure 32-37. (A) A small embolus (*arrow*) shown in a branch of the middle lobe vessel in a patient who had had three previous standard angiograms that failed to reveal emboli. (×3.) (From R. H. Greenspan et al. In vivo magnification angiography. *Invest. Radiol.* 2:419, 1967. Reproduced by permission of the publisher.) (B) Two emboli shown on a magnification pulmonary angiogram. In retrospect, the upper, larger embolus (*large arrow*) could be seen on the standard nonmagnified study. The lower embolus could not (*small arrows*). (Courtesy of Richard H. Greenspan, M.D.)

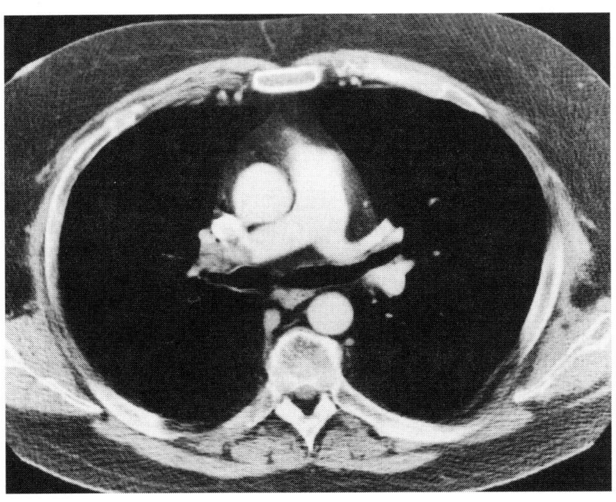

A

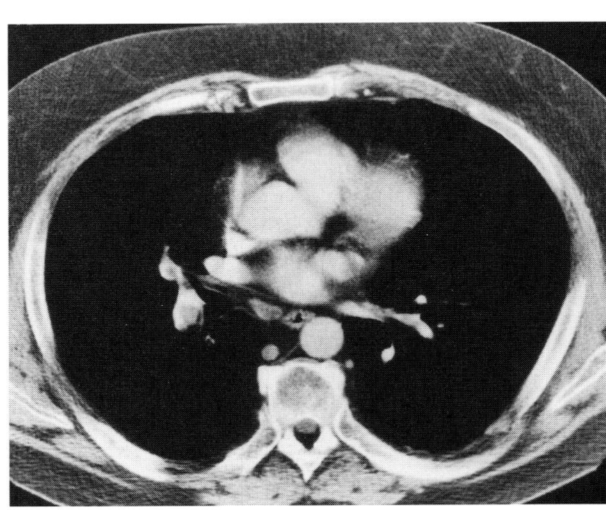

B

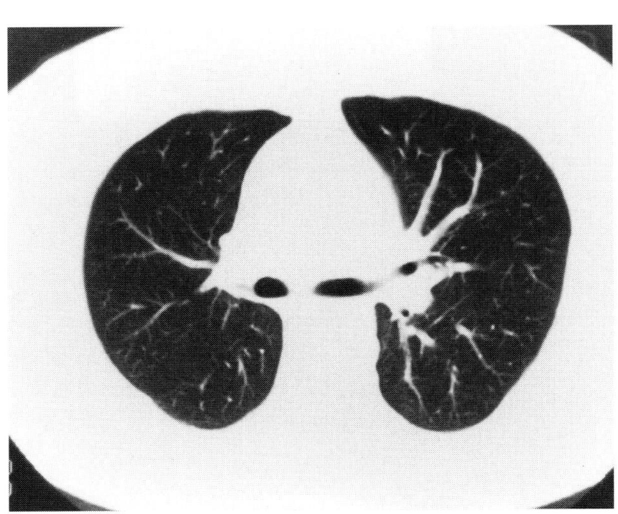

C

Figure 32-38. Pulmonary embolism demonstrated in an asymptomatic 48-year-old man with lymphoma on a routine follow-up CT scan. (A) A low-attenuation filling defect is seen in the right main pulmonary artery at the origin of the descending ramus. (B) Additional defects are evident in the basilar segmental arteries of the right lower lobe. (C) Pulmonary parenchymal windows demonstrate thin, attenuated vessels in the right lobe due to hypoperfusion distal to the central embolus. A subsequent ventilation-perfusion scan demonstrated multiple segmental perfusion defects in the right lower and middle lobes.

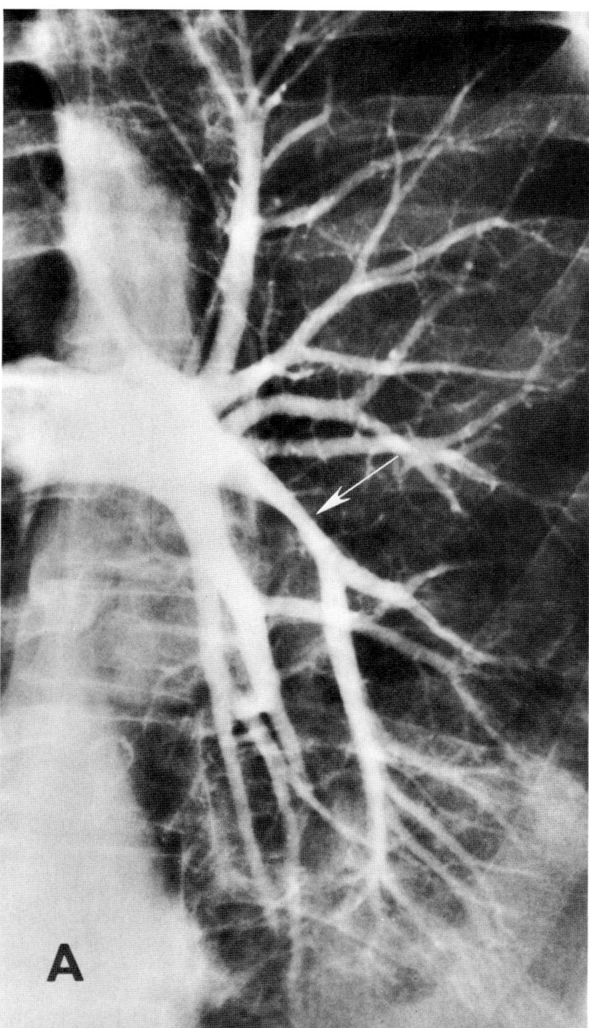

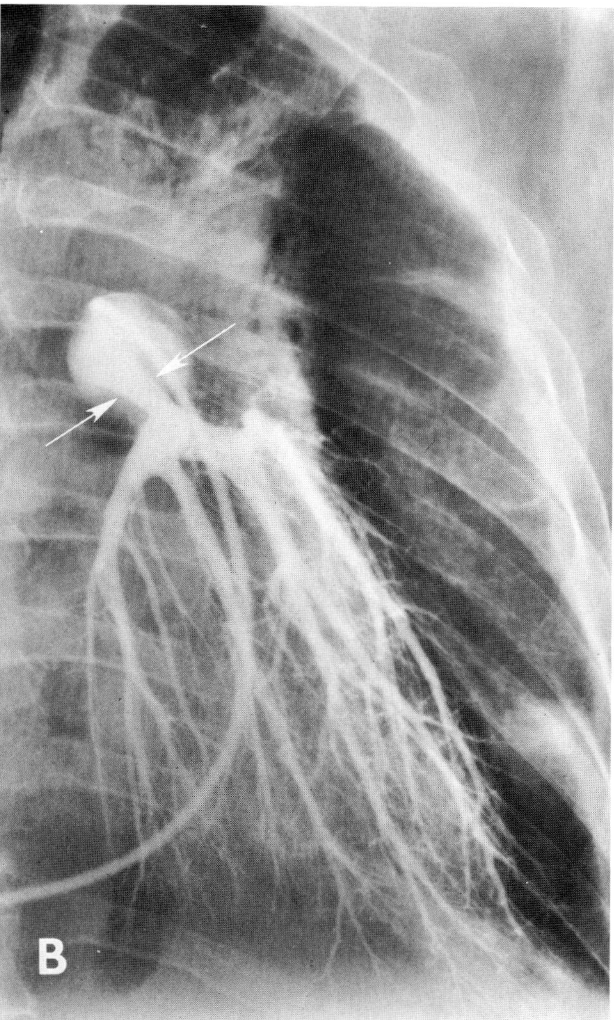

Figure 32-39. Pulmonary artery changes in lung cancer. (A) Biopsy-proved anaplastic left pulmonary malignancy in a 58-year-old man. The pulmonary arteriogram shows a left hilar mass and encasement of the artery (*arrow*) to the partially atelectatic left posterior basal segment. (B) Different patient in whom oat cell carcinoma had been diagnosed 2 years earlier and treated by chemotherapy and radiation therapy. The arteriogram shows a marked contraction of the lung, obvious encasement of the left main artery (*arrows*) and the segmental pulmonary artery, as well as occlusion of the branches to the left upper lobe and the lingula.

Although malignant tumors in the chest often cause characteristic vascular deformities, the absence of such changes may not indicate benignancy. Malignant tumors have been observed to surround pulmonary arteries without causing appreciable changes in their caliber. Pulmonary arteriography can be of diagnostic value and assist in the prognosis as well as in the selection and formulation of a suitable therapeutic approach. Palliation may also be obtained by percutaneous endovascular interventional therapy (Fig. 32-40). Because pulmonary arteriography can provide decisive evidence of unresectability (Fig. 32-41), it may be useful before thoracotomy, especially if the CT or the MRI is equivocal.

Miscellaneous Acquired Pulmonary Vascular Abnormalities

Primary pulmonary hypertension is a poorly understood condition, and the diagnosis rests on the exclusion of all known causes of reactive pressure elevation in the pulmonary artery—of which there are many. Its arteriographic appearance is certainly not specific. Typically, central pulmonary arterial dilatation occurs,

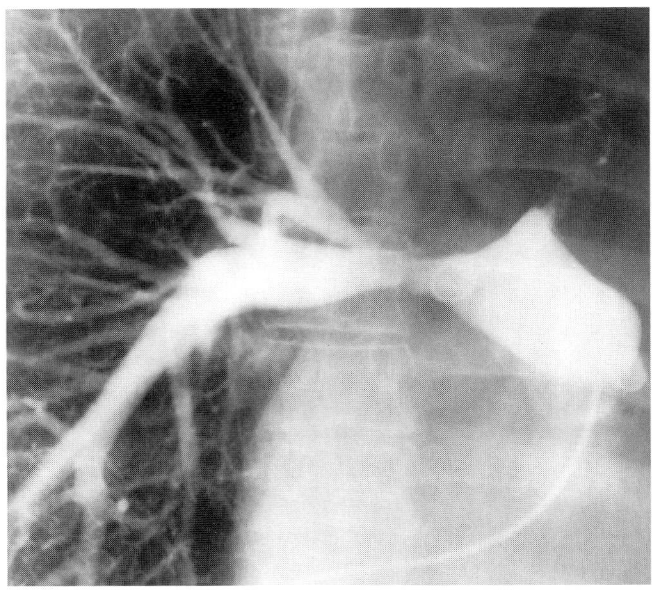

A

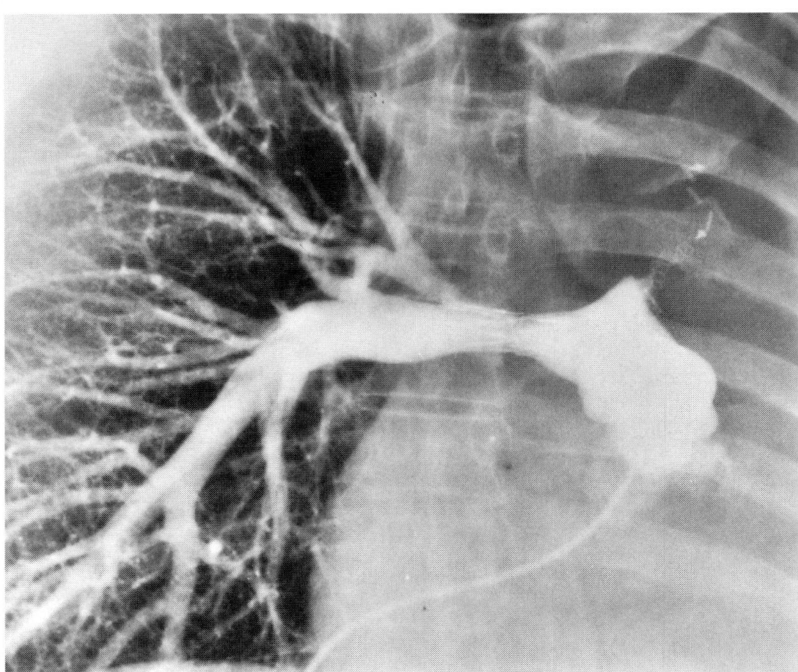

B

Figure 32-40. Recurrent lung adenocarcinoma following left lobectomy with encasement of the right main pulmonary artery. (A) Encasement of the right main pulmonary artery with a 36-mmHg gradient across the stenosis. (B) Following placement of a Gianturco-Rösch Z stent, there is moderate improvement of the stenosis and reduction of the gradient to 12 mmHg. Clinically, the patient had marked improvement in his dyspnea and was able to tolerate a higher level of exertion.

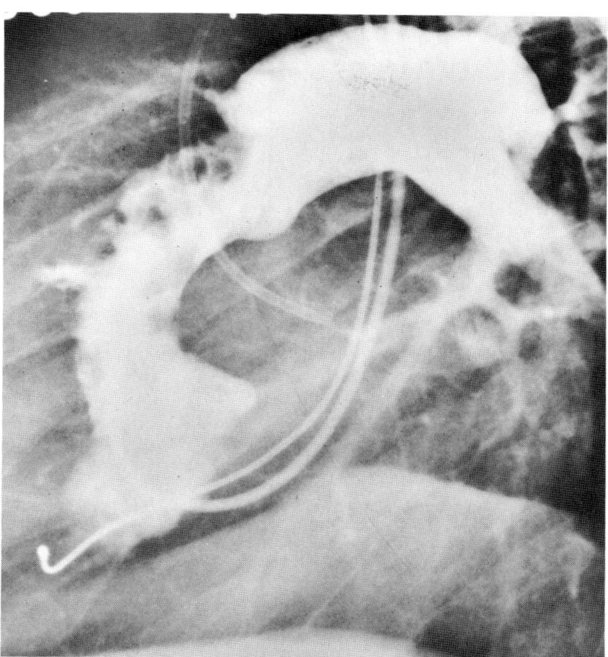

Figure 32-41. Sarcomatous invasion of the main pulmonary artery. An obviously inoperable situation clearly evidenced by pulmonary arteriography.

and, given time, peripheral branches exhibit tapered narrowing with peripheral cutoff (Fig. 32-42). Here, as in better-understood conditions causing cor pulmonale, right ventricular enlargement becomes grossly evident with the onset of chamber dilatation.

Although primary pulmonary hypertension is rare and hard to establish, *secondary pulmonary hypertension* is common and easily documented. Pulmonary hypertension can be a manifestation of increased vascular resistance at the postcapillary level.[100] A prime example is mitral valve stenosis, in which pulmonary venous pressure is elevated and basilar pulmonary vessels are constricted in comparison with upper lobe vessels. The extent to which such distinctions are useful depends on the purity of the mechanism present in a given case. Usually it is not pure in long-standing disease, because secondary degenerative intimal changes, medial hypertrophy, heart failure, pulmonary vascular congestion, embolism, thrombosis, and treatment all serve to produce an amorphous pathologic result.

Pulmonary hypervascularity occurs in response to acquired nonpulmonary diseases, ranging from congestive heart failure to high-output states associated with severe anemia, hyperthyroidism, and systemic ar-

Figure 32-42. Primary pulmonary hypertension in a 26-year-old woman. The patient had a 5-year history of exertional dyspnea, pulmonary hypertension, and right ventricular hypertrophy (shown electrocardiographically). The central pulmonary arteries are dilated, the peripheral branches are small and tapered, and the heart is enlarged. There are incidental small angiomatous changes in the right upper lobe. The pulmonary artery pressure was 105/50 mmHg. The diagnosis was made by exclusion.

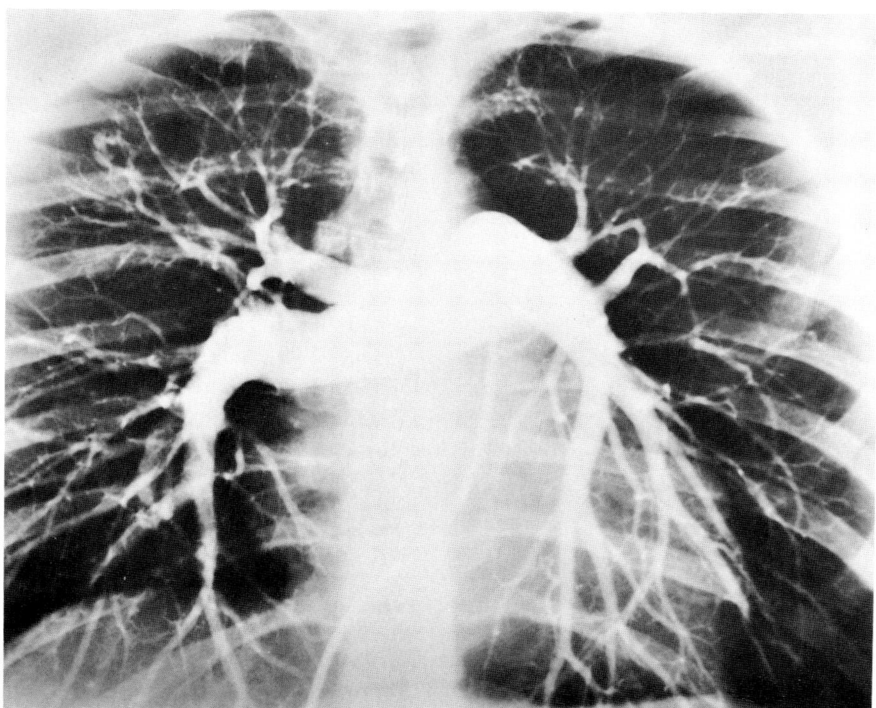

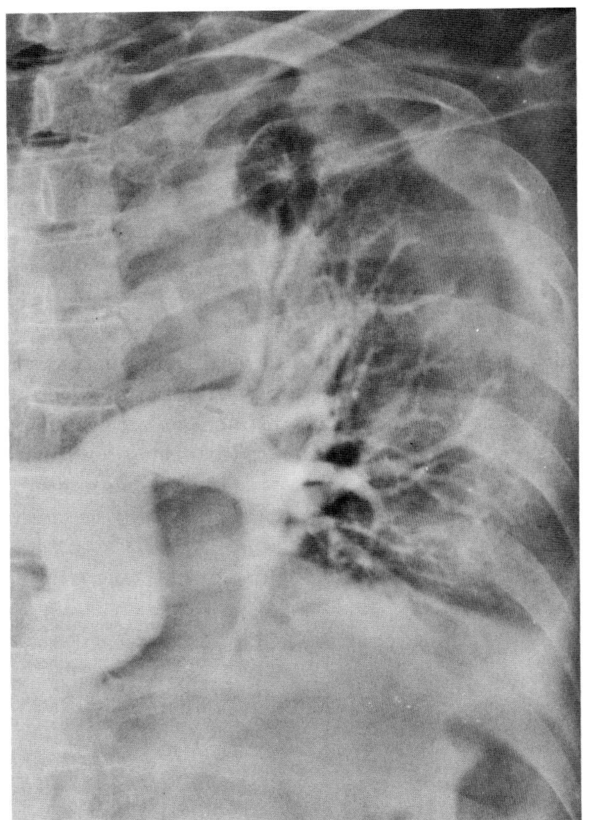

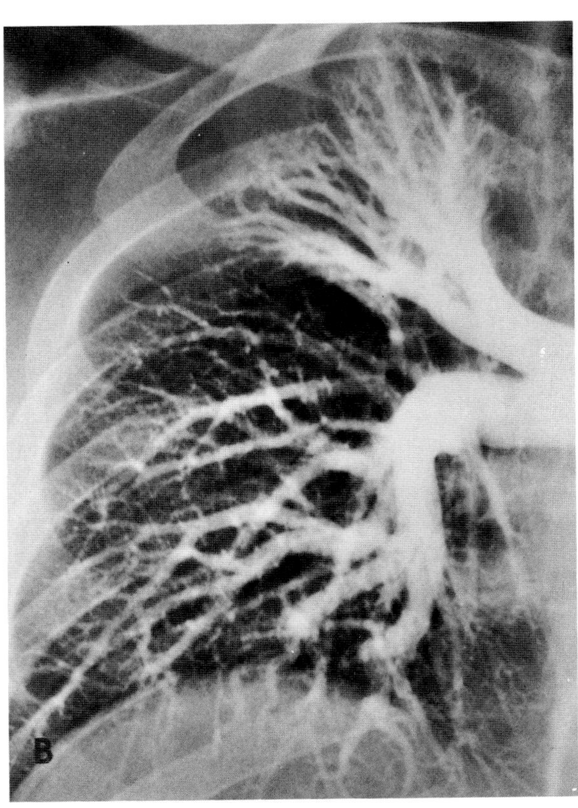

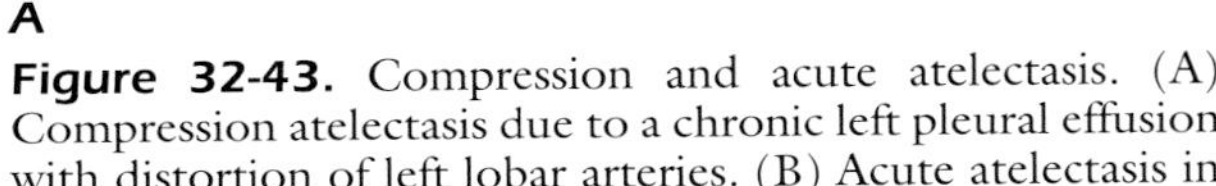

A

B

Figure 32-43. Compression and acute atelectasis. (A) Compression atelectasis due to a chronic left pleural effusion with distortion of left lobar arteries. (B) Acute atelectasis in a patient with a collapsed right upper lobe due to postoperative mucous plugs. The arteries are closely crowded together without any other evident abnormality.

teriovenous fistulas.[101] The resulting general enlargement of pulmonary vessels may be reversible and is not as striking as that often accompanying congenital left-to-right shunts.

Many other conditions cause *pulmonary hypovascularity* in addition to those already discussed. Among these conditions are atelectasis, pneumothorax, thoracoplasty, pulmonary compression, phrenic paralysis, extrinsic pulmonary artery obstruction, thoracic deformity, and possibly protracted respiratory support therapy.

Atelectasis of all or part of a lung causes changes in vessel distribution and blood flow. Vessels are crowded together and tortuous in the area of collapse, tending to make less apparent the moderate, reversible diminution in flow that occurs in acute atelectasis and to a greater degree in chronic pulmonary compression (Figs. 32-43 and 32-44). Similarly, nonselective pulmonary angiograms done before and after the institution of a *pneumothorax*[102,103] show a prompt diminution in vascularity, whereas persistent nonexpansion results in an irreversible reduction in the vascular bed (Fig. 32-45). Selective pulmonary arteriograms in similar clinical circumstances[104] demonstrate patent central arteries with small, withered branches that, although patent, are functionless. Figure 32-46 illustrates the somewhat analogous outcome of chronic occlusion of the left pulmonary artery by extrinsic pressure from

Figure 32-45. Pneumothorax: acute and long-term results. (A) An acute, spontaneous right pneumothorax causing an immediate, unilateral decrease in the pulmonary blood flow. (B) A nonfunctioning lung without evident pulmonary blood flow. The left lung failed to reexpand after long-term "therapeutic" left pneumothorax. The failure of opacification of the left pulmonary artery does not indicate that the vessel is not present; selective angiograms might have shown small, irregular, and patent but useless pulmonary vessels. ▶

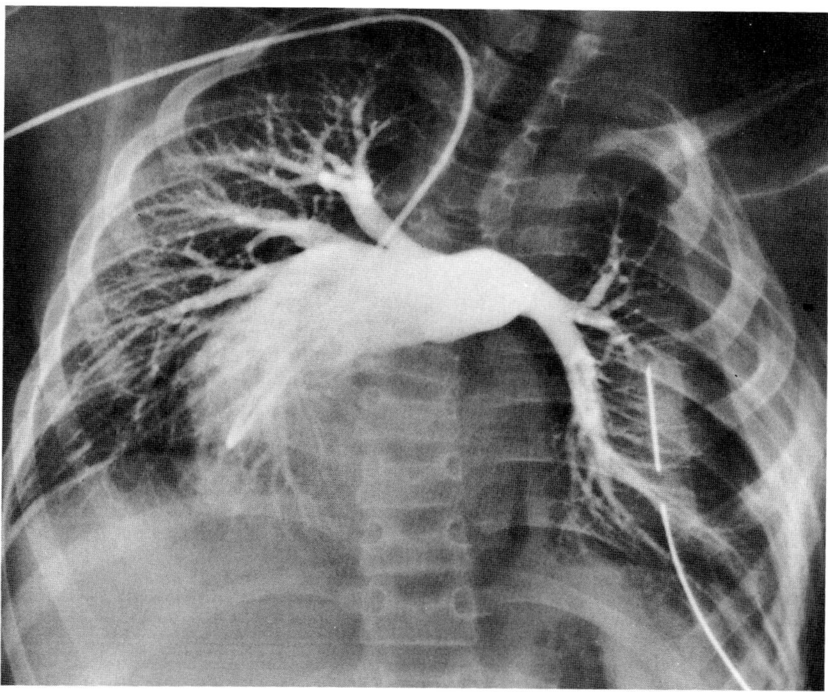

Figure 32-44. Postempyema pulmonary compression. Markedly thickened pleura and an intrapleural gas-filled cavity (complications of prior pneumonia), with gross cardiovascular displacement to the right. The pulmonary arteries to the compressed left lung are open, but most of the pulmonary blood flow goes through the opposite lung. Decortication and subsequent physical therapy led to considerable improvement.

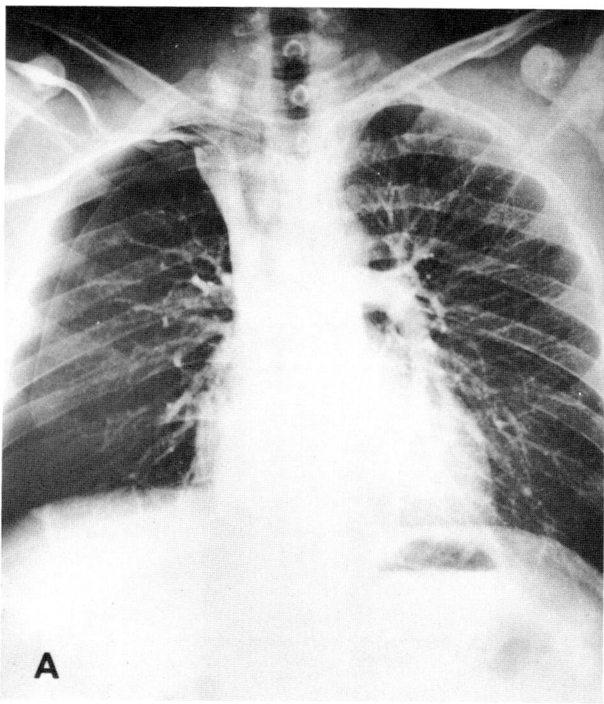

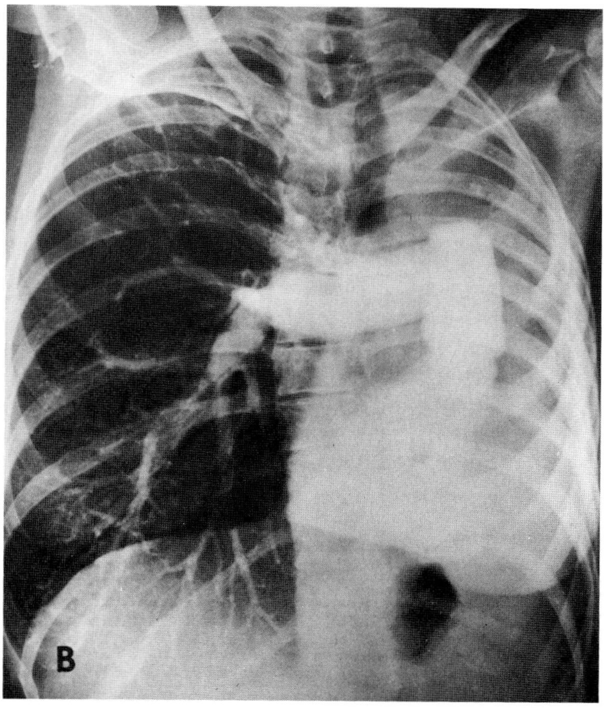

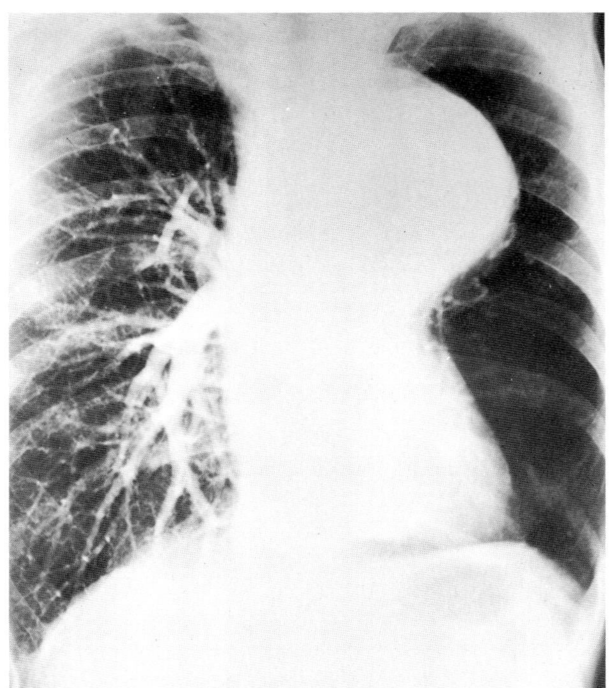

Figure 32-46. Occlusion of left pulmonary artery due to aortic aneurysm. The right pulmonary artery carried the pulmonary flow. Although the left bronchus was still open, its lung was small and its contribution to functioning was virtually nil.

an *aortic arch aneurysm*. Although the left bronchus remained open, ventilation and lung volume on the affected side were markedly lowered.

In *kyphoscoliosis*[105] and other severe thoracic cage deformities, pulmonary arteriography visualizes the resulting bizarre distortion of blood vessels (Fig. 32-47). The severe stretching, buckling, and twisting of the pulmonary vessels, together with gross ventilatory problems, account for the high incidence of death from pulmonary heart disease in these patients. Though rarely indicated or done, pulmonary angiography in patients with *heart failure* shows vascular engorgement, principally venous engorgement, and slow blood flow.[48] Angiocardiograms made during transient vasomotor collapse have revealed an impressive circulatory stasis. For visualizing these hemodynamic alterations this approach might be informative, but in the patient's interest, vasomotor collapse signifies that visualization is best delayed until the peripheral vascular bed has regained its normal composure. Based on a survey done years ago,[106] it seems possible that vasomotor collapse following angiocardiography has led to the unnecessary death of patients given epinephrine instead of more appropriate measures, including atropine, the Trendelenburg position, peripheral vasocon-

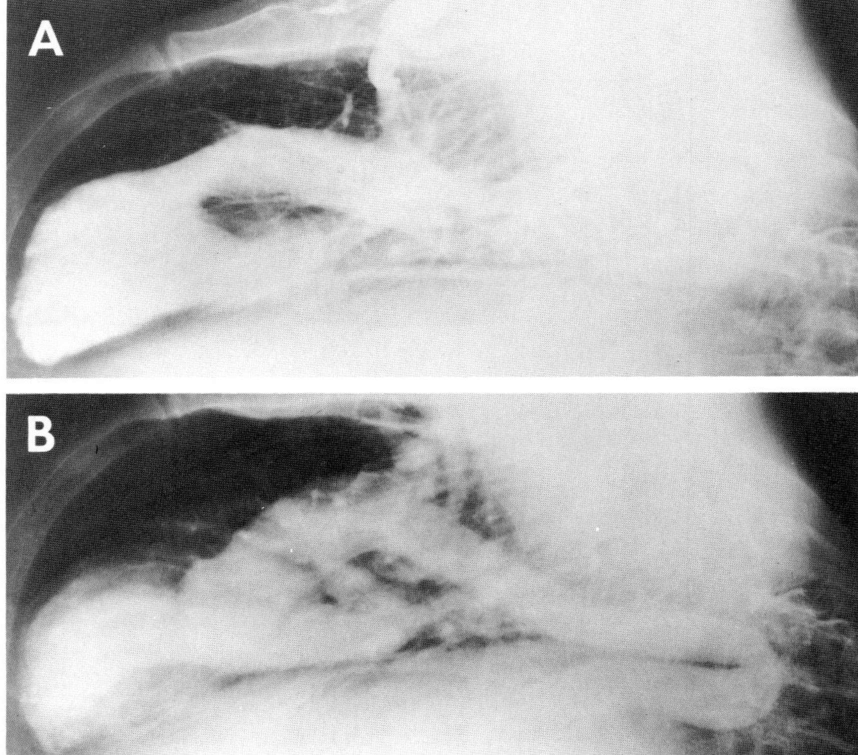

strictors, and intravenous fluid or diuretics, as indicated by individual circumstances.

Takayasu arteritis most often involves the aorta and its brachiocephalic branches, but it also involves the pulmonary arteries.[107–112] Yamada et al.[109] reported an incidence of 70 percent in patients with aortic or brachiocephalic artery involvement who had pulmonary angiograms. The changes seen in the pulmonary arteries resemble those seen in the aorta and its branches. Angiographically, stenotic or occlusive lesions are most commonly evident in the segmental and subsegmental branches of the upper lobe branches, although the peripheral branches may also be involved. Microscopically, marked intimal fibrosis resulting in stenosis or occlusion of the pulmonary elastic arteries is evident. Recanalization with "vessel in a vessel" may be seen.[108]

In *Behçet disease*, a rare multisystem disease of unknown etiology characterized by coexistent oral and genital ulcers, thrombophlebitis, and eye and skin lesions, pulmonary aneurysms are seen in approximately 2 percent of patients. The aneurysms are thought to be due to an obliterative endarteritis of the vasa vasorum of the pulmonary arteries. They have a high propensity to bleed, and perivascular pulmonary hemorrhage is frequently seen. The presence of pulmonary artery aneurysms is a poor prognostic sign, with a 30 percent 3-year mortality rate due to rupture of an aneurysm following the initial diagnosis of an aneurysm.[113,114]

Rasmussen aneurysms may be seen in cavitary tuberculosis secondary to the erosion by the cavity into a pulmonary artery. These pulmonary artery aneurysms may then lead to the formation of arteriovenous fistulas. Both the aneurysms and fistula can be treated by percutaneous intervention if necessary.[115]

Conclusion

Pulmonary angiography remains the "gold standard" for the diagnosis of pulmonary embolism and of many other acquired and congenital pulmonary artery disorders, even though other modalities (CT and MRI) are demonstrating their usefulness. The angiographic catheter also provides an alternative therapeutic approach for the treatment of pulmonary aneurysm, arteriovenous fistula, embolized foreign bodies, and pulmonary embolism.

Acknowledgments

This chapter is dedicated to the memory of Charles T. Dotter, M.D., who authored the chapter in the first three editions of this book. His original chapters served as a guideline, and in many places we merely updated his manuscript and have retained most of his illustrations.

References

1. Heath D, Edwards JE. The pathology of hypertensive pulmonary vascular disease: a description of six grades of structural changes in the pulmonary arteries with special reference to congenital cardiac septal defects. Circulation 1958;18:533.
2. Kjellberg SR, Mannheimer E, Rudhe U, Jonsson B. Diagnosis of congenital disease. Chicago: Year Book, 1955.
3. Castaneda-Zuniga WR, Formanek A, Amplatz K. Radiologic diagnosis of different types of pulmonary stenoses. Cardiovasc Radiol 1978;1:45.
4. deVries HK, van den Berg JW. On the origin of poststenotic dilatations. Cardiologia (Basel) 1958;33:195.
5. Dotter CT. Motion in cardiovascular radiography. Circulation 1955;12:1034.
6. Holman E. The obscure physiology of poststenotic dilatation: its relation to the development of aneurysms. J Thorac Surg 1954;28:109.
7. Dotter CT. Congenital abnormalities of the pulmonary arteries. In: Abrams angiography. 3rd ed. Boston: Little, Brown, 1983.
8. Johnson LW, Grossman W, Dalen JE, Dexter L. Pulmonic stenosis in the adult: long-term follow-up results. N Engl J Med 1972;287:1159.
9. Arvidsson H, Karnell J, Möller T. Multiple stenosis of the pulmonary arteries associated with pulmonary hypertension, diagnosed by selective angiocardiography. Acta Radiol (Stockh) 1955;44:209.
10. Falkenbach KH, Zheutlin N, O'Loughlin BJ. Isolated pulmonary artery coarctation and pulmonary hypertension. Radiology 1958;70:870.
11. Figley MM, Stern AM, Talner NS, Sloan HE. Congenital pulmonary arterial stenosis. Presented at the 44th Annual Meeting of the Radiological Society of North America, November 16–21, 1958.
12. Søndergaard T. Coarctation of the pulmonary artery. Dan Med Bull 1954;1:46.
13. Amplatz K, Moller JH. Radiology of congenital heart disease. St. Louis: Mosby Year Book, 1993:1039–1044.
14. van Son JA, Julsrud PR, Hagler DJ, Sim EK, Puga FJ, Schaff HV, Danielson GK. Imaging strategies for vascular rings. Ann Thorac Surg 1994;57:604.
15. Sisson JH, Murphy GE, Newman EV. Multiple congenital arteriovenous aneurysms in pulmonary circulation. Bull Hopkins Hosp 1945;76:93.
16. Steinberg I, McClenahan J. Pulmonary arteriovenous fistula: angiocardiographic observations in nine cases. Am J Med 1955;19:549.
17. Friedlich AL, Bing RJ, Blount SG Jr. Physiological studies in congenital heart disease: circulatory dynamics in anomalies of venous return to heart including pulmonary arteriovenous fistula. Bull Hopkins Hosp 1950;86:20.
18. Higgins CB, Wexler L. Clinical and angiographic features of

◀ **Figure 32-47.** Severe kyphoscoliosis. (A) Right heart angiocardiogram, lateral projection. (B) Left heart angiocardiogram. The marked, bizarre distortion of the pulmonary vessels and, in particular, of the aorta (which follows the spine in such cases) is obvious. It is little wonder that respiratory disability is frequently the result.

pulmonary arteriovenous fistulas in children. Radiology 1976; 119:171.
19. Castaneda-Zuniga W, Epstein M, Zollikofer C, Nath PH, Formanek A, Ben-Shachar G, Amplatz K. Embolization of multiple pulmonary artery fistulas. Radiology 1980;134:309.
20. Porstmann W. Therapeutic embolization of arteriovenous pulmonary fistulas by catheter technique. In: O. Eklöf, ed. Current concepts in pediatric radiology. Berlin: Springer, 1977:23.
21. Taylor BG, Cockerill EM, Manfredi F, Klatte EC. Therapeutic embolization of the pulmonary artery in pulmonary arteriovenous fistula. Am J Med 1978;64:360.
22. Terry PB, Barth KH, Kaufman SL, White RI. Balloon embolization for treatment of pulmonary artery fistulas. Med Intell 1980;302:1189.
23. Pereiras R, Castellanos A, Viamonte JM, Beguerie RH, Centurion JJ, Peña EG. Aortografia retrograda superior desde la arteria carotida primitiva en el niño y en el adulto. Rev Cubana Cardiol 1950;11:65.
24. Lukas DS, Dotter CT, Steinberg I. Agenesis of the lung and patent ductus arteriosus with reversal of flow. N Engl J Med 1953;249:107.
25. Dotter CT, Steinberg I. The diagnosis of congenital aneurysm of the pulmonary artery. N Engl J Med 1949;240:51.
26. Boijsen E, Kozuka T. Angiographic demonstration of systemic arterial supply in abnormal pulmonary circulation. AJR 1969;106:70.
27. Flynn JE, Siebens AA, Williams SF. Congenital absence of a main branch of the pulmonary artery. Am J Med Sci 1954; 228:673.
28. Oyamada A, Gasul BM, Holinger PH. Agenesis of the lung: report of a case, with a review of all previously reported cases. Am J Dis Child 1953;85:182.
29. Steinberg I. Congenital absence of a main branch of the pulmonary artery: report of three new cases associated respectively with bronchiectasis, atrial septal defect and Eisenmenger's complex. Am J Med 1958;24:559.
30. Steinberg I, Dotter CT, Lukas DS. Congenital absence of a main branch of the pulmonary artery. JAMA 1953;152:1216.
31. Takahashi M, Ohno M, Mihara K, Matsuura K, Sumiyoshi A. Intralobar pulmonary sequestration: with special emphasis on bronchial communication. Radiology 1975;114:543.
32. Luhmer I, Ziemer G. Coarctation of the pulmonary artery in neonates: prevalence, diagnosis and surgical treatment. J Thorac Cardiovasc Surg 1993;106:889.
33. Amplatz K, Möller JH. Radiology of congenital heart disease. St. Louis: Mosby Year Book, 1993:1033–1039.
34. Gebauer PW, Mason CB. Intralobar pulmonary sequestration associated with anomalous pulmonary vessels: a nonentity. Dis Chest 1959;35:282.
35. Gustafson RA, Murray GF, Warden HE, Hill RC, Rozar GE. Intralobar sequestration: a missed diagnosis. Ann Thorac Surg 1989;47:841.
36. Hayashi AH, McLean DR, Peliowski A, Tierney AJ, Finer NN. A rare intrapericardial mass in a neonate. J Pediatr Surg 1992;27:1361.
37. Lager DJ, Kuper KA, Haake GK. Subdiaphragmatic extralobar pulmonary sequestration. Arch Pathol Lab Med 1991; 115:536.
38. Ke FJ, Chang SC, Su WJ, Perng RP. Extralobar pulmonary sequestration presenting as an anterior mediastinal tumor in an adult. Chest 1993;104:303.
39. Silverman JF, Obrez I, Kriss JP. Coronary artery fistula: diagnosis and evaluation by selective contrast and radioisotopic coronary arteriography. J Can Assoc Radiol 1974;25:310.
40. Steinberg I, Baldwin JS, Dotter CT. Coronary arteriovenous fistula. Circulation 1958;17:372.
41. Mukai H, Minemawari Y, Hanawa N, Mita T, Motoe M, Nakata T. Coronary stenosis and steal phenomenon in coronary-pulmonary fistula—assessment with stress thallium tomography after coronary angioplasty and fistulectomy. Jpn Circ J 1993;57:1021.
42. New York Heart Association. Diseases of the heart and blood vessels: nomenclature and criteria for diagnosis. 6th ed. Boston: Little, Brown, 1964.
43. Dotter CT. Diagnostic cardiovascular radiology: a changing scene. Circulation 1956;14:509.
44. Dotter CT. Angiocardiography and "cor pulmonale." Trans Am Coll Cardiol 1957;7:186.
45. Sussman ML, Jacobson G. A critical evaluation of the roentgen criteria of right ventricular enlargement. Circulation 1955;11:391.
46. Chen JTT, Capp MP, Johnsrude IS, Goodrich JK, Lester RG. Roentgen appearance of pulmonary vascularity in the diagnosis of heart disease. AJR 1971;112:559.
47. Miscall L, Duffy RW. Surgical treatment of bullous emphysema: contributions of angiocardiography. Dis Chest 1953; 24:489.
48. Dotter CT, Steinberg I. Angiocardiography: annals of roentgenology. Vol. 10. New York: Hoeber, 1951.
49. Steinberg I, McCoy HI, Dotter CT. Angiocardiographic findings in pulmonary tuberculosis. Dis Chest 1951;19:510.
50. Botenga ASJ. The role of bronchopulmonary anastomoses in chronic inflammatory processes of the lung: selective arteriographic investigation. AJR 1968;104:829.
51. Webb WR, Jacobs RP. Transpleural abdominal systemic artery–pulmonary artery anastomosis in patients with chronic pulmonary infection. AJR 1977;129:233.
52. Dalen JE, Alpert JS. Natural history of pulmonary embolism. Prog Cardiovasc Dis 1975;17:259.
53. Israel HL, Goldstein F. The varied manifestation of pulmonary embolism. Ann Intern Med 1957;47:202.
54. Stein PD, Hull RD, Saltzman HA, Pineo G. Strategy for diagnosis of patients with suspected acute pulmonary embolism. Chest 1993;103:1553–1559.
55. PIOPED investigators. Value of the ventilation/perfusion scan in acute pulmonary embolism: results of the prospective investigation of pulmonary embolism diagnosis (PIOPED). JAMA 1990;263:2753.
56. Oudkerk M, van Beek EJ, van Putten WL, Buller HR. Cost-effectiveness analysis of various strategies in the diagnostic management of pulmonary embolism. Arch Intern Med 1993;153:947.
57. Stein PD, Athanasoulis C, Alavi A, Greenspan RH, Hales CA, Saltzman HA, et al. Complications and validity of pulmonary angiography in acute pulmonary embolism. Circulation 1992; 85:462.
58. Gorham LW. A study of pulmonary embolism: I. A clinicopathologic investigation of 100 cases of massive embolism of the pulmonary artery; diagnosis by physical signs and differentiation from acute myocardial infarction. Arch Intern Med 1961;108:8.
59. Towbin A. Pulmonary embolism: incidence and significance. JAMA 1954;156:209.
60. Williams JR, Wilcox WC. Pulmonary embolism: roentgenographic and angiographic considerations. AJR 1963;89:333.
61. Williams JR, Wilcox WC, Andrews GJ, Burns RR. Angiography in pulmonary embolism. JAMA 1968;184:473.
62. Greenspan RH. Angiography in pulmonary embolism. In: Abrams angiography. 3rd ed. Boston: Little, Brown, 1983.
63. Bookstein JJ. Segmental arteriography in pulmonary embolism. Radiology 1969;93:1007.
64. Allison PR, Dunnill MS, Marshall R. Pulmonary embolism. Thorax 1960;15:273.
65. Ferris EJ, Stanzler RM, Rourke JA, Blumenthal J, Messer JV. Pulmonary angiography in pulmonary embolic disease. AJR 1967;100:355.
66. Hampton AO, Castleman B. Correlation of postmortem chest teleroentgenograms with autopsy findings with special reference to pulmonary embolism and infarction. AJR 1940;43: 305.
67. Bertucci V, Asch MR, Balter MS. Prognosis in a patient with an initial normal pulmonary angiogram. Chest 1994;105:1257.
68. Novelline RA, Baltarowich OH, Athanasoulis CA, Waltman

AC, Greenfield AJ, McKusick KA. The clinical course of patients with suspected pulmonary embolism and a negative pulmonary arteriogram. Radiology 1978;126:561.

69. McIntyre KM, Sharma GVRK. Subselective pulmonary arteriography with balloon occlusion for the detection of pulmonary embolism. Am J Cardiol 1974;33:154.
70. Orta DA Jr, Eisen S, Yergin BM, Olsen GN. Segmental pulmonary angiography in the critically ill patient using a flow directed catheter. Chest 1979;76:268.
71. Wilson JE III, Bynum LJ. An improved pulmonary angiographic technique using a balloon-tipped catheter. Am Rev Respir Dis 1976;114:1137.
72. Soares FA, Landell GA, de Oliveira JA. Pulmonary tumor embolism to alveolar septal capillaries: a prospective study of 12 cases. Arch Pathol Lab Med 1991;115:127.
73. Soares FA, Landell GA, de Oliveira JA. Pulmonary tumor embolism to alveolar septal capillaries: an unusual cause of sudden cor pulmonale. Arch Pathol Lab Med 1992;116:187.
74. Fred HL, Burdine JA Jr, Gonzalez DA, Lockhart RW, Peabody CA, Alexander JK. Arteriographic assessment of lung scanning in the diagnosis of pulmonary thromboembolism. N Engl J Med 1966;275:1025.
75. Sasahara AA, Stein M, Simon M, Littmann D. Pulmonary angiography in the diagnosis of thromboembolic disease. N Engl J Med 1964;270:1075.
76. Schriner RW, Ryu JH, Edwards WD. Microscopic pulmonary tumor embolism causing subacute cor pulmonale: a difficult antemortem diagnosis. Mayo Clin Proc 1991;66:143.
77. Ho KJ. Diffuse fatal pulmonary microembolism of retroperitoneal extravascular origin. Arch Pathol Lab Med 1989;113: 1401.
78. Fleischner F, Hampton AO, Castleman B. Linear shadows in the lung (interlobar pleuritis, atelectasis, and healed infarction). AJR 1941;46:610.
79. Fleischner FG. Radiologic changes in pulmonary embolism. In: Sasahara AA, Stein M, eds. Pulmonary embolic disease. New York: Grune & Stratton, 1965.
80. Freiman DG, Suyemoto J, Wessler S. Frequency of pulmonary thromboembolism in man. N Engl J Med 1965;272:1278.
81. Tardivon AA, Musset D, Maitre S, Brenot F, Dartevelle P, Simonneau G, Labrune M. Role of CT in chronic pulmonary embolism: comparison with pulmonary angiography. J Comput Assist Tomogr 1993;17:345.
82. Teigen CL, Maus TP, Sheedy PF, Johnson CM, Stanson AW, Welch TJ. Pulmonary embolism: diagnosis with electron-beam CT. Radiology 1993;188:839.
83. Remy-Jardin M, Remy J, Wattinne L, Giraud F. Central pulmonary thromboembolism: diagnosis with spiral volumetric CT with the single-breath-hold technique—comparison with pulmonary angiography. Radiology 1992;185:381.
84. Verschakelen JA, Vanwijck E, Bogaert J, Baert A. Detection of unsuspected central pulmonary embolism with conventional contrast-enhanced CT. Radiology 1993;188:847.
85. Grist TM, et al. Pulmonary angiography with MR imaging: preliminary clinical experience. Radiology 1993;189:523.
86. Downing SE, Vidone RA. Pulmonary vascular responses to embolization with autologous thrombi. Surg Gynecol Obstet 1967;125:269.
87. Bookstein JJ, Feigin DS, Seo KW, Alazraki NP. Diagnosis of pulmonary embolism: experimental evaluation of the accuracy of scintigraphically guided pulmonary arteriography. Radiology 1980;136:15.
88. Dotter CT. Acquired abnormalities of the pulmonary arteries. In: Abrams angiography. 3rd ed. Boston: Little, Brown, 1983.
89. Greenspan RH, Steiner R. Radiology and lung scanning in diagnosis of pulmonary embolism. In: Hume M, Sevitt S, Thomas DP, eds. Venous thrombosis and pulmonary embolism. Cambridge: Harvard University Press, 1970.
90. Dotter CT, Rösch J, Seaman AJ, Dennis D, Massey WH. Streptokinase treatment of thromboembolic disease. Radiology 1972;102:283.
91. Dalen JE, Brooks HL, Johnson LW, Meister SG, Szucs MM, Dexter L. Pulmonary angiography in acute pulmonary embolism: indications, techniques, results in 367 patients. Am Heart J 1971;81:175.
92. Steinberg I, Dotter CT. Lung cancer: angiocardiographic findings in one hundred consecutive proved cases. Arch Surg 1952;64:10.
93. Steinberg I, Dotter CT, Andrus DD. Angiocardiography in thoracic surgery. Surg Gynecol Obstet 1950;90:45.
94. Amundsen P, Sorenson E. Angiocardiography in intrathoracic tumors with particular reference to the question of operability. Acta Radiol 1956;45:185.
95. Olsson HE, Spitzer RM, Erston WF. Primary and secondary pulmonary artery neoplasia mimicking acute pulmonary embolism. Radiology 1976;118:49.
96. Roth FJ, Ranninger K, Beachly M, Henry D. Angiographische Darstellung eines Primaren Sarkoms der Arteria Pulmonalis. ROEFO 1975;122:47.
97. Primack SL, Müller NL, Mayo JR, Remy-Jardin M, Remy J. Pulmonary parenchymal abnormalities of vascular origin: high-resolution CT findings. Radiographics 1994;14:739.
98. Liebow AA. Recent observations on pulmonary collateral circulation. Med Thorac 1962;19:609.
99. Viamonte M Jr. Angiographic evaluation of pulmonary neoplasms. Radiol Clin North Am 1965;3:529.
100. Steiner RE. Pulmonary hypertension: a symposium: II. Radiological appearances of the pulmonary vessels in pulmonary hypertension. Br J Radiol 1958;31:188.
101. Chen JTT, Capp MP, Johnsrude IS, Goodrich JK, Lester RG. Roentgen appearance of pulmonary vascularity in the diagnosis of heart disease. AJR 1971;112:559.
102. McCoy HL, Steinberg I, Dotter CT. Angiocardiographic findings in thoracoplasty, artificial pneumoperitoneum, and phreniclasia. J Thorac Surg 1951;21:149.
103. Steinberg I, McCoy HI, Dotter CT. Angiocardiographic findings in artificial pneumothorax. Am Rev Tuberc Pulm Dis 1950;62:353.
104. Cicero R, del Castillo H, Fernandez M, Moulun M. Selective angiopneumography and a correlative study of bronchography and the histopathologic findings in tuberculous fibrothorax. Am Rev Tuberc Pulm Dis 1956;73:61.
105. Dubilier W Jr, Steinberg I, Dotter CT. Kyphoscoliosis: angiocardiographic findings. Radiology 1953;61:56.
106. Dotter CT, Jackson FS. Death following angiocardiography. Radiology 1950;54:527.
107. Kawai C, Ishikawa K, Kato M, Ishii Y, Nakao K. "Pulmonary pulseless disease": pulmonary involvement in so-called Takayasu's disease. Clinical Conference in Cardiology from the Third Medical Division, Kyoto University Hospital, Kyoto, Japan. Chest 1978;73:651.
108. Tamaki M. Angiocardiography: a contribution to its technical and clinical aspects. Presented at the 17th Annual Meeting of the Japan Radiological Society, Fukuoka, Apr. 1–3, 1958.
109. Yamada I, Shibuya H, Matsubara O, Umehara I, Makino T, Numano F, Suzuki S. Pulmonary artery disease in Takayasu's arteritis: angiographic findings. AJR 1992;159:263.
110. Talwar KK, Kumar K, Chopar P, Sharma S, Shrivastava S, Wasir HS, Rajani M, Tandon R. Cardiac involvement in nonspecific aortoarteritis (Takayasu's arteritis). Am Heart J 1991; 122:1666.
111. Liu YQ, Jin BL, Ling J. Pulmonary artery involvement in aortoarteritis: an angiographic study. Cardiovasc Intervent Radiol 1994;17:2.
112. Sharma S, Talwar KK, Rajani M. Coronary artery to pulmonary artery collaterals in nonspecific aortoarteritis involving the pulmonary arteries. Cardiovasc Intervent Radiol 1993;16:111.
113. Numan F, Islak C, Berkmen T, Tüzün H, Cokyüksel O. Behçet disease: pulmonary arterial involvement in 15 cases. Radiology 1994;192:465.
114. International Study Group for Behçet Disease. Criteria for diagnosis of Behçet disease. Lancet 1990;335:1078.
115. Lundell C, Finck E. Arteriovenous fistulas originating from Rasmussen aneurysms. AJR 1983;140:687.

33

Developmental Anomalies of the Pulmonary Arteries

PAUL R. JULSRUD

Congenital abnormalities of the pulmonary arteries include an interesting variety of vascular malformations with important clinical consequences. Classification of the structural aberrations can be approached from our understanding of pulmonary artery development.[1–4] Figure 33-1 illustrates schematically a human embryo at the 4-, 6-, and 11-mm stages of development. The central pulmonary arteries are derived from the sixth aortic arches and division of the truncus arteriosus communis, whereas development of the peripheral pulmonary arteries is intimately related to that of the lung bud. Although development of the central and peripheral pulmonary arteries occurs simultaneously and is closely interrelated, their unique origins account for many of the congenital anomalies encountered. Therefore, organizing pulmonary artery congenital anomalies into two broad categories, central and peripheral, can be helpful in classifying and understanding these malformations.

Congenital Anomalies of the Central Pulmonary Arteries

As Figure 33-1 illustrates, normal development of the central pulmonary arteries results from division of the truncus arteriosus and modeling of the right and left sixth aortic arches. Figure 33-2 presents a schematic representation of the normal asymmetric form of the final product. The point of connection of the postbronchial pulmonary artery is located approximately at the junction of the ventral and dorsal components of the sixth aortic arch. The main pulmonary artery is considered to be derived from fusion of the ventral components of the right and left sixth aortic arches. The left dorsal sixth aortic arch persists as the ligamentum arteriosum. Part of the ventral component of the right sixth aortic arch becomes the central portion of the proximal right pulmonary artery. Normally the dorsal component of the right sixth aortic arch resorbs completely. However, if it persists, either as a right patent ductus or a ligamentum arteriosus, it will connect to the right pulmonary artery at the point of juncture between that part of the right pulmonary artery derived from the ventral component of the right sixth aortic arch and that derived from the right postbronchial pulmonary artery.[2] Thus, in this chapter, the central pulmonary arteries are considered to extend from the level of the pulmonary valve to the ligamentum arteriosum on the left and to the level of the lateral border of the superior vena cava on the right. This also corresponds to the usual point of reflection of the pericardium on the proximal left and right pulmonary arteries.

Truncus Arteriosus

The pulmonary and aortic valves result from normal division of the truncus arteriosus. Persistence of the truncus arteriosus results in an interesting anomaly with multiple variations. Two classification schemes, one by Collett and Edwards and another by Van Praagh and Van Praagh, are commonly used in describing this entity.[5–7] Figure 33-3 illustrates the differences between these two classifications. Note that type IV in the Collett and Edwards classification is not due to the persistence of an undivided truncus arteriosus and that types III and IV of the Van Praagh and Van Praagh classification are not included in the Collett and Edwards classification. The surgical treatment of truncus arteriosus is in large part determined by the pulmonary artery anatomy present in an individual patient.[8,9] The angiographic demonstration of the relevant anatomy is illustrated in Figures 33-4 through 33-7. In addition to the aortic arch and pulmonary artery anatomy, it should be noted that the anatomy of the coronary arteries can be of particular clinical importance.[10,11]

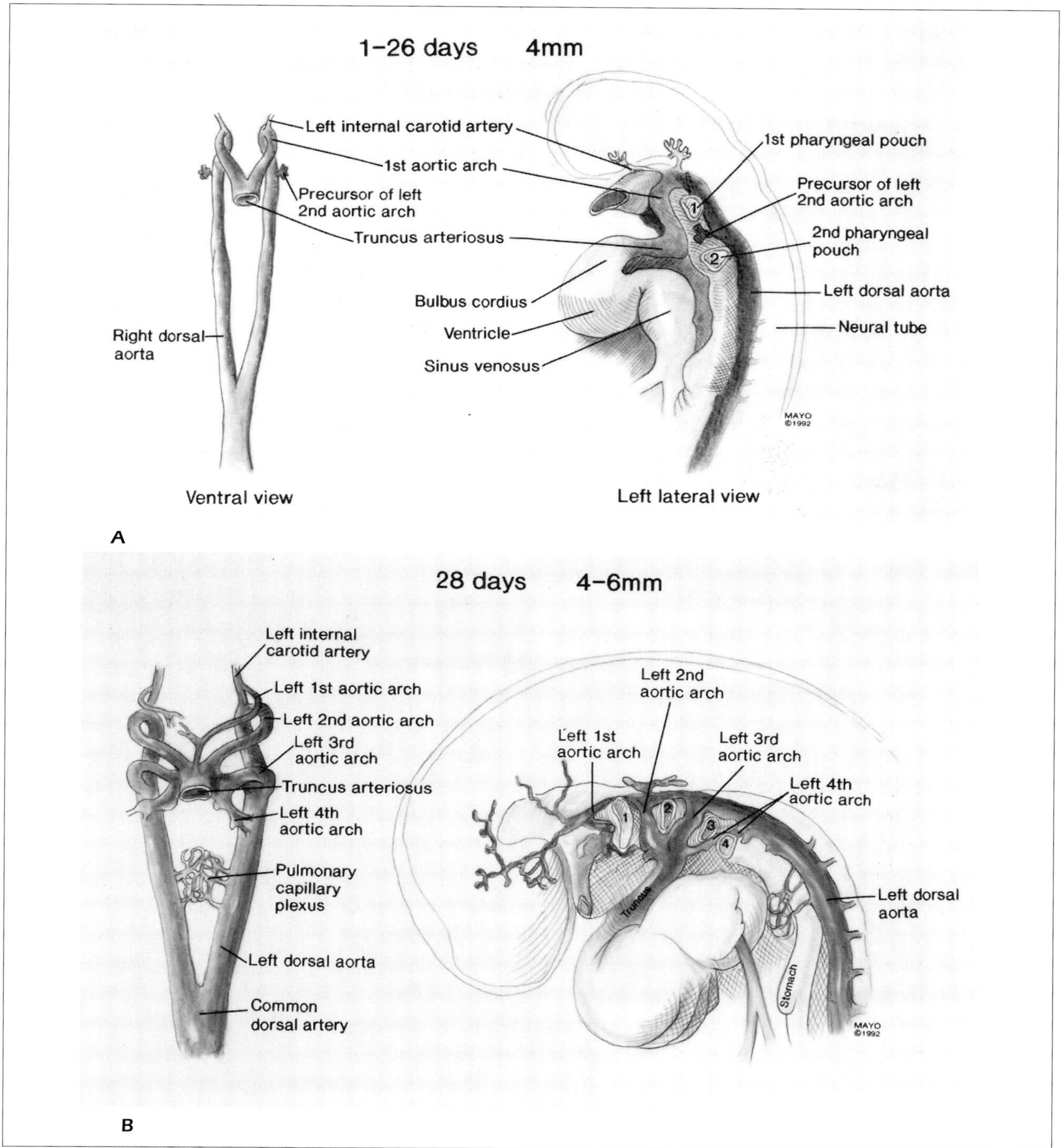

Figure 33-1. Diagram of ventral and left lateral views of the developing cardiovascular system in the human embryo at the 4-, 6-, and 11-mm stages (A, B, and C, respectively). See text for discussion.

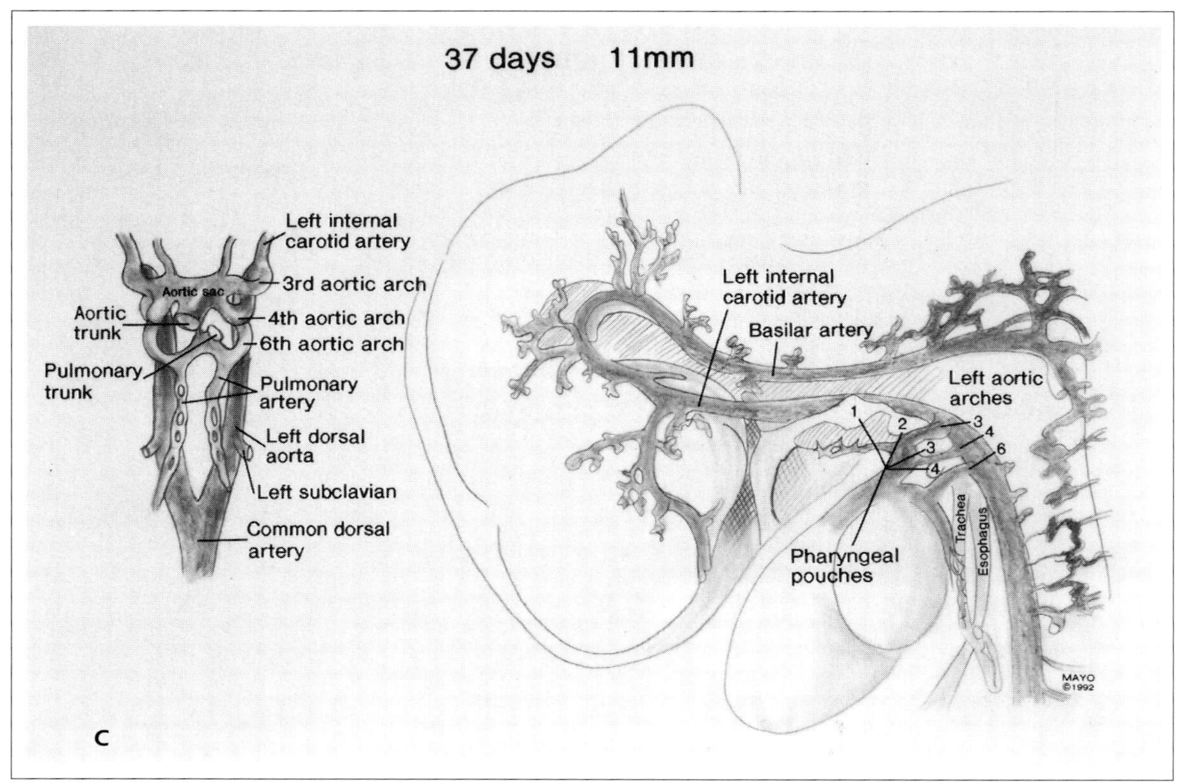

Figure 33-1 (continued).

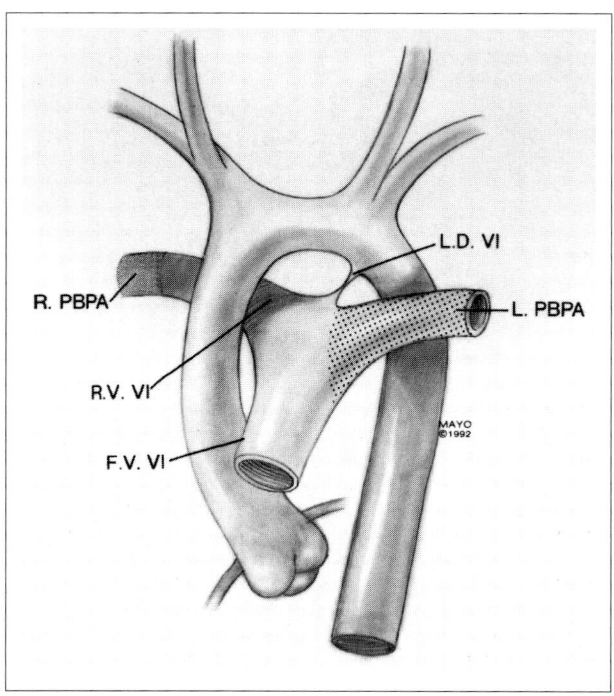

Figure 33-2. Diagram of the fully developed normal proximal pulmonary arteries. *R. PBPA,* right postbrachial pulmonary artery; *L. PBPA,* left postbrachial pulmonary artery; *R.V. VI,* right ventral sixth arch; *F.V. VI,* fused right and left ventral sixth arches; *L.D. VI,* left dorsal sixth arch. See text for discussion. (Adapted from Skidmore FD. The development of the pulmonary circulation. In: Gore DA, Lillihei CW, eds. Congenital malformations of the heart. New York: Grune & Stratton, 1975. Used with permission.)

Figure 33-4. Truncus arteriosus type I (Van Praagh and Van Praagh). (A) Anteroposterior view of truncal root angiogram. Both branch pulmonary arteries are visualized, but their points of origin are not demonstrated. The truncal valve is competent. (B) Lateral view during same injection clearly demonstrates the main pulmonary artery segment and proximal branch pulmonary arteries. *Rpa,* right pulmonary artery; *TRU,* truncus arteriosus; *Lpa,* left pulmonary artery; *Mpa,* main pulmonary artery. (From Yoshizato T, Julsrud PR: Truncus arteriosus revisited: an angiographic demonstration. Pediatr Cardiol 1990;11:36–40. Used with permission.) ▶

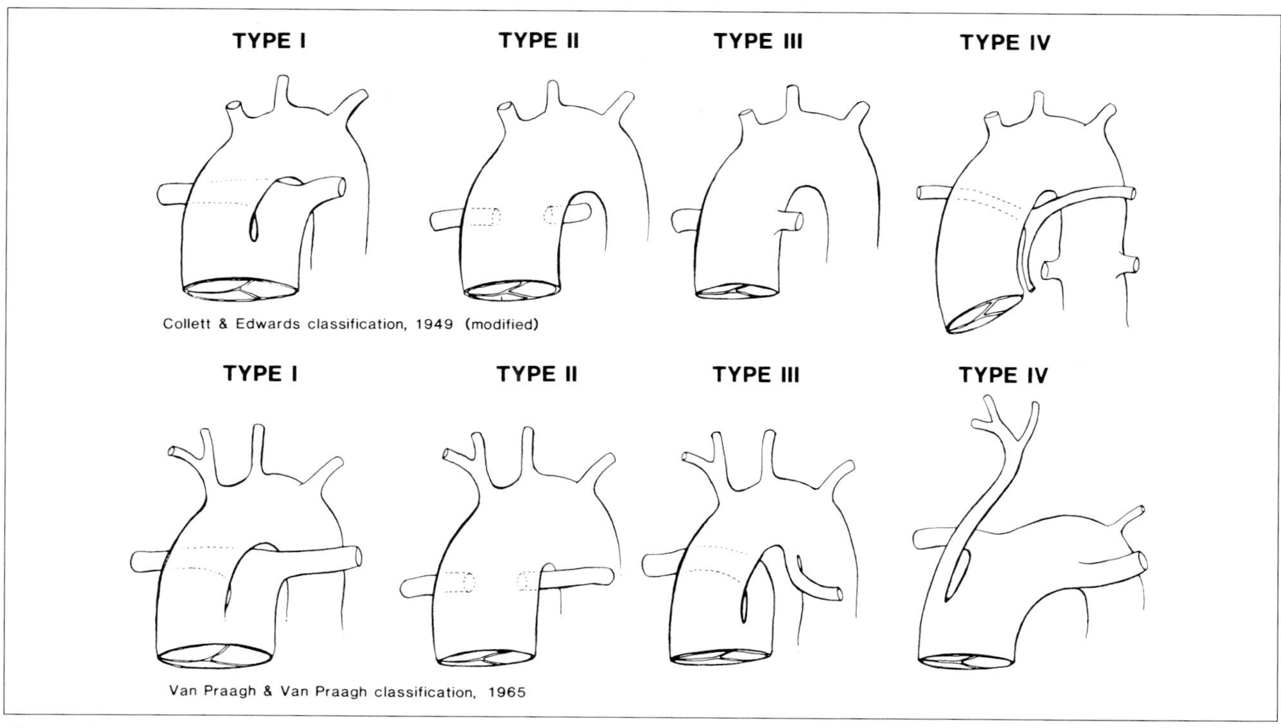

Figure 33-3. Diagrams of different types of truncus arteriosus comparing the Collett and Edwards classification (*above*) and the Van Praagh and Van Praagh classification (*below*) (see text for discussion). (From Yoshizato T, Julsrud PR. Truncus arteriosus revisited: an angiographic demonstration. Pediatr Cardiol 1990;11:36–40. Used with permission.)

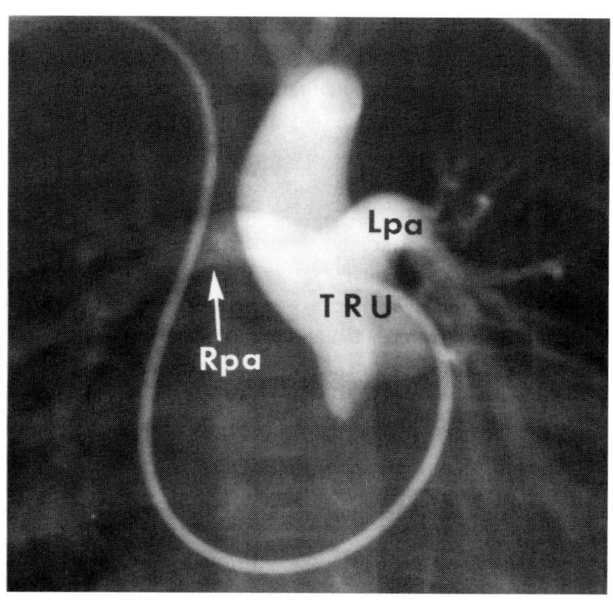

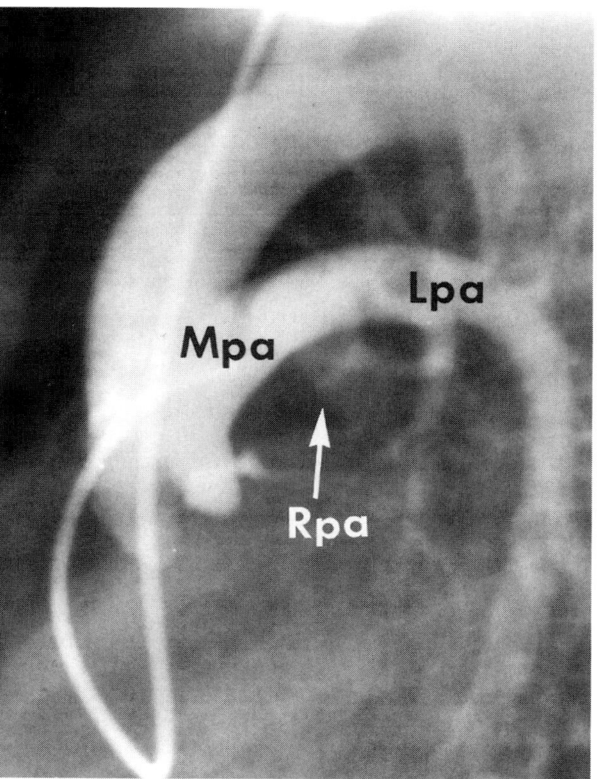

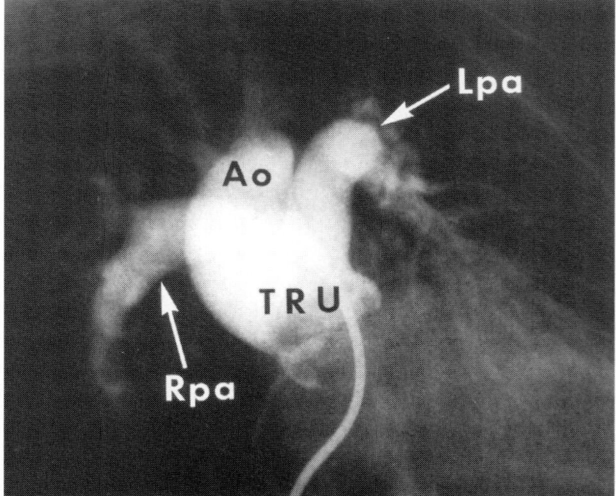

A

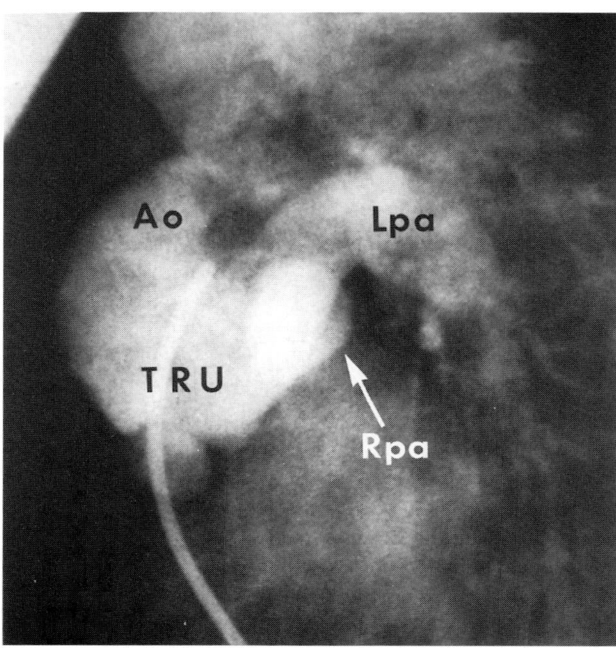

B

Figure 33-5. Truncus arteriosus type II. (A) Truncal root angiogram, anteroposterior view with 30-degree cranial angulation, shows both pulmonary arteries arising from a truncus arteriosus. The truncal valve is competent. (B) Left anterior oblique view with 15-degree caudal angulation confirms the absence of a main pulmonary artery segment and the independent origin of both pulmonary arteries from truncal root. *Ao,* aorta; *Lpa,* left pulmonary artery; *Rpa,* right pulmonary artery; *TRU,* truncus arteriosus. (From Yoshizato T, Julsrud PR. Truncus arteriosus revisited: an angiographic demonstration. Pediatr Cardiol 1990;11:36–40. Used with permission.)

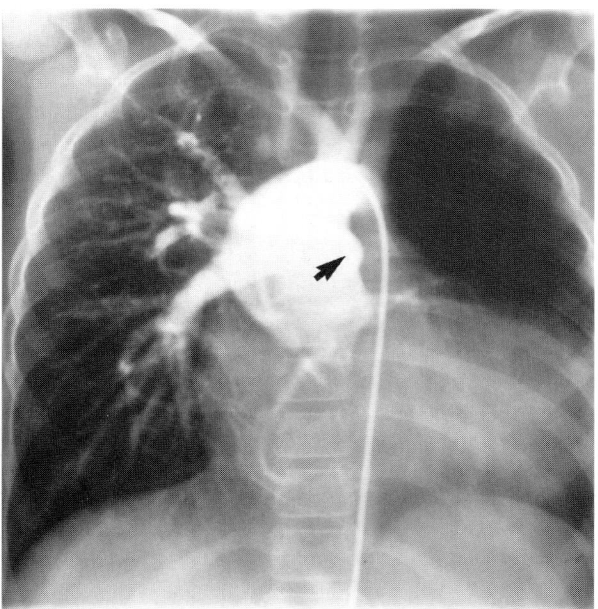

Figure 33-6. Truncus arteriosus type III. Note the site of origin of the right pulmonary artery (*arrow*) and the lack of left pulmonary artery demonstration by this truncal root injection. This is so-called absence of the left pulmonary artery. However, angiography eventually demonstrated a very hypoplastic left pulmonary artery that was supplied by transpleural arterial collateral flow originating from the left subclavian artery.

Pulmonary Valve Stenosis

Although pulmonary valve stenosis may occur in combination with other congenital heart lesions, such as double-outlet right ventricle, tetralogy of Fallot, transposition of the great arteries, tricuspid valve atresia, and so on, this discussion will focus on congenital pulmonary valve stenosis as an isolated anomaly. In contrast to the bicuspid pulmonary valve found in approximately 50 percent of patients with tetralogy of Fallot,[12,13] unicommissural and stenotic tricuspid pulmonary valves are more commonly encountered in the isolated form of congenital pulmonary valve stenosis.[14] Dysplastic pulmonary valves are commonly encountered in patients with Noonan syndrome.[15] Figure 33-8 illustrates the characteristic plain film and angiographic appearance of a 4-year-old patient with isolated congenital pulmonary valve stenosis. Although percutaneous balloon dilatation of pulmonary valve stenosis is currently considered by most the treatment of choice for this lesion, at the time we attempted balloon inflation in the patient shown in Figure 33-8 (January 13, 1981), we were aware of only one previous balloon valvotomy of a stenotic pulmonary valve. In 1979, Semb and associates had reported reducing the gradient across a stenotic pulmonary valve from 20 mmHg to 6 mmHg by pulling an inflated balloon

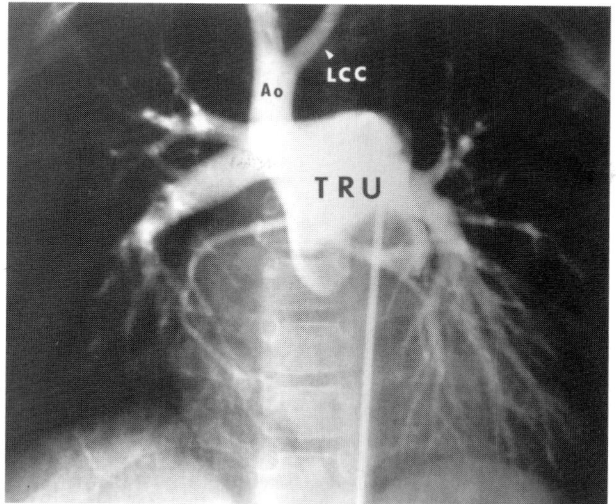

A

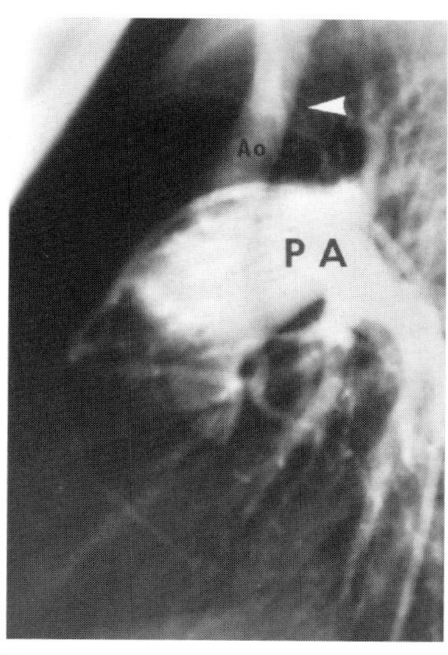

B

Figure 33-7. Truncus arteriosus type IV. (A) Anteroposterior view of truncal root angiogram, with catheter coursing retrograde in descending aorta and through patent ductus arteriosus into the truncal root, demonstrating interruption of the aortic arch beyond the left common carotid artery. The pulmonary artery segment is larger than the aortic segment. The truncal valve is competent. (B) Lateral view during same injection demonstrates a large ductus arteriosus "continuing" as the descending aorta. *White arrowhead* indicates the level of the aortic arch interruption. *Ao,* aorta; *LCC,* left common carotid artery; *TRU,* truncus arteriosus; *PA,* pulmonary artery. (From Yoshizato T, Julsrud PR. Truncus arteriosus revisited: an angiographic demonstration. Pediatr Cardiol 1990;11:36–40. Used with permission.)

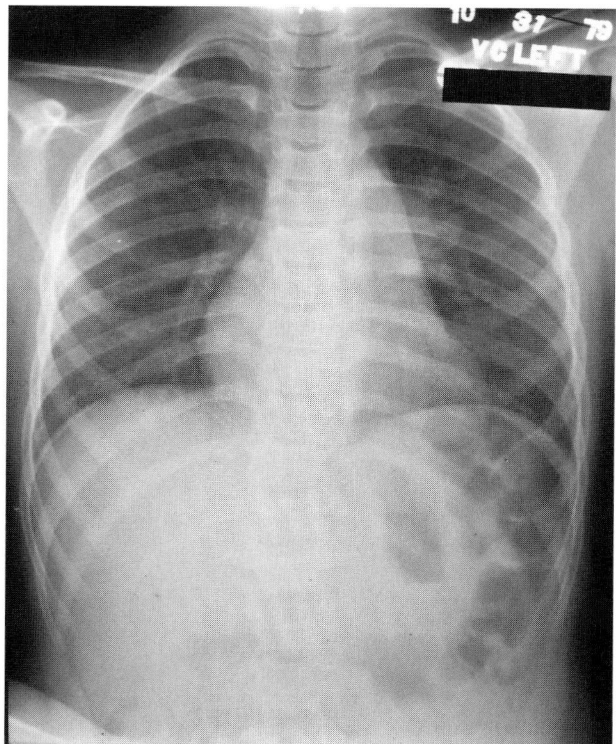

A

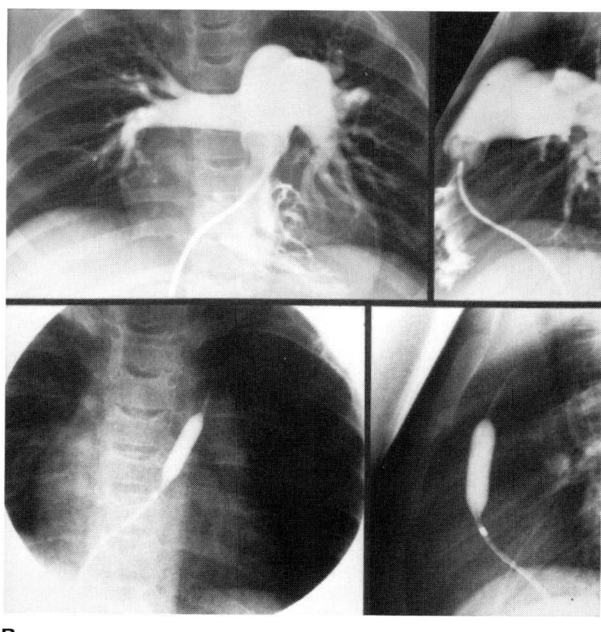

B

Figure 33-8. Pulmonary valve stenosis. (A) Posteroanterior chest radiograph. Note the enlargement of the left pulmonary artery due to the poststenotic dilatation that involves the main and left pulmonary arteries. (B) *Top panel:* Anteroposterior and lateral angiogram for correlation. Note the thickened pulmonary valve, poststenotic dilatation of the main and left pulmonary arteries, and marked narrowing of the right ventricular outflow tract due to narrowing of the right ventricular infundibulum during systole. *Lower panel:* Frames from a cineangiogram during attempted balloon dilatation of the stenotic valve (see text).

through the stenotic valve.[16] Figure 33-8B demonstrates an inflated balloon across the stenotic valve of the 4-year-old patient. Unfortunately, a 6-mm balloon was the largest inflatable balloon we had available at the time, and this being the first known attempt using this technique, we were reluctant to use the "kissing balloon" technique, which had been described in 1980.[17] Although we were not able to adequately relieve the pulmonary valve stenosis in this patient, Kan et al. first described successful balloon dilatation of congenitally stenotic pulmonary valves, and now the procedure is well established.[18–21] Follow-up results after balloon pulmonary valvuloplasty have been gratifying, especially when 30 percent oversized balloons are used.[22] Although this procedure is considered safe, Burrows et al. have documented pulmonary artery dissections following balloon valvotomy for pulmonary valve stenosis.[23]

Pulmonary Valve Atresia

Pulmonary valve atresia is the terminology used to describe conditions in which the heart and the pulmonary arteries do not connect directly via a patent pulmonary valve. Two types of congenital anomalies account for most of the conditions satisfying this definition. Both are relatively uncommon, each totaling 2 to 3 percent of all congenital heart anomalies. Pulmonary valve atresia with an intact ventricular septum is usually associated with a hypoplastic tricuspid valve and a small right ventricle. In addition, coronary artery abnormalities are common.[24–26] The pulmonary blood flow is usually supplied by a patent ductus arteriosus, and, although the pulmonary arteries may be hypoplastic, they are usually otherwise normal.

Pulmonary valve atresia with ventricular septal defect is an entirely different entity and may be considered to represent a severe form of tetralogy of Fallot. In contradistinction to pulmonary valve atresia with intact ventricular septum, patients with pulmonary valve atresia and ventricular septal defect frequently have marked arborization abnormalities of the pulmonary arterial tree. The unusual pulmonary arterial branching patterns that occur in these patients are a consequence of the variations in blood supply to the pulmonary circulation provided by systemic-to-pulmonary collateral arteries.[27–30] These systemic-to-pulmonary collateral arteries originate either directly from the aorta or from one of its branches. Figure 33-9 demonstrates two types of systemic-to-pulmonary collateral artery connections to the pulmonary arterial tree. The difference between the two types depends on whether the peripheral pulmonary arteries supplied by the collateral vessel connect with a central pulmonary artery. The difference between the central pulmonary artery communicating and noncommunicating types of systemic-to-pulmonary collateral arteries has therapeutic implications when surgical or transcatheter embolization procedures are being contemplated.

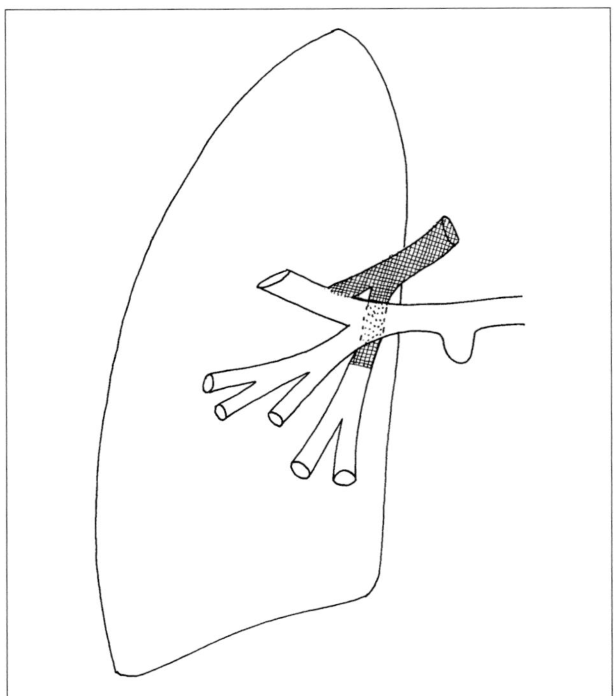

Figure 33-9. Diagram of a systemic-to-pulmonary collateral artery. The cross-hatched vessel identifies the collateral artery, which has two branches. The upper branch of the systemic-to-pulmonary collateral artery connects to the right upper lobe pulmonary artery, which communicates with the central pulmonary artery confluence. The lower branch of the collateral terminates in right lower lobe pulmonary arteries that do not directly communicate with the central pulmonary arteries. (Note the blind ending stump of the main pulmonary artery, frequently present in patients with tetralogy of Fallot and pulmonary valve atresia.) (From Liao PK. Pulmonary blood supply in patients with pulmonary atresia and ventricular septal defect. J Am Coll Cardiol 1985;6:1343–1350. Used with permission.)

Absence of the Pulmonary Valve

Congenital absence of the pulmonary valve usually occurs in patients with tetralogy of Fallot. In addition to little or no pulmonary valve tissue being present, there is marked dilatation of the main and proximal right and left pulmonary arteries (Fig. 33-10). The large pulmonary arteries frequently compress the tracheobronchial tree, resulting in compromised respiratory function.[31,32] Figure 33-11 illustrates another patient with congenital absence of the pulmonary valve and so-called absent left pulmonary artery. In this instance,

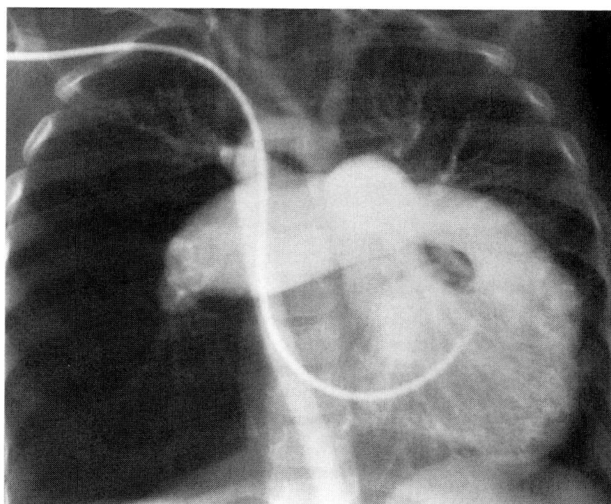

Figure 33-10. Absent pulmonary valve. Right ventricular angiogram in a patient with tetralogy of Fallot and absent pulmonary valve syndrome. Note the markedly enlarged pulmonary arteries. Note also the right aortic arch with mirror-image branching of the brachiocephalic arteries.

the left pulmonary artery does not connect to the main pulmonary artery and most likely was initially supplied by a patent ductus arteriosus.

Aorticopulmonary Window

An aorticopulmonary window is characterized by a defect that is common to the adjacent walls of the ascending aorta and the main pulmonary artery. It is one of the rarest causes of left-to-right shunting. Although this malformation may be associated with other congenital heart defects, it is most commonly an isolated lesion.[33] The defect is usually located 1 to 2 cm above the ostia of the coronary arteries, with its size varying from a "pinhole" to 3 or 4 cm in diameter (Fig. 33-12).

Idiopathic Pulmonary Artery Dilatation

Idiopathic pulmonary artery dilatation most likely has a congenital etiology, although this remains speculative. Figure 33-13 illustrates the plain film, tomographic, and angiographic findings in a 42-year-old man with this condition. Although this patient was asymptomatic, the abnormal chest radiographs prompted further investigations, and no evidence of pulmonary valve stenosis was found. The diagnosis of idiopathic pulmonary artery dilatation depends on excluding structural etiologies, such as poststenotic dilatation due to pulmonary valve stenosis.

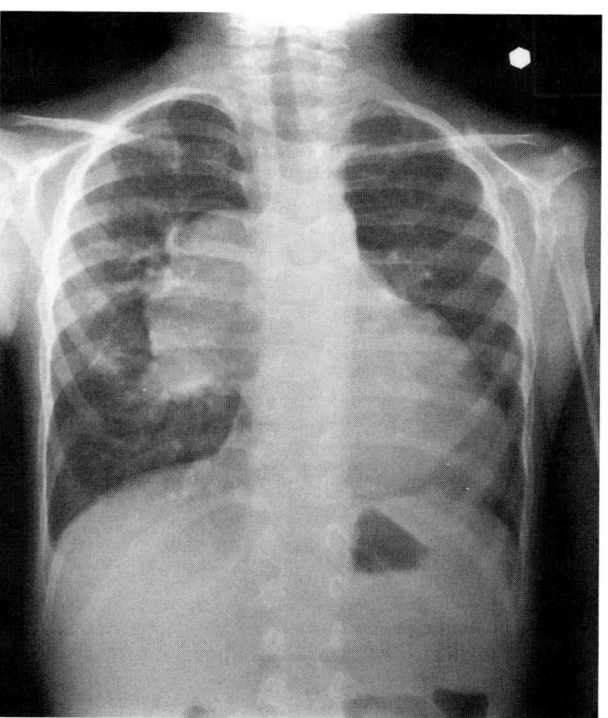

A

B

Figure 33-11. Absent pulmonary valve. (A) Posteroanterior chest radiograph in a patient with tetralogy of Fallot with a masslike density in the right hilar region. (B) Pulmonary angiogram for correlation. Note the marked dilatation of the proximal right pulmonary artery in this patient with tetralogy of Fallot and absent pulmonary valve syndrome. Note also that this patient has so-called absence of the left pulmonary artery in that it does not connect with the main pulmonary artery. Subsequent injections in the left subclavian artery demonstrated a hypoplastic left pulmonary artery that was supplied by transpleural collateral channels originating from the left subclavian artery.

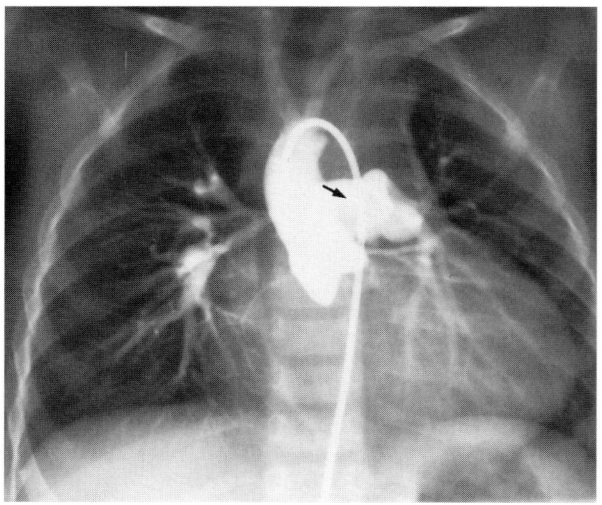

A

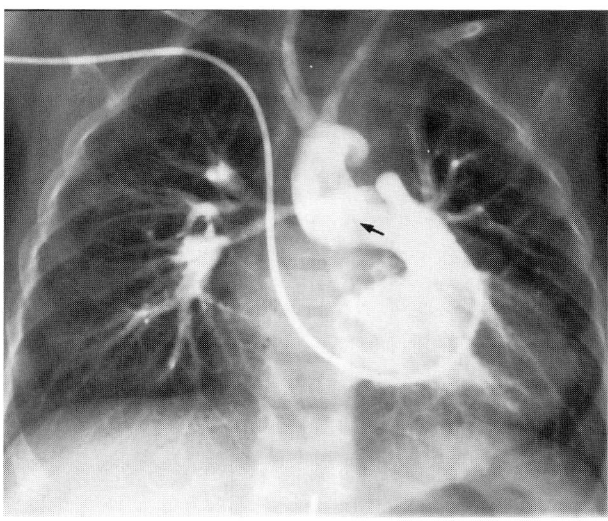

B

Figure 33-12. Aorticopulmonary (AP) window. (A) Aortic root injection in a patient with aorticopulmonary window (*arrow*). Note the opacification of the pulmonary arterial tree, which is hypoplastic, particularly on the right. (B) Right ventricular injection in the same patient. Note the opacification of the aorta through the AP window (*arrow*) due to right-to-left shunting during the injection.

Figure 33-13. Idiopathic pulmonary artery dilatation. (A) Posteroanterior chest radiograph demonstrating marked dilatation of the central pulmonary arteries. (B) Tomogram at the level of the carina demonstrating marked enlargement of the proximal left pulmonary artery. (C) Pulmonary angiogram. Anteroposterior projection demonstrating marked enlargement of the central pulmonary arteries in a patient with no detectable hemodynamic gradient across the pulmonary valve. (D) Lateral view of pulmonary angiogram for correlation.

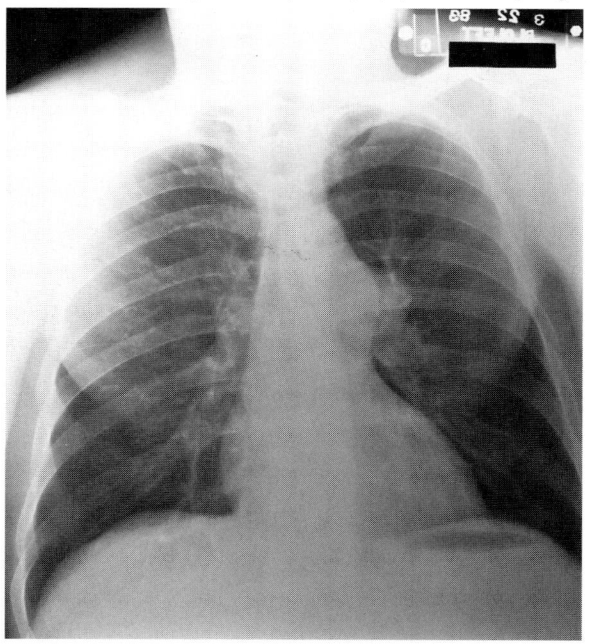

A

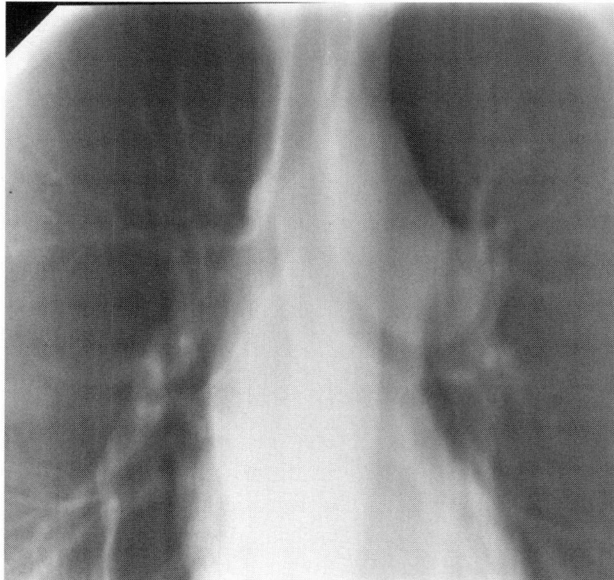

B

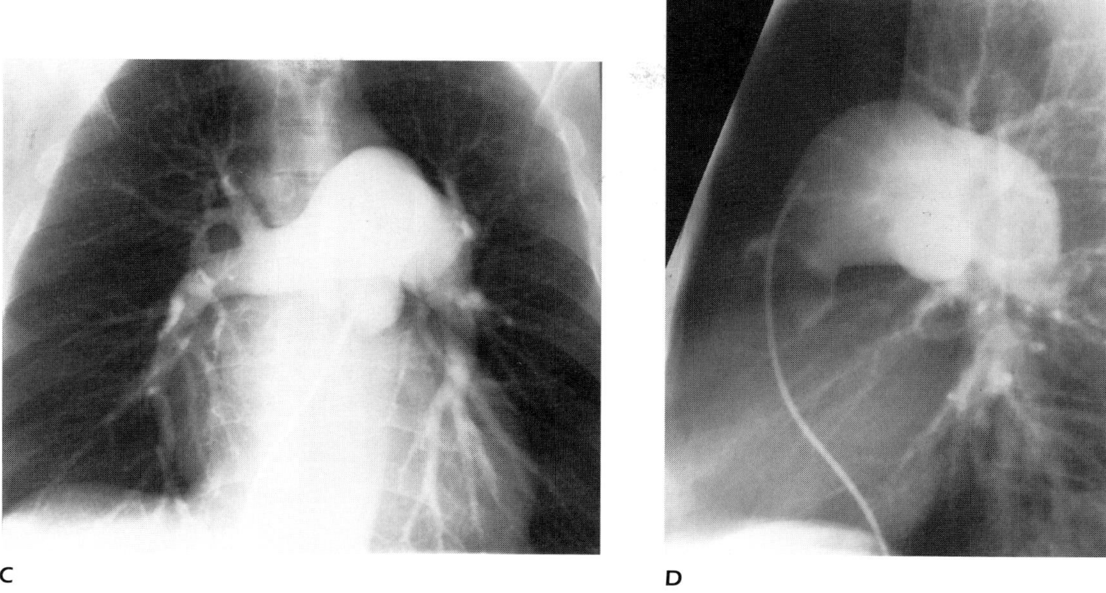

Figure 33-13 (continued).

Hypoplastic Central Pulmonary Arteries

Underdeveloped central pulmonary arteries can be encountered in association with many different congenital anomalies. Frequently, this hypoplasia is generalized and is thought to be due to decreased amounts of pulmonary parenchyma, which results secondarily in a reduction in pulmonary artery size. However, the most common setting in which small central pulmonary arteries are encountered in association with congenital heart disease is in patients with tetralogy of Fallot. Figure 33-14 illustrates the angiographic findings in a 1-year-old with tetralogy of Fallot and hypoplastic pulmonary arteries. The estimated cross-sectional area of the central pulmonary arteries illustrated in Figure 33-14 is 28 percent of expected when indexed to the patient's body surface area.[34] The smallest pulmonary arteries are found in patients with pulmonary valve atresia with or without a ventricular septal defect (VSD). The hypoplastic pulmonary arteries presented in Figure 33-15 are in a patient with tetralogy of Fallot and pulmonary valve atresia; this view was taken using pulmonary vein wedge angiography.[35,36]

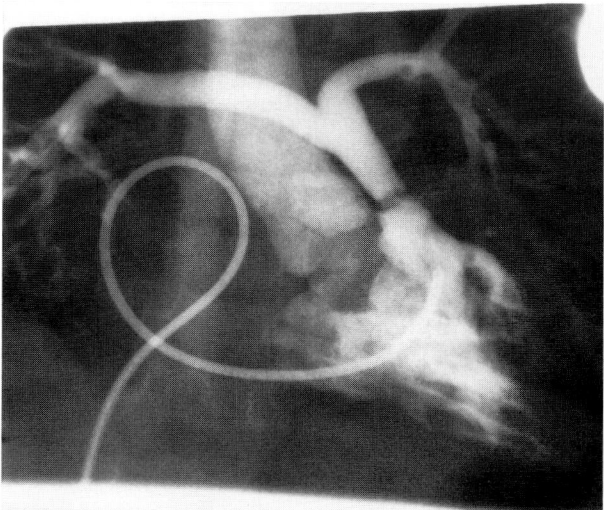

Figure 33-14. Hypoplastic pulmonary arteries. Right ventricular angiogram with 15-degree cranial angulation. The hypoplastic central pulmonary arteries are 28 percent of expected size (see text for discussion). The pulmonary valve annulus is also markedly hypoplastic in this patient with tetralogy of Fallot and a right-sided aortic arch.

Central Pulmonary Artery Stenosis

Localized areas of narrowing in the central pulmonary arteries occur either as isolated anomalies (40 percent) or in association with other congenital cardiovascular diseases.[37] These other associated conditions include pulmonary valve stenosis, atrial septal defect, ventricular septal defect (VSD), tetralogy of Fallot, patent ductus arteriosus, Williams syndrome, rubella, Ehlers-Danlos syndrome, Noonan syndrome, Alagille syndrome, and cutis laxa.[37–46] Figure 33-16 illustrates pulmonary artery stenosis in its isolated form. A murmur was heard early in life, but the patient had been

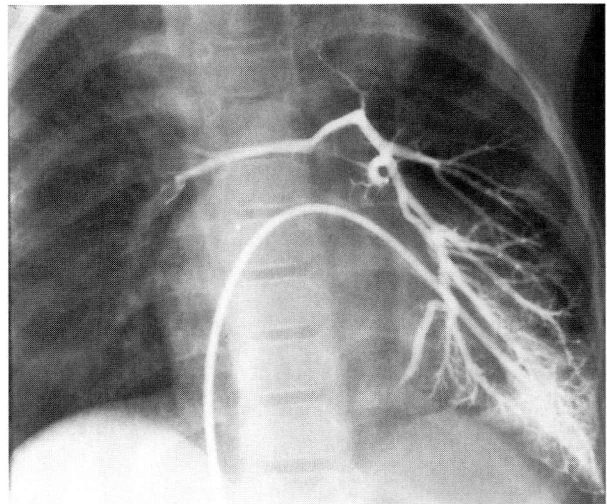

Figure 33-15. Hypoplastic pulmonary arteries. Pulmonary vein wedge angiogram. The venous catheter was introduced into a left lower lobe pulmonary vein via a patent foramen ovale. The hypoplastic pulmonary arteries are opacified by retrograde flow of radiographic contrast media from the pulmonary venous wedge injection.

entirely asymptomatic. At the time of this angiogram, the main pulmonary artery pressure was elevated (56 mmHg systolic, 11 mmHg diastolic, 31 mmHg mean). Figure 33-16B illustrates the fact that stenoses of the central pulmonary arteries may cause hypoplasia of the ipsilateral peripheral pulmonary arterial tree.

An interesting form of central pulmonary artery stenosis involving the proximal left pulmonary artery is thought by some to be related to abnormalities involving the ductus arteriosus (Fig. 33-17). The histologic features of this entity suggest that the left pulmonary artery stenosis is due to aberrant ductal tissue.[47]

Figure 33-18 illustrates a current approach to transcatheter therapeutic management of patients with central pulmonary artery stenosis. Balloon dilation of a proximal left pulmonary artery stenosis was followed by insertion of a wire stent to maintain expansion of the left pulmonary artery.

Figures 33-14 through 33-18 demonstrate that diagnostic views of the central pulmonary arteries can be accomplished using a variety of angiographic projections. Cranial angulation of the anteroposterior projection, sometimes referred to as the "sitting-up" view, has been shown to be useful to accommodate for the "horizontal" course of the main pulmonary artery in patients with tetralogy of Fallot.[48–50] Figure 33-19 illustrates another useful pulmonary artery view, which combines 25 degrees of caudal angulation with 70 degrees of left anterior angulation. This view reliably demonstrates the proximal left pulmonary artery.

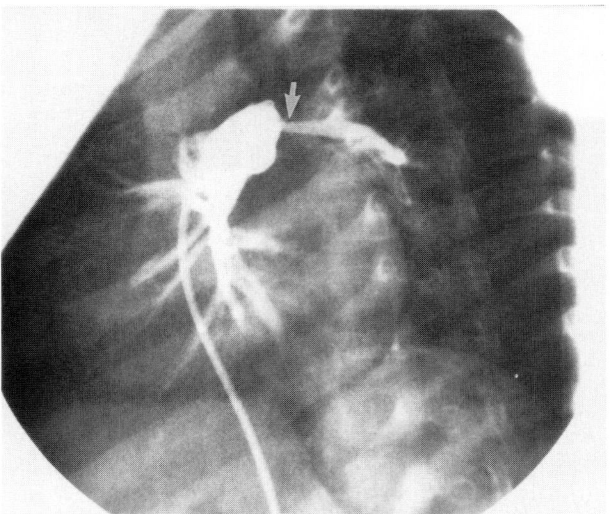

A

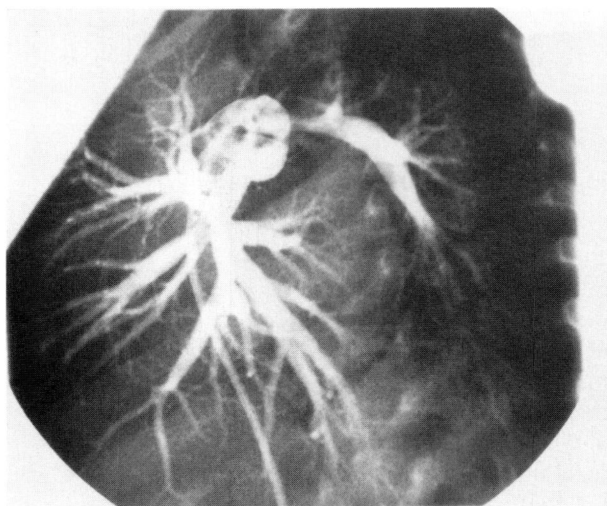

B

Figure 33-16. Central pulmonary artery stenosis. (A) A 70-degree left anterior oblique view of a pulmonary artery angiogram. Note the marked narrowing at the origin of the left pulmonary artery (*arrow*). (B) Later phase of the same pulmonary angiogram demonstrating more of the peripheral pulmonary arteries. Note the small left peripheral pulmonary arteries.

Anomalous Origin of Pulmonary Arteries

The most notable abnormality involving an unusual origin of one of the pulmonary arteries is the so-called pulmonary artery sling.[51] In this anomaly, the left pulmonary artery courses to the right side of the trachea before "swinging" back into its normal position in the left hilum. This abnormal position and course of the left pulmonary artery makes it appear to originate from the proximal right pulmonary artery. As it passes

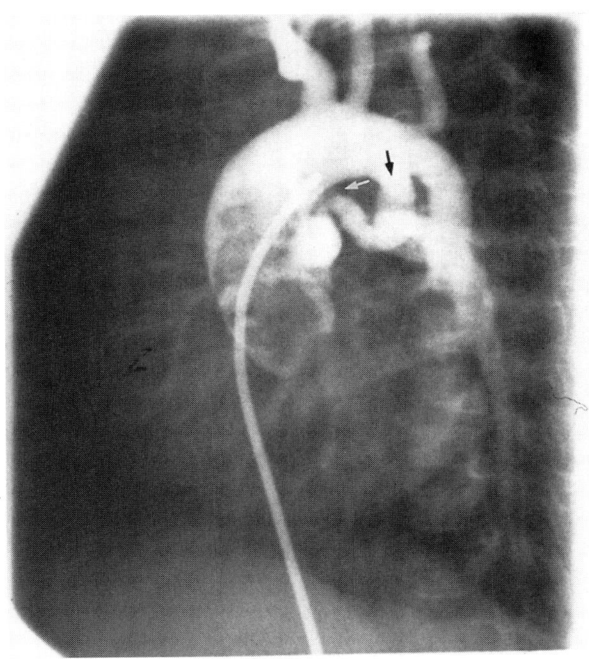

A

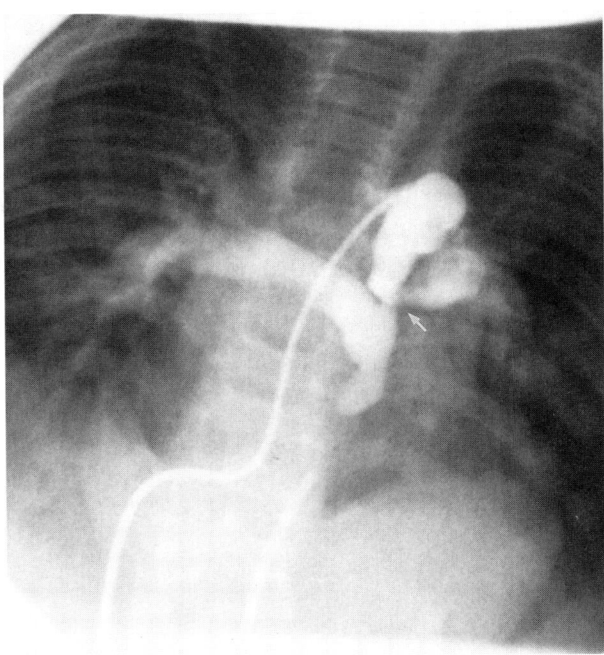

B

Figure 33-17. Stenosis at the origin of the left pulmonary artery. Tetralogy of Fallot with pulmonary valve atresia and patent ductus arteriosus. (A) A 70-degree left anterior oblique view of an aortic arch angiogram demonstrating a vertically oriented patent ductus arteriosus (*black arrow*) and stenosis at the origin of the left pulmonary artery (*white arrow*). (B) Anteroposterior view with 30 degrees of cranial angulation (sitting-up view) during selective injection in the patent ductus arteriosus demonstrating the stenosis at the origin of the left pulmonary artery (*arrow*).

around the trachea, the left pulmonary artery is located anterior to the esophagus (Fig. 33-20). There may be associated partial obstruction of the origin of the right main stem bronchus, resulting in collapse or, more frequently, hyperinflation of the right lung.

The left or right pulmonary artery can also originate from the aorta. It can arise as the first branch of a right aortic arch or from one of the normal branch vessels of the aorta.[52,53] It can also be supplied solely by a ductus arteriosus in so-called congenital absence of the left pulmonary artery (Fig. 33-21). Anomalous origin of the right pulmonary artery is more common than that of the left.

Anomalous Origin of Coronary Arteries

Anomalous origin of coronary arteries from a pulmonary artery is another rare but interesting congenital anomaly involving pulmonary arteries. The most common abnormality in this group is anomalous origin of the left coronary artery from the main pulmonary artery. In this anomaly, a pressure gradient exists between the aorta and the main pulmonary artery, creating the necessary hemodynamic conditions for a "steal phenomenon" to occur in the distribution of the left coronary artery. In fact, this is the most common congenital anomaly causing myocardial infarction in childhood.[54] The right coronary artery can also arise anomalously from the main pulmonary artery. Figure 33-22 illustrates a 5½-year-old with an anomalous origin of a right coronary artery who was entirely asymptomatic. Her abnormality was uncovered by investigations resulting from detection of a heart murmur during her preschool physical examination. Coronary arteries may also arise from either the right or left pulmonary arteries. Daskalopoulos et al. reported a fatal complication due to anomalous origin of the left circumflex coronary artery from the proximal right pulmonary artery in a patient with truncus arteriosus.[11]

Abnormal origin of the coronary artery from a pulmonary artery is to be differentiated from a fistulous connection between a coronary artery and a pulmonary artery.[55,56] Figure 33-23 illustrates a left coronary artery–main pulmonary artery fistula that was the sole source of pulmonary blood supply in a patient with tetralogy of Fallot and pulmonary valve atresia.

Text continues on page 838

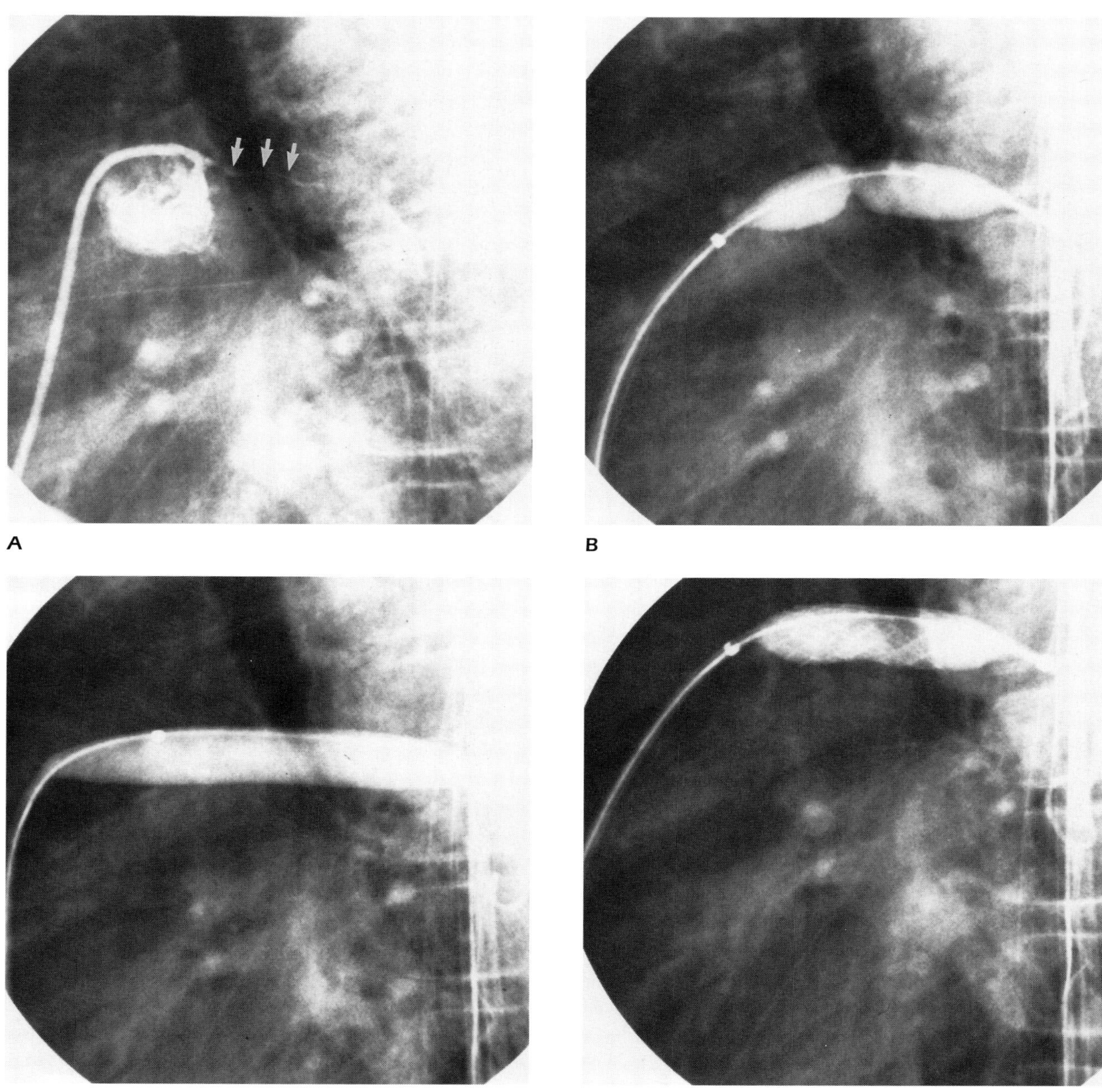

Figure 33-18. Stenosis at the origin of the left pulmonary artery. Percutaneous balloon dilatation and stent placement in a left pulmonary artery. (A) Predilatation pulmonary angiogram in 70-degree left anterior oblique view. Note the extremely hypoplastic left pulmonary artery (*arrows*), which is visualized as a 1-mm "thread" due to the severe stenosis at the origin of the left pulmonary artery. (B) Indentation of the dilating balloon, indicating that the "threadlike" appearance of the proximal left pulmonary artery was due to a discrete stenosis at its origin. (C) Final balloon inflation demonstrating obliteration of the indentation. (D) Placement of stent at the time of balloon expansion of the stent in the proximal left pulmonary artery. (E) Anteroposterior view of the stent in the proximal left pulmonary artery. (F) Lateral view of stent in the proximal left pulmonary artery. (G) Postinterventional pulmonary angiogram in lateral view demonstrating improved flow into the left pulmonary artery.

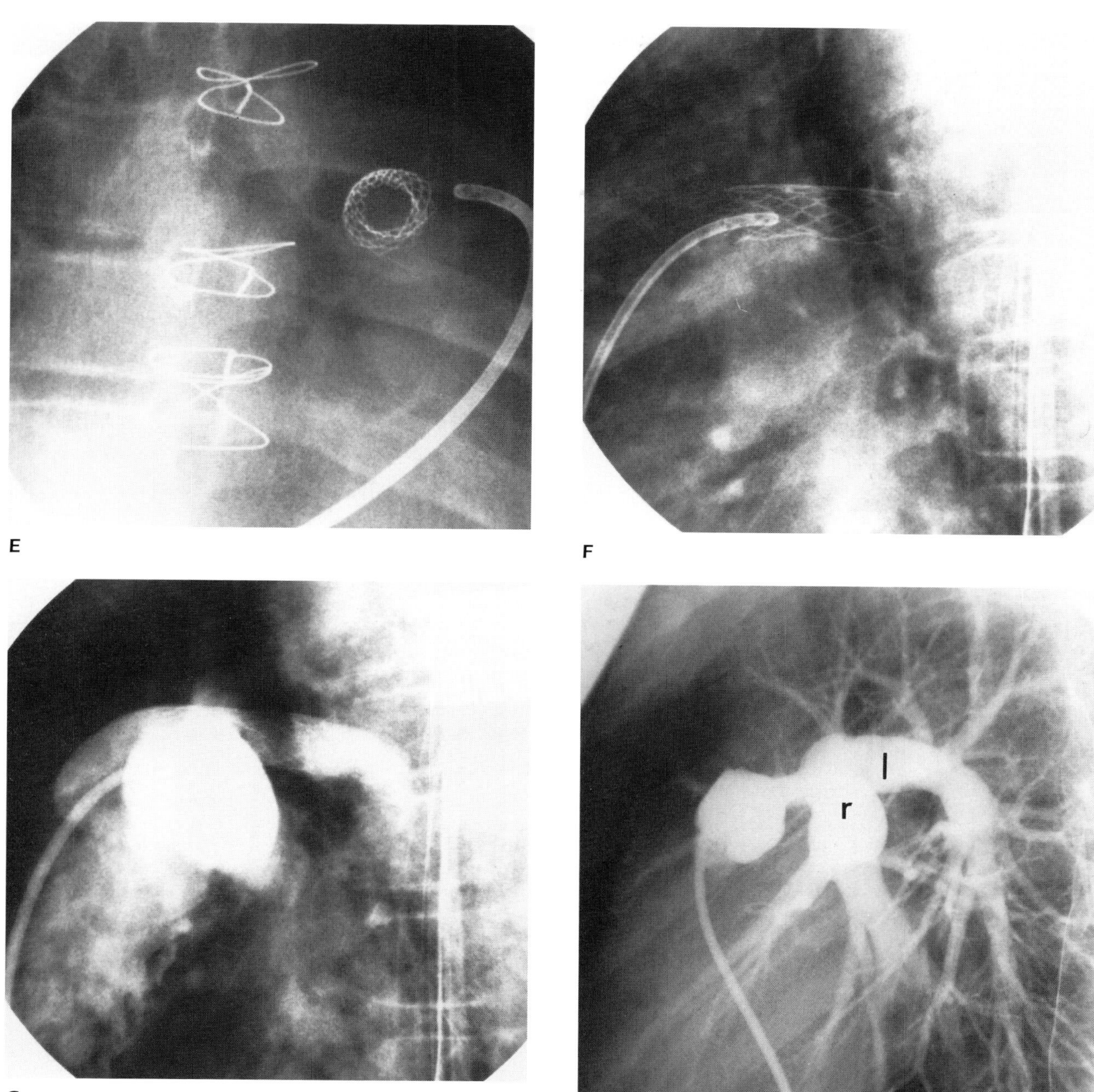

Figure 33-18 (continued).

Figure 33-19. Angiographic view profiling the proximal left pulmonary artery by combining 70 degrees of left anterior oblique angulation with 25 degrees of caudal angulation. The narrowing of the main pulmonary artery is due to previous banding. l, left pulmonary artery; r, right pulmonary artery.

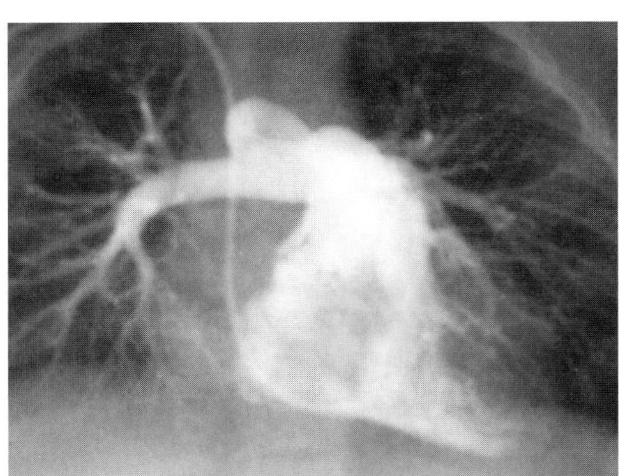

A

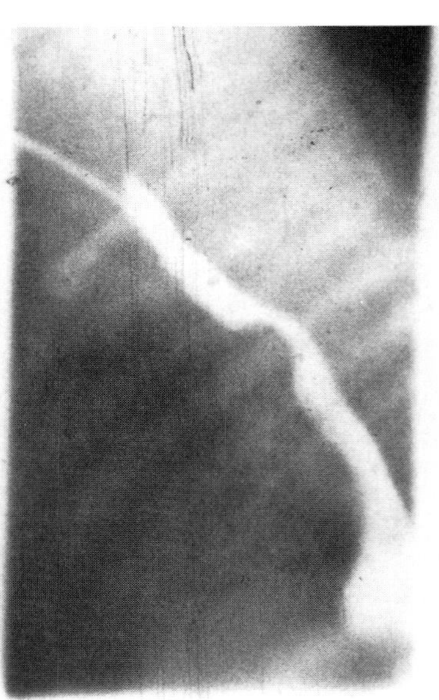

B

Figure 33-20. Pulmonary artery sling. (A) Right ventricular injection demonstrating the pulmonary arteries. The left pulmonary artery initially courses to the right of the trachea before crossing back to enter the left hilum. (B) Lateral view of the esophagogram in this patient. Note the anterior compression on the esophagus due to the left pulmonary artery coursing between the trachea and esophagus. (From Clarkson PM, Ritter DG, Rahimtoola SH, Hallermann FJ, McGoon DC. Aberrant left pulmonary artery. Am J Dis Child 1967;113:373–377. Used with permission.)

Figure 33-21. Anomalous origin of the left pulmonary artery. (A) Right ventricular injection in a patient with tetralogy of Fallot demonstrating a normal origin of the right pulmonary artery and so-called absence of the left pulmonary artery. (B) Later phase of the same right ventriculogram demonstrating origin of the left pulmonary artery from a patent left ductus arteriosus (*arrow*). (From Stewart et al. An atlas of vascular rings and related malformations of the aortic arch system. Springfield, IL: Charles C Thomas, 1968. Used with permission.)

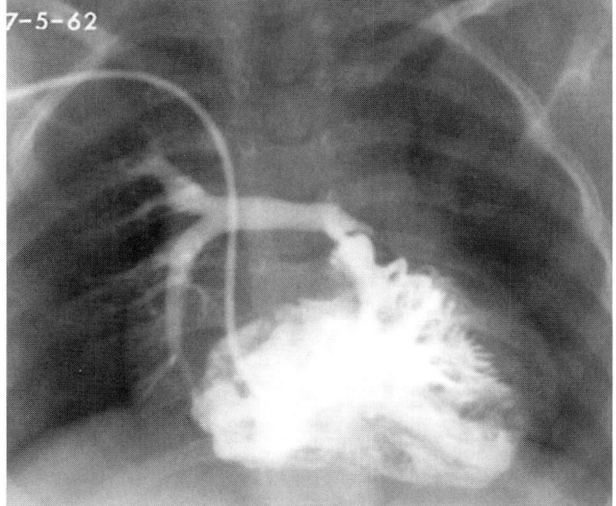

A

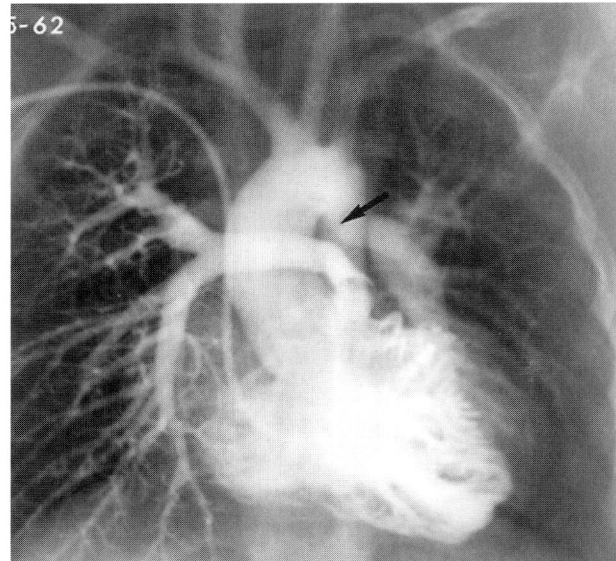

B

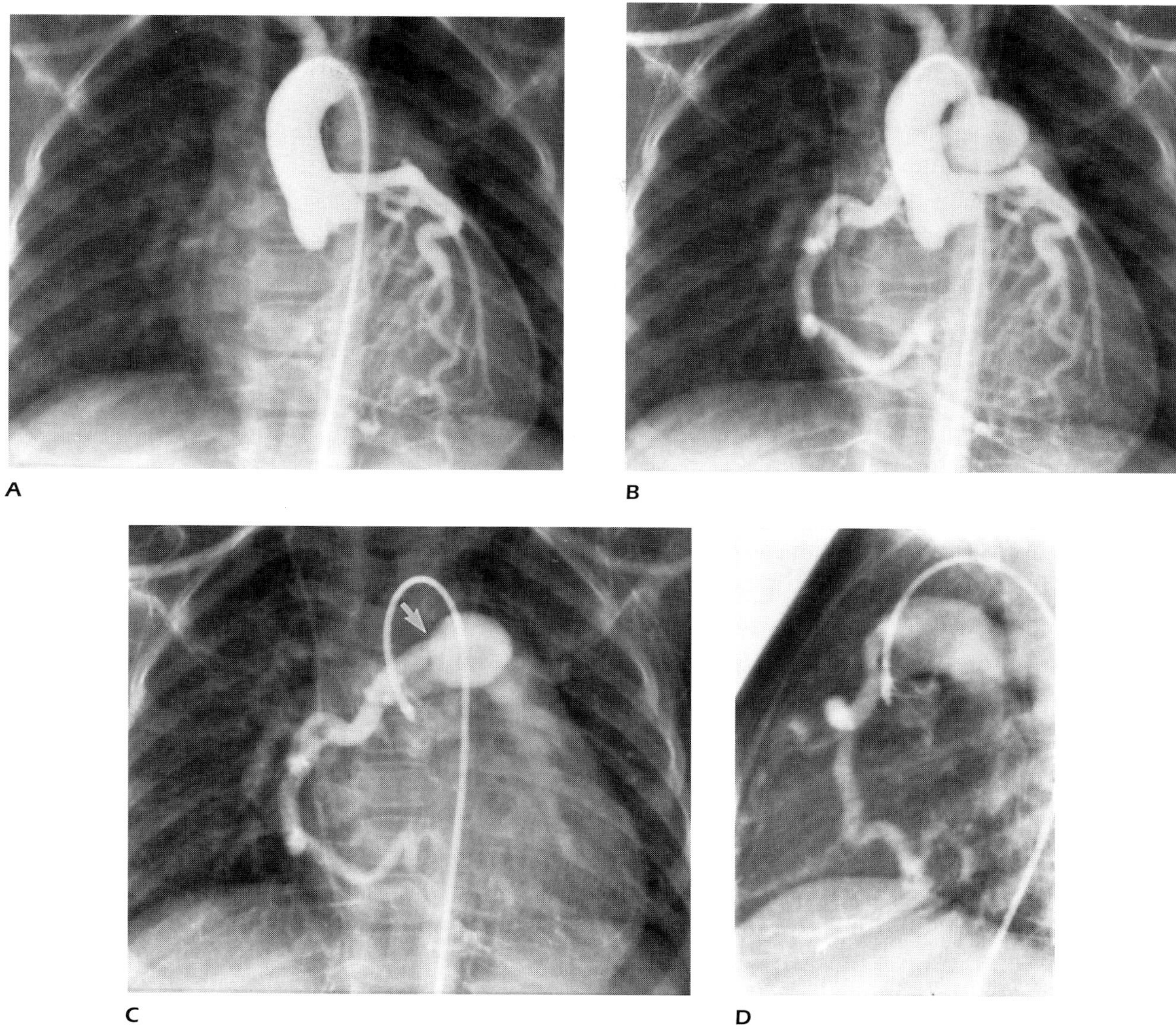

Figure 33-22. Anomalous origin of the right coronary artery from the main pulmonary artery. (A) Early phase of aortogram demonstrating an enlarged left coronary artery system. Note the absence of right coronary artery opacification. (B) Later phase demonstrating opacification of the right coronary artery system from collateral connections with the left coronary artery system. Note opacification of the main pulmonary artery due to the left-to-right shunt via the anomalous right coronary artery. (C) Final phase of angiogram after clearing of the contrast from the aorta and left coronary artery. The site of origin of the right coronary artery from the main pulmonary artery is now clearly identified (*arrow*). (D) Lateral view of the final phase shown in (C) for correlation.

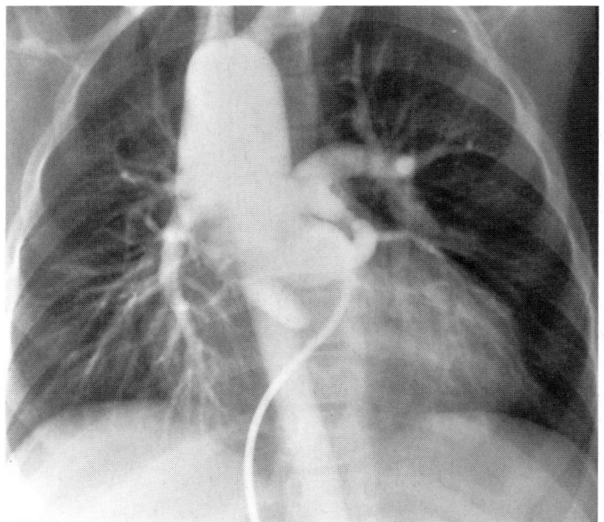

Figure 33-23. Left coronary artery–pulmonary artery fistula. The left coronary artery proximal to the fistulous connection to the main pulmonary artery is dilated because of increased blood flow. Note the right aortic arch with mirror-image branching pattern of the brachiocephalic vessels in this patient with tetralogy of Fallot and pulmonary valve atresia.

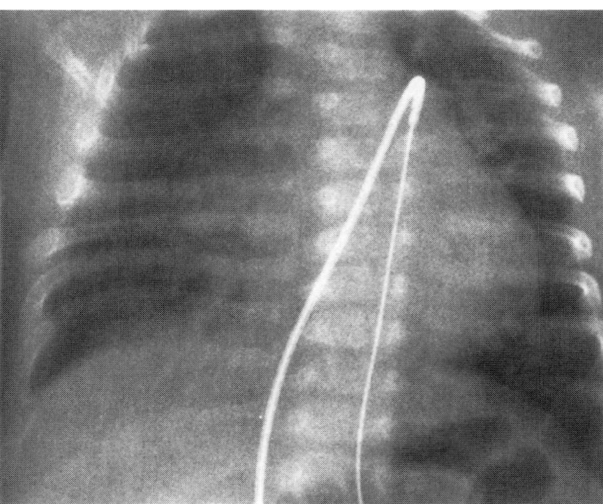

Figure 33-24. Anteroposterior chest radiograph in a patient with patent ductus arteriosus. Note the venous catheter, which has traversed a patent ductus arteriosus. A guidewire has been advanced into the descending aorta.

Patent Ductus Arteriosus

The ductus arteriosus provides the normal connection between the systemic and pulmonary circulation in the fetus. Persistence of a patent ductus arteriosus is a relatively common cause of left-to-right shunting in the newborn. Although it can occur in isolation, a persistently patent ductus arteriosus is frequently associated with other congenital heart defects, such as tetralogy of Fallot and endocardial cushion defect. Echocardiographic assessment of patent ductus arteriosus is possible;[57] however, angiography of this entity remains relevant because of the development of transcatheter techniques for ductal closure. Figure 33-24 demonstrates the radiographic appearance of a catheter that has passed through the ductus arteriosus from the pulmonary artery with a guidewire advanced into the descending aorta. Figure 33-25 illustrates the most common anatomy of a patent ductus arteriosus. Note that it courses in an anterior–superior direction from its aortic end to enter the left pulmonary artery near its origin. Contrast this usual orientation of a patent ductus arteriosus with that illustrated in Figure 33-17, which demonstrates a patient with tetralogy of Fallot and pulmonary valve atresia. In Figure 33-17, the patent ductus arteriosus originates more proximally from the undersurface of the transverse aortic arch and has a vertical orientation. Figure 33-26 illustrates yet another variant of a patent ductus arteriosus. In this instance with a right aortic arch and mirror-image brachiocephalic branching, the patent ductus arteriosus originates near the origin of the left subclavian artery from the left innominate artery.

Calcification in the wall of a patent ductus arteriosus is not uncommon and may cause great difficulty when surgical repair is attempted because of the increased rigidity and/or friability of the tissues. Calcification may occur with or without ductal patency and with or without aneurysmal dilation of a ductus arteriosus. The plain film and CT findings of an aneurysm of a nonpatent ductus arteriosus in a neonate have been described by Slovis et al.[58]

In concluding this discussion of abnormalities involving the central pulmonary arteries, it seems appropriate to revisit the subject of embryologic development. The clinical significance of these developmental errors is underscored by various aortic arch anomalies and their pulmonary artery interrelationships. As thoroughly described by Stewart et al.,[52] there are numerous arch anomalies resulting in vascular rings, depending on the position of the aortic arch and the location of a patent ductus arteriosus or ligamentum arteriosum. For example, virtually all patients with a right aortic arch and an aberrant left subclavian artery have a left-sided ductus arteriosus or ligamentum arteriosum. This left-sided ductus arteriosus or ligamentum arteriosum arises from a posterior remnant of the left aortic arch and results in an anatomic vascular ring (Fig. 33-27).

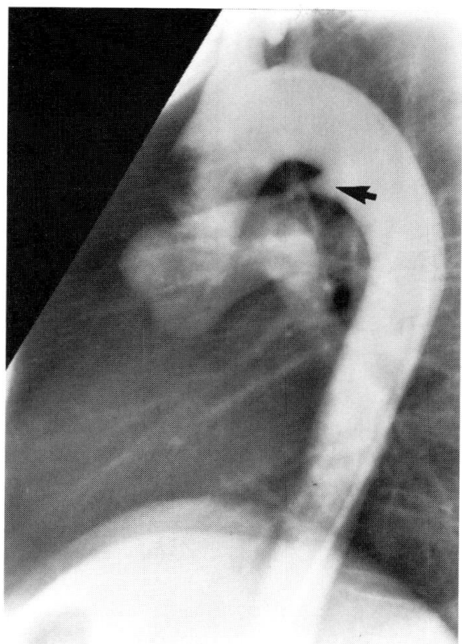

Figure 33-25. Patent ductus arteriosus. Lateral view of a thoracic aortogram demonstrating a patent ductus arteriosus (*arrow*) in a 54-year-old woman.

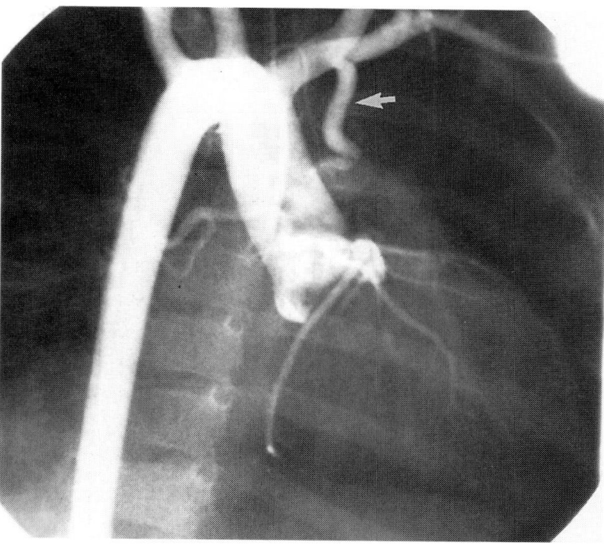

Figure 33-26. Patent ductus arteriosus. Aortogram in patient with tetralogy of Fallot. There is a right aortic arch with mirror-image brachiocephalic branching. A left patent ductus arteriosus (*arrow*) originates as the first branch of the left innominate artery.

Congenital Anomalies of the Peripheral Pulmonary Arteries

The peripheral pulmonary arteries develop in conjunction with the ipsilateral lung bud and therefore have congenital anomalies distinct from those involving the central pulmonary arteries, which derive from the sixth aortic arch (see Figs. 33-1 and 33-2). Although the peripheral pulmonary artery branching pattern normally follows the usual bronchial branching pattern, many minor variations are commonly encountered.[59,60] A detailed description of the segmental and subsegmental pulmonary artery branching patterns, including their radiographic appearance, can be found in an

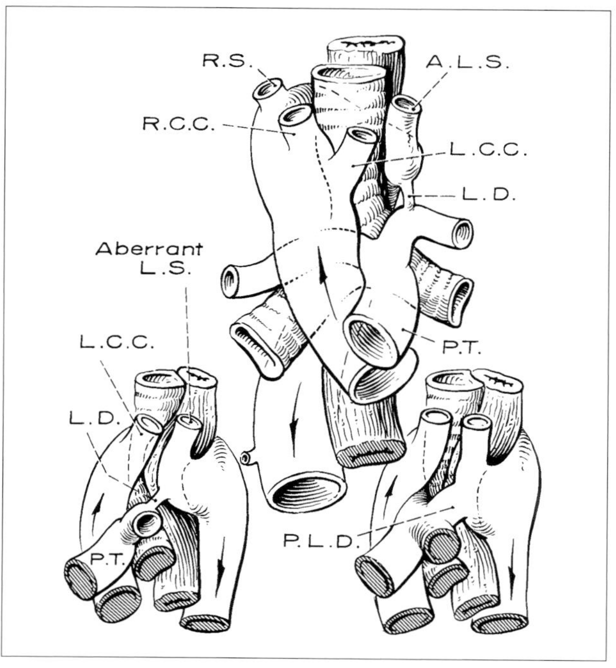

Figure 33-27. Right aortic arch with an aberrant left subclavian artery producing a vascular ring. The main illustration views the malformation from the front. The two smaller drawings, which are left lateral views, illustrate the presence of a nonpatent and a patent left ductus arteriosus. The trachea and esophagus are completely encircled by the pulmonary artery and ascending aorta anteriorly, by the right arch on the right, by the junction of the right arch, left dorsal aortic root, and upper descending aorta posteriorly, and by the left dorsal aortic root and left ductus arteriosus on the left. *R.S.*, right subclavian artery; *A.L.S.*, aberrant left subclavian artery; *R.C.C.*, right common carotid artery; *L.C.C.*, left common carotid artery; *L.D.*, left ductus arteriosus or ligamentum arteriosum; *P.T.*, pulmonary trunk; *P.L.D.*, patent left ductus arteriosus; *aberrant L.S.*, aberrant left subclavian artery.

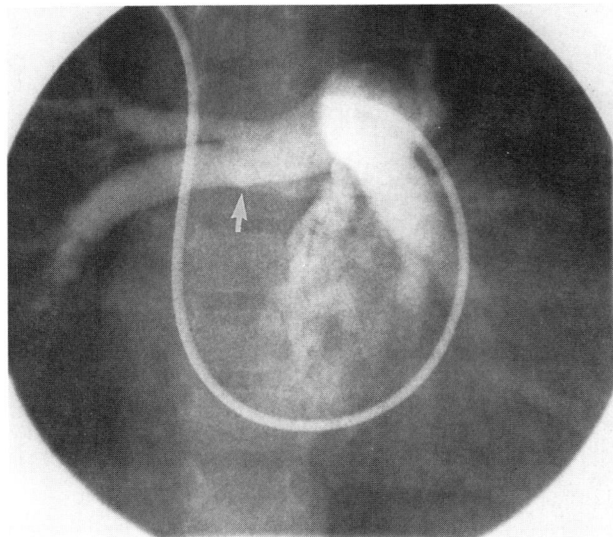

A

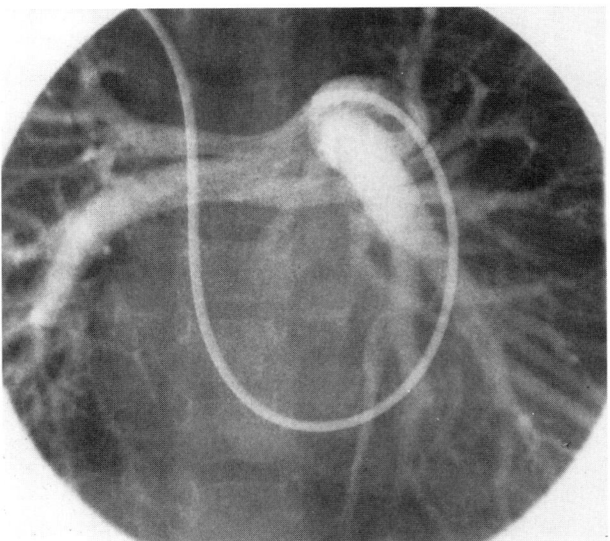

B

Figure 33-28. Anomalous origin of a peripheral pulmonary artery. (A) Early phase of pulmonary angiogram. Note the faint opacification of the anomalously arising segmental left pulmonary artery from the right pulmonary artery (*arrow*). (B) Later phase of pulmonary angiogram. The anomalously arising segmental left pulmonary artery is more densely opacified, and its origin and its branches terminating in the anterior segment of the left upper lobe are more clearly visualized (see text).

excellent text by Yamashita.[61] Lobar or segmental pulmonary arteries originating from the contralateral pulmonary arterial tree are a rare form of peripheral pulmonary artery branching anomaly. Figure 33-28 illustrates an anomalous origin of the pulmonary artery supplying the anterior segment of the left upper lobe from the intermediate branch of the right pulmonary artery. Stewart et al. have postulated an embryologic hypothesis to account for the formation of the previously discussed pulmonary artery sling anomaly and the anomaly depicted in Figure 33-28.[52] Figure 33-29 diagrams this hypothesis.

Peripheral Pulmonary Arteries Supplied by Systemic Arteries

During the early stages of lung bud development, the newly formed peripheral pulmonary arteries receive their blood supply from the intersegmental arteries of the right and left dorsal aorta (see Fig. 33-1B). With normal sixth arch development, the connections between the peripheral pulmonary arteries and the aorta regress, resulting in the normal dichotomous branching pattern beginning with the main pulmonary artery (see Figs. 33-1 and 33-2). However, connections between the peripheral pulmonary arterial tree and systemic arteries can persist; these connecting vessels are presumed to be derivatives of the intersegmental arteries and have been called *systemic-to-pulmonary collateral arteries.*[27] Figure 33-30 illustrates a large systemic-to-pulmonary collateral artery that connects with pulmonary arteries supplying the left lower lobe in a patient with tetralogy of Fallot and pulmonary valve atresia. Figure 33-31 demonstrates another systemic-to-pulmonary collateral artery that, in addition to connecting to the left lower lobe pulmonary artery, also gives origin to an intercostal artery. Figure 33-31 also provides an example of the severe stenosis that is often present at the transition point from the systemic collateral artery to the pulmonary artery. Systemic-to-pulmonary collateral arteries are most commonly found in patients with tetralogy of Fallot with pulmonary valve atresia; however, they can also occur in less severe forms of tetralogy of Fallot as well as in children without any associated congenital heart disease or pulmonary sequestration.

Pulmonary Sequestration

Although the previously described systemic-to-pulmonary collateral arteries are sometimes confused with a pulmonary sequestration, the sine qua non of this latter entity is its tracheobronchial tree abnormality. The term *sequestration* of the lung was introduced by Pryce in 1946 to describe an abnormal area of lung tissue.[62] The abnormal lung tissue was described as being "sequestrated" by virtue of a "bronchial dislocation," that is, an absence of normal airway connections

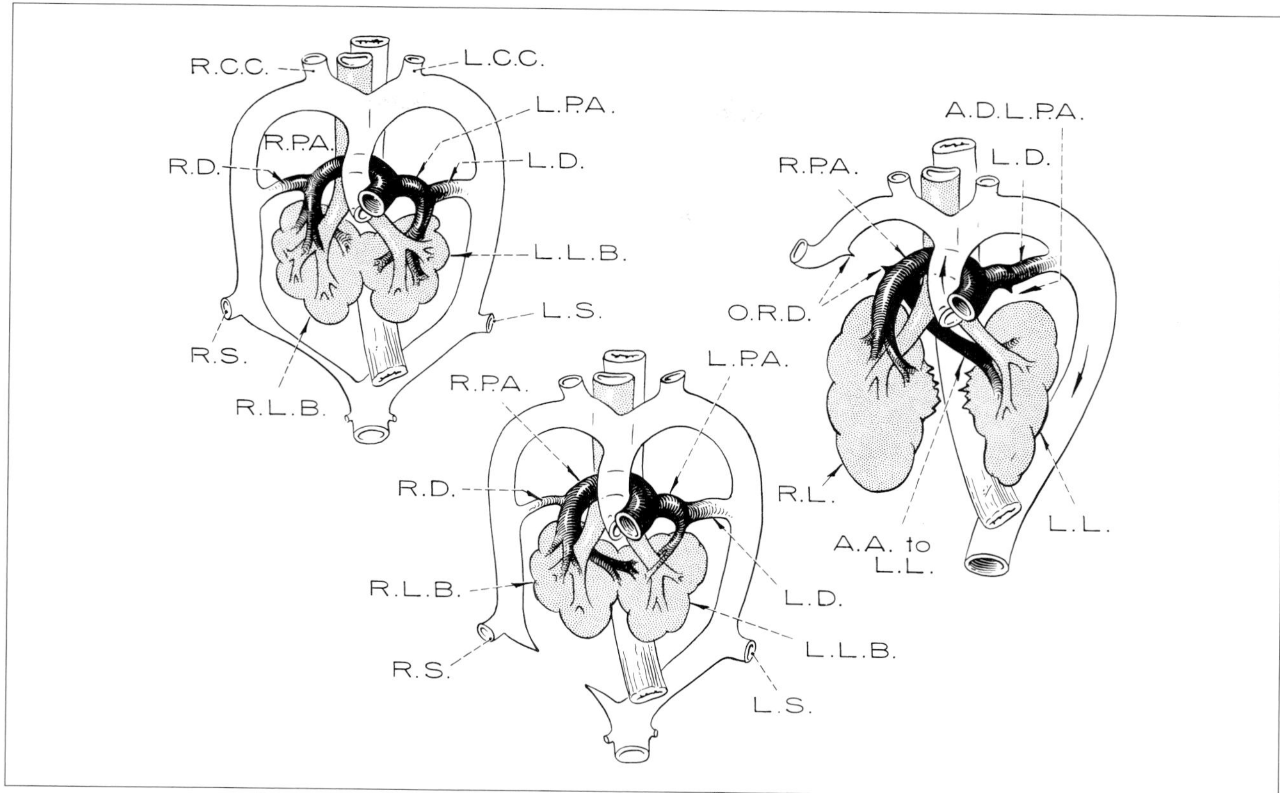

Figure 33-29. (A) Diagram illustrating developing pulmonary arteries and lungs. The primitive lung buds are at first a common mass of developing lung tissue. Normally, both pulmonary arteries are of equal size and supply the respective halves of this tissue. In the development of an anomalous origin of the left pulmonary artery, the events are probably as follows: (B) The left pulmonary artery either fails to develop or regresses distally. Collateral vessels, originating from the right pulmonary artery, are stimulated to develop and vascularize the entire primitive lung tissue, which is undivided at this stage of development. Division of the primitive lung buds and maturation of the hilus stimulate confluence of the collateral vessels and allows one, perhaps the most favorably located artery, to enlarge and assume the function of a left pulmonary artery. (C) As the developing lungs separate completely and enlarge, this vessel compensates by elongating and enlarging. *R.L.B.*, right lung bud; *L.L.B.*, left lung bud; *O.R.D.*, obliterated right ductus arteriosus; *A.D.L.P.A.*, atretic distal part of left pulmonary artery; *L.C.C.*, left common carotid artery; *L.P.A.*, left pulmonary artery; *L.D.*, left ductus arteriosus or ligamentum arteriosum; *L.S.*, left subclavian artery; *R.S.*, right subclavian artery; *R.D.*, right ductus arteriosus or right ligamentum arteriosum; *R.C.C.*, right common carotid artery; *L.L.*, left lung; *A.A.*, ascending aorta; *R.L.*, right lung; *R.P.A.*, right pulmonary artery. (From Stewart et al. An atlas of vascular rings and related malformations of the aortic arch system. Springfield, IL: Charles C Thomas, 1968. Used with permission.)

Figure 33-30. Systemic to pulmonary collateral artery. Descending thoracic aortogram demonstrating a large systemic to pulmonary collateral artery that connects with segmental arteries to the left lower lobe. Note the stenosis at the point of transition between the systemic-to-pulmonary collateral artery and the segmental pulmonary arteries. The peripheral pulmonary arteries supplied by this collateral did not connect with any central pulmonary arteries, making this a so-called noncommunicating systemic-to-pulmonary collateral artery (see Fig. 33-9). There are two smaller systemic-to-pulmonary collateral arteries supplying areas of the right lung.

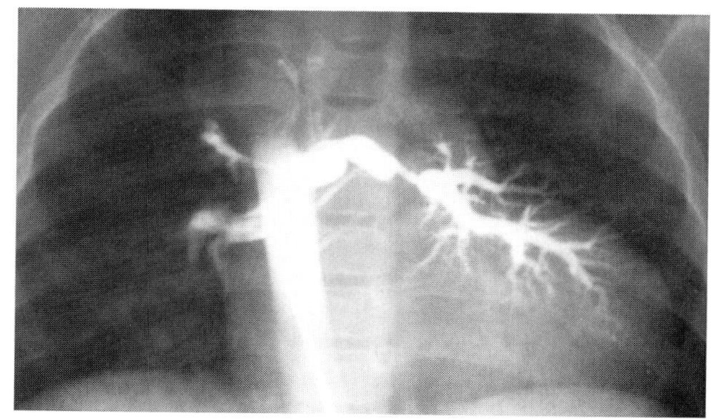

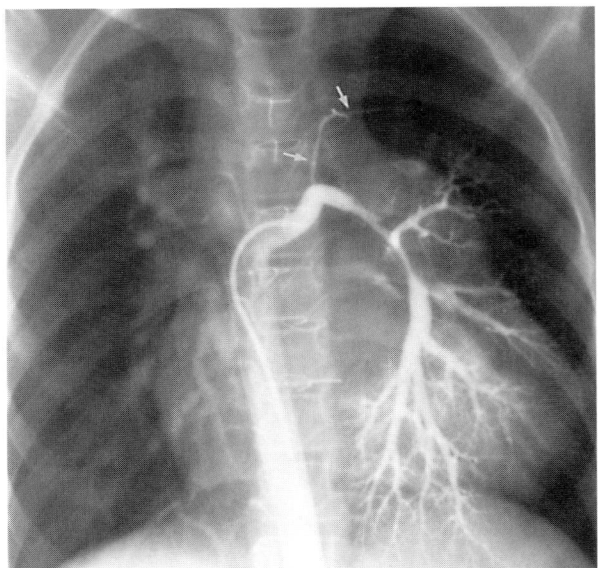

Figure 33-31. Systemic-to-pulmonary collateral artery. Selective injection in a large left-sided systemic-to-pulmonary collateral artery in a patient with tetralogy of Fallot and pulmonary valve atresia with right aortic arch. Note the intercostal artery (*arrows*) arising from the systemic-to-pulmonary collateral artery proximal to its connection to the left pulmonary arteries.

between the abnormal pulmonary tissue and the rest of the tracheobronchial tree. All seven patients described by Pryce also had systemic-to-pulmonary collateral arteries supplying the area of abnormal lung tissue.[62] The importance of making the distinction between a sequestration with an associated systemic-to-pulmonary collateral artery and a systemic-to-collateral artery without an accompanying bronchial abnormality has clinical relevance. The former condition is predisposed to infection and requires surgical excision, whereas the latter is associated with normal lung tissue, and surgery is only indicated if the left-to-right shunt warrants corrective measures. Although angiographic definition of the systemic artery supplying a sequestration has been the traditional method of preoperative evaluation, magnetic resonance imaging (MRI) has also been useful in this regard and may obviate the need for invasive angiography.[63]

Hypoplasia of the Peripheral Pulmonary Arteries

As previously discussed, generalized hypoplasia of the pulmonary arterial tree is commonly associated with certain congenital heart defects, such as tetralogy of Fallot and pulmonary valve atresia with intact ventricular septum. Figure 33-32 illustrates diffuse hypoplasia of the peripheral pulmonary arteries in a patient who

Figure 33-32. Hypoplastic pulmonary arteries, Williams syndrome. (A) A 30-degree right anterior oblique view of a pulmonary angiogram. (B) A 70-degree left anterior oblique view of a pulmonary angiogram. The pulmonary arteries are 30 percent of expected indexed to body surface area (see text).

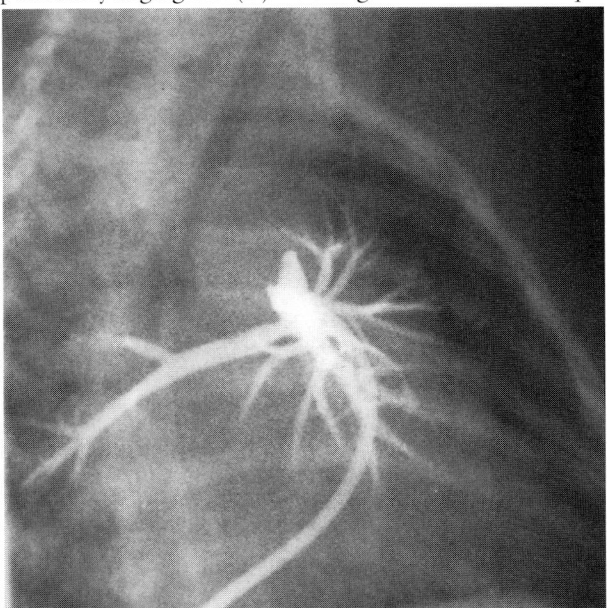

A

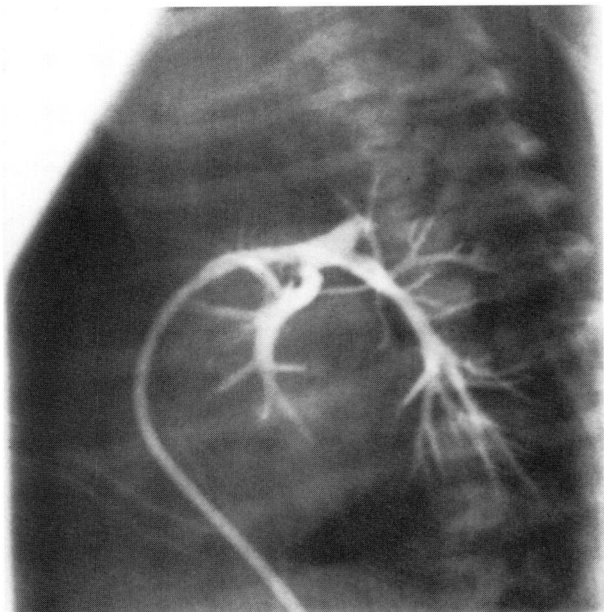

B

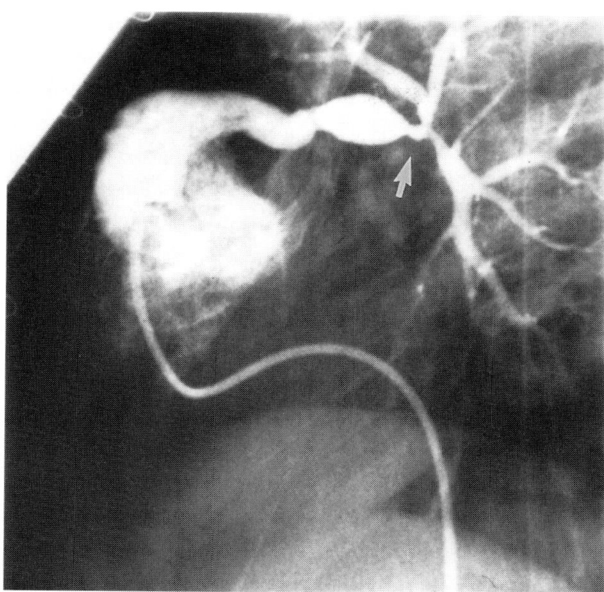

Figure 33-33. Peripheral pulmonary artery stenosis. Lateral view of an injection in the right ventricular outflow tract. Note the severe narrowing of the left pulmonary artery at the hilar level. There is also narrowing of the origins of the branch vessels to the left upper and lower lobes (*arrow*).

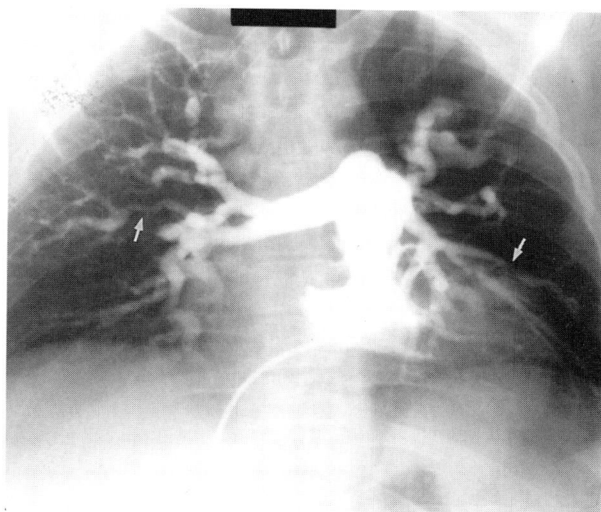

Figure 33-34. Peripheral pulmonary artery stenoses. Right ventricular injection with opacification of the pulmonary arterial tree demonstrating multiple bilateral peripheral pulmonary artery stenoses (*arrows*) (see text for discussion).

also had mild pulmonary valve stenosis. This patient had elfin facies, elevated serum calcium levels, mental retardation, and a normal chromosomal analysis, all characteristic of Williams syndrome. Interestingly, this patient did not have supravalvular aortic stenosis. In this patient with Williams syndrome, the lungs were not hypoplastic; however, the pulmonary artery size was 30 percent of that expected when indexed to her body surface area.[34]

Congenitally hypoplastic peripheral pulmonary arteries accompanying an underdeveloped lung due to defective organogenesis or intrauterine pulmonary infections represent another spectrum of disease that may be considered secondary in nature. Although peripheral pulmonary artery hypoplasia in these instances is secondary to underlying pulmonary problems, these anomalies are still considered congenital because of their presence at the time of birth. This is in contrast to small pulmonary arterial trees caused by acquired pulmonary processes such as postinfectious bronchiolitis obliterans (Swyer-James or Macleod syndrome).[64,65]

Peripheral Pulmonary Artery Stenoses

Discrete areas of narrowing involving the peripheral pulmonary arteries may occur as isolated congenital anomalies but are more commonly associated with other cardiovascular lesions, most frequently with tetralogy of Fallot (Fig. 33-33).[66] Other etiologies for stenoses of the peripheral pulmonary arteries include those previously mentioned as causing stenotic lesions involving the central pulmonary arteries. Figure 33-34 illustrates the angiographic findings in a patient with multiple peripheral congenital pulmonary artery stenoses. At age 17, he had been diagnosed as having idiopathic primary pulmonary artery hypertension. However, at age 42, his disease had not progressed in the typical fashion for primary pulmonary hypertension. This led to further evaluation, including the angiogram shown in Figure 33-34, which established the diagnosis of multiple peripheral congenital pulmonary artery stenoses. One should also be aware that chronic pulmonary emboli may go undetected and present with similar angiographic findings (Fig. 33-35).

Peripheral Pulmonary Artery Aneurysms

Localized dilatation or ectasia of a peripheral pulmonary artery due to a congenitally weakened or defective vessel wall is less common than that of a pulmonary vein. On angiography these aneurysms are indistinguishable from the much more common mycotic aneurysms, which are usually multiple.[67,68] Figure 33-36 illustrates a right pulmonary artery aneurysm in a patient with tetralogy of Fallot and pulmonary valve atresia.

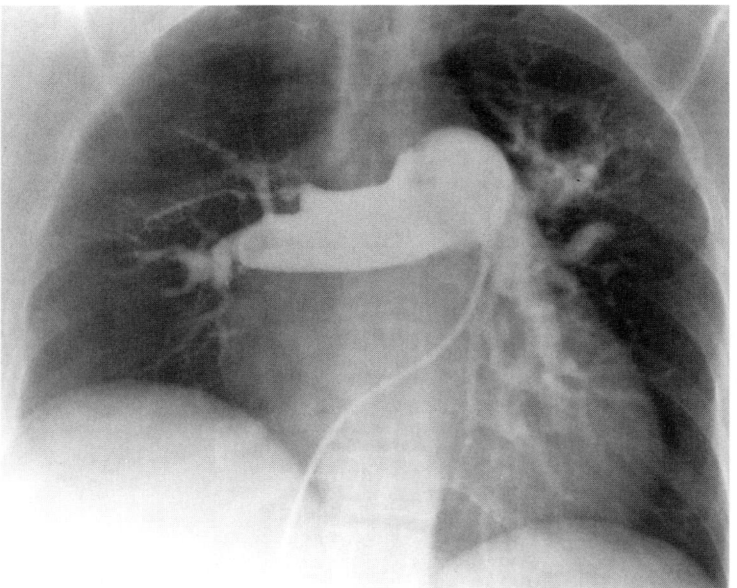

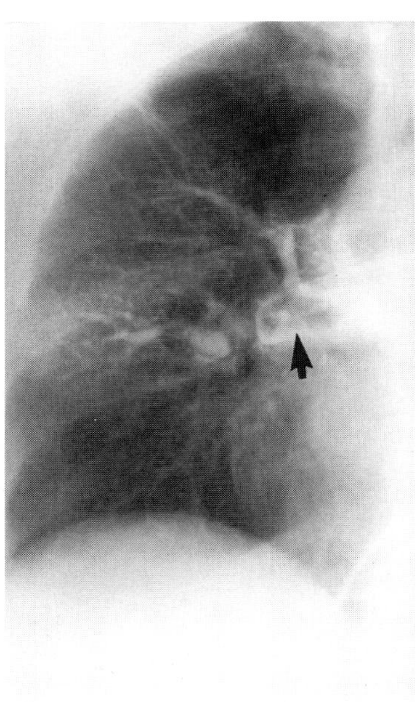

A B

Figure 33-35. Pulmonary artery emboli. (A) Pulmonary angiogram demonstrating bilateral peripheral pulmonary artery stenoses, particularly severe on the right, with lack of opacification of several segmental right pulmonary arteries. (B) Late phase of same angiogram demonstrating large embolus (*arrow*) in the right pulmonary artery.

Pulmonary Arteriovenous Malformations

A much more common cause of localized dilatation involving the peripheral pulmonary arteries occurs with pulmonary arteriovenous (AV) malformations. Most arteriovenous malformations, or fistulas, are congenital, and 60 to 90 percent are found in patients with hereditary hemorrhagic telangiectasia (HHT), also called Osler-Weber-Rendu syndrome.[69,70] HHT is an inherited disease that is autosomal dominant with variable penetrance due to an abnormality in chromosome 9.[71] Approximately one-third to one-half of patients with pulmonary AV fistulas have multiple pulmonary AV malformations, especially those with HHT. The angioarchitecture of these vascular malformations is particularly relevant because transcatheter embolization may be considered the treatment of choice. Although three-dimensional computed tomography has been suggested for pretherapy evaluation, accurate angiographic assessment of these lesions continues to be essential before transcatheter embolization.[72–74] The angiographic findings in a patient with a solitary pulmonary AV fistula are presented in Figure 33-37.

An interesting form of acquired pulmonary AV fistula occurs in patients with congenital heart disease who have undergone a superior vena caval–right pulmonary artery anastomosis (Glenn shunt).[75] The angiographic appearance of these fistulas is shown in Figure 33-38. The multiple pulmonary AV fistulas demonstrated in Figure 33-38 produced a large right-to-left shunt, resulting in clinically significant cyanosis. This patient was treated by transcatheter embolization with excellent results.

Conclusion

Although noninvasive imaging techniques, such as ultrasonography, computed tomography, and magnetic resonance imaging, continue to evolve, pulmonary angiography is the imaging modality most capable of defining pulmonary artery congenital anomalies. As an invasive procedure, pulmonary angiography has attendant risks due to catheter placement, use of radiographic contrast material, and ionizing radiation. However, it is still considered a relatively safe procedure because only 2 percent of patients at highest risk from this procedure—those with elevated pulmonary artery pressures—have major complications related to the use of radiographic contrast media.[76] Hence, angiography of the pulmonary arteries remains the diagnostic technique of choice for most patients with congenital anomalies of the pulmonary arteries.

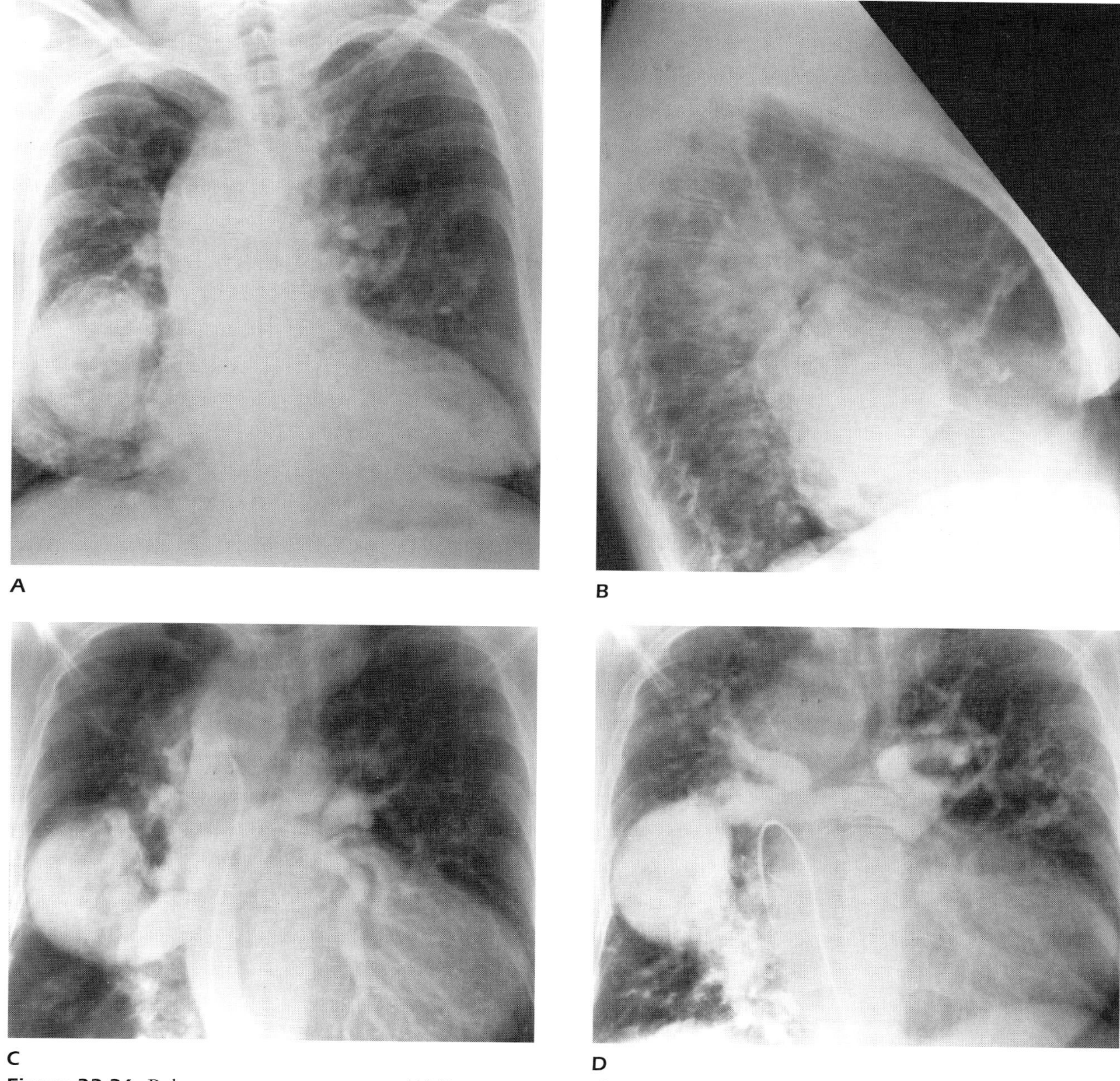

Figure 33-36. Pulmonary artery aneurysm. (A) Posteroanterior chest radiograph in a patient with tetralogy of Fallot with pulmonary valve atresia and a right aortic arch. Note the large mass density in the right lung. (B) Lateral chest radiograph for correlation. (C) Aortogram demonstrating multiple systemic-to-pulmonary collateral arteries and opacification of the large right pulmonary artery aneurysm. (D) Late phase of a selective injection in the systemic-to-pulmonary collateral artery supplying the right pulmonary artery aneurysm. Note that the central pulmonary arteries also connect to the large right pulmonary artery aneurysm.

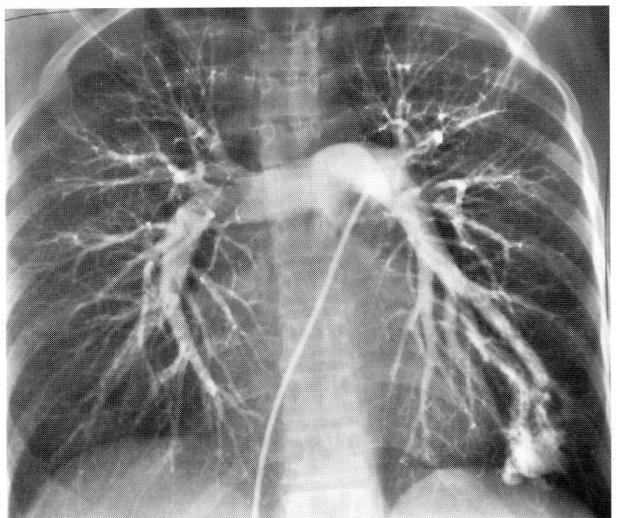

A

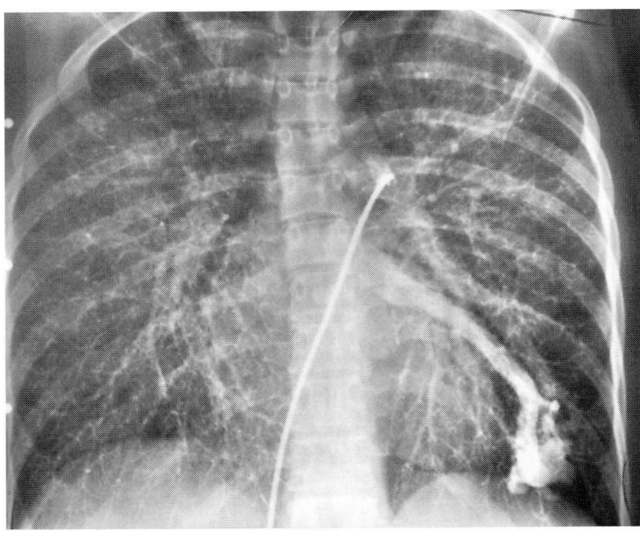

B

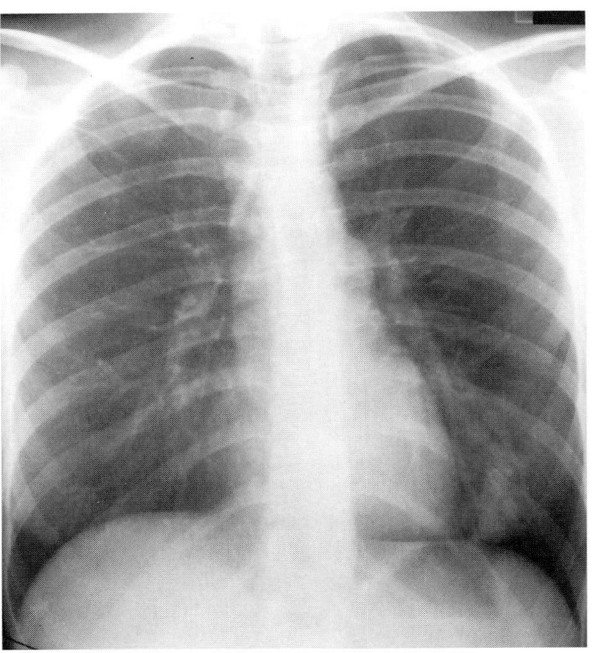

C

Figure 33-37. Pulmonary arteriovenous (AV) fistula. (A) Pulmonary artery angiogram in a patient with a pulmonary AV fistula in the anterior segment of the left lower lobe. (B) Later phase demonstrating the pulmonary vein that drains the AV malformation. (C) Posteroanterior chest radiograph for correlation. Note the masslike density in the left lower lobe.

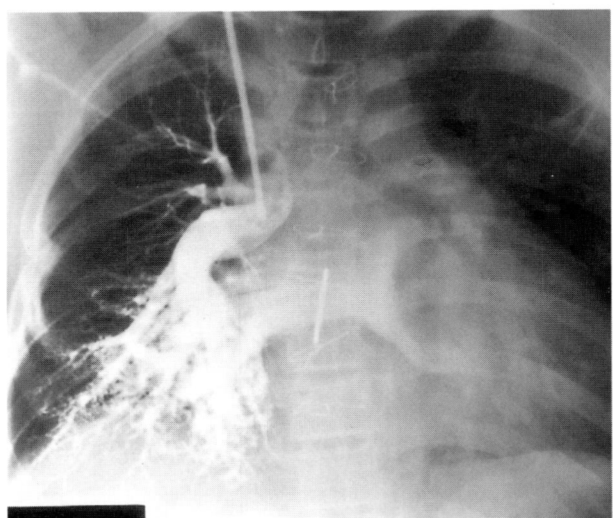

Figure 33-38. Multiple pulmonary AV fistulas secondary to Glenn anastomosis. Right pulmonary angiogram via a transvenous catheter that enters the right pulmonary artery through the superior vena cava via a Glenn shunt (see text). Note the numerous dilated peripheral arteries and veins in the right lower lobe secondary to formation of multiple AV fistulas in the right lower lobe. There is early appearance of contrast media in the left atrium due to the right-to-left shunting through the numerous fistulas.

References

1. Huntington GS. The morphology of the pulmonary artery in the mammalia. Anat Rec 1919;17:165–201.
2. Skidmore FD. The development of the pulmonary circulation. In: Gore DA, Lillihei CW, eds. Congenital malformations of the heart. New York: Grune & Stratton, 1975:89–102.
3. Effmann EL. Development of the right and left pulmonary arteries: a microangiographic study in the mouse. Invest Radiol 1982;17:529–538.
4. de Ruiter MC, Gittenberger-de Groot AC, Rammos S, Poelmann RE. The special status of the pulmonary arch artery in the bronchial arch system of the rat. Anat Embryol 1989;179: 319–325.
5. Collett RW, Edwards JE. Persistent truncus arteriosus: a classification according to anatomic types. S Clin North Am 1949; 29:1245.
6. Van Praagh R, Van Praagh S. The anatomy of common aorticopulmonary trunk (truncus arteriosus communis) and its embryologic implications. Am J Cardiol 1965;16:406–425.
7. Yoshizato T, Julsrud PR. Truncus arteriosus revisited: an angiographic demonstration. Pediatr Cardiol 1990;11:36–40.
8. Ceballos R, Soto B, Kirklin JW, Bargeron LM. Truncus arteriosus: an anatomical-angiographic study. Br Heart J 1983;49: 589–599.
9. Schumacher G, Schreiber R, Lorenz HP, Sebening W, Meisner H, Sebening F, Bühlmeyer K. The angiographic differentiation of the forms of truncus arteriosus communis and its significance for the prognosis. Electromedia 1986;54(2):50–59.
10. Anderson KR, McGoon DC, Lie JT. Surgical significance of the coronary arterial anatomy in truncus arteriosus communis. Am J Cardiol 1978;41:76–81.
11. Daskalopoulos DA, Edwards WD, Driscoll DJ, Schaff HV, Danielson GK. Fatal pulmonary artery banding in truncus arteriosus with anomalous origin of circumflex coronary artery from right pulmonary artery. Am J Cardiol 1983;52:1363–1364.
12. Satyanarayana RBN, Anderson RC, Edwards JE. Anatomic variations in the tetralogy of Fallot. Am Heart J 1971;81:361–371.
13. Anderson RH, Allwork SP, Ho SY, Lenox CC, Zuberbuhler JR. Surgical anatomy of tetralogy of Fallot. J Thorac Cardiovasc Surg 1981;81:887–896.
14. Altrichter PM, Olson LJ, Edwards WD, Puga FJ, Danielson GK. Surgical pathology of the pulmonary valve: a study of 116 cases spanning 15 years. Mayo Clin Proc 1989;64:1352–1360.
15. Rodriguez-Fernandez HL, Char F, Kelly DT, Rowe RD. The dysplastic valve and Noonan's syndrome. Circulation 1972; 46(Suppl II):98.
16. Semb BKH, Tjönneland S, Stake G, Aabyholm G. "Balloon valvulotomy" of congenital pulmonary valve stenosis with tricuspid valve insufficiency. Cardiovasc Radiol 1979;2:239–241.
17. Velasquez G, et al. Nonsurgical aortoplasty in Leriche syndrome. Radiology 1980;134:359–360.
18. Kan JS, White RI, Mitchell SE, Gardner TJ. Percutaneous balloon valvuloplasty: a new method for treating congenital pulmonary-valve stenosis. N Engl J Med 1982;307(9):540–542.
19. Lababidi Z, Wu J. Percutaneous balloon pulmonary valvuloplasty. Am J Cardiol 1983;52:560–562.
20. Tynan M, Baker EJ, Bohmer J, Jones O, Reidy JF, Joseph MC, Ottenkamp J. Percutaneous balloon pulmonary valvuloplasty. Br Heart J 1985;53:520–524.
21. Kveselis DA, Rocchini AP, Snider AP, Rosenthal A, Crowley DC, Dick M. Results of balloon valvuloplasty in the treatment of congenital valvar pulmonary stenosis in children. Am J Cardiol 1985;56:527–532.
22. Masura J, Burch M, Deanfield JE, Sullivan ID. Five-year follow-up after balloon pulmonary valvuloplasty. J Am Coll Cardiol 1993;21(1):132–136.
23. Burrows PE, Benson LN, Moes F, Freedom RM. Pulmonary artery tears following balloon valvotomy for pulmonary stenosis. Cardiovasc Intervent Radiol 1989;12:38–42.
24. Freedom RM, Dische MR, Rowe RD. The tricuspid valve in pulmonary atresia and intact ventricular septum: a morphological study of 60 cases. Arch Pathol Lab Med 1978;102:28.
25. Aboliras ET, et al. Definitive operation for pulmonary atresia with intact ventricular septum: results in 20 patients. J Thorac Cardiovasc Surg 1987;93(Suppl IV):454–464.
26. Burrows PE, Freedom RM, Benson LN, Moes CAF, Wilson G, Koike K, Williams WG. Coronary angiography of pulmonary atresia, hypoplastic right ventricle, and ventriculocoronary communications. AJR 1990;154:789–795.
27. Liao PK, Edwards WD, Julsrud PR, Puga FJ, Danielson GK, Feldt RH. Pulmonary blood supply in patients with pulmonary atresia and ventricular septal defect. J Am Coll Cardiol 1985; 6:1343–1350.
28. Jefferson K, Rees S, Somerville J. Systemic arterial supply to the lungs in pulmonary atresia and its relation to pulmonary artery development. Br Heart J 1972;34:418–427.
29. McGoon MD, Fulton RE, Davis GD, Ritter DG, Neill CA, White RI Jr. Systemic collateral and pulmonary artery stenosis in patients with congenital pulmonary valve atresia and ventricular septal defect. Circulation 1977;56:473–479.
30. Haworth SG. Collateral arteries in pulmonary atresia with ventricular septal defect: a precarious blood supply. Br Heart J 1980;44:5–13.
31. Emmanouilides GC, Thanopoulos B, Siassi B, Fishbein M. "Agenesis" of the ductus arteriosus associated with the syndrome of tetralogy of Fallot and absent pulmonary valve. Am J Cardiol 1976;37:403.
32. Rabinovitch M, et al. Compression of intra-pulmonary bronchi by abnormally branching pulmonary arteries associated with absent pulmonary valves. Am J Cardiol 1982;50:804.
33. Neufeld HN, Lester RG, Adams P Jr, Anderson RC, Lillehei CW, Edwards JE. Aorticopulmonary septal defect. Am J Cardiol 1982;9:12–25.
34. Sievers HH, Onnasch GGW, Lange P, Bernhard A, Heintzen PH. Dimensions of the great arteries, semilunar valve root and right ventricular outflow tract during growth: normative angiographic data. Pediatr Cardiol 1983;4:189–196.
35. Nihill MR, Mullins CE, McNamara DG. Visualization of the pulmonary arteries in pseudotruncus by pulmonary vein wedge angiography. Circulation 1978;58:140.
36. Freedom RM, Pongiglione G, Williams WG, Trusler GA, Moes CAF, Rowe RD. Pulmonary vein wedge angiography: indications, results, and surgical correlates in 25 patients. Am J Cardiol 1983;51:936.
37. Gay BB, Franch RH, Shuford WH, Rogers JV. The roentgenologic features of single and multiple coarctations of the pulmonary artery and branches. AJR 1963;90(3):599–613.
38. Williams JCP, Barratt-Boyes BG, Lowe JB. Supravalvular aortic stenosis. Circulation 1961;24:1311.
39. Black JA, Bonham CRE. Association between aortic stenosis and facies of severe infantile hypercalcaemia. Lancet 1963;2: 745–749.
40. Arvidsson H, Carlsson E, Hartmann A, Tsifutis A, Crawford C. Supravalvular stenoses of the pulmonary arteries: report of eleven cases. Acta Radiol 1961;56:466.
41. Emmanouilides GC, Linde LM, Crittenden IH. Pulmonary artery stenosis associated with ductus arteriosus following maternal rubella. Circulation 1964;29:514.
42. Noonan JA. Hypertension with Turner phenotype: a new syndrome with associated congenital heart disease. Am J Dis Child 1968;116:373.
43. Keith JD, Rowe RD, Vlad P. Heart disease in infancy and childhood. 3rd ed. New York: Macmillan, 1978.
44. Alagille D, Odievre M, Gautier M, Dommergues JP. Hepatic ductular hypoplasia associated with characteristic facies, vertebral malformations, retarded physical, mental and sexual development, and cardiac murmur. J Pediatr 1975;86:63.
45. Hayden JG, Taler NS, Klaus SM. Cutis laxa associated with pulmonary artery stenosis. J Pediatr 1968;72:506.

46. Jue KL, Noren GR, Anderson RC. The syndrome of idiopathic hypercalcemia in infancy with associated heart disease. J Pediatr 1965;47:1130.
47. Elzenga NJ. The ductus arteriosus and stenoses of the adjacent great arteries. Grafisch verzorging, Alblasserdam, Netherlands: Davids Decor, 1986.
48. Freedom RM, Olley PM. Pulmonary arteriography in congenital heart disease. Cathet Cardiovasc Diagn 1976;2:309.
49. Fellows KE, Keane JF, Freed MD. Angled views in cineangiocardiography of congenital heart disease. Circulation 1977; 56(3):485–490.
50. Bargeron LM, Elliott LP, Soto Benigno, Bream PR, Curry GC. Axial cineangiography in congenital heart disease. Circulation 1977;56(6):1075–1092.
51. Wittenborg MH, Tantiwongse T, Rosenberg BF. Anomalous course of left pulmonary artery with respiratory obstruction. Radiology 1956;67:339–345.
52. Stewart JR, Kincaid OW, Edwards JE. An atlas of vascular rings and related malformations of the aortic arch system. Springfield, IL: Charles C Thomas, 1963.
53. Goor DA, Lillehei CW. Congenital malformations of the heart. New York: Grune & Stratton, 1975:352.
54. Garson A. Electrocardiography. In: Anderson RH, Macartney FJ, Shinebourne EA, Tynan M, eds. Paediatric cardiology. London: Churchill Livingstone, 1987:296.
55. Silverman JF, Obrez I, Kriss JP. Coronary artery fistula: diagnosis and evaluation by selective contrast and radioisotopic coronary arteriography. J Can Assoc Radiol 1974;25:310.
56. Steinberg I, Baldwin JS, Dotter CT. Coronary arteriovenous fistula. Circulation 1958;17:372.
57. Smallhorn JF, Hunta JC, Anderson RH, Macartney FJ. Suprasternal cross-sectional echocardiography in assessment of patent ductus arteriosus. Br Heart J 1982;48:321.
58. Slovis TL, Meza MP, Rector FE, Chang CH. Aneurysm of a nonpatent ductus arteriosus in a neonate: CT findings. AJR 1993;160:141–142.
59. Jackson CL, Huber JF. Correlated applied anatomy of the bronchial tree and lungs with a system of nomenclature. Dis Chest 1943;9:319.
60. Boyden EA. Segmental anatomy of the lungs, a study of the patterns of the segmental bronchi and related pulmonary vessels. New York: McGraw-Hill, 1955.
61. Yamashita H. Roentgenologic anatomy of the lung. Tokyo: Igaku-Shoin, 1978.
62. Pryce DM. Lower accessory pulmonary artery with intralobar sequestration of lung: a report of seven cases. J Pathol 1946; 58:457–467.
63. Doyle AJ. Demonstration of blood supply to pulmonary sequestration by MR angiography. AJR 1992;158:989–990.
64. Swyer PR, James GCW. A case of unilateral pulmonary emphysema. Thorax 1953;8:133–136.
65. Macleod EM. Abnormal transradiancy of one lung. Thorax 1954;9:147–153.
66. Gay BA Jr, Franch RH, Shuford WH, Rogers JV. The roentgenologic features of single and multiple coarctations of the pulmonary artery and branches. AJR 1963;90(3):599–613.
67. Deterling RA, Clagett OT. Aneurysm of the pulmonary artery: review of the literature and report of a case. Am Heart J 1947; 34:471–499.
68. Ungaro R, Saab S, Almond C, Kumar S. Solitary peripheral pulmonary artery aneurysms: pathogenesis and surgical treatment. J Thorac Cardiovasc Surg 1976;71:566–571.
69. Dines DE, Arms RA, Bernatz PE, Gomes MR. Pulmonary arteriovenous fistulas. Mayo Clin Proc 1974;49:460–465.
70. White RI Jr, Lunch-Nyhan A, Terry P, et al. Pulmonary arteriovenous malformations, techniques, and long-term outcome of embolo-therapy. Radiology 1988;169:663–669.
71. McDonald MT, Papenberg KA, Ghosh S, et al. A disease locus for hereditary haemorrhagic telangiectasia maps to chromosome. Nature Genet 1994;6:197–204.
72. Remy J, Remy-Jardin M, Giraud F, Wattinne L. Angioarchitecture of pulmonary arteriovenous malformations: clinical utility of three-dimensional helical CT. Radiology 1994;191:657–665.
73. White RI Jr, Mitchell SE, Barth KH, et al. Angioarchitecture of pulmonary arteriovenous malformations: an important consideration before therapy. AJR 1983;140:681–686.
74. Casteneda-Zuniga W, Epstein M, Zollikofer C, et al. Embolization of multiple pulmonary artery fistulas. Radiology 1980;134: 309–310.
75. McFaul RC, Tajik AJ, Mair DD, Danielson GK, Seward JB. Development of pulmonary arteriovenous shunt after superior vena cava–right pulmonary artery (Glenn) anastomosis: report of four cases. Circulation 1977;55:212.
76. Perlmutt LM, Braun SD, Newman GE, Oke EJ, Dunnick NR. Pulmonary arteriography in the high-risk patient. Radiology 1987;162:187–189.

34

The Physiologic and Microstructural Basis for Radiologic Findings in the Normal and Disturbed Pulmonary Circulation

MORRIS SIMON

The pulmonary blood circulation is a striking example of the exquisite relationship between function and structure in a biologic system. A great variety of normal and pathologic hemodynamic states exist, and these are associated with structural changes that can often be recognized by the radiologist. The changes reflect both the type and the severity of the hemodynamic variations.[1–3] It is thus important for the radiologist to understand the physiologic and microstructural basis of the gross vascular changes that may be observed on plain films, traditional pulmonary angiograms, computed tomographic (CT) images, or magnetic resonance images (MRI). This will not only help to explain the nature of the altered vascular morphology but will also enable the radiologist to better detect, diagnose, and assess the severity of many cardiopulmonary disturbances.

Background

Modern concepts of pulmonary blood flow derive from the reports of many animal experiments and human studies scattered through the anatomic, physiologic, clinical, and radiologic literature.[4–45] These reports provide a wealth of factual information, propose a number of useful hypotheses, and formulate some important biologic principles. However, in this brief presentation, which aims to provide the radiologist with a clear, practical, and unified overview of the pulmonary circulation, it has been necessary to isolate those concepts that may affect the radiologic image and to consider only the most reasonable and compatible of many alternative hypotheses. In addition, physiologic data have been reduced to mean values or orders of magnitude, and experimental details are omitted to focus on the essence of a concept, even at the risk of oversimplification.

Early experimental studies of the pulmonary circulation, beginning with the pioneering studies of Poiseuille in 1855,[5,6] were concerned with the effects of ventilation on vascular resistance. It was soon established that lung inflation increased total pulmonary vascular resistance.[7,22,27,28,46] This observation seemed to conflict with later radiologic observations that during inspiration the lung arteries and veins were actually dilated and pulmonary blood volume was increased, as if augmenting the pumping action of the right ventricle.[9,10,30] This paradox was resolved by Macklin and others, who first drew attention to the fundamental differences in behavior between the invisible microcirculation and the macrocirculation visible to the radiologist.[13,15,28–30] This distinction is important in radiologic-physiologic correlation. It is embodied in the compartmental theory, which separates the pulmonary vessels into an alveolar compartment, subject to lung stretch and alveolar pressure, and an extraalveolar compartment, which is responsive to variations in negative interstitial pressure (Fig. 34-1). At full inspiration the radiologically invisible alveolar vessels are constricted and cause increased resistance, whereas the extraalveolar vessels, including those normally seen on the radiograph, become distended.

Before the advent of radiologic methods of studying the pulmonary vessels it was assumed that pulmonary blood flow was uniform in all regions of the lungs. The directly measured arterial and venous pressures, the indirectly measured total blood flow, and the calculated pulmonary vascular resistance were considered representative of all lung regions. This assumption was questioned by Bjure and Laurell in 1927, when they suggested on the basis of chest radiographs of normal upright subjects that the lung apices were relatively underperfused because of the effect of gravity.[8] Regional variations in vessel caliber were also recognized early in radiographs of patients with multifocal emphysema

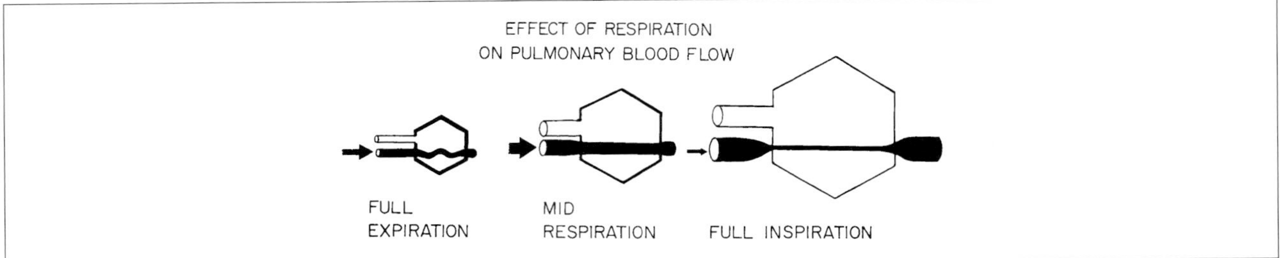

Figure 34-1. Respiration produces contrasting effects on the alveolar and extraalveolar elements of the microcirculation. A single alveolar unit shows that the alveolar capillaries are tortuous and kinked at full expiration, well distended in midrespiration, and stretched thin in full inspiration. Blood flow is thus moderate in expiration, maximal in midrespiration, and minimal in full inspiration. However, the degree of distention of the extraalveolar artery and vein reflects the increasingly negative interstitial pressure, so that these vessels are smallest in expiration, moderate-sized in midrespiration, and largest in inspiration. This explains the appearance of well-distended extraalveolar vessels on the standard radiograph taken in full inspiration, despite the momentarily high vascular resistance and reduced flow.

and pulmonary embolism, but the relationship to regional blood flow differences was not appreciated for some time.[47] In addition, there was early recognition that grossly altered flow states could be correlated with overall vessel caliber changes, and the terms *pleonemia* and *oligemia* came into use for the increased and decreased flow states associated with some types of congenital heart disease.[14,37]

In the mid-1950s rapid developments in cardiac surgery stimulated demands for cardiac catheterization and angiography and provided the opportunity for detailed correlation of radiologic changes with physiologic data in human patients. Specific vascular patterns were identified in association with pulmonary arterial hypertension.[18,24–26,45] A particular pattern of regional redistribution of blood flow was recognized in association with pulmonary venous hypertension in mitral stenosis, and it was shown that the vascular changes varied according to the severity of the hemodynamic disturbance.[20,21] Similar findings were subsequently noted in pulmonary venous hypertension due to left ventricular failure.[32,33,35] It seemed that the plain chest film was becoming a simple and readily available physiologic tool.[31,44] However, as in most uncontrolled clinical studies, the data were cluttered by many clinical variables and proved difficult to analyze. There was clearly a need for a more sophisticated experimental model that could provide simultaneous morphologic, radiologic, and physiologic data from various lung regions under controlled conditions.

The experimental groundwork was laid by Rodbard in 1956 in a prophetic theoretical analysis and in vitro simulation of the pulmonary circulation.[23] A glass-and-rubber-tubing manifold was used to study the alterations of "arterial," "venous," and "alveolar" pressures, as well as the effects of changing the "posture" of the device. A clear-cut regional flow dependence on

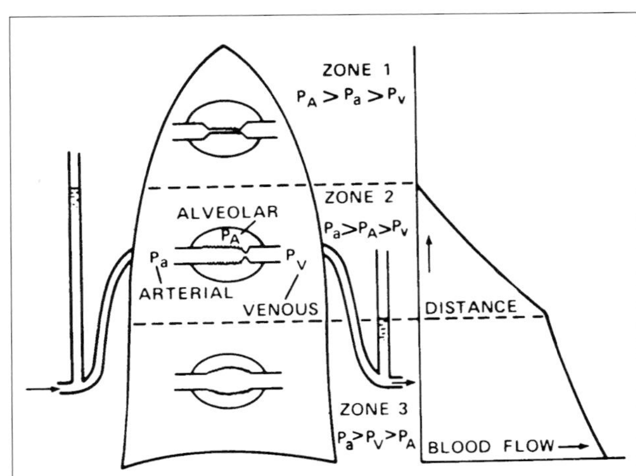

Figure 34-2. West's model of the pulmonary circulation defined three physiologic zones of blood flow in the upright lung. These zones result from a different relationship in each zone between the alveolar pressure, the arterial pressure, and the venous pressure. In the upper zone (zone 1), the alveolar pressure exceeds both the arterial and venous pressures so that the capillaries collapse and there is no blood flow in that zone. (Zone 1 probably does not exist in the normal human lung.) In the midzone (zone 2), the arterial pressure exceeds the alveolar pressure, but the alveolar pressure still exceeds the venous pressure. As a result, flow in zone 2 is determined by the arterial-alveolar gradient. This gradient increases rapidly from above downward because the arterial pressure is rising while the alveolar pressure is unchanging, since air is almost weightless. In the lower zone (zone 3), both arterial and venous pressures exceed alveolar pressure and flow is determined primarily by the arteriovenous gradient, which is constant throughout this zone, and to a lesser degree by the rising capillary pressures, which cause some increasing capillary distention and a slight increase in flow from the top to the bottom of zone 3. (From West JB, Dotter CT, Naimark A. Distribution of blood flow in isolated lung: relation to vascular and alveolar pressures. J Appl Physiol 1964;19:713. Used with permission.)

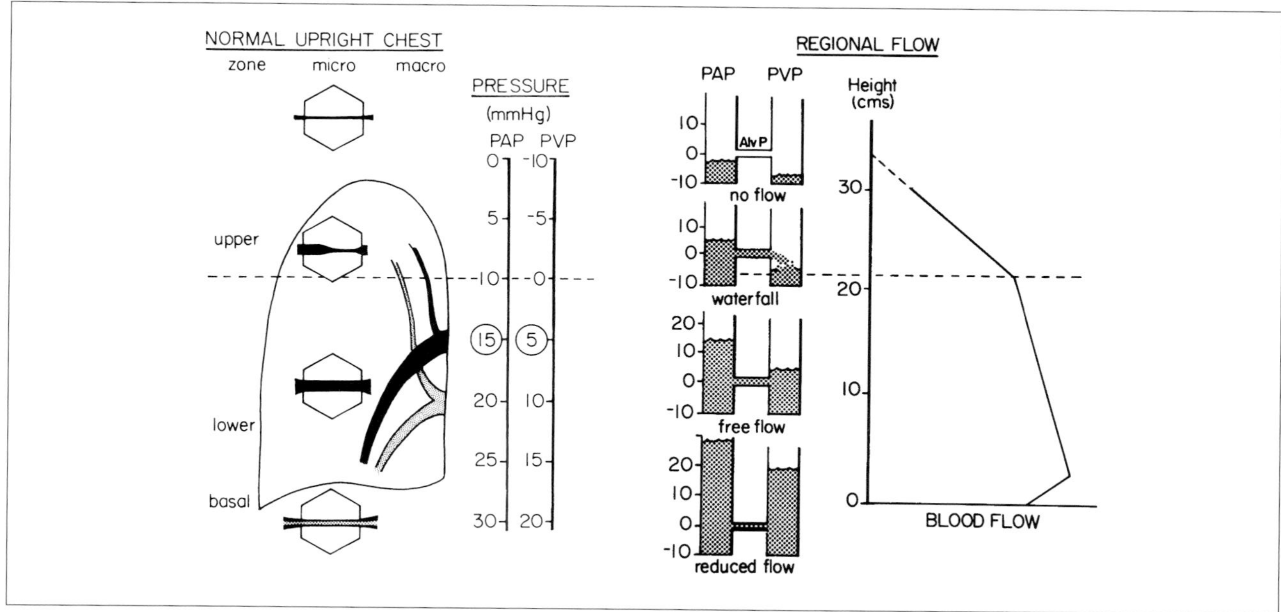

Figure 34-8. Normally, the upright adult lung has only two zones with different regional flow characteristics, an upper zone of "waterfall flow" and a lower zone of "free flow." These zones correspond with West's zone 2 and zone 3. Under exceptional or abnormal circumstances, there may be an apical zone of "no flow," equivalent to West's zone 1, or a basal zone of "reduced flow." The diagram illustrates distinctive effects in each of the four zones on (*left*) the microscopic vessels and the arterial and venous pressures and (*right*) on pressure gradients (*connected reservoirs*) and regional blood flow (*graph*). The top three zones result from differences in the relationships between alveolar pressure, arterial pressure, and venous pressure, and the fourth zone at the base reflects a higher (i.e., a less negative) interstitial pressure, which causes microvascular constriction.

shallow zone of slightly reduced flow, probably due to increasing interstitial pressure caused by the weight of the lung or possibly by excessive transudation of plasma into the interstitium at the lung base, where the normal hydrostatic pressures are greatest.

Thus the normal upright adult lung has essentially only two flow zones, the "waterfall" zone and the "free-flow" zone. Under unusual or abnormal conditions a "no-flow" zone may occur at the apex or an expanded "reduced-flow" zone may occur at the base.

This concept explains the normal upright chest radiographic appearance in which there is a rapid increase in caliber of segmental and other vessels as one moves downward from the apex to the hilar level, and a slower increase from the hilar level to the lung base. It also accounts for the more uniform caliber of pulmonary vessels in all regions when the subject assumes the horizontal position.

Interstitial Pressure

The blood vessels of the lung are surrounded by interstitial tissues.[40,83,84] The interstitial pressure is negative to a greater or lesser degree, depending on the magnitude of the applied respiratory forces acting on the interstitium in opposite directions. On the one hand, during inspiration the muscles of the chest wall and the diaphragm are expanding the lung. On the other hand, this is opposed by the elastic recoil of the lung parenchyma as the result of a combination of the surface tension of the alveolar lining layer and the elasticity of its collagen fibers. In addition, the blood vessels possess substantial muscular tone that is under homeostatic control, which tends to constrict them. These forces account for the varying negative interstitial pressures. These are partly counterbalanced by the weight of the lung and by the positive intravascular pressures. The net negative interstitial pressure keeps the vessels open. If a buffer medium such as edema transudate becomes available, the interstitial pressure becomes less negative and allows the vessels to constrict by their inherent tone. If air or liquid enters the pleural space, the entire lung collapses proportionately, the elastic recoil pressure is reduced, the interstitial pressure becomes less negative, and, once again, the lung vessels are able to constrict. These examples of loss of negative interstitial pressure and reduction of vessel caliber are familiar to radiologists.

Thus some of the forces acting on the interstitium are dynamic (e.g., ventilation and vascular pulsation), and others are static (e.g., the elastic properties of the chest wall and the lung, as well as the weight of the blood and lung tissue). They can be significantly altered by pathologic processes (e.g., pulmonary edema, pneumothorax, or fibrothorax). There is no simple single value for interstitial pressure. Like pleural pressure, it is normally negative but its precise values vary with anatomic location and phase of respiration.

The Flow-Caliber Relationship

Measurement of blood flow by any of the standard clinical methods involves cardiac catheterization and is of limited value because only the *total* blood flow through both lungs is measurable. It is common to have some regions of the lung with locally decreased flow while compensatory increased flow occurs in other regions, resulting in a misleading normal or near-normal net total blood flow. Furthermore, a substantial but localized increase in flow, as in an arteriovenous malformation, may have a negligible effect on the total flow. There is no simple physiologic method of measuring single-vessel or regional blood flow in the lungs. Radionuclide perfusion scans, angiography, and MRI still provide the only effective clinical methods for evaluating the regional distribution of blood flow.[85]

There is the intriguing possibility that the size of a blood vessel, as seen on a standard chest radiograph or an angiogram, actually reflects the magnitude of the blood flow through its lumen. This implies there is a normal biologic balancing mechanism that adjusts the caliber of the vessel lumen in accordance with the volume of blood flow through it, and that this is independent of the intravascular pressure. If this is true and if this flow-caliber relationship could be established experimentally, the radiologist would be in a unique position to measure blood flow in any single vessel by simply measuring its diameter. Until now, the feat of measuring single-vessel blood flow has been confined to the experimental laboratory and then only as a tour de force requiring sophisticated instrumentation.[52,79]

There is substantial naturalistic support for this hypothesis. It is common knowledge that organs with high blood flows are served by large arteries and veins whereas those with low flows have small ones. In a branching arterial tree of an organ such as the lung, successive branches receive a decreasing fraction of the blood flow and become correspondingly reduced in caliber.[12] On the venous side, the flow volume increases as tributaries combine, and venous caliber increases accordingly. The ascending aorta and the pulmonary artery trunk normally carry the same blood flow, the total cardiac output, and are normally identical in caliber despite a marked difference in the intraluminal pressure. The pressure difference is reflected in the thickness of the vessel wall, not its lumen diameter. If pulmonary blood flow is pathologically increased, whether locally (as in an arteriovenous malformation), regionally (as with diversion of blood flow from diseased areas of the lung), or generally (as in an atrial septal defect), the caliber of the affected arteries and veins visibly increases.[37,86,87] Conversely, if blood flow is reduced pathologically, whether locally (as beyond a pulmonary embolus), regionally (as in the lung bases in mitral stenosis), or generally (as in the tetralogy of Fallot), the caliber of the affected vessels decreases.

There is thus an apparent natural adjustment of the caliber of feeding arteries and draining veins in accordance with the flow volume. This is a biologic phenomenon without parallel in the physics of inanimate matter. We know that *flow volume* = *flow velocity* × *lumen cross-sectional area*. In a plumbing or a hydraulic system, the metal or plastic pipes are rigid, and large changes in the flow volumes of water are accommodated by simply varying the flow velocity (Fig. 34-9). However, blood is a tissue with cellular elements suspended in intercellular fluid, the plasma. Sudden

Figure 34-9. In a plumbing system with rigid pipes, the flow velocity varies in accordance with the pipe diameter or the flow volume. (A) If rigid pipes of varying diameter are arranged in a series, then, for any given flow volume, the water velocity varies inversely with the cross-sectional area of the pipe section. (B) If rigid pipes of equal diameter are arranged in a parallel fashion, the water velocity varies directly with the flow in each pipe section, which is controlled by the setting of each faucet.

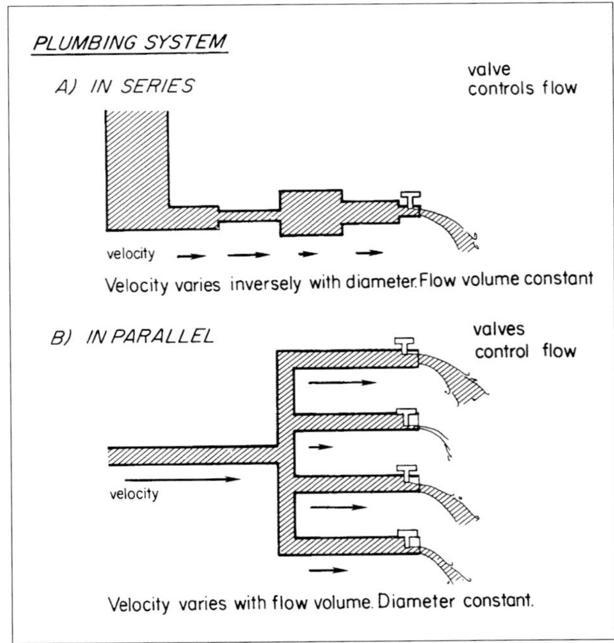

changes in velocity or changes in direction of flow at high velocity would produce shear forces that could disrupt the fragile red blood cells. Teleologically it would seem desirable to maintain a steady blood velocity within a small biologically acceptable range, despite the greatly varying blood flow volume demands of different organs or anatomic regions as well as of the same vessels at times of different physiologic activity, such as with exercise or gravity effects (Fig. 34-10). If blood velocity needs to be maintained at a fairly constant level suitable for transporting blood cells without risk of hemolysis and it seems that the optimal systolic velocity is about 40 to 50 cm per second, and the optimal mean velocity is about 25 to 30 cm per second, there would have to be some way to adjust the cross-sectional area, and thus the diameter, of each vessel according to its mean blood flow volume. In addition, it would also be necessary to be able to modulate this basic vessel size to allow for transient physiologic or pathologic fluctuations of flow volume. The first adjustment mechanism involves vessel wall growth, a slow process that can either enlarge the basic vessel size by cell division or decrease the basic vessel size by atrophy, which can be regarded as reverse growth.

The second mechanism involves the instantaneous vasomotor dilatation or constriction of the vessel caliber in response to transient variations of flow volume, for example, during exercise. A stable caliber is achieved once the new cross-sectional area, or diameter, matches the required blood flow volume so that a "normal" flow velocity is restored. The stimulus for a blood vessel to change its caliber must be a momentary change in blood velocity, but how the vessel wall senses this remains speculative. The phenomenon is clearly not related to changes in pressure, which may be relatively unaltered. Caliber changes may affect vessels quite remote from the site of the lesion that causes the flow disturbance.

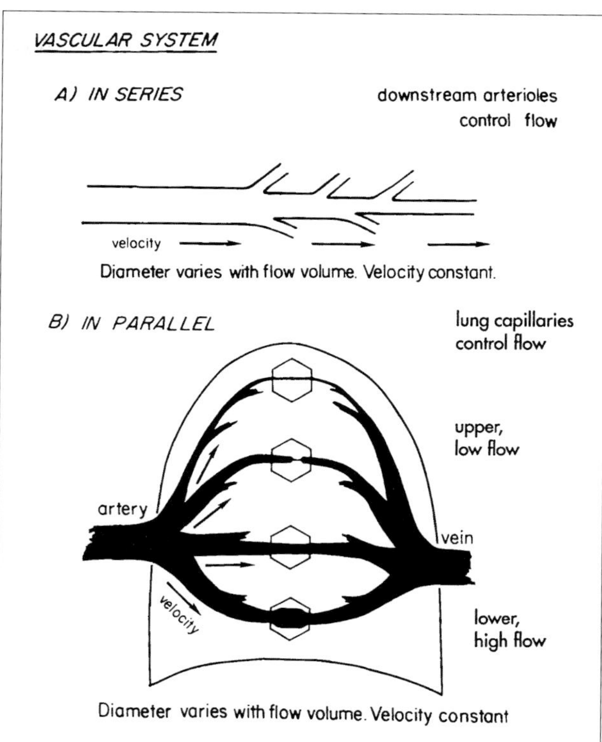

Figure 34-10. In a normal vascular system, the velocity of the blood flow in the vessels visible radiologically is maintained within a small physiologically optimal range. Therefore it is necessary for the vessel's cross section, and thus its diameter, to be adjusted in accordance with the flow volume, which is controlled by the microcirculation. The biologic control of large blood vessel size appears to involve two mechanisms. The first mechanism is a slow adjustment by vessel growth, or atrophy, until its basic size matches its average flow volume and the mean velocity is within the normal range. The second mechanism is a rapid adjustment of caliber by vasomotor dilatation or constriction to allow for transient flow variations without great velocity changes. The vessel caliber adjustments are recognized (A) in series, as in the aorta, and (B) in parallel systems, as in the pulmonary vessels.

The flow-caliber balancing process depends on a few simple and common preconditions:

1. A live patient. A cadaver has no blood flow regardless of vessel caliber. The response depends on functioning homeostatic control mechanisms.
2. Normal blood vessels. Neoplastic or atherosclerotic vessels may not react appropriately to changes in blood velocity.
3. A stable altered hemodynamic state. There must be sufficient time to allow growth adjustments to occur. Transient vasomotor caliber changes may be insufficient to allow for large changes in flow so that short periods of abnormal flow velocity may exist.
4. Matching changes in feeding artery and draining vein. If only an artery or only a vein dilates, this is usually due to a pathologic change in the vessel wall (i.e., an aneurysm or a varix) and does not reflect a change in the flow volume. The flow velocity would be reduced during the blood's passage through a pathologically dilated vessel.
5. Normal pulmonary artery pressures. Arterial hypertension causes competing functional and structural changes in the arteries (see below) and may eventually cause a pathologic reduction in blood flow and an increase in blood velocity.
6. Normal blood viscosity. Polycythemia vera may cause vessel dilatation even with normal or reduced blood flow, probably as a result of an increased total blood volume.

7. Normal blood volume. Hypervolemia and hypovolemia may cause vessel caliber changes independent of changes in blood flow—a capacitance effect.

Given these usual conditions, can the measured vessel caliber be used to quantitate blood flow through a given blood vessel? Is it possible to translate the radiologist's vague impression of increased or decreased blood flow into precise physiologic values? To do this, the radiologist would require a graph relating vessel diameter (in millimeters) to flow volume (in milliliters per minute) for standard chest radiographs and another for angiograms (taken at 40 inches source–image distance). It may become possible to determine this relationship experimentally using newer electromagnetic, ultrasonic, or magnetic resonance flow probes that provide precise and simultaneous measurements of the vessel lumen diameter and mean flow velocity, permitting the calculation of flow volumes.[52]

Figure 34-11. An approximate relationship between the diameter of a pulmonary artery on the standard chest radiograph and the blood flow in that vessel (*solid line*). The measurements obtained from an angiogram must be reduced by one-fifth to correct for additional magnification. The graph is indirectly based on angiographic and polymer cast measurements. Note: Both scales are logarithmic. For vessel diameters above 15 mm the rate of flow increase is reduced, possibly because of lower vessel wall compliance. A close straight-line approximation of this curve is provided by the simple formula $D^2 \times 10$ (*dashed line*), in which D is the measured vessel diameter.

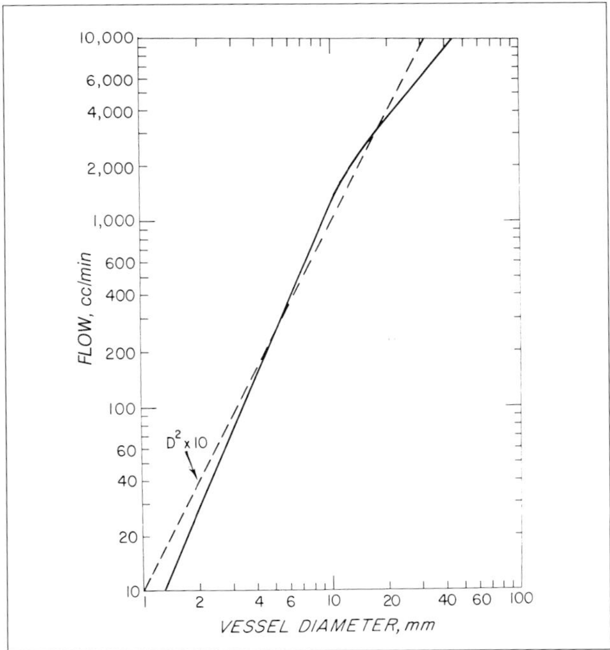

Table 34-1. Flow-Caliber Relationship*

Vessel Diameter (mm)	Flow (ml/min)
1–20	$D^2 \times 10$
21–30	$D^2 \times 8$
31–40	$D^2 \times 6$

*These simplified formulas permit a fairly close approximation of the values shown in Figure 34-11 and will provide a rough estimate of the flow volumes.

Until then a tentative graph has been derived indirectly from angiographic and catheterization measurements in the adult human, as well as from morphometric studies of plastic casts of the pulmonary vessels (Fig. 34-11).[12] Alternatively, a set of simple formulas has been derived from the same data to express this relationship to a close approximation for the standard chest radiograph (Table 34-1). The angiographic measurements must be reduced by one-fifth before the graph or the formulas are used to correct for the additional magnification at 40 inches source–image distance as well as the fact that the vessel lumen diameter rather than the outer vessel wall diameter is being measured. These indirectly derived flow values should be regarded as theoretical approximations.

From the tentative graph it can be shown that a normal pulmonary artery trunk measuring 25 mm in diameter has a blood flow of 5 liters per minute, a segmental artery measuring 5 mm in diameter has a flow of 250 ml per minute, and a subsegmental artery measuring 1.5 mm in diameter has a flow of 12 ml per minute. These appear to be reasonable values by other criteria. The graph can now be used to measure blood flow in an abnormal vessel, such as an artery feeding an arteriovenous malformation (Fig. 34-12). In a region of abnormal flow, it is possible to estimate the regional flow by measuring a representative segmental artery, determining its flow volume, and multiplying that flow volume by the estimated number of segments involved in the abnormal region. Thus if there is a flow redistribution to both upper zones, a total of 10 segments may be assumed. In the case of a left-to-right intracardiac shunt, the flow through one representative segmental artery is determined and is multiplied by 20 to determine the magnitude of the shunt.

Measuring vessel diameter on standard radiographs is not easy with a conventional ruler, but measuring with a caliper with magnified or digital millimeter scales is more reliable. Precise measurements of vessel size can be obtained electronically from CT or MRI, or conventional angiograms, if these are available, because of the greater local contrast between the vessel and the surrounding lung tissue.

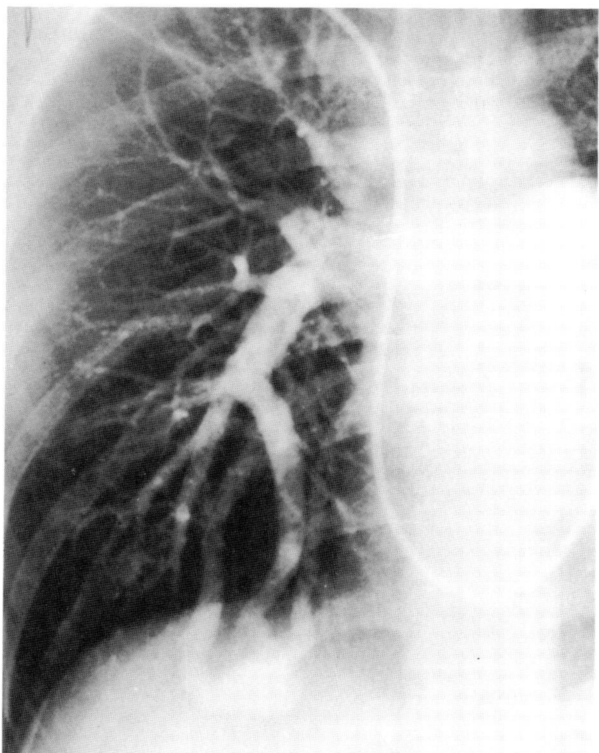

Figure 34-12. Angiogram, taken in supine position, demonstrating an arteriovenous malformation in the right lower lobe with characteristic dilatation of the feeding artery and two draining veins. The contrast medium has filled the dilated feeding artery, the lesion itself, and the large veins, whereas in other regions of the lung it has not even reached the terminal arterial branches. This indicates both increased blood flow as well as some increased velocity. The feeding segmental artery measures 12 mm in diameter, in contrast to the adjacent normal segmental arteries, which measure 4.5 mm in diameter. Reference to the flow-caliber graph in Figure 34-11 suggests that the diameter of the feeding artery represents a blood flow of 1200 ml per minute, and the additional velocity increase would imply an even larger number. The arteriovenous malformation thus carries almost a quarter of the normal cardiac output, greatly in excess of the average segmental flow of 250 ml per minute. This quantitative estimate would strongly favor surgical excision or therapeutic embolization.

Redistribution of Blood Flow

The pulmonary vessels comprise a vast system of parallel arteriovenous pathways with substantial reserve capacity. Blood flow follows the path of least resistance,[2,53] usually the dependent pathways where hydrostatic pressures are greatest and the microvasculature therefore most distended. The effect is most striking at the lung bases of an upright person, particularly a tall person. The reduced apical flow and the increased basal flow represent the normal redistribution of flow pattern of the standard upright chest radiograph. A more uniform distribution is seen in the horizontal position, particularly if the person is prone, since the gravitational effect is equalized between the lung apex and base, and the smaller dorsal-to-ventral differences are not detectable on the frontal projection standard radiograph, though they may be seen on CT or MR axial cross-sectional images.

Focal diseases of the lung parenchyma or the pulmonary vessels may increase the local or regional microvascular resistance and reduce pulmonary blood flow to the affected areas.[74,88,89] The reduced flow, in turn, causes a secondary decrease in caliber of the larger feeding and draining vessels serving these areas. However, the cardiac output remains unaffected until the disease process is extensive because blood flow is simply diverted to newly recruited and thus dilated vessels in the remaining normal lung regions. The combination of regions of abnormal vascular constriction and regions of compensatory dilatation is referred to as *pathologic redistribution of flow*.

The patterns of vascular redistribution thus reflect the localization and magnitude of regional blood flow increase and decrease under varying normal and pathologic circumstances.[21,44,89,90] They range from the largely random patterns of emphysema or pulmonary embolism to the characteristic patterns associated with altered posture or venous hypertension.

Pulmonary Arterial Hypertension

It is well established that the normal very low pulmonary vascular pressures and the high total pulmonary blood flow volumes can be maintained even in the presence of localized or patchy pulmonary disease associated with vascular obstruction or destruction and easily recognized by the radiologist. This is due to the large reserve capacity of the pulmonary vascular bed as well as a variety of homeostatic mechanisms designed to preserve optimal overall physiologic conditions for gas exchange. Unused vascular pathways are available for recruitment, and even channels already perfused can be dilated further.[2,3] Only when these compensatory mechanisms have become overwhelmed by the extent or the severity of the process does the pulmonary artery pressure rise and, later still, does the total pulmonary blood flow decrease, threatening right heart failure and death (see Fig. 34-6).

When chronic pulmonary arterial hypertension develops, a pathognomonic structural change occurs in the pulmonary vessels.[17-19,25,45,89,91] The central pulmonary arteries, characteristically the pulmonary artery

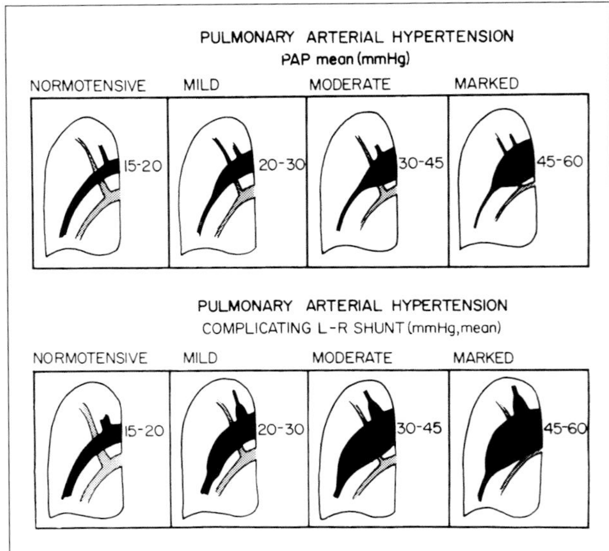

Figure 34-13. Varying degrees of distention of the central pulmonary arteries in association with chronic pulmonary arterial hypertension of increasing severity. The *upper series* shows changes that typify chronic pulmonary hypertension developing in previously normal pulmonary vessels. The *lower series* shows more marked distention in patients with comparable levels of hypertension superimposed on vessels already dilated as a result of a preexisting left-to-right shunt with increased pulmonary blood flow. Acute pulmonary hypertension results in a markedly smaller degree of distention for a given pressure range because it takes time for the changes to develop fully (see Table 34-2). Note that the transition point between central dilatation and peripheral constriction usually occurs at the lobar level if the vessels were previously normal but may be farther out if the arteries were initially dilated.

trunk, the right and left main pulmonary arteries, and the interlobar arteries, become dilated. In abrupt contrast to this, the lobar branches, the segmental branches, and those beyond decrease in caliber. These paradoxical caliber changes are independent of the cause of the pulmonary hypertension. In general, the degree of central distention reflects the severity of the pulmonary arterial hypertension (Fig. 34-13). The radiographic change can be graded subjectively as mild, moderate, or marked. Corresponding ranges of pulmonary artery pressure can be fairly well predicted, but only if allowance is made for the acuteness or chronicity of the process, as well as for the background status of the pulmonary vessels. In practice, therefore, three separate pressure scales are necessary to correlate the radiologic appearances with the severity of the pulmonary arterial hypertension. The clinical categories are (1) acute, as in massive pulmonary embolism; (2) chronic, as in cor pulmonale due to emphysema or interstitial fibrosis; and (3) chronic with a preexisting left-to-right shunt, as in atrial septal defect with reversal of shunt (Table 34-2). It is clear that for a given degree of pulmonary arterial hypertension, the degree of central vessel dilatation is least striking in acute hypertension, "typical" in common chronic hypertension, and exaggerated when superimposed on vessels already dilated as a result of a left-to-right shunt.

The transition point between central dilatation and peripheral constriction is typically at the origin of the lobar artery branches. In patients with prior arterial enlargement due to long-standing left-to-right shunts, the transition point may occur further out, at the segmental artery level. The degree of constriction of the peripheral branches is variable and difficult to grade and thus does not help in the quantitation of hemodynamic severity. For the same reason, the use of a ratio of central vessel caliber to peripheral vessel caliber is unreliable and of little value.

In the presence of pulmonary arterial hypertension, the pulmonary veins usually appear normal or slightly reduced in caliber. Occasionally, when the hypertension is secondary to partial reversal of a left-to-right shunt, the caliber of the veins may still exceed the normal range despite some reduction in their previously increased size.

It must be reemphasized that the criteria for quantitating blood flow in a single vessel according to vessel caliber do not apply in the presence of pulmonary arterial hypertension. The biologic adjustment of caliber

Table 34-2. Correlation of Degree of Central Distention of Pulmonary Arteries with Severity of Mean Pulmonary Artery Hypertension (expressed in mmHg)

	Degree of Distention of Central Arteries*				
Type of Hypertension	**Not Recognizable**	**Mild**	**Moderate**	**Marked**	**Gross**
Acute	30	45	60		
Chronic		30	45	60	
Chronic, with left-to-right shunt			30	45	60

*The radiologic changes are least pronounced in acute pulmonary hypertension, more pronounced in chronic hypertension, and exaggerated when superimposed on a left-to-right shunt.

according to blood flow is in competition with the peripheral arterial constriction and central arterial dilatation resulting from the elevated pulmonary artery pressure. Despite apparent peripheral vascular constriction, patients with pulmonary arterial hypertension may have normal or near-normal total blood flows. This would imply recruitment of a greater number of small-caliber vessels or an abnormal increase in flow velocity despite the added risk of hemolysis. Arterial caliber measurements cannot be used to assess blood flow if pulmonary hypertension exists.

The pathogenesis of the abrupt transition from central dilatation to peripheral constriction in the same arterial tree is a matter of speculation. There is evidence to suggest that in fact the "normal" biologic response to increased intraarterial pressure is vasoconstriction, as manifested by the peripheral arterial branches. This active response is just the opposite of that of rubber tubing, which would passively distend in direct proportion to the intraluminal pressure. On the other hand, the central arteries do indeed seem to behave like rubber tubing, providing the radiologist with a built-in pressure gauge. Laplace's law offers the best explanation of this paradoxical behavior (Fig. 34-14). The tension on the vessel wall is a product of the intraluminal pressure and the radius of the vessel. It seems that when the arterial pressure rises, vessels below 1 cm in diameter have sufficient strength to overcome the increased tension on the wall by muscular constriction. However, in vessels larger than 1 cm in diameter, the wall tension becomes so great that the available muscle power is unable to overcome it. These larger vessels then behave like rubber tubing and distend passively to a degree that reflects the severity of the pulmonary arterial hypertension. The transition point is sharp because in a branching arterial tree the vessel caliber decreases abruptly at each division point.

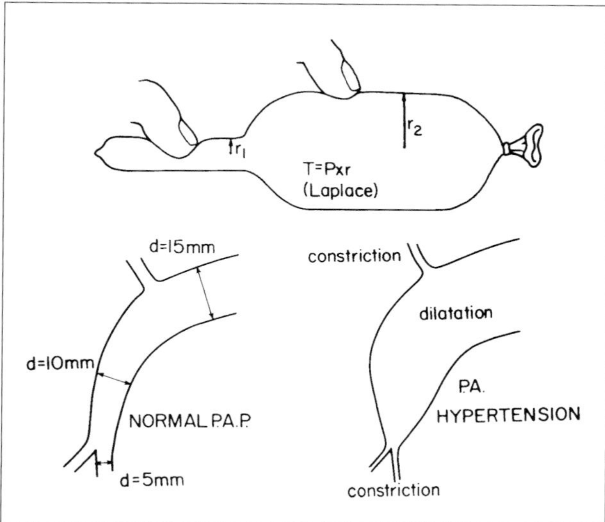

Figure 34-14. Laplace's law offers the best explanation for the paradoxical central dilatation and peripheral constriction that characterize pulmonary arterial hypertension. The tension on the vessel wall is a product of both the intraluminal pressure and the radius of the vessel. In response to an initial rise in pressure, vessels less than 1 cm in diameter, including the normal lobar divisions of the pulmonary artery, are still exposed to a relatively low wall tension and can respond appropriately by vasoconstriction. However, the larger central pulmonary arteries experience such great wall tensions that they are unable to constrict, and they become passively distended. The degree of distention of the central arteries will reflect the severity of the hypertension. In the event that the lobar divisions were initially enlarged above the critical 1 cm diameter, they too will be unable to constrict and will be distended so that the transition point moves outward from the lobar to the segmental level.

Pulmonary Venous Hypertension

Progressive increases in pulmonary venous pressure produce a sequence of striking radiologic changes that reflect both the presence and the severity of this hemodynamic disturbance.[87,88,92–98] Three well-defined stages can be recognized in chronic pulmonary venous hypertension:

1. Flow redistribution
2. Septal interstitial edema
3. Alveolar edema

Each stage can be further subdivided radiologically into mild, moderate, and marked grades of severity. There is a fairly good overall correlation between these categories and the pressure values obtained at cardiac catheterization (Fig. 34-15). In specific patients, the estimated pressures should be adjusted slightly according to the particular clinical circumstances. Thus in long-standing mitral valve disease the values may be slightly higher than shown because adaptive structural changes develop in the pulmonary microvasculature and lymphatics. Conversely, in the recovery phase of pulmonary venous hypertension following myocardial infarction, the values may be somewhat lower than indicated because clearance of edema fluid or pleural effusion may lag behind the pulmonary venous pressure recovery by some hours or even days.

Stage 1: Upper Zone Flow Redistribution

To explain the typical radiologic redistribution pattern found in the first stage of pulmonary venous hypertension, it is important to distinguish what is happening in the pulmonary microcirculation from the visible changes involving the larger vessels (Fig. 34-16). Elevation of the pulmonary capillary pressure increases the

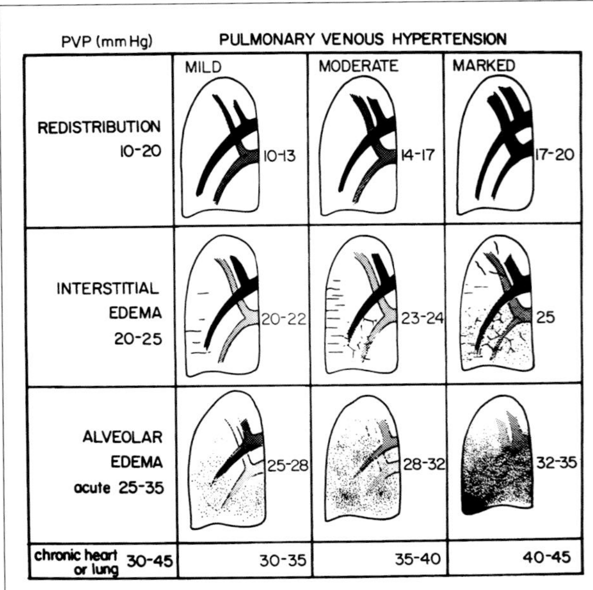

Figure 34-15. There are three clear-cut radiologic stages of subacute or chronic pulmonary venous hypertension. Within each stage, it is possible to distinguish three radiologic grades of increasing severity. Each grade may be correlated with a small range of pulmonary venous pressures. In acute pulmonary venous hypertension, such as after an initial myocardial infarction, the stage of flow redistribution may not be seen. In the stage of septal interstitial edema, the pressure differences are too small to matter. The indicated venous pressure ranges are most reliable in subacute or chronic pulmonary venous hypertension, the most common clinical forms. The values may be higher if there is long-standing severe heart or lung disease, as shown at the bottom of the diagram, because of adaptive changes that develop slowly over time. The values may be slightly less than shown if the patient is in the process of recovering clinically, since clearing of edema fluid may take some hours after the increased venous pressure has come down.

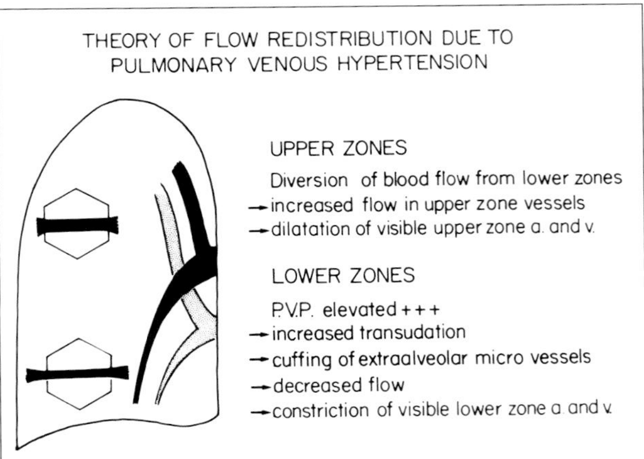

Figure 34-16. Flow redistribution associated with pulmonary venous hypertension is initiated by a series of pathophysiologic events in the microcirculation of the lower zone, causing increased local vascular resistance and decreased flow. The flow decrease results in secondary constriction of the larger vessels serving the lower zones. The cardiac output remains relatively unaffected, and thus the blood flow must be diverted through available vascular channels in the upper zones, where pressures are still within the normal range. The increased flow in the upper zones causes dilatation of the larger vessels serving these regions.

rate of transudation of plasma from the capillaries into the interstitial space. Because the hydrostatic pressures are greatest in the dependent regions of the lungs, transudation is most marked in the lower zones of an upright patient.[21,32,76,99] In stage 1, the initial interstitial transudate moves out of the alveolar walls and into the adjacent extraalveolar interstitial spaces and lymphatic channels that surround the microscopic arteries, veins, and airways. This phenomenon may be due to the effect of inspiration, which simultaneously stretches and squeezes the alveolar walls while distending the extraalveolar interstitium with transudate. The alveolar walls and interlobar septa thus remain thin, and gas exchange proceeds. The increased lymph flow is still within the capacity of the distended lymphatic drainage channels. The sleeve of perivascular edema that forms around the small extraalveolar vessels allows them to constrict because of their inherent tone. This constriction increases vascular resistance at the lung bases and reduces blood flow to these regions. The larger arteries and veins that serve the lung bases and that are visible on the radiograph respond to the decreased blood flow with a reduction in caliber, tending to restore flow velocity. Thus the microcirculation causes the decreased flow, while the macrocirculation reflects it. The radiographic outlines of the visible vessels in the lower zones become blurry as the perivascular and peribronchial edema and lymphatic distention extend centrally toward the hilum of the lung.

Because blood flow to the lower zones is diminished while the total output of the right ventricle remains unchanged, there is recruitment of vascular channels in the upper zones, where the hydrostatic pressures and vascular resistance are lowest. The increased blood flow in the upper zones causes dilatation of the visible arteries and veins serving these regions. These vessels remain sharply defined because there is no interstitial fluid accumulation around them. This completes the characteristic pattern of stage 1 pulmonary venous hypertension, namely, constriction and blurring of the lower zone vessels and dilatation of the upper zone vessels, which remain sharp.

The acuteness or chronicity of the process affect the radiologic appearance. Initially in an acute myocardial infarction, the redistribution pattern may be absent.

Later constricted vessels at the base become blurry because of the perivascular sleeve of edema fluid. This may conceal the constriction to some degree. In chronic mitral valve disease, the vessels are more sharply defined. It seems that in the acute situation, the normal perivascular lymphatic channels are rapidly overloaded and the edema fluid accumulates in the perivascular interstitial tissues. In the chronic case, there has been time for hypertrophy of the perivascular lymph channels, and a large amount of edema fluid can be drained efficiently.

The base-to-apex redistribution pattern is easily recognized on chest radiographs. This pattern constitutes the earliest evidence of left ventricular failure in radiologic practice. It is often encountered in patients who may have no overt clinical symptoms and signs of left heart failure and serves as a warning of impending clinical decompensation or as a sign of incomplete recovery.[32]

The mild grade of the redistribution pattern is the most difficult to recognize since slight basal constriction and slight apical dilatation may appear as equalization of the vessel caliber in the upper and lower zones. This must be distinguished from hyperkinetic flow states, such as with fever or anemia, and also from early pulmonary arterial hypertension. The clue is the blurring of the lower zone vessels, seen in pulmonary venous hypertension in the presence of left-sided heart disease. The moderate grade shows a definite but relatively modest increase in caliber of the upper zone vessels relative to those in the lower zone, and in the marked grade the caliber differences are striking.

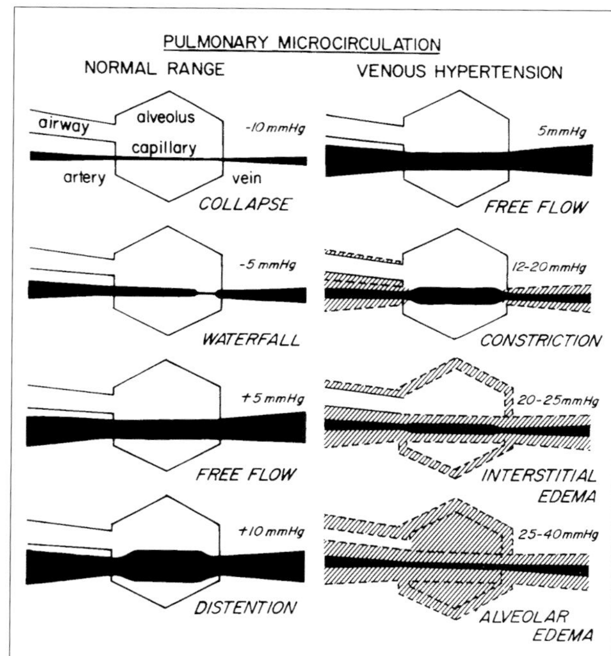

Figure 34-17. Summary of the sequence of changes in the pulmonary microcirculation that reflect increasing pulmonary venous pressure. A range of normal mean venous pressures is shown on the *left*. The hydrostatic pressure increment due to gravity produces a range of venous pressures between the lung apex and the base sufficient to ensure that at least two and up to four different vascular states may exist in the normal lung at any one time. Pathologically increased mean pressures are shown on the *right*. These add three additional and distinctive states of the microcirculation, all appearing first at the lung bases.

Stage 2: Septal Interstitial Edema

Interstitial edema results when the pulmonary capillary pressure exceeds the colloidal osmotic pressure of blood, the primary force holding the plasma in the capillary lumen. The endothelial basement membrane is relatively leaky, and the plasma now spills into the interstitial spaces at a rate that exceeds the drainage capacity of the lymphatics.[100–102] The interstitium of the alveolar walls, the interlobular septa, and the subpleural tissues, which are all in free communication, become swollen with edema fluid and appear on the radiograph as background haze, septal lines, and accentuated interlobar fissures. However, the tight epithelial basement membranes prevent the edema fluid from entering the alveolar sacs, which remain air-filled though diminished in size (Fig. 34-17). These changes are again observed first at the bases, where pressures are highest. They progress upward in accordance with the severity of the venous hypertension. When the perihilar tissues become involved, hilar haze and thickening of bronchial walls seen end on will occur.

Interstitial edema may develop at lower capillary pressures if the plasma colloids are reduced, as in hypoalbuminemia. On the other hand, it may appear only at higher venous pressures in long-standing conditions, such as mitral stenosis, in which lymphatic hypertrophy permits the clearance of large volumes of transudate without difficulty.

Stage 3: Alveolar Edema

Alveolar edema is usually associated with a sudden overwhelming elevation of the pulmonary venous pressure. The edema fluid may initially accumulate in the interstitial tissues before the tight junctions of the epithelial basement membrane disrupt and allow the edema fluid to pour into the alveolar spaces (see Fig. 34-17). However, in some acute cases there may be little or no swelling of the alveolar interstitium before the plasma floods into the air sacs. These two forms appear very different histologically. Plasma fills the alveolar spaces in both situations, but one shows swollen

5. Herrick JF. Poiseuille's observations on blood flow lead to a law in hydrodynamics. Am J Physiol 1942;10:22.
6. Poiseuille JLM (1855). Quoted by Quincke H, Pfeiffer E. Uber den Blutstrom in den Lungen. Arch Anat Phys Wiss Med 1871;39:90.
7. Bowditch HP, Garland GM. The effects of the respiratory movements on the pulmonary circulation. J Physiol (Lond) 1879;2:92.
8. Bjure A, Laurell H. Abnormal static circulatory phenomena and their symptoms; arterial orthostatic anemia as neglected clinical picture. Acta Soc Med Ups 1927;33:1.
9. Robb GP, Steinberg I. Visualization of the chambers of the heart, the pulmonary circulation and the great blood vessels in man: a practical method. AJR 1939;41:1.
10. Steinberg I. Intravenous angiography: the twentieth year. AJR 1959;81:886.
11. Lodge T. The anatomy of blood vessels of the human lung as applied to chest radiology: IV. Changes in the lung vascular tree in disease processes. Br J Radiol 1946;19:77.
12. Cumming G, Hunt LB, eds. Form and function in the human lung. Baltimore: Williams & Wilkins, 1968.
13. Macklin C. Evidence of increase in the capacity of the pulmonary arteries and veins of dogs, cats and rabbits during inflation of the freshly excised lung. Rev Can Biol 1946;5:199.
14. Cournand A. Recent observations on the dynamics of the pulmonary circulation. Bull NY Acad Med 1947;23:27.
15. Westermark N. On the influence of the intraalveolar pressure on the normal and pathological structure of the lungs. Acta Radiol (Stockh) 1944;2(Suppl):874.
16. Westermark N. Roentgen diagnosis of pulmonary embolism. In: Rigler LG, ed. Roentgen studies of the lungs and heart. Minneapolis: University of Minnesota Press, 1948:174–187.
17. Healy RF, Dow JW, Sosman MC, Dexter L. The relationship of the roentgenographic appearance of the pulmonary artery to pulmonary hemodynamics. AJR 1949;62:777.
18. Davies LG, Goodwin JF, Steiner RE, van Leuven BD. Clinical and radiological assessment of pulmonary arterial pressure in mitral stenosis. Br Heart J 1953;15:393.
19. Whitaker W, Lodge T. The radiological manifestations of pulmonary hypertension in patients with mitral stenosis. J Fac Radiol 1954;5:182.
20. Steinbach HL, Keats TE, Sheline AE. The roentgen appearance of the pulmonary veins in heart disease. Radiology 1955;65:157.
21. Simon M. The pulmonary veins in mitral stenosis. J Fac Radiol (Lond) 1958;9:25.
22. Burton AC, Patel DJ. Effect on pulmonary vascular resistance on inflation of the rabbit lung. J Appl Physiol 1958;12,13:239.
23. Rodbard S. Distribution of flow through a pulmonary manifold. Am Heart J 1956;51:106.
24. Doyle AE, Goodwin JF, Harrison CV, Steiner RE. Pulmonary vascular patterns in pulmonary hypertension. Br Heart J 1957;19:353.
25. Steiner RE. Radiological appearances of the pulmonary vessels in pulmonary hypertension. Br J Radiol 1958;31:188.
26. Kerley P. Lung changes in acquired heart disease. AJR 1958;80:256.
27. Permutt S, Howell JBL, Proctor DF, Riley RL. Effect of lung inflation on static pressure-volume characteristics of pulmonary vessels. J Appl Physiol 1961;16:64.
28. Howell JBL, Permutt S, Proctor DF, Riley RL. Effect of inflation of the lung on different parts of the pulmonary vascular bed. J Appl Physiol 1961;16:71.
29. Caro CG. Extensibility of blood vessels in isolated rabbit lungs. J Physiol (Lond) 1965;178:193.
30. Hughes JMB, Glazier JB, Maloney JE, West JB. Effect of extra-alveolar vessels on distribution of blood flow in the dog lung. J Appl Physiol 1968;25:701.
31. Rigler LG. Functional roentgen diagnosis: anatomical image, physiologic interpretation. Caldwell Lecture, 59th Annual Meeting of the American Roentgen Ray Society. AJR 1959;82:1.
32. Simon M. The pulmonary vessels in incipient left ventricular decompensation: radiologic observations. Circulation 1961;24:185.
33. Lavender JP, Doppman J, Shawdon H, Steiner RE. The pulmonary veins in left ventricular failure and mitral stenosis. Br J Radiol 1962;35:293.
34. Fleischner FG. Atypical arrangement of free pleural effusion. Radiol Clin North Am 1963;1:347.
35. Lavender JP, Doppman J. The hilum in pulmonary venous hypertension. Br J Radiol 1962;35:303.
36. Fleischner FG. The butterfly pattern of acute pulmonary edema. Am J Cardiol 1967;20:39.
37. Simon M. The pulmonary vasculature in congenital heart disease. Radiol Clin North Am 1968;6:303.
38. West JB, Dollery CT, Naimark A. Distribution of blood flow in isolated lung: relation to vascular and alveolar pressures. J Appl Physiol 1964;19:713.
39. West JB, Dollery CT. Distribution of blood-flow and the pressure-flow relations of the whole lung. J Appl Physiol 1965;20:175.
40. Permutt S. Effect of interstitial pressure of the lung on pulmonary circulation. Med Thorac 1965;22:118.
41. West JB, Dollery CT, Heard BE. Increased pulmonary vascular resistance in the dependent zone of the isolated dog lung caused by perivascular edema. Circ Res 1965;17:191.
42. Rodbard S, Kira S. The effect of airways pressure on the pulmonary circulation. Jpn Heart J 1966;1:369.
43. West JB, Glazier JB, Hughes JMB, Maloney JE. Recent work on the distribution of pulmonary blood flow and topographical differences in alveolar size. In: Cumming G, Hunt LB, eds. Form and function in the human lung. Baltimore: Williams & Wilkins, 1968.
44. Simon M. The pulmonary vessels: their hemodynamic evaluation using routine radiographs. Radiol Clin North Am 1963;1:363.
45. Simon M, Sasahara AA, Cannilla JE. The radiology of pulmonary hypertension. Semin Roentgenol 1967;2:368.
46. Murray JF. Effects of lung inflation on pulmonary arterial pressure in dogs with pulmonary edema. J Appl Physiol 1978;45:442.
47. Milne ENC, Bass H. The roentgenologic diagnosis of early chronic obstructive pulmonary disease. J Can Assoc Radiol 1969;20:3.
48. Bergofsky EH. Mechanisms underlying vasomotor regulation of regional pulmonary blood flow in normal and disease states. Am J Med 1974;57:378.
49. Smith HC, Butler J. Pulmonary venous waterfall and perivenous pressure in the living dog. J Appl Physiol 1975;38:304.
50. Giuntini C, Mariani M, Barsotti A, Fazio F, Santolicandro A. Factors affecting regional pulmonary blood flow in left heart valvular disease. Am J Med 1974;57:421.
51. Hales CA, Ahluwalia B, Kazemi H. Strength of pulmonary vascular response to regional alveolar hypoxia. J Appl Physiol 1975;38:1083.
52. Kolin A, MacAlpin R, Steckel R. Electromagnetic rheoangiometry: an extension of selective angiography. AJR 1978;130:13.
53. Fishman AP. The pulmonary circulation. JAMA 1978;293:1299.
54. Collins R, Maccario JA. Blood flow in the lung. J Biomech 1979;12:373.
55. Hughes JMB, Glazier JB, Maloney JE, West JB. Effect of interstitial pressure on pulmonary blood flow. Lancet 1967;1:192.
56. Hughes JMB, Glazier JB, Maloney JE, West JB. Effect of lung volume on the distribution of pulmonary blood flow in man. Respir Physiol 1968;4:58.
57. Friedman M, Wanner A. Volume characteristics of extra- and intraparenchymal segments of the canine pulmonary artery. J Appl Physiol 1977;42:519.

58. Malik AB, van der Zee H, Neumann PH, Gertzberg NB. Effects of pulmonary edema on regional pulmonary perfusion in the intact dog lung. J Appl Physiol 1980;49:834.
59. Bachofen H, Bachofen M, Weibel ER. Ultrasound aspects of pulmonary edema. J Thorac Imaging 1988;3(3):1.
60. Staub NC. New concepts about the pathophysiology of pulmonary edema. J Thorac Imaging 1988;3(3):8.
61. Pistolesi M, Miniati M, Giuntini C. State of the art: pleural liquid and solute exchange. Am Rev Respir Dis 1989;140: 825.
62. Milne ENC, Pistolesi M, Miniati M, Giuntini C. The vascular pedicle of the heart and the vena azygos: I. The normal subject. Radiology 1984;152:1.
63. Pistolesi M, Milne ENC, Miniati M, Giuntini C. The vascular pedicle of the heart and the vena azygos: II. Acquired heart disease. Radiology 1984;152:9.
64. Pistolesi M, Miniati M, Milne ENC, Giuntini C. The chest roentgenogram in pulmonary edema. Clin Chest Med 1985; 6:315.
65. Milne ENC. A physiologic approach to reading critical care unit films. J Thorac Imaging 1986;1(3):60.
66. Milne ENC, Pistolesi M, Miniati M, Giuntini C. The radiologic distinction of cardiogenic and non-cardiogenic edema. AJR 1985;144:879.
67. Hedlund LW, Vock P, Effmann EL, et al. Hydrostatic pulmonary edema: an analysis of lung density changes by computed tomography. Invest Radiol 1984;19:254.
68. Cutillo AG, Morris AM, Ailion DC, et al. Quantitative assessment of pulmonary edema by nuclear magnetic resonance methods. J Thorac Imaging 1986;1(3):60.
69. Smith RC, Mann H, Greenspan RH, et al. Radiographic differentiation between different etiologies of pulmonary edema. Invest Radiol 1987;22:859.
70. Milne ENC. Editorial. J Thorac Imaging 1988;3(3):6.
71. Miniati M, Pistolesi M, Paoletti P, et al. Objective radiographic criteria to differentiate cardiac, renal, and injury lung edema. Invest Radiol 1988;23:433.
72. Pistolesi M, Miniati M, Milne ENC, Giuntini C. Measurement of lung edema: the radiographic approach. Appl Cardiopulm Pathophysiol 1988;2:141.
73. Pistolesi M, Miniati M, Milne ENC, Giuntini C. Pulmonary edema. In: Sperber M, ed. Radiologic diagnosis of chest disease. New York: Springer-Verlag, 1990:355.
74. Bone RC, Goheen JR, Ruth WE. Radiographic, hemodynamic and clinical comparison of pulmonary venous hypertension complicating acute respiratory failure in severe chronic airway obstruction. Chest 1977;71(Suppl II):284.
75. Fraser GR, Pare JAP. Diagnosis of diseases of the chest. 3rd ed. Philadelphia: Saunders, 1990; vol. 3, chap. 10.
76. Milne ENC. Correlation of physiological findings with chest roentgenology. Radiol Clin North Am 1973;11:17.
77. Braunwald E. Heart disease: a textbook of cardiovascular medicine. Philadelphia: Saunders, 1980; chaps. 9, 24, 44.
78. Fishman AP. Respiratory gases in the regulation of the pulmonary circulation. Physiol Rev 1961;41:214.
79. McDonald DA. Blood flow in arteries. 2nd ed. Baltimore: Williams & Wilkins, 1974.
80. Anthonisen NR, Milic-Emili J. Distribution of pulmonary perfusion in erect man. J Appl Physiol 1966;21:760.
81. Chest films provide index of dynamic lung compliance. JAMA 1969;208:1782.
82. Milne ENC, Bass H. Relationship between specific dynamic compliance and diaphragmatic excursion. Radiology 1969; 92:615.
83. Beeckman P, Vanclooster R, Michels J, Silver D. A radiological study of the effects of left heart failure on regional lung differences. J Belge Radiol 1978;61:247.
84. Weibel ER, Bachofen H. Structural design of the alveolar septum and fluid exchange. In: Fishman AP, Renkin EM, eds. Pulmonary edema. Bethesda, MD: American Physiological Society, 1979.
85. Bryant LR, Cohn JE, O'Neill RP, Danielson GK, Greenlaw RH. Pulmonary blood flow distribution in chronic obstructive airway disease: lung scintiscanning and pulmonary arteriography. Am Rev Resp Dis 1968;97:832.
86. Farhi A, Burke H, Newman E, Klatte EC, Carwell G, Arnold T. The effect of exercise on the heart and the pulmonary vasculature: a preliminary report. Radiology 1968;91:488.
87. Fouche RF, Beck W, Schrirer V. The roentgenological assessment of left-to-right shunt in secundum type atrial septal defect. AJR 1963;89:254.
88. Milne ENC. The physiologic basis of pulmonary radiologic changes. In: Abrams HL, ed. Angiography. 2nd ed. Boston: Little, Brown, 1971; chap. 31.
89. Milne ENC, Bass H. Roentgenologic and functional analysis of combined chronic obstructive pulmonary disease and congestive cardiac failure. Invest Radiol 1969;4:129.
90. Hublitz UF, Shapiro JH. Atypical pulmonary patterns of congestive failure in chronic lung disease: the influence of preexisting disease on the appearance and distribution of pulmonary edema. Radiology 1969;93:995.
91. Rees S. The chest radiograph in pulmonary hypertension with central shunt. Br J Radiol 1968;41:172.
92. Logue RB, Rogers JV Jr, Gay BB Jr. Subtle roentgenographic signs of left heart failure. Am Heart J 1963;65:464.
93. Fleming PR, Simon M. The haemodynamic significance of intrapulmonary septal lymphatic lines (lines B of Kerley). J Fac Radiol 1958;9:33.
94. Milne ENC. Physiological interpretation of the plain radiograph in mitral stenosis, including a review of criteria for the radiological estimation of pulmonary arterial and venous pressures. Br J Radiol 1963;36:902.
95. Friedman WF, Braunwald E. Alterations in regional pulmonary blood flow in mitral valve disease studied by radioisotope scanning: a simple nontraumatic technique for estimation of left atrial pressure. Circulation 1966;34:363.
96. Milne ENC, Carlssen E. Physiological interpretation of the plain radiograph following mitral valvotomy, valvuloplasty and prosthetic replacement. Radiology 1969;92:1201.
97. Balbarini A, Limbruno V, Bertoli D, et al. Evaluation of pulmonary vascular pressures in cardiac patients: the role of the chest roentgenogram. J Thorac Imaging 1991;6(2):62.
98. Harison MO, Conte PJ, Heitzman ER. Radiological detection of clinically occult cardiac failure following myocardial infarction. Br J Radiol 1971;44:265.
99. Staub NC. The pathogenesis of pulmonary edema. Prog Cardiovasc Dis 1980;23:53.
100. Robin ED, Cross EC, Zelis R. Pulmonary edema (part 1). N Engl J Med 1973;288:239.
101. Robin ED, Cross CE, Zelis R. Pulmonary edema (part 2). N Engl J Med 1973;288:292.
102. Staub NC. Pulmonary edema. Physiol Rev 1974;54:687.
103. Rao BS, Cohn KE, Eldridge FL, Hancock EW. Left ventricular failure secondary to chronic pulmonary disease. Am J Med 1968;45:229.
104. Chinard FP, Enns T, Nolan MR. Indicator-dilution studies with "diffusible" indicators. Circ Res 1962;10:473.
105. Levine OR, Mellins RB, Fishman AP. Quantitative assessment of pulmonary edema. Circ Res 1965;17:414.
106. Van de Water JM, Sheh JM, O'Connor NE, Miller IT, Milne ENC. Pulmonary extravascular water volume: measurement and significance in critically ill patients. J Trauma 1970;10: 440.
107. Baudendistel L, Shields JB, Kaminiski DL. Comparison of double indicator thermodilution measurements of extravascular lung water (EVLW) with radiographic estimation of lung water in trauma patients. J Trauma 1982;22:983.

35

Anomalous Pulmonary Venous Connection

PAUL R. JULSRUD
KENNETH E. FELLOWS

Anomalous pulmonary venous connection is a congenital abnormality in which the pulmonary veins do not anatomically join the left atrium but connect directly to systemic veins, the right atrium, or the coronary sinus. A total anomalous pulmonary venous connection (TAPVC) exists when all pulmonary veins connect anomalously. A partial anomalous pulmonary venous connection (PAPVC) indicates that one or more, but not all, pulmonary veins are involved. In this chapter, the discussion of anomalous pulmonary venous connection does not include abnormalities in the number of pulmonary veins, stenotic but otherwise normal pulmonary connections, or variations in the mode of entrance of pulmonary veins into the left atrium (e.g., cor triatriatum).

Total Anomalous Pulmonary Venous Connection

TAPVC was first described in 1789.[1] The frequency of TAPVC is between 0.04 percent[2] and 2 percent[3,4] in various autopsy series of patients with congenital heart disease. It has accounted for 2.6 percent of the symptomatic cases of congenital cardiac disease in the New England Regional Infant Cardiac Program over a 10-year period.* This represents an incidence of 0.06 per 1000 live births. A male preponderance of 3.6:1.0 has been noted in TAPVC to the portal vein.[5] Anomalous connections to other sites are more evenly divided between the sexes, the male-female ratio being 1.6:1.0.[6] In addition to the presence of an atrial septal defect or a patent foramen ovale, which is necessary to sustain life, TAPVC is frequently associated with other congenital cardiac anomalies. Autopsy series of TAPVC report associated complex congenital cardiac anomalies in as much as 38 percent of cases. In patients with heterotaxy syndrome, TAPVC is frequently associated with other development abnormalities of the cardiovascular system.[6–9] Humes et al., in a study of 49 patients with heterotaxy syndrome who underwent a modified Fontan operation, found that 43 patients (88 percent) had anomalous pulmonary venous return.[10] TAPVC is also the most frequent cardiac malformation in patients with the cat's eye syndrome.[11]

Embryology

TAPVC can be understood best by a review of the developmental phases of normal pulmonary vein formation. Such a review can also help explain the possible pathogenesis of TAPVC. However, the exact etiology of these cardiovascular anomalies has not been proved, and any explanations are offered as likely possibilities rather than accepted facts.

At approximately 3 weeks of age (crown-rump length, 3 mm), the primordium of the respiratory system appears as an outgrowth from the ventral surface of the foregut.[12,13] Being a foregut derivative, the lung bud shares its early arterial and venous blood supply with the splanchnic plexus. The anastomotic venous channels that drain this area provide early continuity between the differentiating pulmonary vasculature and (1) the umbilicoomphalomesenteric (placental-portal) venous system and (2) the anterior and posterior cardinal veins (Fig. 35-1).[12–14]

In preparation for future normal cardiopulmonary circulation, a direct venous connection must be established between the pulmonary venous plexus and the developing heart. There is evidence that initially such

*The New England Regional Infant Cardiac Program includes essentially all infants with significant congenital heart disease in the first year of life who die, undergo cardiac catheterization, or have cardiac surgery at one of the 11 medical centers in New England. Data for TAPVC reported from July 1, 1968, to June 30, 1978.

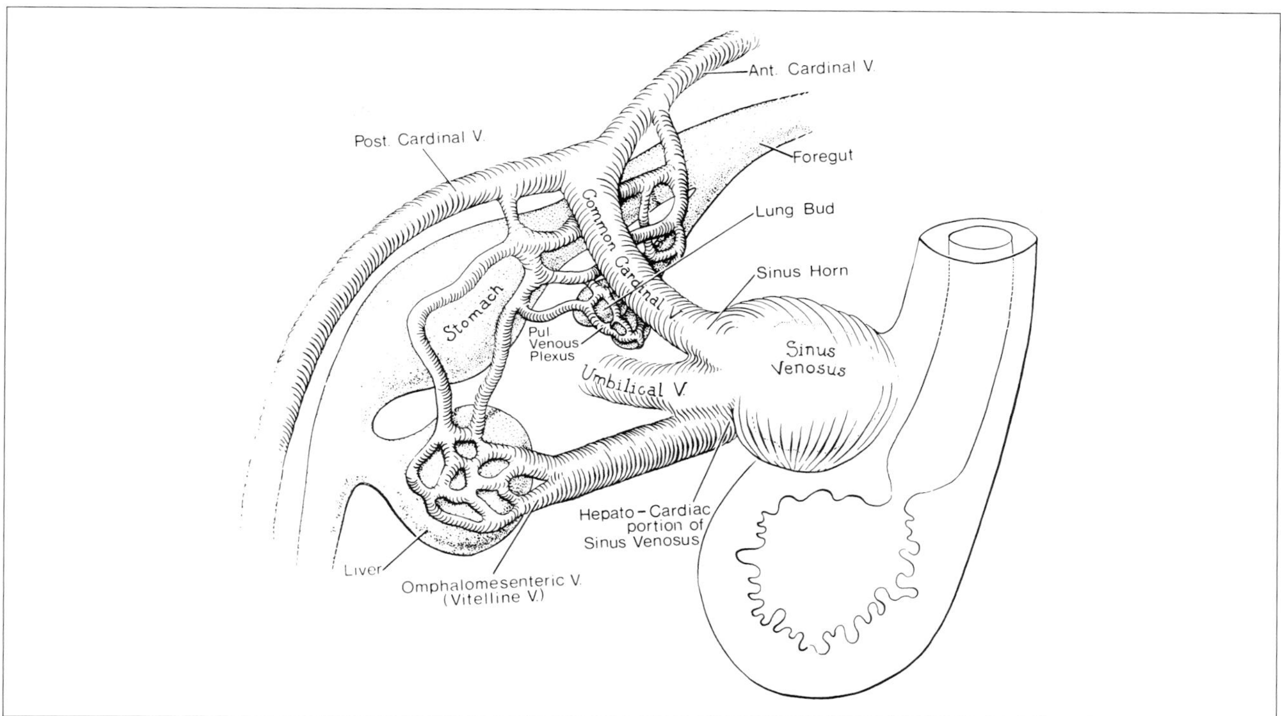

Figure 35-1. Lateral view of human embryo (approximately 3- to 4-mm stage). Venous plexus of the primitive lung buds drains systemically to anterior cardinal, posterior cardinal, and omphalomesenteric veins, which then connect with the heart at the sinus venosus.

venous connections are multiple, arising as evaginations from different areas of the sinus venosus–atrial portion of the developing heart tube.[15,16] Normally, one of them, referred to as the *common pulmonary vein,* originates as an evagination from the dorsal wall of the evolving left atrium, immediately to the left of the primitive interatrial septum.[6,14–18] In addition, there may be one or more similar dorsal evaginations arising from the sinus venosus.[15,16] The evaginations from the sinus venosus are caudal to the common pulmonary vein (Fig. 35-2). The evaginations from the sinus venosus together with the common pulmonary vein form vascular channels that anastomose with the pulmonary venous plexus. The direct cardiac connection thus provided shunts flow away from the earlier venous pathways (Fig. 35-3). Normally all the pulmonary venous connections to the sinus venosus involute. The common pulmonary vein arising from the left atrium persists as the sole conduit of pulmonary blood returning to the heart. The usual anatomic arrangement of four more or less separate pulmonary veins entering the left atrium is thought to result from differential growth that incorporates the common pulmonary vein into the left atrium.[18]

The presence of evaginations from the region of the sinus venosus, which could persist as pulmonary venous connections, helps to explain certain forms of TAPVC. Inasmuch as the differentiating sinus venosus develops several internal folds that partition off portions of the primitive right atrium, the right and left sinus horns, and the hepatocardiac venous channel, any of these structures could be the site of an early pulmonary venous connection.[15] This may account for TAPVC to the right atrium, the coronary sinus (derivative of the left sinus horn), the proximal superior vena cava (SVC) (derivative of the right sinus horn), and the inferior vena cava (IVC) above the hepatic veins (hepatocardiac component of the sinus venosus).

Regarding TAPVC to the right atrium, the postulated persistence of a direct cardiopulmonary venous connection originating from the right atrial portion of the sinus venosus provides an alternative to the theory of malalignment of the atrial septum.[18] If malalignment of the atrial septum to the left of the normal common pulmonary vein were the mechanism for anomalous pulmonary venous connection to the right atrium, one would expect the pulmonary veins to enter the right atrium between the coronary sinus and the interatrial septum. However, this was not found in available specimens, suggesting that the theory of malalignment of the atrial septum is not an entirely satisfactory explanation for this anomaly.

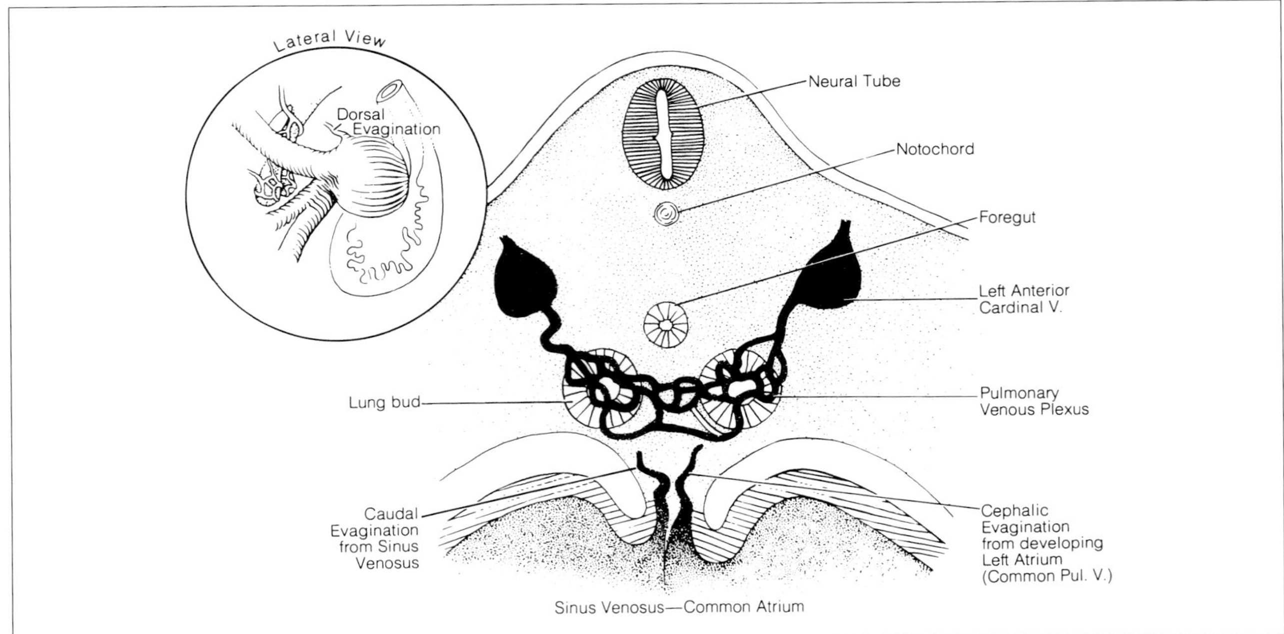

Figure 35-2. Transverse section of human embryo (slightly later than Fig. 35-1). A cephalic evagination (the primitive common pulmonary vein) extends from the developing left atrium toward the pulmonary venous plexus. Caudally, another evagination (which eventually disappears in normal individuals) also arises from the sinus venosus.

Figure 35-3. Transverse section similar to Figure 35-2 (but later stage). The dorsal evaginations (*a* and *b*) of the sinus venosus and left atrium have connected with the pulmonary venous plexus, establishing direct drainage from the lung buds to the heart and short-circuiting earlier (systemic venous) pathways.

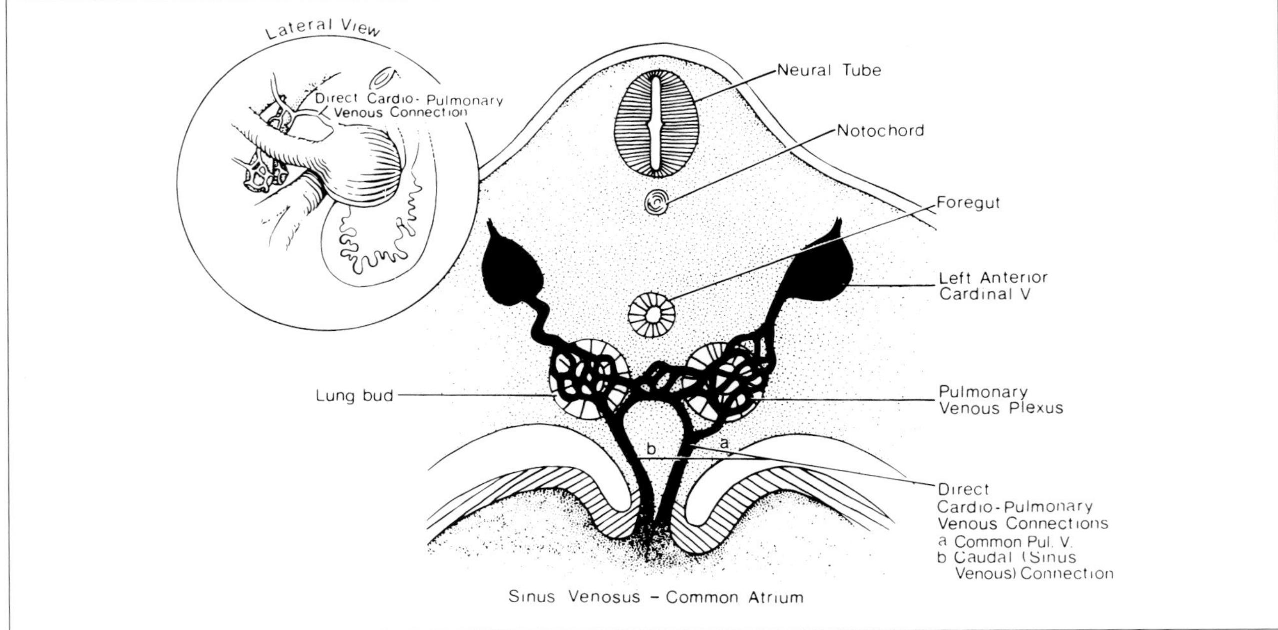

In addition to anomalous pulmonary venous connections directly to the derivatives of the sinus venosus, others may result from persistence of the earlier venous connections to the heart via the cardinal or omphalomesenteric (portal) systems (see Fig. 35-1). Absence of a direct connection between the heart and the primordial pulmonary veins is likely to promote continued flow through existing channels.[19] Depending on which collateral channels become dominant, the anomalous connection may be to the right SVC (above the azygos entrance), the left vertical vein (persistent left anterior cardinal vein draining to the left innominate vein), the left SVC (persistent left anterior cardinal vein draining to the coronary sinus), the proximal azygos vein (derivative of the posterior cardinal system), or to subdiaphragmatic veins (derivatives of the omphalomesenteric system).

Mixed forms of TAPVC exist when there is more than one type of anomalous connection present as a result of the persistence of two or more primitive pulmonary venous pathways in the same individual.

Table 35-1 summarizes the types of total anomalous pulmonary venous connection based on a current understanding of pulmonary vein formation. The various routes of anomalous connection associated with each type of TAPVC are listed with the embryologic structures from which they are derived.

Table 35-1. Types of TAPVC and Their Embryologic Derivatives

Type of TAPVC	Embryologic Analogue
Supracardiac	Cardinal veins
Left vertical vein	Left anterior (distal)
Left SVC	Left anterior (proximal)
Right SVC (cranial to azygos entrance)	Right anterior
Azygos vein	Right posterior
Cardiac	Sinus venosus
Right atrium	Right atrial portion
Coronary sinus	Left sinus horn
Right SVC (caudal to azygos entrance)	Right sinus horn
IVC (cranial to hepatic veins)	Hepatocardiac portion
Infracardiac	Omphalomesenteric veins
Portal vein	Fused vitelline veins
Persistent ductus venosus	Ductus venosus
IVC (caudal to hepatic veins)	Fused subcardinal and vitelline veins
Gastric veins	Splanchnic veins
Hepatic veins	Vitelline veins

Anatomy

TAPVC can be separated into four anatomic types: supracardiac, cardiac, infracardiac, and mixed.[3]

Supracardiac TAPVC

In supracardiac TAPVC, all pulmonary veins join to form a horizontal venous confluence posterior to the left atrium (Fig. 35-4A). In this chapter, a confluence of all the pulmonary veins is referred to as a *common pulmonary trunk* (CPT) rather than a *common pulmonary vein,* because to most students of embryology the latter term implies an origin from the left atrium. Pulmonary venous blood is then channeled via a remnant of the cardinal venous system to the right atrium.

Left-Sided Supracardiac TAPVC. TAPVC to the left vertical vein accounts for approximately one-third of all cases of TAPVC.[6,20] The large left vertical vein (persistent left anterior cardinal vein) usually courses anterior to the left pulmonary arteries, ascends in the superior mediastinum, and connects a horizontal common pulmonary trunk with the left innominate vein (see Fig. 35-4A, 1). Occasionally, the left vertical vein ascends between the left main stem bronchus and left pulmonary artery, creating obstruction to pulmonary venous return (see Fig. 35-4A,1).[21] Another site of obstruction sometimes found in this anomalous pathway is at the junction of the left innominate vein and the right SVC.[6] Less frequently, left-sided supracardiac TAPVC appears as a left SVC connecting a pulmonary venous confluence with the coronary sinus. Because this remnant of the left anterior cardinal system in this case joins the heart, it is properly called a *left SVC* (see Fig. 35-4A, 2).

Right-Sided Supracardiac TAPVC. Persistent pulmonary venous connections to remnants of the right cardinal system are much less common than to the left. In this form of TAPVC, the horizontal common pulmonary trunk connects with the right SVC (persistent right anterior cardinal vein) cranial to the entrance of the azygos vein much more frequently than with the azygos vein (remnant of the right posterior cardinal vein) (see Fig. 35-4A, 3,4).[6,20] The horizontal pulmonary venous confluence tends to be displaced superiorly and to the right as compared to its usual position directly posterior to the left atrium. In TAPVC of the right supracardiac type, there is a high incidence of obstruction caused by hypoplasia and stenosis of the anomalous pulmonary vein.[6]

Cardiac TAPVC

As previously discussed, TAPVC at the cardiac level may result from short-circuiting of pulmonary venous blood flow via direct connections between the sinus venosus and the pulmonary venous plexus. The most common derivatives of the sinus venosus receiving pulmonary veins are (1) the right atrium, (2) the coronary sinus, (3) the SVC below the azygos entrance, and (4) the IVC above the hepatic veins (see Fig. 35-4B). In cardiac forms of TAPVC, there is no confluence of

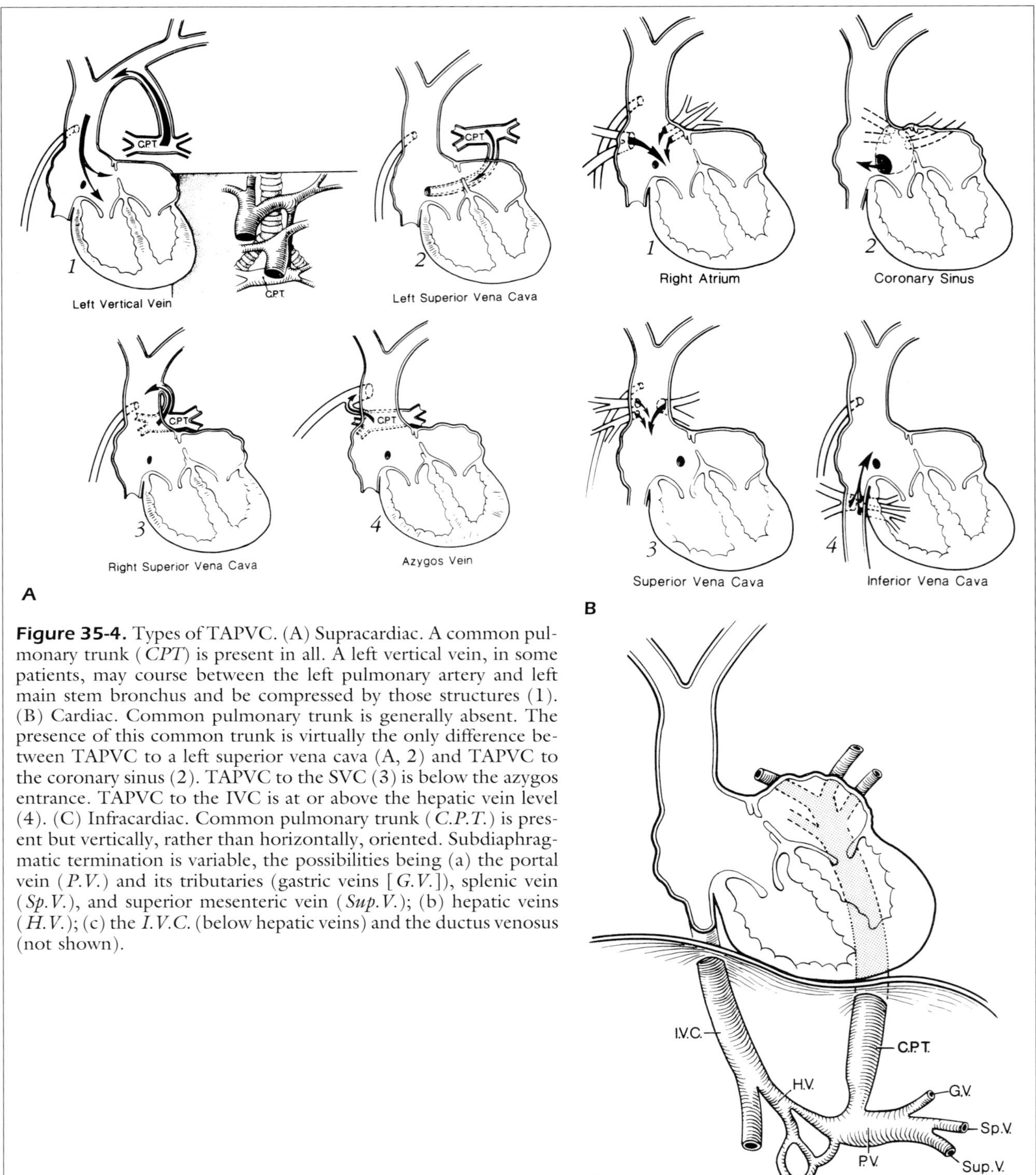

Figure 35-4. Types of TAPVC. (A) Supracardiac. A common pulmonary trunk (*CPT*) is present in all. A left vertical vein, in some patients, may course between the left pulmonary artery and left main stem bronchus and be compressed by those structures (1). (B) Cardiac. Common pulmonary trunk is generally absent. The presence of this common trunk is virtually the only difference between TAPVC to a left superior vena cava (A, 2) and TAPVC to the coronary sinus (2). TAPVC to the SVC (3) is below the azygos entrance. TAPVC to the IVC is at or above the hepatic vein level (4). (C) Infracardiac. Common pulmonary trunk (*C.P.T.*) is present but vertically, rather than horizontally, oriented. Subdiaphragmatic termination is variable, the possibilities being (a) the portal vein (*P.V.*) and its tributaries (gastric veins [*G.V.*]), splenic vein (*Sp.V.*), and superior mesenteric vein (*Sup.V.*); (b) hepatic veins (*H.V.*); (c) the *I.V.C.* (below hepatic veins) and the ductus venosus (not shown).

pulmonary veins forming a horizontal vein before making the anomalous connection.[22]

Infracardiac TAPVC

In TAPVC below the diaphragm, the pulmonary veins join to form a vertical common pulmonary venous trunk that descends through the esophageal hiatus to enter the portal or systemic venous circulation (see Fig. 35-4C).[23,24] A horizontal component in the cephalic segment of the venous confluence is usually not present. Except in rare cases, pulmonary venous return of the infracardiac type is severely obstructed.[25] The anomalous connection is ordinarily with a persistent ductus venosus or the portal vein.[6,20] Less commonly, the connection is with other subdiaphragmatic veins, such as the IVC, gastric, or hepatic veins.

Mixed TAPVC

TAPVC involving more than one anomalous pathway is relatively uncommon, accounting for only 5 to 7 percent of cases of TAPVC submitted to autopsy.[6,20] Patients with mixed TAPVC usually do not have a common pulmonary venous confluence. Mixed forms of TAPVC have been reported to be obstructed when a portion of the pulmonary venous flow drains subdiaphragmatically.[6] The mixed type of TAPVC is generally not associated with other major cardiac anomalies.[6]

Physiology

In TAPVC, all pulmonary veins drain either directly or indirectly to the right atrium, creating a complete left-to-right shunt at the atrial level. Therefore, to sustain life, an obligatory right-to-left shunt must also be present. With the exception of rare cases of TAPVC with right-to-left shunts via multiple ventricular septal defects (VSD) or a patent ductus arteriosus,[6,26] patients with TAPVC have either a patent foramen ovale or an atrial septal defect (ASD). Thus, in the absence of obstruction to pulmonary venous return, pulmonary blood flow is greatly increased, resulting in a large net left-to-right shunt at the atrial level (Fig. 35-5). This left-to-right shunt presents a volume overload to the right side of the heart that may produce dilatation of the right atrium, right ventricle, and main pulmonary artery.[27]

With obstruction either in the course of the anomalous vein or (rarely) at the level of the interatrial communication, the critical factor is the degree to which pulmonary return is impeded. Significant obstruction to pulmonary venous return has three serious consequences: (1) pulmonary venous (and arterial) hypertension, (2) pulmonary edema, and (3) diminished

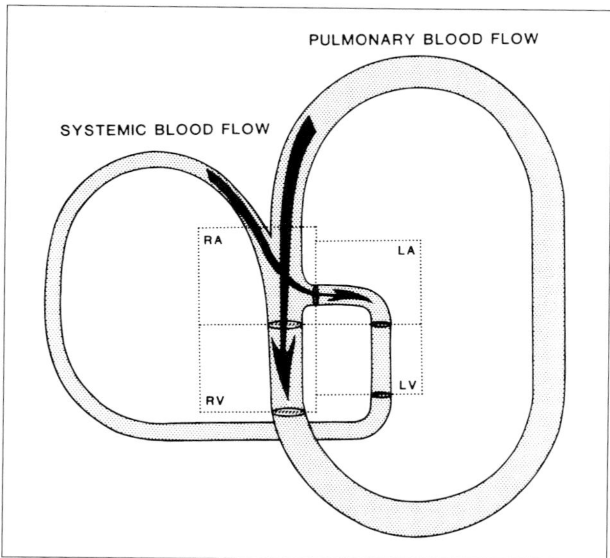

Figure 35-5. Diagram of systemic and pulmonary blood flow in TAPVC. A left-to-right shunt at the atrial level occurs because of the TAPVC; there is also an obligatory right-to-left shunt between the atria. Volume overload causes dilatation of the right heart chambers and increased pulmonary blood flow.

pulmonary return to the heart, which results in low cardiac output.

Thus, TAPVC includes a spectrum of physiologic abnormalities ranging from high pulmonary blood flow and a large net left-to-right shunt in the absence of obstruction to a low-flow state, and frequently pulmonary edema, as a consequence of anatomic obstruction to pulmonary venous return.

Clinical Aspects

The clinical presentation of patients with TAPVC depends on the presence or absence of obstruction. Where there is no pulmonary venous obstruction, the infant is usually asymptomatic at birth. The pulmonary blood flow and net left-to-right shunt increase during the first few weeks of life as the pulmonary vascular resistance decreases with normal maturation of the pulmonary vascular bed. As pulmonary flow increases, ventricular failure may develop and lead to pulmonary congestion and pulmonary edema. The clinical picture of congestive heart failure emerges. The failure is usually accompanied by mild cyanosis[22] and most frequently becomes clinically evident in the first month of life.[28] Mortality in the first year of life for uncorrected TAPVC without obstruction has been reported as low as 22 percent[28] and as high as 75 to 85 percent.[20,22] Because of improved techniques in open heart surgery

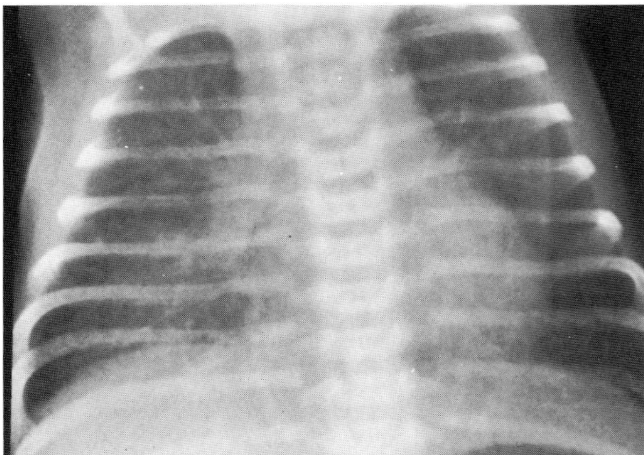

Figure 35-6. Obstructed infracardiac TAPVC in an infant. Heart size is normal. Interstitial pulmonary edema obscures the right hilar vessels. A reticular pattern of interstitial edema exists throughout but is best seen in the right lung.

in infants, immediate surgical correction is generally advocated in the symptomatic infant.[29–31] Surgery may be delayed in an asymptomatic patient.[30,32]

TAPVC with pulmonary venous obstruction presents differently. A cyanotic, tachypneic infant in the early newborn period is commonly seen. Pulmonary edema is usually present at birth, and the clinical appearance is that of congestive heart failure. Increased pressure in the pulmonary vasculature is transmitted to the right ventricle and may ultimately lead to right heart failure and low cardiac output. Deterioration is often progressive and rapid, resulting in death in a matter of days or weeks unless surgical correction is performed immediately.[22,28,33] The radiologist is often the first to suggest the proper diagnosis because of the frequent presence of interstitial pulmonary edema on the initial chest films (Fig. 35-6).

Table 35-2. Plain Film Findings in TAPVC

Feature	Obstructed TAPVC	Nonobstructed TAPVC
Heart size	Normal to decreased	Increased
Pulmonary artery size	Normal	Increased
Characteristic reticular pattern	Present	Absent
Prominent venous density	Rare—may be seen in obstructed supracardiac TAPVC	Frequently present, especially in supracardiac forms of TAPVC

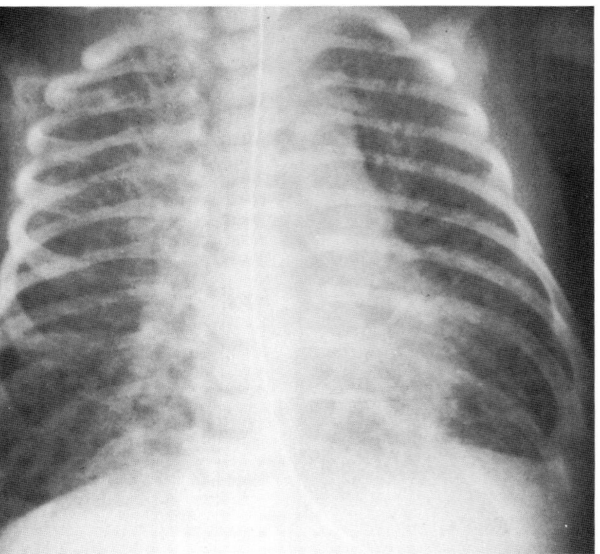

Figure 35-7. Obstructed supracardiac TAPVC (to a left vertical vein). The roentgenographic pattern is similar to that of Figure 35-6. Heart size is normal. Interstitial pulmonary edema obscures the hilar vessels and cardiac borders.

Radiology

Plain Film

The plain film findings vary in cases of TAPVC according to the anatomic and physiologic features that characterize the particular type of TAPVC involved. A summary of the plain film findings in TAPVC is provided in Table 35-2.

Obstructed TAPVC. TAPVC resulting in an acutely symptomatic newborn is almost always due to severe obstruction, which produces pulmonary edema. The great majority of the patients have an anomalous pulmonary venous connection below the diaphragm. High-grade obstruction causes severe pulmonary venous hypertension that presents a roentgen picture of abnormal pulmonary vascular markings and interstitial edema. The appearance is often described as a coarse reticular pattern with nodulolinear streaking, or as a fine mottling (see Fig. 35-6).[33–35] In addition, the individual pulmonary vessels are likely to be obscured by a diffuse haziness caused by perivascular edema. Kerley B septal lines and prominent upper lobe pulmonary veins are rarely seen but have been described in highly obstructed forms of TAPVC.[5] Occasionally, obstruction is found in supracardiac TAPVC and may produce the same plain film appearance[36] (Fig. 35-7).

Because pulmonary blood flow is not increased in obstructed forms of TAPVC, no volume overload is presented to the right heart. This accounts for the common plain chest film findings of a normal-sized

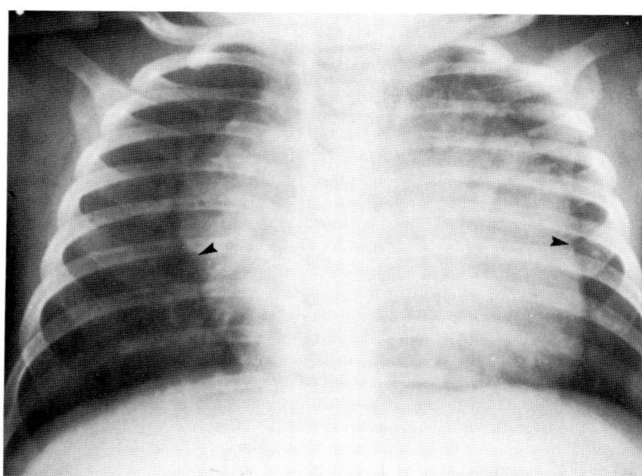

Figure 35-8. Nonobstructed TAPVC (to the coronary sinus). The heart is enlarged and the pulmonary vessels are engorged. There is, however, no pulmonary edema. Notches (*arrows*) along the cardiac borders identify the thymus as the cause of the wide mediastinum.

heart.[37] However, cardiomegaly may develop terminally as a result of hypoxemia and myocardial degeneration.

Nonobstructed TAPVC. The plain chest film findings in a child with nonobstructed TAPVC are quite different. In this form of TAPVC, increased pulmonary blood flow causes a volume overload to the right heart, producing enlargement of the right atrium, right ventricle, and pulmonary outflow tract. The end result is cardiomegaly and pulmonary arteries that are dilated centrally and peripherally (Fig. 35-8).[37] In the newborn, the fetal vascular resistance limits pulmonary flow, but, as the pulmonary resistance falls in the first few weeks of life, the flow increases and may result in pulmonary vascular congestion.

Prominent Venous Structures in TAPVC. In addition to the two general radiographic appearances characterizing obstructed and nonobstructed TAPVC, the presence of an enlarged venous channel may produce a striking plain film finding that is pathognomonic of certain types of TAPVC. Whether such a venous structure is detectable is determined by the site of the anomalous connection and, occasionally, the age of the patient.

The most frequently visualized venous channel occurs on the anteroposterior chest radiograph of a patient with TAPVC to the left vertical vein. The large left vertical vein produces a left superior mediastinal density as it arches cranially to join the left innominate vein. A similar right-sided superior mediastinal density results from dilatation of the right SVC, which receives flow from the left innominate vein. The combined density produced by these dilated venous structures causes a characteristic radiographic appearance that has been described as a "snowman" or a "figure-of-eight" (Fig. 35-9).[38] The presence of this "typical" radiographic configuration is somewhat age-dependent because it may be confused with the thymic shadow (see Fig. 35-8). Therefore, it is rarely a reliable sign in patients under 4 months of age and is usually not present until 4 to 6 years of age.[28,39,40] A lateral view of the chest may show a pretracheal density corresponding to the anomalous pulmonary venous channel and dilated innominate vein before the appearance of the snowman on the anteroposterior chest film.[41] For this reason, a lateral view may be helpful in suggesting the proper diagnosis in a young patient (Fig. 35-10).

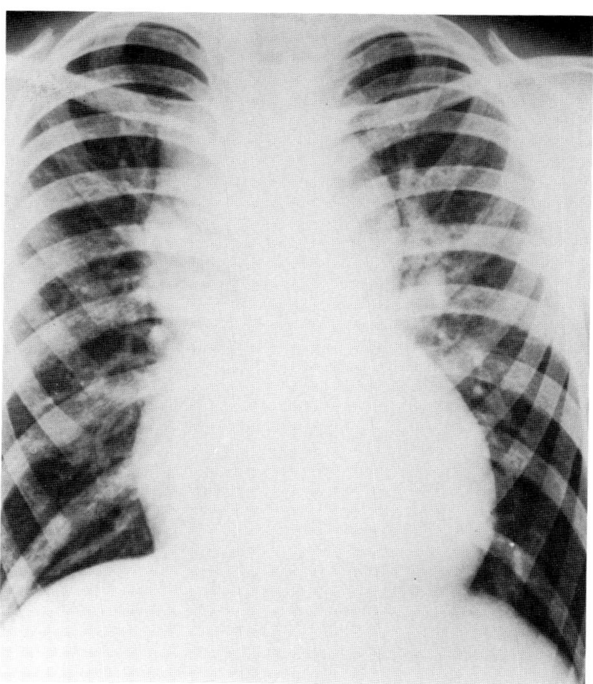

Figure 35-9. TAPVC to a left vertical vein producing a characteristic snowman or figure-of-eight silhouette. The mediastinum is broadened by dilatation of the left vertical vein and the right superior vena cava, which carry an increased volume of blood. The heart is enlarged and the pulmonary flow is increased.

Although TAPVC to the left vertical vein is usually unobstructed, the left vertical vein may be compressed if it ascends between the left pulmonary artery and the left main stem bronchus to enter the left innominate vein (see Fig. 35-4A, 1). In this case, an area of poststenotic dilatation may be identifiable on the plain chest film (Fig. 35-11).

TAPVC to either the right SVC or the azygos vein may produce mass densities on plain films that repre-

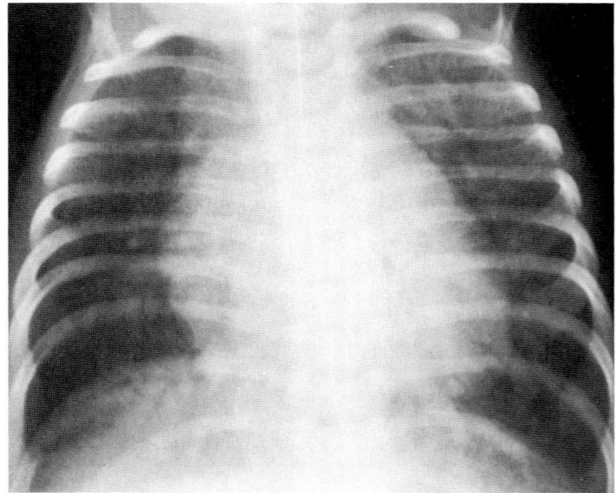

A

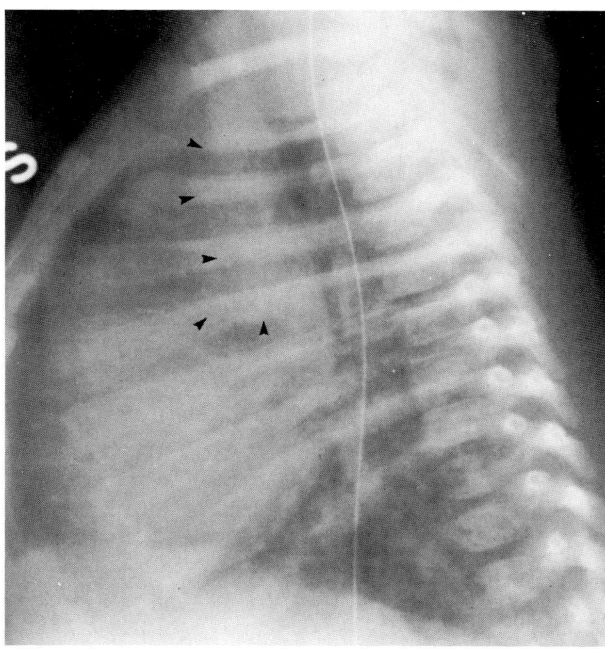

B

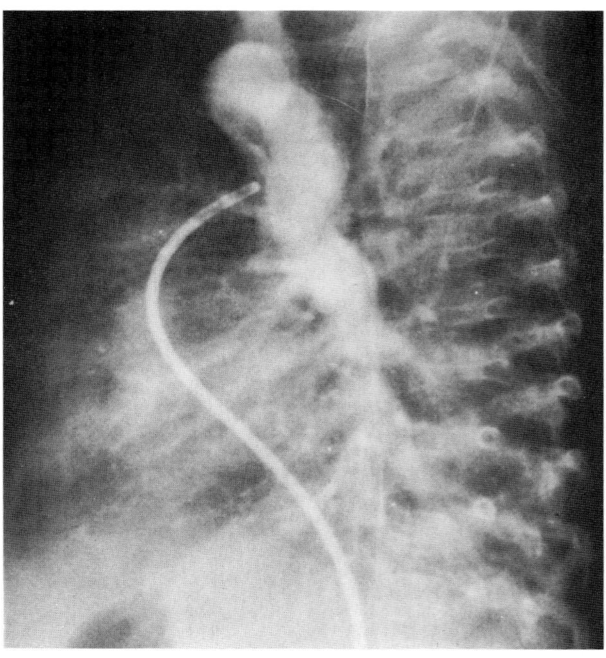

C

Figure 35-10. TAPVC to a left vertical vein in an infant. (A) Frontal chest film. The heart is enlarged, and pulmonary flow is increased. The snowman configuration is not present. The left vertical vein is either obscured by thymus or not dilated enough to be seen. (B) Lateral chest film. A large, pretracheal density (mass) represents superimposition of the left vertical and innominate veins. This density, combined with the findings in (A), suggests the correct diagnosis. (C) Venous phase of pulmonary arteriogram, lateral view. Compare with (B). The superimposed left vertical and innominate veins are opacified by the anomalously draining pulmonary veins.

sent dilatation of those structures receiving the anomalous return.[42,43] This sign is not specific, however, as is illustrated in Figure 35-12. Although plain films (see Fig. 35-12A) were interpreted as displaying a dilated azygos vein, angiocardiography showed that the mass density was actually a tortuous anomalous pulmonary confluence terminating in the right SVC (see Fig. 35-12B).

A detectable plain film density due to an anomalous pulmonary venous pathway is usually associated with supracardiac forms of TAPVC. However, in infracardiac TAPVC, a pulmonary confluence forms a vertical trunk that may produce a density in the clear space posterior to the cardiac shadow on a lateral chest film (Fig. 35-13). The plain film findings can be further extended by the use of a barium esophagram. A localized indentation on the anterior aspect of a barium-filled esophagus can be produced by the anomalous venous channel in TAPVC to the coronary sinus[44] and below the diaphragm.[45] In TAPVC to the coronary sinus, the discrete anterior impression on the esophagus is due to an enlarged coronary sinus.[44] Infracardiac TAPVC produces a broader anterior indentation of the lower esophagus caused by the common pulmonary venous trunk.[45]

Finally, as in all of diagnostic radiology, the entire plain film must be examined for additional information. This is especially pertinent regarding the abdominal situs, because a horizontal, symmetric liver with

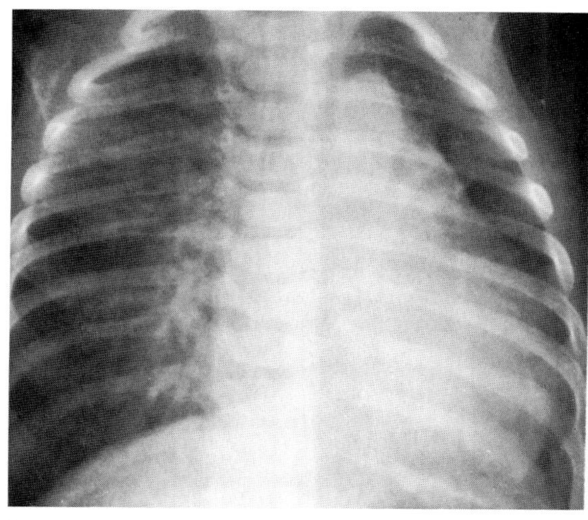

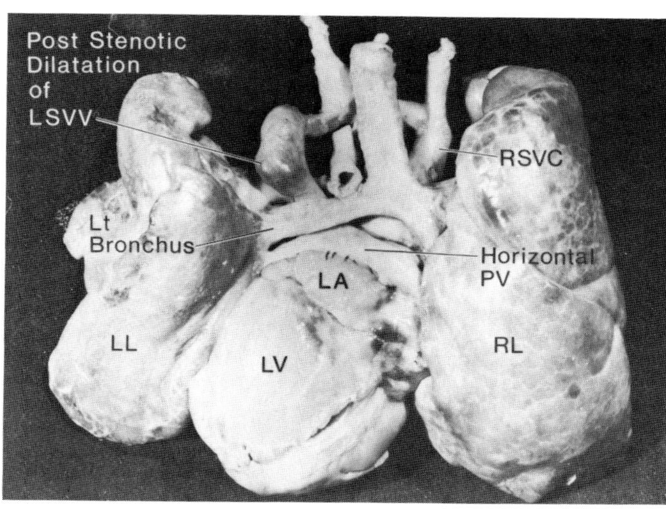

A B

Figure 35-11. TAPVC to a left vertical vein. (A) Frontal chest film displaying a localized left superior mediastinal density. The heart is enlarged, and the pulmonary flow is increased. (B) Posterior view, postmortem specimen of heart and lungs. The left superior vertical vein (*LSVV*) is dilated cranial to its compression between the left main stem bronchus and the left pulmonary artery. *Lt,* left; *LL,* left lung; *LV,* left ventricle; *LA,* left atrium; *RL,* right lung; *PV,* pulmonary vein; *RSVC,* right superior vena cava. (From Delisle G, et al. Total anomalous pulmonary venous connection: report of 93 autopsied cases with emphasis on diagnostic and surgical considerations. Am Heart J 1976;91:99. Used with permission.)

Figure 35-12. TAPVC to superior vena cava. (A) Plain film. In addition to cardiomegaly and increased pulmonary flow, there is a mass density at the right hilus (*arrows*). The findings erroneously suggested TAPVC to a (dilated) azygos vein. (B) The venous phase of a pulmonary artery injection demonstrates a horizontal common pulmonary trunk connecting to the superior vena cava (*SVC*) and accounting for the plain film abnormality. There is reflux into the normal azygos vein (*az*).

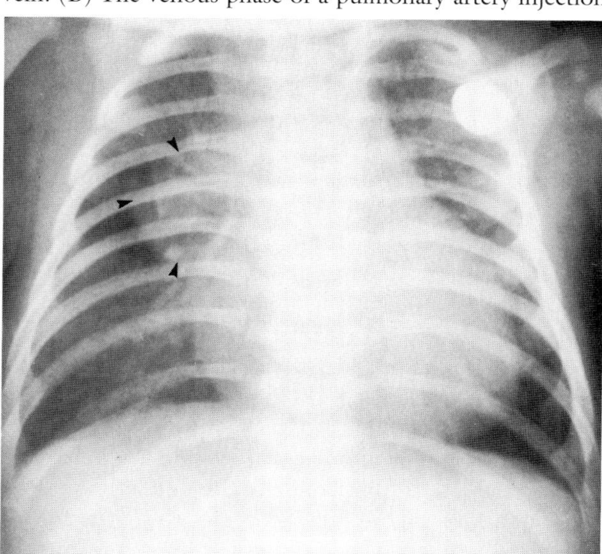

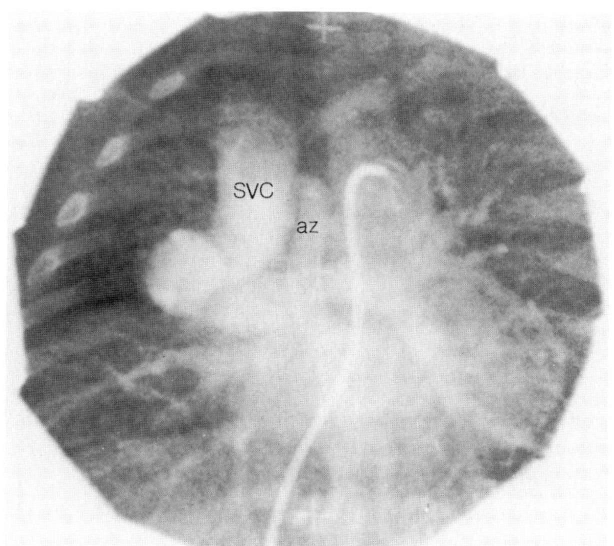

A B

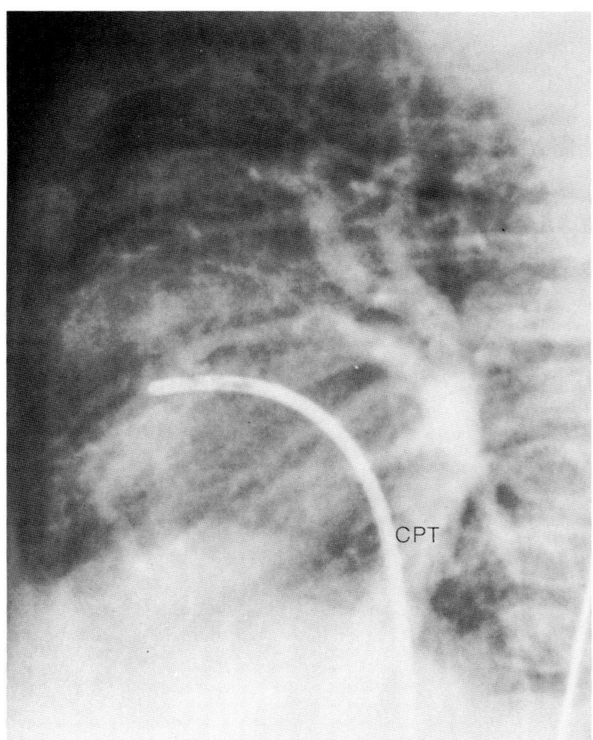

Figure 35-13. TAPVC to the portal vein. Lateral projection (levo phase of a right ventricular angiocardiogram) shows the pulmonary veins joining behind the heart to form a vertical common pulmonary trunk (*CPT*) that descends in the retrocardiac clear space to pass below the diaphragm.

an abnormally located gastric bubble may indicate the presence of a heterotaxy syndrome. Heterotaxy syndromes are found in approximately 25 percent of autopsy cases of TAPVC.[6,46]

Angiography

Although two-dimensional echocardiography with Doppler interrogation and magnetic resonance imaging have been found to be extremely helpful in the diagnosis of TAPVC,[47–55] angiography continues to be a commonly used technique for delineating the pathologic anatomy critical to proper management. In particular, angiographic techniques allow precise demonstration of the site, or sites, of connection of the anomalously draining pulmonary veins. The presence of a mixed form of TAPVC can be identified, alerting the clinician to this serious variety of TAPVC. Localization of the site of an obstruction may also be important and is best accomplished angiocardiographically.

Cardiac Catheterization. Angiocardiography is usually performed in conjunction with a complete cardiac catheterization. Before angiography, catheterization provides valuable information regarding cardiovascular pressures and oxygen saturations. Samples of blood taken from multiple systemic sites during cardiac catheterization often identify the level of an abnormal step-up in oxygen saturation that differentiates supracardiac, cardiac, and infracardiac forms of TAPVC. If, for example, the oxygen saturation step-up is located in the left innominate vein, it is good evidence that a connection exists between it and a left vertical vein receiving the pulmonary venous drainage. If, on the other hand, a step-up in oxygen saturation is found in the right SVC with a normal oxygen saturation in the left innominate vein, a form of right-sided supracardiac TAPVC is probably present with anomalous pulmonary venous drainage directly into the right SVC or the azygos vein. Occasionally, the level of step-up in oxygen saturation may be misleading. In TAPVC directly to the right atrium or coronary sinus, reflex of the right atrial blood may occur into either the SVC or the IVC, in which case an erroneous diagnosis of supracardiac or infracardiac TAPVC may be entertained. In addition, a step-up in oxygen saturation is not always present in infracardiac forms of TAPVC.[56]

Angiographic Technique. The anomalously connecting pulmonary venous channels are usually adequately visualized with biplane angiocardiography during the levo phase of a main pulmonary artery injection. The amount of contrast material injected should be 1.0 to 1.5 ml per kilogram of body weight, and it should be delivered in 1.0 to 1.5 seconds. If there is a patent ductus arteriosus producing a large right-to-left shunt, as is particularly common in obstructive forms of TAPVC,[28,57] much of the contrast material may be lost to the systemic arterial circulation. In this case, selective injections in the proximal right and left pulmonary arteries may be necessary to visualize the pulmonary venous connections adequately. Filming of pulmonary artery injections must continue long enough into the levo phase to allow filling of the anomalous pulmonary venous channels with contrast agent. Filming for 10 to 15 seconds has been recommended.[58] The angiographer must also be ready to make adjustments during cine filming to ensure that the area of interest is located in the field of view, which suddenly may turn out to be below the diaphragm, at the cardiac level, or in the superior mediastinum.

Retrograde injections into the anomalous pulmonary venous channels also provide good anatomic definition, provided that pulmonary blood flow is not so great that it washes out the contrast material too rapidly. Catheter manipulation into a left vertical vein is frequently accomplished without difficulty, and an angiogram may be obtained to demonstrate the anomaly. When angiography is done in conjunction with a pullback pressure tracing, any site of obstruction can be precisely identified. Similarly, retrograde catheterization of an enlarged coronary sinus or anomalous channel draining to the right SVC is often easily performed. A retrograde injection into the portal venous system via umbilical vein catheterization has been advocated in the neonatal period when an infracardiac type of TAPVC is suspected from a clinical presentation and plain chest film findings.[59,60]

Left ventricular angiograms are not routinely necessary but add information regarding left ventricular size and function, left ventricular outflow obstruction, and the status of the ventricular septum. Although the left ventricle may appear small in patients with TAPVC,[61,62] especially relative to the dilated right ventricle, its volume usually does not prohibit corrective surgery.[63]

Finally, because mixed forms of TAPVC are frequently misdiagnosed (hence their grave prognosis[30]), additional modifications in technique to exclude their presence may be needed. If, after the initial angiocardiographic procedure, doubt remains as to the site of drainage of one of the lungs or one of its segments, selective injections either into the appropriate pulmonary artery or into the anomalous pulmonary confluence are indicated to define further the pulmonary venous pathways and to establish the presence or absence of a mixed form of TAPVC.

In supracardiac TAPVC, the confluence of pulmonary veins forms a horizontal trunk before it connects with the systemic circulation. In anomalous return via a left vertical vein, the angiographic appearance demonstrates the prominent venous channel accounting for the snowman seen on plain chest films (Fig. 35-14). Right-sided supracardiac TAPVC to either the azygos vein or right SVC (see Fig. 35-12) is associated with a horizontal pulmonary venous trunk that is often displaced superiorly and to the right of its usual position behind the left atrium. This altered anatomy may be significant when surgical anastomosis of the horizontal trunk to the left atrium is undertaken.[29]

The two forms of TAPVC at the cardiac level, to the coronary sinus and directly to the right atrium, can be differentiated preoperatively with angiocardiography. In TAPVC to the coronary sinus, the contast-filled dilated coronary sinus forms a characteristic oval or egg-shaped density with its long axis oriented vertically (Fig. 35-15A).[64,65] On lateral view, the posterior and inferior wall of the dilated coronary sinus often forms a sharp, curvilinear J-shaped contour before entering the right atrium (see Fig. 35-15B). The anatomy can also be seen on a retrograde injection into the coronary sinus (Fig. 35-16). In TAPVC to the right atrium, the filling of the right atrium also produces an oval density in the frontal projection; but, unlike TAPVC to the coronary sinus, the oval has a horizontally oriented long axis and is more laterally located (Fig. 35-17).

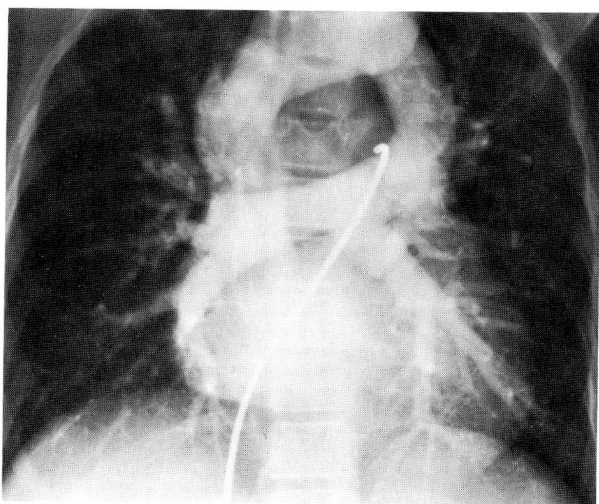

Figure 35-14. TAPVC to a left vertical vein (snowman). The levo phase of a pulmonary artery injection demonstrates the vascular structures responsible for the snowman configuration seen on plain films. The pulmonary veins join to form a horizontal common pulmonary trunk that drains successively to a dilated left vertical vein, an innominate vein, and the right superior vena cava.

Infracardiac TAPVC has a vertically oriented common pulmonary trunk that courses inferiorly in the posterior mediastinum to enter the abdomen (Fig. 35-18). The orientation of this common pulmonary trunk as well as variations that occur in its configuration are of surgical importance.[23] Occasionally, the individual pulmonary veins join at different levels along the common pulmonary trunk. Preoperative knowledge of this type of anatomic variation in infracardiac TAPVC is important to the surgeon.[24,66]

Angiographic visualization of two sites of anomalous drainage in a patient makes the diagnosis of mixed TAPVC. Figure 35-19 illustrates a form of mixed TAPVC involving both supracardiac and infracardiac structures. Since mixed forms of TAPVC usually do not have a horizontal venous confluence, corrective surgery may be more difficult. Thus preoperative planning depends on an adequate demonstration of the anatomy involved.

Partial Anomalous Pulmonary Venous Connection

The true incidence of PAPVC is difficult to estimate because it is likely that a number of patients with PAPVC are clinically unrecognized. Autopsy series of

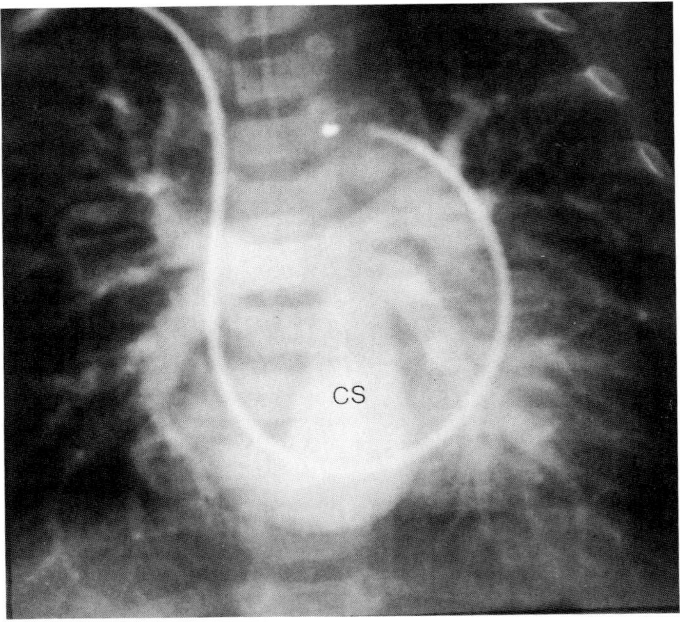

A

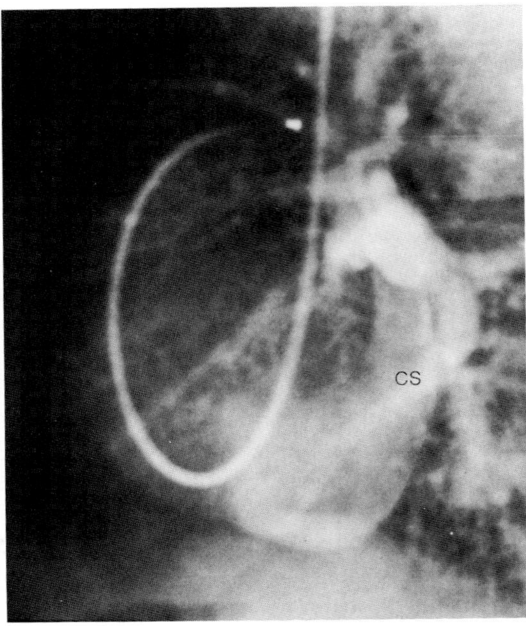

B

Figure 35-15. TAPVC to coronary sinus (levo phase of pulmonary artery injection). (A) Frontal view shows the pulmonary veins draining directly to the coronary sinus (*CS*). Typically, the CS is vertically oriented and slightly oval or egg-shaped. (B) In lateral view the posterior wall of the dilated CS is J-shaped.

patients with congenital heart disease describe frequencies of 0.5 to 7.0 percent[67,68] with no male or female preponderance noted.[69] Atrial septal defects have been reported in approximately 50 percent of cases.[70] However, this finding depends on the site of anomalous connection; a 90 percent incidence of ASD has been reported in PAPVC to either the SVC or the right atrium, whereas only a 15 percent incidence occurs with PAPVC to the IVC.[71] An ASD is almost never associated with PAPVC from the left lung.[72,73] Conversely, 9 percent of 664 patients with an ASD have been found to have associated PAPVC.[74] Other congenital cardiac malformations occasionally associated with PAPVC are VSD, tetralogy of Fallot, pulmo-

Figure 35-16. TAPVC to coronary sinus (retrograde injection into a right pulmonary vein). The coronary sinus (*CS*) is dilated, vertical in its orientation, and oval in shape.

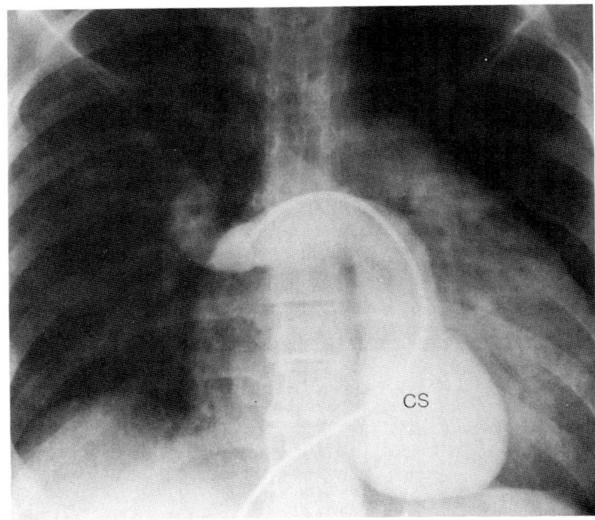

Figure 35-17. TAPVC to right atrium (levo phase of a pulmonary artery injection). Compare with TAPVC to coronary sinus in Figures 35-15 and 35-16. The oval opacification is farther to the right and not vertically oriented. *RA,* right atrium.

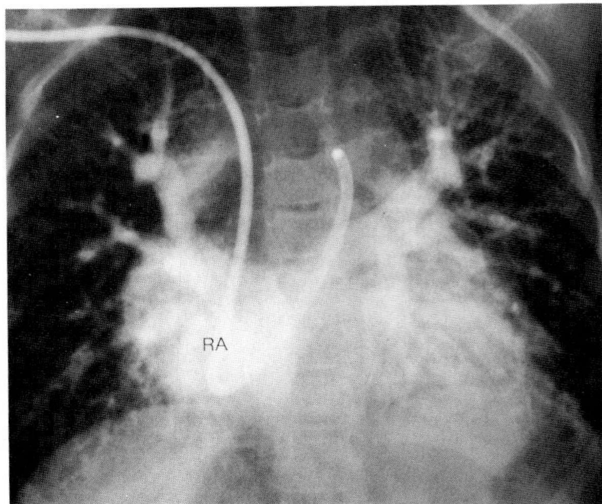

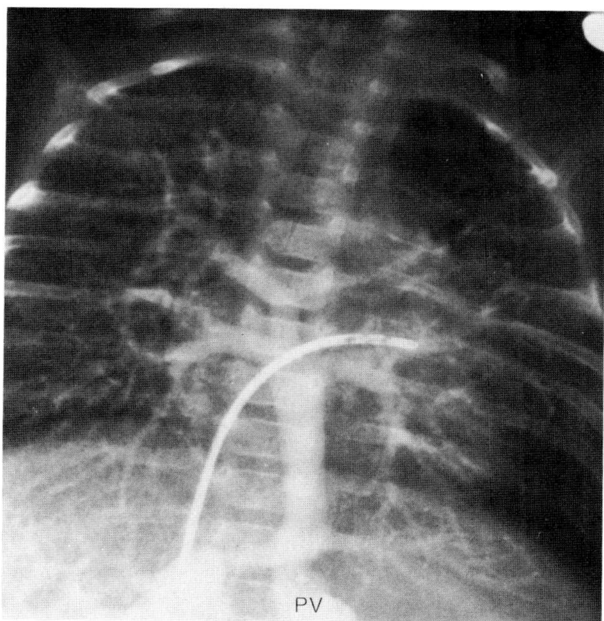

Figure 35-18. TAPVC to portal vein (levo phase of pulmonary artery injection). A treelike confluence of pulmonary veins forms a vertically oriented common pulmonary trunk that penetrates the diaphragm to join the portal vein (*PV*).

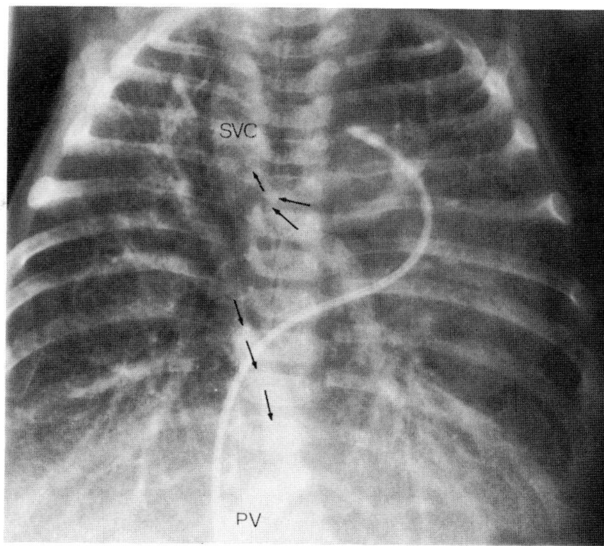

Figure 35-19. Mixed TAPVC (levo phase of pulmonary artery injection). Left pulmonary veins connect to the superior vena cava (*SVC*) and the right pulmonary veins drain to the portal vein (*PV*).

nary valve atresia and VSD, coarctation of the aorta, common atrium, and single ventricle.[70] Mitral valve stenosis and regurgitation, secondary to both congenital and rheumatic heart disease, have also been reported in patients with PAPVC.[75,76]

Embryology

The embryologic abnormalities responsible for PAPVC are thought to be similar to those described for TAPVC, differing primarily in degree. However, several forms of PAPVC deserve special consideration because of their unique developmental anatomy.

In PAPVC of the right lung to the SVC, there is a very high (90 percent) incidence of a sinus venosus ASD.[71] An explanation is that a dorsal evagination takes origin from the sinus venosus in the region of its junction with the right sinus horn. An anomalous pulmonary venous connection arising in this location may prevent closure of the sinus venosus portion of the interatrial septum. An alternative hypothesis has been suggested which postulates that the sinus venosus defect represents persistence of a venous connection normally found in the fetus between the pulmonary veins and the superior caval vein.[77]

Another form of PAPVC that has distinct characteristics and embryologic development is clinically named the *scimitar syndrome*. This multifaceted anomaly, involving much more than the pulmonary veins, appears to be related to abnormal regional development of the right lung and may be due to an early alteration in the epitheliomesenchymal interaction necessary for normal pulmonary organogenesis.[78]

Finally, the persistence of a left pulmonary venous connection to a remnant of the left anterior cardinal system, referred to as the *levo-atrial-cardinal vein* (LACV), results in a rare form of PAPVC.[79,80] See Fig. 35-20.

Anatomy

PAPVC may involve a single pulmonary vein or almost all the pulmonary veins, although rare, mixed forms of PAPVC involving both lungs occur (Fig. 35-21). Anomalous connections from the right lung are much more frequent than from the left.[70,81] The most common sites of anomalous connection from the right lung are to the SVC and the right atrium, the former being twice as frequent as the latter.[70] When the left lung is involved, the connection is usually to a left vertical vein and less commonly to the coronary sinus.[82] Infrequent sites of connection include the inferior vena cava, azygos vein, and left subclavian vein.[70]

The anatomy of PAPVC is similar to that of TAPVC except that not all the pulmonary veins are connected anomalously, and obstruction of the veins involved is

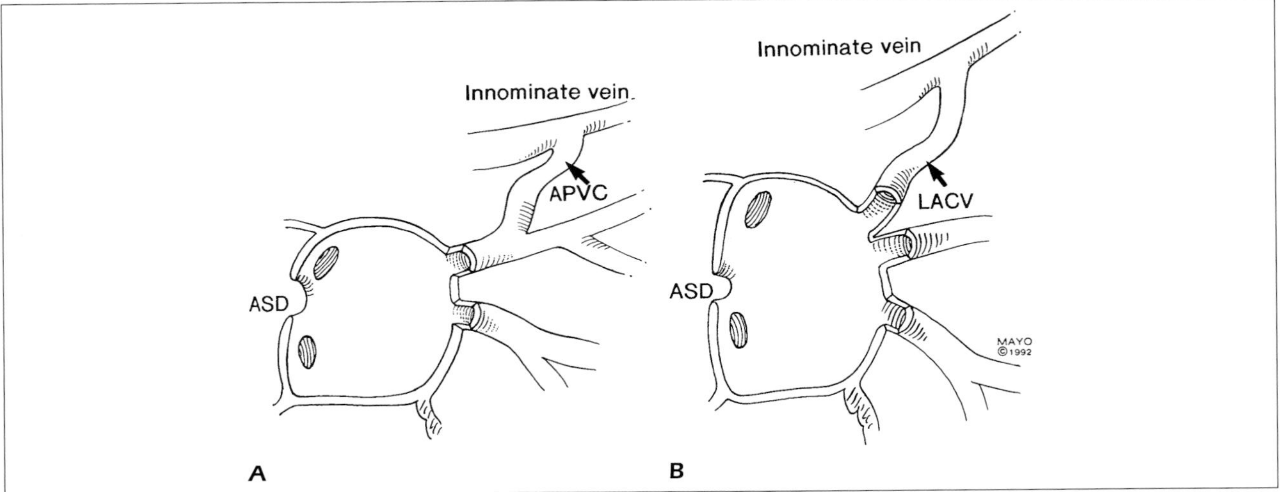

Figure 35-20. (A) Anomalous pulmonary venous connection (*APVC, arrow*) connecting the left upper pulmonary vein to the left innominate vein. (B) Incorporation of part of the left upper pulmonary vein into the left atrium results in the formation of levo-atrial-cardinal vein (*LACV, arrow*). The LACV connects the left atrium to the left innominate vein (a derivative of the anterior cardinal system). Note the absence of the mitral valve and a small atrial septal defect (*ASD*).

rarely present. However, PAPVC of the right lung to either the SVC or the IVC and PAPVC of the left lung to a LACV have anatomic characteristics that deserve mention.

PAPVC of the right lung to the SVC is associated in 90 percent of patients with an atrial septal defect.[71] The type of ASD found in these cases is usually a sinus venosus defect characterized by a location above the fossa ovalis (adjacent to the orifice of the SVC) with its roof formed by the posterior wall of the atria. Given the presence of a sinus venosus ASD, there is an 83 percent incidence of associated PAPVC involving the right lung.[83] In PAPVC from the right lung to the SVC, one-third of cases involve pulmonary venous drainage from the right upper lobe alone, one-third both the right upper and middle lobes, and one-third from the entire right lung.[83]

Figure 35-21. Mixed PAPVC (levo phase of pulmonary artery injection). Pulmonary veins from the right and left lower lobes connect with the left atrium (*LA*). The right upper lobe pulmonary vein connects with the superior vena cava (*single arrow*). The left upper pulmonary vein (*double arrow*) connects with a levo-atrial-cardinal vein (see Fig. 35-27).

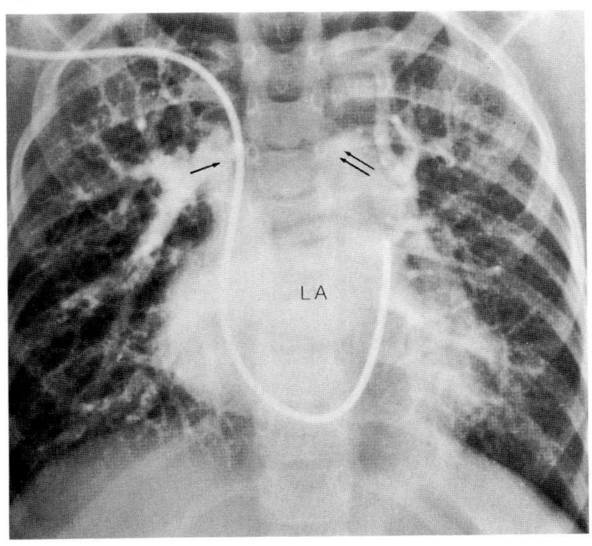

In addition to an associated sinus venosus ASD in cases of PAPVC to the SVC, frequently there is localized dilatation of the SVC just proximal to its junction with the right atrium, although the anomalous veins may connect to the SVC well above the dilated segment.[84]

PAPVC resulting in partial or total right lung drainage to the IVC accounts for approximately 5 percent of cases of PAPVC.[71] Besides being much rarer than PAPVC of the right lung to the SVC, it is accompanied by an intact atrial septum in about 85 percent of the cases.[71] Furthermore, in PAPVC of the right lung to the IVC, there are frequently associated anomalies of the ipsilateral hemithorax involving the bronchopulmonary tree, pulmonary artery, systemic collateral arteries, hemidiaphragm, and adjacent extrapleural tissues. This set of anomalies is commonly referred to as the *scimitar syndrome,* although in any given case not all the associated anomalies need be present.

The scimitar syndrome takes its name from the "scimitar sign," a description of the radiographic finding on an anteroposterior chest film of a broad,

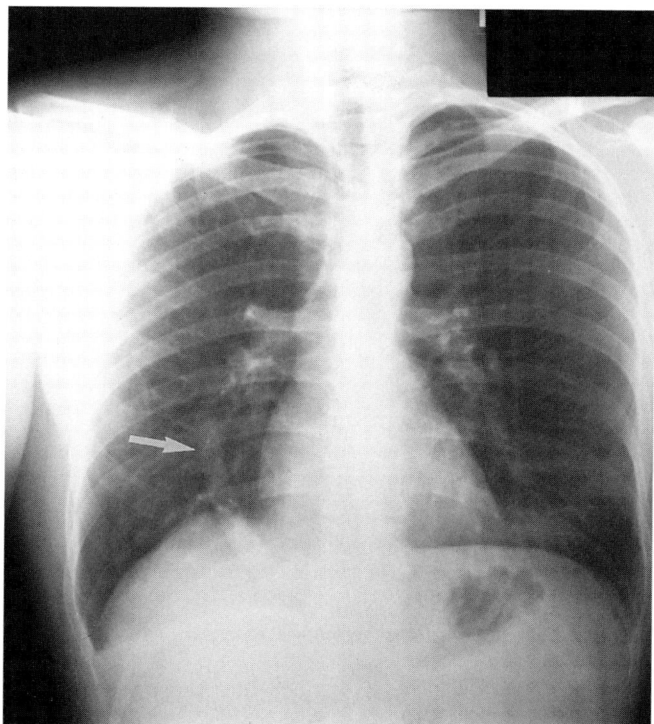

A

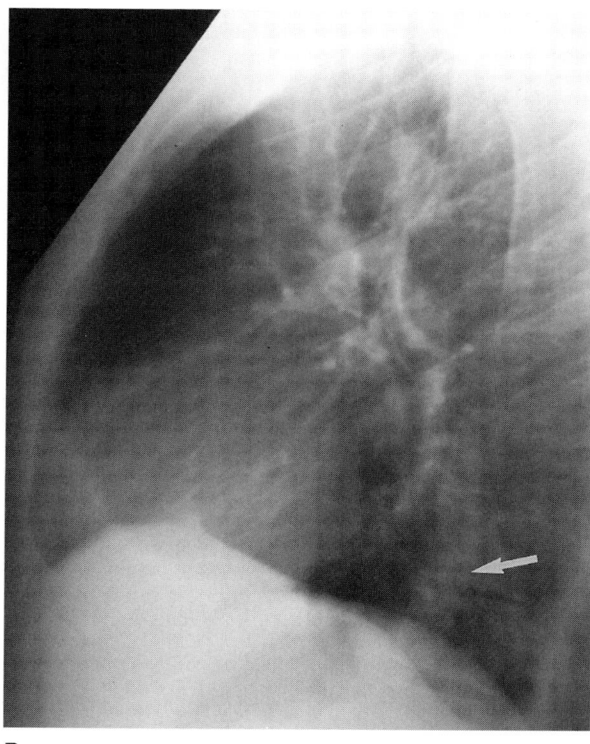

B

Figure 35-22. Scimitar syndrome. (A) Frontal chest film displays a slight shift of the heart to the right due to hypoplasia of the right lung (note that the ribs are closer together on the right). The scimitar sign is produced by the vertically oriented pulmonary vein (*arrow*) as it courses toward the IVC–right atrium junction. (B) Lateral chest (same patient) shows the anomalous vein in the posterior chest (*arrow*). Note the abnormal attachments of the right hemidiaphragm to the thoracic wall.

curvilinear density in the right lung formed by an anomalous pulmonary venous channel as it courses toward the IVC (Fig. 35-22A). Its curvilinear shape and progressive widening as it approaches the diaphragm have the appearance of a Turkish sword, or scimitar.[85] The abnormal pulmonary vein always drains the right lower lobe but may receive tributaries from any part of the right lung as it descends in the major fissure.[86] An interesting associated vascular anomaly, levo-atrial-cardinal vein (LACV), occurs in patients with PAPVC from the left lung, usually with coexisting left atrial outflow obstruction (i.e., mitral atresia). In this situation, an abnormal vessel, the levo-atrial-cardinal vein, provides a vascular connection between the left atrium and a derivative of the anterior cardinal venous system. This abnormal vessel is thought to represent a persistent collateral channel between a pulmonary vein and a systemic vein that would otherwise be identified as an anomalous pulmonary venous connection. However, in the setting of LACV, it is thought that by virtue of incorporation of a portion of the pulmonary venous system into the left atrium, the collateral channel connects the left atrium to a systemic vein (see Fig. 35-20).[87–90]

Physiology

Anomalously connected pulmonary veins direct oxygenated blood into the right atrium and its tributaries, creating a left-to-right shunt. The magnitude of this left-to-right shunt depends on the amount of perfused lung tissue draining anomalously. When a single pulmonary vein is anomalously connected, approximately 20 percent of the total pulmonary blood flow is directed to the systemic circulation.[48] The shunt may be augmented by the presence of an ASD (Fig. 35-23). In addition to a left-to-right atrial shunt, ASDs of the sinus venosus type may have an associated right-to-left shunt (by streaming of blood from the SVC to the left atrium). Thus, the net amount of left-to-right shunt at the atrial level depends not only on the quantity of anomalous pulmonary venous return but also on additional shunting through ASDs.

As in any left-to-right shunt, there is recirculation of pulmonary blood resulting in a volume overload of the right heart and lungs. Whether there is, in addition, a pressure overload imposed on the right-sided chambers depends on the presence of obstruction to the pulmonary venous return (usually absent) or on

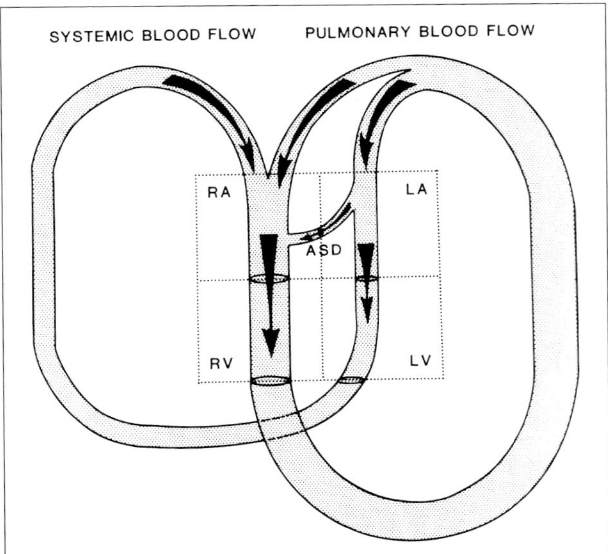

Figure 35-23. Systemic and pulmonary flow in PAPVC. The effect of the anomalously draining veins is a left-to-right shunt at the atrial level. Volume increase in the right heart and pulmonary arteries is additionally augmented in the presence of an atrial septal defect (*ASD*).

pulmonary arteriolar hypertension induced by the left-to-right shunt. In this regard, PAPVC alone usually does not lead to severe pulmonary vascular disease but requires an associated ASD or other complicating defect.[42,91]

Clinical Aspects

The clinical manifestations of PAPVC are similar to those of an ASD and depend primarily on the amount and direction of shunting at the atrial level. If less than 50 percent of the pulmonary venous blood returns to the right atrium, symptoms are uncommon.[92] Patients with more than 50 percent of pulmonary venous draining anomalously may have symptoms of congestive heart failure. In the presence of an ASD, young adults with PAPVC may become cyanotic and then experience dyspnea on exertion if pulmonary hypertension results in reversal of the atrial shunt.[42]

Patients with the scimitar syndrome appear differently from other patients with PAPVC. Most are asymptomatic and discovered accidentally through routine chest films. Recurrent respiratory infection causes symptoms in some patients and is thought to be secondary to the associated pulmonary parenchymal abnormalities. Other respiratory complaints such as coughing, hemoptysis, and dyspnea also occur.[93]

Radiology

Plain Film

In the absence of pulmonary hypertension, PAPVC produces a left-to-right shunt at the atrial level and plain film findings similar to those of an uncomplicated ASD. Unless the shunt results in a QP-QS (pulmonary blood flow–systemic blood flow) ratio of 2:1 or greater, there is usually no plain film indication of an abnormality. When the shunt is greater than 2:1, signs of increased pulmonary flow are generally present. Because the left-to-right shunt causes a volume overload for the right atrium and right ventricle, these structures dilate, as do the pulmonary arteries and veins. The dilatation usually manifests itself on the plain film as a prominent main pulmonary artery, which is accentuated by clockwise rotation of the heart. Moreover, there may be absence of the SVC shadow that normally forms the right border of the superior mediastinum, also a result of clockwise rotation of the heart on its vertical axis in response to enlargement of right-sided chambers. As the heart rotates, the SVC is placed in an anterior and medial position, resulting in its loss as a lateral border-forming structure of the superior mediastinum. Thus the normal, smooth, curvilinear right margin of the superior mediastinum is lost.

Specific plain film signs of PAPVC can be produced by the anomalous pulmonary venous channels. PAPVC to a dilated left vertical vein may result in the figure-of-eight or snowman configuration seen in similar cases of TAPVC. PAPVC from the left upper lobe to the innominate vein may also present a plain film appearance characterized by a rounded shadow extending superiorly and medially from the aortic arch.[94] This curvilinear density is due to the left vertical vein as it courses cranially to join the innominate vein.

The most common form of PAPVC from the right lung involves an anomalous connection between the right upper lobe and the SVC.[70] The vein making this connection may be recognizable on the plain chest film (Fig. 35-24). Another plain film finding that may be present in PAPVC of the right lung to the SVC is dilatation of the SVC just above its junction with the right atrium.[84]

Among the least common receptors of sites of PAPVC are the azygos vein and the coronary sinus. These rare forms of PAPVC usually involve veins of the right lung and left lung, respectively.[70] If either of these normal venous structures becomes dilated, it may produce a density detectable on a plain chest film. In addition, a barium esophagram may help by showing displacement of the esophagus by a dilated coronary sinus.[44]

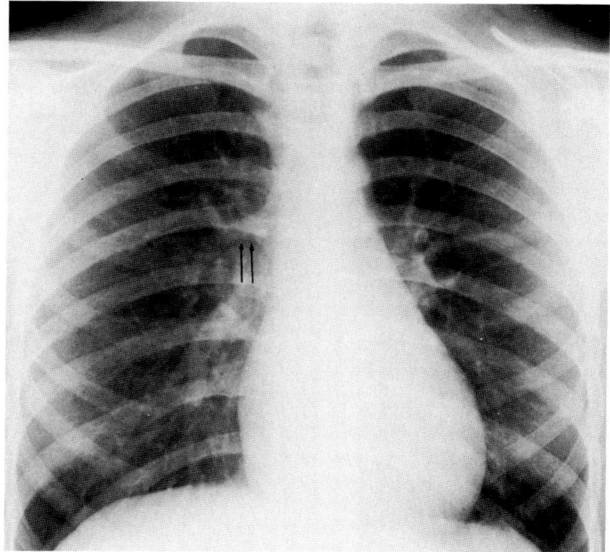

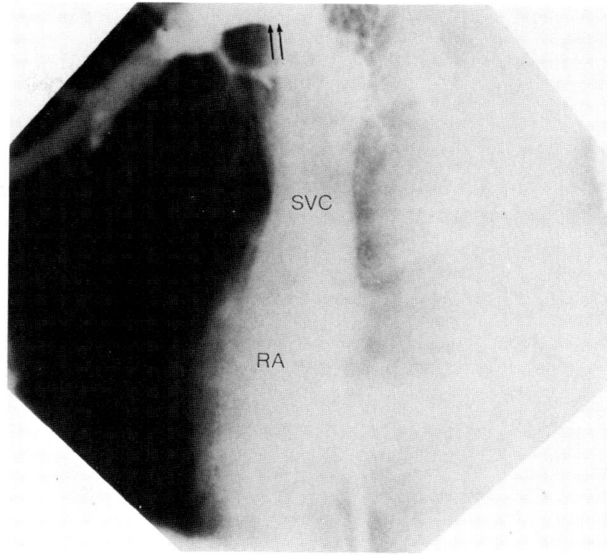

A **B**

Figure 35-24. PAPVC (right upper lobe vein to superior vena cava). (A) The anomalous vein (*arrows*) is identifiable on a frontal film by its location superiorly in the right hilus, its horizontal course, and its merger with the superior vena cava. (B) Angiographic confirmation of the anomalous vein connecting with the superior vena cava (*SVC*). *RA*, right atrium.

Although PAPVC to the IVC represents only 5 percent of all cases of PAPVC,[71] it is of particular interest because it often has a characteristic plain film radiographic appearance. The scimitar sign and syndrome have been well documented in the medical literature.[71,85,92,93,95–102] The scimitar syndrome refers to a constellation of associated anomalies, each having its own plain film manifestations:

1. The hallmark of the syndrome is the scimitar sign (see Fig. 35-22). In addition to having a curved shape, the anomalous vein usually widens medially in frontal view.[85] This prominent venous channel may also be seen on the lateral view in the retrocardiac clear space.
2. Hypoplasia of the right lung decreases the volume of the right hemithorax, producing an ipsilateral shift of the heart and mediastinal structures (see Fig. 35-22A). Pathologically, deficiencies in lobation, bronchial diverticula, and cystic malformations may also be present.
3. Although the right hemidiaphragm may be elevated because of volume loss in the right hemithorax, it often has intrinsic abnormalities such as eventration, abnormally high attachments to the thoracic wall, and accessory leaflets.
4. Thick extrapleural soft tissues may surround the hypoplastic right lung (see Fig. 35-22B).[86,93,97,102,103] This anomaly is often most prominent anteriorly and therefore is seen best in lateral view. Furthermore, the occasional presence of pleuropericardial adhesions may produce an indistinct right heart border.
5. The pulmonary vasculature may be diminished in the right lung because of hypoplasia or absence of the right pulmonary artery. Wide variation exists, and 40 percent of cases are reported to have normal pulmonary arteries.[103] The vascularity of the left lung is often increased because of diminished flow to the right lung and may be additionally enhanced by the presence of a left-to-right shunt (Fig. 35-25).
6. Anomalous systemic arteries arising from the abdominal aorta and supplying the lower lobe of the right lung are usually present, although they are seen rarely on plain roentgenograms. Magnetic resonance imaging can be used to identify these vessels (and the anomalous scimitar vein) in doubtful cases.

Although the plain film findings reflect the associated abnormalities found in this syndrome, not all components need be present in an individual case. It is possible to have the scimitar sign (an anomalous vein) without any other facets of the scimitar syndrome being demonstrable.

The scimitar sign is not always diagnostic. There are reports of a scimitar sign in cases in which PAPVC was

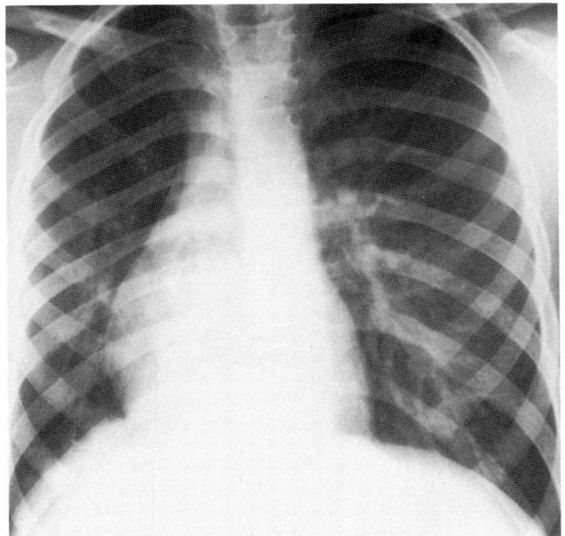

A

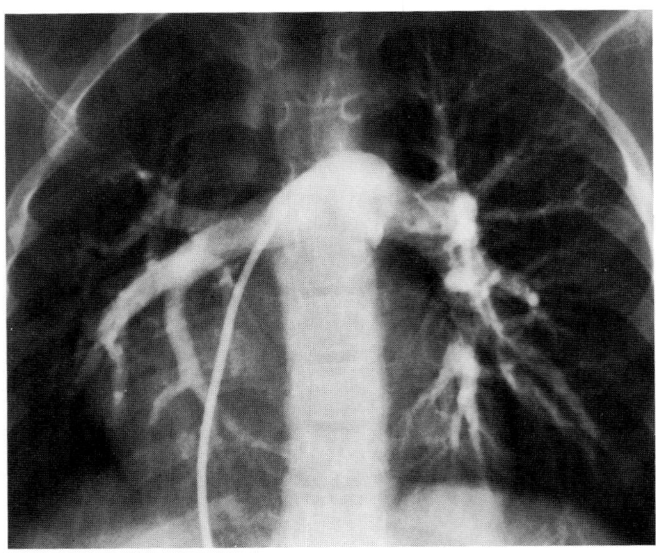

B

Figure 35-25. Scimitar syndrome. (A) There is dextrocardia and mild hypoplasia of the right lung (note decreased width of intercostal spaces on right). A typical scimitar density is not seen, but vertically oriented vascular densities are present in the right lung. Pulmonary flow is diminished on the right and increased on the left. (B) Pulmonary angiography demonstrates mild hypoplasia of the right pulmonary artery. See also Figure 35-28.

lacking. In these cases, a "wandering" pulmonary venous channel courses in the right hemithorax toward the right cardiophrenic angle but eventually enters the left atrium instead of the IVC.[99,104] Other lesions that may produce a scimitarlike appearance are pulmonary arteriovenous fistulas,[105] varicosities of the pulmonary veins,[106,107] and abnormal intrapulmonary segmental veins.[108]

Angiocardiography

Although echocardiography, including a Doppler study, and magnetic resonance imaging have been shown to be useful in diagnosing PAPVC,[50,51,54,55,109,110] angiocardiography continues to play a significant role in defining the anatomic abnormality in many patients with PAPVC. It is most helpful in demonstrating mixed forms of PAPVC. This information is sometimes important in the preoperative planning of a surgical correction.

The angiocardiographic technique is similar to that described for TAPVC. However, it is necessary to do selective pulmonary artery injections to exclude bilateral or mixed forms of PAPVC and to determine the presence of an ASD.[91,111] In PAPVC from the left lung with an intact atrial septum, a right pulmonary artery injection produces opacification of the left atrium only. But, in the presence of an associated ASD, a similar selective injection in the right pulmonary artery results in "spilling over" of contrast into the right atrium from the left atrium. Therefore, if PAPVC is suspected from a main pulmonary artery injection or other cardiac catheterization data (oxygen saturation, indicator dye curves, etc.), a selective pulmonary artery injection ipsilateral to the suspected PAPVC can be done to demonstrate the anomalous pathways. Subsequently, a contralateral selective pulmonary artery injection may be necessary to identify additional contralateral anomalous pulmonary venous connections or an additional ASD. Spurious results with this technique may be due to catheter recoil into the main pulmonary artery; hence the need for proper catheter placement well beyond the bifurcation of the main pulmonary artery.[111]

Occasionally, a pulmonary vein enters the left or right atrium adjacent to the interatrial septum. In the presence of an associated ASD, it may be particularly difficult to identify angiographically the atrial termination of such a pulmonary vein because both atria opacify almost simultaneously.[112] Furthermore, the impression from catheter passage during cardiac catheterization is notoriously misleading. In this situation, angled angiocardiographic views have proven useful in visualizing the interatrial septum tangentially and in demonstrating the atrial connection of the pulmonary vein.[113] A steep (80-degree) left anterior oblique projection, when combined with moderate (20-degree) cranial angulation, permits visualization of the interatrial septum tangential to its surface. Filming in this projection after a retrograde injection into a pulmonary vein (usually right-sided) clearly indicates on which side of the atrial septum the pulmonary vein enters and hence the presence or absence of an anomalous pulmonary venous connection at the atrial level (Fig. 35-26).

Two types of PAPVC have a unique angiographic appearance: (1) LACV and (2) the scimitar syndrome.

The best method of angiographically defining the anatomy and various connections of an LACV is to inject directly into it via a retrograde catheter or to inject a larger amount of contrast material into the left atrium.[114] Figure 35-27 demonstrates the angiocardiographic appearance of an LACV with connections to the innominate vein, multiple left pulmonary veins, and left atrium (see also Fig. 35-21).

Angiocardiography may be used to study any of the vascular anomalies associated with the scimitar syndrome. The procedure of choice for angiographically demonstrating the anomalous pulmonary venous return from the right lung as well as the status of the right pulmonary artery is a main or right pulmonary artery injection (see Fig. 35-25). Late filming must include the right cardiophrenic region to define the number and level of the anomalous venous connections. Certain abnormalities can produce a false scimitar sign, such as pulmonary venous varicosity,[106,107] pulmonary arteriovenous fistula,[105] and other abnormal pulmonary venous structures that do not connect anomalously.[104,108,115] Because other cardiovascular anomalies (i.e., VSD, tetralogy of Fallot, and patent ductus arteriosus) may be present in children with the scimitar syndrome, additional angiocardiography may be necessary.[116]

Figure 35-26. Atrial septal defect. A small secundum defect (*ASD*^{II}, *between arrows*) is well seen on this compound angled projection (10-degree cranial and 80-degree left anterior oblique angulation). The injection is in a right upper lobe pulmonary vein (*RPV*), which clearly is connected to the left atrium (*LA*).

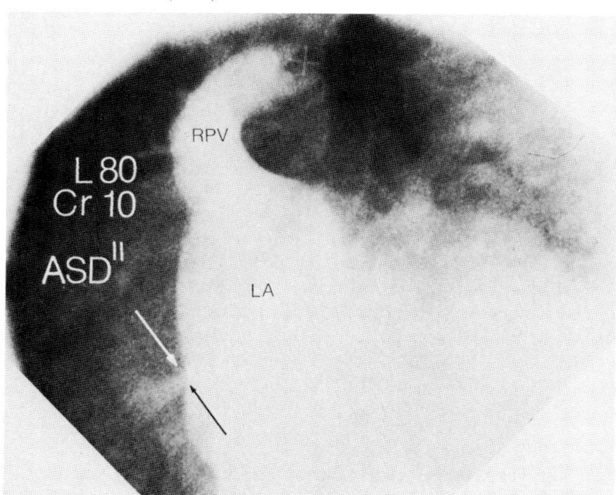

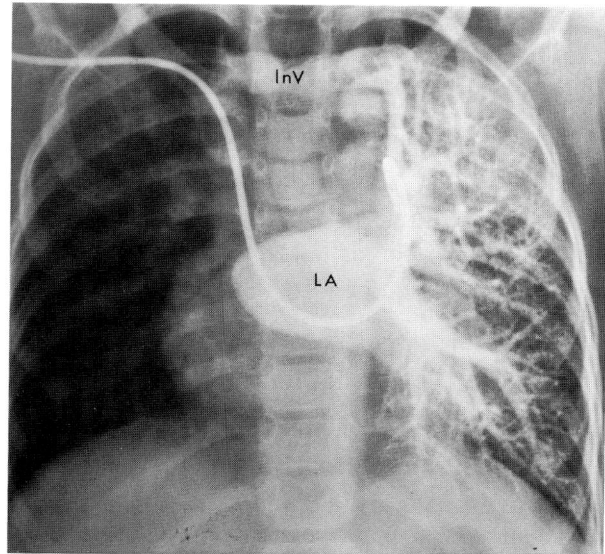

Figure 35-27. PAPVC to a levo-atrial-cardinal vein (same patient as in Fig. 35-21). Levo phase of a left pulmonary arteriogram demonstrates flow from the left upper lobe pulmonary vein superiorly to the innominate vein (*InV*) and inferiorly to the left atrium (*LA*). Lower lobe veins connect directly with the left atrium.

Anomalous systemic arteries supplying the right lung in scimitar syndrome may be faintly demonstrated on the levo phase of a pulmonary artery injection. Better visualization of these arterial connections is provided by an abdominal aortogram (Fig. 35-28).

Figure 35-28. Scimitar syndrome (same patient as in Fig. 35-25). Thoracoabdominal aortography demonstrates an aberrant systemic vessel (*arrow*) supplying part of the right lower lobe.

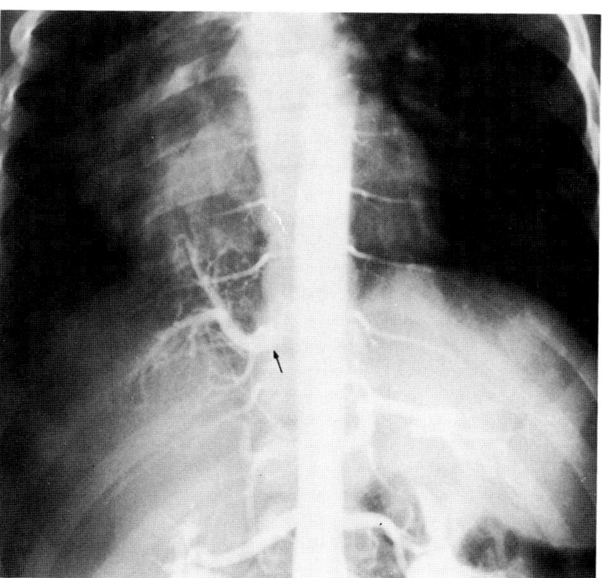

Summary

TAPVC can be divided anatomically and radiographically into four types: (1) supracardiac, (2) cardiac, (3) infracardiac, and (4) mixed, depending on the site of the anomalous connection of the pulmonary veins. The abnormal routes of pulmonary venous return characteristic of these different types of TAPVC can be best understood by retracing primitive pulmonary venous pathways thought to be present in the developing embryo.

Anatomically and physiologically, TAPVC may be divided once more on the basis of the presence or absence of obstruction to pulmonary venous return. This difference accounts for two distinct radiographic and clinical presentations found in TAPVC. If significant obstruction is present, the patient is usually critically ill at birth with symptoms indicating congestive heart failure. A typical plain chest radiograph in this case has a reticular, congested vascular pattern thought to be due to perivascular edema superimposed on dilated lymphatics and pulmonary veins. A similar appearance has been seen in the chest radiographs of patients with transient respiratory distress of the newborn, pulmonary lymphangiectasia, and other forms of congenital heart disease resulting in obstruction to pulmonary venous return (e.g., pulmonary vein atresia, cor triatriatum, supravalvular mitral ring, congenital mitral stenosis, parachute mitral valve, and hypoplastic left heart syndrome). Conversely, if there is no obstruction to pulmonary venous return, immediate symptoms are usually absent and a large net left-to-right shunt at the atrial level is present. In these patients, the plain film findings are those of a large left-to-right shunt. Other radiographic signs due to the presence of an anomalous pulmonary venous pathway (e.g., snowman) may be present.

PAPVC includes a diverse spectrum of lesions. PAPVC is also characterized by a net left-to-right shunt at the atrial level, the size of which reflects the amount of pulmonary venous blood returning anomalously and the presence or absence of an ASD. Depending on the size of the left-to-right shunt, clinical and radiographic findings are similar to those found with an ASD. In addition, certain forms of PAPVC frequently have associated congenital anomalies, such as (1) a high incidence of sinus venosus ASDs in PAPVC from the right lung to the SVC and (2) the scimitar syndrome.

Although noninvasive imaging techniques, particularly magnetic resonance imaging, are increasingly able to diagnose pulmonary venous abnormalities, many still consider angiocardiography the method of choice for demonstrating anomalous pulmonary venous connections. In TAPVC, angiography displays the anatomic features of an individual case and is particularly helpful in identifying variations that have therapeutic and prognostic significance. Included in such variations are (1) sites of obstruction along the anomalous pulmonary venous pathway, (2) the absence of a common pulmonary venous trunk or an unusual orientation of the pulmonary venous confluence, and (3) mixed types of TAPVC. Finally, in all forms of anomalous pulmonary venous connection, angiocardiography provides valuable information regarding associated intracardiac lesions and other congenital vascular anomalies.

References

1. Wilson J. A description of a very unusual formation of the human heart. Philos Trans R Soc Lond (Biol) 1789;88:346.
2. Abbott ME, ed. Atlas of congenital cardiac disease. New York: American Heart Association, 1936.

b3. Darling RC, Rothney WB, Craig JM. Total pulmonary venous drainage into the right side of the heart. Lab Invest 1957;6:44.

4. Mehrizi A, Dekker A, Ottesen OE. Angiocardiographic features of total anomalous venous return into coronary sinus simulating tricuspid atresia or stenosis. J Pediatr 1964;65: 615.
5. Lucas RV Jr, Anderson RC, Amplatz K, et al. Congenital causes of pulmonary venous obstruction. Pediatr Clin North Am 1963;10:781.
6. Delisle G, Ando M, Calder AL, et al. Total anomalous pulmonary venous connection: report of 93 autopsied cases with emphasis on diagnostic and surgical considerations. Am Heart J 1976;91:99.
7. Ivemark BI. Implications of agenesis of the spleen on the pathogenesis of conotruncal anomalies in childhood. Acta Paediatr Scand 1955;104(Suppl):1.
8. Ruttenberg HD, Neufeld HN, Lucas RV, et al. Syndrome of congenital cardiac disease with asplenia: distinction from other forms of congenital cyanotic cardiac disease. Am J Cardiol 1964;13:387.
9. Deshpande JR, Kinare SG. Atresia of the common pulmonary vein. Int J Cardiol 1991;30(2):221–226.
10. Humes RA, Feldt RH, Porter CJ, et al. The modified Fontan operation for asplenia and polysplenia syndromes. J Thorac Cardiovasc Surg 1988;96(2):212–218.
11. Freedom RM, Gerald PS. Congenital cardiac disease and the "cat eye" syndrome. Am J Dis Child 1973;126:16.
12. Langman J. Medical embryology: human development—normal and abnormal. 3rd ed. New York: Longman, 1975.
13. Patten BM. Human embryology. 3rd ed. New York: McGraw-Hill, 1968.
14. Butler H. An abnormal disposition of the pulmonary veins. Thorax 1952;7:249.
15. Auër J. The development of the human pulmonary vein and its major variations. Anat Rec 1948;101:581.
16. Los JA. Cardiac septation and development of the aorta, pulmonary trunk, and pulmonary veins: previous work in light of recent observations. Birth Defects 1978;14:109.
17. Neill CA. Development of the pulmonary veins, with reference to the embryology of anomalies of pulmonary venous return. Pediatrics 1956;18:880.
18. Edwards JE. Pathologic and developmental considerations in anomalous pulmonary venous connection. Mayo Clin Proc 1953;18:441.
19. Becher MW, Rockenmacher S, Marin-Padilla M. Total anomalous pulmonary venous connection: persistence and atresia of the common pulmonary vein. Pediatr Cardiol 1992;13:187–189.

20. Burroughs JT, Edwards JE. Total anomalous pulmonary venous connection. Am Heart J 1960;59:913.
21. Casta A, Wolf WJ. Echo Doppler detection of external compression of the vertical vein causing obstruction in total anomalous pulmonary venous connection. Am Heart J 1088; 116(4):1045–1047.
22. Keith J, Rowe RD, Vlad P, et al. Complete anomalous pulmonary venous drainage. Am J Med 1954;16:23.
23. Clark DR, Paton BC, Stewart JR. Surgical treatment of total anomalous pulmonary venous drainage. Adv Cardiol 1979; 26:129.
24. Kawashima Y, Matsuda H, Nakano S, et al. Tree-shaped pulmonary veins in infracardiac total anomalous pulmonary venous drainage. Ann Thorac Surg 1977;23:436.
25. Whight CM, Barratt-Boyes BG, Calder A, et al. Total anomalous pulmonary venous connection: long-term results following repair in infancy. J Thorac Cardiovasc Surg 1978;75:52.
26. Hastreiter AR, Paul MH, Molthan ME, et al. Total anomalous pulmonary venous connection with severe pulmonary venous obstruction: a clinical entity. Circulation 1962;25:916.
27. Haworth SG, Reid L. A structural study of pulmonary circulation and of heart in total anomalous pulmonary venous return in early infancy. Br Heart J 1977;39:80.
28. Gathman GE, Nadas AS. Total anomalous pulmonary venous connection: clinical and physiologic observations of 75 pediatric patients. Circulation 1970;42:143.
29. Clarke DR, Stack J, DeLeval M, et al. Total anomalous pulmonary venous drainage in infancy. Br Heart J 1977;39:436.
30. Katz NM, Kirklin JW, Pacifico AD. Concepts and practices in surgery for total anomalous pulmonary venous connection. Ann Thorac Surg 1978;25:479.
31. Wukasch DC, Deutsch M, Reul GJ, et al. Total anomalous pulmonary venous return: review of 125 patients treated surgically. Ann Thorac Surg 1975;19:622.
32. Gomes MR, Feldt RH, McGoon DC, et al. Total anomalous pulmonary venous connection. J Thorac Cardiovasc Surg 1970;60:116.
33. Lucas RV, Adams P, Anderson RC, et al. Total anomalous pulmonary venous connection to the portal venous system: a case of pulmonary venous obstruction. AJR 1961;86:561.
34. Carey LS, Edwards JE. Severe pulmonary venous obstruction in total anomalous pulmonary venous connection to the left innominate vein: report of a case. AJR 1963;90:593.
35. Harris GBC, Neuhauser EBD, Giedion A. Total anomalous pulmonary venous return below the diaphragm: the roentgen appearance in three patients diagnosed during life. AJR 1960; 84:436.
36. Kauffman SL, Ores CN, Anderson DH. Two cases of total anomalous pulmonary venous return of the supracardiac type with stenosis simulating infradiaphragmatic drainage. Circulation 1962;25:376.
37. Haworth SG, Reid L, Simon G. Radiological features of the heart and lungs in total anomalous pulmonary venous return in early infancy. Clin Radiol 1977;28:561.
38. Snellen HA, Albers FH: The clinical diagnosis of anomalous pulmonary venous drainage. Circulation 1952;6:801.
39. Paster SB, Swensson RE, Yabek SM. Total anomalous pulmonary venous connection. Pediatr Radiol 1977;6:132.
40. Genz T, Locher D, Genz S, et al. Chest x-ray film patterns in children with isolated total anomalous pulmonary vein connection. Eur J Pediatr 1990;150:14–18.
41. Weaver MD, Chen JTT, Anderson PAW, et al. Total anomalous pulmonary venous connection to the left vertical vein: a plain-film sign useful in early diagnosis. Radiology 1976;118:679.
42. Lucas RV, Schmidt RE. Anomalous venous connections, pulmonary and systemic. In: Moss AJ, Adams FH, Emmanonilides GC, eds. Heart disease in infants, children and adolescents. 2nd ed. Baltimore: Williams & Wilkins, 1977.
43. Moës CAF, Fowler RS, Trusler GA. Total anomalous pulmonary venous drainage into the azygos vein. AJR 1966;98:378.
44. Fellows KE Jr, Sigmann J, Stern AM, et al. Coronary sinus enlargement in infants: a diagnostic note. Radiology 1970; 94:347.
45. Eisen S, Elliot LP. A plain film sign of total anomalous pulmonary venous connection below the diaphragm. AJR 1968; 102:372.
46. Bharati S, Lev M. Congenital anomalies of the pulmonary veins. Cardiovasc Clin 1973;5:23.
47. Paquet M, Gutgesell H. Echocardiographic features of total anomalous pulmonary venous connection. Circulation 1975; 51:599.
48. Tajik AJ, Gau GT, Ritter DG, et al. Echocardiographic pattern of right ventricular diastolic volume overload in children. Circulation 1972;46:36.
49. Van Hare GF, Schmidt KG, Cassidy SC, et al. Color Doppler flow mapping in the ultrasound diagnostic of total anomalous pulmonary venous connection. J Am Soc Echocardiogr 1988; 1:341–347.
50. Seliem MA, Chin AJ, Norwood WI. Patterns of anomalous pulmonary venous connection/drainage in hypoplastic left heart syndrome: diagnostic role of Doppler color flow mapping and surgical implications. J Am Coll Cardiol 1992;19: 135–141.
51. Masui T, Seelos KC, Kersting-Sommerhoff BA, et al. Abnormalities of the pulmonary veins: evaluation with MR imaging and comparison with cardiac angiography and echocardiography. Radiology 1991;181:645–649.
52. Livolsi A, Kastler B, Marcellin L, et al. MR diagnosis of subdiaphragmatic anomalous pulmonary venous drainage in a newborn. J Comput Assist Tomogr 1991;15(6):1051–1053.
53. Sreeram N, Walsh K. Diagnosis of total anomalous pulmonary venous drainage by Doppler color flow imaging. J Am Coll Cardiol 1992;19:1577–1582.
54. Julsrud PR, Ehman RL, Hagler DJ, et al. Extracardiac vasculature in candidates for Fontan surgery: MR imaging. Radiology 1989;173:503–506.
55. Julsrud PR. Magnetic resonance imaging of the pulmonary arteries and veins. Semin Ultrasound CT MR 1990;11(3): 184–205.
56. Higashino SM, Shaw GG, May IA, et al. Total anomalous pulmonary venous drainage below the diaphragm: clinical presentation, hemodynamic findings and surgical results. J Thorac Cardiovasc Surg 1974;68:711.
57. Behrendt DM, Aberdeen E, Waterston DJ, et al. Total anomalous pulmonary venous drainage in infants: I. Clinical and hemodynamic findings, methods, and results of operation in 37 cases. Circulation 1972;47:347.
58. Duff DF, Nihill MR, McNamara DG. Infradiaphragmatic total anomalous pulmonary venous return: reveiw of clinical and pathological findings and results of operations in 28 cases. Br Heart J 1977;39:619.
59. Sneed RC. Total anomalous pulmonary venous return: diagnosis by umbilical vessel catheterization. South Med J 1972; 65:1145.
60. Tynan M, Behrendt D, Urquhart W, et al. Portal vein catheterization and selective angiography in diagnosis of total anomalous pulmonary venous connection. Br Heart J 1974;36:1155.
61. Bove KE, Geiser EA, Meyer RA. The left ventricle is anomalous pulmonary venous return: morphometric analysis of 36 fatal cases in infancy. Arch Pathol 1975;99:522.
62. Graham TP Jr, Jarmakani JM, Canent RJ Jr. Left heart volume characteristics with a right ventricular volume overload: total anomalous pulmonary venous connection and large atrial septal defect. Circulation 1972;45:389.
63. Mathew R, Thilenius OG, Replogle RL, et al. Cardiac function in total anomalous pulmonary venous return before and after surgery. Circulation 1977;55:361.
64. Lester RG, Mauck HP, Grupp WL. Anomalous pulmonary venous return to the right side of the heart. Semin Roentgenol 1966;1:102.
65. Rowe RD, Glass IH, Keith JD. Total anomalous pulmonary venous drainage at cardiac level: angiographic differentiation. Circulation 1961;23:77.
66. Trinkle JK, Danielson GK, Noonan JA, et al. Infradiaphragmatic total anomalous pulmonary venous return. Ann Thorac Surg 1968;5:55.

67. Healy JE Jr. An anatomic survey of anomalous pulmonary veins: their clinical significance. J Thorac Cardiovasc Surg 1952;23:433.
68. Kalke BR, Carlson RG, Ferlic RM, et al. Partial anomalous pulmonary venous connections. Am J Cardiol 1967;20:91.
69. McCormack RJM, Marquis RM, Jullian DG, et al. Partial anomalous pulmonary venous drainage and its surgical correction. Scott Med J 1960;5:367.
70. Brody H. Drainage of pulmonary veins into the right side of the heart. Arch Pathol 1942;33:221.
71. Schumacher HB Jr, Judd D. Partial anomalous pulmonary venous return with reference to drainage into the inferior vena cava and to intact atrial septum. J Cardiovasc Surg (Torino) 1964;5:271.
72. Kittle CF, Crocket JE. Vena cava bronchovascular syndrome: a triad of anomalies involving the right lung. Ann Surg 1962; 156:222.
73. Miller SW, Dinsmore RE, Liberthson RR, et al. Anomalous pulmonary venous connection of entire left lung with intact atrial septum: radiological features and clinical implications. Radiology 1977;122:591.
74. Gotsman MS, Astley R, Parsons CG. Partial anomalous pulmonary venous drainage in association with atrial septal defect. Br Heart J 1965;27:566.
75. Mascarenhas E, Javier RP, Samet P. Partial anomalous pulmonary venous connection and drainage. Am J Cardiol 1973;3: 512.
76. Pritchard DA, Tajik AJ, Rutherford BD, et al. Partial anomalous pulmonary venous connection (intact atrial septum) associated with mitral regurgitation. Am Heart J 1977;94:209.
77. Devine WA, Anderson RH. Superior caval to pulmonary venous fistula—the progenitor of the sinus venosus defect? Pediatr Pathol 1989;9:345–349.
78. Alescio T, Cassini A. Induction in vitro of tracheal buds by pulmonary mesenchyme grafted on tracheal epithelium. J Exp Zool 1962;150:83.
79. Edwards JE, DuShane JW. Thoracic venous anomalies. Arch Pathol 1950;49:517.
80. Taybi H, Kurlander GJ, Lurie PR, et al. Anomalous systemic venous connection to the left atrium or to a pulmonary vein. AJR 1965;94:62.
81. Snellen HA, van Ingen HC, Hoefsmit ECM. Patterns of anomalous pulmonary venous drainage. Circulation 1968;38: 45.
82. Hickie JB, Gimlette TMD, Beacon APC. Anomalous pulmonary drainage. Br Heart J 1956;18:365.
83. Daria JE, Cheitlin MD, Bedynek JL. Sinus venosus atrial septal defect: analysis of fifty cases. Am Heart J 1973;85:177.
84. Dow JD. The radiological diagnosis of the sinus venosus type of atrial septal defect. Guy's Hosp Rep 1959;108:305.
85. Neill CA, Ferencz C, Sabaiston DC, Sheildon H. The familial occurrence of hypoplastic right lung with systemic arterial supply and venous drainage: "scimitar syndrome." Johns Hopkins Med J 1960;107:1.
86. Kiely B, Filler J, Stone S, et al. Syndrome of anomalous venous drainage of the right lung to the inferior vena cava: a review of 67 reported cases and three new cases in children. Am J Cardiol 1967;20:102.
87. Edwards JE, DuShane JW. Thoracic venous anomalies: I. Vascular connection of the left atrium and the left innominate vein associated with mitral atresia and premature closure of the foramen ovale. II. Pulmonary veins draining wholly into the ductus venosus. Arch Pathol 1950;49:517.
88. Abrams HL, ed. Vascular and interventional radiology. 3rd ed. Abrams angiography. Boston: Little, Brown, 1983;2: 883–884.
89. McIntosh CA. Cor triatriatum triloculare. Am Heart J 1926; 1:735–744.
90. Bellet S, Gouley BA. Congenital heart disease with multiple cardiac anomalies: report of a case showing aortic atresia, fibrous scar in myocardium and embryonal sinusoids remains. Am J Med Sci 1932;183:458–465.
91. Frye RL, Krebs M, Rahimtoola SH, et al. Partial anomalous pulmonary venous connection without atrial septal defect. Am J Cardiol 1968;22:242.
92. Thomas TV, Gumucio ML, Premsingh N. Scimitar syndrome: surgical considerations. J Kans Med Soc 1978;79:547.
93. Mathey J, Galley JJ, Logeais Y, et al. Anomalous pulmonary venous return into inferior vena cava and associated bronchovascular anomalies (the scimitar syndrome). Thorax 1968;23: 398.
94. Adler SC, Silverman JF. Anomalous venous drainage of the left upper lobe; a radiographic diagnosis. Radiology 1973; 108:563.
95. Bruwer A. Roentgenologic findings in total anomalous pulmonary venous connection. Mayo Clin Proc 1956;31:171.
96. Dotter CT, Hardisty NM, Steinberg I. Anomalous right pulmonary vein entering the inferior vena cava: two cases diagnosed during life by angiocardiography and cardiac catheterization. Am J Med Sci 1949;218:31.
97. Felson B. Pulmonary agenesis and related anomalies. Semin Roentgenol 1972;7:17.
98. Gwinn JL, Barnes GR. The scimitar syndrome: anomalies of great vessels associated with lung hypoplasia. Am J Dis Child 1967;114:585.
99. Roehm JOF Jr, Jue KL, Amplatz K. Radiographic features of the scimitar syndrome. Radiology 1966;86:856.
100. Sepulveda G, Lukas DS, Steinberg I. Anomalous drainage of pulmonary veins: clinical, physiologic, and angiocardiographic features. Am J Med 1955;18:883.
101. Steinberg I. Roentgen diagnosis of anomalous pulmonary venous drainage of right lung into inferior vena cava: report of three new cases. AJR 1959;81:280.
102. Tomsick TA, Moesner SE, Smith WL. The congenital pulmonary venolobar syndrome in three successive generations. J Can Assoc Radiol 1976;27:196.
103. Farnsworth AE, Ankeney JL. The spectrum of the scimitar syndrome. J Thorac Cardiovasc Surg 1974;68:37.
104. Goodman LR, Jamshidi A, Hipona FA. Meandering right pulmonary vein simulating the scimitar syndrome. Chest 1972;62:510.
105. Steinberg I, McClenahan J. Pulmonary arteriovenous fistula, angiocardiographic observations in nine cases. Am J Med 1955;19:549.
106. Gottsman L, Weinstein A. Varicosities of the pulmonary veins. Dis Chest 1959;35:322.
107. Nelson WP, Hall RJ, Garcia E. Varicosities of the pulmonary veins simulating arteriovenous fistulas. JAMA 1966;195;103.
108. Everhart FJ, Korns ME, Amplatz K, et al. Intrapulmonary segment in anomalous pulmonary venous connection: resemblance to scimitar syndrome. Circulation 1967;35:1163.
109. Julsrud PR, Ehman RL. The "Broken Ring" sign in magnetic resonance imaging of partial anomalous pulmonary venous connection to the superior vena cava. Mayo Clin Proc 1985; 60:874–879.
110. Vesely TM, Julsrud PR, Brown JJ, et al. MR imaging of partial anomalous pulmonary venous connections. J Comput Assist Tomogr 1991;15(5):752–756.
111. Sos TA, Tay D, Levin AR, et al. Angiographic demonstration of the absence of an atrial septal defect in the presence of partial anomalous pulmonary venous connection. AJR 1974; 121:591.
112. Alpert JS, Dexter L, Vieweg WVR, et al. Anomalous pulmonary venous return with intact atrial septum: diagnosis and pathophysiology. Circulation 1977;56:870.
113. Fellows KE Jr, Keane JF, Freed MD. Angled view in cine angiocardiography of congenital heart disease. Circulation 1977;56:485.
114. Blieden LC, Schneeweiss A, Deutsch V, et al. Anomalous venous connection from the left atrium to the cardinal venous system: "levoatriocardinal vein." AJR 1977;129:937.
115. Morgan JR, Forker AD. Syndrome of hypoplasia of the right lung and dextroposition of the heart: "scimitar sign" with normal pulmonary venous drainage. Circulation 1971;43:27.
116. Jue KL, Amplatz K, Adams P. Anomalies of great vessels associated with lung hypoplasia. Am J Dis Child 1966;111:35.

36

The Vertebral and Azygos Veins

HERBERT L. ABRAMS
MICHAEL F. MEYEROVITZ

The venous system of humans, in accord with conventional anatomic description, is divided into two main groups: the pulmonary veins and the systemic veins. With the exception of the cardiac veins, the systemic venous drainage returns to the heart through two great vessels, the superior and the inferior vena cava. From the cranial cavity and the upper extremities, the blood converges on the superior vena cava, and from the abdominal viscera and lower extremities, on the inferior vena cava.

Obstruction of either of these trunks is not incompatible with life in human beings.[1–3] The development of a large bypass mechanism effectively establishing communication between the two vast caval drainage areas can be accomplished by collateral vessels, of which the vertebral veins and the azygos system form an important component.[3–6] In the dog, both venae cavae may be occluded for 30 minutes with survival if the azygos vein is patent.[7] This occlusion is accompanied by a fivefold increase in azygos blood flow. How the increase is possible becomes apparent after consideration of the intercommunications of the vertebral veins.[5,8,9] At the base of the brain, they anastomose extensively with the venous trunks of the cranium; in the neck, with the deep cervical veins; in the thorax and abdomen, with the intercostal and lumbar veins; and in the pelvis, with the large venous plexuses anterior to the sacrum. In turn, the sacral and lumbar veins communicate directly with the inferior vena caval system; the lumbar and intercostal veins, with the azygos system; and the azygos system, with the superior vena cava and its branches.[10]

In the early 1940s, Batson revived interest in this system of veins by demonstrating that a thin, opaque medium injected into the dorsal vein of the penis of a cadaver would spread into the sacral canal, fill the veins in the wings of the bony pelvis, and finally move up the vertebral system as far as the cranial cavity. The mode of spread was similar to that of carcinoma of the prostate, and Batson suggested that in the great venous lakes formed by these plexuses, tumor emboli might well spread from origin to final site of deposition. He also showed that the vertebral veins filled after injection in a live monkey when the inferior vena cava was compressed.[11–13]

Shortly after Batson described the anatomy of the vertebral veins and expounded his theory of their role in metastases, Harris went to great lengths to prove that Batson's ideas were not original.[14] The vertebral venous system was by no means unknown to anatomists before Batson's time, although Franklin, in his monograph on veins written in 1937, did not even mention the vertebral plexuses.[15] Willis in 1664[16] and Winslow in 1732[17] characterized the structure of the spinal veins. Bock in 1823 described the rich venous plexuses within the bony canal, the posterior venous plexus, and the azygos system.[18] Even the suggestion that the vertebral venous system was a storage reservoir as well as a drainage channel goes back a century. Quain pointed out in 1828 that the blood from "the interior of the spine is conveyed into the great spinal veins which are wider in the middle than all their extremities and therefore resemble so many reservoirs."[19] Hilton in 1855 stated,

> The absence of valves in the whole of the venous tubes is a circumstance which is doubtless connected with a wise intention. It enables the blood to pass in either direction, and consequently, greatly increases the freedom of venous circulation; a point of essential importance with an organ, whose functional capacity is so liable to interruption under so slight a disturbance of the balance of its circulating fluid.[20]

Batson's real accomplishments, then, were to recognize that this reservoir might be a channel through which tumor emboli could travel to near or distant foci and to redirect attention to a relatively neglected area of the venous system.

Some years after Batson's original reports, Johnstone attempted to repeat his work.[21] He concluded that there was no evidence that the vertebral veins provided the main route for the spread of metastases in carcinoma of the prostate or the breast, and he was unable to establish effectively that opaque medium injected into the dorsal vein of the penis would actually reach the cranial cavity. Robinson injected Neoprene into eight stillborn infants but was unable to obtain satisfactory roentgenographic studies.[3]

Onuigbo[22] has noted that the metastatic spread of lung cancer does not follow the pattern that would be predicted if the vertebral veins were a major route for tumor spread. Lung cancer only rarely involves the contralateral lung, although there are many vertebral connections between the lungs. In addition, despite the connections between the vertebral veins and thoracic lymph nodes, metastatic lymph node involvement follows lymphogenous pathways and does not appear randomly throughout the thorax.

In 1951 Lawrence and Moore demonstrated experimentally that when the inferior vena cava, the epigastric veins, and the lumbar veins were ligated, the vertebral veins were an effective route for spread of tumor to the vertebrae and lungs in rabbits.[23] In their experiments they injected a suspension of transplantable rabbit carcinoma cells into the femoral vein, which resulted in metastatic spread via the vertebral venous system. Even when the azygos vein was also ligated, pulmonary metastases developed. Coman and DeLong injected viable tumor cells in the femoral vein of 14 animals while abdominal compression was employed; in 12, tumors appeared in the vertebral venous system.[24] Microscopic sections revealed that the growth usually arose from emboli in the larger, thin-walled vertebral veins. The absence of emboli in the arterioles indicated that the tumor had not passed through the lungs and returned via the arterial tree. In 16 control animals that received injections of tumor cells without abdominal pressure, 15 had tumor implants in the lungs alone with no evidence of tumor in the spinal column. These authors agreed that the vertebral veins offered an avenue of transport of tumor emboli for prostatic and breast carcinoma and that perhaps coughing or the Valsalva maneuver—which increases intraabdominal pressure—might suffice to shift blood from the inferior vena cava to the vertebral or azygos system. Others have emphasized the importance of this system as a means of spreading infection.[25]

The use of isotopic bone scanning, which provides an assessment of osseous metastases more sensitive than can be achieved by radiographic studies, has shown a much higher incidence of metastases to bone in colorectal cancer than had been indicated by conventional studies. Nuclear medicine studies have shown a 33 to 61 percent incidence of osseous metastases from colorectal carcinoma.[26–29] Although low-pressure drainage of intraabdominal veins to the liver and lungs serves as the major route of metastatic spread, the higher-pressure vertebral venous system, with drainage to spine and skeleton, must also be involved in the dispersion of metastases.

Thus there is some evidence that the paravertebral and azygos venous networks play an important role in the presence of disease. In some animals, the azygos veins constitute the main venous channels of the thorax,[30] and there may be multiple communications between the lymphatic and azygos systems.[31] Foreign substances in the spinal cord theca drain directly through the vertebral veins into the azygos system.[32] The usefulness of the Queckenstedt sign depends on the free flow of blood into the vertebral veins after occlusion of the internal jugular vein with consequent distention of the vertebral veins and a rise in cerebrospinal fluid pressure in the absence of block.[10] The prominence of the azygos vein may be exaggerated in the presence of congestive heart failure,[33] and it has been mistaken for enlarged lymph nodes or even tumor.[34]

Methods of Study

The radiologic anatomy of these veins has commanded increasing attention. Anderson in 1950 duplicated Batson's work in detail[35] and extended the study to living adults. He succeeded in opacifying the vertebral veins after femoral vein injection of Diodrast when abdominal compression was employed. Mellins reported 70 inferior vena cavograms, in 12 of which the azygos system was opacified.[4] In 6 of these 12 cases the vertebral venous plexus was demonstrated. Nine of the 12 had inferior vena caval obstruction, and in 1 there was increased intraabdominal pressure at the time of examination.

The method described by Anderson of opacifying the vertebral and azygos veins by femoral vein injection with simultaneous inferior vena caval compression was employed by Helander and Lindbom in a study of 70 cases.[36] They inserted polyethylene catheters into both femoral veins in a cranial direction by the Seldinger method for percutaneous catheterization. The tip of the catheter was placed in the iliac vein adjacent to the junction of the external and internal iliac veins. A continuous saline drip helped to prevent clotting in the catheter. The inferior vena cava was blocked with a football bladder pressed tightly against the abdomen with a plastic plate held by a belt. Thirty cubic centimeters of 35 percent Diodrast was injected simultaneously into both tubes in 3 to 6 seconds. The first film was exposed toward the end of the injection, and three to four subsequent exposures were made at intervals of 2 to 4 seconds. The anteroposterior projection with the patient supine was used routinely and was occasionally supplemented by oblique or lateral projections. Nordenstrom modified their method in the experimental animal by using a catheter balloon to obstruct the inferior vena cava and obtained some excellent studies in dogs.[37] Perey et al. have applied the balloon occlusion method to clinical studies.[38]

Intraosseous venography is an alternative method of demonstrating the vertebral veins and the azygos system. Since Fischgold and his coworkers first described this method in 1952,[39] a number of other workers have demonstrated its efficacy.[40–43] Fischgold injected the opaque medium directly into the spinous process and subsequently was able to visualize the vertebral venous system and the azygos veins.[39] Tori injected the spinous process of the thoracic vertebrae or the posterior segment of the last rib and obtained a film during the middle of the examination, one toward the end, and one after 10 seconds.[42] Lessman et al., after administering preliminary sedation and local anesthesia, inserted the bone marrow needle into the medullary cavity until it was fixed securely in place.[40] A preliminary film was obtained after the injection of 1 to 2 ml of the contrast agent. After the position and technique were determined, the injection was begun, and three to four films were obtained during and after the injection. It is also possible to opacify the azygos system by retrograde injection through a catheter inserted from the superior vena cava.[44,45] Ranniger has performed a large series of such studies.[46]

Abrams has studied the lumbar azygos system by selective catheterization.[47] This is a simple, efficacious method and, when combined with cine or rapid filming, permits optimal opacification. The catheter is passed from the right femoral vein into the inferior vena cava and thence directly into the third, fourth, or fifth left lumbar vein. This maneuver may be accompanied by simultaneous catheterization of the ascending lumbar vein from the left common iliac vein. Thirty milliliters of 76 percent Renografin is then injected in 5 seconds if both veins are catheterized, or 15 ml in 2 to 3 seconds if only one vein has been entered. Opacification of the azygos vein is entirely satisfactory.

In most descriptions of the efforts to opacify the vertebral system in vivo—with the exception of intraosseous injection and selective lumbar vein catheterization—obstruction of the inferior vena cava by abdominal pressure, by ligation, or by catheter balloon has figured prominently. It can be clearly shown, however, that the interlinkage between the caval and vertebral systems is so intimate and extensive that caval obstruction is not necessary for opacification of (and hence for blood flow from the lower extremities through) the vertebral venous plexuses in humans. In Abrams's experience[48,49] injection through the saphenous or femoral veins without abdominal pressure has produced significant opacification of the vertebral and azygos systems in about two-thirds of 60 cases. Others have noted the same phenomenon.[38] All patients were in the younger age groups and were being studied for congenital cardiac anomalies.

Serial CT sections will commonly display the azygos and hemiazygos systems, allowing identification of the normal or pathologic anatomy.[50–52] However, because of its multiplanar capabilities, its ability to image vascular structures noninvasively without contrast medium, and its ability to indicate direction of flow, magnetic resonance imaging (MRI) is probably the method of choice for demonstrating these veins.[53] Transesophageal two-dimensional Doppler echography can also demonstrate the azygos vein for most of its length and can be used to identify the direction and velocity of its blood flow.[54–57]

With the current high resolution available with ultrasound, even the normal fetal azygos vein can be imaged sonographically in a high proportion of pregnancies.[58]

The Normal Vertebral and Azygos Venous Systems

These studies of the venous return to the heart not only yielded some remarkably clear radiologic demonstrations of the normal channels but also illustrated some of the variations in venous anatomy and the alternative avenues of venous return to the heart.

The Vertebral Veins

The vertebral venous system is composed of transverse, interconnecting plexuses of veins that anastomose with similar networks above and below by thin-walled longitudinal channels. At a single level, for example, the external plexuses include anterior components in front of the vertebral bodies and posterior components, which surround the appendages. The internal plexuses include the longitudinal sinuses, the dural and spinal veins, and the veins that drain the vertebral bodies (basivertebral veins) (Fig. 36-1). Both the internal and external plexuses drain into the intervertebral veins, which communicate directly with the sacral, lumbar, intercostal, and cervical vertebral veins.

In the sacral region ((Figs. 36-2 and 36-3) the extent to which the sacral plexuses are in continuity with the major channels from the lower extremities is readily demonstrated. The common iliac and internal

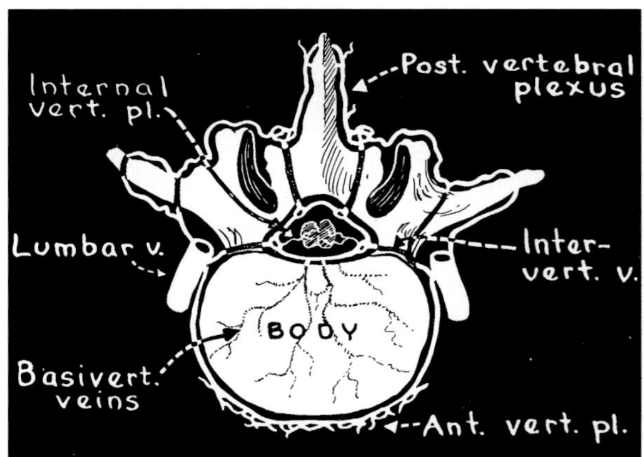

Figure 36-1. Diagrammatic representation of the vertebral plexuses at the lumbar level (seen from above). The external plexuses include anterior components in front of the vertebral bodies and posterior components, which surround the spinous and transverse processes. The internal plexuses include the dural and spinal veins; the longitudinal sinuses; and the basivertebral veins, which drain the vertebral bodies. The internal and external plexuses communicate with the intervertebral veins, which terminate in the lumbar veins. The lumbar veins are connected with both the inferior vena cava and the ascending lumbar veins.

iliac veins communicate by a host of channels with vertebral and ascending lumbar veins. Similarly, the inferior vena cava throughout the lumbar region communicates with the lumbar veins at every level and hence with the ascending lumbar trunks (Figs. 36-4 and 36-5).

The plexiform nature of the lumbar vertebral veins and their segmental arrangement are well illustrated in Figure 36-6. This arrangement is sustained in the thoracic region, where the vertebral drainage is into the intercostal veins (Figs. 36-7 and 36-8).

The Azygos System

The segmental lumbar veins are joined by a longitudinal vessel, the ascending lumbar vein. On either side of the spine there may be one or two ascending lumbar veins. The right ascending lumbar vein becomes the azygos vein as it enters the thorax, and the left ascending lumbar vein is continuous with the hemiazygos chain (Fig. 36-9). The azygos vein, after entering the thorax through the diaphragm, ascends on the anterior surface of the vertebral column up to the level of the fourth thoracic vertebra. It then pursues an anterior course just cephalad to the right main bronchus

Figure 36-2. (A and B) Sacral venous plexuses in a 7-month-old girl, anteroposterior projection. The ramifying channels of the sacral venous plexuses and their connections with both the common iliac veins and the ascending lumbar veins are visible. The common iliac veins unite to form the inferior vena cava at the level of the fourth lumbar vertebra. Double ascending lumbar veins are present, well opacified on the right (the medial ascending lumbar vein on the right is somewhat obscured by the inferior vena cava). Two of the segmental lumbar vertebral plexuses are visualized. *RCIV*, right common iliac vein; *LCIV*, left common iliac vein; *IVC*, inferior vena cava.

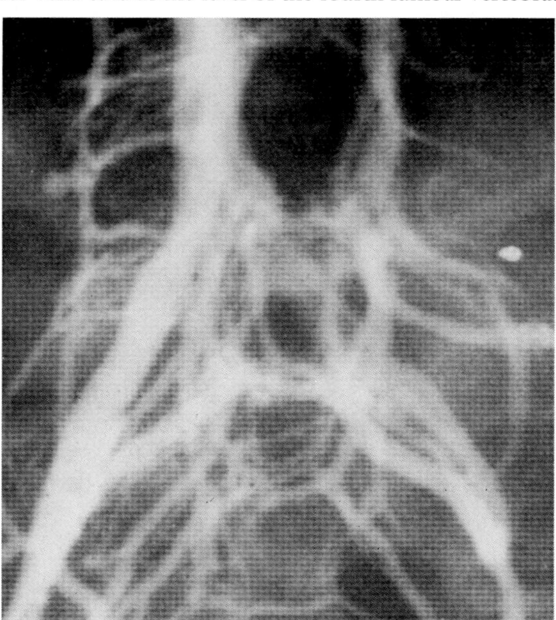

A

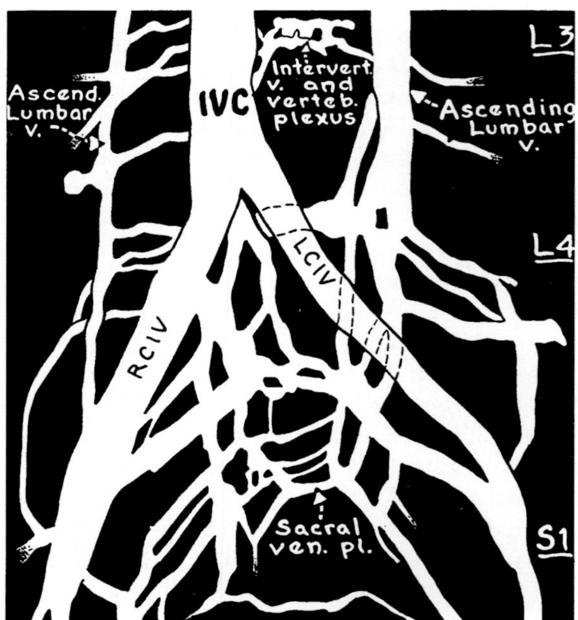

B

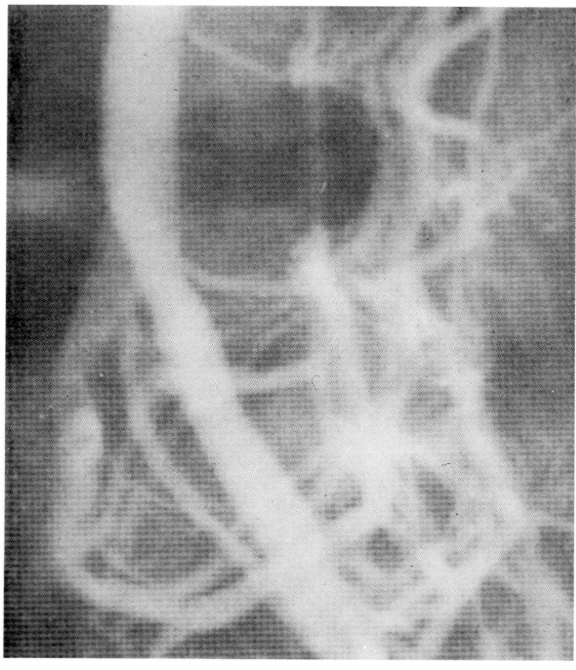

A

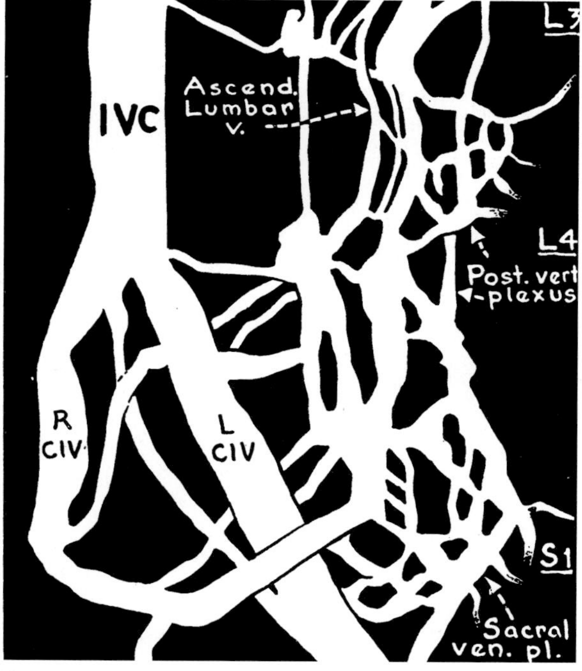

B

Figure 36-3. (A and B) Sacral venous plexuses. A steep right posterior oblique projection brings out the rich anastomoses between the common iliac, sacral, ascending lumbar, and vertebral veins. The ascending lumbar veins communicate with the inferior vena cava by transverse channels. Note how the posterior vertebral plexuses surround the spinous and transverse processes of the vertebra. *LCIV,* left common iliac vein; *RCIV,* right common iliac vein; *IVC,* inferior vena cava.

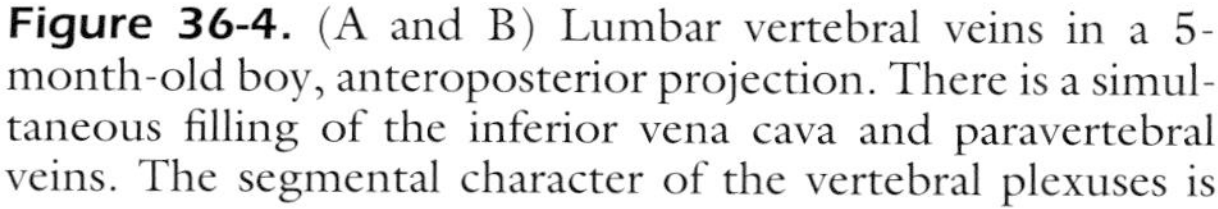

Figure 36-4. (A and B) Lumbar vertebral veins in a 5-month-old boy, anteroposterior projection. There is a simultaneous filling of the inferior vena cava and paravertebral veins. The segmental character of the vertebral plexuses is shown, as well as their relationship to the midportion of the vertebral bodies. This derives from the participation of two somites in the formation of each vertebral body. Ascending lumbar veins are present bilaterally. *IVC,* inferior vena cava.

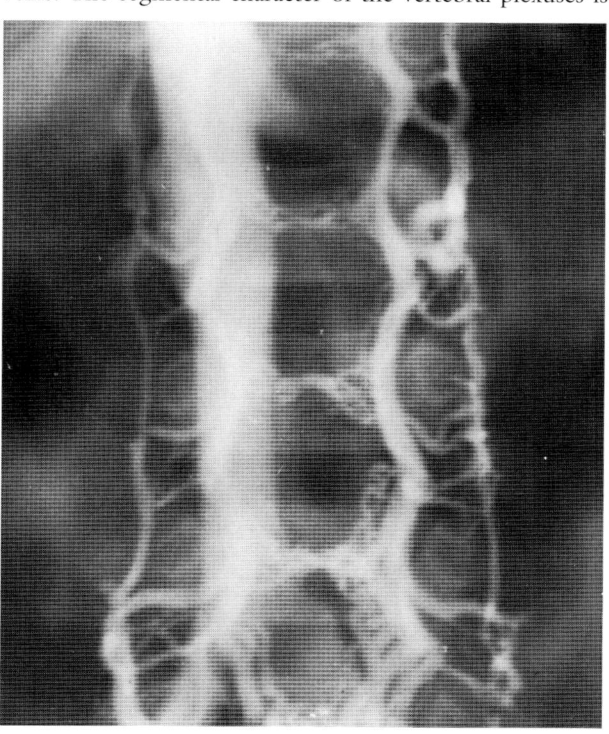

A

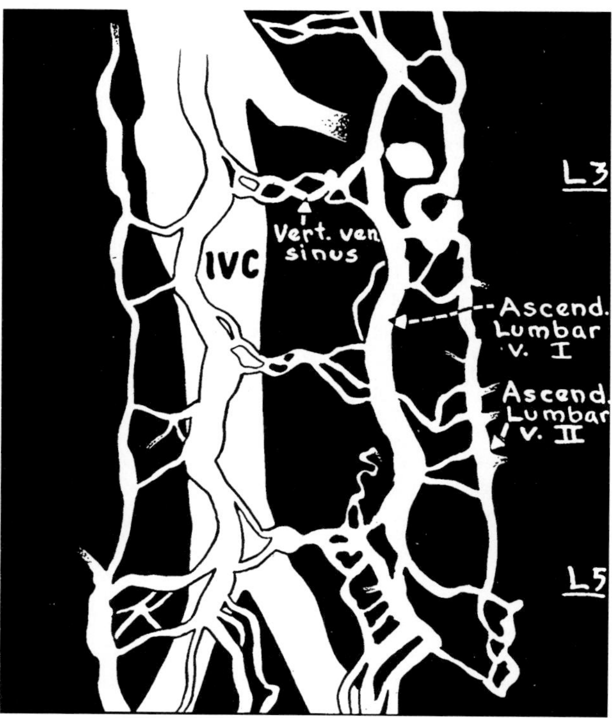

B

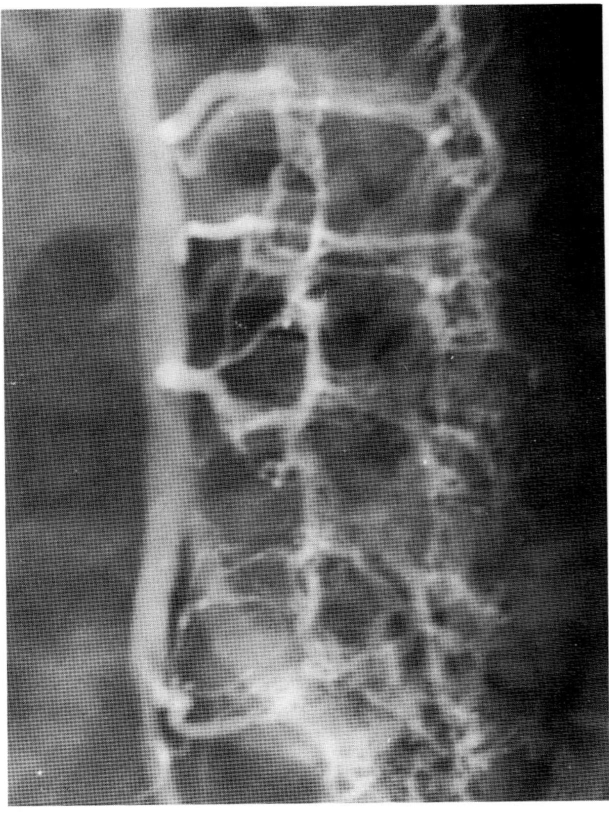

A

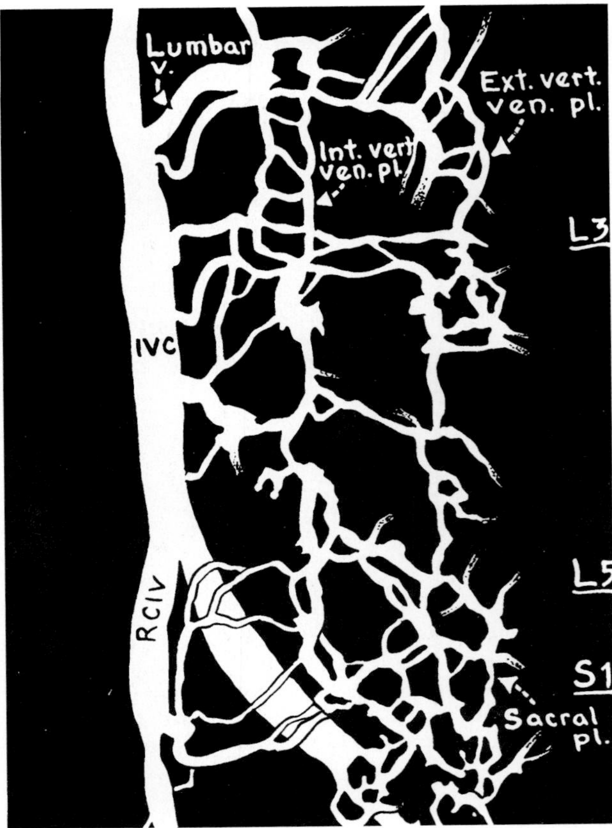

B

Figure 36-5. (A and B) Lumbar vertebral veins, steep right posterior oblique projection. The communications of the lumbar veins on both sides with the inferior vena cava anteriorly, the ascending veins, and the vertebral plexuses posteriorly are clearly shown. *RCIV,* right common iliac vein; *IVC,* inferior vena cava.

and enters the superior vena cava. The posterior intercostal veins, except for the upper three, drain into the azygos vein.

In 0.5 percent of the population, the azygos vein ascends more laterally along the vertebrae and empties into the superior vena cava at a more cranial level. This course gives rise to a so-called azygos lobe—the medial half of the upper right lobe of the lung, which is defined by a venous "mesentery."[59] The azygos vein may resemble a subpleural metastasis in an isolated CT section.

In two-thirds of cases the left renal vein is connected to the ascending lumbar or hemiazygos vein.[8] The hemiazygos vein crosses in front of the vertebral column at the level of the eighth or ninth thoracic vertebra to join the azygos vein. The accessory hemiazygos vein receives the upper thoracic veins on the left and is continuous with the hemiazygos vein below and the left superior intercostal vein above. Figure 36-10 illustrates the technique of intraosseous injection and the degree to which paravertebral and azygos venous filling may be attained in this way.

Some Variations in Systemic Venous Return

No single description of the vertebral and azygos systems can be entirely correct because there is an enormous number of variations in the patterns of systemic venous return.[8,47,48,60–68] Seib described 21 different patterns of the azygos venous system found in dissec-

Figure 36-7. (A and B) Lower thoracic vertebral venous plexus. At this level the vertebral veins are similar to those in the lumbar area and now drain into the intercostal veins, which in turn empty into the hemiazygos and azygos channels. *IVC,* inferior vena cava. ▶

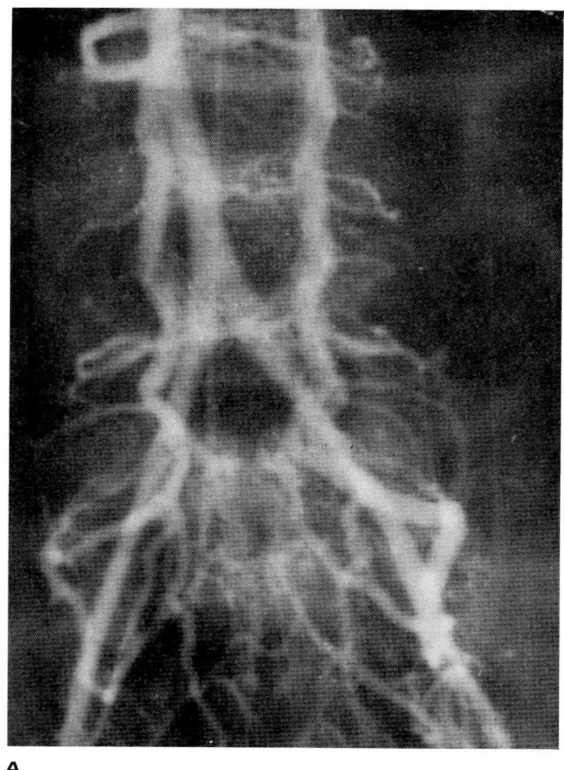

A

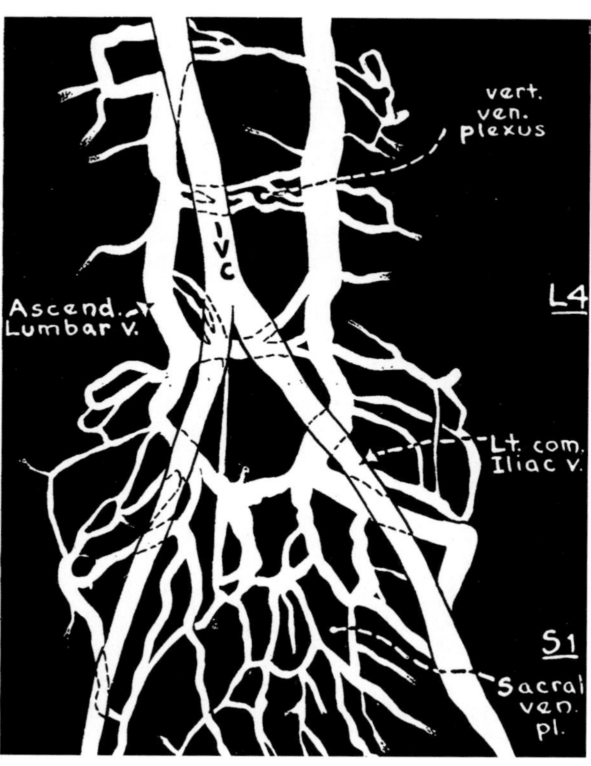

B

Figure 36-6. (A and B) Sacral and lower lumbar vertebral veins in a 2-month-old boy. The plexiform character of the vertebral veins and the profuseness of their ramifications are illustrated in this study. The ascending lumbar channels are occasionally large and almost equal in size to the inferior vena cava (*IVC*), as in this case.

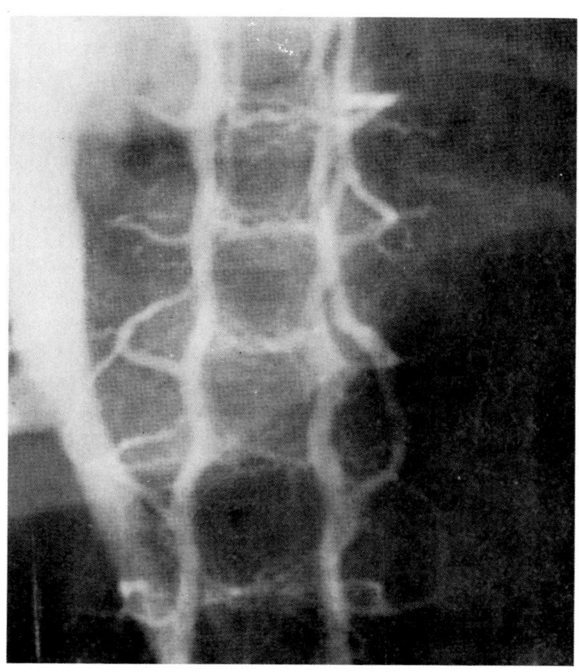

A

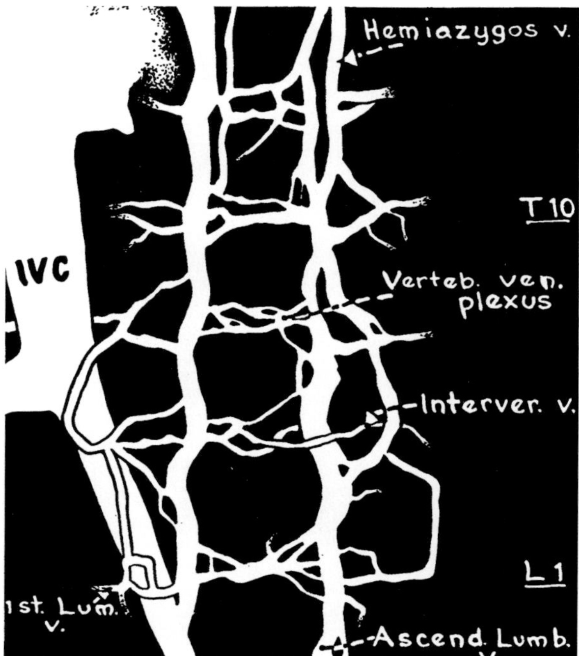

B

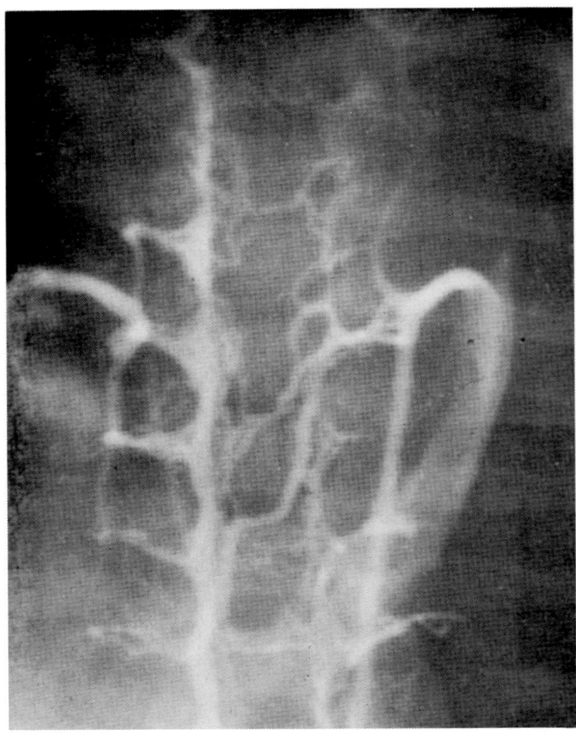

A

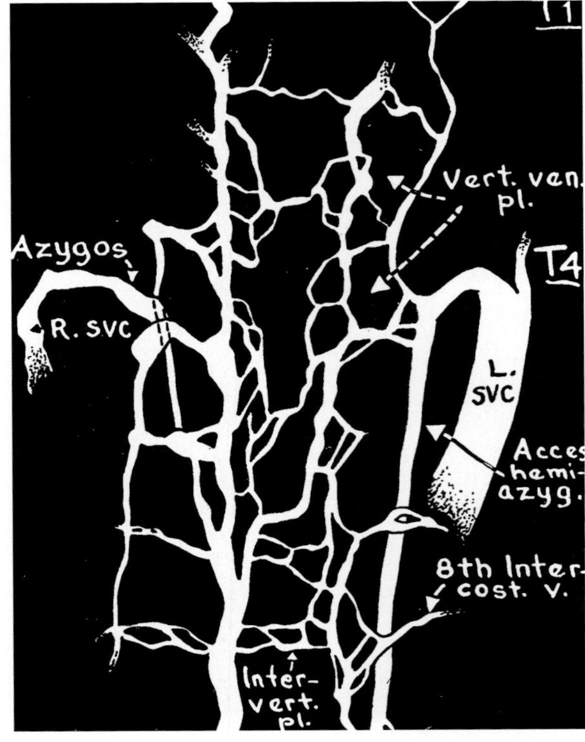

B

Figure 36-8. (A and B) The vertebral veins at the upper thoracic level. The vertebral venous plexuses are opacified following the injection of the opaque medium into the left saphenous vein. The primitive paired arrangement of both the azygos and the superior vena cava veins is preserved, the accessory hemiazygos emptying into the left superior vena cava (*L. SVC*) and the azygos emptying into the right superior vena cava (*R. SVC*). The medial portions of the intercostal veins are opacified.

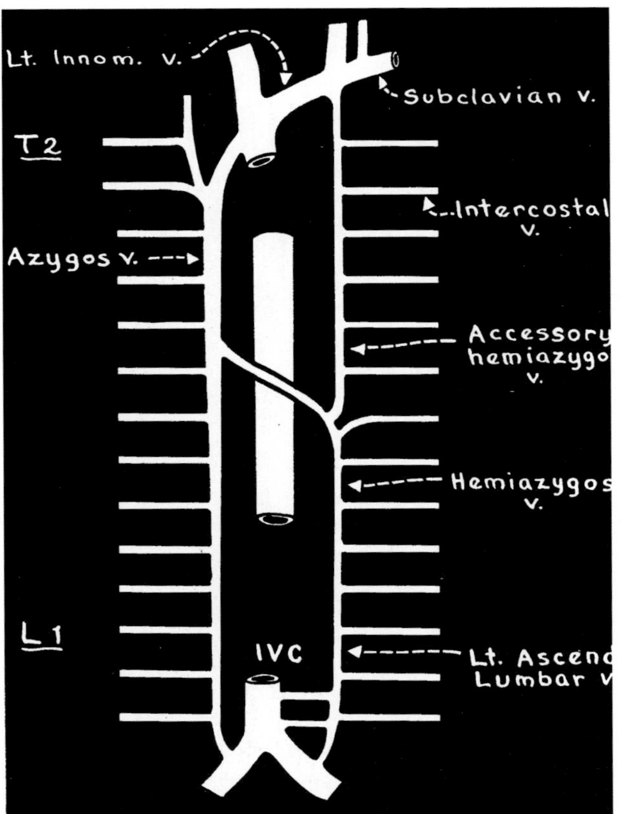

tion of human adult cadavers.[69] Persistence of a left superior vena cava is probably the most common and best-known variation in venous anatomy, occurring in 0.3 percent of people with normal hearts and in 4.4 percent of patients with congenital heart disease[41,70,71]; but absence of the inferior vena cava,[61,65] drainage of the inferior vena cava[63] or superior vena cava[47] into the left atrium rather than the right atrium, and pre-esophageal location of the azygos and hemiazygos veins[62] with resultant stricture have all been described. Partial anomalous pulmonary venous connection with[72] and without[73,74] an atrial septal defect have been described and can be imaged with CT, MRI, and angiography.[75]

Figure 36-9. Diagrammatic representation of the azygos venous system. The segmental lumbar veins are joined to each other by a longitudinal vessel, the ascending lumbar vein. The right ascending lumbar vein as it enters the thorax becomes the azygos vein, and the left ascending lumbar vein is continuous with the hemiazygos vein. The hemiazygos vein crosses in front of the vertebral column at the level of the eighth or ninth thoracic vertebra to join the azygos vein. The accessory hemiazygos vein is continuous with the hemiazygos, receives the upper thoracic veins on the left, and joins the left superior intercostal vein above. *IVC*, inferior vena cava.

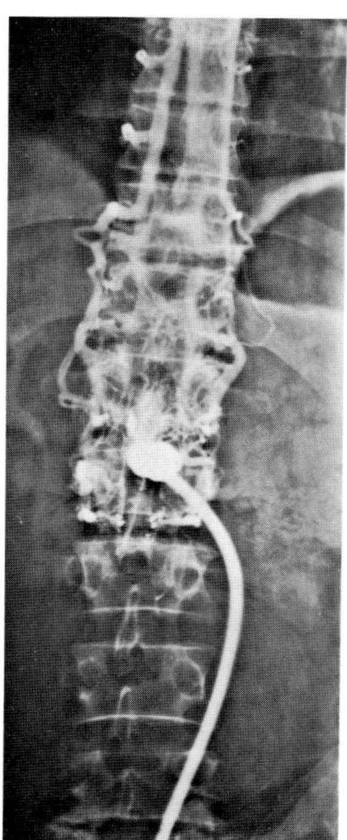

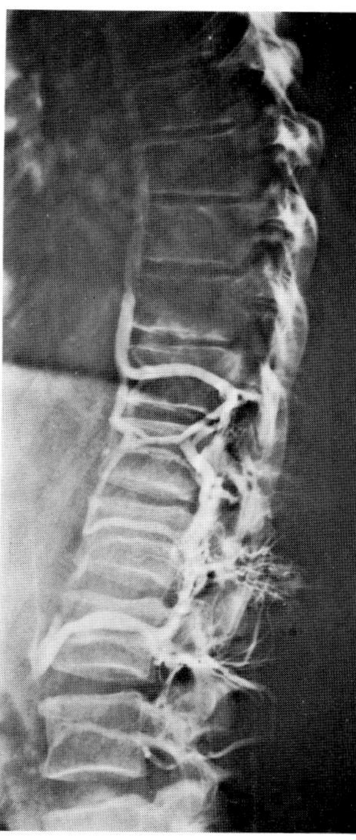

Figure 36-10. Osseous vertebral venography. The opaque medium is injected into the spinous process and rapidly fills the paravertebral plexuses and the azygos system. (Courtesy of Franz P. Lessman, M.D.)

Absence or hypoplasia of the left innominate vein is an anomaly in which blood from the left upper extremity and the left jugular veins cannot reach the superior vena cava and right atrium through the usual channels. At times a persistent left superior vena cava entering the coronary sinus may be present in such cases (Fig. 36-11). Alternatively, an opaque agent injected in the left antecubital vein may flow into the left superior intercostal vein, enter the azygos vein, and thus reach the superior vena cava. A portion of it may enter the paravertebral plexuses, cross the spine, and reach the superior vena cava through collateral channels. In the case illustrated in Figure 36-12, not only was there agenesis of the innominate vein, but also the proximal superior vena cava was absent. The course followed by blood from the upper extremity is similar

Figure 36-11. (A and B) Variations in systemic venous return: hypoplasia of left innominate vein associated with persistent left superior vena cava. After injection of left antecubital vein, the left axillary and subclavian veins are opacified. A persistent left superior vena cava draining into the right atrium via the coronary sinus is noted, and the innominate vein is observed to be hypoplastic. The opaque medium ascends into the internal jugular vein and communicates with the anterior jugular vein, which in turn allows opacification of the right superior vena cava. A communicating vein between right and left superior venae cavae is present. *LAV,* left axillary vein; *LSV,* left subclavian vein; *L. SVC,* left superior vena cava; *R. SVC,* right superior vena cava; *RSV,* right subclavian vein; *RA,* right atrium.

A

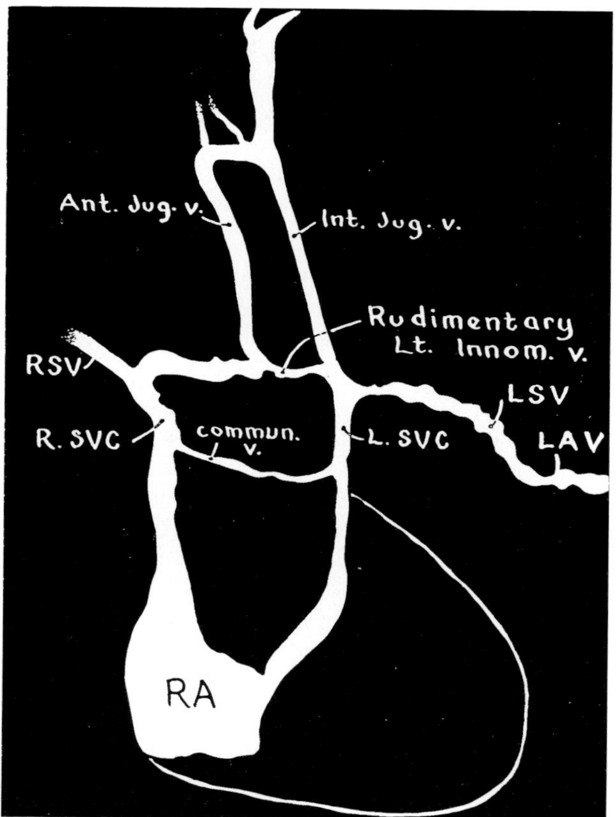

B

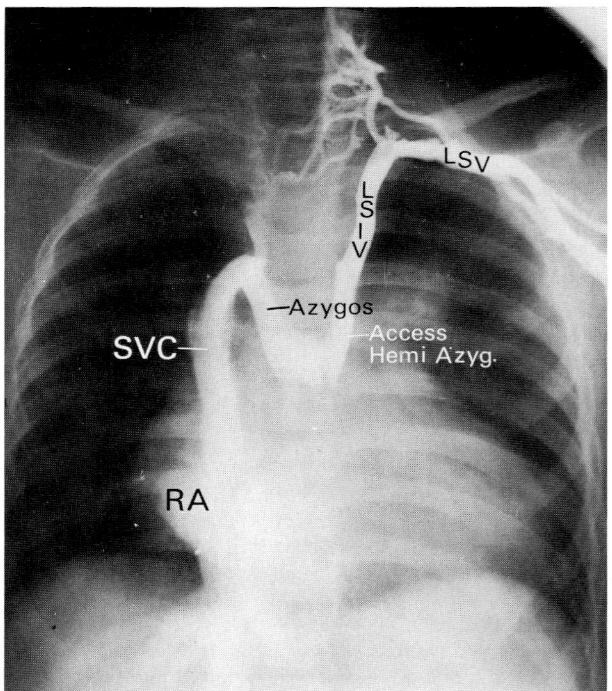

Figure 36-12. Agenesis of the left innominate vein. The opaque medium injected into the left brachial vein opacifies the left subclavian vein (*LSV*) and then flows through the left superior intercostal vein (*LSIV*) to reach the accessory hemiazygos vein. It then joins the azygos flow and finally reaches the superior vena cava (*SVC*). Notice that there is also filling of some of the paravertebral veins in the lower cervical and upper thoracic region. *RA,* right atrium.

to that found in the presence of superior vena caval or left innominate vein obstruction. An additional pathway from the left upper extremity is through a large superior intercostal vein into the accessory hemiazygos vein, the vertebral veins, the inferior vena cava via anastomotic channels, and finally into the caudal portion of the right atrium (Fig. 36-13). In this way blood from the upper part of the body detours to the great caval vein draining the lower portion of the body. There are a number of other available pathways,[76] and the intracranial venous sinuses may participate in the collateral system when an innominate vein is obstructed.[77]

Figure 36-14 demonstrates in anteroposterior and right posterior oblique projections the retrograde filling of the accessory hemiazygos vein in the presence of bilateral superior venae cavae. Figure 36-15 is an example of a persistent left inferior vena cava, a vessel that may be present in a small percentage of cases but is usually small. In the absence of the right inferior vena cava, the left-sided vessel—if present—will be large (see Fig. 36-15).

If the inferior vena cava is occluded, blood from the lower extremities may reach the heart through the paravertebral and azygos systems (Fig. 36-16).[15] If the inferior vena cava is congenitally absent, the same avenues will be utilized. Figure 36-17 demonstrates a huge hemiazygos vein as the major channel from the abdomen emptying into the superior vena cava and thence into the right atrium. In Figure 36-18 the large hemiazygos vein empties into a left superior vena cava, which communicates with the right atrium through the coronary sinus.

Enlargement of the azygos vein (greater than 5 to 7 mm in diameter) usually reflects congestive heart failure, although it may be caused by an increase in azygos blood flow most often due to cirrhosis and increased collateral flow through the esophageal veins or to interruption of the suprahepatic inferior vena cava.[47,48,61,65,78,79] Although this may be an isolated finding,[80–84] inferior vena cava (IVC) interruption is usually associated with congenital cardiac anomalies,[85,86] polysplenia syndrome,[87] or asplenia.[88] The term *IVC interruption* is somewhat of a misnomer because only the hepatic portion of the inferior vena cava is usually absent. In the reported cases the venous drainage of the inferior vena cava reached the heart through the azygos and the superior vena caval systems.

Rarely, one or both of the venae cavae may enter the left atrium.[47,48,63,89–91] In these cases the return of the systemic venous blood to the left heart produces definite peripheral arterial oxygen unsaturation. In the cases shown in Figures 36-19 and 36-20 the left superior vena cava entered the left atrium and the right superior vena cava drained into the right atrium. Figure 36-21 illustrates an instance of hemiazygos venous drainage into the left atrium associated with absence of the inferior vena cava.

Implications and Applications

Batson's concept of the vertebral venous system as a large, low-pressure, intercommunicating reservoir of blood in which alterations in pressure and direction of flow may occur receives some support from the present studies. In some instances the opaque medium traveled well above the termination of the azygos vein and as high as the level of the first thoracic vertebra (see Fig. 36-9). Because the venous drainage from the upper thorax normally runs caudad toward the right atrium, a reversal of direction of flow must be presupposed. A clear demonstration that opacified blood

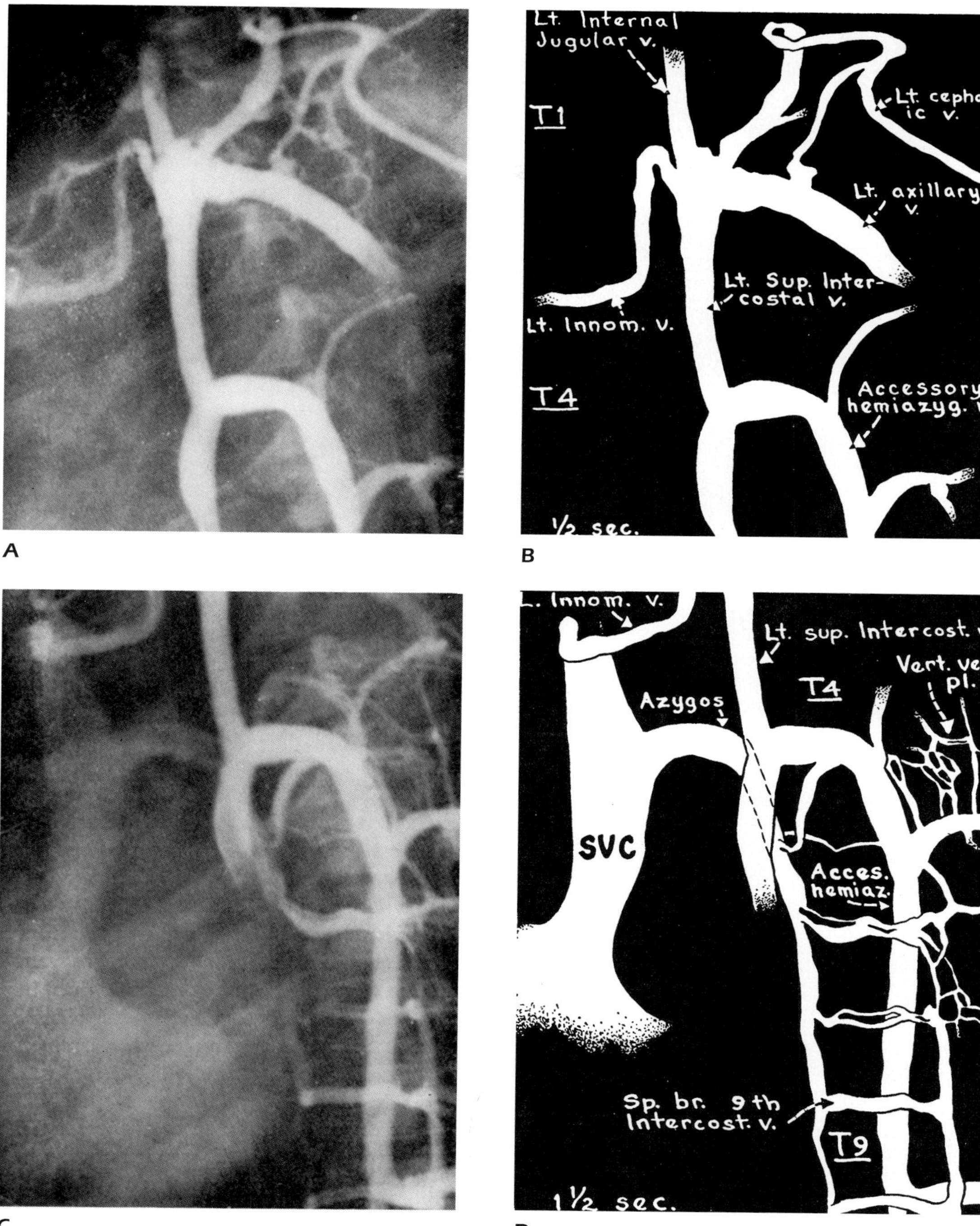

Figure 36-13. Variations in systemic venous return: hypoplasia of the left innominate vein with visualization of the azygos and paravertebral veins from above. The opaque medium was injected into the left cephalic vein with the exposure in the steep right posterior oblique projection. Because the left innominate vein is hypoplastic, no easy communication between the left subclavian vein and the superior vena cava (*SVC*) is possible; the opaque medium enters a large superior intercostal vein to join the hemiazygos system. The spinal branches of the intercostals are opacified from the hemiazygos vein, and cross-communications with the azygos become visible along with filling of the vertebral plexus. Thereafter, the opaque medium flows caudad, reaches the inferior vena cava (*IVC*) through collateral vessels, and then returns cephalad through the inferior vena cava into the right atrium. (A and B) One-half second after injection. Left cephalic, left axillary, and left superior intercostal veins are opacified, as is the accessory hemiazygos. A small left innominate vein is visible. (C and D) One and one-half seconds.

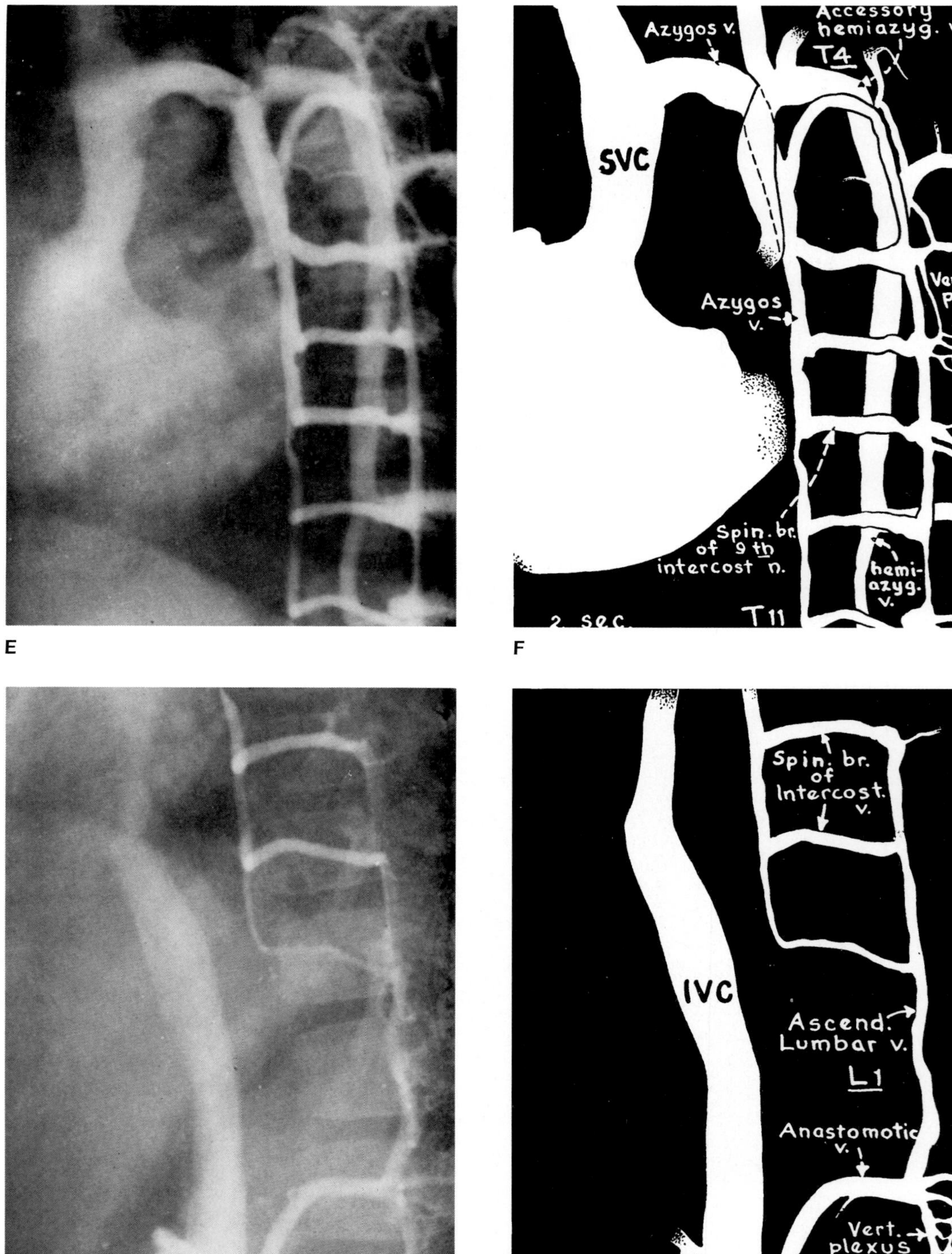

E F G H

Figure 36-13 (continued). The opaque medium has filled the accessory hemiazygos, some of the intercostal veins, and the azygos vein, and opacification of the superior vena cava of moderate degree is now noted. (E and F) Two seconds. The azygos vein is now more densely opacified, as are some of the spinal branches of the lower intercostals and the hemiazygos vein. (G and H) Three and one-half seconds. The inferior vena cava has become opacified following caudad flow of the opaque medium through the hemiazygos vein and thence into collateral channels. The opaque medium is now flowing cephalad through the inferior vena cava into the right atrium.

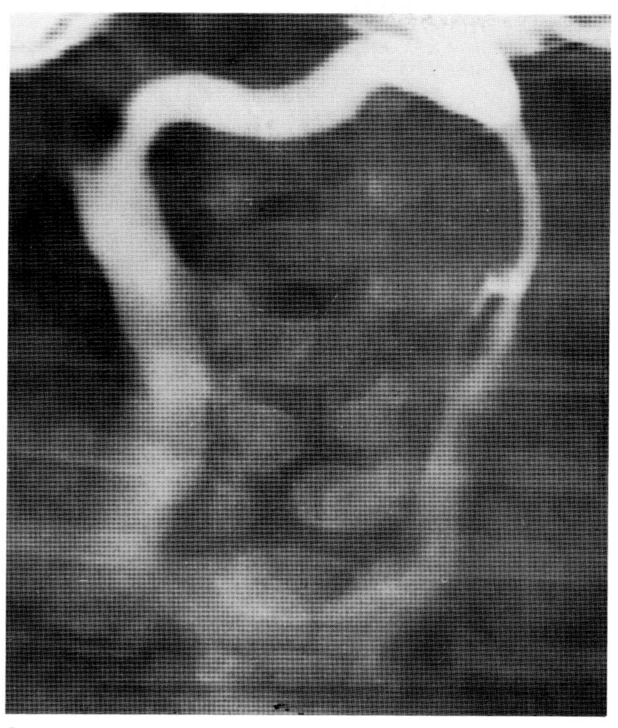

A

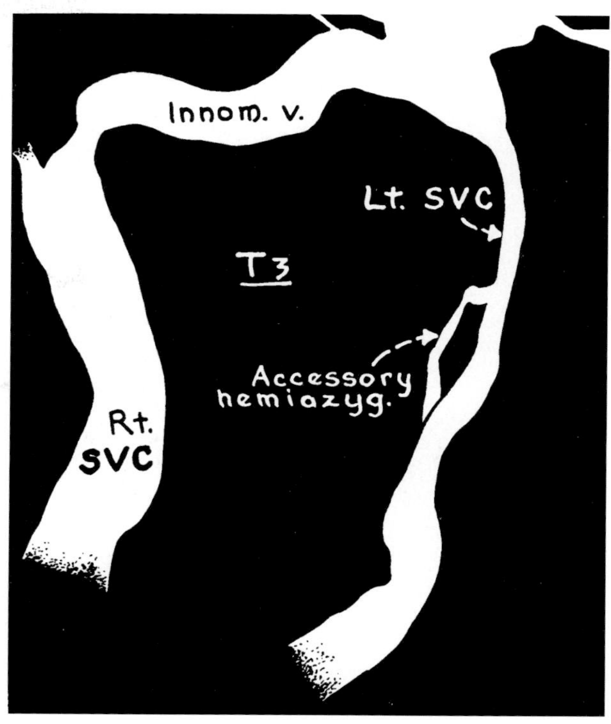

B

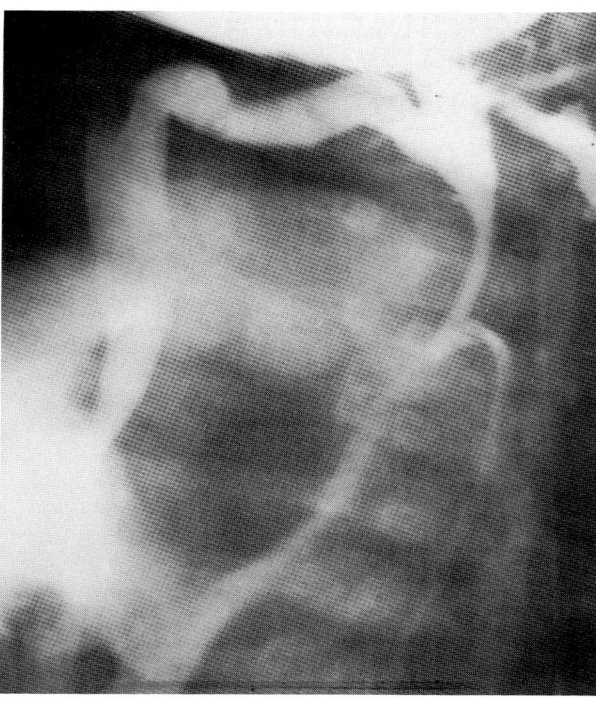

C

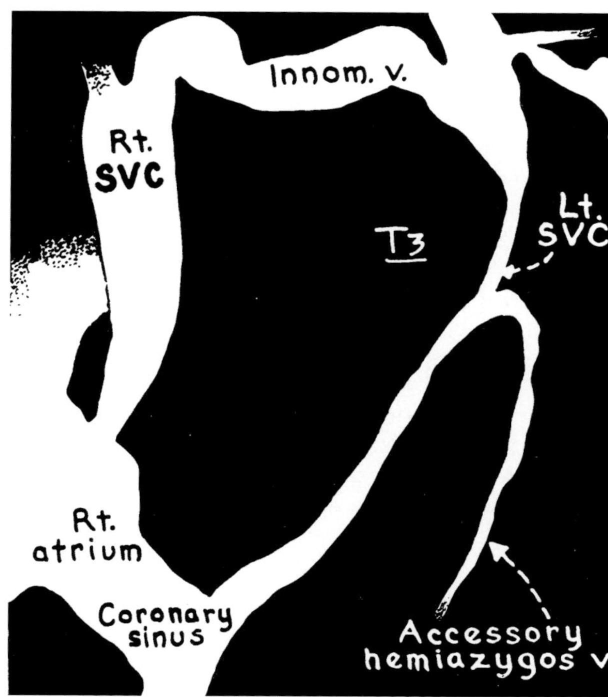

D

Figure 36-14. Variations in systemic venous return: accessory hemiazygos vein entering a left superior vena cava. (A and B) Anteroposterior projection. The left superior vena cava is small by comparison with the right, and the innominate vein is large. (C and D) Right posterior oblique projection. The posterior position of the accessory hemiazygos vein is shown, as well as the entrance of the left superior vena cava into the right atrium through the coronary sinus. *Lt. SVC,* left superior vena cava; *Rt. SVC,* right superior vena cava.

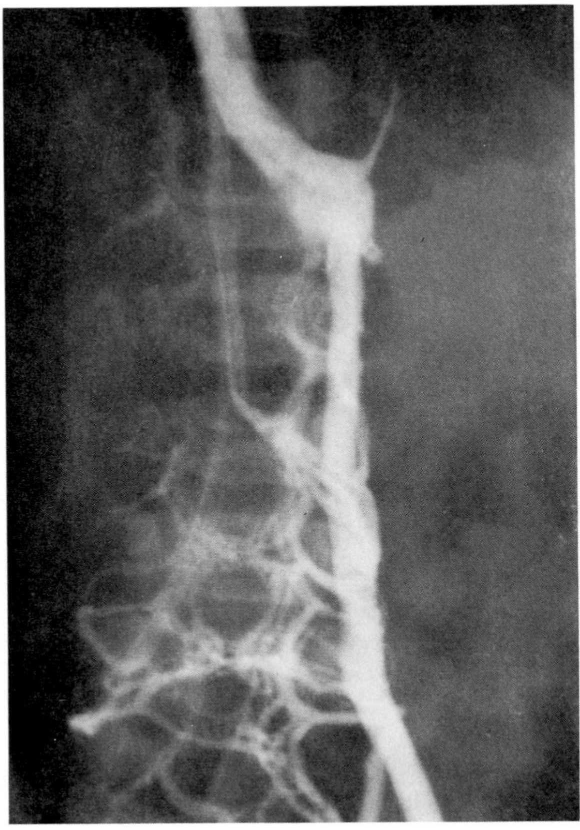

A

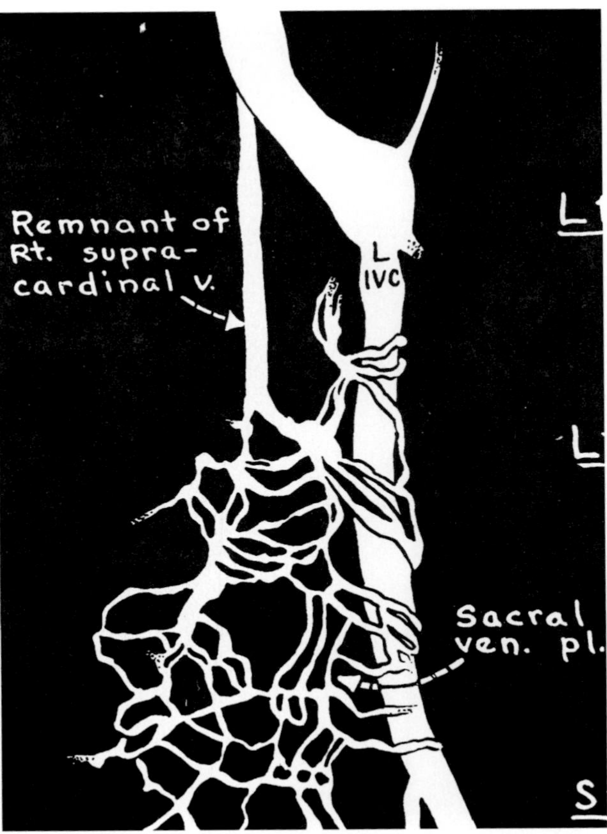

B

Figure 36-15. (A and B) Variations in systemic venous return: left inferior vena cava (*LIVC*). In a small percentage of cases the left inferior vena cava persists as a tiny vessel. In this case it forms the main channel of venous return from the abdomen, and the right inferior vena cava (remnant of right supracardinal vein) is diminutive.

from the left upper extremity can travel through the azygos and paravertebral route into the abdomen, reach the inferior vena cava, and then ascend into the right atrium has also been given (see Fig. 36-13).

The injection of the opaque medium into the respective veins of the lower and upper extremity was, of course, performed under pressure in the preceding studies. But it seems unlikely that the pressure used in manual injection exceeded the pressure at times attained in the thorax by coughing and the Valsalva maneuver or in the abdomen by bearing down. Under the conditions of these injections, the profuseness of the connections between the caval and vertebral venous systems, on the one hand, and between the vertebral and azygos systems, on the other, was clearly delineated.

The plexiform structure of the vertebral veins is in marked contrast to the venous drainage of such viscera as the liver, the spleen, the heart, and the lungs. The arrangement is distinctly primitive and, in a sense, a persistence of the plexoid venous systems of the embryo. Whereas the sinusoidal venous network of an organ such as the liver is transformed early in embryonic life into a congruous, relatively uniform pattern in which small vein confluence forms ever-larger channels of venous return, no such change occurs in the vertebral venous drainage.

In attempting to illustrate some of the normal components of the vertebral and azygos venous systems in human infants, emphasis has been placed on the variability of the patterns observed. That this emphasis is appropriate has frequently been stressed by anatomists.[69] In most instances little clinical significance is attached to the variations in venous return. Occasionally, however, knowledge of these variations may have important practical implications.

Absence of the Inferior Vena Cava

In one instance in which the hepatic portion of the inferior vena cava was absent and the venous drainage from the abdomen reached the right atrium through

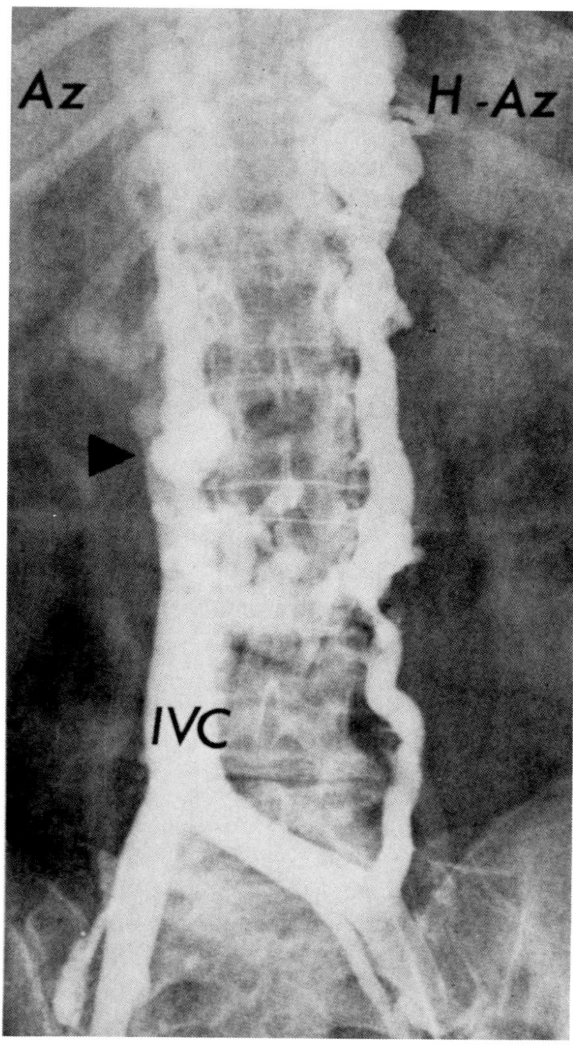

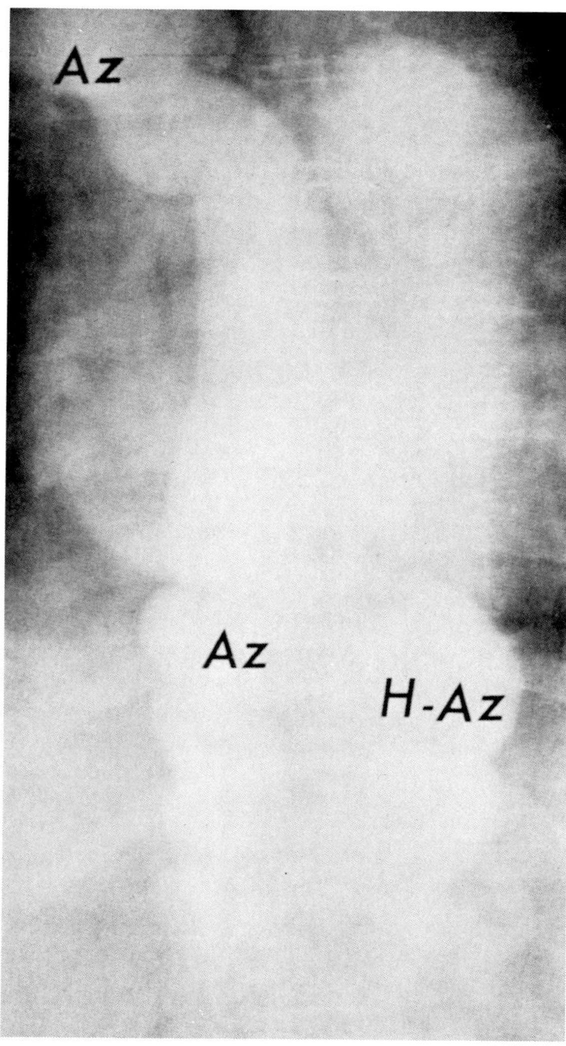

Figure 36-16. Dilated lumbar, azygos, and hemiazygos veins in inferior vena caval obstruction. (A) Anteroposterior view, lumbar region. There is obstruction of the inferior vena cava (*IVC*) at the level of the renal vein (*arrowhead*). Ascending lumbar veins are filled via communicating channels and are in continuity with the azygos (*Az*) and hemiazygos (*H-Az*) veins. (B) Anteroposterior view, later phase, thoracolumbar region. The huge hemiazygos vein crosses the spine to join the azygos at the level of the eighth thoracic vertebra. (Courtesy of Douglass Adams, M.D.)

the azygos system and the superior vena cava, ligation of the azygos vein was followed by retroperitoneal hemorrhage and death.[78] A major dual system of venous return from the lower portion of the body did not exist in the patient. Awareness of this possibility might have forestalled the surgical procedure. The cardiac physiologist, too, should be aware of the variations that occur after right heart catheterization through the femoral vein; the unusual course taken by the catheter in the absence of an inferior vena cava may otherwise be a vexing source of puzzlement. The radiologist who is aware of the azygos vein anatomy may detect congenital absence of the inferior vena cava by the prominence of the azygos vein on conventional films.[92]

An inferior vena cavogram provides unambiguous confirmation of the azygos continuation of the IVC. In most cases, however, the diagnosis can be made on the basis of ultrasonic,[93] computed tomographic,[94,95] radionuclide angiographic,[96] or MRI findings. The sonographic demonstration of what appears to be a vertical IVC draining directly into the right atrium is pathognomonic of IVC interruption. In IVC interruption, the suprahepatic IVC exists only as the hepatic

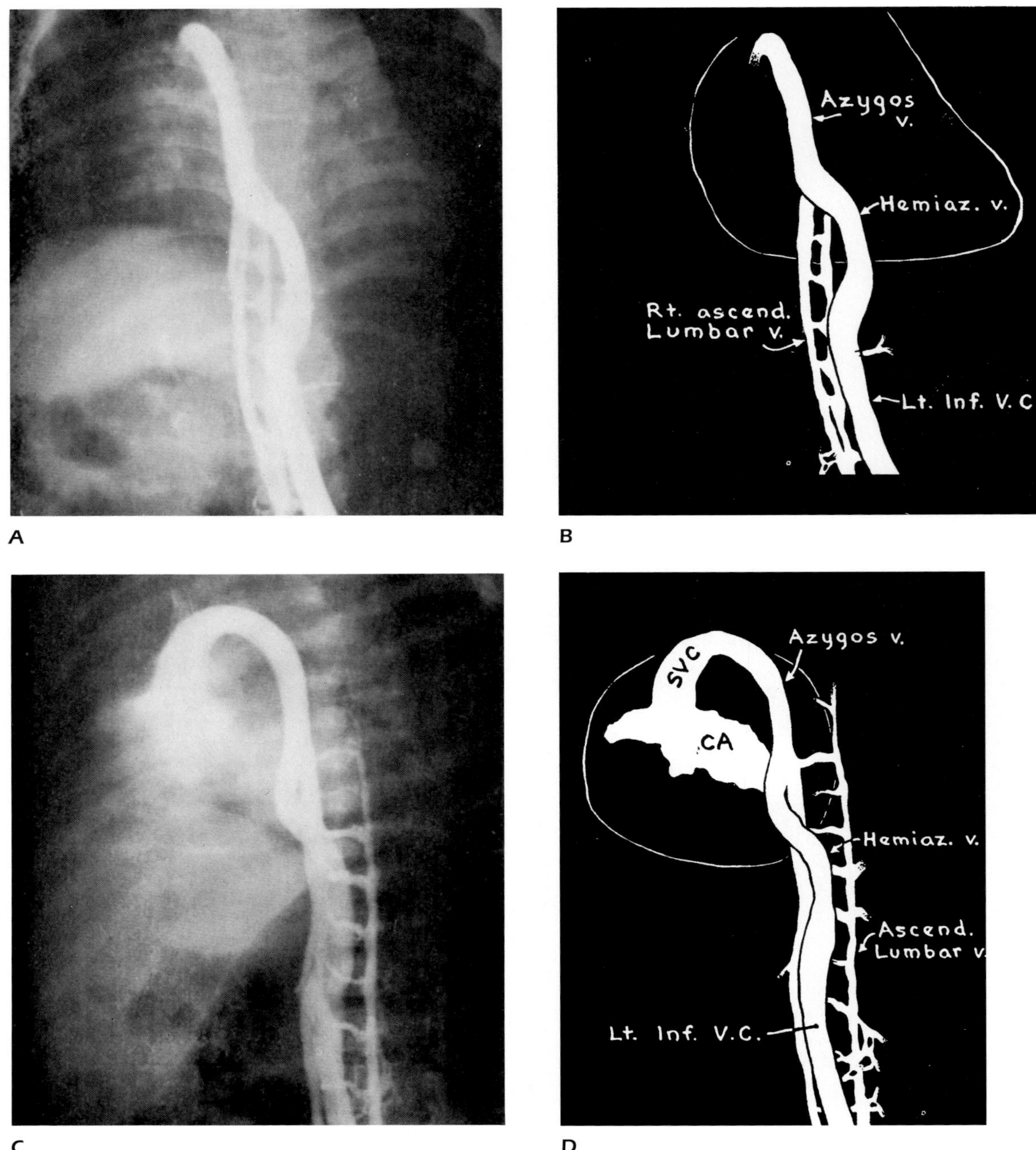

Figure 36-17. Variations in the systemic venous return: absence of the inferior vena cava. The hepatic portion of the inferior vena cava is absent, and the opaque medium has flowed into the hemiazygos vein and thence into the azygos vein. The hemiazygos is a large channel and is continuous with a left inferior vena cava (*Lt. Inf. V.C.*) below. The azygos vein empties into the superior vena cava, and thus blood from the lower extremities and abdomen reaches the right atrium. (A and B) Anteroposterior view. (C and D) Steep right posterior oblique projection. *SVC,* superior vena cava; *CA,* common artery.

Dilatation of the Azygos Vein

The location of the arch of the azygos vein in the right tracheobronchial angle has been carefully described.[100] When enlarged, the arch may resemble a paratracheal tumor.[45,80,83,101,102] In contrast to a tumor, it undergoes significant changes with position, respiration, and hemodynamic alterations.[80,100] It must be kept in mind that varied elements may be associated with azygos vein enlargement (such as portal hypertension, right heart failure, obstruction or absence of the inferior vena cava, and constrictive pericarditis). Local obstruction of the azygos vein can result in its dilatation. In a case reported by Siddorn and Worsornu,[103] compression by enlarged hilar lymph nodes secondary to a chronic lung abscess resulted in an 8 × 6 cm dilatation of the azygos arch. Rarely a congenital aneurysm of the azygos[104,105] or hemiazygos vein[106] may occur. Seebauer et al.[105] describe a 12-cm congenital aneurysm of the azygos vein presenting as a chest mass.

Unexplained Cyanosis

Anomalous systemic venous return to the left atrium may produce cyanosis unaccompanied by murmurs or significant disability. The electrocardiogram may or may not show left ventricular hypertrophy, but the cardiac silhouette is usually normal. On catheterization of the right side of the heart, the hemodynamics are usually normal as well. This lesion may be defined preoperatively by ultrasound, MIR, or angiography. If the anatomy is clearly outlined, surgical correction may then be accomplished.

Fistulas

Fistulas have been reported involving the azygos vein or vertebral system. A congenital fistula with separate connections between the aorta and the azygos vein, superior vena cava, and innominate vein has been described.[107] A posttraumatic aortoazygos fistula with pseudoaneurysm formation was discovered on an examination performed for increasing shortness of breath 6 weeks after the patient had suffered a gunshot wound to the right infrascapular area.[108]

Fistulas between the vertebral artery and vein have increased in frequency with the increase in traumatic injuries[109–116] although such fistulas may also be spontaneous.[117–119] In one case reported by Quatromoni et al.,[44] the fistula was secondary to direct percutaneous carotid angiography. Fistulas most commonly develop in the second and third parts of the vertebral system, where the vertebral vein exists as a plexus of veins rather than a discrete vein. In the interosseous segment, the bony framework prevents fistula closure by swelling or hematoma of adjacent tissues.[44]

Azygos Rupture

Although injuries to the azygos vein are most commonly due to penetrating trauma, this vein may uncommonly be torn from blunt trauma.[120–123] This may be associated with fracture-dislocations of the midthoracic spine where the bony injury directly tears the azygos vein[123] or it may be due to deceleration forces (analogous to deceleration injuries to the thoracic aorta) where the rupture occurs close to its junction with the superior vena cava (SVC).[120,122] Patients usually have persistent hypotension despite resuscitation. Diagnosis is difficult, but a right hemothorax or a widened mediastinum may be evident radiographically. Angiography is essential to exclude an arterial injury.[124]

Azygos Flow in Portal Hypertension

Variceal flow in portal hypertension is most commonly via the azygos vein, and the exact drainage system can be demonstrated by cineportography.[125] This collateral blood flow can be estimated by selectively cannulating the azygos vein from the SVC via either a transfemoral or transjugular approach, and placing a continuous thermodilution catheter into the azygos vein so that its tip is approximately 5 cm from the SVC junction.[126–128] Azygos blood flow rates using this technique are as follows[126]: normal subjects 0.08 to 0.19 liter per minute; cirrhosis and portal hypertension 0.22 to 1.61 liter per minute; extrahepatic portal hypertension 0.45 ± 0.19 liter per minute. When cannulating the azygos vein, a lateral view should be used to confirm the catheter position because internal mammary vein cannulation may mimic azygos vein cannulation on the posteroanterior view[129]; with azygos vein cannulation, a lateral view will show the catheter to be directed posteriorly rather than anteriorly. Azygos flow can also be measured by transesophageal Doppler echography.[56]

Catheter Access

Occasionally patients who need long-term intravenous hyperalimentation have limited venous access because of superior and inferior vena caval thrombosis. In such cases, it is possible to gain catheter access to the azygos vein via a cutdown on an intercostal vein.[130–132] The catheter can then be threaded through the intercostal vein into the azygos vein.

References

1. Aronsson H. Vertebral venous system and its clinical importance. Nord Med 1947;33:268.
2. Norgore M. Clinical anatomy of the vertebral veins. Surgery 1945;17:606.
3. Robinson LS: The collateral circulation following ligation of the inferior vena cava: injection studies in stillborn infants. Surgery 1949;25:329.
4. Mellins HZ. Functions of the vertebral venous system. Bull Univ Minn Hosp and Minn Med Found 1951;22:213.
5. Northway RO, Greenway GD. The vena cava and its collateral circulation. Univ Hosp Bull Univ Mich Sch Med 1944;10:67.
6. Salen EF. Phlebographic study of constrictive processes in superior vena cava area and of accompanying changes in collateral circulation. Acta Radiol 1951;36:81.
7. Andreasen AT, Watson F. Experimental cardiovascular surgery. Br J Surg 1952;39:548.
8. Anson BJ, Caldwell EW. The pararenal vascular system: the study of 425 anatomical specimens. Quart Bull Northwest Univ Med Sch 1947;21:320.
9. Braun JP, Tournade A. Venous drainage in the craniocervical region. Neuroradiology 1977;13:155.
10. Herlihy WF. Revision of venous system; role of vertebral veins. Med J Aust 1947;1:661.
11. Batson OV. The function of the vertebral veins and their role in the spread of metastases. Ann Surg 1940;112:138.
12. Batson OV. The role of the vertebral veins in metastatic processes. Ann Intern Med 1942;16:38.
13. Batson OV. The vertebral vein system as a mechanism for the spread of metastases. AJR 1942;48:715.
14. Harris HA. A note on the clinical anatomy of the veins, with special reference to the spinal veins. Brain 1941;64:291.
15. Franklin KJ. A monograph on veins. Springfield, IL: Charles C Thomas, 1937.
16. Willis T. Quoted by Harris HA. A note on the clinical anatomy of the veins, with special reference to the spinal veins. Brain 1941;64:291.
17. Winslow JB. Quoted by Harris HA. A note on the clinical anatomy of the veins, with special reference to the spinal veins. Brain 1941;64:291.
18. Bock AC. Darstellung der Venen. Leipzig, 1823.
19. Quain J. Elements of descriptive and practical anatomy. London: Simpkin & Marshall, 1828.
20. Hilton J. Quoted by Norgore M. Clinical anatomy of the vertebral veins. Surgery 1945;17:606.
21. Johnstone AS. Experimental study of vertebral venous system; preliminary report. Proc R Soc Med 1946;39:538.
22. Onuigbo WIB. Paradoxical position of vertebral veins in cancer carriage. Med Hypotheses 1977;3:267–269.
23. Lawrence EA, Moore DB. Importance of vertebral venous system in metastasis of neoplasms as demonstrated by transplantable rabbit carcinoma. Surg Forum 1952;2:269.
24. Coman DR, DeLong RP. Role of vertebral venous systems in metastasis of cancer to spinal column: experiments with tumor cell suspensions in rats and rabbits. Cancer 1951;4:610.
25. Cohn TD, Krinsky M, Zarowitz H. Metastatic brain abscess: role of vertebral vein in circulation. Am Practit Dig Treat 1950;1:792.
26. Antoniades J, Cross MN, Walner RJ, et al. Bone scanning in carcinoma of the colon and rectum. Dis Colon Rectum 1976;19:139–143.
27. Fletcher JW, Solaric-George E, Henry RE, et al. Radioisotopic detection of osseous metastases: evaluation of 99m Tc pyrophosphate. Arch Intern Med 1975;135:553–557.
28. Shirazi PH, Rayundu GVS, Fordham EW. 18F bone scanning: review of indications and results of 1500 scans. Radiology 1974;112:361–368.
29. Tofe AJ, Francis MD, Harvey WJ. Correlation of neoplasms with incidence and localization of skeletal metastases: an analysis of 1,355 diphosphonate bone scans. J Nucl Med 1975;16:986–989.
30. Halpern MH. Azygos vein system in rat. Anat Rec 1953;116:83.
31. deFreitas V, Zorzetto NL, Prates JC, et al. Experimental study of lymphatico-venous communications after thoracic duct ligature in dogs. Anat Anz 1979;146:27–38.
32. Howarth F, Cooper ERA. Departure of substances from spinal theca. Lancet 1949;2:937.
33. Fleischner FG, Udis SW. Dilatation of azygos vein: roentgen sign of venous enlargement. AJR 1952;67:569.
34. Burke DT, Goldberg L. Azygos veins in tomography. Can Med Assoc J 1949;60:271.
35. Anderson RK. Diodrast studies of the vertebral and cranial venous systems. J Neurosurg 1951;8:411.
36. Helander CG, Lindbom A. Sacrolum-bar venography. Acta Radiol 1955;44:410.
37. Nordenstrom B. Method of angiography of the azygos vein and the anterior internal venous plexus of the spine. Acta Radiol 1955;44:201.
38. Perey O, Lind J, Wegelius C. Phlebography of the intervertebral plexus. Acta Orthop Scand 1956;25:228.
39. Fischgold H, Adam H, Ecoiffier J et al. Opacification of spinal plexuses and azygos veins by osseous route. J Radiol Electrol Med Nucl 1952;33:37.
40. Lessman FP, Schobinger von Schowingen RS, Lasser EC. Intraosseous venography in skeletal and soft tissue abnormalities. Acta Radiol 1955;44:397.
41. Susse HJ, Aurig G. Das transossale Venogramm der Venae intercostales, der Vena azygos und der Vena thoracica interna. ROEFO 1954;81:335.
42. Tori G. Demonstration of azygos, hemiazygos and lumbar veins by means of intraosseous phlebography. Nuntius Radiol 1953;19:724.
43. Tori G. The radiological demonstration of the azygos and other thoracico-abdominal veins in the living. Br J Radiol 1954;27:16.
44. Quatromoni JC, Johnson JM, Wood M. Vertebral arteriovenous fistulas. Am J Surg 1979;138:907–911.
45. Stauffer HM, LaBree JW, Adams FH. Normally situated arch of azygos vein: roentgenologic identification and catheterization. AJR 1951;66:353.
46. Ranniger K. Retrograde azygography. Radiology 1968;90:1097–1104.
47. Abrams HL. Selectivity in the study of the cardiovascular system. Calif Med 1962;96:149.
48. Abrams HL. The vertebral and azygos venous systems, and some variations in systemic venous return. Radiology 1957;69:508.
49. Abrams HL. The relationship of systemic venous anomalies to the paravertebral veins. AJR 1958;80:414.
50. Smathers RL, Buschi AJ, Pope TL Jr, et al. The azygos arch: normal and pathological CT appearance. AJR 1982;139:477–483.
51. Takasugi JE, Godwin JD. CT appearance of the retroaortic anastomoses of the azygos system. AJR 1990;154:41–44.
52. Dudiak CM, Olson MC, Posniak HV. CT evaluation of congenital and acquired abnormalities of the azygos system. Radiographics 1991;11:233–246.
53. Hansen ME, Spritzer CE, Sostman HD. Assessing the patency of mediastinal and thoracic inlet veins: value of MR imaging. AJR 1990;155:1177–1182.
54. Sukigara M, Takamoto S, Omoto R. Downhill azygos vein secondary to occlusion of the superior vena cava in Bechet's disease. Chest 1988;94:1308–1309.
55. Caletti G, Brocchi E, Baraldini M, et al. Assessment of portal hypertension by endoscopic ultrasonography. Gastrointest Endosc 1990;36:521–527.
56. Sukigara M, Komazaki T, Ohata M. Transesophageal real-time two-dimensional Doppler echography—a new method for the evaluation of azygos venous flow. Gastrointest Endosc 1988;34:125–128.

57. Sukigara M, Matsumoto T, Takeuchi M, et al. Doppler echography for hemodynamic studies of the azygos vein. Surg Endosc 1989;3:21–28.
58. Belfar HL, Hill LM, Peterson CS. Sonographic imaging of the fetal azygos vein: normal and pathologic appearance. J Ultrasound Med 1990;9:569–573.
59. Kolbenstvedt A, Kolmannskog F, Aakhus T. The appearance of an anomalous azygos vein on computed tomography of the chest. Radiology 1979;130:386.
60. Butler H, Balankura K. Preaortic thoracic and azygos veins. Anat Rec 1952;113:409.
61. Downing DF. Absence of the inferior vena cava. Pediatrics 1953;12:675.
62. Flynn R. Congenital stricture of esophagus (case with two aberrant veins crossing in front of esophagus). Med J Aust 1946; 1:701.
63. Gardner DL, Cole L. Long survival with inferior vena cava draining into left atrium. Br Heart J 1955;17:93.
64. Hamilton HB, Meader RG. Anomalous single azygos-hemiazygos vein associated with retroaortic left renal and accessory renal veins. Yale J Biol Med 1942;14:463.
65. Stackelberg B, Lind J, Wegelius C. Absence of inferior vena cava diagnosed by angiocardiography. Cardiologia (Basel) 1952;21:583.
66. Winter FS. Persistent left superior vena cava: survey of world literature and report of 30 additional cases. Angiology 1954; 5:90.
67. Mayo J, Gray R, St. Louis E, et al. Anomalies of the inferior vena cava. AJR 1983;140:339–345.
68. Mezzogiorno A, Passiatore C. An atypic pattern of the azygos venous system in man. Anat Anz 1988;165:277–281.
69. Seib GA. Azygos system of veins in American whites and American Negroes, including observations of inferior caval venous system. Am J Phys Anthropol 1934;19:39.
70. Faer MJ, Lynch RD, Evans HO, et al. Inferior vena cava duplication: demonstration by computed tomography. Radiology 1979;130:707–709.
71. Cha MC, Khoury GH. Persistent left superior vena cava. Radiology 1972;103:375–381.
72. Mullen JC, Razzouk AJ, Williams WG, et al. Partial anomalous pulmonary venous connection to the azygos vein with atrial septal defect. Ann Thorac Surg 1991;52:1164–1165.
73. Yabek SM, Akl BF, Berman W Jr. Partial anomalous pulmonary venous connection to the azygos vein with intact atrial septum. Chest 1979;76:486–487.
74. Jennings JG, Serwer GA. Partial anomalous pulmonary venous connection to the azygos vein with intact atrial septum. Pediatr Cardiol 1986;7:115–117.
75. Thorsen MK, Erickson SJ, Mewissen MW, et al. CT and MR imaging of partial anomalous pulmonary venous return to the azygos vein. J Comput Assist Tomogr 1990;14:1007–1009.
76. Katz S, Hussey HH, Oveal JR. Phlebography for the study of obstruction of veins of the superior vena caval system. Am J Med Sci 1947;214:7.
77. Schwartz A, Fraenkel M. Diversion of venous blood flow through transverse sinuses in one sided innominate vein obstruction. Radiology 1952;58:728.
78. Effler DB, Greer AE, Sifers EG. Anomaly of the vena cava inferior: report of fatality after ligation. JAMA 1952;146:1321.
79. Latimer HB, Virden HH. A case of complete absence of the inferior vena cava. J Kans Med Soc 1944;45:346.
80. Batistich AT. Dilatation of azygos vein stimulating mediastinal tumor. Australas Radiol 1976;20:329–332.
81. Ginaldi S, Chuang VP, Wallace S. Absence of hepatic segment of the inferior vena cava with azygous continuation. J Comput Assist Tomogr 1980;4:112–114.
82. Abrams HL, Kaplan HS. Angiocardiographic interpretation in congenital heart disease. Springfield, IL: Charles C Thomas, 1956.
83. Kahn ZM, Adour KK. Azygos continuation of the inferior vena cava mimicking mediastinal mass. Ear Nose Throat J 1976;55:369–372.
84. Schrader DL, Miller WT. Right paratracheal shadow in an asymptomatic young man. Chest 1977;72:647–648.
85. Garris JB, Kangarloo H, Sample WF. Ultrasonic diagnosis of infrahepatic interruption of the inferior vena cava with azygos (hemiazygos) continuation. Radiology 1980;134:179–183.
86. Jacob T, Ablett M, Stark J. Transposition of the great arteries, primum atrial septal defect, azygos continuation of the inferior vena cava, bilateral superior venae cavae and dextrocardia with centrally placed liver. Am Heart J 1977;93:623–625.
87. Naraval RC, Weiner CI. Radiological case of the month: polysplenia syndrome with azygos continuation. Md State Med J 1976;25:69–70.
88. Ivemark BI. Implications of agenesis of spleen on pathogenesis of conotruncus anomalies in childhood: analysis of heart malformations in splenic agenesis syndrome, with 14 new cases. Acta Pediatr 1955;44(Suppl 104):590.
89. Campbell M, Deuchar DC. The left sided superior vena cava. Br Heart J 1954;16:423.
90. Taussig HB. Congenital malformations of the heart. New York: Commonwealth Fund, 1947.
91. Tuchman H, Brown JF, Huston JH, et al. Superior vena cava draining into left atrium: another cause for left ventricular hypertrophy with cyanotic congenital heart disease. Am J Med 1956;21:481.
92. Berdon WE, Baker DH. Plain film findings in azygos continuation of the inferior vena cava. AJR 1968;104:452–457.
93. Huhta JC, Smallhorn JF, Macartney FJ. Cross-sectional echocardiographic diagnosis of azygos continuation of the inferior vena cava. Cathet Cardiovasc Diagn 1984;10:221–232.
94. Webb WR, Gamsu G, Speckman JM, et al. Computed tomographic demonstration of mediastinal venous anomalies. AJR 1982;139:157–161.
95. Breckenridge JW, Kinlaw WB. Azygos continuation of inferior vena cava: CT appearance. J Comput Assist Tomogr 1980;4:392–397.
96. Roguin N, Lam M, Frenkel A, et al. Radionuclide angiography of azygos continuation of inferior vena cava in left atrial isomerism (polysplenia syndrome). Clin Nucl Med 1987;12: 708–710.
97. Sardi A, Minken SL. The placement of intracaval filters in an anomalous (left-sided) vena cava. J Vasc Surg 1987;6:84–86.
98. Castellino RA, Blank N, Adams DF. Dilated azygos and hemiazygos veins presenting as paravertebral intrathoracic masses. N Engl J Med 1968;278:1087–1091.
99. Ferris EJ, Vittimberga J, Byrne JJ, et al. Inferior vena cava ligation and plication: study of collateral routes. Radiology 1967;89:1.
100. Doyle FH, Read AE, Evans KT. Mediastinum in portal hypertension. Clin Radiol 1961;12:114.
101. Magbitang MH, Hayford FC, Blake JM. Dilated azygos vein simulating mediastinal tumor: report of a case. N Engl J Med 1960;263:598.
102. Sayer WJ, Parmley LF Jr, Morris J de LS. Mediastinal tumor simulated by azygos phlebectasia. Ann Intern Med 1954;40: 175.
103. Siddorn JA, Worsornu L. Dilatation of the azygos vein simulating a mediastinal tumour. Thorax 1979;34:117–119.
104. Barret D, Barraine R, Cabrol C, et al. Les aneurysmes de la veine azygos. J Radiol 1980;61:125–129.
105. Seebauer L, Prauer HW, Gmeinwieser J, et al. A mediastinal tumor simulated by a sacculated aneurysm of the azygos vein. Thorac Cardiovasc Surg 1989;37:112–114.
106. Hayward I, Forrest JV, Sagel SS. A case of an idiopathic aneurysm of the hemiazygos vein diagnosed by CT is presented. Then a patient with hemiazygos vein dilatation due to a known etiology is shown for comparison. J Comput Assist Tomogr 1989;13:1072–1074.
107. Soler P, Mehta AV, Garcia OL, et al. Congenital systemic arteriovenous fistula between the descending aorta, azygos vein, and superior vena cava. Chest 1981;80:647–649.
108. Shin MS, Soto B, Baxley WA. Azygos dilatation due to traumatic aortoazygos fistula. AJR 1979;133:758–759.

109. Avellanosa AM, Glasauer FE, Oh YS. Traumatic vertebral arteriovenous fistula associated with cervical spine fracture. J Trauma 1977;17:885–888.
110. Binkley FM, Wylie EJ. A new technique for obliteration of cerebrovascular arteriovenous fistulae. Arch Surg 1973;106: 524–527.
111. Kornmesser TW, Bergan JJ. Anatomic control of vertebral arteriovenous fistulas. Surgery 1974;75:80–86.
112. Nagashima C, Iwasaki T, Kawanuma S, et al. Traumatic arteriovenous fistula of the vertebral artery with spinal cord symptoms: case report. J Neurosurg 1977;46:681–687.
113. Rockett JF, Moinuddin M, Robertson JT, et al. Vertebral artery fistula detected by radionuclide angiography: case report. J Nucl Med 1976;17:24–25.
114. Sherk HH, Giri N, Nicholson JT. Gunshot wound with fracture of the atlas and arteriovenous fistula of the vertebral artery: case report. J Bone Joint Surg (Am) 1974;56:1738–1740.
115. Waga S, Handa J, Teraura T, et al. Traumatic vertebral arteriovenous fistula. Surg Neurol 1974;2:279–281.
116. Weinberg PE, Flom RA. Traumatic vertebral arteriovenous fistula. Surg Neurol 1973;1:162–167.
117. Geraci AR, Upson JF, Greene DG. Congenital vertebral arteriovenous fistula. JAMA 1969;210:727–728.
118. Markham JW. Spontaneous arteriovenous fistula of the vertebral artery and vein: case report. J Neurosurg 1969;31:220–223.
119. Rothman SLG, Pratt AG, Kier EL, et al. Traumatic vertebral-carotid-jugular arteriovenous aneurysm: case report. J Neurosurg 1974;41:92–96.
120. Thurman RT, Roettger R. Intrapleural rupture of the azygos vein. Ann Thorac Surg 1992;53:697–699.
121. Sherani TM, Fitzpatrick GJ, Phelan DM, et al. Ruptured azygos vein due to blunt chest trauma. Br J Surg 1986;73: 885.
122. Walsh A, Snyder HS. Azygos vein laceration following a vertical deceleration injury. J Emerg Med 1992;10:35–37.
123. Shkrum MJ, Green RN, Shum DT. Azygos vein laceration due to blunt trauma. J Forensic Sci 1991;36:410–421.
124. Baldwin JC, Oyer PE, Guthaner DF, et al. Combined azygos vein and subclavian artery injury in blunt chest trauma. J Trauma 1984;24:170–171.
125. Kimura T, Moriyasu F, Kawasaki T, et al. Relationship between esophageal varices and azygos vein evaluated by cineaortography. Hepatology 1991;13:858–864.
126. Lebrec D. Methods to evaluate portal hypertension. Gastroenterol Clin North Am 1982;21:41–59.
127. McCormick PA, Burroughs AK. Hemodynamic evaluation of portal hypertension. Hepatogastroenterology 1990;37:546–550.
128. Bosch J, Groszmann RJ. Measurement of azygos venous blood flow by a continuous thermal dilution technique: an index of blood flow through gastroesophageal collaterals in cirrhosis. Hepatology 1984;4:424–429.
129. Lee SS, Hadengue A, Braillon A, et al. A pitfall in azygos vein cannulation in cirrhotic patients: mistaken cannulation of the mammary vein. Angiology 1990;41:942–945.
130. Meranze SG, McLean GK, Stein EJ, et al. Catheter placement in the azygos system: an unusual approach to venous access. AJR 1985;144:1075–1076.
131. Pokorny WJ, McGill CW, Harberg FJ. Use of azygos vein for central catheter insertion. Surgery 1985;97:362.
132. Newman BM, Cooney DR, Karp MP, et al. The intercostal vein: an alternate route for central venous alimentation. Pediatr Surg 1983;18:732–733.

37

The Superior Vena Cava

MICHAEL A. BETTMANN

Angiography of the superior vena cava (SVC) is undertaken for several major indications. Although it is most commonly performed in patients with the SVC syndrome for evaluation of both anatomy and cause, cavography may also be helpful for evaluation of mediastinal abnormalities that do not obstruct the SVC and for suspected anatomic variants, such as left-sided SVC.

The use of superior vena cava angiography has been modified by the emergence of other diagnostic tools such as computed tomography (CT),[1] radionuclide flow studies,[2,3] ultrasonography,[4-6] oculoplethysmography, and even MRI and MRA.[7] These modalities may establish the diagnosis, allow evaluation of superior mediastinal masses, define involvement of adjacent structures, and determine the presence of collateral channels. Thus it is possible to use these techniques to help define the causes of mediastinal abnormalities as well as to help outline appropriate therapy. There are still, however, many indications for angiographic evaluation. Angiography is frequently the only method that can define the exact vascular anatomy, so it is of practical use both in the assessment of anatomic variants and in the evaluation of patients with the SVC syndrome in whom the site of obstruction may be anywhere along the length of the cava. Collateral channels can be demonstrated by radionuclide flow studies, but both the location of the collaterals and their relative importance are best demonstrated by angiography.[7a] These factors are important in planning therapy for malignant mediastinal masses, the chief cause of the SVC syndrome.[8-11] Angiography is very helpful in deciding on the most appropriate therapy: surgical excision, bypass of the SVC, chemotherapy, radiation therapy, or, more recently, treatment endovascularly by placement of a stent. Cavography is particularly useful in determining the proper field for radiation therapy.[8,12] Further, angiographic evaluation, in concert with CT, ultrasound, or MRI, may be able to give a definitive diagnosis and thus avoid unnecessary radiation therapy.

SVC angiography is also useful subsequent to therapy to define its adequacy, since certain patients may develop collateral channels sufficient to alleviate the SVC syndrome, despite failure of resolution of the cause of the syndrome. In other patients, SVC obstruction may be due to thrombosis, and catheter study of the SVC may be used before as well as for follow-up of thrombolytic therapy.[13] In still others, cavography may be able to demonstrate patency of patch or bypass grafts.[14,15] Noninvasive methods, particularly CT and ultrasound, may, however, be preferable in such situations.

Anatomy

The superior vena cava, which is about 70 mm long in normal adults, is formed by the junction of the two innominate veins. It lies within the fibrous pericardium in its lower half and terminates in the posterior superior portion of the right atrium. Collateral emptying of the blood from the area of drainage of the SVC is via several main pathways.[16-20] Which of these collaterals predominates is determined in part by the level of the obstruction.

If obstruction is low in the SVC, drainage may be primarily via the azygos and hemiazygos systems to the ascending lumbar veins and then to the renal veins or common iliac veins and the inferior vena cava. Obstruction above the level of the azygos vein may lead to drainage retrograde from the innominate veins via three major pathways. One is via the internal thoracic veins (which anastomose across the midline both anterior and posterior to the sternum) to the superior and then to the inferior epigastric veins, which in turn empty into the external iliac veins. A second innominate pathway is via the lateral thoracic veins to the superficial epigastric veins, which anastomose below the inguinal ligament to the greater saphenous veins into the common femoral veins and then into the iliac systems. In the third pathway, drainage may proceed from the innominate veins to the highest intercostal and first posterior intercostal and then into the azygos/hemiazygos system, or via the anterior intercostals to the internal thoracic and then to the superior and inferior epigastric veins. Multiple interconnections exist among these collateral channels; for example, there are anastomoses between the anterior and posterior intercostal veins, allowing drainage of the azygos/hemiazygos system into the internal thoracic veins. There may also be flow retrograde via the internal thoracic veins to the inferior epigastric veins and then through the umbilical veins in the falciform ligament into the left branch of the portal vein.[18] "Retrograde varices" may occur, caused by flow through the upper esophageal veins into the portal circulation. These varices have been reported to bleed.[21] A final posterior pathway is via the jugular and intercostal veins to the vertebral plexuses and then to the ascending lumbar veins.

Technique

Many techniques have been used for SVC evaluation.[22–27] The simplest approach is infusion of contrast via an arm vein with sequential filming of the thorax. For cut-film imaging, 50 ml of contrast media, usually at a concentration of 280 mg iodine per milliliter, is used; satisfactory visualization is more often obtained if 50 ml is injected simultaneously via an 18- or 19-gauge needle in each antecubital fossa. The contrast is ordinarily injected manually over 8 to 10 seconds, and films are then exposed over the mediastinum at a rate of one per second for 12 seconds. This bilateral-needle method is rapid and simple and gives good visualization of the axillary, subclavian, and innominate veins, and frequently the SVC as well. A major drawback, however, is that in the presence of collateral channels or partial occlusion of the venous system proximal to the SVC the exact site of obstruction may not be well seen. It is, therefore, often necessary to use a 4 to 7 French end-hole or multi-side-hole catheter. Under fluoroscopic control and with small injections of contrast, the catheter is advanced into the innominate vein and, if clear, into the proximal portion of the SVC. Then pressure injection of 45 ml of contrast at 15 ml per second can be made. Once again, sequential filming at one per second for 8 to 12 seconds is sufficient to give excellent definition of the SVC and of collateral channels.

This catheter method is also useful in evaluation of anatomic variants. If that is a consideration in the study, it is preferable to use an approach from the left arm, because most variations occur on the left. Further, access via catheter facilitates subsequent percutaneous interventions.

Digital subtraction angiography is generally preferable to cut film, particularly if a 12-inch or larger image intensifier is available, because a lower concentration of contrast can be used (150–200 mgI/ml), less film is necessary, and images can be reviewed immediately and postprocessed for improved information. Cut-film angiography is actually rarely necessary.

Superior Vena Cava Syndrome

The SVC syndrome was first described by Hunter in 1747[28] in a patient with an aortic aneurysm. It consists of swelling of the head and neck, orbital edema, proptosis, distention of the veins of the neck and trunk, cyanosis, headache, and occasionally restlessness, dizziness, syncope, or somnolence. These symptoms develop as a result of partial or complete obstruction of the SVC with resultant stasis, venous engorgement, and anoxia. In most cases, the syndrome is secondary to mediastinal neoplasms[8–10]; the vast majority of these are malignant, about three-fourths primary or metastatic lung carcinoma and one-fourth lymphoma. The SVC syndrome is due to obstruction, although the obstruction may be incomplete. The incidence of obstruction varies with the disease. In one series of 225 patients with small-cell anaplastic bronchogenic carcinoma, 11.5 percent had SVC obstruction at the time of diagnosis.[29] Thrombosis due to an indwelling line is increasing as a cause of the SVC syndrome, with the continuing increase in the use of such lines.

The degree to which obstruction correlates with symptoms varies widely and depends on the underlying disease, the rate of onset of obstruction, and the development of collateral channels. Thus patients with lung or mediastinal tumors may have high-grade obstruction with no symptoms of the SVC syndrome. Cavography in such patients may provide important information in regard to resectability (Figs. 37-1 through 37-3). Conversely, incomplete obstruction may cause significant symptoms, as illustrated in Figure 37-4. This patient had right lung carcinoma and venous distention in the neck. The chest radiograph demonstrated mild mediastinal widening, and cavography showed incomplete obstruction with few collateral vessels. Similarly, the patient shown in Figure 37-5 had syncopal episodes, facial edema, and venous distention in the neck and thorax. Cavography via the right brachial vein demonstrated incomplete obstruction. Open thoracotomy showed an unresectable bronchogenic carcinoma. Symptoms resolved for several months following mediastinal irradiation to a field defined by angiography and surgery. Symptoms recurred, however. Perhaps because of prior treatment and slow recurrence, they were now accompanied by extensive collateral formation, as seen in Figure 37-5C. Complete SVC occlusion was noted at autopsy.

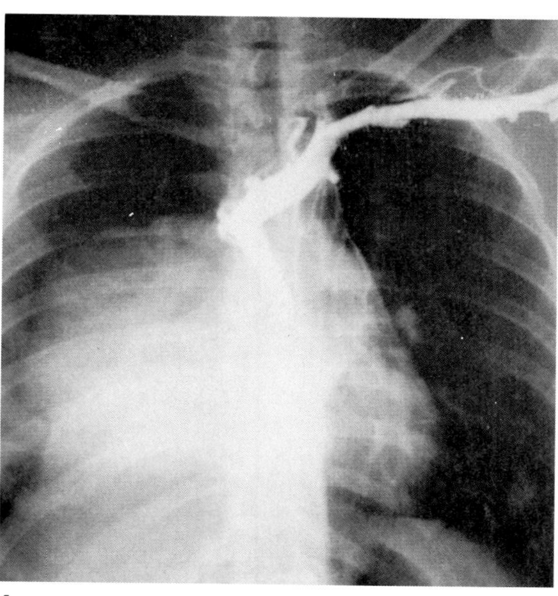

A

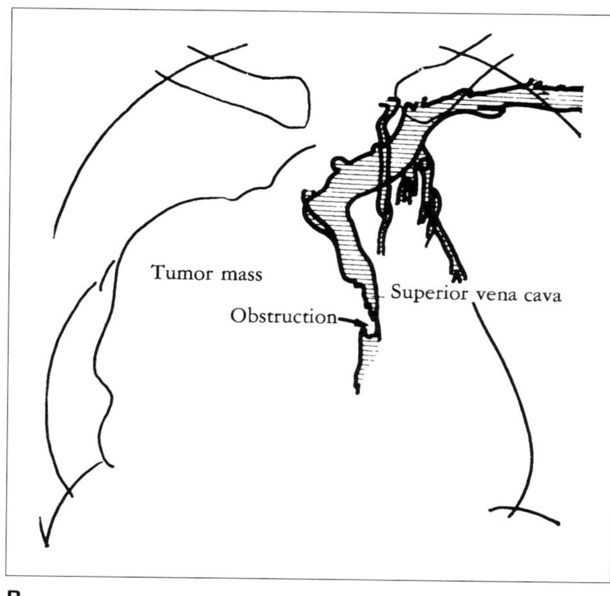

B

Figure 37-1. Large malignant mediastinal teratoma in a 22-year-old woman. (A) Left subclavian vein injection shows high-grade obstruction of the SVC, secondary to the mass. (B) Schematic representation of (A). Circumferential involvement of the SVC suggests unresectability. (From Dotter CT, Steinberg I. Angiocardiography [Annals of Roentgenology, Vol. 20]. New York: Paul B. Hoeber, 1951. Used with permission.)

Figure 37-2. High-grade obstruction of the SVC by metastatic thyroid carcinoma, with long, ragged-appearing invasion. (From Dotter CT, Steinberg I. Angiocardiography [Annals of Roentgenology, Vol. 20]. New York: Paul B. Hoeber, 1951. Used with permission.)

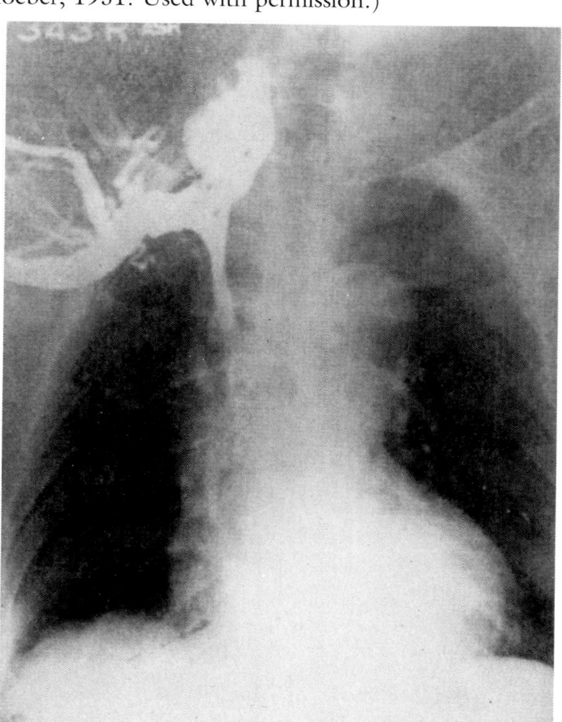

Polypoid invasion of the SVC (Fig. 37-6) is almost invariably secondary to malignancy, either mediastinal lymphoma or, more frequently, lung carcinoma.

The most common benign cause of SVC obstruction is sclerosing (also called fibrosing) mediastinitis. This entity accounts for about 3 percent of the cases of SVC syndrome. It is secondary to mediastinal granulomas, which in most cases rupture, causing a fibrotic reaction and slowly developing obstruction of the SVC.[30,31] It has been stated that sclerosing mediastinitis is always secondary to histoplasmosis, although this supposition has not been proved.[32] The slow onset of SVC obstruction usually leads to development of extensive collateral channels, and frequently the SVC syndrome does not occur. CT may be satisfactory in defining SVC obstruction, but cavography may be useful in defining the extent of the obstruction and the nature of the collateral flow. Treatment is often not necessary, but if symptoms occur, surgical bypass with an autologous vein graft has been used. Percutaneous stent placement is an appealing alternative. As illustrated in Figure 37-7, complete occlusion with a relatively smooth contour is the typical angiographic appearance. Drainage in this case was via the highest intercostal veins into the azygos and hemiazygos systems. The patient had an interposition graft placed between the right innominate vein and the right atrium. Because of fibrotic involvement of the left innominate

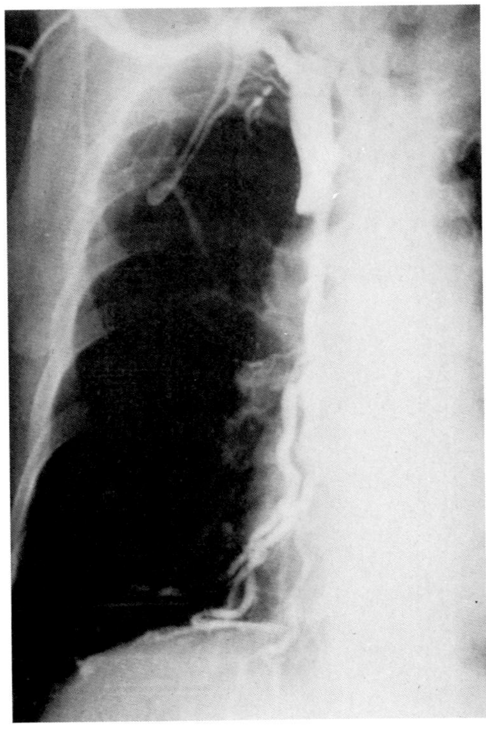

A

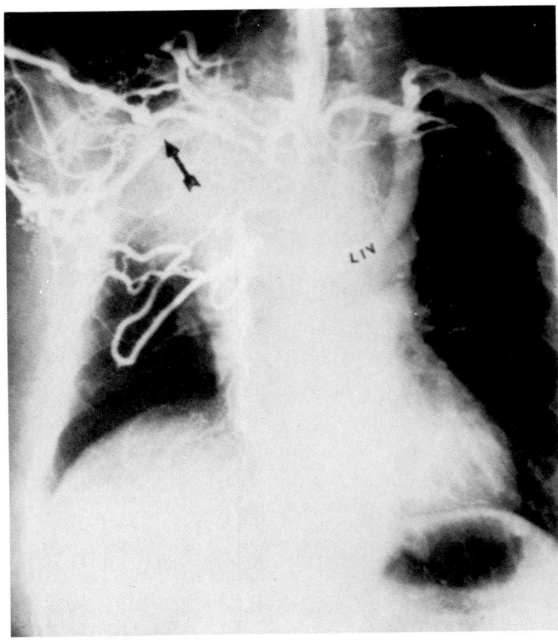

B

Figure 37-3. Superior vena cava obstruction caused by lung carcinoma. (A) Complete SVC occlusion in a 49-year-old man with drainage via the azygos vein. (B) Right subclavian (*arrow*), left innominate (*LIV*), and SVC occlusion in a 63-year-old woman. Note marked distortion of vessels. Drainage on right is primarily via internal thoracic system.

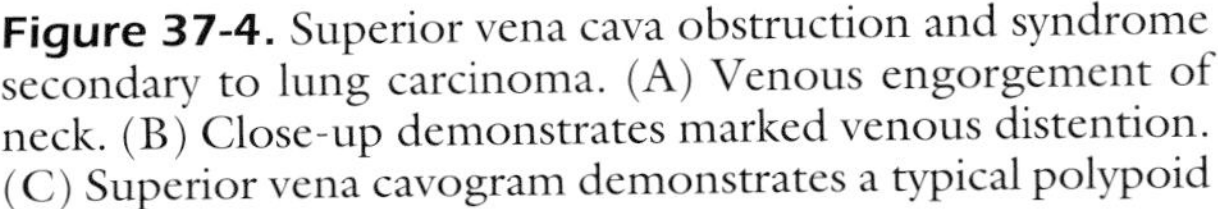

Figure 37-4. Superior vena cava obstruction and syndrome secondary to lung carcinoma. (A) Venous engorgement of neck. (B) Close-up demonstrates marked venous distention. (C) Superior vena cavogram demonstrates a typical polypoid malignant invasion. SVC syndrome developed despite incomplete obstruction because of the lack of development of collaterals.

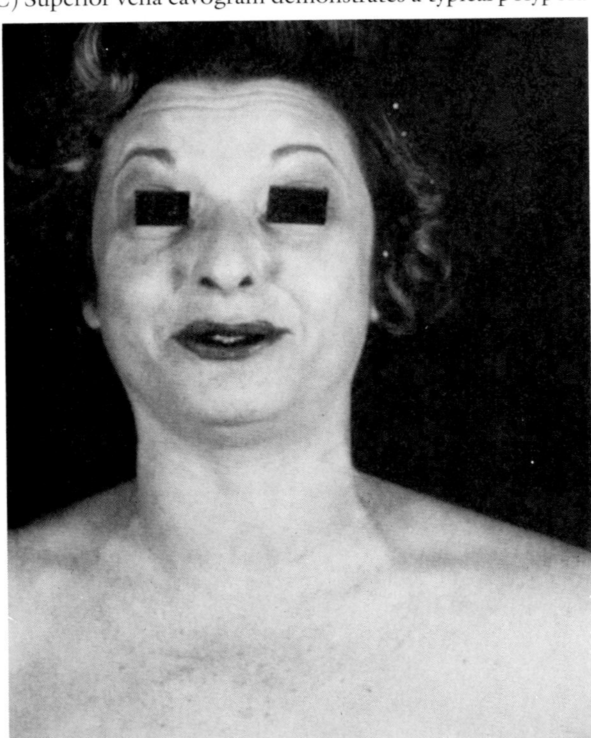

A

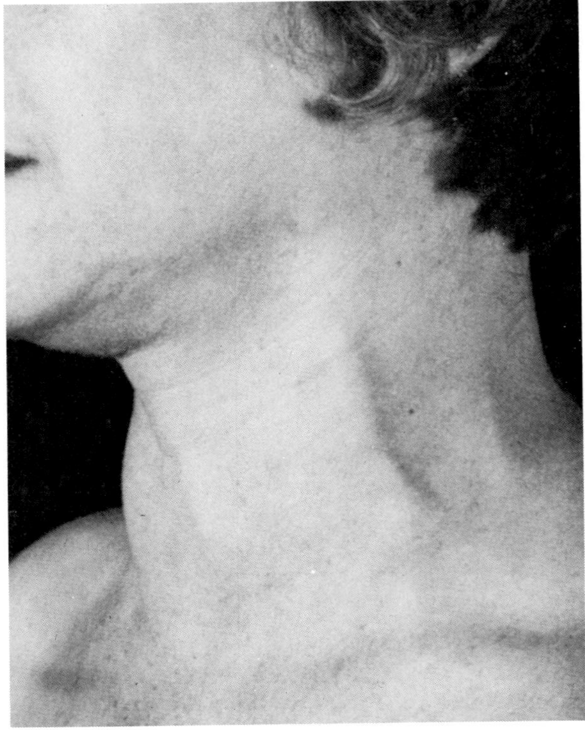

B

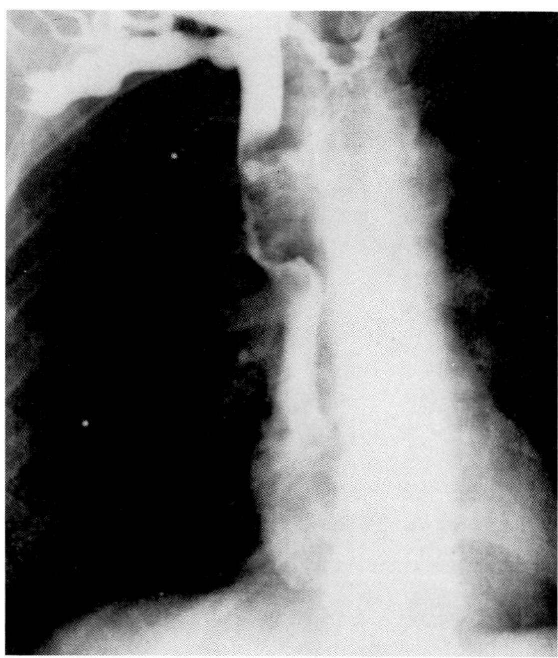

C

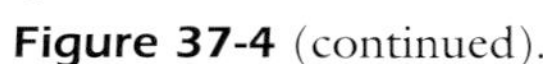

Figure 37-4 (continued).

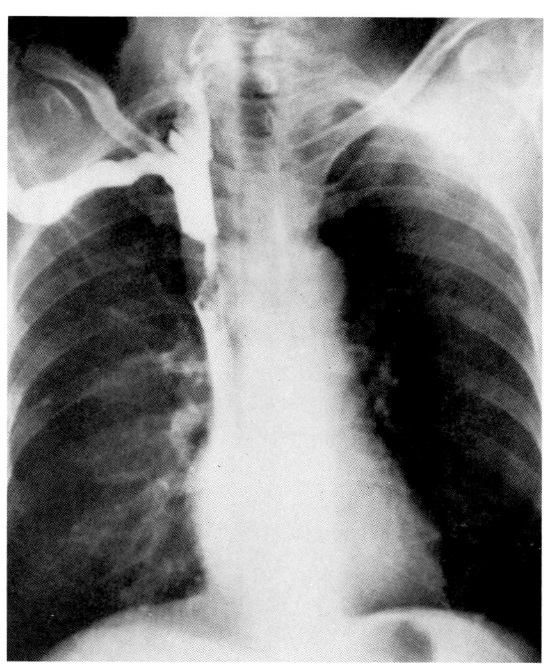

B

Figure 37-5. Superior vena cava invasion by lung carcinoma. (A) Posteroanterior chest film showing only mild widening of superior mediastinum. (B) Superior vena cavogram demonstrating typical polypoid invasion and incomplete obstruction. (C) Infrared photographs of trunk 10 months later, after development of SVC syndrome, demonstrating multiple subcutaneous collateral channels.

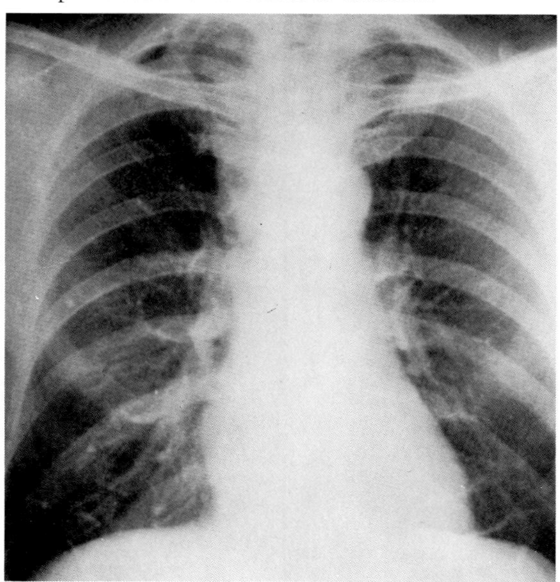

A

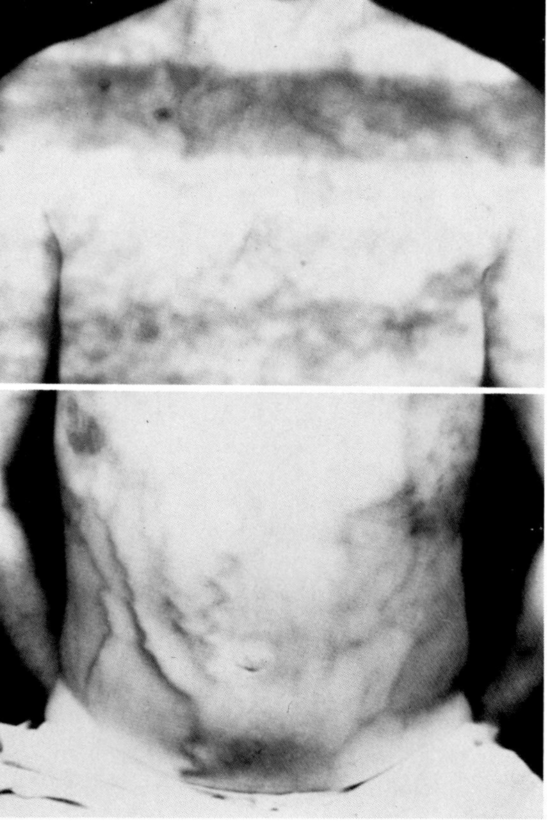

C

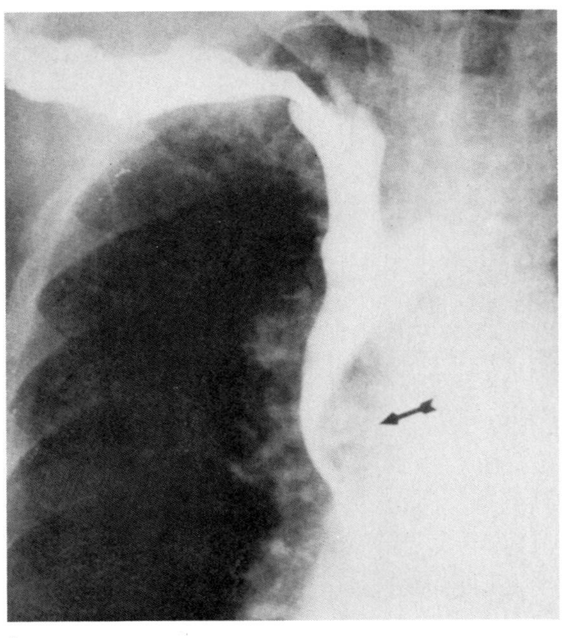

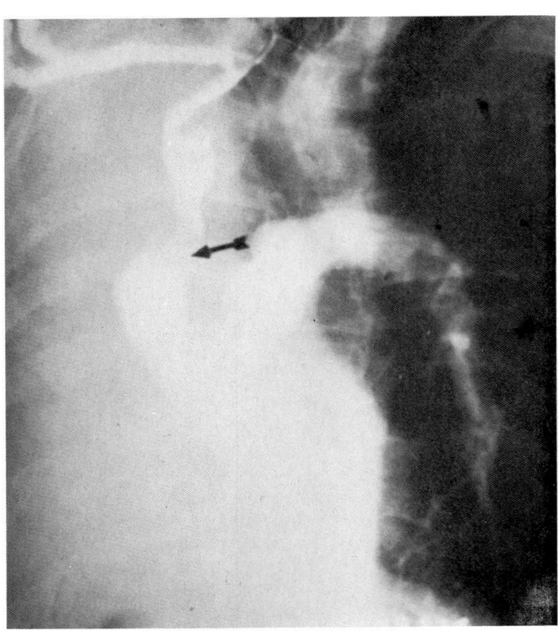

A B

Figure 37-6. Polypoid invasion of SVC by malignant lesions (*arrows*). (A) Secondary to mediastinal lymphoma. (B) Secondary to recurrent lung carcinoma after right pneumonectomy.

vein, the left subclavian and jugular veins continued to drain via collaterals to the hemiazygos system and the inferior vena cava.

There are many other known causes of the SVC syndrome. Obstruction secondary to thrombosis has been seen after surgery for repair of tetralogy of Fallot[13] and in patients with ventriculoatrial shunts for hydrocephalus.[33] Obstruction in a patient with a ventriculopleural shunt is shown in Figure 37-8. Obstruction caused by fibrosis without thrombosis has been reported in patients with transvenous endocardial pacing wires, particularly if two wires cross in the SVC.[34–36] Many other entities have been reported to cause SVC obstruction, by thrombosis, fibrosis, compression, or invasion. These include peritoneal venous (LeVeen) shunts,[37] cutaneous arteritis,[38] Behçet disease,[39] the Mustard procedure,[40] release of pericardial tamponade,[41] substernal goiter,[19] developmental processes such as bronchogenic cysts,[42] and aneurysms of the ascending or descending aorta or right subclavian artery.[28,43–45] Obstruction of both innominate veins and the SVC secondary to a luetic aneurysm is demonstrated in Figures 37-9 and 37-10. This etiology is very unusual; more prevalent is obstruction due to atherosclerotic or dissecting aneurysms. Neoplasms that have been shown to cause the SVC syndrome include thyroid adenoma,[11] thymoma,[46] neuroblastoma,[47] plasmacytoma,[48] and liposarcoma,[49] as illustrated in Figure 37-11. Other infectious and granulomatous processes may also cause SVC obstruction. Tuberculosis (Fig. 37-12) is now rare, but sarcoidosis,[50] actinomycosis,[51] and cryptococcosis[52] have all been reported.

Persistent Left Superior Vena Cava

The persistent left SVC is thought to be the most common anomalous systemic vein-to-cardiac connection, higher in incidence than anomalous pulmonary venous drainage. The overall incidence is 0.3 percent, but it rises to 4.3 percent in patients with other congenital heart disease.[53,54] This anomaly is most frequently found in conjunction with a right-sided SVC. It may also be solitary, or it may be associated with drainage into the left atrium,[55] with atrial septal defect, or with a variety of other lesions.[56]

In the embryo, the right and left anterior cardinal veins join the right and left posterior cardinal veins to form the ducts of Cuvier. These drain into the sinus venosus. Normally, the left duct of Cuvier regresses, as does the left anterior cardinal vein, leaving the oblique cardiac vein of Marshall inferiorly and the highest intercostal vein superiorly. The oblique cardiac vein drains into the coronary sinus. Early in development

Text continues on page 926

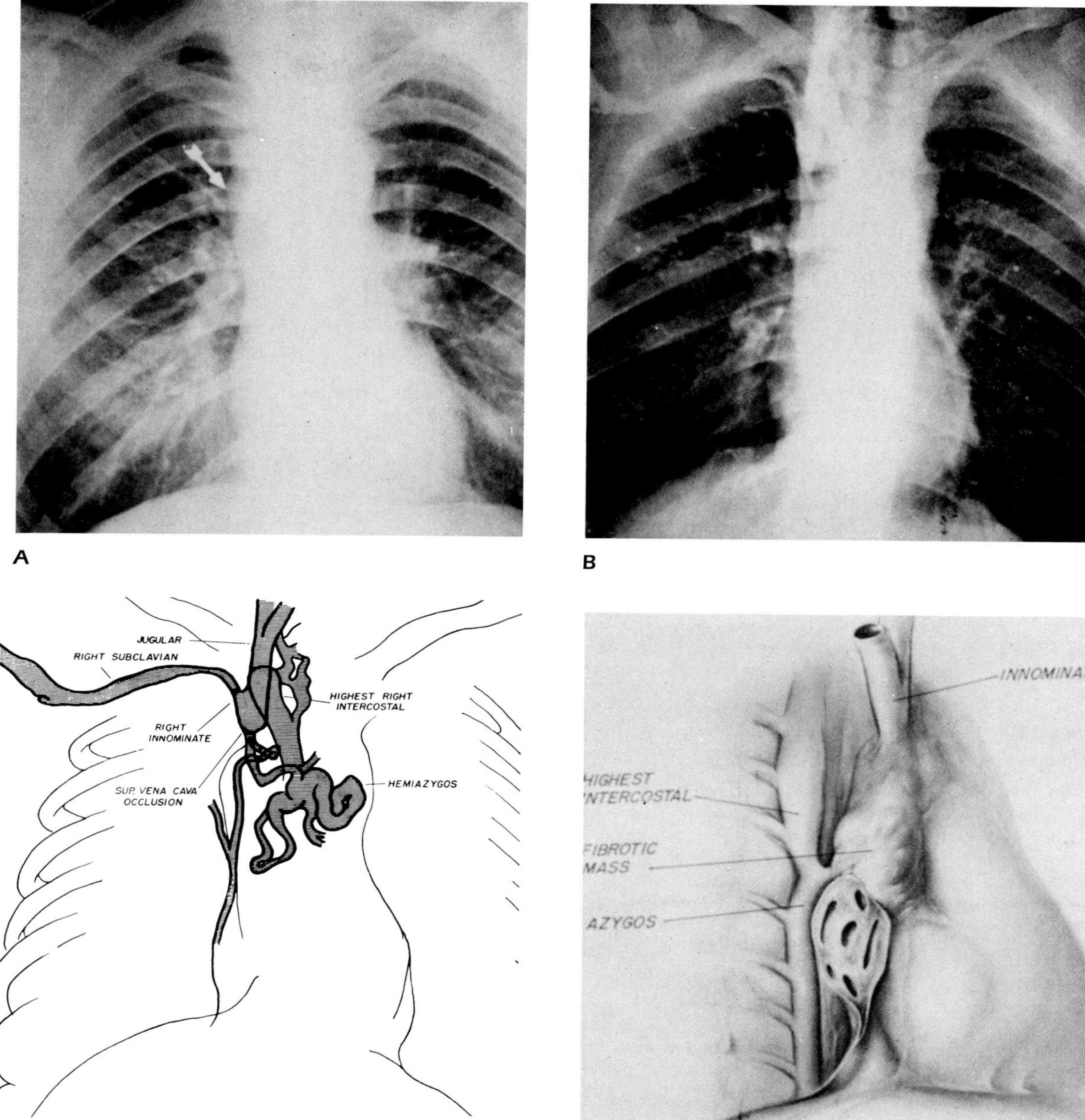

Figure 37-7. Superior vena cava occlusion secondary to sclerosing mediastinitis. (A) Frontal chest film demonstrating slight mediastinal widening (*arrow*). (B) Superior vena cavography via right subclavian vein demonstrates smooth, tapered SVC occlusion and suggests left innominate vein occlusion, with drainage via the highest right intercostal into the hemiazygos system. (C) Schematic representation of (B). (D) Cross-sectional sketch of operative findings. (E) Sketch of interposition graft from right innominate vein to central SVC. (F) Cross section of mass (H&E, ×250) showing extensive, fairly well-ordered fibrous tissue. (G) Postoperative study demonstrating drainage via the right innominate vein and the SVC graft, as well as via the left subclavian vein and the hemiazygos system. (C, D, and E from Holman CW, Steinberg I. Treatment of superior vena caval occlusion by arterial graft. JAMA 1954;155:1403. Used with permission.)

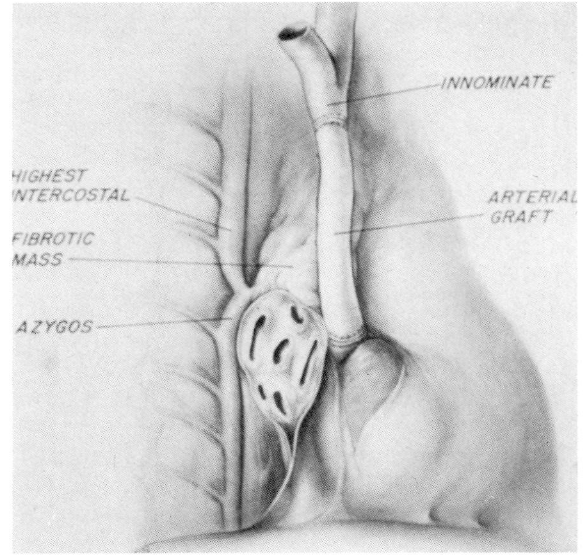

E

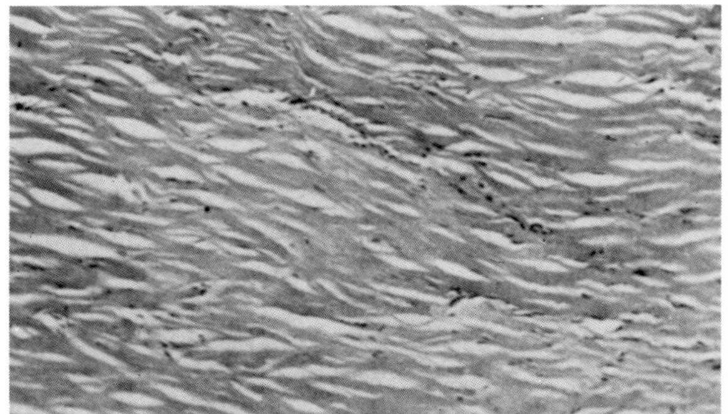

F

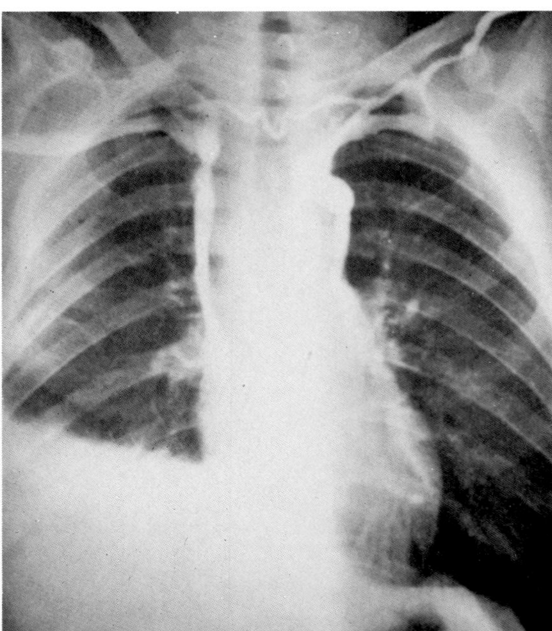

G

Figure 37-7 (continued).

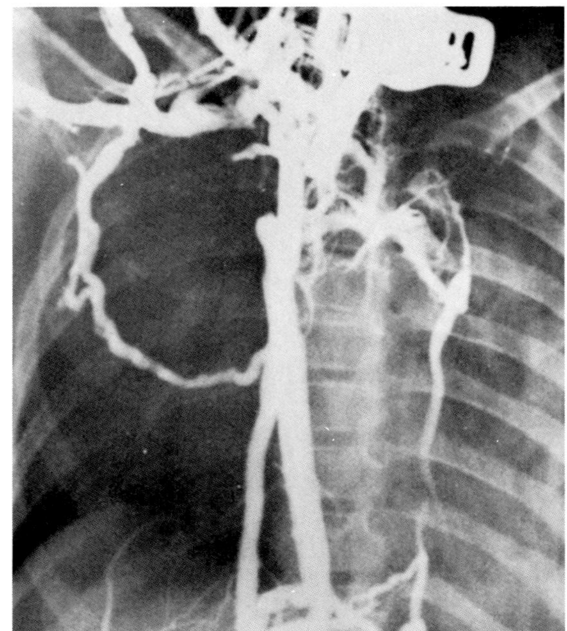

A

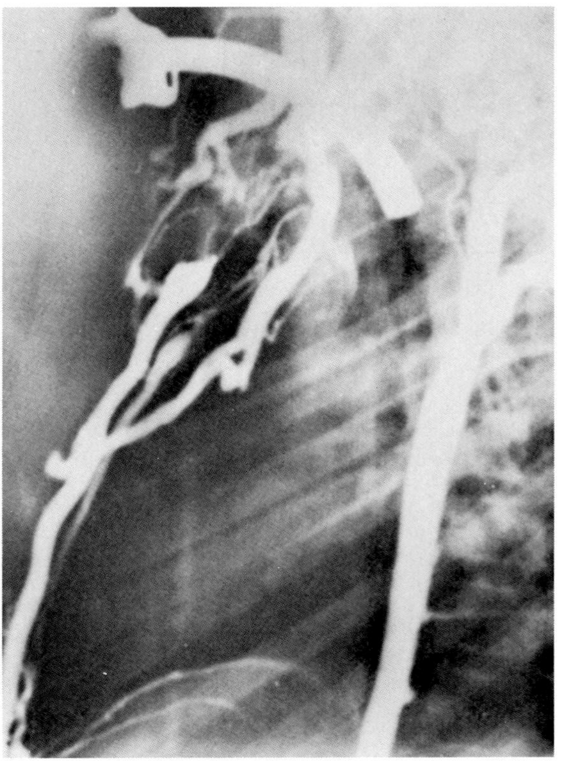

B

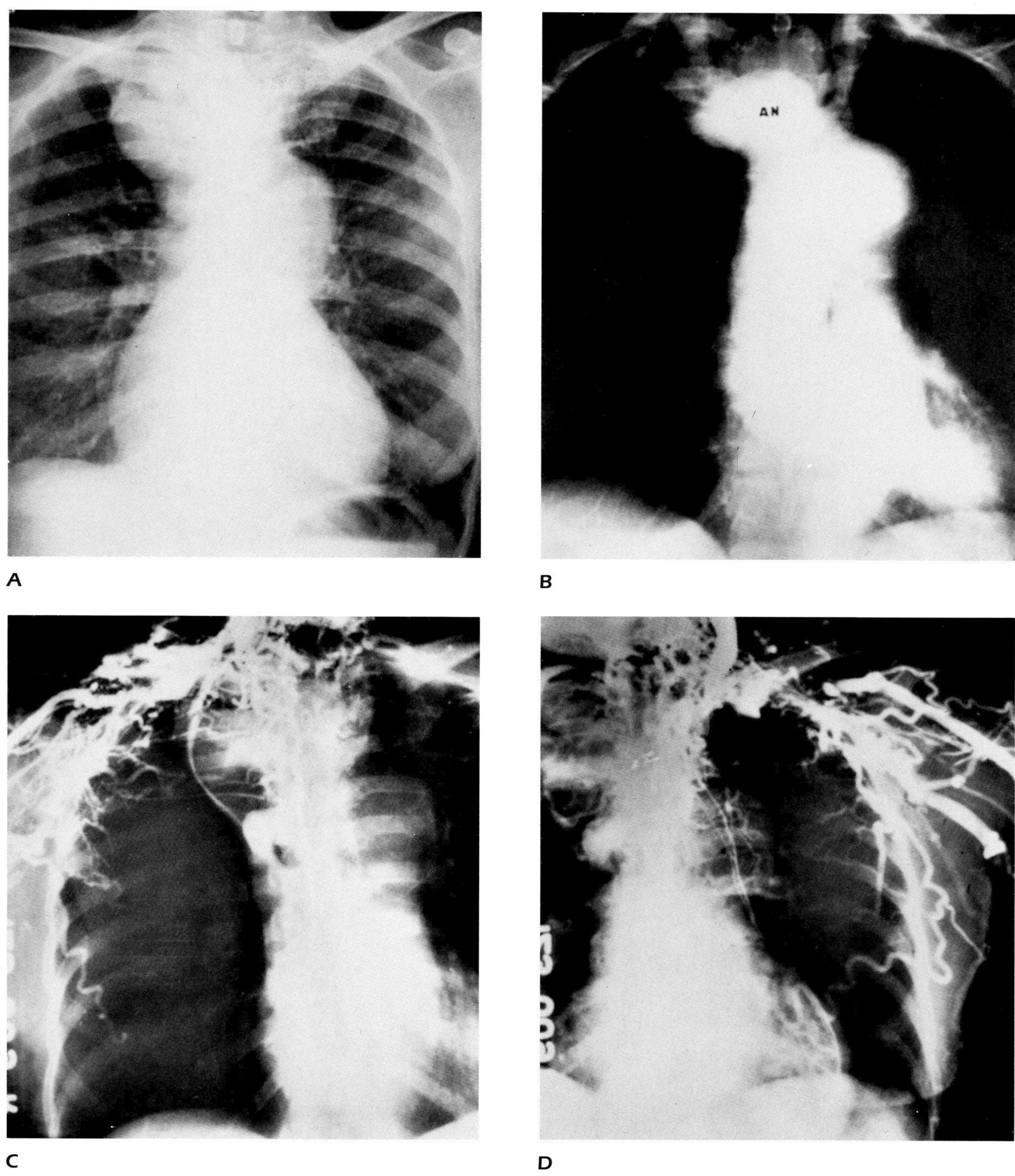

Figure 37-9. Syphilitic aneurysm of the aorta and innominate artery in a 63-year-old woman. (A) Chest film suggests aneurysm and tracheal compression from the right. (B) Aortogram demonstrates dilated ascending aorta and frank aneurysm of the innominate vein (*AN*). Right (C) and left (D) subclavian vein studies demonstrate complete bilateral innominate vein obstruction with drainage via the azygos system on the right and lateral thoracic and intercostal collaterals on both sides.

◀ **Figure 37-8.** Superior vena cava syndrome after ventriculopleural shunt for hydrocephalus in an 8-year-old girl. (A) Frontal and (B) lateral views of right subclavian vein injection demonstrating right innominate and mid-SVC occlusion with drainage via (1) the anterior intercostal veins on the right to the internal thoracic vein, (2) collaterals on the right to the azygos vein, and (3) collaterals on the left to the hemiazygos vein.

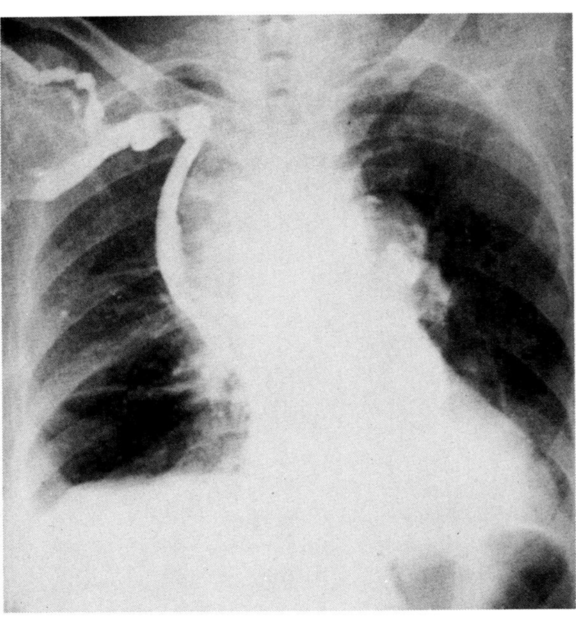

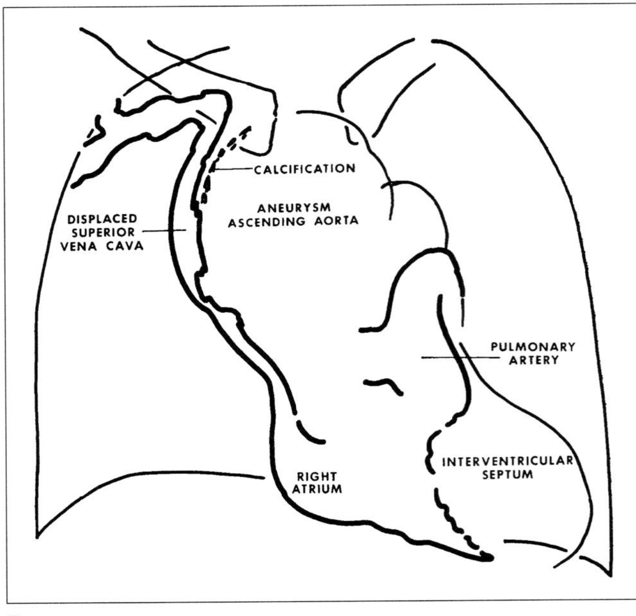

A B

Figure 37-10. (A) Huge syphilitic aneurysm in a 53-year-old woman causing displacement and narrowing of the SVC. (B) Schematic representation. (From Dotter CT, Steinberg I. Angiocardiography [Annals of Roentgenology, Vol. 20]. New York: Paul B. Hoeber, 1951. Used with permission.)

Figure 37-11. Large mediastinal myoliposarcoma in a 29-year-old woman. (A) Left subclavian vein injection showing smooth but marked displacement of the SVC, without obstruction. Note also the distortion of the pulmonary outflow region. (B) Schematic representation. (From Dotter CT, Steinberg I. Angiocardiography [Annals of Roentgenology, Vol. 20]. New York: Paul B. Hoeber, 1951. Used with permission.)

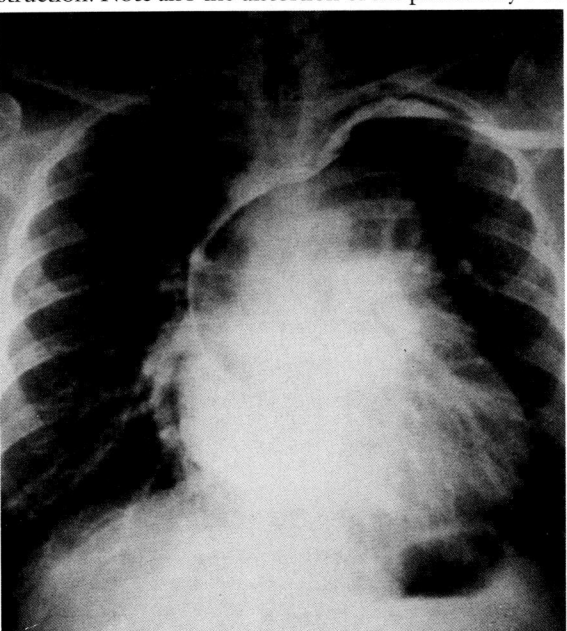

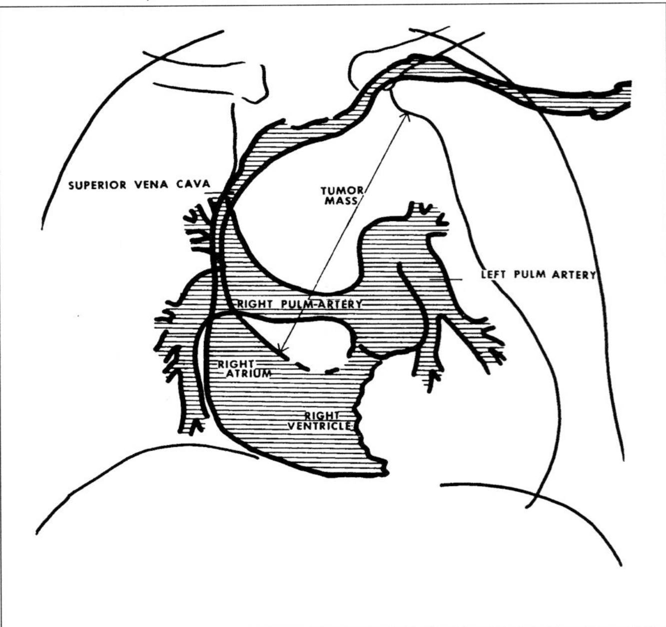

A B

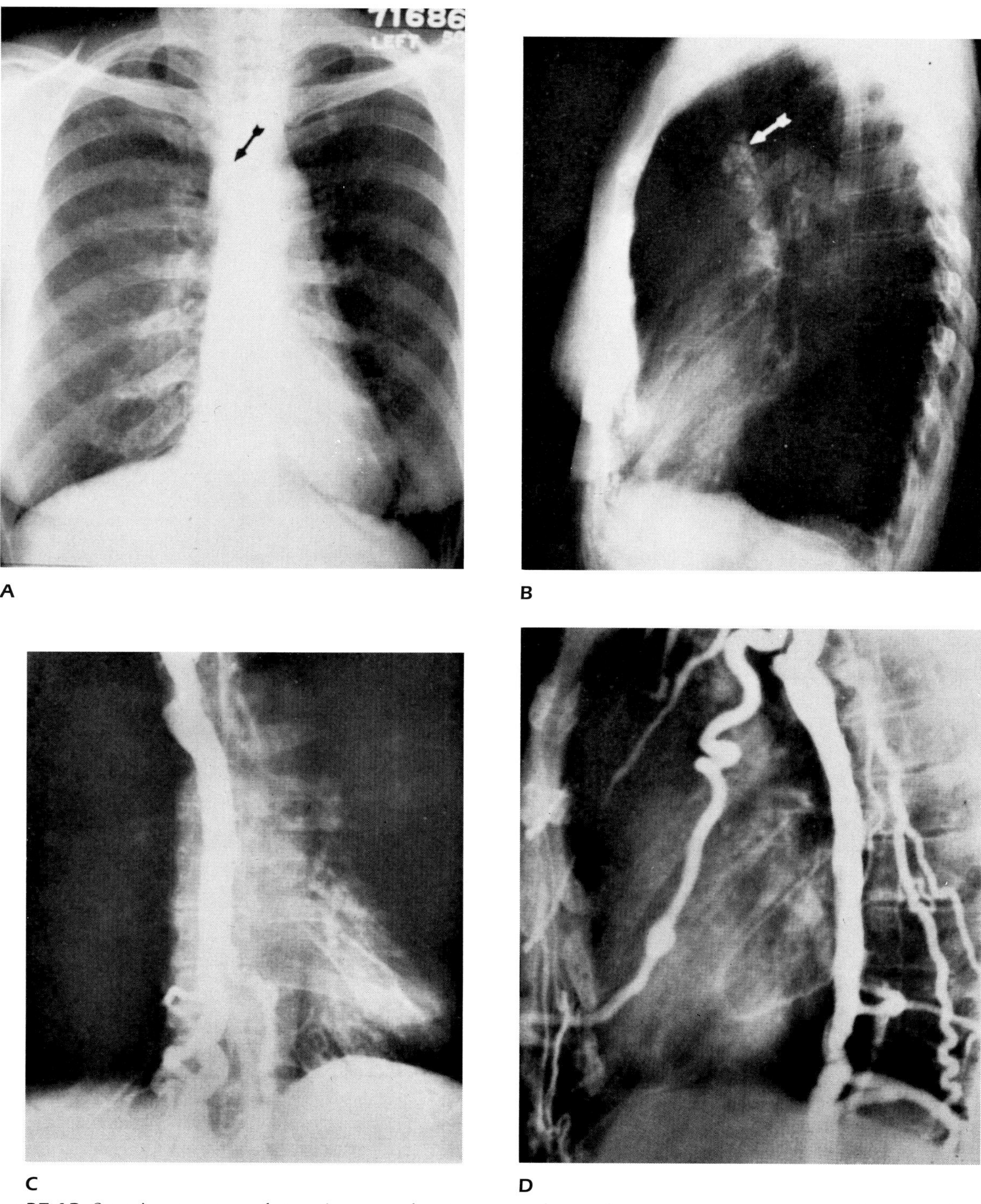

Figure 37-12. Superior vena cava obstruction secondary to tuberculosis. (A and B) Posteroanterior and lateral chest radiographs demonstrate a partially calcified 2 × 5-cm right superior mediastinal mass (*arrows*). (C) Frontal and (D) lateral views from superior vena cavogram show complete SVC obstruction, with drainage largely via the azygos vein to the IVC. (From Steinberg I. Superior vena caval syndrome due to tuberculosis. AJR 1966;98:440. Used with permission.)

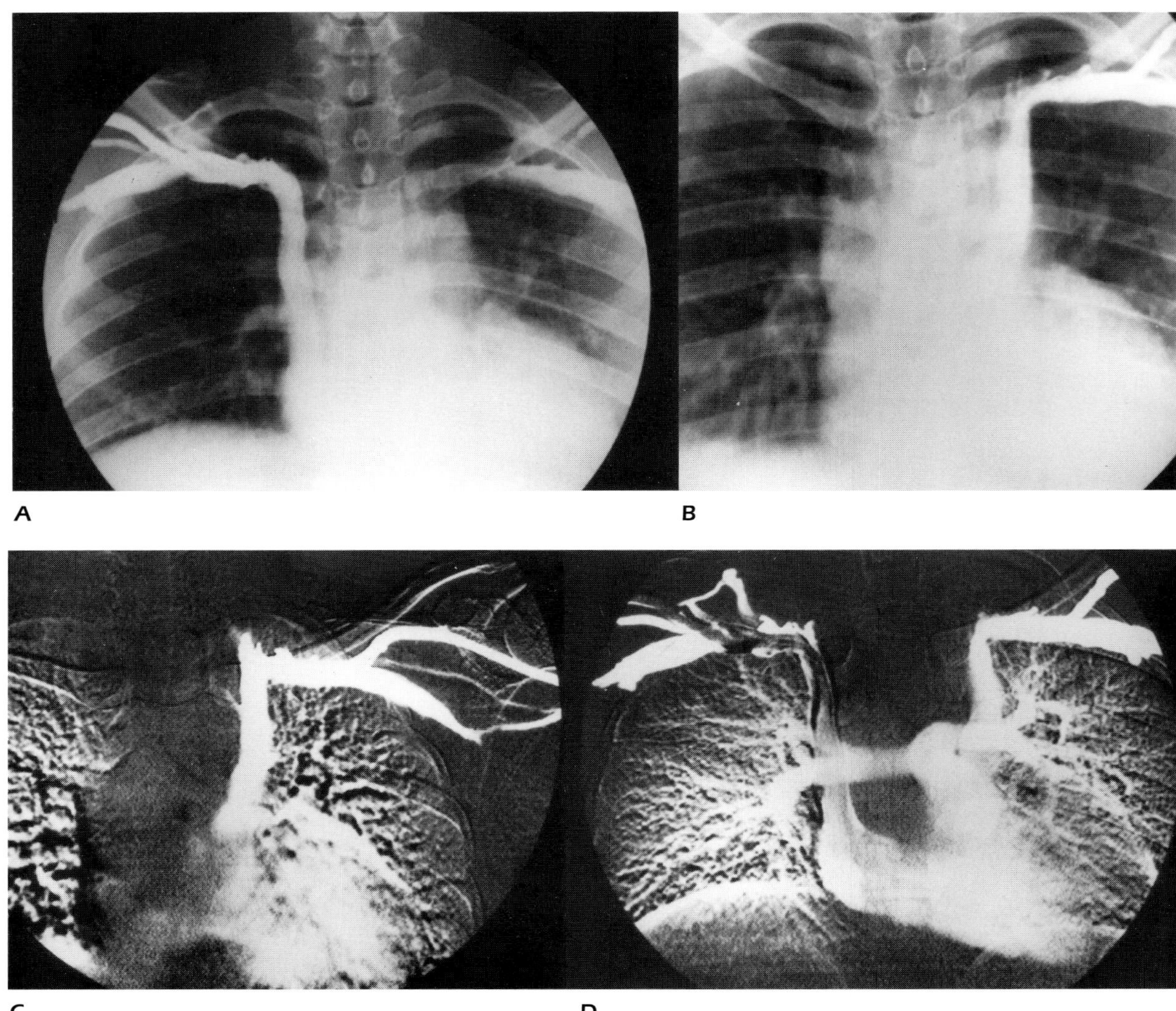

Figure 37-13. Young, asymptomatic white woman with widened mediastinum on chest radiograph. (A) Right brachial vein injection shows normal right innominate and SVC, without inflow from left. (B) Left brachial vein injection demonstrates the left innominate and persistent left superior vena cava. (C) Subtracted view of (B). Note early drainage into coronary sinus and right atrium. (D) Simultaneous injection of both brachial veins and both cavae.

the left subclavian vein drains into the left anterior cardinal vein, but subsequently the left innominate vein forms and enlarges and the subclavian vein migrates cephalad to join the left jugular vein and empty into the left innominate vein. If the left innominate vein fails to form, a separate left SVC will persist, draining into the right atrium via the coronary sinus. Alternatively, the right anterior cardinal vein may regress, leaving a single left SVC emptying into the coronary sinus.

At the time of development of the primitive venous plexuses of the lung, at the third to fourth embryonic week, the drainage is into the anterior cardinal veins. Later the pulmonary veins migrate to empty directly into the left atrium. Remnants, however, may lead to partial anomalous pulmonary venous return via the left vertical pulmonary vein, which empties into the left innominate vein.[20] This variant is to be distinguished from the persistent left superior vena cava, with which it may be confused.[56]

On plain radiographs, the left SVC may appear as widening in the area of the aortic arch, a bulge below the aortic arch, or a left paramediastinal density. On catheterization, this structure is seen to run inferiorly toward the right. It begins anterior to the aortic arch, then runs along the posterior heart border and empties into the coronary sinus and right atrium. Although plain film diagnosis is frequently possible, angiographic evaluation via the left brachial system is definitive, rapid, and safe (Fig. 37-13).

On a lateral radiograph of the chest, the left vertical pulmonary vein usually appears as a linear density running from the pulmonary artery region toward the aorta.[57] Seen on angiography, it is clearly distinguishable from a persistent left SVC.

Treatment of SVC Occlusion

Over the last few years there have been impressive advances in the percutaneous treatment of diseases of the SVC, as in other areas of the vascular system. Advances in treating the SVC have consisted primarily of treatment for occlusion (rather than of causes of occlusion), in the form of techniques to reestablish and then maintain patency. Currently, occlusion is essentially the only major SVC disease which benefits from the techniques and tools of the interventional radiologist. The etiology is generally extrinsic compression due to adjacent disease, such as primary or metastatic malignancy in the chest, or thrombosis, related to indwelling lines for cardiac pacing, drug delivery, or hyperalimentation. Rarely, occlusion is due to a hypercoagulable state, to trauma, or to radiation. The treatment used depends on the etiology of the occlusion; if occlusion is due to extrinsic compression or radiation, it is unlikely to be truly acute in onset, and thrombus in the SVC is likely to be of relatively minor importance. If occlusion is secondary to an indwelling line, or in certain cases to localized strictures, then dissolution of thrombus is the first approach.

Success in thrombolysis in the SVC, as in other uses of this approach, depends on the age and the extent of the thrombus, and the technique utilized. In general, although experience is relatively limited, good results have been achieved with direct, prolonged infusion of urokinase into the occlusion.[58,59] In symptomatic patients, essentially the only ones requiring this therapy, it is usual to encounter occlusion of not only the SVC, but also one or both innominate veins and, depending on the entry site of the intravenous line, more peripheral veins as well. There are two major questions that must be addressed in all such cases. First, which access should be used for treatment, and second, should the line be removed, either before or after treatment? In practice, all such lines should be removed as they are likely to be nonfunctional and, having caused thrombosis and occlusion, re-occlusion is likely to occur. It is more difficult to define when the line should be removed. Due to fear of embolization, it is the author's practice to remove the line only after partial or complete thrombus dissolution. This has the added practical advantage of allowing planning for and placement of a new central line, using veins which are patent, or ones in which patency has been reestablished.

Regarding technique, the author's usual approach has been to attempt to access the SVC via the vein in which the line has been placed. A puncture is made, for example, into a vein of the upper arm if a subclavian line has led to subclavian, innominate, and SVC occlusion (Fig. 37-14). This is done either with ultrasound guidance or with fluoroscopic control during infusion of contrast into a more peripheral vein in the hand or forearm. A 4 or 5 French angled catheter is used, generally with a straight or 15-mm J guidewire; as in other situations, an angled hydrophilic wire is also often helpful. The peripheral extent of the occlusion is defined (and documented radiographically) and the occlusion is then traversed with a guidewire and catheter, both to define the extent of the thrombosis and, as in other uses of catheter-directed thrombolysis, as a predictor of the likelihood of success.[60] If the occlusion can be traversed, infusion of the thrombolytic agent is begun using a multi-side-hole system, either coaxially (e.g., guidewire and catheter) or with a straight multi-side-hole catheter directly. It has not been our practice to work through a sheath since it may be helpful in preventing peripheral propagation of thrombosis to use as small a catheter system as possible. In general, systemic heparinization is also instituted, although it is not clear that this is necessary. Similarly, the ideal dose of urokinase is not clear. Our approach is to use a total dose of 120,000 units per hour, diluted to a concentration of 2000 or 4000 units/ml with normal saline (60 or 30 ml/hr). This is of practical consideration, since each vial contains 250,000 units, and monitoring of the infusion may fall to personnel without particular experience or expertise. Reevaluation of progress is carried out at 12 to 24 hours, and prolonged infusions ranging from 24 to 72 hours may be necessary. As in all other situations in which thrombolysis is used, once there is complete or near complete thrombus dissolution, it is imperative that the underlying cause of the occlusion be addressed. Usually, as noted, this requires removal of an indwelling central line. If the line cannot be removed because it is essential and there is no other access site, anticoagulation (heparin followed by warfarin) and antiplatelet medications (such as aspirin and/or ticlopidine) can be employed. The likelihood of long-term patency, however, is low. In the unusual situation in which thrombosis is due to an underlying stricture, angioplasty is the least invasive treatment, although its long-term success is not yet well established in benign central venous strictures.

Treatment of SVC obstruction which is nonthrom-

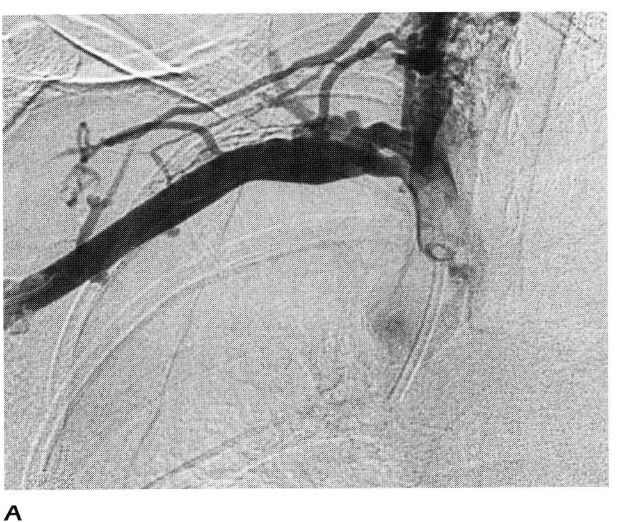

A

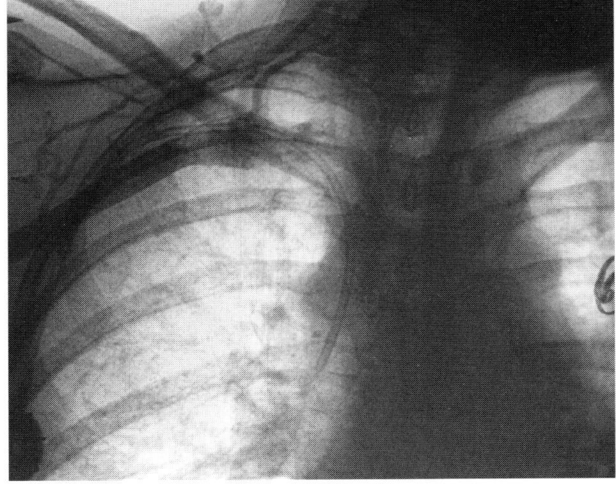

B

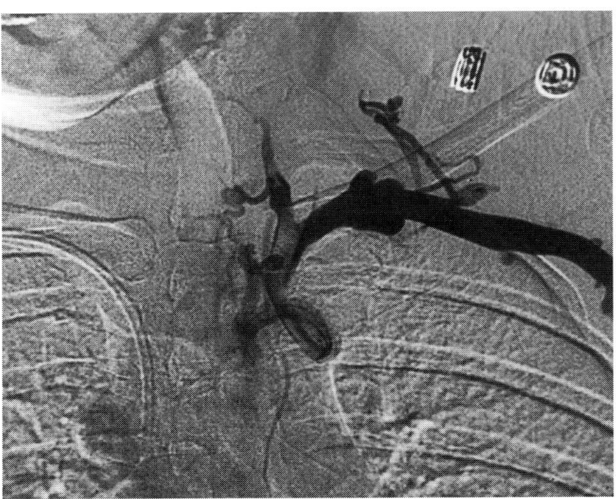

C

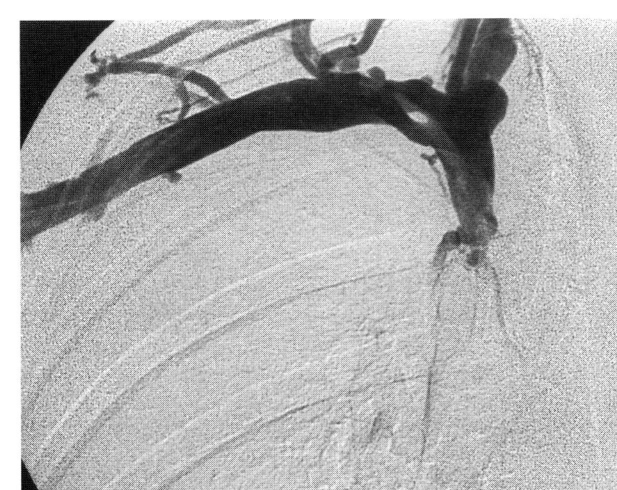

D

Figure 37-14. Thirty-five-year-old man with port catheter for long-term antibiotic therapy presented with painful, swollen right arm and neck. (A) Film from initial right arm venogram demonstrates thrombus in right innominate and collateral filling into the right jugular. (B) Nonsubtracted film obtained at the same time shows position and extent of catheter. (C) Left arm venogram shows thrombus in the left innominate vein, which is essentially completely obstructed. (D) After 24 hours of urokinase infusion, the right innominate is free of thrombus, but the SVC remains occluded. The catheter was then removed. Urokinase infusion was continued for an additional 24 hours, without change. Balloon angioplasty was then performed at the innominate SVC junction, also without change. Placement of a stent was therefore undertaken. (E) Deployment of a Wallstent in the right innominate and SVC, via the right internal jugular vein. Stent was dilated to 15-mm diameter. (F) Right jugular vein injection after deployment shows excellent flow in the innominate and SVC, to the right atrium.

botic has, in the past, required surgery, radiation therapy, chemotherapy, or a combination of these. All are accompanied by substantial morbidity, and radiation and chemotherapy generally lead to symptom resolution relatively slowly. Over the last several years, there has been a growing experience with treatment of symptomatic SVC occlusion by percutaneous stent placement. Several types of metallic stents have been employed, all with relatively high technical and clinical success rates, and a low incidence of complications.[61-64] One or more stents can be placed utilizing either the upper extremity approach or a retrograde approach from the femoral vein (see Fig. 37-14). Stent placement is usually done following angioplasty, to facilitate initial deployment. Angioplasty alone is unlikely to provide long-term patency because of the elas-

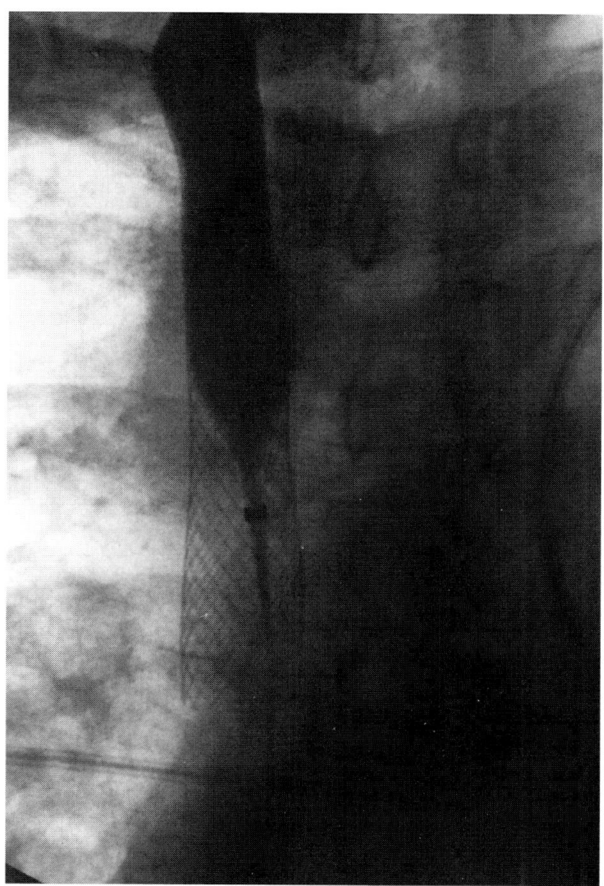

E

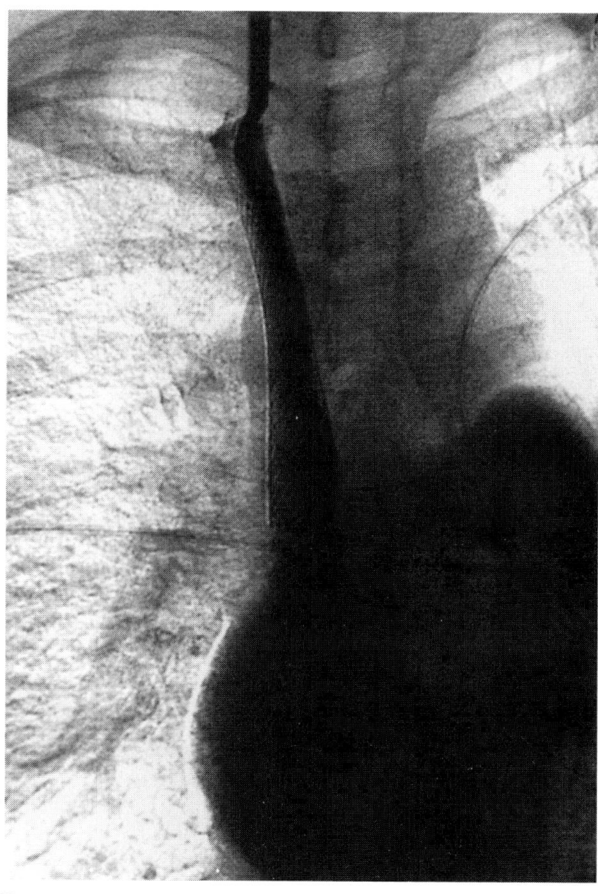

F

Figure 37-14 (continued).

tic nature of benign strictures and the marked compressive effect of malignant ones. In this regard, the hoop strength of the stent used—the ability to resist extrinsic compression—is important. The ability to resist ingrowth through the interstices may also be relevant, but stent grafts or coated stents have not yet been used clinically in the SVC.[65,66] The ability to resist thrombosis is also an important consideration, but to date there is little information to suggest that any particular stent provides advantages in this regard. Although all types of stents have been used, the greatest experience to date, largely due to ease of placement and appropriate sizing, has been with the Wallstent.

Conclusion

Angiography is an important tool in the evaluation of the SVC. For diagnostic purposes, sufficient information can be gained from CT, ultrasound, and MRI in most cases, but angiography remains important in defining the anatomy and extent of vascular compromise, and in resolving confusing noninvasive findings. Percutaneous treatment using angiographic techniques is increasingly important. Thrombolysis to resolve intrinsic occlusions and angioplasty and stent placement to treat underlying and extrinsic lesions (benign strictures, adjacent malignancy) are key therapeutic options for symptomatic SVC occlusion. Angiography, then, plays a central role in the evaluation and treatment of diseases of the superior vena cava and its branches.

References

1. Rosenberger A, Adler O. Superior vena cava syndrome: a new radiologic approach to diagnosis. Cardiovasc Intervent Radiol 1980;3:127.
2. Son YH, Wetzel RA, Wilson WJ. ^{99m}Tc pertechnetate scintiphotography as diagnostic and follow-up aids in major vascular

obstruction due to malignant neoplasm. Radiology 1968;91:349.
3. Gollub S, Hirose T, Klauber J. Scintigraphic sequelae of superior vena caval obstruction. Clin Nucl Med 1980;5:89.
4. Wyse RK, Haworth SG, Taylor JF, MacArtney FF. Obstruction of superior vena caval pathway after Mustard's repair: reliable diagnosis by transcutaneous Doppler ultrasound. Br Heart J 1979;42:162.
5. Stevenson JG, Kawabori K, Guntheroth WG, et al. Pulsed Doppler echocardiographic detection of obstruction of systemic venous return after repair of transposition of the great arteries. Circulation 1979;60:1091.
6. Canedo MI, Otken L, Stefadouros MA. Echocardiographic features of cardiac compression by a thymoma simulating cardiac tamponade and obstruction of the superior vena cava. Br Heart J 1977;39:1038.
7. Prager BC, Gross WS, Behrendt DM. Oculoplethysmography in diagnosing obstruction of the superior vena cava. South Med J 1980;73:442.
7a. Richard HM, Selby JB, Gay SB, Tegtmeyer CJ. Normal venous anatomy and collateral pathways in upper extremity venous thrombosis. Radiographics 1992;12:527–534.
8. Lochridge SK, Knibbe WP, Doty DB. Obstruction of the superior vena cava. Surgery 1979;85:14.
9. Case records of the Massachusetts General Hospital. Weekly clinicopathological exercises. Case 33-1976 N Engl J Med 1976;295:381.
10. Goodman R. Superior vena cava syndrome: clincial management. JAMA 1975;231:55.
11. Gomes MN, Hufnagel CA. Superior vena cava obstruction: a review of the literature and report of two cases due to benign intrathoracic tumors. Ann Thorac Surg 1975;20:344.
12. Davenport D, Ferree C, Blake D, Raben M. Radiation therapy in the treatment of superior vena caval obstruction. Cancer 1978;42:2600.
13. Mearns AJ, Davies JA, Hoggard CA, Watson DA. Thrombotic superior vena caval obstruction after repair of tetralogy of Fallot. Thorax 1977;32:623.
14. Tanabe T, Kubo Y, Hashimoto M, Sugie S. Patch angioplasty of the superior vena caval obstruction (case reports with long follow-up results). J Cardiovasc Surg (Torino) 1974;20:519.
15. Arai T, Inagaki K, Hata E, Hirata M, Onoue Y, Morimoto K. Reconstruction of the superior vena cava in a patient with a thymoma. Chest 1978;73:230.
16. Okay NH, Bryk D. Collateral pathways in occlusion of the superior vena cava and its tributaries. Radiology 1969;92:1493.
17. Wilson ES. Systemic to pulmonary venous communication in the superior vena caval syndrome. AJR 1976;127:247.
18. Lee KR, Preston DF, Martin NL, Robinson RG. Angiographic documentation of systemic-portal venous shunting as a cause of a liver scan "hot spot" in superior vena caval obstruction. AJR 1976;127:637.
19. Ulreich S, Lowman RM, Stern H. Intrathoracic goitre: a cause of the superior vena cava syndrome. Clin Radiol 1977;28:663.
20. Kjellberg SR, Mannheimer E, Rudhe U, Jonsson B. Development of the great veins. In: Kjellberg SR, Mannheimer E, Rudhe U, Jonsson B, eds. Diagnosis of congenital heart disease. Chicago: Year Book, 1955:1–14.
21. Johnson LS, Kinnear DG, Brown RA, Mulder DS. "Downhill" esophageal varices: a rare cause of upper gastrointestinal bleeding. Arch Surg 1978;113:1463.
22. Robb GP, Steinberg I. Visualization of the chambers of the heart, the pulmonary circulation and the great blood vessels in man: a practical method. AJR 1939;41:1.
23. Katz S, Hussey HH, Veal JR. Phlebography for study of obstruction of veins of superior vena caval system. Am J Med Sci 1947;214:7.
24. Roberts DJ Jr, Dotter CT, Steinberg I. Superior vena cava and innominate veins: angiocardiographic study. AJR 1951;66:341.
25. Hudson G. Venography in superior vena caval obstruction. Radiology 1957;68:499.
26. Howard N. Phlebography in superior vena caval obstruction. Radiology 1963;81:380.
27. Webb WR, Gamsu G, Rohlfing BM. Catheter venography in the superior vena cava syndrome. AJR 1977;129:146.
28. Hunter W. History of aneurysm of aorta with some remarks on aneurysm in general. Med Observ Inquiries 1747;1:323.
29. Dombernowsky P, Hansen HH. Combination chemotherapy in the management of superior vena caval obstruction in small-cell anaplastic carcinoma of the lung. Acta Med Scand 1978;204:513.
30. Mahajan V, Strimlau V, Van Ordstrand HS, et al. Benign superior vena cava syndrome. Chest 1975;68:32.
31. Feigin DS, Eggleston JC, Siegelman SS. The multiple roentgen manifestations of sclerosing mediastinitis. Johns Hopkins Med J 1979;144:1.
32. Dines DE, Bernatz PE, Pairolero PC, Payne WS. Mediastinal granuloma and fibrosing mediastinitis. Chest 1979;75:320.
33. Kuffer F. Prophylactic long-term anticoagulant treatment of hydrocephalic patients with ventriculo-atrial shunts. Dev Med Child Neurol 1976;37(Suppl):74.
34. Youngson GG, McKenzie FN, Nichol PM. Superior vena cava syndrome: case report. A complication of permanent transvenous endocardial cardiac pacing requiring surgical correction. Am Heart J 1980;99:503.
35. Paulett M, Pingitore R, Contini C. Superior vena cava stenosis at site of intersection of two pacing electrodes. Br Heart J 1979;42:487.
36. Matthew DM, Forfar JC. Superior vena caval stenosis: a complication of transvenous endocardial pacing. Thorax 1979;34:412.
37. Eckhauser FE, Strodel WE, Knol JA, Turcotte JG. Superior vena caval obstruction associated with long-term peritoneovenous shunting. Ann Surg 1979;190:758.
38. Dorrington WP, McIvor J, Woodrow D, Cream JJ. Cutaneous arteritis with superior vena cava obstruction. Br J Dermatol 1979;100:439.
39. Roguin N, Haim S, Reshet R, Peleg E, Riss E. Cardiac involvement and superior vena caval obstruction in Behçet's disease. Thorax 1978;33:375.
40. Cumming GR, Ferguson CC. Obstruction of superior vena cava after the Mustard procedure for transposition of the great arteries. J Thorac Cardiovasc Surg 1975;70:242.
41. Comyn DJ. Cardiac tamponade with superior vena caval obstruction. S Afr Med J 1978;54:750.
42. Miller DC, Walter JP, Guthaner DF, Mark JB. Recurrent mediastinal bronchogenic cyst: cause of bronchial obstruction and compression of superior vena cava and pulmonary artery. Chest 1978;74:218.
43. Farrer PA, Kloiber R. Combined superior vena cava and pulmonary artery obstruction by an ascending aortic aneurysm. Clin Nucl Med 1979;4:495.
44. Morris AL, Barwinsky J. Unusual vascular complications of dissecting thoracic aortic aneurysms. Cardiovasc Radiol 1978;1:95.
45. Saw HS, Yar SN, Sivanesan S. Aneurysm of the right subclavian artery: an unusual cause of superior vena caval obstruction. Aust NZ J Surg 1979;49:241.
46. Canedo MI, Otken C, Stefadouros MA. Echocardiographic features of cardiac compression by a thymoma simulating cardiac tamponade and obstruction of the superior vena cava. Br Heart J 1977;39:1038.
47. Familusi JB, Sanuel I, Jaiyesimi T, Aderele WI. Superior vena cava occlusion in a 12-year-old girl with neuroblastoma. Clin Pediatr (Phila) 1977;16:1160.
48. Torstveit JR, Bennett WA, Hinchliffe WA, Cornell WP. Primary plasmacytoma of the atrium. J Thorac Cardiovasc Surg 1977;74:563.
49. Schweiter DL, Aguam A. Primary liposarcoma of the mediastinum: report of a case and review of the literature. J Thorac Cardiovasc Surg 1977;74:83.
50. Gordonson J, Trachtenberg S, Sargent EN. Superior vena cava obstruction due to sarcoidosis. Chest 1973;63:292.

51. Schmidt G, Fuessl H. Thoracic actinomycosis with superior vena cava obstruction. Dtsch Med Wochenschr 1979;104:1607.
52. Menon A, Rajamani R. Giant "cryptococcoma" of the lung. Br J Dis Chest 1976;70:269.
53. Mitchell SE, Clark RA. Complications of central venous catheterization. AJR 1979;133:467.
54. Campbell M, Deuchar DC. Left-sided superior vena cava. Br Heart J 1954;16:423.
55. Hairston P. Left superior vena cava to left atrial draining associated with double outlet right ventricle. Arch Surg 1969;98:344.
56. Cha ME, Khoury GH. Persistent left superior vena cava: radiologic and clinical significance. Radiology 1972;103:375.
57. Moes CAF, Goldman BS, Mustard WT. Anomalous pulmonary venous return from the left lung into a left vertical vein. J Can Assoc Radiol 1967;18:377.
58. Rantis P, Littooy F. Successful treatment of prolonged superior vena cava syndrome with thrombolytic therapy: a case report. J Vasc Surg 1994;20:108–113.
59. Edwards RD, Cassidy J, Taylor A. Superior vena cava obstruction complicated by central venous thrombosis—treatment with thrombolysis and Gianturco-Z stents. Clin Radiol 1992;45:278–282.
60. Shortell C, Ouriel K. Thrombolysis in acute peripheral arterial occlusion: predictors of immediate success. Ann Vasc Surg 1994;8:59–65.
61. Rösch J, Uchida BT, Hall LD, et al. Gianturco-Rosch expandable Z-stents in the treatment of superior vena cava obstruction. Cardiovasc Intervent Radiol 1992;15:319–327.
62. Furur S, Sauada S, Kuramoto K, et al. Gianturco stent placement in malignant caval obstruction: analysis of factors for predicting the outcome. Radiology 1995;195:147–152.
63. Hennequin LM, Fade O, Fays JG, et al. Superior vena cava stent placement: results with the Wallstent endopresthesis. Radiology 1995;196:353–361.
64. Hall LD, Murray JD, Boswell GE. Venous stent placement as an adjunct to the staged, multimodal treatment of Paget-Schroetter syndrome. J Vasc Intervent Radiol 1995;6:565–570.
65. Veith FJ, Abbott WM, Yao JST, et al. Guidelines for development and use of transluminally placed endovascular prosthetic grafts in the arterial system. J Vasc Intervent Radiol 1995;6:477–492.
66. Aggaruval RK, Ireland DC, Azrin MA, Ezevourtz MD, DeBoao DP, Gershlich AT. Antithrombotic properties of stents eluting platelet glycoprotein IIb/IIIa antibody. Circulation 1995;92:I–488(abs).

38

The Inferior Vena Cava

ERNEST J. FERRIS
HEMENDRA R. SHAH

The inferior vena cava (IVC), the largest vein in the body, drains blood from the abdomen and lower extremities. Anatomically, it is a continuation of the femoral veins as they enter the abdominal cavity. Each common femoral vein enters the abdominal cavity beneath the inguinal ligament and continues as the external iliac vein. The external iliac veins lie medial to the external iliac arteries, although on the right the external iliac vein passes behind the artery as it ascends to the brim of the minor pelvis and terminates by joining the internal iliac vein. The internal iliac veins, as demonstrated in Figure 38-1, drain numerous pelvic structures.[1]

The external iliac veins continue at the confluence of the internal iliac veins opposite the sacroiliac joint as the right and left common iliac vein. The common iliac veins join at about the level of the fourth to fifth lumbar vertebra to form the inferior vena cava. The IVC ascends in the retroperitoneum (posterior perirenal space) and penetrates the right leaflet of the diaphragm to enter the right atrium. Although it has a host of tributaries, the main ones are the common iliac veins, lumbar veins, right ovarian or testicular vein, renal veins, right suprarenal vein, and hepatic veins.

The IVC is related to many intraperitoneal and extraperitoneal structures (Fig. 38-2). Anteriorly, it is separated by a coat of peritoneum. Crossing anterior to the IVC are anterior lymph nodes, the right gonadal artery, branches of the aortic plexus of the sympathetic chain, the root of the mesentery duodenum, and the pancreas. As the IVC ascends superiorly, it enters the sulcus venae cavae on the posterior surface of the liver. Here, the tail of the caudate lobe separates the IVC from the portal vein and porta hepatis (Fig. 38-3). Bordering on the right of the IVC are the peritoneum, ureter, kidney, and liver; periaortic nodes and the aorta form its left margin. Posteriorly lie the psoas muscle and the right renal artery (Fig. 38-4). In the region of the sulcus venae cavae, the medial crus of the right diaphragmatic leaflet borders the IVC posteriorly.

After diaphragmatic penetration, a sleeve of pericardium envelops the IVC immediately before its entrance into the right atrium. On the endocardial side of the IVC-cardiac junction is the valve of the inferior vena cava.

Techniques of Visualizing the IVC

With the current host of imaging modalities, the IVC can be visualized in numerous ways. Not only the lumen, as was the case with venography, but the entire structure, even with differentiation of the endothelial coat, muscle, and adventitial covering, may be delineated with modern techniques. The following are the current methods available:

1. Inferior vena cavography
2. Capnocavography
3. Ultrasound: (Doppler)-duplex and intravascular ultrasound
4. Computed tomography
5. Magnetic resonance imaging, MR angiography
6. Angioscopy, surgical or percutaneous
7. Radionuclide cavography

The technique used for visualization depends on the clinical question to be answered, the interventional therapy to be applied, and, in the present era of cost containment, the cost of the study.

Inferior Vena Cavography

Roentgenographic visualization of the inferior vena cava in vivo dates back to 1935, when dos Santos[2] injected radiopaque material into a saphenous vein cutdown. Twelve years later (1947) Fariñas[3] modified the technique of dos Santos by applying external pressure over the epigastrium in an attempt to obtain better contrast density of the IVC. In the same year, O'Lough-

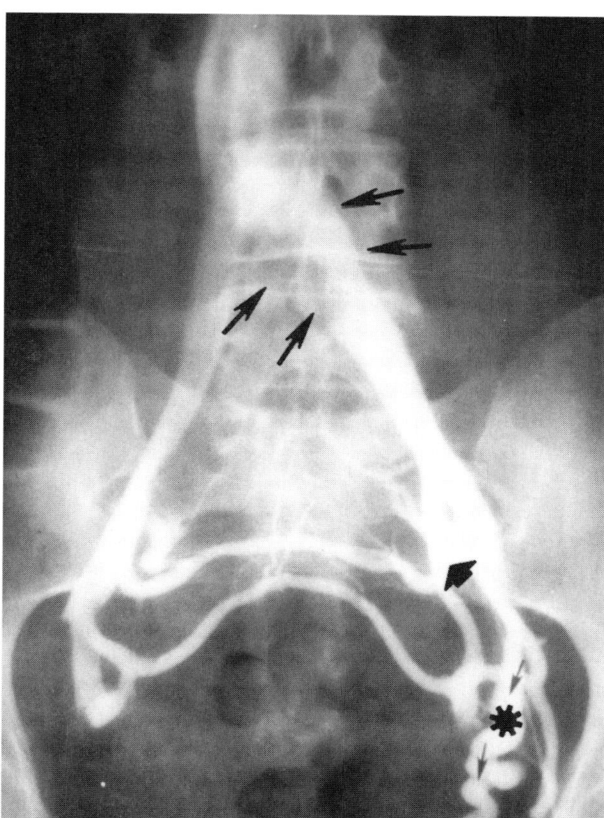

Figure 38-1. Inferior vena cavogram showing reflux into the internal iliac vein. Contrast material was injected into the left external iliac vein in a young woman. There is slight deformity of the left common iliac vein (*arrows*) from the overlying right common iliac artery. Reflux of the contrast material fills the left internal iliac vein (*large arrowhead*) and traverses across the midline to fill the contralateral internal iliac vein as well. The asterisk denotes the left gonadal vein filling from the left internal iliac vein, presumably from either too large a volume of contrast material with retrograde gonadal vein flow, partial obstruction of the left common iliac vein secondary to arterial compression with resultant stasis, or a combination of both.

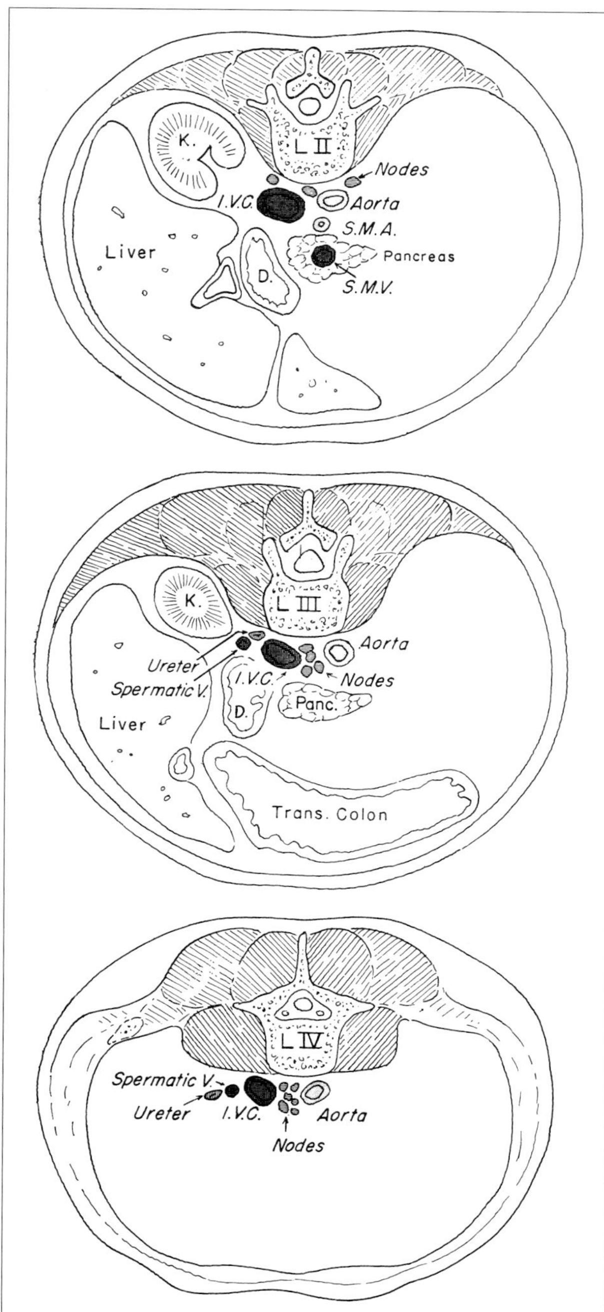

Figure 38-2. Diagrams at the level of the second, third, and fourth lumbar vertebrae showing the relationship of the inferior vena cava in cross section to other retroperitoneal and intraperitoneal structures. *I.V.C.*, inferior vena cava; *D.*, duodenum; *S.M.V.*, superior mesenteric vein; *S.M.A.*, superior mesenteric artery; *K.*, kidney. (From Ferris EJ, Hipona FA, Kahn PC, et al, eds. Venography of the inferior vena cava and its branches. Baltimore: Williams & Wilkins, 1969. Used with permission.)

lin[4] perfected the technique by the percutaneous injection of contrast material into the femoral veins with 18-gauge needles. To prevent streaming from the lower extremities, he applied blood pressure cuffs to both thighs below the puncture sites. O'Loughlin[4] also introduced the Valsalva maneuver to cavography to slow circulation as well as to cause reflux into the IVC tributaries. Kaufman et al.[5] in 1956 attempted translumbar cavography with 17-gauge needles. Although this met with limited success, it was the forerunner of translumbar cavography, now used primarily for long-term chemotherapy catheter placement.[6] Kaufman also used a modified Seldinger technique by

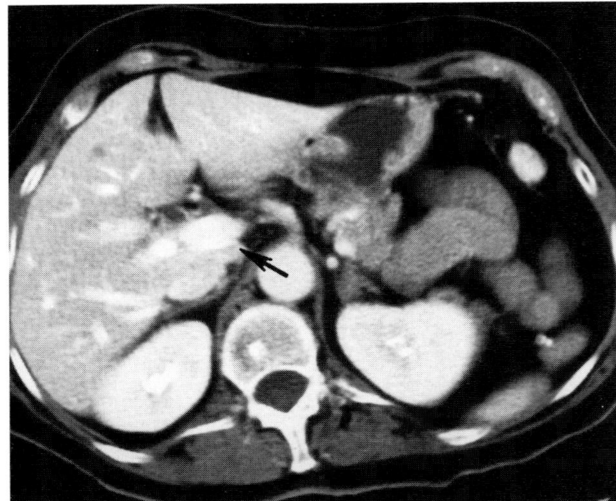

Figure 38-3. CT scan of the upper abdomen with IV contrast showing caudate lobe (*arrow*) between the IVC and the portal vein.

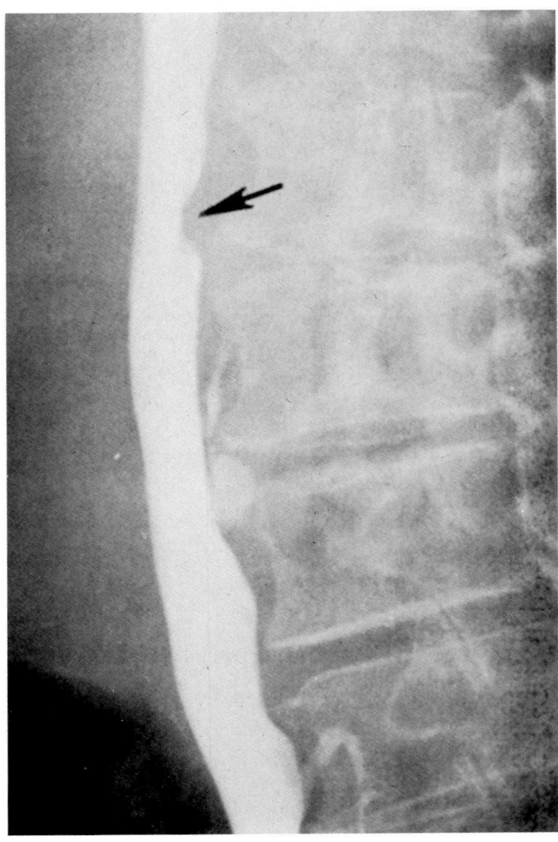

Figure 38-4. Inferior vena cavogram in the right posterior oblique projection. *Arrow* indicates the impression made by the right renal artery.

threading polyethylene tubing through 13-gauge needles percutaneously positioned in the femoral veins. Helander and Lindbom[7] employed the Seldinger technique of catheterizing the femoral veins. Extrinsic abdominal compression caused reflux into the vertebral venous plexus and hence allowed study of spinal canal diseases. Without abdominal compression, there was excellent visualization of the IVC.

Marcozzi and Messinetti[8] advocated transsomatic vertebral angiography of the IVC in patients in whom other methods proved unsuccessful. Transsomatic vertebral angiography is performed by injecting 50 ml of contrast material into the third or fourth lumbar vertebra.[9] Alternatively, the spinous apophyses of the lumbar or sacral vertebrae may be injected. Injection into the greater trochanters of the femur also results in good opacification of the IVC. However, with the advent of more sophisticated and less invasive imaging procedures, intraosseous venography is now essentially of historic diagnostic value.

Retrograde catheterization from the antecubital vein through the superior vena cava and right atrium has also been performed. With the use of digital angiography, one can now obtain excellent opacification of the IVC from the injection of contrast material into the dorsal veins of both feet.

For venography of the lumbar spinal plexus, one can catheterize the lumbar ascending veins from the femoral veins. With compression of the abdomen, excellent delineation of the lumbar spinal plexus has been seen.[10–12]

Standard Technique

Inferior vena cavography is done in a variety of ways. Obviously, the areas of interest dictated by the indications for the study determine, to a great degree, the technique used. For example, cavography to evaluate possible extension of a right renal tumor into the IVC may be performed by positioning a catheter in the lower cava. Conversely, if one is performing cavography as a preliminary step to insertion of a prophylactic caval filter, the technique may include injection into both lower external iliac veins to prevent overlooking a double IVC. Alternatively, one may use the right femoral approach and deflect the catheter retrograde down into the left common iliac vein. An injection at that point will provide for an excellent cavogram and will not overlook a double IVC.

After the inguinal areas are prepared and draped, the femoral artery is located by palpation. The femoral vein is slightly medial to the artery. By keeping the palpating fingers on the artery during insertion of a 4-inch, 18-gauge, thin-walled Seldinger needle into the

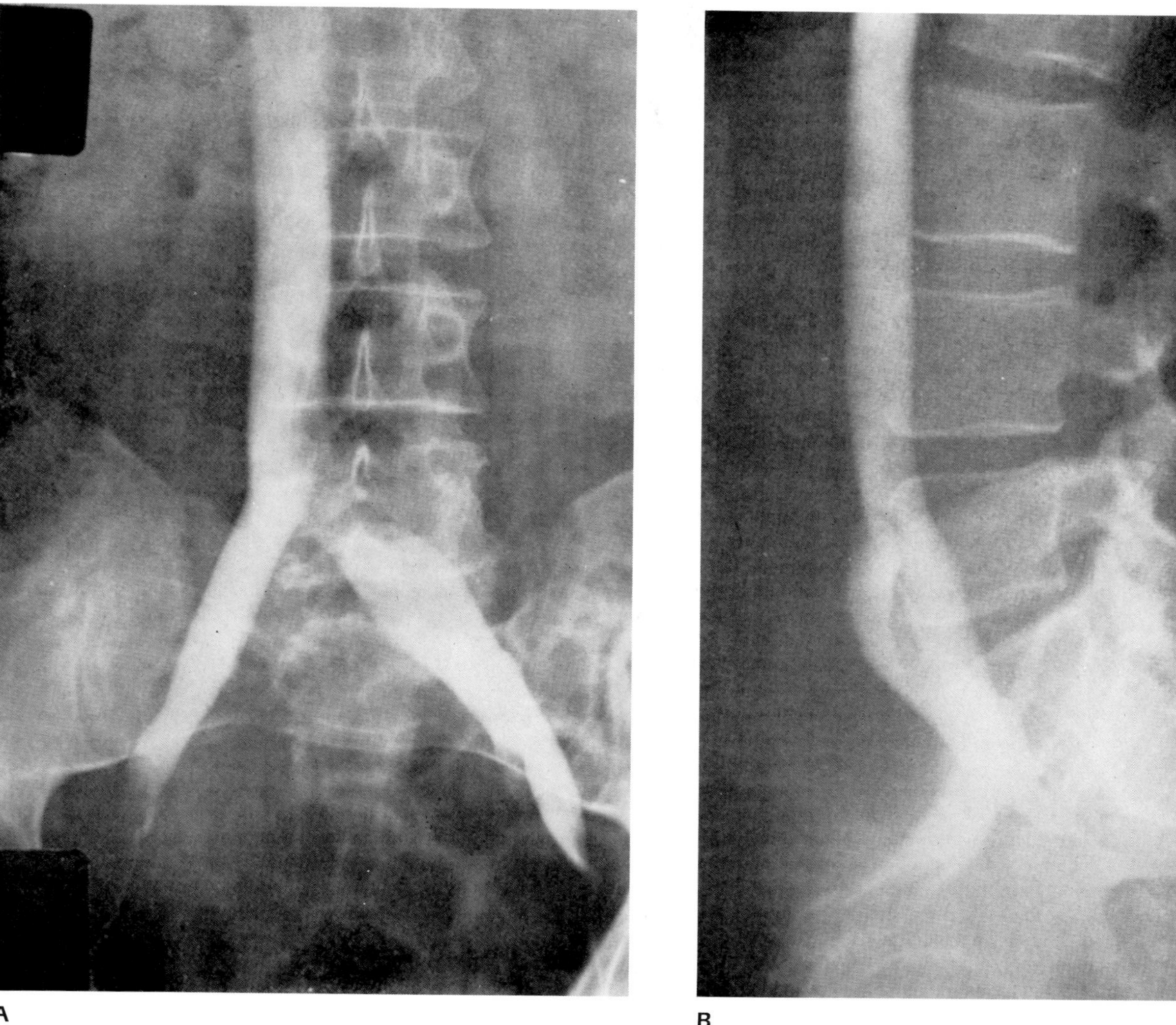

Figure 38-5. Normal inferior vena cavogram. Simultaneous anteroposterior (A) and translateral projection (B).

vein, one diminishes the possibility of accidentally puncturing the femoral artery. Alternatively, a beveled needle may be used to attempt a single-wall puncture. With aspiration during percutaneous penetration of the needle, one-wall puncture is feasible. An appropriate guidewire (e.g., 0.035 French through an 18-gauge thin-walled needle) is advanced and an end-hole introductory catheter (5 French) with side holes is inserted. A short tubing is attached to the sheath or catheter. Once the lumen is entered and free flow is obtained, the sheath is threaded superiorly with a short 0.035 French guidewire. To ensure the position in the external or low common iliac vein, fluoroscopic verification of the catheter tip with a test injection of 3 ml of contrast material is advisable. If both femoral veins have been catheterized, the catheters are suitably attached to a Y connector and 50 ml of 60 percent contrast material is delivered in 3 seconds. With the development of various preshaped catheters, most angiographers now prefer a ring-shaped end with multiple side holes positioned in the lower IVC or right (or, less commonly, left) common iliac vein. Twelve ml per second of 60 percent contrast material for a total of 40 to 50 ml with serial filming in one or two planes is the customary approach. When digital studies are used, 5 ml per second for a total of 15 to 20 ml of 30 percent contrast material is usually sufficient to obtain a satisfactory inferior vena cavogram (IVC gram). Filming is in the anteroposterior and lateral projections with biplane technique using a serial changer (Fig. 38-5). Ordinarily two films per second for 5 seconds are followed by a delayed series of one film every

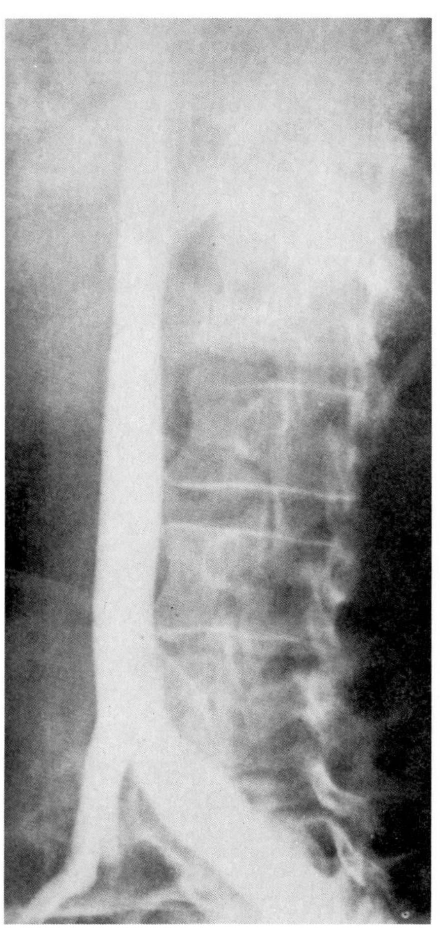

A

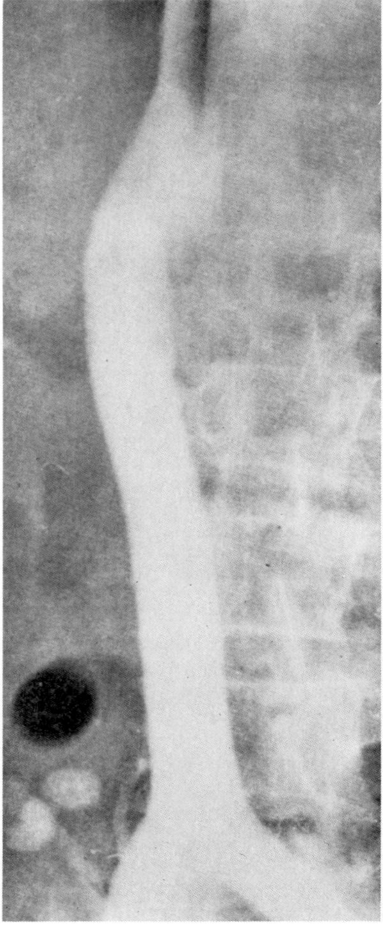

B

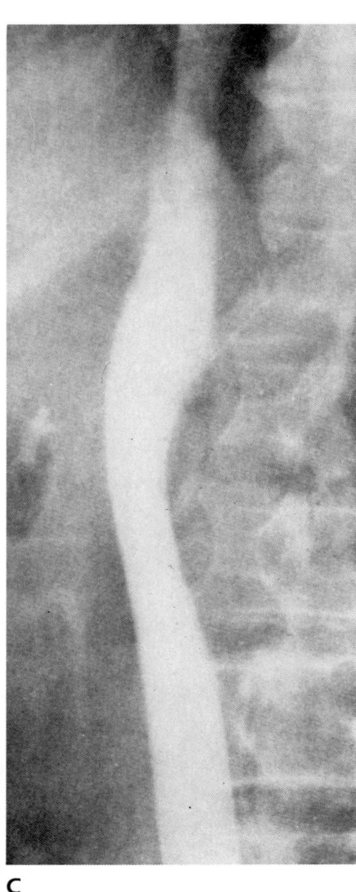

C

Figure 38-6. (A) Normal inferior vena cavogram, right posterior oblique projection. Note how the IVC is slightly separated from the spine at the level of the first and second lumbar vertebrae. (B) Frontal projection of the IVC illustrating some diminution in density of the opaque column and slight lateral displacement at the level of the first and second lumbar vertebrae. (C) Right posterior oblique projection clearly delineates the retroperitoneal neoplastic nodal involvement (metastatic disease from adenocarcinoma of the colon). (From Ferris EJ, Hipona FA, Kahn PC, et al, eds. Venography of the inferior vena cava and its branches. Baltimore: Williams & Wilkins, 1969. Used with permission.)

third second for 21 seconds so as to record the position of the aorta during the levo phase of the study. Furthermore, the arterial phase may show abnormal vessels and corroborate or clarify IVC abnormalities seen during the venous phase. Depending on the indication for the study, venous pressure may be obtained and circulation time measured (the latter if an arterial phase is deemed to be important). When venous pressure is high, the programming of the serial films is adjusted appropriately. If one is studying patients whose disease process might be manifested by extrinsic pressure deformity of the IVC, a right posterior oblique projection will demonstrate external deformity to the best advantage (Fig. 38-6). A postangiographic roentgenogram of the kidneys should be obtained at the end of the examination.

Capnocavography

Capnocavography (Fig. 38-7A) is a study that would rarely be performed today. However, if an IVC gram is indicated, and there is a major or intermediate allergic response history to iodine and/or contrast agents, carbon dioxide may be used.[13] With the patient in a secured left lateral decubitus position, 60 to 100 ml of pure carbon dioxide is injected into the left femoral vein (see Fig. 38-7A). With digital studies, the examination is comparable to a positive contrast IVC gram.

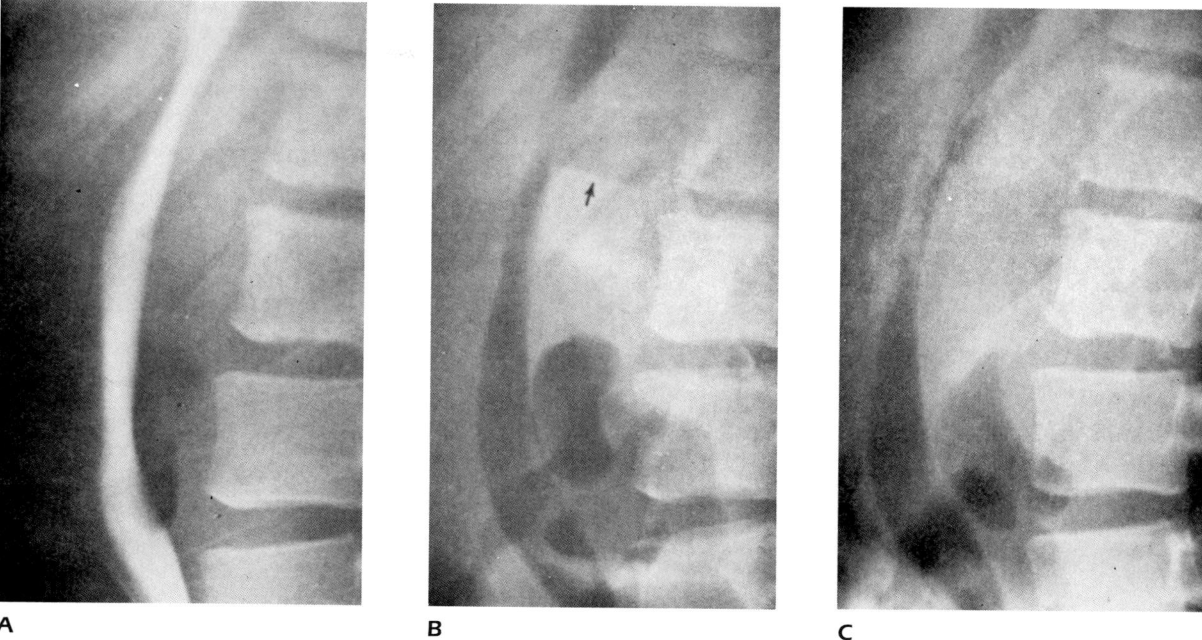

Figure 38-7. (A) Lateral projection of the inferior vena cava filled with opaque contrast material. (B) This study was followed by the capnocavogram, which depicts the IVC clearly. The *small arrow* points to carbon dioxide in the right renal vein. The gas study is performed with the patient's left side down to prevent gas embolism to the pulmonary arteries. This patient had a lymphoma with marked anterior displacement of the cava. (A and B from Hipona FA, Ferris EJ, Pick R. Capnocavography: a new technique for examination of the inferior vena cava. Radiology 1969;92:606–609. Used with permission.) (C) Double-contrast cavogram in the same patient.

Double-contrast IVC cavography may be performed in patients without an allergic history by preceding the carbon dioxide injection with several milliliters of iodinated contrast material (see Fig. 38-7B).

Ultrasound

The IVC can be easily evaluated by static (Fig. 38-8) or real-time ultrasound. The IVC below the level of the liver, however, can be more difficult to evaluate because of either bowel gas or the deep position of the cava due to the patient's size.[14–16] The IVC is usually evaluated in the supine or left lateral decubitus position. The latter position is particularly helpful in patients with a large amount of bowel gas. Axial, longitudinal, and coronal images are usually obtained. Scanning is performed using 3.5- or 5-MHz transducers. In very obese patients, however, one may need 2.5 MHz, and in infants, 7 MHz may be helpful. Most scanning is performed using sector transducers, but linear transducers can evaluate a longer segment whenever possible.

The IVC is seen as an anechoic tubular structure in longitudinal or coronal scanning and as an oval or

Figure 38-8. Ultrasound of inferior vena cava (*arrows*) in longitudinal axis. *Asterisk* denotes lumen.

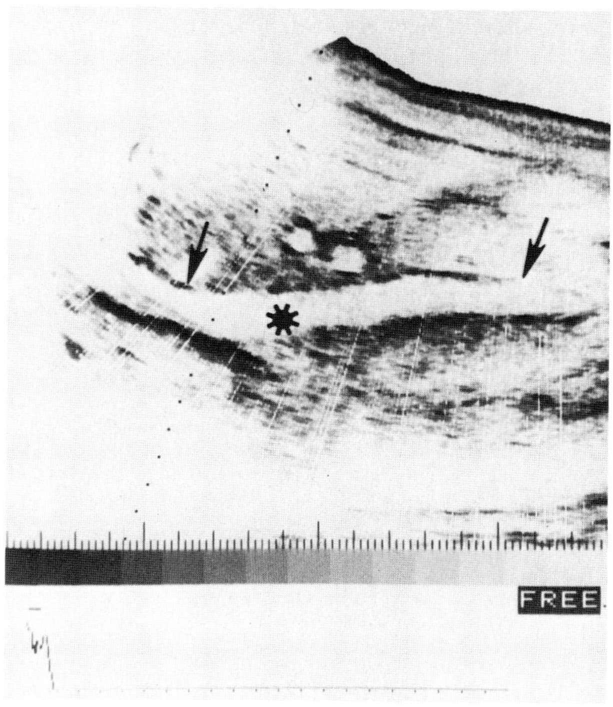

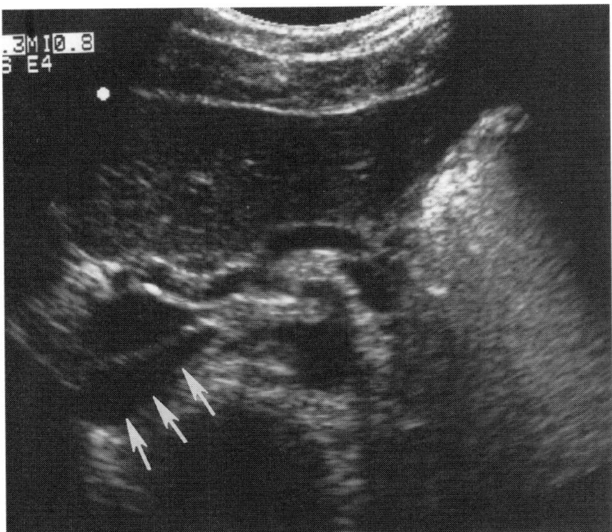

Figure 38-9. Axial real-time ultrasound of the upper abdomen showing oval IVC (*arrows*).

round structure in axial or transverse scanning (Fig. 38-9). In longitudinal scanning, the IVC is seen entering the right atrium, so it is possible to evaluate tumor thrombus extension into the heart in patients with renal cell carcinoma (Fig. 38-10).[17] The hepatic veins are easily seen entering the IVC in practically all (except very obese) patients. In most patients, the left renal vein can be seen passing between the aorta and superior mesenteric vessels and then joining the IVC (Fig. 38-11). The right renal vein can be seen in some patients. In real-time sonography one can detect changes in the IVC caliber with respiration and transmitted pulsation from the heart.[16]

Duplex and Color Sonography

With the advent of duplex sonography, we can now obtain waveform recordings from the inferior vena cava. The waveform from the IVC near the heart usually shows a zigzag pattern related to transmitted pulsation from the right atrium, compared with the low-velocity phasic waveform away from the heart similar to that in the extremity veins (Figs. 38-12 and 38-13).[17] With color Doppler ultrasound, one can evaluate the IVC quickly. One can determine the direction of flow and masses within the lumen of the IVC, as well as obtain waveforms at specific sites, such as at the level of obstruction.[18]

Intravascular Ultrasound

With the advent of small ultrasound probes, it has become feasible to design a method for performing endoluminal ultrasound of small and large tubular structures, including blood vessels.[19–21] The great advantage of this technique is that one can visualize all coats of the vessel, rather than simply the confines of opposing intimal borders as seen in angiography.[22,23]

A 20-MHz transducer specifically designed for intravascular use has been the developing standard wavelength used. The transducer is contained in a catheter 95 cm long (Boston Scientific). Whereas the catheter

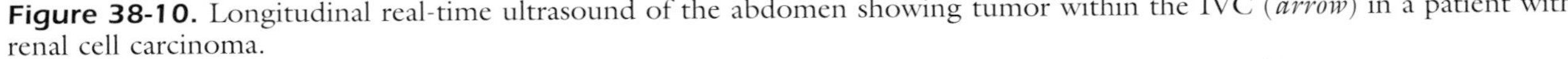

Figure 38-10. Longitudinal real-time ultrasound of the abdomen showing tumor within the IVC (*arrow*) in a patient with renal cell carcinoma.

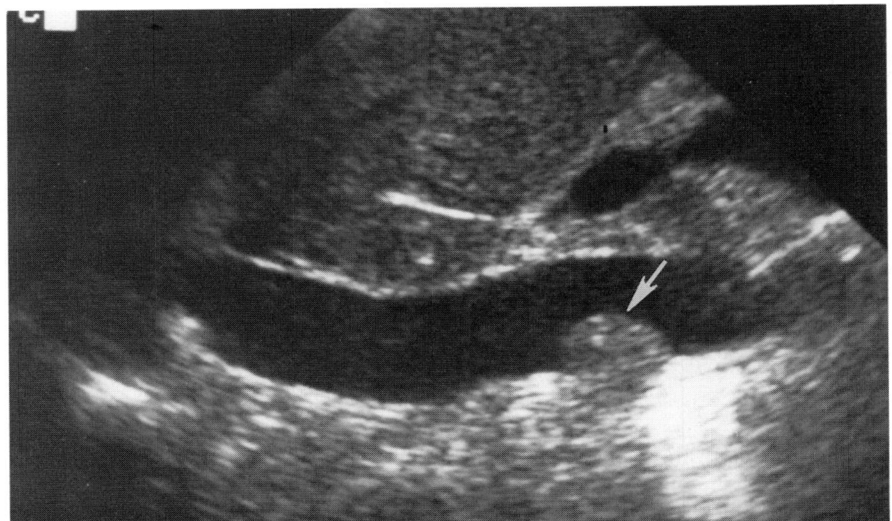

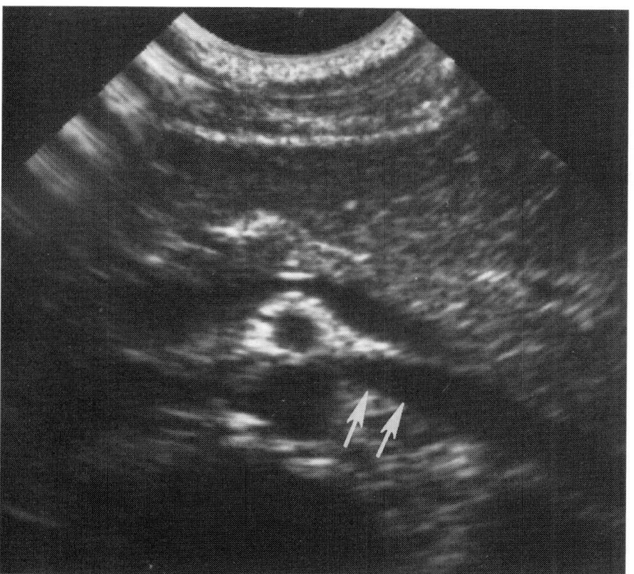

A

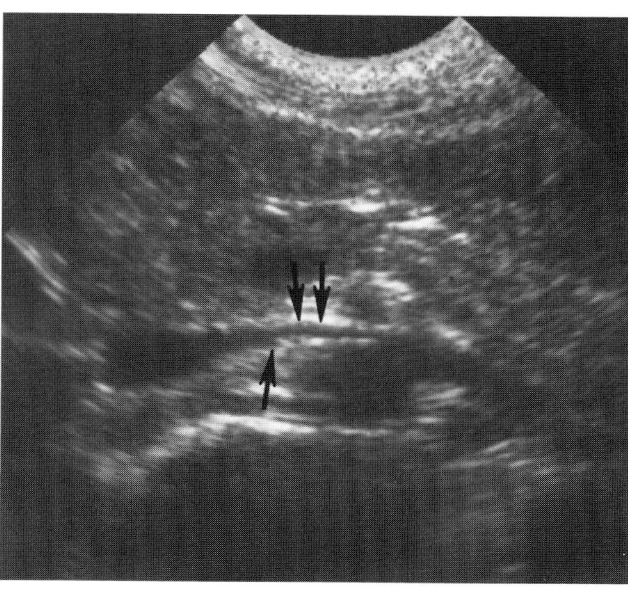

B

Figure 38-11. (A and B) Two axial real-time ultrasounds showing the left renal vein (*arrows*) passing between aorta and superior mesenteric artery.

is designed for single use, the transducer core is movable and can be reused. Two configurations of catheters are available: either a blunt tip design of a 6.2 F catheter that will traverse a 7 F sheath or a variable-size catheter on a monorail system. The intravascular ultrasound transducer is interfaced to an imaging console designed for high-frequency imaging and 360-degree scan capability for image display and processing (Diasonics; Hewlett Packard). Studies are recorded on videotape, and the hard copies are available via an ancillary thermal printer.

The value of intravascular ultrasound in the venous system is varied, but the presence of intraluminal defects such as tumor (Fig. 38-14) or sterile thrombi (Fig. 38-15) can be well delineated using this method.[24] Interventional ultrasound in assessing inferior vena caval filter thrombi in patients with recurrent emboli has been reported (see Fig. 38-15).[25,26]

Figure 38-12. Doppler waveform from the inferior vena cava near the right atrium showing pulsatile (zigzag) pattern.

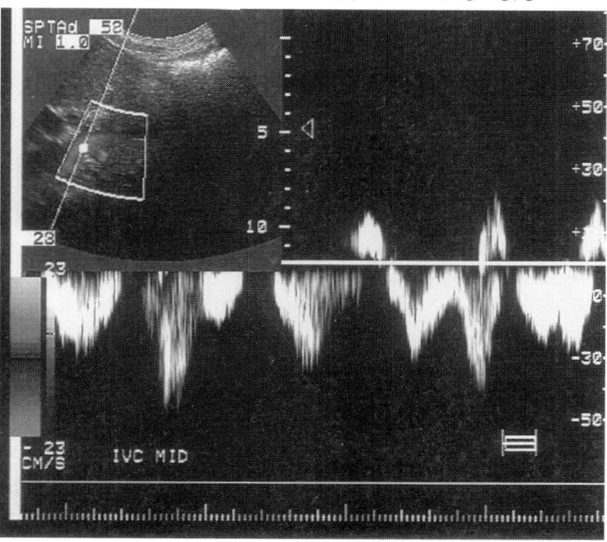

Figure 38-13. Low-velocity phasic waveform from a normal inferior vena cava below the liver.

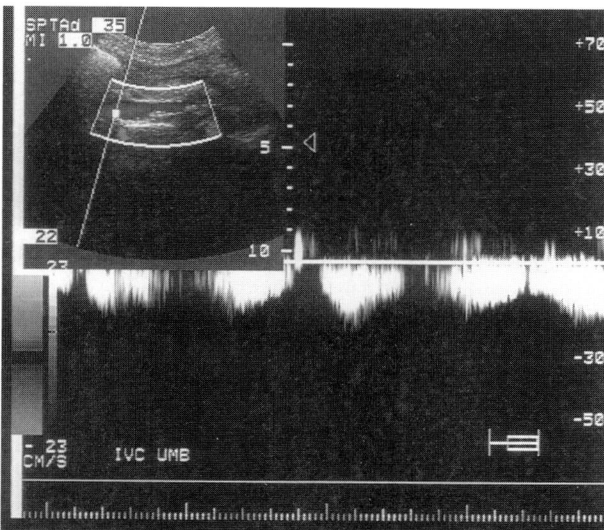

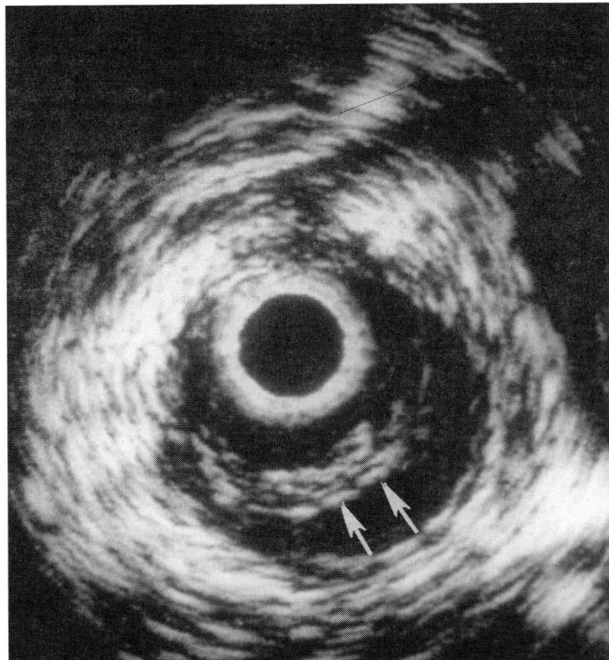

Figure 38-14. Tumor thrombus. Intravascular ultrasound shows a filling defect in the suprarenal inferior vena cava (*arrows*) secondary to tumor extension from a left renal carcinoma invading the inferior vena cava.

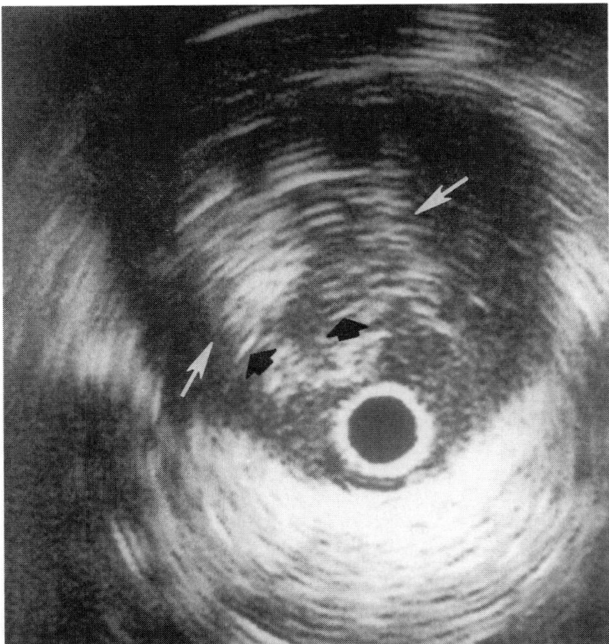

Figure 38-15. Caval thrombus. Intravascular ultrasound illustrates thrombus (*arrows*) trapped in an inferior vena caval Bird's Nest filter at L3-L4. *Arrowheads* depict the echogenic mesh of wires.

Computed Tomography (CT)

The inferior vena cava is easily seen on CT scans, even without intravenous contrast.[27] It is usually round, oval, or flat, but may vary in appearance in the same individual. Often the appearance varies with the phase of respiration (large or distended with inspiration or Valsalva maneuver) or the state of the patient's circulation (distended in patients with congestive heart failure, slitlike in patients with hypovolemia) (Fig. 38-16).[28] The usual anteroposterior diameter is 2 to 3 cm.

Intravenous contrast material is helpful in evaluating a thrombus or mass within the IVC.[29–34] The thrombus presents as low density within the IVC. Dynamic scans may show enhancement of the tumor thrombus. Intravenous contrast is usually administered in the peripheral vein of the upper extremity. If contrast is injected in the foot vein, low-density artifacts related to flow phenomenon from the noncontrasted blood from the noninjected lower extremity can cause confusion, and a diagnosis of thrombus may be made erroneously. Also, with the use of power injection and rapid scanners, the IVC usually shows similar changes in the upper abdomen due to mixing of contrast blood from the hepatic and renal veins and noncontrasted blood from the lower extremities (Fig. 38-17).[29,35,36] CT is helpful in evaluating unsuspected thrombus within the IVC and also common congenital anomalies, the knowledge of which may be critical for patient management. These are discussed under the section on anomalies.

Magnetic Resonance Imaging (MRI)

MRI is as good as CT for evaluating the IVC. Added advantages of MRI include no need for intravenous contrast, no radiation, and the ability to obtain sagittal and coronal images (Fig. 38-18). Usually there is no signal within the IVC, because flowing blood has no signal. However, there is presence of signal within the IVC related to slower flow or entry slice phenomenon.[37] The IVC is usually evaluated in axial planes, but coronal and sagittal planes are useful in the case of a mass within the IVC or outside of the IVC (Fig. 38-19). Congenital anomalies are more easily identified on MRI when compared with CT because MRI can differentiate between dilated vessels and lymph nodes.

Percutaneous Angioscopy

Percutaneous angioscopy is technically feasible[38] and has been used in assessing such abnormalities as the iliac vein spur. The clearing of blood with balloon oc-

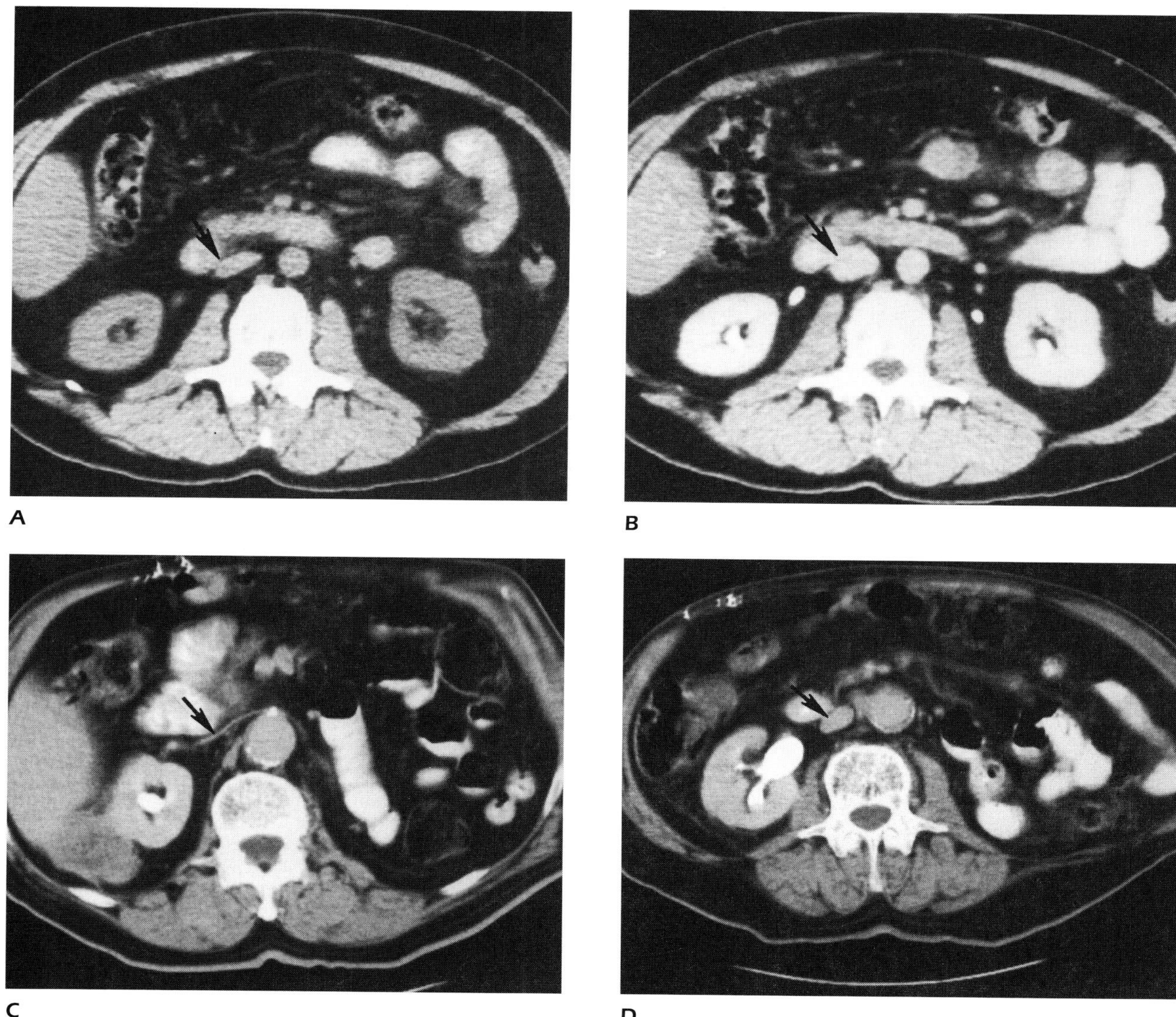

Figure 38-16. (A and B) CT scans of the abdomen in a patient showing changes in caliber of IVC (*arrows*) during pre- and postcontrast scans. (C and D) Another patient showing changes in caliber of IVC (*arrows*) at different levels during the same examination. These examples show change in caliber of IVC in different phases of respiration. There is a metastatic lesion in the right perinephric space.

clusion and rapid saline injection to visualize through small spaces has proven too tedious to be of practical use. With surgical control and large endoscopes, it may be of some value. In the past, venous angioscopy has been used for control of valvulotomies in in-site venous graft procedures in the lower extremities.[39,40]

Radionuclide Cavography

Angioscanning has been applied to the IVC, and multiple nuclear agents have been used. When tagged albumin is injected into the dorsal vein of both feet during a radionuclide venogram for the evaluation of deep venous thrombosis, one may also assess the patency of the IVC.[41,42]

Abnormal Anatomy

Embryogenesis

To understand the anomalies of the IVC, one must understand its embryogenesis.[1,43] The IVC originates from three paired veins: the posterior cardinal, the subcardinal, and the supracardinal networks.[44]

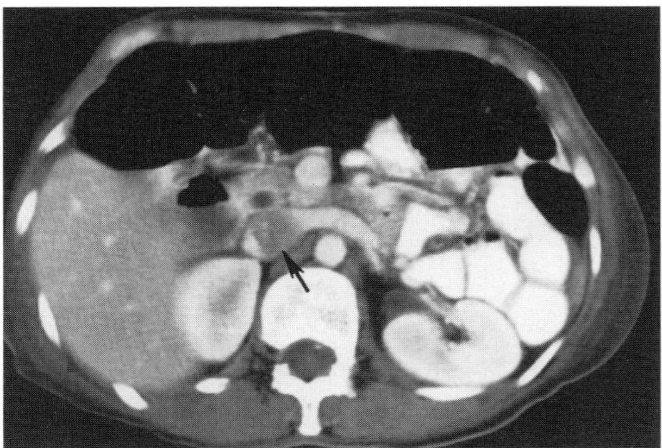

A

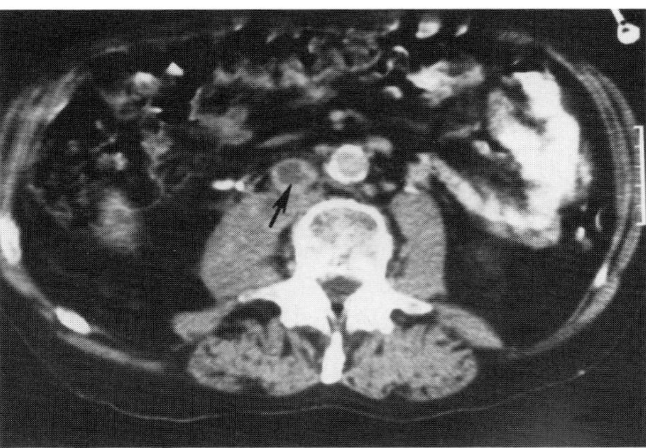

B

Figure 38-17. (A) Postintravenous contrast scan of the upper abdomen showing pseudothrombus in the IVC (*arrow*) due to rapid scanning using an injector. (B) Postintravenous contrast scan of the midabdomen showing low-density thrombus in the IVC (*arrow*) in a patient with obstruction of the IVC at a higher level by a retroperitoneal sarcoma.

In the young embryo the main venous channels of the mesonephroi are the paired posterior cardinal veins, which join cranially with the precardinal veins (anterior cardinal) to form the duct of Cuvier. In the early stages the paired subcardinal veins are small and lie in a ventral position. Anastomotic channels exist between the two (Fig. 38-20A). As the mesonephroi enlarge, the subcardinal veins become larger and develop intersubcardinal anastomoses (Fig. 38-20B). Subsequently, the cephalic portion of the left posterior cardinal vein and the cranial subcardinal and posterior cardinal veins begin to atrophy (Fig. 38-20C). The newly developed intersubcardinal anastomosis assumes importance now as the flow direction begins to shift from the left side to primarily the right via the intersubcardinal channels. In the interim there is a

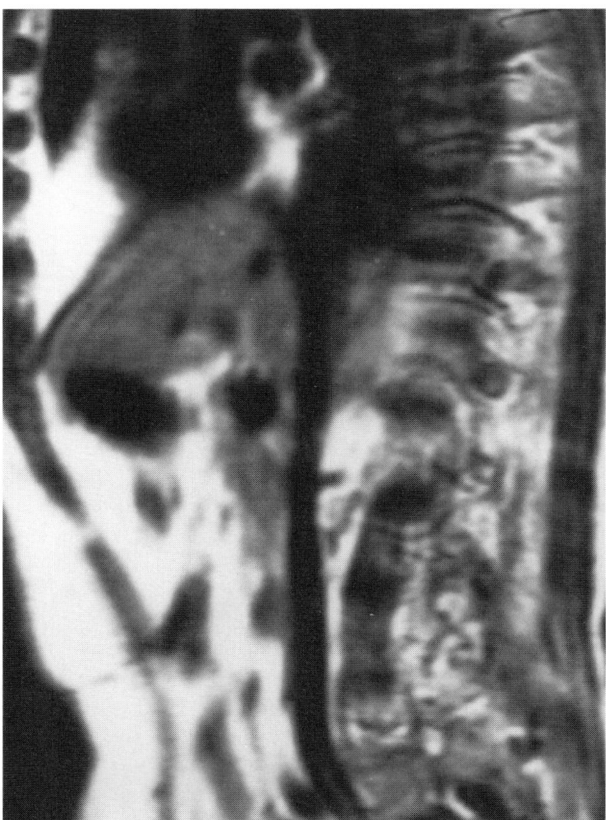

A

Figure 38-18. (A and B) Sagittal and coronal MR images of the abdomen showing the longitudinal course of the IVC.

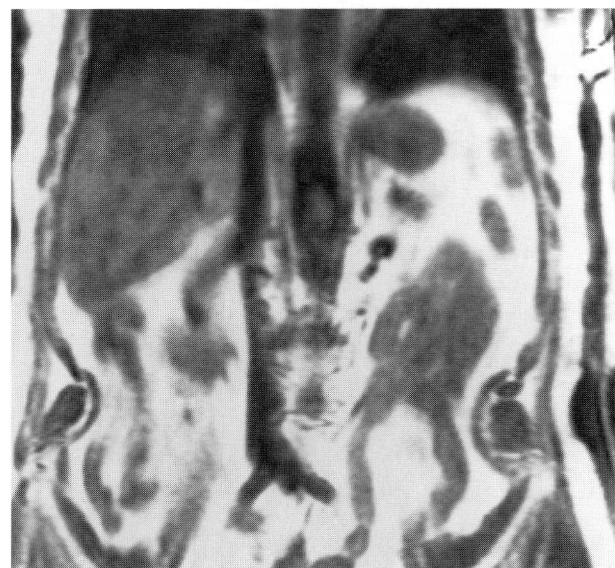

B

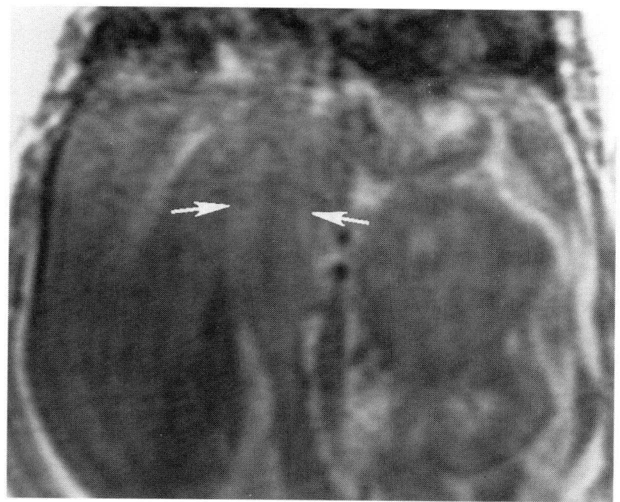

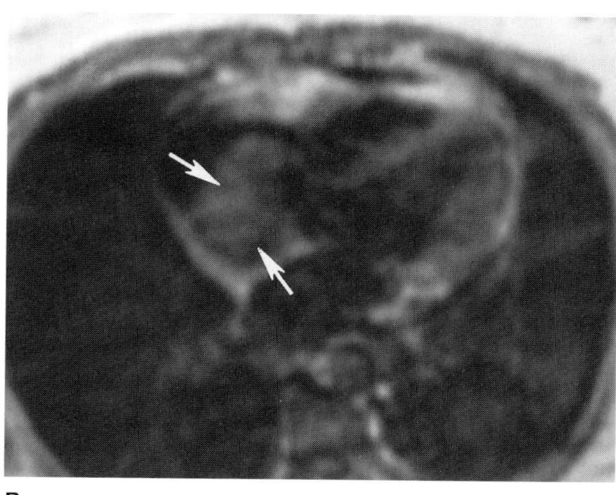

Figure 38-19. (A) Coronal MR image of the abdomen showing a left kidney mass with tumor expanding the IVC (*arrows*) and extending into the right atrium. (B) Axial MR image showing mass in right atrium (*arrows*).

union between developing hepatic sinusoids, the vena hepatic communication of Hochstetter, and a portion of the right subcardinal vein to form the prerenal division of the IVC. Anastomosis between the posterior cardinal veins caudally develops to a great degree (Fig. 38-20D). Thus the presence of the prerenal segment, the intersubcardinal anastomosis, and the caudal connections between the two posterior cardinal veins, along with left and subsequently right posterior cardinal vein atrophy, allows for more drainage on the right side and shunting of left-sided flow to the right. This situation thus tends toward the adult characteristics (Fig. 38-20E).

The posterior cardinal veins continue to atrophy gradually while the pars subcardinalis and intersubcardinal anastomoses increase, leading to flow from the left postcardinal system into the prerenal segment of the IVC. In the thoracic and lumbar regions, paired supracardinal veins appear dorsolaterally to the aorta. Cranially, the supracardinal veins anastomose with the posterior cardinal veins. Caudally, the supracardinal veins anastomose with the subcardinal veins. The supracardinal-subcardinal anastomosis thus allows for the eventual postrenal (subcardinalis)–prerenal (supracardinalis) continuity. Furthermore, each subcardinal-supracardinal communication forms the lateral margin of the embryonic renal collar (which forms a short segment of the IVC at the renal vein level) and on the right participates in the formation of the pars renalis. Figure 38-20C shows the prerenal division (pars hepatica and pars subcardinalis) and the postrenal division (pars renalis and pars supracardinalis) approaching the configuration of the adult IVC.

A perimetonephric ring forms on the right between the union of the right posterior cardinal and supracardinal veins. Because the counterparts on the left are atrophying, no left ring is formed. The renal collar in the form of a circumaortic venous ring develops, atrophies, and leaves some components to form, with the perimetonephric ring, the renal-level margins of the IVC. The left subcardinal vein (left-sided inferior vena cava) is the last one to regress.

Anomalies

In categorizing anomalies, the classifications of Huntington and McClure[45] and McClure and Butler[43] are probably the simplest and are based on defects in embryogenesis. Philips, in Ferris et al.,[1] has clarified the classification and included paraembryonic defects in the overall congenital defects of the inferior vena cava and associated anomalies. The following classification is based on that of Philips.[1] If one takes into account the four major trunks that constitute the original embryonic venous plan of the postrenal division, they fall into four groups:

A. Right posterior cardinal vein
B. Right supracardinal vein
C. Left supracardinal vein
D. Left posterior cardinal vein

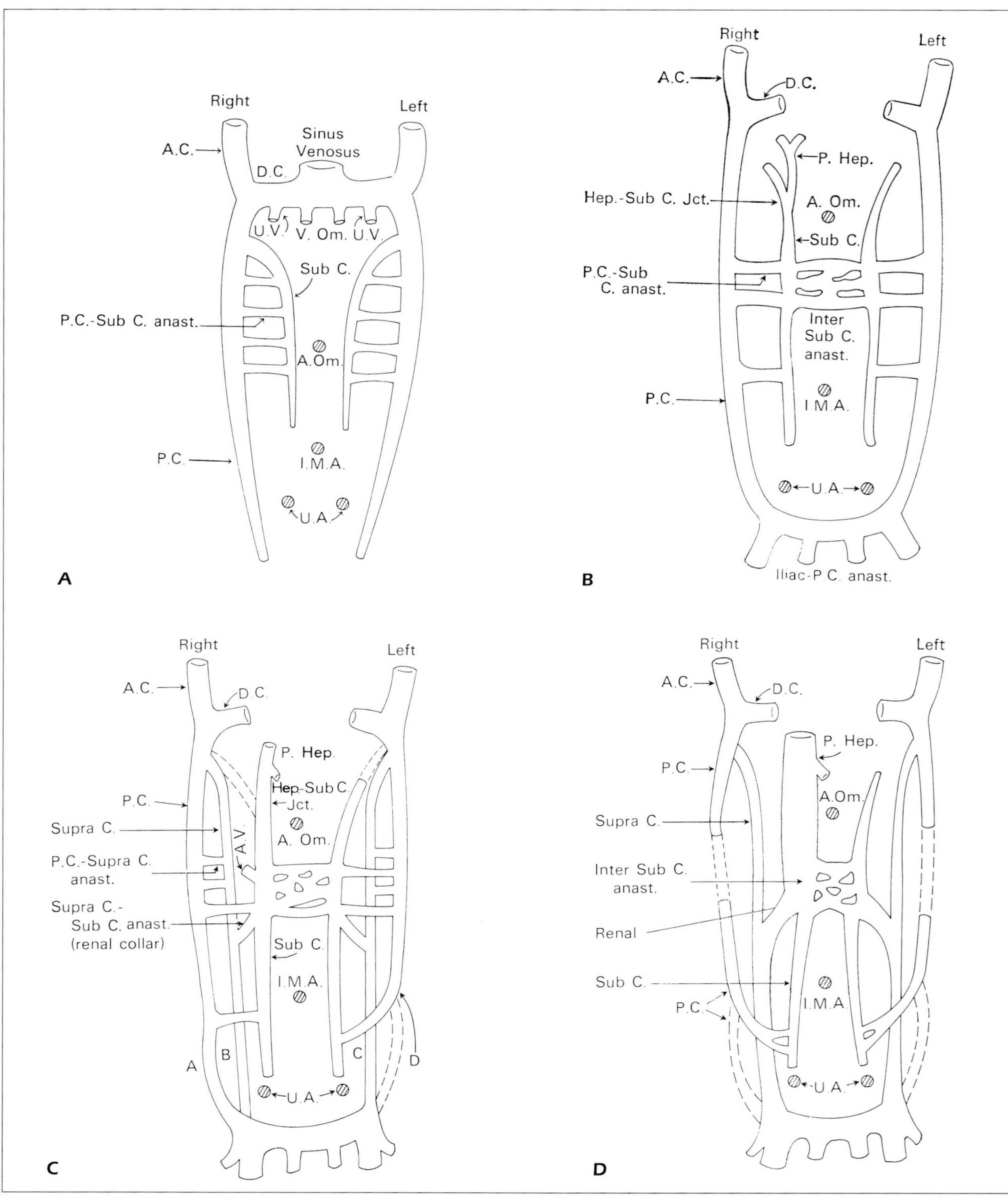
Right
Left
A.C.
Sinus Venosus
D.C.
U.V.
V. Om.
U.V.
Sub C.
P.C.-Sub C. anast.
A.Om.
P.C.
I.M.A.
U.A.
A
Right
Left
A.C.
D.C.
P. Hep.
Hep.-Sub C. Jct.
A. Om.
Sub C.
P.C.-Sub C. anast.
Inter Sub C. anast.
P.C.
I.M.A.
U.A.
Iliac-P.C. anast.
B
Right
Left
A.C.
D.C.
P. Hep.
Hep-Sub C. Jct.
P.C.
Supra C.
A.V.
A. Om.
P.C.-Supra C. anast.
Supra C.-Sub C. anast. (renal collar)
Sub C.
I.M.A.
A
B
C
D
U.A.
C
Right
Left
A.C.
D.C.
P. Hep.
P.C.
A.Om.
Supra C.
Inter Sub C. anast.
Renal
Sub C.
I.M.A.
P.C.
U.A.
D

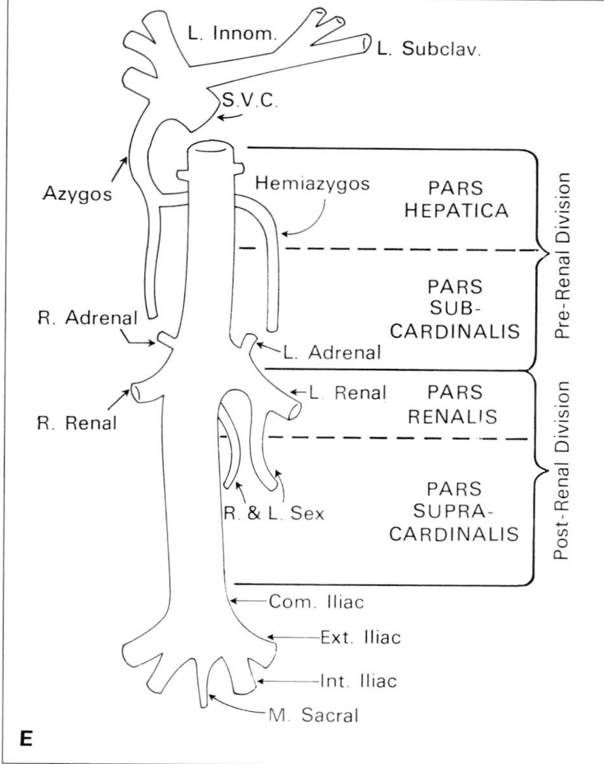

Figure 38-20. (A) Early embryo demonstrating the primitive state of the paired venous complex. All the blood caudal to the duct of Cuvier reaches the right heart by way of the posterior cardinal veins. *A.C.*, anterior cardinal vein; *D.C.*, duct of Cuvier; *U.V.*, umbilical vein; *V.Om.*, omphalomesenteric vein; *Sub C.*, subcardinal vein; *P.C.*, posterior cardinal vein; *P.C.-Sub C. anast.*, anastomosis between subcardinal and posterior cardinal veins; *A.Om.*, omphalomesenteric artery; *I.M.A.*, inferior mesenteric artery; *U.A.*, umbilical artery. (B) Embryo at the 11- to 15-mm stages showing dimunition in size of the posterior cardinal veins, particularly the left. Anastomoses develop between the subcardinal veins. The intrahepatic component and its anastomoses with the right subcardinal vein presage the development of the prerenal segment of the inferior vena cava. *P.Hep.*, pars hepatica of the inferior vena cava; *Hep.-Sub C.Jct.*, hepatic-subcardinal junction, posterior cardinal vein; *Inter Sub C. anast.*, intersubcardinal anastomosis; *Iliac-P.C. anast.*, iliac-posterior cardinal anastomosis. (C) Further stage of evolution shows the formation of the postrenal division of the inferior vena cava with development of the supracardinal veins and continued atrophy of the left posterior cardinal vein. The origin of the embryonic renal collar appears with the development of the supracardinal-subcardinal anastomosis. *Supra C.*, supracardinal vein; *A.V.*, adrenal vein. (D) Atrophy of most of the posterior cardinal component with persistence of the iliac-posterior cardinal anastomosis. Blood returns to the right heart by way of large lumbar supracardinal veins. The adult right-sided inferior vena cava is now seen with the prerenal and postrenal divisions intact. (E) Final divisions of the adult right-sided normal inferior vena cava. *S.V.C.*, superior vena cava. (Adapted from Ferris EJ, Hipona FA, Kahn PC, et al, eds. Venography of the inferior vena cava and its branches. Baltimore: Williams & Wilkins, 1969. Used with permission.)

When single or multiple combinations of the above persist, IVC variations occur. In humans, the known variations of the postrenal division of the IVC are as listed in the following paragraphs.

Type A

A persistent right posterior cardinal vein is an uncommon anomaly and is known as a retrocaval or circumcaval ureter.[46,47] The ureter lies dorsal to the IVC in its proximal portion. As a rule, the diagnosis is made by intravenous pyelography, which shows a medial displacement of the ureter in the midlumbar region and a dorsal position of the ureter on lateral roentgenograms (Fig. 38-21). In the event of obstruction to a significant degree, reparative surgery is indicated.

Type B

A persistent right supracardinal vein is a normal IVC (i.e., the postrenal segment).[48,49]

Type AB

A persistent right posterior cardinal vein and a right supracardinal vein will be manifest as a right periureteric venous ring. The ureter passes through, with the right supracardinal vein forming the roof and the right posterior cardinal vein forming the floor of the ring.[50] This anomaly, also called a *transcaval ureter,* is rare, with only two cases reported.[51]

Type AD

There has been only one case of persistent right and left posterior cardinal veins (bilateral retrocaval ureters), and this was reported by Gladstone[52] in an acardiac monster.

Type D

A persistent left posterior cardinal vein would theoretically be manifest as a left retrocaval ureter. A true left retrocaval ureter has never been reported except in a case with complete situs inversus.[53]

Type BC

Persistence of the right and left supracardinal veins is the etiology of the so-called double postrenal vena cava. The two IVCs may be of equal size, but usually the right IVC is larger (Fig. 38-22). The left IVC drains ventral to the aorta and uses the renal vein segment for prerenal continuity. The frequency of duplication varies between 0.2 and 3.0 percent.[54,55] Although the frequency is low, anatomic demonstration of the anomaly is important if one is to consider a surgical procedure on the IVCs for the prevention of pulmonary embolism.

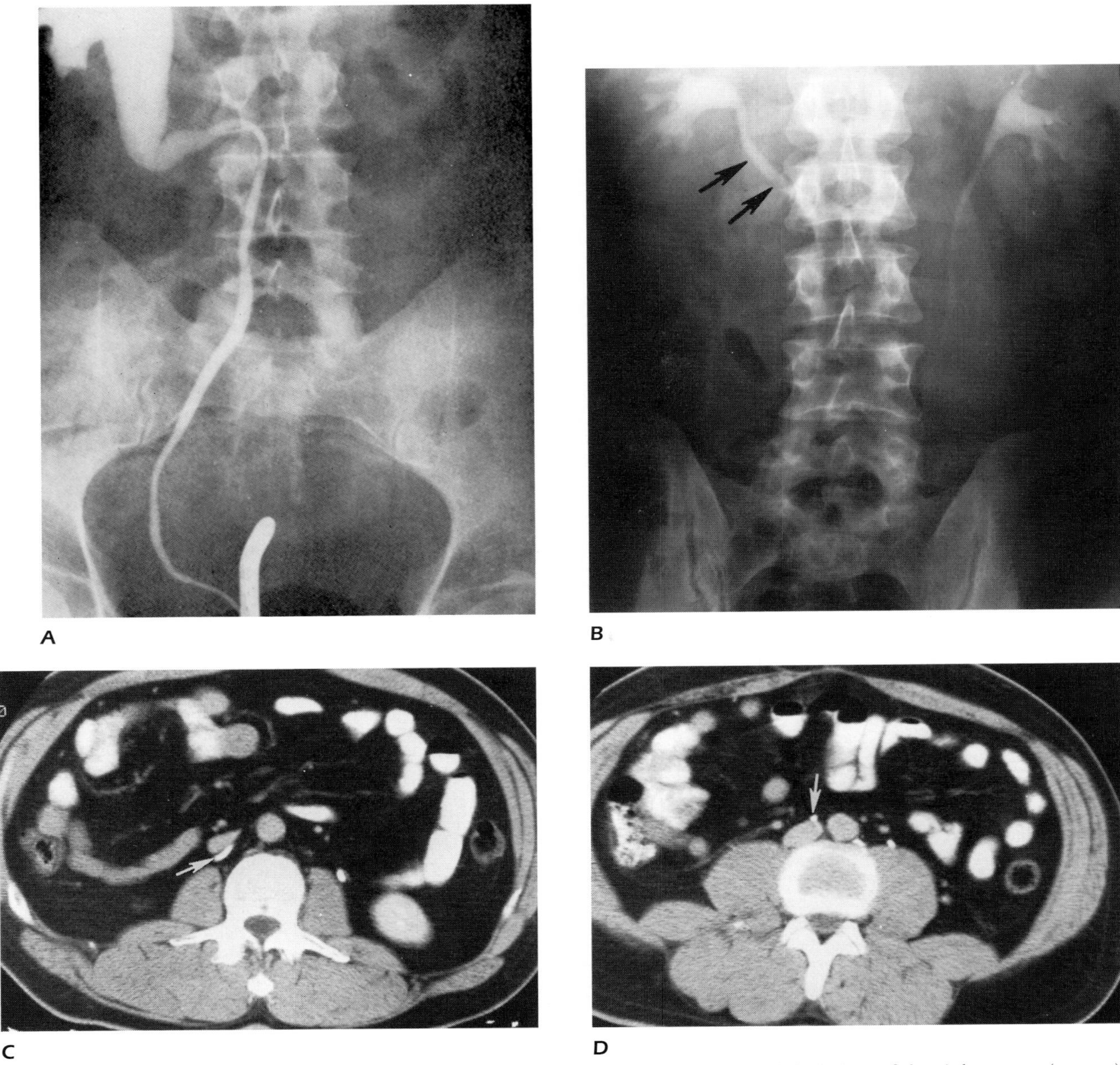

Figure 38-21. (A) Retrocaval ureter; retrograde pyelogram showing the characteristic medial angulation of the middle portion of the ureter. There is a low-grade element of obstruction present. (B) Intravenous urogram of another patient showing medial deviation of the right ureter (*arrows*). (C) CT scan of the midabdomen showing ureter (*arrow*) posterior to IVC. (D) CT scan in the lower abdomen showing ureter (*arrow*) anterior to IVC.

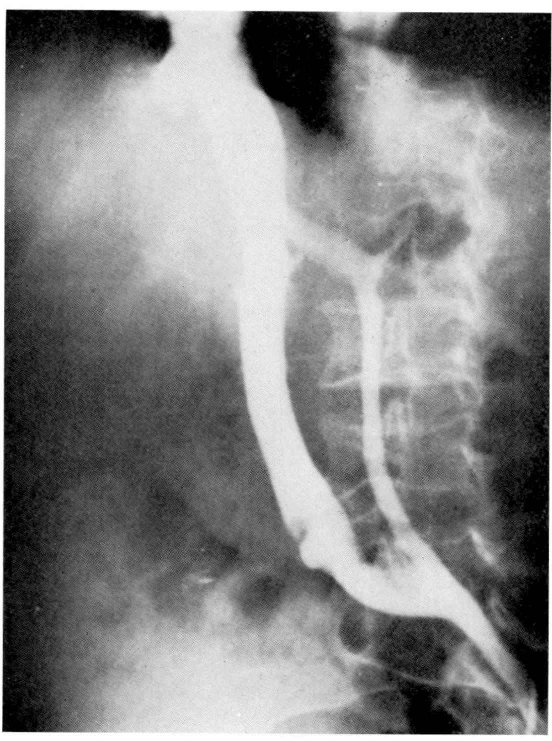

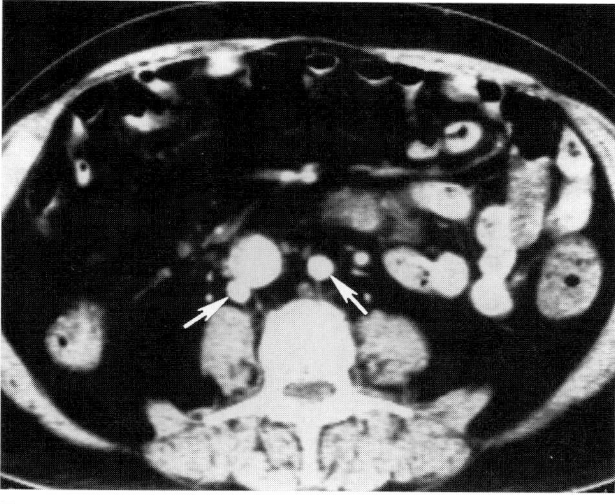

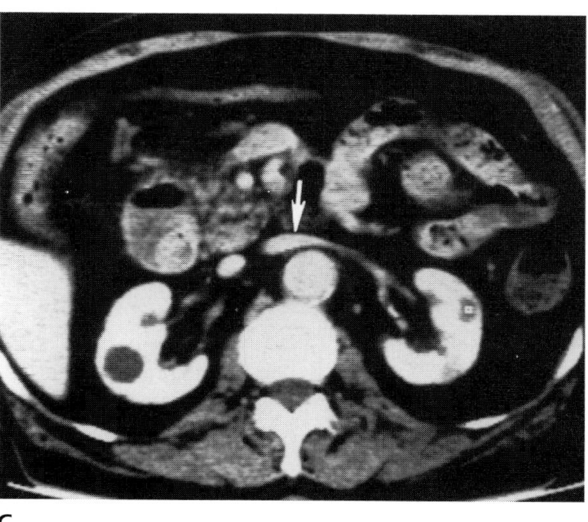

A B C

Figure 38-22. Double inferior vena cava. (A) As a rule, the left IVC is smaller than the right. (Courtesy of R. Nebesar, M.D.) (B) CT scan of another patient showing double IVC (*arrows*). (C) CT scan of the upper abdomen in the same patient showing left IVC crossing over to the right (*arrow*) at the level of the left renal vein.

Type C

Persistent left lumbar supracardinal vein resulting in a left-sided IVC is reported to occur with an incidence of 0.2 to 0.5 percent.[47,55,56] The left-sided IVC drains the left renal vein, crosses acutely to the right of the spine, and continues cranially as the normal prerenal portion of the IVC (Fig. 38-23). The left renal and adrenal veins empty directly into the left-sided IVC, whereas the right adrenal and right gonadal veins drain into the right renal vein and subsequently into the normal right-sided prerenal division of the left-sided IVC complex. This, in essence, is the mirror image of a normal IVC, analogous to an anterior right aortic arch. Another interesting variation is a retroaortic left renal vein (Fig. 38-24).

Miscellaneous Anomalies

Some anomalies cannot be neatly categorized into the system of McClure and Butler.[43] One may have an absence of the prerenal segment of the IVC with azygos (persistent supracardinal system) (Fig. 38-25). This anomaly is usually of academic interest only but is occasionally associated with transposed viscera and often with dextrocardia or congenital heart disease.[57–59] Plain roentgenograms of the chest will show a dilated azygos vein simulating a tumor. These anomalies are discussed in detail in Chapter 36.

Persistence of a circumaortic venous ring (renal collar) is another anomaly not easily classified (Fig. 38-26). The incidence is said to be 8.7 percent.[55]

In asplenia the IVC has a characteristic reaction to the abdominal aorta, which Elliot et al.[60] describe and categorize into two types. In type 1 the thoracic aorta, regardless of the side that the IVC is on, descends on the opposite side of it in the chest, angles across the spine in the abdomen, and descends adjacent to the IVC. In type 2 the thoracic aorta descends on the same side as the IVC and maintains this relationship within the abdomen.

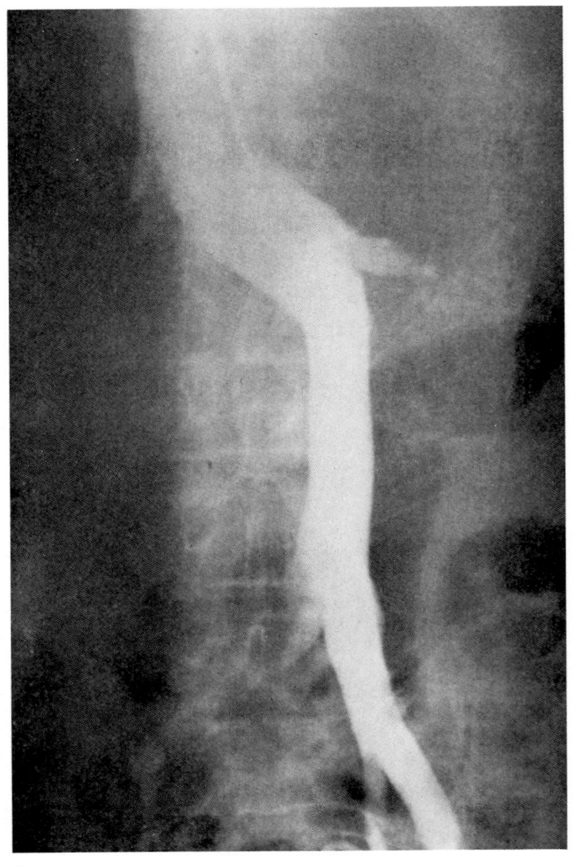

A

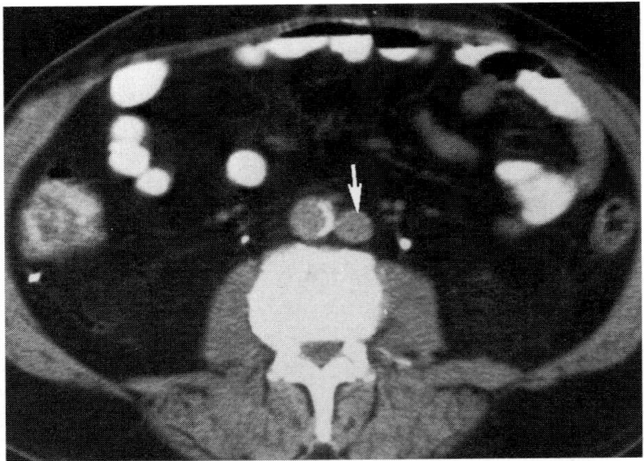

B

C

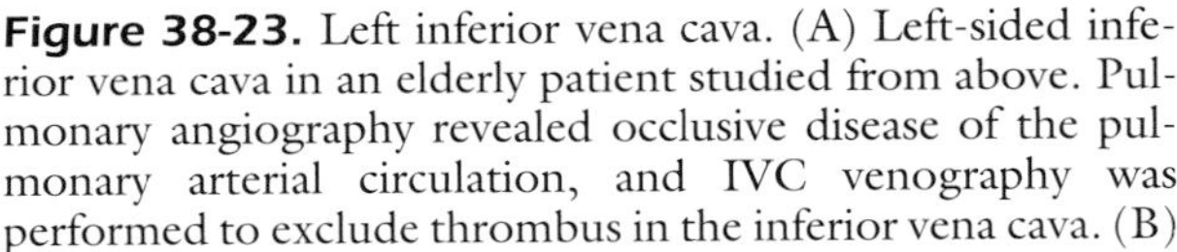

Figure 38-23. Left inferior vena cava. (A) Left-sided inferior vena cava in an elderly patient studied from above. Pulmonary angiography revealed occlusive disease of the pulmonary arterial circulation, and IVC venography was performed to exclude thrombus in the inferior vena cava. (B) CT scan of another patient showing left IVC (*arrow*). The aorta, with calcification within the wall, is to the right of the cava. (C) CT scan of the upper abdomen in the same patient showing left IVC crossing over to the right (*arrow*) at the level of the left renal vein.

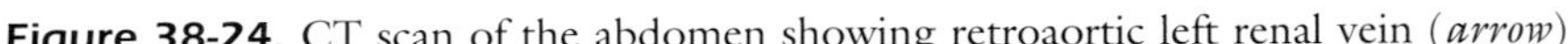

Figure 38-24. CT scan of the abdomen showing retroaortic left renal vein (*arrow*).

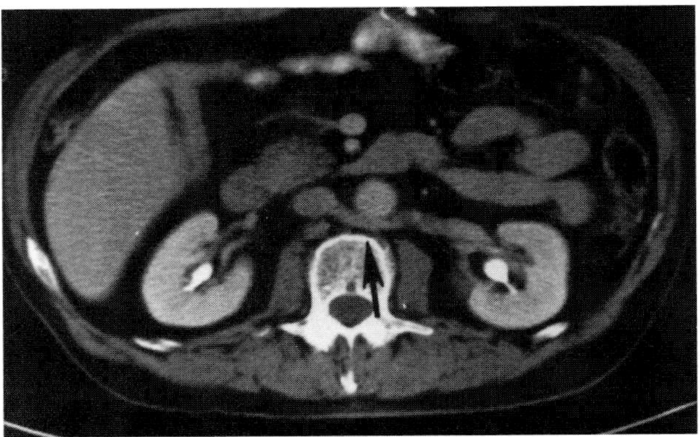

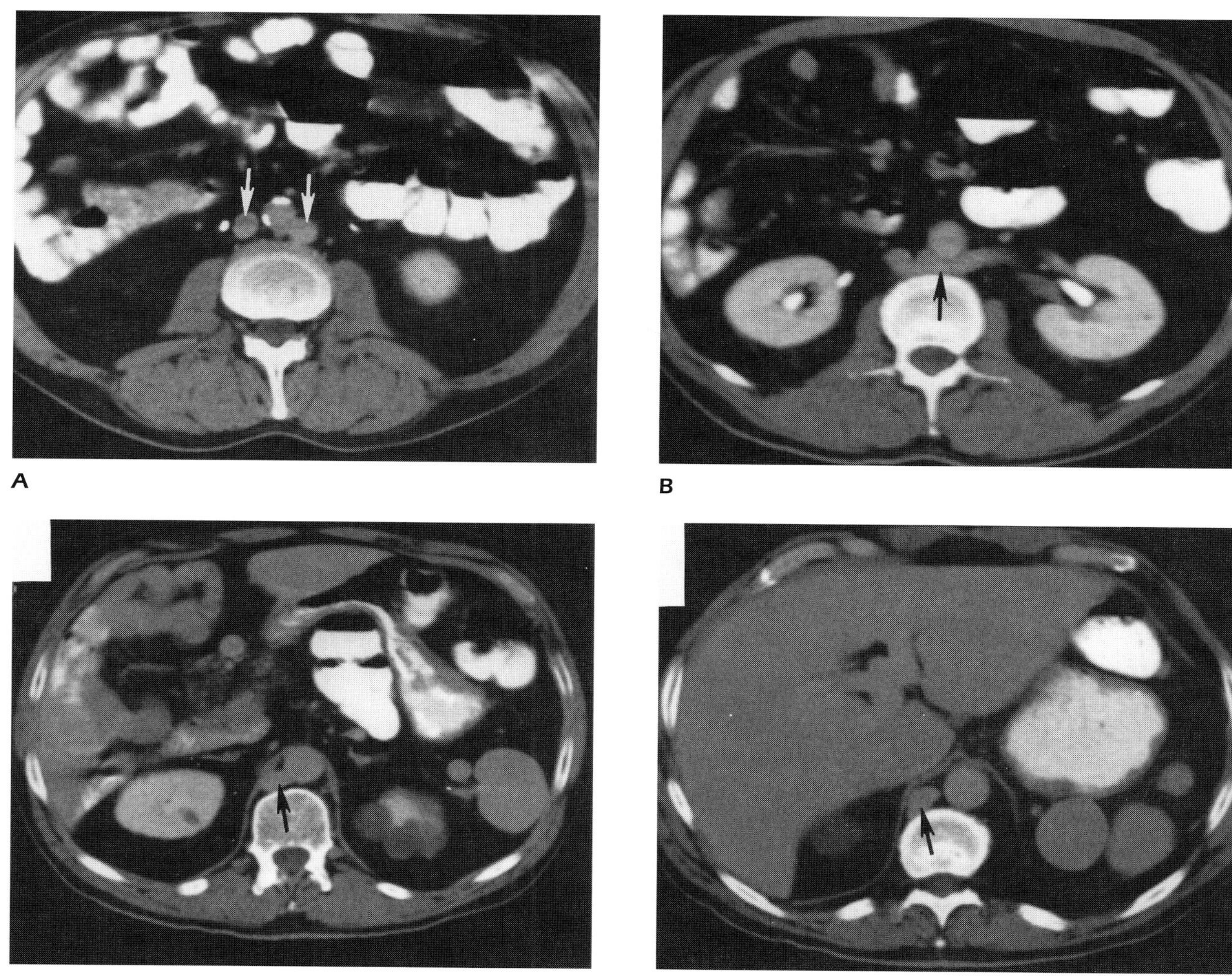

Figure 38-25. Azygos continuation of IVC in a patient with polysplenia syndrome. (A) CT scan of the abdomen showing double IVC (*arrows*). The small bowel is on the right side of the abdomen. (B) CT scan showing left IVC crossing to the right behind the aorta at the level of the left renal vein (*arrow*). (C) CT scan showing no IVC in its regular position, but a large azygos vein (*arrow*). Note the position of the cecum in the midabdomen (malrotation). (D) CT scan showing large azygos vein (*arrow*) and multiple spleens. Azygos continuation is usually seen with a single cava—not with a double cava, as in this case.

Collateral Circulation

The study of collateral circulation of the partially or completely obstructed IVC has intrigued anatomists and pathologists for years. Morgagni[61] was among the first to recognize IVC occlusion and the development of extensive collateral pathways. In 1911 Pleasants[62] compiled the world literature in a classic review and stressed the categorization of venous return. This was based on the level of obstruction (i.e., the upper, middle, or lower division of the IVC). When cavography was introduced in 1935 by dos Santos,[2] a great surge of interest developed in many aspects of the IVC, in particular its collateral channels. Circulatory dynamics and flow patterns of the partially or completely obstructed IVC were studied.

It appeared that the collateral channels were categorized into those seen on injection and dissection (potential) and those seen on cavography in the living (practical). We might, then, conveniently divide the collateral pathways into those commonly seen in IVC obstruction by inferior vena cavography and those potentially available but not usually seen in vivo. These might logically be called *practical routes* and *potential*

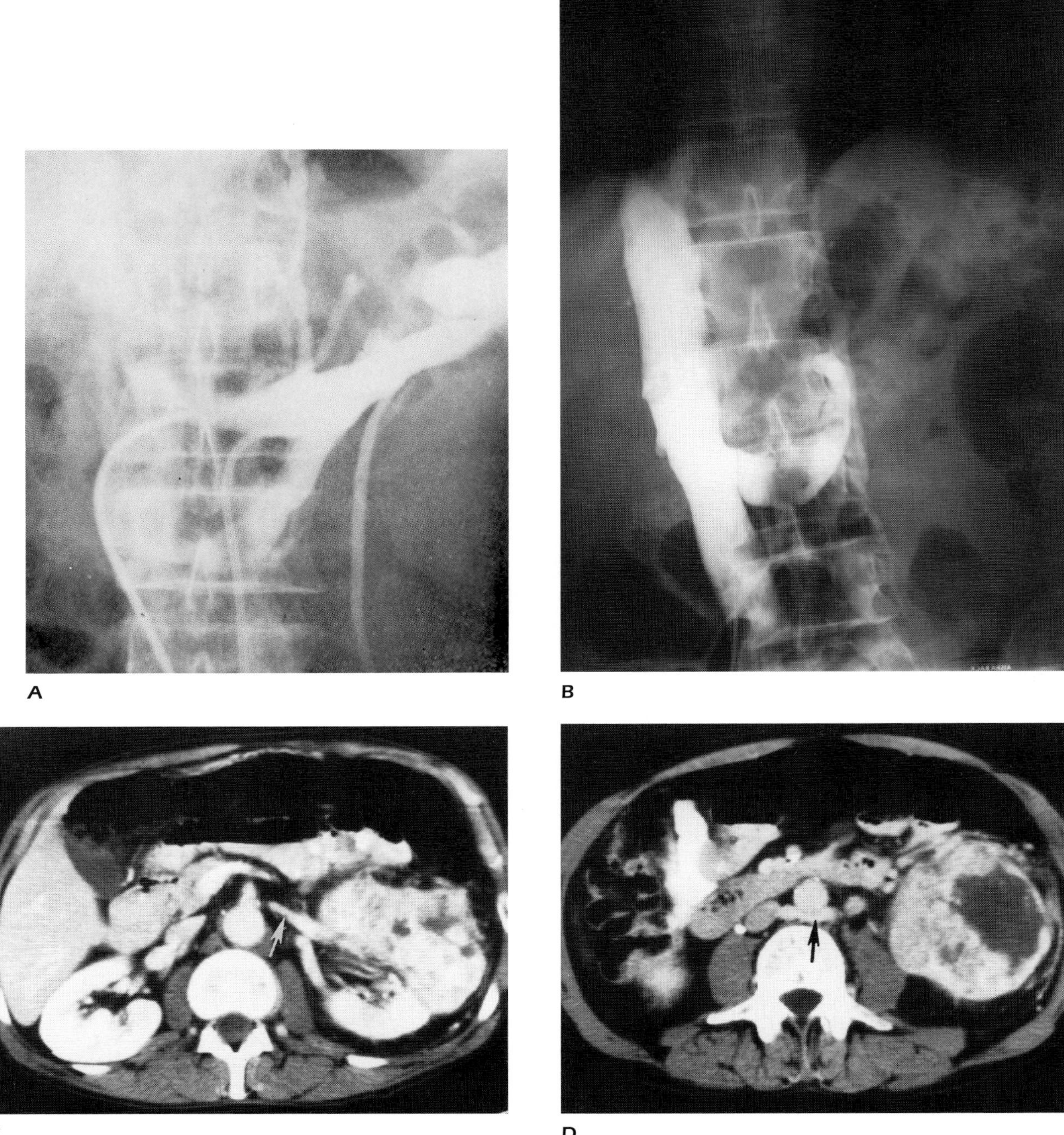

Figure 38-26. IVC collar, circumaortic left renal veins. (A) Circumaortic renal venous ring. A catheter is in position in the anterior vein. The posterior vein is directed medially and downward. The left kidney is involved by tumor and is distorting the peripheral renal vein. (From Ferris EJ, Hipona FA, Kahn PC, et al, eds. Venography of the inferior vena cava and its branches. Baltimore: Williams & Wilkins, 1969. Used with permission.) (B) Another patient showing an IVC collar on venography. (C) CT scan of the same patient showing the left anterior renal vein (*arrow*). (D) CT scan of the abdomen 4 cm below (C) showing the left retroaortic renal vein (*arrow*). The patient has a left renal cell carcinoma. (Knowledge of this anomaly is crucial for the urologist in planning nephrectomy.)

routes on the basis of in vivo venography and injection and dissection techniques, respectively.[63] Because the collateral circulation is further modified by the level of obstruction, we can subdivide and classify collateral circulation of the IVC as follows[1]:

Infrarenal obstruction
  A. Practical routes
  B. Potential routes
Middle IVC obstruction
  A. Practical routes
  B. Potential routes
Upper IVC obstruction
  A. Practical routes
  B. Potential routes

In studying these routes, three principles of the availability of collateral pathways advanced by Edward A. Edwards[64] deserve special mention.

1. *Course of Communicating Vessels.* All vessels that parallel the axis of an obstructed vessel are potential collateral pathways if they are directly or indirectly linked to the trunk above and below the level of obstruction.
2. *Presentation and Orientation of Valves.* If a vein is valved against the necessary direction of the collateral flow, it cannot act as a collateral channel immediately. Once the vein undergoes dilatation to approximately twice its diameter, the valves become incomplete and flow can occur in either direction.
3. *Size of the Communicating Stoma.* A single large channel is more effective in collateral circulation than multiple small channels. This principle is in conformity to Poiseuille's law: The volume of flow is proportional to the fourth power of the diameter of the vessel.

Infrarenal Obstruction

Practical Routes

Because this level of the IVC is more commonly involved with occlusive disease than are the remaining segments of the IVC, it has been well studied by cavography. There are four pathways available[1]: the central, intermediate, portal, and superficial.

The *central channels* (Fig. 38-27A and B) comprise the ascending lumbar veins, the internal and external vertebral venous plexuses, the azygos-hemiazygos complex, and the IVC above the obstructed segment. Figure 38-27C, a cross section of the central channels, shows the intricate interplay of communication channels. The ascending lumbar veins, usually single on either side, freely and regularly communicate with the IVC via the caval division of the lumbar veins. The ascending lumbar veins, acting somewhat as a fulcrum, also are intimately connected to the vertebral venous plexus via the intervertebral veins (Fig. 38-27C). The azygos vein arises from the dorsal aspect of the IVC at the level of the second lumbar vertebra; the hemiazygos vein originates from the left renal vein via the hemiazygos-lumbar plexus. Both veins pass cranially through the diaphragm and continue on into the thorax, where a subcentral anastomosis exists at the level of the azygos-superior vena cava junction.

The vertebral venous system is a complex, intricate network situated outside the abdominal cavity. It has free exchange of flow via valveless connections to the cavity system of veins. Only the intradural component of the internal vertebral venous plexus is equipped with valves. The external vertebral venous plexus of veins seen anteriorly and posteriorly communicates with the ascending lumbar veins as well as the internal vertebral venous network. Anatomically, the extradural plexus is illustrated in Figure 38-27C. There are cross-communications between the paired posterior and paired anterior sinuses at almost every vertebral body level. At the foramen magnum free communication exists between the vertebral sinuses and the cranial sinuses via the basilar plexus, the occipital sinuses, and the internal jugular vein via a venous rete in the hypoglossal canal.[65] Intervertebral veins originate from the longitudinal sinuses and emerge through each intervertebral and anterior sacral foramen.

The IVC, above the level of obstruction, serves as a collateral channel in a sense because it is endowed with so many anastomotic channels.

The *intermediate channels* (Fig. 38-28) include the gonadal veins, the ureteric veins, and the left renal-azygos venous system. The left sex vein drains into the left renal vein, whereas the right sex vein usually empties directly into the inferior vena cava below the right renal vein. In some cases (8.0–21.7 percent)[66–68] the right sex vein drains into the right renal vein. The entrance of the sex veins when they merge with the renal vein is distal to the adrenal vein on the left and is at a corresponding location on the right. Duplication of the sex veins occurs in 6 to 40 percent of cases.[1] This situation is much more common in males. In approximately 50 percent of the cases in females and about 25 percent in males, the valves of the gonadal veins are not competent and hence allow bidirectional flow.[69]

Through the ovarian-parametrial venous complex there is flow from one side of the pelvis to the other and hence an intimate, although indirect, communication between both ovarian veins (see Fig. 38-28). Because of the morphology, the same situation does not

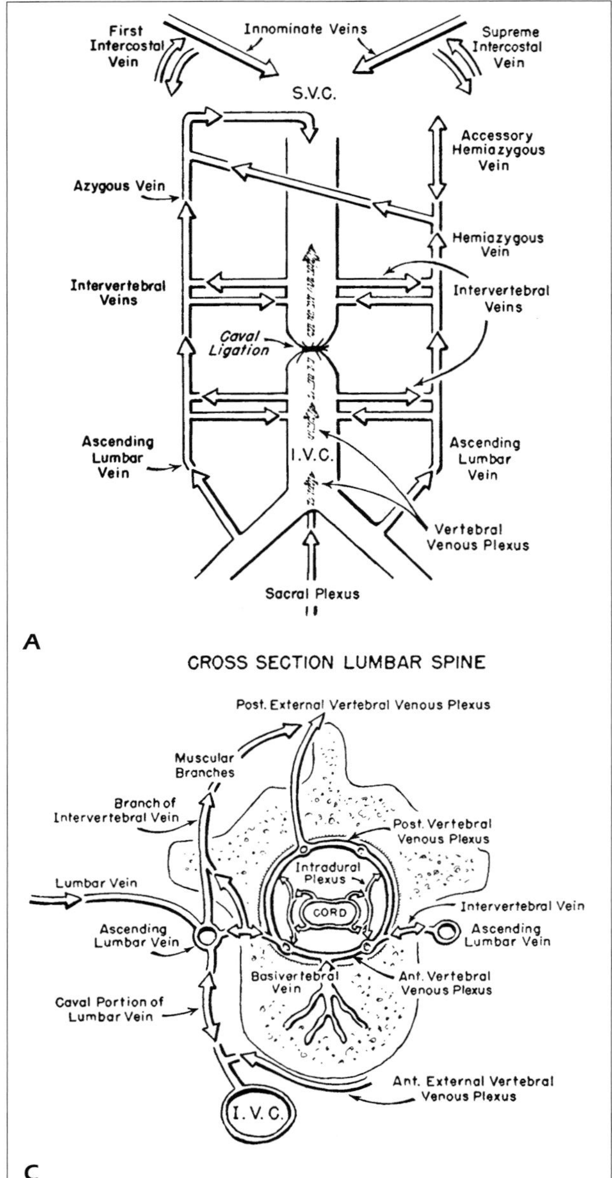

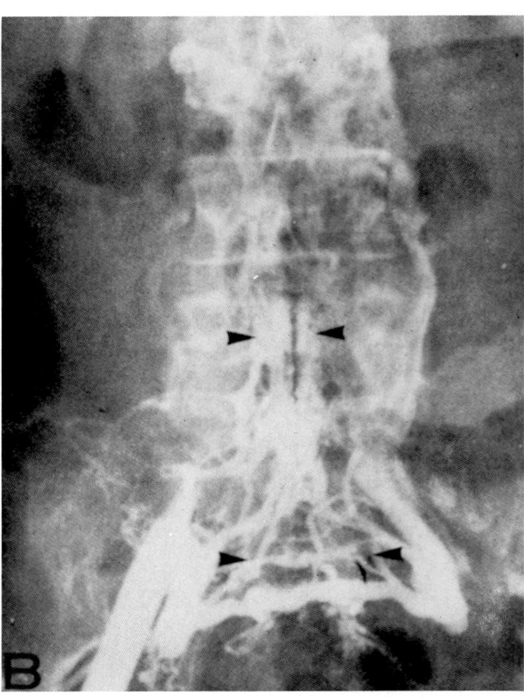

B

Figure 38-27. (A) Semidiagram of central collateral channels in obstruction of the infrarenal segment of the inferior vena cava. The valveless intervertebral veins connect the vertebral venous plexus with the ascending lumbar veins. There is a rich anastomosis between the internal iliac and sacral plexus that drains into the vertebral venous plexus. This is illustrated in (B), in which thrombosis of the lower cava deploys blood into the sacral plexus (*lower arrowheads*) and then to the internal vertebral venous plexus (*upper arrowheads*). (C) A semidiagram in cross section of the spine and associated veins. Notice the communication between the ascending lumbar veins and the inferior vena cava by way of the caval portion of the lumbar vein. The intricate connections between the external and internal vertebral venous networks can also be appreciated. (From Ferris EJ, Vittimberga FJ, Byrne JJ, et al. The inferior vena cava post ligation and plication. Radiology 1967;89:1–10. Used with permission.)

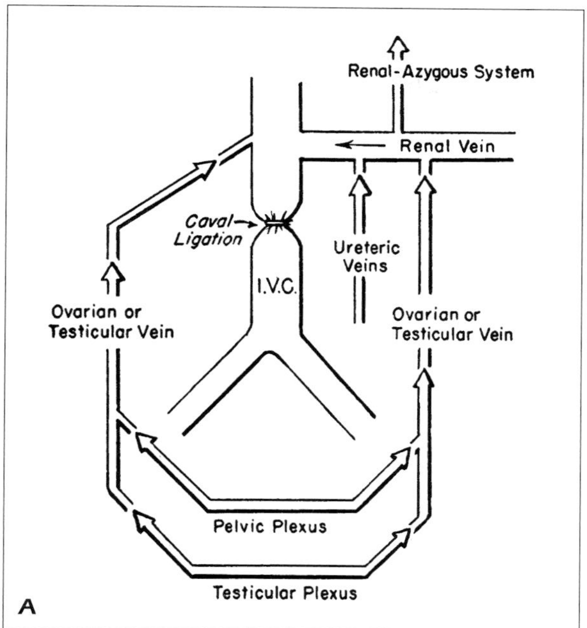

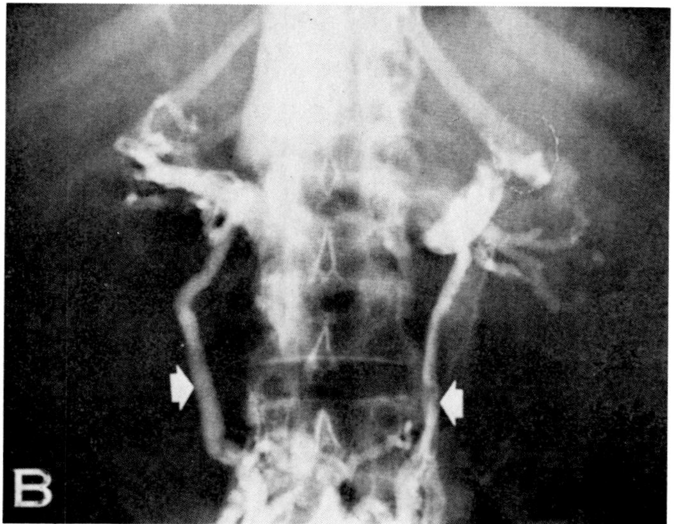

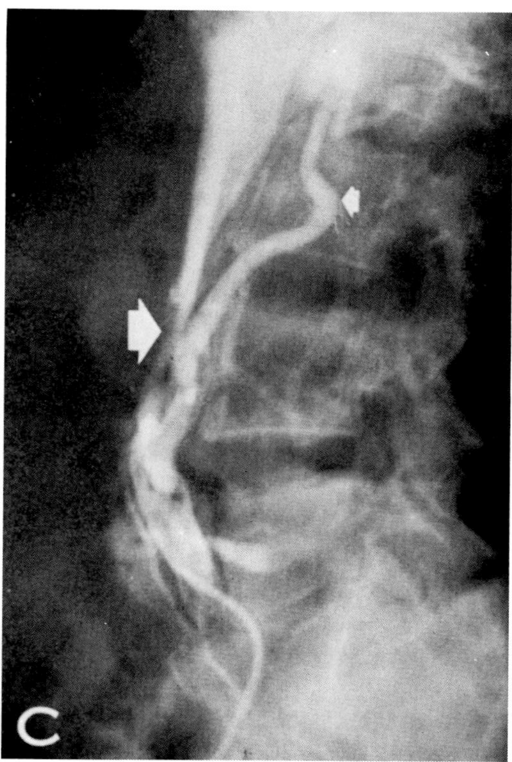

Figure 38-28. (A) Intermediate route of collateral circulation in infrarenal obstruction of the inferior vena cava, illustrated in semidiagrammatic form. (B and C) Frontal and lateral projections of intermediate type of collateral circulation in a female with ligation of the inferior vena cava. *Arrows* note the ovarian veins, which in this case both drain into the renal veins. (From Ferris EJ, Vittimberga FJ, Byrne JJ, et al. The inferior vena cava post ligation and plication. Radiology 1967;89:1–10. Used with permission.)

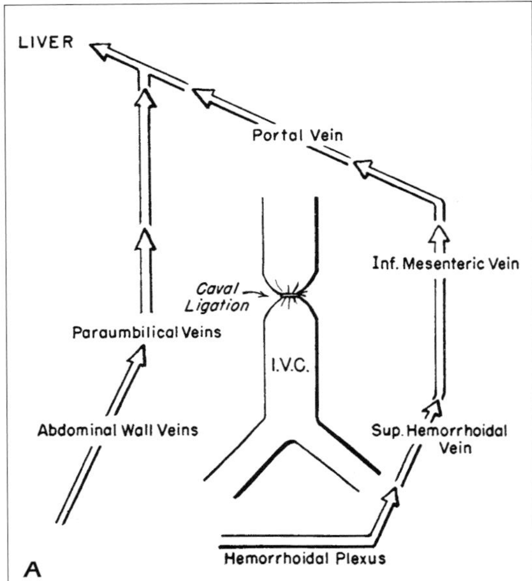

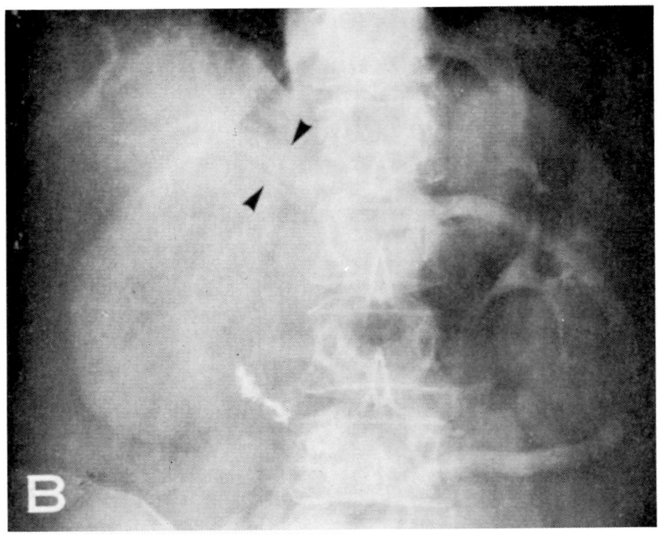

B

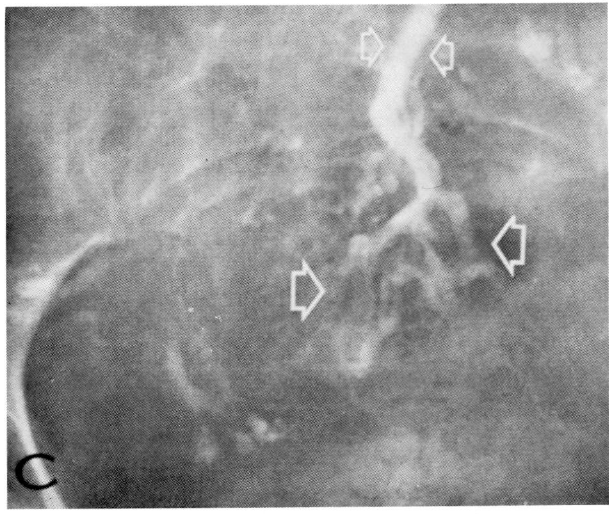

C

Figure 38-29. (A) Diagram showing the method of portal vein filling in infrarenal obstruction of the inferior vena cava. (B) The portal vein (*arrowheads*) fills via the inferior mesenteric vein. The patient, a middle-aged woman, had occlusion of the lower IVC from gynecologic cancer spread. Bilateral femoral vein injections were performed in this case. (C) The hemorrhoidal plexus of the inferior mesenteric vein (same patient) is clearly demonstrable (*lower arrows*). The *upper arrows* point to the inferior mesenteric vein. (From Ferris EJ, Vittimberga FJ, Byrne JJ, et al. The inferior vena cava post ligation and plication. Radiology 1967;89:1–10. Used with permission.)

hold regarding the testicular veins, although there is some intercommunication at the testicular level.

Ureteric veins may become huge in IVC occlusion and may be mistaken for the sex veins, particularly on the left side. Notching of the ureter may occur somewhat as in renal artery occlusion or narrowing with ureteric arterial collateral circulation.[70] One of the authors (EF) noted in three cases that there is slightly more pronounced notching of the ureter with ureteric venous collaterals when a marked Valsalva maneuver is performed or when the venogram and subsequent pyelogram are obtained in the upright position, and in his experience, this is particularly appreciated on cinepyelography. However, it is questionable whether notching due to arterial or venous collaterals can definitively be differentially diagnosed in this fashion.

The left renal vein drainage of the ureteric sex veins may spill over into the hemiazygos system when the patient is in the upright position or performs a Valsalva maneuver.

The *portal system* was once thought to be a rare route of collateral venous return in infrarenal IVC occlusion but is now seen with increasing frequency (Fig. 38-29). Filling is via the superior hemorrhoidal anastomosis with the middle and inferior hemorrhoidal plexuses of the internal iliac venous system. When abdominal wall veins are transporting large volumes of blood in a collateral fashion, there may be drainage into a patent umbilical vein, another pathway for the portal vein to transport blood. It should be stressed that large-volume cavography (60–80 ml of 60 percent contrast material) is usually required to opacify the portal venous collateral route.

The *superficial routes* are numerous but are not always prominent in infrarenal obstruction of the IVC except in those cases in which there is occlusion of one or both of the common iliac veins (Fig. 38-30). It is true that when conventional cavography is performed,

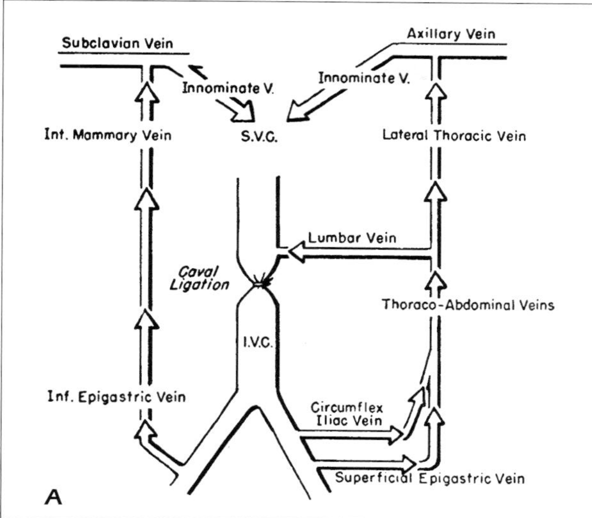

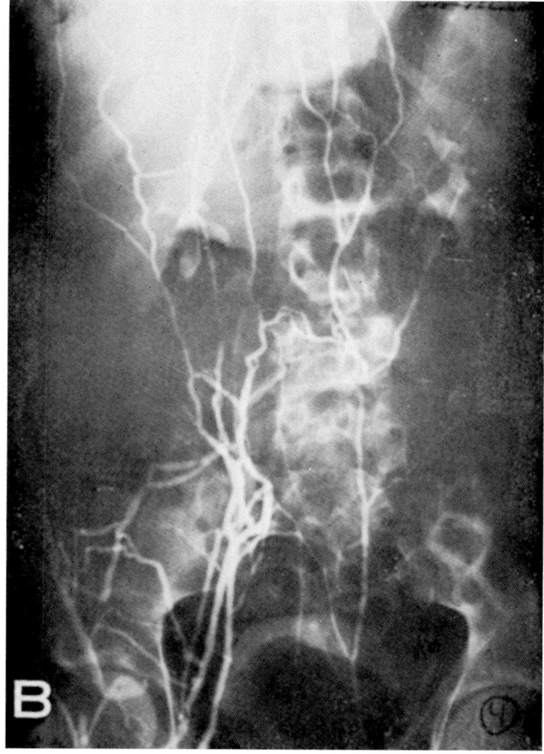

B

Figure 38-30. Superficial routes can be numerous. (A) Diagram presenting a relatively simplified picture of these routes. (B) A case of infrarenal caval occlusion; superficial routes are delineated. Injection could be performed in the right femoral vein only. (From Ferris EJ, Hipona FA, Kahn PC, et al, eds. Venography of the inferior vena cava and its branches. Baltimore: Williams & Wilkins, 1969. Used with permission.)

the needle or catheter position in the external or common iliac vein would naturally not opacify the abdominal wall collaterals. In saphenous vein studies the superficial routes, if in actual use, will be demonstrated. It takes several weeks to overcome the valve function in the superficial routes; in the interim, other routes (e.g., intermediate, central, and portal) may accommodate the increase in flow and hence diminish the need for further collateral transport from the superficial system. The inferior epigastric veins drain superiorly into the internal mammary veins. Internal mammary-phrenic anastomosis may redirect blood in a centripetal fashion to the IVC at the unobstructed diaphragmatic level. The circumflex iliac and superficial epigastric veins drain into the thoracoabdominal veins, and the lateral thoracoabdominal veins drain cranially into the axillary vein. At any point in the superficial system, communications between the lumbar veins may deploy blood flow to the ascending lumbar-vertebra venous plexus or, in some cases, into the IVC above the obstructed segment.

Potential Routes

The potential routes of alternate return and combinations of collateral channels after infrarenal obstruction of the inferior vena cava are numerous. Pleasants's description in 1911[62] of collateral circulatory patterns emphasized those seen in infrarenal obstruction. These channels were discovered by injection and dissection techniques (Fig. 38-31).

The portal route, more commonly seen when the obstruction is at the level of the middle or upper IVC, has many other pathways of filling not described above. The portosystemic communications have been studied extensively. After ligating the IVC in the thorax of a cadaver and concomitantly tying the azygos system, Edwards[64] injected contrast material into the IVC below the obstruction and demonstrated innumerable communications between the systemic and portal systems. These are listed below from Edwards[64]:

1. Posterior mediastinal, superior phrenic, pericardiophrenic, and internal mammary communications to esophageal veins result in drainage into the portal system.
2. The inferior phrenic, left suprarenal, and left renal veins have normal small communications to the hemiazygos system. By way of the epiploic veins of the stomach, the hemiazygos vein communicates with the splenic and hence the portal systems.
3. The inferior and superior phrenic veins and the suprarenal and renal veins may communicate with the liver via the portal system through splenorenal and phrenic-liver capsular portal branches. This route,

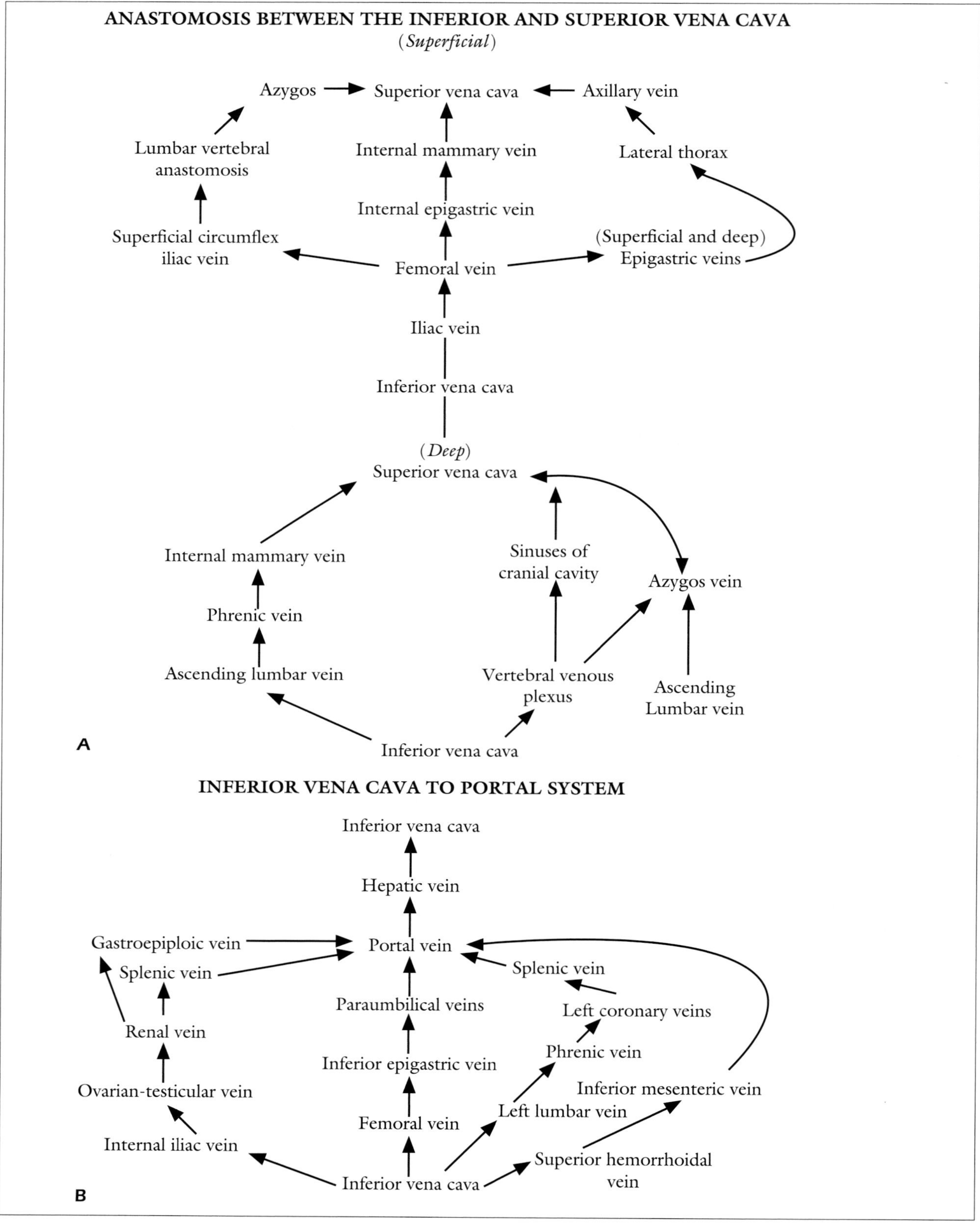
ANASTOMOSIS BETWEEN THE INFERIOR AND SUPERIOR VENA CAVA
(Superficial)
Azygos
Superior vena cava
Axillary vein
Lumbar vertebral anastomosis
Internal mammary vein
Lateral thorax
Internal epigastric vein
Superficial circumflex iliac vein
(Superficial and deep) Epigastric veins
Femoral vein
Iliac vein
Inferior vena cava
(Deep)
Superior vena cava
Internal mammary vein
Sinuses of cranial cavity
Azygos vein
Phrenic vein
Ascending lumbar vein
Vertebral venous plexus
Ascending Lumbar vein
A
Inferior vena cava
INFERIOR VENA CAVA TO PORTAL SYSTEM
Inferior vena cava
Hepatic vein
Gastroepiploic vein
Portal vein
Splenic vein
Splenic vein
Paraumbilical veins
Left coronary veins
Renal vein
Phrenic vein
Inferior epigastric vein
Ovarian-testicular vein
Inferior mesenteric vein
Left lumbar vein
Femoral vein
Internal iliac vein
Superior hemorrhoidal vein
B
Inferior vena cava

because of the small size of the communicating channels, is unlikely to be seen in vivo.

4. Renal or paraaortic tributaries may communicate with the pancreas, duodenum, and proximal jejunal veins and hence drain into the portal vein.
5. Derivatives of the subcardinal veins—the suprarenal, gonadal, ureteric, periureteric, and paraaortic veins—may communicate with veins of the distal ileum and the ascending colon. Embryologically the distal ileum and ascending colon are in communication with the subcardinal derivatives. It is likely, therefore, that the adult communications are persistent embryonic remnants.
6. Subcardinal derivatives on the left communicate with the descending and sigmoid colon and hence communicate with the portal system via the inferior mesenteric vein.
7. Renosplenic shunts, left renal vein–inferior mesenteric shunts, and left gonadal–inferior mesenteric shunts were also seen.

Middle IVC Obstruction

Obstruction of the IVC between the renal and hepatic veins is an uncommon problem usually caused by invasion into the lumen of the cava by a renal vein tumor thrombus. The collateral pathways are those seen on venography—practical routes—and those usually seen with injection and dissection techniques—potential routes.

Practical Routes

These are essentially similar to those seen in infrarenal obstruction of the IVC, but some modifications are inherent, as listed below:

1. Central routes (see Fig. 38-27).
2. Intermediate routes (see Fig. 38-28). Because the renal veins cannot drain directly into the obstructed IVC at this level, there is spilling into the hemiazygos and azygos systems on the left and right, respectively.
3. Portal system (see Fig. 38-29), which assumes more importance.
4. Superficial channels (see Fig. 38-30).

If the renal vein is patent to the cava, there may be ureteric retrograde flow to the iliac-sacral plexus and thence to the vertebral venous system of veins. Retrograde filling of the gonadal or ovarian veins, particularly on the left, may occur to the pelvis, where ovarian-sacral plexus-vertebral venous plexus anastomoses occur. The hemiazygos-azygos system contributes to drainage from the kidneys. Adrenal vein–phrenic vein circulation to the cephalic unobstructed portion of the IVC also becomes important.

Potential Routes

Potential routes of venous return in occlusion of the midportion of the IVC are similar, with minor modifications, to those outlined under infrarenal obstruction. They may be classified as listed below:

1. Anastomosis between the IVC and the superior vena cava (see Fig. 38-31A).
2. IVC to the portal system (see Fig. 38-31B).
3. Left renal to spermatic-ovarian to internal pudendal plexus to inferior hemorrhoidal to superior hemorrhoidal to inferior mesenteric vein to portal venous systems. The parietes-retroperitoneal portal collateral potentials are essentially those described by Edwards.[64]
4. The lower IVC collateral circuit to the cava above the obstructed segment is similar to that in infrarenal IVC occlusion except that there is renal escape in the azygos-hemiazygos system in occlusion of the middle IVC.

Upper IVC Obstruction

This is an extremely uncommon site of IVC occlusion. The routes of collateral return have not been as carefully studied as the middle and lower IVC collateral channels.

Practical Routes

The central (see Fig. 38-27), superficial (see Fig. 38-30), and, to a lesser degree, intermediate routes (see Fig. 38-28), the last modified by renal azygos-hemiazygos escape, are the channels seen by IVC cavography. If there is associated or physiologic hepatic vein obstruction in association with the upper IVC occlusion, there is hepatofugal flow. This retrograde drainage of the liver prevents the portal route from being effective in antegrade drainage of the lower abdominal systemic-portal shunts (Fig. 38-32).

◀ **Figure 38-31.** (A) Potential routes (superficial and deep) of venous return in infrarenal obstruction of the inferior vena cava. (B) Simplified potential routes of venous return to the portal system. (From Ferris EJ, Hipona FA, Kahn PC, et al, eds. Venography of the inferior vena cava and its branches. Baltimore: Williams & Wilkins, 1969. Used with permission.)

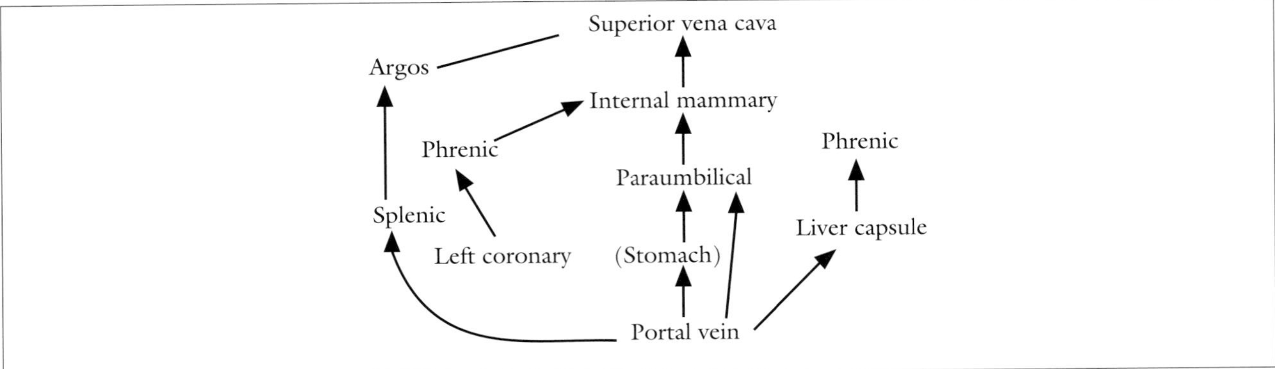

Figure 38-32. Portal route to the inferior vena cava. The potential routes are not visualized as a rule because of the circumvented, long pathways involved. Unopacified blood with its diluting effect is one reason for failure of visualization in vivo. (From Ferris EJ, Hipona FA, Kahn PC, et al, eds. Venography of the inferior vena cava and its branches. Baltimore: Williams & Wilkins, 1969. Used with permission.)

Potential Routes

These include the following:

1. IVC to superior vena cava (see Fig. 38-31A).
2. IVC to IVC—limited because of high caval obstruction.
3. Parietes-portal systemic collaterals from the portal to the systemic circulation and thence to the vertebral venous plexus and deep ascending lumbar group. This assumes an intricate network whereby systemic blood traverses the portal system and reverts back to the systemic system because of an obstruction of the upper IVC hepatic pathway.
4. Portal vein to superior vena cava as previously described under Infrarenal Obstruction, Potential Routes (see Fig. 38-32).

Extrinsic Obstruction

Because of the intimate contiguity of the IVC with so many regional structures, extrinsic compression can occur in a host of disease processes affecting the abdomen. Extrinsic pressure can occur along the entire perimeter of the vessel, but for anatomic localization,[1] pressure defects may be considered with respect to their posterior, anterior, medial, and lateral relations.[1]

Anterior

The right spermatic artery, branches of the aortic plexus of the sympathetic nervous system, and the transverse colon, root of the mesentery, duodenum, head of the pancreas, portal vein, liver, right common iliac artery, and right lumbar lymphatic nodes all bear an anterior relationship to the IVC. Enlargement or posterior displacement of these structures can cause extrinsic pressure deformity of the anterior margin of the IVC.

Posterior

The lumbar vertebrae, right renal artery, right celiac (semilunar) ganglion, and right medial crus of the diaphragm, because of their peculiar location, may indent the posterior wall of the IVC.

Right

The peritoneum, liver, and right psoas muscle can impress the right wall of the IVC. Because retroperitoneal lymph nodes occur alone or in conglomerate masses and are difficult to place in any one location, they are arbitrarily placed in this group by Shapiro (in Ferris et al.).[63]

Left

The aorta and the right medial crus of the diaphragm have their effect on the left caval wall.

Other Sources

Another orderly approach to extrinsic-pressure deformity is to consider each organ in the abdomen when it is involved by pathology. The liver may compress the IVC merely by diffuse or local enlargement in the

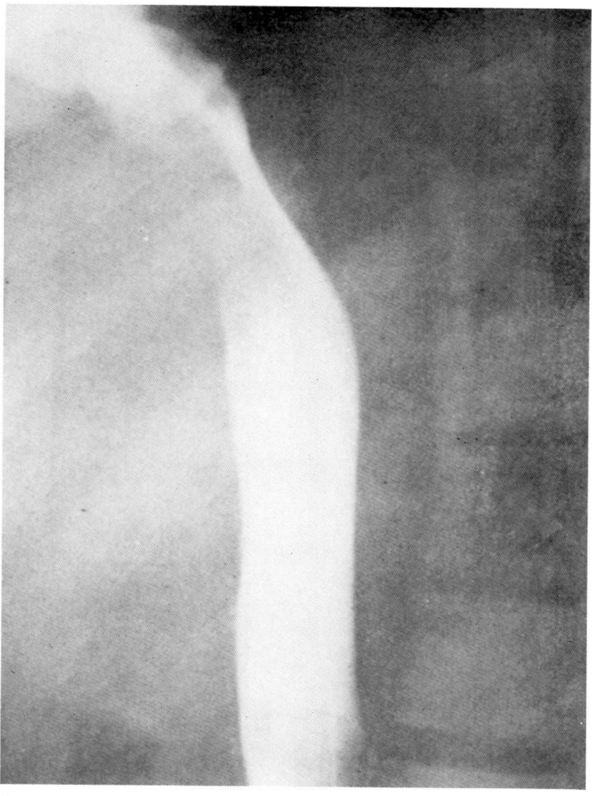

A

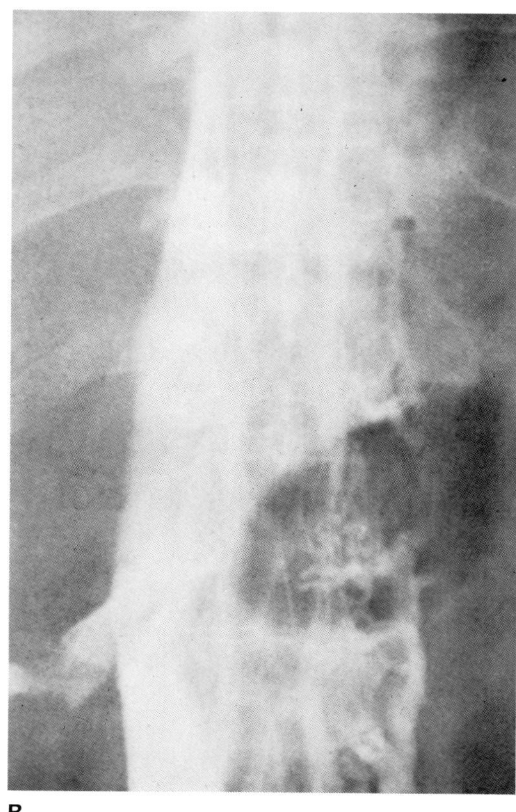

B

Figure 38-33. Frontal (A) and lateral (B) projections of inferior vein cava showing compression of the anterior wall of the IVC secondary to a regenerating nodule in a patient with cirrhosis (who also had hepatic vein occlusion). (From Ferris EJ, Hipona FA, Kahn PC, et al, eds. Venography of the inferior vena cava and its branches. Baltimore: Williams & Wilkins, 1969. Used with permission.)

region of the fossa, where the IVC passes over the posterior wall of the liver. Because the left lobe is remote from the course of the upper IVC, caval deformity from a mass in the left lobe is unlikely. Almost any type of liver mass (neoplastic, infectious, hemorrhagic, cystic) can compress the IVC (Fig. 38-33). It is interesting to note, however, that in cirrhosis the pressure of obstruction implies a regenerating nodule because cirrhosis is said not to cause compression of the IVC.[71]

Kidney and adrenal gland involvement by neoplastic disease may cause extrinsic deformity of the IVC by direct contiguity of the expanded organ with the cava or by periaortic lymph node involvement (Figs. 38-34 and 38-35). Lymphatic extension is very characteristic of carcinoma of the kidney. A ptosis of the kidney and renal ectopia, particularly on the right, can affect the course of the IVC. In our experience, routine visualization of the IVC by some imaging method on all patients with adrenal and particularly renal tumors is invaluable and helps determine the extent of the neoplasm, its operability, and, in the opinion of some, the prognosis.

Gastrointestinal Tract and Pancreas

Abnormalities of the duodenum and pancreas, because of their anatomic proximity to the IVC, may produce caval pressure deformity. At the root of the mesentery, a favorite location for metastatic lymph node disease from the colon, the cava may be distorted or displaced.

Aorta

A tortuous aorta arching to the right displaces the IVC (Fig. 38-36). Aneurysms of the aorta on the right iliac artery, depending on their direction of expansion, can compress the cava or even erode into it, with a resultant aortocaval fistula (Fig. 38-37).

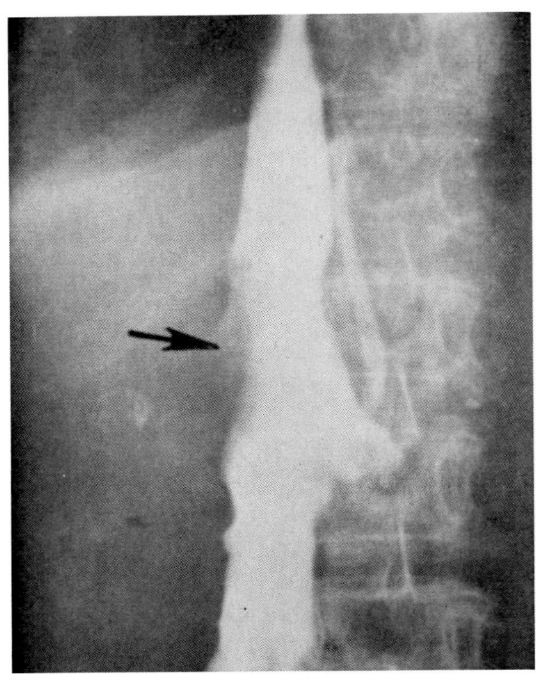

A

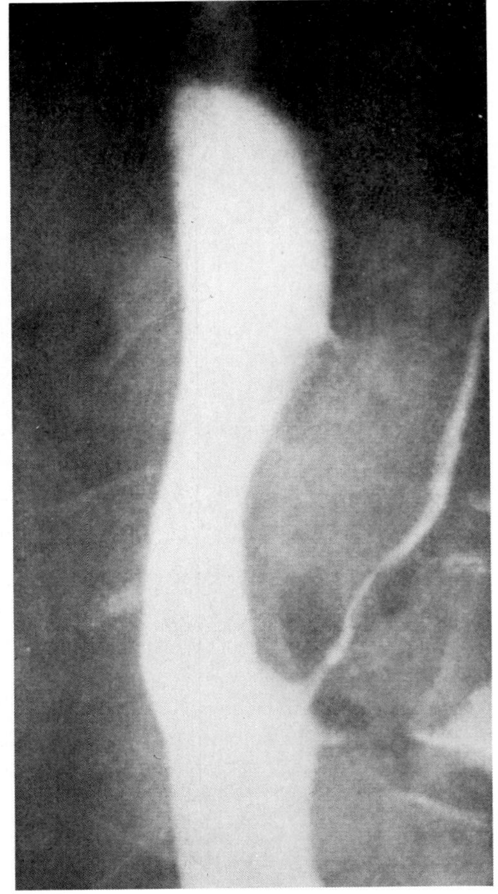

B

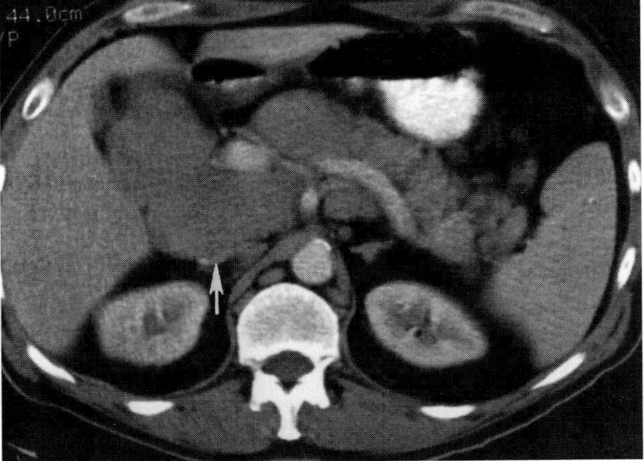

C

Figure 38-34. Cavogram in the frontal and lateral projections. (A) *Arrow* indicates nodal involvement (proved at surgery) for a hypernephroma of the right kidney. (B) Lateral projection shows the compressive effect of the nodes on the posterior wall. (C) CT scan showing compression of IVC (*arrow*) by portocaval nodes.

Lymph Nodes

Computed tomography (CT) is being used to a significant degree in primary and secondary lymph node abnormalities (Fig. 38-38). However, because of limitations not inherent in the lymphogram (i.e., internal architectural changes), lymphography—particularly in Hodgkin disease—is still used occasionally.

Soft Tissue Masses and Inflammatory Diseases

Retroperitoneal infections with an abscess or a large intraperitoneal mass may cause extrinsic deformity of the IVC. Tuberculous extension from lumbar spine involvement and retroperitoneal fibrosis (Fig. 38-39) may distort the IVC.

Pregnancy

Compression of the IVC from a large uterus secondary to pregnancy is seen when the visualization of the cava

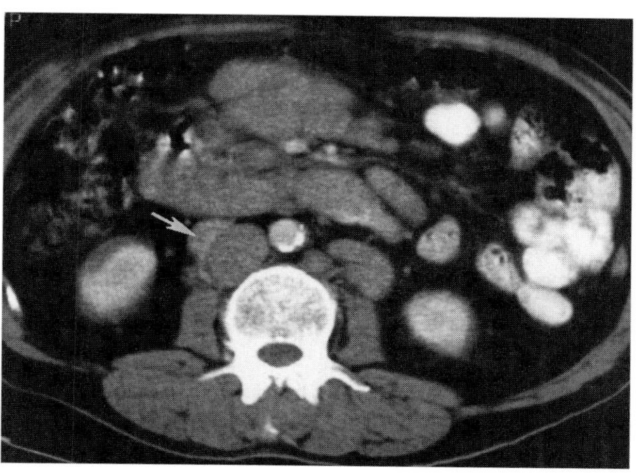

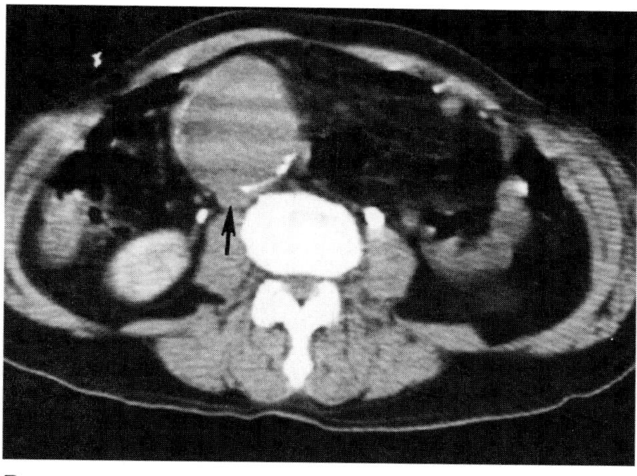

Figure 38-35. (A) CT scan showing compression of IVC (*arrow*) by retrocaval node. (B) CT scan showing large abdominal aortic aneurysm anterior to IVC and compressing it (*arrow*).

Figure 38-36. (A) Cavography raised the question of an aortic aneurysm or a nonvascular extrinsic process at the level of the second to third lumbar vertebrae. The levo phase of the cavogram was unsuccessful. (B) Aortogram performed for renal hypertension shows that the tortuous aorta swinging to the right is the cause of the defect noted on cavography.

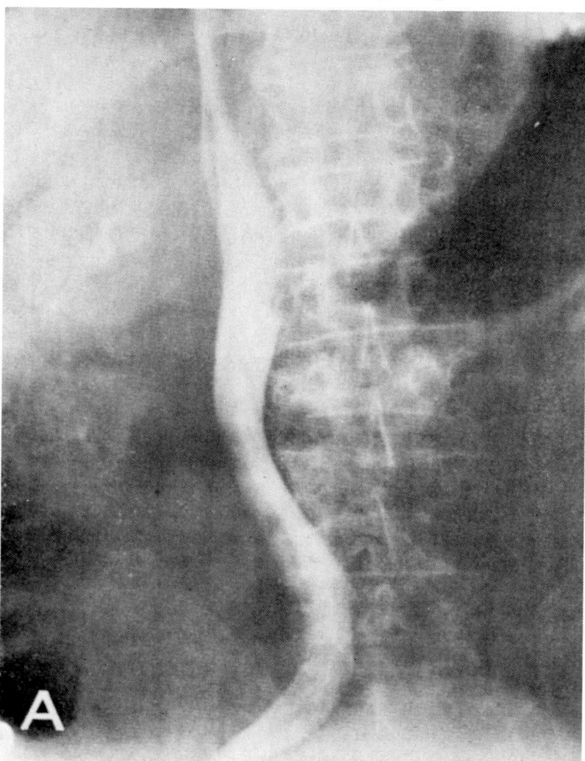

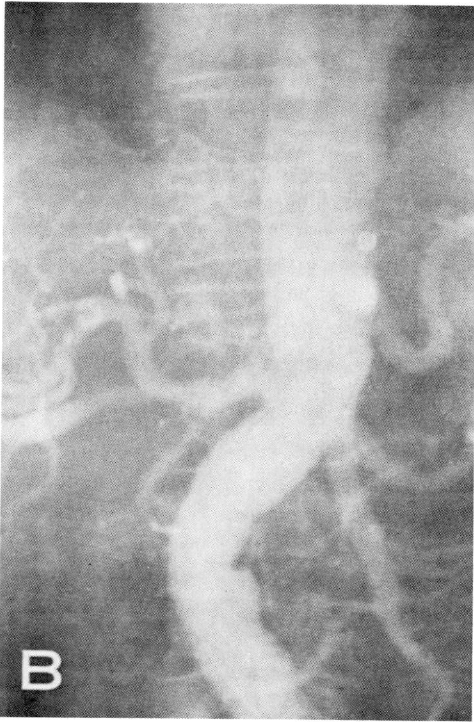

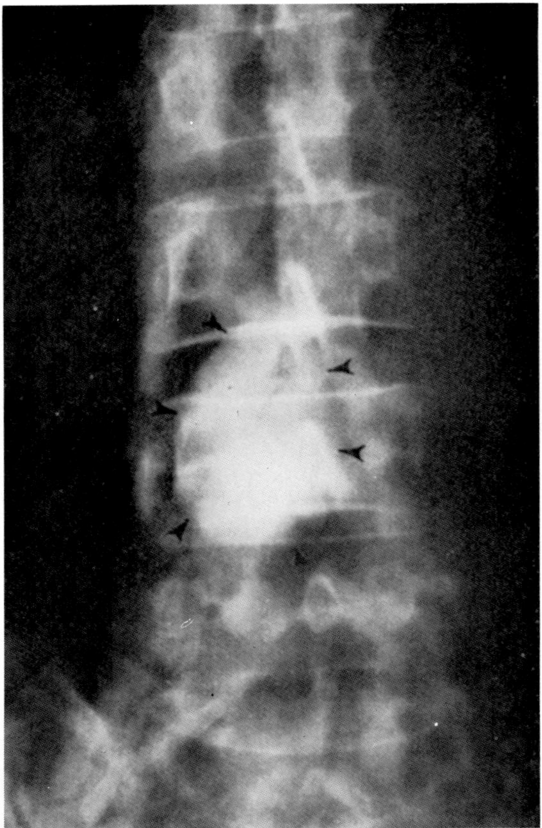

Figure 38-37. Aortocaval fistula. Aortogram shows a mycotic aneurysm (*arrowheads*) with rupture into the inferior vena cava. (From Ferris EJ, Hipona FA, Kahn PC, et al, eds. Venography of the inferior vena cava and its branches. Baltimore: Williams & Wilkins, 1969. Used with permission.)

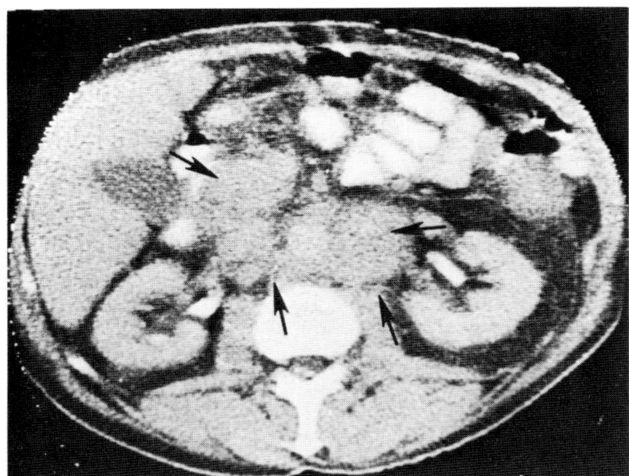

Figure 38-38. CT scan at the level of the kidneys illustrating massive paraaortic adenopathy (*arrows*) in a patient with widespread lymphosarcoma.

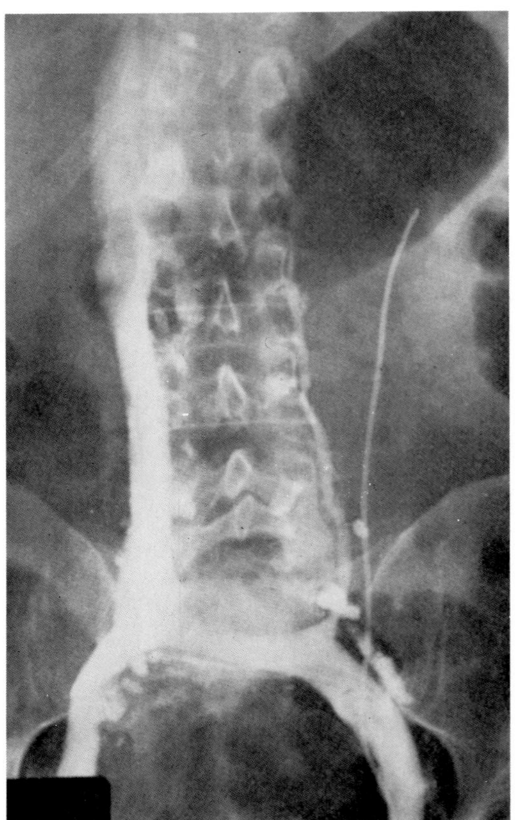

A

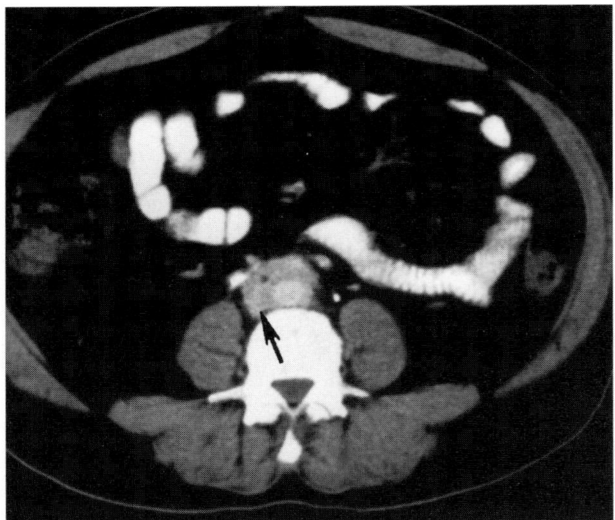

B

Figure 38-39. (A) Inferior vena cavogram in a patient with retroperitoneal fibrosis. A diffuse constrictive effect on the lower inferior vena cava and the left common iliac vein is seen. (From Ferris EJ, Hipona FA, Kahn PC, et al, eds. Venography of the inferior vena cava and its branches. Baltimore: Williams & Wilkins, 1969. Used with permission.) (B) Another case of retroperitoneal fibrosis. CT scan of the abdomen shows a soft tissue mass surrounding the aorta and compressing the IVC (*arrow*).

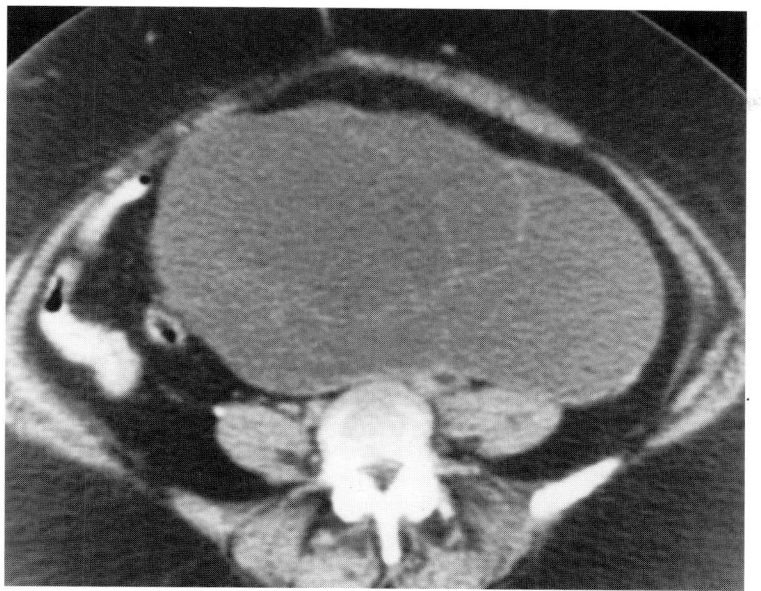
A

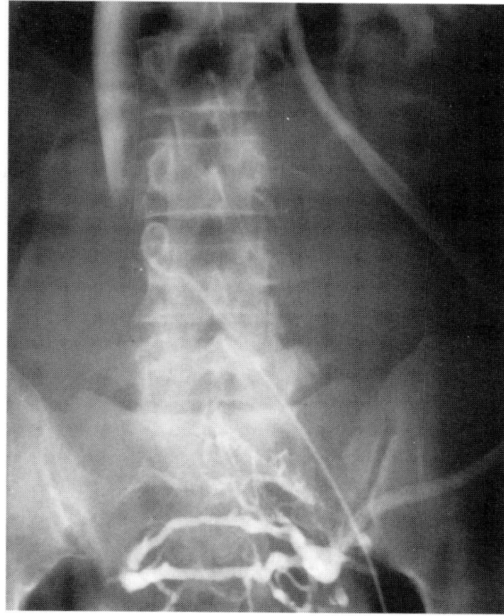
B

Figure 38-40. (A) CT scan of the lower abdomen showing a large ovarian mass causing compression of the IVC. (B) Inferior vena cavogram with catheter in the left common iliac vein showing compression of the IVC with a large left ovarian vein. This condition simulates what occurs in pregnancy.

is performed with the patient in the supine position (Fig. 38-40).[72,73] Prone visualization of the cava will illustrate a normal contour as the gravid uterus dependently moves anteriorly and the pressure on the IVC diminishes.

Intrinsic Obstruction

In considering intrinsic obstruction of the IVC, several points are worthy of note. Intrinsic obstruction of the cava is usually secondary to long-standing extrinsic pressure on the cava with resultant stasis and thrombosis. Over 90 percent of IVC obstructions occur in the lower IVC.[62] Rarely calcification of thrombi in the IVC occurs.

It is perhaps most convenient to discuss intrinsic obstructions relative to upper, middle, or infrarenal segments of the IVC.

Upper IVC Occlusion

This is an unusual site for intrinsic obstruction of the IVC. Usually there is an abnormality in the liver causing compression of the IVC, which then predisposes the cava to thrombus. Hepatic vein occlusion may extend into the IVC, or, more commonly, renal vein occlusion extends into the upper IVC and often even into the right atrium (Fig. 38-41). Kimura et al.[74] have

Figure 38-41. Huge tumor thrombus (*arrows*) in the upper inferior vena cava that had extended from a tumor thrombus in the right renal vein (renal cell carcinoma). This study is the venous phase of a right selective renal angiogram.

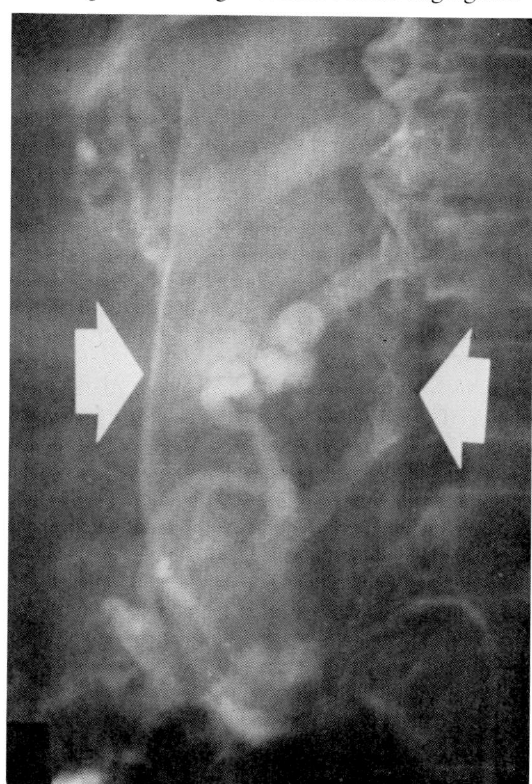

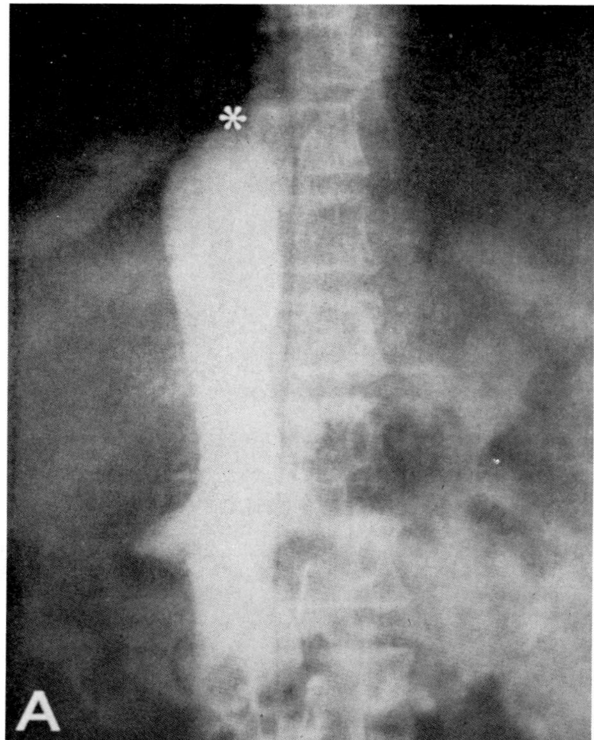

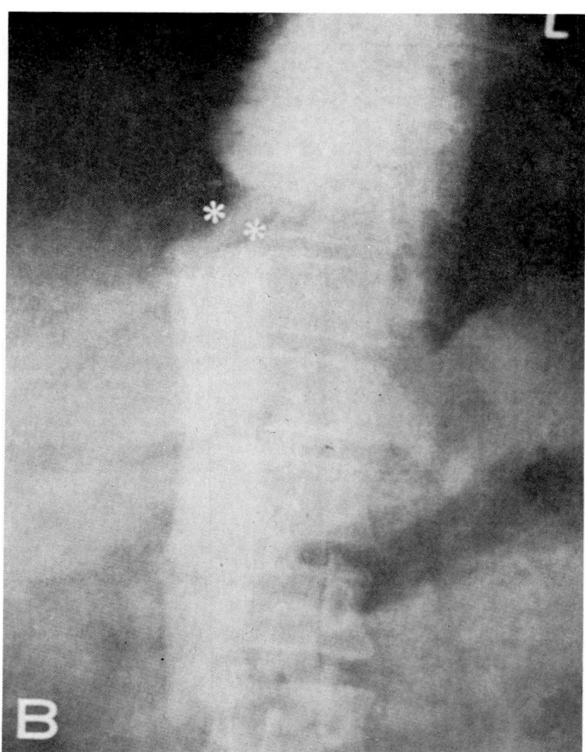

Figure 38-42. (A) Inferior vena cava study showing a membrane (*asterisk*) at the level of the diaphragmatic leaflet. The clinical symptoms and signs were those of IVC obstruction. (B) Cavogram after commissurotomy. Improvement in the size of the orifice (*asterisks*) and flow-rate dynamics was better appreciated on cineangiography. (From Ferris EJ, Hipona FA, Kahn PC, et al, eds. Venography of the inferior vena cava and its branches. Baltimore: Williams & Wilkins, 1969. Used with permission.)

described a membrane thought to be of congenital origin in the upper cava (Fig. 38-42). The patients present with edema. The explanation for onset of the symptomatology later in life from a supposedly congenital process is not clear. One can make the diagnosis by cavography—MRI, CT, or Doppler scanning.[75] Transcardiac membranotomy is the definitive therapy. Metal stents, now available, hold promise.

Middle IVC Occlusion

The most common cause of midcaval occlusion is carcinoma of the kidney with extension of renal vein tumor into the IVC.[76] Occasionally, extrinsic pressure from paracaval lymph nodes involved with metastatic hypernephroma causes enough stasis of the middle IVC to initiate thrombosis.[76a] Usually, however, caval thrombus in association with carcinoma of the kidney is actually tumor thrombus (Fig. 38-43A). Because of the shorter length of the right renal vein, it is said that renal thrombus can be delineated often by selective renal angiography[77] (see Fig. 38-43A). Alternatively, CT

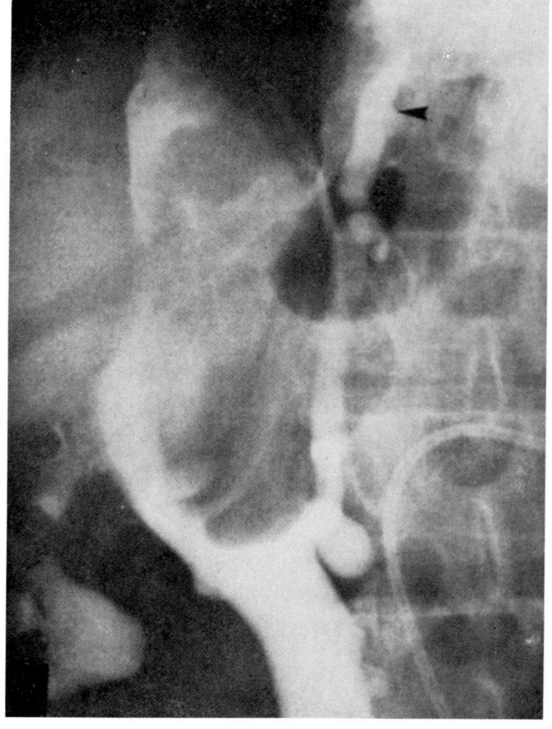

A

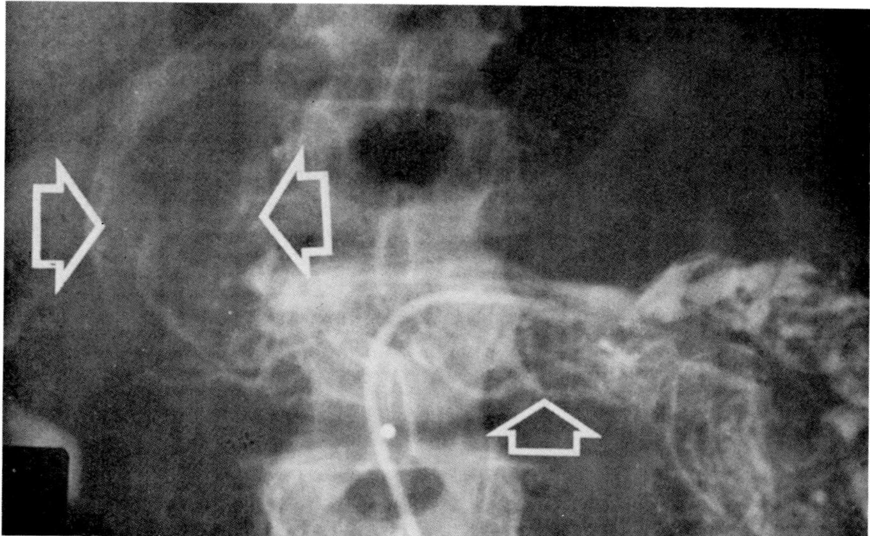

B

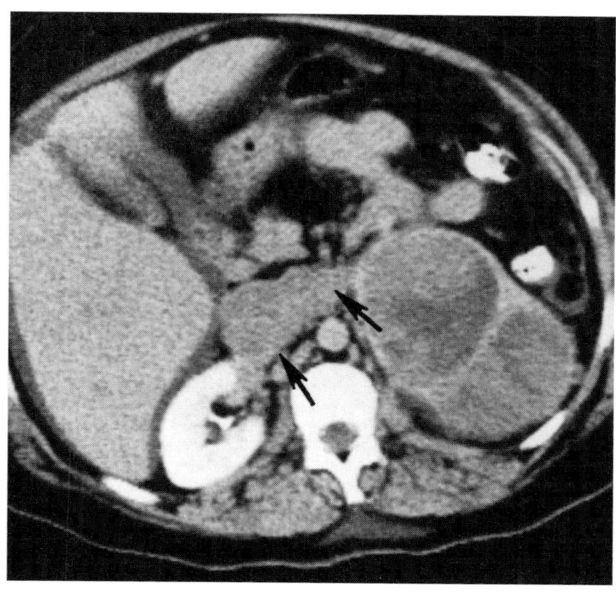

C

Figure 38-43. (A) Cavogram in a patient with a left renal carcinoma that had extended into the inferior vena cava. Note collateral venous filling (*arrowhead*). (B) Renal angiogram on same patient. "Tumor vessels" are seen in the neoplastic thrombus (*arrows*) extending from the left renal vein into the inferior vena cava. (A and B from Ferris EJ, Hipona FA, Kahn PC, et al, eds. Venography of the inferior vena cava and its branches. Baltimore: Williams & Wilkins, 1969. Used with permission.) (C) CT scan of another patient showing left renal cell carcinoma with enhancing tumor in the left renal vein and IVC (*arrows*).

or ultrasound, as well as MRI, can be used (Figs. 38-43B and C). Extension upward to the hepatic segment of the IVC and to the right atrium is common. Pulmonary emboli are frequent. One can observe that, in spite of extension of thrombus into the upper IVC, hepatic vein occlusion is seldom seen because the obstruction is rarely complete.

Infrarenal Occlusion

Phlebothrombosis of the iliofemoral venous system may extend upward to involve the infrarenal segment of the IVC (Fig. 38-44). Usually, however, thrombus of the lower IVC is seen with stasis secondary to extrinsic pressure.

Transcatheter brush biopsy for intraluminal caval masses may be of some assistance if the occlusion is thought to be neoplastic.[78]

The Inferior Vena Cava Postoperatively

Inferior vena cavography is useful in studying patients after ligation, plication, or clipping procedures, when recurrent embolization is suspected.[63,79,80] Of 148 patients evaluated, in one of the author's personal experience, thrombi have been seen above the surgical site in 12 patients (Fig. 38-45). However, only 3 of these patients had clinical suggestion of recurrent pulmonary thromboembolism. The cava is so richly endowed with collaterals that stasis above the level of the surgical site is probably not as common as anticipated.

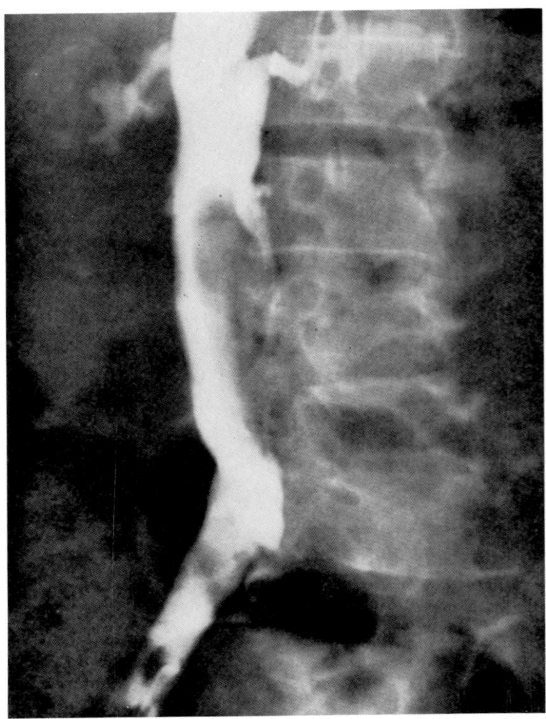

Figure 38-44. Inferior vena cavogram in a patient with a huge thrombus in the inferior vena cava. The left femoral vein was not cannulated. (From Ferris EJ, Hipona FA, Kahn PC, et al, eds. Venography of the inferior vena cava and its branches. Baltimore: Williams & Wilkins, 1969. Used with permission.)

It is common to have thrombi below the operative site, as occurred in over 50 percent of one series (Fig. 38-46). Although early in venographic evaluation (i.e., 3 to 6 months) clips and plications seemed to have a higher patency rate than ligations, the patients were virtually identical with respect to caval occlusion after 24 months. The collateral channels, such as the ascending lumbar and gonadal veins, may be the route of recurrent embolization. In 5 patients (total 148 patients) who had symptoms of recurrent pulmonary embolism with a positive perfusion scan and a positive pulmonary angiogram, large collateral channels were seen. None of these patients had obvious thrombi above the surgical site. In three instances the ovarian veins appeared to be the logical route for recurrent embolization (Fig. 38-47), and in two cases huge lumbar veins (one containing thrombi) were observed. Nevertheless, it is extremely difficult to be certain of the significance of excessively large collateral channels because they have been seen in many patients who have

Figure 38-45. (A) Inferior vena cavogram in a patient several days after placement of a Teflon clip for prevention of pulmonary embolism. There is a thrombus above the operative site (*upper arrow*) as well as a thrombus in the ascending lumbar vein (*lower arrow*). (B) Close-up of (A). (From Ferris EJ, Vittimberga FJ, Byrne JJ, et al. The inferior vena cava post ligation and plication. Radiology 1967;89:1–10. Used with permission.)

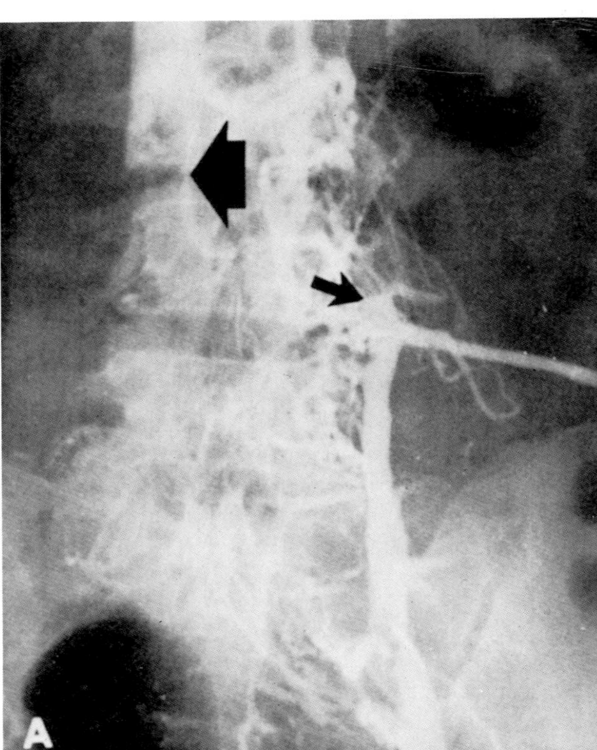

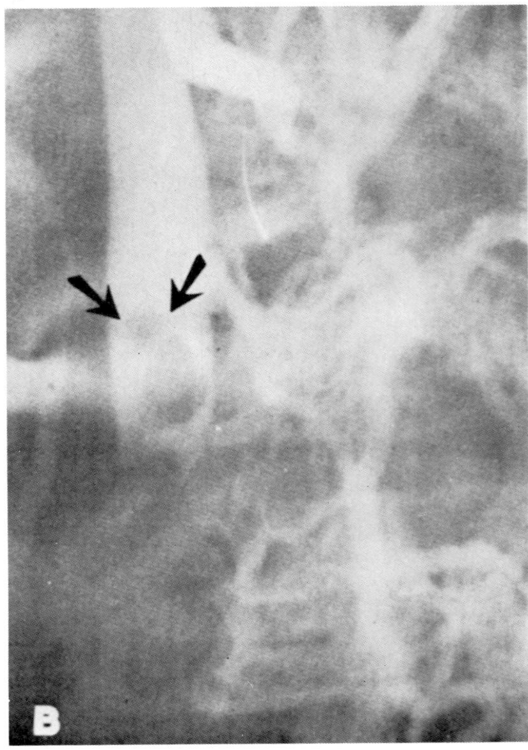

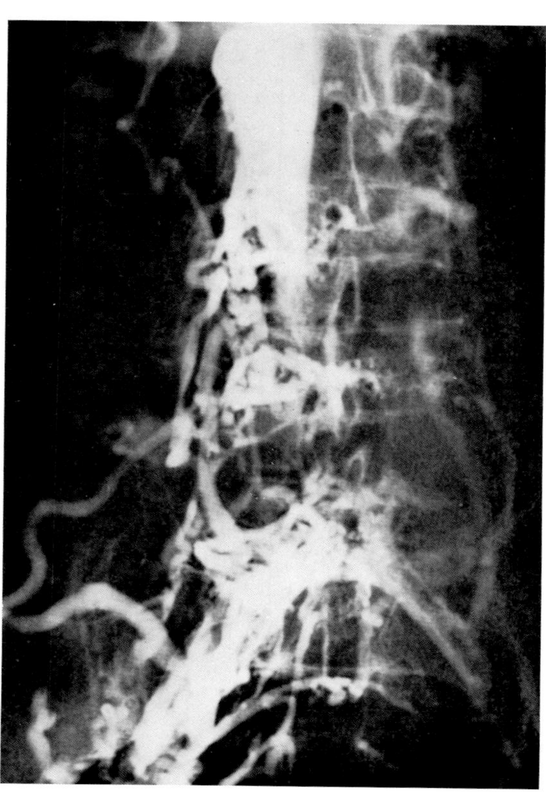

Figure 38-46. Cavogram showing thrombosis below the operative site of ligation. There is also a thrombus in the left common iliac vein. (From Ferris EJ, Vittimberga FJ, Byrne JJ, et al. The inferior vena cava post ligation and plication. Radiology 1967;89:1–10. Used with permission.)

Figure 38-47. (A) Inferior vena cavogram in a woman who had IVC surgery for prevention of pulmonary emboli. The ovarian veins (*arrow*) are huge and presumably could transport large emboli. This patient did have pulmonary symptoms of recurrent emboli. (B) The pulmonary angiogram was positive. The patient refused surgery to interrupt her ovarian veins but did well on heparin therapy. (From Ferris EJ, Vittimberga FJ, Byrne JJ, et al. The inferior vena cava post ligation and plication. Radiology 1967;89:1–10. Used with permission.)

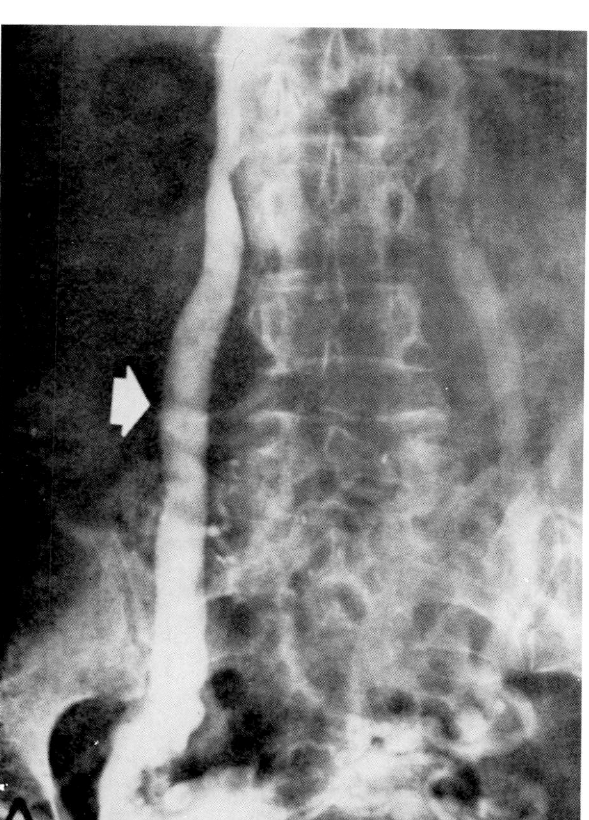

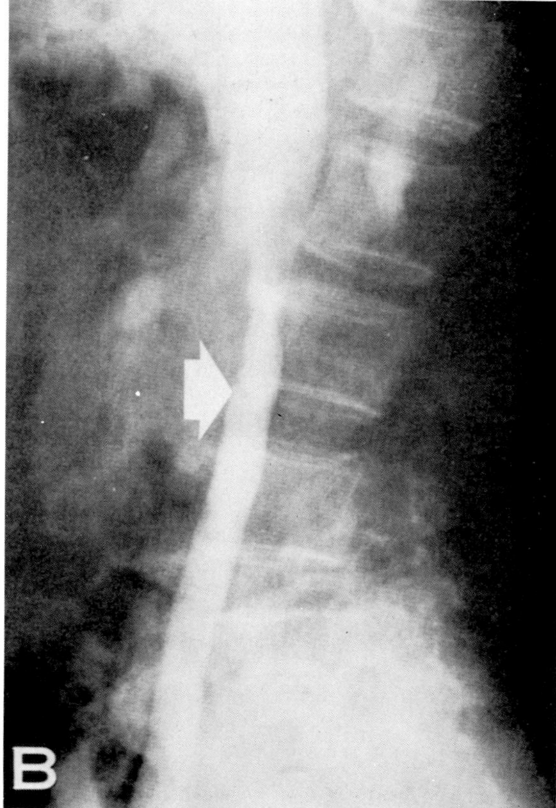

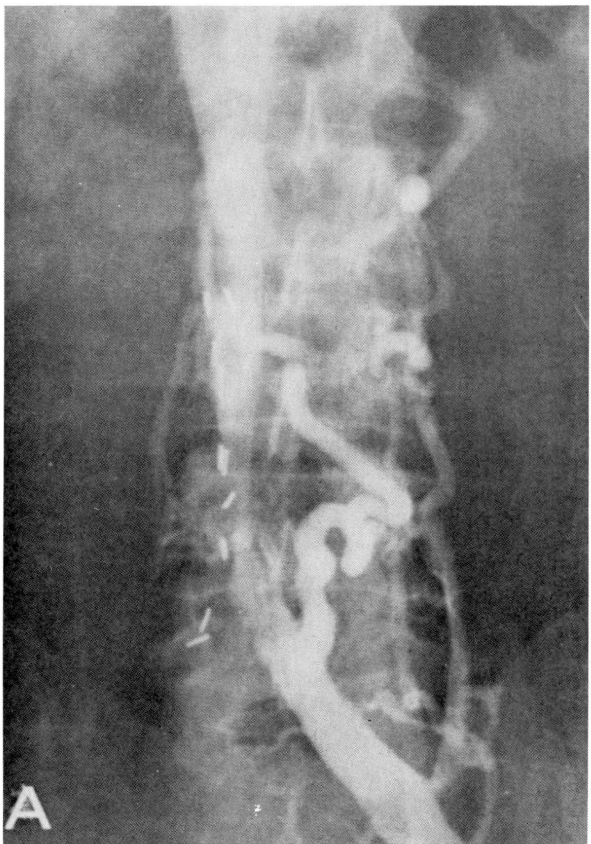

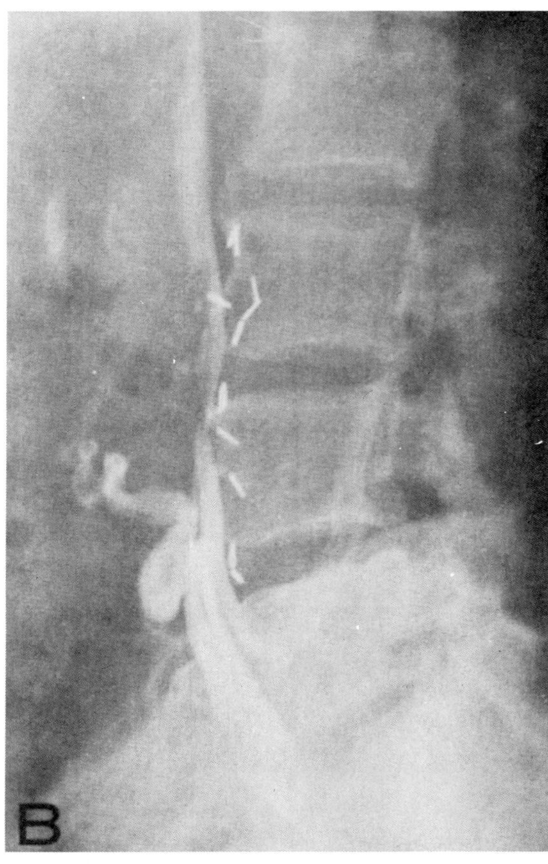

Figure 38-48. Recanalized inferior vena cava 2 years after ligation for prevention of pulmonary emboli. (A) Anteroposterior projection. (B) Lateral projection. Note that the IVC is filled above the third lumbar vertebra, the operative site, before contribution by collateral circulation. Filling is particularly evident on the lateral projection. (From Ferris EJ, Vittimberga FJ, Byrne JJ, et al. The inferior vena cava post ligation and plication. Radiology 1967;89:1–10. Used with permission.)

been free from obvious recurrent emboli for over 5 years.

In the past several years six cases of so-called recanalization of the IVC after ligation have been seen (Fig. 38-48). None of the patients died, nor were the recanalized lumina large enough to advocate intervention.

In 47 patients studied 2 years after plication, it was possible to verify patency at the operative site in 24 (Fig. 38-49), whereas the remaining 23 had completely thrombosed the plication site. These findings are in general agreement with those of Bergan et al.,[81] who also found a high incidence of eventual closure of plications. However, it is interesting to note that in the series of 47 patients studied, only 12 had closure at the operative site during the first 6 months. It seems, therefore, that between 6 months and 2 years after surgery there is a progressive increase in rate of closure in patients who have undergone a plication procedure.

Inferior Vena Cava Filters

It is not the purpose of this chapter to discuss the treatment aspects of the percutaneous inferior vena caval filters; this is found in Chapter 59 of *Abrams' Angiography: Interventional Radiology.* In many instances, however, one may be requested to evaluate the IVC postfilter insertion for a variety of reasons. Hence some comments about the postfilter appearance of the cava, particularly in long-term follow-up, might be important.

Since 1985, 324 percutaneous inferior vena caval filters in 320 patients have been placed at the University of Arkansas for Medical Sciences. Long-term follow-up on these patients was successful in 88 percent of cases. One hundred twenty are known dead (38 percent), 8 of whom were proven by autopsy to have died from pulmonary emboli. Fifteen patients of 280

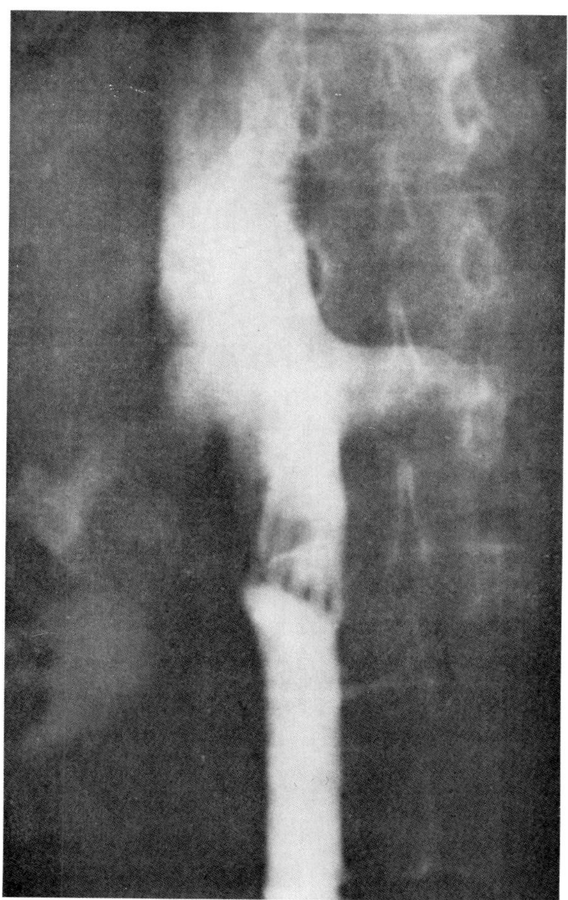

A

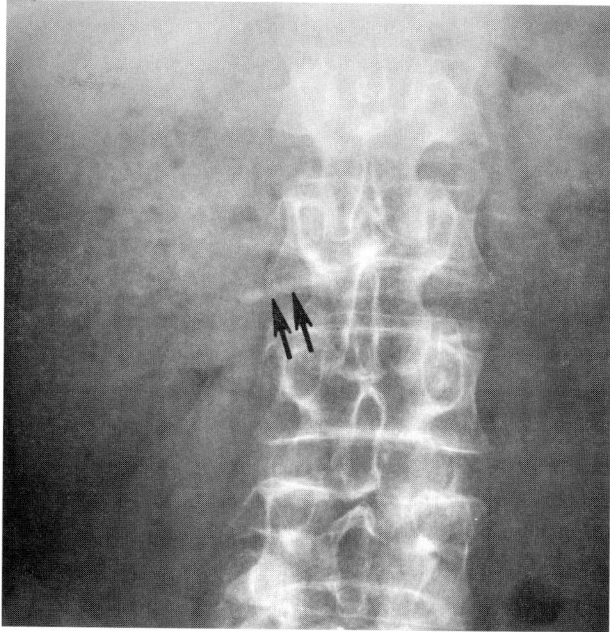

B

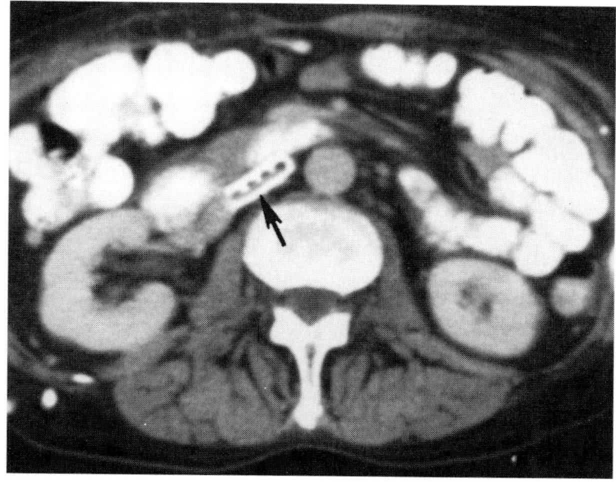

C

Figure 38-49. (A) Plication several weeks after placement of a Teflon clip. Cavography confirms patency. (B) Plain film of another patient showing IVC clip (*arrows*) overlying the right inferior second lumbar vertebra. (C) CT scan of the same patient showing the IVC clip (*arrow*) and collateral vessels on the right side of the abdominal wall.

(5 percent) followed by clinical and radiologic means had recurrent or new significant pulmonary emboli. Thirty-eight patients of 280 (14 percent) developed inferior vena caval thrombosis. Twenty patients of 320 treated had significant filter penetration through the wall of the IVC, with 4 instances of communication with a regional organ. Migration to the right heart or pulmonary artery occurred in 3 of 192 patients (2 percent). Inferior vena caval stenosis was seen in 9 of 192 patients (5 percent) evaluated with various imaging modalities. Asymptomatic fracture of a strut was noted in 5 of 280 patients (2 percent). New or extension of old deep venous thrombosis was noted in 37 of 280 patients (13 percent). Examples of several filter placements are demonstrated in Figure 38-50.

Physiologic Aspects of Cavography and Pitfalls in Diagnosis

Venous flow in the IVC is phasic and pulsatile and therefore is affected by normal and abnormal cardiac changes. Hipona (personal communication) has demonstrated that peak blood flow velocity (normally 30 to 45 cm per second) in the IVC may slow, come to a momentary standstill, or paradoxically reverse its direction. This latter sitaution of systolic reversal of IVC flow is seen in tricuspid insufficiency. In long-standing cases of cardiac failure or constrictive pericarditis, the

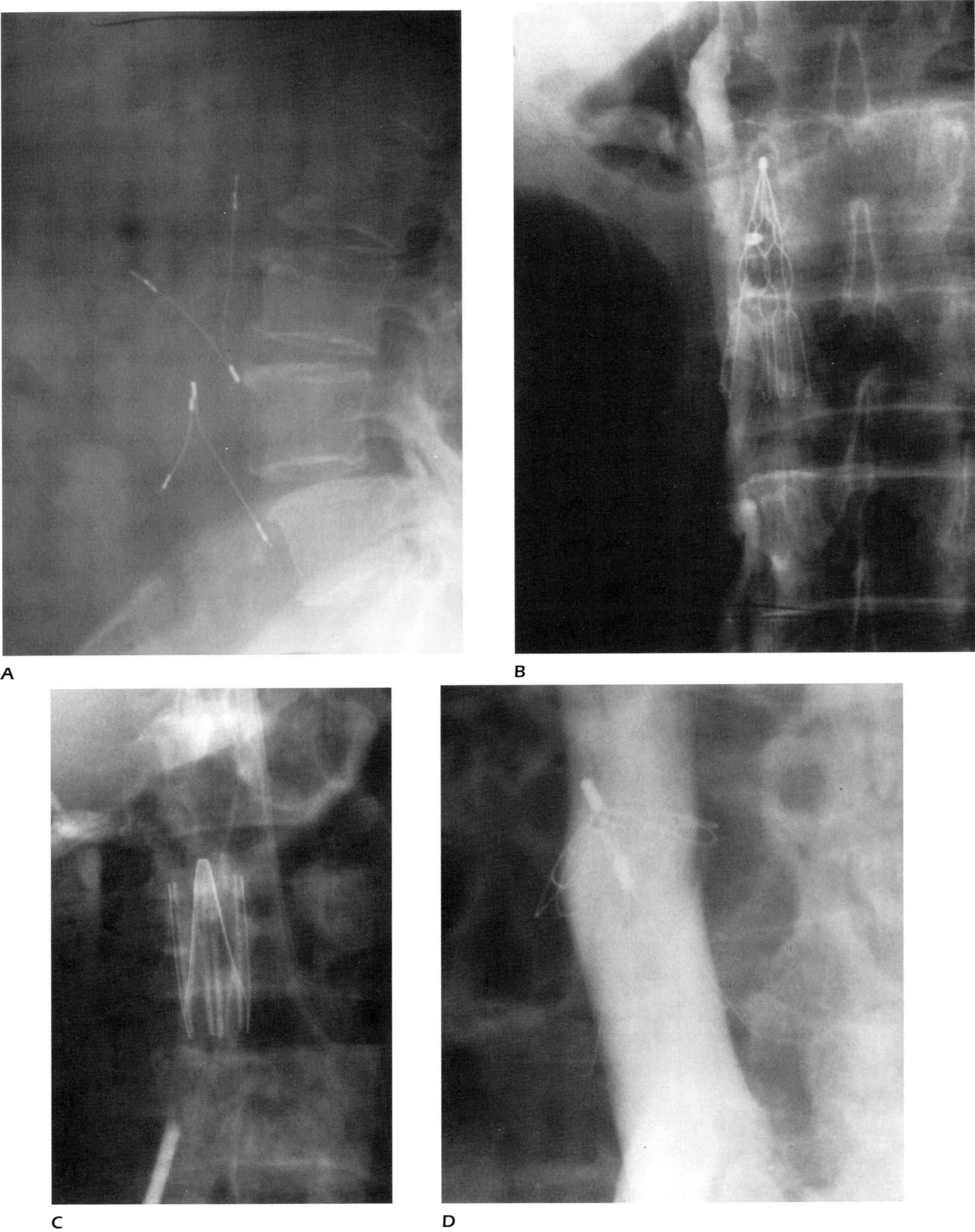

Figure 38-50. Four different types of percutaneous inferior vena caval filters. (A) Bird's Nest, lateral projection. (B) Titanium Greenfield M.H. (modified hook). (C) Vena Tech or L.G.M. (D) Palestrant-Simon Nitinol Filter.

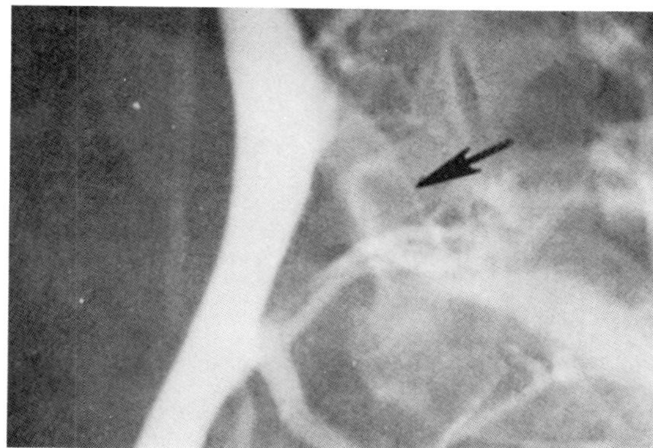

Figure 38-51. Streaming from the left common iliac vein simulates a thrombus (*arrow*) at the caval bifurcation with an injection into the right femoral vein only. The left common iliac vein is normal.

IVC enlarges to what could be called a megacava. Respiratory variations in IVC flow are apparent with a simple Valsalva maneuver, which causes a reduction in IVC flow rate. Contrariwise, a slow, deep inspiration causes an increase in IVC flow rate. Exercise of the lower extremities causes an increase in arterial flow and hence in the speed of circulation in the IVC.

Pitfalls in diagnosis are multiple and are chiefly due to poor technique. Injection into a single femoral vein instead of a bilateral femoral vein injection will often cause such a dilution effect of the IVC from the side not punctured that thrombus of the lower cava will be overlooked or unjustly invoked (Fig. 38-51). Slight straining or a Valsalva maneuver during cavography may cause marked to moderate filling of central collateral channels, particularly in children. Abrams found that in 67 percent of normal cavograms collateral channels were opacified to varying degrees (see Chapter 36). If the patient is instructed to hold his or her breath and not to bear down during the injection, collateral channels do not readily fill and IVC opacification is much improved.

In the lumbar, hepatic, and renal veins, so-called washout must not be interpreted as an organic filling defect. In serial cavography this is uncommon because one can note the changing configuration of the jet of unopacified blood. With the single-exposure technique the dynamics necessary to evaluate washout are not present.

Anatomic factors such as severe lordosis and osteophytes can cause diminution in contrast density of the opacified IVC, particularly along the medial margin (Fig. 38-52).

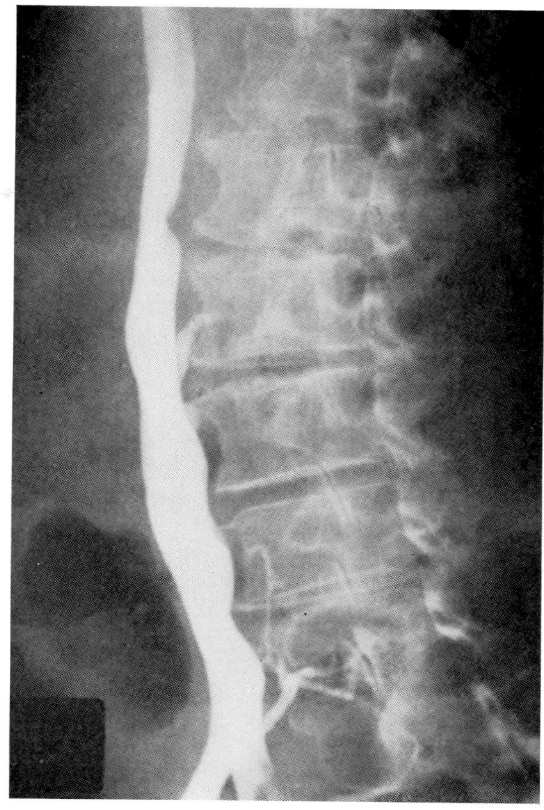

Figure 38-52. Inferior vena cavogram in an elderly patient with posterior indentation secondary to osteophyte formation. (From Ferris EJ, Hipona FA, Kahn PC, et al, eds. Venography of the inferior vena cava and its branches. Baltimore: Williams & Wilkins, 1969. Used with permission.)

Primary Tumors of the Cava

Primary tumors of the IVC are rare.[82] Leiomyoma, endothelioma, sarcoma (leiomyosarcoma), and enchondroma have been reported.[83–85] Most of these are found at postmortem examination, although severe cases have been resected.[83,85] Figure 38-53 illustrates a leiomyosarcoma of the infrarenal IVC.

Ultrasound and CT have more recently been shown to be of value in assessing tumors of the IVC (Fig. 38-54).

Complications

Complications following inferior vena cavography performed by the standard method are uncommon. If a guidewire is used to thread Teflon sheaths up the femoroiliac venous system, a perforation of the iliac vein or the IVC secondary to a penetrating injury from the guidewire is possible. This is usually without sequelae.

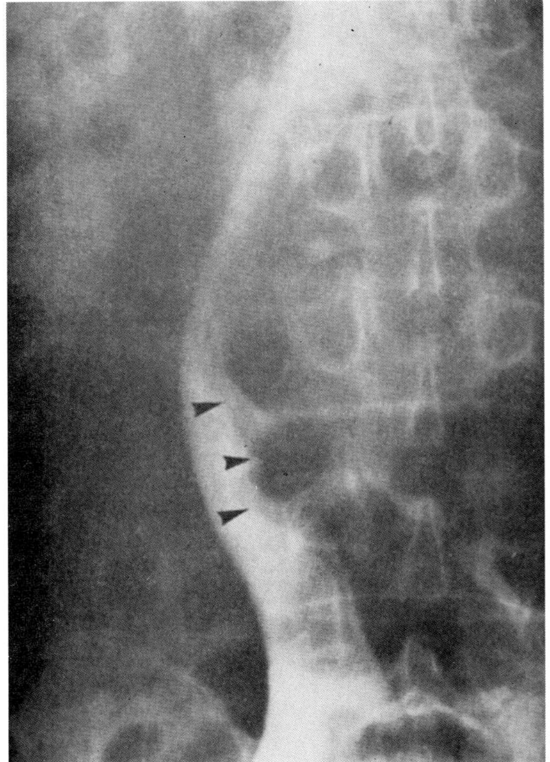

Figure 38-53. Leiomyosarcoma (*arrows*) appearing as an irregular, bilobed deformity of the inferior vena cava.

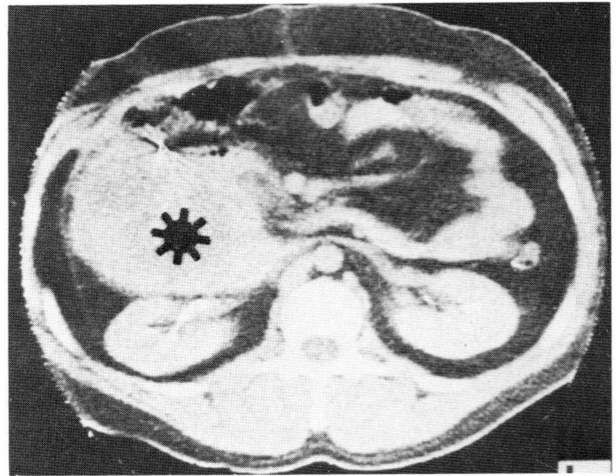

A

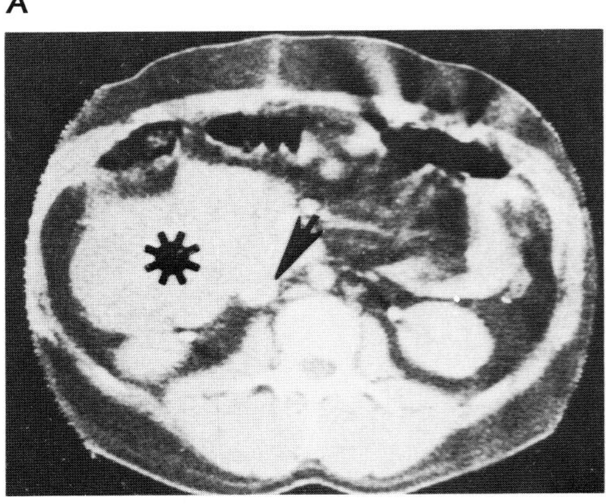

B

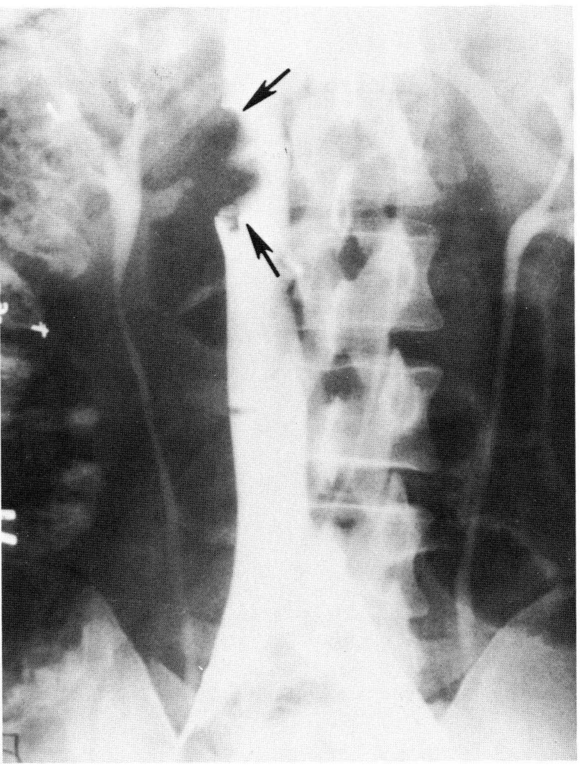

C

Extravasation of contrast material occasionally occurs, particularly when the patient is turned for an oblique projection, but as a rule is innocuous. Doumanian and Amplatz[86] have reported that the IVC can rupture when high-velocity injections are performed.

Iliac Vein Spurs

An entity that has received much emphasis over the past several years is the development of an irritative intimal "spur" of the left common iliac vein secondary to the compressive pulsatile force of the aortic bifurcation and right common iliac artery that transverse an-

Figure 38-54. (A) CT scan showing a leiomyosarcoma of the inferior vena cava (*asterisk*). (B) Slightly lower section shows the massive extent of this tumor (*asterisk*). *Arrowhead* denotes the IVC partially filled by contrast material. (C) Inferior vena cavogram of this patient illustrating a bilobed filling defect in the inferior vena cava (*arrows*). One does not really appreciate the extensive exophytic component of the tumor without other imaging modalities such as the CT scan (A and B).

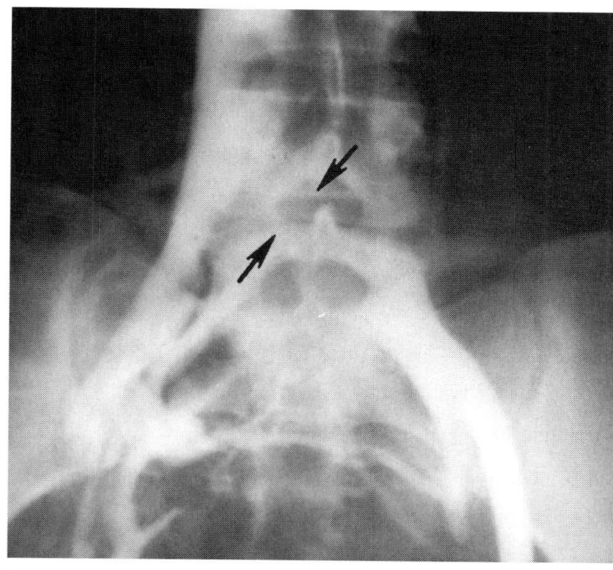

A

Lateral Spur

Medial Spur

Diaphragm

B

Figure 38-55. May-Thurner syndrome. (A) Inferior vena cavogram. This 19-year-old woman with long-standing left leg edema has marked compression of her left common iliac vein (*arrows*) by the overlying right common iliac artery. This resulted in stasis with a gradient of 3 to 5 mmHg across this area. Surgery revealed a lateral spur—one of three types of intimal reactive hyperplasia as demonstrated in the diagrammatic sketch in (B). (From Ferris EJ, Lim WN, Smith PL, et al. May-Thurner syndrome. Radiology 1983;147:29–31. Used with permission.)

terior to the iliocaval junction (Fig. 38-55). Weber and May[87] have classified these "spurs" into a lateral type, a medial type, and an obliterative type. They present as eccentric or central filling defects or complete obstruction of the left common iliac vein just short of the iliocaval junction. If pressure measurements are made of the left common iliac vein in comparison with the right iliac vein, as well as the cava, one may note a slight pressure difference on the left.[88] Furthermore, in significant obstruction, exercise of the left leg will usually increase the pressure gradient by several millimeters of mercury. Interestingly enough, occasionally there will be a significant pressure difference, yet venography will still not delineate the intimal abnormality. Because the patients do indeed have swelling of the left leg with a negative left venogram except for the defect at the iliocaval junction, pressure measurements are important in evaluation for potential surgical intervention. One method of surgical correction is to strip the right long saphenous vein and to bridge this vein from the right to the left iliac vein. In this fashion the leg edema is frequently alleviated.

References

1. Philips, EV. In: Ferris EJ, Hipona FA, Kahn PC, et al., eds. Venography of the inferior vena cava and its branches. Baltimore: Williams & Wilkins, 1969.
2. dos Santos R. Phlébographie d'une veine cave inférieure suture. J Urol Med Chir 1935;39:586.
3. Fariñas PL. Abdominal venography. AJR 1947;58:599–602.
4. O'Loughlin BJ. Roentgen visualization of the inferior vena cava. AJR 1947;58:617–619.
5. Kaufman JJ, Burke DE, Goodwin WE. Abdominal venography in urological diagnosis. J Urol 1956;75:160–168.
6. Denny DF Jr, Greenwood LH, Morse SS, et al. Inferior vena cava: translumbar catheterization for central venous access. Radiology 1989;172:1013–1014.
7. Helander CG, Lindbom A. Sarcolumbar venography. Acta Radiol (Stockh) 1955;44:410–416.
8. Marcozzi G, Messinetti S. An original technique of transsomatic vertebral angiography of the inferior vena cava. Angiology 1966;17:710–717.
9. Batson OV. Vertebral phlebography. In: Schobinger RA, Ruzicka FF, eds. Vascular roentgenology. New York: Macmillan, 1961.
10. Bucheler E, Janson R. Combined catheter venography of the lumbar venous stem and the inferior vena cava. Br J Radiol 1973;46:655–661.
11. Gargano FP, Meyer JJ. Transfemoral ascending lumbar catheterization of the epidural veins in lumbar disk disease. Radiology 1974;111:329–336.
12. Miller MH, Handel SF, Coan JD. Transfemoral lumbar epidural venography. AJR 1976;126:1003–1009.
13. Hipona FA, Ferris EJ, Pick R. Capnocavography: a new technique for examination of the inferior vena cava. Radiology 1969;92:606–609.
14. Gooding GAW. The abdominal great vessels. In: Rumack CM, Wilson SR, Chauboneau JW, eds. Diagnostic ultrasound. St. Louis: Mosby–Year Book, 1991;1:335–352.
15. Mintz GS, Kotler MN, Parry WR, et al. Real time inferior vena caval ultrasonography: normal and abnormal findings and its

use in assessing right-heart function. Circulation 1981;64: 1018–1024.
16. Needleman L, Rifkin MD. Vascular ultrasonography: abdominal applications. Radiol Clin North Am 1986;24:461–484.
17. Mellins HZ. Inferior vena cava obstruction. In: Pollock HM, ed. Clinical urology: an atlas and textbook of urological imaging. Philadelphia: Saunders, 1990:2105–2111.
18. Zweibel WS. Color-duplex and Doppler spectrum analysis: principle, capabilities, and limitations. Semin Ultrasound CT MR 1990;11(2):84–96.
19. Crowley RJ, von Behren PL, Couvillon LA Jr, et al. Optimized ultrasound imaging catheters for use in the vascular system. Int J Card Imaging 1989;4:145–151.
20. Meyer CR, Chiang EH, Fechner KP, et al. Feasibility of high-resolution, intravascular ultrasound imaging catheters. Radiology 1988;168:113–116.
21. Pandian NG, Kreis A, Brockway B, et al. Ultrasound angioscopy: real-time, two-dimensional, intraluminal ultrasound imaging of blood vessels. Am J Cardiol 1988;62:493–494.
22. Tobias J, Mallery J, Gessert J, et al. Intravascular ultrasound cross-sectional arterial imaging before and after balloon angioplasty in vitro. Circulation 1989;80:873–882.
23. Yock PG, Johnson EL, Linker DT. Intravascular ultrasound: development and clinical potential. Am J Card Imaging 1988; 2:185–193.
24. Marx MV, Tauscher JR, Williams DM, et al. Diagnosis of caval thrombus with intraluminal US: animal model and clinical studies. Radiology 1990;174:1061–1062.
25. McCowan TC, Ferris EJ, Carver DK. Inferior vena caval filter thrombi: evaluation with intravascular US. Radiology 1990; 177:783–788.
26. McCowan TC, Ferris EJ, Carver DK. IVUS explores details of venous structures. Diagn Imaging 1990:107–108.
27. Patten RM, Shuman WP, Jeffrey RB Jr. Retroperitoneum and lymphovascular structures. In: Moss AA, Gamsu G, Grenant HK, eds. Computed tomography of the body with magnetic resonance imaging. 2nd ed. Philadelphia: Saunders, 1992: 1091–1138.
28. Jeffrey RB Jr, Federle MP. The collapsed inferior vena cava: CT evaluation of hypovolemia. AJR 1988;150:431–432.
29. Glazer GM, Callen PW, Parker JJ. CT diagnosis of tumor thrombus in the inferior vena cava: avoiding false positive diagnosis. AJR 1981;137:1265–1267.
30. Marks WM, Korobkin M, Callen PW, et al. CT diagnosis of tumor thrombosis of the renal vein and inferior vena cava. AJR 1978;131:843–846.
31. Schmitz L, Jeffrey RB, Palubinskas AJ, et al. CT demonstration of septic thrombosis of the inferior vena cava. J Comput Assist Tomogr 1981;5:259–261.
32. Steele JR, Sones PJ, Heffner LT. The detection of inferior vena caval thrombosis with computed tomography. Radiology 1978;138:385–386.
33. Weyman PJ, McClennan BL, Stanley RJ, et al. Comparison of computed tomography and angiography in the evaluation of renal cell carcinoma. Radiology 1980;137:417–424.
34. Zerhouni EA, Barth KH, Siegelman SS. Demonstration of venous thrombosis by computed tomography. AJR 1980;134: 753–758.
35. Fagelman D, Lawrence LP, Black KS, et al. Inferior vena cava pseudothrombus in computed tomography using a contrast medium power injector: a potential pitfall. J Comput Assist Tomogr 1987;11:1042–1043.
36. Vogelzang RL, Gore RM, Nieman HL, et al. Inferior vena cava CT pseudothrombus produced by rapid arm-vein contrast infusion. AJR 1985;144:843–846.
37. Hricak H, Amparo E, Fisher MR, et al. Abdominal venous system: assessment using MR. Radiology 1985;156:415–422.
38. Ferris EJ, Ledor K, Ben-Avi DD, et al. Angioscopy—a percutaneous technique. Radiology 1985;157:319–322.
39. Fleisher HL, Thompson BW, McCowan TJ, et al. Angioscopically monitored saphenous vein valvulotomy. J Vasc Surg 1986; 4(4):360–364.
40. McCowan TC, McAlister MK, Ferris EJ, et al. Angioscopic evaluation of vascular anastomoses of the lower extremities in the canine model. J Ark Med Soc 1988;84(9):373–376.
41. Ferris EJ. George W. Holmes Lecture. Deep venous thrombosis and pulmonary embolism: correlative evaluation and therapeutic implications. AJR 1992;159:1149–1155.
42. Son YH, Wetzel RA, Wilson WJ. ^{99m}Tc pertechnetate scintiphotography as diagnostic and follow-up aid in major vascular obstruction due to malignant neoplasm. Radiology 1968;91: 349–357.
43. McClure EF, Butler EG. The development of the vena cava inferior in man. Am J Anat 1925;35:331.
44. Arey LB. Developmental anatomy. 6th ed. Philadelphia: Saunders, 1954.
45. Huntington GS, McClure CFW. The development of the veins in the domestic cat (*Felis domestica*). Anat Rec Phila 1920–1921;20:1–19.
46. Bolooki H, Margulies M, Yermakov VM, et al. Portal hypertension with anomalies of inferior vena cava and hepatic veins. Arch Surg 1967;94:267–270.
47. Gladstone RJ. A case of left inferior vena cava occurring in a female subject in whom the left superior intercostal vein joined the vena azygos major and the 12th ribs were absent. J Anat Physiol 1912;46:220–227.
48. Gladstone RJ. A case in which the right ureter passed behind the vena cava: with a short note upon a case in which the left renal vein passed behind the abdominal aorta, and the bearing of these abnormalities on the development of abdominal veins. J Anat Physiol 1911;45:225–231.
49. Milloy FJ, Anson BJ, Cauldwell EW. Variations in the inferior vena caval veins and in their renal and lumbar communications. Surg Gynecol Obstet 1962;115:131–142.
50. Wicke A. Quoted by Ferris EJ, et al. The inferior vena cava post ligation and plication. Radiology 1967;89:1–10.
51. Dharman K. Transcaval ureter. J Urol 1980;123:575–576.
52. Gladstone RJ. An acardiac foetus (acephalus-omphalositicus). J Anat Physiol 1905;40:71–80.
53. Brooks RE Jr. Left retrocaval ureter associated with situs inversus. J Urol 1962;88:484–487.
54. Hirsch DM Jr, Chan KF. Bilateral inferior vena cava. JAMA 1963;185:729–730.
55. Seib GA. The azygous system of veins in American whites and American Negroes, including observations on the inferior caval venous system. Am J Phys Anthropol 1934;19:39–163.
56. Reis RH, Esanther G. Variations in the pattern of renal vessels and their relation to the type of posterior cava in man. Am J Anat 1959;104:295–318.
57. Anderson RC, Heilig W, Novick R, et al. Anomalous inferior vena cava with azygos drainage: so-called absence of the inferior vena cava. Am Heart J 1955;49:318–322.
58. Campbell M, Deuchar DC. The left-sided superior vena cava. Br Heart J 1954;16:423–439.
59. Downing DF. Absence of the inferior vena cava. Pediatrics 1953;12:675–680.
60. Elliot LP, Cramer GG, Amplatz K. The anomalous relationship of the inferior vena cava and abdominal aorta as a specific angiocardiographic sign in asplenia. Radiology 1966;87:859–863.
61. Morgagni JB. Seats and causes of disease investigated by anatomy. London: Miller & Cadell, 1769; vol. 3.
62. Pleasants JH. Obstruction of the inferior vena cava with a report of 18 cases. Johns Hopkins Hosp Rep 1911;16:363–548.
63. Ferris EJ, Vittimberga FJ, Byrne JJ, et al. The inferior vena cava post ligation and plication. Radiology 1967;89:1–10.
64. Edwards EA. Functional anatomy of the portasystemic communications. Arch Intern Med 1951;88:137–154.
65. Batson OV. The function of the vertebral veins and their role in the spread of metastases. Ann Surg 1940;112:138–149.
66. Ahlberg NE, Bartley O, Chidekel N. Right and left gonadal veins: an anatomical and statistical study. Acta Radiol (Stockh) 1966;4:593–601.
67. Ahlberg NE, Bartley O, Chidekel N, et al. An anatomic and roentgenographic study of the communications of the renal

vein in patients with and without renal carcinoma. Scand J Urol Nephrol 1967;1:43–51.
68. Pick JW, Anson BJ. Renal vascular pedicle: anatomical study of 430 body-halves. J Urol 1940;44:411–434.
69. Ahlberg NE, Bartley O, Chidekel N. Retrograde contrast filling of the left gonadal vein: a roentgenologic and anatomical study. Acta Radiol (Stockh) 1965;3:385–392.
70. Berland LL, Maddison FE, Bernhard VM. Radiologic follow-up of vena cava filter devices. AJR 1980;134:1047–1052.
71. Bergstrand I, Ekman CA, Kohler R. IVC obstruction in hepatic cirrhosis. Acta Radiol (Stockh) 1964;2:1–8.
72. Kerr MG, Scott DB, Samuel E. Studies of the inferior vena cava in late pregnancy. Br Med J 1964;1:532–533.
73. Samuel E. The inferior vena cavogram in pregnancy. Proc R Soc Med 1964;57:702–704.
74. Kimura C, Shirotani H, Hirooka M, et al. Membranous obliteration of the inferior vena cava in its hepatic portion. J Cardiovasc Surg (Torino) 1963;4:87–98.
75. Jae Hoon Lim, Jae Hyung Park, Yong Ho Auh. Membranous obstruction of the inferior vena cava: comparison of findings at sonography, CT, and venography. AJR 1992;159:515–521.
76. Leiter E. Inferior vena caval thrombosis in malignant renal lesions. JAMA 1966;198:1167–1170.
76a. Ney C. Thrombosis of inferior vena cava associated with malignant renal tumors. J Urol 1946;55:583–590.
77. Ferris EJ, Bosniak MA, O'Connor JF. An angiographic sign demonstrating extension of renal carcinoma into the renal vein and vena cava. AJR 1986;108:384–391.
78. Mills SR, Doppman JL, Head GL, et al. Transcatheter brush biopsy of intravenous tumor thrombi. Radiology 1978;127:667–670.
79. Alpert J, Steinman C, Haimovici H. Suture plication of the inferior vena cava: a long-term experimental evaluation of plication channels. Arch Surg 1966;93:388–391.
80. Surington CT, Jonas AF Jr. Intraabdominal venography following inferior vena cava ligation. Arch Surg 1952;65:605–609.
81. Bergan JJ, Kinnaird DW, Koons K, et al. Prevention of pulmonary embolism: comparison of vena cava ligation, plication and filter operation. Arch Surg 1966;92:605–610.
82. Missal ME, Robinson JA, Tatum RW. Inferior vena cava obstruction: clinical manifestations, diagnostic methods and related problems. Ann Intern Med 1965;62:133–161.
83. Cope JS, Hunt CJ. Leiomyosarcoma of inferior vena cava. Arch Surg 1954;68:752–756.
84. Haug WA, Losi EJ. Primary leiomyosarcoma within the femoral vein. Cancer 1954;7:159–162.
85. Melchior E. Sarkom der vena cava inferior. Dtsch Z Chir 1928;213:135–140.
86. Doumanian HO, Amplatz K. The significance of the Bernoulli effect in selective angiocardiography. Presented at 14th Annual Meeting of the Association of University Radiologists, Little Rock, AK, May 12, 1966.
87. Weber J, May G von R. Phlebographie und Venendruckmessungim Abdomen und Becken. Baden-Baden: Gerhard Witzstrock, 1978:109.
88. Ferris EJ, Lim WN, Smith PL, et al. May-Thurner syndrome. Radiology 1983;147:29–31.

Section E: **THE THORACIC OUTLET**

39

Parathyroid Angiography

MARCELLE J. SHAPIRO
JOHN L. DOPPMAN

More than 90 percent of patients with primary hyperparathyroidism (PHPT) are cured by the first operation.[1] When arteriography and venous sampling were the only techniques available, localization was clearly reserved for patients with prior unsuccessful cervical exploration or prior thyroid surgery.[2] Over the past 15 years, newer imaging modalities, including nuclear medicine scanning, ultrasound (US), computed tomography (CT), and magnetic resonance imaging (MRI), have been introduced. Their noninvasiveness and reported efficacies have attracted attention and have tempted some to consider routine preoperative localization. However, none of the currently available studies approaches the ability of an experienced parathyroid surgeon in localizing hyperfunctioning glands and curing 92 to 98 percent of patients with the initial operation.[3–7a] In addition, the cost of this workup may be substantial. We therefore still maintain that "the only localizing study indicated in a patient with untreated primary hyperparathyroidism is to localize an experienced parathyroid surgeon."[8,8a] When is it then appropriate to consider preoperative localization studies, and where do parathyroid arteriography and venous sampling fit in this scheme?

Experienced surgeons have reported success rates of 89 to 91 percent with parathyroid reoperation.[9–11] However, the procedure may be more technically demanding, and success rates diminish with each additional procedure.[9] Complications, especially vocal cord paralysis, also increase with reoperation.[11,12] Moreover, because most abnormal glands in a juxtathyroid location tend to be excised with initial surgery, the incidence of ectopic glands, especially mediastinal glands, is increased with persistent hyperparathyroidism.[9,10,13–15] Given this background, it is uniformly agreed that preoperative localization is beneficial when reoperation is contemplated.[7–8a]

Because of the greater risk and potential discomfort with invasive procedures, noninvasive procedures are initiated first. In patients with persistent hyperparathyroidism following prior unsuccessful surgery, the reported sensitivities for noninvasive imaging modalities[7,7a,16–20] are as follows: thallium-technetium scintigraphy: 26 to 68 percent; sonography (US): 36 to 76 percent; CT: 46 to 55 percent; and MRI: 50 to 78 percent. False-positive rates[7,7a,16–19] have been reported as high as 23 percent with thallium-technetium scintigraphy; 44 percent with US; 57 percent with CT; and 30 percent with MRI, all of which are substantial. Technetium 99m sestamibi, a newer agent initially introduced for myocardial perfusion imaging as an alternative to thallium 201, has been applied to parathyroid imaging alone and in combination with iodine 123 subtraction imaging of the thyroid.[21–25] Preliminary experience suggests that this agent, especially in combination with iodine 123 subtraction imaging of the thyroid,[25] may be more sensitive and have lower false-positive rates than those encountered with other noninvasive modalities. However, larger prospective, comparative studies are needed before this newer agent and technique may be universally recommended. It is therefore held that the results of at least two noninvasive examinations should agree for definitive localization.[7,7a] In an earlier series by Miller et al., when CT, US, and scintigraphy were performed, adenoma localization was successful on at least one study in 78 percent.[16] However, only 31 percent had an adenoma identified on at least two studies.[16] If the results of noninvasive studies remain discordant, invasive procedures should be considered, beginning with percutaneous CT- or US-guided aspiration before moving on to arteriography or selective venous sampling.

Percutaneous Aspiration for Parathyroid Hormone (PTH) Assay

Doppman initially aspirated 14 parathyroid adenomas, the adjacent thyroid gland, and sternocleidomastoid muscle at the time of surgical exposure and showed that elevated parathyroid hormone levels were found only in parathyroid glands.[26,26a] This subsequently led to percutaneous aspiration under US or CT guidance as a means of localization.[26,26a] Several gentle to-and-fro motions of a 23-gauge needle are made into the suspicious gland identified by US or CT followed by aspiration of saline through the needle to a total volume of 1 ml. PTH assay is performed on this sample; gradients have ranged from 10 to greater than 1 million in the National Institutes of Health (NIH) experience.[8,8a] Percutaneous aspiration is therefore recommended as the initial invasive technique for confirming an adenoma when a mass is demonstrated by US or CT.[7–8a] Doppman has reported greater than 50 percent successful localization in reoperative patients when this combination is used.[8,8a,26,26a] However, if localization remains unreliable, arteriography and venous sampling should be considered.

Parathyroid Arteriography

Digital subtraction arteriography (DSA) has simplified the approach to parathyroid arteriography over the past 15 years.[27] In general, diagnostic studies may be performed with injection of the innominate, subclavian, and carotid arteries while imaging over the neck and mediastinum. In an early series from the NIH, over 70 to 80 percent of glands seen on conventional selective arteriography were seen on intraarterial DSA imaging.[27] However, the area in which glands were frequently missed with DSA was the anterior mediastinum.[28] When intraarterial DSA is unrevealing, conventional selective arteriography of bilateral thyrocervical

Figure 39-1. (A) A selective left inferior thyroid arteriogram produces a dense thyroid staining with fleeting opacification of a deep mediastinal adenoma (*arrow*). Without reflux this adenoma might not have been opacified. (B) More proximal injection reveals an early branch of the inferior thyroid artery (*small arrows*) supplying a typical anterior mediastinal adenoma (*large arrow*).

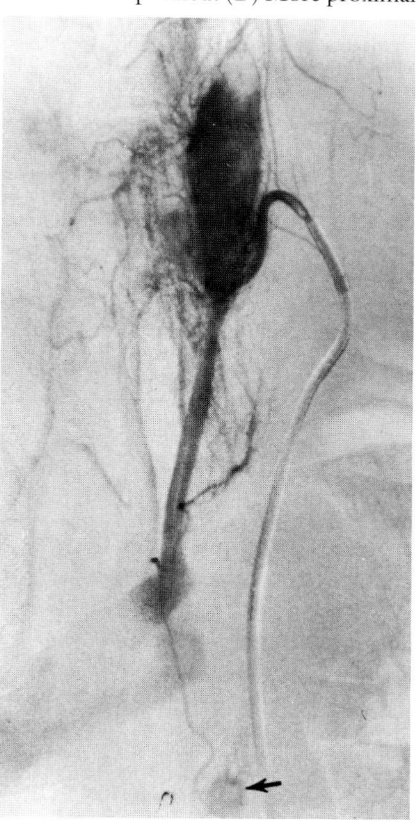

A

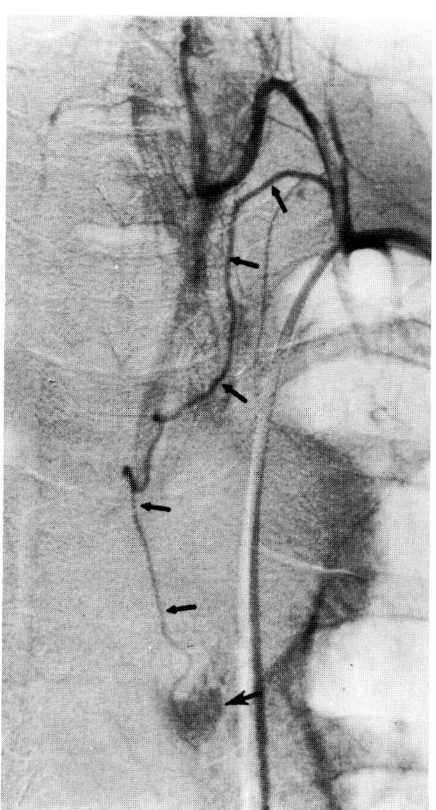

B

trunks, internal mammary, and superior thyroid arteries should be performed because the glands not seen on DSA will be identified.[27] In elderly patients, uncoiling of the aorta and tortuosity of the innominate and subclavian arteries may render selective thyrocervical and internal mammary catheterization from a transfemoral route extremely difficult. Under such circumstances, a transbrachial or transaxillary approach should be considered.

Advancing the catheter deep into the inferior thyroid artery may cause excessive staining of the thyroid lobe and may obscure parathyroid pathology. In addition, the blood supply to a mediastinal adenoma may arise quite proximally from the inferior thyroid artery (Fig. 39-1) or thyrocervical trunk (Fig. 39-2) and be missed by a distal injection.

An inferior thyroid artery may supply the contralateral thyroid lobe and a contralateral parathyroid adenoma (Fig. 39-3), especially when the ipsilateral inferior thyroid artery has been ligated or when thyroid tissue has been resected.

The internal mammary artery sometimes arises from a common stem with the thyrocervical trunk off the anterior rather than the inferior margin of the subclavian artery (Fig. 39-4). Multiple anterior intercostal arteries arise from the medial margin of the internal mammary artery and arc laterally to supply anterior intercostal spaces. A prominent pericardiophrenic

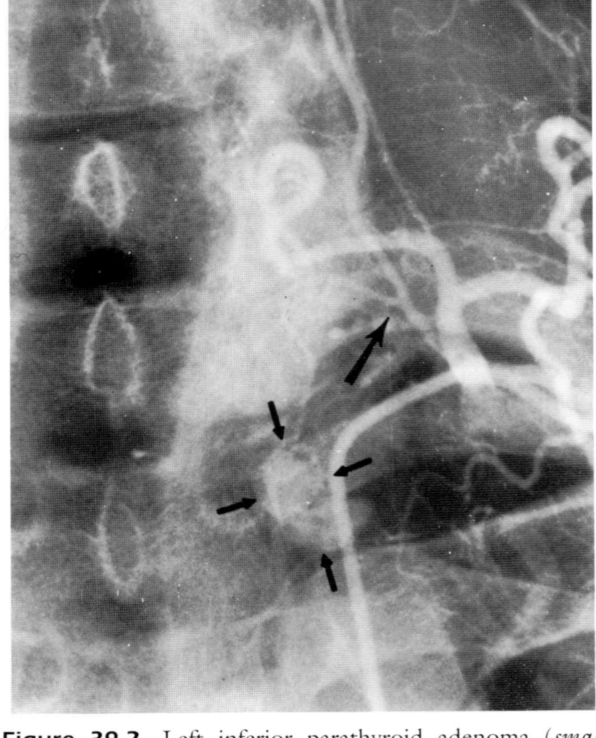

Figure 39-2. Left inferior parathyroid adenoma (*small arrows*) supplied by ascending cervical branch (*large arrow*) of thyrocervical trunk. A selective inferior thyroid injection would miss this adenoma.

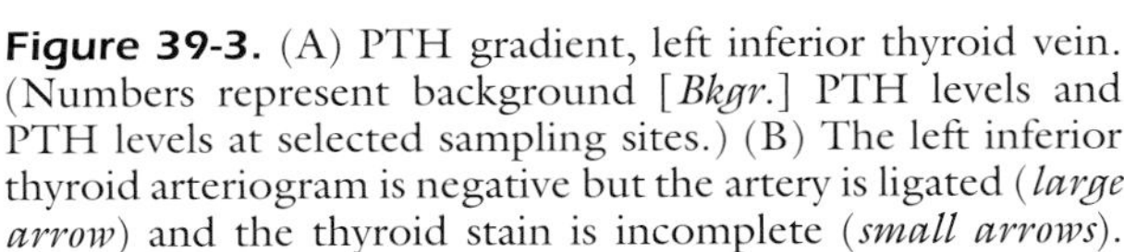

Figure 39-3. (A) PTH gradient, left inferior thyroid vein. (Numbers represent background [*Bkgr.*] PTH levels and PTH levels at selected sampling sites.) (B) The left inferior thyroid arteriogram is negative but the artery is ligated (*large arrow*) and the thyroid stain is incomplete (*small arrows*). (C) The right inferior thyroid artery supplies the medial part of the left thyroid lobe (*small arrows*) and a left inferior parathyroid adenoma (*large arrows*). Arteriography based solely on venous sampling results might have failed to inject the right inferior thyroid artery.

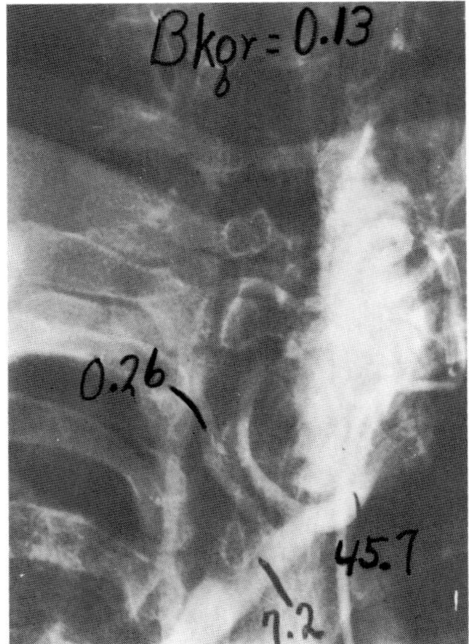

A

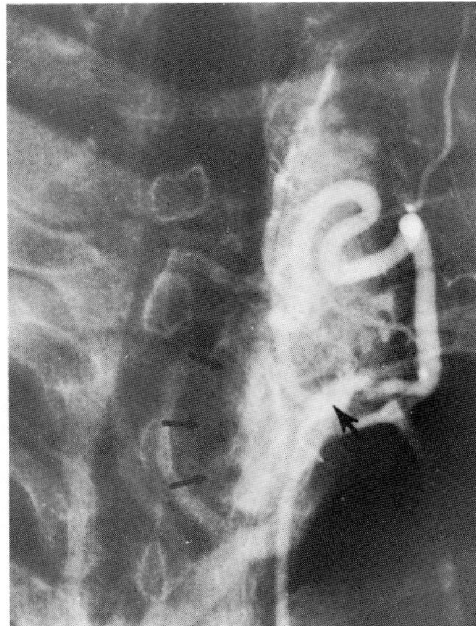

B

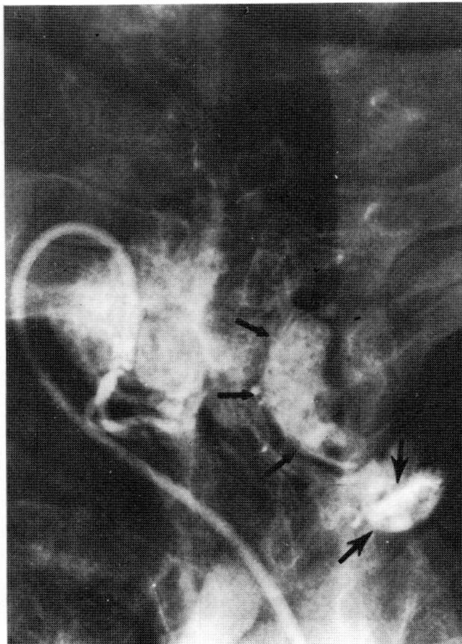

C

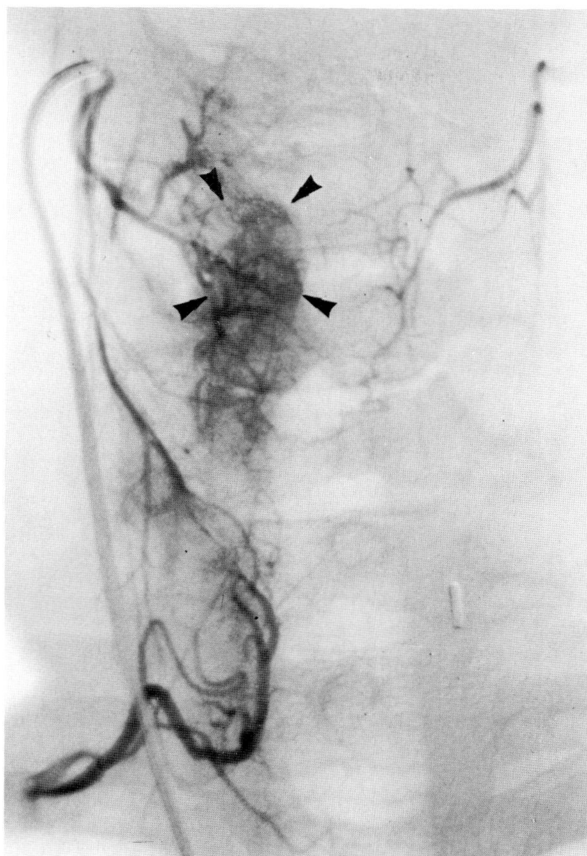

Figure 39-10. Normal stain of endolarynx and vocal cords (*arrowheads*) during superior thyroid arteriography. Note that the wedged selective injection of the right superior thyroid artery fills the right inferior and left superior thyroid arteries by reflux, thereby expediting arteriographic studies.

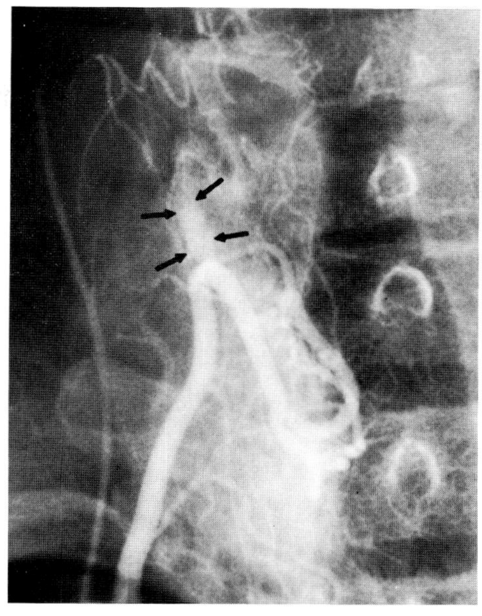

A

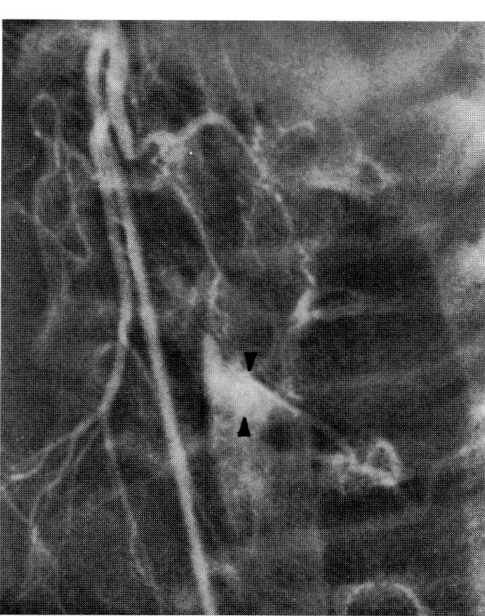

B

Figure 39-11. Small—3 × 6 mm in (A), 3 × 3 mm in (B)—hyperplastic parathyroid glands (*arrows,* A; *arrowheads,* B) demonstrated by selective arteriography. Both cases were surgically verified.

◀ **Figure 39-9.** (A) PTH gradient in left inferior thyroid vein suggests posterior mediastinal adenoma (*arrows*). (Numbers represent PTH levels at selected sampling sites.) (B) Left inferior thyroid arteriogram fails to reveal adenoma because of ligated thyroid artery (*arrow*). (C) Superior thyroid arteriogram opacifies the distal inferior thyroid artery and reveals a small branch (*arrows*) leading to (D) a parathyroid adenoma in the posterior superior mediastinum (*arrows*).

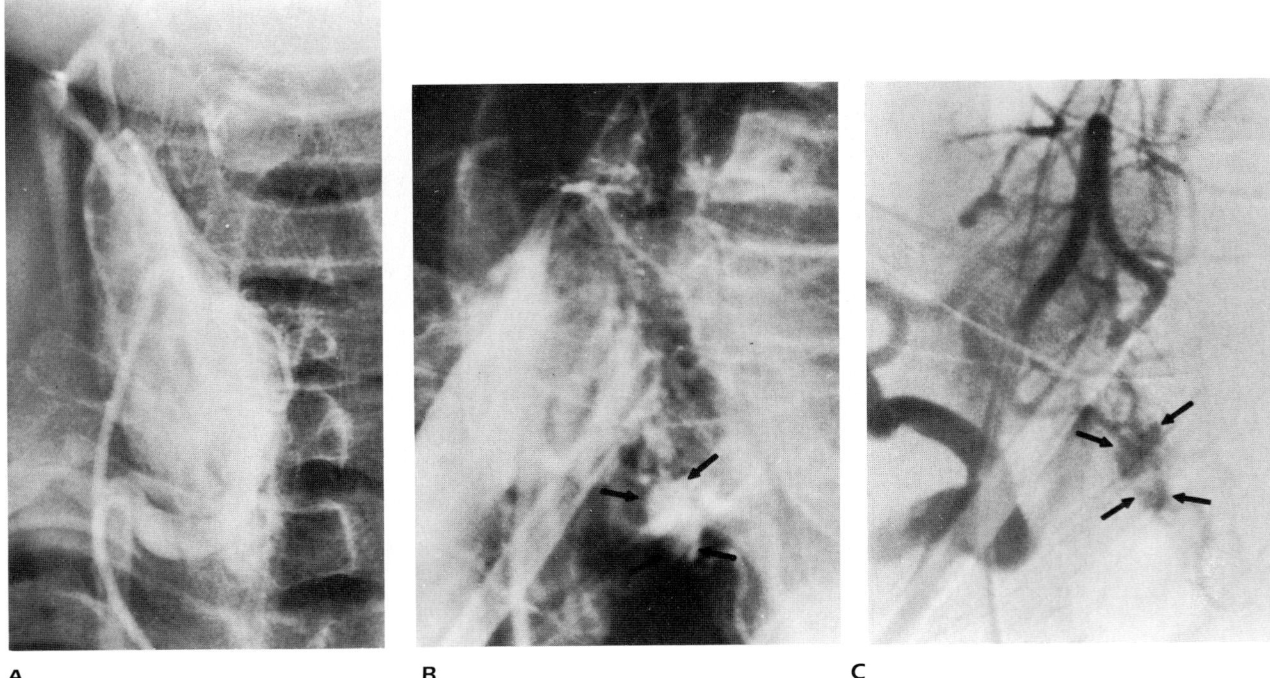

Figure 39-12. (A) Posterior mediastinal adenoma almost completely obscured by overlying thyroid gland on anteroposterior projection. (B) Oblique projection demonstrates adenoma (*arrows*), seen still better (C) on subtraction film (*arrows*).

Complications

The principal risk of parathyroid arteriography is damage to the spinal cord with resultant quadriplegia. This results from excessive quantities of contrast material selectively injected into the costocervical trunk, which commonly provides a major radiculomedullary branch to the anterior spinal artery at the cervicothoracic level. Wedging of the catheter in this small vessel is difficult to avoid, and injection in a wedged position may be particularly likely to damage the cord. Although often incriminated in these accidents, the thyrocervical trunk rarely supplies vessels to the cord. In more than 1000 thyrocervical trunk injections, subtracted and scrutinized for spinal cord blood supply, one of the authors (JLD) has encountered only three convincing examples. However, the costocervical trunk may be confused with the thyrocervical trunk on anteroposterior fluoroscopy, especially when the inferior thyroid artery has been ligated at the initial operation. In the large NIH experience with parathyroid arteriography no spinal complications have occurred.[2]

Parathyroid Venous Sampling

Selective venous sampling requires extensive experience[2] and may be time-consuming even in the best of hands because sampling from small veins is necessary to provide useful information. The need for venous sampling has been substantially reduced since percutaneous aspiration under CT or US guidance has come into use. In the rare circumstance when all other noninvasive and invasive studies are indeterminate, venous sampling may help to define a region for reexploration.[36]

Parathyroid glands in the neck drain into the ipsilateral inferior thyroid veins, which generally join to form a common inferior thyroid vein before entering the left innominate vein (Fig. 39-15).[35–38] As elsewhere, variations in venous anatomy are almost routine, and accessory inferior veins, especially on the left side, are common. In addition, the inferior thyroid veins are frequently ligated as the thyroid gland is mobilized during the initial unsuccessful operation. For these reasons, a road map of the venous drainage patterns

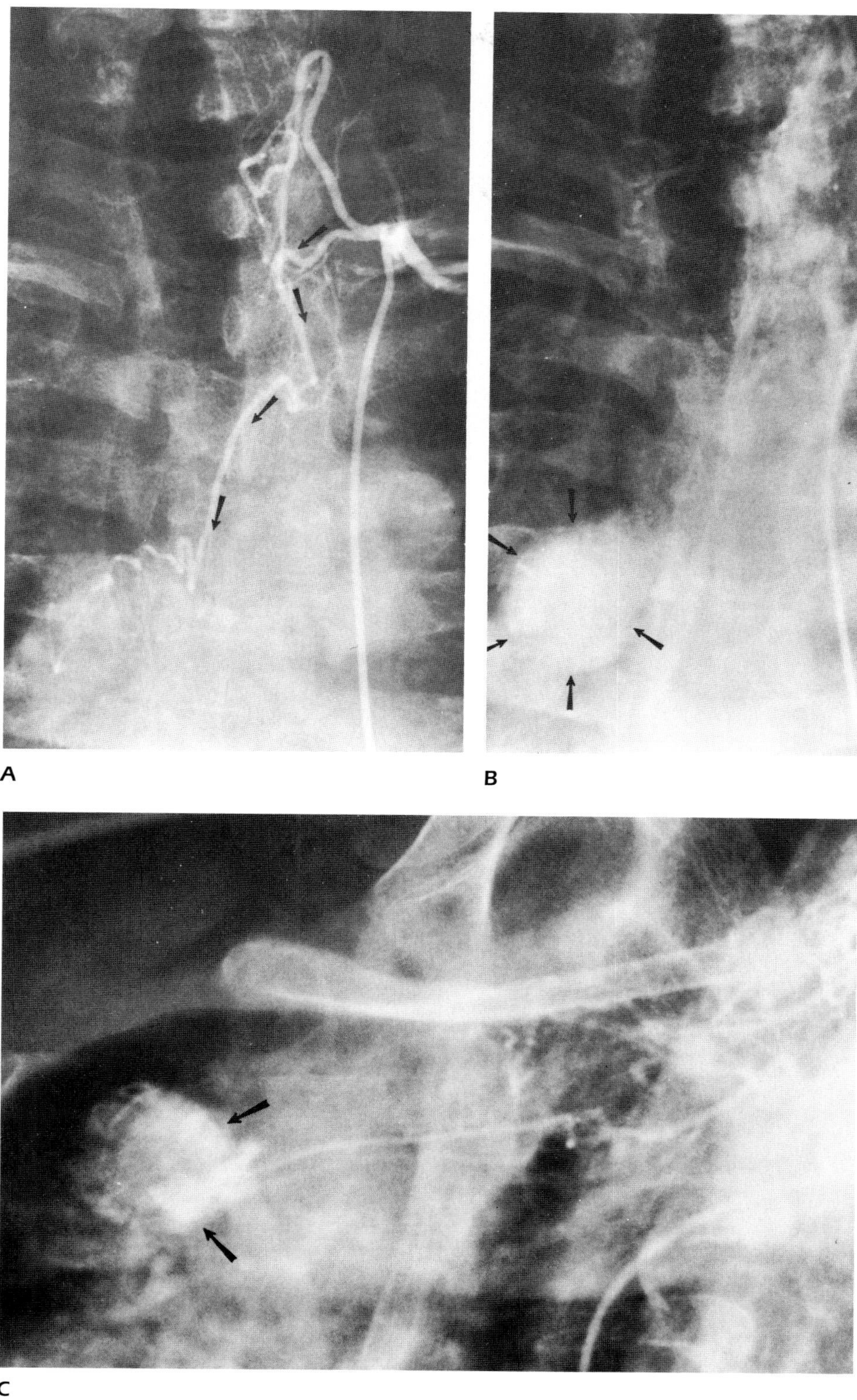

Figure 39-13. Blood supply (*arrows,* A) descending from the left inferior thyroid artery to an anterior mediastinal parathyroid adenoma (*arrows,* B). Note on steep oblique projection (C) the far anterior position of the gland (*arrows*).

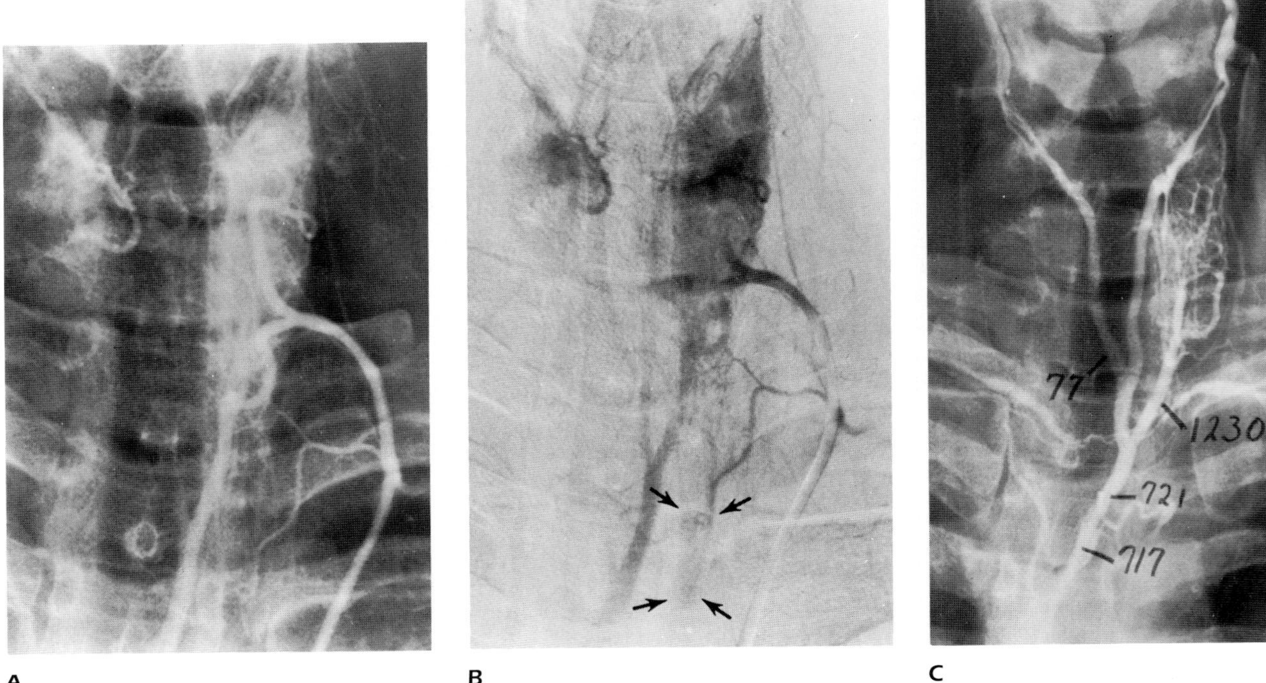

A B C

Figure 39-14. Unsubtracted inferior thyroid arteriogram (A) fails to reveal left inferior adenoma easily identified on subtracted studies (*arrows,* B). (C) Note the excellent correlation with venous sampling. (Numbers represent PTH levels at selected sampling sites.)

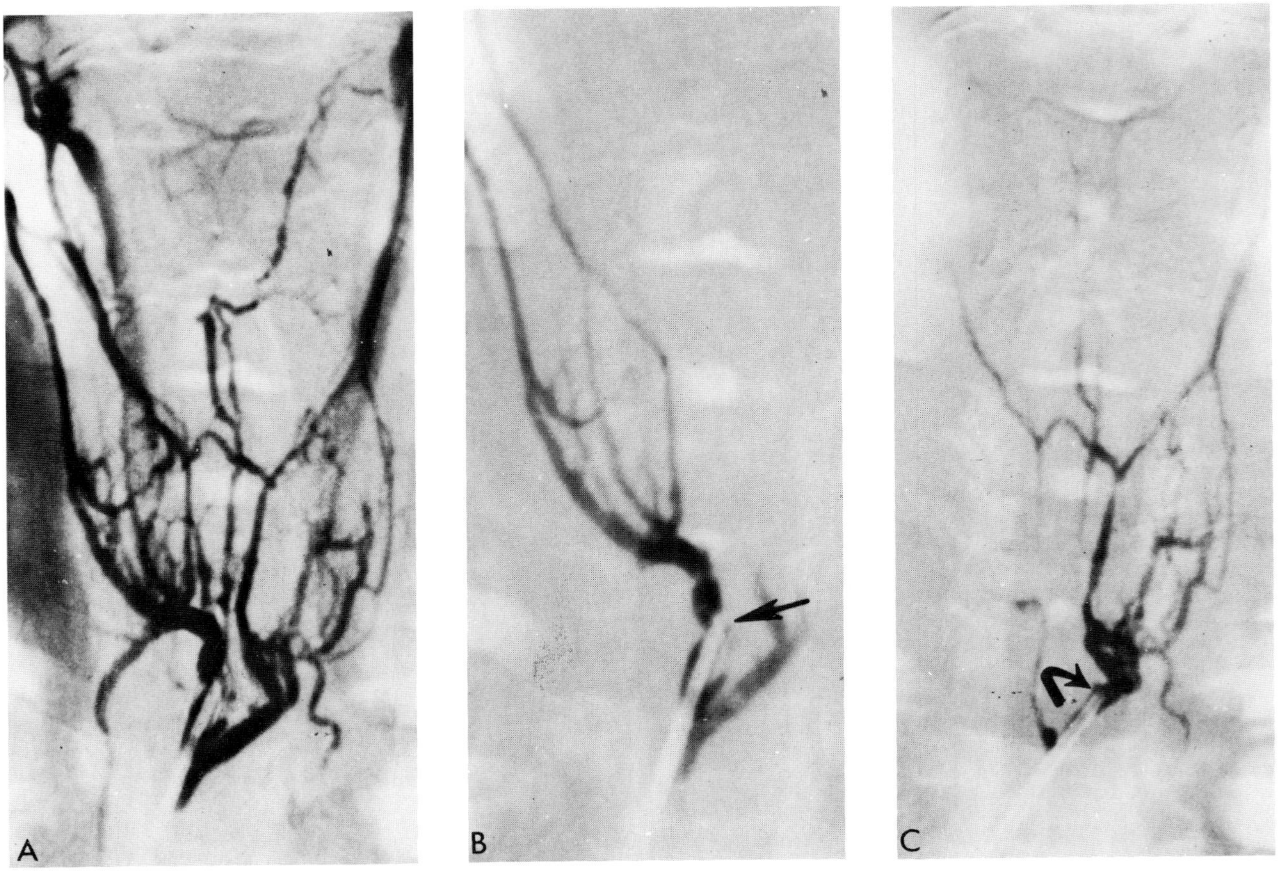

derived from delayed arteriographic films is an invaluable aid when one is undertaking venous sampling. Knowing precisely where to look greatly expedites this often tedious investigation.

The common inferior thyroid vein drains into the superior margin of the left innominate vein, often quite close to the junction with the right innominate vein. The catheter must be advanced into the right and left inferior thyroid veins to obtain samples of lateralizing value. Parathyroid glands always drain into the thyroid veins descending along the lateral margin of the thyroid lobe[38]; samples from medial lobar and isthmic veins are of no value (Fig. 39-16).

Parathyroid adenomas produce unilateral PTH gradients[35,39–42]; samples from the contralateral inferior thyroid vein are background (inferior vena cava, IVC) level, because the remaining normal parathyroid glands are suppressed. Primary hyperplasia results in bilateral but often unequal PTH gradients, since hyperplasia is generally an asymmetric process. Elevations of PTH more than two times background (IVC) level are considered significant, but much higher gradients are not unusual in selective thyroid veins.[43]

Valves guard the ostia of most thyroid veins, and negotiating the catheter through these leaflets may be very time-consuming. Although appearing rather delicate, they cannot be deliberately perforated with the catheter tip without a major risk of venous wall perforation. When veins are particularly tortuous in elderly patients, drinking will momentarily straighten them as the thyroid gland ascends and may permit catheter advancement. Once a catheter is well positioned, aspirating a blood sample can be equally frustrating. Gentle suction to avoid venous collapse, turning the head, the Valsalva maneuver, and siphonage may all prove helpful. A single radiograph with minimal contrast injection should be obtained with each sample to record catheter position. A forceful large-volume retrograde venogram (see Fig. 39-16) at this stage will display the complete thyroid venous bed and expedite the subsequent catheterizations.

The thymic vein of Keynes drains into the inferior margin of the left innominate vein. A PTH elevation in this vein suggests a parathyroid adenoma in the anterior mediastinum. However, major anastomoses between the inferior thyroid and the thymic veins are common, especially on the left side (Fig. 39-17). PTH elevations in the thymic vein with cervical adenomas as well as PTH elevations in cervical veins with mediastinal adenomas have been noted. Venous drainage patterns from the arteriographic study usually help to clarify such problems.

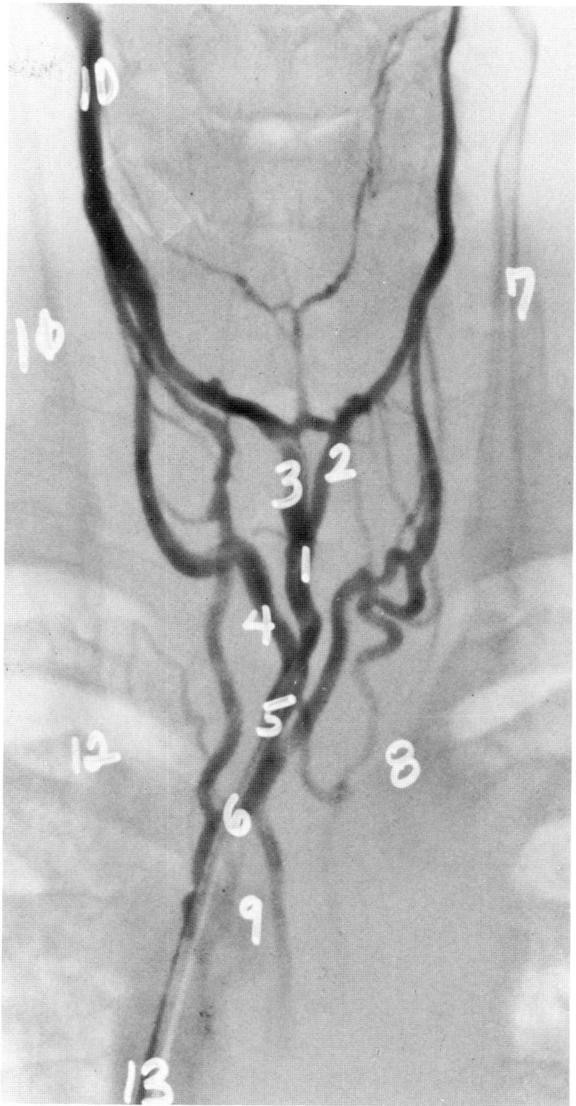

Figure 39-16. Typical "road map" of venous samples. Midline isthmic samples (*1, 2, 3*) never provide useful information. Samples *4, 5, 6,* and *8* reflect drainage along lateral thyroid lobes and usually provide the significant information because of lateral drainage of parathyroid glands.

Samples from the middle and superior thyroid veins are rarely helpful unless all inferior veins have been ligated and venous drainage from the thyroid bed is pre-

◀ **Figure 39-15.** Normal thyroid venous anatomy (A) with selective samples from the right (B) and left (C) inferior thyroid veins (*arrows*).

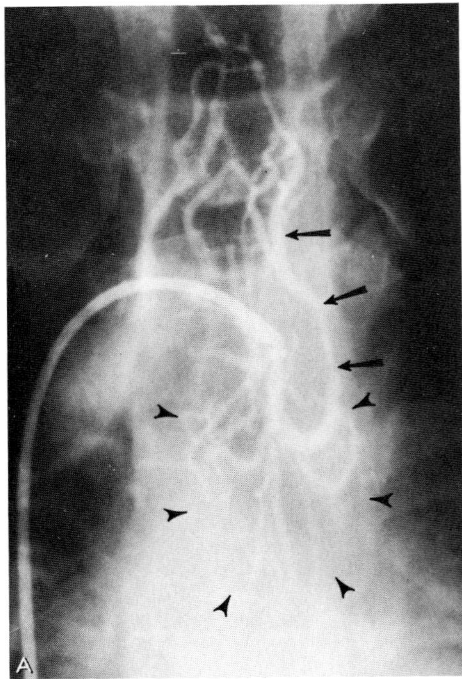

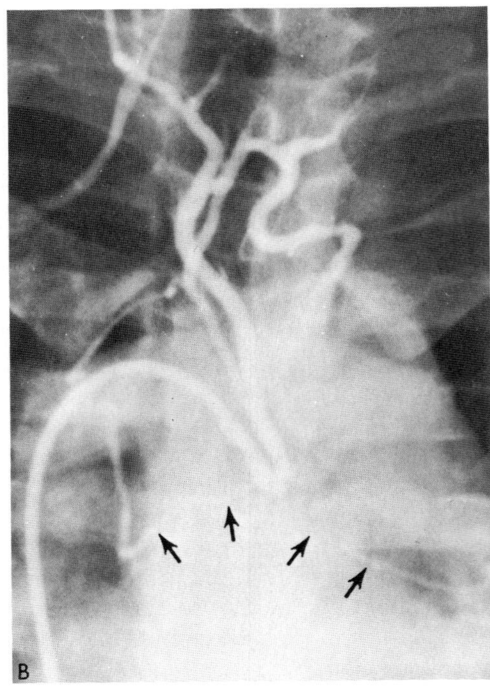

Figure 39-17. Left (A) and right (B) inferior thyroid veins draining into thymic vein. *Arrowheads* (A) and *arrows* (B) show intrathymic branches; *arrows* (A) show left inferior thyroid vein.

dominantly craniad. Even under such circumstances, the vertebral veins are the more common collateral channels, and these veins frequently have elevated PTH levels when the overlooked adenoma is in the neck or tracheoesophageal groove, the most common site for an ectopic superior gland.

Large-vein samples (jugular veins, innominate veins, superior vena cava) are generally unhelpful.[44] Elevations of PTH in these veins are often equivocal and difficult to interpret in comparison to the unequivocal gradients in selective veins. Interpreting PTH gradients in the left innominate vein is particularly treacherous because the mediastinum and both sides of the neck drain into this same vessel. Looking for peripheral PTH gradients after unilateral neck massage is also of no value in this group of patients undergoing repeat surgery.[45,46]

Adenomas are occasionally stained by forceful retrograde venous injections. More frequently helpful than staining has been the demonstration of a capsular or circumscribing vein surrounding the adenoma.[47] When the appropriate artery cannot be catheterized, a forceful injection into the appropriate vein containing the elevated PTH level may reveal the site of the occult gland. Intrathyroid parathyroid glands, the surgeon's justification for resecting thyroid tissue, are rare and are usually identified by intraoperative ultrasound.[48]

Mediastinal Adenomas

The most notorious of the ectopic parathyroid sites and the one immortalized by the case of Captain Martel lies in the *anterior* mediastinum[49]; however, the posterior superior mediastinum is the site of the most frequently overlooked parathyroid glands. For embryologic, arteriographic, and surgical considerations, it is helpful to divide mediastinal adenomas into these two categories.[30,49,50]

Posterior Superior Mediastinal Adenomas

The posterior superior mediastinum is bounded anteriorly by the trachea, inferiorly by the transverse aorta, and posteriorly by the upper four thoracic vertebrae. Although glands in this compartment may appear on anteroposterior arteriograms to lie above the manubrium, and thus in the neck, they are actually posterior in the tracheoesophageal groove. This is the most common site for an overlooked parathyroid gland both in Wang's experience[10,50–52] and in the NIH experience.[53] Such glands are *ectopic superior* parathyroids. Their arterial supply always arises from the inferior thyroid artery; they can usually be recovered from the neck because they never descend deeply. Because these adenomas lie behind the trachea, they may overlap the

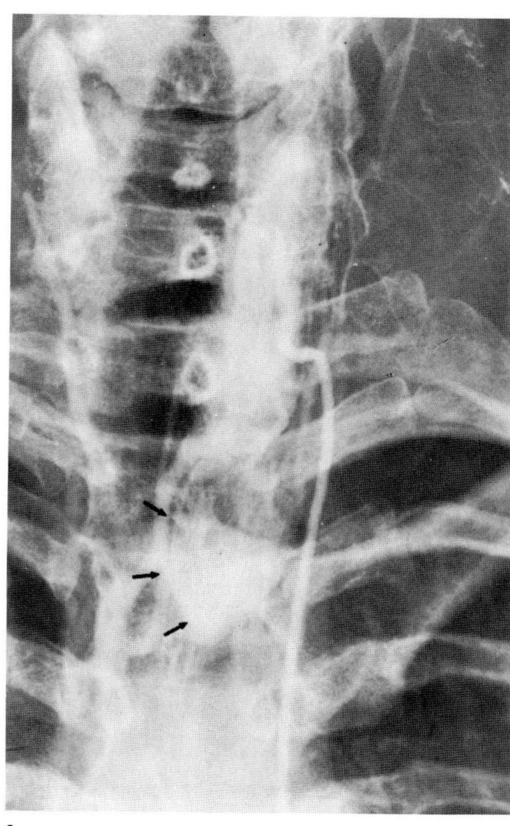

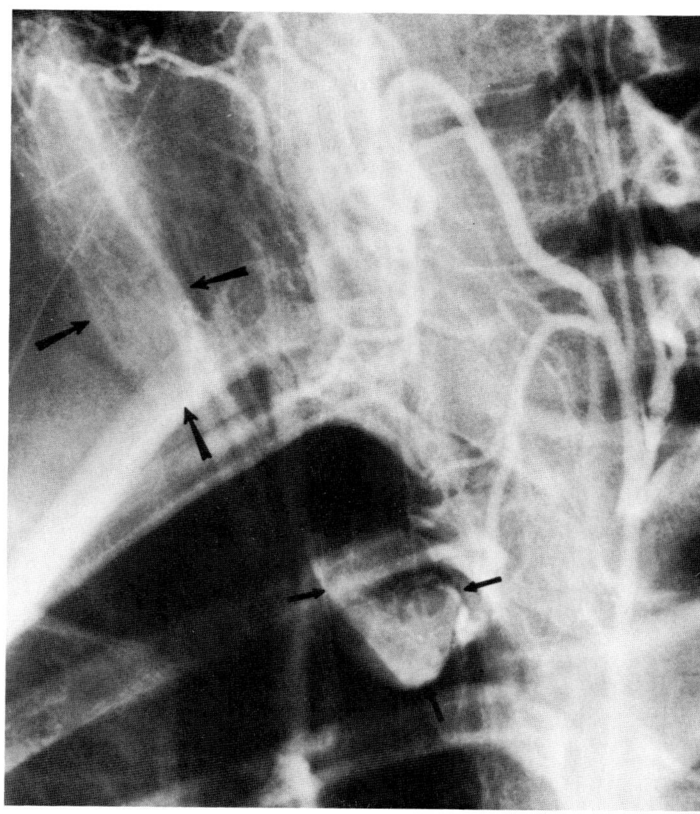

A B

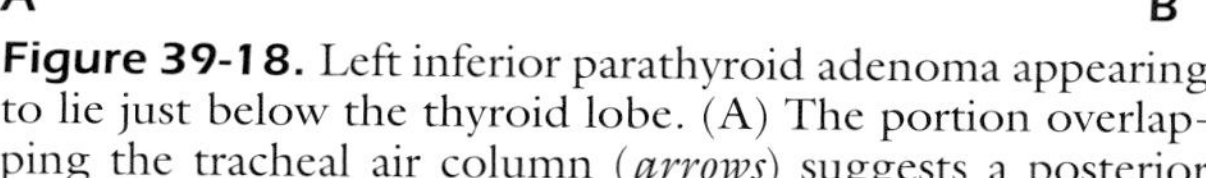

Figure 39-18. Left inferior parathyroid adenoma appearing to lie just below the thyroid lobe. (A) The portion overlapping the tracheal air column (*arrows*) suggests a posterior mediastinal location. (B) The site is verified on steep oblique projection (*small arrows*); note the anterior location of the thyroid lobe (*large arrows*).

tracheal air column on anteroposterior angiograms (Fig. 39-18), thereby providing a clue to their posterior location.[54]

Anterior Mediastinal Adenomas

Ectopic parathyroid glands in the anterior mediastinum are inferior glands that originate and descend with the thymus.[51] They may lie as low as the pulmonary artery in the aorticopulmonary window. Their blood supply either descends from the inferior thyroid artery or arises from the thymic branch of the internal mammary artery. Venous drainage parallels the arterial supply either into the neck (inferior thyroid vein) or into the thymic vein (never into the internal mammary vein). Glands with an inferior thyroid vascular leash tend to be extracted with the thymus from the cervical incision.[29,30] Deeper glands with an internal mammary blood supply resist extraction and often require a median sternotomy. These glands are rarely visualized on chest radiographs but are frequently demonstrated on CT[32] and MRI[19] because of the contrast provided by the fat-filled mediastinum (Fig. 39-19), especially in older patients.

Figure 39-19. CT scan demonstrating a parathyroid adenoma (*arrowhead*) of the anterior mediastinum. Note the contrast provided by mediastinal fat.

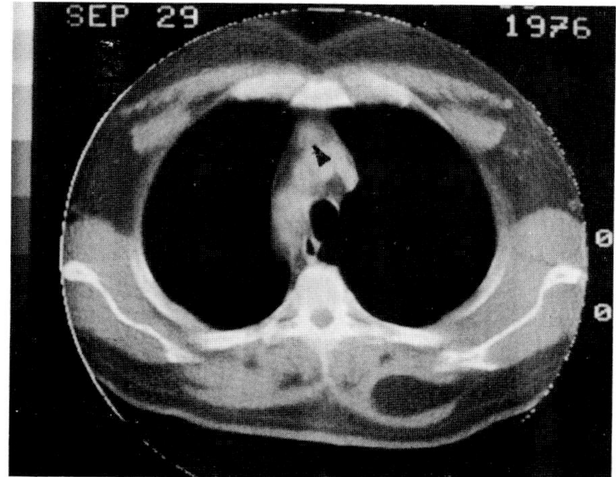

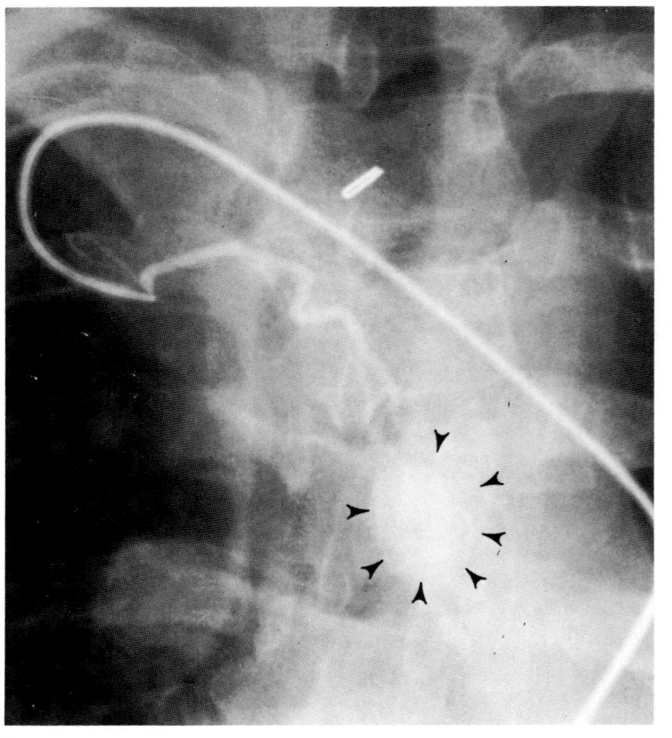

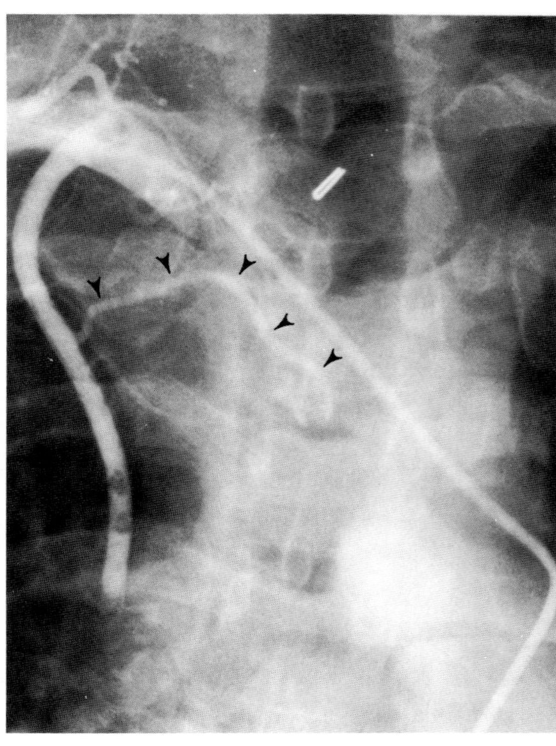

Figure 39-20. (A) Selective arteriogram of thymic branch supplying an anterior mediastinal adenoma (*arrowheads*). (B) Because wedging is unavoidable, the gland was densely stained prior to Gelfoam embolization (*arrowheads*) of the feeding artery.

In a review of the NIH experience with patients who had undergone prior surgery, invasive procedures permitted successful localization of adenomas in 95 percent of patients in whom noninvasive tests were unrevealing.[13] The combination of noninvasive and invasive studies provided correct localization in 96 percent of reoperated patients.[13]

Transcatheter Therapy

In addition to parathyroid localization, radiologic techniques may be used to ablate abnormal glands. Doppman et al. pioneered the angiographic approach to parathyroid adenoma ablation in the early 1970s after recognizing that occasional spontaneous infarction of an adenoma can occur with resolution of hypercalcemia.[55] A variety of embolic agents were initially employed[55–57]; however, success was limited by incomplete glandular infarction with persistent hypercalcemia. A single patient cured by embolization had her gland inadvertently stained with contrast medium during catheter placement for embolization (Fig. 39-20). Because several additional patients became temporarily hypocalcemic after accidental staining during arteriography, a study of deliberate contrast medium extravasation as a method of ablating parathyroid function was initiated.[58] The technique of parenchymal staining involved deliberately extravasating contrast medium into the interstitium of a gland by controlled hyperfusion.[59–61] The catheter should be wedged into the feeding artery to achieve the perfusion pressure required to accelerate transcapillary passage of opaque contrast medium. According to the original NIH experience, wedging was vital to the success of the procedure because ablation failed in 75 percent of patients in whom wedging could not be achieved but was successful in 85 percent of patients in whom it was achieved.[61] Once a catheter is wedged, the manual injection of 15 to 20 ml of contrast medium produces maximal capillary dilatation, reflected by early and intense venous filling. This is followed by increased opacification of the adenoma as undiluted contrast agent transudes into the interstitial spaces (Fig. 39-21). Cellular damage is caused by a combination of hyperosmotic and chemotoxic effects of the undiluted contrast medium. In the presence of a capsule, such as that seen around the parathyroid gland, acute

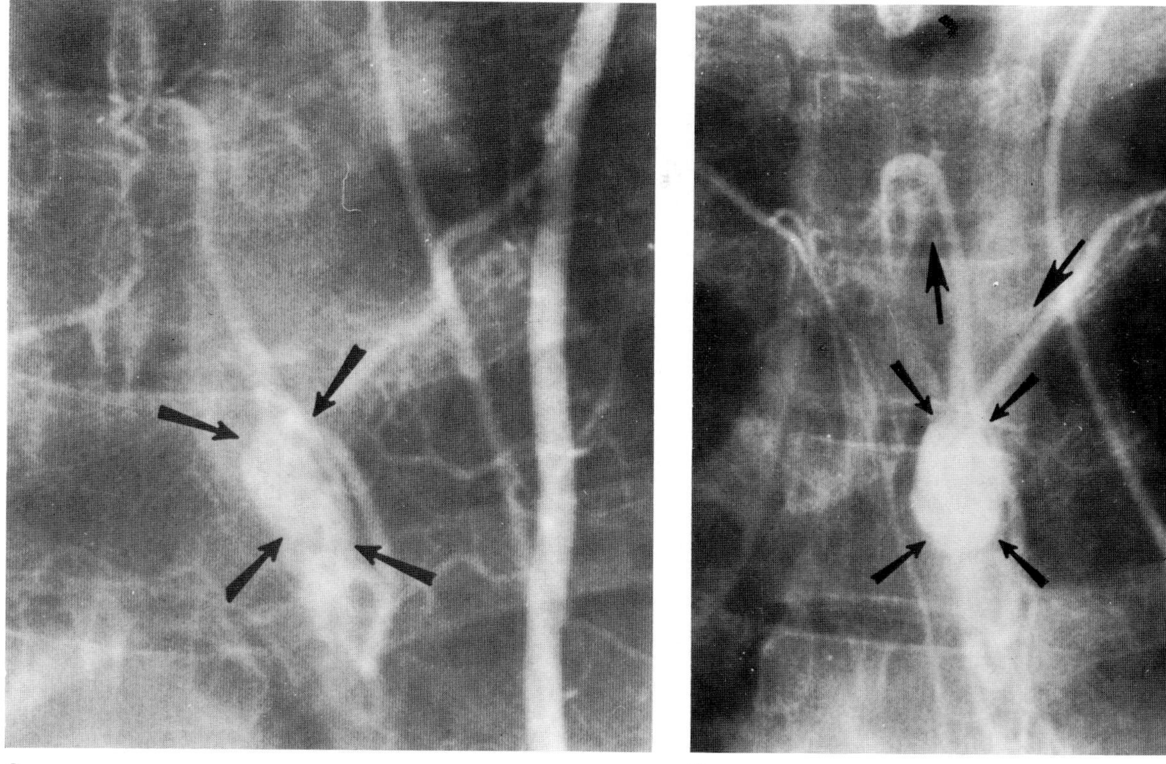

Figure 39-21. (A) Anterior mediastinal adenoma (*arrows*) with blood supply from the left internal mammary artery. (B) Staining (*small arrows*) during selective injection of 15 ml contrast material. Note the dense opacification of the vein as well as of the artery (*large arrows*).

edema induced by contrast extravasation may also temporarily decrease blood flow to the gland, adding an ischemic injury as well.[62] Retrosternal burning is experienced during perfusion but rapidly disappears as soon as the catheter is withdrawn. Local anesthetics may be added to the perfusate.

Although conventional wedging is essential when staining "from a distance" with conventional catheters the use of a Tracker catheter has enabled the angiographer to place the catheter tip very close to the adenoma and staining can be accomplished without wedging. A prolonged perfusion of ionic contrast through the Tracker positioned close to the adenoma will stain as effectively as the old "wedged" technique and spares extensive staining of the ipsilateral thymic lobe.

When properly stained, the gland remains opaque up to 24 hours (Fig. 39-22), and residual intraglandular iodine by CT scanning has been detected as late as 72 hours. With successful ablation, serum levels of calcium drop within the ensuing 24 to 48 hours, a response similar to that following surgical excision.

The largest series with the longest follow-up published using this technique is from the NIH.[14,61] In this series of 24 patients who had undergone at least one prior unsuccessful surgical resection, the success rate at 1 month after ablation was 83 percent and 71 percent at 5 and 9 years after ablation.[61] Twenty-three of the adenomas were in the mediastinum. Acute complications were not encountered when glands supplied by a thymic artery arising from the internal mammary artery were ablated. However, vasovagal reactions and/or acute thyroiditis were seen when ablation of neck glands was performed via the superior or inferior thyroid artery.[61]

Objections to staining as an alternative to sternotomy center about the lack of tissue for (1) histologic examination and (2) transplantation.[63,64] Parathyroid carcinoma is rare,[65] and a suggestion of malignancy is often available from other modalities. Concerning the lack of tissue for transplantation, when the patient has already undergone surgical exploration, the number of remaining glands and adequacy of their blood supply are not completely known. Therefore, ablation of the only remaining functioning gland will likely cause irreversible hypoparathyroidism. In the NIH series,[61] permanent hypocalcemia developed in 8 percent of pa-

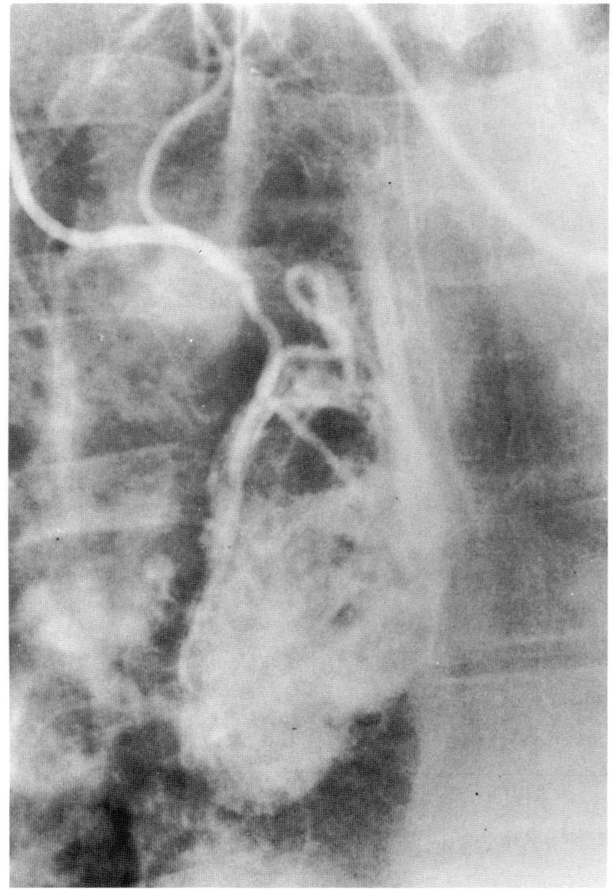

A

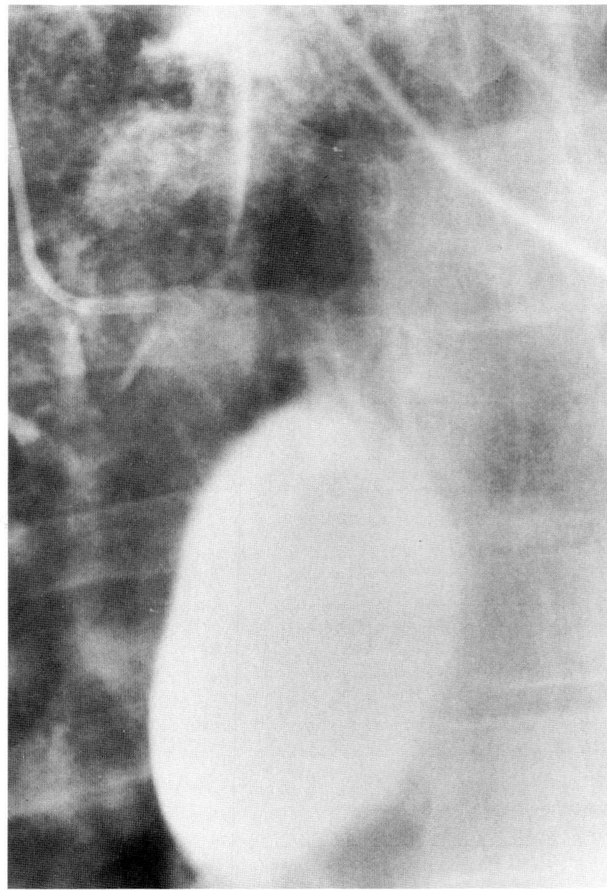

B

Figure 39-22. (A) Large anterior mediastinal adenoma supplied by right internal mammary artery. (B) Two hours after staining, the gland is intensely opacified. (C) At 24 hours, lateral chest film shows persistent staining.

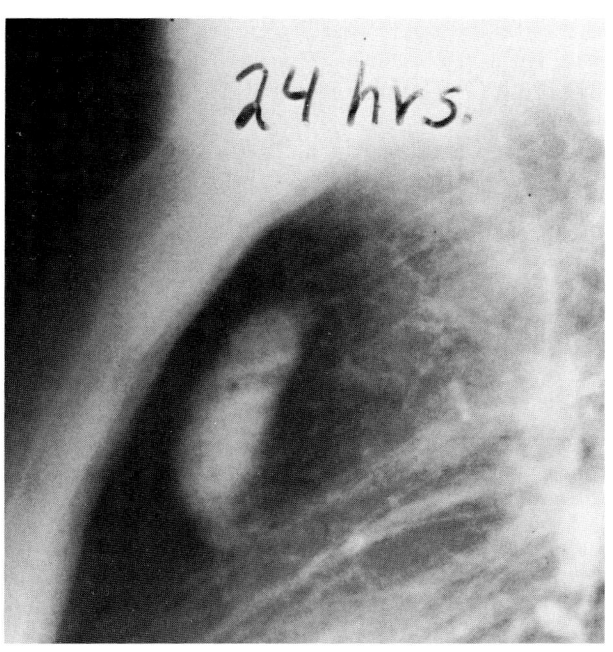

C

tients treated with ablation, which is comparable to the incidence reported after parathyroid reoperation *without* autotransplantation.[66] Therefore, when it is known that three or more glands have been resected, surgery with cryopreservation of the resected glands, with an option for delayed autotransplantation, is recommended.[7,7a] Ablation is reserved only for poor surgical candidates. In addition, the location of the gland is an important consideration. Only glands in the mediastinum are considered for ablation with contrast because of the risk of injury to the recurrent laryngeal nerve with ablation of glands in the neck.[7,7a]

References

1. Satava RM, Beahres OH, Scholz DA. Success rate of cervical exploration for hyperparathyroidism. Arch Surg 1975;110:625–628.
2. Doppman JL. Parathyroid localization: arteriography and venous sampling. Radiol Clin North Am 1976;14:163–188.
3. van Heerden JA, James EM, Karsel PR, et al. Small part ultrasonography in primary hyperparathyroidism. Ann Surg 1982;195:774–780.
4. Attie JN, Khan A, Rumancik WM, et al. Preoperative localization of parathyroid adenomas. Am J Surg 1988;156:323–326.
5. Thompson NW. Localization studies in patients with primary hyperparathyroidism. Br J Surg 1988;75:97–98.
6. Russell CF, Edis AJ. Surgery for primary hyperparathyroidism: experience with 500 consecutive cases and evaluation of the role of surgery in the asymptomatic patient. Br J Surg 1982;69:244–247.
7. Miller DL. Pre-operative localization and interventional treatment of parathyroid tumors: when and how? World J Surg 1991;15:706–715.

7a. Doppman JL, Miller DL. Localization of parathyroid tumors in patients with asymptomatic hyperthyroidism and no previous surgery. J Bone Min Res 1991;6(2):S153–S158.

8. Doppman JL. Reoperative parathyroid surgery: localization procedures. Prog Surg 1986;18:117–132.

8a. MacFarlane MP, Fraker DL, Shawker TH, et al. Use of preoperative fine-needle aspiration in patients undergoing reoperation for primary hyperparathyroidism. Surgery 1994;116:959–965.

9. Norton JA. Reoperative parathyroid surgery: indication, intraoperative decision making and results. Prog Surg 1986;18:133–145.
10. Wang CA. Parathyroid re-exploration: a clinical and pathological study of 112 cases. Ann Surg 1977;186:140–145.
11. Grant CS, van Heerden JA, Charbonneau JW, et al. Clinical management of persistent and/or recurrent primary hyperparathyroidism. World J Surg 1986;10:555–565.
12. Patow CA, Norton JA, Brennan MF. Vocal cord paralysis and reoperative parathyroidectomy. Ann Surg 1986;203:282–285.
13. Miller DL, Doppman JL, Krudy AG, et al. Localization of parathyroid adenomas in patients who have undergone surgery: Part II. Invasive procedures. Radiology 1987;162:138–141.
14. Doherty GM, Doppman JL, Miller DL, et al. Results of a multidisciplinary strategy for management of mediastinal parathyroid adenoma as a cause of persistent primary hyperparathyroidism. Ann Surg 1992;215(2):101–106.
15. Fraker DL, Doppman JL, Shawker TH, et al. Undescended parathyroid adenoma: an important etiology for failed operations for primary hyperparathyroidism. World J Surg 1990;14:342–348.
16. Miller DL, Doppman JL, Shawker TH, et al. Localization of parathyroid adenomas in patients who have undergone surgery: Part I. Noninvasive imaging methods. Radiology 1987;162:133–137.
17. Erdman WA, Breslau NA, Weinreb JC, et al. Noninvasive localization of parathyroid adenomas: a comparison of x-ray computed tomography, ultrasound, scintigraphy, and magnetic resonance imaging. Magn Reson Imaging 1989;7:187–194.
18. Levin KE, Gooding GAW, Okerlund MD, et al. Localizing studies in patients with persistent or recurrent hyperparathyroidism. Surgery 1987;102:917–925.
19. Auffermann W, Gooding GAW, Okerlund MD, et al. Diagnosis of recurrent hyperparathyroidism: comparison of MR imaging and other imaging techniques. AJR 1988;150:1027.
20. Doppman JL, Shawker TH, Krudy AG, et al. Parathymic parathyroid: CT, US, and angiographic findings. Radiology 1985;157:419–423.
21. Coakley AJ, Kettle AG, Wells CP, et al. $^{99}Tc^{m}$ sestamibi—a new agent for parathyroid imaging. Nucl Med Commun 1989;10:791–794.
22. O'Doherty MJ, Kettle AG, Wells CP, et al. Parathyroid imaging with technetium-99m sestamibi: preoperative localization and tissue uptake studies. J Nucl Med 1992;33:313–318.
23. Taillefer R, Boucher Y, Potvin C, et al. Detection and localization of parathyroid adenomas in patients with hyperparathyroidism using a single radionuclide imaging procedure with Technetium-99m sestamibi (double-phase study). J Nucl Med 1992;33:1801–1809.
24. Wei JP, Burke GJ, Mansberger AR. Prospective evaluation of the efficacy of technetium 99m sestamibi and iodine 123 radionuclide imaging of abnormal parathyroid glands. Surgery 1992;112:1111–1117.
25. Weber CJ, Vansant J, Alazraki N, et al. Value of technetium 99m sestamibi iodine 123 imaging in reoperative parathyroid surgery. Surgery 1993;114:1011–1018.
26. Doppman JL, Krudy AG, Marx SJ, et al. Aspiration of enlarged parathyroid glands for parathyroid hormone assay. Radiology 1983;148:31–35.

26a. Doppman JL. Percutaneous aspiration for hormone levels in the diagnosis of functioning endocrine tumors. Cardiovasc Intervent Radiol 1991;14:73–77.

27. Krudy AG, Doppman JL, Miller DL, et al. Abnormal parathyroid glands: comparison of nonselective arterial digital arteriography, selective parathyroid arteriography, and venous digital arteriography as methods of detection. Radiology 1983;148:23–29.
28. Krudy AG, Doppman JL, Miller DL, et al. Detection of mediastinal parathyroid glands by nonselective digital arteriography. AJR 1984;142:693–696.
29. Doppman JL, Mallette LE, Marx SJ, et al. The localization of abnormal mediastinal parathyroid glands. Radiology 1975;115:31–36.
30. Doppman JL, Marx SJ, Brennan MF, et al. The blood supply of mediastinal parathyroid adenomas. Ann Surg 1977;185:488–490.
31. Krudy A, Doppman JL, Brennan MF. The significance of the thyroidea ima artery in arteriographic localization of parathyroid adenomas. Radiology 1980;136:51.
32. Edis AJ, Purnell DC, van Heerden JA. The undescended "parathymus": an occasional cause of failed neck exploration in hyperparathyroidism. Ann Surg 1979;190:64.
33. Newton TH, Eisenberg E. Angiography of parathyroid adenomas. Radiology 1966;86:843–850.
34. Seldinger SI. Localization of parathyroid adenomata by arteriography. Acta Radiol (Stockh) 1954;42:353.
35. Doppman JL, Hammond WG. The anatomic basis of parathyroid venous sampling. Radiology 1970;95:603–610.
36. Sugg SL, Fraker DL, Alexander R, Doppman JL, et al. Prospective evaluation of selective venous sampling for parathyroid hormone concentration in patients undergoing reoperations for primary hyperparathyroidism. Surgery 1993;114(6):1004–1010.
37. Doppman JL, Melson GL, Evens RG, et al. Selective superior and inferior thyroid vein catheterization: venographic anatomy and potential applications. Invest Radiol 1969;4:97.
38. Shimkin PM, Doppman JL, Pearson KD, et al. Anatomic considerations in parathyroid venous sampling. AJR 1973;118:654–662.
39. Hjern B, Almqvist S, Granberg PO, et al. Pre-operative localization of parathyroid tissue by selective neck vein catheterization and radioimmunoassay of parathyroid hormone. Acta Chir Scand 1975;141:31.
40. In Der Maur GAP. Preoperative Localisatie Van Vergrote Buschildklieren. Groningen: Verenigde Reproduktie Bedrijven, 1975.
41. O'Riordan JLH, Kendall BE, Woodhead JS. Preoperative localization of parathyroid tumors. Lancet 1971;2:1172.

42. Wells SA Jr, Ketcham AS, Marx SJ, et al. Preoperative localization of hyperfunctioning parathyroid tissue: radioimmunoassay of parathyroid hormone in plasma from selectively catheterized thyroid veins. Ann Surg 1973;177:93–98.
43. Powell D, Shimkin PM, Doppman JL, Wells S, et al. Primary hyperparathyroidism: preoperative tumor localization and differentiation between adenoma and hyperplasia. N Engl J Med 1972;286:1169–1175.
44. Reitz RE, Pollard JJ, Wang CA, et al. Localization of parathyroid adenomas by selective venous catheterization and radioimmunoassay. N Engl J Med 1969;281:348–351.
45. Reiss E, Canterbury JM. Application of radioimmunoassay to differentiation of adenoma and hyperplasia and to preoperative localization of hyperfunctioning parathyroid glands. N Engl J Med 1969;280:1381–1385.
46. Spiegel AM, Doppman JL, Marx SJ, et al. Preoperative localization of abnormal parathyroids: neck massage vs. arteriography and selective venous sampling. Ann Intern Med 1978;89:935.
47. Doppman JL, Brennan MF, Kahn CR, et al. The circumscribing or periadenomal vessel: a helpful angiographic finding in certain islet cell and parathyroid adenomas. AJR 1981;136: 163–165.
48. Spiegel AM, Adamson RH, Mallette LE, et al. Intrathyroid parathyroid tumors: a seldom recognized cause of surgical failure in primary hyperparathyroidism. JAMA 1975;234: 1029.
49. Cope O. Surgery of hyperparathyroidism: the occurrence of parathyroids in the anterior mediastinum and the division of the operation into two stages. Ann Surg 1941;114:706.
50. Nathaniels EK, Nathaniels AM, Wang C. Mediastinal parathyroid tumors: a clinical and pathological study of 84 cases. Ann Surg 1970;171:165–170.
51. Wang CA. The anatomic basis of parathyroid surgery. Ann Surg 1976;183:271.
52. Wang CA, Mahaffey J. Hyperfunctioning supernumerary parathyroid glands. Surg Gynecol Obstet 1979;148:711.
53. Brennan MF, Doppman JL, Marx SJ, et al. Reoperative parathyroid surgery for persistent hyperparathyroidism. Surgery 1978;83:669–676.
54. Doppman JL, Brennan MF, Brown EM. Tracheal overlap: arteriographic sign of parathyroid adenomas in the posterior superior mediastinum. AJR 1978;130:1197–1199.
55. Doppman JL, Marx SJ, Spiegel AM, et al. Treatment of hyperparathyroidism by percutaneous embolization of a mediastinal adenoma. Radiology 1975;115:37–42.
56. Marx SJ, Doppman JL, Spiegel AM, et al. Embolization of mediastinal parathyroid adenoma. J Clin Endocrinol Metab 1974;39:1110–1114.
57. Geelhoed GW, Doppman JL. Embolization of ectopic parathyroid adenomas: a percutaneous treatment of hyperparathyroidism. Am Surg 1978;44:71–80.
58. Doppman JL, Brown EM, Brennan MF, et al. Angiographic ablation of parathyroid adenomas. Radiology 1979;130:577–582.
59. Doppman JL, DiChiro G. Paraspinal muscle infarction: a painful complication of lumbar artery embolization associated with pathognomonic radiographic and laboratory findings. Radiology 1976;119:609–613.
60. Rapoport SL. Blood-brain barrier opening by isotonic saline infusion in normotensive and hypertensive animals. Acta Radiol (Stockh) 1978;19:921.
61. Miller DL, Doppman JL, Chang R, et al. Angiographic ablation of parathyroid adenomas: lessons from a 10 year experience. Radiology 1987;165:601–607.
62. Doppman JL, Popovsky M, Girton M. The use of iodinated contrast agents to ablate organs: experimental studies and histopathology. Radiology 1981;138:333–340.
63. Brennan MF, Brown EM, Spiegel AM, et al. Autotransplantation of cryopreserved parathyroid tissue in man. Ann Surg 1979;189:139–142.
64. Wells SA Jr, Ellis JG, Gunnells JC, et al. Parathyroid autotransplantation in primary parathyroid hyperplasia. N Engl J Med 1976;295:57–62.
65. van Heerden JA, Weiland LH, ReMine WH, et al. Cancer of the parathyroid glands. Arch Surg 1979;114:475–480.
66. Saxe A. Parathyroid transplantation: a review. Surgery 1984; 95:507–526.

40

Arteriography of Thoracic Outlet Syndrome

ERICH K. LANG
JANIS GISSEL LETOURNEAU
DEBORAH G. LONGLEY

The presenting symptoms of thoracic outlet syndrome—pain, numbness, paresthesia, sensory deficit, motor weakness, muscle atrophy, and even gangrene of the upper extremity—are attributable to intermittent and positional compression of the neurovascular structures passing through the thoracic outlet and the complications that sometimes follow.[1-11] A variety of underlying conditions, such as cervical rib syndrome, costoclavicular syndrome, scalenus anticus syndrome, hyperabduction syndrome, and pectoralis minor syndrome, have been suspected of causing compression of the brachial plexus, the subclavian or axillary artery and/or vein, or all three.[1,2,4,5,8,9,11-21] Functional stress such as excessive exercise during sports may aggravate underlying conditions or, in fact, cause the complex.[6,22-24] However, vascular complications of thoracic outlet syndrome are uncommon and are estimated to occur in less than 5 percent of patients with this diagnosis.[21,25,26]

Because both vascular and neural structures are subject to compression, symptoms may be neurologic, vascular, or both.[16] Symptoms attributable to neural compression are encountered more often.[2] They consist of pain, paresthesia, and numbness involving fingers and hand and commonly follow an ulnar nerve distribution.[4,17] Impairment of arterial or venous flow may be attributable to compression of the arteries or veins by extrinsic structures or through a process afflicting the lumen. Computed tomography (CT) (Fig. 40-1) and magnetic resonance imaging (MRI) both before and after intravenous contrast enhancement, as well as myelography and in some instances diskography, are the procedures of choice for diagnosis and localization of such lesions as cervical disks, neoplasms, or spurs encroaching on nerve roots.[27,28] Color Doppler sonography is a noninvasive technique that has proved extremely useful in the triage of patients presenting with this often clinically confusing symptom complex.[29-31] Arteriography is the accepted gold standard for diagnosing arterial lesions and for identifying coexisting multiple lesions and complicating factors such as mural thrombi and dissection.[1,12,32-37] Moreover, arteriography can be expanded to therapeutic interventions such as transluminal angioplasty or thrombolytic perfusion.[38-40] Venography is the procedure of choice for detailed assessment of lesions afflicting venous structures.[6,41] Magnetic resonance angiography (MRA), two- or three-dimensional time-of-flight sequences, phase contrast, and echo-planar sequences, offer a noninvasive modality for detailed assessment of arterial and venous structures.[42,43] Faster scan sequences obviating gating, more sophisticated gradient-echo coils, and particularly larger apertures permitting varied positions of the upper extremities may make this the definitive examination technique in the near future.[44]

Anatomy

The subclavian arteries arise from the innominate artery on the right side and directly from the aortic arch on the left side. They exit from the thorax behind the sternoclavicular joints and traverse laterally, arching across the pleural cupula. When passing over the first rib, the subclavian artery goes through the scalene tunnel formed by the scalenus anticus muscle in front and the scalenus medius behind. In rare instances, the scalenus anticus muscle may pass behind the left subclavian artery.[45] Further laterally the subclavian artery passes under the subclavius muscle and clavicle and finally enters the axilla, where it crosses beneath the tendon of the pectoralis minor muscle.[5,16] The segment of the artery traversing the axilla is referred to as the *axillary artery;* the segment distal to the pectoralis tendon is called the *brachial artery.*

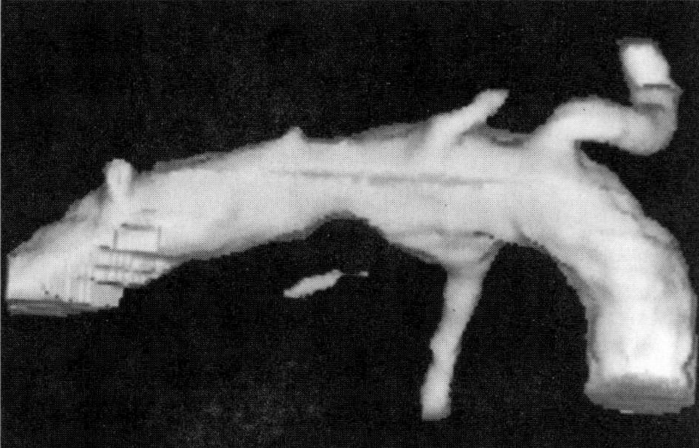

Figure 40-1. Spiral CT angiography of the subclavian artery. Siemens, 80 ml nonionic contrast medium, 5 ml-per-second flow, 20-second delay. Slice thickness 2 mm. Tail movement 3 mm per second. Postprocessing by maximum intensity projection and three-dimensional surface shaded display. Note the accurate morphologic documentation of the right subclavian artery with the ridgelike impression due to the first rib. (Courtesy of Dr. P. Farres, AKH, Vienna.)

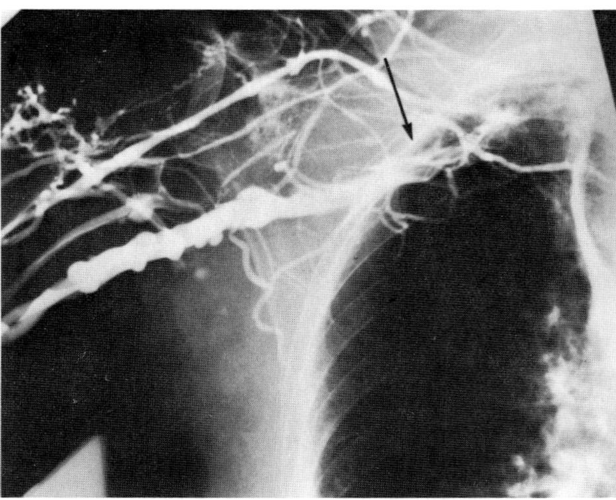

Figure 40-2. This 76-year-old woman with mediastinal lymphoma developed swelling of her right upper extremity. Venography demonstrated occlusion of the subclavian vein (*arrow*). Note filling of collateral vessels. (Courtesy of A.M. Palestrant, M.D.)

Arteries, veins, and the brachial plexus are at variable risk of intrinsic compression at the following anatomic sites:

1. The point of exit from the intervertebral foramina (nerves)
2. The space medial to the interscalene triangle and on top of the pleural cupula (artery, vein, and nerves)
3. The interscalene triangle (artery and nerves); in particular, rami from C8 and T1, forming the lower neural trunk that runs parallel and posterior to the subclavian artery, and causing the groove in the first rib[16,46]
4. The space between the scalenus anticus muscle and the clavicle (vein)
5. The costoclavicular space; space between the first rib and clavicle (artery, vein, and nerves)[33]
6. The space defined by the costocoracoid fascia (artery, vein, and nerves)
7. The space beneath the pectoralis minor tendon (artery, vein, and nerves—particularly the median nerve, whose heads encircle the artery in a scissorlike fashion at this point)[16]

Pathophysiology

Compression of the artery, vein, and nerves can be caused by inherent tightness of the above-described anatomic spaces, accentuated by hypertrophied muscles encroaching on these spaces, or pathologic conditions such as osteoarthritic spurs, abundant callus formation, tumors, or congenital abnormalities.[24]

Osteoarthritic spurs are undoubtedly the most common cause of compression of exiting nerve roots.[47] Pancoast tumors or upper mediastinal tumors are most prone to affect the more easily compressible subclavian veins (Fig. 40-2).[4,22,25]

Cervical ribs can compromise the costoclavicular space. The frequent association of a cervical rib with a fibrous band attaching itself to the undersurface of the first rib further compromises the space and compresses the subclavian artery against the first rib.[7,8,18,22,48–50] An abnormally long transverse process of C7 may function like a cervical rib.

Congenital or acquired lesions of the clavicle or first rib, such as abundant callus, a pseudoarticulation or pseudoarthrosis after a fracture, chondromatous tumors, or fibrous dysplasia, can severely compromise the costoclavicular space (Fig. 40-3).[5,12,13]

Hypertrophy, fibrosis, or myositis ossificans involving the subclavius muscle may cause diminution of the costoclavicular space.

Primary arterial disease, such as giant-cell arteritis, Takayasu or Sjögren disease, fibrosis attendant upon radiation therapy, intimal hyperplasia, traumatic intimal flap formation and subintimal hematoma formation, and aneurysms may significantly influence blood flow to the upper extremity (Figs. 40-4 through 40-6).[3,8,17,35,37,51–53]

The presence of collateral anastomotic channels be-

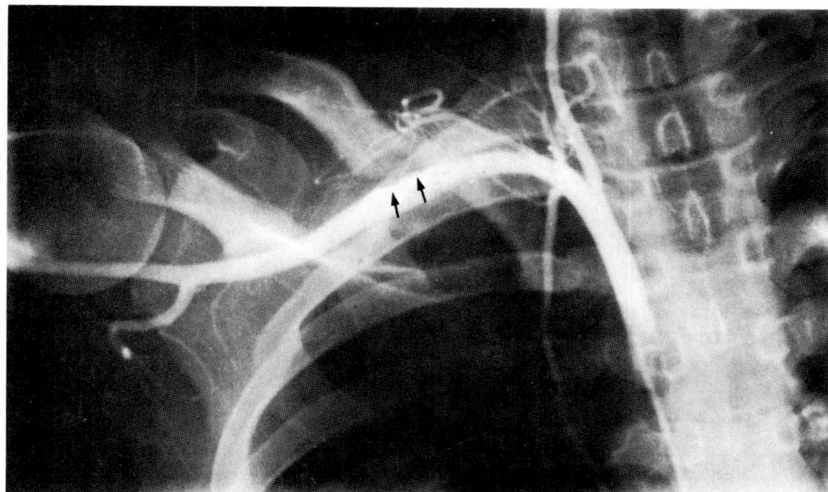

Figure 40-3. The fractured and overriding fragments of the clavicle encroach on the costoclavicular space and compress the subclavian artery. Note the irregularity of the superior circumference of the subclavian artery, reflecting intimal injury (*arrows*). The hemodynamic significance of the lesion is indicated by a mild poststenotic dilatation.

Figure 40-4. Arteriogram (in neutral position) demonstrating a fusiform dilatation of the subclavian artery distal to the scalene tunnel. A weblike filling defect extends across the inferior circumference of the vessel (*arrow*). Histologically, the lesion was found to represent intimal hyperplasia with cytoplasmic degeneration of the endothelium of the artery. (From Lang EK. Arteriographic diagnosis of the thoracic outlet syndrome. Radiology 1965;84:296. Used with permission.)

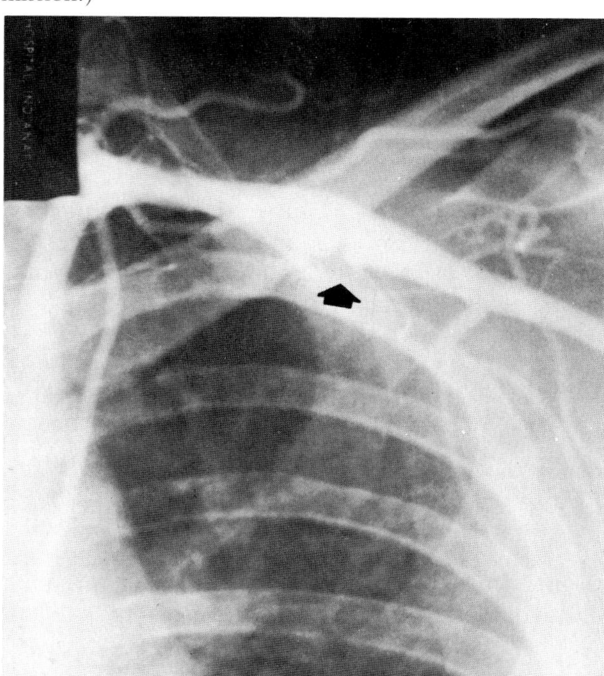

Figure 40-5. High-grade stenosis of the right subclavian artery distal to the scalene tunnel. The changes are attributable to intimal proliferation, adventitial fibrosis, and sometimes organized thrombi within the lumen in response to injury by radiation therapy. (From Budin JA, Casarella WJ, Harisiadis L. Subclavian artery occlusion following radiotherapy for carcinoma of the breast. Radiology 1976;118:169. Used with permission.)

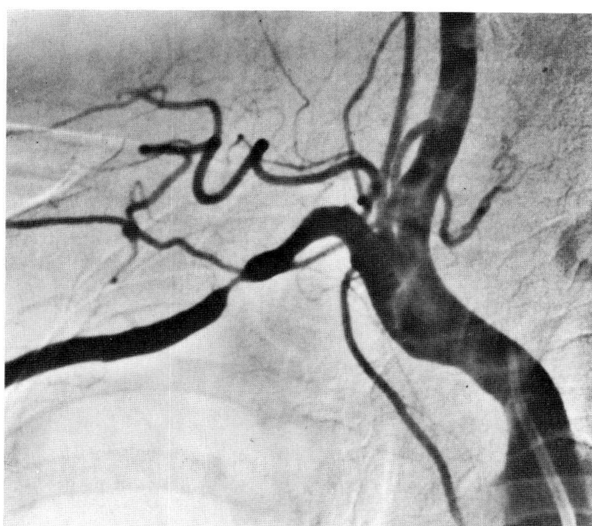

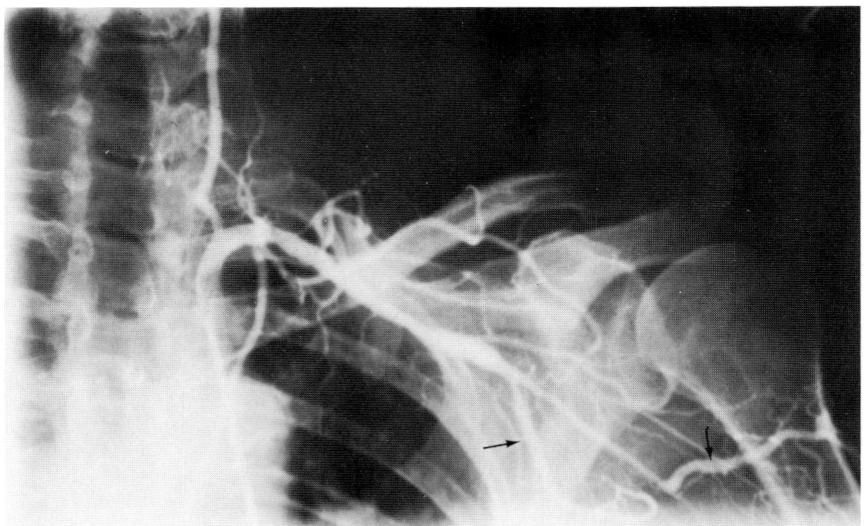

Figure 40-6. Left subclavian arteriogram demonstrating fusiform narrowing of the axillary artery as well as dilated collateral channels (*arrow*). The pathologic examination revealed evidence of giant-cell granulomatous arteritis. In conjunction with the clinical history and elevated alpha$_2$, beta$_2$, and gamma globulins, a diagnosis of polymyalgia rheumatica was established. (From Thompson JR, Simmons CR, Smith LL. Polymyalgia arteritica with bilateral subclavian artery occlusive disease. Radiology 1971;101:595. Used with permission.)

tween the suprascapular, circumflex scapular, subscapular, and posterior circumflex humeral arteries, and also between the transverse cervical and posterior circumflex humeral arteries, ensures blood supply to the periphery in case of occlusion of the subclavian artery while it passes through the thoracic outlet (Fig. 40-7).[12,36,54]

Figure 40-7. Tapered cutoff of the left subclavian artery at its point of exit from the scalene tunnel is demonstrated in the Lang position. Prominent antegrade collateral flow via the suprascapular and subscapular arteries into the posterior circumflex humeral artery reconstitutes flow in the axillary and brachial arteries (*arrows*). (From Lang EK. Arteriographic diagnosis of the thoracic outlet syndrome. Radiology 1965;84:296. Used with permission.)

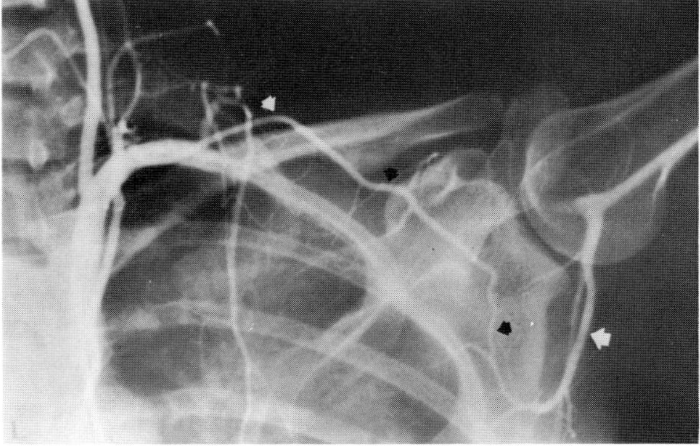

Clinical Examination

A number of clinical tests have been introduced that attempt to differentiate between the diverse pathologic conditions grouped together as neurovascular compression syndromes and presenting with similar symptoms.[47]

1. The Adson test was once thought to be specific for compression by the scalenus anticus muscle.[1] For this test the patient sits in an upright position and is instructed to retain deep inspiration, elevate the chin, and rotate the symptomatic side while the radial pulse rate and blood pressure are monitored. A reduction or obliteration of the radial pulse or change in blood pressure is interpreted as a positive test result. A bruit audible over the clavicle is said to be frequently associated with a cervical rib.[55]
2. The Allen maneuver has been designed to test for the so-called hyperabduction and pectoralis minor syndrome.[4,19,20,56] Abduction and elevation of the upper extremity above the head causes diminution of the costoclavicular space and stretches the axillary artery and nerve at a point where they pass beneath the coracoid process behind the pectoralis minor muscle tendon. The test has therefore been advocated for the assessment of both hyperabduction and pectoralis minor syndrome. However, plethysmographic observation of obliteration of the

pulse in 94 percent of patients with a true compression syndrome but also in 86 percent of asymptomatic patients has cast doubt on the specificity of the test.[11]

3. The claudication test, which consists of exercising both forearms for 60 seconds while assuming the just-outlined position, has been advocated to confirm test results.[24]

It is difficult to establish an accurate diagnosis by clinical examination.[57,58] For example, rudimentary or complete cervical ribs are seen on the routine chest x-ray films in 0.5 percent of all patients, only a very few of whom are symptomatic.[4] In many of these asymptomatic patients the Allen test will produce positive findings.[11] The diagnosis often depends on invasive angiography or is made retrospectively on the basis of clinical response to attempted surgical correction.[59]

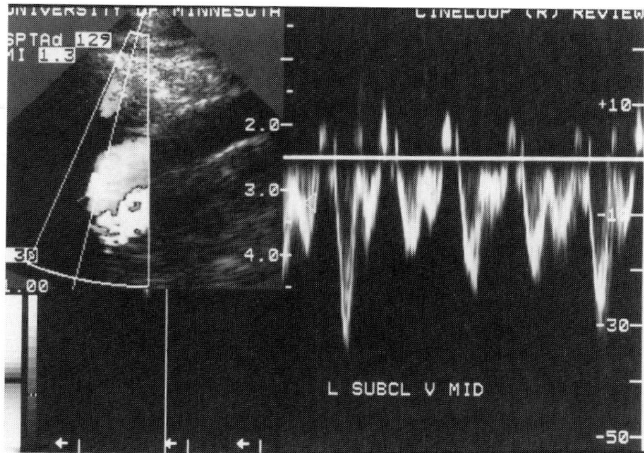

Figure 40-8. Normal spectral tracing from the midportion of the subclavian vein with the arm held in a neutral position. This patient has numbness and pain with partial abduction of the left arm; further abduction to 180 degrees is limited by these symptoms. His right arm is asymptomatic.

Color Doppler Sonography

Examination Technique

Patients are examined in the supine position with the head rotated away from the side being studied; the arms are held in a neutral position. A complete duplex survey of the brachycephalic veins is performed; this survey includes the internal jugular, medial, mid- and lateral segments of the subclavian, proximal axillary, and distal innominate veins bilaterally.[29] Features sought include occlusive or nonocclusive thrombosis, venous stenosis, aneurysmal dilatation, collateral vessels, and flattening or turbulence of venous flow as demonstrated by spectral analysis. The subclavian artery is also studied in the neutral position with specific attention directed to potential areas of focal stenosis or aneurysmal dilatation.

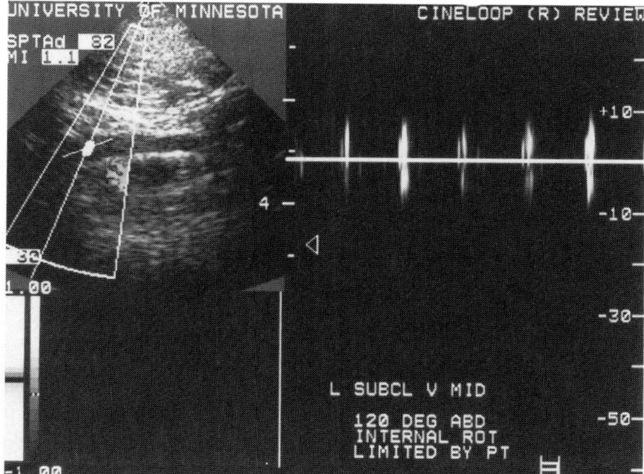

Figure 40-9. With partial arm abduction (120 degrees), there is complete cessation of flow in the left subclavian vein. The "signal" seen is an artifact transmitted from the subclavian artery. (Same patient as in Fig. 40-8.)

The subclavian vein is then restudied at 90 degrees, 135 degrees, and 180 degrees of shoulder abduction, with the elbow supported to eliminate the possibility of voluntary muscular effort contributing to false-positive studies. This maneuver produces more narrowing in the costoclavicular space. Diagnostic criteria for significant venous compression include total cessation of flow through the subclavian vein or complete loss of the normally transmitted atrial and respiratory dynamics (Figs. 40-8 through 40-11).[41] The subclavian artery is also reinterrogated with varying degrees of abduction, with cessation of flow or a doubling of peak systolic velocity over that in the neutral position considered significant (Figs. 40-12 through 40-14). Patients are routinely examined after surgical release procedures, including surgical resection of the first rib, and after any radiologic interventions, such as thrombolysis, venoplasty, or venous stent placement. This routine examination provides a hemodynamic baseline should the patient present once again with symptoms.

Findings

The ultimate utility of duplex sonography in patients with suspected thoracic outlet syndrome has not been defined.[30] Moreover, the role of this technology in this clinical setting will likely never be totally clarified be-

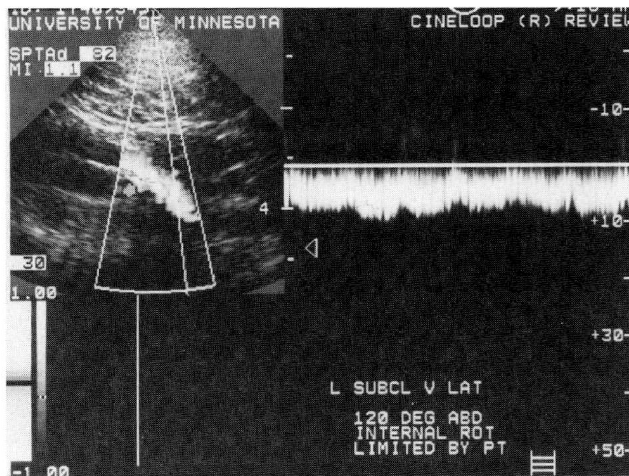

Figure 40-10. Lateral to the more proximal subclavian vein obstruction planar venous flow is identified, indicating that this segment of vein is patent with abduction but that flow courses proximally by collateral channels. (Same patient as in Fig. 40-8.)

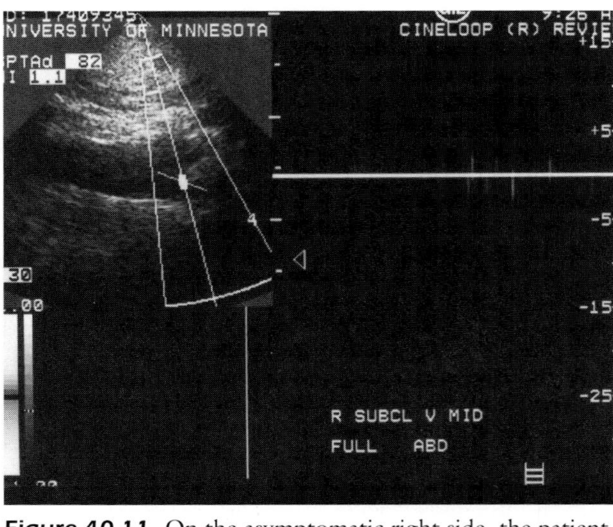

Figure 40-11. On the asymptomatic right side, the patient can attain full arm abduction. Complete cessation of flow is seen with this maneuver. (Same patient as in Fig. 40-8.)

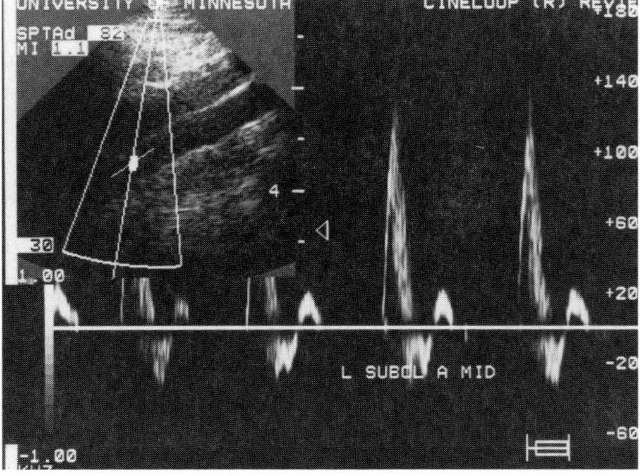

Figure 40-12. This same patient also has a positive arterial study on the left side with an arterial velocity of 130 cm per second with the arm in a neutral position.

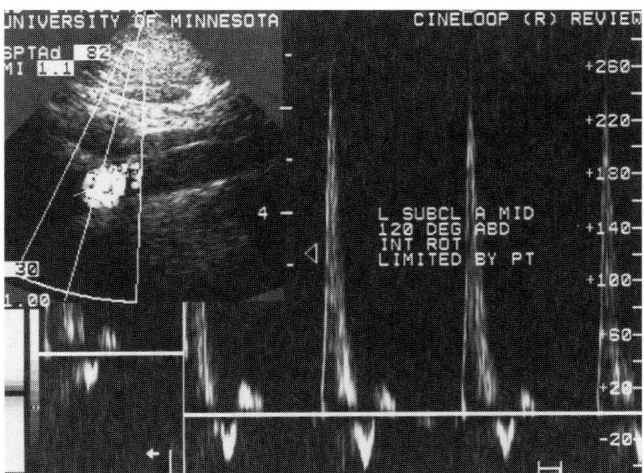

Figure 40-13. With partial abduction (120 degrees), the peak systolic velocity doubles to 260 cm per second.

cause of the overlap in duplex findings in "normal," asymptomatic volunteers with those of patients with angiographically proven disease.

In a study of 20 asymptomatic volunteers, 10 percent satisfied the venous criteria and 20 percent satisfied the arterial criteria for the duplex diagnosis of thoracic outlet syndrome. Although one might assume that overlap of positive findings in normal and affected subjects could be minimized, or even eliminated, by using more stringent diagnostic criteria, this is not entirely possible. Complete cessation of venous or arterial flow, the most stringent of possible diagnostic criteria, can be frequently documented in asymptomatic volunteers.[31] Correlation of color Doppler sonographic findings in patients suspected of having thoracic outlet syndrome with angiographic data and results of related surgery has indicated that the technology provides good diagnostic accuracy for venous obstruction or compression. A sensitivity of 92 percent and a specificity of 95 percent can be attained

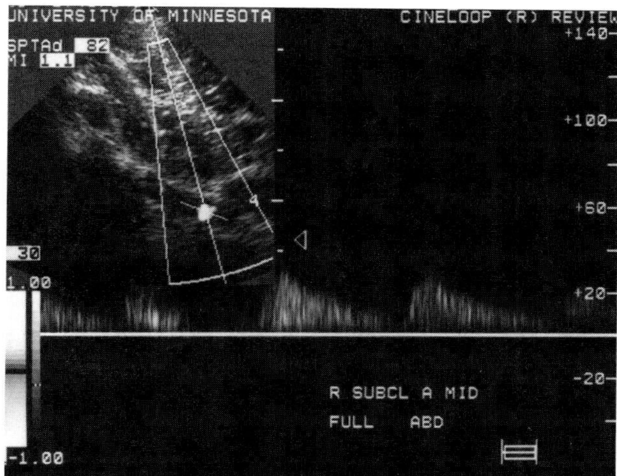

Figure 40-14. A postocclusive arterial waveform is seen in the right subclavian artery with complete abduction, demonstrating positional arterial occlusion on the asymptomatic side.

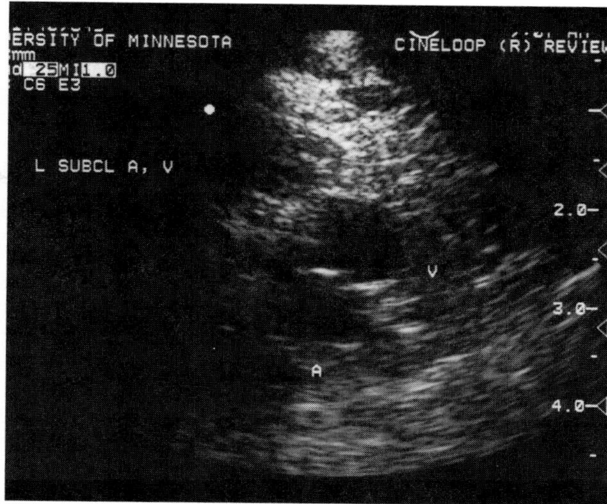

Figure 40-15. Definitive identification of the subclavian vein is critical for an accurate study. The vein (*V*) lies anterior to the artery (*A*) in a parasagittal scan plane at the level of the midclavicle. This scan plane is perpendicular (transverse) to the course of the vessels. The artery and vein lie immediately adjacent to each other.

with this diagnostic technique.[31] However, care must be taken to not misidentify a collateral vein for the subclavian vein and therefore err in the diagnosis of subclavian thrombosis. In subclavian vein thrombosis, collateral veins can enlarge substantially, course in the expected location of the subclavian vein, and maintain spectral waveform characteristics not too dissimilar from that of the subclavian vein. This potential for false-negative studies can be minimized by carefully defining the anatomic relationship between the subclavian artery and vein; this is accomplished by scanning transversely to the expected course of these vessels. The vein should lie anterior to the artery; the relationship of the artery and vein in a cephalocaudal plane is more variable (Fig. 40-15). Insufficient data do not permit one to assess the accuracy of color Doppler sonography in the diagnosis of significant subclavian artery compression.

Conclusion

Clinical diagnosis of thoracic outlet syndrome is difficult and fraught with many inaccuracies. Definitive traditional radiologic diagnosis has required invasive imaging techniques. Color Doppler sonography is a promising technology for the noninvasive diagnosis of vascular causes of thoracic outlet syndrome, including significant venous or arterial compression and venous thrombosis.

Magnetic Resonance Angiography

Magnetic resonance angiography using 2D or 3D time of flight, phase contrast, or echo sequences can produce acceptable images of arterial and venous structures. Magnetic resonance angiography makes use of the so-called flow void in which the flowing blood within vessels emits little or no signals and the lumen appears black. The dephasing phenomenon that records differences in precessional frequencies among protons in a flowing blood column offers another opportunity for demonstrating the vessels. Lastly, movement of relatively large volumes of blood relative to the imaged plane can be exploited to generate an image of the vessel by a process known as time-of-flight effect (Fig. 40-16).[43] However, multiple directional changes in the path of the subclavian artery cause problems in depicting the true lumen of the vessel. Fictitious images may result from changes in velocity, from turbulent or laminar flow, and particularly from alteration in the direction of flow in the vessels in respect to the *x-y* axes. Particularly bothersome artifacts may result when the position of the arms and shoulders is changed and a change in the flow direction in relation to the magnetic field results. Though time-consuming, phase contrast sequences in multiple planes, eliminate this difficulty, and the technique may be use-

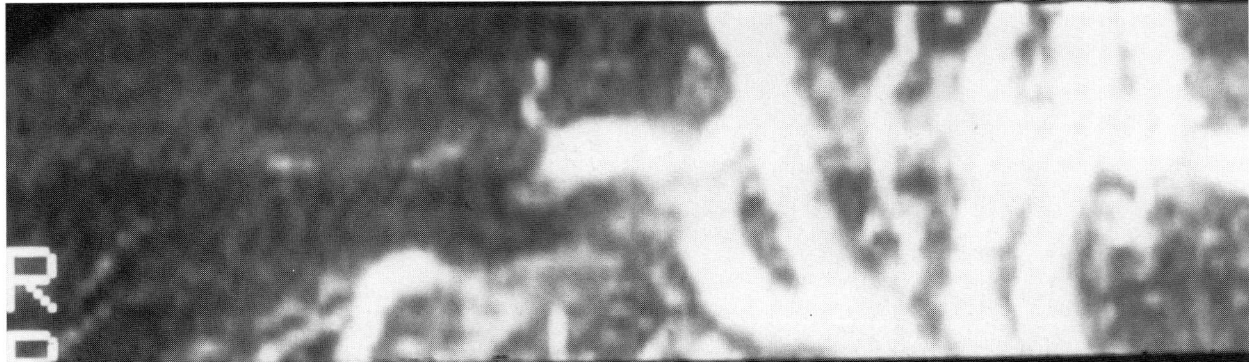

Figure 40-16. Two-dimensional time-of-flight magnetic resonance angiogram demonstrates cessation of antegrade flow in the subclavian artery at the point of exit from the interscalene tunnel. Because of potential "flow-nils" in the x-y axes, this must be interpreted with caution and confirmed by digital angiography.

ful for noninvasive screening, allowing one to assess arterial and venous structures at the same time.

Arteriography

Technique

Selective subclavian arteriography via the transfemoral approach is favored because it permits examination in various stress positions and because antegrade injection of contrast medium simulates conditions of normal blood flow.[17,26,39,45]

The examination is carried out using digital or standard arteriographic techniques. From 2 to 8 ml 50 percent dilute to 8 to 12 ml nondilute nonionic contrast medium is injected for each series, and serial roentgenograms are exposed at a rate of two and one frames per second, respectively, covering the first 2 seconds as well as the period from the 4th to the 12th second. The latter portion of the run is designed to demonstrate reconstitution of flow in collateral channels in patients with complete or near-complete obstruction of the subclavian artery.

The known aggravation of symptoms attendant upon exercise suggests a relationship to the tonus of the involved muscle groups and emphasizes the importance of isometrics contraction and tonus of muscles in the production of the lesion. To assure normal muscle tonus, examinations should be done under local anesthesia.[17,56]

Practically all lesions can be demonstrated on arteriograms in at least one of three different positions.

1. A baseline study is done with the patient in the neutral position (i.e., the patient is placed supine on the examination table and instructed to assume a relaxed position). This series is for the assessment of intrinsic arterial lesions, thrombosis of the artery, and aneurysmal or poststenotic dilatation of the artery heralding a hemodynamically significant obstruction (Figs. 40-17 and 40-18).[35,60]
2. The second series is carried out with the patient supine on the examination table and the arm to be examined abducted 90 degrees and lifting a 2-lb weight 2 cm above the tabletop. The head is turned sharply to the contralateral side and the injection of contrast medium recorded while the patient maintains deep inspiration (Lang maneuver). The maneuver causes tightening of the scalene muscles and diminution of the costoclavicular and costocoracoid space beneath the pectoralis minor ten-

Figure 40-17. Selective left subclavian arteriogram in neutral position demonstrates the normal noncompromised lumen of the vessel.

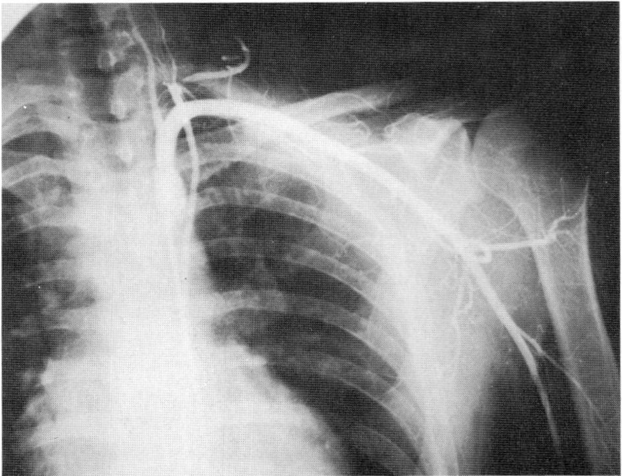

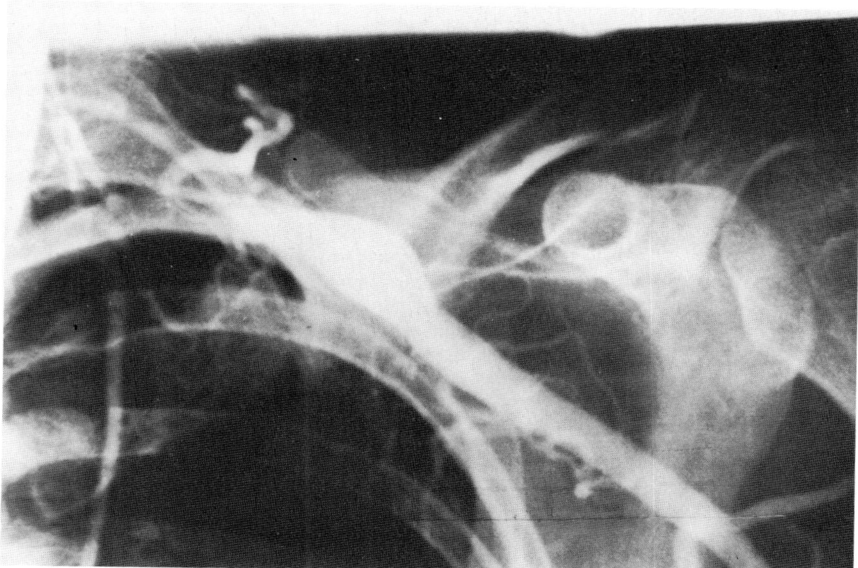

Figure 40-18. The marked compression of the subclavian artery at its point of exit from the scalene tunnel is followed by a poststenotic dilatation, which attests to the hemodynamic significance of the lesion. (From Lang EK. Arteriographic diagnosis of the thoracic outlet syndrome. Radiology 1965;84:296. Used with permission.)

don. It is used to assess compression sites in the interscalene triangle, the costoclavicular space, and the costocoracoid space beneath the pectoralis minor tendon.[11,35,36] One must be cautious in interpreting minor compression effect in the costoclavicular space because even normal asymptomatic patients may show findings under this severe stress condition (Figs. 40-19 and 40-20).[55]

3. The third series is done with the patient sitting and abducting the arm while turning the head to the contralateral side. The mere weight of the shoulder girdle may be an important factor in producing compression, and some lesions may therefore be best demonstrable in the erect position (Fig. 40-21).[5,33,35]
4. Occasionally, the patient should be evaluated under the conditions producing complaints. In most instances, the position simulates occupational maneuvers.[35,52]

Because the stress maneuvers frequently result in compression of the artery and reduction of flow, the amount of contrast medium per injection is reduced for these series to 4 or 8 ml of 50 percent dilute nonionic contrast medium for digital studies, and 6 to 8 ml of contrast medium for standard arteriography. This is to avoid excessive flow of contrast medium into the vertebral artery.[52]

Findings and Interpretation

Demonstration of poststenotic dilatation distal to the classic points of compression (interscalene tunnel, costoclavicular space, or below the pectoralis minor muscle tendon) in the neutral position is a persuasive angiographic finding of a hemodynamically significant obstructive lesion.[60]

Demonstration of an oblique compression defect or twist of the subclavian artery in the scalene tunnel generally does not indicate a hemodynamically significant lesion.[32,56,61] Fibrous bands originating from a cervical rib and inserting along the superior circumference of the tuberculum of the first rib may cause this twist effect when the median scalene muscle contracts (activated by turning the head to the contralateral side (Fig. 40-22).

A characteristic ridgelike compression of the inferior circumference of the subclavian artery while it passes the interscalene triangle indicates compression of the vessel against the anterior first rib (see Fig. 40-20).

An impression on the superior circumference of the subclavian artery coupled with the characteristic ridgelike compression of its inferior circumference indicates diminution of the costoclavicular space with the subclavian artery compressed by the subclavius muscle against the anterior first rib (see Fig. 40-20).

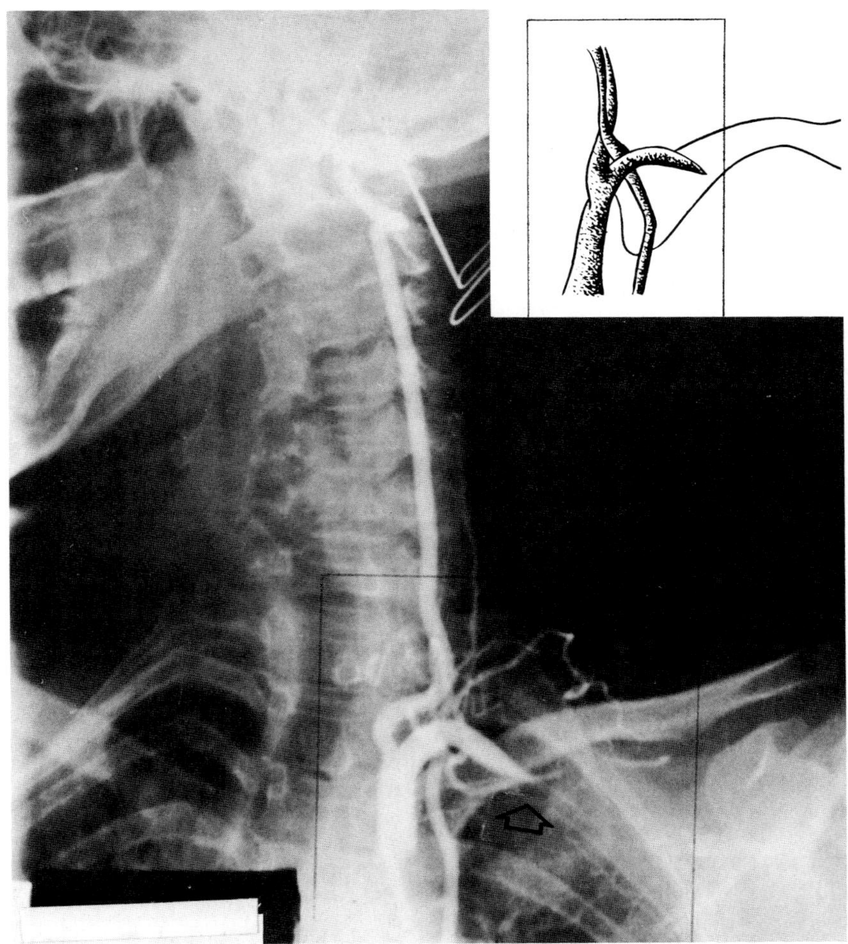

Figure 40-19. Left subclavian arteriogram (recorded in the Lang position) demonstrates a complete cutoff of the subclavian artery at its point of exit from the scalene tunnel (*arrow*). Note the marked filling of the vertebral artery. (From Lang EK. Arteriographic diagnosis of the thoracic outlet syndrome. Radiology 1965;84:296. Used with permission.)

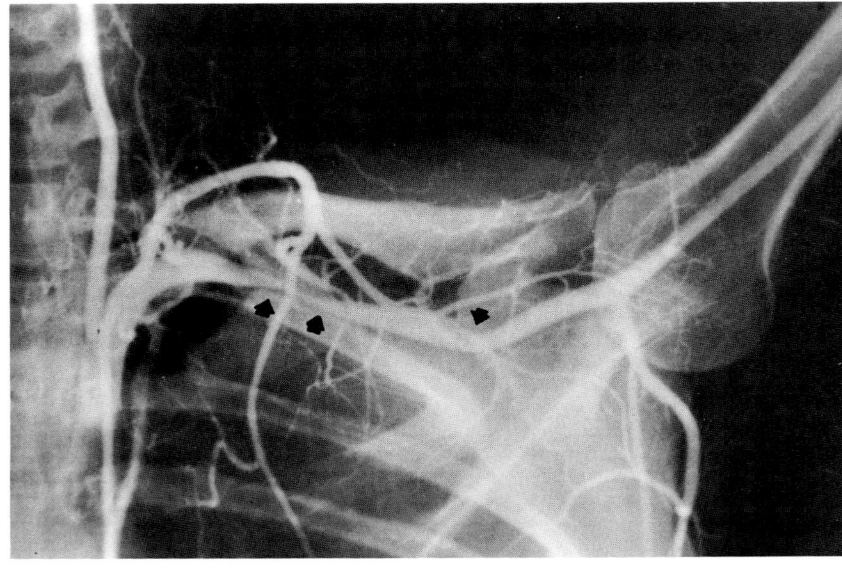

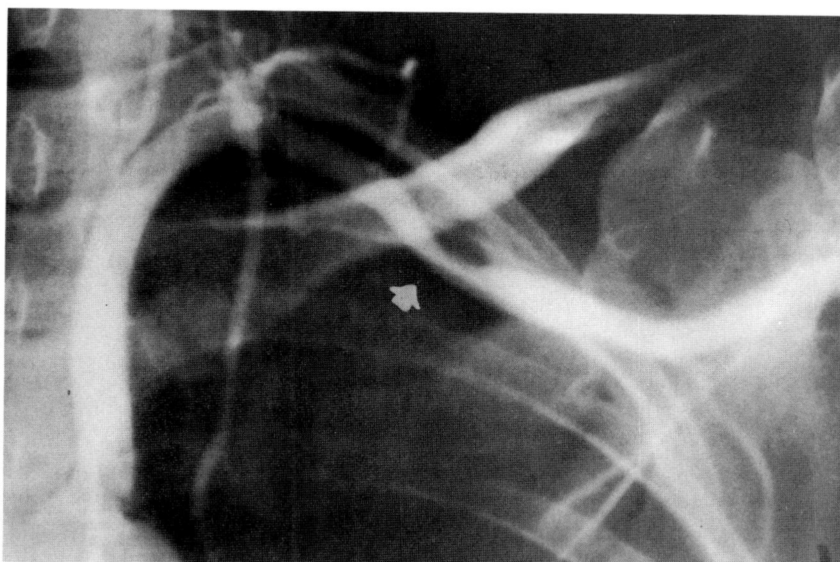

Figure 40-21. Left subclavian arteriogram (recorded with patient in erect position and exercising Adson maneuver) demonstrates compression of the subclavian artery at its point of emergence from the interscalene triangle (*arrow*). The weight of the shoulder girdle is the important factor producing compression.

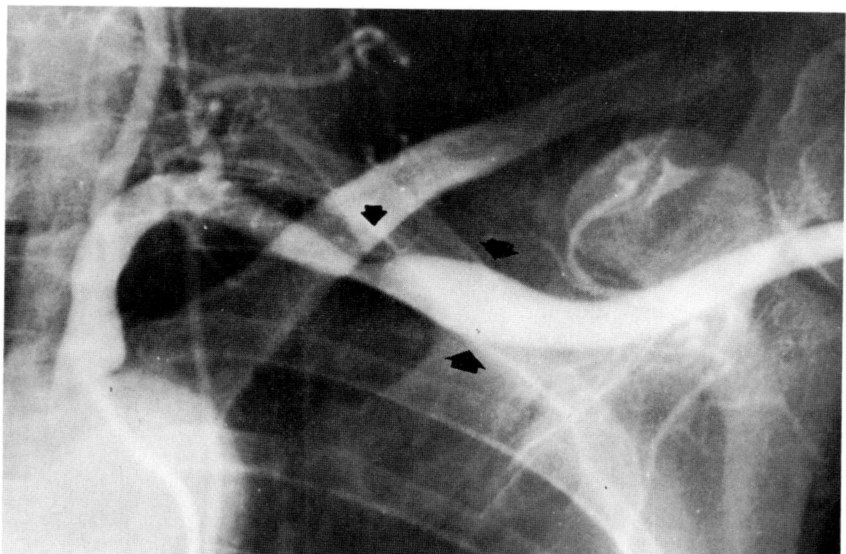

Figure 40-22. The subclavian artery appears twisted at its point of exit from the scalene tunnel. Fibers originating from the cervical rib and attaching to the first anterior rib and the median scalene muscle cause the compression (*medial arrow*). A significant poststenotic dilatation of the artery attests to the hemodynamic significance of the lesion (*lateral arrows*). (From Lang EK. Arteriographic diagnosis of the thoracic outlet syndrome. Radiology 1965;84:296. Used with permission.)

◂ **Figure 40-20.** Marked compression of a long segment of the subclavian artery while it traverses the interscalene triangle and costoclavicular space is demonstrated on an arteriogram recorded in the modified Allen position (Lang position). The artery is compressed against the first rib (*two arrows on left*). The long segment of effacement of the superior circumference reflects a pressure effect by the scalenus medius and subclavius muscles. A second area of compression is noted at a point where the artery crosses beneath the tendon of the pectoralis minor muscle (*arrow on right*). The undue prominence of the suprascapular, circumflex scapular, subscapular, and posterior circumflex humeral arteries suggests that this antegrade collateral system is frequently activated. (From Lang EK. Arteriographic diagnosis of the thoracic outlet syndrome. Radiology 1965;84:296. Used with permission.)

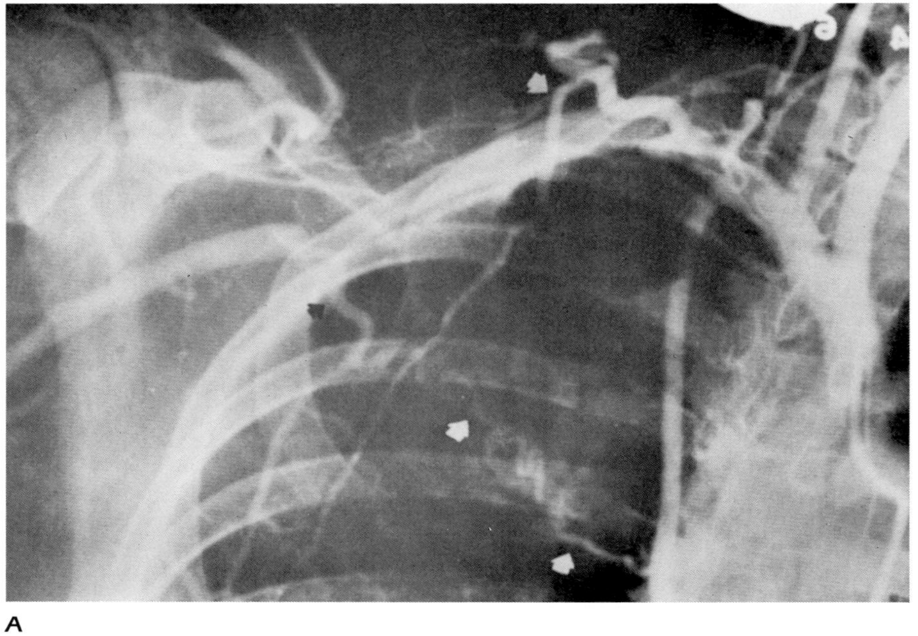

A

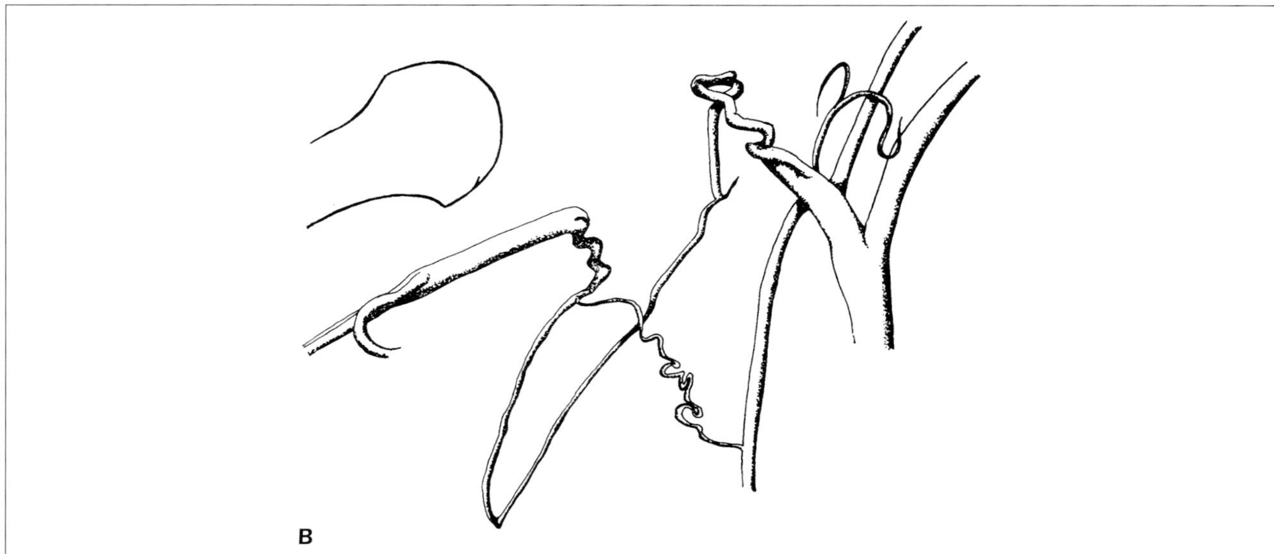

B

Figure 40-23. (A and B) A 10-cm-long segment of the subclavian artery is obliterated as a result of posttraumatic thrombosis. The flow in the axillary artery is reconstituted via collaterals (*arrows*) from the transverse cervical, internal mammary, intercostal, posterior circumflex humeral, and subscapular arteries. (From Lang EK. Quantitative assessment of flow in antegrade and retrograde collateral channels serving the brachiocephalic area. Radiology 1966;87:457. Used with permission.)

A tapered and complete cutoff of the subclavian at its point of emergence from the scalene tunnel indicates compression of the vessel in the interscalene triangle and scalene tunnel (see Fig. 40-19).

Demonstration of a ridgelike compression of the inferior margin of the subclavian artery coupled with an impression on the superior circumference indicates a tightness in both the costoclavicular space and the interscalene triangle.

Compression of the axillary artery at the point of crossing beneath the pectoralis minor tendon indicates tightness in the costocoracoid space and is usually best demonstrated in the Lang position (see Fig. 40-20).

Hemodynamically significant lesions are usually de-

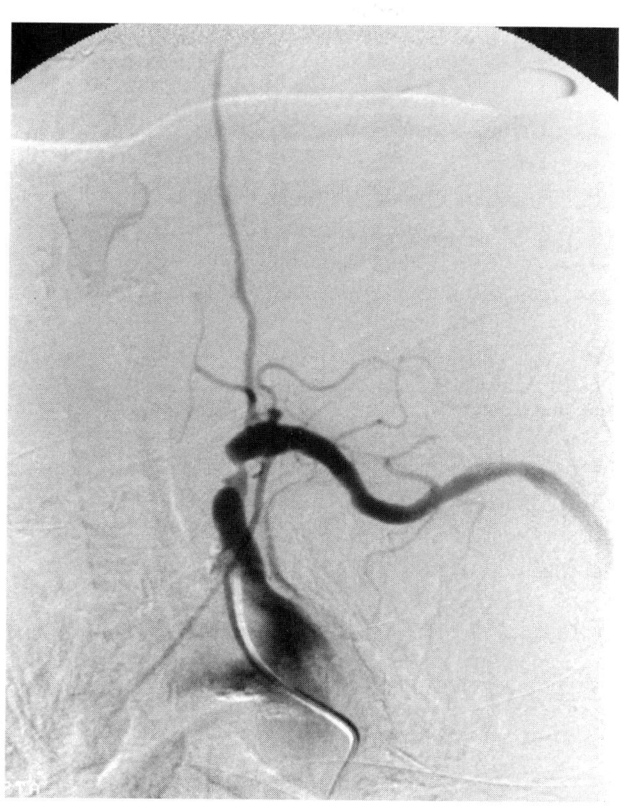

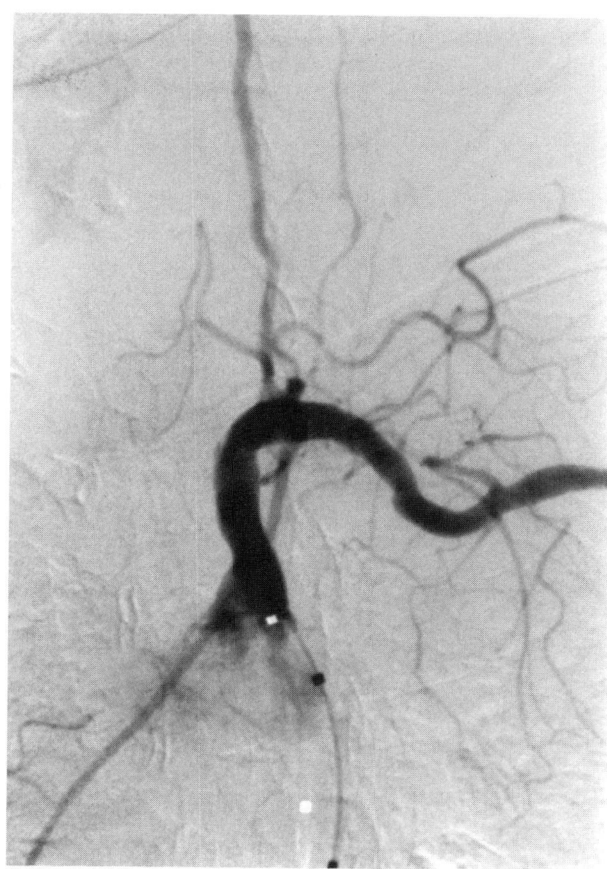

A B

Figure 40-24. (A) Digital arteriogram showing a 95 percent stenosis of the first segment of the subclavian artery by an eccentric arteriosclerotic plaque. (B) After transluminal balloon dilatation, there has been excellent reconstitution of the lumen with no residual stenosis.

monstrable both in the erect position, while performing an Adson maneuver, and in the Lang position and will frequently show a poststenotic dilatation of the subclavian artery distal to the site of obstruction in the neutral position.[60] Reconstitution of flow distal to the site of obstruction via antegrade collaterals is a strong argument for a hemodynamically significant obstruction (Fig. 40-23).

Mural thrombi may form at the site of compression or turbulence.[17,32,34] Such thrombi can propagate distally and lead to complete occlusion of the lumen or can give rise to emboli causing embolization of the distal arterial runoff.[17] Temporary or permanent occlusion of the subclavian and axillary arteries results in immediate activation of an antegrade collateral pathway (see Fig. 40-23).[35,54] This antegrade collateral pathway by the suprascapular, circumflex scapular, subscapular, and posterior circumflex humeral arteries or the transverse cervical and posterior circumflex humeral arteries can retain a perfusion and flow rate of about 10 percent of normal.[54]

Obviously, in the presence of diagnosed thrombotic disease, the arteriogram can be expanded into a therapeutic procedure. Intraarterial urokinase infusion in the treatment of thromboembolism or thrombotic occlusion can be readily instituted.[40] Underlying obstructing lesions can then be treated by percutaneous transluminal angioplasty (Fig. 40-24).[38,39]

The ability to document multiple coexisting lesions is one of the major contributions of arteriography (see Fig. 40-20).[35,36,52] Documentation of the precise point of reconstitution of flow in patients with complete obstruction is of great importance in the choice of corrective surgical intervention (see Fig. 40-23).[52]

Venography

Venography is an excellent method of pinpointing the site of obstruction and of characterizing the nature of the obstruction (i.e., an intrinsic or extrinsic pro-

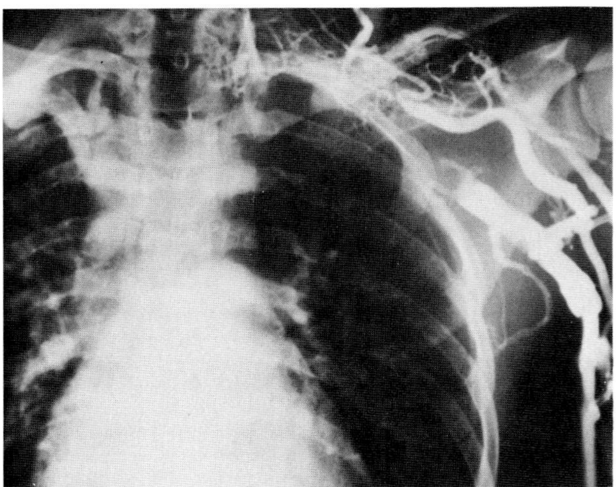

Figure 40-25. Antegrade venogram demonstrates lack of filling and flow in the axillary and subclavian veins. Note the extensive bypass collaterals via the cervical and intercostal veins. A neoplastic process and fibrosis attendant upon radiation therapy resulted in total occlusion of the axillary and subclavian veins. (From Lang EK. Quantitative assessment of flow in antegrade and retrograde collateral channels serving the brachiocephalic area. Radiology 1966;87:457. Used with permission.)

cess).[26] On the basis of characteristic appearance and historical information the underlying etiology (i.e., hematoma, neoplasm, cicatricial encasement such as caused by radiation therapy or mediastinal collagenosis) is usually diagnosable (Figs. 40-25 and 40-26).[3,16,25,50] Interventional techniques such as thrombolysis, balloon angioplasty, and placement of metallic stents can then be used to correct the underlying condition.[25]

Summary

In addition to clinical examination, color Doppler sonography and possibly magnetic resonance angiography are the principal triage examinations to exclude the diagnosis of a vascular thoracic outlet syndrome.[31,41–43,47,62] Digital angiography, standard angiography, and venography are the definitive examinations to affirm the diagnosis and in many instances can be expanded to provide therapeutic interventions.

References

1. Adson AW, Coffey JR. Cervical rib: a method of anterior approach for relief of symptoms by division of the scalenus anticus. Ann Surg 1927;85:839.
2. Bateman JE. Neurovascular syndromes related to the clavicle. Clin Orthop 1968;58:75.
3. Budin JA, Casarella WJ, Harisiadis L. Subclavian artery occlusion following radiotherapy for carcinoma of the breast. Radiology 1976;118:169.
4. Ferguson TB, Burford TH, Roper CL. Neurovascular compression at the superior thoracic aperture: surgical management. Ann Surg 1968;167:573.
5. Lord JW, Rosati LM. Neurovascular compression syndromes of upper extremities. Ciba Clin Symp 1958;10:35.
6. McCleery RS, Kesterson JE, Kirtley JA, Love RB. Subclavius

Figure 40-26. (A) Marked anterior and downward displacement of the axillary artery by a large hematoma contained behind the costocoracoid fascia. The posterior circumflex humeral artery is compressed at its point of exit through the costocoracoid fascia. (B) Basilic venogram demonstrates complete cessation of flow in the axillary vein at the point of crossing by the pectoralis minor tendon, reflecting the greater vulnerability of venous structures to compression.

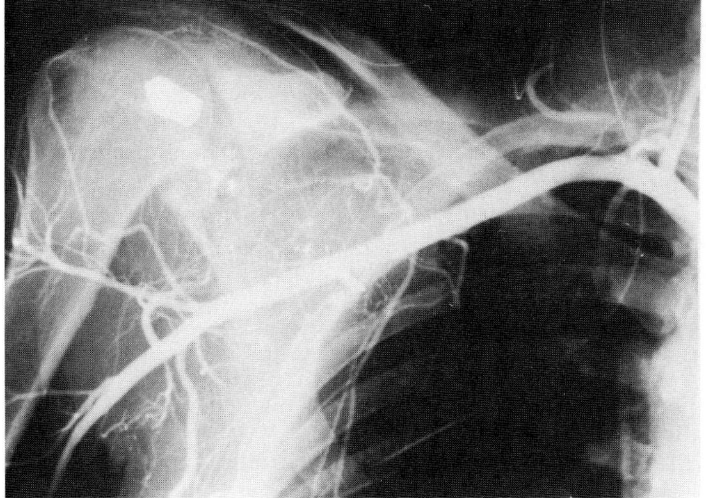

A

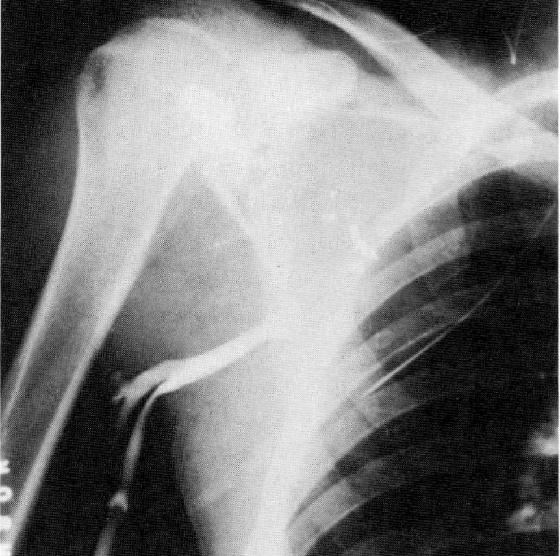

B

and anterior scalene muscle compression as a cause of intermittent obstruction of the subclavian vein. Ann Surg 1951;133: 588.
7. Naffziger HC, Grant WT. Neuritis of the brachial plexus, mechanical in origin: the scalenus syndrome. Surg Gynecol Obstet 1938;67:722.
8. Neviaser JS. Musculoskeletal disorders of the shoulder region causing cervicobrachial pain. Surg Clin North Am 1963;43: 1703.
9. Overton LM. The causes of pain in the upper extremities: a differential diagnosis study. Clin Orthop 1967;51:27.
10. Schlesinger EB. The thoracic outlet syndrome from a neurosurgical point of view. Clin Orthop 1967;51:49.
11. Windsor T, Brow R. Costoclavicular syndrome: its diagnosis and treatment. JAMA 1966;196:697.
12. Bocquet M, Foli-Desjardins R, Batioese R, Garreta L. Dynamic arteriography in the costoclavicular syndrome. Ann Radiol (Paris) 1970;13:827.
13. Davis JM, Golinger D. Cervical rib, subclavian artery aneurysm, axillary and cerebral emboli. Proc R Soc Med 1966;59:1002.
14. DeBruin TR. Costoclavicular space enlargement: eight methods for relief of neurovascular compression. Int Surg 1966;46: 340.
15. DeVilliers JC. A brachiocephalic vascular syndrome associated with cervical rib. Br Med J 1966;2:140.
16. Falconer MA, Weddell G. Costoclavicular compression of the subclavian artery and vein: relation to the scalenus anticus syndrome. Lancet 1943;2:539.
17. Haimovici H, Caplan LH. Arterial thrombosis complicating the thoracic outlet syndrome: arteriographic considerations. Radiology 1966;87:462.
18. Nichols HM. Anatomic structures of the thoracic outlet. Clin Orthop 1967;51:17.
19. Riddell DH. Thoracic outlet syndrome: thoracic and vascular aspects. Clin Orthop 1967;51:53.
20. Roos DB, Owens JC. Thoracic outlet syndrome. Arch Surg 1966;93:71.
21. Scher LA, Beith FJ, Sanson RH, Gupta SK, et al. Vascular complications of thoracic outlet syndrome. J Vasc Surg 1986;3(3): 565–568.
22. Aquino BC, Barone EJ. "Effort" thrombosis of the axillary and subclavian vein associated with cervical rib and oral contraceptives in young woman athlete. J Am Board Fam Pract 1989; 2(3):208–211.
23. Friedman SG, Crystal K. Axillary artery thrombosis from handball. JVIR 1991;2:1–5.
24. Nuber GW, McCarthy WJ, Yao JJ, Schaefer MF, et al. Arterial abnormalities of the shoulder in athletes. Am J Sports Med 1990;18(5):514–519.
25. Aburahma AF, Sadler DL, Robinson PA. Axillary-subclavian vein thrombosis: changing patterns of etiology, diagnostic and therapeutic modalities. Am Surg 1991;57(2):101–107.
26. Jamieson CW. Venous complications of the thoracic outlet syndrome. Eur J Vasc Surg 1987;1(1):123.
27. Fox AJ, Lin JP, Pinto RS, et al. Myelographic cervical nerve root deformities. Radiology 1975;116:355–361.
28. Stark DD, Bradley WG Jr. Magnetic resonance imaging. In: Haughton VM, Daniels DL, Gzervionke LF, Williams AL, eds. Cervical spine. St. Louis: Mosby, 1988.
29. Falk RL, Smith BF. Thrombosis of upper extremity thoracic inlet veins: diagnosis with duplex Doppler sonography. AJR 1987;149:677–682.
30. Longley B, Yetlicka JW, Molina E, et al. Color Doppler ultrasound of thoracic outlet syndrome. Semin Intervent Radiol 1990;7:230–235.
31. Longley B, Yetlicka JW, Molina E, et al. Thoracic outlet syndrome: evaluation of subclavian vessels by color Doppler duplex sonography. AJR 1992;158:623–630.
32. Adler J, Hooshmand I. The angiographic spectrum of the thoracic outlet syndrome: with emphasis on mural thrombosis and emboli and congenital vascular anomalies. Clin Radiol 1973; 24:35.
33. Benzian SR, Mainzer F. Erect arteriography: its use in the thoracic outlet syndrome. Radiology 1974;111:275.
34. Dick R. Arteriography in neurovascular compression at the thoracic outlet, with special reference to embolic patterns. AJR 1970;12:110–141.
35. Lang EK. Arteriographic diagnosis of the thoracic outlet syndrome. Radiology 1965;84:296.
36. Lang EK. Neurovascular compression syndrome. Dis Chest 1966;50:572.
37. Thompson JR, Simmons CR, Smith LL. Polymyalgia arteritica with bilateral subclavian artery occlusive disease. Radiology 1971;101:595.
38. Farina C, Mingoli A, Schultz RD, et al. Percutaneous transluminal angioplasty vs. surgery for subclavian artery occlusive disease. Am J Surg 1989;158(6):511–514.
39. Hebrang A, Maskovic J, Tomac B. Percutaneous transluminal angioplasty of the subclavian arteries: longterm results in 52 patients. AJR 1991;156(5):1091–1094.
40. Sullivan KL, Minken SL, White RI Jr. Treatment of a case of thromboembolism resulting from thoracic outlet syndrome with intraarterial urokinase infusion. J Vasc Surg 1988;7(4): 568–571.
41. Schubard PJ, Haeberlin JR, Porter JM. Intermittent subclavian venous obstruction: utility of venous pressure gradients. Surgery 1986;99:365–368.
42. Azarow KS, Pearl RF, Hoffman MA, et al. Vascular ring: does magnetic resonance imaging replace angiography? Ann Thorac Surg 1992;53(5):882–885.
43. Zerhouni EA. MR imaging applications in chest disease: present and future applications. RSNA, Chicago, Nov. 29–Dec. 4, 1992.
44. Edwards FH, Wing G, Thompson L, Bellamy RF, et al. Three dimensional image reconstruction for planning of complex cardiovascular procedure. Ann Thorac Surg 1990;49(3):486–488.
45. Inuzuka N. A case of scalenus anterior muscle passing behind the left subclavian artery. Okajimas Folia Anat Jpn 1989;66(5): 229–240.
46. Gilroy J, Meyer JS. Compression of the subclavian artery as a cause of ischemic brachial neuropathy. Brain 1963;86:733.
47. Colon E, Westdorp R. Vascular compression in the thoracic outlet: age dependent normative values in noninvasive testing. J Cardiovasc Surg 1988;29:166–171.
48. Baumgarten F, Nelson RJ, Robertson JM. The rudimentary 1st rib: a case of thoracic outlet syndrome with arterial compromise. Arch Surg 1989;124(9):1090–1092.
49. Brannon EW Jr, Wickstrom J. Surgical approaches to neurovascular compression syndromes of the neck. Clin Orthop 1967; 51:65.
50. Pittan MR, Darke SG. The place of first rib resection in the management of axillary-subclavian vein thrombosis. Eur J Vasc Surg 1987;1(1):5–10.
51. Bar-Ziv J, Eger M, Feuchtwanger M, Hirsch M. Angiography in diagnosis of subclavian vessel injury. Clin Radiol 1972;23: 471.
52. Lang EK. Roentgenographic diagnosis of the neurovascular compression syndromes. Radiology 1962;79:58.
53. Persaud V. Subclavian artery aneurysm and idiopathic cystic media necrosis. Br Heart J 1968;30:346.
54. Lang EK. Quantitative assessment of flow in antegrade and retrograde collateral channels serving the brachiocephalic area. Radiology 1966;87:457.
55. Weibel J, Fields WS. Arteriographic studies of thoracic outlet syndrome. Br J Radiol 1967;40:676.
56. Wright IS. Neurovascular syndrome produced by hyperabduction of the arms: the immediate changes produced in 150 normal controls, and the effects on some persons of prolonged hyperabduction of arms, as in sleeping, and in certain occupations. Am Heart J 1945;29:1.
57. Stanton PE, McClusky DAM, Richardson HD, Larius PA. Thoracic outlet syndrome: a comprehensive evaluation. South Med J 1978;71:1070–1073.

58. Warrens AN, Heaton JM. Thoracic outlet compression syndrome: the lack of reliability of its clinical assessment. Ann R Coll Surg 1987;69:203–204.
59. Daskalakis E, Bouhoutsos J. Subclavian and axillary vein compression of musculoskeletal origin. Br J Surg 1980;67:573–576.
60. Wellington JL, Martin P. Post-stenotic subclavian aneurysms. Angiology 1965;16:566.
61. Urschel HC Jr, Razzuk MA. Management of the thoracic outlet syndrome. N Engl J Med 1972;286:1140.
62. Grassi CJ, Polak JF. Axillary and subclavian venous thrombosis: follow-up evaluation with color Doppler flow US and venography. Radiology 1990;175:651–654.

Index

Index